Potter's Pathology of the Fetus, Infant and Child

Potter's Pathology of the Fetus, Infant and Child

SECOND EDITION

EDITOR

Enid Gilbert-Barness, AO,
MD, MBBS, FRCPA, FRCPath, DSci(hc), MD(hc)

Professor of Pathology and Cell Biology, Pediatrics and
Obstetrics and Gynecology
University of South Florida College of Medicine
Tampa General Hosptial
Tampa, FL, USA
Professor Emeritus, Pathology, Laboratory Medicine and
Pediatrics,
Distinguished Medical Alumni Professor Emeritus
University of Wisconsin Medical School
Madison, WI, USA

FOREWORD BY

John M. Opitz, MD, MD(hc), DSci(hc), MD(hc), MD(hc)

Professor of Pediatrics (Medical Genetics)
Human Genetics, Pathology, and Obstetrics & Gynecology
University of Utah Health Sciences Center
Salt Lake City, UT, USA

ASSOCIATE EDITORS

Raj P. Kapur, MD, Ph.D.

Department of Laboratories
Children's Hospital and Regional Medical Center
Associate Professor of Pathology
University of Washington
Seattle, WA, USA

Luc L. Oligny, MSc, MD

Associate Professor and Vice-Chairman
Département de Pathologie et Biologie Cellulaire
Faculty of Medicine
Université de Montréal
Chief
Department of Pathology
Centre Hospitalier Universitaire Sainte-Justine
Montreal, Quebec, Canada

ASSISTANT EDITOR

Joseph R. Siebert, Ph.D.

Department of Laboratories
Children's Hospital and Regional Medical Center
Professor of Pathology
University of Washington
Seattle, WA, USA

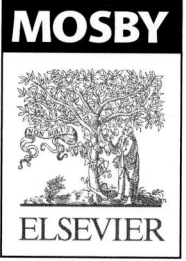

MOSBY

ELSEVIER

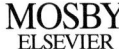

MOSBY
ELSEVIER

Mosby is an affiliate of Elsevier Inc.

ISBN: 9780323034036

British Library Cataloguing in Publication Data
A catalogue record for this book is available from the British Library

Library of Congress Cataloging in Publication Data
A catalog record for this book is available from the Library of Congress

Printed in China
Last digit is the print number: 9 8 7 6 5 4 3 2

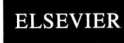

ELSEVIER your source for books, journals and multimedia in the health sciences
www.elsevierhealth.com

Working together to grow libraries in developing countries

www.elsevier.com | www.bookaid.org | www.sabre.org

ELSEVIER   BOOK AID International   Sabre Foundation

Commissioning Editor: Michael Houston and William Schmitt
Development Editor: Claire Bonnett
Editorial Assistant: Elizabeth MacSween
Project Manager: Gemma Lawson
Design Manager: Sarah Russell
Illustration Manager: Bruce Hogarth
Illustrator: Martin Woodward
Marketing Manager(s) (USA/UK): Leontine Treur/Ethel Cathers

Table of Contents

VOLUME ONE

PART I: Pathogenesis of Fetal and Infantile Disorders

PART II: Examination of the Fetus and Infant

Contributors list

Virginia M. Anderson, MD
Department of Pathology
SUNY Downstate Medical Center
New York, NY, USA

Frederic B. Askin, MD
Professor of Pathology
The Johns Hopkins University School of
Medicine
Director of Pathology
The Johns Hopkins Bayview Medical
Center
Baltimore, MD, USA

Lewis A. Barness, MD, DSci(hc)
Distinguished University Professor
Professor of Pediatrics
Tampa General Hospital
Professor of Public Health
College of Public Health
College of Medicine and Department of
Community and Family Health
University of South Florida College of
Medicine
Tampa, FL, USA
Professor Emeritus, Pediatrics
University of Wisconsin Medical School
Madison, WI, USA

Jay Bernstein, MD
Director of Research and Associate
Medical Director Emeritus
William Beaumont Hospital
Royal Oak, MI, USA
Clinical Professor of Pathology Emeritus
Wayne State University School of
Medicine
Detroit, MI, USA

Fouad Boulos, MD
Breast Research Fellow
Department of Pathology
Vanderbilt Medical Center
Nashville, TN, USA

Theonia K. Boyd, MD
Assistant Professor of Pathology
Harvard Medical School
Department of Pathology
Children's Hospital Boston
Boston, MA, USA

Edward B. Clark, MD
Wilma T. Gibson Presidential Professor
& Chair
Department of Pediatrics
University of Utah
Salt Lake City, UT, USA

Cheryl M. Coffin, MD
Professor of Pathology
Department of Pathology
Primary Children's Medical Center
Salt Lake City, UT, USA

**M. Michael Cohen Jr, DMD, MScD,
PhD, FCCMG**
Professor Emeritus of Pediatrics
Faculty of Medicine
Dalhousie University
Halifax, Nova Scotia, Canada

Beverly Barrett Dahms, MD
Professor of Pathology and Pediatrics
Department of Pathology
University Hospitals of Cleveland
Case Medical Center
Case-Western Reserve University School
of Medicine
Cleveland, OH, USA

**Diane Debich-Spicer, BS,
PA(ASCP)**
Department of Pathology
Tampa General Hospital
Tampa, FL, USA

**Derek J. deSa, MBBS, DPhil(Oxon),
FRCPath, FRCPC**
Professor Emeritus of Pathology
University of British Columbia
Children's and Women's Health Centre
Vancouver, BC, Canada

Sherman Elias, MD
John J. Sciarra Professor and Chair
Department of Obstetrics and
Gynecology
Feinberg School of Medicine
Northwestern University
Chicago, IL, USA

Ferechté Encha-Razavi, MD
Department of Pathology
Henri Mondor Hospital
Créteil, France

Philip M. Farrell, MD, PhD
Professor of Pediatrics and Population
Health Sciences
Dean and Vice President Emeritus
University of Wisconsin Medical School
Madison, WI, USA

Jaime L. Frías, MD
Visiting Scientist – McKing Consulting
Corporation
Division of Birth Defects and
Developmental Disabilities
National Center on Birth Defects and
Developmental Disabilities
Center for Disease Control and
Prevention
Atlanta, GA, USA

Michael K. Fritsch, MD, PhD
Assistant Professor of Pathology
Department of Pathology
University of Wisconsin-Madison
Madison, WI, USA

Mary Milne Gilbert Lawrence, MD, MPH
Associate Professor of Ophthalmology
University of Minnesota Medical School
Associate Chief of Ophthalmology
Minneapolis Veterans Affairs Medical Center
Glaucoma, Cataract, and Visual Rehabilitation
Minneapolis, MN, USA

Enid Gilbert-Barness, AO, MD, MBBS, FRCPA, FRCPath, DSci(hc), MD(hc)
Professor of Pathology and Cell Biology, Pediatrics and Obstetrics and Gynecology
University of South Florida College of Medicine
Tampa General Hospital
Tampa, FL, USA
Professor Emeritus, Pathology, Laboratory Medicine and Pediatrics
Distinguished Medical Alumni
Professor Emeritus
University of Wisconsin Medical School
Madison, WI, USA

Allan M. Goldstein, MD
Assistant Professor of Surgery
Harvard Medical School
Massachusetts General Hospital
Department of Pediatric Surgery
Boston, MA, USA

Fiona Graeme-Cook, MB, FRCPI
Assistant Professor of Pathology
Department of Pathology
Massachusetts General Hospital
Boston, MA, USA

Sivaselvi Gunasekaran, MD
Clinical Associate Professor
University of South Florida
Department of Pathology
Tampa General Hospital
Tampa, FL, USA

Hart Isaacs Jr, MD
Clinical Professor of Pathology
Children's Hospital
University of California
San Diego, CA, USA

Dagmar K. Kalousek, MD, FRCPC
Professor Emeritus
Department of Pathology
University of British Columbia
Vancouver, BC, Canada

Raj P. Kapur, MD, PhD
Department of Laboratories
Children's Hospital and Regional Medical Center
Associate Professor of Pathology
University of Washington
Seattle, WA, USA

R.O.C. Kaschula, MB ChB, MMed(Path)
Department of Pathology
Red Cross Children's Hospital
Rondebosch, Cape Town, South Africa

Vikram Krishnasetty, MD
Department of Radiology
Massachusetts General Hospital
Harvard Medical School
Boston, MA, USA

Atilano Lacson, MD
Affiliate Professor, Pathology and Pediatrics
University of South Florida
Tampa, FL, USA

Jeanne-Claudie Larroche, MD
Emeritus Directeur de Recherche au CNRS
Hôpital de Port-Royal
Paris, France

Geoffrey A. Machin, MD, PhD, FRCPath, FRCP(C)
Victoria, BC, Canada

Jennifer L. Root Mayer, MD, FAAP
Assistant Professor of Pediatrics
University of South Florida College of Medicine
Tampa, FL, USA
Medical Director
All Children's Hospital at Sarasota Memorial Hospital
Sarasota, FL, USA

Richard L. Naeye, MD
University Professor of Pathology Emeritus
Chairman Emeritus
Department of Pathology
The Milton S. Hersey Medical Center
The Pennsylvania State University College of Medicine
Hersey PA, USA

Christian Nezelof, MD
Emeritus Professor of Pathology
Université de Paris V
Paris, France

G. Petur Nielsen, MD
James Homer Wright Laboratories
Department of Pathology
Massachusetts General Hospital
Harvard Medical School
Boston, MA, USA

Luc L. Oligny, MD, MSc
Associate Professor
Département de Pathologie et Biologie Cellulaire
Faculty of Medicine
Université de Montréal
Chief
Department of Pathology
Center Hospitalie Universitaire Sainte-Justine
Montreal, Quebec, Canada

Janice J. Ophoven, MD
Assistant Medical Examiner
St Louis County
Woodbury, MN, USA

John M. Opitz, MD, MD(hc), DSci(hc), MD(hc), MD(hc)
Professor of Pediatrics (Medical Genetics)
Human Genetics, Pathology, and Obstetrics & Gynecology
University of Utah Health Sciences Center
Salt Lake City, UT, USA

Sherrie L. Perkins, MD, PhD
Professor of Pathology
Department of Pathology
University of Utah Health Sciences Center
Salt Lake City, UT, USA

Elizabeth J. Perlman, MD
Professor of Pathology
Northwestern University
Pathologist-in-Chief
Children's Memorial Hospital
Chicago, IL, USA

M. Halit Pinar, MD
Director of Perinatal and Pediatric Pathology
Women and Infants Hospital of Rhode Island
Professor
Department of Pathology and Laboratory Medicine
Brown Medical School
Providence, RI, USA

Raymond W. Redline, MD
Professor of Pathology and
Reproductive Biology
Case Western Reserve School of Medicine
Co-Director, Pediatric and Perinatal
Pathology
University Hospitals of Cleveland
Cleveland, Cuyahoga-East, OH, USA

Drucilla J. Roberts, MD
Associate Professor of Pathology
Harvard Medical School
Massachusetts General Hospital
Department of Pathology
Boston, MA, USA

Stephen G. Romansky, MD
Pediatric Pathologist
Department of Pathology
Long Beach Memorial and Miller
Children's Hospital
Long Beach, CA, USA

Lucy B. Rorke-Adams, MD
Professor of Pathology, Neurology and
Pediatrics
Department of Pathology –
Neuropathology
The Children's Hospital of Philadelphia
Philadelphia, PA, USA

Andrew E. Rosenberg, MD
James Homer Wright Laboratories
Department of Pathology
Massachusetts General Hospital
Harvard Medical School
Boston, MA, USA

Daniel I. Rosenthal, MD
Department of Radiology
Massachusetts General Hospital
Harvard Medical School
Boston, MA, USA

Pierre Russo, MD
Director
Division of Anatomic Pathology
The Children's Hospital of Philadelphia
Professor
Department of Pathology and
Laboratory Medicine
University of Pennsylvania School of
Medicine
Philadelphia, PA, USA

Melinda E. Sanders, MD
Assistant Professor of Pathology
Vanderbilt University Medical Center
Nashville, TN, USA

Robert E. Scully, MD
Emeritus Professor of Pathology
Harvard Medical School
Department of Pathology
Massachusetts General Hospital
Boston, MA, USA

Thomas A. Seemayer, MD
Emeritus Professor of Pathology
University of Nebraska Medical Center
Omaha, NE, USA

Joseph R. Siebert, PhD
Department of Laboratories
Children's Hospital and Regional
Medical Center
Research Associate Professor of
Pathology
University of Washington
Seattle, WA, USA

Don B. Singer, MD
Professor Emeritus of Pathology
Brown University School of Medicine
Providence, RI, USA

Glenn P. Taylor, MD, FRCPC
Head, Division of Pathology
Department of Paediatric Laboratory
Medicine
The Hospital for Sick Children
Toronto, Ontario, Canada

Margot I. Van Allen, MD
Professor
Medical Genetics Program
British Columbia's Children's Hospital
Vancouver, BC, Canada

Linda de Vries, MD, PhD
Professor in Neonatal Neurology
Department of Neonatology
University Medical Centre
Wilhelmina Children's Hospital
Utrecht, The Netherlands

Frances V. White, MD
Assistant Professor
Department of Pathology and
Immunology
Division of Anatomic Pathology
Washington University School of
Medicine
St. Louis, MO, USA

Golder N. Wilson, MD, PhD
Clinical Professor of Pediatrics
Texas Tech University and Kinder
Genome Pediatric Genetic Practice
Dallas, TX, USA

Foreword–second edition

It is a great privilege and pleasure to welcome and to introduce this new edition of *Potter's Pathology of the Fetus, Infant and Child* edited with her usual energy and enthusiasm by my friend and most distinguished colleague of 35 years, Dr. Enid Gilbert-Barness. I do not know how many autopsies Enid has performed by now. Also, I cannot hold her responsible for the fact that I never completed a formal training program in pathological anatomy during those glorious years between 1970 and 1979 when we worked together on a daily basis at the University of Wisconsin, and when I learned most of what I know about developmental pathology. But I do know for a fact, that with her unparalleled experience and as the undisputed world-leader in fetal and pediatric pathology, Enid brought to the challenge of this revision a wealth of knowledge and discerning wisdom as to the *essentials* of the field, gained after decades of fruitful collaboration with other pathologists, pediatricians, anatomists, embryologists, geneticists, teratologists, and all of the clinical specialists who work with pregnant women.

Enid's efforts do great honor to the work of her distinguished predecessor, Edith L. Potter (1901-1993), late Professor of Pathology at Chicago Lying-in-Hospital and at the University of Chicago Medical School. It can be said that the first three editions of the Potter Book (1952, 1961, and 1977 with John Craig) laid the foundation of fetal and pediatric pathology in North America with magisterial, one is tempted to say old testamentary, authority, focusing exclusively on human pathology with all of the anatomical, histological, radiological, and infectious disease methods then available. The book was beautifully illustrated on the basis of well over 10,000 autopsies that Dr. Potter had done before writing the book.

When Enid undertook the two-volume edition of the Potter book in 1997, a new era was ushered in. The massive increase in knowledge since the last edition made multi-authorship mandatory and demonstrated conclusively that it is not possible anymore to practice fetal-pediatric pathology without concomitant expertise in at least molecular-diagnostic methods, cytogenetics, genetics, ultrasonography, developmental biology, and all of the other approaches we use daily to test causal and pathogenetic hypotheses in the dead fetuses and infants entrusted to us for final diagnosis.

In the early 1960s when we were studying the Zellweger syndrome (independently discovered in Madison), we noted multiple renal cysts in the affected infants. And having just read with tremendous enthusiasm the second edition of Potter's "Bible," I suggested to David W. Smith we discuss these findings with Dr. Potter, the world's greatest authority on renal cysts and easily accessible by a short train ride from Madison to Chicago. After arrival in her office, she glanced up briefly, said, "Ah, Smith, Opitz," returned to work at her microscope, finally turned around and said, "Slides." And then: "Multiple cortical cysts! Liver normal?" When she looked at the slides of hepatic tissue, we heard her mutter, "Well, well, well…" under her breath. This is when she had noticed profuse amounts of a golden brown pigment, especially in Kupffer cells and other reticuloendothelial cells, concluded that it might be iron and encouraged us to stain with Prussian blue, thus confirming her hypothesis. Mightily impressed, Dave Smith and I were about to take our leave when she suddenly became downright voluble, recalling that recently she had been consulted on a similar case in an inbred Dutch family from Holland, Michigan. Thus, we were able to add another family to our 1968/1969 review of the Zellweger syndrome and to stimulate our colleagues in Madison, Shahidi and Vitale, to study the iron defect in that condition. This resulted in the 1969 *New England Journal of Medicine* paper, which in turn stimulated the research of Sidney Goldfischer and his coworkers at Albert Einstein Medical School that led to the discovery of the peroxisomal defect in Zellweger syndrome and large group of related disorders. Dr. Potter was then shortly before her retirement and her work on the Michigan case was completed by her successor, Douglas R. Shanklin.

Enid Gilbert-Barness is a very different person from the late Edith Potter, but no less brilliant, astute and insightful with an almost unequaled breadth of knowledge and experience. I was present at the University of Wisconsin when she assigned her future husband, Lew Barness, an exceptionally difficult CPC discussion pertaining to some thesaurismosis or another. Appearing stumped, Dr. Barness tried the clever trick of parsing Enid's bibliography for her favorite disease and, throwing up his hands in amazement and frustration, explained, "Why, she has written on *all* of them." Nevertheless, Lew made the correct diagnosis.

This edition of *The Pathology of the Fetus, Infant and Child* is the culmination of a marvelous period in the history of pathology, which can be said to have begun properly with the epochal 1779 publication of Giovanni Battista Morgagni's *De sedibus et causis morborum* ... (translated by the Sydenham

Society). However, the introduction of embryological-developmental and comparative notions to the study of malformed fetuses and infants was largely due to Johann Friedrich Meckel the Younger (1781–1833), who in a scholarly outpouring almost as prolific as that of my favorite pediatric pathologist, was the first to relate human malformations to *normal* homologous anatomical conditions in other animals, accepted heredity as cause of malformations, was the founder of genetic syndromology (e.g., Meckel syndrome), anticipated the concept of pleiotropy, heterogeneity, developmental constraint, and reduced penetrance, and showed that the duck-billed platypus was a mammal after all when he discovered its mammary glands on Christmas Day 1825. And whereas Meckel's legacy is sadly forgotten, largely because of the virtually total lack of illustrations in his books and monographs, Enid has stressed all of her professional life, like her illustrious predecessor Edith Potter, that *pathology is a visual art* and has been at great pains to illustrate with over 2500 excellent figures alone in the present volumes.

Immediately after Meckel's death, his profound insights into developmental and constitutional pathology were forgotten. Karl (von) Rokitansky (1804-1878) dissected more than 30,000 bodies and his four-volume *Manual of Pathological Anatomy* (1842-1846, translated by the Sydenham Society), became the standard text until Virchow. However, instead of Meckel's recapitulationist view of human malformations vis-a-vis the normal anatomical states in "lower" animals, Rokitansky accepts the similarities as examples of maternal impression (*Versehen*).

It was the great merit of the French comparative anatomists of the 19th and 20th century to have founded the science of teratology (*Tératologie* as Isidore Geoffroy St-Hilaire called it in 1832) referring not only to the environmental production of malformations in animals, but *sensu lato* to the study of *all* congenital anomalies. In Italy, Cesare Taruffi (1821–1902) of Bologna compiled a multivolume compendium of malformations, incomplete at the time of his death. In Germany, Ernst Schwalbe's *Die Morphologie der Missbildungen des Menschen und der Tiere* (*The Morphology of Malformations of Human and Animals*), begun in 1906, was not completed until 1958 by Georg B. Gruber, the same year in which Rupert A. Willis of Leeds published his *Borderland of Embryology and Pathology* with his cranky denigration of the concept of atavisms, which Meckel had labored to document so exhaustively. This edition of the Potter book, a little over a half-century since its first publication, truly is a monument to the art and science of fetal and pediatric pathology and will continue to have a profound impact on the rejuvenation and development of the specialty. And for this accomplishment, we owe Enid Gilbert-Barness a profound debt of gratitude.

May I also suggest that reference to the Potter book be supplemented by the Gilbert-Barness and Debich-Spicer texts: *Embryo and Fetal Pathology, Color Atlas with Ultrasound Correlation* (Cambridge University Press, 2004), and the *Handbook of Pediatric Autopsy Pathology* (Humana Press, 2005).

John M. Opitz
Salt Lake City, Utah
Professor of Pediatrics (Medical Genetics), Human Genetics,
Pathology, Obstetrics & Gynecology

Foreword–first edition

There will be few today, when textbooks are as plentiful as apples on trees and we are up to our knees in journals, reprints, and faxes, who can appreciate the impact that Edith Potter's book made on us in 1952. To pediatricians and others who were beginning to come to grips with diseases of neonates and to "would be" pediatric pathologists it came as literal enlightenment. Edith Potter was one of that small group of highly intelligent and very able women, such as Dorothy Anderson in New York, Agnes MacGregor in Edinburgh, and Maude Abbott in Toronto, who applied themselves to children's pathology long before it had any financial rewards.

I will never forget my first visit to Edith Potter. I had met Sidney Farber in his emporium at the newly built Jimmy Fund Building and I had sat with Dorothy Anderson and bathed in nicotine as she chain-smoked around me, but Edith Potter was quite different. Her office was a new experience. It was a small room where she sat behind a desk in an immaculate white coat. Every bench, chair, and floor space was covered with piles of papers, and on the top of every pile there was a cactus, all of different shapes and sizes. She rose to greet me, "How nice to meet you at last, do move that plant off that chair onto the desk and sit down." She had the rare quality of the very few, very great people of grace and charm, being at complete ease with herself and having the self-confidence that makes modesty and arrogance redundant. She was very happy to be a woman.

Her book was the product of her own great experience. She had performed approximately 10,000 autopsies, and it contained the basic data and tables on which she had based her opinions. She was a pioneer and an honest observer, and this shone through her simple, direct writing and her photographs. Her book contained descriptions of conditions that had not already reached medical literature and this, to some extent, separated it from most other textbooks, most of which are now largely compiled using multiple authors from published sources. I remember sitting beside Edith Potter at a meeting in New York, listening to someone describing what he claimed to be a new syndrome. At the end of the talk we looked at each other and I raised an eyebrow at her. She replied, "Yes." It was in the character of Edith Potter that she did not get up and tell that young man where he would find the original description of this new syndrome.

What has happened to "Potter's" book over the years? She did not feel like being strangled by continual re-editing. The next two editions had considerable additions. The book maintained its high standards in both writing and illustration. But now, with this edition, it has gone full circle. It has now come to an editor who in many ways is very like Edith Potter, both in philosophy related to work and life, in breadth and extent of experience. Enid Gilbert-Barness took on where Edith Potter left off, notably in her work on heart development and in concepts of malformations together with John Opitz. She is an ideal person to create a new fresh and live "Potter" to take us into the next century. I am itching to get my hands on the new edition.

JOHN L. EMERY

Enid Gilbert-Barness has produced an entirely new two-volume text of the *Pathology of the Fetus and Infant* which retains the name of Potter. As a foundation, it incorporates Edith Potter's expertise and vast experience to illustrate the pathology of the period of life most vital to the developing child. It is the most comprehensive and most modern text on the subject and includes state-of-the-art developments in genetic and developmental pathology. Pediatric pathology comes alive under Gilbert-Barness' creative guidance and explanation. The 21st century has found a successor to Edith Potter. This book should be the ultimate authoritative text for pediatricians, pathologists, developmentalists, geneticists, and pediatric scientists to understand the pathology that they may encounter in the years ahead.

FRANK OSKI, MD

Preface–second edition

Ten years have elapsed since the first edition of **Potter's Pathology of the Fetus and Infant** was published. During that time great advances have been made, particularly in molecular genetics, developmental pathology, immunopathology and DNA technology. In this second edition I have been ably assisted by two associate editors, Luc L. Oligny and Raj Kapur and an assistant editor, Joseph Siebert. We welcome new contributors who include Frederic Askin, Theonia Boyd, Fouad Boulos, Cheryl Coffin, Michael Cohen, Edward Clark, Sherman Elias, Philip Farrell, Jaime Frías, Michael Fritsch, Fiona Graeme-Cook, Allan Goldstein, Raj Kapur, Atilano Lacson, Jennifer Maer, Christian Nezelof, Luc L. Oligny, Sherri Perkins, Elizabeth Perlman, Halit Pinar, Ray Redline, Drucilla Roberts, Lucy Rorke, Andrew Rosenberg, Pierre Russo, Melinda Sanders, Thomas Seemayer, Joseph Siebert, Don Singer, Glenn Taylor, Fran White. We have encouraged the new contributors to respond to the challenge in our specialty to retain pertinent information from the first edition while incorporating advances in molecular and genetic sciences. Our aim is to provide a timely and comprehensive textbook of pediatric pathology of the embryo, fetus, infant and child.

The number of chapters has been increased from 35 to 41. The total group of contributing authors has increased from 34 to 43. In order to provide more detail some of the chapters have been divided into three or more sections. New chapters have been included on Ancillary Tests, Thoraco-abdominal Defects, Back, Perineum and Cloaca, Breast, Salivary glands, and Overgrowth Syndromes.

We feel that there are few books comparable to these volumes in which one will find a general overview and up-to-date information including genetic and molecular aspects of diseases.

Molecular advances hold promise of effectively addressing new and emerging diseases in children. Our goal is for this text to be comprehensive, concise and reader friendly, embracing the art and science of pediatric pathology. This book is a substantial revision and reorganization of the original text based on a complete review of current knowledge. Every subject has been scrutinized and all chapters have been improved and updated.

The text is divided into four parts in two volumes.

Volume 1 includes:

Part I - Pathogenesis of Fetal and Infantile Disorders

Part II - Examination of the Fetus and Infant

Part III - Major Anomalies of External Anatomy or In-situ Relationships

Volume 2 includes:

Part IV - Systemic Pathology

Numerous tables, diagrams, and line drawings in color and color illustrations enhance the text in order to make the material esthetically pleasing and more easily read.

To meet the requirements of the new generation a CD-ROM version is included.

With the addition of several new chapters and a complete revision of the original chapters, thousands of new references and color photographs and drawings have added new information in bringing these volumes into the present millennium.

It is our hope that the subject of Pediatric Pathology will open new avenues and vistas for our readers and that they will share with us the interest, excitement and enthusiasm as was first generated by Edith Potter.

Enid Gilbert-Barness
Editor

Preface–first edition

Edith Potter, a pioneer in pediatric pathology, collected and meticulously described a host of malformations and diseases affecting the fetus and infant. It is 20 years since the third edition of the *Pathology of the Fetus and Infant* was published with Dr. John Craig as co-author. She died in 1993 aware of, and pleased with, the germination of this new edition of her book.

We have attempted to preserve her unique contributions, including the spectacular illustrations that made her book so valuable. Dr. Potter had performed over 10,000 perinatal autopsies at the Chicago Lying-In Hospital. So convincing was her appeal for the performance of a perinatal autopsy that the medical examiner made it mandatory in Chicago for autopsies to be performed on all perinatal deaths.

In the preface of the first edition of her book Edith Potter stated

The description of the body of a dead infant is of no value as an isolated piece of information, but if it is integrated with the various aspects of heredity, conception, development, intrauterine and extrauterine environment and behavior, it becomes part of an important chronicle.

We have attempted to preserve this philosophy, and the material in this book represents not only Dr. Potter's contributions and her experience with several thousand autopsies but also the expertise of 34 other contributing authors whose specialties encompass pediatric and developmental pathology, molecular and cytogenetics, and pediatric specialties. In addition to information obtained from new techniques, sections on genetic influences on mechanism of growth and development, prenatal diagnosis, and placental pathology, are included.

The explosion of new diagnostic methods in the past decade has been coupled with increased understanding of molecular genetics and its role in mechanisms of growth. As we approach the 21st century, traditional morphologic descriptions of pathologic processes will be, at least in part, replaced by in-depth understanding of molecular genetics and by the use of newer techniques for diseases and conditions that affect the development and function of the embryo, fetus, and infant. This has stimulated my interest in developing a contemporary source of embryo, fetal, and infant pathology while preserving our homage to Edith Potter, the mother of perinatal pathology.

From the long available study of pathologtic products of conception, too frequently has a wealth of information been overlooked. My hope is that this volume will stimulate a pursuit of knowledge that can be gleaned from this source of material with enthusiasm and thoroughness and will be a ready reference source for pediatric and general pathologists, pediatricians, obstetricians, geneticists, and those engaged in reproductive medicine as well as the practical application of these techniques.

The first half of the book includes chapters devoted to developmental and genetic pathology and the second half to system pathology. As pathology is a visual art, over 2500 illustrations with more than 140 in color have been included. Most of the tables include McKusick numbers, a six-digit number used in McKusick's *Catalog of Genetic Diseases: Mendelian Inheritance in Man*, for which there is a computerized version, OMIM (Online Mendelian Inheritance in Man), available 24-hours-a-day for consultation and references.

Over the past 25 years I have had the extraordinary good fortune of collaborating with Dr. John Optiz, distinguished master of medical genetics, a scholar, a gentleman, and a treasured friend. This rewarding experience has been beyond all measure the highlight and most important influence in my professional career.

I am indebted to all contributors to this volume for their dedication and hard work; to the many friends and colleagues with whom I have worked and who have reviewed chapters and made invaluable suggestions, including: Jeanne Ackerman, Frederic Askin, Daniel Batten, John Bell, Kurt Benirschke, Orestes Borrego, Stephen Brantley, Irwin Browasky, Harold Bruyere, Sunita Chandra, Jacob Churg, John Curran, Salvatori Di Mauro, Monica and Ricardo Drut, Doug England, Phillip Farrell, Jaime Frías, Kennedy Gilchrist, Robert Good, Americo Gónzalvo, Sivaselvi Gunasekaran, Robert Huntington, Reza Hafez, Richard Hodach, Sonia Hofman, Edward Howes, Shizen Ishikawa, Sarah Jackson, Bernard Kaplan, Ringer Kemble, George and Steve Kargas, Boris Kousseff, Robert and Mabel Marshall, Rumiko Matsuoka, Robert McCord, Lorraine Meisner, Beverly Middleton, Carl Muus, Richard Naeye, Toshio Nishikawa, Terry Oberly, Frank Oski, Herbert Pomerance, Allen Root, Suzanne Sage, Robert Scully, William Segar, Thomas Stocker, Tom Warner, Thomas Wiedrich, Fred Zugibe, and Lewis Barness who has reviewed the entire volume. My gratitude is also extended to Irwin Browarsky, Eugene Ruffolo, Santo Nicosia, and John Balis, my colleagues, for their support during the preparation of this volume.

I wish to express my deep gratitude to Robert Gorlin who has been most generous in making available many illustrations and who has critically reviewed many of the chapters and made invaluable suggestions. I am indebted to Diane Debich-Spicer for her superb photographic illustrations and helpful advice. The untiring dedication of my secretary, Kay Wolfe, throughout the preparation of this volume has exceeded all expectations and has made this book possible. She is ever-cheerful and with an always smiling face has made this effort exciting and a real joy. Also, I extend my thanks to librarians Margaret Petro and Gerda Anderson of Tampa General Hospital for their invaluable assistance.

I am profoundly grateful to my mentors Lewis Barness, Sydney Gellis, Gace Guin, Sidney Farber, Stanley Inhorn, Charles Janeway, John Opitz, Henry Pitot, Gabriele Zu Rhein, and others for their profound influence on my career in pediatrics and pedatric pathology; and to the great pioneers in pediatric pathology who have made sentinel contributions in that field: Maude Abbott, Dorothy Andersen, James Arey, Robert Bolande, Jay Bernstein, Kurt Benirschke, Colin Berry, Wiliam Blanc, Bruce Beckwith, John Craig, Louis Dehner, Renata Dische, John Emery, Sidney Farber, Daria Haust, George Fetterman, John Kissane, Benjamin Landing, Rickard Naeye, William Newton, Gene Perrin, Edith Potter, Harvey Rosenberg, Tom Stocker, Gordon Vawter, and others including the contributors to this volume. As has been said, advances are made by individuals standing on the shoulders of giants.

Finally, words fall short in expressing my gratitude to Mosby–Year Book and, in particular, to Lynne Gery, the guiding light of this book, Susan Gay, and Allan Kleinberg, for their helpful suggestions and support and for far exceeding my expectations in meeting all my requests and much more.

ENID GILBERT–BARNESS

DEDICATION

To Lew for teaching me the art of pediatrics and
for his love and encouragement,

To Mary, Elizabeth, Jennifer and Rebecca
and the memory of James, and to the grandchildren
Alexandra, Louis, Christian, James, Thomas, Blake, Spencer,
Curtis, Kiara, Rebecca and Nathaniel

ACKNOWLEDGEMENTS

The value of this book is due to its expert contributors and we are indebted to their hard work, knowledge, thoughtfulness and good judgment. Our sincere appreciation also goes to all our colleagues, friends and associates from around the world who have been so generous in their knowledge, support and suggestions as well as providing many illustrations.

Last but most importantly we especially thank our families for their patience and understanding and for the Editors of Elsevier, in particular, Michael Houston, Claire Bonnett, William Schmitt and Gemma Lawson who most graciously have met all our requests and more. We also acknowledge with gratitude the superb artwork of Diane Debich-Spicer. Of paramount importance we are especially indebted to Kathy Lonkey for her enduring and untiring efforts in assembling and coordinating the entire text with her ever present smile.

Enid Gilbert-Barness
Raj Kapur
Luc L. Oligny
Joseph Siebert

Pathogenesis of fetal and infantile disorders

PART I

Mechanisms of development and growth: molecular genetics

Golder N. Wilson   Luc L. Oligny

'We cannot doubt that the most urgent need of modern embryology is a series of advances of a purely theoretical, even mathematico-logical nature. Only by something of this kind can we redress the balance which has fallen over to observation and experiment; only by some such effort can we obtain a theoretical embryology suited in magnitude and spaciousness to the wealth of facts which contemporary investigators are accumulating day by day.'   Joseph Needham, 1959[1]

Role of genetics in developmental pathology

The fetal pathologist stands at the crossroads of two exciting disciplines. Molecular technology has opened entire genomes for dissection and streamlined investigation of many diseases. In situ hybridization and microarray analysis add new dimensions to tissue pathology that should revitalize morphologic work. DNA analysis has revealed novel inheritance mechanisms that bring many 'sporadic' fetal anomalies under the scrutiny of a genetic approach. Gene and genome analysis have revealed the molecular architecture behind complex developmental pathways, illuminating new parallels between birth defects and cancer. The scope of human genetic variation is so extensive, and the tools for analyzing it so powerful, that every pregnancy loss or fetal anomaly has potential for new pathogenetic insights. As recognized so presciently by Edith Potter, phenotypic analysis is now the limiting factor in human developmental understanding. A close interaction between fetopathology, medical genetics, and molecular biology provides an unprecedented venue to relate organ/tissue phenotypes to DNA base pairs (Fig. 1.1). What a remarkable opportunity!

Some pathologists, particularly those inundated with the demands of a pediatric/obstetric service, may feel somewhat alien to genes and molecules. For them, this chapter is intended to be like the Wizard of Oz – granting by proclamation what they already possess. The linear concepts of genes and DNA are far simpler than the three-dimensional complexities of anatomy and histology, and this chapter seeks to provide an update and review. For most, skimming the sections on gene structure and expression should restore the brains, heart, and courage to be an active partner in developmental genetic analysis. A new hierarchy of developmental regulation is evident, extending from DNA amplification (genomics) to chromatin conformation/modification (epigenetics) to the myriad variations in RNA, protein, and metabolite expression (proteomics, integromics, systems biology). The landslide of unsuspected genetic mechanisms and developmental relationships can only be skirted in one chapter, but these examples should inspire every fetal pathologist to refashion old anomalies in the fabric of newly discovered molecules.

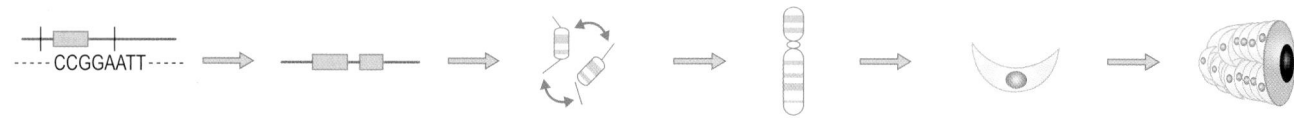

Nucleotide DNA motif	Gene/DNA genome	Chromatin region/band Gene families/networks	Chromosome	Cell/enzymes Proteome/transcriptome	Tissues/organs
(Sequencing/PCR/ASO/SNP)	(DNA blots/arrays)	(Fish/DNA blots/arrays)	(Karyotype)	(Enzymes,expression arrays)	(Histology/ISH)
Primary mutation Altered methylation "First hit"	Secondary mutations Multifactorial changes "Second hit"	DNA instability Tumor progression Microdeletions	Aneuploidy Tumor spread	Altered cell growth/death Vascular proliferation	**Neoplasia**
Primary mutation Altered imprinting	Secondary mutations Multifactorial changes	Altered epigenesis Microdeletions	Aneuploidy	Altered cell growth/death Uteroplacental changes Fetal changes	**Birth defects**

FIGURE 1.1 Molecular characterization in development and neoplasia. A developmental pathway from DNA sequence to complex structure is envisioned, with parallel regulatory steps contributing to neoplasia (middle panel) or birth defects.

An important preface to developmental pathology is an appreciation of the enormous role of genetics in producing birth defects. A parallel to be given recurring emphasis is neoplasia, an area in which pathology has made enormous contributions. Figure 1.1 illustrates this relationship, highlighting the genetic hierarchy from base pair to organ structure in its top panel. Cytogenetic and molecular techniques, available at each level of the genetic hierarchy (upper panel of Fig. 1.1), continue to unveil the remarkable genetic contribution to neoplasia (middle panel) and developmental anomalies (lower panel). Boveri's chromosomal hypothesis paralleled Lejeune's recognition of trisomy 21 in Down syndrome, predicting the many steps at which altered gene expression can produce abnormal tissue growth (neoplasia) or development (congenital anomalies). The similarities between molecular embryology and molecular oncology are strengthened by anomaly patterns (syndromes) that include cancer predisposition [e.g. Beckwith-Wiedemann syndrome (BWS), neurofibromatosis-1], the dual roles of many **proto-oncogene/ tumor suppressor** genes as developmental genes (e.g. *PAX/C-KIT* genes (see 'Gene notation' in glossary) in Waardenburg syndrome/ Piebald trait), and the stepwise progression from primary mutation, environmental factor, **epigenetic** change to multi-factorial result (e.g. *HOX* genes in human leukemias and limb defects).

The number of chromosomal rearrangements and gene mutations associated with tumors is now so great that almost every cancer patient undergoes some sort of molecular or cyto-genetic testing. The same progression from chromosome anomaly to causative breakpoint to cancer/tumor suppressor gene can now be followed for most developmental anomalies, and epigenesis is a central factor in both neoplasia and development.[2,3] This stepwise evolution provides a clear analytic strategy, illustrated here by application to insect segmentation, human limb defects, and cancer syndromes.

Direct evidence of the genetic contribution to fetal malformation is available from the compendium of Mendelian diseases compiled by Victor McKusick.[4] This single most useful reference in genetics is now accessible on the Web, together with laboratory, genome, and literature databases that integrate information on phenotype and genotype. About one-half of the 6422 Mendelian and multifactorial disorders in the literature involve altered morphogenesis, including over 800 with neoplasia.[5] These Mendelian causes of altered development can be viewed as extremes that provide routes to more common defects, just as rare children with hypercholesterolemia elucidated one factor in atherosclerotic heart disease. Alleles of major effect would reach endpoints (cross thresholds) regardless of genetic background; weaker alleles would require interaction to influence phenotype as defined by **multifactorial determination**.

Complementing genetics as a most important companion to fetal pathologists are parallel advances in developmental biology. This newly revised chapter gives equal time to the revolution in development, emphasizing new mechanisms and molecules and again emphasizing commonalities between neoplasia and birth defects. Indeed, molecular diagnosis of birth defects is as powerful as that for neoplasia, even if commercial testing is not always available. Fluorescent karyotyping and gene expression profiling of single cells[6] is a reality for both fields, and molecules diagnostic for diseases and predispositions are expanding in both arenas.

Diagnostic testing has always been within the realm of pathology, and applications to single blastomeres or embryo/ fetal therapy may allow fetal pathologists to join their surgical colleagues in guiding management. The importance of growth-regulating genes in developmental aberrations foretells of a 'gestational endocrinology' where predisposition is recognized and anomaly averted by appropriate maternofetal treatment. Congenital adrenal hyperplasia provides the prototype.[7] Full participation in the molecular revolution falls within the ability of all pathologists, whose unique skills in morphologic charac-terization need only be supplemented by simple methods for immortalized cell culture and DNA banking.[8] Even missed opportunities can be redeemed with techniques for in situ hybridization or DNA extraction using paraffin blocks.[9] With appreciation of the potential for genetic and developmental

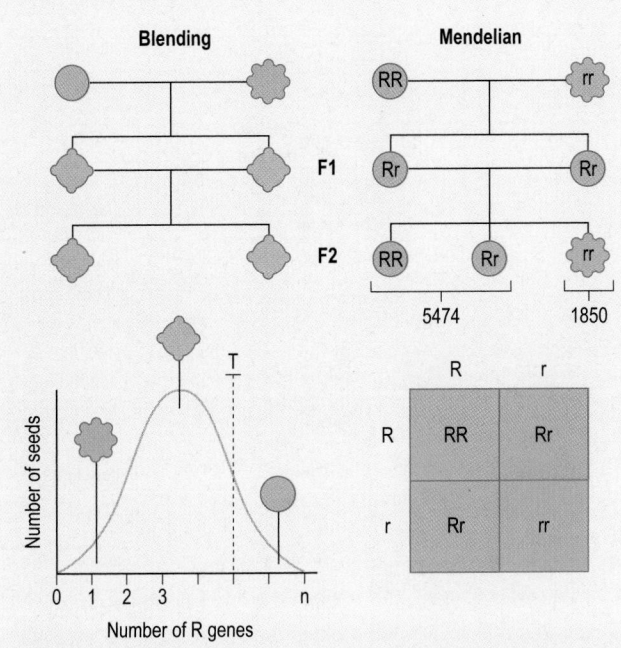

FIGURE 1.2 Blending versus Mendelian inheritance. The right panel shows Mendel's classic breeding experiment with round and wrinkled-seed peas. First-generation offspring (F1) were interbred to produce a second generation (F2) with the genotypes of RR or Rr leading to round seeds and that of rr leading to wrinkled seeds. Mendel deduced that random segregation of R and r alleles with dominance of R over r would explain the 3/1 ratio of phenotypes he observed. On the left, a conceptual experiment illustrates the result of blending inheritance if several genes with alternative alleles R and r interact to determine the number of seed wrinkles. Averaging of seed wrinkles would occur in the F1 generation and remain relatively constant after further crosses. Note the difference from Mendelian inheritance where the full wrinkled phenotype (genotype rr) re-emerges in the F2 generation. Discrete phenotypes can be produced by polygenic inheritance if a threshold T is postulated where a transition from wrinkled to round occurs at a given number of R alleles.

analyses, fetopathology departments can revitalize their domain of scientific treasure.

Basic genetics

The classic genetic approach begins with a pedigree and proceeds with interpretation based on Mendelian, multifactorial, or chromosomal constructs. The goal of this approach is a specific diagnosis that allows prognostic and reproductive counseling. The textbook of Scriver et al[10] provides a good introduction to basic genetics and that of Kumar et al[11] integrates classical pathology with molecular advances in genetic, metabolic, and neoplastic disorders. Italicized terms are defined in a glossary at the end of this chapter (note that the names of genes are also italicized).

Mendelian, multifactorial, and chromosomal inheritance

Figure 1.2 contrasts the Galtonian and Mendelian models of inheritance that achieved prominence at the beginning of the twentieth century. Mendelian theory explained inheritance by assuming **segregation** of particles called genes. Traits (**phenotype**) such as round versus wrinkled seeds in pea plants were determined by a pair of *alleles* (**genotype**); the genotypes of offspring were predictable from those of the parents given the ideas of independent assortment and **dominance.** Given that R is a form of the gene (**allele**) that determines round seeds, and that r encodes wrinkled seeds, a 3/1 ratio of offspring can be predicted from an Rr versus Rr cross (Fig. 1.2).[10] Of particular note in Mendel's remarkable model was the ability of an r allele to emerge intact after two generations to restore the wrinkled-seed phenotype; here was the mechanism needed to explain natural selection and the magical appearance of disease after normal or 'skipped' generations in human genetics.

Galton took the old notion of blending inheritance and designed a quantitative model that accounted for traits such as intelligence or stature. Here numerous alleles at several **loci** produced an aggregate trait. For the alternate alleles A and a, B and b, and so forth, the degree of stature or intellect would depend on the combinations of 'good' alleles, so that genotype AaBbCcDdEeFfGg would be much taller or smarter than genotype aabbccDdeeffgg. Extremes would be rare, since offspring would tend to inherit an average number of 'good' alleles and have intermediate phenotypes. In Figure 1.2 an alternative model for inheritance of round versus wrinkled seeds is shown where the number of seed wrinkles might be determined by the number of r alleles at several loci; breeding of extreme $(RR)_n$ and $(rr)_n$ individuals would yield mostly $(Rr)_n$ offspring with intermediate numbers of wrinkles on their seeds. When environmental modifications are factored into the equation, this polygenic or **multifactorial** model becomes quite useful to explain inheritance of **quantitative traits** such as intelligence, stature, and blood pressure.

Although many rare syndromes exhibit **Mendelian inheritance,**[5] most common birth defects do not. By modifying the polygenic model to include a **threshold** (Fig. 1.2), Carter[12] was able to explain recurrence risks for anomalies such as cleft lip/cleft palate and neural tube defects. Individuals with an unusually large number of 'bad' alleles plus a suitable fetal environment would cross a threshold and suffer the defect; Fraser[13] gave experimental validation to such models by showing interaction of embryogenetic mechanisms in murine cleft palate. Genes determining such factors as facial width, palatal height, and jaw growth would constitute an additive genotype that approached the cleft palate threshold. Environment was represented by steroid treatment that increased susceptibility to cleft palate in certain mouse strains.

The different implications of Mendelian versus polygenic/threshold models are readily understood by considering the simplified pedigree in Figure 1.3. The probability of relatives sharing a particular allele with the **proband** (arrow) can be estimated according to degree of relationship. Identical twins

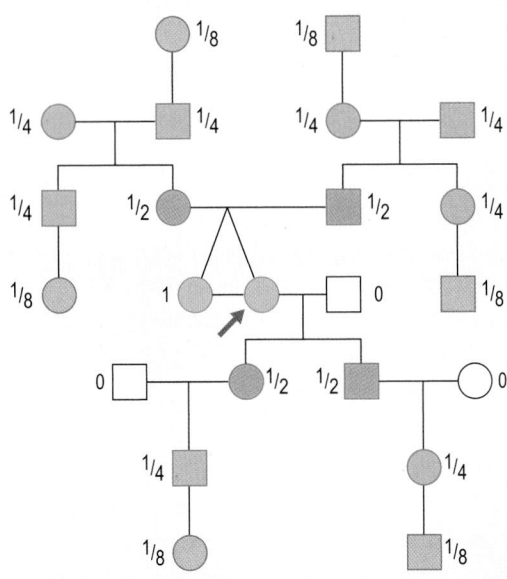

FIGURE 1.3 Genetic relationships, showing the fraction of genes shared by various relatives of a proband (arrow). First-degree (primary), second-degree (secondary), and third-degree (tertiary) relatives are indicated in orange, blue and lavender, respectively. The spouses, being genetically unrelated with the proband, share essentially no genes with her and her relatives.

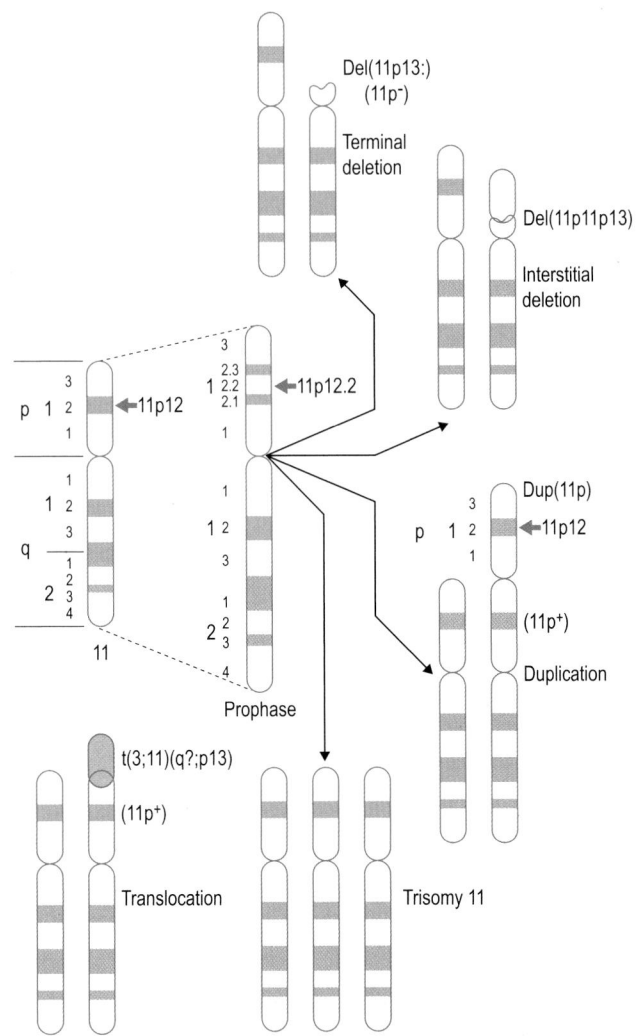

FIGURE 1.4 Cytogenetic notation illustrated with a hypothetical chromosome 11. At the left, short arm (p), long arm (q), and band nomenclature are illustrated. Extended length of the chromosome in prophase and notation for various rearrangements or trisomy are shown to the right.

have a probability of 1, **first-degree** relatives (dizygotic twins, parents, sibs, children) a probability of 1/2, second-degree relatives (grandchildren, grandparents, half-sibs, aunts, nieces) a probability of 1/4, and so on. The dependence of Mendelian traits on single alleles may sustain high recurrence risks to distant relatives, even if **variable expressivity** or **incomplete penetrance** masks the allele in certain individuals. For polygenic traits, the risk falls off sharply with degree of relationship. The probability of receiving five A alleles from a parent with five Aa loci is only 1/32; it is 1/1096 from a grandparent. The background 1 per 1000 incidence of many common birth defects rises to a 2–3% empiric recurrence risk in the sibling or child of an affected individual but returns toward background in second- or third-degree relatives. Empiric risk figures vary somewhat according to the type of defect, but the above estimates provide a simple guide for counseling.

Although Mendel was fortunate to pick traits that confirmed his idea of independent assortment, co-transmission or **linkage** of alleles at different loci was soon observed. Chromosomes provide the physical explanation for segregation and linkage, with **meiosis** ensuring transmission of one allele from each parental pair. Chromosomes also undergo maldistributions and rearrangements that establish a separate category of genetic disease (Schinzel[14] is a useful reference for disease phenotypes, Wyandt and Tonk[15] for variations and new techniques). Figure 1.4 illustrates the conventions for **cytogenetic notation** using a hypothetical chromosome 11 as an example. The short (**p**) and long (**q**) chromosome arms are divided into regions and sub-

regions according to bands. The designation 11p12 refers to chromosome 11s short arm, band 2 of the first large region; this band may split into sub-bands when cells are arrested in prophase to produce extended chromosomes. The smallest sub-band resolved by **prophase analysis** is equivalent to at least 10^6 **base pairs** (bp), enough to encode 20 to 25 genes of 40 **kilobases** (kb). **Chromosomal rearrangements** can include parts of chromosomes (terminal or **interstitial deletions**, partial duplications) or entire extra/missing chromosomes (**trisomies/monosomies** – Fig. 1.4 and Ch. 5).

Cytogenetic notation has been standardized to specify the number, sex, and rearrangements involved in any given karyotype – i.e. 47,XY,+11 for the trisomy 11 depicted in Figure 1.4. Exact breakpoints demarcating partial deletions and duplications can be indicated – e.g. *del(11)(p11p13)* – or shorthand terminology – e.g. 11p⁻ – can be used. In Figure 1.4, note that extra un-identified material on the chromosome 11 short arm could be indicated on the basis of its location as 11p⁺; if the extra material can be identified (by fluorescent technology described below), it is specified as accurately as possible – e.g. t(3;11)g(q?;p13). Chromosomal anomalies often present as **sporadic** (isolated) events in pedigrees, although **translocation carriers** can present with several affected children or abortuses/stillbirths as shown in Figure 1.5E.

Molecular technology has added a new level of resolution to chromosome analysis through the use of fluorescent in situ hybridization (FISH, described in more detail and illustrated in Ch. 5). Variously colored fluorescent tags can be added to single or multicopy DNA segments, using these molecules to target their complementary sequences in chromosomal DNA. Single locus probes can reveal gene dosage in interphase nuclei, allowing rapid diagnosis of trisomies (e.g. three signals due to three copies of 21q in Down syndrome) or submicroscopic deletions (e.g. only one signal, due to deletion within 15q in Prader-Willi syndrome). Repetitive DNAs specific to one chromosome become multilocus probes that fluoresce or 'paint' two entire homologues, allowing identification of small fragments (e.g. fluorescing blue like its normal X homologues) or complex rearrangements (e.g. pink, green, blue segments within a chromosome arm indicates exchange among three different chromosomes). Chromosome analysis is now merging with DNA chips to provide telomere or array analyses, capable of defining subtle deletion/duplication of any chromosome segment by its altered fluorescent pattern or chip representation.

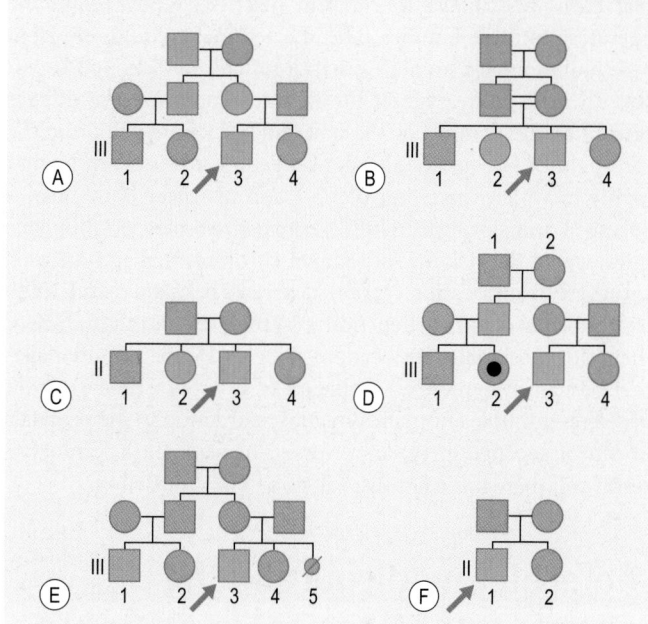

FIGURE 1.5 Pedigrees illustrating various mechanisms of inheritance (see text). Affected individuals are shown in blue.

Interpretation of pedigrees

Distinction among classic inheritance mechanisms depends on prior knowledge about a disease or the interpretation of pedigrees. Figure 1.5 illustrates six pedigrees that represent different modes of inheritance. The individual who has prompted evaluation is called the proband or **propositus** and is highlighted by an arrow to establish a frame of reference for the pedigree. Generations and individuals may also be labeled for easy reference. In pedigree A the vertical pattern and male-to-male transmission are strongly suggestive of autosomal dominant inheritance. Note that X-linked inheritance is ruled out by father–son transmission since males transmit their X chromosome only to daughters. Autosomal dominant inheritance implies that individual III-3 has a 1/2 chance of an affected child with each pregnancy. Barring late-onset disease or incomplete penetrance, individual III-4 is unaffected and would have negligible risk.

Pedigree B in Figure 1.5 is suggestive of autosomal recessive inheritance because of the horizontal pattern of affected individuals and the double line indicating consanguinity. The risk for the parents of III-3 to have another affected child is 1/4; that for III-1 or III-4 to be a carrier is 2/3, given the fact that they are not affected. The risk for affected or unaffected sibs to have an affected child depends on the incidence of the particular recessive disease. Under the assumptions of Hardy and Weinberg, **carrier frequency** in the general population is twice the square root of disease incidence (i.e. about 1/20 for cystic fibrosis given an incidence of 1/1600 in whites). Individuals III-1 or III-4 in

pedigree B in Figure 1.5 would then have a (2/3)(1/20)(1/4) = 1/120 risk of having a child with cystic fibrosis, given that their spouse is Caucasian and unrelated.

Pedigree C in Figure 1.5 is again consistent with autosomal recessive disease but it represents children with spina bifida. On the basis of **empiric risks** for neural tube defects, multifactorial inheritance is far more likely than autosomal recessive inheritance. Had the family been counseled after individual II-2 was born, a 2% risk appropriate for **primary** or first-degree relatives would have been given. After the second affected child, the risk becomes 4–5% on the basis of empirical studies. Multifactorial disorders are unique in adjusting risks according to the number of affected members in a family. The adjustments reflect knowledge that the family's genes must be shifted toward the threshold for neural tube defects in comparison with the population mean. Folic acid is an environmental factor that can be supplemented to lower susceptibility to this disease.

Pedigree D in Figure 1.5 is suggestive of X-linked recessive inheritance because of affected males and transmission through females. Note that the grandmother and mother of III-3 must be carriers since two affected males having spontaneous mutations would be extremely unlikely to occur in one family. Both women thus face a 1/4 overall risk for affected children in their next pregnancy, or a 1/2 chance that a male fetus will be affected. This risk also applies to individual III-2 since she must have received her father's X chromosome with its abnormal allele (she is thus an **obligate carrier**, shown on the pedigree with a dot). Individual III-1 had no risk of being affected and no risk of transmitting the disease.

Pedigrees E and F in Figure 1.5 are the most frequently encountered in actual medical practice. It is essential to realize that each inheritance mechanism discussed above could be operating in these families. The affected males could represent new mutations for an autosomal dominant or X-linked recessive disorder, homozygotes for an autosomal recessive disease carried by the parents, or the first family members to cross the threshold of polygenic inheritance. Pedigree E is taken from a family in which the father of III-1 and his sister both carry a balanced translocation. Unlike simple trisomies or monosomies, where the risk for subsequent chromosomal anomalies is about 1%, translocation carriers face risks between 5 and 100% for abnormal offspring depending on their sex and the nature of their chromosomal translocation. Appropriate medical management of family E requires suspicion of a chromosome disorder based on multiple anomalies/mental retardation in the proband or the associated pregnancy loss. The proband's karyotype result will then guide family evaluation and counseling.

Molecular medicine and the language of DNA

Classic genetics viewed genes as abstract particles or factors that segregate to produce Mendelian or polygenic traits. Direct information about genes was first based on their products via the one gene–one enzyme hypothesis of Beadle and Tatum. After DNA structure and the genetic code were elucidated, molecular cloning and sequencing technologies allowed characterization of individual genes, gene products (e.g. mRNA and other types of RNAs), and their associated molecules (e.g. transcription factors, RNA-polymerase and other enzymes involved in transcription). Iterative, robotic, and imaging techniques can rapidly define populations of genes, RNAs, or proteins, visualizing their changes in extracts or real time. Cascades of interacting molecules can be examined all along the route from signal to factor to DNA–RNA–protein expression, and this section reviews steps in the genome's 'second code' for gene expression.[16]

DNA structure and the central dogma of gene expression

The fundamental unit of both DNA structure and genetic information is the **base pair** (bp). With the exception of certain bacteriophages, native DNA consists of antiparallel **complementary strands** joined by phosphodiester bonds between the 3'-hydroxyl and 5'-hydroxyl groups of deoxyribose (Fig. 1.6). DNA replication and transcription are directional, in that the first nucleotide of the complementary DNA or RNA will have a triphosphate at the **5′ end** and a hydroxyl at the **3′ end**. For proper base pairing to occur, the two strands of DNA must be oriented in opposite directions so that the 5'-nucleotide of one strand pairs with the 3'-nucleotide of its complement. The phosphate groups are on the outside of the DNA double helix, while the paired bases are stacked on the inside like steps on a spiral staircase (Fig. 1.6). This clustering of hydrophobic aromatic rings on the inside with hydrophilic phosphates and hydroxyl groups on the outside combines with hydrogen bonding to stabilize the helix. The thermodynamic advantages of the DNA duplex are indicated by the tendency of complementary DNA strands to associate spontaneously when placed in appropriate solutions, a reaction known as **DNA hybridization**. Conversely, the duplex can be subjected to increased temperature or ionic strength until the strands dissociate, a characteristic known as the T_m or melting temperature of the duplex. The role of hydrogen bonding in helix stability is illustrated by the higher melting temperatures of DNA duplexes with abundant GC base pairs (three hydrogen bonds) rather than the two hydrogen bonds between AT base pairs (Fig. 1.6). The role of base stacking is indicated by the lowering of T_m, which can be achieved by organic (more hydrophobic) solvents such as formamide. As shown in Figure 1.6, the dimension of a base pair in DNA is about 3.4Å long and 20Å wide; a complete helical turn is achieved every 34Å [approximately 10 nucleotides (or bp) per turn].

The central dogma

The flow of information from DNA to RNA to protein became known as the **central dogma** (see Fig. 1.8B), the basis for gene expression in all organisms. It was a remarkable milestone in biology, explaining how gene structure related to gene function.

The sequence of base pairs in DNA serves as a template for replication, as well as a template for protein synthesis. Correspondence of 3 bp codons in DNA with amino acids in protein proved to be the coding mechanism, implying redundancy based on 64 possible nucleotide triplets encoding 20 amino acids and 3 **termination signals** (Fig. 1.7).[17] Genes were then defined as linear sequences of codons with initiation signals (recognized by transcription factors – Fig. 1.8A, B) and intervening or termination signals (recognized by different sets of factors – Fig. 1.8 C, D). Note that punctuation signals are needed to establish the reading **frame;** otherwise a DNA strand could be read in three ways depending on which nucleotide was chosen to initiate the first codon. When a specified frame of reading contains no stop codons, that DNA region is called an **open reading frame** (ORF), which may potentially encode a protein. The absence of stop signals provides a useful way to recognize coding regions in randomly isolated DNA sequences.

Elegant experiments in bacteria and bacteriophage confirmed the colinearity of DNA and protein sequences, and showed the existence of three types of RNA molecules that were involved in protein synthesis (Fig. 1.8). A messenger RNA (mRNA) is transcribed from the coding or sense strand of DNA and used as a template to join amino acids by base pairing with unique adaptor or transfer RNAs (tRNA). The adaptor function is a critical aspect of information transfer since it adapts the bp language of DNA/RNA to the amino acid language of proteins. Protein synthesis occurs on ribosomal complexes composed of numerous proteins and RNAs. The mRNA provides DNA-encoded information, the ribosome provides movement and catalysis, and tRNA provides the link between mRNA codons and specific amino acids.

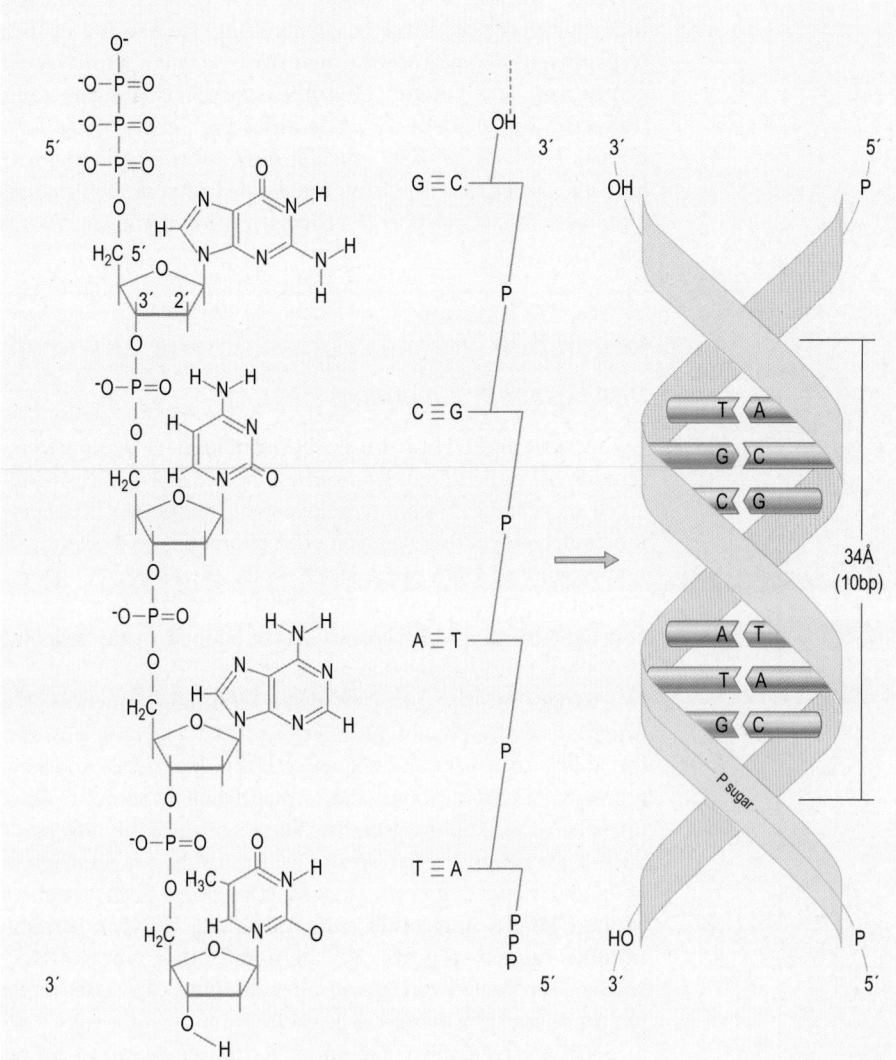

FIGURE 1.6 The structure of DNA. Three ways of representing DNA structure are shown, with 5′ representing ends of DNA strands having a terminal 5′-triphosphate on deoxyribose (initiation site for replication) and 3′ the ends with a terminal 3′-hydroxyl on deoxyribose. In the middle is a linear drawing indicating base pairs, and to the right is a representation of the double-stranded DNA helix where each 10 base pairs measure 34Å

Modifications to the central dogma

While the central dogma has been exhaustively verified in its main outline, **recombinant DNA** technology has highlighted some shortcomings. Modifications include:

- the possibility to convert RNA into DNA; and
- the fact that non-coding introns need to be **spliced** out to make mRNA.

They are illustrated in Figure 1.8 A–D, which also introduces the convention of representing DNA double strands by a single line, with boxes signifying important regions. In such diagrams, it is understood that DNA is double-stranded as shown in the upper part of Figure 1.8B, but only a single strand (usually the coding or **sense strand**) is represented. Such conventions allow direct comparison of the sense strand of DNA with single-strand RNA and are used throughout the literature of molecular biology. A first modification of the central dogma, one that was to be very useful for gene cloning, is based on the fact that information flow can be bidirectional: certain RNA viruses possess an enzyme called reverse transcriptase, which can synthesize a **complementary DNA** (cDNA) using mRNA as a template (Fig. 1.8D). **Reverse transcriptase** (RT) is employed in nature by RNA viruses to convert their RNA-based genome into DNA, which they can subsequently insert into the host genome. RT has proven extremely useful in the laboratory, where it is used to make cDNA copies of mRNAs for gene cloning and expression studies.

Figure 1.8B–D illustrates another modification of the central dogma prompted by the discovery of **splicing**. Comparison of cDNAs with their respective genes revealed that intervening sequences within genes (called **introns**) are present in the nascent RNA which is exactly homologous with its DNA template. The introns are excised (spliced) from the high molecular weight nuclear RNA (HnRNA) during RNA processing; the intronic RNA is then discarded and degraded. The segments of RNA between the introns (the **exons**) are then joined to one another. The exons are thus the segments of RNA which code for protein

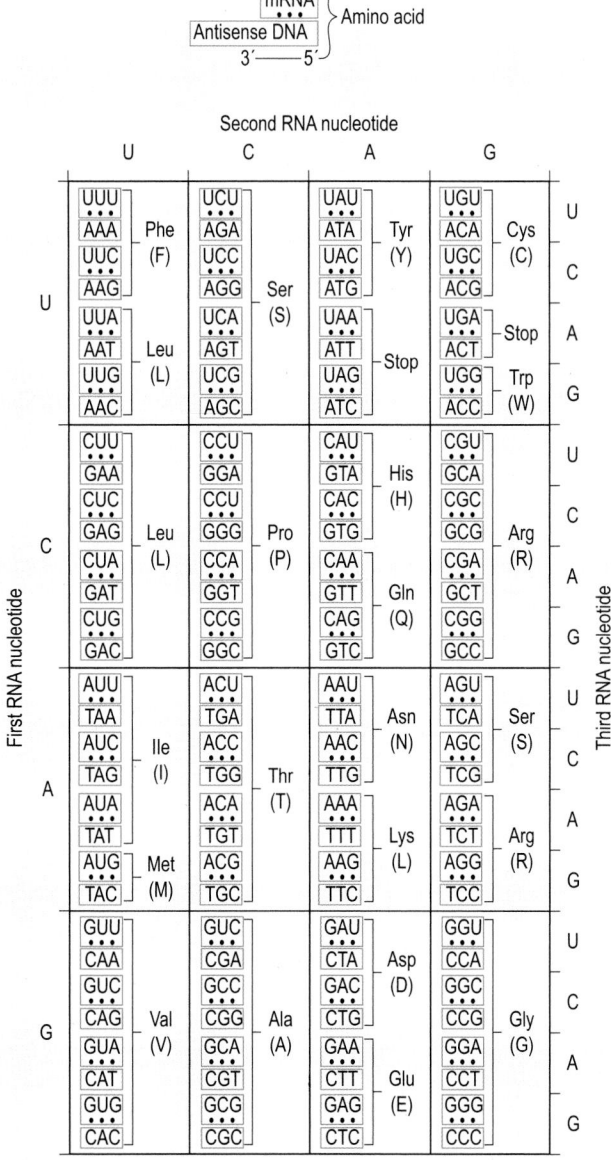

FIGURE 1.7 The genetic code. Amino acid three-letter and one-letter abbreviations are indicated beside the appropriate codons. (After Beaudet et al 1990,[17] with permission.)

extremely variable in size among different genes; it is postulated that they may play a role in determining the half-life of their respective RNA, and thus the quantity of protein a mRNA can synthesize. The kinetics of mRNA synthesis indicate rapid transcription at about 50 nucleotides per second (80 s for a typical HnRNA of 4000 nucleotides), slower splicing with half-lives of nuclear RNA intermediates from 3 to 30 min, and extremely rapid transport of processed mRNA from nucleus to cytoplasm.[18]

Regulation of gene expression: the DNA level

DNA dosage and rearrangement

Cytogenetic and DNA hybridization studies have demonstrated remarkable structural differences among DNA sequences within a cell or genome. Highly repetitive (satellite, heterochromatin), moderately repetitive (centromeric, telomeric) and slightly or non-repetitive DNA sequences were identified; a general correlation between lower copy number, transcriptional activity, and light-banding on trypsin-Giemsa stained metaphases has been observed (discussed in more detail in Ch. 5).

Changes in the primary gene (coding) sequences (i.e. mutations with a phenotypic effect) are relatively rare. However, the ability to isolate and sequence individual genes and large segments of chromosomes and to map whole genomes revealed unexpected variations within the two sets of alleles of individuals. Such a variation is even greater within groups of individuals, including populations of different ethnicities. Such variations include **single nucleotide polymorphisms** (SNPs), **variable number tandem repeats** (VNTRs), and other types of DNA sequences repeated variable numbers of times (discussed in the DNA polymorphism section below).

SNPs are relatively frequent, affecting on average 1 bp per 300–600 nucleotides in humans (the frequency depends on the type of DNA analyzed, such as promoter sequences, exonic DNA, intronic DNA, etc). SNPs may play a role in the efficiency with which a gene is transcribed (e.g. promoter SNPs), and in the activity of a gene's protein (e.g. exonic SNPs).[19]

Throughout the genome, repeated di- and trinucleotides organized in tandem are present, and the number of times that they are repeated can be different from one to another, leading to **VNTR polymorphisms**. Certain families of repeated DNA can spontaneously expand by an average of 11 DNA segments (repeats) within each human meiosis (i.e. they are meiotically unstable, whereas other DNA polymorphisms tend to remain stable from one generation to the next).[20] This variability in DNA segment repeats is accompanied by frequent rearrangements within repetitive DNA, producing human chromosome heteromorphisms; these variably repeated segments of DNA are required for programmed gene rearrangements as in immunoglobulin or olfactory genes.

DNA polymorphisms such as SNPs and VNTRs also provide an extremely powerful means to track alleles from one generation to the next (e.g. to identify mutant alleles in the course of prenatal diagnoses); to compare sets of alleles between individuals (e.g. for

synthesis. Characterization of numerous genes has established that exons often correspond to specific domains of the protein: e.g. leader sequences and cofactor binding regions (Fig. 1.8D).

Four different classes of introns exist (Fig. 1.8C); those within mRNA are the most abundant and are demarcated by a 5′ GU and a 3′ AG. **RNA splicing** is catalyzed by small nuclear RNAs (**Snurps**) and proteins, which form a complex termed a **spliceosome**. Other aspects of RNA processing include addition of a methylated G cap and a **poly A region** at the termini of HnRNA and of mRNA. Like introns, the 5′ and 3′ untranslated regions (UTRs) of mRNA that bracket the coding exons are

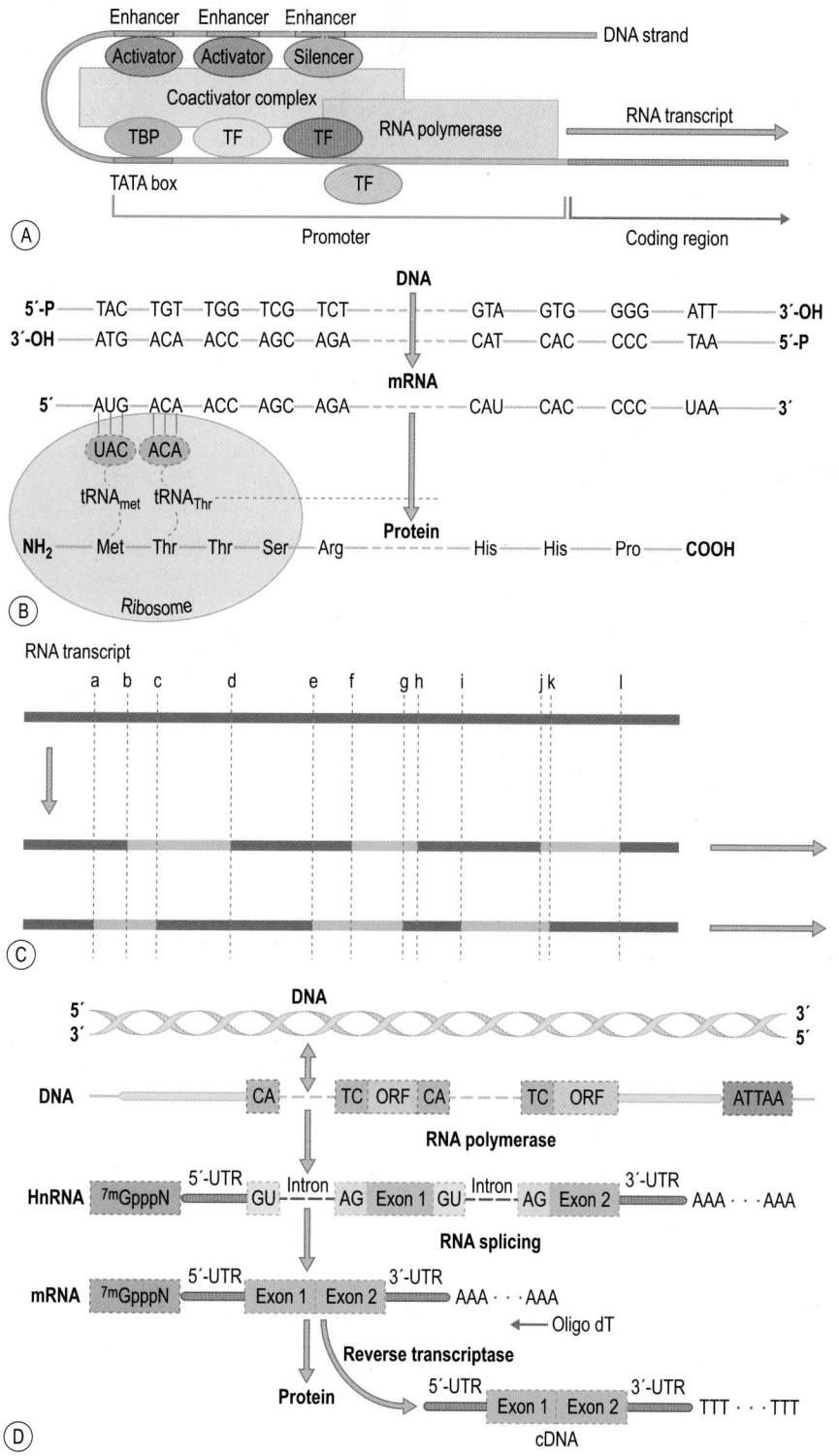

FIGURE 1.8 Modern central dogma. (A) Gene expression is regulated by the coordinated action of gene regulatory proteins that bind to control regions in DNA. First, transcription factors (TF) bind the promoter, stimulating the TATA box binding protein (TBP) to bind the TATA box. This causes multiple proteins to coalesce with the TBP to form a co-activator complex. The formation of co-activator complex will be modulated by the binding of activators and silencers (also transcription factors) onto enhancers to facilitate or inhibit the formation of the co-activator complex. Once this machinery is in place, RNA polymerase starts transcription of RNA. (B) Genetic flow of information begins with the complementary double strands of DNA, which are transcribed into mRNA and translated into protein. Note the 5′ to 3′ direction of RNA transcription, the amino- to carboxy-terminus direction of protein synthesis, and the use of transfer RNAs with specific anticodons to adapt from nucleotide to amino acid language. (C) RNA processing allows the same RNA transcript to be processed differently in different cells (through poorly understood mechanisms), or even in the same cell, thus coding for two distinct proteins. Note that non-coding exons are in green. (D) Additional complexity of the modern central dogma is shown by DNA open reading frames (ORF), protein-encoding exons, introns (dotted lines), splice signals for splicing out introns (CA, TC in DNA; GU, AG in RNA), 5′ and 3′ untranslated regions (UTR) in mRNA, methylguanine cap sites (GpppN) and polyadenylate tracts added during RNA maturation, and the complementary DNA (cDNA) that is synthesized by the reverse transcriptase of retroviruses. [(A) and (C) from 'Essentiel d'embryologie humaine et principes d'embryogenèse moléculaire', © Luc L. Oligny 2005, with permission.]

paternity ascertainment, or for comparing DNA found at a crime scene with that of suspects); and to compare different ethnicities and species to determine how closely linked they are genetically, and when they separated and became genetically isolated.

Other means of controlling gene expression which do not follow the central dogma have recently been found. Examples include:

- increasing gene expression by increasing the number of DNA copies of that gene (gene amplification), as is the case for amphibian ribosomal RNA, some silkworm genes, human folate-resistant cell cultures, and in aggressive neuroblastomas which amplify *NMYC*;
- gene inactivation by trinucleotide repeat expansion in diseases like fragile X syndrome, Huntington disease and myotonic dystrophy.

These new controlling mechanisms offer novel means for understanding and manipulating developmental gene regulation. The relevance of new, non-classical pathways which control gene expression is reinforced by progressive DNA expansions/contractions and myriad gene rearrangements characteristic of most cancers.

Furthermore, DNA dosage/arrangement changes may combine with DNA/chromatin modifications in the regulation of gene expression: a prototype is provided by repetitive sequences along eukaryotic chromosomes that bind **small interfering RNAs** (siRNAs). Binding can activate:

- the enzyme Met1, which methylates cytosines; and
- histone methylation.

Together, these epigenetic modifications can cause heterochromatinization and inactivation of the involved segment of DNA. Variation in the numbers or arrangements of these receptor DNA sequences could therefore alter which genes are inactivated as heterochromatin.[21, 22]

DNA methylation

DNA methylation, which is accomplished by the DNA methyltransferases, occurs on the cytosine residues of CG dinucleotides (also commonly called 'CpG,' for 'cytosine-phosphate-guanine').[23, 24] CpG dinucleotides are clustered together as **'CpG islands'** rather than being distributed in a haphazard fashion. It is thought that this island formation plays a role in the activation of DNA methyltransferases (DNMTs) during cellular differentiation (cytosine is methylated into 5-methyl-cytosine, or 'm5C') as methylation preferentially occurs in such islands. In humans, approximately 80% of CpG are methylated (3–8% of all cytosines are methylated).

Once a CG is methylated in a cell, it will remain methylated in all its descendants, as a result of the action of DNMTs (Fig. 1.9A, B). As cytosines are methylated only when immediately followed by a guanine (5′ → 3′), the complementary strand also reads CG in the 5′ → 3′ direction. As a new strand of DNA is polymerized from the template ('old') strand, the methylated CGs on the 'old' strand very efficiently activate the DNMT which then methylates the CG on the new strand, to ensure a faithful transmission of methylation.

It is believed that methylation of promoters inhibits their recognition by transcription factors and enzymes, as methylated cytosines bind MeCP, a methyl-cytosine binding protein (Fig. 1.9C); hence, if an enhancer region normally recognized by an activating transcription factor is methylated, transcription will be inhibited, whereas methylation of enhancers normally recognized by silencing transcription factors promotes transcription (see Fig. 1.8 for overview).[23, 24, 25] In some instances, when an inactive gene must be reactivated, nuclear demethylases will remove the methyl groups from its promoter; this appears to be the mechanism by which a cut plant in water will reactivate the mechanisms responsible for growing roots. No definitive cytosine demethylase has been identified in mammals.

Eukaryotes use methylation to inhibit the expression of genes which are not needed by a given cell.[23–24] Methylation contributes to cell differentiation, since the changes in DNA structure and expression will be transmitted to all the daughter cells of a progenitor cell. Methylation of promoters probably plays a major role in cellular differentiation during embryogenesis: cells eliminate the transcription of unwanted genes by methylating their promoters. Oocytes and spermatozoa are more differentiated than the totipotent cells of the zygote, containing large numbers of inactivated genes that are not available to the embryo. To remedy this situation, the morula (16-cell embryo, third day post conception) undergoes global demethylation to reactivate most genes; those genes subject to **parental (genomic) imprinting** escape this demethylation as discussed later. Cell differentiation occurs through methylation of key gene promoters in a strict sequence that depends on cell type.

DNA methylation also plays a role in the adult host's defense against micro-organisms. When viruses or plasmids infect a plant, their DNA configuration is recognized as foreign and inactivated by DNA methyltransferases. The foreign sequence may become integrated within the host's genome, but sustains 'biological death' through lack of transcription; it can no longer replicate independently of the host's genome and becomes 'junk' DNA within all descendants of the initially infected cell. Retroviruses undergo similar inactivation in mice, and it is conceivable that this phenomenon could be exploited in the treatment of AIDS.

Cytosines can lose their 5-methyl groups in a non-specific fashion, a process that occurs slowly and constantly in the human genome. A majority of promoter CG sites must be demethylated before transcription is restored, so this slow, spontaneous demethylation contributes little to gene reactivation. However, 5-methylcytosine can spontaneously be oxidized to uracil or thymine, producing cytosine to thymine (C to T) point mutations; loss of the methyl group leads to cytosine deamination and conversion to thymine. Similar deamination of non-methylated cytosine converts C to uracil (U), causing a C to U point mutation; the cell can methylate uracil to produce thymine or replace uracil with thymine during DNA replication. In any event, the end results are C to T point mutations that play a major role in genetic diseases. For example, a survey of 139 genetic diseases caused by a point mutation showed a third to be secondary to a cytosine or 5-methylcytosine to thymine deamination. Furthermore, in large

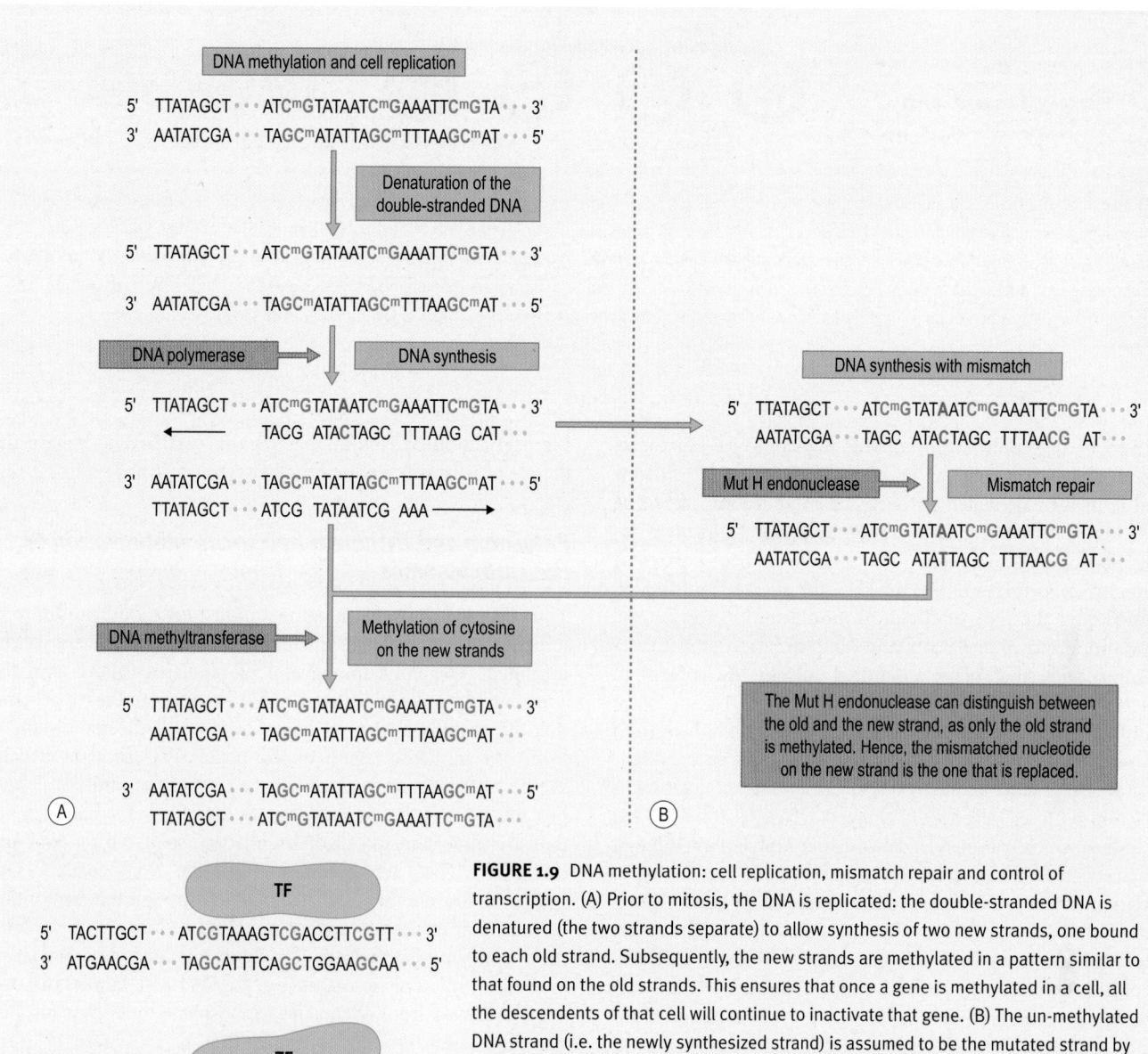

FIGURE 1.9 DNA methylation: cell replication, mismatch repair and control of transcription. (A) Prior to mitosis, the DNA is replicated: the double-stranded DNA is denatured (the two strands separate) to allow synthesis of two new strands, one bound to each old strand. Subsequently, the new strands are methylated in a pattern similar to that found on the old strands. This ensures that once a gene is methylated in a cell, all the descendents of that cell will continue to inactivate that gene. (B) The un-methylated DNA strand (i.e. the newly synthesized strand) is assumed to be the mutated strand by the enzymes involved in mismatch repair. Once the mismatch is repaired, the cytosines on the new strand are methylated according to the template of the old strand. (C) The un-methylated sequence on the left can bind a transcription factor to activate transcription. On the right, the same sequence in another cell cannot bind with this transcription factor, because it has been methylated and the methyl groups interfere with this recognition. (From 'Essentiel d'embryologie humaine et principes d'embryogenèse moléculaire', © Luc L. Oligny 2005, with permission.)

series of patients, over 50% of all the point mutations affecting the anti-oncogene P53, and 45% of all the mutations of hemophilia B's factor IX were of this type.[26]

Methylation inhibits (and occasionally activates) a very large number of genes, including some proto-oncogenes.[27] In cancers, there is often a decreased expression of DNA methyltransferase which leads to a non-specific demethylation of 5-methylcytosine. It appears that this demethylation can reactivate the expression of proto-oncogenes which thus act as unregulated growth-promoting agents (e.g. oncogenes, telomerases, etc.) and of genes involved in cell migration, leading to the emergence of progressively more aggressive clones (clonal evolution). Abnormal methylation (hence inactivation) of anti-oncogenes similarly plays a major role in cancer.

Histones and acetylation

Until recently, histones were thought to have an exclusively mechanical and structural role, to 'protect' DNA from injurious agents, and to allow DNA compaction. Recent evidence shows

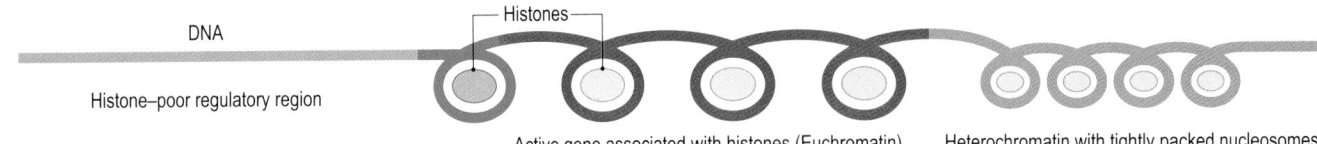

DNA

Histone-poor regulatory region

Histones

Active gene associated with histones (Euchromatin)   Heterochromatin with tightly packed nucleosomes

FIGURE 1.10 Role of histones in gene transcription. Nucleosomes are DNA–histone complexes (the first nucleosome is shown in dark blue). Regions with active transcription, such as promoters and enhancers of non-silenced genes, are histone-poor. This allows optimal recognition of these sequences by transcription factors. Transcriptionally-silenced regions are histone-rich, in order to prevent their recognition and stimulation by transcription factors which could otherwise bind and activate them. The presence of histones in lesser numbers in transcriptionally-active genes does not hinder the transcription machinery. (From 'Essentiel d'embryologie humaine et principes d'embryogenèse moléculaire', © Luc L. Oligny 2005, with permission.)

that histones also control transcription, regulating accessibility of genes to RNA polymerases and transcription factors.[28–30] Histone action is in turn regulated by chemical modification including acetylation, methylation (not to be confused with DNA methylation), phosphorylation, and ubiquitination. The particular histone involved (H1, H2, H3, or H4), the specific amino acid modified, and the type of chemical modification (acetylation, methylation, phosphorylation, and ubiquitination) constitutes a 'histone code', that plays a seminal role in the control of transcription.[24]

All four types of histones are subject to acetylation of their positively charged lysines. Acetylation of each lysine decreases the electrical charge of a histone by one electron, thus modulating its interaction with the electrically-charged DNA. Histone H4 has four lysines which can be acetylated; hyper-acetylation (three or four acetylated sites) enhances transcription, while hypo-acetylation (one or zero sites) tends to inhibit it. Whereas acetylation of histones always facilitates transcription, the other histone modifications are more complex. For example, methylation of histone H3 on its lysine-9 residue allows it to bind to a Polycomb protein (see below), blocking transcription. However, methylation of other lysines within histones can change the chromatin configuration to enhance, rather than repress, transcription.

Histone modification can modulate nucleosome formation and DNA compaction into chromatin. For example, a gene's rate of transcription is proportional to the acetylation of its H4 histones. H4 acetylation (by histone acetyltransferases) influences the conformation of DNA/chromatin, thus modulating RNA polymerase binding and initiation of transcription (Fig. 1.10). Histone acetylation correlates with gene transcription, and certain transcription factors contain histone acetyltransferases to modify histones of the promoters they control. As expected, the H4 histones of inactive X chromosomes in females are hypo-acetylated, and their DNA is methylated.

During DNA synthesis, DNA strands are denatured and freed from their histones: when histones are hyper-acetylated at a given site, these acetylated histones remain near the replication fork, and are immediately integrated in the two new strands of DNA. Therefore, acetylated H4s are decreased by approximately 50% in each strand at that site. Acetylases will subsequently increase the acetylation of H4s in that region, so that H4s regain the degree of acetylation which they possessed prior to mitosis.

Polycomb and Trithorax: heterochromatinization of the chromosomes

The effects of DNA methylation and histone modifications tend to be local: only genes in the vicinity of these modifiers will be inhibited. The Polycomb group of repressors (PcG) and the Trithorax group of activators (TrxG) are large families of proteins that affect transcription of genes over much greater distances, from one insulator region to the next.[31] PcG proteins usually inhibit transcription whereas TrxG proteins promote it. These proteins control the expression patterns of developmental genes that are important in cell differentiation, stem cell renewal and cancer.[32–34] They are recruited to specific DNA sequences to inhibit or activate their associated genes through the recognition of transcription factors and/or modified histones. PcG proteins may condense chromatin by blocking histone acetylating enzymes, while TrxG proteins (e.g. the SWI/SNF family) may use energy derived from adenosine triphosphate hydrolysis to open up chromatin into euchromatin that is accessible to transcription factors, RNA polymerase and other factors necessary to transcribe genes.

Once recruited, TrxG proteins (e.g. Swi proteins in yeast) have been shown to change nucleosome positioning relative to the DNA strand by sliding nucleosomes along DNA.[34, 35] These changes facilitate the binding of transcription factors with DNA and activate gene expression. It is likely that the association of TrxG proteins with chromatin prevents PcG proteins from binding in that region. Conversely, PcG proteins exclude the transcription machinery from promoters and tilt the equilibrium towards heterochromatin. When many adjacent chromatin sites are recognized by PcG proteins, adjacent proteins may join together into a large polymer that compacts the chromatin into heterochromatin, to block transcription.[22, 34–35]

The mechanisms by which descendent cells retain the chromatin positioning of their PcG/TrxG proteins are unclear. Although some PcG proteins remain bound to their chromatin during chromosome replication, cytosine methylation and histone modifications probably play a greater role in this clonal transmission. In any event, specific patterns of heterochromatin are faithfully transmitted from progenitor to daughter cells, as are methylation and histone modifications.

Epigenesis and gene expression – an integrated view

Epigenetic transmission does not alter genome sequence but plays a major role in the transmission of differentiation factors from one cell to all its descendants. 'Epigenetic memory', i.e. heritable changes in chromatin transmitted in a cell lineage, is certainly not the result of a single, simple mechanism. Its multiple aspects include DNA methylation, histone modifications, nucleosome positioning within gene and promoter sequences, the PcG and TrxG protein interactions, all culminating in the regulation of transcription through chromatin conformation.

Interactions among these levels of regulation are complex and can be divided into antagonistic processes. Factors repressing transcription include:

- recruitment of DNA methylating enzymes by inhibitory transcription factors to inactivate promoters;
- direct inhibition of genes by other transcription factors, secondarily recruiting PcG proteins and histone de-acetylation;
- recruitment of methyl-cytosine binding proteins and histone de-acetylating enzymes to form chromatin-inactivating complexes;
- recruitment of histone de-acetylases by PcG proteins;
- binding of PcG proteins by methylated histone H3 to initiate heterochromatinization; and
- stimulation of DNA methylation by PcG proteins.
Factors activating transcription include:
- recruitment of histone acetyltransferases by transcription factors to promote euchromatinization and gene transcription;
- recruitment of TrxG proteins by acetylated histones;
- re-orienting nucleosomes and exposing promoters and TATA boxes to allow the initiation of transcription; and
- recruitment of histone acetyltransferases by TrxG proteins to promote transcription.

Note that the factors that repress transcription act in synergy, causing a positive feedback loop which assures co-activation of all the repressive machinery. Likewise, factors that activate transcription also activate a positive feedback loop to co-activate all of the activating machinery.

These systems are so intrinsically linked in embryonal cell differentiation that it is very difficult to determine which is the primary epigenetic mark (e.g. cytosine methylation, histone modification, PcG/TrxG protein binding), and to distinguish this primordial marking from its related changes. It is likely that an epigenetic transmission can be initiated by any one of these transcription factor-driven mechanisms. Once initiated, these mechanisms stimulate one another, acting as a 'fail-safe' system because of their genetic redundancy.

Regulation of gene expression: the RNA level

If the hypothesis of an early RNA world is true, (i.e. that primordial life arose through RNA, with DNA developing sub-sequently), then it is not surprising that the major RNA players in the central dogma have more complex and diverse fates than anticipated. This section will highlight the complexity of an RNA-based regulation of gene expression, which can occur at least at six levels:

- Depending on the relative potency of the various factors affecting a gene's promoter/silencers/inhibitors (cumulative effects of all of the activating/inhibiting transcription factors), transcription of RNA can range from null to very high (discussed previously).
- Regulatory elements are present within the mRNA which determine the efficiency with which it will be translated into protein.
- Such regulatory elements also determine the half-life of the mRNA, and thus the amount of times a mRNA can be translated into protein before it decays.
- **Alternative splicing,** through which identical RNA molecules may be spliced in different ways, hence producing proteins which differ from one another (in some cases, one gene can produce more than 10 000 different proteins; for example, the gene *DSCAM* can be spliced to form ~ 38 000 different proteins, thus generating by itself a huge number of different cell adhesion molecules (CAM) required for the proper migration of neurons).[36]
- RNA can associate with DNA to cause its heterochromatinization.
- tRNA mutations at the level of anticodons alter the translation of mRNA into protein.
- tRNA mutations outside of the anticodons can alter its interaction with mRNA.
- double-stranded RNA can recognize homologous sequences on mRNA, causing its degradation through the enzyme DICER, effectively silencing this mRNA.
- Ribosomes are composed of RNA.
- Some RNAs, called **ribozymes,** have intrinsic enzymatic function.

Messenger RNAs, like their encoding DNA, are associated with proteins from birth to death. Some 570 proteins in yeast have RNA-binding domains, making possible unique pathways for specific mRNAs as they proceed from the stages of synthesis by RNA polymerase, splicing, terminal cleavage, sublocalization with similar mRNAs, to mRNA degradation (the 'exonuclease death') in the cytoplasm.[37] RNA-binding proteins include general chaperones recognizing general features like the 7-methylguanosine cap or polyadenosine (polyA) tail as well as regulators of individual mRNA fates that recognize individual mRNA sequences. Some of these proteins are involved in shuttle of heterogenous mRNAs from the nucleus; others regulate packaging and consequent ribosome targeting, translational activity, and protection from nuclease breakdown.

Specific localization of RNA within a particular region of an embryo (fly or human) can be instrumental in the segmentation of that organism; the cells which produce this RNA are controlled by region-specific transcription factors. For example, in *Drosophila* embryos, only the posterior-most cells transcribe the *oskar* mRNA, which is thus localized exclusively in this region; hence, translation of oskar mRNA to oskar protein occurs exclusively in the posterior-most cells of the embryo, but this protein can diffuse anteriorly. This segmentation of oskar synthesis (expression), coupled with its ability to diffuse, generates a caudo-cephalic concentration gradient which is essential to induce to the formation of the embryonic germline and abdomen.

Control of transcription can also be achieved by specific microRNAs (miRNAs) that associate through complementary base pairing with 3'-untranslated regions of their parent mRNA, inhibiting protein synthesis.[37]

Studies of ribosomal and transfer RNAs also reveal variability in their types of protein associations, nuclease cleavage, and yields of small RNA products. Primary transcripts of mRNA, rRNA, and tRNA are all cleaved by endonucleases to yield free 3'-ends, causing them to be routed differently (e.g. the polyA tail is added only to mRNAs).

The mammalian mRNA 3'-endonuclease reaction involved in mRNA maturation requires at least 15 proteins; some of these protein factors are shared with a less characterized complex that cleaves tRNA, but the major endonucleases required appear to be different.[38] For example, endonuclease specificity is illustrated by the fact that the ELA2 endonuclease that cleaves tRNA is a susceptibility factor for prostate cancer; this endonuclease is also essential for yeast cell survival.

In addition to the protein complexes which can modulate and cleave RNA, structural motifs within the various RNA molecules also have regulatory roles. For example, mutations in the anticodon of tRNAs cause mRNA to be misread, with the normal amino acid being substituted by the mutated tRNA; tRNA mutations outside of the anticodon can also alter the way tRNAs translate mRNA. For example, some tRNA suppressors contain mutations outside the anticodon sequence (e.g. the 'Hirsh suppressor' tryptophanyl tRNA that can override terminator codons). This tRNA has a mutant RNA element that alters proofreading constraints at the ribosome, foretelling other regulatory mechanisms where ribosomal RNA/aminoacyl-tRNA elements and elongation factors modulate synthesis of individual proteins.[39]

The importance of small RNA molecules, 21–30 nucleotides in length, extends far beyond their influence on major RNA classes. miRNAs, siRNAs, and repeat-associated small interfering RNAs function throughout biology, having the ability to silence chromatin, interfere with cell division, maintain stem cells in their undifferentiated state, negotiate viral/nuclear DNA competition, and even promote DNA degradation. A database for miRNA-encoding genes now has 1650 members, including 227 from humans and 21 from human viruses. Repositories of miRNAs are commercially available as reagents which efficiently inhibit the expression of specific genes, acting variously at transcriptional, RNA processing, or translational levels.[37–40]

The discovery of miRNAs has promoted the study of non-coding RNA in general: miRNAs show an enormous diversity (> 75 000 small RNA species in certain plants), a striking evolutionary conservation, and significant origin by antisense transcription – e.g. allowing both strands of cDNA strands to be read in the same segment.[37] The unexpected abundance of non-coding, polyadenylated RNAs, processed into various types of small RNAs, likely explains why early human genome sequence estimates of gene number (85 000–150 000) were so high; current estimates of 25 000 genes are based on matches with protein sequences rather than counting of potential transcription units.

The ability of RNA molecules to act as **ribozymes,** catalyze their own splicing or yield complex secondary structures, adds even more potential steps to RNA regulation. The idea of RNA regulatory factors, long overshadowed by protein transcription factors, has now been resuscitated.[37, 38]

Regulation of gene expression: the protein level

The regulation of gene expression by proteins adds another layer of complexity/control onto RNA-based regulation, to allow fine-tuning of gene expression. For example, proteins can act as morphogens to control the promoters of developmental genes, or to activate protein-based cascades to control the expression of such genes. A perfectly controlled activation/inhibition is crucial for the regulation of cell pathways and cell differentiation. For example, retinoic acid receptors control multiple critical developmental pathways; severe malformations arise when their ligand (e.g. Accutane®) is present in pharmaceutical rather than natural amounts.

Transcription factors

Transcription factors are molecules (proteins, RNA, retinoic acid, etc.) that directly bind DNA to activate or inhibit the expression of gene(s) under their control. This action is generally mediated through a direct interaction with the transcriptional control machinery (promoters, enhancers, silencers, and protein–protein interactions, including RNA polymerase) of those genes. The fundamental transcriptional complex containing RNA polymerase II, DNA, and global transcription factors like TFIIA-F has now been characterized in three dimensions.[41, 42] A large number of transcription factors can interact simultaneously with this machinery (Fig. 1.11, Box 1.1), and their cumulative activating and inhibiting forces determine gene expression. Some 1850 transcription factors have been identified in humans, many associated with developmental disorders.[43] Various mutations can affect transcription factors, and their nature (e.g. point mutations, splice mutations, deletions, etc.) can result in phenotypes of varying severity. Some transcription factors can also bind mRNA, to activate or inhibit their translation into proteins.

A relevant group of transcription factors are those encoded by **master switch** or selector genes. Master switch genes all code for transcription factors which can regulate cell cycles, differentiation, and morphogenesis through the activation and inhibition of subordinate genes (Fig. 1.11). Hence, by definition, the activation of a single master switch gene allows the synchronous regulation of a large battery of subordinate genes necessary for the differentiation of a cell or tissue.

The expression of genes by different types of cells during various stages of development (i.e. at various states of differentiation) and after stimulation with different signals can be assessed through **DNA chip** technology. Such experiments have revealed that whole regions of chromosomes (regulons) can have genes

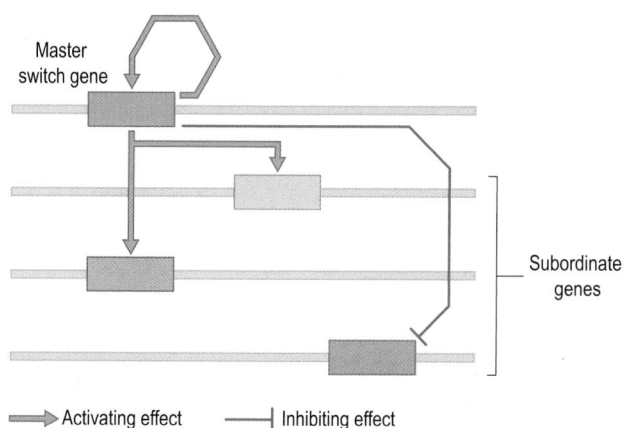

Activating effect ⊣ **Inhibiting effect**

FIGURE 1.11 Master switch genes. As a general rule, master switch genes tend to auto-activate their promoters in a positive feedback manner, to ensure a constant state of activation in expressing cells and their descendants. Master switch genes can activate or inhibit their subordinate genes, to control their downstream cascades. (From 'Essentiel d'embryologie humaine et principes d'embryogenèse moléculaire', © Luc L. Oligny 2005, with permission.)

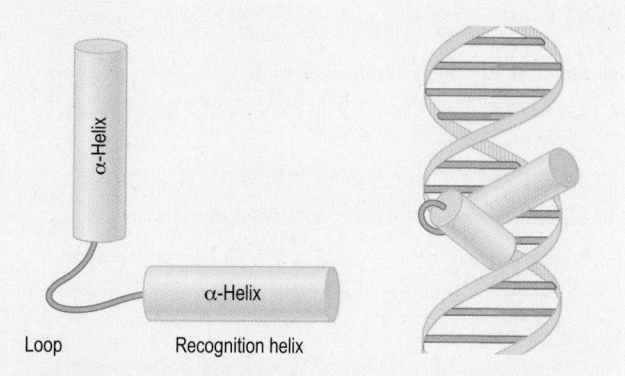

FIGURE 1.12 Helix-loop-helix (HLH) type transcription factors. The figure to the left shows the structure of the HLH protein. The helical portions are tightly coiled spirals of amino acids, whereas the loop joins the two α-helices to provide optimal DNA interaction. The figure to the right shows how the HLH protein binds a major groove of the DNA molecule. Note that subtle changes in the amino acid sequence of the recognition helix causes HLH to recognize different DNA sequences, and to thus bind and activate or repress the control sequences of a whole series of different genes. (From 'Essentiel d'embryologie humaine et principes d'embryogenèse moléculaire', © Luc L. Oligny 2005, with permission.)

that are co-expressed. Sequence comparisons have shown that regulons share upstream binding motifs specific for the same transcription factor (i.e. one transcription factor can activate all the genes of a regulon), thus acting as a master switch gene. In yeast, these regulons can extend for 20–30 kb, defining regions comparable to the puffs of high gene activity seen on *Drosophila* chromosomes.[42]

Many transcription factors have major roles in developmental and fetal pathology. The proteins coded for by master switch genes can belong to several classes of transcription factors (homeodomain, PAX, zinc fingers, etc.).

More than 100 homeodomain transcription factors exist. They are characterized by a 'homeobox' of 180 nucleotides (60 amino acids). These developmental genes have been remarkably conserved throughout evolution, and are virtually identical in yeast, *Drosophila* and humans (discussed below). Many of these homeodomain proteins also share a unique region of secondary structure called a 'helix–loop–helix' (HLH) motif (Fig. 1.12). A subfamily of HLH proteins have alkaline or 'basic' domains (the β-HLH proteins), including the MYF-3 and MYF-5 transcription factors involved in myogenesis. β-HLH transcription factors need to dimerize with other β-HLH proteins to bind DNA in order to control transcription; the alkaline nature of these proteins allows peculiar interactions with DNA, which is acidic.

Another group of master switch genes was also identified by sequence similarity in *Drosophila* – the PAX or PAired boX genes. Nine families of PAX genes are known, some demarcating larger developmental fields into specific regions like limbs, others activating specific transcription factors like MYF-3 within these regions to form specialized cell types (e.g. myoblasts). The *PAX-6* gene is crucial for eye development in humans (involved in aniridia) and other organisms (e.g. *Drosophila*). Some PAX-6

gene mutations exhibit dominant inheritance because of **haploinsufficiency:** one active allele does not produce enough PAX-6 protein to activate and inhibit the cascades of downstream promoters, leading to ocular maldevelopment. If both copies are mutated, craniofacial, cerebral, and more severe ocular abnormalities are produced.

A third class of transcription factors are those with a zinc-finger motif: zinc molecules cause these proteins to have a tertiary structure resembling fingers. The 'fingers' bind the promoters of the genes under their control, so as to activate or inhibit them. Zinc finger proteins illustrate the multiple domains that can exist within transcription factors, allowing them to coordinate multiple different expression pathways. They can contain:

- a DNA-binding domain consisting of at least two highly conserved zinc fingers;
- a ligand-binding domain that modifies the transcriptional activity of the factor;
- transactivation domain(s) whose function may or not be modulated by binding of the ligand;
- in many, an associated homeodomain.

WT-1 (the Wilms tumor-1 gene product), the fly developmental gene *hunchback*, certain hormone and retinoic acid receptors belong to the zinc-finger class of transcription factors.

Other proteins and the promise of proteomics

The translation of the 4 bp code into a ≥ 20 amino acid code enables the synthesis of an astronomical number of proteins

BOX 1.1 SOME INHERITED HUMAN DISORDERS DUE TO MUTATIONS IN GENES ENCODING TRANSCRIPTION FACTORS.

Nuclear receptor family of zinc fingers (ZNF):
- Androgen receptor (AR): androgen insensitivity syndromes, and spinal / bulbar muscular atrophy
- Estrogen receptor (ER): estrogen resistance
- Glucocorticoid receptor (GR): glucocorticoid resistance
- Thyroid hormone receptor Δ (TRΔ): thyroid hormone resistance
- Vitamin D receptor (VDR): hereditary vitamin D resistant rickets type II
- *DAX1:* X-linked adrenal hypoplasia congenita; dosage-sensitive sex-reversal

Other zinc fingers:
- Wilms tumor-1 (*WT-1*): WAGR syndrome; Denys-Drash syndrome
- GLI-3: Greig cephalopolysyndactyly syndrome; Pallister-Hall syndrome

PAX (paired box):
- *PAX2:* optic nerve coloboma and renal hypoplasia
- *PAX3:* Waardenburg syndrome types I and III; craniofacial-deafness-hand syndrome
- *PAX6:* aniridia; Peter's anomaly; isolated foveal hypoplasia; autosomal dominant keratitis

bHLH (helix–loop–helix):
- MITF: Waardenburg syndrome type II
- TWIST: Saethre-Chotzen syndrome

Homeodomain:
- *MSX-1:* autosomal dominant tooth agenesis
- *MSX-2:* Boston-type craniosynostosis
- *HOX-D13:* synpolydactyly
- *HOX-A13:* hand-foot-genital syndrome
- RIEG: Rieger syndrome
- SHOX: short stature
- *IPF1:* pancreatic agenesis

HMG (high mobility group):
- SRY: sex reversal
- SOX9: camptomelic dysplasia; sex reversal
- SOX10: Hirschsprung disease

POU (named from PIT1-OCT1-UNC86 and pronounced 'pow'):
- PIT1: hypopituitary dwarfism
- POU3F4: X-linked deafness type 3

Others:
- TBX1: DiGeorge syndrome
- TBX3: ulnar-mammary syndrome
- TBX5: Holt-Oram syndrome
- RFX5: bare lymphocyte syndrome
- RFXAP: bare lymphocyte syndrome
- CIITA: bare lymphocyte syndrome
- OSF2: cleidocranial dysplasia
- HNF1α: maturity-onset diabetes of the young
- HNF4α: maturity-onset diabetes of the young

Co-activators:
- ATRX: X-linked α-thalassemia and mental retardation
- CBP: Rubenstein-Taybi syndrome

General transcription factors:
- ERCC2: xeroderma pigmentosa
- ERCC3: xeroderma pigmentosa
- ERCC6: Cockayne syndrome
- CSA: Cockayne syndrome
- P44T: Werdnig-Hoffman spinal muscular atrophy

Tumor suppressors:
- RB: retinoblastoma, osteosarcoma
- P53 (also referred to as TP53): Li-Fraumeni syndrome
- NF-1: neurofibromatosis type 1

After Semenza 1999,[25] with permission. The reader is referred to that text for more details

which exhibit a great variability in their three-dimensional structure, and generates a nearly infinite level of complexity with respect to gene regulation and genetic diseases. Diversity of protein function includes the binding of DNA by transcription factors, contractile proteins in muscles, structural proteins in collagen, and cell adhesion proteins so important for development (see below). As with DNA chip profiling of gene sequences or transcripts, a particular protein population (proteome) can be profiled by shotgun sequencing techniques, microcapillary or two-dimensional electrophoresis, laser technologies, micro-arrays and mass spectroscopy.[43–45] This field of study is called proteomics.

Most proteins are compartmentalized, with the cytoplasm resembling a crystal more than a fluid, and protein localization/ trafficking can be visualized by fluorescent or electron microscopy in vivo, or used to isolate specific proteomes in vitro.[44] An example of the latter approach characterized the integrated membrane proteins of the nuclear envelope by shotgun sequencing, and then used their derived encoding sequences to match them with gene loci of interest in muscular dystrophy families.

The use of proteomic technology links the enormous variability in protein populations and structures to the nucleic acid language of genome and RNA. The laborious work of isolating enzymes and the more modern dilemma of predicting protein function from identified genes can now be simplified by characterizing protein groups: proteins defined by housekeeping, signal-response, cell cycle phase, compartment, or differentiation state can be sequenced en masse, then correlated with their gene struc-

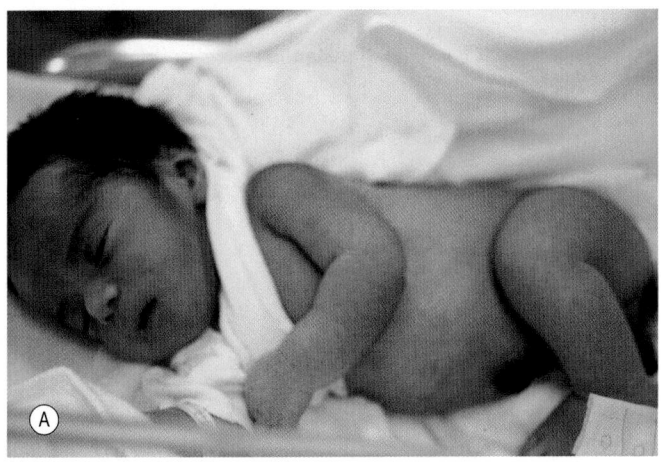

FIGURE 1.13 Infant with type II osteogenesis imperfecta (A) showing severe deformities of limbs, and bones (B).[18, 20]

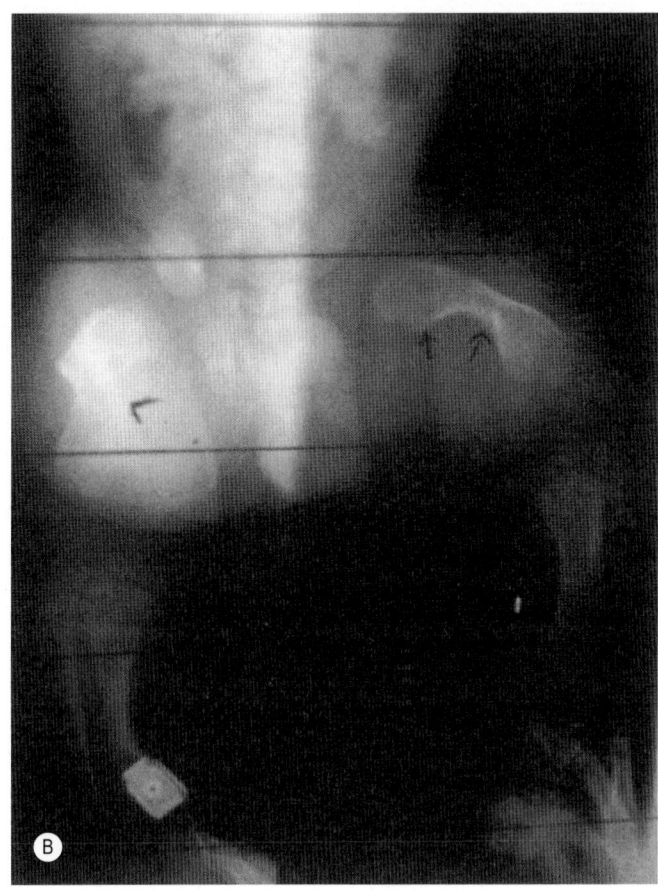

ture and expression. Protein–protein interactions can be predicted by looking for encoding sequences within cDNAs that predict shared protein motifs; two-hybrid and multiassay methods for determining all protein interactions in yeast or *Drosophila* have been developed.[46] As with ubiquitous single nucleotide polymorphisms, proteomes involved in particular pathways or cell types can provide fingerprints of disease or susceptibility. Examples include variations in tumor or insulin signaling proteomes that may guide and monitor chemotherapy or diabetes.[47]

Molecular basis of disease: example of osteogenesis imperfecta

The basic elements of DNA structure and expression summarized above provide an approach to all single gene disorders. If a particular gene or its product protein can be implicated in the disease, the pathology can be understood by characterizing the pathway of gene expression. Severe forms of osteogenesis imperfecta offer dramatic examples of altered fetal development that exhibit Mendelian inheritance (Fig. 1.13).[48] In these children the affliction of sclerae and long bones matched the known distribution of type I collagen (Table 1.1). Genes encoding this protein became candidates for the abnormal alleles implied by Mendelian inheritance. Complex biochemical

studies were required to characterize the two *polypeptide chains* that made up type I collagen, known as α_1 and α_2. Protein electrophoresis demonstrated an altered mobility of these polypeptides in certain patients with osteogenesis imperfecta. Antibodies to these polypeptides were then employed to isolate the genes encoding type I collagen synthesis.[48]

Figure 1.14 depicts the gene for the α_1 chain of type I procollagen.[48] The gene contains 41 exons (green) separated by larger introns (white). The gene coding for the α_2 chain of type I procollagen is very similar, with one additional exon. Collagen proteins have a modular structure that is reflected by their coding exons. The requirements of triple-helix formation mandate the occurrence of glycines, the smallest amino acid, at every third amino acid residue. Collagen proteins are composed of amino acid triplets in the form of glycine-X-Y, and their exons are assembled from 54 bp units (i.e. 18 codons) as illustrated in the upper portion of Figure 1.14. In this case, the X and Y are variables standing for any amino acid rather than specific designations using the amino acid code in Figure 1.7. After transcription of a large pre-mRNA, the introns are spliced out to yield mRNA of two different sizes. Such **alternative splicing** emphasizes that the same gene may be utilized to encode multiple mRNAs and proteins, although the significance of these two procollagen I mRNAs is unknown. After translation, two procollagen I α_1 chains associate with one of the α_2 chains to form a triple helix. Amino acids at the N- and C-terminal ends are

TABLE 1.1 COLLAGEN TYPES, DISTRIBUTIONS, AND MUTATIONS IN CONNECTIVE TISSUE DISEASES

Collagen (chains)	Tissue distribution	Type of mutation	Diseases
I α_1(I)	Skin, tendons, bones, arteries	Deletions, splicing defects	OI types I, II; EDS type VII
		Point mutations	OI types II, III, IV
I α_2(I)	Skin, tendons, bones, arteries, tumors	Deletions, splicing defects	OI type II; OI types I, IV; EDS type VII
		Point mutations	OI types II, III, IV
II α_1(II)	Cartilage, vitreous of eye	Point mutations	Stickler, Kneist syndromes; SED
III α_1(III)	Skin, arteries, uterus	Deletions, point mutations	EDS types I, IV
IV α_1(III)	Basement membranes	Point mutations	Alport syndrome
V α_1(V)	Skin, placenta, blood vessels	Point mutations	EDS types I, II
α_2(V)	Skin, placenta, blood vessels	Point mutations	EDS type I
VII α_1(VII)	Chorioamniotic membranes, skin	Point mutations	Epidermolysis bullosa
IX α_1(IX)	Hyaline cartilage	Point mutations	Multiple epiphyseal dysplasia
X α_1(X)	Columnar, calcifying cartilage	Point mutations	Schmid metaphyseal dysplasia
XI α_1(XI)	Fibrillar collagen in bone, cartilage	Point mutations	Stickler syndrome type III

EDS, Ehlers-Danlos syndrome; OI, osteogenesis imperfecta; SED, spondyloepiphyseal dysplasia.
After OMIM 2006,[4] with permission.

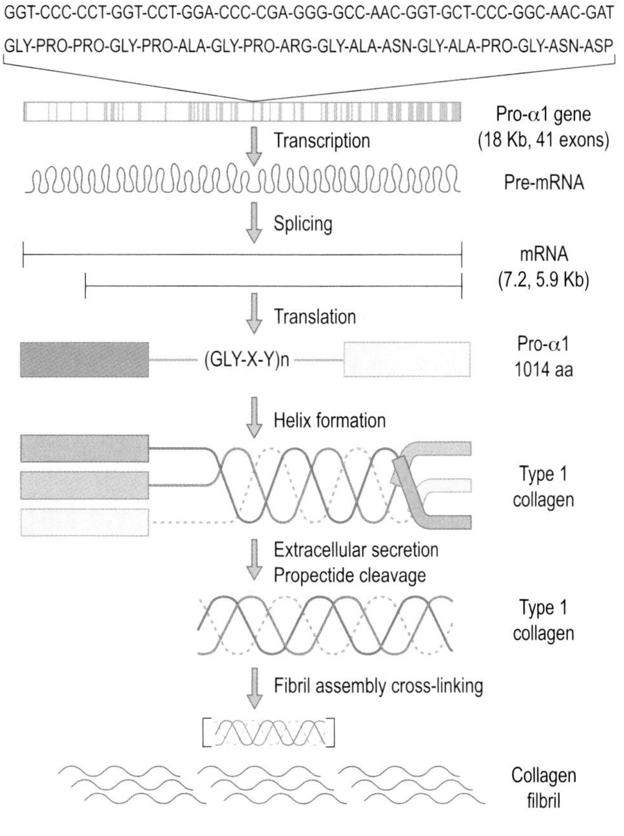

GGT-CCC-CCT-GGT-CCT-GGA-CCC-CGA-GGG-GCC-AAC-GGT-GCT-CCC-GGC-AAC-GAT
GLY-PRO-PRO-GLY-PRO-ALA-GLY-PRO-ARG-GLY-ALA-ASN-GLY-ALA-PRO-GLY-ASN-ASP

Transcription — Pro-α1 gene (18 Kb, 41 exons)

Pre-mRNA

Splicing — mRNA (7.2, 5.9 Kb)

Translation — Pro-α1 1014 aa — (GLY-X-Y)n

Helix formation — Type 1 collagen

Extracellular secretion Propeptide cleavage — Type 1 collagen

Fibril assembly cross-linking — Collagen fibril

FIGURE 1.14 Type I collagen gene expression. The sequences at the top represent a single exon unit that has been duplicated to produce the 41 exons (dark regions) of various sizes in the gene. Note transcription to a pre-mRNA, RNA splicing, translation, helix formation (two molecules of α_1, one of α_2 beginning at C-terminus), extracellular secretion, and fibril assembly by cross-linking.

removed and the processed protein is secreted into the extracellular space. Each triple-helix protein is then assembled into a larger fibril by cross-linking between lysine residues. The final product is an interlaced collagen fiber that plays a major role in connective tissue strength.[48, 49] Mutations which alter the tertiary structure of either the α_1 or α_2 chain prevent this crystallization; the severity of the phenotype is proportional to the extent to which crystallization is impeded (see below).

Nature of mutations

At the level of DNA, types of mutation are fairly limited as depicted in Figure 1.15. It is the particular context of gene structure, expression, and function that gives a mutation its unique character. DNA alterations may be classified as **nucleotide substitutions,** deletions, or duplications. Causes include ionizing radiation, chemicals, and interactions between DNA strands guided by complementary nucleotide sequences. Each of these processes may be opposed by cellular repair and suppression mechanisms. The ubiquitous and frequent occurrence of mutations in DNA is indicated by diseases such as xeroderma pigmentosum in which DNA repair is abnormal. The nature and frequency of mutations seems different among organisms, genomes, and gene regions within organisms. Very high mutation rates are associated with certain mobile DNA sequences in *Drosophila* and with mitochondrial genomes. Until recently the highest mutation rates known in man were in diseases such as Duchenne muscular dystrophy or neurofibromatosis where large genes are involved. Rates of 100 mutations per 10^6 gametes were viewed as high until the fragile X syndrome was characterized. As discussed below, mutations of the 'trinucleotide repeat' type, such as the fragile X mutation, may have rates of one per gamete.

Single base changes are collectively known as **point mutations**. As shown in Figure 1.15, the number of **transversions**

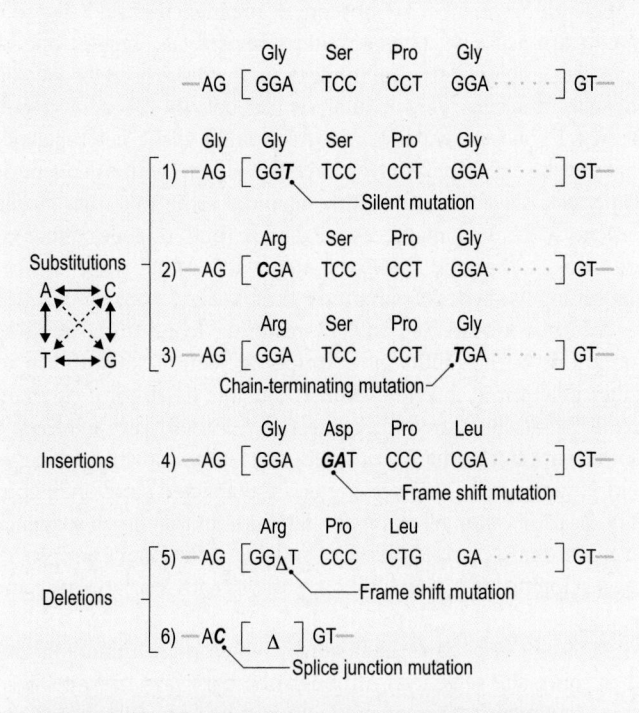

FIGURE 1.15 Consequences of point mutations (nucleotide substitutions) in DNA codons for transcribed RNA or translated protein. Deletions (E), transitions (◄——►), and transversions (◄----►) are shown.

should be twice that of **transitions**, but the actual numbers are about equal. Transitions appear to be the preferred mechanism, perhaps reflecting the frequent methylation of cytosine in animal cells. When a substituted nucleotide does not change the amino acid code or alter protein function, it may be called a silent mutation (example 1, Fig. 1.15). Mutations may occur within or outside functional DNA regions. When they are devoid of any effect, they are called **DNA sequence polymorphisms,** including:

- the **SNPs,** which can be within coding regions, or within introns; and
- those with **VNTRs** discussed above.

Amino acid substitutions with benign effects result in **protein polymorphisms** (example 2, Fig. 1.15). Examples include blood group proteins that are not associated with maternofetal incompatibility. Substitutions that exchange similar amino acids, such as the hydrophobic residues valine and leucine, are called conservative mutations and usually have minimal effects on protein function and organismal phenotype. Those replacing valine with a larger or differently charged amino acid such as glutamine would have a greater impact. For these reasons, the pattern of nucleotide and amino acid substitutions occurring over evolutionary time can give considerable insight into the function of a gene or protein as highly conserved coding regions reflect the segments of that protein which are crucial to function.

Other consequences of nucleotide substitutions include production of a stop codon (**chain-terminating mutation;** example 3, Fig. 1.15) and creation/obliteration of regulatory signals

such as **splice junction** donor or acceptor sites (example 6). Insertions or deletions of nucleotides may change the reading frame of the genetic code and produce a different amino acid sequence distal to the mutation (frame shift or nonsense mutations; examples 4 and 5). Sometimes DNA regions containing thousands of nucleotides are inserted or deleted during processes such as viral DNA insertion, programmed rearrangements of immunoglobulin genes, or amplification of *dihydrofolate reductase* and *NMYC* genes in response to folate depletion and development of certain neuroblastomas, respectively. Amplification of di- and trinucleotide repeating units are of recent interest because of their utility in **gene mapping** and their involvement in several genetic diseases (see below).

Mutation to phenotype: the basis of molecular medicine

A classic example includes the effects of DNA nucleotide changes on type I collagen. As with any protein-coding gene, the phenotype depends on the nature of amino acid alterations produced, their position within the protein chain, and their effects on protein function or localization. Some of the mutations affecting type I collagen are depicted in Figure 1.16.[49] Note the shorthand nomenclature for mutations, using a number that denotes the position of the mutation from the N-terminus and the change in terms of the amino acid code (see Fig. 1.7). For example, $G_{391}R$ indicates a glycine to arginine transition 391 amino acids from the N-terminal amino acid. The corresponding nucleotide transversion could be similarly represented as $G_{1171}C$ – note from the genetic code (Fig. 1.7) that a G to C transversion in the first position of the codon is the only change that would convert glycine to arginine. Another convention is to indicate deletions by Δ; for example, the ΔA_{1172} nucleotide deletion shown in example 5 of Figure 1.15 would also produce a $G_{391}R$ amino acid substitution with a **frameshift** of subsequent codons.

This terminology indicates a common language for mutations in terms of DNA structure, but the interpretation of that language depends on the hierarchy of expression and function for each gene product. Since the presence of a small uncharged amino acid (glycine) at the beginning of each (gly-X-Y)ₙ repeat in collagen is crucial, changes from glycine to arginine should be devastating for the molecule (e.g. a large, charged amino acid which does not cause the protein to rotate; see example 2, Fig. 1.15). Several mutations changing glycine to arginine have been detected, and each produces severe osteogenesis imperfecta (darker circles, Fig. 1.16A).[49] When smaller amino acids such as cysteine are substituted for glycine, the phenotype is usually milder (lighter circles, Fig. 1.16A). However, position in the collagen chain is also a factor, since helix formation among the α_1 and α_2 chains is initiated at the C-termini. Mutations affecting glycine residues near the C-terminus are even more severe than those near the N-terminus and cause early neonatal death; G to C amino acid substitutions are also more severe when they occur near the carboxyl terminus of the α_1 chain (Fig. 1.16A). Another factor is the stoichiometry of triple-helix formation, since:

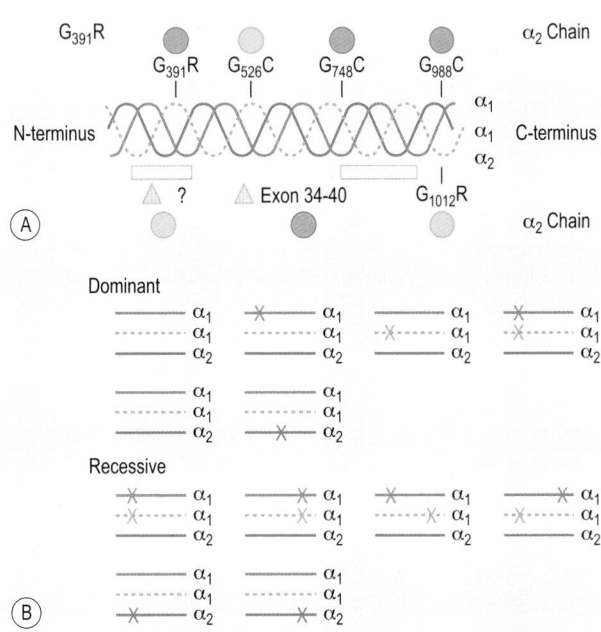

FIGURE 1.16 Mutations in type I collagen. (A) Amino acid changes producing severe (○1) or milder (●2) osteogenesis imperfecta are shown above (α1 chain) or below (α2 chain) the triple helical type I collagen molecule. Letters represent the amino acid code (see Fig. 1.7), Δ represents deletions. (B) Interaction of mutant (×) α₁ or α₂ chains to produce different proportions of abnormal collagen triple helices based on their 2:1 stoichiometry. (From Sykes 1987,[49] with permission.)

- two α₁ chains are incorporated for each α₂ chain; and
- collagen is formed from the crystallization of the normally perfectly linear triple helix molecule.

As illustrated in the upper portion of Figure 1.16B, a mutation in one of the two α₁ genes will affect 3/4 of type I collagen triple helices, as opposed to 1/2 when a mutation occurs in one of the two α₂ genes. Mutations in the α₂ genes thus tend to produce milder phenotypes unless deletions of entire exons occur (Fig. 1.6A).

Mutations in type I collagen illustrate three important properties of human genetic diseases. First, the terms **dominant** and **recessive** are sometimes misleading when a phenotype is traced to the molecular level. The milder cases of osteogenesis imperfecta were all considered dominant because of obvious vertical transmission. Before molecular analysis, severe type II patients were thought to have recessive disease since the parents were unaffected. However, most of these cases are also heterozygotes with only one of two genes mutated. By encoding a defective collagen molecule, the abnormal allele interferes with normal allele function by infiltrating the triple helix, a mechanism known as **protein suicide**. Recurrence of osteogenesis imperfecta in siblings has now been traced to **germline (or germinal) mosaicism** – a portion of parental gametes carry the abnormal allele even though their somatic tissues are normal. Germinal mosaicism is

sufficiently frequent that subsequent pregnancies are assigned a 6% recurrence risk of osteogenesis imperfecta. This is one of several examples of atypical inheritance that have been discovered through molecular genetic analysis (see below). A second lesson of type I collagen mutations is the striking allelic heterogeneity that may be encountered. No unrelated patients with osteogenesis imperfecta have been found to have the same mutation. Some patients with autosomal recessive disease (both α₁ genes mutated) are thus compound heterozygotes with some triple helices containing two types of variant α1 chains (Fig. 1.16B).

Another unexpected insight resulting from study of these mutations is the ability of a single nucleotide substitution to cause deletion of multiple exons. Thus the deletion of α₂ chain exons 34–40 illustrated in Figure 1.16A actually resulted from a point mutation in the AG splice donor site as shown in example 6 of Figure 1.15.[49] This finding was unexpected since analogous mutations in other genes caused retention of the intron sequence in mature mRNA due to lack of splicing; additional examples of exon skipping have been found in patients with Marfan syndrome and gyrate atrophy.[50] Type I collagen mutations can now be used to study the implied mechanism by which point mutations can alter splice site selection. Although the pathways from collagen gene mutation to osteogenesis imperfecta phenotype are extremely variable and complex, they provide a road map for many disorders of fetal development and growth. Note that an entire category of connective tissue disease can now be understood on the basis of collagen gene mutations (Table 1.1) and that characterization of these genetic extremes has led to understanding of a common form of degenerative arthritis.[48]

DNA diagnosis and genomics: new approaches to embryology and dysmorphology

What governs the number and arrangement of genes and how do they interact to produce organismal form and function? It is this direction that the physician must follow to attain sufficient understanding of the human organism to explain all diseases, particularly complex ones such as those affecting fetal development. McKusick[4] has called this approach a **'genomics'** of medicine, explaining predisposition and disease on the basis of the structure and organization of human genes. An emerging genomics of connective tissue disease is summarized in Table 1.1. With the osteogenesis story as a template, one can approach any complex disease by defining the molecular alterations that allow objective and predictive testing.

DNA polymorphism: genetic and physical mapping

Genes are grouped into a standard arrangement called a **genome** that is characteristic of each organism. A genome is a consensus DNA sequence that is unique but not invariant for species. The human genome is characterized by a DNA sequence of about 3×10^9 base pairs packaged into 22 autosomal and two sex (X and Y) chromosomes. Gene maps of complex organisms such as humans must therefore localize over 100 000 gene-sized DNA segments. Two types of gene maps are employed: genetic and physical. **Genetic** (or **linkage**) **maps** concentrate on the order of genes along a DNA segment or chromosome, while **physical maps** correlate gene loci with chromosomal landmarks and define distances in terms of DNA base pairs. The human genome sequence, published at 90% accuracy in 2001, now confirmed at 99.9% accuracy, provides a human physical map for the human genome.[51] Complete and accurate sequences for entire human chromosomes are now available.[52]

Traditionally, **linkage** maps are derived by documenting how frequently two traits are transmitted together in families – the more frequently they are transmitted together, the less meiotic *recombination* between them, and the closer together their loci must be on the chromosomal DNA. As mentioned previously, Mendel was lucky to choose traits that were on separate pea chromosomes and showed no linkage (independent segregation). Progress with linkage maps was exceedingly slow until DNA polymorphisms could be evaluated (e.g. **SNPs,** microdeletions, microduplications and **VNTRs**); wholesale expansions or contractions of repetitive DNA families are now known to be extremely common, upsetting prior notions of a stable and constant genome.[18] This variability may not make sense until the three-dimensional structure and functioning of DNA in the nucleus is understood; it is possible that some DNA regions/repetitive elements must be conserved to preserve function, in the same way that proline amino acids are critical in the folding of the collagen protein.[53]

Single nucleotide polymorphisms occur every 300–600 bp, more frequently in non-coding or intervening DNA, providing multiple alleles that have unique versions in any particular family. A 'Hap-Map' or haplotype map project is underway to catalogue the estimated 5.3 million SNPs in humans, each with a frequency of 10–50% in the population.[54] SNPs can be characterized rapidly and simultaneously due to their simple allele structure (i.e. A vs C at a particular nucleotide position), exemplified by characterization of 1.58 million SNPs in each of 71 individuals in a recent study.[54, 55] The abundance of SNPs and the ability to examine numerous SNPs in single experiments means that any inherited trait can be linked to a specific chromosome region and thereby positioned on the physical map. Even multifactorial traits like diabetes mellitus or schizophrenia can be associated with particular SNPs using whole-genome analysis, establishing these SNPs as **DNA markers** for enhanced susceptibility in families or subpopulations. Complicating such analyses and providing new insights are comparisons of recombination frequencies (genetic distance) and nucleotide (physical) distances between loci; these vary between sexes, among individuals, within gene/chromosome regions (conferring mutational hotspots), and among organisms.

The approach to genetic mapping can be illustrated by one its first examples in humans, the demonstration that the polymorphic ABO blood group locus was linked to that for nail-patella syndrome. The pedigree in Figure 1.17 demonstrates a vertical pattern typical of autosomal dominant inheritance, and blood typing shows individuals I-2, II-2, and II-3 all to have type A blood types – i.e. genotypes AA or AO. Since the presumed father was type O and the couple had a child (II-4) who was type O, the type A individuals must all be AO **heterozygotes.** Note that individual II-5 is type O but affected with nail-patella syndrome. If the ABO blood group and nail-patella syndrome are linked, this individual must represent a **cross-over,** i.e. has a recombinant chromosome 9 where one paternal O allele was transferred next to the maternal nail-patella allele. Individual II-5 has transmitted her recombinant chromosome to her daughter, causing her to be both type O and affected. From studies of many families, it is known that **recombination** occurs between the ABO and nail-patella loci about 10% of the time, i.e. a genetic distance of about 10 **centimorgans** between the two loci. In the average individual or organism, 1 centimorgan will correspond to a physical distance of about 10^6 bp.

Besides the risk for recombination, there are additional problems with using the ABO blood group as a diagnostic test for nail-patella syndrome. First, one must test several family members to determine the **phase** of blood group and nail-patella alleles before the blood group becomes predictive of nail-patella status within that family. Note that type A is predictive of nail-patella in the left side of the family, while type O becomes predictive for the right side of the pedigree (Fig. 1.17A). Also, the limited number of ABO alleles makes linkage analysis **uninformative** for certain matings. For example, if prenatal diagnosis had been attempted on individual III-1 of Figure 1.17A, the type A result would not distinguish whether he received his maternal or paternal A allele. Much greater precision can be obtained using a DNA-based test, such as linkage studies through polymorphisms of DNA sequences much closer to the nail-patella gene than the ABO group or through directly analyzing the nail-patella gene for mutations.

Beneath the pedigree in Figure 1.17 (left panel) are diagrammed polymorphisms based on variable restriction endonuclease sites [restriction fragment length polymorphisms **(RFLPs)**] or variable numbers of tandem repeats **(VNTRs)** between restriction endonuclease sites. The black rectangle indicates the DNA region that is available as a probe to hybridize with patient DNAs on **Southern blots.** Hypothetical autoradiograms generated by digestion of patient DNA through restriction enzymes, size fractionation of the DNA by gel electrophoresis, transfer of size-fractionated DNA to **nitrocellulose** or **nylon membranes,** and hybridization with radioactive probes are shown in Fig. 1.17 (right panel). Current analysis would substitute alternative SNP alleles for DNA fragment lengths 1 and 2 displayed beneath the pedigree, visualized after polymerase chain reaction (*PCR*) amplification and spectral detection of the alternative nucleotide alleles (e.g. A vs C).

For the upper **autoradiogram,** the nail-patella allele is clearly linked to the larger allele 1 generated by the lack of restriction site E_2. For the lower autoradiogram it is the smallest allele (1) with the fewest number of interspersed repeating units that is linked with the nail-patella phenotype. Note that Southern analysis using either DNA polymorphism would be completely informative for

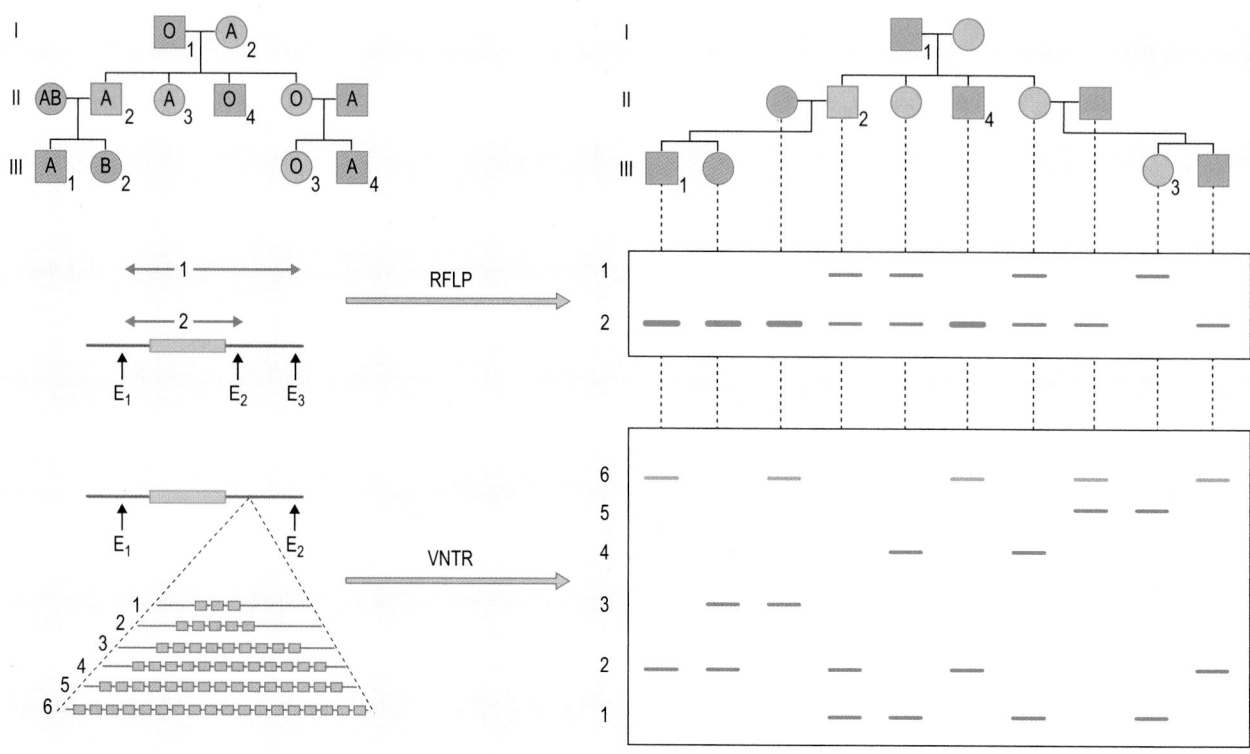

FIGURE 1.17 Hypothetical analysis of autosomal dominant nail-patella syndrome using blood type or DNA polymorphisms. The left panel shows the family pedigree above with affected individuals (in blue) and ABO blood types. Note the segregation of the abnormal nail-patella allele with ABO allele A except for individual II-5, where a cross-over has occurred. Below the pedigree are shown examples of restriction fragment length polymorphisms (RFLPs – alleles 1 and 2 based on the presence/absence of restriction site E_2) or variable number of tandem repeats (VNTRs – alleles 1 to 6 based on the number of intervening repeats). The right panel illustrates the use of each type of DNA marker to analyze the pedigree after DNA restriction, Southern blotting, and hybridization with DNA probes indicated by lines (orange representing normal alleles, and blue the mutated alleles). Note the segregation of the abnormal nail-patella allele with RFLP allele 1 and VNTR allele 1.

prenatal diagnosis (i.e. individuals III-1, III-3) and that no cross-overs between the polymorphism and disease-associated mutation are evident. If the low recombination frequency were verified using many families, these polymorphic loci could be placed closer to the nail-patella locus than the ABO blood group on a map of chromosome 9. It is easy to see how family studies employing a large number of DNA polymorphisms could produce a detailed genetic map of chromosome 9, easily compared to the physical map in this region by aligning each polymorphic DNA sequence with that from the genome project. Besides providing linkage/susceptibility markers and causes of genetic disease, the remarkable variability of human DNA also establishes a unique 'genetic fingerprint' for each individual that can be used for identity or paternity testing.

Functional and positional cloning

For the more common Mendelian disorders, causative genes are readily identified by linkage in affected families and examining regional genes for suggestive nucleotide mutations. Rarer genetic disorders, including reproductive lethals that preclude familial transmission, required karyotypic clues, i.e. the identification of the exceptional patient with the disease associated with a chromosomal anomaly, such as a translocation or a deletion to reveal the location of the responsible genes.[56] FISH technology discussed previously allows use of DNA probes with different fluorescent labels (orange and blue in Fig. 1.18) to determine that a particular DNA segment lies within a chromosome deletion (D) or **translocation breakpoint** (T); control probes (excepting sex chromosome segments) should give two fluorescent signals in diploid cells, while those to deleted or transected loci may give one or three fluorescent signals, respectively; see Figure 1.18 (lower right and Ch. 5). FISH can aid gene mapping by allowing direct physical visualization of gene order: in Figure 1.18 the cell labeled M shows two-color FISH with probes for loci a and b, demonstrating that locus a is proximal.

These positional approaches to gene isolation can be contrasted with functional approaches that follow the traditional route from enzyme deficiency or protein alteration to the corresponding gene (Fig. 1.18). Each approach culminates in the isolation of a **candidate gene** that can be cloned by recombinant

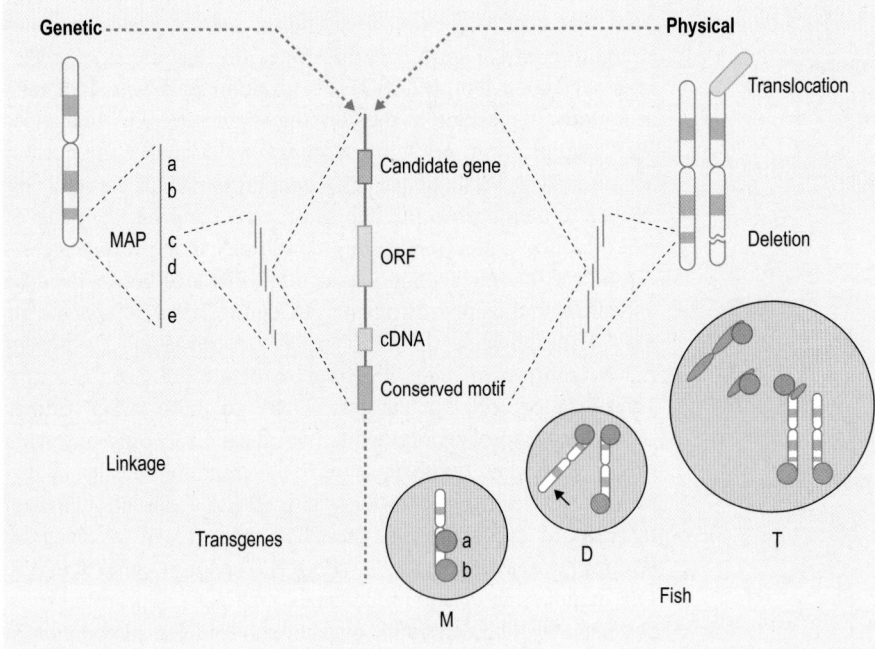

FIGURE 1.18 Genetic and physical mapping. Genetic analysis employs linkage or expression systems (cells, transgenic mice) to associate traits or cell/organism properties with particular genes or chromosome regions. Linkage units are based on recombination (centimorgans) and thus are relative, varying by sex and chromosome region. Physical analysis allows direct visualization of chromosome regions utilizing translocations or deletions. Fluorescent in situ hybridization (FISH) bridges these methods by using gene probes to visualize their precise locus on the chromosome. Use of two gene probes will reveal their order on the chromosome (M), demonstrate deletion of one gene relative to another (D) by showing a single spot of orange fluorescence, or localize a gene at a translocation breakpoint (T) by showing three blue spots caused by transection of the region recognizing the blue probe. Physical mapping allows direct measure of distances in terms of chromosome bands or DNA base pairs. The approaches are usually combined to produce a precise map (center) of expressed DNA regions (presumptive genes) identified on the basis of possible functional relationships (candidate genes) or evidence suggestive of RNA transcription. ORF, open reading frames; cDNA, complementary DNA; conserved motifs, regions of DNA sequence shared by other proteins.

DNA technology and examined for mutations in affected patients. The first diseases to be characterized by functional approaches had obvious candidate genes: i.e. globin genes for hemoglobino-pathies, type I collagen genes in osteogenesis imperfecta. In these disorders, **functional cloning** was accomplished by using antibodies to pick out recombinant bacteriophage or plasmids that expressed the candidate protein. Before the characterization of abundant DNA polymorphisms, positional cloning (reverse genetics) was labor-intensive due to the slow progress of linkage analysis (e.g. cystic fibrosis) or dependence on chromosomal rearrangements that signaled gene location (e.g. Duchenne muscular dystrophy). Functional cloning of rarer or unknown proteins was hindered by the need to use transforming DNA segments to mimic disease attributes in cells or animals (e.g. complementation assays for peroxisomal proteins deficient in Zellweger syndrome). Now arrays of DNA fragments or complementary RNAs on microchips can highlight which DNA regions or transcripts are present at altered dosage in cells from an affected patient. Such techniques will find fruitful application in deciphering altered genes within tissues of limited abundance, such as early embryos, blighted ova, or early tumors/cancers.

DNA diagnostic techniques

When genetic diseases have been related to mutations in characterized DNA molecules, as described above for certain connective tissue diseases, diagnostic testing is available with a simple set of laboratory techniques. Figure 1.19 illustrates use of the **PCR** to amplify a particular gene region that is known to be the site of disease mutations. The enormous increase in sensitivity afforded by PCR can be appreciated by considering that 100–200 μg of DNA is routinely obtained from 10 mL of peripheral blood or 200–300 mg of frozen tissue. For Southern blotting, 10 μg is often used for each restriction analysis in order to obtain adequate hybridization signals in 1–3 days. PCR requires only 1 μg for routine analysis and yields up to 0.5 μg of specific gene product from the less than 1 pg of specific gene sequences in the 1 μg of genomic DNA. Hybridization signals with colorimetric, fluorescent, or radioactive probes can then be detected in a few minutes when necessary. Alternatively, PCR can be used to analyze DNA from neonatal blood spots or single cells.[57]

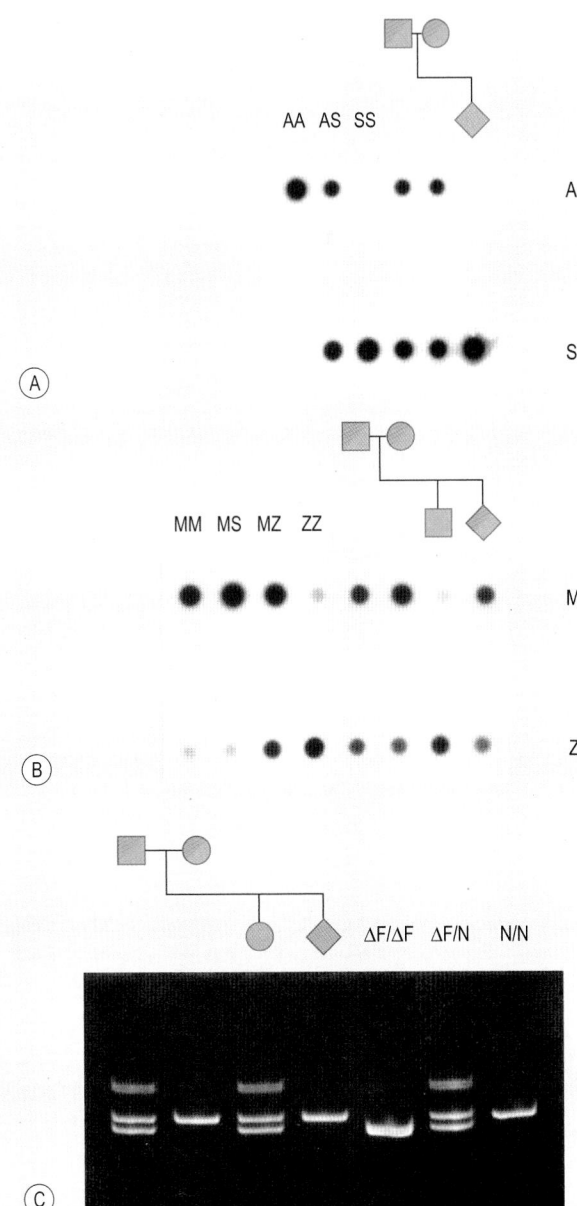

By using amplified DNA that is enriched some 10^6-fold for a particular gene sequence, screening for mutant alleles becomes straightforward. Figure 1.19 illustrates the technique of allele-specific oligonucleotide (**ASO**) hybridization for diagnosis of gene mutations. In addition to the flanking oligonucleotides that allow PCR amplification, ASOs are synthesized that match the normal or mutated gene sequence. PCR-amplified patient samples are applied to membranes and hybridized to the appropriate panel of ASO probes under **stringency** conditions that prevent hybridization if there is a single nucleotide difference between probe and allele. In the upper two panels of Figure 1.19, ASO specific for the A and S alleles of the β-globin locus or the M and Z alleles of the α_1-antitrypsin locus are used to determine patient status. Hybridization of the patient's DNA to both ASO probes establishes heterozygosity, while hybridization to only one ASO probe establishes homozygosity. If the mutation results in duplicated or deleted nucleotides, as in the Δ F mutation that is frequent in cystic fibrosis, the PCR product can be sized by electrophoresis on polyacrylamide gels. The lower panel of Figure 1.19 demonstrates faster mobility of amplified PCR products from patients with 3 bp deletions caused by rho F alleles, allowing rapid DNA diagnosis. Note that two patients do not have rho F mutations despite the implications of the pedigree; other cystic fibrosis mutant alleles must be present, emphasizing that most DNA diagnostic tests give very sensitive and specific detection – they do not provide general screens for disease. Over 20 additional cystic fibrosis mutations have now been characterized, allowing routine prenatal screening of expectant couples with good sensitivity.

Automated detection of mutant alleles in amplified patient DNA is now readily available.[58] Different color-coded ASO probes that become fluorescent upon hybridization can also be added to patient DNA samples, with colored spectra indicating allele content. The DNA diagnostic laboratory is now highly mechanized; limitations include large genes without common mutant alleles (e.g. Marfan syndrome, neurofibromatosis-1) and disorders characterized by research laboratories that are not sufficiently common to stimulate commercial laboratory interest. The molecular revolution has remarkable triumphs in genome sequencing, characterizing gene mutations, and automated mutation detection, but significant ethical concerns remain.[59] Limited access to DNA diagnosis because of disease rarity or inadequate insurance, potential for employment or insurance discrimination, and inadequate counseling before or after testing are ongoing dilemmas.[59]

FIGURE 1.19 Examples of PCR/ASO to diagnose sickle cell anemia (A) or (B) α1-antitrypsin deficiency (genotype ZZ) (C). In each case, duplicate dot blots from controls or families are shown after hybridization to probes specific for A or S (above) and M or Z alleles. Prenatal testing shows that the fetus in (A) is homozygous for the sickle allele, whereas the fetus in (B) is a carrier for α1-antitrypsin deficiency. (C) DNA diagnosis for cystic fibrosis transmembrane regulator gene. The DNA fragments are separated on a polyacrylamide gel to demonstrate the smaller band resulting when the 3-bp ΔF deletion is present. Since the affected individual and her mother do not have a smaller band, they must have a cystic fibrosis mutation different from ΔF. Absence of the father's ΔF mutation in the sib of unknown sex (e.g. prenatal diagnosis) excludes disease if paternity is correct. (These analyses were performed by Dr C. Sue Richards at GeneScreen, Dallas, TX.)

Examples of genetic mapping: X-linked hydrocephalus and mental retardation syndromes

As the first example of genetic linkage (color blindness), the X chromosome provides a good beginning for the appreciation of molecular genetic analysis. More than 80 forms of mental retardation have been mapped to specific regions of the X chromosome.[60] Many of these have dramatic morphologic or metabolic phenotypes (e.g. Lowe syndrome, Lesch-Nyhan syndrome), but the 40 or so that lack distinctive features (non-specific X-linked mental retardation) emphasize the power of genetic linkage analysis. The characterization of gene expression (through gene profiling and proteomics) in brain tissue indicates that the success met with X-linked disorders can also be achieved for those with autosomal inheritance. The outlook for conditions, like autism, that are undoubtedly genetic, usually heterogeneous, and which provide few phenotypic clues to etiology can now be optimistic.

The upper panel of Figure 1.20A illustrates the DNA linkage analysis of a MASA syndrome family. This disorder falls into the non-specific group and is named for its characteristic features of *m*ental retardation, *a*phasia, *s*pasticity, and *a*dducted thumbs.[61, 62] In the absence of an obvious candidate gene for the condition, a panel of X-chromosome DNA polymorphisms was used to analyze MASA families; the representative Southern blot in Figure 1.20A demonstrates linkage with the upper restriction fragment allele revealed by the **anonymous DNA probe** F8C located at chromosome band Xq28 (see Fig. 1.20A, lower panel).[61] Results of Southern blot analysis with the probes **DXS14** (D, DNA marker; X, X chromosome; S, single copy; No. 14 to be registered) and DXS72 did not show linkage with MASA alleles as summarized in the diagram beneath the F8C blot. Other investigators had also shown linkage of X-linked hydrocephalus (hydrocephalus due to congenital stenosis of aqueduct of Sylvius – HSAS, MIM 307000) to the Xq28 region. Although there was no obvious clinical link between X-linked hydrocephalus and MASA syndrome, their co-occurrence in one family and linkage to the same Xq28 region raised suspicion that different alleles at the same genetic locus might be involved. Focus on the Xq28 region revealed an L1 cell adhesion molecule (*L1CAM*) that became a plausible candidate gene for these two conditions. The family analyzed in Figure 1.20 proved to have a gene deletion that obliterated the carboxy terminus of the L1CAM protein, allowing rapid identification of the *L1CAM* gene.[62]

The demonstration of *L1CAM* mutations in MASA and X-linked hydrocephalus individuals allowed distinction between **syndrome variability** and **genetic heterogeneity,** two causes of variation that complicate medical genetics. Linkage analysis refined clinical delineation by distinguishing MASA syndrome from other X-linked mental retardation disorders with spasticity, and mutational analysis substantiated clinical suspicion that MASA and X-linked hydrocephalus could result from mutations at the same genetic locus. Study of the developmental expression and cerebral distribution of the L1CAM molecule now offers an approach to understanding the hydrocephalus and spasticity associated with these mutant alleles.[61, 62]

Examples of physical mapping: fragile X syndrome

Another type of non-specific X-linked mental retardation was described in 1943 by Martin and Bell (Fig. 1.21A).[63] In 1969, Lubs defined a cytogenetic marker in cells from a patient with Martin-Bell syndrome. This 'fragile' site on the X chromosome was related to low folic acid concentrations in the culture medium by Sutherland, and soon found to be diagnostic of Martin-Bell or fragile X syndrome. As a definitive marker became available, it was realized that there were some specific features such as megalotestes, prominent jaw, and lax joints that were characteristic of fragile X-syndrome patients.

Characterization of the gene responsible for fragile X syndrome was guided by the physical marker – the 'fragile' site at Xq27 (Fig. 1.21).[64] Preliminary linkage studies using the nearby marker DXS548 confirmed that the fragile site was close to the responsible gene, rather than being a secondary manifestation of a gene elsewhere on the X chromosome. Successively smaller DNA segments were cloned from the Xq27 region using yeast artificial chromosomes (50- to 100-Mb DNA inserts), cosmids (20–40 kb DNA inserts), and plasmids (1–10 kb DNA inserts). Mapping of smaller DNA segments to larger ones was facilitated by sequence-tagged sites (**STS** – @, #, and * symbols in Fig. 1.21B – reference points on the DNA sequence); yield of the expected STS PCR product from a particular recombinant clone registered that cloned segment on the larger map.

DNA segments from the candidate region were tested for hybridization with brain cDNA and variation in fragile X families, and some with brain expression exhibited size variation: fragile X boys had DNA segment sizes of 6–7.5 kb, while normal individuals averaged 5.2 kb. DNA sequencing of the region showed variable numbers of a trinucleotide CGG repeat to be the cause, with normals having 5–45 repeats, fragile X carriers 60–200 repeats, and fragile X males and females having between 200 and more than 1000 repeats. DNA diagnosis could then be performed by quantifying the number of CGG triplet repeats (see Ch. 5 for discussion on fragile X diagnosis).

Fragile X syndrome became a prototype for a group of expanding nucleotide repeat diseases, including Huntington chorea (abnormal expansion of the CAG trinucleotide) and Steinert myotonic dystrophy (abnormal expansion of the CTG trinucleotide). These disorders share several characteristics, including:

- in abnormally long alleles, there is progressive meiotic and mitotic increase in the size of the repeat region once it is amplified, with broad size ranges in tissues of affected individuals;
- greater amplification during meiosis of one sex (females in fragile X, males in Huntington chorea);
- more severely affected offspring with each generation (anticipation);
- abnormally repeated CGG and CTG lead to an inhibition of the synthesis of the gene's protein.

CAG expansion results in an increase in the number of repeated glutamines within the protein; cytotoxicity is proportional to the length of the abnormally-repeated polyglutamine tract.

Experience with DNA testing and multiple fragile X syndrome families has revealed a new phenotype for those with intermediate expansion: these individuals are said to have a premutation and exhibit an adult degenerative disorder called the fragile X-associated tremor/ataxia syndrome.[63]

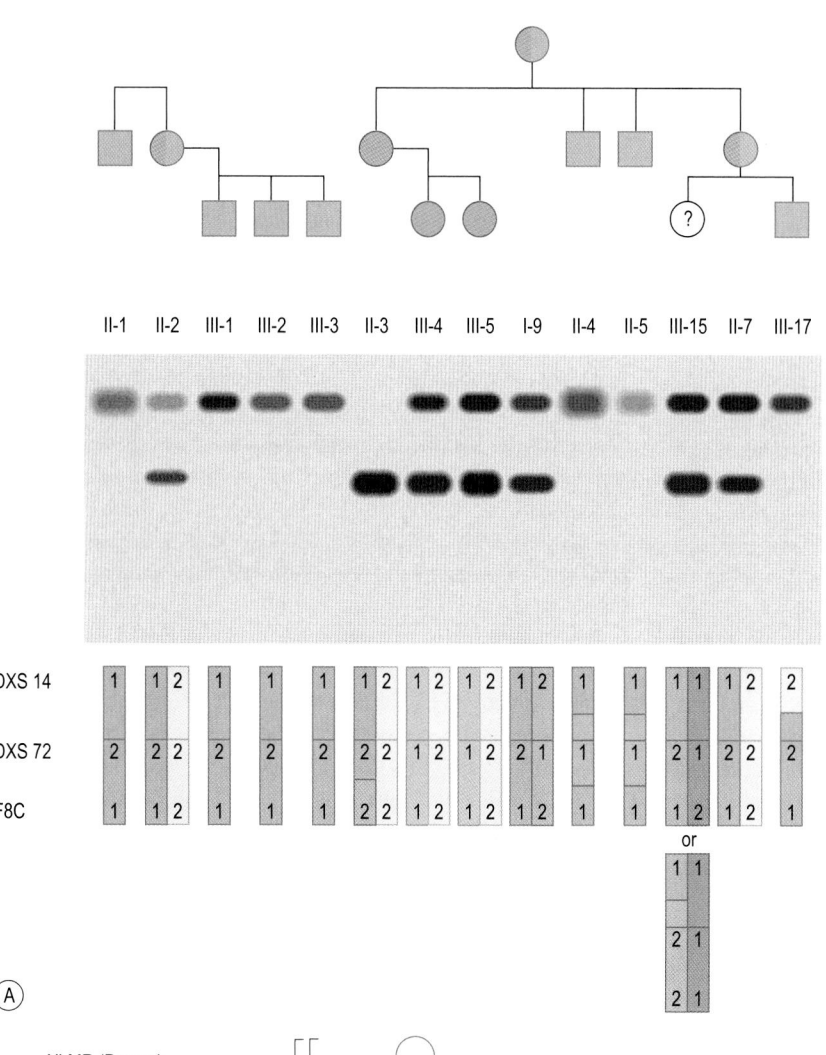

FIGURE 1.20 Relation of mental retardation, aphasia, shuffling gait, adducted thumbs (MASA) syndrome and X-linked hydrocephalus (HSAS) to a single locus encoding the L1 cell adhesion molecule (*L1CAM*). (A) A Southern analysis showing segregation of the MASA allele with the larger restriction fragment length polymorphism (RFLP) allele from the F8C locus at band Xq28. (B) The many types of non-specific X-linked mental retardation (XLMR) loci that have been linked to specific areas of the X chromosome are shown, with particular mutations in the *L1CAM* gene demonstrated in MASA syndrome and X-linked hydrocephalus.

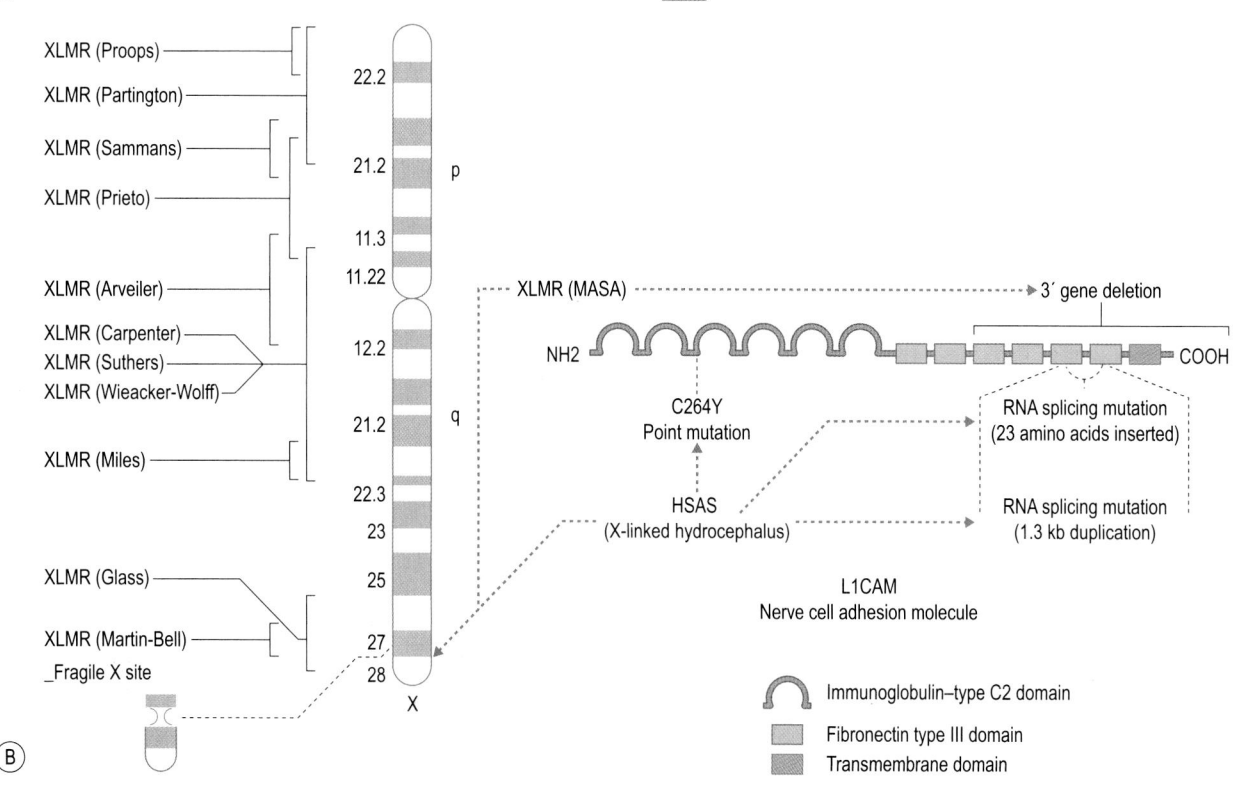

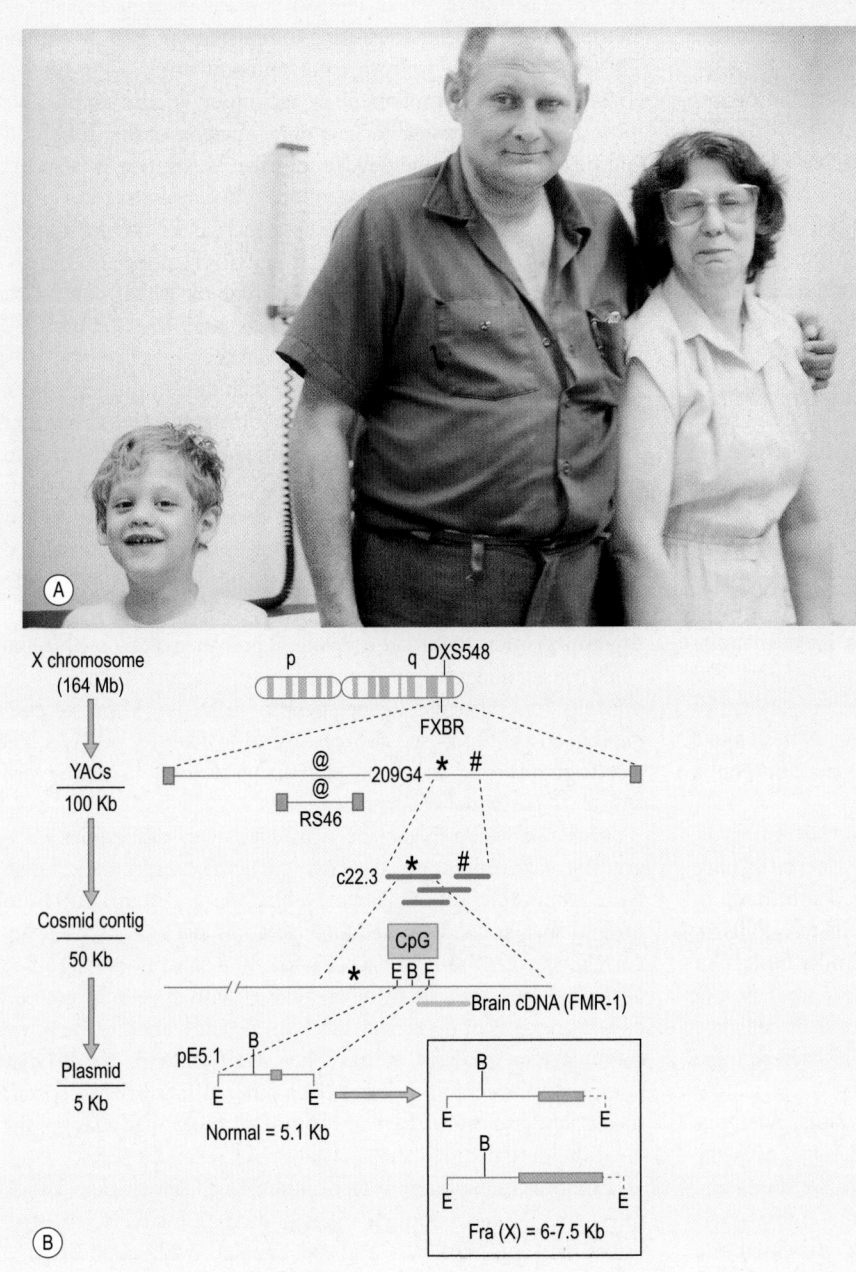

FIGURE 1.21 (A) Family with fragile X syndrome showing an affected child, his mother, and the maternal uncle. (B) Cloning of the fragile X (*FMR1*) gene. Genetic analysis first confirmed the fragile X breakpoint region (FXBR) was causative of disease by showing linkage to a marker (DXS548) in the same region, then yeast artificial chromosomes (YACs) were isolated that contained the marker region. Sequence-tagged sites (@, *, #), meaning regions that yield PCR products with unique primers, allow rapid matching of YACs with cosmid and plasmid contigs (contiguous cloned DNA fragments) that had successively smaller regions of the FMBR. Because the *FMR1* gene was expected to be expressed in brain, cDNA clones from this organ were tested against FMBR fragments until one that contained an expressed sequence was identified (cosmid c22.3). A derived plasmid (pE5.1) was used as a DNA probe against Southern blots containing DNAs from normal and fragile X patients, demonstrating a larger *Eco*R1 restriction fragments in affected individuals; orange rectangles represent the variably repeated CGG trinucleotide. (From Verkerk et al 1991,[64] with permission.)

Molecular embryology: new approaches to human embryogenesis and oncogenesis

In February 1997, the world was not prepared for the cover of *Time* magazine: a ewe had been cloned. Up to then, the scientific community thought that it would be decades before a mammal, and especially a human, could be cloned; ethicists were not ready for this reality. Now there can be no question that developmental biology is a clinically relevant discipline, particularly in the area of pediatric pathology. This section will review some basic principles of molecular embryology so as to foster molecular thinking when pathologists are confronted with a fetal malformation.

Experimental developmental biology

Commonly used model organisms

The fruit fly (*Drosophila melanogaster*) is by far the most studied and best understood organism in molecular embryology. The genes and cascades discovered in this organism are generally similar to those of vertebrates; some are virtually identical and more than half have significant molecular homology. The molecular cascades found in *Drosophila* are thus extremely valuable for the study of vertebrates.

The worm *Caenorhabditis elegans* is a valuable model organism because its development is absolutely constant in both males and females. At various developmental stages, each worm cell follows an identical differentiation sequence and lineage that have been precisely mapped in this transparent organism. There is little plasticity in that ablation of one worm cell or group of cells always leads to the same anomaly. This reproducibility provides a precise template for study of cellular interactions during development. The study of programmed cell death (see below) was greatly facilitated by the discovery of *ced* (*cell death* gene) mutations in *C. elegans*.

Recent research has provided a vertebrate model for developmental studies in the zebrafish (*Danio rerio*). This 3–4 cm fish is inexpensive to maintain, has a short, three-month life cycle, and produces hundreds of offspring at weekly intervals. The zebrafish has a relatively small genome which can be 'mutated' relatively easily, including the ability to make haploid and diploid, androgenetic, or gynogenetic organisms. Its embryos are also quite transparent, allowing easy study of internal development. The ability to modify the genome and the gene expression patterns of zebrafish at will, together with their transparent tissues, make these fish ideal models for simulation of human developmental disorders.

More traditional vertebrate models include chick embryos, with particular value of chick/quail chimeras. The two birds have histologically distinct nuclei, with coarsely clumped chromatin in chicks and an open chromatin with a prominent nucleolus in quails (including a prominent nucleolus). Their similar molecular embryogenesis makes grafting possible, allowing manipulation of specific embryonal regions. The easy identification of cell type allows precise observation of cell migration and has been seminal in understanding the migration of neural crest cells.

The frog (*Xenopus*) has been historically important, because its large transparent eggs are easily manipulated. *Xenopus* was the organism in which the Spemann organizer was defined, and proved to be crucial for the understanding of the embryologic concepts of induction and developmental fields; the Spemann organizer is the homologue of the mammalian Hensen's node.

Finally, the mouse (*Mus musculus*) has been invaluable for genetic studies, with many Mendelian and transgenic phenotypes that simulate human developmental disorders. The ability to create 'knock-out' and 'knock-in' mouse models by inserting or disrupting genes of interest is a major strength of this model. Rodents have also been valuable for studies of teratogens and fetoplacental interactions.

Methods employed in developmental biology

Methods for studying embryology include tissue manipulation and application of the same molecular techniques discussed in prior sections. The ability to manipulate embryos in vivo or in various artificial situations (like the exposed chick embryo or large frog egg/blastula) has been invaluable. In ablation experiments, the region of interest is resected or destroyed (e.g. Hensen's node), and the resulting malformation(s) is/are studied. The ablation can be performed at different times, with different consequences. A complementary technique is grafting of structures at abnormal sites. For example, ablation of Henson's node will prevent neural tube development while grafting of a second Hensen's node from another embryo will cause a second neural tube to form. Embryologic concepts such as gradient fields (see below), competence (ability of tissue to respond to signals), inducers/organizers (key embryonic regions which control the differentiation of surrounding tissues), and fate (endpoint of tissue differentiation) have resulted from such experiments.

Molecular analysis of embryos includes immunohistochemistry or protein electrophoresis to determine the chronology and topography of protein expression, and Northern blotting for characterizing gene expression (using electrophoresis to separate RNA gene fragments by size), then identify those of interest by transfer to membranes and hybridization with fluorescent or radioactive probes. Reverse transcriptase PCR (RT-PCR) also identifies actively transcribed (expressed) genes, using oligothymine primers to initiate copying of polyadenylated mRNA into cDNA; subsequent amplification and analysis can measure mRNA diversity or particular gene-specific mRNAs. More recently, expression profiling (see above) is used to identify mRNAs, and electrophoresis or shotgun sequencing is used to define proteomes of particular embryonic tissues.

Molecular analysis can be combined with tissue ablation or grafting experiments to associate particular molecular changes with embryonic mechanisms. Depletion of certain mRNA or protein species can be noted after ablation of Henson's node and correlated with those in excess when a second node is grafted. Differentiation stages can be correlated with specific proteomes and with excess or deficiency of key molecules. Despite the power of molecular analysis, it has been very difficult to associate complex embryonic processes (like differentiation) with specific molecules. Too often, there are abundant molecular changes that are difficult to distinguish as causal versus secondary effects.

Embryo manipulation techniques (e.g. **knock-ins, knock-outs,** and usage of **reporter genes** such as luciferase or green fluorescent protein) can also be coupled with application of extrinsic substances, as with experiments showing that application of retinoic acid to the lateral aspect of chick embryos causes the development of an extra limb. Signals and gene products can also be varied intrinsically by constructing **transgenic organisms.** Parents or embryos are infected by a virus expressing a gene of interest, and appropriate vectors are now available that target the gene to its proper chromosome location and replace its naturally occurring allele. Incorporation of transgenes with appropriate high-expression (ubiquitous) promoters can define developmental consequences of overexpression, while coupling with signal responsive, tissue- or time-specific promoters can evaluate timed or tissue-specific overexpression. The insertion of defective or down-regulated genes can evaluate consequences of underexpression. Transgenic experiments can target particular tissues or regions of the embryo for somatic mutations or stem cells for germline expression. Suitable breeding of germline transgenics can produce mouse lineages with the desired gene alteration, or produce cultured cell lines like mouse embryonic stem cells with stable transgenic mutations.

Developmental processes

Cellular differentiation (epigenetic control of gene expression)

With exceptions of selective rearrangements in certain genes (e.g. T-cell receptor genes), all cells of an organism have the same genetic information. Differentiation is characterized by the activation of certain genes, and the inactivation of other genes to address specific developmental needs of cells and tissues (e.g. to specify whether ectoblastic cells will become brain, neural crest or epidermis).[65–67] Cellular differentiation is the result of the activation of genes which cause a more primitive cell to specialize, e.g. the evolution of a pluripotent mesoblastic cell into a muscle cell.[68, 69] It is associated with the inactivation of the genes which are not necessary for that cell's function (e.g. inactivation of the bilirubin-synthesizing machinery by myocytes). For example, *HOX* genes play a major role in cellular differentiation: their proteins bind promoters of developmental genes and activate or inhibit their transcription; this effect is generally irreversible, but in **cancer,** a loss of inhibition of transcription of these genes can cause cells to **de-differentiate.**[27]

Until recently, the fact that all adult mammalian somatic cells are differentiated prevented their cloning: these cells have inactivated a large subset of genes indispensable for the formation and normal growth of an embryo. This can be contrasted with the cells of mammalian zygotes and blastulas, whose genes are all potentially active and available for transcription.[26] At the stage of the 'inner cell mass', cells are still omnipotent, since cellular separation at this stage will produce monozygotic twins. As the embryo develops into a morula and a blastocyst, asymmetric division of 'mother' cells will produce differently programmed daughter cells that exhibit progressive differentiation with subsequent cell divisions (Fig. 1.22). In some tissues, this ongoing increase in differentiation continues into childhood.

The molecular cascades which control cellular differentiation are still generally poorly understood, but some basic principles are starting to emerge:

- Inhibition of gene transcription is usually initially achieved through the action of inhibiting transcription factors (silencers, on Fig. 1.8A); due to largely unknown mechanisms, these inhibited promoters then become methylated, and this methylation, in conjunction with other epigenetic marks, results in a permanent state of inhibition (see prior discussion of DNA methylation).
- As methylation is passed from one cell to its descendants, gene inactivation (which leads to differentiation) is generally irreversible. Other means of stable gene regulation (e.g. histone modifications, heterochromatinization) are also passed on to daughter cells, to further ensure irreversibility.
- Many developmentally important genes activate their own promoter (positive feedback), causing the gene to be perpetually active in all descendants of the cell within which it was initially

expressed. The perpetuated expression again leads to an irreversible state of differentiation.
- Molecular differentiation is a gradual, stepwise process, explaining progressive changes in morphologic appearance as differentiation proceeds from the totipotent blastic cells of the inner cell mass to terminal differentiated states.
- Differentiation and mitotic activity tend to be inversely proportional (the greater the differentiation of a cell population, the lower its proliferation rate); this is also true in cancer (Fig. 1.23).
- Oncogenesis can be thought of as a de-regulation of basic embryologic mechanisms, which explains the similarities between molecular embryology and molecular oncology.

The **master switch** or **selector genes** discussed previously (Fig. 1.11) control fundamental aspects of development; they do so by activating or repressing batteries of subordinate genes. The expression of a selector gene at different moments of embryonal development may result in different effects, as the promoters of subordinate genes are not all available for modulation at the same time. One master switch gene may be used at different times and/or in different regions to perform different tasks. Their pleiotropic activity increases genome efficiency because fewer genes are necessary than if each function required a designated, single-purpose gene.

In humans, the actions of master switch genes are illustrated by the *MYOD1/MYF5* genes, as shown in Figure 1.24. Subdivision of embryonic domains by homeotic proteins (PAX, HOX) defines which primitive cells will become a certain tissue (e.g. skeletal muscle). When the gene 'Myoblast Differentiation-1' (*MYOD1*) is expressed in primitive mesenchymal cells, it causes them to differentiate into skeletal myocytes. MYOD1 (the gene product) is a transcription factor that binds multiple promoters specific to skeletal muscular differentiation. Thus, a single gene is sufficient to activate and inactivate a whole cascade of subordinate genes (Fig. 1.24A). Furthermore, MYOD1 recognizes its own promoter, and therefore activates its own transcription in a positive feedback loop fashion. Once a cell activates the transcription of MYOD1, auto-activation causes this cell and its descendants to express MYOD1 forever. From then on, these cells can take no other differentiation path than that of a myocyte.

Vertebrates cannot survive without myocytes, and a 'double insurance' or redundant mechanism ensures muscular development in the event MYOD-1 dysfunction. A second gene is available (called *MYF5*) that performs similar functions to those of MYOD1; both are normally expressed (two alleles of *MYOD1* and two of *MYF5*), and each can substitute for the other in the event of a mutation (Fig. 1.24B). In addition, MYOD1 and MYF5 bind and cross-activate their promoters. Similar double insurance phenomena are found in many developmentally critical molecular cascades, ensuring an adequate development but also complicating the study of developmental cascades.

In oncologic states cellular differentiation inhibits mitotic activity. This is also true for the embryo: MYOD1 expression is inversely proportional to myocyte proliferation. Fibroblast growth factor (FGF) acts as a growth factor (proto-oncogene) in myoblasts; FGF down-regulates myoblastic differentiation (without inhibiting it totally), by down-regulating the transcription of

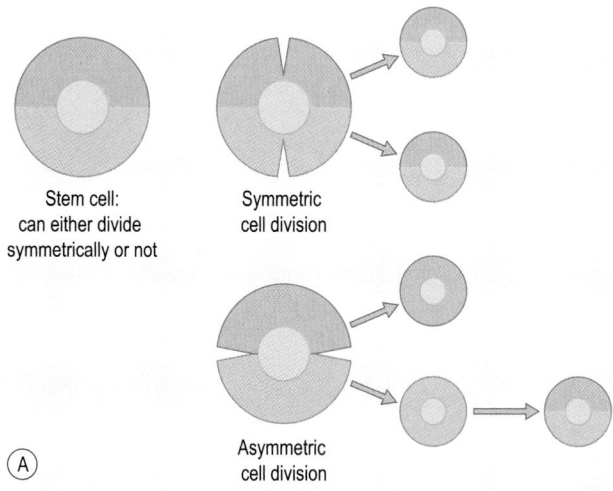

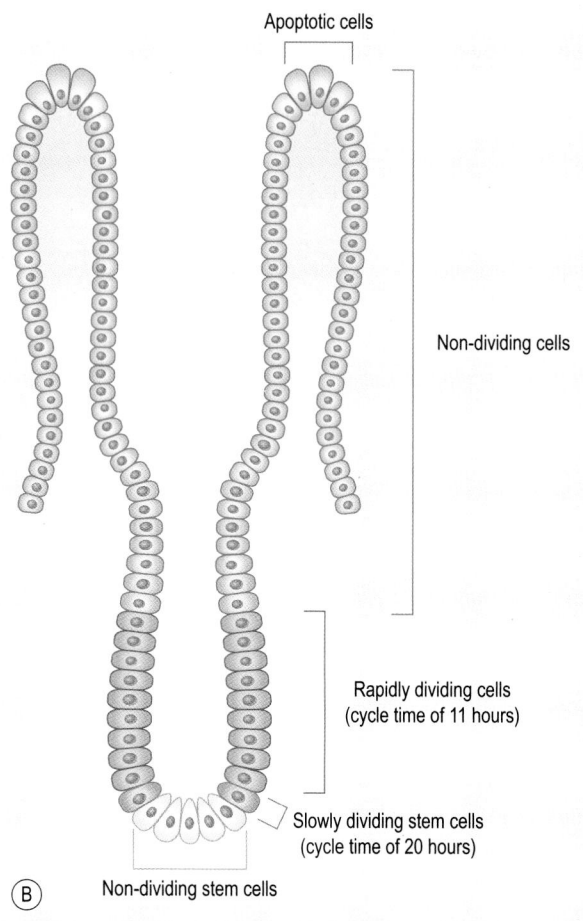

FIGURE 1.22 Differentiation and cell proliferation. (A) In symmetric cell divisions, a stem cell gives rise to two identical stem cells; each symmetric division doubles the number of stem cells in an organ. In asymmetric divisions, two different daughter cells are produced: one stem cell identical to the original stem cell, and one differentiated daughter cell. Asymmetric divisions keep the number of stem cells constant. Symmetric cell divisions separate a differentiating factor equally within both daughter cells, which are thus molecularly identical to their precursor. In asymmetric divisions, this molecule is divided unequally. For example, if 'pinkness' is a stem cell characteristic, the blue cell is determined to differentiate, whereas the pink cell will remain a stem cell that will eventually resegment itself. In any event, the stem cell population can replenish itself, so as not to become depleted. This mechanism is used by embryonic cells and by adult organs alike (e.g. intestinal crypt cells). (B) Renewal of the villi stem cells in the small intestine. The rapidly dividing cells are increasingly more differentiated as they ascend in the crypts. (From 'Essentiel d'embryologie humaine et principes d'embryogenèse moléculaire', © Luc L. Oligny 2005, with permission.)

MYOD1 and *MYF5,* thus partially inhibiting the stimulation of their downstream cascades. Once the concentration of FGF returns to baseline levels its inhibition of *MYOD1* and *MYF5* relaxes allowing their transcription to resume to higher levels and further muscular differentiation (e.g. increase the synthesis of myofilaments).

Gamete differences, maternal molecules and genomic imprinting

Oocytes are larger than spermatozoa by several thousand-fold, regardless of species. Both types of gametes contain the same haploid genome (23 chromosomes in humans), but spermatozoa are essentially devoid of cytoplasm and nucleoplasm. The oocyte provides these components to the embryo as well as mitochondria, mRNA and most proteins – mitochondria of the future adult are thus of maternal origin. After fertilization the zygote and early embryo relies on nucleoplasmic stocks of maternal RNA and protein during its initial mitotic divisions.[70]

In embryos of certain organisms, like frogs, gravity causes a cytoplasmic gradient of the mRNA and proteins: the heaviest sink in the cytoplasm, the lightest 'float' to the top. This gradient allows a division of the zygote into a ventral pole (corresponding approximately to the heaviest portion) and a dorsal pole (the lightest). Evidently, mammals had to evolve other means of segmentation, to accommodate shaking and rotation by the uterus. Segmentation in the cephalo-caudal, dorso-ventral and medio-lateral axes is discussed below.

Another difference between parental gametes is that they contain different 'marks' or 'imprints' on select regions of their haploid genomes. Genomic imprinting was discovered in the 1980s, and is now recognized to be very important clinically.[71–73] Imprinting is characterized by the differential activation of alleles according to their parental origin, associated with dif-

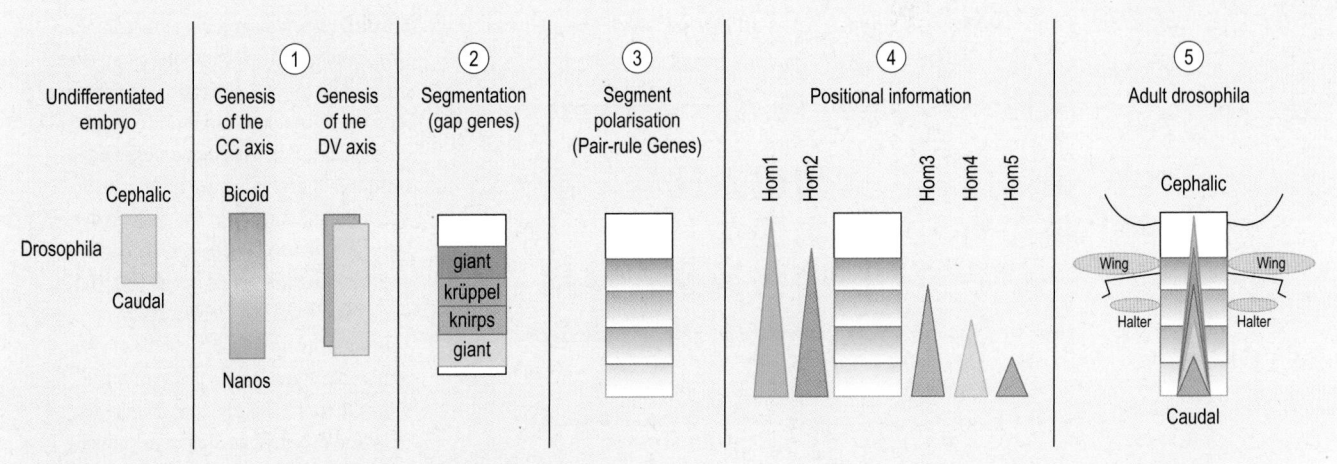

FIGURE 1.27 Sequential action of the segmentation genes in Drosophila. The caudo–cephalic (C–C) and dorso–ventral (D–V) axes are initially established; then, the embryo is segmented by the Gap genes in the C–C axis, followed by a C–C segmentation by the Pair-rule genes. The subsequent segment-polarity segmentation in the C–C axis is not shown. Finally, each of these segments is oriented with respect to the other segments by the hom genes, so as to determine if they are to form a cephalic, thoracic or abdominal segment. This segmentation cascade resembles that of vertebrates. (From 'Essentiel d'embryologie humaine et principes d'embryogenèse moléculaire', © Luc L. Oligny 2005, with permission.)

Each gap domain is then partitioned by differential expression of nine pair-rule genes. Pair-rule genes encode transcription factors that are virtually identical to the *PAX* genes of humans. Differential expression of pair rule genes like fushi-tarazu, even-skipped, and hairy produces differential development of each gap domain, dividing them into segments. Bordering each gap domain are cells without pair-rule gene expression, allowing separation of each gap region. As their expression divides and distinguishes gap domains, the pair-rule transcription factors induce segment-polarity genes that will further segment the embryo along its C–C axis. These segments are given structural diversity through action of homeotic gene complexes (Figs 1.27 and 1.28).

In summary, interacting gap, pair-rule, and homeotic complex proteins divide and differentiate the embryonic syncytium and its resulting cells. Each cell group has its unique exposure and coordinated response to combinations of master-switch transcription factors. The system provides a powerful model for vertebrate embryogenesis including segmentation, since *Drosophila* transcription factors and their downstream cascades have significant homologies with vertebrate molecules.[94]

Segmentation: homeotic genes and homeoproteins

Homeotic genes control the basic architecture of *Drosophila* development, specifying which segments will become abdomen and which will become antennae. By definition, homeotic gene mutations cause one body segment to differentiate into the structures of another, losing their 'positional identity'. For example, mutation of the homeotic gene *antennapedia* results in the replacement of antennae by legs. Likewise, mutation of the homeotic gene *bithorax* produces two identical winged

segments by transforming one segment's smaller appendages into wings.

The homeotic genes are translated into transcription factors called homeoproteins. These proteins share a sequence of approximately 60 amino acids which allows them to bind DNA (and also RNA in some cases). This shared sequence is called the homeodomain, and it has been highly conserved in yeasts, flies, worms, and vertebrates during evolution. By definition, homeoproteins are proteins containing a homeodomain sequence.

Over 100 homeoproteins exist, and all have helical tertiary structures that allow sequence-specific DNA binding within major and minor grooves.[91] Subtle differences in the homeodomain's 60 amino acids mediate selective binding to the regulatory sequences controlled by these homeoproteins. Thus, each homeoprotein acts on multiple promoters, enhancers, and inhibitors to regulate expression of its subordinate genes. The cumulative effects of multiple activating and inhibitory transcription factors on these subordinate genes determine their extent of expression. In *Drosophila*, some homeotic genes are intimately linked as two homeotic complexes, containing 6 and 3 homeotic genes (Fig. 1.28). As discussed below, the topographic arrangement of homeotic complex genes plays a crucial role in the anatomic and temporal expression of these genes.

Segmentation: vertebrate HOX genes

In vertebrates, homeoproteins are detected as early as the blastocyst stage. When the primitive streak begins gastrulation at about 14 days post conception, the embryo is already demarcated into dorso–ventral, medio–lateral, and cephalo-caudal regions. The gastrula is molecularly segmented by unique combinations of

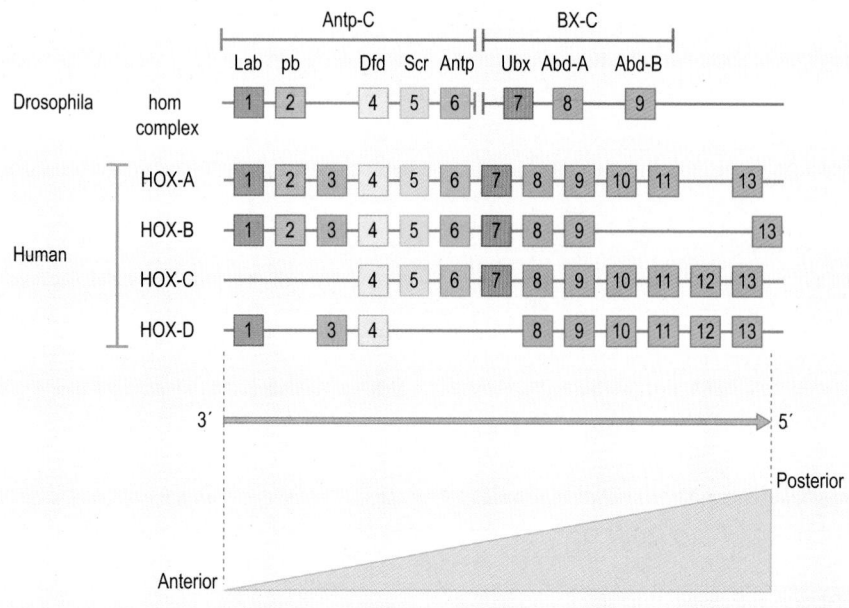

Retinoic acid concentration gradient within the embryo. The 3′ most HOX genes are activated at very low levels of RA, with each subsequent gene in the 5′ direction requiring greater concentrations of RA to become activated

FIGURE 1.28 Homeotic domains of *Drosophila*. The two homeotic complexes of drosophila (Antp-C and BX-C) are compared with the four human homeotic complexes. In vertebrates, Hox 9–13 arose from Abd-B. Note that these genes are transcribed sequentially, starting at the 3′-most gene of the complex (HOX-A1/B1/C4/D1), and ending with the 5′-most genes (HOX-A9/B-13/C-13/-D13). The retinoic acid concentration gradient probably plays a major role in the transcription of these genes. (From 'Essentiel d'embryologie humaine et principes d'embryogenèse moléculaire', © Luc L. Oligny 2005, with permission.)

expressed homeoproteins, even if morphologic segments are not obvious. As in the fly, combinations of homeoproteins control expression of specific master switch and subordinate genes, coordinating differentiation based on cell position. Homeotic genes are now recognized to be involved in the embryogenesis of most mammalian organs, including the nervous system.[94]

During evolution, the primordial eight-gene homeotic complex found in ancestral insects was duplicated and rearranged, so as to form four homeotic complexes, each on a different chromosome in mammals (Fig. 1.28). Each complex (HOX-A, HOX-B, HOX-C, and HOX-D) contains 9–12 *HOMEOBOX* (or *HOX*) genes; these homeotic complexes are highly homologous to their insect ancestor and, as a result, to each other. The HOX genes are designated according to their complex and sequential location (e.g. *HOX-A13*, *HOX-B9*, etc). Genes of concordant position (e.g. *HOX-A9*, *HOX-B9*, *HOX-C9*) have derived from the same insect homeotic gene and are more homologous than those at different positions within the same complex (e.g. *HOX-A9* versus *HOX-A2*).

Their tandem locations are partially responsible for the temporal expression of homeotic genes. Expression of each *HOX* gene activates expression of its 5′ neighbor: activation changes hetero- to euchromatin and the euchromatin state spreads beyond to the next gene in the cluster. Transcription starts at the first gene of each complex (*HOX-A1*, *-B1*, etc.) and migrates through the cluster. Retinoic acid is a regulator of spatiotemporal expression of HOX genes; promoters of proximal genes like *HOX-A1* require small concentrations to become active, while distal genes like *HOX-A13* require larger concentrations or retinoic acid for activation of transcription.

Retinoic acid gradients contribute to anteroposterior segmentation in mammals, the varied concentrations activating particular combinations of *HOX* cluster genes. Expression of genes along the *HOX* complexes, simultaneous among clusters, successive within clusters, differentiates the embryo along its C–C axis. *HOX-A1*, its homologues (*HOX-B1* and *-D1*) and *HOX-C4* are the first to be expressed, and their expression initially appears within the caudal embryonic pole and caudal regions of the limbs. This *HOX-1* group expression gradually 'migrates' toward the cephalic pole. Increasing concentrations of retinoic acid and spread of euchromatin from *HOX-A1* and homologues stimulate expression of adjacent genes (e.g. *HOX-A2*), their products appearing where *HOX-A1* was initially expressed. As *HOX-A2* is expressed, it stimulates transcription of *HOX-A3*, and proceeds along the cluster. A migration or 'wave' of expression proceeds through the HOX complexes, eliciting corresponding gradients in gene product expression. Proximal *HOX* genes (e.g. A1, B1), initially expressed caudally, will be the only genes expressed in cephalic embryonic segments. Middle segments will have increasing numbers of HOX genes expressed (e.g. *HOX-A1/A2*, *B1/B2*, etc.), while caudal-most regions will express all cluster members (e.g. *HOX-A1* through *-A13*, *-B1* through *-B13*, etc.).

Examples of developmental analysis

Approaches to neural development (the four phases)

The nervous system is by far the most architecturally complex human organ. Nevertheless, a few basic molecular tools enable embryos to form the neural tube, divide it into segments, generate thousands of neuron types, and guide their axons and dendrites to proper destinations. The molecular concepts discussed above provide insights into how embryos can achieve such complex differentiation.

The development of the central nervous system (CNS) can be divided into four phases.[94–97] In the first phase, neuroblasts proliferate very rapidly throughout the length of the neural tube. The second phase is characterized by the migration of the newly generated neurocytes; they migrate from the central germinal layer towards the periphery. The third phase is characterized by the growth of neurites toward their targets, through attraction by chemotactic and trophic factors. During the final phase, which continues until adulthood, neural connections are adjusted and refined by the electrical stimulations which they receive. Note that the embryonic CNS produces everything in excess and later eliminates its surplus by apoptosis; this system insures against hypoplasia of vital structures in a system devoid of proliferative reserves.

The first phase of neural development begins through neuroblastic proliferation: each cell division generates a neuroblast which remains adjacent to the ependymal canal, and one neurocyte which cannot proliferate. As differentiated neurons can no longer undergo mitosis, each has a 'date of birth' (Fig. 1.29). The birth of same-type neurons occurs during a very limited time period, after which the production of that type of neuron can no longer occur. Hence, neuroblasts of different generations will be exposed to different types and concentrations of morphogens, accounting for their variable differentiation pathways.

In the second phase, the neural tube contains glial cells that extend from the center of the tube (the ependymal canal) to its periphery, as with the spokes of a wheel. The germinal neurons (the neuroblasts) are located adjacent to the lumen of the tube. As they proliferate, they generate maturing neurons which migrate (under the influence of CAMs and chemotactic factors) to more peripheral positions with each new generation. The first cells to be generated migrate the shortest distance, the last ones the longest. The first and second phases of neural development overlap, with cell proliferation continuing until the last generation of neuroblasts are produced and begin to migrate.

The birth place of a neuron is as important as its birth date, for its position controls the expression of HOX genes and other segmentation-specific morphogens. These specific patterns of expression are essential for orchestrating orderly intercellular connections. Once arrived at its definitive location, a neuron develops projections called neurites (the future axons and dendrites).

The distal extremity of each neurite develops a growth cone with cytoplasmic projections. These processes advance and retreat, attracted by CAMs and extracellular matrix molecules for which they share affinities, repelled by CAMs at inappropriate locations. Neurite migration is promoted by a combined interaction of chemotaxis and CAMs. Because similar groups of neurites share the same CAMs, and thus are attracted to one another, they migrate together; similar neurites associate to form homogenous tracts rather than mingling into other tracts.

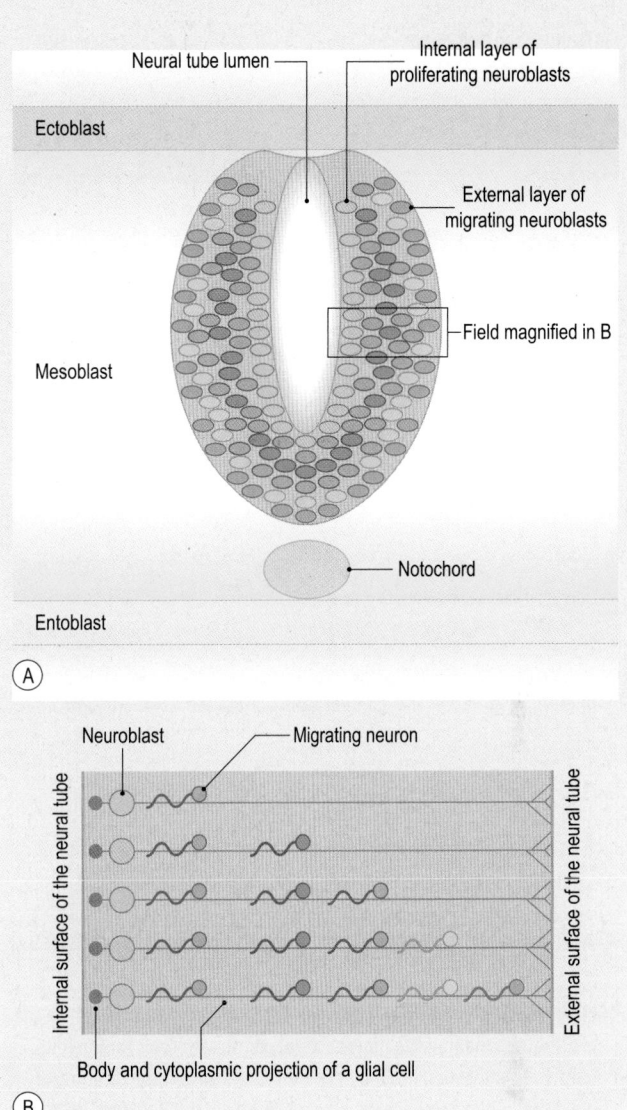

FIGURE 1.29 Neural tube formation. (A) Neural tube formation, with neuroblastic proliferation and migration of neurocytes. (B) Migration of primitive neurons, as guided by the cytoplasmic projections of the radially-arranged glial cells. (From 'Essentiel d'embryologie humaine et principes d'embryogenèse moléculaire', © Luc L. Oligny 2005, with permission.)

Many different guidance proteins are involved, including REELINs, EPHRINs, SEMAPHORINs, and NETRINs. Other intercellular signals, including those that interact with receptor tyrosine kinases or G-protein-coupled receptors, contribute to nerve migration and tract formation.[98]

In the third phase of neural development, neurites arriving at their target positions are stimulated by trophic substances. Some substances, like nerve growth factor, are chemotactic molecules secreted by and attracting neurites to their targets.[96–98] Without such stimulation, the neuron dies. Targets produce enough substance to support an appropriate number of neurons;

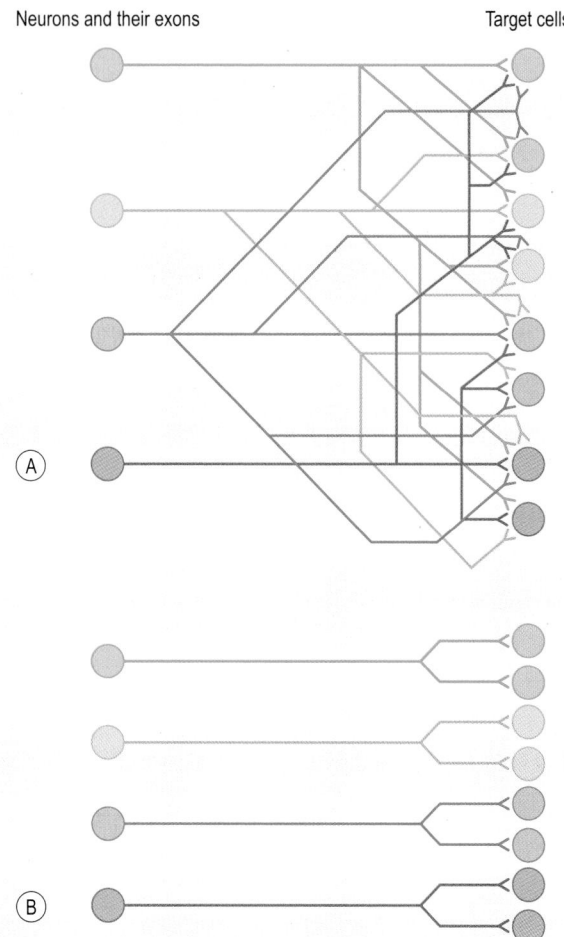

Neurons and their exons   Target cells

(A)

(B)

FIGURE 1.30 Increase in specificity of neural connections.
(A) Neurons making their initial connections with their target cells (neurons, myocytes, etc.). Each neuron innervates a large number of targets. Once the neurons have reached all of the targets in the vicinity of their final destination, the non-specific connections are eliminated. This results in the loss of large numbers of neurons and axons. (B) Final connections: the non-specific connections have been eliminated through the harmful effect of retrograde depolarization. (From 'Essentiel d'embryologie humaine et principes d'embryogenèse moléculaire', © Luc L. Oligny 2005, with permission.)

its synapses. This depolarization is not harmful to the synapse when it proceeds from the neurite to the target cell (physiologic depolarization), but is harmful in the reverse direction (retrograde depolarization). Thus, synapses that specifically trigger a target's depolarization survive unharmed while others with non-specific connections are resorbed. Physiologic nerve conduction thus eliminates non-specific synapses.

Similarities between the embryo and cancer

As suggested in Figure 1.1, embryos share many features with cancerous cells.[99-102] Implantation of the embryo and progression of neoplasia both involve:

- invasion of tissues through enzymatic proteolysis;
- guidance of cell migration (tumor invasion) by fibronectins, integrins and other molecules of the extracellular matrix; and
- secretion of angiotrophic factors to avoid growth-stunting hypoxia.

It has been speculated that cancer cells may modulate their adjacent mesenchyme in ways that favor their metastasis.

Embryos and cancer cells both show rapid cell growth. As mentioned previously, blasts double their cell number every 2–4 days in their first 4 weeks, mostly stimulated by proto-oncogenes. Neoplastic growth rates may be less dramatic but have similar signals: regulation of cell growth is lost due to mutations activating proto-oncogenes or disrupting tumor suppressors. In carcinogenesis, the disturbed cell growth can result from:

- overproduction of growth factors;
- reduced enzymatic degradation of growth factors;
- mutated oncogene receptors that resist inactivation or become autonomous without need for ligand (the oncogene protein);
- mutations in other components of signal transduction cascades, as when increased expression of MYC or CDK-4 proteins in the P53-RB cascade stimulates DNA synthesis (Fig.1.25).

Other common characteristics include extended cell longevity/immortality through activation of telomerase; this enzyme replicates DNA sequences that are unique to ends (telomeres) of chromosomes. The telomeric clusters tend to shorten with each cell division, encoding a timetable for senescence that causes cells to die after a programmed number of cycles. Immortalized cells, like those of neoplastic or germline tissues, activate telomerase, which preserves their telomere length and avoids programmed cell death. Cancer cells become like embryonic cells or the stem cells of adult tissues; they outlive and overgrow neighboring somatic cells that cannot replicate their telomeres.[100, 101]

Neoplastic cells and embryos are also protected from immunologic responses that would hasten their elimination. The mechanisms responsible for this tolerance are largely unknown, but fibrin may act as an 'insulator'. Hypercoagulability states, common in paraneoplastic syndromes, would benefit intravascular tumor cells; Nitabuch's fibrin layer could also act as a barrier at the placental insertion site. The hypercoagulable state of pregnancy has also been postulated to play a role in eluding the immunologic destruction of the embryo.

The use of the blood circulation for cell migration is used by the germ cells of birds and by hemopoietic cells in mammals.

excess neurons are eliminated by apoptosis. At this stage, persisting neurites establish non-specific connections with the largest possible number of targets. As a result, each target is initially innervated non-specifically by large numbers of neurites.

The fourth phase is characterized by a process unique to the CNS. Temporary but well-regulated connections form among various CNS regions by growth of axons and dendrites along specific tracts (Figs 1.29 and 1.30).[97, 98] Cells that were initially distant can now start to interact with one another. Once a target is stimulated (by a synaptic depolarization), it depolarizes all of

Migrating cells bind to 'homing molecules' localized on the surface of endothelial cells. These endothelial molecules are specific to each organ, exemplified by homing molecules in liver endothelial cells that are different from those of other tissues. Only cells with receptors for a specific homing molecule will bind endothelium at that particular site, eventually penetrating the vessel through diapedesis (invasion). Homing molecules are exploited advantageously in bone marrow grafting, where they direct intravenously injected marrow cells to repopulate the marrow. Malignant cells also possess homing receptors, explaining the predilection of tumoral metastasis: colonic adenocarcinomas preferentially spread to liver, breast carcinomas spread to bone, liver, and brain. Despite its vascular perfusion (20% of cardiac output), the kidney is rarely a metastatic target; perhaps cancer cells do not possess the appropriate receptors for renovascular homing molecules.

Another parallel concerns the epigenetic mechanisms of DNA methylation and histone modification, regulating differentiation in the embryo and reactivation of silenced genes in cancer.[101, 102] Epigenetic deregulation of developmentally important genes can also affect imprinted genes; for example, altered imprinting in an adrenocortical carcinoma can lead to overexpression of IGF2 and a loss of H19 expression.[103] Proto-oncogenes may lose silencing signals, being 'mutated' to become unregulated oncogenes. Tumor suppressor genes can be pathologically methylated, and thereby inactivated, during the clonal evolution of tumor cells to malignancy. DNA methylation or demethylation can aid tumor progression, prompting 'de-differentiation' as a reverse embryology, and these epigenetic alterations can be reversed by drugs in the treatment of cancer.[100] Epigenetic modulation is an early event in colorectal carcinoma, occurring at the early adenoma stage of cancer progression. Though the mechanisms for epigenetic alterations in cancer are poorly understood, they enable neoplastic progression by expression of specific cell adhesion molecules, proteases, angiotrophic factors, telomerase, and apoptotic-inhibiting molecules.

It is apparent that the molecular cascades so perfectly well regulated in embryogenesis can be hijacked by cancer cells to favor their growth, invasion, and dissemination. Several 'developmental cancer syndromes' are known. For example, in Bloom syndrome, the dosage of the BLM protein is crucial to somatic changes in that disorder and to genome instability of those patients' intestinal cells.[104] Inactivation of one BLM allele (**haploinsufficiency**) causes defective DNA repair with production of a cancer syndrome that predisposes to colorectal cancers. Haploinsufficiency of tumor suppressor genes has been demonstrated in other developmental/cancer syndromes, including *ATM* in ataxia-telangiectasia, *PTCH* in basal cell nevus syndrome, and *PTEN* in Ruvalcaba or Cowden syndrome.[104] The SHH cascade is also crucial to both development and neoplasia, as exemplified by the fact that in humans, abnormal cholesterol synthesis yields an abnormal development of the forebrain, and the basal cell nevus syndrome associated with the development of large numbers of basal cell carcinomas. The addition of cholesterol to promote SHH action in forebrain, in addition to the basal nevi is paralleled by farnesylation of RAS which regulates cell proliferation by controlling mitogen-activated protein kinase (MAPK).[105]

The link between CAMs, development, and neoplasia is exemplified by aberrant cell adhesion resulting from the COLLAGEN VII mutations that cause the epidermis–dermis fragility in epidermolysis bullosa.[106] When such mutations preserve the anchoring domains of COLLAGEN VII, COLLAGEN VII promotes squamos cell cancer and allows dermal invasion through its interaction with laminins.

Epilogue

This discussion of molecular embryology emphasizes the ubiquitous processes that govern animal development, each reducible to a few molecular concepts. Advances in developmental biology, like those in genetics, are now applicable to all fields of medicine. Their impact is nowhere greater than on pathology, with new laboratory tests and new approaches to birth defects and tumors. The fetal pathologist in particular must consider molecular mechanisms behind each step of classical embryogenesis, for these are the vulnerabilities that can be exploited for understanding, diagnosis, prevention, and therapy.

Novel inheritance mechanisms revealed by molecular developmental technology

Molecular and developmental advances have catalyzed a genuine scientific revolution. The simple rules for loci, alleles, and segregation derived by Mendel have been outgrown, and new genetic paradigms have emerged. While Mendelian reasoning could be stretched to accommodate multifactorial and threshold traits, newer embryologic and genetic findings force new concepts. Novel mechanisms for allele expression differences, triplet repeat expansion, and mitochondrial or maternal inheritance have transcended Mendelian boundaries (Fig. 1.31). These new mechanisms provide many additional reasons why the patient with no family history may reflect a genetic change.

Contiguous gene deletions

Contiguous gene deletions are chromosomal microdeletions which result in the loss of several genes that are contiguous within this chromosomal region. They can be identified by FISH, but are too small to be visualized by conventional cytogenetic techniques (discussed in Ch. 5). These disorders bridge the gap between obvious chromosomal anomalies and Mendelian disease.[107] Submicroscopic deletions are important avenues for positional

TABLE 1.2 CONTIGUOUS GENE DELETION SYNDROMES AND RELATED DELETIONS

Deletion	Phenotype	Significant genes in region
Del(4)(q12)	Piebald trait	c-kit proto-oncogene (signal transduction)
Del(8)(q24)	Langer-Giedion syndrome	
Del(11)(p13)	WAGR	WT1 tumor suppressor gene paternal origin
Del(15)(q11)	Prader-Willi syndrome	
Del(15)(q11)	Angelman syndrome	UBE3A maternal origin
Del(16)(p13.3)	Rubinstein-Taybi syndrome	*CREBBP* transcription factor
Del(17)(p11.2)	Miller-Dieker syndrome	LIS-1 G protein (signal transduction)
Del(17)(p11.2)	Smith-Magenis syndrome	
Del(22)(q11)	Shprintzen-DiGeorge spectrum including isolated conotruncal defects	TBX gene
Del(X)(p22.3)	Kallmann syndrome, ichthyosis	KAL gene (?cell adhesion), steroid sulfatase
Del(X)(p22.3)	Kallmann syndrome, ichthyosis, chondrodysplasia punctata	KAL gene, ?gene for chondrodysplasia
Del(X)(p21)	Duchenne muscular dystrophy, glycerol kinase deficiency, adrenal hypoplasia	Dystrophin gene, glycerol kinase
Del(X)(q28)	Adrenoleukodystrophy (ADLP), color blindness	ADLP PMP

PMP, Peroxisomal membrane protein; WAGR, Wilms tumor, aniridia, genitourinary defects, retardation.
See text for references.

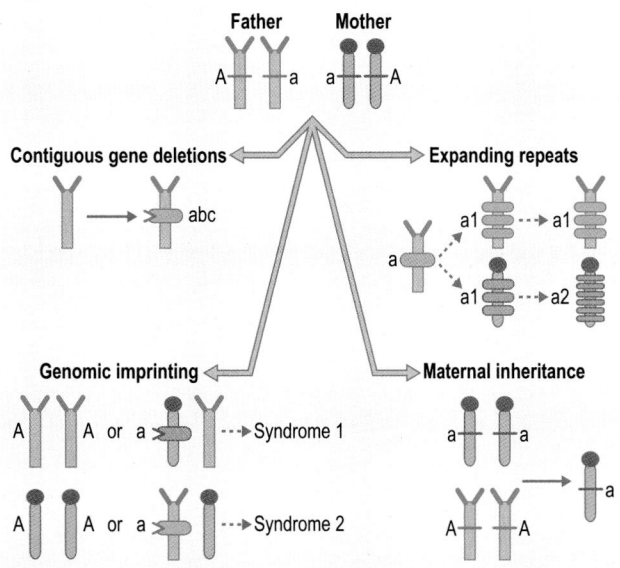

FIGURE 1.31 Atypical inheritance mechanisms. Mendelian segregation of normal (A) or abnormal (a) alleles is not sufficient to explain certain types of disease. Deletion of contiguous genes to produce composite phenotypes, expansion of triplet repeats, genomic imprinting where disease may depend on parental origin of the abnormal region/allele, and mitochondrial or maternal effect mutations that may produce maternal inheritance are illustrated.

cloning as depicted in Figure 1.18. They also identified important master switch molecules, and reinforce the importance of molecular developmental thinking.

High-resolution (prometaphase) banding can resolve 1000–2000 bands in the haploid chromosome complement as opposed to the 550-band routine karyotype. Small deletions can thus be visualized that encompass a few genetic loci (less than 1000 kb) and produce a unique phenotype due to the combined deficiency of several genes (Table 1.2). FISH technology has supplanted laborious prometaphase techniques by demonstrating submicroscopic deletions by their absence of fluorescent signals. One of the first contiguous gene syndromes to be recognized was the Wilms tumor, aniridia, genitourinary defect and mental retardation (WAGR, MIM 194072) syndrome which results from a microdeletion of the 11p13 region and which is transmitted as an autosomal dominant trait. Some families, with a similar deletion, show only aniridia and Wilms tumor, resulting respectively from **haploinsufficiency** of *PAX6* and *WT1*, the latter also responsible for the genitourinary defects (it is thought that a mutation other than that of *PAX6* is responsible for the mental retardation).[108]

Duchenne muscular dystrophy (DMD, MIM 310200) is another prototype of contiguous gene deletion syndromes. This X-linked recessive gene spans more than two megabases; the very rare cases of DMD which show an associated deletion of band Xp21.2 were extremely helpful in cloning this gene.[109] Families in which adrenal hypoplasia, chronic granulomatous disease or retinitis pigmentosa were transmitted along with DMD were likewise helpful in linking these three diseases to Xp21.2, and in cloning their genes.

Other contiguous gene deletions (Table 1.2) include Langer-Giedion syndrome (mental retardation and bony exostoses), Prader-Willi and Angelman syndromes, Miller-Dieker syndrome (mental retardation with lissencephaly), Smith-Magenis syndrome (mental retardation with absent rapid eye movement during sleep, and self-mutilation), and Shprintzen-DiGeorge spectrum that can include patients with isolated heart defects.[110, 111]

The 22q11 deletion responsible for Shprintzen-DiGeorge spectrum is inherited in about 10% of cases, and these are striking for their phenotypic variability. Affected children may have the complete DiGeorge sequence of branchial arch defects, including cardiac anomalies, thymic aplasia, and parathyroid agenesis. Yet parents with the same deletion may only have behavior problems (including schizophrenia) or never come to medical attention. In order to explain this variable expressivity, one turns to the molecular developmental thinking discussed previously. What master switch genes are involved, and do their variable effects result from variable extents of haploinsufficiency, variable epigenetic regulation (including parental origin of the deleted chromosome), or variable regulation of subordinate genes (e.g. cell proliferation, apoptosis, or CAMs)?

A *TBX* gene has been identified within the 22q11 deletion area, and knock-out of its homologue in mice produces similar alterations of branchial arch development.[111] The *TBX* transcription factor may provide insights into Shprintzen-DiGeorge syndrome and insights into pharyngeal, cardiac, and thymus development. Current progress suggests that some deletion phenotypes are related directly to the genes deleted (e.g. LIS-1 in Miller-Dieker lissencephaly),[112] while others depend on deletion position and its effects on chromatin structure. The recently defined 1p36 deletion[113] may be an example of the latter process, and illustrates that comparative genome hybridization techniques should rapidly augment the list of submicroscopic deletions in humans (Table 1.2).

Genomic imprinting

Analysis of microdeletions on chromosome 15 revealed that human phenotypes are subject to modification by the developmental mechanisms of genomic imprinting (see above). Named by analogy to the behavioral 'imprinting' of young animals on their mothers, a number of germline chromosome regions are marked according to their sex of origin.[71, 72, 114, 115] Molecular analysis demonstrated why the same 15q11 deletion could be found in patients with Prader-Willi or Angelman syndrome: patients with Prader-Willi syndrome always had deletions in the paternally derived chromosome 15, while patients with Angelman syndrome always had deletions in the maternally derived chromosome 15 (Table 1.2). These observations correlated with pioneering experiments in mice that demonstrated the need for pronuclei derived from both parents to produce an intact fetus (Fig. 1.32).[115] Although fusion of two maternal or two paternal pronuclei produced zygotes with normal genetic material, their uniparental origin prohibited normal differentiation. Interestingly, human triploidy with two paternal genomes also produces placental tissue (hydatidiform mole), while triploidy with two maternal genomes biases toward fetal tissues (e.g. ovarian teratomas). Now human diseases are being scrutinized for imprinting effects to discern how many human chromosomes will be imprinted compared with murine chromosomes 2, 6, 7, 11, and 17 (see Ch. 5, and Table 5.4).[116]

Imprinted chromosome regions can produce disease by several mechanisms. As illustrated in Figure 1.33 (left panel), the usual biparental contribution results in one chromosome from the mother (in pink) and one from the father (in blue). If

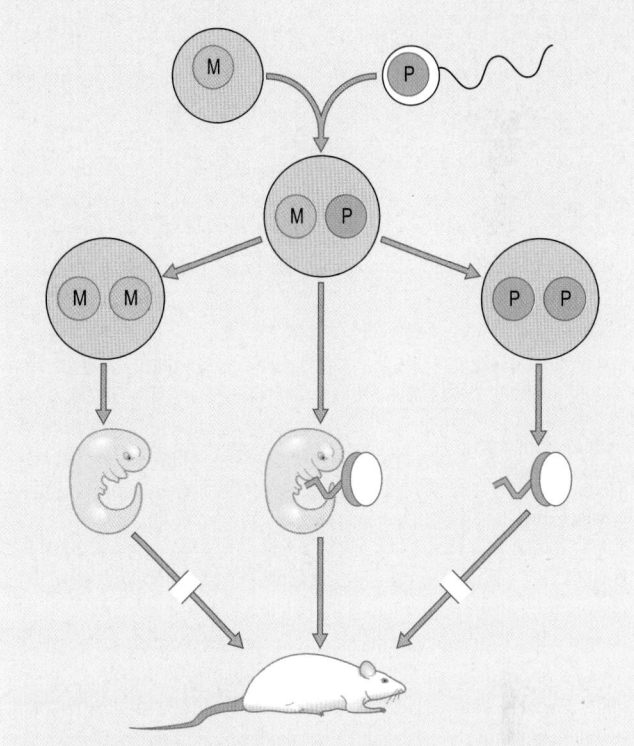

FIGURE 1.32 Mouse pronuclear transfer demonstrates normal pregnancy when maternal and paternal pronuclei are present in the fertilized egg. Absence of maternal or paternal pronuclei results in abortion despite a normal amount of genetic material.

there is non-disjunction during meiosis, a trisomic zygote may be produced with two maternal (left) or two paternal (right) chromosomes. If one cell of the morula loses one of its extra chromosomes (i.e. reverts from a trisomic to a disomic state), it will generate mosaic embryos with two cell lines, one with a normal number of chromosomes. However, such loss yields a 1/3 chance that both chromosomes of a pair are derived from one parent (uniparental disomy). If one considers an abnormal allele or deletion on one of the parental chromosomes, then two types of **uniparental disomy** may be considered: disomy for the same parental chromosome (**uniparental isodisomy,** right) or disomy where both parental chromosomes are represented (**uniparental heterodisomy,** left). Effects of uniparental isodisomy thus include homozygosity for abnormal alleles, as in the two cases of cystic fibrosis that have been reported in which only one parent is a carrier (see diagram for paternal isodisomy, Fig. 1.33).[115] Another way of generating uniparental disomy is with **Robertsonian translocations** or **isochromosomes.** In the right panel of Figure 1.33, a maternal Robertsonian translocation can be transmitted to produce maternal uniparental isodisomy for that chromosome or a trisomy containing two maternally derived and one paternally derived chromosome. These mechanisms for uniparental inheritance emphasize that every Mendelian disease or chromosomal disorder must be

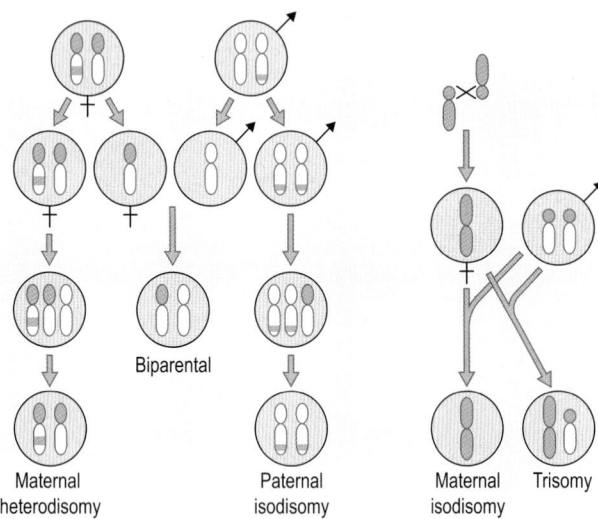

Biparental

Maternal
heterodisomy

Paternal
isodisomy

Maternal
isodisomy

Trisomy

FIGURE 1.33 Consequences of chromosome segregation for regions subject to genomic imprinting. (Left) Disomic gametes with two maternal (pink) or two paternal chromosomes will produce a trisomy when fertilized. If the non-disjunction occurs at meiosis I, both maternal chromosomes will be present in the disomic gamete; meiosis II non-disjunctions would produce two copies of the same paternal chromosome. Correction of the trisomic zygote produces uniparental disomy in one third of cases, heterodisomy (homozygosity of mutations unlikely – dark blue band) or isodisomy (homozygous mutations much more likely – light blue band). (Right) Robertsonian translocations can be transmitted to produce offspring where both chromosomes derive from one parent (uniparental isodisomy). DNA polymorphisms must be employed to prove uniparental origin since translocations occurring after fertilization may have biparental origin.

evaluated for imprinting effects – i.e. whether there is a difference in offspring phenotype that results from maternal versus paternal transmission of abnormal alleles or, in the case of chromosome disorders, from predominance of maternally versus paternally derived chromosome material.[114]

In humans, one of the best understood examples of imprinting is the couple *IGF2/H19*.[73, 117] Both genes reside on the 11p15.5 imprinted domain, along with more than 10 other imprinted genes. *IGF2* (insulin-like growth factor 2) is a growth factor (proto-oncogene) expressed in a large number of embryonic tissues (placenta, adrenals, kidneys, tongue, liver, etc).[117] Methylation of the maternal and paternal alleles of *IGF2* is different, accounting for the paternal allele of *IGF2* being preferentially expressed. This contrasts with *H19* which is maternally expressed. *H19* is not translated into protein, but apparently acts as a RNA transcription factor to inhibit genes under its control (e.g. *IGF2*).[117] In normal cells, H19 down-regulates IGF2, and the equilibrium between these two genes leads to normal growth (for simplicity, the other imprinted genes on 11p15.5 and throughout the genome have been omitted from this discussion, although they certainly play a major role in this phenomenon). In BWS, partial moles, complete moles, and many

cancers, this equilibrium is altered, leading to *IGF2* over-expression and overgrowth. For example, *IGF2* overexpression has been documented in Wilms tumor, Ewing sarcoma, rhabdomyosarcoma, adrenocortical tumors, hepatoblastoma and hepatocellular carcinoma, and pheochromocytoma; note that the incidence of these tumors is greatly increased in BWS, and that placentas of BWS fetuses can show mole-like changes. *IGF2* is also overexpressed in partial and complete moles, choriocarcinoma, leukemias, germ cell tumors, as well as in bladder, breast, cervical, esophageal, gastric, colorectal, pulmonary, ovarian, prostatic, renal cell, and other carcinomas and tumors.

What is the purpose of imprinting? The concept of 'selfish genes' is now generally accepted in biology, and it seems that imprinting could have evolved as such a mechanism.[118] Indeed, many imprinted genes are growth factors, with the activated paternal alleles acting as growth factors (e.g. *IGF2*), and activated maternal alleles acting as growth suppressors (e.g. *H19*). This is rationalized through a Darwinian natural-selection argument: fathers benefit from having large offspring, even at the expense of the mother, whereas mothers are not advantaged in having too large a baby. Molecularly, fathers stimulate the growth of their offspring, and mothers slow down this stimulation.

The importance of imprinting in human reproduction is supported by the estimated 1% of human genes that are imprinted, and this frequency has raised concerns about imprinting changes with artificial reproductive technology.[114, 119] Imprinting may be a factor that selects against fetal aneuploidy, illustrated by **confined placental mosaicism** that can correct from trisomy to two chromosomes from one parent (see Ch. 5). Maternal uniparental disomy 16 produced in this manner has produced growth-retarded fetuses, and confined chorionic trisomy 15 mosaicism has corrected to paternal uniparental disomy 15 with a phenotype of Angelman syndrome.[120]

Many genetic disorders exhibit peculiarities of onset or transmission that may indicate a role for abnormal genomic imprinting. These include Huntington disease, neurofibromatosis 1 and 2, tuberous sclerosis, Cowden syndrome, polycystic kidney disease, myotonic dystrophy, diabetes mellitus, psoriasis, and many single birth defects (cleft palate, neural tube defects, congenital heart disease) that exhibit parental sex-dependent recurrence risks. Imprinting may influence mental development, since girls with Turner syndrome who receive a paternal X chromosome develop speech faster than those with a maternal X.[121] DNA methylation patterns may one day supplement DNA polymorphisms as markers for risk factors in human disease.

DNA duplication and triplet repeat expansion

The idea of 'selfish DNA' was proposed to explain the significant fraction of the human genome that is repetitive and apparently non-functional.[118] Replication advantage through polymerase affinity, or replication slippage, could amplify DNA copy number without requiring phenotypic advantage. Molecular technology has now defined numerous examples of DNA duplication, sometimes of particular genes,[122, 123] sometimes of repeating units underlying the VNTR diagrammed in Figure 1.17, and sometimes with novel expansions of repetitive DNA elements.[53] Gene duplication is dramatic even in close evolutionary relatives, with 30% of human duplications not present in chimpanzees.[124] Diseases involving gene duplication include one type of Charcot-Marie-Tooth disease caused by an extra 1.5 megabase segment from chromosome 17. Disease symptoms can be nicely related to the extra amounts of 22-kilodalton myelin protein (PMP22), encoded by a gene defective in the *trembler* mouse. The complexity of gene dosage–phenotype relationships is indicated by the fact that some patients with similar (type I) Charcot-Marie-Tooth disease have point mutations in the PMP22 gene.[124] The role of gene duplication in human trisomies is complex, illustrated by the recent production of mice trisomic for their homologue of the Down syndrome critical region: no developmental abnormalities were noted.[125]

Another form of DNA duplication does have dramatic effects, illustrated by trinucleotide repeat amplification in fragile X syndrome (see above and Ch. 5).[63] Inhibition of fragile X gene expression and its clinical effects correlate with the number of trinucleotide repeats upstream of the gene (see Fig. 1.21 and discussion). Triplet repeat amplification in fragile X syndrome is a prototype for several diseases, allowing DNA diagnosis by PCR amplification and sizing of fragments to count numbers of repeats. Steinert myotonic dystrophy is another example: the disorder exhibits autosomal dominant inheritance with increasing severity in subsequent generations (**anticipation**) and in offspring of affected females (**maternal effect**). DNA probes targeting the Steinert gene on chromosome 19 disclosed a variable CTG repeat near a protein kinase gene expressed in muscle.[126]

As in fragile X, myotonic dystrophy repeats are more susceptible to expansion during female meiosis. Even females with mild disease can undergo sufficient meiotic amplification to cause severe congenital myotonic dystrophy in their offspring. Unstable trinucleotide repeats have also been found in Huntington chorea, spinobulbar muscular atrophy (SMA), and spinocerebellar ataxia type 1 (SCA1). Probes directed to various types of trinucleotide repeats have detected over 40 such loci in the human genome, hence many more diseases are likely to be explained by triplet repeat instability.[127]

Trinucleotide repeat disorders have also revealed new disease mechanisms, appreciated by considering the pathways of genetic information discussed in this chapter.[128] Myotonic dystrophy cells accumulate transcribed repeats as ribonucleoprotein complexes in muscle cells, perhaps disrupting synthesis of RNAs and proteins. Nerve cells in Huntington chorea produce polyglutamines from the CAG triplet repeats, forming aggregates of the protein HUNTINGTIN, which can be demonstrated using immunohistochemical staining directed at polyglutomine tracts. Similar aggregates are found in nine other neurologic disorders with CAG repeat expansion, forming a novel category of polyglutamine diseases (e.g. SMA, SCA1, SCA2, etc).[128] The proteins with a polyglutamine tract expansion are cytotoxic. The pathology may overlap with that caused by porphyrin accumulation in homozygous porphyria; accumulations of neurotransmitter-like molecules can activate programmed cell death through the activator protein-1/ JNK/ MAP kinase cascade.[129] Once again the steps of chromatin, transcription, protein factors, signal transduction, and cell process can be invoked to envision the molecular pathology.

Mitochondrial and Maternal Effect Mutations

The term **maternal effect** has been used loosely in disorders such as myotonic dystrophy, maternal phenylketonuria, and neurofibromatosis, to describe enhanced severity in offspring caused by maternal disease. Several mechanisms may produce a maternal effect, including teratogenic action of metabolites, genomic imprinting, or female meiotic instability of trinucleotide repeats. Of pertinence to developmental pathology are two genetic mechanisms that should receive increasing attention. Mitochondrial inheritance reflects the presence of mitochondrial DNA in germ cells that are transmitted only through the oocyte.[130] Mutations affecting the mitochondrial genome will thus exhibit maternal inheritance, showing transmission to all children of affected females but to no children of affected males. Disorders such as Kearns-Sayre syndrome, Leber hereditary optic neuropathy, and several mitochondrial encephalopathies have been related to specific mutations in mitochondrial DNA. Of interest is the phenomenon of **heteroplasmy,** whereby different numbers of abnormal mitochondria may exist in certain cells and cell lineages. Variable expression as a consequence of heteroplasmy can complicate recognition of maternal inheritance; it also opens the possibility of mitochondrial defects in selected organs or tissues and extends the phenotypic spectrum for mitochondrial diseases. A maternally transmitted form of diabetes mellitus is one example.[130]

Less appreciated but of great potential for disorders affecting development of the early embryo are maternal effect mutations.[131, 132] After fertilization the maternal and paternal genomes do not fuse as naked DNA molecules but are clothed by an egg cytoplasm rich in maternally encoded molecules. The dowry of **maternal RNAs** and proteins brought to fertilization by the oocyte contrasts mightily with the limited materials injected with the sperm head. Alleles altering these maternal molecules can have a double effect: not only may the altered maternal allele be transmitted to the zygote (1/2 chance), but 1/2 of its product in the egg cytoplasm will be abnormal. Until **zygotic expression** takes over from maternal control (i.e. several days post conception in humans), maternal alleles encoding molecules in the egg cytoplasm can have tremendous influence. Maternal effect mutations are very frequent in simpler organisms such as *Drosophila* but are not yet recognized in mammals. Higher transmission rates of congenital heart disease from affected mothers may represent an example.[133] Infertility, abortion, or early embryonic defects will be the most common presentation of human maternal effect mutations, and alleles with severe consequences may not be transmitted to reveal obvious maternal inheritance. If operative in higher mammals, this category of genetic diseases would provide another exciting opportunity for fetal pathology.

Molecular approaches to growth and development

Developmental categories

Several frameworks can be used for classification of abnormal development. From an organismal perspective, the four Hs of hierarchy, homology, heterochrony, and homeostasis can be mentioned. Hierarchy reflects the network properties of developing pathways, where single aberrations can have numerous consequences due to a cascade of derivative tissues. The peroxisomal disorders discussed below emphasize the hierarchy extending from metabolic alterations (e.g. **plasmalogen** deficiency) to altered neurogenesis (e.g. cerebral heterotopias) to surface aberrations from fetal hypotonia (e.g. single palmar creases, clubfoot). Homology means similarity among developmental structures, e.g. the similarity of right/left limb bud development implied by vertebrate symmetry. Homology among structures of different species brings in a phylogenetic perspective, and homology between birth defect and primordial structure (developmental arrest) underlies the idea of altered developmental timing (heterochrony).[134]

Anomalies such as holoprosencephaly, single ventricle, and tubular stomach can all be viewed as developmental arrests with the implication that molecules controlling subsequent stages are good candidates for exploration. Implied by the threshold model for inheritance of common birth defects and the reparative potential of embryos is the idea of developmental homeostasis invoked by Waddington and, with regard to the effects of aneuploidy, by Shapiro.[135] Each concept implies experimental strategies for defining molecular developmental events, and together they illustrate the many facets of development that must be unified by any comprehensive theory.

More specific classification schemes concern the mechanisms of normal and abnormal development. Chapters 2 and 3 discuss the differences between intrinsic abnormalities of developing tissues (malformations, dysplasias) and extrinsic forces that perturb them (deformations, disruptions). Distinction among isolated anomalies (e.g. cleft palate), single anomalies with serial consequences (e.g. Robin or Potter sequence), and multiple anomalies (syndromes, associations) is important, as are relationships between certain developing organs (e.g. ear and kidney) that cause them to be jointly involved across many syndromes (developmental fields, shared transcription factors, etc). The value of clinical categories lies in recognition of increasing genetic impact in the progression from mechanical defect (disruption, deformation) to isolated anomaly (sequence, association) to syndrome. Unfortunately, a morphologic concept such as disruption does not immediately reveal a molecular strategy, although vascular pathogenesis could have anticipated mutations such as the Mov13 mouse with transgenic disruption of the type I collagen α_1 chain.[136] Perhaps the best route toward a molecular understanding lies in defining classic developmental processes (e.g. blastogenesis, gastrulation, neurulation) in terms of specific cell types and molecular processes (e.g. growth, differentiation, migration, adhesion) discussed previously. Progress in defining mechanisms for cell lineage (e.g. neural crest), tissue interaction (e.g. FGF in amphibian induction), and differentiation (e.g. cell adhesion, signal transduction) is a beginning toward an understanding of something as complex as the primitive streak. As the basic elements of developmental processes are understood, broader perspectives such as homology or homeostasis can be given cellular and molecular definition.

An intermediate classification of development that has virtue for molecular exploration is that formulated by Steele.[137] Developmental processes can be explained in terms of growth, differentiation, or **pattern formation** in the way that pathologists have classified congenital tumors. Hamartomas (e.g. a cartilaginous pulmonary hamartoma) are composed of an abnormal mixture of tissue elements or an abnormal proportion of a single element, but these elements are normally present in that site; choristomas (e.g. ectopic adrenal tissue under the renal capsule) are normal tissues that grow at inappropriate locations – i.e. altered pattern. 'Primitive' undifferentiated tumors (e.g. Wilms tumor) have altered growth and differentiation. Developmental examples might include adrenal hypoplasia (abnormal growth), lissencephaly (abnormal differentiation), and situs inversus or polydactylies (normal structures at abnormal locations, i.e. abnormal pattern formation). Examples within each category will be presented to show the high road from pathologic description to developmental genetic analysis, an approach that can elevate routine autopsy to important discovery.

Molecular analysis of growth

Growth alterations can be proportionate (symmetric in terms of the fetus) or dysharmonic. The latter category applies to most congenital syndromes, and intrauterine growth retardation is a red flag for syndrome consideration. Standard curves for overall, regional, and organ growth are available for late embryonic and fetal periods; harmony of fetal growth can thus be quantified using standard protocols for surface measurements and organ weights (Ch. 16). Proportionate growth alteration suggests excess or deficiency of global factors – e.g. insulin excess in offspring of diabetic mothers or nutrient insufficiency with placental anomalies. Perhaps the purest example would be symmetric pituitary dwarfism, of which many types exist, all caused by postnatal growth hormone deficiency in contrast with the markedly disproportionate dwarfism caused by skeletal dysplasia. In fact, most growth alterations involve some disproportion based on variable tissue susceptibility to the offending agent or sparing of important organs. Brain sparing underlies the prominent heads seen in many types of growth delay. Strikingly disproportionate growth acceleration or delay implies effects on particular tissues or organs (e.g. decreased neural tissue in fetal alcohol or Cockayne syndrome, decreased bone density in osteogenesis imperfecta) and focuses attention on molecules regulating the growth of that tissue.

TABLE 1.3 SELECTED PROTO-ONCOGENES AND TUMOR SUPPRESSOR GENES

Gene class	Gene	Origin	Type	Locus	MIM #
Tyrosine protein kinases	V-SRC	Rous sarcoma virus	Onc	20q12	190090
	ABL1	Abelson leukemia virus	Onc	9q34	189980
	KIT	Feline sarcoma virus	Onc	4q22	164920
GTP-binding or GTP-activating proteins	HRAS	Harvey sarcoma virus	Onc	11p15	190020
	ERAS	Harvey sarcoma virus	Onc	Xp11.2	300437
	NF1	Neurofibromatosis-1	TS	17q11	162200
Growth factor related	PDGFB	Simian sarcoma virus	Onc	22q12	190040
	EGFR	Avian erythroblastosis virus	Onc	7p12	131550
	CSF1R	McDonough sarcoma virus	Onc	5q33	164770
Nuclear proteins	MYC	Myelocytomatosis virus	Onc	8q24	190080
	MYCN	Neuroblastoma	Onc	2p23	164840
	RB1	Retinoblastoma	TS	13q14	180200
	WT1	Wilms tumor	TS	11p13	607102

CSF-1R, Colony stimulating factor-1 receptor; EGFR, epidermal growth factor receptor; GTP, guanosine triphosphate; ONC, oncogene; PDGF, platelet-derived growth factor; TS, tumor suppressor.
Modified from Knudson 1986,[138] with permission.

Example: sequential gene expression in growth and neoplasia

Molecular analysis has defined many growth-related molecules through their alteration in tumors.[77, 85, 99, 102–106] As mentioned in the introduction to this chapter, the sporadic nature of most tumors masked the enormous genetic contribution to neoplasia that was uncovered by molecular analysis. Table 1.3 lists several examples under the categories of oncogenes and tumor suppressor genes that were discussed previously. It has been emphasized that tumors are frequently the endpoints in a series of genetic changes, involving both positive and negative regulation (Fig. 1.1). The definition of molecular changes that fulfill Knudson's two-hit or two-stage hypothesis has also been reviewed.[138] While Knudson's explanation involved one abnormal *RB1* allele from the germline (predisposition or first hit), followed by somatic Rb1 gene mutations in susceptible tissue (second hit in retina), epigenetic changes can also be placed on this pathway to neoplasia. This is reflected in the fact that most germline *RB1* mutations originate on the paternal chromosome, implying a role for genomic imprinting/DNA methylation. Characterization of the *RB1* gene as a cell cycle regulatory element places it within cell proliferation/cell death pathways discussed in the section on molecular embryology (see Fig. 1.25). Analogous cascades can be imagined for many developmental anomalies.

Example: Russell-Silver syndrome

Russell-Silver syndrome is a disorder of growth that illustrates the approach for molecular analysis. The phenotype of prenatal growth retardation with prominent forehead (pseudohydrocephaly), triangular facies, fifth finger clinodactyly, multiple nevi or café au lait spots, and hemihypertrophy is undoubtedly heterogeneous but has value in predicting catch-up growth and normal intelligence. Most cases are sporadic, but occasional families have exhibited autosomal dominant inheritance. Although karyotyping is usually normal, a group of patients with Russell-Silver characteristics and ring 15 chromosome abnormality have been described.[139, 140] The ring 15 patients were atypical in having mental retardation, and only a subset of ring 15 cases have characteristics reminiscent of the Russell-Silver phenotype.

Using molecular reasoning, a growth-regulating gene is suggested within the deleted region of chromosome 15 that is mutated in non-chromosomal cases of Russell-Silver syndrome. Heterogeneous phenotypes in ring 15 patients might reflect genomic imprinting – perhaps the ring 15 chromosomes that mimicked Russell-Silver phenotypes were all of maternal (or paternal) origin, or a contiguous gene syndrome. Mostly sporadic cases with occasional autosomal dominant inheritance could imply interaction with another gene or somatic mutations – lateral asymmetry of growth and particularly examples of crossed asymmetry that occur in Russell-Silver syndrome would be consistent with the latter.

Investigators have pursued these speculations with mixed results. The *IGF1R* (IGF1 receptor) is located in the appropriate chromosome 15 region and is deleted in ring 15 patients with Russell-Silver characteristics.[139] This locus is also known to be imprinted in the mouse. Although examination of Russell-Silver patients for uniparental origin of the distal chromosome 15 region has been negative, a telomeric cluster responsible for imprinting in the 11p15 region has been found.[139] As discussed above, the imprinted *IGF2* of BWS is in the same region; all the more intriguing because of the nearby Wilms tumor locus (*WT1* in 11p13) and occurrence of Wilms tumor in patients with hemihypertrophy. A Russell-Silver phenotype was observed in the patient with cystic fibrosis and isodisomy 7, and imprinting changes are supported by its occurrence after in vitro fertilization.[140] This transition from growth disorder to molecular causation should be indelibly engraved in the minds of fetal pathologists; it can be applied to every fetal growth abnormality that exhibits genetic predisposition (see Ch. 41).

Molecular analysis of differentiation

Although growth and differentiation are inextricably linked, anomalies such as cerebral polymicrogyria or lissencephaly are most remarkable for their abnormal differentiation. Two diseases associated with these anomalies are the Zellweger and Miller-Dieker lissencephaly syndromes, offering contrasting examples of molecular analyses using functional versus positional cloning.

Example: Zellweger syndrome and peroxisome assembly

Zellweger syndrome (Fig. 1.34A) is a lethal autosomal recessive condition associated with severe hypotonia, unusual facies, neuromigration defects (Fig. 1.34B), micronodular cirrhosis, renal cysts, and bone dysplasia. Numerous metabolic abnormalities are associated with this syndrome, including excess of very long chain fatty acids, pipecolic acid and phytanic acid, and deficiency of plasmalogens, myelin, and certain bile acids.[141] Multiple enzymes responsible for degradation or synthesis of these chemicals, united by their location in peroxisomes, were shown to be deficient in Zellweger patients. Peroxisomes (Fig. 1.34C) were thought to be absent until antibodies to peroxisomal membrane proteins **(PMPs)** of the peroxisomal membrane identified 'ghost' structures in affected tissues, implying normal membrane synthesis with aberrant assembly of numerous matrix proteins **(PMaPs)**. Attention was thus focused on the membrane proteins as candidates for mutation in Zellweger syndrome, and defects in several have been characterized.[142]

A scheme for peroxisome assembly can be hypothesized as illustrated in Figure 1.34D, showing predominance of PMP synthesis in early embryonic tissues or brain that have scanty matrices with minimal catalase staining. Import of PMaPs leads to easily visualized peroxisomes in liver and kidney, with surprising variation in peroxisome morphology from tissue to tissue.[142]

Interesting regions of PMP genes include DNA- and ATP-binding sites similar to those of the cystic fibrosis transmembrane regulator.[142] These molecules can be added to the many discussed in the section on neural development, relating neuron migration and cerebral differentiation to signal molecules and adhesive proteins defined through genetic mutations. They are also involved in limb differentiation, causing one form of chondrodysplasia punctata (see below).

Example: lissencephaly in Miller-Dieker syndrome

The submicroscopic deletion of chromosome band 17p13 provided a positional target for studies leading to isolation of the *LIS1* gene (Table 1.2). This gene is expressed in brain and shows homology to G proteins that are known to be involved in nerve cell signaling.[143] There is also a β-transducin-like repeat in the *LIS1* gene that is homologous to a cell cycle regulator in yeast and to the *Drosophila* groucho protein that is involved in neurogenesis. Once again an abnormal developmental process can be explained by stepwise changes in chromatin, signal molecules, and cell differentiation (to nerve tracts and gyri).

Molecular analysis of pattern formation

In addition to growth and differentiation, development results in a particular arrangement of organs and tissues, a body plan typical for each organism. Questions of pattern range from the spacing of bristles on the insect cuticle to the fascinating stripes of zebras. Theories of pattern formation have included gradients derived from properties of chemical solutions, cell repulsion/attraction models to explain bristle spacing, and polar coordinate theories of limb formation. The text of Gilbert[68] provides elegant and well-illustrated review of historical, theoretical, evolutionary, and molecular aspects of pattern formation.

Molecular aspects of pattern formation will include **targeting sequences** that direct proteins to various regions of the cell – e.g. the amino-terminal charged amino acids targeting to mitochondria and the carboxy-terminal amino acids targeting to peroxisomes.[130, 141] Cell surface and signaling molecules must direct **topogenesis** of cells: the positional information or 'address' of cells discussed by Wolpert.[69] Cardiac topogenesis has been modeled on the basis of cell surface properties, and Edelman has discussed a 'topobiology' based on properties of cell adhesion molecules such as the *L1CAM* locus implicated in MASA syndrome.[144] As discussed above, analysis of segmentation in *Drosophila* has provided an approach and candidate genes that will be extremely useful for defining the anomaly patterns seen in developmental pathology.

Example: piebald trait

Molecular characterization of the autosomal dominant condition known as piebald trait illustrates the value of molecular and developmental homology in genetic analysis. As shown in Figure 1.35, ventral depigmentation observed in human piebald trait is remarkably similar to the appearance of mice with the trait **dominant spotted**.[145] Characterization of mutations in the proto-oncogene *Kit* in affected mice drew attention to the fact that the human homologue had been mapped to chromosome band 4q12. Several piebald trait patients had been recognized with deletions of the 4q12-15 region (Fig. 1.35), leading to scanning of the human *KIT* gene for deletions (Southern blotting) or point mutations (SSCP) in piebald patients.[145] Relation of depigmentation to a tyrosine kinase involved in signal transduction implies that normal *KIT* signaling is required for melanoblast migration. The ventral, usually midline patterning of white patches merely reflects the longer distance that dorsally derived melanoblasts must travel to reach these positions. Molecular, cellular, and embryologic knowledge thus combines to provide a genetic explanation for altered pattern formation.

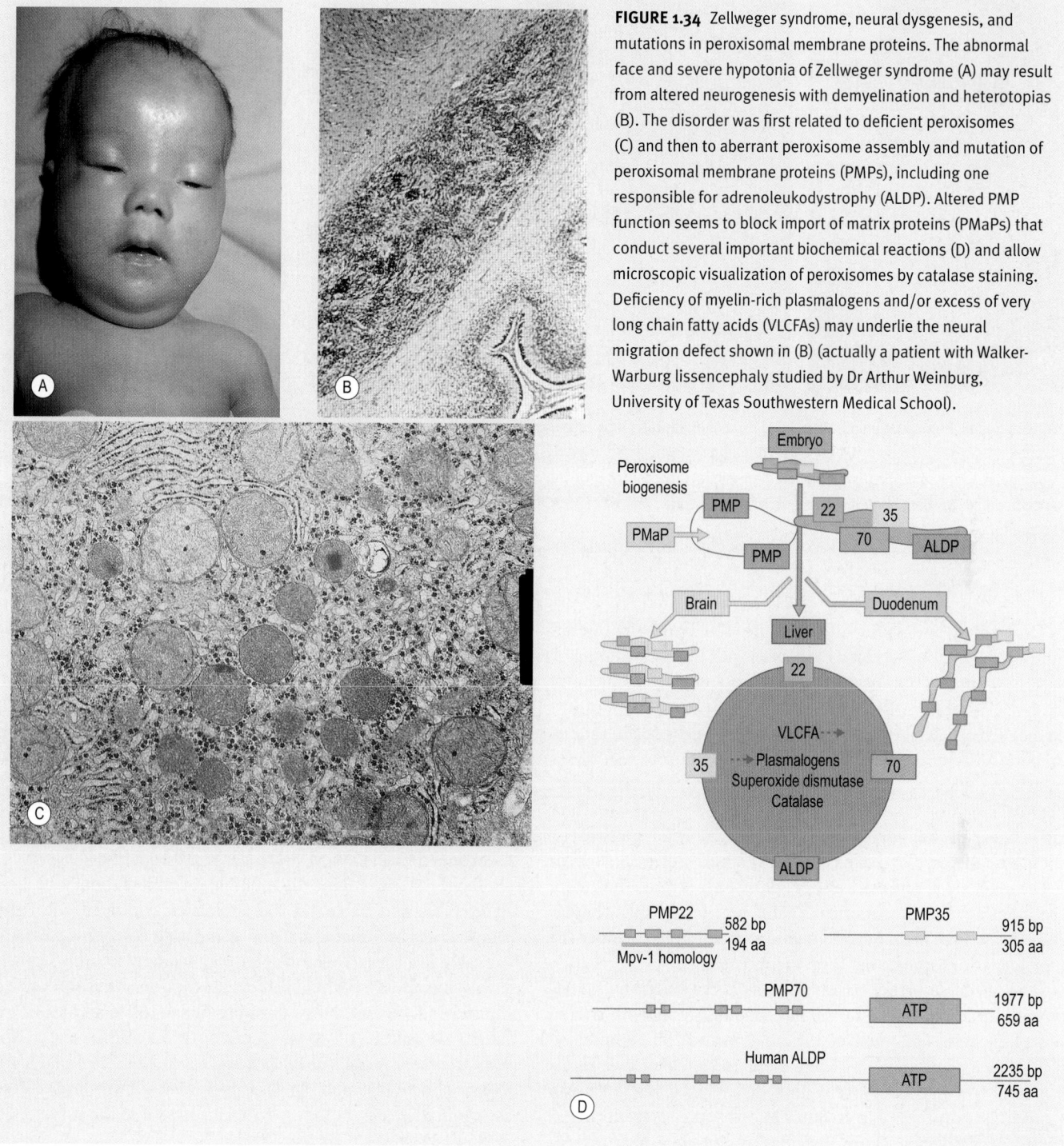

FIGURE 1.34 Zellweger syndrome, neural dysgenesis, and mutations in peroxisomal membrane proteins. The abnormal face and severe hypotonia of Zellweger syndrome (A) may result from altered neurogenesis with demyelination and heterotopias (B). The disorder was first related to deficient peroxisomes (C) and then to aberrant peroxisome assembly and mutation of peroxisomal membrane proteins (PMPs), including one responsible for adrenoleukodystrophy (ALDP). Altered PMP function seems to block import of matrix proteins (PMaPs) that conduct several important biochemical reactions (D) and allow microscopic visualization of peroxisomes by catalase staining. Deficiency of myelin-rich plasmalogens and/or excess of very long chain fatty acids (VLCFAs) may underlie the neural migration defect shown in (B) (actually a patient with Walker-Warburg lissencephaly studied by Dr Arthur Weinburg, University of Texas Southwestern Medical School).

Example: Human limb deficiencies – comparison of defect patterns

Limb development has been a favored area of experimentation with ease of grafting/ablation (with regeneration) and of defining morphology (with skeletal staining). Such experiments also generated theories of pattern formation, including the polar coordinate system for limb formation/regeneration. These morphologic approaches have defined molecules important for limb patterning, and provide a last example of the exciting interface between molecular discovery and clinical delineation.

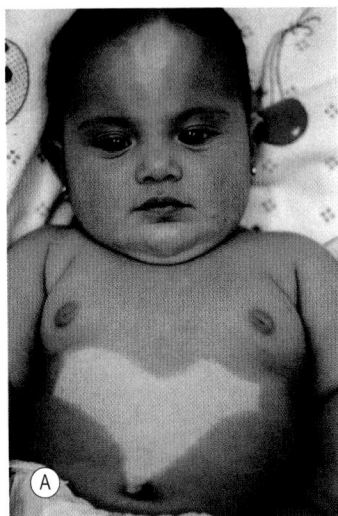
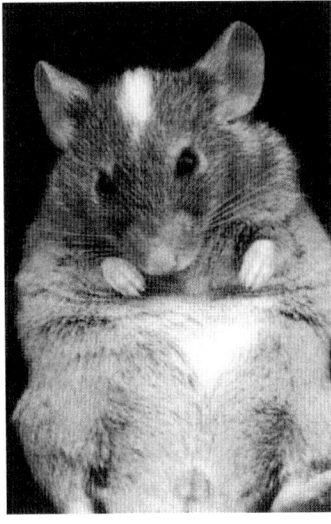
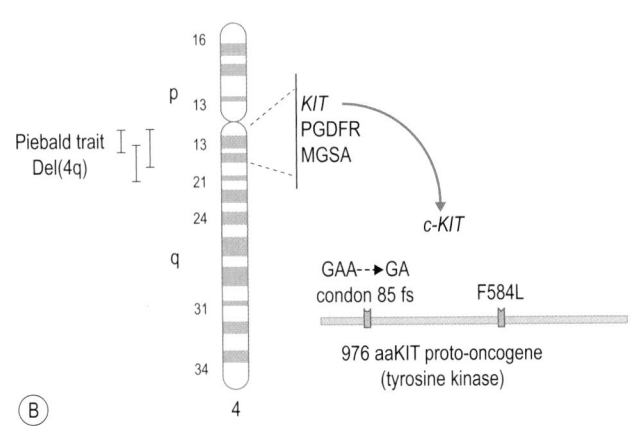

FIGURE 1.35 (A) Human piebald trait and the 'dominant spotting mouse' have mutations of the c-kit proto-oncogene.[83, 84] Characterization of the mouse mutation allowed recognition that the corresponding location of the human c-kit gene was deleted in several patients with the piebald trait. (B) Deletion of c-kit gene as opposed to the platelet-derived growth factor receptor (PDGFR) or melanoma growth stimulatory activity (MGSA) gene was demonstrated by Southern analysis; then, point mutations were demonstrated using PCR/SSCP (see Fig. 1.19).[83, 84] The c-kit gene encodes a tyrosine kinase that presumably is required for melanoblast migration. [(A) Courtesy RA Fleischman.[145]]

Congenital anomalies affecting the 120 bones in human limbs include global skeletal dysplasias with limb shortening or deformity, limb duplications like the frequent postaxial polydactyly (1% of live births), and limb deficiencies (0.6% of live births). The skeletal dysplasias often involve general alterations in bone differentiation, illustrated by the stippled epiphyses shown in Figure 1.36A. Limb deficiencies provoke more medical attention because of their startling phenotype and their challenges for habilitation (Fig. 1.36B, C). Fetal pathologist should be inspired by Lenz's alertness to limb defect clusters in 1961, and by Frances Kelsey's prescient action that kept thalidomide out of America.[146] The lessons of this chapter should also take them beyond public attribution to consider the (epi-)genetic cascades that fashion limb defects.

The heritable nature of limb defects is evidenced by review of the McKusick catalogue: among 1836 disorders with altered morphogenesis, 652 involved the skeleton and 205 of these had limb deficiencies alone.[147] There were 165 skeletal dysplasias, but only two had concurrent limb deficiencies (e.g. Ellis-van Creveld syndrome). Limb duplications were present in 57 (28%) of the genetic limb deficiencies, anticipating compensatory mechanisms discussed below. Patterns of bony defects and associated anomalies in genetic limb deficiencies also reflect molecular cascades, further emphasized by similar patterns among limb defects from a population survey.[148] Each anomaly pattern fits with the spatiotemporal gradients deduced from experimental manipulation of model embryos.

A rather confusing nomenclature exists for limb deficiencies, with terms like amelia, (absence of limbs); hemimelia, longitudinal, pre- or postaxial deficiencies (selective absence of medial vs lateral components); ectrodactyly (absence of central components – Fig. 1.36B); and phocomelia or intercalary deficiencies (absence of middle segments with retention of distal segments – Fig. 1.36C). Froster and Baird[148] used a hierarchical classification for their population-based study that follows limb segment ontogeny: upper extremity before lower, proximal segment before distal. A patient with absent humeri, radioulnar fusion, and hypoplastic femur would thus be classified under humeral defects, with the other limb defects classified as additional musculoskeletal anomalies. The 205 heritable limb deficiencies ascertained from OMIM[4] were classified similarly.

Table 1.4 shows the distribution of absent bones in limb deficiencies and Table 1.5 the anomalies associated with limb deficiencies by organ system, comparing survey cases and heritable disorders. Distal bias in the hierarchy of limb segment involvement was evident in survey cases and genetic disorders: e.g. humerus (2.4% and. 2.9%) to radius–ulna (16.5% and 19.3%) to hand (39% and 33%); so was anterior (preaxial) bias: e.g. radius (54% and 13%), versus ulna (33% and 6.3%), tibia (25% and 5.4%) versus fibula (14% and 3.4%). Upper versus lower limb defects took precedence in both, e.g. 57% versus 18% in the survey, 32% versus 7.3% in the database.[146, 148]

Not shown was the expected high frequency of unilateral cases in the survey (86%) and their rarity (2%) in the genetic database. The 15% of survey cases with symmetrical involvement establishes a minimal estimate of their genetic contribution, recognizing that mutations may impact laterality as well. Associated anomalies were significant (53%) among survey cases and more so in genetic disorders (80%), being most frequent in amelia (61% and 91%) and upper limb deficiencies (38% and 73%), less frequent when lower limb defects were present alone (20% and 33%). Among the syndromic cases or genetic disorders, the

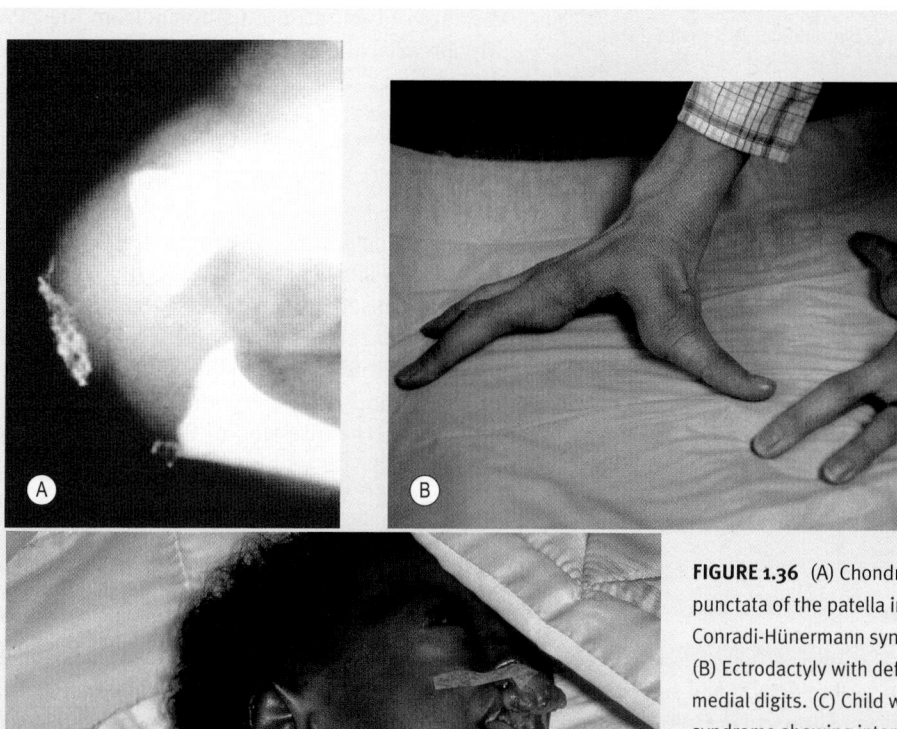

FIGURE 1.36 (A) Chondrodysplasia punctata of the patella in a child with Conradi-Hünermann syndrome. (B) Ectrodactyly with deficiency of the medial digits. (C) Child with Roberts syndrome showing intercalary deficiency (phocomelia) of the upper limb and cleft lip/cleft palate.

TABLE 1.4 DISTRIBUTION OF LIMB DEFICIENCIES IN A POPULATION SURVEY AND IN HEREDITABLE DISORDERS

Limb deficiencies	British Columbia survey*			Heritable disorders#		
	Cases*	Fraction (%)	Syndromic$	Total (No.)	Fraction (%)	Syndromic$
All limb deficiencies	6.0	100	53	205	100	80
Amelia	0.15	2.5	61	11	5.4	91
Upper limb	3.4	57	38	66	32	73
Lower limb	1.1	18	20	15	7.3	33
Amniotic bands	0.19	3.2	25	0	0	0
Humerus	0.090	1.5	64	6	2.9	83
Radius	0.92	15.3	54	26	13	96
Ulna	0.074	1.2	33	13	6.3	77
Femur	0.26	4.3	16	9	4.4	89
Tibia	0.07	1.2	25	7	5.4	71
Fibula	0.06	1.1	14	11	3.4	82

*Cases per 10 000 live births compiled from data of Froster and Baird.[131, 147, 148]

#Heritable disorders from OMIM.[147]

$Only cases or disorders with anomalies outside of the limbs are included as syndromes – many had deficiency at several limb sites; recognizable syndromes like Ellis van Creveld were excluded by Froster and Baird, so concurrent anomalies represent unknown syndromes or associations.

TABLE 1.5 SPECTRUM OF ASSOCIATED ANOMALIES IN SYNDROMIC LIMB DEFICIENCIES

Associated anomalies by system	British Columbia survey* (%)	Heritable disorders# (%)
Limb deficiencies	348 cases (100)$	164 disorders (100)$
Craniofacial	28	79
Cardiovascular	18	40
Nervous	14	36
Integumentary	12	26
Genitourinary	20	20

*Cases per 10 000 live births compiled from data of Froster and Baird.[131, 147, 148]
#Heritable disorders from OMIM.[147]
$Only cases or disorders with anomalies outside of the limbs are included as syndromes – many had deficiency at several limb sites; recognizable syndromes like Ellis van Creveld were excluded by Froster and Baird, so concurrent anomalies represent unknown syndromes or associations.

frequencies of associated organ system defects had similar order – craniofacial (28% and 79%), cardiovascular (18% and 40%), etc. – except for genitourinary anomalies (20% in both groups) that likely reflects cases with VATER association in the survey.[147]

Example: Human limb deficiencies – molecular mechanisms for pattern formation

The molecular mechanisms involved in the normal development of limbs in humans are starting to be rather well understood (Figs 1.37 and 1.38). This knowledge explains the patterns of human limb anomalies described above, and should soon allow a molecular approach to the classification and diagnosis of limb malformations.[149] In the near future, i.e. as soon as the molecular cascades are better unraveled for the given systems, such classifications should be available for all congenital anomalies.

The role of the apical-ectodermal ridge (AER) in regulating proximodistal limb development was first revealed by ablation experiments in the chick: removal of the AER from the distal limb bud produced transverse deficiency, more severe with earlier times of AER removal (Fig. 1.37). The proximodistal sequence and longer period of AER extension explains why distal anomalies are more common (Table 1.4). Transplantation experiments also demonstrated a posterior region on each limb bud that governed cephalocaudal differentiation, the zone of polarizing activity (ZPA – Fig. 1.37). Grafting of a second ZPA onto a more cephalic region produced mirror-image duplication, suggesting that it set up a gradient across the limb bud, producing postaxial bones near the ZPA and preaxial bones away. By human analogy, the ZPA would be by the armpit, setting up gradients that produce near ulna-pinkie (posterior, postaxial) and far radius-thumb (anterior, preaxial). Greater

distance of their primordial tissue from the ZPA could explain why preaxial anomalies are more common among human limb deficiencies.[66, 147–149]

Molecular signals have now been associated with these limb organizers (Fig. 1.37). FGFs could substitute for AER when applied to chick limb buds, and their receptors (like FGFR3) are mutated in human skeletal dysplasias (like achondroplasia). Excess or deficiency of exogenous FGF can cause complex duplication/deficiencies of chick limbs, reminiscent of their combinations in human defects (see above). Applications to the ZPA revealed some old friends to this discussion, retinoic acid and SHH protein. Both molecules could produce mirror limbs in chicks, and further experiments showed that retinoic acid induced SHH expression in the limb, equivalently producing a second ZPA. It will be no surprise, when thinking of limb segment differences, to learn that the HOX gene families are involved in limb patterning. Their involvement is complex, but it appears that the HOX-A cluster is active in proximodistal patterning, the HOX-D cluster in anteroposterior differentiation (Fig. 1.38).[149]

Genes discovered through study of human limb defects have joined with those from chick embryologic studies to define sequential steps in human limb patterning. At the DNA level are epigenetic regulators of chromatin conformation and expression, illustrated by the causative genes in Roberts syndrome (Fig. 1.36C). An unusual chromosome finding called premature centromere separation and susceptibility to DNA damaging agents indicate abnormal chromatin structure in this condition, linking this to its severe limb defects. At the transcription level, *SHH* gene deletions at 7q11 cause one form of split hand-split foot anomaly, and its pathway members are implicated by *PTCH1* mutations (basal cell nevus syndrome with short metacarpals) and *GLI3* (Grieg syndrome, Pallister-Hall syndrome, isolated polydactyly). HOX transcription factors are implicated by mutations of synpolydactyly (*HOX-D13*) and hand-foot-uterus syndrome (*HOX-A13*).[150] Other transcription factor motifs like the T-box are found in *TBX3* (Holt-Oram syndrome) and *TBX5* (ulnar mammary syndrome). Proteins mediating limb extension include fibroblast growth factors (acrocephalosyndactylies), collagens (osteogenesis imperfecta – Fig. 1.13), fibrillins (Marfan syndrome), and peroxisomal proteins (chondrodysplasia punctata – Fig. 1.36A).[66]

These same molecular participants can explain several of the limb deficiency associations shown in Table 1.5. Craniofacial associations are highlighted by *FGF* or *GLI3* phenotypes (acrocephalosyndactylies), heart by the *TBX* phenotypes (Holt-Oram), and brain by SHH (holoprosencephaly) or *GLI3* (Pallister-Hall) phenotypes. If these genes are keys, then the sporadic defects of Froster and Baird and thalidomide play a similar tune of limb, craniofacial and cardiac defects.[146–148]

Finally, the ectodermal origin of AER explains limb defects and integumentary system associations, with one form of ectrodactyly-ectodermal dysplasia-clefting syndrome (EEC1) mapped to 7q11 near the *SHH* locus and another (EEC3) caused

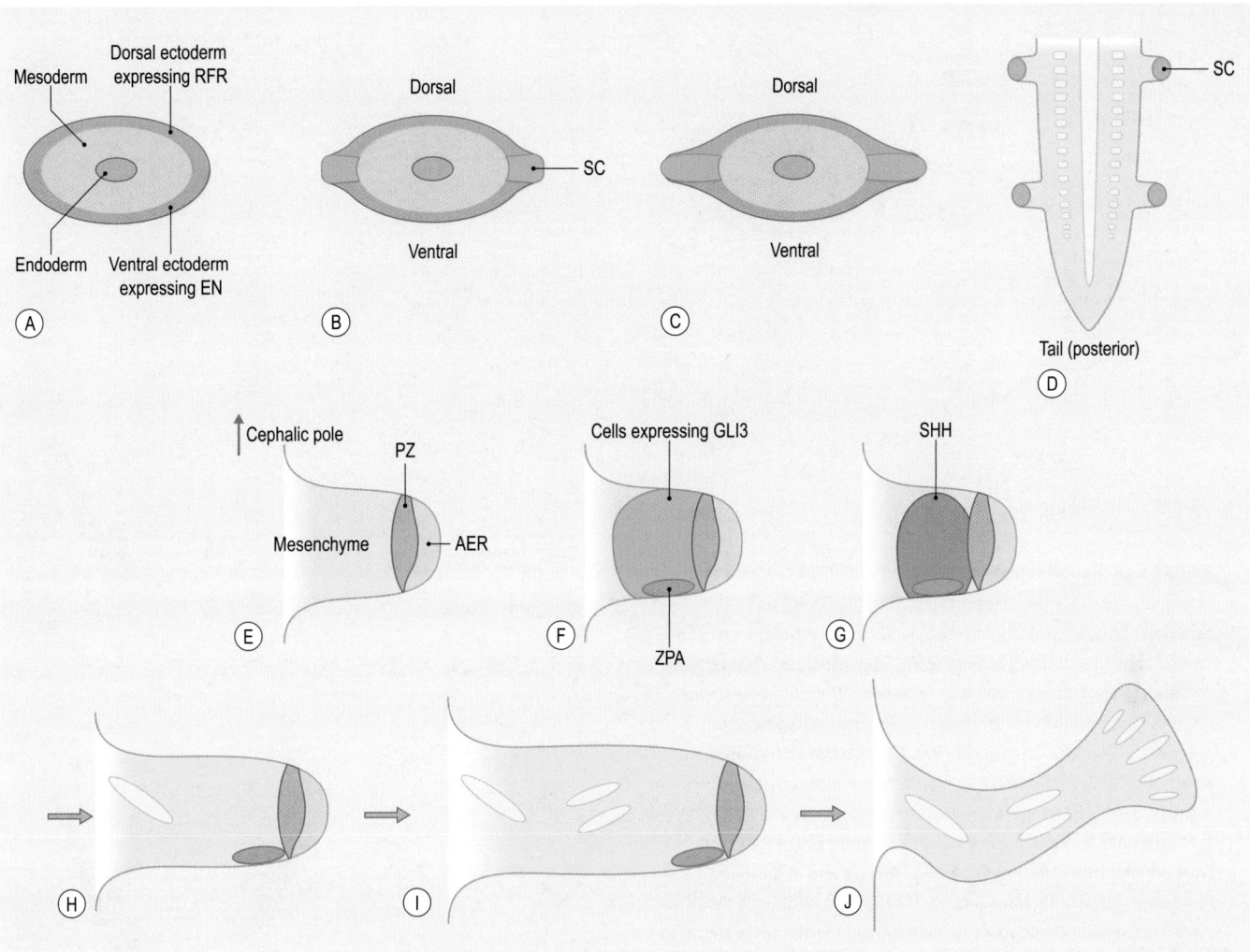

FIGURE 1.37 Normal limb bud development. (A) RFR is expressed in dorsal ectoderm, whereas EN is expressed in the ventral ectoderm, thus establishing dorso–ventral (DV) axis polarity. Note that many other poorly understood genes are involved in DV patterning. (B) The regions of the embryo exposed to both RFR and EN (i.e. the lateral-most portions) are stimulated to express SC. (C) The cells expressing SC proliferate rapidly, causing the limb buds to grow laterally, forming an expansion called the progress zone. (D) Same embryo as in (C), sectioned in the medio-lateral (coronal) plane. (E) The limb becomes segmented in the medio–lateral axis. The distal-most portion is referred to as the apical ectodermal ridge (AER). The cells of the AER stimulate the cells of the proliferating zone to proliferate rapidly, causing the limb to grow laterally. (F) and (G) A group of mesenchymal cells appears in the posterior margin of limb buds, forming the zone of polarizing activity (ZPA). Retinoic acid (RA) stimulates the cells of the ZPA to express *HOX-B8*; *HOX-B8* stimulates these cells to secrete a diffusible morphogen called sonic hedgehog (SHH). On the other hand, *GLI3*, expressed everywhere but in the ZPA, inhibits *SHH* production. The end result is the creation of a SHH concentration gradient along the caudo–cephalic axis. (H) As the limb grows, the mesenchyme furthest from the AER condenses to form the future humerus/femur. (I) and (J) As the PZ extends further laterally, the limb mesenchyme condenses to form the radius-ulna/tibia-fibula and eventually, the phalanges develop under the influence of *HOX-A* and *HOX-D*. [(A) through (J): redrawn from Manouvrier-Hanu et al 1999,[149] with permission.]

by a *P63* gene homologous to the *P53* proto-oncogene. This disorder returns full circle to Figure 1.1 and the dual roles of master-switch genes in development and neoplasia. Involvement of *GLI* in glioblastoma and rhabdomyosarcoma, *PTCH* in basal cell carcinomas, and *HOX* families in leukemias[151] again emphasize the ability of molecular pathways to unify pathologic phenomena.

Future prospects: developmental pathology, genomics, and the second codes

A molecular approach to abnormal growth and development has been summarized. Regulatory processes are now defined from

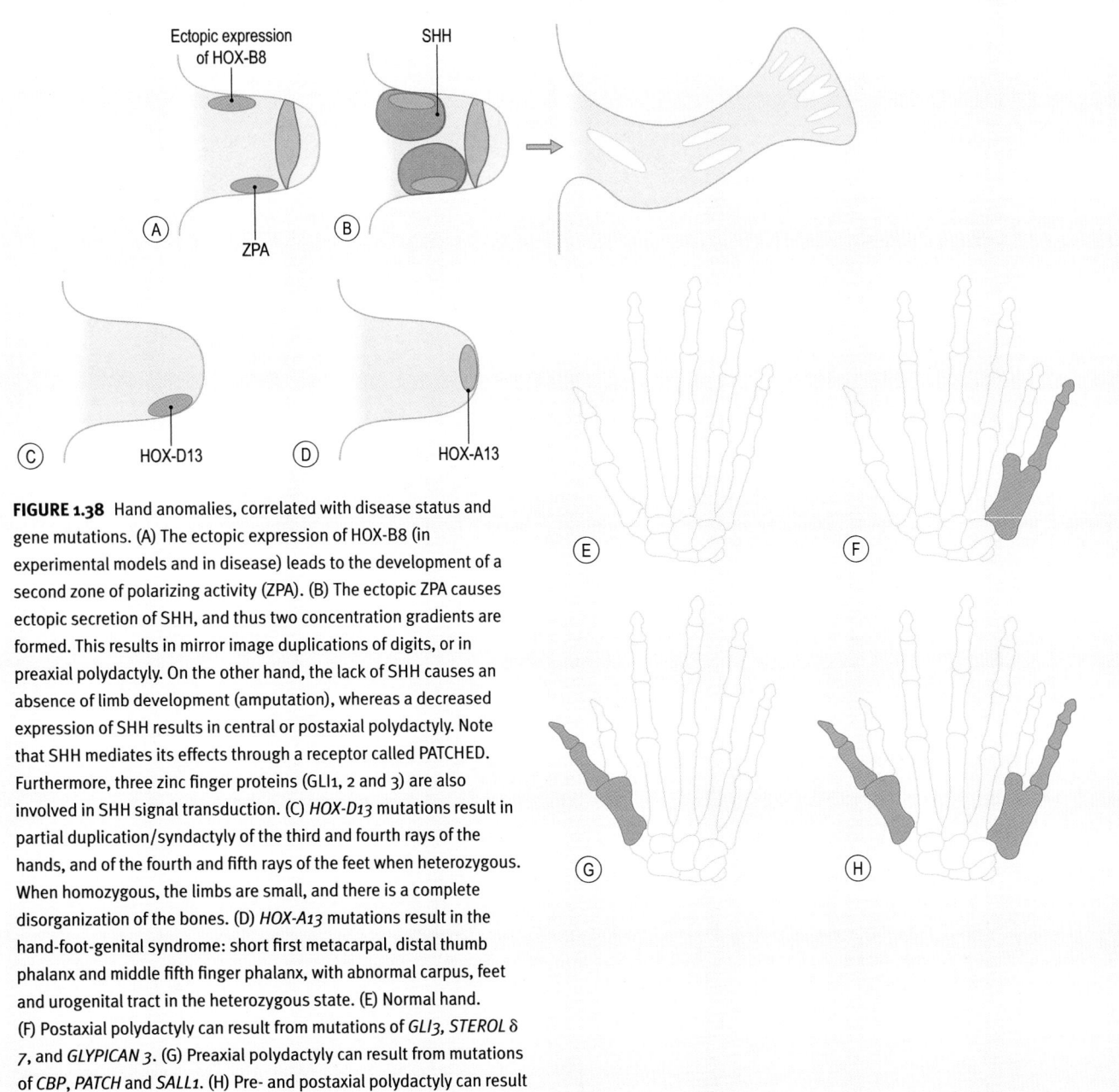

FIGURE 1.38 Hand anomalies, correlated with disease status and gene mutations. (A) The ectopic expression of HOX-B8 (in experimental models and in disease) leads to the development of a second zone of polarizing activity (ZPA). (B) The ectopic ZPA causes ectopic secretion of SHH, and thus two concentration gradients are formed. This results in mirror image duplications of digits, or in preaxial polydactyly. On the other hand, the lack of SHH causes an absence of limb development (amputation), whereas a decreased expression of SHH results in central or postaxial polydactyly. Note that SHH mediates its effects through a receptor called PATCHED. Furthermore, three zinc finger proteins (GLI1, 2 and 3) are also involved in SHH signal transduction. (C) *HOX-D13* mutations result in partial duplication/syndactyly of the third and fourth rays of the hands, and of the fourth and fifth rays of the feet when heterozygous. When homozygous, the limbs are small, and there is a complete disorganization of the bones. (D) *HOX-A13* mutations result in the hand-foot-genital syndrome: short first metacarpal, distal thumb phalanx and middle fifth finger phalanx, with abnormal carpus, feet and urogenital tract in the heterozygous state. (E) Normal hand. (F) Postaxial polydactyly can result from mutations of *GLI3, STEROL δ 7,* and *GLYPICAN 3*. (G) Preaxial polydactyly can result from mutations of *CBP, PATCH* and *SALL1*. (H) Pre- and postaxial polydactyly can result from mutations of *GLI3*.

genome change to epigenesis and expression as second code. Their medical application is dependent on clinical delineation and molecular thinking by physicians. Grouping of anomalies to sequences of gene expression has led to understanding of insect pattern formation and mammalian limb defects; universal roles for such genes are emphasized in Table 1.6. Sometimes chromosomal changes or unusual transmission (parental origin, anticipation) can focus attention on particular loci or inheritance mechanisms; sometimes families with several affected members allow positional focus through linkage studies. Increasingly, the developmental genetics of simpler organisms provide ideas for investigation. When a candidate gene is found, its election as a disease gene can be accomplished by relatively simple techniques. Characterized mutations become known steps in a sequence of genetic change, allowing extension from Mendelian extremes to polygenic defect and environmental modification. Table 1.6 is the beginning in a new science of human development: a science based on molecules rather than on terms borrowed from psychology (e.g. 'fate' or 'potential').[152] The contributions of human syndrome

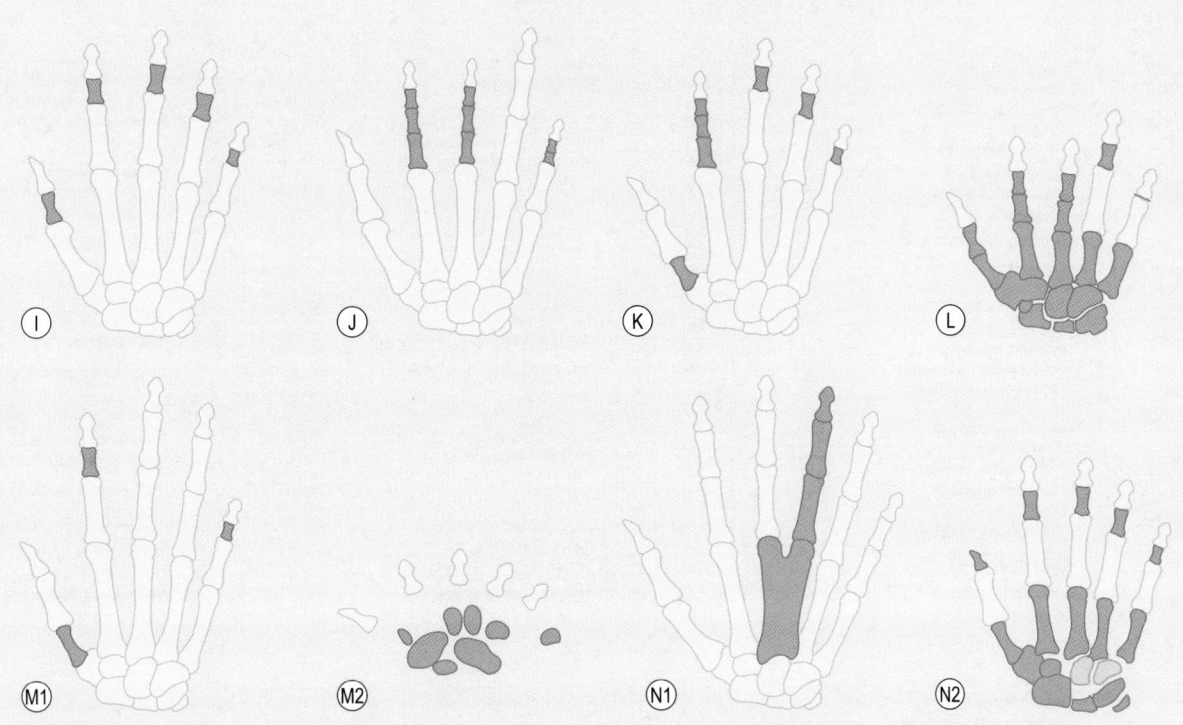

FIGURE 1.38 (*cont'd*) (I) The genes involved in brachydactyly type A1 are unknown. (J) Haw-type brachydactyly type C: note hypersegmented phalanges; genes unknown. (K) CDMP-type brachydactyly type C: *CDMP1* (= growth differentiation factor 5) affects chondrogenesis and joint positioning. (L) Acromesomelic dysplasia, Hunter-Thompson type: in this case, the *CDMP1* mutation results in nine rather than eight abnormally shaped carpal bones, short metacarpal and phalanges, and absent fifth middle phalanx. (M) Grebe syndrome: M1 shows the effect of a heterozygous mutation of *CDMP1*, whereas M2 corresponds to the homozygous mutation of the same gene. In homozygotes, carpal bones are short and fused, metacarpals are rudimentary or absent, only the distal phalanges develop, including a postaxial distal phalanx. (N) Synpolydactyly: N1 shows the mesoaxial polydactyly due to either a *HOX-D13* or a *GLI3* heterozygous mutation. N2, the effects of a homozygous *HOX-D13* mutation are shown: note the abnormally shaped carpal bones, including two supernumerary carpal bones (in blue), and very short carpal-like metacarpals. [(A) through (G) and (I) to (N) redrawn from Manouvrier-Hanu et al 1999,[149] with permission.]

TABLE 1.6 GENE HOMOLOGY IN ANIMAL DEVELOPMENT

Gene	Discovery	Mouse phenotype	Human phenotype	Mechanisms
VG1	*Xenopus* pattern formation			Axis formation
WNT1	*Drosophila* segmentation	Mouse breast tumor	Cerebellar hypoplasia	Signal transduction (axis duplication)
PAX 3	*Drosophila* segmentation	Splotch	Waardenburg Sx.	Signal transduction
PAX 6	Drosophila segmentation	Small eye	Aniridia	Transcription factor
HOX	*Drosophila* segmentation	Segmentation defects	Segmentation defects	Transcription factor
WT1	Human tumor (Wilms)	Tumors, urogenital defects	Tumors, urogenital defects	Transcription factor
KIT	Feline sarcoma virus	Dominant spotted	Piebald trait	Signal transduction
GLI	*Drosophila* segmentation	Extra toes	Greig syndrome	Transcription factor (human glioma)
LIS1	Miller-Dieker syndrome		Lissencephaly	Signal transduction
NF1	Neurofibromatosis		Neurofibromas	Signal transduction
KAL1	Kallmann syndrome		Olfactory, genital	Chemotactic and growth factor
L1CAM	Human birth defects		Hydrocephalus, MASA syndrome	Cell adhesion
CCRL	Human birth defects		Lowe syndrome	Signal transduction
ATP7A	Human birth defects	Mottled	Menkes syndrome	Transport (ATPase)

MASA, Mental retardation, aphasia, shuffling gait, adducted thumbs.
See OMIM 2006,[4] and listed references[10, 68]

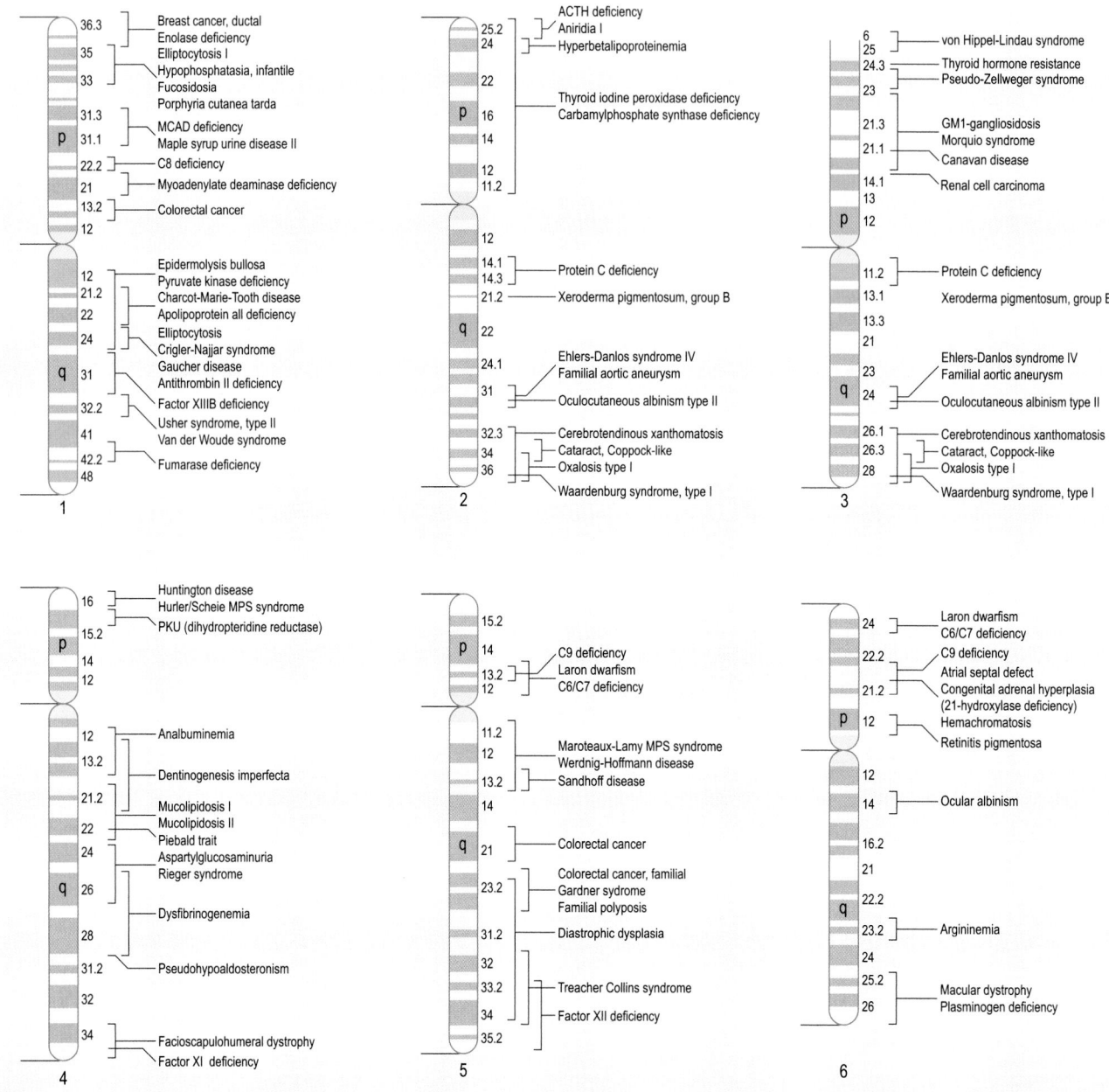

FIGURE 1.39 The human genome map. Selected loci relevant to growth, development and cancer are shown, particularly those discussed in this chapter. Because cancer and single birth defects are multifactorial disorders, designated loci are for susceptibility rather than simple Mendelian inheritance. The complete human genome map can be accessed at Entrez Genome (http://www.ncbi.nlm.nih.gov/entrez/query.fcgi?db=Genome) and other academic sites.

delineation and phenotype–genotype correlation in this new science should not be forgotten.

An extensive human gene map and complete genome sequence is now available for guidance of developmental studies (Fig. 1.39). The synergy of analytic and recombinant technology promises to accelerate this exploration, with the sequences and

expression profiles of entire chromosomes now known. Complete genome sequences have been tabulated for many organisms, and the expression profiles and proteomes of many tissue, differentiation, or temporal states are known. For yeast, a systems biology approach has identified all major protein–protein interactions. A library of genetic, epigenetic, and gene product information is now available for scholars to peruse for new meaning. These repositories are also toolboxes for working on clinical problems. Though this explosion of molecular information can have tremendous application to fetal pathology, clinical and autopsy studies remain underfunded and underappreciated. Perhaps the very majesty of molecular information will stimulate interest in morphologic characterization, for this elegant physique will soon be embarrassed by shabby clothes. If the exigencies of clinical correlation revitalize morphologic studies, then the rewards for fetal pathology and developmental biology will be rich indeed.

Acknowledgements

Dr Oligny: Many students and colleagues have given their time to read portions of this manuscript critically. They offered suggestions to make it clearer, and corrected some errors which had eluded me. I thank them all. Special thanks must go to Karine Jacob, for insightful suggestions.

Dedications

Dr Wilson: This chapter is dedicated to the pediatric geneticists and pathologists whose clinical skills made it possible.
Dr Oligny: This chapter is dedicated to my mentors, Drs Tom Seemayer, Glenn Taylor, Jim Dimmick and Dagmar Kalousek, and to the Society for Pediatric Pathology, for ongoing support.

Glossary of genetic and developmental terms

These brief definitions should be supplemented by consulting general references as listed.

Acrocentric chromosome: Chromosome with very small short (p) arms (13, 14, 15, 21, 22) as opposed to metacentric chromosomes with approximately equal short and long (q) arms.

Allele: Alternative gene structure, e.g. S and A alleles of the β-globin gene.

Anonymous DNA probe: Randomly cloned DNA segment used for hybridization.

Anticipation: Worsening of phenotype with subsequent generations.

Alternative splicing: Some RNAs possess various splicing codes, which can be interpreted differently by the splicing machinery. Hence, one gene can generate more than one mRNA, i.e. more than one protein.

Apoptosis: the genetically programmed death of a cell. It is characterized by the intracytoplasmic and intranuclear activation of an enzymatic cascade which digests the cell from inside-out. It results in cellular 'dropout' without an associated inflammatory reaction.

ASOs: Allele-specific oligonucleotides used to detect various alleles of a gene, in DNA diagnosis.

Autoradiogram: Detection of radioactivity using X-ray film.

Base pairs (bp): Adenine–thymine (A–T) or guanine–cytosine (G–C) pairing in DNA; also the basic unit for DNA strand length.

Candidate gene: Gene implicated in pathogenesis based on protein function, chromosomal location, or sequence homology.

Carrier frequency: Population frequency of carriers, estimated for autosomal recessive disease by the Hardy-Weinberg law.

c DNA: See complementary DNA.

Centimorgan: Unit of genetic mapping equal to 1% meiotic recombination.

Central dogma: Universal pathway for gene expression from DNA to RNA to protein.

Chain-terminating mutation: Change of one codon normally coding for an amino acid to one of the three codons which signal for termination.

Chromation: DNA with its associated proteins and various other molecules. See *Euchromatin.*

Chromosomal rearrangements: Aberration where chromosomes are broken and rejoined as opposed to numerical excess or deficiency.

Chromosome painting: Use of repetitive DNA FISH probes to fluoresce entire chromosomes or chromosome regions.

Codon: Three base pairs encoding an amino acid or termination signal.

Complementary DNA (cDNA): DNA synthesized from mature mRNA using viral reverse transcriptase; cDNA will have no intronic sequences.

Complementary strands: Partner strands in the DNA double helix, able to reunite (hybridize) when separated by matching A–T, G–C base pairs.

Confined placental mosaicism: Different karyotype in placenta as opposed to other fetal tissues.

Contig: Overlapping array of DNA fragments.

Contiguous gene deletions: Deletion encompassing neighboring genes to produce a composite phenotype.

CpG islands: CpG (or CG) are cytosine–guanine dinucleotides that can be modified by DNA methyltransferases; methylated CpGs occur non-randomly in clusters or islands within the genome.

Cross-over: Breakage and reunion of chromosomes that realign parental loci during meiosis.

Cytogenetic notation: Formal nomenclature describing karyotypes and chromosome location, e.g.:

47,XY,+11: Extra copy of chromosome 11 (trisomy 11)

45,XY,-11: Loss of one copy of chromosome 11 (monosomy 11)

46,XY,11q-: Deletion of a segment of unspecified length, up to the telomere, on the long arm of one chromosome 11 (the other chromosome 11 of that pair is normal)

46,XY,11q+: Extra material of unknown origin on the terminal portion of one of the long arm of chromosome 11

46,XY,del(11)(p11p13): Interstitial deletion between bands p11 and p13 of the short arm of one chromosome 11

46,XY,dup(3q): Duplication of a segment of the long arm of chromosome 3 onto that long arm.

Determination: A blast becomes determined when it is still morphologically blastic but its molecular characteristics are altered so that one or both of its daughter cells are forced to produce more differentiated cells. These daughter cells are already programmed to become one cell type or another. For example, a primitive myeloblast looks like any other hemopoietic blast, but can only produce other myeloblasts or more differentiated myeloid cells.

Differentiation: The phenotypic expression of molecular changes following determination. One must remember that 'phenotypic' has a different connotation for different specialties. For example, a 'myeloblast' will appear totally undifferentiated using a Giemsa stain at ? 40, but may show granules (i.e. signs of differentiation) under oil immersion. Furthermore, even if no sign of differentiation can be seen at this magnification, an immunophenotype through flow cytometry will allow distinction from a lymphoblast. Molecular techniques allow an even finer 'phenotypic' distinction. Hence, 'differentiation' does not have the same meaning for everyone, and this must be kept in mind.

DNA chip: Hundreds to thousands of cDNAs or oligonucleotides which can hybridize to alleles or genes of interest are spotted onto a slide, each with its own address within this matrix (or array). Such arrays can then be hybridized either with DNA, RNA or cDNA from cells of interest (e.g. a primordial embryonic limb bud or a cancer cell), to see which genes are lost/duplicated, or to quantify their expression.

DNA cloning: Isolation of a DNA segment by insertion into a simple genome (plasmid, bacteriophage or YAC – yeast artificial chromosome) and production of multiple copies.

DNA diagnostic techniques: Use of DNA-modifying enzymes, hybridization, and size separation technologies for diagnosis of identity, genetic disease, or predisposition.

DNA hybridization: Rejoining (reannealing) of complementary DNA or RNA stands.

DNA marker: DNA segment, often anonymous, that exhibits sufficient sequence variation to be useful in genetic linkage and DNA diagnosis.

DNA sequence: Order of nucleotides in a DNA segment, usually displayed from the 5′-triphosphate (5′end) to the 3′-hydroxyl (3′ end) nucleotides.

DNA sequence polymorphism: Variation in nucleotide sequence at a locus; allele frequencies greater than 1% and phenotypic neutrality are usually implied.

Domains: Functional amino acid sequence regions within a protein that often correspond with exons in genomic DNA (i.e. leader or transmembrane domains).

Drosphilia: Fruit fly, an extensively studied organism is classical and molecular genetics.

DXS14: Standard nomenclature for anonymous DNA fragments whereby D = DNA, X = chromosome of origin, S, Z = single or multiple copies in genome, 14 = number based on order of isolation (E may be appended for expressed fragments).

Empiric risks: Recurrence risk based on epidemiologic survey of affected families.

Epigenesis: Heritable changes in gene function that do not alter the DNA coding sequence. Epigenetic mechanisms include changes in chromatin structure, cytosine methylation, histone modification, or protein binding (e.g. Polycomb/Trithorax binding to chromatin). Epigenetic changes activate or inhibit gene transcription, and are faithfully transmitted from a cell to all its descendants.

Euchromatin: Cytologically, euchromatin is the genetically active unstained DNA, in contrast to heterochromatin. In cytogenetics, euchromatin appears as light bands in trypsinized Giemsa-stained metaphases, euchromatin has a propersity to be more genetically active than the DNA on the dark bands of heterochromatin, but this rule is not absolute (e.g. in routine G-banded karyotypes, the active and inactive X chromosomes in women have identical morphology). In molecular biology, euchromatin refers to an open-state chromatin which allows transcription and cleavage by nucleases, whereas heterochromatin in inactive as it is too tightly condensed to allows to access to transcription factors nor to nucleases.

Exon: Portion of gene that encodes protein.

First-degree relative: Those with 50% of genes in common (child, parent, siblings).

FISH: Fluorescent in situ hybridization, a technique by which fluorochromes are attached to DNA probes and hybridized with cytogenetic or cell preparations.

Frame: Reading frame by which a DNA sequence encodes amino acids.

Frameshift: Mutations that alter the reading frame by deleting/adding nucleotides.

Functional cloning: Isolation of gene segments based on gene function, i.e. using antibodies to a characterized protein or expression assays where traits are deleted or restored to cultured cells.

Gene map: Order of genes within a chromosome or entire genome.

Gene notation: By convention in molecular biology, genes are referred to by italics, whereas proteins are designated by a standard case. Furthermore, human genes and proteins are written in large case, non-human vertebrate genes and proteins are written with the first letter in uppercase, and invertebrate genes and proteins are referred to in small case. To refer specifically to the gene or protein of a given species, one may use the first letter of that species as the first letter of the gene or protein. Therefore, 'hox' refers to the hox gene found in an invertebrate (such as *Drosophila* or C. elegans), Hox to the hox protein of a vertebrate, Mhox (or mHox) to the Hox protein of the mouse and HOX to the human hox gene. This nomenclature will be used throughout this text, although it is not adopted by all authors or journals.

Genetic heterogeneity: Multiple loci/genes can produce a similar phenotype when mutated, such as autosomal dominant or X-linked Charcot-Marie-Tooth disease.

Genetic mapping: Use of genetic linkage to determine the position and distance of genes with respect to one another, based on recombination distances (centimorgans = approximately 1 megabase).

Genome: Complete set of genes (DNA) in an organism.

Genomic DNA: DNA isolated from an organism or tissue, containing transcription signals (e.g. promoters, enhancers, silencers) and introns that will be absent from cDNA.

Genomic imprinting: See parental imprinting.

Genomics: Study of function and disease based on gene structure and organization.

Genotype: Genetic constitution, often with reference to particular alleles at a locus.

Germinal mosaicism: Mosaicism within the germline, whereby a fraction of eggs or sperm may contain a particular mutation or chromosomal aberration.

GLI: Gene family discovered in human gliomas that has homology to the *Drosophila* segmentation gene krüppel.

Haploinsufficiency: There is haploinsufficiency when the loss of half of the normal activity of a protein causes disease; these mutations are thus manifest in the heterozygous state, but often show reduced penetrance and variable expressivity as the residual normal allele may be more or less active, and the upstream and downstream cascades may be more or less efficient (e.g. due to polymorphisms). Diseases of haploinsufficiency have been reported with mutations involving genes encoding certain transcription factors, structural proteins and cell surface receptors. The malformations tend to be much more severe when these mutations are present in the homozygous state.

Heterochromatin: See euchromatin.

Heteroplasmy: Different mitochondrial genomes in the same cell, a mechanism by which the proportions of altered mitochondria may increase in specific tissues to cause disease.

Heterozygote: Individual with different alleles at a locus.

Histones: Proteins associated with DNA within the nucleus, to allow compaction and the control of transcription.

Homeobox: DNA sequence shared by numerous segmentation genes, characterized by an extremely conserved sequence of 180 nucleotides/60 amino acids (see *HOX*).

Homeotic mutations: Mutations altering segment identity in *Drosophila*. In a broader sense, a developmental switch analogous to that replacing one homologous insect segment with another.

HOX, Hox: Gene clusters in humans and mice that exhibit homology to the structure and expression of *Drosophila* homeotic loci. HOX genes all belong to the homebox family, but only those arranged on a cluster which controls their timing and their site of expression are designated as HOX.

Hybridization: Recognition and pairing of two single-stranded DNA (ssDNA) segments or of one ssDNA segment with its complementary RNA strand.

IGF: Insulin-like growth factor.

Incomplete penetrance: Absence of phenotypic expression in a person known from a pedigree to have an abnormal genotype.

Induction: During embryogenesis, certain tissues influence the behavior and development (e.g. differentiation, migration, apoptosis, etc.) of adjacent tissues. One says that they induce that response. From this, it is evident that cells communicate, one with another.

Insulators: DNA sequences which functionally separate large segments of DNA, each containing many genes. Insulators allow each of these segments to be activated or repressed 'en bloc', so that the genes which they contain can all be expressed or repressed as a single unit.

Interstitial deletions: Chromosomal deletion removing regions between termini.

Introns: Non-coding intervening sequences between coding regions of genomic DNA.

Isochromosomes: Duplicate long or short chromosome arms that result in segmental trisomies and monosomies – e.g. Turner syndrome patients with i(Xq) are monosomic for Xp and trisomic for Xq.

Junk DNA: DNA that has no known coding or regulatory function; note the difference between junk (collected and treasured) as opposed to garbage.

Kilobases (kb): Unit of DNA/RNA length = 1000 bp; megabase = 1 million bp.

Knock-in and *knock-out:* The stem cells of mice can be manipulated by adding or removing a gene of interest, resulting respectively in a knock-in and in a knock-out mouse. Knock-ins may include the insertion of a 'reporter gene' such as 'green fluorescent protein' which allows the determination of when and where a gene is active in the developing embryo. Such constructs have proven extremely powerful in the elucidation of patterns of gene expression and function during mammalian embryogenesis.

L1CAM: L1 cell adhesion molecule implicated in X-linked hydrocephalus.

Linkage: Tendency for neighboring genes to segregate together in families.

Linkage maps: See genetic maps.

Locus (pl. *Loci*): Unique location on a chromosome, generally used to designate the position of a gene and its alleles.

Master switch gene: Genes that code for a transcription factor (e.g. MYO-D) which can by itself cause a cell (e.g. a primitive myoblast) to activate a battery of genes necessary to initiate differentiation along one path (e.g. actin, desmin), and also inactivate some of the genes which are not required for that path's function (e.g. factor VIII).

Maternal effect: Increased severity in offspring of affected mothers as compared with those of affected fathers.

Maternal effect mutations: Mutations of genes encoding maternal molecules that are present in egg cytoplasm.

Maternal inheritance: Inheritance mechanisms that exhibit maternal transmission based on abnormal mitochondria or maternal RNAs.

Maternal RNAs: RNAs in the egg cytoplasm (e.g. mRNA, ribosomal RNA) that accomplish protein synthesis before activation of the zygotic genome.

Meiosis: Process of germ cell division that randomly allots one chromosome of each pair to gametes.

Mendelian inheritance: Classic autosomal dominant, autosomal recessive and X-linked inheritance mechanisms derived from Mendel's observations in peas.

Microdeletions: Chromosome deletions requiring prometaphase banding or FISH for visualization.

Mitosis: Process of somatic cell division that produces identical genomes in daughter cells.

Morphogen: A substance which, in a concentration-dependent manner, determines the future identity of a cell. Morphogens can act within a cell (e.g. transcription factors) or between cells (e.g. cell signaling molecules, such as SHH and retinoic acid).

Mosaicism: Variation in DNA sequence or chromosome constitution among different cells of an organism.

Multifactorial inheritance: Dependence of traits on multiple genes plus the environment.

Multipoint linkage: Linkage analysis that examines multiple traits or markers in a pedigree and orders them relative to one another.

Murine: Referring to mice (*Mus musculus*).

Nitrocellulose membranes: Paper used to bind DNA (Southern), RNA (Northern), or protein (Western) during capillary transfer (blotting) from gels.

Nucleosome: The human genome of 3×10^9 base pairs per cell is longer than one meter when unraveled; however, it is compacted in a nucleus only 10 μm in diameter. This feat is achieved partly through wrapping DNA around special proteins called histones. A nucleosome comprises this protein core and the segment of DNA between two histone cores. The DNA segment contained in a nucleosome is wrapped twice around each histone core and there are generally between 180 and 200 nucleotides between each histone core (i.e. within each nucleosome).

Nucleotide substitutions: Mutations substituting one nucleotide for another.

Nylon membranes: Similar to nitrocellulose but with amino groups for stronger binding.

Obligate carrier: Carrier deduced by pedigree structure.

Oligonucleotide: Short nucleotide sequence often obtained by chemical synthesis.

Oncogene: A gene which encodes for a protein which stimulates a cell to proliferate in an abnormal fashion. Oncogenes can be transmitted to a cell by a virus containing an oncogene, but in humans, oncogenes usually arise from mutations activating a proto-oncogene into an oncogene. Proto-oncogenes are genes which stimulate embryonal (and adult) cell proliferation in a very precise fashion, contrary to anti-oncogenes (also called tumor suppressor genes) which inhibit this proliferation. The equilibrium between the expression of proto-oncogenes and anti-oncogenes at the cell and tissue levels determines their mitotic activity.

Open reading frame: DNA sequence with no termination codons in a particular reading frame.

Paired box: DNA sequence motif found in the *paired* gene of the fruit fly (see PAX).

Parental (genomic) imprinting: A gene is said to be imprinted when the allele received from one parent is transcribed more or less than that received from the other parent. A 'partial paternal imprint' means that the paternal allele of that gene is silenced relative to the maternal allele. Similarly, a gene with a 'complete maternal imprint' shows a complete inhibition of its maternal allele. Parental imprints can be manifested in only some tissues or in all cells of the body, and they can be complete or partial, depending on the gene involved.

Pattern formation: Specification of cell, tissue, or organ arrangement.

PAX: Family of nine developmental genes conserved across all species, which contain *paired* boxes.

pc: Post conception, i.e. from the time of fertilization of the zygote. Not to be confused with Pc which denotes Polycomb proteins.

PCR: Polymerase chain reaction by which individual gene segments are amplified through sequential cycles of polymerization, heat denaturation, and reannealing.

Phase: Arrangement of alleles on parental chromosomes; e.g. A NP/B np (i.e. the presence of the blood-group allele. A linked to the normal allele for nail patelle syndrome on one chromosome, the other chromosome having the allele B linked to the mutated np allele) rather than A np/B NP in a parent with nail-patella syndrome. Determination of the phase of a mutated allele with its linked allele is essential for prenatal counselling.

Phenotype: Individual traits or characters.

Physical mapping: Gene order based on actual physical measurements in terms of chromosome bands or DNA base pairs.

Plasmalogen: Type of glyceroetherlipid abundant in myelin.

Plication: Folding of the embryo, from a flat to a tubular structure.

PMaPs: Peroxisomal matrix proteins such as catalase or urate oxidase.

PMPs: Peroxisomal integral membrane proteins.

Point mutations: Nucleotide substitutions.

Poly A region: 3′-Terminal string of adenines added to mRNA during processing and thought to regulate cytoplasmic transport and/or stability.

Polymorphism: Multiple alleles at a locus, producing amino acid or DNA sequence variation.

Polypeptide chains: Proteins or, in the case of multiple subunits, components of proteins formed by peptide bonds between amino acids.

Positional cloning: Isolation of gene segments based on chromosome location.

Primary relative: First-degree relative, i.e. those sharing 50% of genes.

Primer: Oligonucleotide used to begin nucleic acid polymerization at a particular site on a DNA strand, e.g. with PCR or reverse transcriptase.

Proband: Individual bringing family to attention, affected or not, indicated by arrow in pedigrees.

Prometaphase analysis: Karyotype prepared from synchronized cells arrested in early prophase to optimize the number of bands that can be visualized and thus analyzed; largely supplanted by FISH.

Propositus: Same as proband.

Protein polymorphism: Products of alternate alleles at a locus exemplified by the ABO or HLA systems.

Quantitative traits: Incremental phenotypes such as height or blood pressure.

Recombinant DNA: Chimeric DNA molecules produced by joining of segments from different species, often using the complementary 'sticky ends' produced by restriction endonucleases.

Recombination: Breakage and reunion of DNA strands.

Repetitive DNA: DNA sequences that have multiple copies in a genome.

Restriction endonuclease: Bacterial enzyme designed for defense against bacteriophage that recognizes and cleaves at specific nucleotide sequences.

Reporter genes: Genes which are included in a knock-in construct, and which can be readily identified when the knocked-in gene is activated. Such genes include green fluorescent protein (GFP), which fluoresces when exposed to ultraviolet light, and the firefly luciferase gene, which spontaneously emits visible light without harming the cells expressing it.

Reverse genetics: Genetic analysis proceeding from chromosomal location to cloned gene; *positional cloning* is now the preferred term.

Reverse transcriptase: Enzyme isolated from retroviruses that synthesizes a DNA copy (cDNA) from mRNA using a 3′-primer (e.g. oligo dT complementary to the polyA tail).

RFLPs: Restriction fragment length polymorphisms, appearing as alleles of different sizes when DNA is cut with restriction enzymes. May result from alterations of the sequence cleaved by the restriction enzyme, or more commonly, by variable numbers of repeats within the DNA fragment.

Ribozymes: Protein-free RNAs with intrinsic enzymatic activity.

RNA splicing: Genes are made of a DNA segment which codes for a linear homologous segment or RNA. This RNA contains protein-coding segments called exons, separated from each other by intervening segments of non-coding RNA called introns. Introns need to be spliced out of the RNA, and each exon must be fused with its 3′ immediate exonic neighbor to make mRNA. Indentical segments of RNA can be spliced in different fashions (alternative splicing) to make different mRNAs which will code for different proteins. Hence, one gene can code for up to thousands of proteins.

Robertsonian translocations: Joining of two chromosomes of a pair to produce a single recombined chromosome comprised of either two short or two long arms.

Selector gene: See master switch gene.

Sense strand: Strand of DNA that encodes a protein product, as opposed to the complementary anti-sense strand.

Single nucleotide polymorphism: See SNP.

SNP: Single nucleotide polymorphism, a single base pair difference in DNA sequence. Once characterized, multiple SNPs can be analyzed by PCR and DNA sequencing; SNPs occur every 300–600 bp in humans and provide abundant DNA markers for linkage and disease association/ susceptibility studies.

Snurps: Small nuclear ribonucleoproteins involved in RNA splicing.

Somatic mosaicism: Variation in DNA sequence or karyotype among different somatic cells of an organism.

Southern blots: Technique for capillary transfer of DNA to membranes devised by Southern; Northern (RNA) and Western (protein) blots are puns on Southern's name.

Splice junction: Exon-intron junctions that join sequentially to eliminate introns.

Spliceosome: The complex of RNAs and proteins that accomplishes RNA splicing.

Splicing: See RNA splicing and alternative splicing.

Sporadic: Isolated case, often implying lack of inheritance or genetic causation.

SSCP: Single-strand conformational polymorphism, resulting in sequence-dependent electrophoretic migration of DNA sequences to differentiate between alleles as their tertiary structure is altered, causing them to migrate differently even when of identical size and differing by only one base pair.

Stringency: The ionic strength and temperature conditions employed for nucleic acid hybridization that determines the specificity of probes for target sequences. Hybridization in conditions of high stringency occurs only when complementary strands match perfectly or are unmatched only at one or very few base pairs.

STS: Sequence-tagged site, a site of known DNA sequence that can be amplified using PCR to show its presence in a given cloned segment.

Submicroscopic deletion: Small chromosome deletions that can be visualized only by DNA analysis.

Syndrome variability or expressivity: Differing phenotypic manifestations among individuals with the same syndrome.

Targeting sequences: Amino acid regions that direct proteins to particular cellular locations.

TATA box: DNA segment rich in thymine and adenine, allowing initiation of transcription.

Termination signals: Three different DNA trinucleotides (codons) act as stop or termination signals, to indicate to the transcription machinery that RNA synthesis must stop at that point.

Transgenic organism: A genetically manipulated organism which contains genes derived from another species. Bacteria, yeasts and knocked-in mice are common transgenics.

Threshold: Theoretical barrier at which an individual's combination of genes and environmental exposure crosses from predisposition to actual defect.

Tm (melting temperature): Temperature that separates or 'melts' a double-strand nucleic acid.

Topogenesis: Genesis of topology or pattern – targeting for proteins, pattern formation for cells and tissues.

Transcription factors: Molecules (proteins, RNA and other molecules such as retinoic acid) which bind DNA directly to activate or inhibit the expression of gene(s) under their control. This action is generally through a direct interaction with the promoter/enhancer/silencer regions of those genes. By extension, molecules which activate or inhibit transcription by binding proteins bound to DNA are also called transcription factors.

Transitions: Purine-purine or pyrimidine-pyrimidine nucleic acid substitutions (adenine and guanine are purines, cytosine, thymine and uracil are pyrimidines).

Translocation breakpoint: Region of recombination between two chromosomes.

Translocation carriers: Individuals with 'balanced' translocations that have no extra or missing chromosome material, thus yielding no phenotypic anomaly.

Transversions: Purine-pyrimidine or pyrimidine-purine nucleic acid substitutions (adenine and guanine are purines, cytosine, thymine and uracil are pyrimidines).

Triplet repeat amplification: Increased number of tandemly repeating 3-bp units that can alter gene expression, as in fragile X syndrome, and myotonic dystrophy, or that can alter its protein protein function, as in Huntington disease.

Trisomies/monosomies: Cells or tissues with extra or missing entire chromosomes.

Uninformative: Genetic linkage study in which parental alleles, and therefore the risk for disease transmission, cannot be distinguished.

Uniparental disomy: Two copies of a chromosome pair derived from one parent.

Uniparental heterodisomy: Both chromosomes of a single parent are represented.

Uniparental isodisomy: Two identical copies of the same parental chromosome are represented.

Variable expressivity: Variable phenotypes among affected individuals in a family (i.e. in individuals with identical mutations).

VNTRs: Variable number of tandem repeats, a type of DNA polymorphism where alleles differ in size due to differences in their number of tandemly repeated units. VNTRs have no phenotypic or pathologic impact, but are extremely useful in molecular diagnosis as they yield RFLPs.

YACs: See yeast artificial chromosomes.

Yeast artificial chromosomes: Recombinant DNA molecules that contain yeast centromeric and telomeric sequences, allowing cloning of large DNA segments via replication as yeast chromosomes.

Zoo blots: Southern or Northern blots comparing multiple species to assess phylogenetic conservation of a particular gene segment.

Zygotic expression: Synthesis of gene products from zygotic DNA rather than maternal RNA molecules.

References

NOTE: Commentary accompanies references recommended for general background or key points.

Role of genetics in developmental pathology

1. Needham J. A history of embryology. New York: Arno Press; 1975. Reprint of 1959 edn.
2. Lengauer C. An unstable liaison. Science 2003; 300:442–443.
3. Kinzler KW, Vogelstein B. Familial cancer syndromes: the role of caretakers and gatekeepers. In: Scriver CR, Beaudet AL, Sly WS et al, eds. The metabolic & molecular bases of inherited disease. 8th edn. New York: McGraw-Hill; 2001:675–677.
4. McKusick VA. Mendelian inheritance in man. 11th edn. Baltimore: The Johns Hopkins University Press; 1994. This legendary catalogue of genetic diseases is now accessible by web as Online Mendelian Inheritance in Man (OMIM): www.ncbi.nlm.nih.gov/entrez/. It is the Human Genome Organization's (HUGO) official catalogue, and can be searched by eponym, disorder, or key findings (e.g. it will retrieve all the syndromes combining polydactyly and imperforate anus).
5. Wilson GN. Genomics of human dysmorphogenesis. Am J Med Genet 1992; 42:187–196. Numbers from 2005 update, in preparation.
6. Levsky JM, Shenoy SM, Pezo RC, et al. Single-cell gene expression profiling. Science 2002; 297:836–840. The authors provide a platform for the fusion of genomics and cell biology: 'cellular genomics'.
7. Pang S, Pollack MS, Marshall RN, et al. Prenatal treatment of congenital adrenal hyperplasia due to 21-hydroxylase deficiency. N Engl J Med 1990; 322:111–115.
8. Wilson GN, Richards CS, Katz K, et al. Nonspecific X-linked mental retardation with aphasia exhibiting genetic linkage to chromosomal region Xp11. J Med Genet 1992; 29:629–633.
9. Goelz SE, Hamilton SR, Vogelstein B. Purification of DNA from formaldehyde fixed and paraffin embedded human tissue. Biochem Biophys Res Commun 1985; 130:118–126.

Basic genetics

10. Scriver CR, Beaudet AL, Sly WS et al, eds. The metabolic & molecular bases of inherited disease, 8th edn. New York: McGraw-Hill; 2001. Multi-authored by disease experts with comprehensive discussion of molecular pathogenesis.
11. Kumar V, Abbas AK, Fausto, eds. Robbins and Cotran pathologic basis of disease. 7th edn. Philadelphia: Elsevier Saunders; 2005. Multi-authored and superbly illustrated with CD-ROM and website links.
12. Carter CO. Genetics of common disorders. Br Med Bull 1969; 25:52–57.
13. Fraser FC. The multifactorial threshold concept – uses and misuses. Teratology 1976; 14:267–280.

14. Schinzel A. Catalogue of unbalanced chromosome aberrations in man. 2nd edn. New York: de Gruyter; 2001.
15. Wyandt HE, Tonk VS, eds. Atlas of human chromosome heteromorphisms. Dordrecht: Kluwer Academic; 2004.

Molecular medicine and the language of DNA

16. Hood L, Heath JR, Phelps ME, et al. Systems biology and new technologies enable predictive and preventative medicine. Science 2004; 306:640–643. Part of a section on new genome-scale technologies for gene expression and regulation.
17. Beaudet AL, Scriver CR, Sly WS, et al. Introduction to human molecular and biochemical genetics. New York: McGraw-Hill; 1990:10.
18. Darnell JE Jr. Variety in the level of gene control in eukaryotic cells. Nature 1982; 297:1818–1819.
19. Bélanger H, Beaulieu P, Moreau C, et al. Functional promoter SNPs in cell cycle checkpoint genes. Hum Mol Genet 2005; 14:2641–2648.
20. Sebat J, Lakshmi B, Alexander J, et al. Large-scale copy number polymorphism in the human genome. Science 2004; 305:525–528.
21. Volpe TA, Kidner C, Hall IM, et al. Regulation of heterochromatic silencing and histone H3 lysine-9 methylation by RNAi. Science 2002; 297:1833–1837.
22. Allshire R. RNAi and heterochromatin – a hushed up affair. Science 2002; 297:1818–1819.
23. Bird A. DNA methylation patterns and epigenetic memory. Genes Dev 2002; 16:6–21.
24. Jones PA, Takai D. The role of DNA methylation in mammalian epigenetics. Science 2001; 293:1068–1069. Part of a special section on epigenetics.
25. Semenza GL. Transcription factors and human disease Oxford: Oxford University Press; 1999.
26. Russo VEA, Martienssen RA, Riggs AD. Epigenetic mechanisms of gene regulation. Plain view NY: Gold Spring Harbor Laboratory Press, 1996.
27. Feinberg AP. The epigenetics of cancer etiology. Semin Cancer Biol 2004; 14:427–432 .
28. Goll MG, Bestor TH. Histone modification and replacement in chromatin activation. Genes Dev 2002; 16:1739–1742.
29. Li E. Chromatin modification and epigenetic reprogramming in mammalian development. Nat Rev Genet 2002; 3:662–673.
30. Jenuwein T, Allis CD. Translating the histone code. Science 2001; 293: 1074–1080.
31. Felsenfeld G, Burgess-Beusse B, Farrell C, et al. Chromatin boundaries and chromatin domains. Cold Spring Harb Symp Quant Biol 2004; 69:245–250.
32. Mohd-Sarip A, Verrijzer P. A higher order of (chromatin) silence. Science 2004; 306:1484–1485.
33. Goll MG, Bestor TH. Histone modification and replacement in chromatin activation. Genes Dev 2002; 16:1739–1742.
34. Fitzgerald DP, Bender W. Polycomb group repression reduces DNA accessibility. Mol Cell Biol 2001; 21:6585–6597.
35. Mahmoudi T, Verrijzer, CP. Chromatin silencing and activation by Polycomb and trithorax group proteins. Oncogene 2001; 20:3055–3066.
36. Rougon G, Hobert O. New insights into the diversity and function of neuronal immunoglobulin superfamily molecules. Annu Rev Neurosci 2003; 26:207–238.
37. Moore MJ. From birth to death: the complex lives of eukaryotic mRNAs. Science 2005; 309:1514–1518. Part of a special section on RNA structure, small RNAs, and roles of non-coding RNA.
38. Wickens M, Gonzalez TN. Knives, accomplices, and RNA. Science 2004; 306:1299–1300.
39. Daviter T, Murphy FV, Ramakrishnan V. A renewed focus on transfer RNA. Science 2005; 308:1123–1124.
40. Bernstein E, Allis CD. RNA meets chromatin. Genes & Dev 2005; 19:1635–1655.
41. Klug A. A marvellous machine for making messages. Science 2001; 292: 1844–1846. Commentary on X-ray crystallography of RNA polymerase II and its transcription complex pp. 1847–1882.
42. Francis N J, Kingston RE. Mechanisms of transcriptional memory. Nat Rev Mol Cell Biol 2001; 2:409–421.
43. Shannon MF, Roa S. Of chips and chIPs. Science 2002; 296:666–669.

44. Gietta G, Deerinck TJ, Adams SR et al. Multicolor and electron microscopic imaging of connexin trafficking. Science 2002; 296:503–506.

45. Schirmer EC, Florens L, Guan T, et al. Nuclear membrane proteins with potential disease links found by subtractive proteomics. Science 2003; 301:1380–1382.

46. Giot L, Bader JS, Brouwer C, et al. A protein interaction map for *Drosophila melanogaster*. Science 2003; 302:1727–1736.

47. Liotta LA, Kohn EC, Petricoin EF. Clinical proteomics. Personalized molecular medicine. JAMA 2001; 286:2211–2214.

48. Byers PH. Disorders of collagen biosynthesis and structure. In: Scriver CR, Beaudet AL, Sly WS et al, eds. The metabolic & molecular bases of inherited disease. 8th edn. New York: McGraw-Hill; 2001:5241–5286.

49. Sykes B. Genetics cracks bone disease. Nature 1987; 330:607–608.

50. Dietz HC, Vallee D, Francomano CA, et al. The skipping of constitutive exons in vivo induced by nonsense mutations. Science 1993; 259:680–683.

DNA diagnosis and genomics: new approaches to embryology and dysmorphology

51. Collins FS, Guttmacher AE. Genetics moves into the medical mainstream. JAMA 2001; 286: 2322–2323. Has references to the first human genome data, now accessible online with tutorials at www.ncbi.nlm.nih.gov/genome/guide/human/

52. Scherer SW, Cheung J, MacDonald JR, et al. Human chromosome 7: DNA sequence and biology. Science 300: 767–772.

53. Kosak ST, Groudine M. Gene order and dynamic domains. Science 2004; 306:644–647.

54. Patil N, Berno AJ, Hinds DA, et al. Blocks of limited haplotype diversity revealed by high-resolution scanning of human chromosome 21. Science 2001; 294:1719–1722.

55. Altshuler D, Clark AG. Harvesting medical information from the family tree. Science 2005; 307:1052–1053. Commentary on Hinds DA, Stuve LL, Nilsen GB, et al. Whole-genome patterns of common DNA variations in three human populations. Science 2005; 307:1072–1079.

56. Vortkamp A, Gessler M, Grzeschik K-H. GLI3 zinc-finger gene interrupted by translocations in Greig syndrome families. Nature 1991; 352:539–540.

57. Yan H, Kinzler KW, Vogelstein B. Genetic testing – present and future. Science 2000;1890–1892.

58. Strom C. Mutation detection, interpretation, and applications in the clinical laboratory setting. Mutat Res 2005; 573:160–167.

59. Ojha RP, Thertulian R. Health care policy issues as a result of the genetic revolution: implications for public health. Am J Public Health 2005; 95:385–388.

60. Kleefstra T, Hamel BC. X-linked mental retardation: further lumping, splitting and emerging phenotypes. Clin Genet 2005; 67:451–467.

61. Macias VR, Day DW, King TE, et al. Clasped-thumb mental retardation (MASA) syndrome: confirmation of linkage to Xq28. Am J Med Genet 1992; 43:408–414.

62. Vits L, Van Camp G, Coucke P, et al. MASA syndrome is due to mutations in the neural cell adhesion gene L1CAM. Nat Genet 1994; 7:408–413.

63. Willemsen R, Mientjes E, Oostra BA. FXTAS: a progressive neurologic syndrome associated with fragile X premutation. Curr Neurol Neurosci Rep 2005; 5:405–410.

64. Verkerk JMH, Pieretti M, Sutcliffe JS, et al. Identification of a gene [FMR-1] containing a CGG repeat coincident with a breakpoint cluster region exhibiting length variation in fragile X syndrome. Cell 1991; 65(5):905–914.

Molecular embryology: new approaches to human embryogenesis and oncogenesis

65. Alberts B, Johnson A, Lewis J, et al. Molecular biology of the cell. 4th edn. New York: Garland Science; 2002.

66. Epstein CJ, Erickson RP, Wynshaw-Boris A. Inborn errors of development – the molecular basis of clinical disorders of morphogenesis. Oxford Monographs on Medical Genetics, no. 49. Oxford: Oxford University Press; 2004.

67. Reik W, Dean W, Walter J. Epigenetic reprogramming in mammalian development. Science 2000; 1293:1089–1093.

68. Gilbert SF. Developmental biology. 8th edn. Sunderland: Sinauer; 2006.

69. Wolpert L. Principles of development. Oxford: Oxford University Press; 1998.

70. Wassarman PM. Mammalian fertilization: molecular aspects of gamete adhesion, exocytosis, and fusion. Cell 1999; 96:175–283.

71. Falls JG, Pulford DJ, Wylie AA, et al. Genomic imprinting: implications for human disease. Am J Pathol 1999; 154:635–647. A review article.

72. Hall JG. Genomic imprinting: review and relevance to human diseases. Am J Hum Genet 1990; 46:857–873.

73. Hark AT, Schoenherr, CJ, Katz DJ, et al. CTCF mediates methylation-sensitive enhancer-blocking activity at the H19/Igf2 locus. Nature 2000; 405: 486–489.

74. Scotting PJ, Walker DA, Perilongo G. Childhood solid tumors: a developmental disorder. Nat Rev Cancer 2006; 5:481–488.

75. Yelon D, Stainier DYR. Pattern formation: swimming in retinoic acid. Curr Biol 2002; 12:R707–R709.

76. Bolande RP. Benignity of neonatal tumors and concept of cancer repression in early life. Am J Dis Child 1971; 122:12–14.

77. Levine AJ. P53, the cellular gatekeeper for growth and division. Cell 1997; 88:323–331.

78. Vaux DL, Korsmeyer SJ. Cell death in development. Cell 1999; 96:245–254. A review article.

79. Zhang L, Zhou W, Velculescu VE, et al. Gene expression profiles in normal and cancer cells. Science 1997; 276:1268–1272.

80. Shintani T, Klionsky DJ. Autophagy in health and disease: A double-edged sword. Science 2004; 306:990–995.

81. Oligny LL. Human molecular embryogenesis – an overview. Pediatr Dev Pathol 2001; (4)4:324–343.

82. Gumbiner BM. Cell adhesion: the molecular basis of tissue architecture and morphogenesis. Cell 1996; 84:345–357. A review article.

83. Lauffenburger DA, Horwitz AF. Cell migration: a physically integrated molecular process. Cell 1996; 84:359–369. A review article.

84. Takeichi M. The cadherins: cell–cell adhesion molecules controlling animal morphogenesis. Development 1988; 102:639–655. A review article.

85. Villavicencio EH, Walterhouse DO, Iannaconne PM. The sonic hedgehog-patched-gli pathway in human development and disease. Am J Hum Genet 2000; 67:1047–1054.

86. Hooper JE, Scott MP. Communicating with hedgehogs. Nat Rev Mol Cell Biol 2005; 6:306–317. A review article.

87. Nüsslein-Volhard C. Of flies and fishes. Science 1994; 266:572–574.

88. Beddington RSP, Robertson EJ. Axis development and early asymmetry in mammals. Cell 1999; 96:195–209.

89. Casey B. Two rights make a wrong: human left-right malformations. Hum Mol Genet 1998; 7:1565–1571. A review article.

90. Conlon RA. Retinoic acid and pattern formation in vertebrates. Trends Genet 1995; 11:314–319.

91. Gehring WJ, Affolter M, Bürglin T. Homeodomain proteins. Ann Rev Biochem 1994; 63:487–526. A review article.

92. Johnson KR, Sweet HO, Donahue LR, et al. A new spontaneous mouse mutation of Hoxd13 with a polyalanine expansion and phenotype similar to human synpolydactyly. Hum Mol Genet 1998; 7:1033–1038.

93. Lohmann I, McGinnis W. Hox genes: it's all a matter of context. Curr Biol 2002; 12:R514–R516.

94. Akin ZN, Nazarali AJ. Hox genes and their candidate downstream targets in the developing central nervous system. Cell Mol Neurobiol 2005; 25:697–741.

95. Odenwald WF. Changing fates on the road to neuronal diversity. Dev Cell 2004; 5:133–134 .

96. Placzek M, Briscoe J. The floor plate: multiple cells, multiple signals. Nat Rev Neurosci 2005; 6:230– 240.

97. Hinck L. The versatile roles of 'axon guidance' cues in tissue morphogenesis. Dev Cell 2005; 8:783– .

98. Poliakov A, Cotrina M, Wilkinson DG. Diverse roles of eph receptors and ephrins in the regulation of cell migration and tissue assembly. Dev Cell 2004; 7:465– 480.

99. Guo W, Giancotti FG. Integrin signaling during tumor progression. Nat Rev Mol Cell Biol 2004; 5:816–826.

100. Esteller M. DNA methylation and cancer therapy: new developments and expectations. Curr Opin Oncol 2005; 17:55– 60.

101. Valk-Lingbeek ME, van Bruggeman SW. Stem cells and cancer; the Polycomb connection. Cell 2004; 118:409– 418.

102. Grier DG, Thompson A, Kwasniewska A, et al. The pathophysiology of HOX genes and their role in cancer. J Pathol 2005; 205:154– 171.

103. Wilkin F, Gagne N, Paquette J, et al. Pediatric adrenocortical tumors: molecular events leading to insulin-like growth factor II gene over-expression. J Clin Endocrinol Metab 2000; 85:2048–2056.

104. Fodde R, Smits R. Cancer biology: A matter of dosage. Science 2002; 298: 761–762.

105. Meder D, Simons K. Ras on the roundabout. Science 2005; 307:1731–1733.

106. Yuspa SH, Epstein EH Jr. An anchor for tumor cell invasion. Science 2005; 307:1727–1728.

Novel inheritance mechanisms revealed by molecular developmental technology

107. Schmickel RD. Contiguous gene syndromes: a component of recognizable syndromes. J Pediatr 1986; 109:231–241.

108. Fischback BV, Trout KL, Lewis J, et al. WAGR syndrome: a clinical review of 54 cases. Pediatrics 2005; 116:984–988.

109. Francke U, Harper JF, Darras BT, et al. Congenital adrenal hypoplasia, myopathy, and glycerol kinase deficiency: molecular evidence for deletions. Am J Hum Genet 1987; 40:212– 227.

110. Smith ACM, McGavran L, Robinson J, et al. Interstitial deletion of (17)(p11.2p11.2) in nine patients. Am J Med Genet 1986; 24:393– 414.

111. Baldini A. Dissecting contiguous gene defects: TBX1. Curr Opin Genet Dev 2005; 15:279–284.

112. Leventer R J. Genotype–phenotype correlation in lissencephaly and subcortical band heterotopia: the key questions answered. Child Neurol 2005; 20:307–312.

113. Redon R, Rio M, Gregory HG. Tiling path resolution mapping of constitutional 1p36 deletions by array-CGH: contiguous gene deletion or 'deletion with positional effect' syndrome? J Med Genet 2005; 42:166–171.

114. Swales AK, Spears N. Genomic imprinting and reproduction. Reproduction 2005; 130:389–399.

115. Wilson GN, Hall JG, de la Cruz F. Genomic imprinting: summary of an NICHD conference. Am J Med Genet 1993; 46:675–680.

116. O'Brien SJ, Womack JE, Lyons LA, et al. Anchored reference loci for comparative mapping in mammals. Nat Genet 1993; 3:103– 112.

117. Sparago A, Cerrato F, Vernucci M, et al. Microdeletions in the human H19 DMR result in loss of IGF2 imprinting and Beckwith-Wiedemann syndrome. Nat Genet 2004; 36:958–960.

118. Orgel LE, Crick FHC, Sapienza C. Selfish DNA. Nature 1980; 288:645–646.

119. Thompson JR, Williams CJ. Genomic imprinting and assisted reproductive technology: connections and potential risks. Semin Reprod Med 2005; 23:285–295.

120. Stetton G, Escallon CS, South ST, et al. Reevaluating confined placental mosaicism. Am J Med Genet A 2004; 131:232–239.

121. Skuse JH, James RS, Bishop DVM, et al. Evidence from Turner's syndrome of an imprinted X-linked locus affecting cognitive function. Nature 1997; 387:705–708.

122. Hu X, Worton RG. Partial gene duplication as a cause of human disease. Hum Mutat 1992; 1:3–12.

123. Lupski JR, Wise CA, Kuwano A, et al. Gene dosage is a mechanism for Charcot-Marie-Tooth disease type 1A. Nat Genet 1:29, 1993.

124. Cheng Z, Ventura M, She X. A genome-wide comparison of recent chimpanzee and human segmental duplications. Nature 2005; 437:88–93.

125. Olson LE, Richtsmeier JT, Leszl J, et al. A chromosome 21 critical region does not cause specific Down syndrome phenotypes. Science 2004; 306:687–690.

126. Redman JB, Fenwick RG, Fu Y-H, et al. Relationship between parental trinucleotide GCT repeat length and severity of myotonic dystrophy in offspring. JAMA 1993; 269:1960–1965.

127. Riggins GJ, Lokey LK, Chastain JL, et al. Human genes containing polymorphic trinucleotide repeats. Nat Genet 1992; 2:186–191.

128. Taylor JP, Hardy J, Fischbeck KH. Toxic proteins in neurodegenerative disease. Science 2002; 296:1991–1995.

129. Wilson GN. Tales form the neural genome: the lessons of homozygous porphyria. Arch Neurol 2004; 61:1650–1651.

130. Dimauro S, Davidzon G. Mitochondrial DNA and disease. Ann Med 2005; 37:222–232.

131. Wilson GN, Stout JP, Schneider NR, et al. Balanced translocation 12/13 and situs abnormalities: Homology of pattern in man and lower organismss? Am J Med Genet 1991; 38:601–607.

132. Wilson GN. Mutational risks in females: genomic imprinting and maternal molecules. Mutat Res 1992; 296:157–165.

133. Nora JJ, Nora AH. Maternal transmission of congenital heart diseases: new recurrence risk figures and the question of cytoplasmic inheritance and vulnerability to teratogens. Am J Cardiol 1987; 59:459–463.

Molecular approaches to growth and development

134. Wilson GN. Heterochrony and human malformation. Am J Med Genet 1989; 29:311–321.

135. Wilson GN. Karyotype/phenotype controversy: genetic and molecular implications of alternative hypotheses. Am J Med Genet 1990; 36:500– 505.

136. Jaenisch R. Transgenic animals. Science 1988; 240:1468–1474.

137. Steele R. Oncogenes, proto-oncogenes, and development. In: Malacinski GM, ed. Developmental genetics of higher organisms: a primer in developmental biology. New York: MacMillan; 1988.

138. Knudson AG Jr. Genetics of human cancer. Annu Rev Genet 1986; 20: 231–251.

139. Gicquel C, Rossignol S, Cabrol S, et al. Epimutation of the telomeric imprinting center region on chromosome 11p15 in Silver-Russell syndrome. Nat Genet 2005; 37:1003–1007.

140. Svensson J, Bjornstahl A, Ivarsson SA. Increased risk of Silver-Russell syndrome after in vitro fertilization? Acta Paediatr 2005; 94:1163–1165.

141. Wilson GN. Structure–function relationships in the peroxisome: implications for human disease (minireview). Biochem Med Metab Biol 1991; 46:288– 298.

142. Gould SJ, Raymond GV, Valle D. The peroxisome biogenesis disorders. In: Scriver CR, Beaudet AL, Sly WS, et al, eds. The metabolic & molecular bases of inherited disease. 8th edn. New York: McGraw-Hill; 2001:3181–3217.

143. Reiner O, Carrozzo R, Shen Y, et al. Isolation of a Miller-Dieker lissencephaly gene containing G protein a-subunit-like repeats. Nature 1993; 364:717–721.

144. Edelman GM. Topobiology: an introduction to molecular embryology. New York: Basic Books; 1988.

145. Fleischman RA, Saltman DL, Stastny V, et al. Deletion of the c-kit proto-oncogene in the human developmental defect piebald trait. Proc Natl Acad Sci U S A 1991; 88:10885–10889.

146. Newman CGH. Teratogen update: clinical aspects of thalidomide embryopathy – a continuing preoccupation. Teratology 1985; 32:133–144.

147. Wilson GN. Heritable limb deficiencies. In: Herring JA, Birch JG, eds. The child with a limb deficiency. Rosemont: American Academy of Orthopedic Surgeons; 1998:39–49.

148. Froster UG, Baird PA. Congenital defects of the lower limbs and associated malformations. A population-based study. Am J Med Genet 1993; 45:60–64.

149. Manouvrier-Hanu S, Holder-Espinasse M, Lyonnet S. Genetics of limb anomalies in humans. Trends Genet 1999; 15: 409–417.

150. Goodman FR. Congenital abnormalities of body patterning: embryology revisited. Lancet 2003; 362:651–662.

151. Dube ID, Kamel-Reid S, Yuan CC, et al. A novel human homeobox gene lies at the chromosome 10 breakpoint in lymphoid neoplasias with chromosomal translocation t(10;14). Blood 1991; 78:2996–3003.

Future prospects: developmental pathology, genomics, and the second codes

152. Bonner JT. On development. The biology of form. Cambridge: Harvard University Press; 1974.

Causes and pathogenesis of birth defects

2

John M. Opitz   Golder N. Wilson   Enid Gilbert-Barness

Felix qui potuit rerum cognoscere causas (Lucky is he who could understand the causes of things)

Practical approach to classification

As initially defined by the March of Dimes – Birth Defects Foundation, the term **birth defects** included all '… anatomic or functional variant(s) from the normal range in homo sapiens (sic) …'. Here, birth defects are treated from a narrower, primarily morphogenetic perspective; however, functional correlates must be kept in mind at all times 'even' in a dead fetus or stillborn infant. It is likely that fetuses with structural defects have prenatal death rates equal to or greater than those of unaffected fetuses; indeed, there is good reason to expect higher death rates of abnormal fetuses. Fetal autopsy is at least as important for medical counseling as is postnatal autopsy, and rarity is no excuse for substandard investigation.

Birth defects cover a vast range of anatomic abnormalities. They may occur singly or multiply; they may represent minor anomalies, mild or severe malformations. They are mostly non-neoplastic but at times involve tumor formation, as in congenital teratomas with anal and sacrococcygeal anomalies. They may or may not involve the placenta; they may occur in singletons or multiple fetuses, conjoined or non-conjoined twins, minute embryos or giant fetuses; and they may represent primary defects of morphogenesis, secondary (exogenous) disruptions of development, or later gestational 'bending out of shape' of something that was primarily normally developed (deformities). Accurate documentation of the pattern and mechanisms of birth defects is required before causal analysis is possible (Fig. 2.1).

Correct interpretation of the biologic nature of birth defects requires knowledge of morphology, a discipline of zoology that concerns itself at once with the form, formation, and transformation of living beings. It also requires knowledge of genetics, primarily with respect to the causes of birth defects, and of teratology as the science of developmental disruptions. Since 'nothing in biology makes sense except in the light of evolution,' a phylogenetic perspective of development is essential.[1] Everything that is developed (whether normal or abnormal) has evolved; hence, what we may consider abnormal developmental results may be normal from an evolutionary perspective. Cleft palate or midline cleft of the upper lip, webbing of digits, persistence of tail, presence of cloaca, bicornuate uterus, absence of thumbs, and so forth, are abnormal states in humans, but normal states in other vertebrates, mammals, or closely related primates. Nothing can occur in development (ontogeny) that evolution (phylogeny) has not 'permitted' or made possible; hence, with some exceptions, it may be necessary in the future to regard all primary malformations in humans as atavisms (developmental states normal in phylogenetic ancestors but abnormal in their descendants).

Correct interpretation of the biologic nature of birth defects likewise is predicated on a thorough history; making simultaneous study of the placenta; careful anatomic and histologic studies; and photos, measurements, and radiographs supplemented by special laboratory tests as indicated (Fig. 2.2).[2–4] The study of fetal development and its abnormalities, prenatal detection, postnatal study, and final assessment and counseling represent a multidisciplinary activity with teaching and research

65

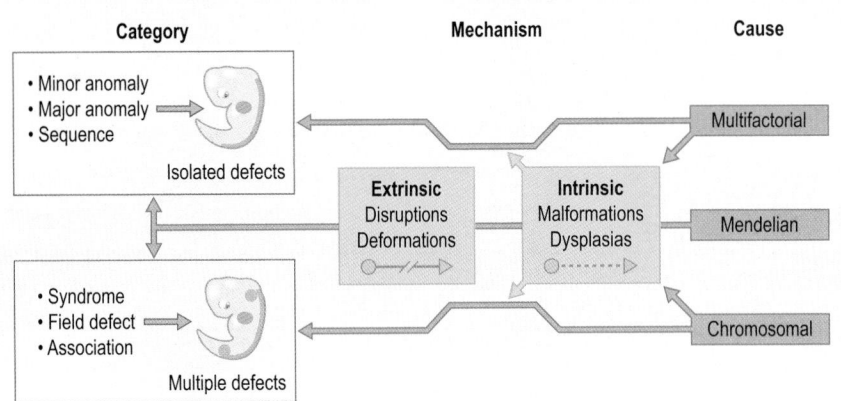

FIGURE 2.1 Categories of birth defects. Isolated defects, sequences, and field defects are more likely to be multifactorial, while malformation syndromes are more likely to be mendelian or chromosomal.

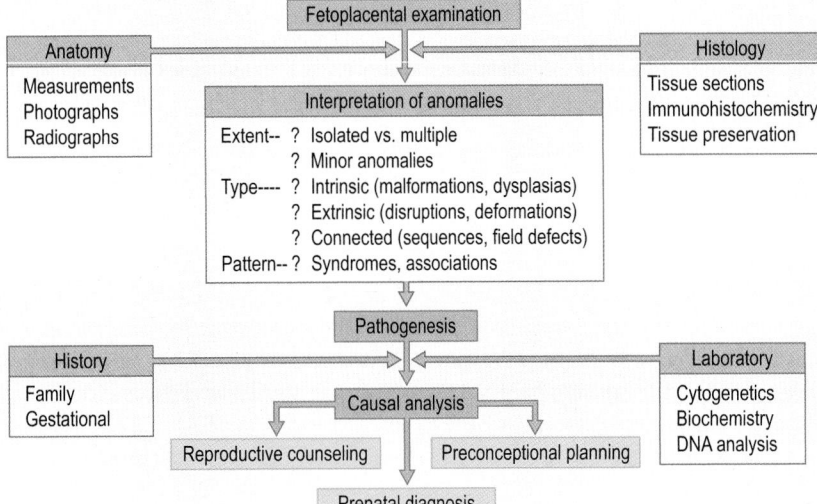

FIGURE 2.2 The fetoplacental examination and the path to primary cause.

missions subordinated to its first responsibility, which is to the family. It is imperative for the various services and centers working in the field of fetal pathology to attain a consensus on methodologic standards; quality assurance and peer review programs are vital for attaining the highest levels of quality and reliability.[5–8]

Reproductive counseling and prenatal options for families with birth defects often depend on the accuracy of pathologic diagnosis (see Fig. 2.2). Thorough documentation of fetoplacental anatomy and histology, and subsequent correct interpretation of the anomalies, are integral steps in the diagnostic process.[1–8] Often, tissue must be preserved in a form suitable for karyotyping (sterile, non-frozen, non-fixed tissue or blood), DNA/ biochemical analysis (fresh or frozen tissue, fresh blood), or long-term storage (tissue frozen at –70°F or below).

Principles for classification of birth defects by type, cause, and pathogenesis (developmental stage and mechanism) will now be discussed, followed by sample cases that illustrate application of these principles.

Terminology: types of birth defects

Figure 2.1 demonstrates the importance of birth defect categories in causal analysis. **Isolated defects** (cleft palate, spina bifida) affect a single body region and are usually considered due to **multifactorial determination. Multiple defects** are more likely to be due to **chromosomal or mendelian inheritance,** particularly if they comprise the pattern expected for syndromes. Classification by mechanisms is also useful, with extrinsic disturbances of development (disruptions, deformations) having less serious genetic implication than those in which organ or cell development is abnormal from the beginning (malformations, dysplasias). These correlations of defect type with cause highlight the need for accurate terminology. For the most part, the terminology of the International Working Group (IWG)[9] and the Berlin group[10] is stressed.

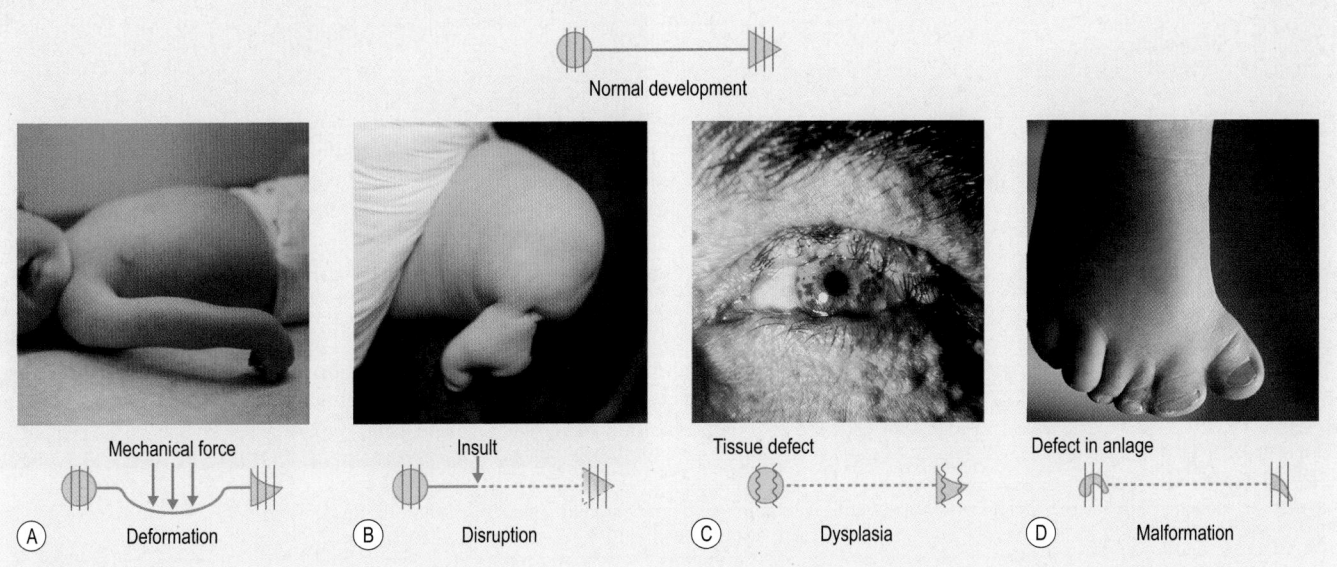

FIGURE 2.3 Mechanisms of dysmorphogenesis. The drawing at the top represents normal development *(horizontal line)* of a primordial structure *(circle)* and its surrounding tissue *(vertical lines)* to produce a mature structure *(triangle)*. Deformation (A, policeman's tip position of the hand) and disruption (B, amniotic band constriction of the lower limb) represent extrinsic interruptions of normal development. Dysplasias (C, Lisch modules and neurofibromas in a patient with neurofibromatosis) and malformations (D, bifid great toe) represent intrinsic abnormalities of the respective surrounding tissue or primordium. (C, courtesy of Dr. Harold Falls.)

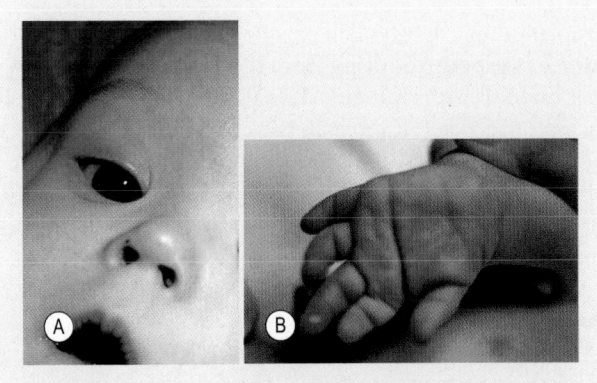

FIGURE 2.4 Minor anomalies in a patient with Down syndrome. (A) Epicanthal folds and anteverted nares. (B) Single palmar crease and clinodactyly (with absent middle crease) of the fifth finger.

Isolated birth defects

Definitions of the kinds of birth defects are given first, followed by terms that are used for birth defect combinations (see Fig. 2.1).

Anomaly

'[Any] deviation from the expected or average type in structure, form and/or function which is interpreted as abnormal.'[9, 10]

Characterization of anomalies as 'abnormal' distinguishes them from normal variants (e.g., mongolian spot) that are both more frequent (arbitrarily, more than 4% of the population) and less noxious than anomalies. **Major anomalies** are those with cosmetic or surgical consequences: e.g., the deformed wrist, limb defect, neurofibromas, and duplicated great toe shown in Figure 2.3. **Minor anomalies,** despite their diagnostic importance, have little impact on individual well-being: e.g., anteverted nares, epicanthal fold (Fig. 2.4A); clinodactyly, single palmar crease (Fig. 2.4B).

Malformation

'... a morphological defect of an organ, or larger region of the body resulting from an intrinsically abnormal developmental process.' 'Intrinsically abnormal' implies a genetic cause (e.g., chromosome abnormality, mendelian mutation, or genetic predisposition/multifactorial determination). These *vitiae primae formationis* are also referred to as primary malformations. 'Defect of an organ' generally refers to a **defect of organogenesis,** whereas one involving a 'larger region of the body' refers to an **abnormality of blastogenesis.** Since embryonic anatomy is dynamic, a localized error in one primordium may produce malformations in several derived structures (see definitions of sequences and field defects below). **No trait in humans is purely genetically determined; the attributes of penetrance (presence or absence of the malformation in a gene carrier) and expressivity (severity) are not attributes of**

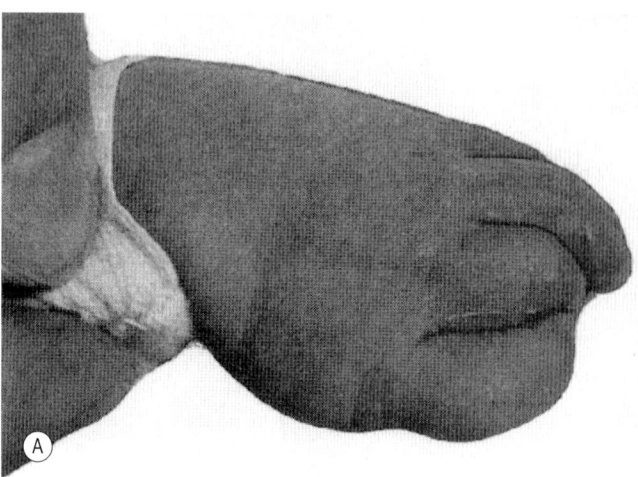 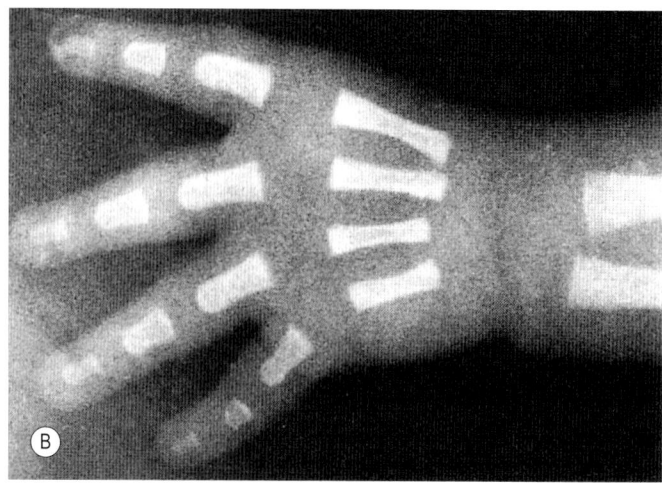

FIGURE 2.5 Absence of the thumb and first metacarpal bone with apparently normal radius. (A) External view. (B) Radiograph.

the mutant gene, but of alleles and genes elsewhere (epistasis). Environmental modulation is also frequent, especially evident in dominant traits with striking right–left asymmetry of expression of the developmental defect.

Absence of the thumb (Fig. 2.5) is an example of a malformation. Intrinsic abnormality of limb bud development would be suspected, just as for the duplicated toe shown in Figure 2.3D. Malformations are field defects (see below) and may occur as components of various syndromes. **Malformations,** as field defects, are **causally heterogeneous** – diverse gene or chromosomal mutations may shift development to the final common pathway that results in absent thumb. The distinction may be one of degree, exemplified by the absent thumb that accompanies more extensive agenesis of the radial ray. Radial agenesis is a malformation in the sense of intrinsic abnormality and genetic or multifactorial causation, but it reflects abnormality of a larger developmental field. Once the anomaly extends to radial aplasia and bone marrow defects, as in the thrombocytopenia–absent radius (TAR), Aase, or Fanconi syndromes,[11, 12] it is necessary to speak of a limb-marrow field defect.

Dysplasia

'… **an abnormal organization of cells into tissue(s) and its morphologic result(s).**' In other words: a dysplasia is the process (and the consequence) of dyshistogenesis.' The IWG comments further: in diagnostic histopathology the term dysplasia usually connotes neoplastic tissue development; its present use is broader and applies to all **abnormalities of histogenesis,** regardless of neoplastic potential. For instance, osteogenesis imperfecta and the Marfan syndrome are dysplasias because the abnormalities in each condition can be reduced to a defect in connective tissue. Gross clinical abnormalities in these conditions are the result of functional tissue defects which are probably related to defects in collagen (or fibrillin) metabolism. Since the defect involves all anatomic sites in which the affected

tissue element is present, these, and many other dysplasias, show widespread involvement. In contrast to malformations, disruptions and deformities, dysplastic lesions are frequently not confined to single organs. In the case of localized dysplasias such as hemangiomata, the abnormal tissue elements occupy part of an organ.[9]

Disruption

'… **morphologic defect of an organ, part of an organ or larger region of the body resulting from the extrinsic breakdown of, or an interference with, an originally normal developmental process.**' A classic example is the amniotic band that wraps around a developing limb and produces distal hypoplasia or amputation (Figs 2.3B and 2.6).[13] Disruptions are sometimes called secondary malformations. Disruption may be extended to include all birth defects caused by environmental agents, if the exposure will interfere with an originally normal developmental process.

There is no genetic disorder that is not environmentally modified, and no environmental factor that is not genetically modified. For example, no two thalidomide children have the identical condition given identical dosages at identical times; one needs also to take into account the mother's metabolism and other modifications by the placenta. Pure exposure is virtually never seen; mothers of fetal alcohol syndrome (FAS) infants frequently smoke, and those who take hydantoin for seizures may also have taken asthma medication. The broader sense of disruptions as environmental defects is thus useful in explaining why anomalies can be so variable, even among patients with the same genetic syndrome.

Deformation

'… **abnormal form, shape or position of a part of the body caused by mechanical forces.**' Deformities are a normal response to abnormal forces (or inability to resist normal forces,

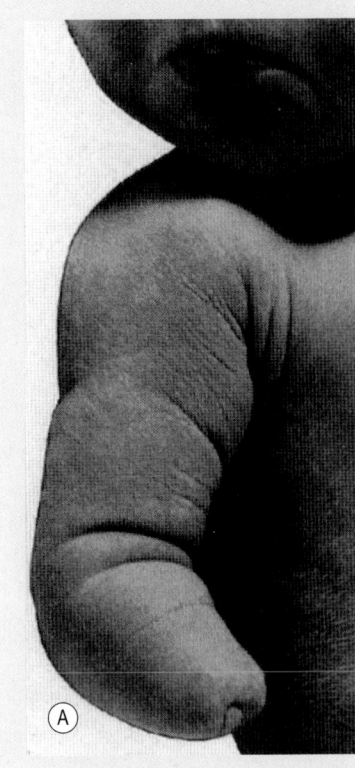

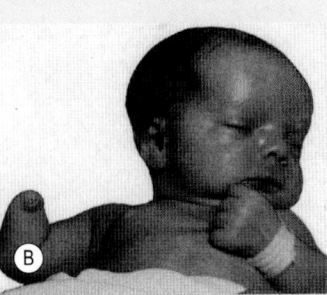

FIGURE 2.6 (A) and (B) Amniotic band disruptions of the forearm.

e.g., in a weak or paralyzed limb) and affect structure after initial development. Many deformities are potentially remediable in the postnatal period or may correct spontaneously. The deformed lower limbs associated with constraint due to oligohydramnios are illustrated in Figure 2.7; a deformed wrist associated with fetal hypotonia is shown in Figure 2.3A. Common deformities include plagiocephalies of all kinds with or without torticollis, scoliosis without vertebral defects, palmar flexion crease abnormalities, arthrogrypotic defects of hands and/or feet, bowing of legs, club feet, and so forth. Deformities may also be acquired postnatally, as in the contractures of limbs or scoliosis in those with central nervous system (CNS) malformations, or plagio- or brachycephaly in those with congenital hypotonia. The **congenital hypotonia sequence** may involve deformities of skull; the facial consequences of chronic mouth breathing such as micrognathia, inverted 'V' shape of upper lip, and long upper lip; flat chest with or without respiratory pectus excavatum; sloping shoulders; winging of scapulae; protuberant abdomen; undescended testes; hyperextensible knees; flat feet; and chronic constipation. Malformed parts of the body may become deformed (radial club hand in radius aplasia); most deformed parts of the body are not malformed. Deformed parts of the body, especially limbs, may be smaller in size, i.e., suffer a growth deceleration, presumably primarily because of disuse. Lack of use may affect growth prenatally as in micrognathia, small hands and feet (micromelia), and the short gastrointestinal tract seen in those born after prolonged oligohydramnios.

Sequence

'... pattern of multiple anomalies derived from a single known or presumed prior anomaly or mechanical factor,' which may be referred to as a *complex* or *anomaly*. Individuals with sequences may be mistakenly categorized as having a multiple defect syndrome if the embryologic connection between the defects is not recognized. **A sequence represents a cascade of primary and secondary events that are consequences of a single primary malformation or a disruption.** Sequences, like isolated malformations, are most often associated with sporadic or multifactorial inheritance. Examples follow.

Malformation Sequence X-linked spina bifida/myelomeningocele sequence with secondary neurohypotrophy of lower limbs, club feet, neurogenic bladder with chronic urinary tract infection; DiGeorge sequence (anomaly, complex) due to del(22)(q11) with presumed primary defect of the neural crest involved in the differentiation of face, branchial arches, and conotruncal area of the heart with secondary hypoparathyroidism, immune defect, and cyanotic congenital heart defect.[14]

Dysplasia Sequence Sacrococcygeal teratoma complex with defective sacrum and coccyx, imperforate anus, rectovaginal fistula, and urinary tract obstruction.

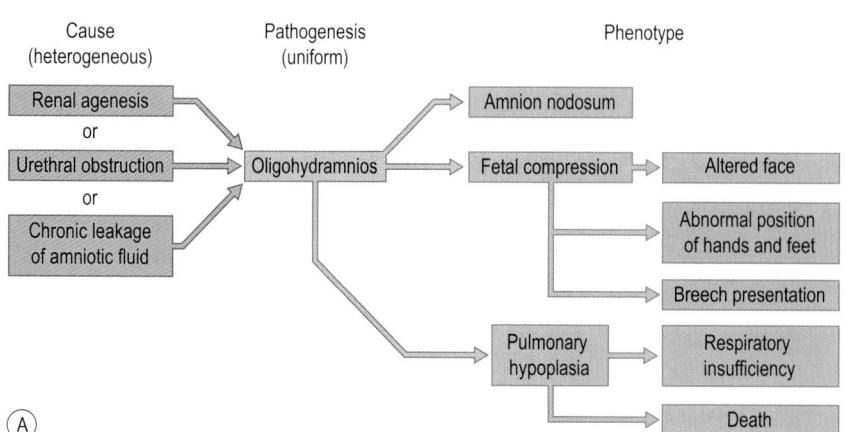

Cause (heterogeneous) → Pathogenesis (uniform) → Phenotype

FIGURE 2.7 (A) Diagram of Potter sequence. (B and C) Infant with renal agenesis deformations (Potter sequence, in Potter syndrome). Note the redundant skin, exaggerated facial creases, and bowing of legs (B). (C) Recreation of the intrauterine position caused by constraint from decreased fetal urine and oligohydramnios.

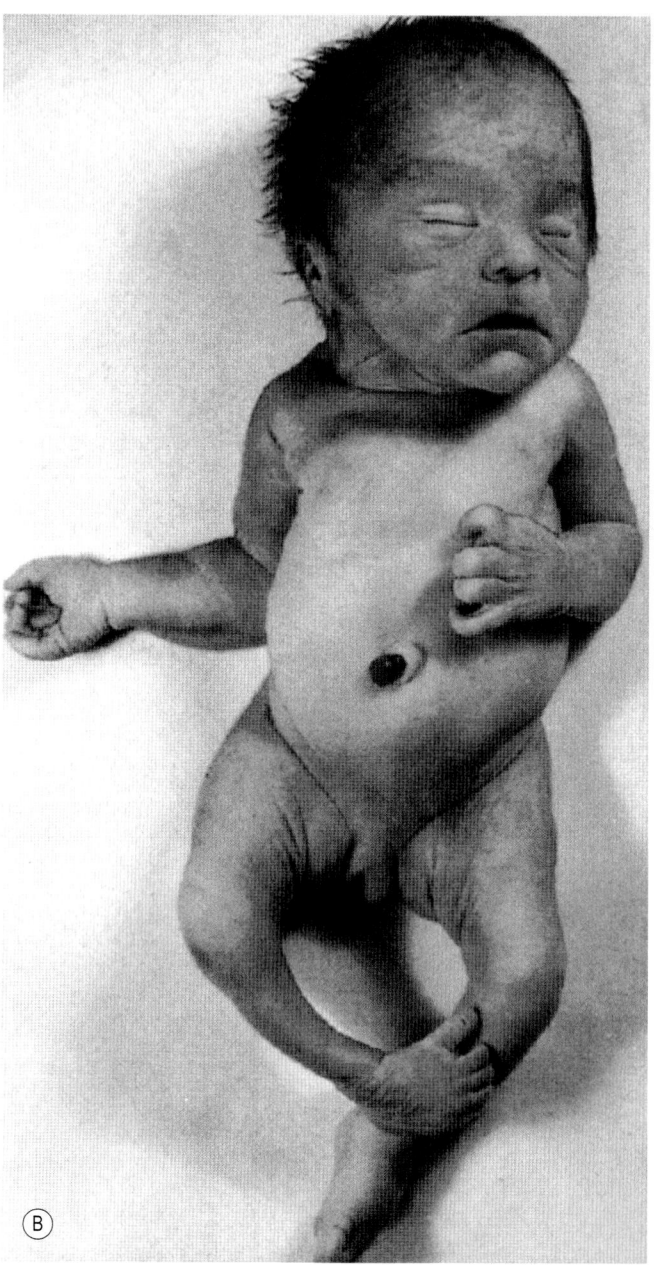

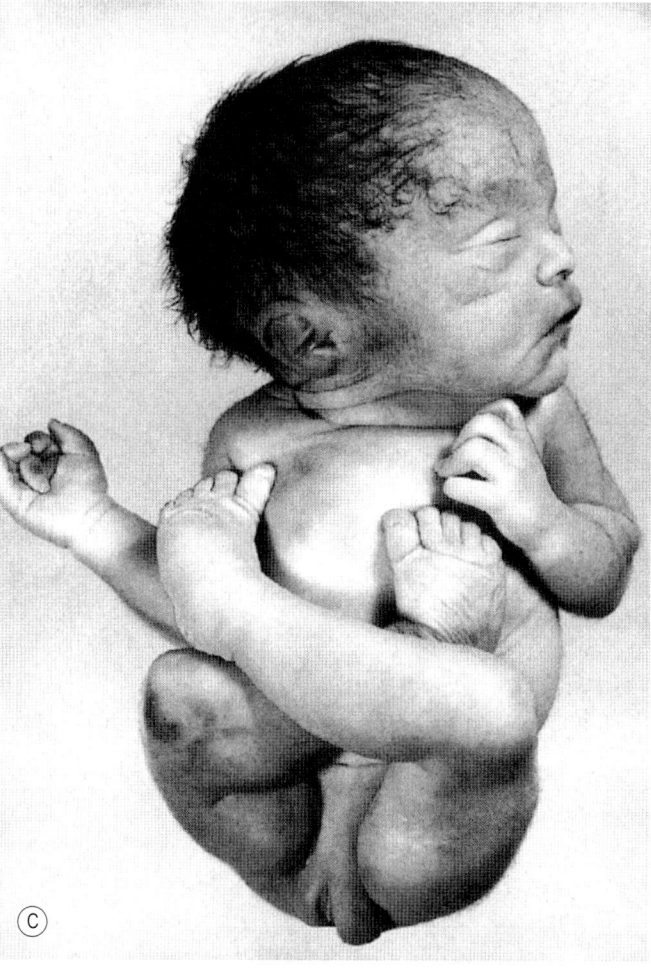

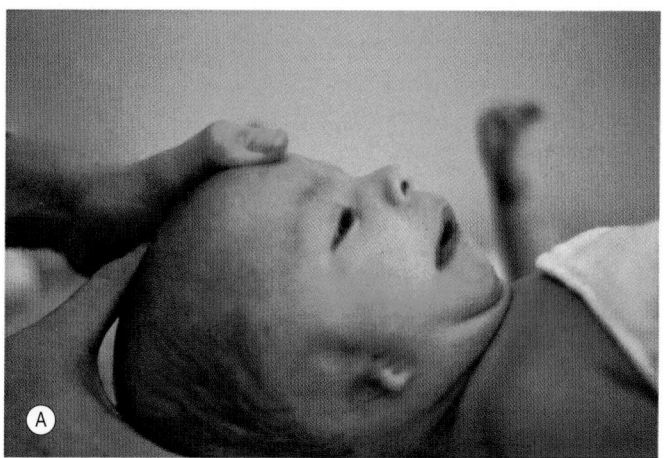 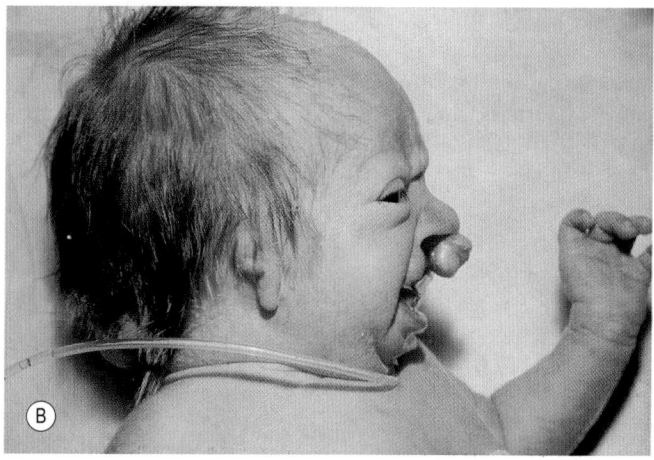

FIGURE 2.8 Patients with hemifacial microsomia (A, abnormal ear, asymmetric jaw) versus the more extensive Goldenhar syndrome (B, malformed ear, bilateral cleft lip and palate, micrognathia, and agenesis of the thumb).

Deformity Sequence Bilateral renal agenesis (Potter syndrome) (see Fig. 2.7) with absence of Müllerian and Wolffian duct derivatives, leading to the oligohydramnios sequence (Potter sequence); hypoplasia or absence of the bladder; oligohydramnios with subsequent deceleration of fetal growth; redundant skin; deformed limbs, nose, ears, and face; and pulmonary hypoplasia.

Birth defect combinations

The distinction between patients with isolated versus multiple congenital anomalies is fundamental for causal analysis. Crucial in this distinction is the recognition of minor anomalies that may shift the patient with one major defect into the syndrome category and to distinguish associations from syndromes. Associations are relatively common and usually have a more optimistic medical and genetic prognosis.

Syndrome

'Multiple anomalies thought to be pathogenetically related and not representing a sequence.' 'Syndrome implies a lower level of understanding of a given pattern of pathogenetically related anomalies than sequence. In the latter, we know the initiating event and the ensuing cascade of secondary effects. With time, a syndrome may become a sequence.'

Syndromes, like sequences, may involve different mechanisms. Malformation syndromes are exemplified by disorders such as **Goldenhar syndrome** (see Fig. 2.8B) that involves multiple orofacial, cardiac, limb, and vertebral malformations. Note the involvement of several embryologically independent regions in a syndrome (eye, ear, heart, vertebrae, thumb) in contrast to the localized branchial arch error in hemifacial microsomia sequence (see Fig. 2.8A). One patient may display several mechanisms: e.g., open lesions such as the scalp defect in trisomy 13 patients may

adhere to amnion and produce amniotic band disruptions. Syndromes may consist only of disruptions, e.g., FAS or twins with multiple emboli from death of a co-twin. As stated, **dysplasias are much more likely to occur as syndromes because tissues contribute to multiple organs.**

Because of the fundamental difference between the processes of morphogenesis and histogenesis (see Ch. 3), most malformed organs are histologically normal and are rarely predisposed to the development of tumors (e.g., Wilms' tumor in a horseshoe kidney). The **metabolic dysplasia syndromes** (the Zellweger syndromes and related conditions, Smith-Lemli-Opitz [RSH] syndrome, mevalonic acidemia, and glutaric aciduria type II) currently represent still very unusual exceptions to the rule that malformation syndromes are not (Garrodian) inborn errors of metabolism. In these cases the malformations can probably be attributed to the interference with normal morphogenesis and histogenesis by metabolic defects that are only partially or not at all corrected by the mother.

Association

The concept of associations was coined by Quan and Smith in 1973,[15] specifically with respect to the VATER association. In 1982, the IWG[16] defined an association as a 'nonrandom occurrence in two or more individuals of multiple congenital anomalies not known to be a polytopic defect, sequence or syndrome.' The IWG commented that *association* is 'synonymous with syntropy [a concept that] refers solely to statistically, not pathogenetically or causally related anomalies. With increasing knowledge a given association will ideally come to be broken apart into one or more sequences, syndromes or field defects.' Thereafter, many investigators came to regard associations as a form of pleiotropy and referred to them as *syndromes* (such as the caudal regression 'syndrome'); others thought that associations were purely statistical, not biologic, entities. Since the late 1980s it has become clear that associations are in fact real biologic entities of great clinical and epidemiologic importance. Several important association entities have been described, among them first and foremost the **VATER association,** and then the **MURCS association,** the **CHARGE association, tracheal agenesis association, otocephaly associations,** and so forth. The following statements summarize our knowledge of associations.[17–20]

1. An association is a biologic entity that constitutes a legitimate diagnosis in a child or fetus. This is particularly important to remember in fetal pathology.
2. The definition of **individual** associations is potentially arbitrary, since associations have no diagnostic boundaries and, except for a cluster of highly correlated core anomalies, they overlap in a large three-dimensional web with many similar entities. Thus, VATER may be difficult, if not impossible, to distinguish from the 'caudal regression syndrome,' which in turn overlaps with the sirenomelia sequence and the abnormal face–femoral–deficiency sequence, and so forth.
3. Associations have a **high frequency.**[15] The total prevalence is 1.22 cases per 1000 live and stillbirths (1 out of 820 births); associations constitute approximately 29% of all multiple congenital anomaly cases and 41% of those with unidentified multiple congenital anomaly patterns.
4. Associations tend to be **sporadic** cases with a low empiric recurrence risk when syndromal diagnoses have been excluded.
5. Associations appear to be **causally nonspecific,** i.e., heterogeneous, and thus by definition are not syndromes.
6. Associations appear to represent 'hits' involving several vulnerable primordia at the same time; Lubinsky[19, 20] has shown that heart defects occur with developmental timing similar to that of other anomalies in the VACTERL association. This simultaneous occurrence is an extremely valuable developmental attribute that rather usefully separates associations from pleiotropic syndromes.
7. Associations mostly, but not exclusively, **affect midline structures.**[21, 22] However, in this context it must be made clear that not all midline anomalies arise during blastogenesis, but all associations and other anomalies of blastogenesis by definition arise in the midline. Thus, any midline anomaly in a newborn infant should alert the clinician to search for others to be sure that the child does not have a graver combination of blastogenetic midline anomalies or even an association.
8. **Teratogens** such as alcohol, cocaine, and retinoic acid and maternal–fetal interactions such as diabetes can disrupt blastogenesis, leading to severe anomalies frequently incompatible with life, or to less severe disturbances of development.

At this point a new definition of 'association' can be offered to replace the 1982 IWG definition: '**Associations represent the idiopathic occurrence of multiple congenital anomalies during blastogenesis.**' Genetic background may play a role in some cases, as demonstrated by a slightly increased risk of individual anomalies in close relatives. A careful chromosome examination is indicated in all cases, as well as a searching analysis of the family history. For example, it is well known that the apparent VACTERL association with hydrocephalus may constitute an X-linked recessive disorder; in all such cases a 25% recurrence risk should be offered as a maximal risk for the next pregnancy.

Developmental Field Defects

'**The result of (non-disruptive) disturbed development of a morphogenic field or of a part thereof,**' or a '... dysmorphogenetically reactive unit, i.e., a set of embryonic primordia that reacted identically to different dysmorphogenetic causes.'[23–26] An example is the **holoprosencephaly spectrum of anomalies,** varying from premaxillary agenesis to cyclopia and occurring in isolation, in numerous syndromes, and in over 30 different chromosomal aneuploidies. Another example concerns the **dextropulmonary isomerism and pulmonic stenosis** that occur together with **asplenia (bilateral right-sidedness)** as opposed to the **levopulmonary isomerism and azygous venous return** that occur with **polysplenia (bilateral left-sidedness).** The connections between primary cause and multiple consequences are less well defined than for sequences, but field defects have more limited and reproducible consequences than are typical in syndromes. Single malformations are causally heterogeneous field defects; **seemingly independent structures can be joined in the same complex pathway of abnormal development: e.g., prechordal plate, frontonasal process, forebrain vesicle, eyes, and palate in holoprosencephaly.**

Recognition of developmental field defects offers the same benefit as recognition of sequences in relating seemingly independent anomalies to a single primary event. **Most field defects, if seen in isolation, carry a low genetic risk.** However, the more complex string of events in field defects mandates caution, as shown by the relation of DiGeorge anomaly in Shprintzen syndrome or CHARGE association patients to deletions of chromosome 22.[27] Field defects emphasize the large amount of gene interaction that must govern the development of even the smallest embryonic regions. Developmental fields are the heritage of ancient experiments in morphology, unifying studies of simpler organisms with those of man; they are designated by particular insect genes (e.g., PAX, HOX loci).[24]

Qualitative terms

The terms **hypoplasia** and **hyperplasia** refer to underdevelopment and overdevelopment of an organism, organ, or tissue resulting from a decreased or increased number of cells, respectively. **Hypotrophy** and **hypertrophy** refer to a decrease and increase, respectively, in size of cells, tissue, or organ. The term **agenesis** connotes the absence of a part of the body caused by an absent anlage (primordium), whereas in **aplasia** the absence of a part of the body results from a failure of the anlage to develop. The term **atrophy** is used when a normally developed mass of tissue(s) or organ(s) decreases because of a decrease in cell size and/or cell number.[9,10]

Causal analysis: classification by cause

Many physicians think of cause as synonymous with pathogenesis, or if in doubt, with *etiology*. A more precise tradition of usage distinguished between the use of *causal genesis* to refer to cause and *formal genesis* to refer to pathogenesis. Recalling the preceding discussion of terminology, it can be seen that radial aplasias due to disruption (thalidomide) or malformation (TAR syndrome) have the same formal genesis but differ in cause. Where the initiating factor or event of a birth defect is a mendelian mutation, chromosome abnormality, virus, form of ionizing radiation, or teratogenic chemical, the word **cause** (not etiology) should be used. Where it is necessary to refer to the known or presumed cascade of effects of the cause during pre- and postnatal development, the word **pathogenesis** (not etiology) should be used. Where it is impossible to distinguish cause from pathogenesis (as in associations), i.e., where cause is unknown and pathogenesis may involve more than one dysmorphogenetic mechanism (as in the infants of diabetic mothers), the word *etiology* may be used.

Although the autopsy examination is designed to elucidate formal genesis (pathogenesis) of disease through the maneuvers diagrammed in Figure 2.2, the ultimate goal is to define a primary cause. It is frustrating when the pathologic diagnosis is not causal, exemplified by diagnoses such as arthrogryposis, skeletal dysplasia, and demyelinating disease. Well-defined causes of birth defects must serve as models that allow presumptive conclusions or lines of investigation to be formulated in ambiguous cases.

Chromosomal abnormalities

Chromosome abnormalities, arising as defects of male or female meiosis, of fertilization, or of the first cell division(s) of the zygote, are the most common causes of death and developmental abnormalities in humans.[28–32] Mutations affecting the meiotic process, although well known in other organisms, remain essentially unexplored in humans. However, the method of fluorescent in situ hybridization (FISH) for individual chromosomes has been applied successfully to sperm, documenting, for example, a non-disjunction rate of 0.31–0.34% for each chromosome[32] Gamete and early zygote lethality rarely come to the attention of the fetal pathologist, but are more likely studied by the reproductive biologist–geneticist and in vitro fertilization specialists. In early embryonic growth disorganization, chromosome abnormalities are very common (see Ch. 4).[33, 34]

The hallmarks of chromosomal disease are **mental retardation and multiple congenital anomalies.** The first cannot be recognized in the perinatal period and the second may be subtle. Karyotyping is freely applied to suspect cases. If a patient has the **multiple minor and major malformations** illustrated in Figure 2.9, a karyotype is mandated.[28–32] Chromosome abnormalities are sometimes found in apparently normally developed embryos. At other times they occur in embryos with

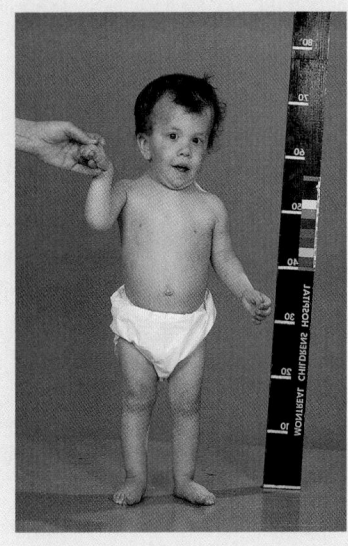

FIGURE 2.9 Patient with 92,XXXX/90,XX tetraploidy mosaicism (7.2% of lymphocytes, 26% of fibroblasts), showing short stature, pterygium colli, hypoplastic nipples, and broad chest. (From Wilson GN, Vekemans MJJ, Kaplan P. MCA/MR syndrome in a female infant with tetraploidy mosaicism: review of human polyploidy phenotype. Am J Med Genet 1988; 30:953, with permission.)

single major anomalies such as large nuchal blebs, limb anomalies, clefts, or holoprosencephaly. The earlier the stage of development, the less specific is the phenotype. The most common prenatal effects of aneuploidy are on **growth** and **phenogenesis** (Table 2.1), but patients with identical chromosomal anomalies may vary greatly in phenotype.[35, 36] **Mosaicism** (see Fig. 2.9) is one confounding factor, and the extent of mosaicism in both somatic and placental tissues has only recently been appreciated. **Confined placental mosaicism** may explain why some children with trisomy 13 exhibit fetal growth retardation while others have normal or increased birth weights.

The conspicuous and well-known effects of aneuploidy on phenogenesis are responsible for unique combinations of non-specific minor anomalies.[37–39] Clinical diagnosis is usually easier in later stages of fetal development. Since many of these defects of phenogenesis are subtle, more or less subjective changes are lost with increasing maceration after fetal death. However, one aspect of phenogenesis that does not change after death is the dermatoglyphic configuration of palms, soles, fingers, and toes. Desquamated skin can be unwrinkled carefully in fixative and examined under the dissecting microscope, allowing the diagnosis of Down syndrome when the soft facial tissues have virtually liquefied. Dermatoglyphic changes in Down syndrome include distal axial triradii, large hypothenar ulnar loop, third interdigital distal loop, and radial loops on the fourth and/or fifth fingers.

Mendelian mutations

Gene mutations, in heterozygous or homozygous state, are recognized with increasing frequency as causes of fetal death.[40, 41] Among these fetuses must be many with previously undescribed

TABLE 2-1 CHARACTERISTICS OF ANEUPLOIDY AND POLYPLOIDY[18–23, 32]

Defects of growth[24] (see Chapter 4)	GD-1 stage: anembryonic sac
	GD-2 stage: nodular embryo (no landmarks)
	GD-3 stage: cylindrical embryo (no landmarks, retinal pigment)
	GD-4 stage: stunted embryo, distorted body shape
	Fetal stage: microcephaly, growth retardation
Defects of blastogenesis	Increased monozygotic twinning; Higher frequency midline anomalies
Defects of organogenesis	Vestigia: Meckel diverticulum, persistent urachus; Atavisms: sesamoid bones, taurodontism; Other variants: colic; vertebral, renal arteries; cervical and spinal ganglia; persistence of platysma muscle
Defects of phenogenesis	Multiple minor anomalies; Loss of family resemblance
Defects of postnatal life	Neoteny: fetal facial characters, clinodactyly
	Functional defects: mental retardation, infertility
	Dysplasias: cancer susceptibility, weak connective tissue
	Altered homeostasis[34]: accelerated aging, immune defects

mendelian diseases that are not postnatally viable and present either in sporadic form (as new mutation) or as recurrent fetal losses due to segregation of an autosomal or X-linked lethal gene. Sublethal mutations may result in fetal death in one pregnancy or the birth of a defective child in another pregnancy.[42, 43]

Autosomal Dominant Inheritance

Autosomal dominant mutations are less common than autosomal recessives and on the whole less deleterious. Virtually none is completely dominant; however, the homozygous state of autosomal dominant mutations is so rare that it is difficult to predict their phenotypic effects. In homozygous achondroplasia the genetic hypothesis is based on the fact that both parents are evidently affected and the fetus/infant is much more severely involved than the most severe heterozygous case. The hypothesis is now capable of verification on the basis of molecular testing with appropriate probes from the mutation of the fibroblast growth factor receptor 3 gene at the tip of the short arm of chromosome 4.

In humans it has also been demonstrated that small deletions, responsible for contiguous gene syndromes, may segregate as dominant mutations; a striking example is the velo-cardiofacial syndrome due to deletion of 22q11. If the deletion is sufficiently extensive, the patient may have a more severe condition, including the DiGeorge sequence. More extensive deletions can be detected by high-resolution (prometaphase) chromosome analysis; smaller deletions require 22q11-specific DNA probes or FISH, and appear as one rather than two signals (see Ch. 6). Small deletions visible by prometaphase analysis are called microdeletions, while those visible only with DNA probes are submicroscopic deletions. High-resolution karyotyping and DNA studies have causally unified a range of phenotypes (including some cases of CHARGE association, Shprintzen syndrome, and isolated conotruncal heart defects) by the presence of deletions in the 22q11 region. This group of disorders is now known as CATCH spectrum, derived from common but variable affliction with cardiac defects, abnormal

face, thymic hypoplasia, cleft palate, and hypocalcemia. Their variable phenotype is illustrated by the patients in Figure 2.10: the girl in Figure 2.10A and B has the prominent nose, high palate, pulmonic stenosis, and long fingers typical of Shprintzen syndrome, while the boy in Figure 2.10C and D has the choanal atresia, colobomas, and micropenis typical of CHARGE association. Although both had standard karyotypes that were normal, neither underwent FISH studies of the 22q11 region.

The multiple effects of such mutations are designated **pleiotropy**: autosomal dominant cases frequently represent relational pleiotropy, i.e., a cascade of effects due to a basic underlying abnormality. **Connective tissue disorders such as Marfan syndrome, Erdheim syndrome, or Kniest dysplasia** illustrate this concept. However, autosomal dominant mutations also involve malformations and malformation syndromes that are not solely dysplasias: **receptor defects, regulator mutations, and preneoplastic conditions such as Beckwith-Wiedemann syndrome, neurofibromatosis, or Gardner syndrome.**[11,12] Some dominant cancer mutations may cause cancer at one site earlier in life and at another later on (e.g., retinoblastoma with subsequent osteosarcoma). It is now apparent that **all cancers involve genetic and/or epigenetic changes,** and it is prudent practice to preserve cancerous and non-cancerous tissue for subsequent molecular studies. This maxim applies particularly in *sporadic cases* that can represent **either two somatic defects or one somatic defect plus a germline defect.** A patchy lesion, rather than generalized involvement, may reflect a somatic mutation (e.g., segmental neurofibromatosis); occurrence in two or more offspring born to phenotypically normal parents may represent germinal mosaicism.

Autosomal Recessive Inheritance

Autosomal recessive disorders are a frequent class of mendelian mutations in humans. All persons must be heterozygous carriers of at least a half-dozen disease-causing autosomal recessive mutations. Because of their hidden nature and the present constraints on human reproduction, it is difficult to

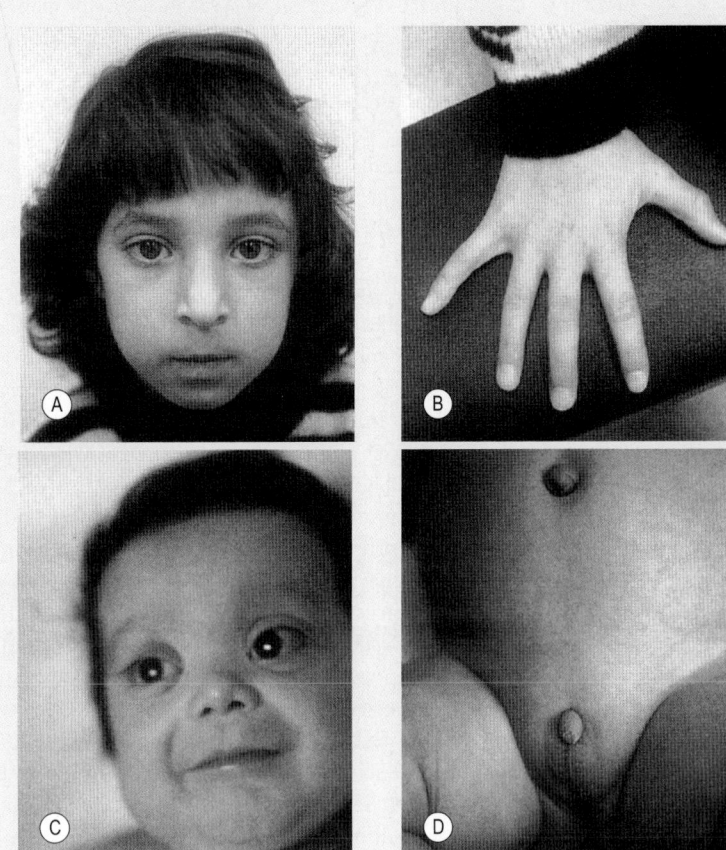

FIGURE 2.10 Patient with Shprintzen syndrome, illustrating the prominent nose (A) and thin fingers (B). Patient with CHARGE association, illustrating (C) a slightly unusual face with corrected choanal atresia, abnormal ears (not shown), and (D) micropenis.

determine whether the high gene frequency in certain cases (e.g., cystic fibrosis) is due to a past or present selective advantage, as has been demonstrated convincingly in the case of several hemoglobinopathies with respect to malaria. The rarer the autosomal recessive disorder, the higher is the rate of parental consanguinity and the greater the chance of confined ethnic occurrence. Only a small fraction of all autosomal recessive disorders have been described, and many of these (perhaps several thousand) are likely to be discovered by fetal genetic pathologists. When the segregation ratio in a given disorder is less than 25% (with equal sex ratio), prenatal lethality must be expected in cases of prenatal loss. In general, **autosomal recessive disorders are more severe, more commonly lethal, and more complexly pleiotropic than autosomal dominant mutations;** they often affect growth, intellect, and fertility adversely.

Unusual mechanisms for expression of autosomal recessive traits include **loss of heterozygosity and uniparental disomy.**[43] Deletion of a locus on one chromosomal homologue may make an autosomal recessive mutation manifest, i.e., hemizygous. Inheritance of identical mutant alleles (autozygosity) may occur by **uniparental isodisomy,** where both chromosome homologues of the offspring derive from a single parental chromosome (maternal or paternal isodisomy). In these situations, the effects of autozygous recessive alleles must be distinguished from the effects of genomic imprinting. Two examples of cystic fibrosis produced by uniparental isodisomy for chromosome 7 have been reported (see Ch. 1).

Some autosomal recessive disorders, such as the short rib polydactyly syndromes, are seen predominantly by the fetal pathologist; others after long postnatal care by such specialists as neonatologists, pediatricians, and oncologists. Many autosomal recessive disorders are inborn errors of metabolism; however, in many complexly pleiotropic conditions, e.g., Ellis–van Creveld syndrome, no metabolic defect has been found (yet). The examples of Zellweger syndrome, mucopolysaccharidoses and mucolipidoses, RSH (Smith-Lemli-Opitz) syndrome, mevalonic acidemia, and glutaric acidemia type II should serve as encouragement to search for metabolic defects in more autosomal recessive conditions. **In the autosomal recessive DNA repair/ chromosome breakage syndromes such as ataxia telangiectasia, xeroderma pigmentosum, Fanconi syndrome, Bloom syndrome, and Nijmegen breakage syndrome, there may be growth disturbances, malformations, and a greatly increased cancer risk.** A cancer risk may also be present in a non-breakage condition such as Perlman syndrome. **Cancer risks are probably greater in autosomal dominant than in autosomal recessive mutations.** At times, the homozygous state of an autosomal recessive disorder in the mother may adversely affect the development of all her fetuses, as in maternal phenylketonuria (PKU) or hypothyroidism.

X-linked Inheritance

X-linked mutations exert their deleterious effects primarily in a hemizygous state, although the vagaries of lyonization may cause some heterozygotes to manifest recessive traits. In **X-linked dominant disorders, all carriers are affected,** but, on the average, less than the hemizygotes. Some X-linked dominant mutations are viable only in heterozygotes; hemizygotes of such conditions may present as stillborn (abnormal) fetuses. These presumed **X-linked lethal defects include incontinentia pigmenti, Aicardi syndrome, focal dermal hypoplasia, orofaciodigital syndrome type I, and possibly also Rett syndrome.** It is perhaps not surprising that so many X-linked mutations affect the structure and function of the CNS, given that the CNS is the largest and most complex organ system with the longest developmental period, and that the X chromosome may be the site of over 6% of all human genes. Many genes on the X chromosome are also involved in CNS, eye, and gonadal development and function in various metabolic paths.

Unique to the X chromosome is the *cis*-acting **X inactivation center** on the long arm and its central role in the process of **lyonization,** with subsequent effects on the expression of X-linked structural or functional mutations. The second X is probably inactivated at different times in different tissues early during embryogenesis, and if one of the two X chromosomes carries a deleterious mutation, **developmental selection** may eliminate from a given tissue or organ the cell line in which the X with the mutant gene is active. Otherwise, the expectation is of a random, patchy distribution of mutant and non-mutant sectors of chromosome expression.

Considering its relatively large size and genetic density, the 'X-and-sex connection' of the X chromosome is not primary but rather supportive, in that ovaries develop in the absence of the Y, and the gonadal dysgenesis of the 45,X constitution most likely represents an aneuploidy effect. X-linked gonadal dysgenesis in 46,XY individuals (Swyer syndrome) points to genes of importance in gonadal–genital development after primary sex determination in males. The gonadal dysgenesis seen in 46,XX individuals with various X deletions in part represents an aneuploidy effect, and in part may indicate the location on the X of specific genes involved in ovarian and other developmental processes. 46,XX males represent a heterogeneous group of individuals who may have material from the short arm of the Y chromosome translocated to the short arm of the X, or who may have autosomal mutations that may also express themselves (sometimes in a sib) as hermaphroditism, i.e., development of ovarian and testicular tissue.

Y-Linked Inheritance

Because individuals without Y chromosomes have the traits of Ullrich-Turner syndrome (45,X), this small chromosome must 'cure' 46,XY individuals of their single-X-ness. Y chromosome loci may offset a relatively non-specific aneuploidy effect, or include genes that were formerly homologous to X chromosome loci but were later rearranged so as to prevent side-by-side pairing of the X and Y. Prevention of X/Y side-by-side pairing and crossover is necessary to preserve stability of the human sex-determining mechanism.

The SRY gene on the short arm of the Y chromosome needs help in effecting primary sex determination, i.e., in causing the medulla of the primitive gonad to differentiate into a testis. This need for additional genes to effect male sex determination is shown by the existence of (rare) 46,XX males and hermaphrodites without translocated Y material, of several forms of 46,XY gonadal dysgenesis in phenotypic females, and of many different syndromes with associated gonadal dysgenesis in genetic males (e.g., the campomelic and Smith-Lemli-Opitz syndromes).[44] One of the most dramatic demonstrations of the epistatic role of autosomal genes in the human sex-determining process is the case of an adolescent 46,XY woman who presented with Swyer syndrome and bilateral gonadoblastomas, and whose 46,XY brother with pseudovaginal perineoscrotal hypospadias and a phenotypically apparently normal father shared the same mutation of the SRY gene. Among the 'extra' genes involved in male sex differentiation are those responsible for müllerian duct suppression, 5 α-reductase expression, adrenal–gonadal steroidogenesis, and hypothalamic regulation of gonadotropins.

Abnormalities That Exhibit Atypical Inheritance Mitochondrial mutations, genomic imprinting, somatic or germline mosaicism, and triplet repeat amplification challenge conventional assumptions about gene action and transmission; a normal family history and normal results of biochemical–cytogenetic testing do not rule out a genetic cause. As with tumors, storage of tissues from perinatal cases with unexplained and unusual anomalies may yield future benefits.

Atypical Inheritance

Normal mitochondrial DNA (mtDNA) is a circular molecule of 16 569 base pairs (bp) that contains 37 genes encoding 22 types of tRNA, two types of ribosomal RNA, and 13 enzymes involved in oxidative phosphorylation.[45] Because spermatozoa do not contribute mitochondria to the zygote, **mitochondrial mutations are inherited only from the mother,** giving a striking inheritance pattern. If the mutation arose in the mother and her egg cytoplasm also contains non-mutant mtDNA molecules, the variable (heteroplasmic) distribution of the two types of mtDNA in different tissues in the body may make for extremely variable expression of the mutant phenotype, ranging from imperceptible degrees of involvement to lethality in given cases. To date, the known effects of mtDNA mutations are mostly metabolic and apparently degenerative diseases (such as MELAS: *m*itochondrial myopathy, *e*ncephalopathy, *l*actic *a*cidosis, and *s*troke-like episodes) that have an A to G substitution at position 3243 of leucine tRNA. A fraction of Japanese patients with insulin-dependent diabetes mellitus, non-insulin-dependent diabetes mellitus (NIDDM), and diabetes and deafness also carry this mutation, at times with a risk for MELAS in a relative.[46] Compared with maternal diabetes predisposition to malforma-

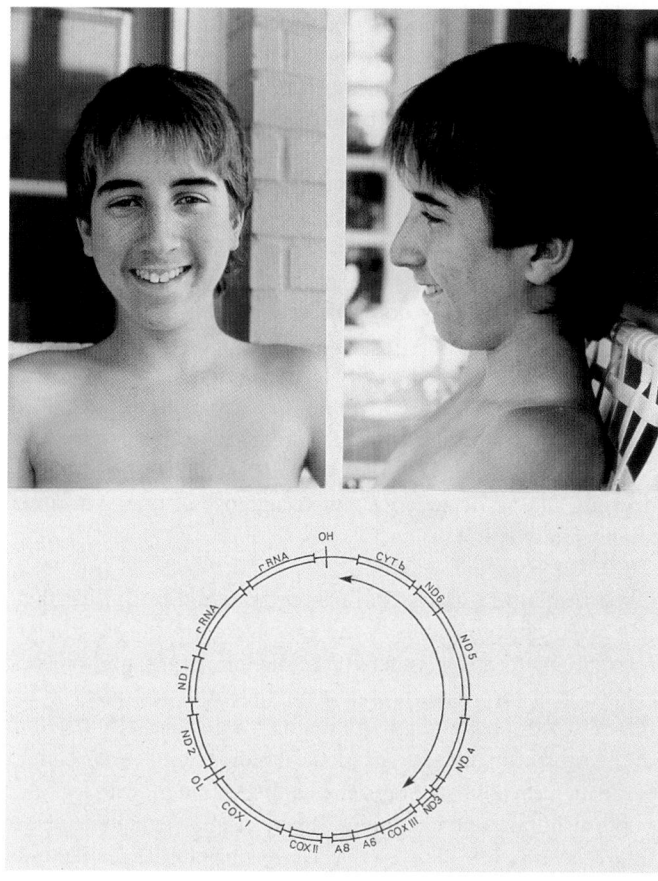

FIGURE 2.11 Patient with Pearson syndrome and a diagram of mitochondrial DNA illustrating his deletion.

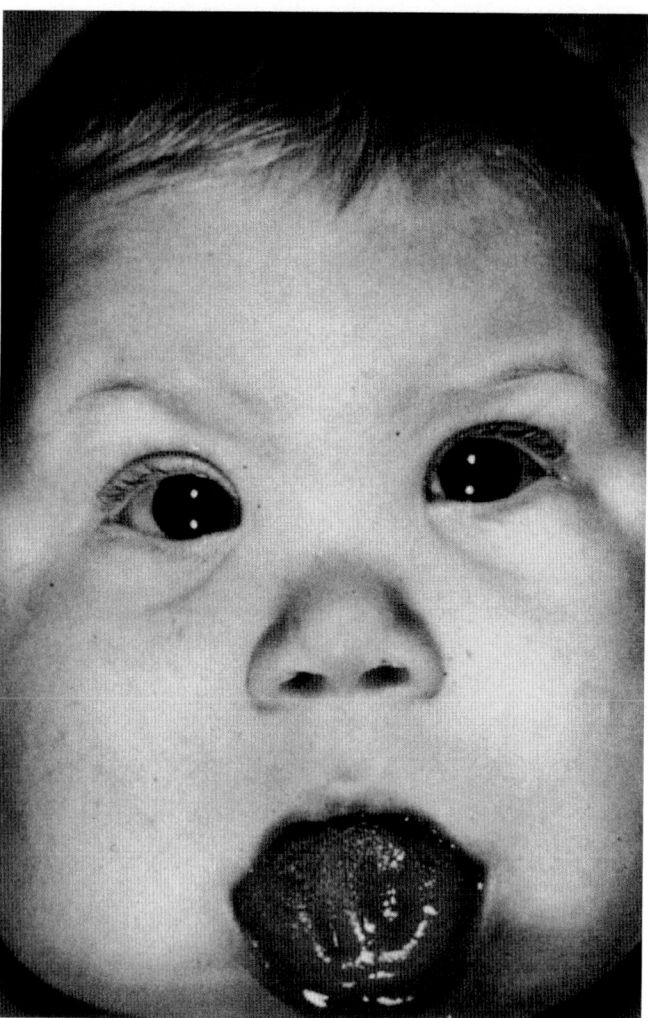

FIGURE 2.12 Patient with Beckwith-Wiedemann syndrome with macroglossia.

tion in their infants, mitochondrial mutations are a rare cause of birth defects. Figure 2.11 shows a child with Pearson syndrome and the extent of his mitochondrial deletion. He presented with anemia and marrow failure but also has ataxia and muscle weakness. There has been an increase in his normal mitochondria with age, perhaps because the deletion encompasses the mtDNA replication region.

Genomic Imprinting Like those described for the del(22)(q11) group, microdeletions at chromosome band 15q11 were detected in both the Prader-Willi and Angelman syndromes (see Ch. 1). **Molecular analysis resolved this dilemma, using DNA restriction polymorphisms to demonstrate that patients with Prader-Willi syndrome always had deletions in the paternally derived chromosome 15, while patients with Angelman syndrome always had deletions in the maternally derived chromosome 15.** Extensive experiments in mice had identified the phenomenon known as genomic imprinting. Mouse eggs were reconstituted to contain two maternal or two paternal pronuclei. In contrast to normal zygotes formed from one maternal and one paternal pronucleus, uniparental zygotes formed only embryonic tissue or only placental tissue. These experiments explained why parthenogenesis does not occur in

mammals, and demonstrated that the parental source of genetic material may be as important as its quantity and quality.[47]

As expected from the mouse experiments, some patients with Prader-Willi or Angelman syndromes have no deletions at the chromosomal or DNA level. Rather, they have uniparental disomy for the 15q11.2 region when evaluated using DNA polymorphisms. As discussed in Chapter 1, the **Beckwith-Wiedemann syndrome (BWS)** of hypoglycemia, omphalocele, and visceromegaly also exhibits imprinting effects (Fig. 2.12).[48] **Duplications of paternally derived chromosome region 11p15** are observed in BWS, and these cases have **increased expression of the insulin-like growth factor 2 (IGF2) locus** that lies in this region. **Euploid BWS cases exhibit paternal uniparental disomy for region 11p15** and also have increased expression of IGF2. Completing the story is homology of the 11p15 region to a portion of mouse chromosome 7 that is known to be imprinted. Mouse *Igf2* alleles are expressed when inherited from the father but inactive when inherited from the mother. Demonstration that *Igf2* imprinting can be relaxed after fibroblast culture provides another potential cause of BWS

– either there is germline uniparental disomy/deletion or the imprinted expression of paternal *IGF2* genes is lost in certain tissues (relaxation of imprint, deletion). The same phenomenon of **relaxed imprinting has been observed for the nearby WT1 (Wilms' tumor suppressor) locus** in Wilms' tumor cells, which may explain why some BWS patients are predisposed to Wilms' tumor.[48]

Triplet Repeat Expansion The **amplification of tandem 3-bp repeats** from several to many thousand copies in the DNA of individuals with **fragile X syndrome** provided a new model for inheritance.[49] Not only did triplet repeat instability yield unprecedented mutation rates (virtually one per gene per generation in female fragile X carriers), but progressive repeat expansion in successive generations vindicated the genetic phenomenon of **anticipation.** Worsening of phenotype as a function of vertical transmission is being sought in numerous disorders, since 50–100 loci have runs of triplet repeats. Instability may be greater in female (fragile X, myotonic dystrophy) or male (Huntington disease) meiosis. Various pedigree patterns can be expected that will vie with imprinting and mitochondrial inheritance in their distortion of mendelian rules. Normal 'transmitting' grandfathers of fragile X males present a graphic example of a genetic cause of 'sporadic' cases.[49]

Multifactorial Abnormalities

Most human malformations occur per se, i.e., are non-syndromal conditions, are relatively common, represent anomalies of incomplete development, and usually occur sporadically with a low recurrence risk, generally in the 3–5% range. They may show deviations from a normal sex ratio and differences in prevalence in different ethnic groups or geographic areas. Recurrence risk may be affected by severity of the lesion in the proband and by family history, so that the greater the number of affected relatives, the higher is the recurrence risk. This evidently non-mendelian behavior is explained in several different ways, the most widely accepted model being biparental inheritance of predisposing genes of additive effect; these genes interact with environmental factors to reduce the probability that a given developmental process will successfully cross a threshold toward completion. This polygenic environmental interaction model is referred to as multifactorial determination (not inheritance). It has been challenged through alternative suggestions of modified single-gene inheritance; the mutation rates involved and/or selective advantages keep such deleterious genes in the population at remarkably high frequencies.

The model of single-gene predisposition to malformations has found its most powerful and best developed expression in the work of Kurnit and co-workers,[50] who successfully simulated continuously distributed liability curves with thresholds under the assumption of a single, major predisposing gene with stochastic properties. Such a gene–defect association is demonstrated in non-syndromal cleft lip, with or without cleft palate, and the transforming growth factor-α (*TGF-α*) gene on the basis of a highly significant association between a *Taq*I RFLP and such

clefting.[51] **All familial occurrence of presumed multifactorial traits must be scrutinized carefully for potential evidence of segregation, given that uncommon mendelian forms of all these malformations have been described.**

Some of these malformations are associated with a paradoxically high rate of fetal death. Nishimura and colleagues[52] and Shiota[53] demonstrated prenatal mortality rates as high as 97.6% for neural tube defects, almost 100% for cyclopia/holoprosencephaly, and 88–94% for cleft lip. These rates were observed in apparently non-syndromal therapeutic termination cases (without chromosome analysis), suggesting that a second threshold may involve lethality. **Environmental factors contributing to multifactorial anomalies** have been identified, especially in the case of neural tube defects where preconceptional addition of **0.4–0.8 mg/day of folic acid to the diet can prevent 70% of occurrence and recurrence of non-syndromal anencephaly/spina bifida.**[54]

Environmental Causes 'Pure' environmental birth defects do not exist, and considering the massive exposure of modern populations to drugs, other chemicals, infections, and physical agents, it is surprising how few birth defects are more or less directly attributable to environmental causes (see Ch. 10). One of the most difficult tasks of medical biology and epidemiology is the identification of teratogens, a process fraught with legal and political implications and attended by a considerable degree of imprecision unless the case is as clear-cut as in the thalidomide, iodine deficiency, and retinoic acid embryopathies. The case for human teratogenicity is bolstered by successful induction of the same or pathogenetically similar pattern of anomalies in one or more than one species of experimental animals. Radiation, hyperthermia, infection, and teratogen (chemical) disruption sequences are the most striking environmental causes; metabolic disruptions constitute disorders in the mother that present relative (maternal diabetes) or absolute (maternal PKU) risks to the fetus. However, maternal metabolism is amenable to environmental control measures.

By stringent criteria, few drugs and chemicals in common use can be proved to be human teratogens.[55] Considerably more are teratogenic in two or more animal species.[55] Numerous reports in humans have related teratogenic effects to drugs and chemical exposure during pregnancy (see Ch. 10). Schardein[55] and Shepard[56] offer excellent guides to the teratogenic literature, which may be supplemented by calling telephone hotlines at certain governmental or academic centers,[57] and by reviews on the teratogenic disruptions.[58–60] Only one environmental chemical – methyl mercury – has proved to be a teratogen.

Pathogenesis – developmental classification

For too long in medical history the terms monster (or monstrosity), malformation, and funny-looking kid (FLK) served to distinguish defects of blastogenesis, organogenesis, and phenogenesis, respectively. The only one of these terms still serving a useful but less specific function is malformation. This term, by formal definition and common use, now refers to any primary (intrinsically caused) defect of development, whether of blastogenesis or organogenesis. There has been a recent tendency to refer to the minor anomalies of phenogenesis as 'dysmorphic features.' This term should be avoided, since it is undefined and indefinable; in common use it is indiscriminately applied to the mild malformations of blastogenesis and organogenesis and to the minor anomalies of phenogenesis. Before these periods of human development and their abnormalities are reviewed, it is necessary to provide a brief historical summary of development.[61–68]

Historical notes

1. **Epigenesis** is the correct view of the **formal** events of the development of individuals.

2. The threefold parallelism of the structure of the earth and its fossils, of adult organisms, and of their prenatal stages has a historical explanation in the theory of **evolution,** i.e., of descent with modification through the action of natural selection.

3. **Genetics,** an intellectual child of embryology, is the science of the causal analysis of development and is the twentieth-century answer to the nineteenth-century question of the mechanisms of transmission of species characteristics from parent to offspring. Through the work of Galton, Johannsen, Fisher, and Wright[69] it also provides a basis for understanding darwinian 'continuous' variability in mendelian terms.

4. **Epigenetics,** a term coined by Waddington, also refers to the causal analysis of development; however, it does so in terms of the **epigenotype:** 'the **total** developmental system consisting of a series of interrelated developmental pathways through which the adult form of an organism is realized. It comprises the **totality** of interactions among genes and between genes and the non-genetic … environment resulting in the phenotype.'[70] Since evolution represents a series of ontogenies, i.e., gradual changes of epigenetic pathways not primarily reflecting genetic differences between generations, epigenetics may be viewed as the twentieth-century answer to the nineteenth-century question regarding the origin of phylogenetic novelty. Thus, a useful distinction must be made in developmental biology between the two adjectives **epigenetic** and **epigenesis,** one referring narrowly to the events of ontogeny from conception to sexual maturity, the other referring broadly to the developmental events that make evolutionary changes possible. In **molecular biology**, epigenetic refers to the chromatin-based control of gene expression (see Ch. 1).

5. The observations and inferences drawn by von Baer relate development and evolution in a correct, non-recapitulationist manner. Those of Meckel,[71, 72] relating malformations in humans to normal stages of development in 'lower' animals, were recapitulationist but also founded in scientific study of **atavisms.**

6. The distinction drawn by Owen between (biologic) analogy and **homology** became one of the most powerful concepts in the analysis of phylogenetic relatedness on the basis of similarity of structure and development by descent, with modification, from an ancestor with a prototypic developmental plan.

7. The **teratogenic** modifiability of development was the most important discovery of a distinguished French tradition of morphology, highlighting the environmental component of epigenetic systems and complementing the observations of corresponding or developmentally homologous malformations in different species.

8. The discoveries of **induction/determination** and **gradient fields** by experimental embryologists, operating largely without genetic theory or concepts, defined certain morphogenetic regions of the embryo in which developmental processes are spatially coordinated, temporally synchronized, and epimorphically hierarchical. This was as true of the **primary field,** i.e., the entire embryo at the beginning of gastrulation, as it was of the secondary, **epimorphic fields** that are established in the embryo near or at the end of gastrulation.

9. The discovery of the dysmorphogenetically reactive units of the embryo on the basis of (causal) **heterogeneity** also established the existence of developmental fields, i.e., regions or (dys)morphogenetic units of the embryo, in which the events are also spatially coordinated, temporally synchronized, and epimorphically hierarchical. The complementary nature of these two concepts of the developmental field is reinforced by the observation of corresponding malformations in different vertebrate species due to the homology of developmental processes (and occasionally of genetic mutations, as in the *splotch* mouse and human Waardenburg syndrome).

10. Since evolutionary changes of morphology represent changes of morphogenesis, and since all morphogenesis occurs in developmental fields, it seems evident that **the developmental field is the fundamental unit of development and of evolution.**

11. Separation of the disciplines of embryology and genetics occurred early in the twentieth century, as exemplified by the career of the American embryologist Morgan, who became a leading geneticist. This separation had disastrous effects on both disciplines, leading to the near-extinction of morphology and the loss by genetics of half its biologic basis. The replacement of morphology by biochemistry did not repair the loss; however, it did prepare the way for the present triumphant reunion of morphology and genetics through molecular biology.[24]

12. While the methods and results of molecular biology have provided extraordinarily gratifying confirmation of the concepts underlying the developmental field and its phylogenetic universality, its use of reductionism tends to unbalance the epigenetic (organicist) view of development, which is so strongly supported by teratology.

13. Thus, the **study of abnormal human development** demands at once an evolutionary perspective on life and a knowledge of anatomy, embryology, pathology, genetics, teratology, and molecular biology, reaffirming strongly the validity of a science of **morphology** as the study of form (normal or abnormal), and the causes of formation and transformation.

Developmental stages

The five stages of human development are outlined in Table 2.2 and illustrated in Figure 2.13.[73]

TABLE 2-2 PERIODS OF HUMAN DEVELOPMENT

Period	Description
Pregenesis (predevelopment, progenesis, pro-ontogenesis)	All stages of development from "separation of germline" early in parental embryogenesis, migration of primordial germ cells to primitive gonadal ridges with subsequent corticomedullary differentiation; division, growth, differentiation, maturation, and release of germ cells to moment of fertilization (GONADOGENESIS, GAMETOGENESIS, SYNGAMY, KARYOGAMY)
Embryogenesis (broadly speaking)	Development from fertilization until end of 8th developmental (10th menstrual or gestational) wk.
Blastogenesis	All stages of development from time of karyogamy until end of gastrulation (stage 12, days 27–28, closure of caudal neuropore, and end of formation of embryonic mesoderm from primitive streak); at this stage the entire embryo is "the primary field"
Organogenesis (or embryogenesis narrowly speaking)	Development from stage 13 (day 28) until end of stage 22 (8th wk, or days 55–56, with crown-rump length of almost 30 mm). Marked by two processes: MORPHOGENESIS (formation of organs in SECONDARY, EPIMORPHIC FIELDS) and HISTOGENESIS (differentiation of cells and tissues); end of 8th wk, i.e., of embryonic period, marks metamorphosis, transition to fetal period
Phenogenesis	Developmental period from metamorphosis until birth (38 wks); PHENOGENESIS involves growth and final attainment of all those qualitative and quantitative traits constituting family resemblance and racial affiliation
Postnatal Life	Growth, psychomotor development, physiologic maturation, puberty, reproduction, senescence, death

From Opitz JM: Blastogenesis and the "primary field" in human development, *Birth Defects* 29(1):3–37, 1993; with permission.

Pregenesis

Synonyms include predevelopment, progenesis, and pro-ontogenesis. This is a developmental process that extends from the origin of the primordial germ cells in the parental yolk sac to the moment of karyogamy creating the new offspring. The process of gonadogenesis involves migration of the primordial germ cells to their final destination around T10 where they settle in the loose connective tissue below the coelomic epithelium and adjacent to the mesonephroi. Interaction between dividing germ cells and mesonephric and coelomic epithelia leads to the formation of the primitive bipotential gonad. In both sexes, this comprises cortex and medulla containing germ cells invested with follicle cells, which become granulosa cells in the female and Sertoli cells in the male.

It is important to realize that the male and female gametes that fuse at karyogamy have a long pregenetic history (see Fig. 2.13). The new embryo is established from parental germ cells that developed while the parent was within the grand-maternal womb. Genetic or teratogenic effects on the grand-maternal gestation may thus alter the differentiation or migration of parental primordial germ cells; these alterations may then be expressed in the grandchild rather than in the parents (see Fig. 2.13). These **transgenerational** effects may include gene mutations that alter stem cells, or epigenetic changes that delay imprint erasure or alter reprogramming of the germ cell

genome to match the genetic sex (see Ch. 1 for discussion of imprinting).

A complex genetic interaction between the product of the **SRY gene** on the short arm of the Y chromosome and numerous autosomal gene products is required for successful **transformation of the primitive gonad into the testis;** in the absence of the SRY gene product, the cortex becomes the ovary. In the male, **gametogenesis** does not begin until puberty and may continue into old age; in the female, meiosis begins in the fifth month of development and ends at menopause (see Fig. 2.13). Meiosis in the offspring represents the final 'consummation' of the mating of the parents; it is at this time that the maternal and paternal homologues of each chromosome pair undergo synapsis (pairing) before recombination and germ cell formation.

The many possible combinations of maternal and paternal homologues in the diploid, developing zygote are illustrated in Figure 2.14. These combinations are further augmented by crossovers during first meiosis. Thus, the greatest source of genetic novelty in offspring is not mutations but the reshuffling of the genome that occurs during parental meiosis. Female gametogenesis provides germ cells radically different in structure and function; the large amount of cytoplasm in the secondary oocyte contains a multitude of proteins and other gene products that have a dramatic impact on the initial development of the zygote, i.e., those stages before the genome of the zygote begins to be transcribed. Contribution of maternal

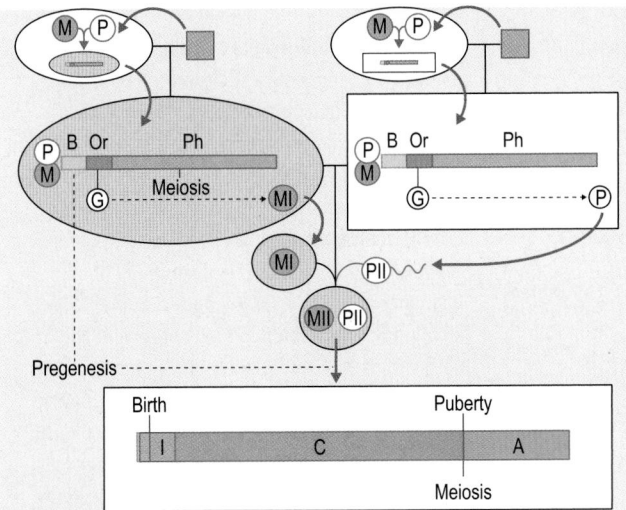

FIGURE 2.13 Developmental stages illustrated in a three-generation pedigree. Pregenesis begins as the primordial germ cells separate from the yolk sac, and continues to the moment when the gametes combine to form a new offspring (karyogamy). Blastogenesis (B: up to 4 weeks), organogenesis (Or: 4–8 weeks), and phenogenesis (Ph: 8–40 weeks) proceed to birth, followed by infancy (I), childhood (C), and adulthood (A). Note that development of the primordial germ cells and gonad (G) that will accomplish conception of the male child (*lower square*) actually occur during the grandparental pregnancy (*circles, upper row*). Germline defects (e.g., failure of imprint erasure, abnormal imprinting, gene mutations) that are expressed in grandchildren may derive from grandmaternal events (transgenerational effects). Note also the different timing in onset of meiosis in males (*squares*) versus females (*circles*).

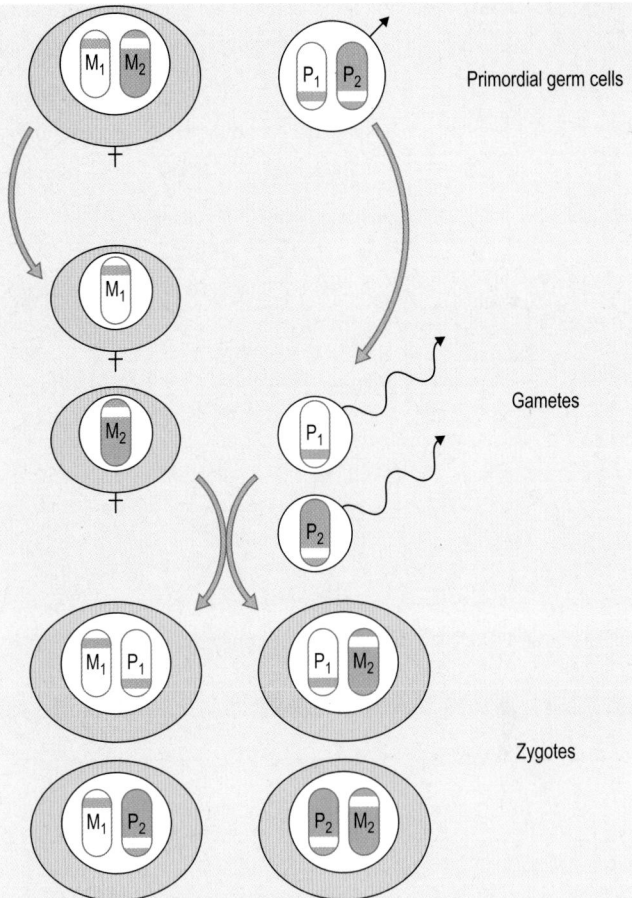

FIGURE 2.14 Karyogamy. The assortment of 23 pairs of chromosomes from each parent (M, mother, P, paternal) into haploid gametes leads to numerous combinations in zygotes. Note that the mother contributes cytoplasm to zygotes, and that genotype combinations would be amplified many times if all 23 chromosome pairs and additional recombinations (*bars*) were diagrammed.

cytoplasm to the zygote (see Fig. 2.14) accounts for two types of genetic diseases: 'maternal effect' mutations that are not yet described in humans, and **mitochondrial diseases** that are well documented.

Blastogenesis

This refers to all stages of development from the time of karyogamy and the first cell division to the end of gastrulation (stage 12, days 27–28, the time of closure of caudal neuropore, and the end of formation of intraembryonic mesoderm from primitive streak). The events during these **first 4 weeks of development** are illustrated in Figure 2.15 and summarized as follows:[61, 62, 64–66]

WEEK 1: Formation of a **'unilaminar' embryo**, i.e., of the inner cell mass within the blastocyst, 'hatching' of the blastocyst, and beginning implantation (stages 1–4, beginning stage 5).

WEEK 2: Formation of the **'bilaminar' embryo** (epiblast/hypoblast) with amniotic cavity and secondary yolk sac; appearance of primary villi and primitive streak (stages 5 and 6).

WEEK 3: Formation of the **'trilaminar' embryo** (ectodermal, mesodermal and endodermal) at the beginning of gastrulation, extending from stage 7 to stage 9. Embryos of the third week are

characterized by the appearance of a primitive streak with notochordal process and notochord; the first somites in the paraxial mesoderm; neural plate, neural folds, and neuromeres in presumptive brain vesicles; primitive heart tube and intraembryonic coelom; and primitive blood vessels and villi.

WEEK 4: The **final stages of blastogenesis** are very complex as they merge into definitive organogenesis (Figs 2.16 and 2.17). At the cephalic end, development is more advanced than at the caudal end. The fourth week includes Carnegie stages 10–13 and involves fusion of neural folds with ultimate closure of rostral (first) and caudal neuropores; formation of the branchial arches (see Fig. 2.15); formation of myocardium with beginning heartbeats (days 21–22) and later formation of the cardiac septa see (Fig. 2.17); beginning formation of the gastrointestinal tract with rupture of the buccopharyngeal plate (see Fig. 2.16); appearance of hepatic plate and of dorsal pancreatic bud and spleen; formation of the urorectal septum and appearance of ureteric buds (see Fig. 2.16); appearance of lung buds and optic vesicles with later lens placode

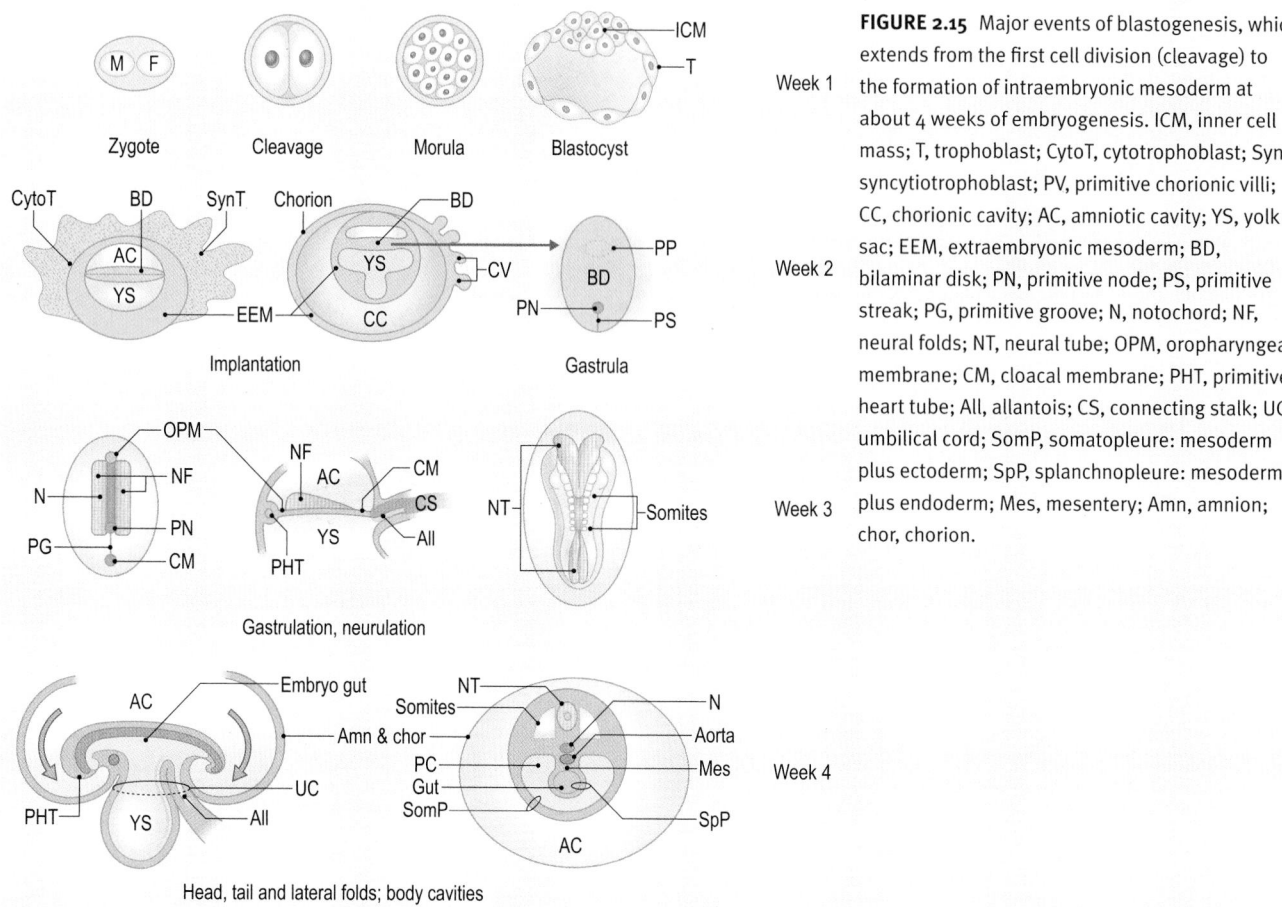

FIGURE 2.15 Major events of blastogenesis, which extends from the first cell division (cleavage) to the formation of intraembryonic mesoderm at about 4 weeks of embryogenesis. ICM, inner cell mass; T, trophoblast; CytoT, cytotrophoblast; SynT, syncytiotrophoblast; PV, primitive chorionic villi; CC, chorionic cavity; AC, amniotic cavity; YS, yolk sac; EEM, extraembryonic mesoderm; BD, bilaminar disk; PN, primitive node; PS, primitive streak; PG, primitive groove; N, notochord; NF, neural folds; NT, neural tube; OPM, oropharyngeal membrane; CM, cloacal membrane; PHT, primitive heart tube; All, allantois; CS, connecting stalk; UC, umbilical cord; SomP, somatopleure: mesoderm plus ectoderm; SpP, splanchnopleure: mesoderm plus endoderm; Mes, mesentery; Amn, amnion; chor, chorion.

(see Fig. 2.17); closure of the otic vesicle with beginning detachment from the overlying ectoderm; and formation of limb buds and extension of somites to number 28 to 30.

Thus, blastogenesis is characterized by four important processes:

1. **Gastrulation** with the formation of mesoderm and the appearance of the midline, cranial/caudal, right/left, and dorsal/ventral body axes; segmentation; and neurulation.
2. **Initiation of all developmental processes** and establishment of the mosaic of secondary epimorphic fields including neurogenesis, angiogenesis, and (meso) nephrogenesis.
3. **Initiation of laterality.**
4. **Initiation of placentation.**

The specific morphogenetic events of blastogenesis can be summarized as follows:

1. **Fusions,** involving the neural tube, cardiac tubes, and müllerian ducts (see Figs 2.15 to 2.17).
2. **Lateralizations** such as the optic fields or nasal placodes (see Fig. 2.17).
3. **Decussations,** e.g., corpus callosum, optic chiasma.
4. Segmentation of neuromeres, rhombomeres, paraxial mesoderm into somites, and pronephros (see Fig. 2.16).
5. **Lateral asymmetry formation** involving heart, situs, vitelline vessels, and tail curl (see Figs 2.15 and 2.16).
6. **Resorptions** such as endodermal lumina, buccopharyngeal and anal membranes, and pro- and mesonephroi.
7. **Fissions** such as division of the lung bud into right and left mainstem bronchi and lungs.
8. **Morphogenetic movements** including shifts in structural relationships; re-entry and rotation of the gut; migration of neural crest cells and primordial germ cells; endocardial cushion and septal cells (see Fig. 2.17).

William Harvey in 1651 referred to chick embryogenesis: '... the generation of the chick from the egg is the result of epigenesis, rather than of metamorphosis, and that all of its parts are not fashioned simultaneously, but emerge in their due succession and order; it appears, too, that its form proceeds simultaneously with its growth, and its growth with its form; also that the generation of some parts supervenes on others previously existing, from which they become distinct; lastly, that its origin, growth and consummation are brought about by the method of nutrition, and that at length the foetus is thus produced.'[74] No better summary of the process was possible in that era, and even now it can hardly be bettered.

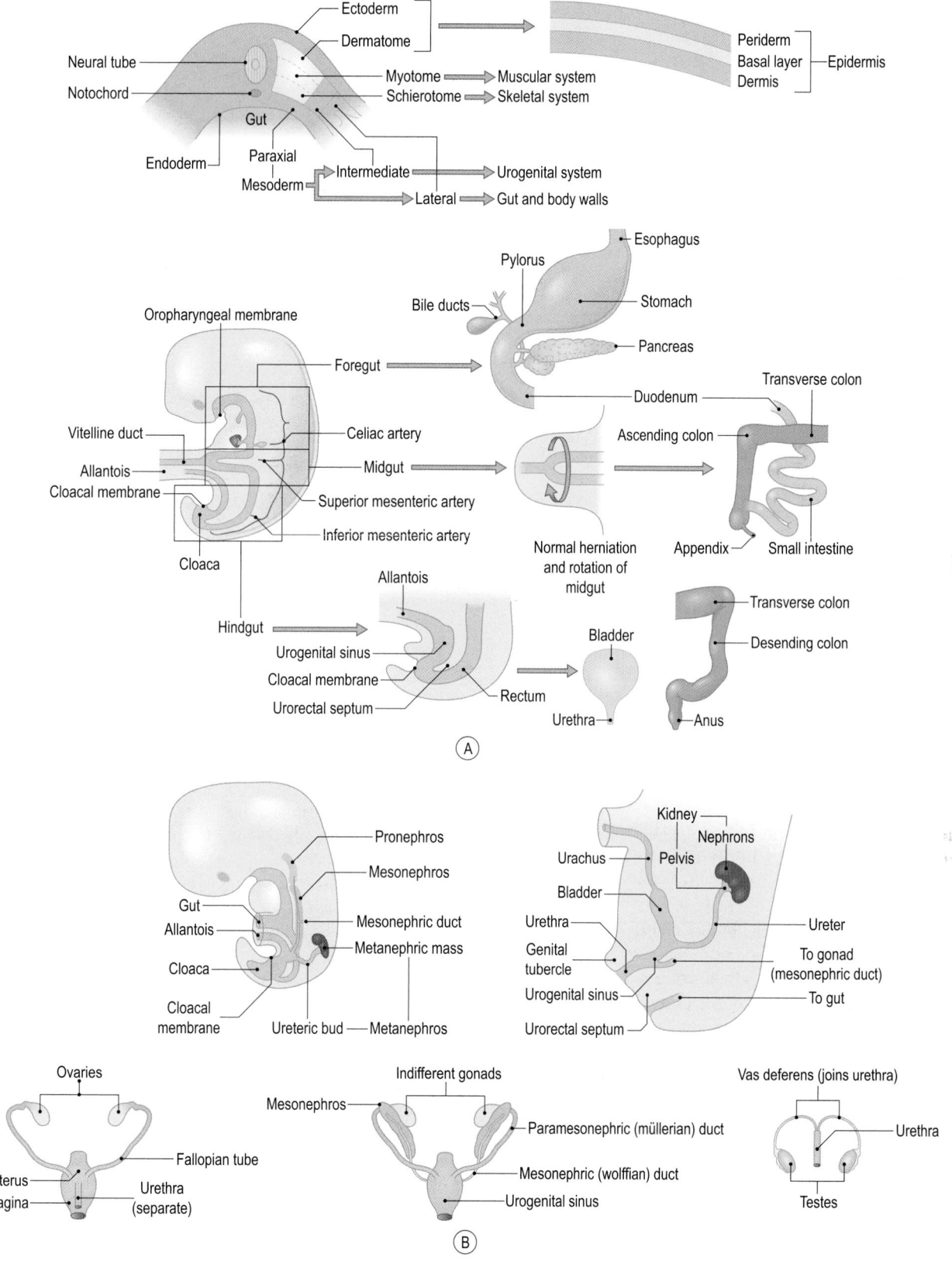

FIGURE 2.16 Organogenesis: derivatives of three germ layers. (A) Upper drawing shows major derivatives of the ectoderm, mesoderm (paraxial, intermediate, and lateral), and endoderm of each somite. Cranial development differs in that ectoderm combines with branchial arch mesoderm (ectomesenchyme) to form the craniofacial structures. The lower drawing illustrates gut development from foregut, midgut, and hindgut regions. Diverticula of the gut include the laryngotracheal tube, liver, pancreas, and spleen primordia. (B) Differentiation of intermediate mesoderm to produce the urogenital system.

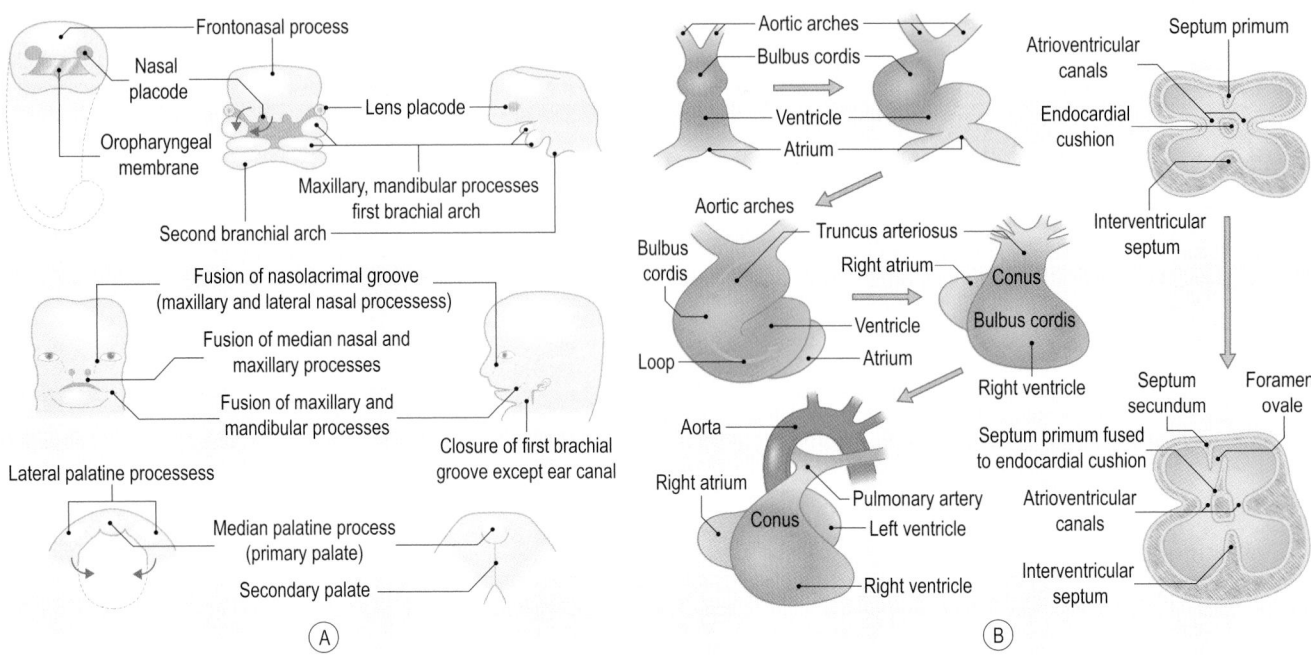

FIGURE 2.17 Organogenesis: differentiation of two important midline structures, the face and heart. (A) Facial development involves fusion of frontonasal processes and branchial arches to produce the face and palate. (B) Major events in cardiac development include dextral looping, splitting of the truncus to form the great arteries, and fusion of the endocardial cushions/cardiac septa *(right)*. Branchial derivatives include the aortic arches (major arteries) and conotruncal regions.

Organogenesis (or Embryogenesis)

This represents development from late stage 13 (day 28) and early stage 14 till the end of stage 23 (end of the eighth week, day 56), when the embryo has attained a crown–rump length (CRL) of 3 cm (see Fig. 2.13; Table 2.2). This stage is marked by three major processes: **growth, morphogenesis** (formation of organs and body parts in secondary, epimorphic fields), and **histogenesis** (differentiation of cells and tissues). Early during this second half of embryonic life the embryo continues active morphogenesis, but by the 'end of the fifth week the developmental history of the human embryo reaches a veritable turning point.'[75] Construction of the body has come to an end, and the embryo embarks on a period of extensive rebuilding of laid-out parts, designed as **metamorphosis.** At this stage the embryo has the generalized structure of fish and amphibian larvae, with striking resemblances among reptiles, birds, and mammals. In the human embryo the arm buds have shifted caudally, with the upper edge now at the root of the ninth somite. They and the leg buds are still flipper shaped. The prominent heart bulge contains the coiled, but still single, tubular heart. The arrangement of the aortic arches resembles most closely that of the frog larva. At this stage of development a transitory formation of gill rudiments may occur on the visceral arches of birds, and rarely even in mammals, e.g., the third branchial arch of the rabbit.[16,75]

Except for marsupials, the process of metamorphosis does not lead to actual terrestrial life, but to an extended fetal period during which locomotion, pulmonary respiration, oral food intake, and urinary excretion are partly or completely suspended. Witschi pointed out a serious and widespread form of heterochronism at this stage of development of the mammalian embryo, i.e., the appearance of traits not expected until much later when the embryo/fetus has reached a much more mammalian (rather than amphibian or fish-like) stage of development. A particularly striking example is the very early appearance of the mammary ridge and of the primordia of mammary glands, which appear during the early stages of embryonic metamorphosis even though in the evolution of mammals they must have originated at the late reptilian or at the mammalian level. According to Witschi, heterochronies at this stage of development are so numerous that the human embryo at the end of metamorphosis is a chimera of amphibian, reptilian, and mammalian characteristics.[75] Restructuring of the branchial arches leads to the formation of a new face (see Fig. 2.17), and conversion of the bilaterally symmetric aortic arch system leads to a single coordinated aortic arch system characteristic of the mature organism (except for functional ductus arteriosus). At the end of the eighth week, metamorphosis is complete and the embryo has become a fetus.

Phenogenesis

This is the developmental process that characterizes the human fetal period from the **beginning of the ninth week** (embryo/fetus with **30 mm CRL**) to the **time of birth at 38 weeks** (fetus with

500 mm CRL) (see Fig. 2.13; Table 2.2). The process of phenogenesis involves growth, ongoing differentiation, and functional maturation of organs and other parts of the body; return of the gut to the abdomen with simultaneous rotation (see Fig. 2.16); and the gradual acquisition of the body shape and proportions appropriate to a mature human fetus at birth. During this period also, the fetus attains all of those qualitative and quantitative characteristics that identify it as a primate mammal and also as a member of an ethnic group and a specific family. It is this more or less complete absence of family resemblance at birth, best identified by experienced older relatives, that may be the most sensitive and poignant initial indicator of aneuploidy.

Postnatal life is a continuation of phenogenesis after completion of the dramatic changes in adaption to extrauterine life. Many organs continue to undergo structural and functional differentiation, growth, and maturation, most notably the CNS, lungs, gut, kidneys and excretory system, and endocrine system, which results in dramatic changes of genitalia and secondary sexual characteristics in both sexes at puberty. Ears and nose continue to grow even into senescence. There is about a 25% lifetime risk of developing a cancer, and a much higher likelihood of developing carcinoma in situ of the prostate in men. Carcinogenesis in humans is attended by many genetic changes of oncogenes that have important functions in normal development, and thus the occurrence of cancer is a developmental process in reverse. The cumulative effects of other multifactorially determined processes such as atherosclerosis, diabetes, hypertension, chronic obstructive pulmonary disease, and Alzheimer's disease combine to bring about a cessation of life in humans between the ages of 80 and 100 years. However, recorded examples of male reproduction in the tenth decade of life, effective repair of fractures and wound healing, and high creativity after the age of 100 certainly confirm the old adage that it serves one well to pick one's parents with the utmost care.

Abnormalities of pregenesis, blastogenesis, and phenogenesis

Abnormalities characteristic of each human developmental period will now be outlined, followed by a summary and case examples illustrating causal and developmental analysis. More comprehensive discussion of abnormalities in each developmental category will be presented in Chapter 3.

Defects of pregenesis – aneuploidy

Although aneuploidy is usually established during pregenesis, it has effects throughout human development, which can be summarized as follows:
1. **Defects of growth (and organization) in early embryos.**[76] These include later intrauterine growth retardation and/or highly suggestive dyssynchronies of developmental processes – some on

schedule, many delayed to various degrees, rarely any that are advanced in developmental timing. To what extent fetuses with intrauterine growth retardation with or without anomalies are to be tested for confined placental mosaicism and uniparental disomy must await the outcome of further research.
2. **Defects in blastogenesis.** These begin with **monozygotic twinning,** which is increased in frequency in the Ullrich-Turner and Down syndromes.[77] Monozygotic or polar body twinning in the acephalus-acardia anomaly is associated with a high frequency (10/14 cases) of chromosome defects in the abnormal twin and a lesser, not necessarily concordant role of non-disjunction in the normal (pump) twin.
3. **Defects of organogenesis.** Malformations in aneuploidy syndromes are all non-specific and non-obligatory; **most are anomalies of incomplete development, few are anomalies of abnormal development** such as polydactyly. *Vestigia* are defined as (rudimentary) persistence into postnatal life of embryonic structures that are regularly present only in a transient manner in prenatal life. Well-known examples are persistent urachus, Meckel diverticulum, webbing of the second and third toes, persistence of tail, and branchial arch fistulas. It may ultimately become obvious that all anomalies of incomplete development are vestigia. **Atavisms** are a (rudimentary) development of an anatomic structure known or presumed to have been present in a phylogenetic ancestor and homologous to that observed in a living relative of that ancestor.[78, 79] The appearance of legs in whales and 'atavistic' polydactyly in horses and guinea pigs are well-known examples. Atavisms are frequent in aneuploidy, with the best-documented examples including several atavistic muscles in trisomies 21, 13, and 18; taurodontism and extra sesamoid bones in Down syndrome; and rare developmental variants in the Wolf-Hirschhorn (4p⁻), cat cry (5p⁻), del(18q), or mono-/polysomy X syndromes. These rare developmental variants include absence of muscles, unusual variations of the arteries (colic, vertebral, renal), striking variations of the first cervical and spinal accessory nerve ganglia, persistence of the occipital platysmal muscle (probably responsible for the unique physiognomy of Down syndrome children), and frequent biphalangy or brachymesophalangy of toes in Down syndrome, which seems to be an accentuation of an uncommon developmental variant that may be present in the normal population. These variants are probably examples of the reduced buffering of developmental paths first postulated by Shapiro.[79, 80]
4. **Defects of phenogenesis.** Most anomalies in aneuploidy and polyploidy syndromes are not gross defects of blasto- or organogenesis but rather of phenogenesis. These defects are called **minor anomalies,** and it is these that put the most characteristic stamp on aneuploid or polyploid individuals.[31, 32] Aneuploidy results during phenogenesis in multiple minor anomalies with abolition of family resemblance, and frequently reduced means and increased variances of morphometric traits.[79] This lack of family resemblance is a highly reliable diagnostic indicator of aneuploidy. It suggests the presence of other subjective anomalies not usually identified in clinical phenotype analysis and anthropometric assessment of the affected individual. Minor anomalies are not only the most common anomalies in aneuploid

individuals, but frequently the only anomalies, unless later dissection turns up clinically inapparent anatomic variations. Without question, the most important minor anomalies in aneuploidy and polyploidy syndromes are the highly quantifiable dermatoglyphic traits, which increase in diagnostic value to the extent that they are compared with the non-aneuploid first-degree relatives of the baby.

5. **Postnatal defects.** Even without gross or histologically demonstrable abnormalities, aneuploidies and polyploidies may alter the CNS, gonads, and growth so that mental retardation, hypotonia, seizures, behavior disturbances, infertility, and more rapid aging are present. Females with Ullrich-Turner syndrome lack normal ovarian differentiation, while males with Down syndrome are usually sterile because of abnormal spermatogenesis. The high incidence of Alzheimer-like changes in Down syndrome is well documented. Some of the manifestations of aneuploidy syndromes may be designated **neoteny,** i.e., retention of fetal developmental ('unfinished') characteristics in postnatal life. In Down syndrome, conspicuous examples of neotenic traits are persistence of fetal facial characteristics, brain structure, and fifth and second fingers. Aneuploid individuals are predisposed to malignancies, a trait that may be reflected in the increased rate of transformation of Down syndrome fibroblasts with SV40 virus.

Defects of pregenesis – gene interactions

As with chromosome aberrations, mutations in developmentally significant genes are established during pregenesis but may be expressed during one or more developmental periods. Gene mutations can act singly or through metabolic complexes and signaling pathways; the former exhibit mendelian patterns of transmission, the latter mendelian or multifactorial determination according to their individual impact. Some are modified by atypical mechanisms such as triplet repeat expansion or imprinting, others modulate the effects of intrauterine environment. Most examples are illustrated in discussion of later developmental periods or in Chapter 3, but a few principles are mentioned here:

1. Of particular interest in human pregenesis are the fruit fly genes that control gametogenesis and early pattern formation,[24] including those expressed in egg cytoplasm that exhibit maternal effect. Certain androgen receptor or Y chromosome mutations can alter spermatogenesis as discussed above, and these many genes that control gametogenesis, fertilization, pronuclear fusion, and oocyte function provide an intriguing area for exploration.

2. Genes with key roles in early pattern formation are likely to produce abnormalities of blastogenesis, illustrated by a number of X-linked genes listed in Chapter 1. The remarkable dissection of early development in simpler organisms provides many candidate genes for testing in humans since a large fraction of early pattern genes are conserved (30–50% from flies to humans; see Ch. 1).

3. Many mendelian mutations impact organogenesis as shown by skeletal disorders such as the brachydactylies and occasional mendelian inheritance of single anomalies such as cleft palate or isolated heart defects. Some ostensible organ defects may actually derive from blastogenesis through the agency of developmental fields (see below). The Holt-Oram syndrome is one of over 150 mendelian disorders that affect heart and hand, implying a common developmental pathway for genes such as TBX-3 that cause these disorders.[81]

4. Less devastating Mendelian mutations can accumulate and act with the environment to produce evolutionary change (long term) or multifactorial defects (short term); such interactions produce species-specific morphology on the one hand and abnormalities of phenogenesis on the other;[70] no wonder that taxonomy and dysmorphology are so similar.

5. Teratogens such as retinoic acid or thalidomide can act throughout gestation to produce anomalies of blastogenesis (brain anomalies), organogenesis (limb defects), and phenogenesis (minor external ear anomalies). As emphasized above, environmental agents are likely to be modified by genetic factors. A frontier analogous to that of maternal effect/gametogenesis mutations is to define teratogenic effects on early development. Maternal diethylstilbestrol can definitely impact fetal genital development and produce adult dysplasias, and it will be interesting to look for effects on egg constituents once these molecular profiles are sufficiently characterized. Characteristic molecular 'fingerprints' from teratogens would open an additional window on the high rates of embryonic death discussed above.

Anomalies of blastogenesis

Defects of earliest cell division, the formation of morula and blastula and of hatching and implantation, so far as they are incapable of spontaneous repair or result in viable forms of twinning, can be presumed to be lethal. However, there are probably defects of subcellular organization with incipient effects on the subsequent 3 weeks of embryonic development that constitute blastogenesis proper and that may lead, for example, to dysmorphogenetic effects largely confined to one side of the body. An impressive example of such a condition is a severe form of hemifacial microsomia that may be associated with hemivertebrae, ipsilateral defects of lung lobulation, renal and radial abnormality, eye defect, and mental retardation. Most lethal defects of the second week of human development probably represent chromosome aberrations; however, lethal or other grave impairments of development at that stage must be due to autosomal or X-linked mutations. The formation of the trilaminar disk and development of the midline during early gastrulation may be impaired by aneuploidy, polyploidy, a large number of known X-linked defects of blastogenesis, environmental factors, maternal–fetal metabolic disturbances such as diabetes, and all the common 'idiopathic' events that lead to the formation of **(sporadic) associations** (see Ch. 3 for examples).

Inductive–determinative processes occurring in developmental fields were discussed earlier.[73] Events occur in a spatially coordinated, temporally synchronized, and epimorphically hierarchical manner in morphogenetic fields.[35] The primary field is the entire embryo during the early stages of gastrulation. Secondary epimorphic fields appear at the end of blastogenesis.[23]

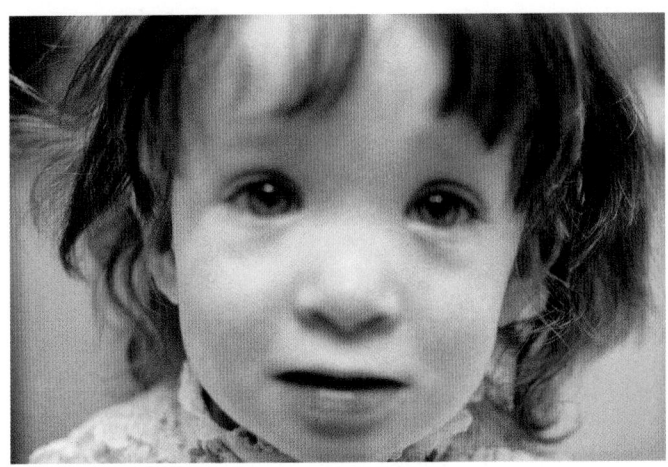

FIGURE 2.18 Patient with fetal alcohol syndrome showing telecanthus, absent philtrum, and thin vermilion border of the upper lip.

Heterogeneity defines dysmorphogenetically reactive units (DRUs), applying equally to the primary field and to the secondary fields (see above). The DRU concept complements the concept of morphogenetic units (MUs) or gradient fields of the experimental (molecular) embryologists so perfectly that they can be considered one and the same.[23, 82] It is remarkable that these developmental entities are shared by all vertebrates, and that there are so few. This extraordinary conservatism of developmental paths and mechanisms gives hope that ultimately their ontogenetic and phylogenetic aspects may be understood.[82, 83]

Blastogenetic abnormalities include monozygous twinning, malformations such as cyclopia or sirenomelia, associations, mendelian phenotypes, and some of the defects caused by teratogens such as maternal diabetes (patient 5B, below) or alcohol (Fig. 2.18). Examples will be presented in Chapter 3.

Anomalies of organogenesis

The later the stage of development, the greater is the number of secondary epimorphic fields, each probably having its own time of maximal sensitivity to endogenous or exogenous dysmorphogenetic causes. Examples include **localized limb defects, renal defects,** and **ear anomalies.** Determination of the latest time an abnormality could have come into being during ontogeny is not the equivalent of determining when the dysmorphogenetic cause acted or began to act. Many malformations appearing to have arisen during organogenesis were evidently determined during blastogenesis. Differential rates of development between sexes, between the two body halves (or identical twins!), and, more important, between the rostral and caudal parts of the embryo lead to the phenomena of abnormal sex ratios, unilaterality or right–left discordance (and non-concordance in identical twins), and involvement of upper or lower limbs with sparing of the others.

Also, the limbs depart from the rest of the body in one important (dys)morphogenetic peculiarity: deficiency of one limb segment may be associated with excess formation in another segment, an equivalent to excess formation in a homologous contralateral structure. Thus, tibial agenesis (a mesomelic defect) is frequently associated with preaxial polydactyly in the acromelic segment, at times to spectacular degrees.[83, 84] Autosomal dominant tibial agenesis/polydactyly may also show striking right–left discordance. Absence of a thumb (on one hand) may be associated with a contralateral triphalangeal or duplicated thumb. Thus, an agenesis in a paired body part can be a true malformation when it is the equivalent of an abnormally formed contralateral structure. Epistasis and epigenetic modifications of dysmorphogenetic potential can be spectacular, so that autosomal recessive radius aplasia may in one relative lead to virtual upper limb amelia (even with severe hypoplasia of the pectoral girdle), in another to mild thumb involvement, and in yet another to 'classic' radius/thumb aplasia with radial clubhand.

Regardless of how restricted, a part of an embryo remains a field so long as a dysmorphogenetic cause can still exert an obvious effect on its final development. The duration of such interactions can sometimes be inferred from clinical documentation, as shown by the anomaly spectrum/time of ingestion studies with thalidomide[85] discussed in Chapter 3. Epistasis can also be recognized though correlations among patients and families. In some members of families with autosomal recessive radius aplasia (discussed above) the only visible effect of the mutation may be on the distal phalanx of the thumb with broad and fenestrated distal phalangeal bone, mild abnormality of nail, and obvious effect on dermatoglyphic pattern.

The following is an attempt to contrast the types of anomalies that arise in the primary field with those that arise in the secondary fields:

1. Anomalies of blastogenesis tend to be severe, those of organogenesis less severe.
2. Anomalies of blastogenesis tend to be complex, those of organogenesis less complex.
3. Anomalies of blastogenesis tend to be multisystem anomalies or complex polytopic field defects such as the acrorenal field defect; those of organogenesis are more likely to be localized, monotopic field defects.
4. Anomalies of blastogenesis are frequently lethal, those of organogenesis less commonly lethal.
5. Anomalies of blastogenesis frequently involve defects of placentation or cord formation; except for the presence of a single umbilical artery, the umbilical cord, placenta, and body wall are usually normal in defects of organogenesis.
6. Defects of blastogenesis are frequently associated with MZ twinning, which is, by definition, an abnormality of blastogenesis; twinning is less common or not a factor in organogenetic malformations.
7. Sex differences in occurrence appear to be less conspicuous in blastogenetic malformations; in organogenetic malformations there are frequently striking sex differences, an apparent indicator of multifactorial determination.
8. Anomalies of blastogenesis are defects of the embryonic midline; defects of organogenesis are not confined to the midline.

9. Abnormalities of blastogenesis may constitute a cancer risk such as teratomas anywhere along the midline from skull to tip of coccyx; organogenetic malformations are rarely associated with a cancer risk.

10. Multiple congenital anomalies of blastogenesis are usually associations; multiple congenital anomalies of organogenesis are more likely to be syndromes representing pleiotropy due to mendelian mutations and/or chromosome abnormalities.

11. Mild 'hits' in blastogenesis may not produce grave defects or associations but may 'linger' in effect into organogenesis, as in mildly affected infants of diabetic mothers or those with the fetal alcohol or retinoic acid (Accutane) syndromes; thus, some apparent organogenetic anomalies may in fact represent mild defects of blastogenesis.

12. Primitive, initially poorly hemoglobinized, short-lived, permanently nucleated red blood cells of yolk sac origin do not appear in the villous capillaries until 4.5 weeks after fertilization;[86] even though the embryonic heart starts beating at 21 days after fertilization, vascular abnormalities are probably less likely a pathogenetic abnormality of blastogenesis than of organogenesis.

Abnormalities of phenogenesis

The later the stage of development, the clearer will be the developmental expression of normal ethnic traits and of family resemblance in the fetus. Thus, phenogenesis (fetal life) is the stage of development when humans acquire the metric attributes recorded in tables of hundreds of different anthropometric measurements of means and standard deviations, medians and centiles, and variances. In a normal fetus the attainment of these traits proceeds in a harmonious, synchronized manner so that at term (266 days) most fetuses have a length of 50 cm, a weight of 3500 g, and an occipitofrontal head circumference of 35 cm. These values vary somewhat according to ethnicity and sex. The methods of physical anthropology and human genetics have established the heritability of many of these traits. However, in addition to the anthropometric traits, less objective attributes of physical development are present in the facial appearance and ear structure of every fetus and infant; these are of equal value in determining family resemblance. It is these subtle, subjective traits that are of such great importance to the relatives of the infant when they perform their analysis of family resemblance and to clinicians when they are asked to evaluate an infant or fetus with an unusual appearance.[87]

Abnormalities of phenogenesis are minor anomalies and are to be distinguished clearly from mild malformations, which are defects of blastogenesis and organogenesis.[27] Any minor anomalies may occur as normal variants, and vice versa. At times it may be difficult to determine at first glance if a given fetus or infant has a syndrome of multiple minor anomalies (as in an aneuploidy syndrome) or a VFDP. A VFDP is a variant familial developmental pattern of several unusual but normal physical variants that may suggest the presence of a syndrome. However, when parents, siblings, half-siblings, and other close relatives are examined, similar physical traits will be found in

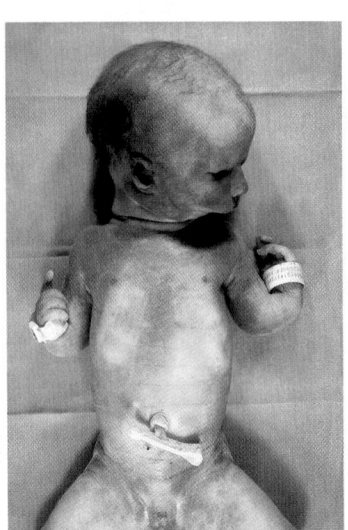

FIGURE 2.19 Patient 1.

them in various combinations, suggesting that these unusual variants behave no differently from those variants that may be regarded as normal ethnic attributes. Additional examples of minor anomalies and methods for documenting them are presented in Chapter 3.

Examples of causal and pathogenetic analysis
Case presentations

The following patients are offered to illustrate the classification of birth defects by cause (causal analysis) and developmental stage (pathogenesis).

PATIENT 1: A term pregnancy yielded an appropriately grown stillborn infant (Fig. 2.19). Family history and parental ages were unremarkable. Autopsy demonstrated a ventricular septal defect.

PATIENT 2: A premature delivery yielded an anomalous stillborn infant (Fig. 2.20). This was the first pregnancy to non-consanguineous parents; family and gestational history were normal. Mother had a severe asthma attack and received several medications during the fourth month of gestation.

PATIENT 3: A term gestation yielded a stillborn infant with intrauterine growth retardation (Fig. 2.21). The parents were first cousins with an otherwise normal family history.

PATIENT 4: A first pregnancy exhibited fetal growth retardation, prompting ultrasonography at 30 weeks' gestation (Fig. 2.22). Oligodactyly and an unusual head shape were demonstrated. After additional studies and perinatal counseling, the infant was delivered and found to have craniosynostosis, oligodactyly, normal body proportions, normal limb lengths, and an unusual facial appearance (see Fig. 2.22C). Death occurred before age 6 months.

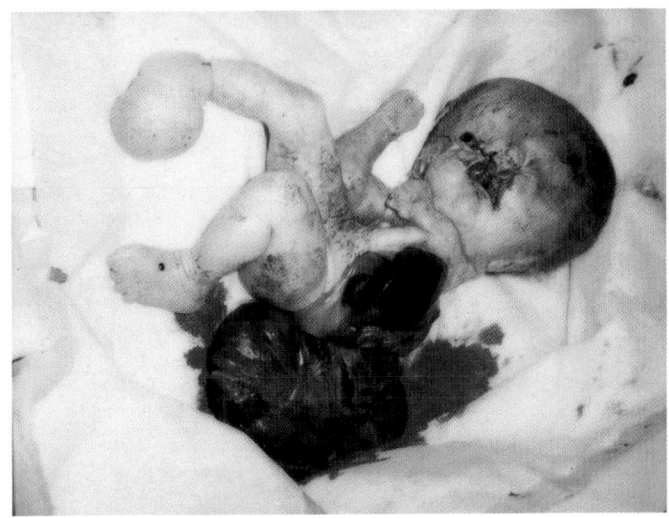

FIGURE 2.20 Patient 2.

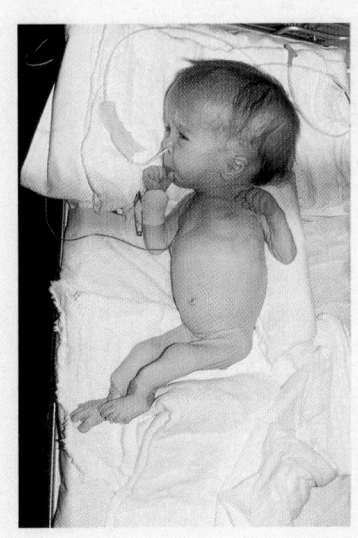

FIGURE 2.21 Patient 3.

PATIENTS 5: Two children with unusual facial findings were born after term gestations (Fig. 2.23). One child (Fig. 2.2A) was the infant of a diabetic mother with a normal family history. This infant had no additional anomalies but did have hypoglycemia, hypocalcemia, and hypernatremia. The other child (Fig. 2.23B) resulted from a second pregnancy in a woman with a previous spontaneous abortion. Anomalies outside the facial region included postaxial polydactyly of the hands, prominent heels, and hypoplastic labia majora.

PATIENT 6: An infant with severe hypotonia, feeding problems, and mild clubfeet was the offspring of a mother with mild mental retardation (Fig. 2.24). The family history was normal except for the maternal grandfather, who had developed cataracts later in life.

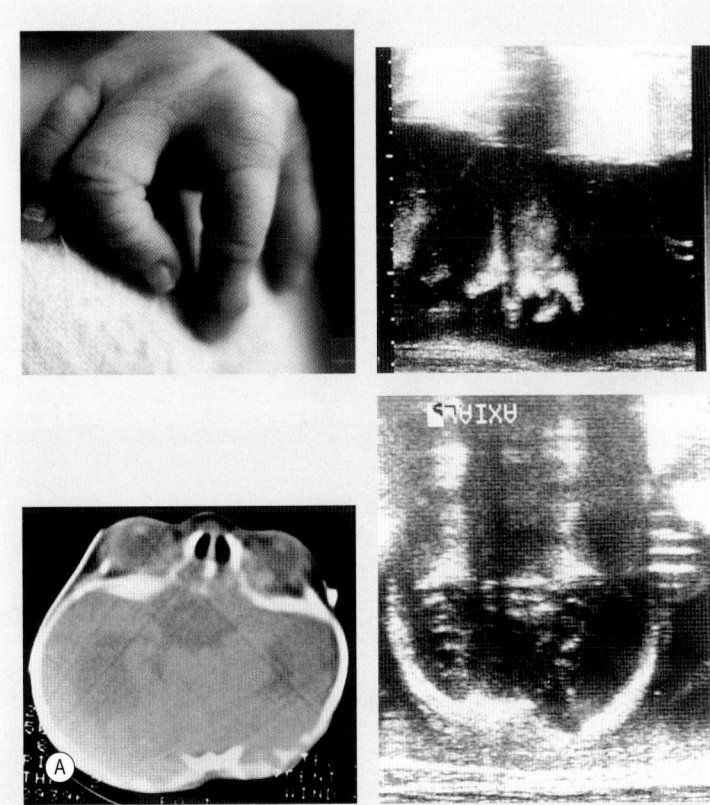

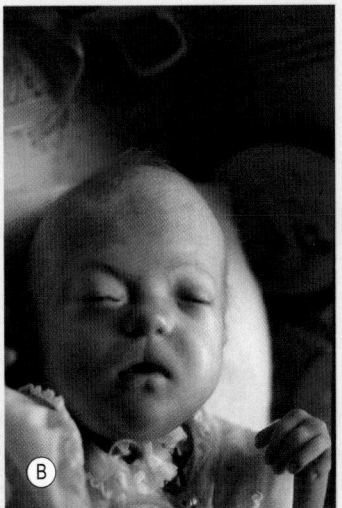

FIGURE 2.22 Patient 4. (A) Prenatal ultrasound image of the head (with postnatal CT scan) and hands (with postnatal photograph). (B) Frontal view of the face.

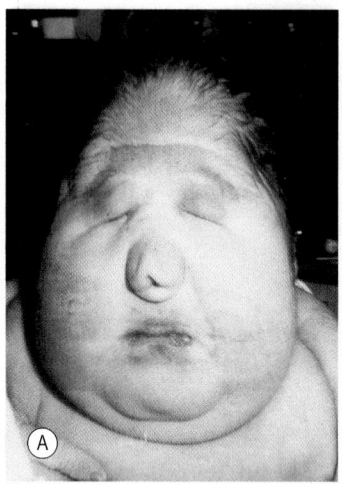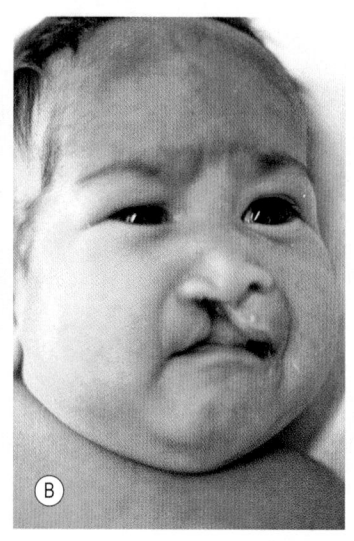

FIGURE 2.23 Patients 5.

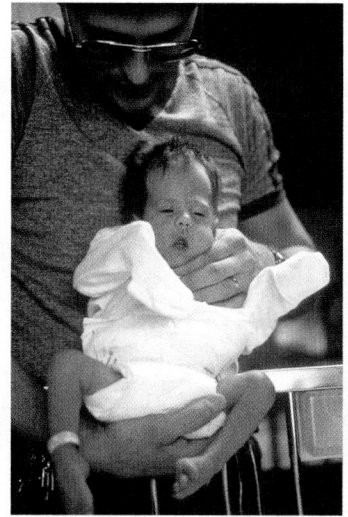

FIGURE 2.24 Patient 6.

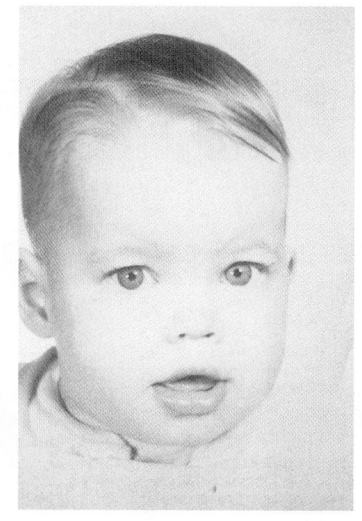

FIGURE 2.25 Patient 7.

PATIENT 7: A male child had a normal gestation and delivery but exhibited developmental delay by age 12 months (Fig. 2.25). Family history demonstrated that the mother's sister also had a son with developmental delay.

PATIENT 8: A female child presented for evaluation of delayed development at age 9 months after being treated for congenital hip dislocation (Fig. 2.26). Family history was normal.

PATIENT 9: A newborn male presented with an absent thumb as shown in Fig. 2.5. Severe respiratory distress leaded to imaging studies that documented tracheoesophageal atresia, and abdominal ultrasound demonstrated an absent kidney. The facial appearance was normal, and no minor anomalies were noted. The family history was normal.

Analysis of patients

PATIENT 1: Figure 2.19 demonstrates severe micrognathia with malar hypoplasia and an unusual ear (large concha, hypoplastic inner helix). Inspection of the mouth showed a U-shaped cleft of the soft palate. Fig. 2.19 demonstrates radial deviation of the hand that is typical of radial aplasia (confirmed by radiography). A ventricular septal defect was also noted. Although the micrognathia and cleft palate are characteristic of Pierre Robin sequence, the additional major and minor anomalies suggest a malformation syndrome. This is why the older term 'Pierre Robin syndrome' is misleading: the Robin sequence can occur as part of many different syndromes (e.g.,

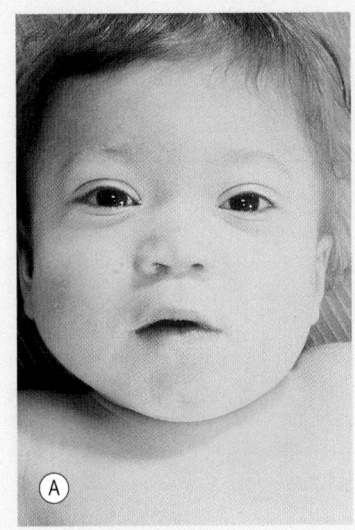
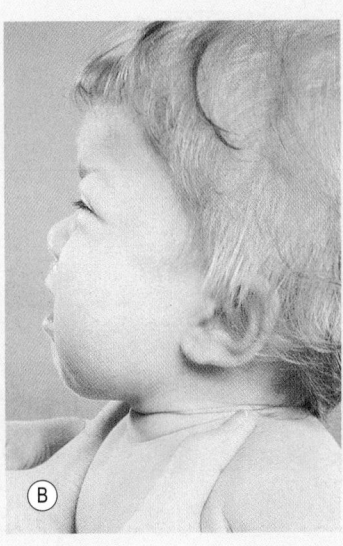

FIGURE 2.26 Patient 8. (A) frontal view. (B) lateral view.

Stickler, Rubinstein-Taybi). Radial aplasia and heart defects can occur in VATER association, but the pattern of anomalies suggests action of a gene or chromosome beyond the period of blastogenesis. Tissue samples for karyotyping would have been appropriate but were not obtained. Consultation of the appropriate references[11, 12] provided a causal diagnosis of autosomal recessive **Nager syndrome** and a recurrence risk of 25%.

PATIENT 2: At first glance the infant in Figure 2.20 appears to have a severe malformation syndrome. However, recognition of the band-like constriction of one ankle and the non-embryonic, topologic distribution of the facial cleft strongly suggests **amniotic band disruption** with minimal recurrence risk. The body wall defects go beyond organ boundaries, suggesting that this disruption sequence began during blastogenesis (before 4 weeks' gestation). This timing provides reassurance that the asthma attack and medications were not causal.

PATIENT 3: Figure 2.21 illustrates a fetus with obvious skeletal dysplasia: the proximal upper limbs are short (rhizomelia), while the lower limbs are short with deviation of their middle (mesomelic) segments. There is arthrogryposis, with ulnar deviation of the hands and inversion of the feet. The facial abnormalities are typical of many types of skeletal dysplasias, showing a prominent forehead, broad and shallow nasal root, and anteverted (upturned) nose. The skeletal defects and minor anomalies imply abnormal development during the periods of organogenesis and phenogenesis, such as would occur with an abnormal gene. Diagnostic radiography (Fig. 2.27) confirmed the causal diagnosis by showing the typical bent femurs of **autosomal dominant campomelic dwarfism.**

PATIENT 4: The additional perinatal studies included a cordocentesis for karyotyping, with the result shown in Figure 2.28. The face in Figure 2.22C is abnormal, with unusual eyebrows, broad nasal root, and down-turned corners of the mouth. The

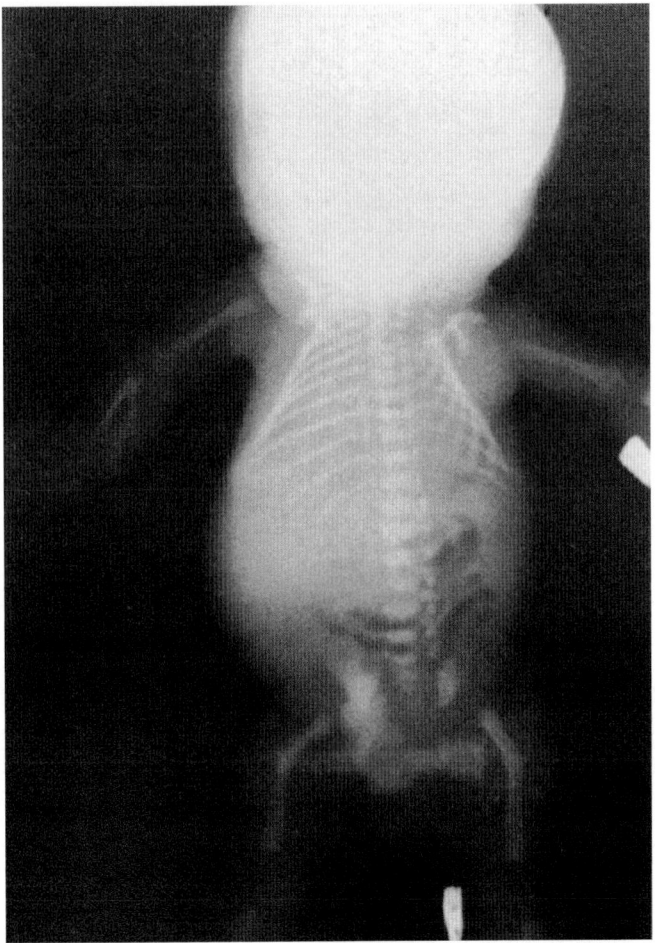

FIGURE 2.27 Radiograph of case similar to Patient 3, showing bent femurs typical of campomelic syndrome.

KARYOTYPE

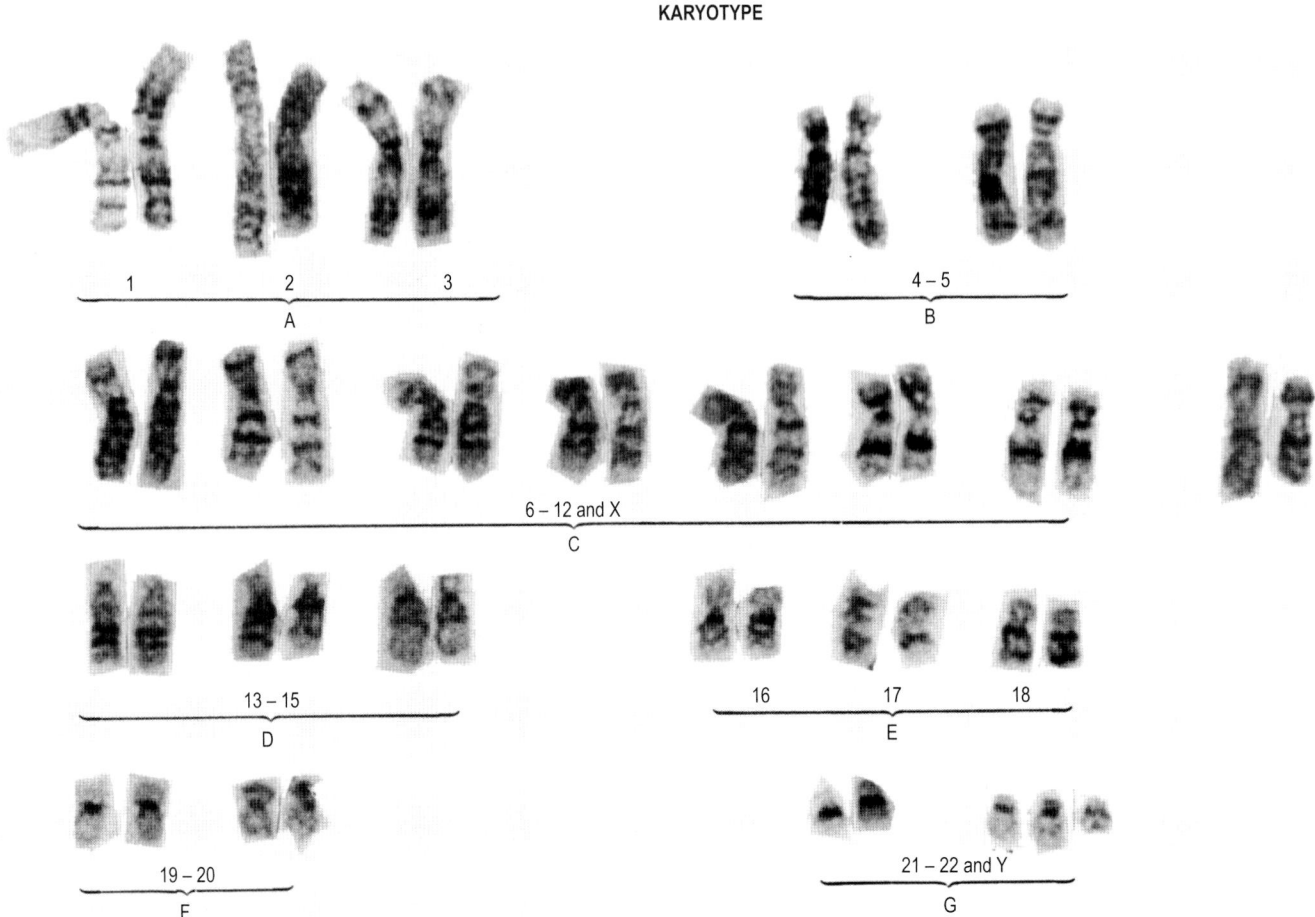

FIGURE 2.28 Karyotype of Patient 4; the extra fragment is grouped with chromosomes 22.

multiple major and minor anomalies suggest a malformation syndrome combining anomalies of organogenesis and phenogenesis. Chromosome analysis showed an extra fragment derived from chromosome 22 based on cytogenetic (see Fig. 2.28) and clinical findings,[28] but definitive identification of the extra fragment would have required **FISH studies** that were not available. Parental chromosome studies are required when a child has a chromosome rearrangement, and the normal result in this instance predicts an empiric 1% recurrence risk for chromosomal anomalies in future pregnancies.

PATIENTS 5: Both children in Figure 2.23 have variations of the **holoprosencephaly field defect ('the face predicts the brain').** Midline clefts (see Fig. 2.23B) should always arouse suspicion of underlying brain anomalies, as should hypernatremia, an uncommon occurrence in infants of diabetic mothers. A computed tomographic scan of the child in Figure 2.23B showed arrhinencephaly; the **diabetes insipidus** reflected presumed **hypothalamic dysfunction. An isolated developmental field defect does not mandate a karyotype,** particularly when maternal diabetes is known to increase the risk of cranial and caudal defects. **When holoprosencephaly occurs with other anomalies,** as in

patient 5A (see Fig. 2.23A), **a karyotype is necessary** and in this case showed **partial trisomy 13.** These patients illustrate that field defects are causally heterogeneous, and that their context must guide the step from pathogenesis to cause. Parental karyotyping, indicated because of the extra, partial chromosome 13, was declined. If a balanced translocation were present in one parent, perhaps accounting for the previous spontaneous abortion, **the recurrence risk could be as high as 10–20%.**

PATIENT 6: After death of the infant shown in Figure 2.24, detailed autopsy, including neuromuscular histologic views, was not helpful in assigning a primary cause of the hypotonia and arthrogryposis. The key to diagnosis was evaluation of the mother (Fig. 2.29), who had difficulty relaxing her fingers after a handshake. Mild affliction of the maternal grandfather (cataracts, frontal baldness, percussion myotonia), moderate disability in the mother, and severe disease in the infant are classic for anticipation related to **expansion of trinucleotide repeats.** Blood lymphocytes or postmortem tissue from the infant should be saved to document repeat expansion near the **Steinert myotonic dystrophy gene by DNA analysis.** This would establish a 50% recurrence risk for the mother and allow prenatal diagnosis.

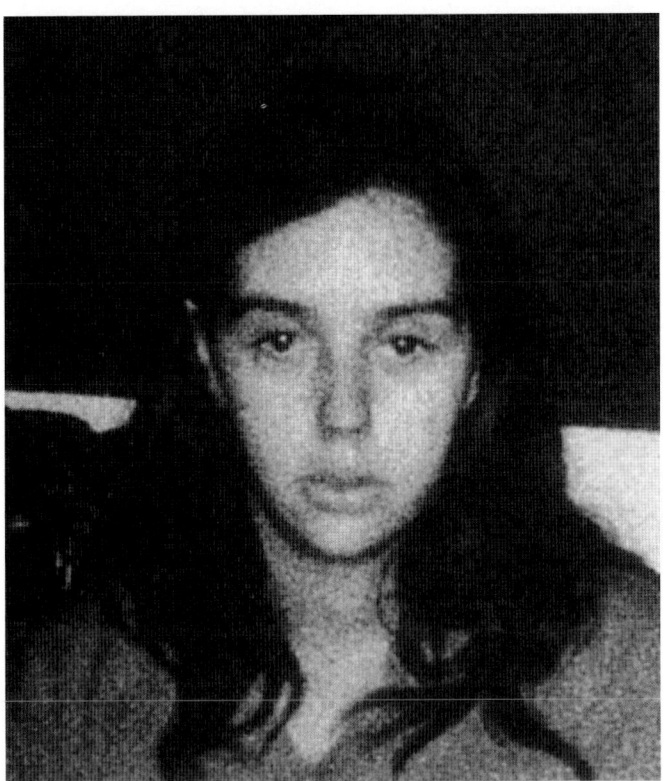

FIGURE 2.29 Mother of Patient 6, showing a myopathic face.

PATIENT 7: The child in Figure 2.25 is quite attractive but has a frontal hair whorl (cowlick) that was also found in his affected cousin. The family history suggests X-linked mental retardation, which was later confirmed by the birth of a third affected male to the patient's sister. Chromosomal studies including fragile X were appropriately performed but yielded normal results. Of more than 80 X-linked disorders that involve mental retardation, over half are 'non-specific' and lack a characteristic facial appearance or definitive anomalies. DNA linkage studies are sorting out these different non-specific disorders according to locus position, and this family was studied to see whether prenatal diagnosis could be offered in view of the sister's 25% recurrence risk. **The overall phenotypic spectrum in this family (frontal cowlick, gastrointestinal problems) suggests the X-linked FG syndrome.**

PATIENT 8: A common clinical error is to focus on one anomaly while neglecting the overall constellation of major and minor anomalies that suggest a syndrome. This child has a 'coarse' face (Fig. 2.26A and B), and additional physical manifestations included prominent abdomen (large liver), short tapered fingers, and gibbous deformity of the spine. A metabolic dysplasia syndrome should be considered, and in this case the urine screen demonstrated mucopolysacchariduria. Enzyme assay of lymphocytes showed the typical deficiency of autosomal recessive **Hurler syndrome,** implying a recurrence risk of 25%.

PATIENT 9: Associations typically involve major anomalies with similar embryologic timing. The child's three anomalies fit the VATER association of vertebral, anorectal, tracheoesophageal, radial, and renal defects that involve mesodermal derivatives that begin differentiation at 20–25 days of embryogenesis. Associations lack minor anomalies, since there is no persistent influence such as an extra chromosome to alter fine tuning of development. Individuals with associations do not have a characteristic facial appearance. The major anomalies documented for patient 9 are also common in trisomy 18, but there were no minor anomalies such as the disproportionately small face, fawn-like ears, broad nasal root, and other manifestations of patients with Edwards syndrome.

Summary

The terminology, causal analysis, and pathogenesis of birth defects have been discussed as they relate to pathologic examination of the fetus and infant. Documentation of anomalies by inspection and histology is the first step, followed by interpretation of their pattern, mechanism, and developmental timing.

The developmental approach to pathogenesis allows classification by life stages. **Pregenesis** begins with the differentiation and migration of parental primordial germ cells and ends with karyogamy; aneuploidies are the major defects of pregenesis so far recognized, but effects on maternal cytoplasm and transgenerational effects can be expected. **Blastogenesis** comprises the first 4 weeks of embryogenesis, a time when the primary embryonic field differentiates into secondary developmental fields. An extensive range of defects – twinning, field defects, and associations – occur during blastogenesis. **Organogenesis** extends from week 4 to week 8 of embryogenesis and accounts for many isolated birth defects, although some localized defects such as anencephaly begin during blastogenesis. **Phenogenesis** constitutes the remaining prenatal period when interference with 'fine tuning' of development produces minor anomalies and growth disturbances. These phenotypically benign but diagnostically significant indicators are extremely helpful in distinguishing **syndromes** (chromosomal, genetic) from **associations. Deformities** and **dysplasias** usually become evident during phenogenesis.

These classifications should guide the pathologist to specific genetic and environmental causes that allow definitive causal diagnoses. Developmental defects also disturb postnatal development, and each syndrome has its natural history that will influence the ease of pathologic recognition. *Postnatal effects* are dramatically illustrated by the altered growth, maturation, reproduction, immunity, and aging that occur in chromosomal syndromes. Because many diagnostic categories are heterogeneous (e.g., skeletal dysplasia, arthrogryposis), delineation of pathogenesis by developmental stage or mechanism (formal genesis) is often insufficient to define cause (causal genesis). It is the great opportunity and responsibility of the pediatric pathologist to document, interpret, and preserve the clinical material that will close these gaps.

Dedication

Dedicated to the immortal memory of my son, Felix Benjamin Opitz (January 3, 1971– June 9, 1994) who, in his enthusiasm, shared with all who knew him a inexhaustible love always with a song in his heart and on his lips. *John M. Opitz*

References

Practical approach to classification

1. Opitz JM. Editorial comment: the developmental field concept. Am J Med Genet 1985; 21:1–11.
2. Opitz JM, Gilbert EF. Pathogenetic analysis of congenital anomalies in humans. In: Ioachim HI, ed. Pathobiology annual, Vol. XII, New York: Raven Press; 1982:301–349.
3. Opitz JM, Herrmann J, Petterson JC, et al. Terminological, diagnostic, nosological and anatomical-developmental aspects of developmental defects in man. In: Harris H, Hirschhorn K, eds. Advances in human genetics, Vol 9. New York: Plenum Press; 1979:71–164.
4. Gilbert-Barness EF, Opitz JM, Barness LA. The pathologist's perspective of genetic disease. Pediatr Clin North Am 1989; 36:163–187.
5. Winter RM, Knowles SAS, Bieber FR, et al. The malformed fetus and stillbirth, a diagnostic approach. Chichester UK: Wiley; 1988.
6. Bruyere HJ, Arya S, Kozel JS, et al. The value of examining spontaneously aborted human embryos and placentas. Birth Defects 1987; 23:169–178.
7. Byrne JM. Fetal pathology laboratory manual. New York: Wiley-Liss for The March of Dimes Birth Defects Foundation; 1983.
8. Opitz JM, Fitzgerald JM, Reynolds JF, et al. The Montana fetal genetic pathology program and a review of prenatal death in humans. Am J Med Genet Suppl 1987; 3:93–112.

Terminology: types of birth defects

9. Spranger J, Benirschke K, Hall JG, et al. Errors of morphogenesis: concepts and terms. Recommendations of an International Working Group. J Pediatr 1982; 100:160–165.
10. Opitz JM, Czeizel A, Evans JA, et al. Nosologic grouping in birth defects. In: Vogel F, Sperling K, eds. Human genetics. Berlin: Springer-Verlag; 1987:382–385.
11. Gorlin RJ, Cohen MM, Hennekam RCM. Syndromes of the head and neck, 4th edn. New York: Oxford University Press; 2001.
12. Jones KL. Smith's recognizable patterns of human malformation, 6th edn. Philadelphia: WB Saunders; 2005.
13. Bamforth JS. Amniotic band sequence: Streeter hypothesis revisited. Birth Defects Orig Artic Ser 1993; 29:279–289.
14. Lammer EJ, Opitz JM. The DiGeorge anomaly as a developmental field defect. Am J Med Genet Suppl 1986; 2:113–127.
15. Quan L, Smith DW. The VATER association, vertebral defects, anal atresia, tracheoesophageal fistula with esophageal atresia, radial and renal dysplasia: a spectrum of associated defects. J Pediatr 1973; 82:104–107.
16. Spranger J, Benirschke K, Hall JG, et al. Errors of morphogenesis: concepts and terms. Recommendations of an international working group. J Pediatr 1982; 100:160–165.
17. Evans JA, Reggin J, Greenberg C. Tracheal agenesis and associated malformations: a comparison with tracheoesophageal fistula and the VACTERL association. Am J Med Genet 1985; 21:21–38.
18. Evans JA, Vitez M, Czeizel A. On the biological nature of associations: evidence from a study of radial ray deficiencies and associated malformations. Birth Defects Orig Artic Ser 1993; 29:63–81.
19. Lubinsky M. Current concepts: VATER and other associations: historical perspectives and modern interpretations. Am J Med Genet Suppl 1986; 2:9–16.
20. Lubinsky M. Midline developmental 'weakness' as a consequence of determinative field properties. In: Topics in pediatric genetic pathology. The Enid Gilbert-Barness Festschrift. Am J Med Genet Suppl 1987; 3:23–28.
21. Czeizel A. Schisis association. Am J Med Genet 1981; 10:25–35.
22. Opitz JM, Gilbert-Barness EF. Editorial comment: CNS anomalies and the midline as a 'developmental field.' Am J Med Genet 1982; 12:443–455.
23. Opitz JM. The developmental field concept in clinical genetics. David W. Smith Festschrift. J Pediatr 1982; 101:805–809.
24. Opitz JM, Gilbert SF. Editorial comment: developmental field theory and the molecular analysis of morphogenesis: a comment on Dr. Slavkin's observations. Am J Med Genet 1993; 47:687–688.
25. Martínez-Frías ML. Developmental field defects and associations: epidemiological evidence of their relationship. Am J Med Genet 1994; 49:45–51.
26. Curran AS, Curran JP. Associated acral and renal malformation: a new syndrome. Pediatrics 1972; 49:716–725.
27. Hall JG. Editorial: Catch 22. J Med Genet 1993; 30:801–802.

Causal analysis: classification by cause

28. Schinzel A. Catalogue of unbalanced chromosome aberrations in man, 2nd edn. Berlin: de Gruyter; 2001.
29. Opitz JM. The Farber lecture: prenatal and perinatal death: the future of developmental pathology. Pediatr Pathol 1987; 7:363–394.
30. Gilbert EF, Arya S, Laxova R, et al. Pathology of chromosome abnormalities in the fetus – pathologic markers. Birth Defects Orig Artic Ser 1987; 23:293–306.
31. Gilbert-Barness EF, Opitz JM. Chromosome anomalies. In: Wigglesworth JS, Singer DB, eds. Textbook of fetal and perinatal pathology, vol I. Boston: Blackwell; 1991:339–379.
32. Gilbert-Barness EF, Opitz JM. Chromosome anomalies. In: Stocker JT, Dehner LP, eds. Pediatric pathology, vol I. Philadelphia: JB Lippincott; 1992:41–71.
33. Guttenbach M, Schakowski R, Schmid M. Incidence of chromosome 18 disomy in human sperm nuclei as detected by nonisotopic in situ hybridization. Hum Genet 1994; 93:421–423.
34. Braude P, Johnson M, Pickering S, et al. Mechanisms of early embryonic loss in vivo and in vitro. In: Chapman M, Grudzinskas G, Chard T, eds. The embryo, normal and abnormal development and growth. London: Springer-Verlag; 1991:1–10.
35. Witschi E. Teratogenic effects from overripenness of the egg. In: Fraser FC, McKusick VA, eds. Congenital malformations – proceedings of the Third International Conference. New York: Excerpta Medica; 1970;157–169.
36. Boué J, Boué A. Anomalies chromosomiques dans les avortements spontanés. In: Boué A, Thibault CD, eds. Les accidents chromosomiques de la reproduction. Paris: INSERM 29; 1973.
37. Warburton D, Bryne J, Canki N. Chromosome anomalies and prenatal development: an atlas. New York: Oxford University Press; 1991.
38. Simpson JL. Aetiology of pregnancy failure. In: Chapman M, Grudzinskas G, Chard T, eds. The embryo, normal and abnormal development and growth. London: Springer-Verlag; 1991:11–34.
39. Nicolaides KH, Snijders RJM, Gosden CM. The role of echography in the diagnosis of fetal chromosome defects. In: Chapman M, Grudzinskas G, Chard T, eds. The embryo, normal and abnormal development and growth. London: Springer-Verlag; 1991:101–121.
40. Gilbert-Barness EF, Opitz JM. Congenital anomalies and malformation syndromes. In: Stocker JT, Dehner LP, eds. Pediatric pathology, vol I. Philadelphia: JB Lippincott; 1992:73–115.
41. Gilbert-Barness EF, Opitz JM. Congenital anomalies and malformation syndromes. In: Wigglesworth JS, Singer DB, eds. Textbook of fetal and perinatal pathology, vol I. Boston: Blackwell; 1991:381–427.
42. McKusick VA. Mendelian inheritance in man, 11th edn. Baltimore: Johns Hopkins; 1994 (www.ncbi.nlm.nih.gov/entrez).
43. Freire-Maia N. A heterozygous expression of a 'recessive' gene. Hum Hered 1975; 25:302–304.
44. Bialer MG, Penchaszadeh VB, Kahn E, et al. Female external genitalia and müllerian duct derivatives in a 46,XY infant with the Smith-Lemli-Opitz syndrome. Am J Med Genet 1987; 28:723–731.

45. Wallace DC. A mitochondrial paradigm of metabolic and degenerative, diseases, aging, and cancer: A dawn for evolutionary medicine. Annu Rev GenetMed 2005; 39:359–407.

46. Kadowaki T, Kadowaki H, Mori Y, et al. A subtype of diabetes mellitus associated with a mutation of mitochondrial DNA. N Engl J Med 1994; 330:962–968.

47. Wilson GN, Hall JG, de la Cruz F. Genomic imprinting: summary of an NICHD conference. Am J Med Genet 1993; 46:675–680.

48. McCowan LM, Becroft DM. Beckwith-Wiedemann syndrome, placental abnormalities, and gestational proteinuric hypertension. Obstet Gynecol 1994; 83:813–817.

49. Bear MF, Huber KM, Warren ST. The mGluR theory of fragile X mental retardation. Trends Neurosci 2004; 27:370–377.

50. Kurnit DM, Aldridge JF, Matsuoka R, et al. Increased adhesiveness of trisomy 21 cells and atrioventricular canal malformations in Down syndrome: a stochastic model. Am J Med Genet 1985; 20:385–399.

51. Cox TC. Taking it to the max: the genetic and developmental mechanisms coordinating midfacial morphogenesis and dysmorphology. Clin Genet 2004; 65:163–176.

52. Nishimura H, Takano K, Tanimura T, et al. Normal and abnormal development of human embryos: first report of the analysis of 1213 intact embryos. Teratology 1968; 1:281–290.

53. Shiota K. Teratothanasia: prenatal loss of abnormal conceptuses and the prevalence of various malformations during gestation. Birth Defects Orig Artic Ser 1993; 29:189–199.

54. Seller MJ. Vitamins, folic acid and the cause and prevention of neural tube defects. In: Bock G, Marsh J, eds. Neural tube defects. Ciba symposium 181. Chichester: Wiley; 1994:161–173.

55. Schardein JL. Chemically induced birth defects, 3rd edn. New York: Marcel Dekker; 2000; see also Reprotox online database (www.reprotox.org).

56. Shepard TH. Catalog of teratogenic agents, 8th edn. Baltimore: Johns Hopkins; 1995.

57. Friedman JM, Politka JE. Teratogenic effects of drugs: a resource for clinicians (TERIS). Baltimore: Johns Hopkins; 1994 (depts.washington.edu/~terisweb/teris/).

58. Ornoy A. The effects of pharmacological agents on the human fetus. Pediatr Pathol 1991; 11:807–812.

59. Persaud TVN. Environmental causes of human birth defects. Springfield IL: Charles C Thomas; 1990.

60. Holmes LB. Fetal environmental toxins. Pediatr Rev 1992; 13:364–369.

Pathogenesis-developmental classification

61. England MA. Color atlas of life before birth – normal fetal development. Chicago: Year Book; 1983.

62. Gilbert SF. Developmental biology, 8th edn. Sunderland, MA: Sinauer Associates; 1994.

63. Hinrichsen KV, ed. Humanembryologie. Lehrbuch und Atlas der vorgeburtlichen Entwicklung des Menschen. Berlin: Springer-Verlag; 1990.

64. Larsen WJ. Human embryology, 3rd edn. New York: Elsevier; 2001.

65. Moore KL, Persaud TVN. The developing human: clinically oriented embryology, 6th edn. Philadelphia: WB Saunders; 2000.

66. Lash JW. Normal embryology and teratogenesis. Am J Obstet Gynecol Suppl 1964; 90:1193–1207.

67. Wolff E. La science des monsters. Paris: Gallimard; 1948.

68. Moore JA. Problems facing the decision maker in the risk assessment process. Teratog Carcinog Mutagen 1987; 7:205–209.

69. Wright S, Eaton ON. Factors which determine otocephaly in guinea pigs. J Agric Res 1923; 26:161.

70. Waddington CH. Evolutionary adaptation. Perspect Biol Med 1959; 2:379–401.

71. Clark OE. The contributions of JF Meckel, the younger, to the science of teratology. J Hist Med Allied Sci 1969; 24:310–322.

72. Seidler E. Johann Friedrich Meckel the younger. Am J Med Genet 1984; 18:571–576.

73. Opitz JM. Blastogenesis and the 'primary field' in human development. Birth Defects Orig Artic Ser 1993; 29:3–37.

74. Harveo GH (Harvey W). Exercitationes de generatione animalium. London: Pulleyn; 1657; Amsterdam: Elsevier.

75. Witschi E. Development of vertebrates. Philadelphia: WB Saunders; 1956.

Abnormalities of pregenesis, blastogenesis, and phenogenesis

76. Gilbert EF, Opitz JM. Developmental and other pathological changes in syndromes caused by chromosomal abnormalities. In: Rosenberg HS, Bernstein J, eds. Perspectives in pediatric pathology, vol VII. New York: Masson; 1982:1–63.

77. Nance W, Uchida I. Turner's syndrome, twinning, and an unusual variant of G-6-PD. Am J Hum Genet 1964; 16:380–392.

78. Hall BK. Developmental mechanisms underlying the formation of atavisms. Biol Rev Camb Philos Soc 1984; 59:89–124.

79. Shapiro BL. Down syndrome – a disorder of homeostasis. Am J Med Genet 1983; 14:241–269.

80. Opitz JM, Gilbert-Barness EF. Reflections on the pathogenesis of Down syndrome. Am J Med Genet Suppl 1990; 7:38–51.

81. Wilson GN. Correlated heart/limb anomalies in mendelian syndromes provide evidence for a cardiomelic developmental field. Am J Med Genet 1998; 76:297–305.

82. DeRobertis EM, Morita EA, Cho KWY. Gradient fields and homeobox genes. Development 1991; 112:669–678.

83. Opitz JM, Lewin SO. The developmental field concept in pediatric pathology – especially with respect to fibular a/hypoplasia and the DiGeorge anomaly. Birth Defects Orig Artic Ser 1987; 23:277–292.

84. Freire-Maia N, Quelce-Salgado A, Amundsen-Kohler. Hereditary bone aplasias and hypoplasias of the upper extremities. Acta Genet Statist Med 1959; 9:33–40.

85. Delahunt CS, Lassen LT. Thalidomide syndrome in monkeys. Science 1964; 146:1300–1305.

86. Szulman AE. Examination of the early conceptus. Arch Pathol Lab Med 1991; 115:696–700.

87. Leppig KA, Werler MM, Cann CI, et al. Predictive value of minor anomalies. I. Association with major malformations. J Pediatr 1987; 110:531–537.

Analysis of developmental pathology

3

John M. Opitz   Golder N. Wilson   Enid Gilbert-Barness

*I should like to work like the archeologist who pieces together the fragments …
These fragments are parts of a whole which, however, is unknown to him. He must
be enough of an artist to recreate the work of the master, but he dare not build
according to his own ideas. Above all, he must keep the broken edges of the
fragments; in that way only may he hope to fit new fragments into their proper
place and thus ultimately achieve a true restoration of the master's creation.*

Hans Spemann, 1936

In Chapter 2, a classification of birth defects was presented according to type (single anomaly, syndrome, association), mechanism (malformation, disruption, deformity), cause (genetic, environmental) and developmental period (pregenesis, blastogenesis, phenogenesis). Here, examples of these categories will be discussed to preview later chapters and to reinforce morphologic approaches to causal analysis and pathogenesis. The classifications are of course overlapping, since the genetic heritage of pregenesis often affects later processes. Abnormalities are presented by developmental period, then sorted according to cause, pattern, and mechanism. They illustrate routes to pathologic diagnosis and its benefits for management, prediction, and prevention of developmental abnormalities.[1]

Defects of pregenesis

As discussed in Chapter 2, pregenesis is a developmental process that extends from the origin of the parental primordial germ cells to the moment of karyogamy creating the new offspring.[2] The process of gonadogenesis involves migration of the primordial germ cells and their interaction with epithelia to form the primitive gonad. The unique chromosomes with their genes and maternal cytoplasm can cause various developmental abnormalities that confront the pediatric pathologist. Some causal categories are presented here, but many disorders are associated with the developmental stage at which they manifest.

Aneuploidy (see also Chapter 5)

Eighty to 90% of potential human beings die before, not after, birth.[2-7] This presents reproductive pathology with its greatest challenge. Most of this loss in earliest stages is due to **chromosome abnormalities**, mostly aneuploidies (abnormalities of individual numbers and pieces of chromosomes) and polyploidies (abnormalities of haploid sets of chromosomes). The pathology associated with this large class of human loss is mostly at the microscopic level, involving ova incapable of fertilization, or of implanting after successful fertilization, and other losses before the first missed period, so that the *12–15%* **spontaneous abortion rate after the first missed period represents less than 2% of the total loss rate** (Table 3.1).[8,9]

Thus, the estimates of Witschi,[9] regarded with considerable distrust by most clinicians until recently, turn out to have been gross underestimates (58% vs. 88% loss before the first missed period). Some 60–84% of all spontaneous abortions after the first missed period have a gross chromosome abnormality, depending on gestational age. In stillbirths (more than 20 gestational weeks), the rate of chromosome abnormalities is between 6.6% and 11.7%. In fetuses between 9 and 20 weeks, the rate of chromosome abnormalities is around 7%, and in

TABLE 3.1 DEVELOPMENTAL EFFECTS OF ANEUPLOIDY ON MIDLINE STRUCTURES IN TRISOMIES 21, 18, AND 13

Anomaly (N)	Trisomy 21 (357)	Trisomy 18 (55)	Trisomy 13 (38)
Neural tube defects	–	3	–
Oral clefts	5	6	22
Omphalocele	2	3	2
Tracheoesophageal defects	–	6	–
Imperforate anus	4	–	–
Conotruncal heart defect	4	3	8
Diaphragmatic hernia	1*	3	2

From Khoury MJ, Cordero JF, Rasmussen S. Ectopia cordis, midline defects and chromosomal abnormalities: an epidemiological perspective. Am J Med Genet 1988; 30:811; with permission.
All cases except * show significant differences ($p<0.05$, Poisson distribution) from mean US population incidence.

TABLE 3.2 BLASTOGENETIC MALFORMATIONS IN HUMANS

Monozygotic twins: non-conjoint
Monozygotic twins: conjoint
Sacrococcygeal teratoma, with or without imperforate anus and sacral/coccygeal defect
Sirenomelia and all forms of caudal 'regression,' including sacral dysgenesis (Fig. 3.6)
Otocephaly (Fig. 3.7)
Anencephaly (Fig. 3.8), encephaloceles, spina bifida
Renal agenesis restricted to unilateral or bilateral forms (Fig. 3.9) or as part of an extensive defect as gross as sirenomelia
Anal/rectal atresia
Tracheoesophageal fistula, tracheal agenesis, esophageal atresia
Pentalogy of Cantrell (involving upper abdominal wall, lower sternum, diaphragm, pericordium, heart, ectopia cordis)
Conotruncal septation defects
Vertebral segmentation defects (Fig. 3.10)
DiGeorge anomaly
Ectopia cordis
Limb–body wall complexes (Fig. 3.11)
Acrorenal field defects
Exstrophy of bladder/cloaca including OEIS complex (omphalocele-exstrophy-imperforate anus-spinal defects)
Polyasplenia field defect (Fig. 3.12)
Acrofacial dysostoses
Agenesis of cloacal membrane
Holoprosencephaly with or without otocephaly
Diaphragmatic defects (Fig. 3.13)
Anomalies of body stalk/wall, umbilical cord formation, and placentation (Fig 3.14; see also Fig. 20.16)
Prune-belly syndrome (Fig. 3.15)
Goldenhar complex (Fig. 3.16)

From Opitz JM. Blastogenesis and the 'primary field' in human development. Birth Defects Orig Artic Ser 1993; 29:3–37, with permission.

perinatal deaths about 6%, the rate being higher in those with severe congenital malformations (28.6%) and in macerated stillbirths (11.6%). For embryos of less than 8 weeks, the rate of chromosome anomalies can be as high as 78% (Table 3.2).[10] Thus, it seems reasonable to assume (as did Witschi) that some **50% of all human conceptions are aneuploid or polyploid**. At the time of birth, some 0.6–0.9% of all liveborn infants have a chromosome abnormality – mostly 47,XXX, 47,XXY, and 47,XYY cases – and seem to suffer little or no prenatal mortality.

In their study of some 3300 karyotyped spontaneous abortions, Warburton and colleagues[11] established a useful classification (see Table 2.1 of Ch. 2) of morphologic classes of spontaneous abortions. (Kalousek, however, uses a different classification [see Ch. 4].) Many aneuploid embryos or fetuses appear normally developed. In **triploid** cases, placentas are either molar (partial moles), or extremely hypoplastic (see Ch. 5); in cases of **complete moles**, chromosomes may appear normal (46,XX) but **represent total androgenesis with both sets of chromosomes being paternally derived (with retention of maternal mitochondrial DNA)**. Simpson[12] summarized the chromosome abnormalities in spontaneous abortions recognized clinically in the first trimester, assuming an overall 46% aneuploidy and polyploidy rate.

Aneuploid phenotypes are more distinctive but still highly variable in the fetal and neonatal periods. There is a well-known relationship between **maternal age** and aneuploidy in liveborn infants, increasing exponentially from 0.5% at maternal age 35 to 1.6% at 40 years and 5.3% at 45 years; the corresponding incidences at the time of amniocentesis for maternal age are 0.8%, 2.5%, and 8.3%, respectively.[13] In a series of 1262 fetuses with malformations or growth retardation studied ultrasonographically,[13] chromosome defects were found in 6% of fetuses with an isolated defect and in 42% of those with more than one malformation (overall rate of 16%).

Since normal morphogenetic events at the midline during blastogenesis seem to be rather unstable, it can be predicted that one developmental effect of aneuploidy is an increased number of **blastogenetic midline anomalies in chromosomally abnormal infants and fetuses**.[14] This was demonstrated in trisomy 21, 18, and 13 (see Table 3.1) from the Greater Atlanta Birth Defects Registry.[15] This association is certainly also known in triploidy. Table 3.1 documents that virtually all midline anomalies occur with a greater than expected frequency in these three syndromes.[16] In this respect, Down syndrome is primarily characterized by oral clefts, omphalocele, imperforate anus, and conotruncal heart defects; however, tracheoesophageal fistulas, duodenal atresias, annular pancreas, neural tube defects, and alobar holoprosencephaly have also been documented. Comparison of the three trisomies suggests that the midline, as a developmental landmark, seems fairly well buffered in Down syndrome, less so in trisomy 18, and weakly buffered in trisomy 13.

Despite some overlap in aneuploid phenotypes due to such factors, the changes produced during phenogenesis discussed in Chapter 2 frequently confer a unique external appearance for many aneuploid disorders. With experience, the diagnostic hypothesis of monosomy X (Fig. 3.1), trisomy 13 (Fig. 3.2), or triploidy in very small fetuses or embryos is easily confirmed by FISH or cytogenetic methods. Mosaicism can pose challenges for diagnosis, but partial trisomies or monosomies often have recognizable phenotypes.

Placental mosaicism with its potential correction to disomy is another factor complicating the aneuploid phenotype. In some fetuses with apparently normal chromosomes, **isodisomy** of a chromosome may be present; this is especially true in cases of **confined placental mosaicism**, most notably **trisomy 16**. It has also been observed in cases of trisomy 15 with **maternal isodisomy of chromosome 15**, leading to **Prader-Willi syndrome**. The frequency of confined placental mosaicism is in the order of 1% in normal newborns, and of 15% IUGR.[16a] If a chromosome abnormality is suspected but cells fail to grow in tissue culture for cytogenetic analysis, an extensive array of **fluorescent probes for in situ hybridization (FISH)** studies on interphase nuclei is available and can be applied in fresh and formalin-fixed material.

TABLE 3.3 EXAMPLES OF METABOLIC DYSPLASIA SYNDROMES

Mucopolysaccharidoses	Hurler, Hunter, and Morquio diseases
Mucolipidoses, sialidoses	I-cell disease, sialidosis
Glycoprotein degradation diseases	Fucosidosis, aspartylglycosaminuria
Lipid storage disease	Wolman disease
Lipidoses	Farber, Gaucher, and Tay-Sachs diseases
Peroxisomal disorders	Zellweger syndrome, adrenoleukodystrophies
Cholesterol metabolism	Mevalonic acidemia, Smith-Lemli-Opitz syndrome

See Scriver and colleagues[136] and the text for details.

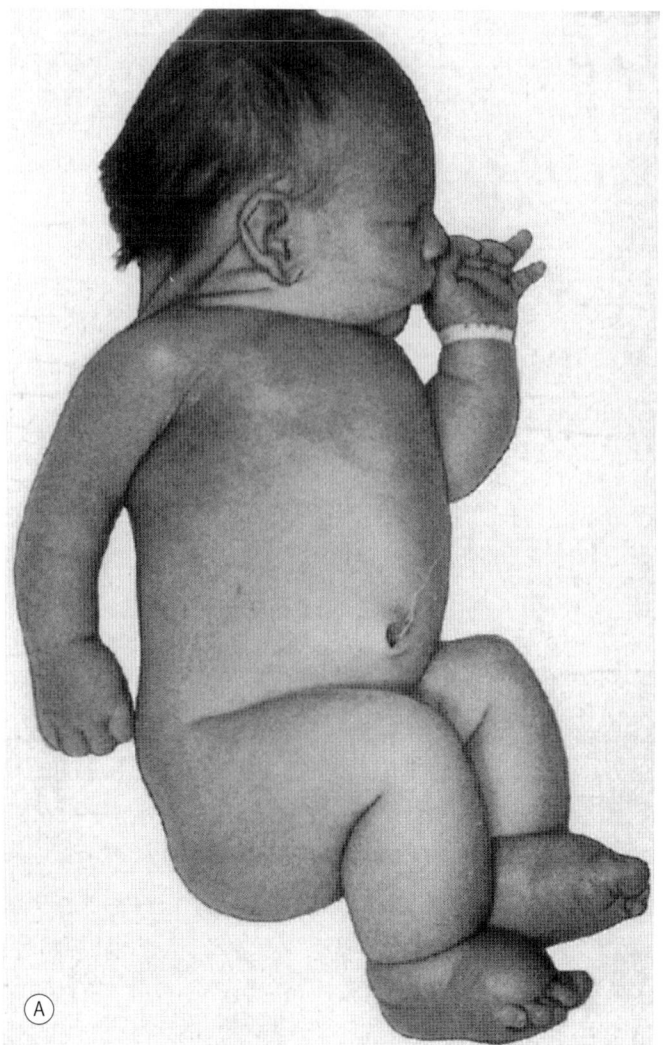

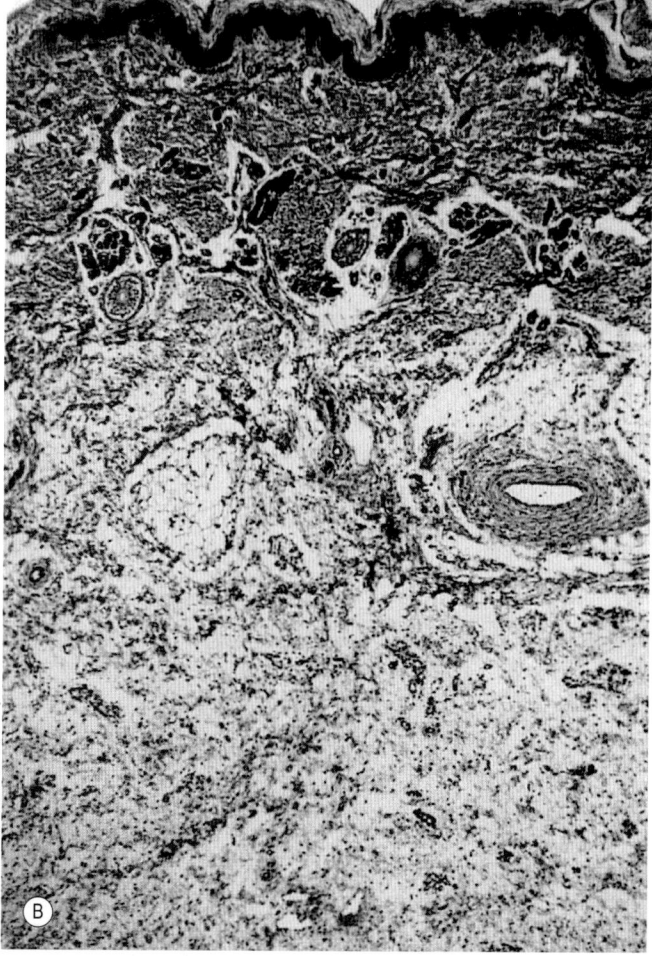

FIGURE 3.1 (A) Patient with Turner syndrome demonstrating pterygium colli and pedal edema. (B) Skin of the patient showing increased thickness of subcutaneous connective tissue without increase in lymphatic channels.

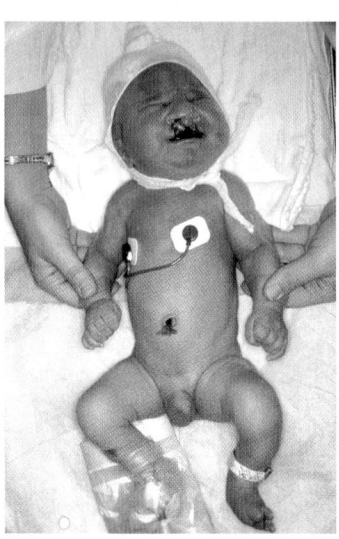

FIGURE 3.2 Patient with trisomy 13 demonstrating bilateral cleft lip/palate, postaxial polydactyly of the hands, and penile chordee.

Mendelian inheritance, multifactorial determination, and atypical mechanisms

Of the more than 4000 disorders listed in Online Mendelian Inheritance in Man (OMIM, www.ncbi.nlm.nih.gov/entrez), about 50% involve alterations of morphology.[17] An additional 1200 multifactorial disorders can be assembled from OMIM and other sources, and 70% of these (mostly isolated birth defects) are errors of morphogenesis.[17] Except for advanced paternal age, causes of human mendelian mutations have not been defined. Searches for increased mutation rates, even in Japanese atomic bomb survivors, have not been revealing. Molecular technology has revealed striking expansions and rearrangements that differ among individuals,[18] but genetic or environmental influences on these variations have not been identified. A growing repertoire of DNA tests does allow demonstration of mendelian mutations in a few defects or syndromes, and it is hoped that array and chip technologies will soon provide test panels for categories defined by morphologic analysis. Some markers for defect susceptibility, such as TGF-α for cleft palate,[19] offer hope that marker DNA chips will one day be coupled with nutritional strategies for prevention or modification of multifactorial defects.

Mendelian mutations expressed during blastogenesis are illustrated by the action of a **number of XLB** (X-linked blastogenesis) **genes on the development of midline organs** (Table 3.2).[20] Others, such as mutations in the sonic hedgehog (*SHH*) gene, can disrupt blastogenesis to cause holoprosencephaly (which again through SHH can cause cyclopia) or, through defective addition of cholesterol moieties to its protein, contribute to problems throughout gestation as in the Smith-Lemli-Opitz syndrome (see below). *SHH* exemplifies the many human homologues to fly-pattern genes that act during blastogenesis,[21] including *HOX* and nodal genes that cause blastogenetic defects such as poly/asplenia (see Table 3.2).

Mendelian mutations can accumulate and act with the environment to produce multifactorial defects; these and modifying influences on mutant genes (imprinting – triplet repeat expansion – compartmentalization and complexing of products in mitochondria or peroxisomes) produce anomalies at every developmental stage. Such interactions probably underlie the many minor anomalies and individual variations produced during phenogenesis, and have substantial contributions to the metabolic and oncogenic dysplasias that appear after birth.

Environmental factors acting during pregenesis are poorly defined in humans. Early miscarriage, particularly in view of the high rates of spontaneous loss (see above), is an insensitive indicator of early teratogen action. Numerous environmental agents cause abnormalities at later developmental periods; some examples are discussed below.

Anomalies of blastogenesis

The period of blastogenesis extends from karyogamy, the earliest cell divisions to the formation of morula, blastula, implantation, and organ primordia by week 4. As mentioned in Chapter 2, the formation of the trilaminar disk and midline during early gastrulation can be impaired by chromosome aberrations, mendelian disorders (Table 3.2 lists a number of X-linked defects of blastogenesis), environmental factors (diabetic and alcohol embryopathies are discussed below), and as yet 'idiopathic' disorders such as associations.

Twinning

Monozygotic (MZ) and conjoint twinning are quintessential defects of blastogenesis.[1,22] Non-conjoint MZ twinning is an abnormal event that may have a normal outcome, but it is attended by a high risk of death of one of the twins, an increased rate of malformations of blastogenetic origin, and a risk of placental vascular connection with twin-to-twin transfusion complications. Thus, many apparent singletons are survivors of a twinning process, and all placentas of singletons deserve careful examination for remnants of a twin.[22] Even a barely recognizable small *fetus papyraceus* attached to the placental surface may lead to a risk of disseminated intravascular coagulation with all its complications. The biology and pathology of twinning is described in Chapter 9.

Malformations

Table 3.2 lists the blastogenetic malformations known in humans,[2] and Figures 3.1 to 3.11 provide examples. In a given case of gross malformation, e.g., tetraphocomelia, otocephaly, sirenomelia, or cyclopia, there is no question as to the blastogenetic origin of the malformation. However, the possibility exists that certain mild malformations, apparently of later origin, may

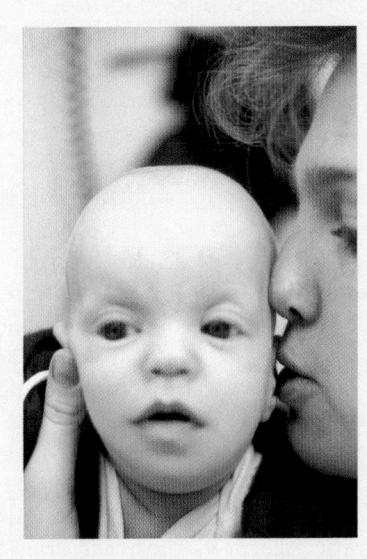

FIGURE 3.3 Child with Wolf-Hirshhorn syndrome (terminal deletion of chromosome 4p) showing prominent forehead and glabella that resembles the prong of a Greek warrior helmet; patients frequently have cleft palate, heart, and renal anomalies.

also represent blastogenetic defects. These milder anomalies may have been 'compensated' during subsequent morphogenesis, yet they retain the potential for severe recurrence, e.g., variable expression of autosomal dominant alobar holoprosencephaly that may be limited to a single upper central incisor. In cases of the apparently single malformation anencephaly, occurrence of other midline anomalies suggests a more generalized defect of blastogenesis.[23] Such a view of neural tube defects seems supported by the fact that dietary folic acid supplementation reduced occurrence and recurrence not only of neural tube defects, but also of other malformations. The fact that neural tube defects carry a recurrence risk not only of neural tube defects, but also of other anomalies (e.g., diaphragmatic defect), also argues for the broader view of neural tube defects as a disturbance of blastogenesis.

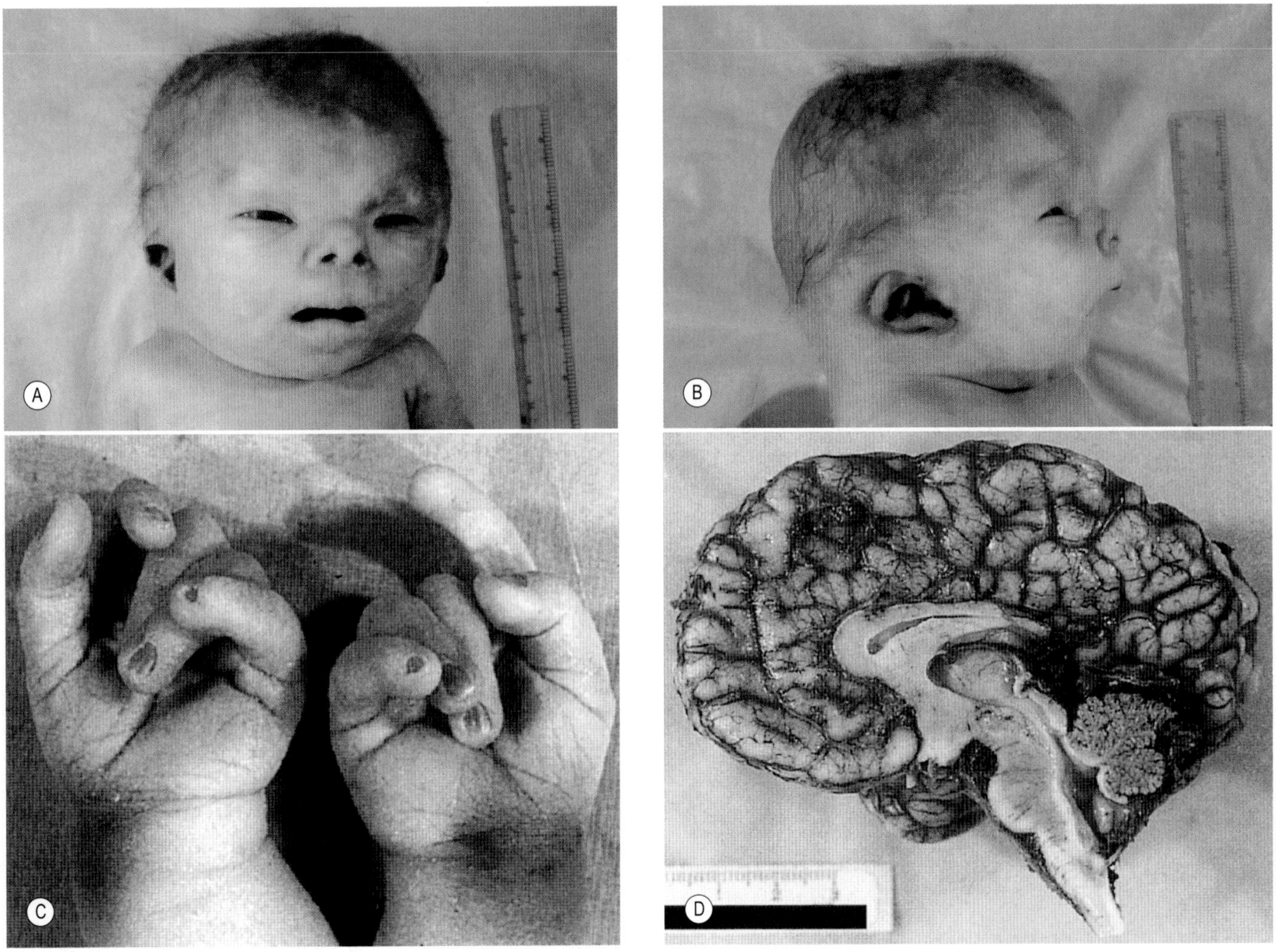

FIGURE 3.4 Patient with dup(3q) syndrome demonstrating an unusual face and head shape (A and B) with broad nasal root, right epicanthal fold, anteverted nares, long philtrum, thin upper lip, down-turned corners of the mouth, micrognathia, posteriorly angulated and malformed ears, and short neck. The patient had clenched fists with overlapping fingers (C) and brain malformations (D), including polymicrogyria, hypoplastic olfactory bulbs, and increased hindbrain-midbrain angulation. (From Wilson GN, Dasouki M, Barr M Jr. Further delineation of the dup(3q) syndrome. Am J Med Genet 1985; 22:117; with permission.)

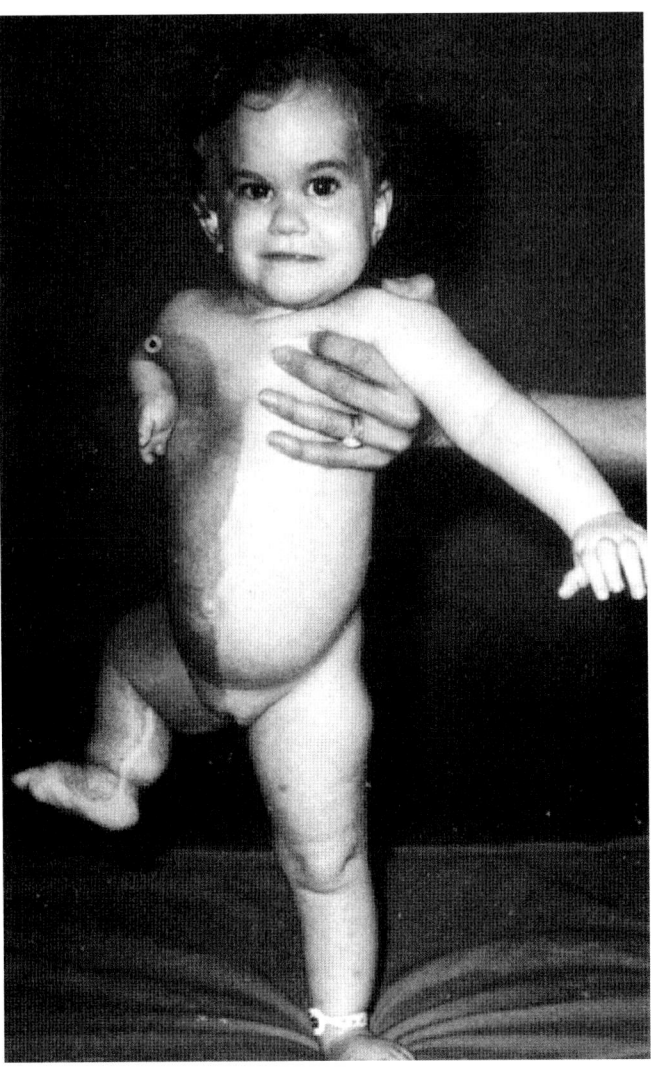

FIGURE 3.5 Infant with congenital unilateral psoriasis, hemiatrophy, and ectromelia. (Courtesy Dr. C.S. Shear.)

Sirenomelia

This **sporadic defect** occurs in about 1 of 60 000 newborn infants, more often in males, and it is more common in one of identical twins.[24] It is a severe **developmental field defect of the posterior axis caudal blastema**, resulting in apparent fusion of the lower limb buds. It occurs in the primitive streak stage during week 3 of gestation before development of the allantois, and the allantoic vessels are usually absent. In many cases there is a single umbilical artery that arises directly from the aorta. Other defects of the caudal axis include imperforate anus, lower vertebral defects, and genitourinary anomalies.[24] Cardiovascular, respiratory, and upper gastrointestinal tract malformations occur in 20–35% of cases.[24] The radial agenesis, esophageal atresia, and tracheoesophageal fistula in some cases suggest that the VATER association (see later for explanation) may represent

a lesser degree of the caudal regression sequence. This sequence is a defect most commonly seen in infants of diabetic mothers. Ectopic renal tissue has been observed within the wall of the gastrointestinal tract. Renal agenesis or cystic renal dysplasia occurs in virtually all cases leading to the Potter sequence, including pulmonary hypoplasia.[24]

Because of the close contiguity of primordia and sites of morphogenesis in blastogenesis and because of the overlap of inductive mechanisms and paths, there is developmental correlation or even integration of ontogeny of structures ordinarily not considered developmentally related and anatomically non-contiguous in the mature organism.[25] The first such **'polytopic' field**[1] discovered was the **acrorenal field defect**,[26] with experimental confirmation[27] of the developmental relationship between the limbs and mesonephros that had been postulated on the basis of clinical and epidemiologic data. Other well-known polytopic field defects are the **DiGeorge anomaly** with associated third and fourth branchial arch, craniofacial and cardiac defects all presumed to be due to defective cranial neural crest action,[28, 29] and the **Wyers type of acrofacial dysostosis** (MIM 193530) that combine mandibulofacial dysostosis and pre- and/or postaxial limb defects through mutations of *EVC* or *EVC2*.[30]

Hanhart and Poland-Möbius complexes

These are examples of polytopic field defects. The Hanhart syndrome (MIM 103300) usually includes severe limb defects of at least one hand or foot and is frequently associated with severe oral abnormalities (Fig. 3.17). The form of the condition associated with cranial nerve palsy (or palsies) is called the Hanhart-Möbius complex.[31] Most cases are reported as aglossia-adactylia syndrome, aglossia-hypomelia syndrome, or glossopalatine ankylosis or ankyloglossia superior-Möbius syndrome. The condition should be separated from the Poland-Möbius syndrome, which involves the Poland anomaly (i.e., chest defect and/or symbrachydactyly) and cranial nerve palsies.

Bersu and colleagues postulated a common ectodermal pathogenic disturbance for the oral and limb defects in Hanhart complex, suggesting that the manifestations represent a single anomaly rather than a syndrome.[32] Splenogonadal fusion may be related to limb deficiency and complex ectromelia conditions such as Hanhart syndrome. Hanhart complex should be considered an example of *Ektodermring* developmental disturbance, the *Ectodermring* involving the sides of the body, limbs, tail ridge (of Grüneberg), and anal membrane; hence, the combination in some cases of typical oral, tongue, tooth, and limb defects with imperforate anus.

Regardless of how improbable it may appear at first glance, a given pair of combinations of anomalies of blastogenesis is a field defect if it can be demonstrated conclusively to be causally heterogeneous. This challenge by clinicians to the developmental biologists will be an indicator of future productivity in the field and of the need for multi- and interdisciplinary approaches to the problems of birth defects in humans.[33,34]

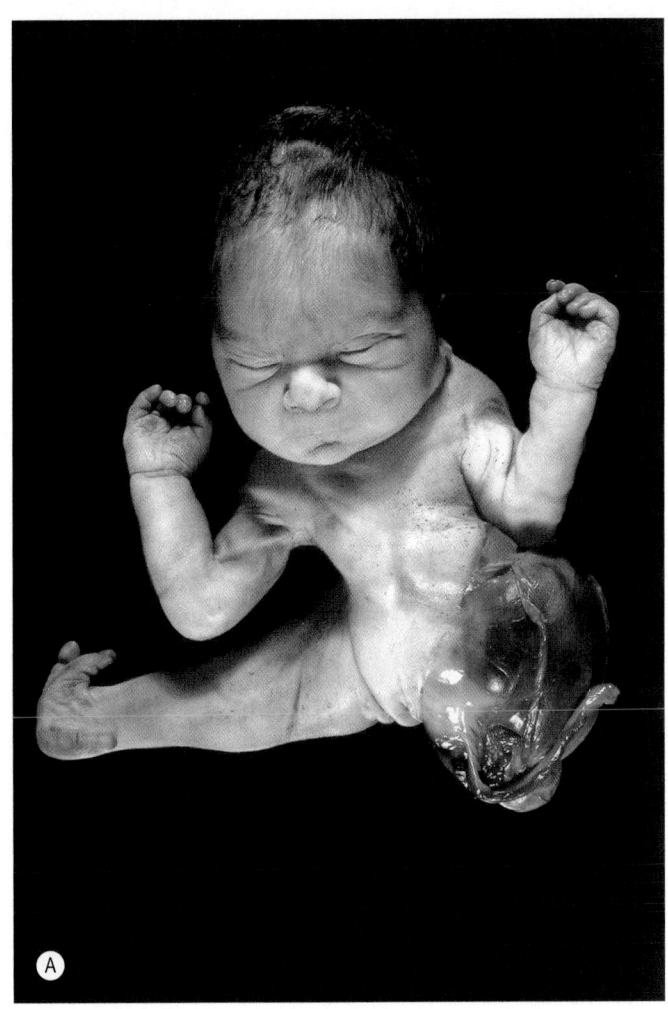

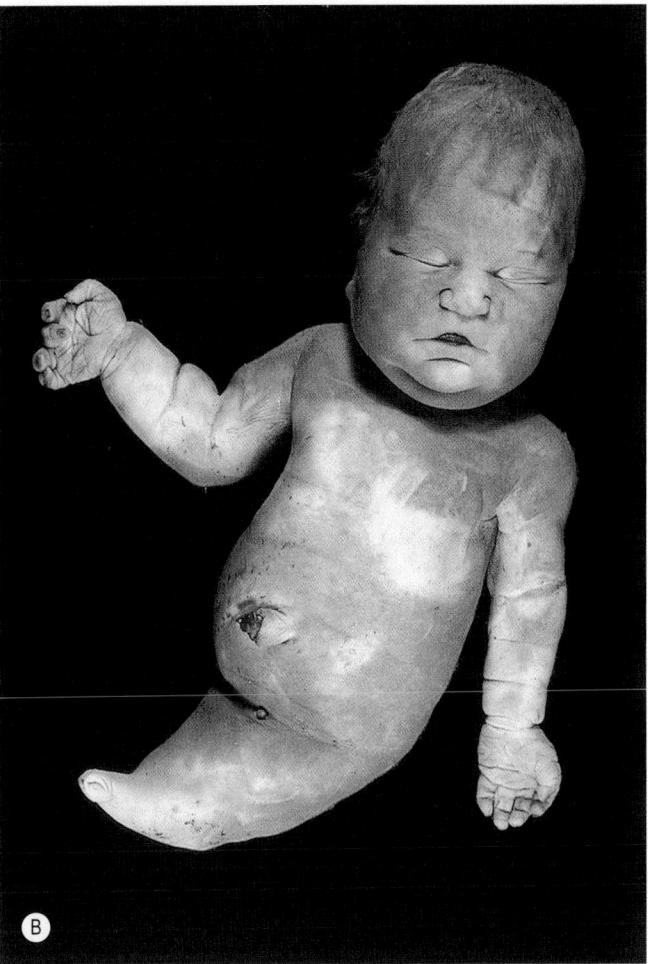

FIGURE 3.6 Sirenomelia showing fusion and varying degrees of hypoplasia of the lower extremities. In (A) the structure extending posteriorly from the buttocks resembles a penis except for absence of a urethra.

Associations

VATER association

This association involves *v*ertebral defects, *a*nal atresia, *t*racheoesophageal fistula, *e*sophageal atresia, and *r*adial and *r*enal abnormalities.[35] Cardiac defects, a single umbilical artery, and prenatal growth deficiency were included by Temtamy and Miller, who used the acronym VATERS association.[36] Other less frequent defects include prenatal growth deficiency, ear anomalies, large fontanelles, defects of lower limbs, and rib anomalies. This pattern of malformations occurs sporadically. The concept of an **expanded VATER** association suggests that the common VATER association may represent a less severe degree of the sirenomelia malformation sequence.

VACTERL is one of many VATER expansions that includes *c*ardiac and *l*imb defects. There is also an overlap caudally with an association of müllerian duct, renal, and cervicothoracic somite malformations (MURCS) (see below) and a cephalic overlap with tracheal agenesis, hemifacial microsomia, and other facial asymmetry defects. The genitourinary defects include renal dysplasia or agenesis; renal ectopia; persistent urachus; hypospadias; and caudally displaced, hypoplastic penis.[37]

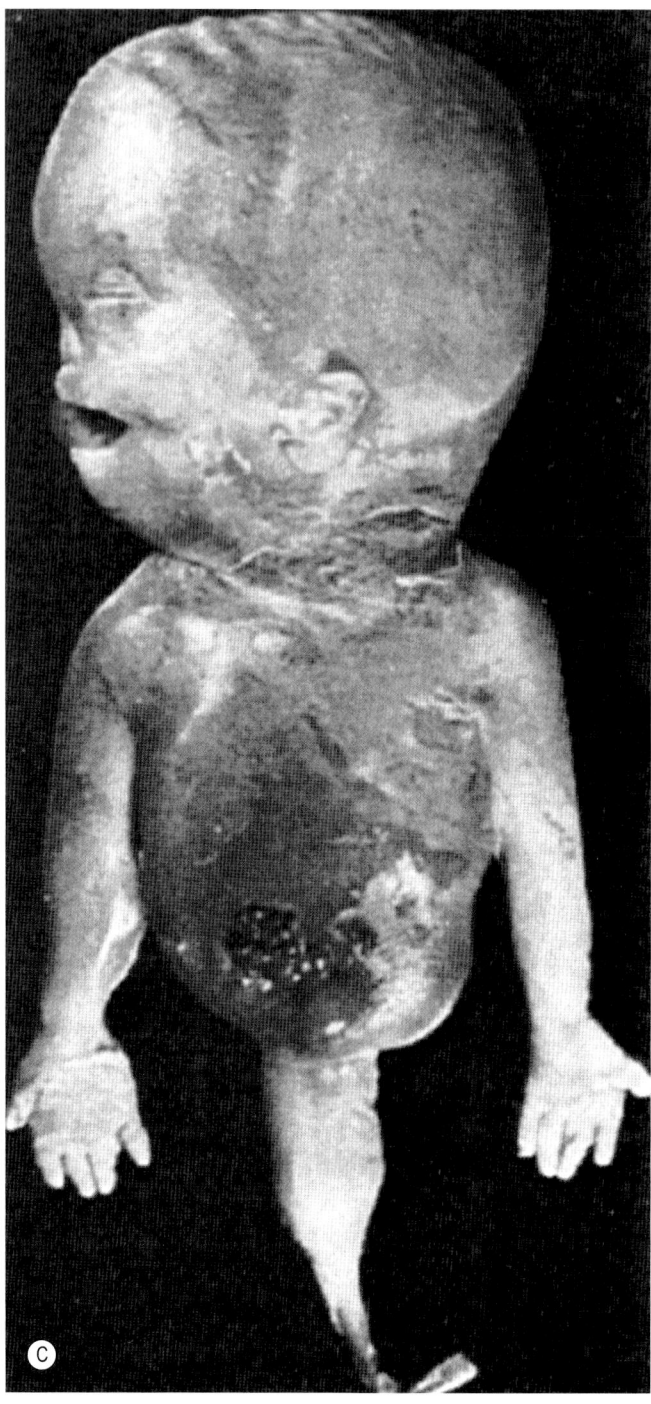

FIGURE 3.6 *(cont'd)*

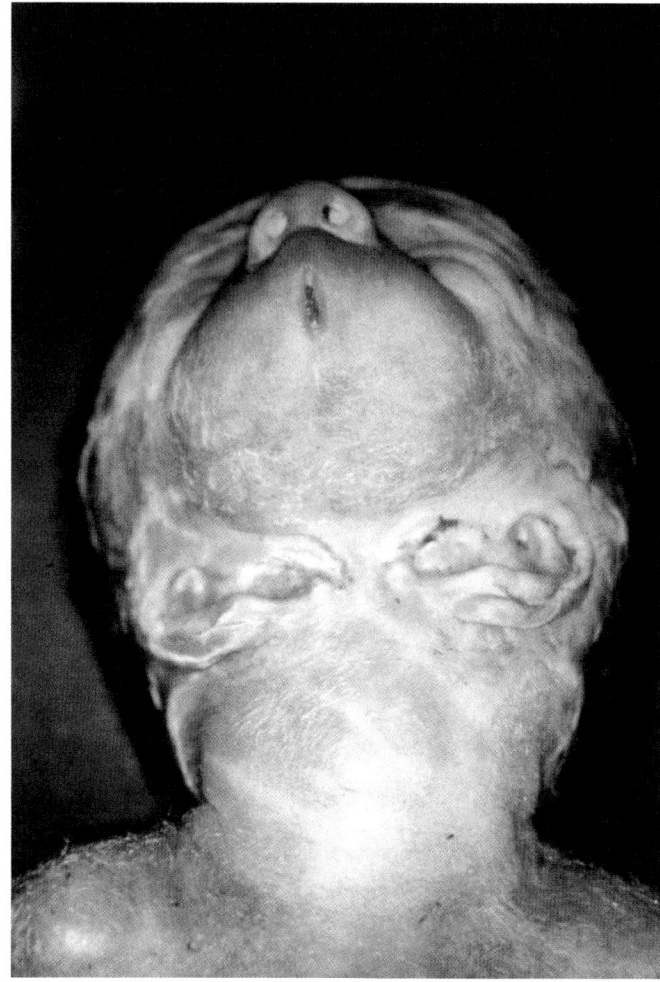

FIGURE 3.7 Otocephaly: extreme mandibular hypoplasia and microstomia associated with synotia.

The non-random VATER association derives from a common developmental pathogenesis, a **defect in blastogenesis that occurs before day 35 of gestation**. All of the following occur before 35 days:

1. The rectum and anus are formed by a mesodermal shelf that divides the cloaca into the urogenital sinus and rectum and anus.
2. A mesodermal septum separates the trachea from the esophagus.
3. The radius is formed by a condensation of mesenchymal tissue in the limb bud.
4. The vertebrae are formed by migration and organization of somite mesoderm.

Lubinsky et al. have suggested that all the VATER associations present **disruption sequences**, as exemplified in the common metabolic disruptive condition of maternal diabetes in infants with the VATER association.[38]

MURCS association

MURCS is an acronym for *mü*llerian duct aplasia, *r*enal aplasia, and *c*ervicothoracic *s*omite malformation, which cause cervico-

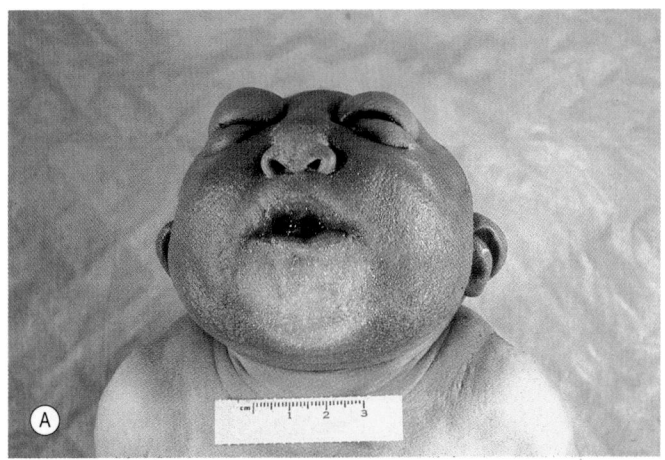 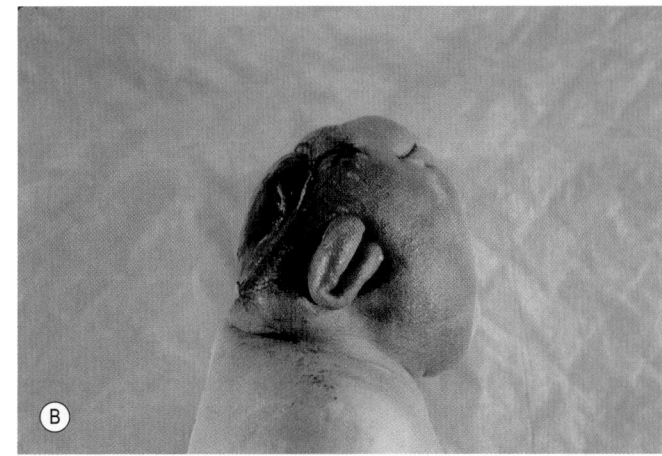

FIGURE 3.8 Anencephaly: frontal (A) and lateral (B) views. (Courtesy Dr. Mason Barr, University of Michigan.)

thoracic vertebral defects, especially from C5 to T1.[39, 40] This condition is **sporadic**. **Absence of the vagina, absence or hypoplasia of the uterus, and renal abnormalities, including agenesis and ectopy**, also occur.

CHARGE association

CHARGE (coloboma, heart disease, atresia choanae, and retarded growth and development) association anomalies include genital and ear anomalies, tracheoesophageal fistula, facial palsy, micrognathia, cleft lip, cleft palate, omphalocele, congenital cardiac defects, and holoprosencephaly.[41, 42] The CHARGE association shows some phenotypic overlap with the VATER association. A few familial cases have been observed; since these may be genetic, the designation CHARGE syndrome may be more appropriate in these cases (such as the locus on chromosome band 8q14).

Heart defects seen in the CHARGE association include tetralogy of Fallot, patent ductus arteriosus, double-outlet right ventricle with a common atrioventricular canal, ventricular septal defect, atrial septal defect, and right-sided aortic arch. **Ear anomalies** and deafness may also occur. All anomalies are produced by altered morphogenesis. The choanae are formed **between days 35 and 38 of gestation**; colobomas results from failure of the fetal choroid fissure to close during week 5 of gestation; cardiac septation begins on day 38 of gestation and is reasonably complete by day 45; holoprosencephaly may reflect altered morphogenesis between gestational weeks 4 and 5. Familial occurrence of some of the associated anomalies has suggested a genetic cause in some cases.[42] With normal parents of an affected child, there appears to be a low recurrence risk.[43]

Schisis association and variants

Czeizel[44] has shown that schisis, or **midline defects** such as neural tube defects (i.e., anencephaly, encephalocele, meningomyelocele) (Fig. 3.18), **oral clefts, omphalocele**, and **diaphragmatic hernia** associate with one another far more frequently than expected.

The schisis association is frequently a lethal abnormality. It occurs more often in girls, in twins (4.6%), and in breech presentations (13.7%) and is associated with lower mean birth weight and a shorter gestational period. **Congenital cardiac defects, limb deficiencies, and defects of the urinary tract**, mainly renal agenesis, have a high association.[44] Schisis-type abnormalities appear to occur non-randomly.

Teratogenic disruptions of blastogenesis

Infants of diabetic mothers (see also Chapter 4)

The subject of infants of diabetic mothers is of cardinal importance in this context because it is now clear that **the major cause of morbidity and mortality in these infants consists of malformations arising during blastogenesis**. In a landmark paper entitled 'Malformations in infants of diabetic mothers occur before the 7th gestational week – implications for treatment,' Mills and colleagues[45] pooled data from 48 studies of anomalies in infants of diabetic mothers published between 1920 and 1964, previously reviewed by Kucera.[46] These data were compared with the birth defect prevalences of the World Health Organization World Wide Survey. Malformations that were significantly more common in infants of diabetic mothers than in those of non-diabetic mothers were analyzed with respect to known embryologic time periods. Under the assumption that no organ will develop malformations after differentiation has occurred, the authors estimated the latest gestational date for the induction of different types of malformations in infants of diabetic mothers. The estimated dates varied from **week 3 (caudal dysplasia) to week 6 (ventricular septal defects)** after conception.[47] Malformations of all kinds are increased in infants of diabetic mothers; **congenital heart defect and neural tube defects are the most common and caudal 'regression' the most specific.**[47]

Association between **high maternal serum levels of hemoglobin A1c (HbA1c)** and congenital anomalies in infants of diabetic mothers was soon demonstrated.[48] In 1988, Mills and

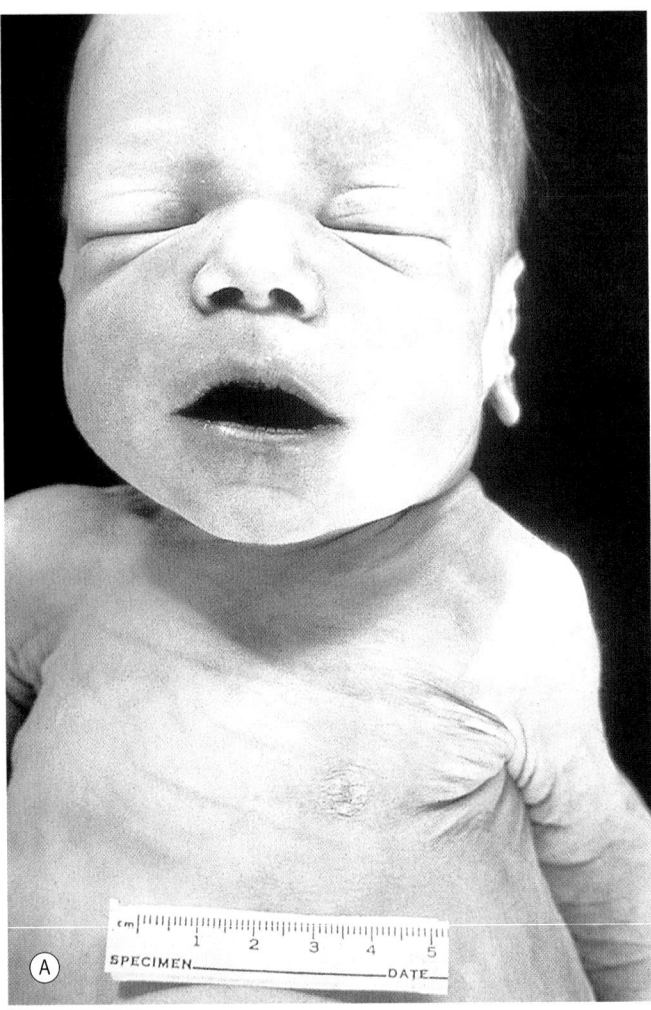

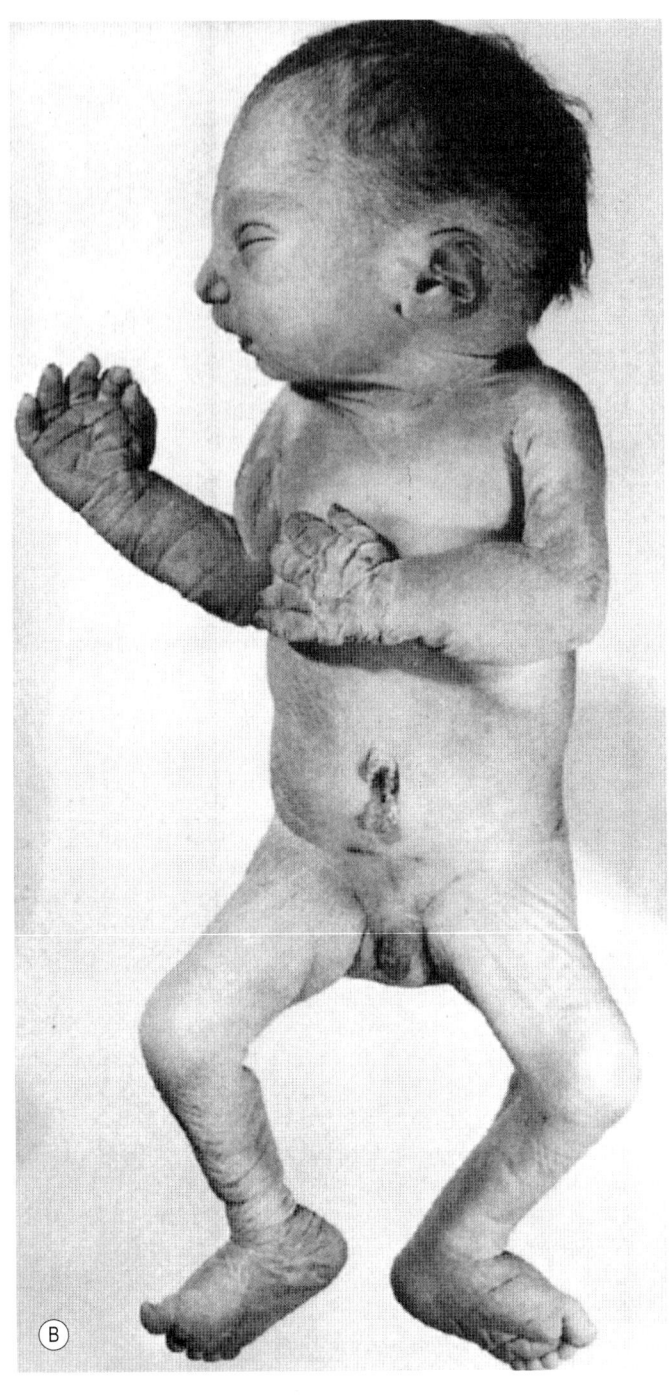

FIGURE 3.9 Infant with renal agenesis. (A) Potter face characteristic of renal agenesis. The inner canthus is covered by a V-shaped fold, the nose is flattened, and a prominent depression is present below the lower lip. (B) Total body showing cutis laxa, especially marked on the hands. The facial profile is characteristic. The ear is less upright than normal, the tragus is absent, the lobe and antitragus are abnormally broad, and the crura of the antitragus are malformed.

colleagues published a controversial paper on the Diabetes in Early Pregnancy (DIEP) study citing the apparent lack of relationship between increased malformation rates in infants of diabetic mothers and glycemic control during organogenesis.[49] As may be guessed from the provocative title, this article created considerable controversy and must be read in conjunction with the article by Greene and colleagues[50] who followed over 300 diabetic women prospectively in the Joslin Clinic. These data, summarized in Table 3.4, show that major fetal anomalies do not increase significantly in rate until first-trimester HbA1c values are 12 or more standard deviations above the mean, and the rate of abortions increases if the HbA1c values are 9 standard deviations above the mean. The authors conclude: 'To keep malformations and spontaneous abortions to a minimum among diabetic women does not require "excellent" control; there seems to be a fairly broad range of "acceptable" control.'

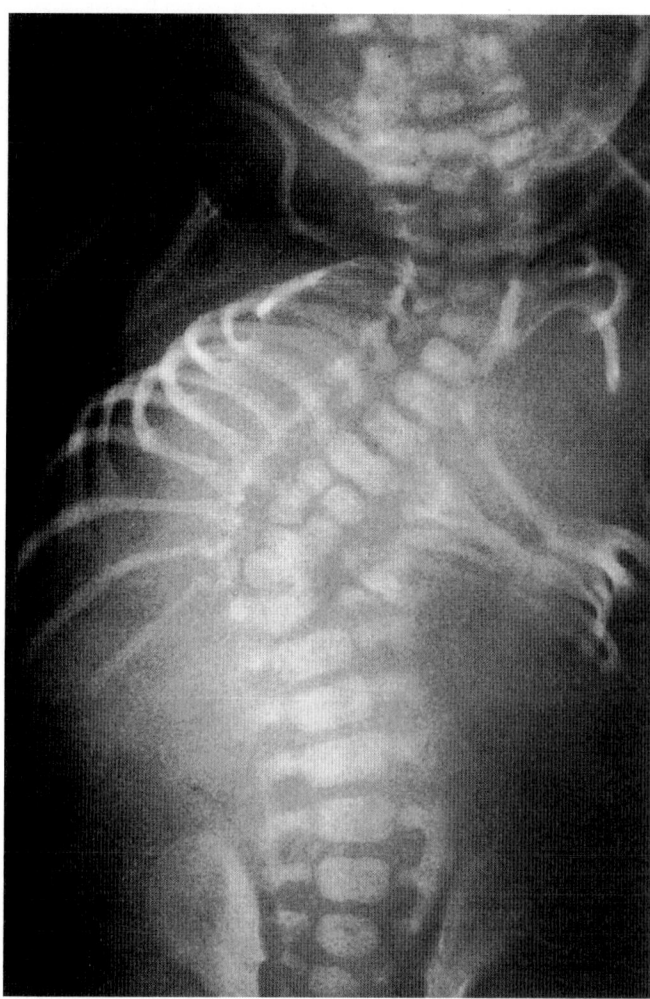

FIGURE 3.10 Radiograph of vertebral segmentation defect. There are abnormalities and reduction in the number of ribs on the left side of the chest associated with scoliosis and kyphosis from hemivertebrae accompanying spina bifida.

TABLE 3.4 OUTCOME OF DIABETIC PREGNANCY RELATIVE TO HEMOGLOBIN A1C LEVEL

HbA1c level (%)	Rate of abortions (%)	Rate of malformations (%)
<9.3	12.4	3.0
>14.4	37.5	40.0

From Greene MF, Hare JW, Clohertz JP, et al. First-trimester hemoglobin A1 and risk for major malformation and spontaneous abortion in diabetic pregnancy. Teratology 1989; 39:225; with permission.

Commenting on the study of Greene and colleagues, Mills[51] concludes that it is now clear that diabetic women in good control are not at increased risk for spontaneous abortions, whereas those in poor control clearly are …Glycemic control as measured by glycosylated hemoglobin explains the malformations in infants of women with very poor control but does not explain the excess of malformations seen in women who maintain fair to good control during organogenesis. Glucose is not an extremely potent teratogen except in high concentrations.

The answer to the question regarding what causes the excess of malformations in the moderately well controlled group of diabetic women is perhaps other metabolic derangements that, on the basis of animal data, include **excessive concentrations of somatomedin inhibitors, ketones such as β-hydroxybutyric acid, hypoglycemia, hyperglycemia, and/or a derangement of arachidonic acid metabolism**. To this must be added the possible synergistic effect of **genetic predisposition**, particularly of the **HLA-DR3** and **HLA-DR4 haplotypes**. In a comment on the paper by Greene and colleagues,[50] Gabbe[52] notes that sacral agenesis, anencephaly, complex cardiac defects, and holoprosencephaly are the most characteristic 'stigmata' of diabetic embryopathy. The concept of 'fuel-mediated teratogenesis' coined by Freinkel[53] appears to be a valuable perspective on the complex pathogenesis of congenital anomalies in infants of diabetic mothers that must clearly arise during blastogenesis. He also notes the known teratogenic roles, in experimental animals, of hypoglycemia, hyperglycemia, β-hydroxybutyrate and somatomedin inhibitors that act synergistically.

It was Pedersen of Copenhagen[54] who first noted or confirmed an impression that women with the best glycemic control during early pregnancy had a lower incidence of infants with birth defects. In the former German Democratic Republic, Fuhrmann and colleagues[55] performed a pioneering study between 1977 and 1981 on 420 women who were in excellent control before conception and maintained glucose levels at less than 100 mg/dL. In this population, the authors were able to demonstrate that the probability of malformation could be reduced to that of the general population.

With respect to genotype, Erikson[56] reported studies involving two outbred strains of Sprague-Dawley rats: strain H (Hanover) and strain U (Uppsala). In H animals there was a low incidence of skeletal malformations in offspring, and in U animals a high incidence. Diabetic H mothers who had H/H or H/U offspring showed the lowest frequency of resorptions (8–9%) and a negligible incidence of skeletal malformations. U/U or H/U diabetic mothers with H/U offspring had 16–20% of resorptions and a 3–5% incidence of skeletal malformations. Most impressive, however, were the data on U/U or H/U mothers who had U/U offspring, in whom there was a 23–30% rate of resorptions and a 17–19% incidence of skeletal malformations. Thus, the teratogenicity in the diabetic mother is potentiated in the presence of genetically predisposed embryos; this requires inducing factors other than D-glucose and β-hydroxybutyrate.

Thus, the infants of diabetic mothers are another dramatic witness to the consequences of disturbed blastogenesis, and the first and still the most striking example (after the fetal alcohol syndrome and folic acid prophylaxis of neural tube defects) of how environmental modification before conception can modify the outcome of these early developmental processes. Hersh and colleagues[57] demonstrate how the variable blastogenetic ano-

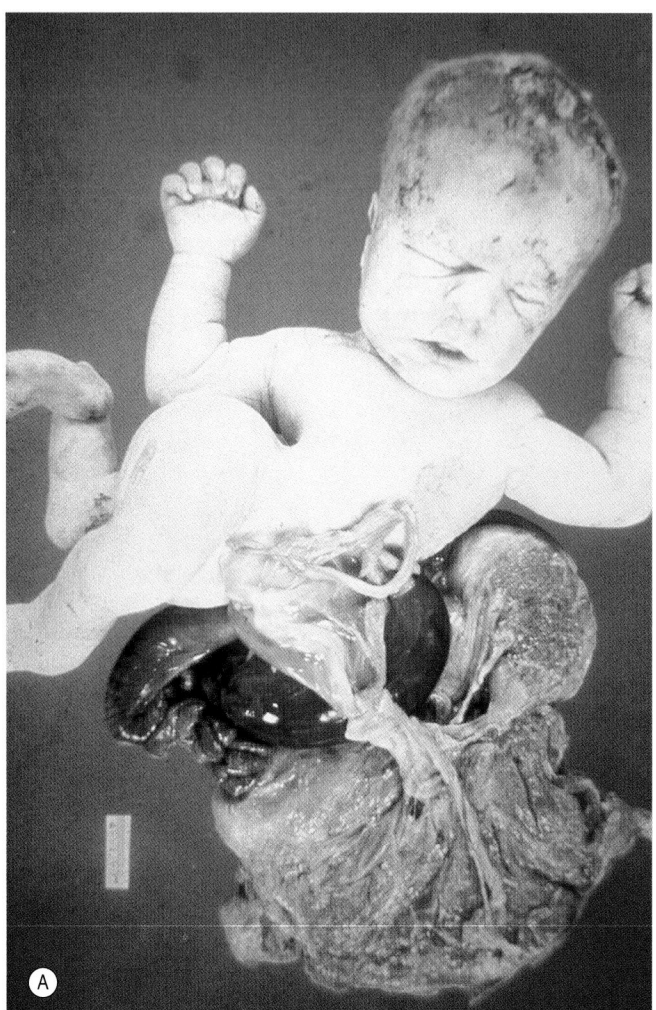
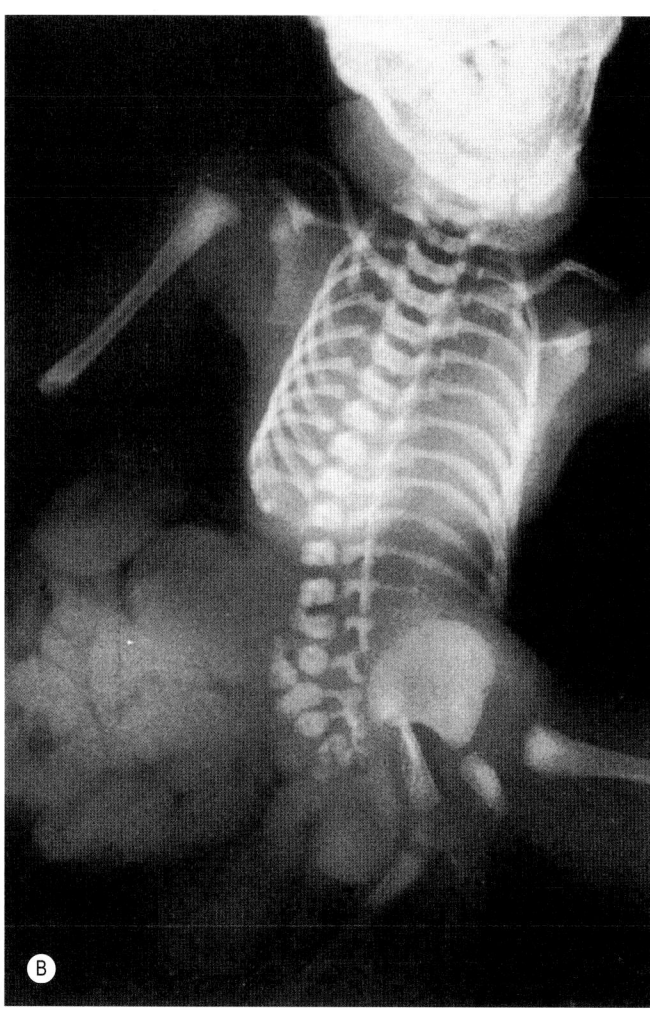

FIGURE 3.11 Limb-body wall complex. Scoliosis of the spine and other skeletal and visceral abnormalities usually accompany eventration caused by abnormal formation of the body stalk. (A) External view. The placenta is attached 4 cm from the edge of the liver. (B) Radiograph showing abnormalities of spine, ribs, and pelvis.

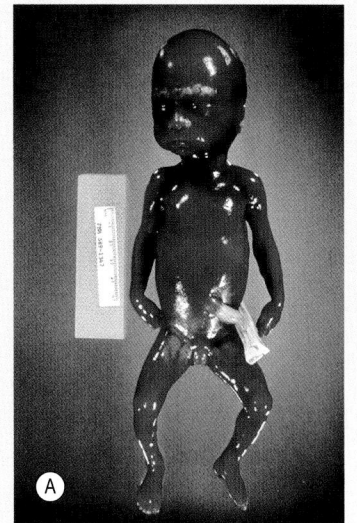
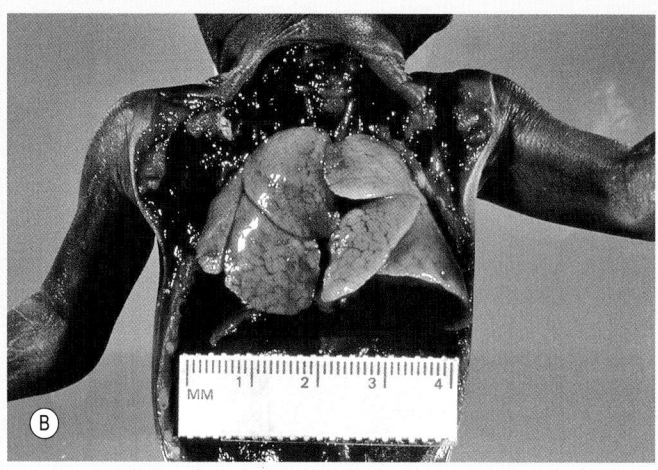

FIGURE 3.12 Polyasplenia field defect. Whole body (A) and chest (B) of a fetus with asplenia, dextropulmonary isomerism, and bowel malrotation, showing bilateral trilobed lungs. (From Wilson GN, Stout JP, Schneider NR, et al. Balanced translocation 12/13 and situs abnormalities: homology of early pattern formation in man and lower organisms? Am J Med Genet 1991;38:601; with permission.)

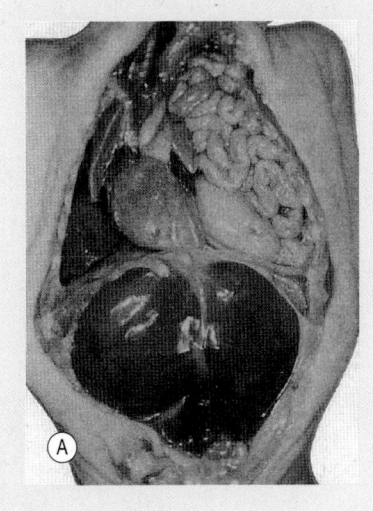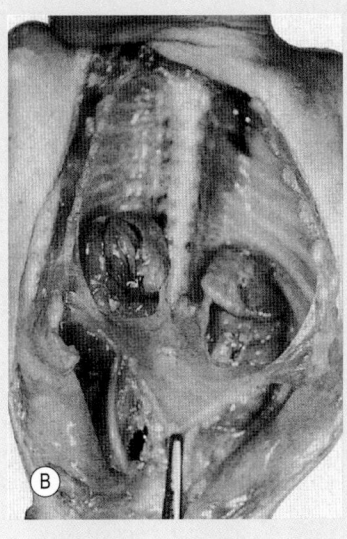

FIGURE 3.13 Bilateral diaphragmatic hernia. (A) Interior of body exposed showing the stomach and intestine in the left side of the chest, and part of the right lobe of the liver in the right side of the chest. (B) All viscera removed except adrenal glands and kidneys, and the diaphragm drawn forward to show defects on both sides. Adrenal glands and upper poles of the kidneys lie in the thoracic cavity because of absence of the posterior portions of the diaphragm.

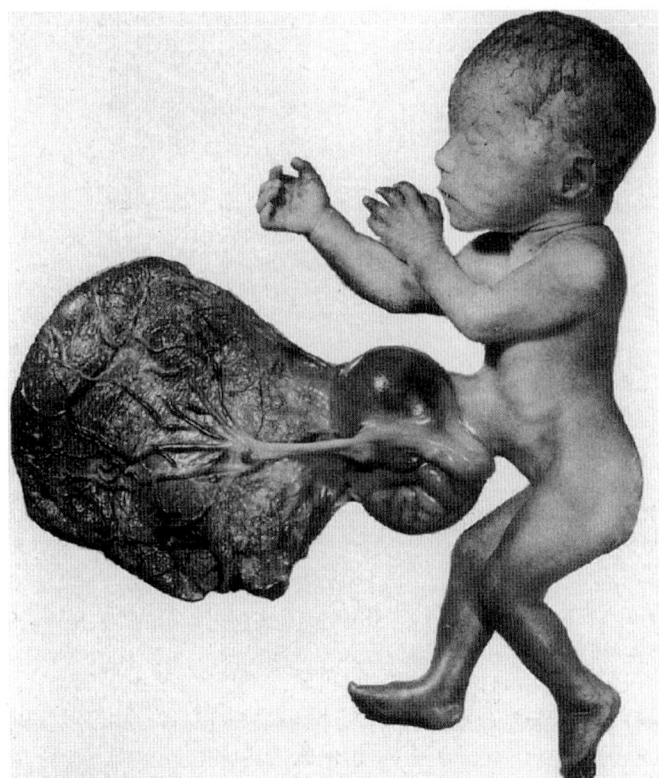

FIGURE 3.14 Intestine and liver outside the abdominal cavity as a result of abnormal formation of the body stalk and umbilical cord. The viscera are covered on one surface by amnion and on the other by chorion.

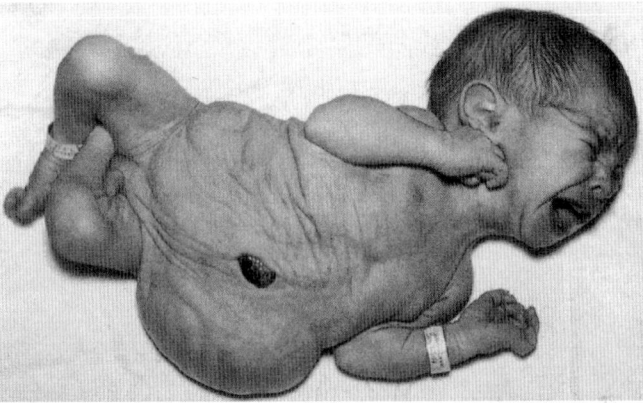

FIGURE 3.15 Prune-belly syndrome. Absence of abdominal muscles associated with hypoplastic right kidneys and persistent urachus attached to the umbilicus. The intestines are in the protuberant mass to the left of the umbilicus. Postoperative death occurred at 9 weeks.

Fetal alcohol syndrome

The most common teratogenic disruption sequence seen in many North American populations is fetal alcohol syndrome (FAS, see Ch. 10), which may also have a prenatally lethal effect. **The condition can affect blastogenesis with resultant holoprosencephaly, complex heart defects, severe limb anomalies, spina bifida, and renal agenesis. It may predispose to tumor formation.** FAS may be difficult to recognize during the fetal or neonatal period, yet it is estimated to be **the most common cause of mental retardation** (1.9 per 1000 births).[58] Since smoking is very common in cases of maternal alcohol abuse, the severe intrauterine growth retardation that may accompany FAS probably represents a component of placental ischemia. In Native American populations these risks are compounded by the high incidence of

malies of diabetic embryopathy – holoprosencephaly, neural tube defects, polyasplenia – reflect the timing and severity of this alteration to the maternofetal environment. Apoptosis is likely a major factor in hyperglycemic embryopathy, and folic acid and vitamin E appear to be protective.[57a]

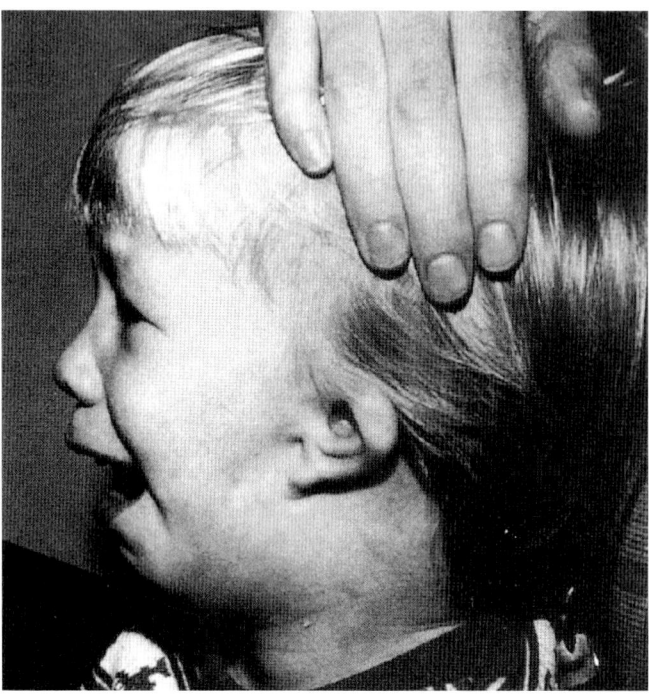

FIGURE 3.16 Ear malformation and mandibular hypoplasia in a child with Goldenhar syndrome. (From Gilbert-Barness and Opitz;[51] courtesy Blackwell Scientific Publications, Inc.)

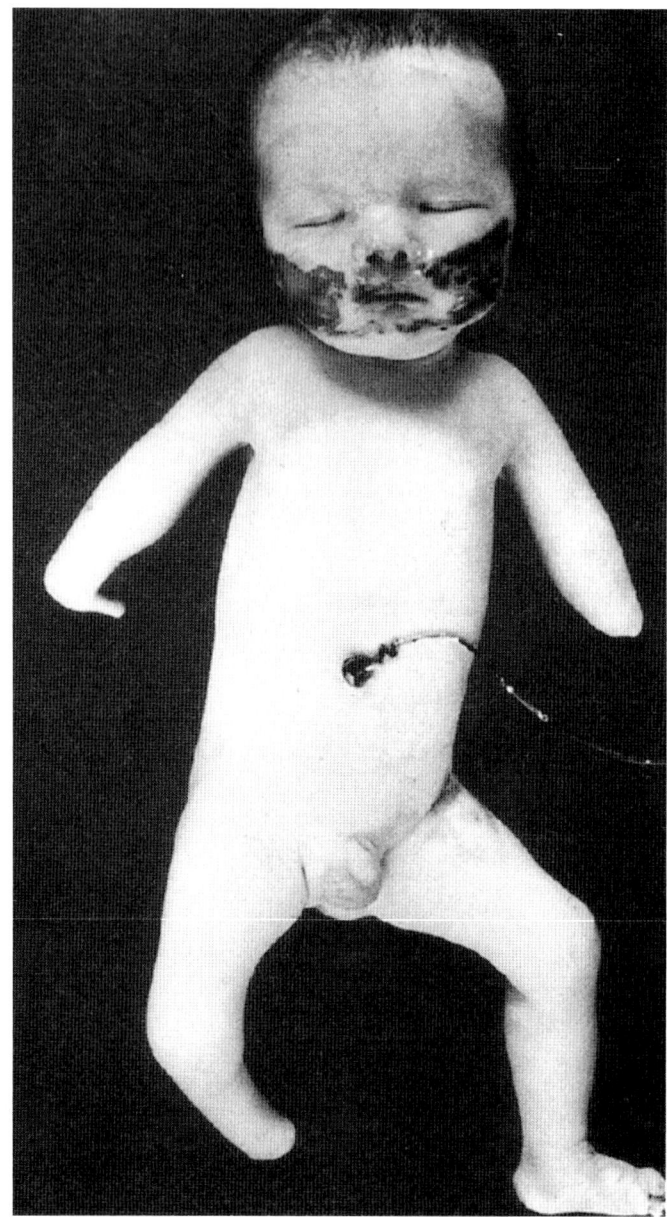

FIGURE 3.17 Infant with Hanhart complex: severe oral involvement and micrognathia with limb defects. Facial marks were caused by tape from a feeding tube. (From Gilbert-Barness and Opitz;[51] courtesy of Blackwell Scientific Publications, Inc.)

non-insulin-dependent diabetes mellitus (NIDDM). Near term, severe maternal alcoholism may be lethal for the fetus.[59]

The fetal brain is a major target of alcohol, and neuropathologic studies in humans demonstrate **smaller brains with abnormal gyri and heterotopias (abnormal cell migration)**. Brain defects are documented in several animal models, including rodents and non-human primates.[59] Intraperitoneal injection of mice with ethanol on gestational day 7 produced decreased embryo size, abnormal neuroepithelium, and facial changes similar to those observed in humans.[60] Genetic susceptibility was suggested in these mice, since the C57BL/6J strain exhibited a disproportionately high incidence of eye anomalies in response to ethanol.[60] Studies of alcohol teratogenesis provide a prototype for approaching other disruptions (see Table 3.3). Genetics and metabolic susceptibilities are also in the process of characterization in humans.[60a]

Anomalies of organogenesis

During the period of organogenesis, the primordial embryonic regions sculpted by blastogenesis develop into specific organs. Abnormalities of these primordia include **localized limb defects** (Figs. 3.19 and 3.20), **renal defects** (Fig. 3.21), and **ear anomalies** (Fig. 3.22). As mentioned in Chapter 2, abnormal processes of organogenesis may build upon abnormal developmental fields that began in blastogenesis.[61] The disastrous experience with thalidomide in humans, subsequently confirmed experimentally in several types of monkeys, led to an extremely accurate deter-

mination of the periods of sensitivity of several organ primordia and body parts, as summarized in Table 3.5.[62]

Defects of phenogenesis

Phenogenesis, the stage of fetal life from 8 weeks to birth, completes the molding of large blastogenetic fields and defined primordia into the recognizable appearance of newborns. Morphologic detail is refined and individual variation is created, subject to the varieties of anthropometric measurements described in Chapter 2. Abnormalities of phenogenesis include

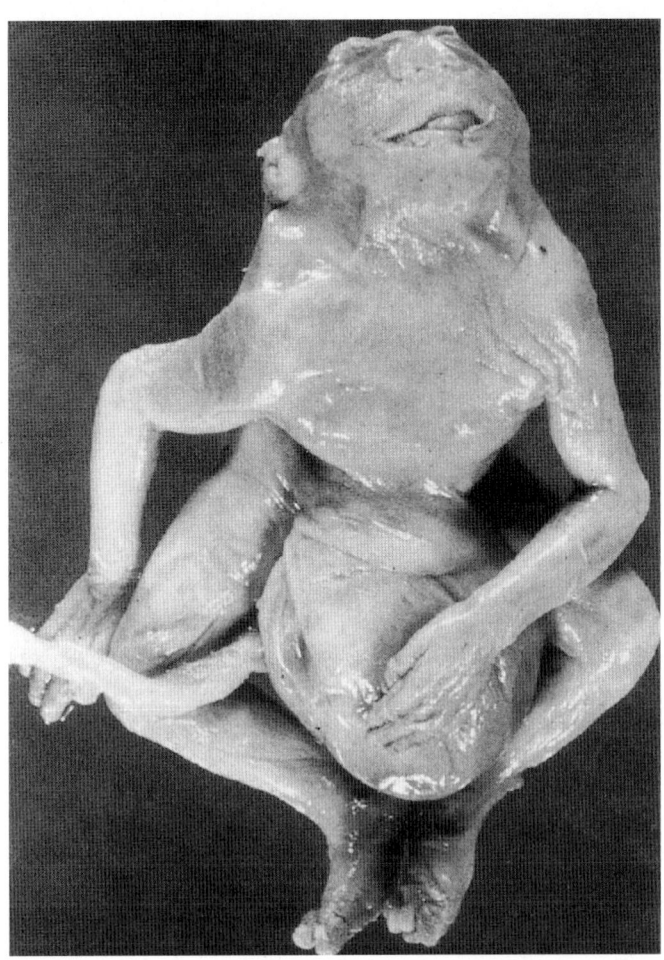

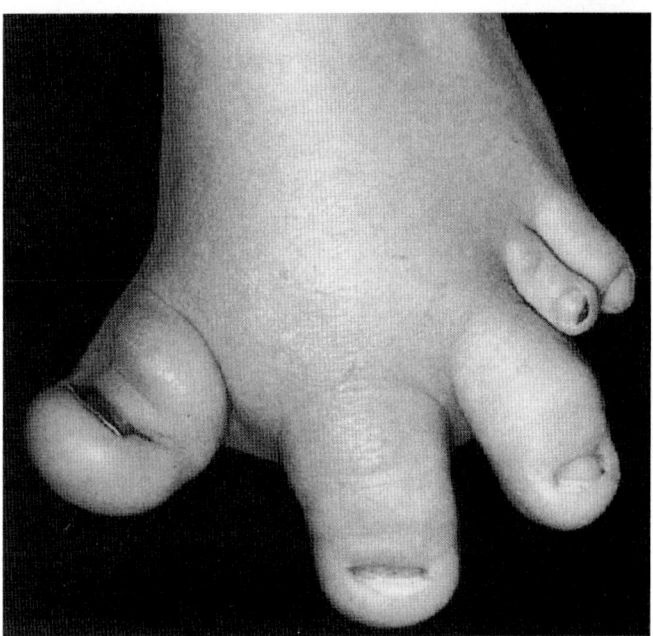

FIGURE 3.19 Congenital gigantism of three toes of one foot in an infant aged 8 months. This was thought to be due to neurofibromatosis.

FIGURE 3.18 Fetus with schisis association: note anencephaly and omphalocele. (From Gilbert-Barness and Opitz;[51] courtesy Blackwell Scientific Publications, Inc.)

FIGURE 3.20 Phocomelia in a macerated fetus. (A) External view. (B) Radiograph.

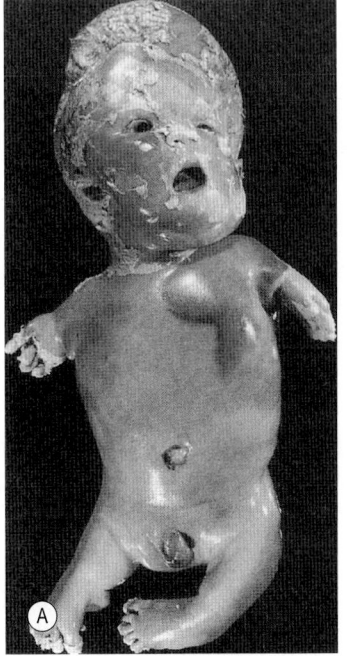

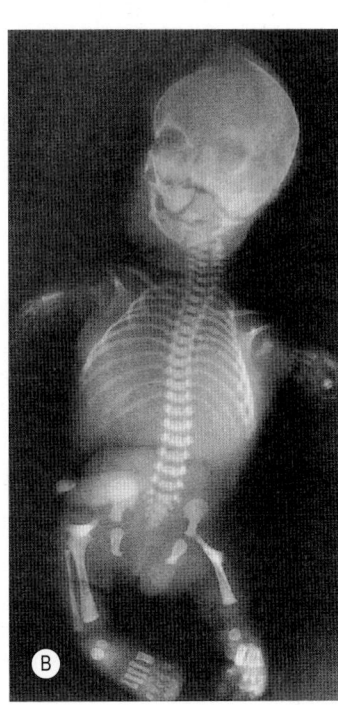

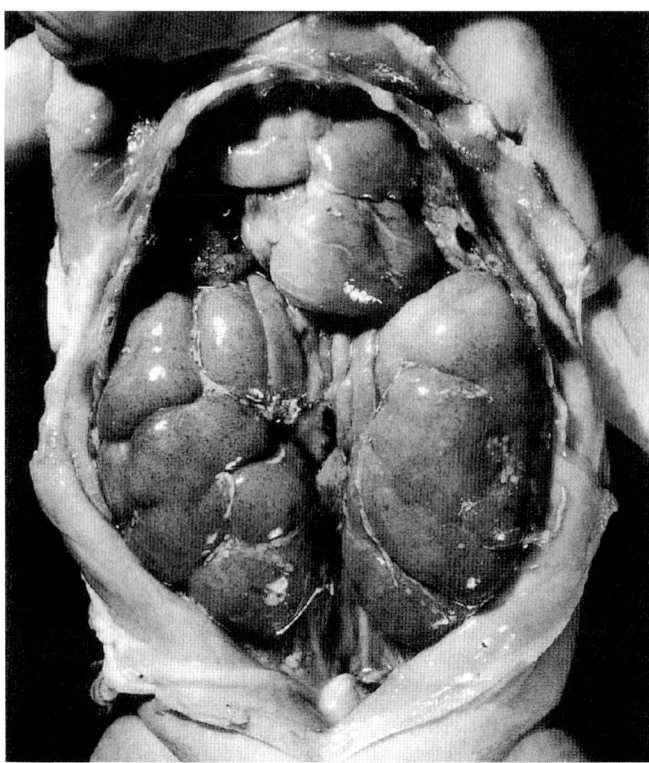

FIGURE 3.21 Autosomal recessive polycystic kidneys exhibiting bilateral enlargement and retention of fetal lobulation. They are covered with punctate dark areas that are the ends of dilated terminal branches of collecting tubules.

TABLE 3.5 EFFECTS OF THALIDOMIDE ON DEVELOPMENT

Days after fertilization	Effects
21	Anotia, facial paralysis, ocular palsies
23	Absent thumbs with intact radii
24–26	(Partial) absence of upper limbs
27–29	Anal atresia, renal anomalies, vaginal atresia
29–31	Severe arm malformations, cardiac defects, duodenal atresia/stenosis
30–33	Severe lower limb defects, heart malformations
33–34	Triphalangeal thumbs, anal stenosis

From Delahunt CS, Lassen LT. Thalidomide syndrome in monkeys. Science 1964; 146:1300; with permission.

deviations in these anthropometric measurements, catalogued as abnormal when beyond certain centiles or distinguished as morphologic variants of little medical or cosmetic consequence (minor anomalies). Measures within two standard deviations (3rd–97th centiles) and variants of incidence more than 4–5% (stork bites, sacral spots) are considered within normal limits (standard range, normal variations). Many dysmorphologists and pediatric pathologists have a set of standard measurements they obtain during examination[63] and charts like that in Figure 3.23 may assist the documentation of minor anomalies.

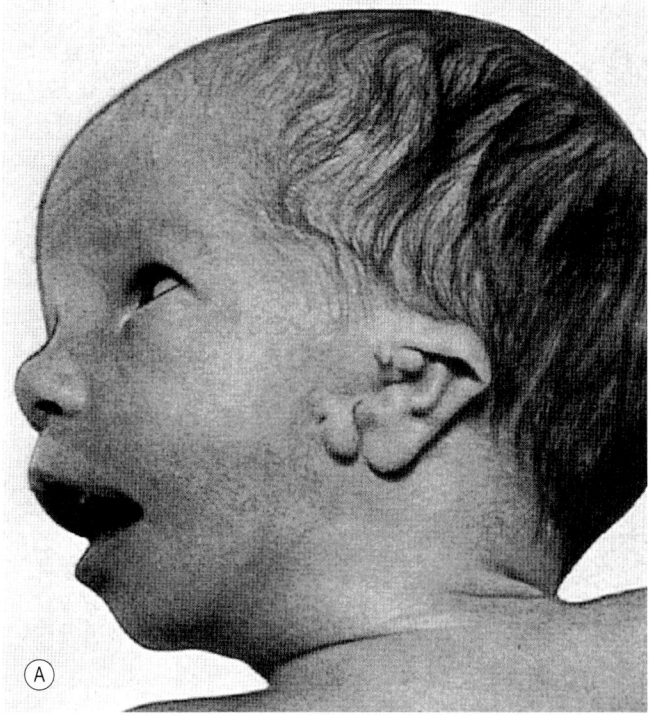

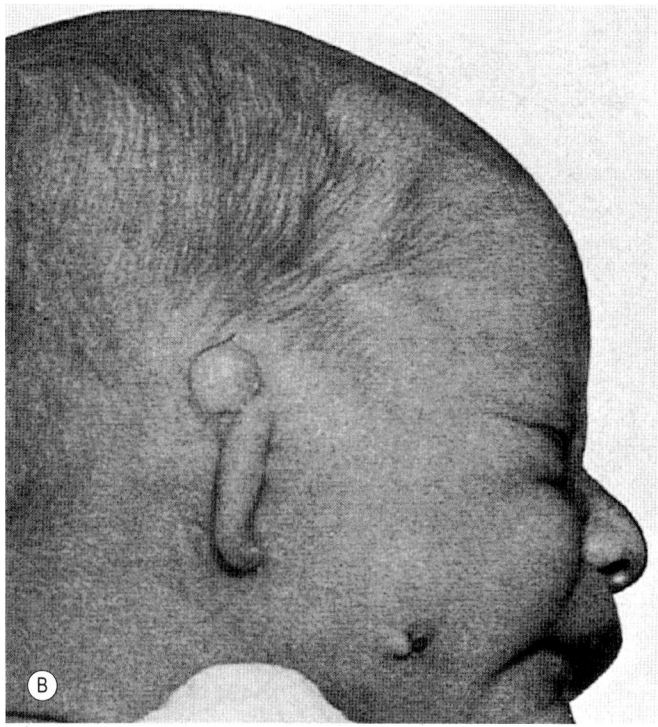

FIGURE 3.22 Ear anomalies. (A) 'Satyr' ear associated with papillomas and an aural fistula caused by abnormal closure of the first branchial groove. (B) Hypoplasia of the pinna with absence of the external auditory meatus associated with a papilloma and an aural fistula located midway between the ear and mouth.

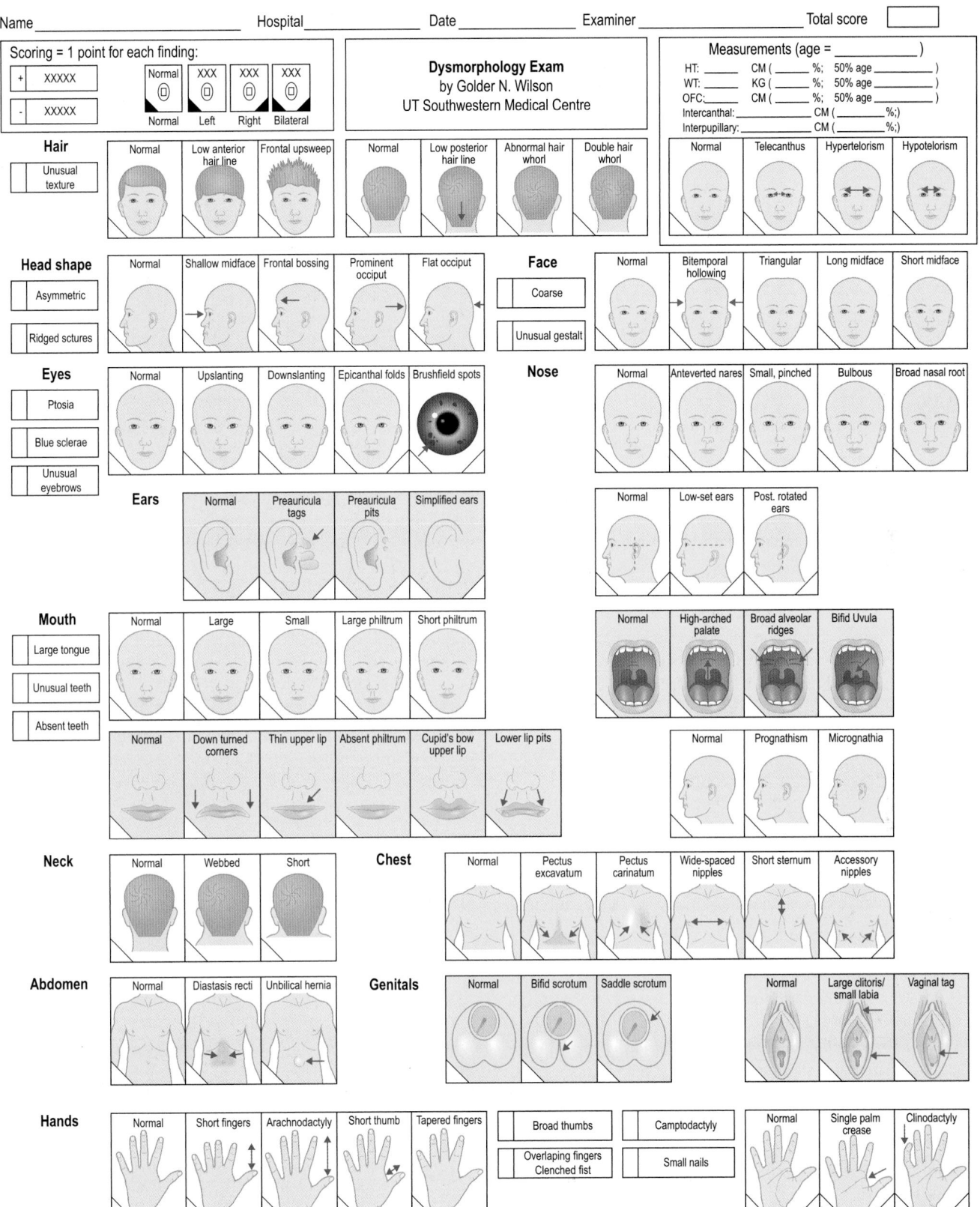

FIGURE 3.23 Minor anomalies as listed in a pictorial checklist devised by Dr. Golder Wilson, Texas Tech University.

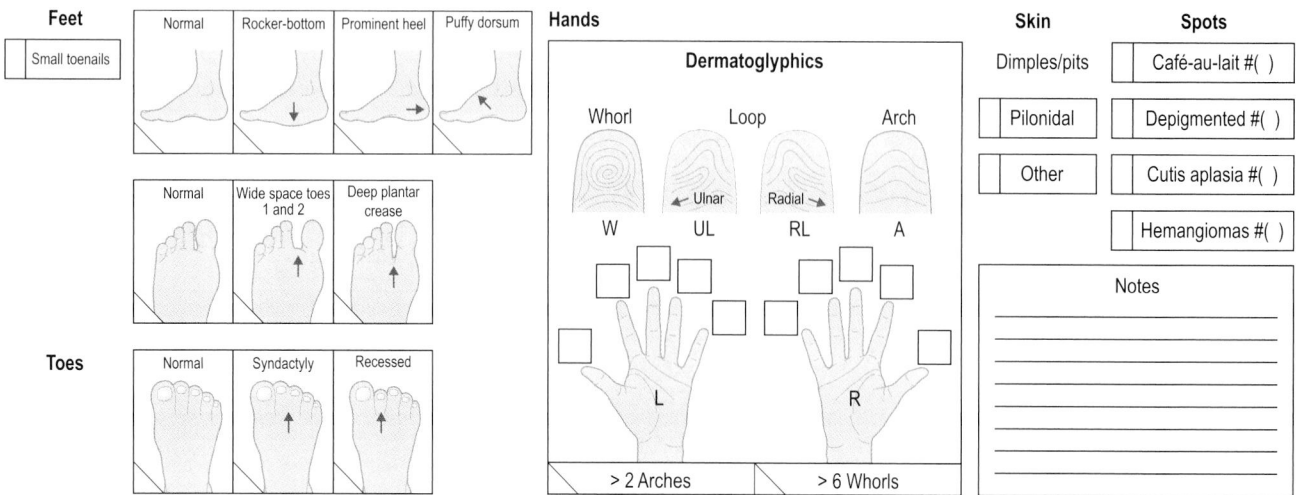

FIGURE 3.23 The examiner should proceed item by item, marking the appropriate normal or abnormal boxes. Normal newborn infants average less than three abnormal findings, while individuals with syndromes (e.g., Down syndrome) often score 15–20 abnormal findings. Dermatoglyphics are read using a magnifying glass.

Pathologists rarely have the opportunity to examine the relatives of dead fetuses and infants entrusted to them for final care; thus, photographs are mandatory and a later aid to the clinical geneticists who will be counseling the family. If the fetus or infant has an appearance or constellation of anomalies that is quite different from the family background, then a chromosome study is indicated. Infants with syndromes often have a characteristic facial appearance that differs from that of close relatives, as illustrated in Figures 3.24 to 3.27 below.

Characteristic facial phenotypes: the example of Cornelia de Lange syndrome

The phenotype of Cornelia de Lange syndrome (CDLS, MIM 112470) is characterized by growth and mental retardation and hirsutism with extreme variability in expression.[64, 65] Major manifestations include mental retardation (100%), synophrys (94%), hirsutism (84%), and thin, down-turned vermilion borders (80%) (Fig. 3.24). Other common anomalies include dental abnormalities with late eruption of widely spaced teeth (93%), and male genital abnormalities such as cryptorchidism and hypospadias (94% of males).

Occasional anomalies include myopia, microcornea, astigmatism, optic atrophy, coloboma of the optic nerve, strabismus, proptosis, choanal atresia, low-set ears, cleft palate, congenital heart defects (most commonly ventricular septal defect), hiatus hernia, duplication of the gut, malrotation of the colon, brachyesophagus, pyloric stenosis, inguinal hernia, small labia majora, radial hypoplasia, short first metacarpal, distal limb defects of the upper extremities and digits, absent second to third interdigital triradius, and diaphragmatic hernia.[65]

A recurrence risk of 2–5% has been reported and there have been case reports of concordance in monozygotic twins. It appears to be an autosomal dominant mutation. Several cases of familial occurrence in mildly affected individuals confirm domi-

nant inheritance. Although there is some phenotypic overlap of CDLS and the dup(3q) syndrome, these entities are distinct[66] and distinguishable. Recently, linkage studies excluded the 3q region and localized CDLS to the 5q31 region where there is a highly conserved Nipped-B-like gene with homologues in flies, worms, plants, and fungi.[67] Mutations were found in nine patients, and the product protein (named DELANGIN by the authors) assists sister chromatid cohesion. Early embryonic expression of *DELANGIN* in limb bud, branchial arch, and craniofacial regions correlates with major defects in Cornelia de Lange syndrome, and continuing disruption of cell division may explain the alterations of phenogenesis (minor anomalies) that are so characteristic of this syndrome.[68]

Minor anomalies and phenogenesis

Minor anomalies are the most common manifestations of aneuploidy; in contradistinction to malformations, they may change considerably during later postnatal development. Thus, an infant with the Beckwith-Wiedemann syndrome may have a striking constellation of minor anomalies that distort facial dimensions and proportions, together with conspicuous glabellar capillary hemangioma and macroglossia (Fig. 3.25). Through processes of maturation and normal and differential growth, the facial appearance in these individuals may change so dramatically that adolescents and adults with the condition who were conspicuously involved earlier in life now have not only a normal, but an even highly attractive appearance. Figures 3.26 and 3.27 illustrate the natural history of facial changes in the Noonan and Williams syndromes. Thus, when performing an autopsy on a child who has died of metastatic Wilms' tumor without evidence of macroglossia or the scar of repaired omphalocele, it is important to check behind the auricles for the semilunar pits on the posterior rim of the helix, the only one of the minor anomalies in the Beckwith-Wiedemann

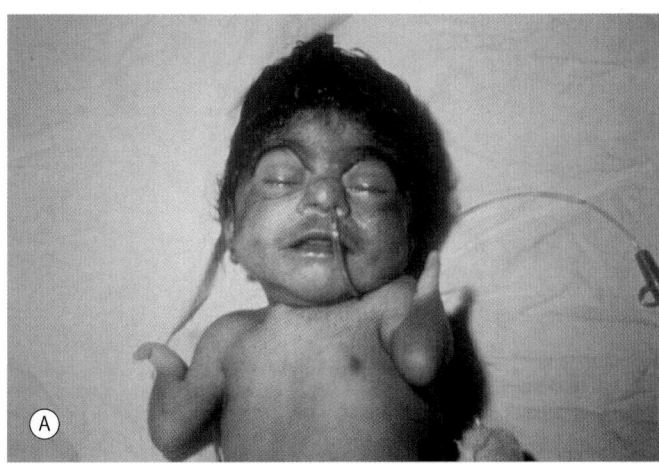

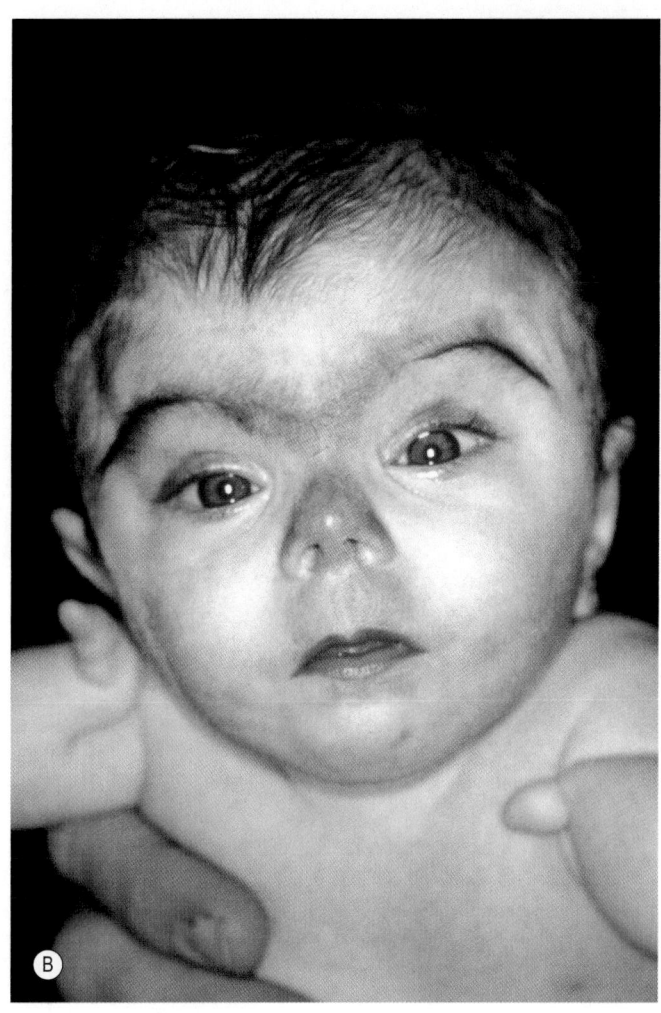

FIGURE 3.24 Cornelia de Lange syndrome. (A) Infant showing oligodactyly, abnormal face with synophrys, anteverted nares, long philtrum, and down-turned corners of the mouth. (B) Child showing the same clinical findings. (Courtesy Dr. Robert Gorlin, University of Minnesota.)

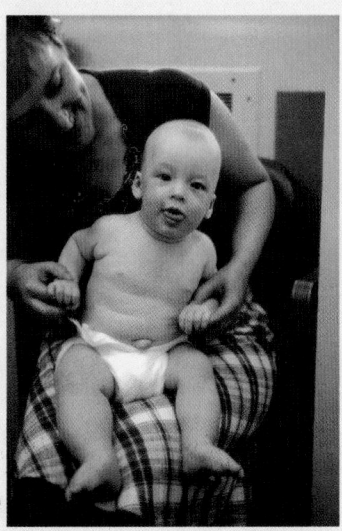

FIGURE 3.25 Child with Beckwith-Wiedemann syndrome: large size, hemihypertrophy (note right leg), large organs, and umbilical hernia.

syndrome that does not change over time (Fig. 3.34B). In case of suspected Smith-Lemli-Opitz syndrome (see below), a check of the fingertips may document presence of ten whorls as a valuable diagnostic sign; such minor anomalies will not change over the life of the patient.

Deformities

Deformities result from a bending out of shape of structures that are otherwise developing normally. The deformation may be due to excessive extrinsic pressure (e.g., uterine fibroid), weakness (contractures due to congenital myopathies), or lack of movement (contractures due to spinal muscular atrophy or rodent curare treatment – Figs 3.28 and 3.29). However, deformed structures frequently are also small, indicating that pressure deformities may reduce normal growth, or inhibit movement of limbs and other body parts. **Movement is essential to normal fetal growth**. Figure 3.30 illustrates an infant who

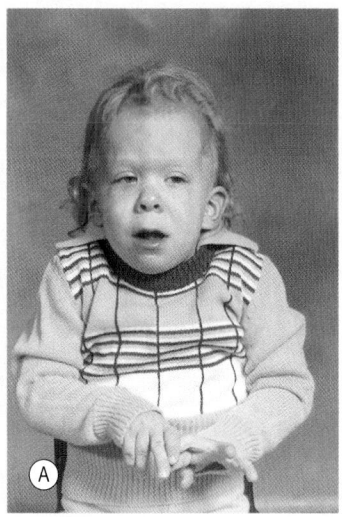
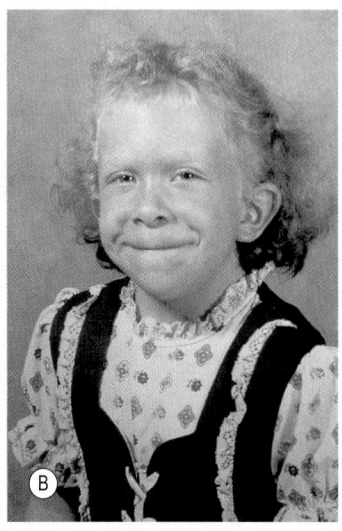

FIGURE 3.26 Same patient with Noonan syndrome at different ages. (A) Young child with broad face, bilateral ptosis, epicanthal folds, anteverted ear lobules, and short neck. (B) Older child with sparse hair, broad face, and unusual ears.

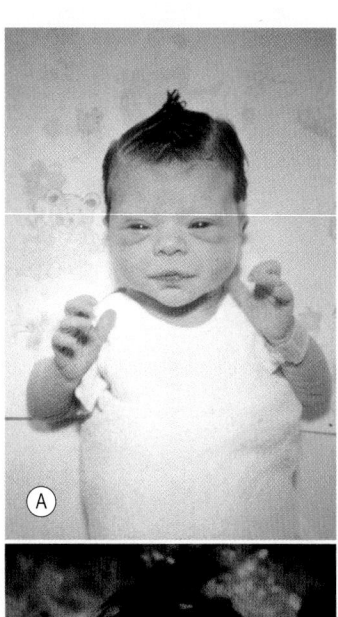
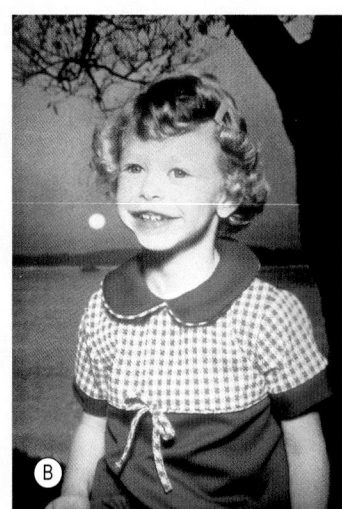
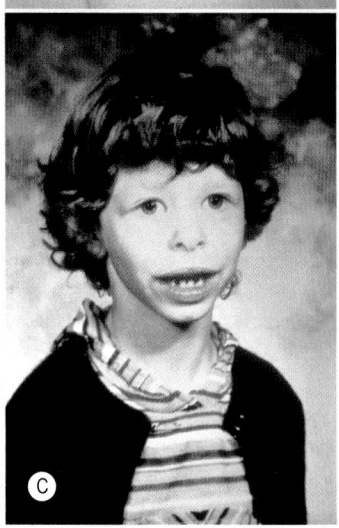
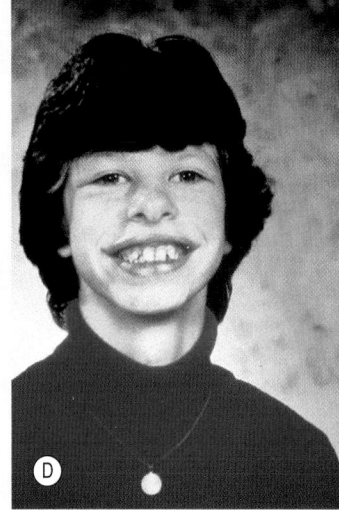

FIGURE 3.27 Patient with Williams syndrome at different ages. (A) Infant with puffy face who had a hoarse cry and hypercalcemia. (B) Child with elfin appearance and loquacious personality. (C and D) Older child and young adult with 'coarse' face, malar flattening, large mouth, thick lips, and less-striking personality.

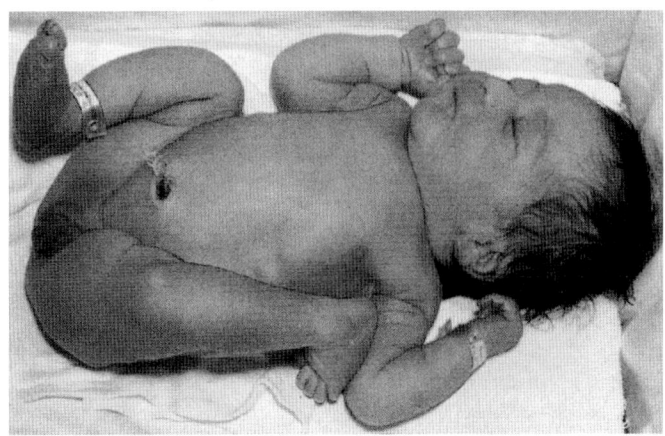

FIGURE 3.28 Genu recurvatum in an otherwise normal infant.

presumably had severe fetal constraint, with secondary adherence of limbs to amnion and disruptive amputation. Sometimes it is easy to identify the source of pressure and/or limitation of movement, e.g., **twinning, septate or bicornuate uterus, uterine myomata, and abdominal implantation. Oligohydramnios** is an important and common source of deformities designated **Potter sequence** after the distinguished initial author of this textbook. It may be due to renal agenesis or failure of fetal urine to enter the amniotic cavity.

Another common type of deformity is that due to **intrinsic weakness or hypotonia** as in the **arthrogryposes or hypotonia sequence**. Collectively, these disorders are referred to as **fetal akinesia (or hypokinesia) sequences**. Their pathogenesis is fairly well understood on the basis of animal models and may

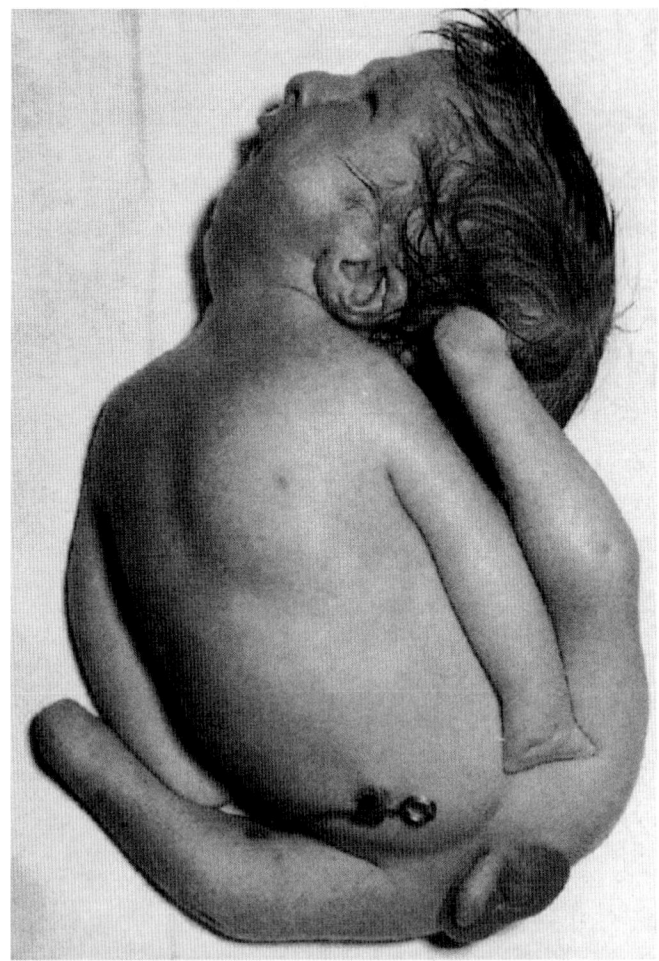

FIGURE 3.30 Infant with arthrogryposis and absence of digits involving all four limbs. The vertebrae are normal but the head is dorsiflexed.

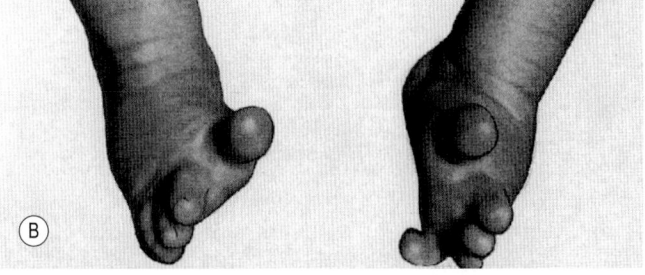

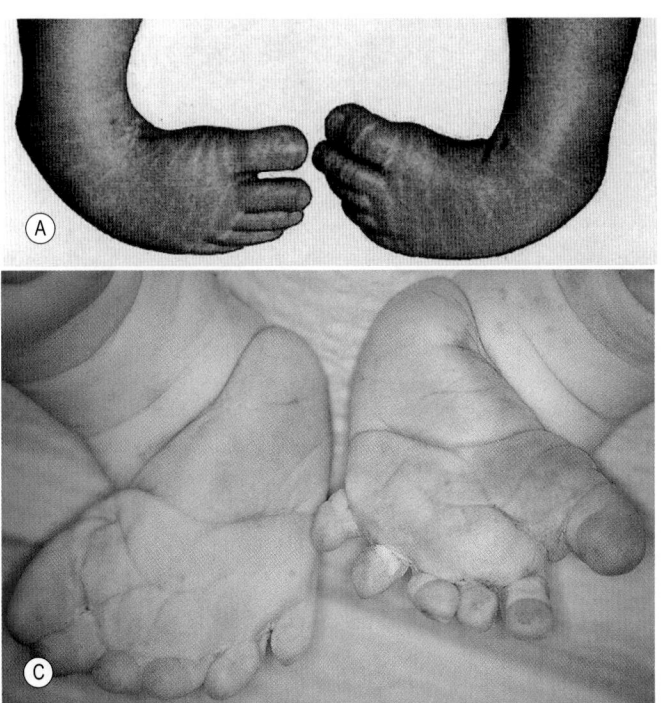

FIGURE 3.29 Clubfoot. (A) Talipes varus, most common form. (B) Mild equinovarus. (C) Severe equinovarus.

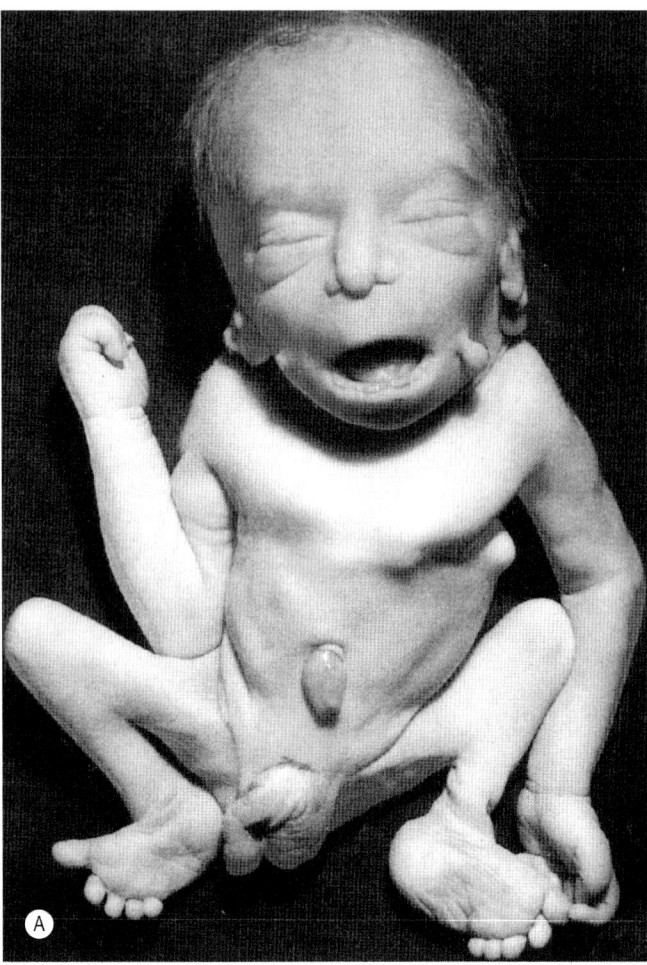

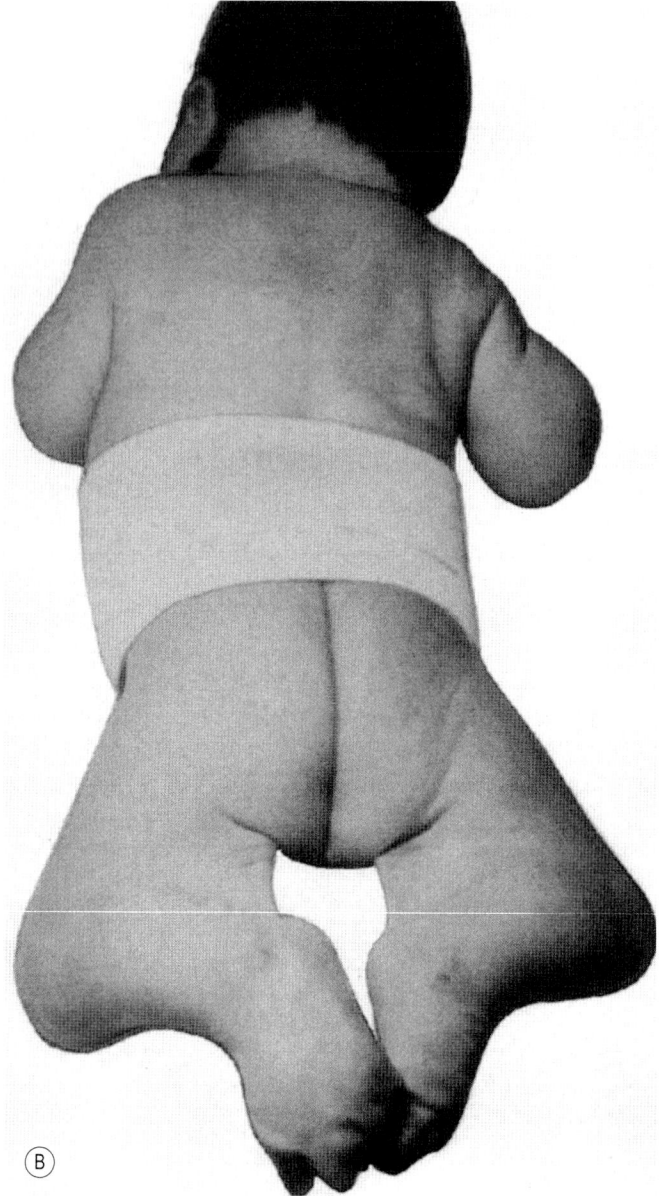

FIGURE 3.31 Webbed knees. (A) Stillborn fetus with multiple malformations. (B) Living infant, normal except for soft tissue deformity of the lower limbs.

involve cerebral, spinal cord, muscle, or peripheral nerve abnormalities. **When amotility is severe, webbing across joints may occur (pterygia),** as in Fig. 3.31. **Dimpling at the joints** is also frequent in immotility and arthrogryposis. Jones[42] outlines an excellent approach to the difficult category of arthrogryposis. The pathogenesis and pathology has been discussed by Porter.[69]

Pena and Shokeir first described early **lethal neurogenic arthrogryposis and pulmonary hypoplasia** as the Pena-Shokeir phenotype (**Pena-Shokeir I syndrome, or fetal akinesia deformation MIM 208150**).[70] Facial abnormalities include prominent eyes, hypertelorism, telecanthus, epicanthal folds, malformed ears, depressed tip of the nose, small mouth, high arched palate, and micrognathia. Polyhydramnios, small placenta, and relatively short umbilical cord are frequent findings. Infants are small for their gestational age; approximately 30% are stillborn. Most die of the complications of pulmonary hypoplasia within the first few weeks. All die before 6 months of age.

This autosomal recessive syndrome has an estimated frequency of 1 in 12 000 births, with a heterozygote frequency of 1 in 55. The phenotypic malformations appear to be nonspecific (genetic heterogeneity) and phenotypic manifestations are caused by decreased or absent movements in utero resulting in the fetal akinesia deformation sequence.[71] There is genetic heterogeneity. One-half of the cases are sporadic. An X-linked form of fetal akinesia syndrome also exists (MIM 300073). Therefore, Hall proposed the term Pena-Shokeir phenotype, because it has been recognized that this is not a specific syndrome but a description of a phenotype produced by fetal akinesia.[71]

The polyhydramnios is due to failure of normal deglutition. Neuromuscular deficiency in the function of the diaphragm and intercostal muscles causes pulmonary hypoplasia. Multiple ankyloses at elbows, knees, hips, and ankles, rocker-bottom feet, talipes equinovarus, and camptodactyly are present. Absence of the flexion creases on the fingers and palms and sparse dermatoglyphic ridges are frequent, as is the formation of pterygia. The lethal form of recessive multiple pterygium syndrome may represent a severe form of the phenotype. The phenotype may resemble that of trisomy 18, from which it should be distinguished.

Neuropathologic findings include thin cerebral and cerebellar cortices, polymicrogyria, and multiple foci of encephalomalacia, with loss of neurons and gliosis. There is usually spinal cord involvement, with reduction in the anterior motor horn cells. Skeletal muscles show diffuse and group atrophy consistent with neurogenic atrophy.

In women with polyhydramnios, the diagnosis should be entertained and hypokinesia should be sought at ultrasonography and in their newborn infants. Pulmonary hypoplasia may be detected by prenatal ultrasonography.

Pena-Shokeir type II syndrome (cerebro-oculo-facioskeletal syndrome [COFS, MIM 214150]) is recognized as an autosomal recessive disorder with degenerative brain and spinal cord defects that are usually manifest at birth. Reduced white matter of the brain with mottling of the gray matter, associated with generalized hypotonia and hypo- or areflexia, is characteristic. It is characterized by progressive psychomotor deterioration, and death usually occurs before 5 years of age.[71]

Deformity may also occur as a result of malformation, as in the paralytic talipes equinovarus deformity due to meningomyelocele or scoliosis due to hemivertebrae. Cervical vertebral anomalies or abnormalities of the sternocleidomastoideus may cause more or less severe facial deformities with plagiocephaly and conspicuous asymmetries (note the head dorsiflexion in Fig. 3.30).

Many deformities improve with age, differential growth, and (more) normal use. Thus, the dramatic 'campomelic' bowing of the tibiae, plagiocephaly, and disuse micrognathia of various types may disappear completely. However, dysostotic micrognathia, as in the **Hanhart syndrome**, will not. Other deformities may worsen with age, especially those associated with brain damage, such as severe CNS malformations and functional impairment of a genetic nature (e.g., **Krabbe disease**), as they cause recumbency and disuse of joints. Having been born without deformities, at death such a child may have severe plagiocephaly, the dramatic facial–oral changes of lifelong mouth breathing, scoliosis, cortical thumbs, rigid fisting, clubfoot, and flexion contractures at other joints.

Defects of differentiation: dysplasias

Dysplasias, as defined in Chapter 2, are defects of cellular and **tissue differentiation**. As such, they may arise at any time in the life of the fetus and infant **after** initial morphogenesis. Since morphogenesis involves fields, i.e., morphogenetic units consisting of **several** types of tissues or their precursors, and occurs 10–14 days **before** tissue differentiation, most malformations are histologically normal, and few dysplasias disrupt morphogenesis. Teratomas are an important exception.

Non-metabolic dysplasia syndromes

These include neurofibromatosis (NF), tuberous sclerosis, von Hippel-Lindau disease, Beckwith-Wiedemann and Perlman syndromes, and vascular dysplasias, including Klippel-Trenaunay-Weber and Sturge-Weber dysplasia.

Neurofibromatosis (von Recklinghausen disease) NF is inherited as an autosomal dominant trait, of which two distinctive forms have been recognized.[72–73] These are discussed below.

TYPE I, PERIPHERAL NEUROFIBROMATOSIS. The peripheral neurofibromatosis (MIM 162200) is an autosomal dominant disease and affects 1 in 4000 live births; the disease is caused by a mutation of the *NEUROFIBROMIN* gene localized to **chromosome 17**.[73a] Diagnostic criteria include the presence of six or more **café-au-lait spots** more than 5 mm in diameter in children, **neurofibromas and plexiform neurofibromas** occurring along nerves (Fig. 3.32) in subcutaneous tissues and sometimes in eyes and meninges.[72] Other manifestations are lipomas, angiomas, optic gliomas, iris hamartomas, sphenoid dysplasia, and frequently local overgrowth and hemihypertrophy. Malignant change occurs in approximately 3–15% of patients, and arise as a result of homozygous deficiency of a tumor-suppressor gene (see Ch. 1). There is a history of first-degree relatives with neurofibromatosis in 50%; 50% represent a new mutation. Patients with more severely affected mothers have more severe disease than those born to affected fathers. About half of the patients who have NF with **hypertension** have **pheochromocytomas**,[72] and **hypertrophic cardiomyopathy** has been observed. An intestinal form may involve the entire length of the gastrointestinal tract. Patients with **vascular neurofibromatosis** may develop infantile gangrene of the limbs.[73]

TYPE 2, CENTRAL NEUROFIBROMATOSIS: This autosomal dominant disease (MIM 101000) occurs in only 1 in 50 000. It is caused by a mutation of the gene NEUROFIBROMIN 2, also called *Merlin*, which is located on **chromosome 22q12.2**.[73b] Diagnosis is established by the presence of **acoustic schwannomas**, frequently bilateral; first-degree relatives with central neurofibromatosis plus a unilateral acoustic schwannoma; or a first-degree relative with central neurofibromatosis plus any two of the following: neurofibromas, meningiomas, gliomas, schwannomas, and lenticular opacity.

A wide range of dysplastic or hamartomatous lesions include heterotopias of neurons, astrocytes, and ependymal cells and proliferation of Schwann cells, meningothelial cells (meningiomatosis), endothelial cells (angiomatosis), and glial cells (glial nodules), as well as macrocephaly.

Tuberous sclerosis This is an autosomal dominant condition (MIM 191090) which shows genetic heterogeneity (mutations of *TSC1, TSC2, TSC3* and *TSC4* can all cause this syndrome). Tuberous sclerosis is characterized by **seizures, mental retardation, and facial angiofibromas** as well as other manifestations listed below.[74] Diagnostic criteria for tuberous sclerosis include two of the following major manifestations or one major plus

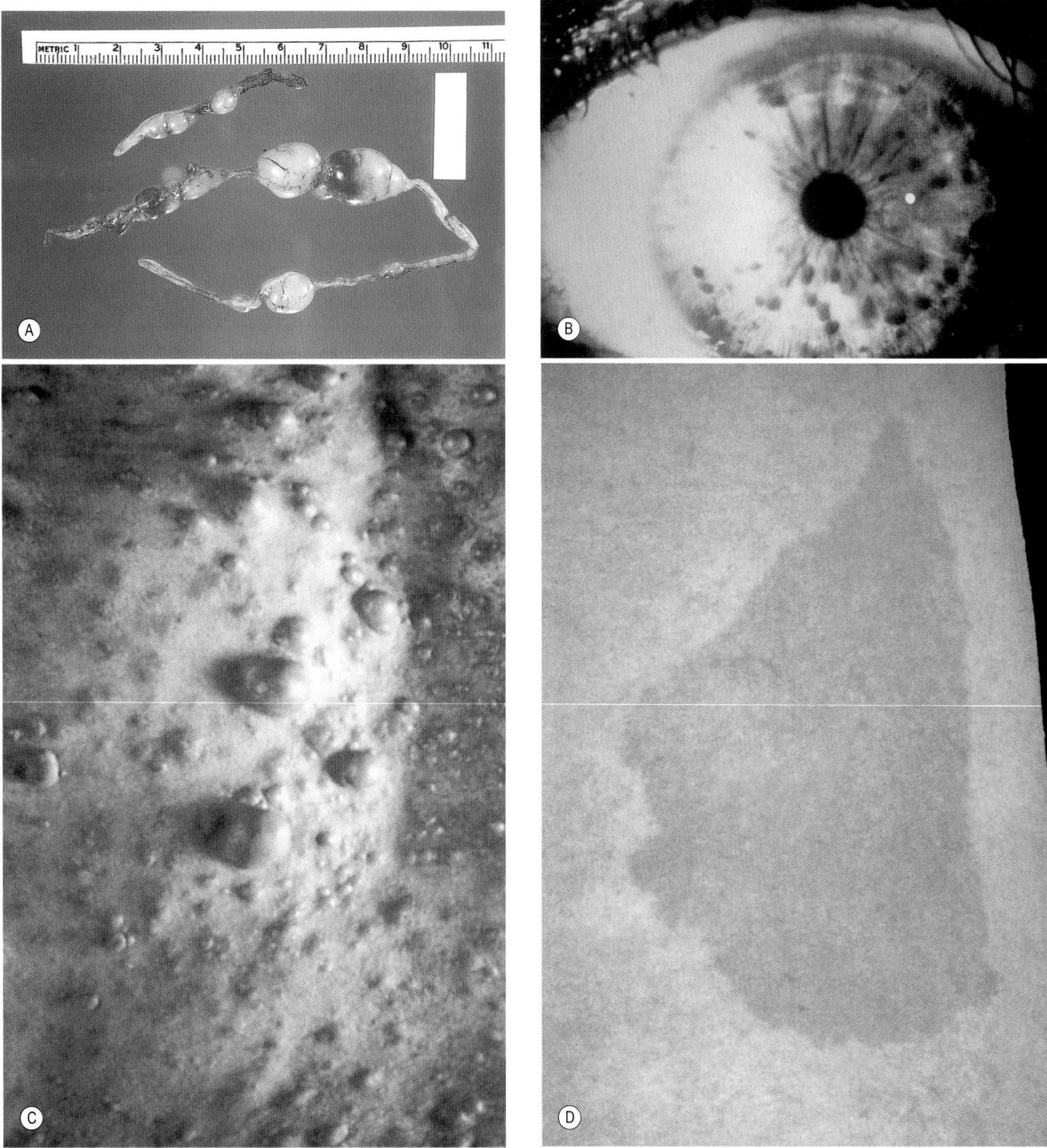

FIGURE 3.32 (A) Neurofibromas along a peripheral nerve. (B) Lisch nodules of iris of eye in neurofibromatosis. (C) Multiple neurofibromatosis of skin. (D) Café-au-lait lesion in neurofibromatosis-coast of California. (3.32B–D from Gilbert-Barness E, Debich-Spicer D, Embryo and Fetal Pathology, Cambridge University Press, with permission.)

two minor manifestations. Since many of these findings are not present in early childhood, periodic assessment is required to diagnose individuals at risk. Major criteria include facial angio-fibromas of forehead plaque, nontraumatic ungula or periungual

fibroma, hypomelanotic macules (ash-leaf spots), shagreen patch (connective tissue nevus), multiple retinal nodular hamartomas, cortical tuber, giant cell astrocytoma, cardiac rhabdomyoma, lymphangiomyomatosis, or renal angiomyolipoma. Minor

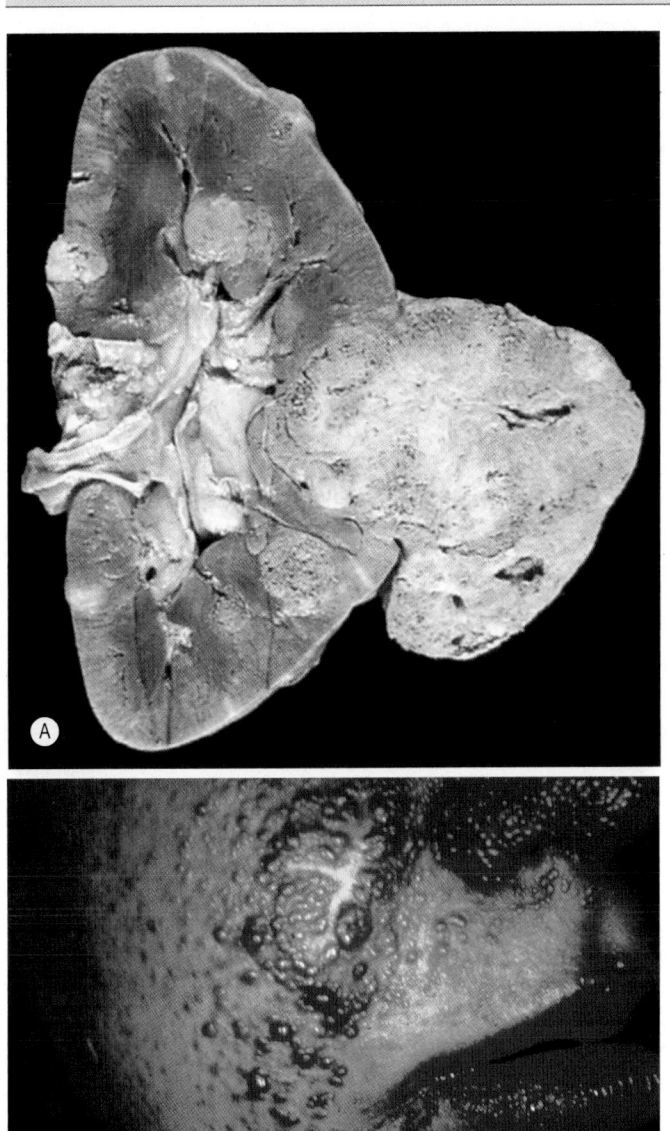

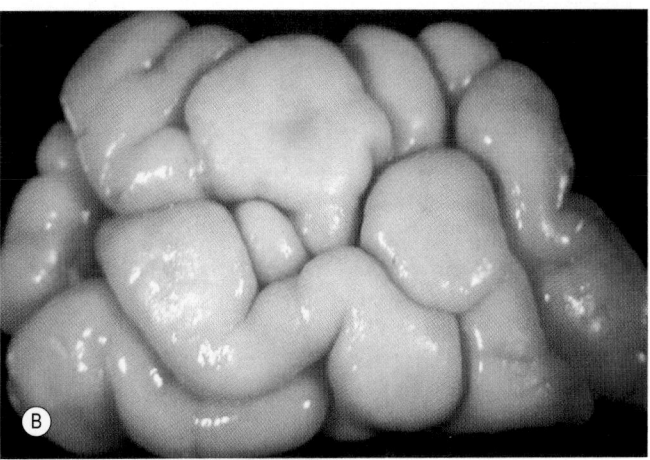

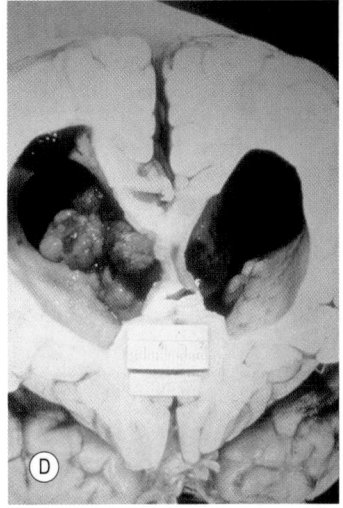

FIGURE 3.33 Tuberous sclerosis. (A) Renal involvement with multiple angiomyolipomas. (B) Cerebrocortical tubers with pachygyria. (C) Angiofibromas of the face. (D) Glial nodules in the ventricles.

criteria include dental enamel pits, hamartomatous rectal polyps, bone cysts, cerebral white matter migration lines, gingival fibromas, nonrenal hamartoma, retinal achromatic patch, "confetti"; skin lesion, or multiple renal cysts.[74, 75]

Imaging of the brain characteristically shows **pachygyria** with cortical tubers. **Subependymal candle gutterings** are seen along the wall of the lateral ventricles with orientation of the glial processes perpendicular to the pial surface. The glial cells are atypical and frequently fail to react immunohistochemically with antisera to GFAP. On electron microscopy, they do not contain the bundles of intermediate filaments that can normally be identified in large astrocytes. Whether these cells are of glial or neuronal origin is not clear. Irregular neuronal lamination, giant multinucleated cells and gliomas may occur, and may progress to malignant glioblastoma.[75] Two genes have been identified. TSC1-9q34 encodes for the protein hamartin, which

complexes with tuberin to negatively regulate the cell cycle. TSC2-16p13.3 encodes for the protein tuberin. It participates in normal brain development and cardiomyocyte terminal differentiation.[75a] It is located near the PKD1 gene. There is a subset of patients with polycystic kidney disease and tuberous sclerosis.

von Hippel-Lindau disease (see also Chapter 22) This 'disease' (MIM 608537) is an autosomal dominant trait caused by a mutation of the gene *VHL*. It has an estimated penetrance of 80–90%. It is characterized by angiomatosis retinae with a beaded artery leading into a tortuous dilated vein, and hemangioblastoma of the cerebellum that may calcify. Hemangiomas may involve the face, adrenal, lung, and liver, and multiple cysts of the pancreas, kidney, and epididymis may occur.[76] The renal cysts are lined by plump clear cells that

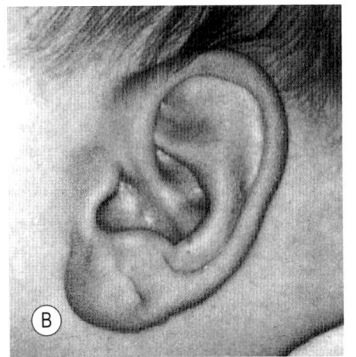

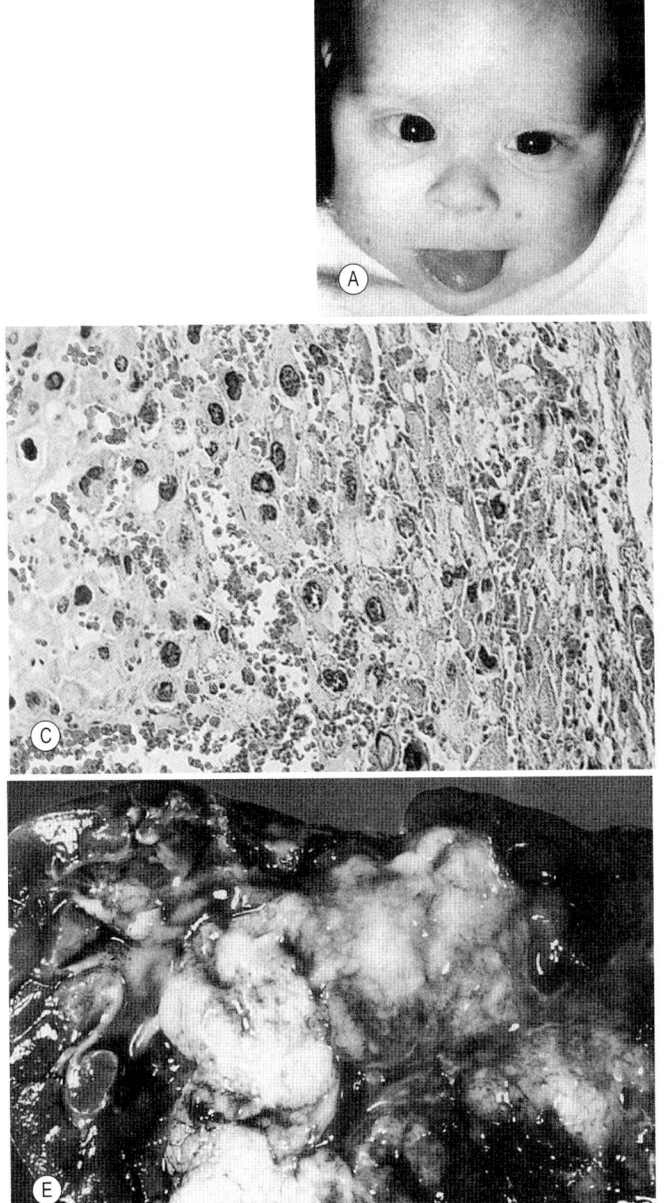

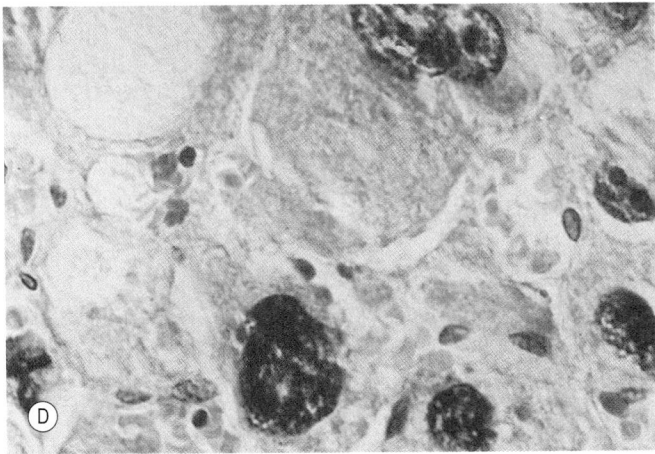

FIGURE 3.34 (A) Wiedemann-Beckwith syndrome with macroglossia, prominent eyes, and infraorbital hypoplasia. (B) Grooves on the lobule. (C and D) Cytomegaly of the adrenal cortex. (E) Wilms' tumor in Beckwith-Wiedemann syndrome. (From Gilbert-Barness and Opitz;[51] courtesy of Blackwell Scientific Publications, Inc.)

may proliferate and result in renal cell carcinoma in 25% of cases.[77] The renal cysts may be diffuse, resembling autosomal dominant polycystic kidneys. It has been hypothesized that the lesions represent an abnormality in the integration between blood vessels and parenchyma, but the cysts are notably associated with epithelial hyperplasia.

Beckwith-Wiedemann syndrome Models to explain Beckwith-Wiedemann syndrome (BWS) (Fig. 3.34) typically include more than one gene and aberrations of imprinted domains.[78] Genetic heterogeneity is demonstrated in this condition by the variety of cytogenetic and molecular alterations of the 11p15 region.[79] Patients can have **normal chromosomes** and underlying gene or imprinting mutations that exhibit sporadic occurrence or autosomal dominant inheritance (expression is often limited to individuals born to female carriers); or they may have **chromosome anomalies** involving duplication or microdeletion of the 11p15.5 region. Linkage to the 11p15.5 region was demonstrated in families with informative RFLP markers, followed by demonstration of gene, imprinting, and/or chromosomal changes. Increased insulin-likegrowth factor-2 (*IGF2*) expression promoted by microdeletion or altered methylation of the *H19* gene within 11p15.5 is a common theme in these various genetic causes of BWS.[80] Mutations of *CDKNIC*, a gene contiguous to *H19* and *IGF2*, can also result in BWS. Mutations at other loci such as the *NSD1* gene at 5q35 also cause BWS, presumably by influencing imprinting and gene expression in the 11p15.5 region. *NSD1* gene mutations and

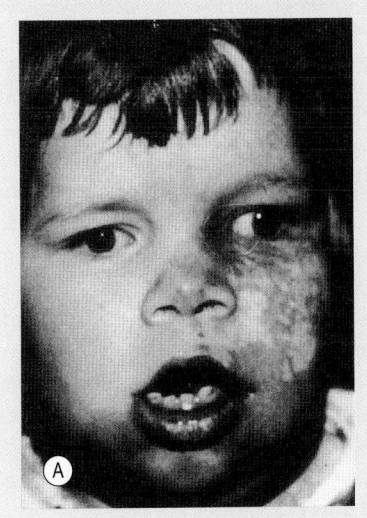 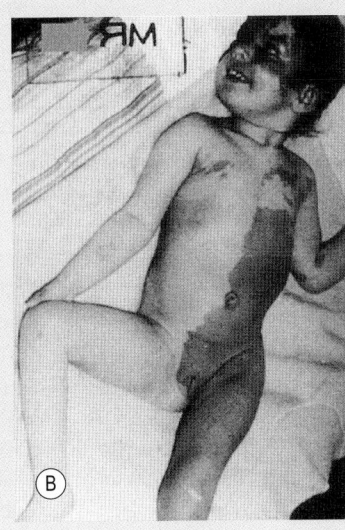

FIGURE 3.35 Sturge-Weber dysplasia. (A) Large vascular malformation of the left side of the face in the distribution of the trigeminal nerve. (B) Predominantly unilateral vascular malformations of the face, trunk, and leg. (From Gilbert-Barness and Opitz;[51] courtesy of Blackwell Scientific Publications, Inc.)

11p15.5 changes also are seen in Sotos syndrome, illustrating the overlap among BWS and related overgrowth/malignancy syndromes.[79] (see Ch. 41).

The classic triad of BWS consists of neonatal hypoglycemia, hemihypertrophy (asymmetric limb overgrowth) and organomegaly with resultant omphalocele. Craniofacial abnormalities include macroglossia, prominent eyes with relative infraorbital hypoplasia, capillary nevus flammeus of the central forehead and eyelids, a metopic ridge in the central forehead, large fontanelles, prominent occiput, malocclusion with a tendency toward mandibular prognathism. Linear fissures in the lobule of the external ear and semilunar indentations of the posterior rim of the helix are characteristic.

Mild microcephaly, hemihypertrophy, clitoromegaly, large ovaries, hyperplastic uterus and bladder, bicornuate uterus, hypospadias, and immunodeficiency may also be present. Nucleocytomegaly of the adrenocortical cells is an almost constant histologic finding, albeit non-specific, and nucleocytomegaly of the pancreatic islets of Langerhans is also frequent. During childhood, these patients show a marked **predisposition to the development of malignant tumors** such as Wilms tumor, adrenocortical carcinoma, hepatoblastoma, gonadoblastoma, and brainstem glioma. Wilms tumor may be bilateral when associated with this syndrome.

Perlman syndrome This is an autosomal recessive condition of renal dysplasia, Wilms tumor, hyperplasia of the endocrine pancreas, fetal gigantism, multiple congenital anomalies, and mental retardation (MIM 267000).[81] The responsible gene appears to be close to the imprinted portion of the short arm of chromosome 11. The responsible gene appears to be close to the imprinted portion of the short arm of chromosome 11. The kidneys show persistent fetal lobation, nephrogenic rests, immature glomeruli, sclerotic glomeruli, primitive tubular structures, and medullary hamartomatous dysplasia. The pancreas shows an increase in the number of islet cells. The frequent

occurrence of Wilms tumor has led to the speculation that persistent foci of renal blastema or nephroblastomatosis constitute predisposing lesions. The condition has some similarity to BWS and is easily differentiated from it on the basis of inheritance, striking differences in minor specific anomalies and appearance, different natural histories, and different constellations of associated malformations.

Klippel-Trenaunay-Weber malformation dysplasia Hypertrophy of usually one, but occasionally more than one, limb, vascular malformations that may be capillary or cavernous, phlebectasias and varicosities characterize the Klippel-Trenaunay-Weber vascular malformation dysplasia.[82] The legs, buttocks, abdomen and lower trunk are the usual sites of the vascular lesions. Less common abnormalities include arteriovenous fistulas, lymphangiomas, macrodactyly, syndactyly, polydactyly, hyperpigmented nevi and telangiectasia. Craniofacial abnormalities include asymmetric facial hypertrophy, hemangiomas, intracranial calcifications and eye abnormalities. Visceromegaly and hemangiomas of the intestinal tract, urinary system and mesentery may be present. Mental deficiency and seizures may occur with facial hemangiomatosis. This condition is sporadic.

Sturge-Weber syndrome This is a non-familial disorder consisting of facial, retinal, and cerebral angiomatoses.[83] The embryonic continuity of the vascular supply of the skin, eye, and telencephalon suggests that an abnormality of the embryonic vascular plexus causes the simultaneous existence of these separate lesions (Fig. 3.35). The facial angiomatosis is usually localized to one side of the face, is confined to the territory of the trigeminal nerve, and involves the distribution of the ophthalmic branch. In the brain, leptomeningeal venous angiomatosis is striking and affects the parieto-occipital region but does not extend into the cortex. The underlying cerebrum contains extensive calcification with or without involvement of the white matter. Some of the calcification is orientated around blood vessels, but most lies in the neuropil unrelated to obvious vasculature.[83] Despite the extensive calcification, gliosis is surprisingly minimal. The pathogenesis of the calcification is unknown.

The clinical manifestations in Sturge-Weber syndrome most frequently include seizures, hemiparesis and mental retardation. Treatment is directed at seizure control, which may involve hemispherectomy. Hemispherectomy in children under the age of 6 months appears to be associated with less severe neurologic deficit than would be expected, presumably because of the increased plasticity of the brain at the younger age.[83]

Teratomas

A particularly instructive example of **dysplastic disruption** of morphogenesis was reported some years ago by Durkin-Stamm and colleagues[84] in two unrelated infants with malformations, benign tumor at birth in the malformed structures, malignant transformation at 3 and 7 months, and death due to metastases at 14 and 12 months, respectively. The second infant had severe hypoplasia of one hind limb with rudimentary foot and two toe structures. There was imperforate anus, with absence of rectum and lower colon; sacral meningomyelocele with malformed sacrum and coccyx; a pseudovaginal perineoscrotal hypospadias-like malformation of the external genitalia, cleft scrotum, histologically normal descended testes; and tumor tissue in all soft tissues of the posterior aspect of the malformed hind limb and the entire sacral, perineal, and pelvic area with relative obstruction of one ureter and unilateral hydronephrosis. The initial biopsy demonstrated, within the dermis, clusters of small, dark, round cells resembling neuroblasts; some cells formed rosettes, but without the mitotic activity and evidence of hemorrhage and necrosis typical of neuroblastoma. After amputation, the tissue consisted predominantly of neuroblastic components, forming typical rosettes in some places. In many areas neuroblastic elements were seen, with maturation into ganglion cells and glial tissue, and with neurofibrillary stroma; less frequent elements were derived from other germ layers, including mesodermal/connective components, small nests of squamous epithelium, pseudostratified, and respiratory ciliated epithelium. The metastatic tissue consisted of medulloepitheliomatous tumor.

Thus, in this fetus, a single cell event apparently gave rise to a teratomatous cell line early during embryogenesis; this cell line infiltrated soft tissues of one hind limb, the pelvis, perineogenital area, hindgut, and caudal neural tube/canal. It interfered with the morphogenesis of these structures, causing hypoplasias, aplasias, and anomalies of incomplete differentiation. The intrinsic tissues of the hindquarter, including the malformed coccyx, were histologically normal. The malformations in these infants can be regarded as secondary rather than intrinsic primary developmental field defects, a conclusion supported by the fact that the anomalies involved the derivatives of many primordia in an anatomically irregular manner, extended beyond and across anatomic boundaries defined by normal embryogenesis, and actively involved processes evolving over a long prenatal period.

Much more common tumors are the more **circumscribed**

teratomas of the sacrococcygeal area, mediastinum, and oropharyngeal (epignathus) and pituitary regions. These tumors, if associated with sacrococcygeal defects and imperforate anus, occasionally represent an autosomal dominant trait. Congenital malignant tumors are thought to be derived from embryonic tissues of germ cell origin, including **yolk sac tumors, teratomas with embryonal carcinoma and choriocarcinoma**, malignant melanomas, Wilms' tumor, neuroblastoma, fibrosarcomas, and rhabdomyosarcomas. There exist numerous types of congenital non-malignant tumors of either pure or mixed cell types, including the **congenital hypothalamic hamartoblastomas of Pallister-Hall syndrome, vascular malformations of all types (e.g., capillary, cavernous, Klippel-Trenaunay-Weber), lymphangiomas and cystic hygromas, pigmented and epidermal nevi, the congenital cardiac rhabdomyoma seen in tuberous sclerosis, and congenital cystic lesions of lungs, gastrointestinal tract, and kidneys**.[85]

Genetic dysplasia syndromes

In many **genetic dysplasia syndromes** the infant may appear normal at birth but develops one or more dysplastic manifestations later. Examples include all the **dysplasias of Gardner syndrome (epidermoid cysts, osteomas, odontomas, multiple intestinal polyposis, abdominal or retroperitoneal desmoids, mesenteric and retroperitoneal fibromatosis) with a high incidence of other tumors** including glioma, medulloblastoma, papillary carcinoma of the thyroid, adrenal carcinoma, hepatocellular carcinoma, osteosarcoma and basal cell carcinomas. Later occurrence of acanthosis nigricans and nasal polyps may delay the diagnosis in **Costello syndrome**. The same is true for the **nevoid basal cell carcinoma (Gorlin) syndrome**; however, in that condition family history and associated anomalies (megalencephaly, hypertelorism, multiple rib anomalies, spina bifida occulta, short metacarpals, kyphoscoliosis and other malformations) may be a clue to early diagnosis. Progression of latent or incipient dysplastic lesions is characteristic of many of the other so-called **hamartoneoplastic syndromes, including tuberous sclerosis, Peutz-Jeghers syndrome, the neurofibromatoses, multiple endocrine neoplasia syndromes, and Maffucci hemangiomatosis/enchondromatosis syndrome**.[86]

The term **dysplasia** is used in three other contexts. The first and most trivial is the misnomer **hip dysplasia** of orthopedic origin, referring to congenital luxation or subluxation of the head of the femur at the acetabular joint. Usually no dysplasia is involved, but a combination of genetic–environmental factors that result in hypoplasia or abnormal angulation of the acetabular roof, loose tendons, ligaments or joint capsule, and hypotonia.

The second context involves the large and important biologic group of the skeletal and connective tissue dysplasias (see Chs 1 and 2). Many of these patients have an external appearance that allows rapid diagnosis. Figure 3.36 illustrates a patient with lethal thanatophoric dwarfism; Figure 3.37 shows a patient with spondyloepiphyseal dysplasia. As discussed in Chapter 2, radiographic evaluation is particularly useful for the skeletal dysplasias, and molecular testing is increasing rapidly. DNA analysis is now

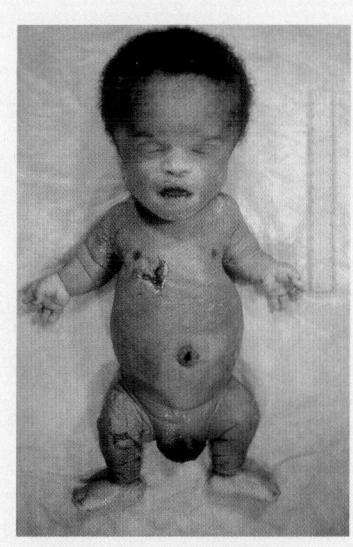

FIGURE 3.36 Newborn infant with thanatophoric dysplasia showing prominent forehead, shallow nasal bridge, and rhizomelic limbs. The wound is from costochondral biopsy. (Courtesy of Dr. Mason Barr, University of Michigan.)

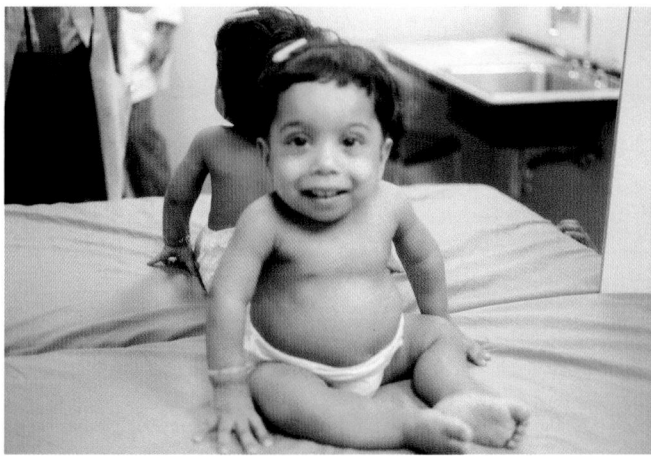

FIGURE 3.37 Child with spondyloepiphyseal dysplasia showing hypoplastic chest and rhizomelia.

available, at least on a research basis, for osteogenesis imperfecta, **Marfan syndrome**, spondyloepiphyseal dysplasia, achondroplasia, and certain of the Ehlers-Danlos syndromes. Texts are available for guidance with this group of disorders.[86, 87]

Marfan syndrome Marfan syndrome[88] (see Ch. 18) is characterized by tall stature with long slender limbs, joint laxity and scoliosis, and little subcutaneous tissue and hypotonia. Eye abnormalities, including dislocation of the lens (Fig. 3.38A), myopia, and retinal detachment, and cardiovascular complications are rarely apparent in infancy. The disorder is caused by autosomal dominant mutations of the *FIBRILLIN* gene at chromosome band 15q21 (MIM 154700), decreasing connective tissue strength with resulting long face and high palate, ligamentous laxity (lens and joint dislocations), dilation of blood vessels and valves (particularly the aorta and mitral valve), ectasias of the spinal dura and pulmonary lining (pneumothorax), scoliosis, hernias, and flat feet (Table 3.6). The extracellular matrix

changes include accumulation of glucosamine glycans in the skin, lung, kidney, cartilage, tendon, muscle, cornea, ciliary zonule, and vascular smooth muscle. The classic change of cystic medionecrosis (Fig. 3.38B) accompanies the aortic dilation and dissection (Fig. 3.38C). Recognition of transforming growth factor-β (TGF-β) receptor mutations in the Shprintzen-Goldberg and Loeys-Dietz connective tissue dysplasia syndromes places the fibrillin/extracellular matrix changes within a pathway potentially impacted by TGF-β receptor ligands such as the antihypertensive drug losartan. The latter drug is under study as an alternative to β-blocker (e.g., propranalol) therapy of aortic dilatation.

Stickler syndrome First described by Stickler and colleagues and later documented by Spranger and by Herrmann and associates, Stickler syndrome (Fig. 3.38D), or hereditary arthroophthalmopathy, is characterized by anomalies such as a depressed nasal bridge, epicanthal folds, midface hypoplasia, cleft of the hard palate, micrognathia, deafness, myopia with frequent retinal detachment, and wedge and fleck cataracts.[89] Hypotonia, marfanoid habitus, prominence of large joints, spondyloepiphyseal dysplasia, and sometimes mental retardation and mitral valve prolapse are also present in Stickler syndrome. This syndrome should be considered in every newborn infant with the **Pierre Robin sequence**. Variability may reflect heterogeneity that is demonstrated by linkage to *COL2A1* in some cases (Stickler type 1, MIM 108300), to *COL11A1* in other cases (Stickler type II, MIM 604841) or to *COL11A2* (Stickler type III, MIM 184840).

Metabolic dysplasia syndromes

A third group of dysplasias are the metabolic dysplasia syndromes.[90] This is a large group of entities if individual genetic mutations and complementation groups are counted; the group is smaller if only clinical phenotypes are taken into account. With the exception of Fabry disease, neonatal adrenoleukodystrophy, and Hunter syndrome, these are all autosomal recessive conditions. Most involve large molecular weight inborn errors of metabolism that, in contradistinction to most low molecular weight inborn errors, cannot be compensated before birth through the fetal–placental exchange mechanism.

In small molecule disorders, e.g., galactosemia or phenylketonuria, the infant is born apparently normally developed but may develop more or less acute manifestations of the metabolic defect shortly after birth. In large molecule disorders, storage is occasionally noted neonatally but usually progresses with facial coarsening and/or organ enlargement over months or years. In both cases, it is presumed that the cells differentiated normally but that their function is more or less impaired or disrupted by the storage phenomenon. Storage may lead to secondary changes such as enlargement and dysfunction of organs, clouding of corneae, stiffness of joints with clawing of fingers, infiltration of skin with facial 'coarseness' and hirsutism, and marrow/skeletal involvement manifested most characteristically as dysostosis multiplex (see Fig. 2.26 in Ch. 2).

Several of the small molecular weight inborn errors can be treated satisfactorily; most of the high molecular weight

TABLE 3.6 MARFAN SYNDROME

Clinical manifestations

Tall with marfanoid habitus	Celft palate sometimes
Ligamentous laxity leading to joint hypermobility	Inguinal hernias
Arachnodactyly	Atrophic striae distensae
Scoliosis	Retinal detachment, glaucoma
Ectopia lentis	Myopia, keratoconus, megalocornea, hypoplasia of iris
Dilatation of the ascending aorta	Spontaneous pneumothorax

Main phenotypic manifestations

Skeletal system

Anterior chest deformity, especially asymmetric pectus excavatum/carinatum

Dolichostenomelia not due to scoliosis

Arachnodactyly

Vertebral column deformity

Scoliosis

Tall stature, especially compared to unaffected parents and sibs

High, narrowly arched palate

Crowding of teeth

Protrusio acetabulae

Abnormal joint mobility

Congential flexion contractures

Hypermobility

Skin and integument

Striae distensae without obvious cuase

Hernia

Cardiovascular system

Dilatation of the ascending aorta*

Aortic dissection*

Aortic regurgitation

Mitral regurgitation

Mitral valve prolapse

Pulmonary system

Spontaneous pneumothorax

Ocular system

Ectopia lentis*

Elongated globe

Retinal detachement

Myopia

Central nervous system

Dural ectasia*

Widening of the lumbosacral canal and neural foramina

Diagnostic criteria

With a first-degree relative with Marfan syndrome

1. Involvement of at least two systems
2. At least one major manifestation (although this requirement is age dependent and occasionally depends on peculiarities of the family's phenotype)

With no first-degree relative afftected by Marfan syndrome, the proband must have

1. Involvement of the skeleton
2. Involvement of at least two other systems
3. At least one major manifestation

*Major manifestations

Source: Gilbert-Barness E, Barness LA: *Metabolic Diseases: Foundations of Clinical Management, Genetics and Pathology,* Vol. II, Natick, MA, Eaton Publishing, 2000.

disorders cannot. In the former entities, the manifestations tend to reflect more specific involvement and impairment, i.e., liver, heart, kidney, or brain. In the latter, e.g., I-cell disease, virtually every organ system and tissue may be affected. Prenatal diagnosis of most of these conditions is possible, and the (mutant) genes responsible for many of these conditions have been mapped or cloned (see OMIM, www.ncbi.nlm.nih.gov/entrez). Details of these conditions are found in the work of Scriver and colleagues,[91] which must be supplemented by OMIM and other reference searches because of the very rapid advances in the field. Several metabolic dysplasia syndrome categories are listed in Table 3.4.

Recent progress has blurred the definition between malformation syndromes and metabolic dysplasia syndromes, raising hopes that discrete metabolic alterations can be defined in other 'classic' syndromes. Peroxisomopathies offer one example, where a diverse spectrum of manifestations first identified as Zellweger syndrome can now be related to organellar assembly (see Ch. 1). Figure 3.39 illustrates some of these manifestations, ranging from the severe hypotonia (causing clubfoot deformity) and dysostosis of Zellweger syndrome to the milder developmental effects of neonatal adrenoleukodystrophy.[92]

Two additional entities that may be considered prototypic of syndromes with metabolic defects are mevalonic acidemia and the Smith-Lemli-Opitz (SLO) syndrome.

Mevalonic acidemia Mevalonic acidemia[93] is an autosomal recessive **inborn error of cholesterol synthesis** discovered in 1986. It is due to deficiency of mevalonate kinase and is associated with a striking facial appearance with multiple minor anomalies of telecanthus, flat bridge of the nose, small nose with anteverted nostrils, long upper lip with flat philtrum, thin vermilion border of lips, relatively small mouth with downturned angles, mild micrognathia, and other hypotonic mouth-

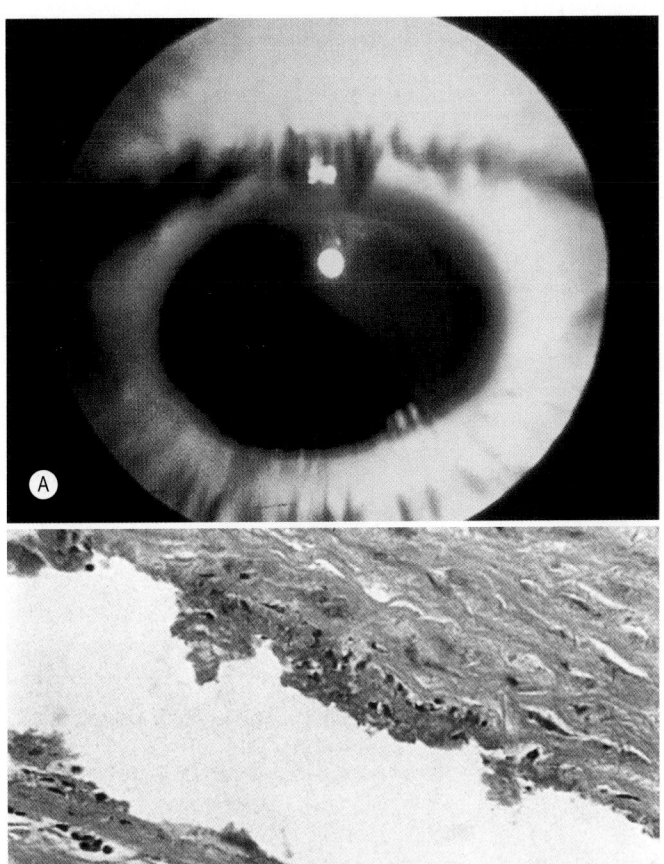

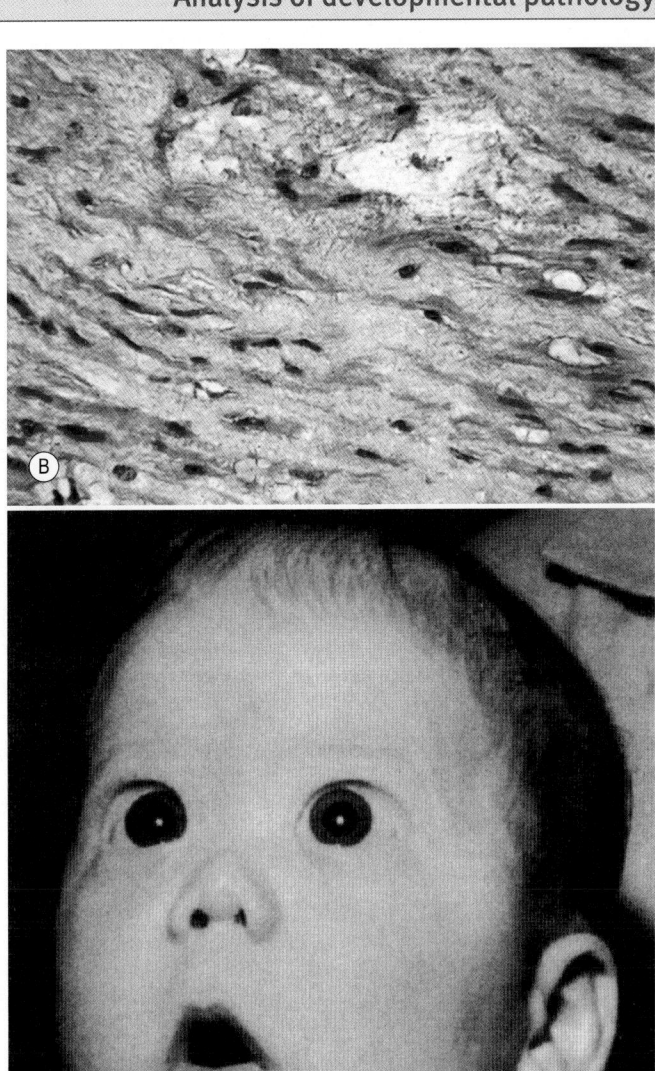

FIGURE 3.38 (A) Dislocation of the lens of the eye in Marfan syndrome. (B) Microscopic appearance of cystic medionecrosis in Marfan syndrome. (C) Dissection of aortic wall. (D) Infant with Stickler syndrome. The facial appearance is due to severe myopia, epicanthic folds, depressed bridge of the nose, anteverted nostrils, and severe micrognathia. (3.38A–C from Gilbert-Barness E, Debich-Spicer D. Embryo and Fetal Pathology. Cambridge University Press, with permission. 3.38D from Gilbert-Barness and Opitz;[51] courtesy of Blackwell Scientific Publications.)

breathing facial changes. It is a sublethal disorder of severe mental retardation with progressive cerebellar atrophy; recurrent crises of high fever, vomiting, and diarrhea (with some patients also manifesting mucocutaneous rashes, edema, and arthritis); failure to thrive; congenital hypotonia; and ataxia. Hepatosplenomegaly with cataracts occurs in less than half of the cases. In lethally affected cases, death occurs between 6 months and 4 years. The diagnosis is confirmed biochemically on the basis of gross elevation of mevalonic acid in all body fluids and in urine, with absence of mevalonate kinase in fibroblasts. Cholesterol levels in plasma are normal or only slightly reduced.

Smith-Lemli-Opitz (RSH) syndrome This autosomal recessive disorder (MIM 270400, Fig. 3.40A) is due to a defect of cholesterol synthesis resulting in low to extremely low cholesterol (and desmosterol) levels and greatly increased plasma concentrations of the immediate precursors of 7-dehydrocholesterol (7DHC) and cholest-5,7,24-trien-3a-ol.[94, 95] These elevations reflect mutations in the sterol delta-7-reductase gene that maps to 11q12-q13.[95] This enzyme reduces the C-7,8 double bond of 7DHC and the precursor of desmosterol, and it has now been shown that provision of cholesterol to affected patients can lower levels of 7-dehydrocholesterol that can be toxic.[95] In contradistinction to mevalonic acidemia, in which no gross malformations have been reported, the SLO syndrome is a true multiple congenital anomalies (MCA) syndrome with protean manifestations ranging from a perinatally lethal form to one of normal growth, multiple minor anomalies and mild mental retardation, allowing school attendance.

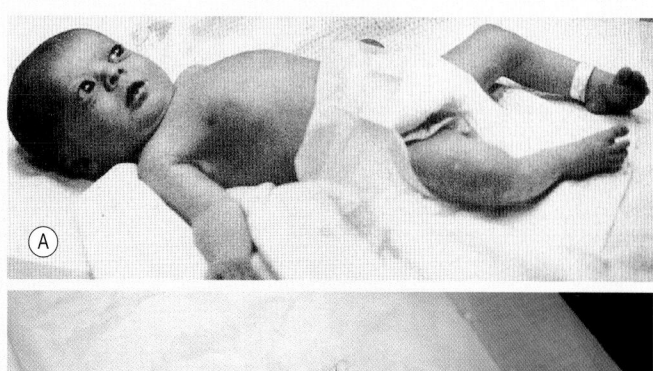

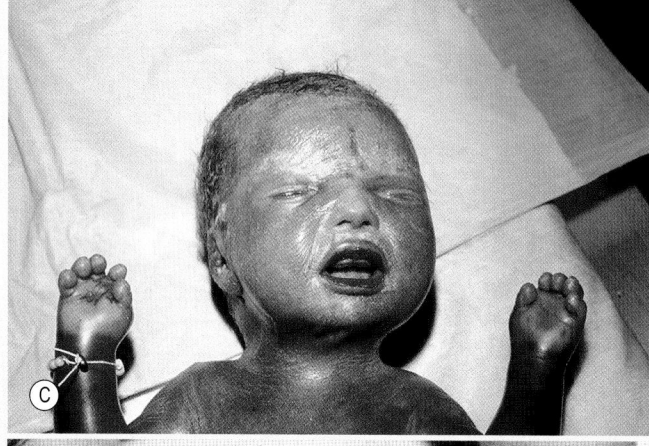

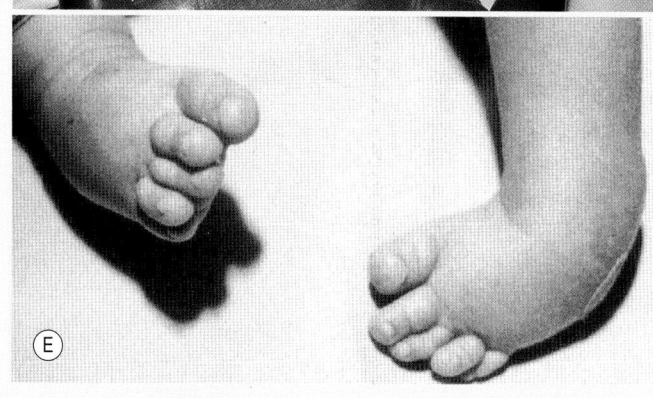

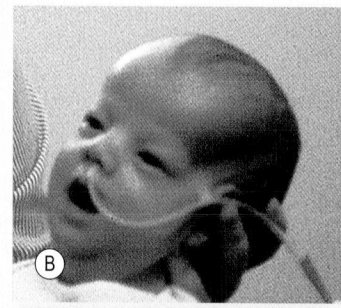

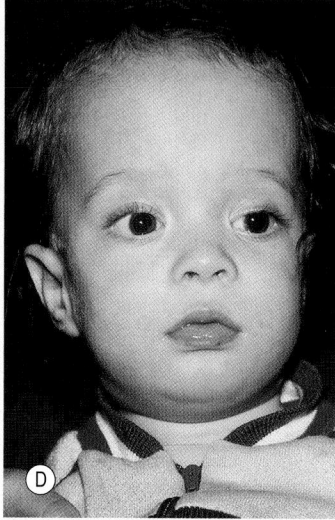

FIGURE 3.39 Range of severity exhibited by peroxisomal metabolic dysplasias. (A) Infant with congenital icthyosis typical of some peroxisomal disorders. (B) Newborn infant with Zellweger syndrome showing prominent forehead, bitemporal hollowing, broad nasal root, and anteverted nares. (C) Stillborn infant with probable infantile Refsum syndrome showing collodion skin as precursor to ichthyosis. (D) Child with probable infantile adrenoleukodystrophy showing mild facial changes, including prominent forehead, epicanthal folds, and anterverted nares. (E) Bilateral club foot deformation caused by in utero hypotonia in an infant with Zellweger Syndrome. (From Wilson GN, Holmes RD, Hajra AK. Peroxisomal disorders: clinical commentary and future prospects. Am J Med Genet 1988; 30:771; with permission.)

A distinct craniofacial appearance with microcephaly, anteverted nostrils, ptosis of eyelids, inner epicanthal folds, strabismus, micrognathia, syndactyly of the second and third toes, hypospadias, cryptorchidism and mental deficiency are the main characteristics. Defects in brain morphogenesis include microencephaly, hypoplasia of the frontal lobes, cerebellar and brainstem hypoplasia, dilated ventricles, irregular gyral patterns and irregular neuronal organization.[94, 95] Atypical mononuclear giant cells in pancreatic islets have been described (see Fig. 3.40C). Less frequent anomalies are postaxial hexadactyly, congenital heart defect, and multiple anomalies of renal and spinal cord development. Cystic renal disease (see Fig. 3.40B), renal

hypoplasia, hydronephrosis and abnormalities of the ureters are frequent. Rarely, severe perineoscrotal hypospadias may be seen. The reported higher frequency of affected males compared with females may be related to a bias in ascertaining the genital anomaly.

The neonatally lethal entity formerly defined as 'type II' by Curry and colleagues[96] results from allelic or variably expressed delta-7-reductase gene mutations; indeed, such cases may be sibs of less severely affected children.[96] Figure 3.41 shows a newborn infant with the severe form of SLO syndrome. On a clinical basis, there is only a unimodal distribution of Bialer severity scores, which argues against the existence of two phenotypically

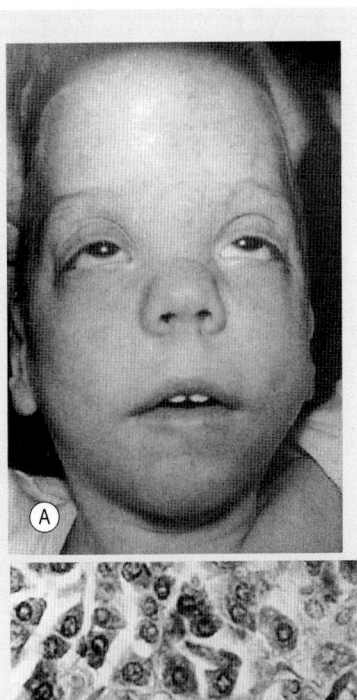

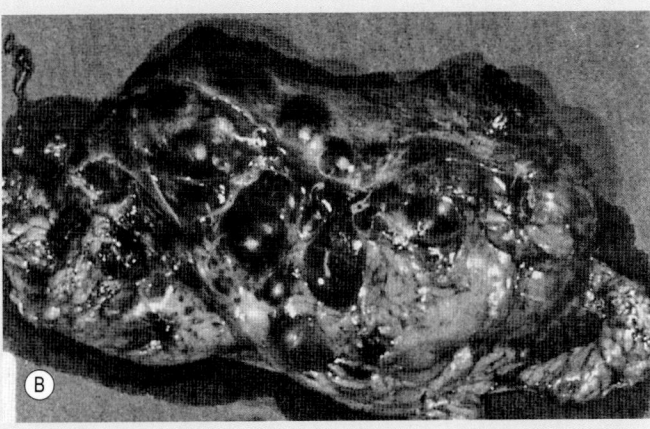

FIGURE 3.40 Smith-Lemli-Opitz syndrome. (A) Characteristic facial appearance with micrognathia, ptosis, and microcephaly. (B) Gross appearance of cystic kidney. (C) Pancreatic giant cells. (From Gilbert-Barness and Opitz;[51] courtesy of Blackwell Scientific Publications, Inc.)

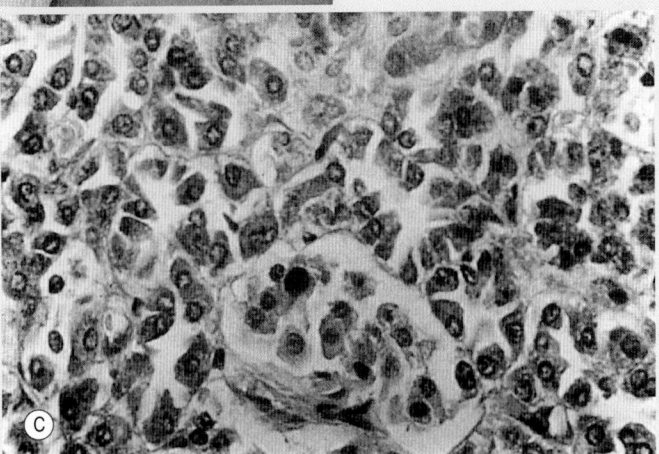

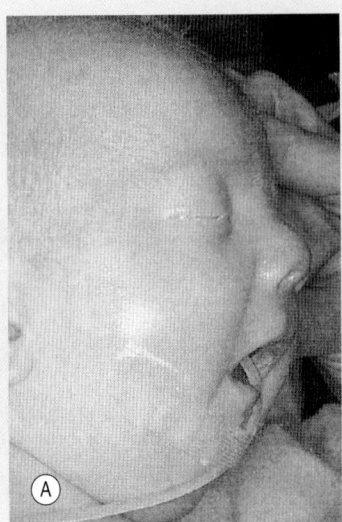

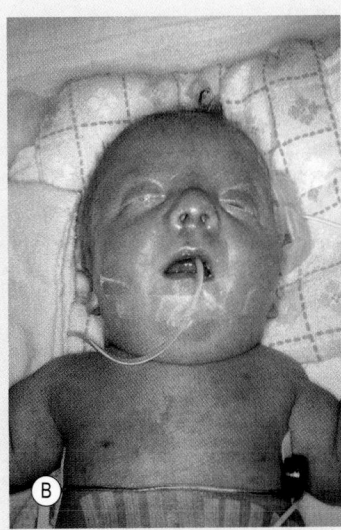

FIGURE 3.41 Newborn infant with the severe form of Smith-Lemli-Opitz syndrome showing bilateral ptosis, anteverted nares, and micrognathia. Nasogastric feeding was required because of hypotonia.

discontinuous or minimally overlapping, genetically distinct entities. A striking aspect of the history and biology of SLO syndrome is the existence of an animal (rat) model known for as long as the syndrome itself. This model was developed by Roux and colleagues[97] in Paris and is effected through an inhibitor of either desmosterol synthesis (triparonol) or 7-dehydrocholesterol conversion (AY9944). Use of these compounds results in embryo lethality and some of the same anomalies seen at times in humans with SLO syndrome, including holoprosencephaly/pituitary agenesis (prevented by a hypercholesterolemia-provoking diet of the pregnant mother rat), edema, hydronephrosis, testicular and ocular abnormalities, and hydrocephalus.

Lethally affected fetuses with SLO syndrome may be small for gestational age and may manifest variable combinations of congenital heart defects, renal anomalies (hypoplasia, agenesis), male pseudohermaphroditism, syndactyly of the second and third toes, postaxial polydactyly (in one case there was 'paradoxical' ulnar oligodactyly!), unilobed lungs, cleft palate, and cataracts. Indicators of a metabolic disease are male pseudohermaphroditism, indicating in this case an apparent defect of steroid synthesis; cystic renal dysplasia; pancreatic islet giant cells with reduced quantities of somatostatin in pancreas; hepatomegaly; ascites; bile duct proliferation, biliary stasis with jaundice and severe hepatocyte cholestasis with or without fibrosis of extra hepatic bile ducts; and large adrenal glands with apparent complete absence of lipid in the adrenal cortex by oil red O staining and electron microscopy. A striking associated phenomenon is the suppression of maternal estriol excretion in late pregnancy (estriol being of fetal origin).[94–96]

Lethal cases of SLO syndrome in infancy and childhood may have any or all of the above findings, a rather striking silvery-platinum blond color of hair, microcephaly, ptosis of the upper eyelids, relatively large ears with minor anomalies of the auricles, anteverted nostrils, striking mouth-breathing facial changes, broad alveolar ridges, submucous cleft of the palate, short sternum, and diastasis recti. There is a highly characteristic appearance of the thumbs, which are smaller than usual, more tapered, proximally set, and webbed into the palm. Additionally present are an increased number of whorls on the fingertips, dorsal dislocation of the halluces, talipes equinovarus, dislocated hips and hamstring contractures. The diagnosis can be confirmed through demonstration of very high tissue levels of 7-dehydrocholesterol (even in formaldehyde-fixed material!).

In fetal pathology it is very important to have a high index of suspicion for SLO syndrome because of its atypical presentation. Indeed, since the segregation ratio in living cases is only 17–18% (and not 25%), many cases are prenatally lethal and require correct diagnosis to prevent recurrence.

Sequences

Potter sequence

In the Potter sequence the initiating event is oligohydramnios of any cause, genetic or otherwise. The oligohydramnion can either be due to a malformation (e.g., bilateral renal agenesis, autosomal recessive or obstruction-induced renal dysplasia, posterior urethral valves as in polycystic kidney) or an extrinsic defect (e.g., amniotic fluid leakage). Lack of amniotic fluid restricts fetal movement and causes fetal compression, producing the typical changes of Potter sequence (see Fig. 2.7 in Ch. 2).

Pierre Robin sequence

The defects in Pierre Robin sequence, also known as Robin sequence, include micrognathia, glossoptosis, and cleft soft palate. Hypoplasia of the mandibular area before week 9 of gestation causes the tongue to be posteriorly located, presumably preventing closure of the posterior palatal shelves.[98] It may also be a result of early mechanical constraint in utero, limiting growth before palatine closure. The Pierre Robin sequence should alert the clinician to the possible presence of Stickler syndrome and the possibility of blindness due to high myopia.

Prune-belly sequence and related defects

Prune-belly sequence occurs sporadically as a triad of apparent absence of abdominal muscles, urinary tract defects, and cryptorchidism. There is cephalad displacement of the umbilicus, flaring of rib margins, Harrison grooves, and pectus deformities, all apparently secondary to the muscle defect. The associated severe oligohydramnios leads to Potter sequence.[99]

A presumed early mesenchymal maldevelopment between weeks 6 and 10 of gestation causes a developmental field defect. Burton and Dillard speculate that splitting of the abdominal wall in prune-belly sequence occurs because of massive bladder dilatation.[100] This hypothesis is supported by the demonstration of attenuation of smooth muscle elements, without differentiation into circular and longitudinal orientations within the bladder, and with replacement by collagen. Renal dysplasia may occur due to severe hydrouretero-nephrosis secondary to urethral or bladder neck obstruction. Neonatal death occurs in 20% of infants; however, there may be long-term survival without significant renal impairment. Megalourethra, megacystis, megaureters, renal hypoplasia, and hydronephrosis have been described, as well as decreased spermatogenesis, absence of spermatogonia, and salt-wasting nephritis.

DiGeorge sequence

The primary defect in DiGeorge syndrome (MIM 188400) is in the development of the fourth branchial arch and derivatives of the third and fourth pharyngeal pouches, probably due to a mutation of TBX1.[100a] (CATCH-22, an autosomal dominant disease with reduced penetrance and variable expressivity has been discussed in Chapter 1.) It includes defects of the thymus, parathyroids, and great vessels. Facial anomalies include hypertelorism, short philtrum, down-slanting palpebral fissures, and ear anomalies. Thymic hypoplasia or aplasia results in a deficit of cellular immunity. Hypoplasia or absence of parathyroids results in hypocalcemia and tetany in early infancy. Cardiovascular defects include aortic arch anomalies, such as right aortic arch, interrupted aorta, conotruncal anomalies (truncus arteriosus and ventricular septal defect), patent ductus arteriosus, and tetralogy of Fallot. Esophageal atresia, choanal atresia, imperforate anus, and diaphragmatic hernia may be accompanying abnormalities. Death usually occurs in early infancy owing to the cardiovascular defects, tetany, or infection related to the defect of cellular immunity. Impairments of the inductive and morphogenetic functions of the neural crest cells are responsible for the defects of the epithelial organ derivatives of the third and fourth pharyngeal pouches and of the corresponding branchial arteries. Because of the role played by cephalic neural crest in morphogenesis of the heart, conotruncal heart defects are commonly seen in infants with DiGeorge sequence. Because of the neural crest–midline pathogenetic origin of DiGeorge sequence, this condition is frequently associated with other midline anomalies, schisis associations, and arrhinencephaly. It may be related causally to the fetal alcohol, fetal accutane disruptions, as well as to the effects of maternal diabetes.[101] It is often caused by a microdeletion of the proximal long arm of chromosome 22q11.2.

Useful websites

1. POSSUM. Subscription service through Murdoch Research Institute, Royal Children's Hospital Melbourne; diagnostic and resource reference for multiple anomaly disorders and skeletal dysplasias, www.possum.net.au/about.htm
2. Online Mendelian Inheritance in Man (OMIM). Catalog of human genes and genetic disorders, contains textual information, references, and links developed at Johns Hopkins University www.ncbi.nlm.nih.gov.omim/
3. GeneClinics. National Institutes of Health (NIH) teaching website, sponsored by the University of Washington, Seattle, WA, with access to genetic testing, www.geneclinic.org
4. The Fetus. Ultrasound diagnosis of anomalies, postdelivery photos, index of disorders by name; www.thefetus.net; accessed through www.sonoworld.com/
5. Genetic Information and Patient Services, Inc. (GIPS); includes glossaries of syndromes and malformations with features; www.icomm.ca/geneinfo/index.html

References

Analysis of developmental pathology

1. Opitz JM. The developmental analysis of human congenital anomalies. In: Papadatos CJ, Bartsocas CS, eds. Skeletal dysplasias. New York: Alan R Liss; 1982:15–43.

Aneuploidy

2. Opitz JM. Blastogenesis and the 'primary field' in human development. Birth Defects 1993: 29:3.

3. Gilbert EF, Opitz JM. Developmental and other pathological changes in syndromes caused by chromosomal abnormalities. In: Rosenberg HS, Bernstein J, eds. Perspectives in pediatric pathology, vol VII. New York: Masson; 1982:1–63.
4. Gilbert EF, Arya S, Laxova R, et al. Pathology of chromosome abnormalities in the fetus – pathologic markers. Birth Defects 1987; 23(1):293.
5. Schinzel A. Catalogue of unbalanced chromosome aberrations in man, 2nd edn. Berlin: de Gruyter; 2001.
6. Gilbert-Barness EF, Opitz JM. Chromosome anomalies. In: Stocker JT, Dehner LP, eds. Pediatric pathology, vol I. Philadelphia: JB Lippincott; 1992:41–71.
7. Kalousek DK, Fitch N, Paradice BA. Pathology of the human embryo and previable fetus: an atlas. Berlin: Springer-Verlag; 1990.
8. Braude P, Johnson M, Pickering S, et al. Mechanisms of early embryonic loss *in vivo* and *in vitro*. In: Chapman M, Grudzinskas G, Chard T, eds. The embryo, normal and abnormal development and growth. London: Springer-Verlag; 1991:1–10.
9. Witschi E. Teratogenic effects from overripenness of the egg. In: Fraser FC, McKusick VA, eds. Congenital malformations – proceedings of the Third International Conference. New York: Excerpta Medica; 1970:157–169.
10. Boué J, Boué A. Anomalies chromosomiques dans les avortements spontanés. In: Boué A, Thibault CD, eds. Les accidents chromosomiques de la reproduction. Paris: INSERM 29; 1973.
11. Warburton D, Bryne J, Canki N. Chromosome anomalies and prenatal development: an atlas. New York: Oxford University Press; 1991.
12. Simpson JL. Aetiology of pregnancy failure. In: Chapman M, Grudzinskas G, Chard T, eds. The embryo, normal and abnormal development and growth. London: Springer-Verlag; 1991:11–34.
13. Nicolaides KH, Snijders RJM, Gosden CM. The role of echography in the diagnosis of fetal chromosome defects. In: Chapman M, Grudzinskas G, Chard T, eds. The embryo, normal and abnormal development and growth. London: Springer-Verlag; 1991:101–121.
14. Opitz JM, Gilbert EF. Pathogenesis analysis of congenital anomalies in humans. In: Ioachim HI, ed. Pathobiology annual, vol XII. New York,: Raven Press; 1982:301–349.
15. Khoury MJ, Cordero JF, Rasmussen S. Ectopia cordis, midline defects and chromosomal abnormalities: an epidemiological perspective. Am J Med Genet 1988; 30:811.
16. Opitz JM, Gilbert-Barness EF. Reflections on the pathogenesis of Down syndrome. Am J Med Genet 1990; 7(suppl):38.
16a. Wilkins-Haug L, Quade B, Morton CC. Confined placental mosaicism as a risk factor among newborns with fetal growth restriction. Prenat Diagn 2006; 26:428–432.

Mendelian inheritance, multifactorial determination, and atypical mechanisms

17. Wilson GN. Genomics of human dysmorphogenesis. Am J Med Genet 1992; 42:187–196.
18. Sebat J, Lakshmi B, Troge J, et al. Large-scale copy number polymorphism in the human genome. Science 2004; 305:525–528.
19. Cox TC. Taking it to the max: the genetic and developmental mechanisms coordinating midfacial morphogenesis and dysmorphology. Clin Genet 2004; 65:163–176.
20. Opitz JM. The developmental field concept in clinical genetics. David W. Smith Festschrift. J Pediatr 1982; 101:805.
21. Opitz JM, Gilbert SF. Editorial comment: developmental field theory and the molecular analysis of morphogenesis: a comment on Dr. Slavkin's observations. Am J Med Genet 1993; 47:687.

Twinning

22. Landy HJ, Weiner S, Corson SL, et al. The 'vanishing twin': ultrasonographic assessment of fetal disappearance in the first trimester. Am J Obstet Gynecol 1986; 155:14.

Malformations

23. Opitz JM, Gilbert-Barness EF. Editorial comment: CNS anomalies and the midline as a 'developmental field.' Am J Med Genet 1982; 12:443.

24. Stocker JT, Heifetz SA. Sirenomelia: a morphological study of 33 cases and review of the literature. Perspect Pediatr Pathol 1987; 10:7.

25. Gilbert-Barness E, Opitz JM. Congenital anomalies and malformation syndromes. In: Stocker JT, Dehner LP, eds. Pediatric pathology. Philadelphia: JB Lippincott; 1993:73.

26. Dieker H, Opitz JM. Associated acral and renal malformations. Birth Defects Orig Artic Ser 1969; 5:68.

27. Geduspan JS, Solursh M. A growth promoting influence from the mesonephros during limb outgrowth. Dev Biol 1992; 151:242.

28. Lammer EJ, Opitz JM. The DiGeorge anomaly as a developmental field defect. Am J Med Genet Suppl 1986; 2:113.

29. Thomas RA, Landing BH, Wells TR. Embryologic and other developmental considerations of thirty-eight possible variants of the DiGeorge anomaly. In: Topics in pediatric genetic pathology: the Enid Gilbert-Barness Festschrift, Am J Med Genet Suppl 1987: 3:43.

30. Opitz JM, Mollica F, Sorge G, et al. Acrofacial dysostoses: review and report of a previously undescribed condition: the autosomal or X-linked dominant Catania form of acrofacial dysostosis. Am J Med Genet 1993; 47:668.

31. Herrmann J, Pallister PD, Gilbert EF, et al. Studies of malformation syndromes of man, XXXXIB. Nosologic studies in the Hanhart and the Möbius syndrome. Eur J Pediatr 1976; 122:19.

32. Bersu ET, Pettersen JC, Charboneau WJ, et al. Studies of malformation syndromes of man XXXXIA. Anatomical studies in the 'Hanhart syndrome' – a pathogenetic hypothesis. Eur J Pediatr 1976; 122:1.

33. Gilbert-Barness EF, Opitz JM. Congenital anomalies – malformation syndromes. In: Wigglesworth JS, Singer DB, eds. Textbook of fetal and perinatal pathology, vol I. Boston: Blackwell; 1991:381–427.

34. Opitz JM, Editorial comment: on the paper by de la Monte and Hutchins on familial polyasplenia. Am J Med Genet 1985; 21:175.

Associations

35. Quan L, Smith DW. The VATER association, vertebral defects, anal atresia, tracheoesophageal fistula with esophageal atresia, radial and renal dysplasia: a spectrum of associated defects. J Pediatr 1973; 82:104.

36. Temtamy SA, Miller JD. Extending the scope of the VATER association: definition of the VATER syndrome. J Pediatr 1974; 85:345.

37. Uehling DT, Gilbert EF, Chesney RW. Urologic implications of the VATER association. J Urol 1983; 129:352.

38. Lubinsky M. Current concepts: VATER and other associations; historical perspectives and modern interpretations. Am J Med Genet Suppl 1986; 2:9.

39. Duncan PA. Embryologic pathogenesis of renal agenesis associated with cervical vertebral anomalies (Klippel-Feil phenotype). Birth Defects Orig Artic Ser 1977; 13:91.

40. Duncan PA, Shapiro LR, Stangel JJ, et al. The MURCS association: müllerian duct aplasia, renal aplasia, and cervicothoracic somite dysplasia, J Pediatr 1979; 95:399.

41. Pagon RA, Graham JM, Zonana J, et al. CHARGE association: coloboma, congenital heart disease, and choanal atresia with multiple anomalies, J Pediatr 1981; 99:223.

42. Jones KL Jr. Recognizable patterns of human malformation, 6th edn. Philadelphia: WB Saunders; 2005.

43. Gilbert-Barness E, Opitz JM. Congenital anomalies and malformation syndromes. In: Stocker JJ, Dehwer LP, eds. Pediatric pathology. Philadelphia: JB Lippincott; 1992:73.

44. Czeizel A. Schisis association. Am J Med Genet 1981; 10:25.

Teratogenic disruptions of blastogenesis

45. Mills JL, Baker L, Goldman AS. Malformations in infants of diabetic mothers occur before the seventh gestational week: implications for treatment. Diabetes 1979; 28:292.

46. Kucera J. Rate and type of congenital anomalies among offspring of diabetic women. J Reprod Med 1971; 7:61.

47. Becerra JE, Khoury MJ, Cordero JF, et al. Diabetes mellitus during pregnancy and the risks for specific birth defects: a population-based case-control study. Pediatrics 1990; 85:1.

48. Miller E, Hare JW, Cloherty JP, et al. Elevated maternal hemoglobin A1c in early pregnancy and major congenital anomalies in infants of diabetic mothers. N Engl J Med 1981; 304:1331.

49. Mills JL, Knopp RH, Simpson JL, et al. Lack of relation of increased malformation rates in infants of diabetic mothers to glycemic control during organogenesis. N Engl J Med 1988; 318:671.

50. Greene MF, Hare JW, Clohertz JP, et al. First-trimester hemoglobin A1 and risk for major malformation and spontaneous abortion in diabetic pregnancy. Teratology 1989; 39:225.

51. Mills JL. Commentary on Greene MF, et al, 1989. In: Metzger BE, Buchanan JA, eds. Diabetes and birth defects. Diabetes Spectrum 1990; 3(3):165.

52. Gabbe SG. Commentary on Greene MF, et al, 1989. In: Metzger BE, Buchanan JA, eds. Diabetes and birth defects. Diabetes Spectrum 1990; 3(3):166.

53. Freinkel N, Cockcroft DL, Lewis NJ, et al. The 1986 McCollum Award Lecture: fuel-mediated teratogenesis during early organogenesis. The effects of increased concentrations of glucose, ketones, or somatomedin inhibitor during rat embryo culture. Am J Clin Nutr 1986; 44:986.

54. Pedersen LM, Tygstrup I, Pedersen J. Congenital malformation in newborn infants of diabetic women (correlation with maternal vascular complications). Lancet 1964; 1:1124.

55. Fuhrmann K, Reiher H, Semmler K, et al. Prevention of congenital malformations in infants of insulin-dependent diabetic mothers. Diabetes Care 1993; 6:219.

56. Erikson UJ. Importance of genetic predisposition and maternal environment for the occurrence of congenital malformations in offspring of diabetic rats. Teratology 1988; 37:365.

57. Hersh JH, Angle B, Fox TL, et al. Developmental field defects: Coming together of associations and sequences during blastogenesis. Am J Med Genet 2002; 110:320–323.

57a. Gareskog M, Eriksson UJ, Wentzel P. Combined supplementation of folic acid and vitamin E diminishes diabetes-induced embryotoxicity in rats. Birth Defects Res A Clin Mol 2006; 76:483–490.

58. Abel EL, Sokol RJ. Fetal alcohol syndrome is now leading cause of mental retardation. Lancet 1986; 2:1222.

59. Streissguth AP, Landesman-Dwyer S, Martin JC, et al. Teratogenic effects of alcohol in humans and laboratory animals. Science 1980; 209:353.

60. Sulik KK, Johnston MC, Webb MA. Fetal alcohol syndrome: embryogenesis in a mouse model. Science 1981; 214:936.

60a. Gemma S, Vichi S, Testai E. Metabolic and genetic factors contributing to alcohol induced effects and fetal alcohol syndrome. Neurosci Biobehav Rev [Epub ahead of print]. 2006 Aug 12.

Anomalies of organogenesis

61. Opitz JM, Lewin SO. The developmental field concept in pediatric pathology – especially with respect to fibular a/hypoplasia and the DiGeorge anomaly. Birth Defects Orig Artic Ser 1987; 23:277.

62. Delahunt CS, Lassen LT. Thalidomide syndrome in monkeys. Science 1964; 146:1300.

Defects of phenogenesis

63. Leppig KA, Werler MM, Cann CI, et al. Predictive value of minor anomalies. I. Association with major malformations. J Pediatr 1987; 110:531.

Characteristics facial phenotypes: the example of Cornelia de Lange syndrome

64. Kousseff BG, Newkirk P, Root AW. Brachmann-de Lange syndrome: 1993 update. Arch Pediatr Adolesc Med 1994; 148:749–755.

65. Van Allen MI, Filippi G, Siegel-Bartelt J, et al. Clinical variability within Brachmann-de Lange syndrome: a proposed classification system. Am J Med Genet 1993; 47:947.

66. Opitz JM. Editorial: Brachmann-de Lange syndrome – a continuing enigma. Arch Pediatr Adolesc Med 1994; 148:1206.

67. Krantz I D, McCallum J, DeScipio C, et al. Cornelia de Lange syndrome is caused by mutations in NIPBL, the human homolog of *Drosophila melanogaster* Nipped-B. Nature Genet 2004; 36:631–635.

68. Tonkin ET, Wang T-J, Lisgo S, et al. NIPBL, encoding a homolog of fungal Scc2-type sister chromatid cohesion proteins and fly Nipped-B, is mutated in Cornelia de Lange syndrome. Nature Genet 2004; 36:636–641.

Deformities

69. Porter HJ. Fetal arthrogryposis multiplex congenita (fetal akinesia deformation sequence [FADS]). Ped Path Lab Med 1995; 15:617.

70. Pena SDJ, Shokeir MHK. Syndrome of camptodactyly, multiple ankyloses, facial anomalies and pulmonary hypoplasia: a lethal condition. J Pediatr 1974; 85:373.

71. Hall J. Analysis of the Pena-Shokeir syndrome. Am J Med Genet 1985; 25:99.

Defects of differentiation: dysplasias

72. Rubenstein AE. Neurofibromatosis: a review of the clinical problem. Ann NY Acad Sci 1986; 486:1.

73. Kousseff BG, Gilbert-Barness EF. Vascular neurofibromatosis and infantile gangrene. J Med Genet 1989; 34:221.

73a. Trovo-Marqui AB, Tajara EH. Neurofibromin: a general outlook. Clin Genet 2006; 70:1–13.

73b. Chen Z, Fadiel A, Xia Y. Functional duality of merlin: A conundrum of proteome complexity. Med Hypotheses 2006 Jul 3; [Epub ahead of print].

74. Bender BL, Yunis EJ. The pathology of tuberous sclerosis. Pathol Annu 1982; 17:339.

75. Crino PB, Nathanson KL, Henske EP. N Engl J Med 2006; 355:1345–1356.

75a. Vinaitheerthan M, Wei J, Mizuguchi M, et al. Tuberous sclerosis: immunohistochemistry expression of tuberin and hamartin in a 31-week gestational fetus. Fetal Pediatr Pathol 2004; 23:241–249.

76. Potter EL, Craig JM. Pathology of the fetus and the infant, 3rd edn. Chicago:Year Book Medical Publishers; 1975:434.

77. Gilbert-Barness EF, Opitz JM, Barness LA. Heritable malformation of the kidney and urinary tract. In: Spitzer A, Avner ED, eds. Inheritance of kidney and urinary tract diseases. New York: Kluwer Academic Press; 1990:327–400.

78. Catchpoole D, Smallwood AV, Joyce JA, et al. Mutation analysis of H19 and NAP1L4 (hNAP2) candidate genes and IGF2 DMR2 in Beckwith-Wiedemann syndrome. J Med Genet 2000; 37: 212–215.

79. Cerrato F, Sparago A, Di Matteo I, et al. The two-domain hypothesis in Beckwith-Wiedemann syndrome: autonomous imprinting of the telomeric domain of the distal chromosome 7 cluster. Hum Mol Genet 2005; 14:503–511. (*Editor's note: in the mouse, 7qter corresponds to the imprinted human 11p15.5.*)

80. Maher ER, Reik W. Beckwith-Wiedemann syndrome: imprinting in clusters revisited. J Clin Invest 2000; 105:247–252.

81. Neri G, Martini-Neri ME, Katz BE, et al. The Perlman syndrome: familial renal dysplasia with Wilms' tumor, fetal gigantism and multiple congenital anomalies. Am J Med Genet 1984; 10:195.

82. Lindenauer SM. Congenital arteriovenous fistula and the Klippel-Trenaunay syndrome. Ann Surg 1971; 174:248.

83. Hoffman HJ, Hendrick EB, Dennis M, et al. Hemispherectomy for Sturge-Weber syndrome. Childs Brain 1979; 5:233.

84. Durkin-Stamm MV, Gilbert EF, Ganick DJ, et al. An unusual dysplasia-malformation-cancer syndrome in two patients. Am J Med Genet 1978; 1:279.

85. Herrmann J, Gilbert EF, Opitz JM. Dysplasia, malformations and cancer, especially with respect to the Wiedemann-Beckwith syndrome. In: Nichols WW, Murphy DG, eds. Regulation of cell proliferation and differentiation. New York: Plenum Press; 1977:1–64.

86. Beighton P, ed. McKusick's heritable disorders of connective tissue, 5th edn. St. Louis: CV Mosby; 1992.

87. Royce PM, Steinmann B, eds. Connective tissue and its heritable disorders. Molecular, genetic, and medical aspects. New York: Wiley-Liss; 1993.

88. Loeys BL, Schwarze U, Holm T, et al. Aneurysm syndromes caused by mutations in the TGF-β receptor. N Engl J Med 2006; 355:788–798.

89. Priestley L, Kumar D, Sykes B. Amplification of the COL2A1 3 prime variable region used for sequestration analysis in a family with the Stickler syndrome. Hum Genet 1990; 85:525.

90. Clayton PT, Thompson E. Dysmorphic syndromes with demonstrable biochemical abnormalities. J Med Genet 1988; 25:463.

91. Scriver CR, Beaudet AL, Sly WS, et al. The metabolic and molecular basis of inherited disease, 8th edn. New York: McGraw-Hill; 2001.

92. Wilson GN, Holmes RD, Hajra AK. Peroxisomal disorders: clinical commentary and future prospects. Am J Med Genet 1988; 30:771.

93. Hoffmann G, Gibson KM, Brandt IK, et al. Mevalonic aciduria – an inborn error of cholesterol and nonsterol metabolism. N Engl J Med 1986; 314:1610.

94. Opitz JM. RSH/SLO ('Smith-Lemli-Opitz') syndrome: historical, genetic and developmental considerations. Am J Med Genet 1994; 50:344.

95. Kelley RI. A new face for an old syndrome (Editorial). Am J Med Genet 1997; 65:251–256.

96. Curry CJR, Carey JC, Holland JS, et al: Smith-Lemli-Opitz syndrome – type II: multiple congenital anomalies with male pseudohermaphroditism and frequent early lethality. Am J Med Genet 1987; 26:45.

97. Roux C, Horvath C, Dupuis R. Teratogenic action and embryo lethality of AY9944: prevention by a hypercholesterolemia-provoking diet. Teratology 1979; 19:35.

Sequences

98. Hanson JW, Smith DW. U-shaped palatal defect in the Robin anomaly: developmental and clinical relevance. J Pediatr 1975; 87:30.

99. Wigger JH, Blanc WA. The prune-belly syndrome. Pathol Annu 1977; 12:17.

100. Burton BK, Dillard RG. Brief clinical report: prune-belly syndrome: observations supporting the hypothesis of abdominal overdistention. Am J Med Genet 1984; 17:669.

100a. Yagi H, Furutani Y, Hamada H, et al. Role of TBX1 in human del22q11.2 syndrome. Lancet 2003; 362:1366–1373.

101. Edwards MJ. The experimental production of clubfoot in guinea pigs by maternal hyperthermia during gestation. J Pathol 1971; 103:49.

Disruptions

4

PART 1   *Jaime L. Frías and Enid Gilbert-Barness*

Teratogenic disruptions

'The dose makes a poison.'   Paracelsus (1493–1541)

Approximately 1 in 250 newborn infants has structural defects caused by a teratogenic exposure and, presumably, a larger number of children have growth retardation and/or functional abnormalities resulting from the adverse effects of environmental agents on prenatal development. Studies of environmentally induced malformations are important to further our understanding of gene–environment interactions in abnormal development, and to provide clues for the prevention of human congenital malformations.[1,2]

A teratogen is defined as any environmental agent that can produce a permanent abnormality in structure or function, restriction of growth, and/or death of the embryo or fetus. Some authors believe that there are no teratogens as such, but that teratogenicity is a function of the exposure.[3] The effects on the embryo or fetus depend of the chemical or physical nature of the agent and a number of other factors such as the dose, route and length of exposure, the developmental stage at which the exposure occurs, the susceptibility of the mother and embryo or fetus, and the presence and nature of concurrent exposures.

Environmental factors that may adversely affect the development of the embryo and fetus account for approximately 15% of all malformations in infants. However, of the estimated 50–70% of human concepti lost in the first 3 weeks of gestation and of the 78% lost before term, some may be due to teratogenic agents.[4] The causes of congenital abnormalities are shown in Table 4.1.1.[5–10]

Teratogenic exposures may result in infertility or pregnancy loss, prenatal onset growth deficiency, structural defects and/or functional central nervous system (CNS) abnormalities. The structural defects generally consist of patterns of congenital anomalies. No single malformation is pathognomonic of a given teratogenic insult, although in some cases the pattern of anomalies caused by a specific teratogen is characteristic enough to be clinically recognizable. However, the range of phenotypic expression can be highly variable, depending on the factors mentioned above. Because teratogens have a multicellular mode of action, both the incidence and the severity of the defects they induce increase with the dose. By the same token, there is a threshold dose below which they exert no adverse effects on morphogenesis.[11,12]

Critical periods in human development and the most common sites of action of teratogens are depicted in Figure 4.1.1.[13]

Teratogenic agents cause **disruptions** during development regardless of the developmental stage or site of action. From fertilization through the early postimplantation period, the effect of a teratogenic insult may be an all-or-none phenomenon. Severe damage may cause the death of the product of conception or, because of the pluripotential nature of the cells, the damage may be compensated allowing development to continue in a normal fashion. Most authors believe that the all-or-none rule applies to the first 2 weeks of development,[3,14] but this is debatable. Crucial morphogenetic processes ongoing during the **blastogenesis** period can be altered and result in a number of structural abnormalities. The stage of **blastogenesis** extends throughout the first 4 weeks of development, from fertilization until the end of the gastrulation stage (days 27–28 post conception).[15]

Most major structural defects resulting from teratogenic exposures occur during the embryonic period, which is when

TABLE 4.1.1 CAUSES OF CONGENITAL DEFECTS

Cause	Percentage
Environmental teratogenic agents	15
Monogenic	15
Chromosomal	15
Unknown (include multifactorial)	55

Based on data from Holmes[5], Wilson[6], Fraser[7], Kalter and Warkany[8], Shephard[9], and Brent and Beckman.[10]

many critical developmental events are taking place and most organs are being formed. The effect of teratogens on human development follows a limited repertoire of pathogenic mechanisms which includes excessive or reduced cell death, interference with cell signaling and differentiation, decreased biosynthesis, alteration of morphogenetic movements, and disruption of tissues.[16–18]

The fetus is less susceptible to morphologic alterations, and teratogenic events cause mainly mild errors of morphogenesis (abnormalities of phenogenesis) such as epicanthic folds, single palmar crease, clinodactyly, and others. However, major abnormalities also can have their origin during the fetal period, as

critical developmental events are still occurring. Development of the urogenital system and the CNS continue beyond the eighth postfertilization week and make the fetus sensitive to late teratogenic exposures that may result in structural or functional abnormalities. Environmental exposures during the fetal period may affect cell growth, decreasing cell population and thus causing fetal growth retardation. In addition, other insults, primarily those mechanical in nature, can produce deformation or destruction of organs or parts of the body that have been normally formed during the embryonic period.[19]

The relationship between the time when an exposure occurs and the resulting pattern of altered morphogenesis has been well defined for several pharmacologic and chemical agents (critical 'window'). For example, exposure to thalidomide at teratogenic levels (≥ 50 mg) between days 20 and 24 post conception produces eye (anophthalmia, coloboma) and ear defects, while exposure between days 24 and 33 results in reduction defects of the upper limbs, and between days 28 and 36, in reduction defects of the lower limbs.[12, 20, 21] The time of action of some human teratogens is shown in Table 4.1.2.

Sensitivity to a potentially teratogenic agent is highly variable, and only a relatively small proportion of exposures during preg-

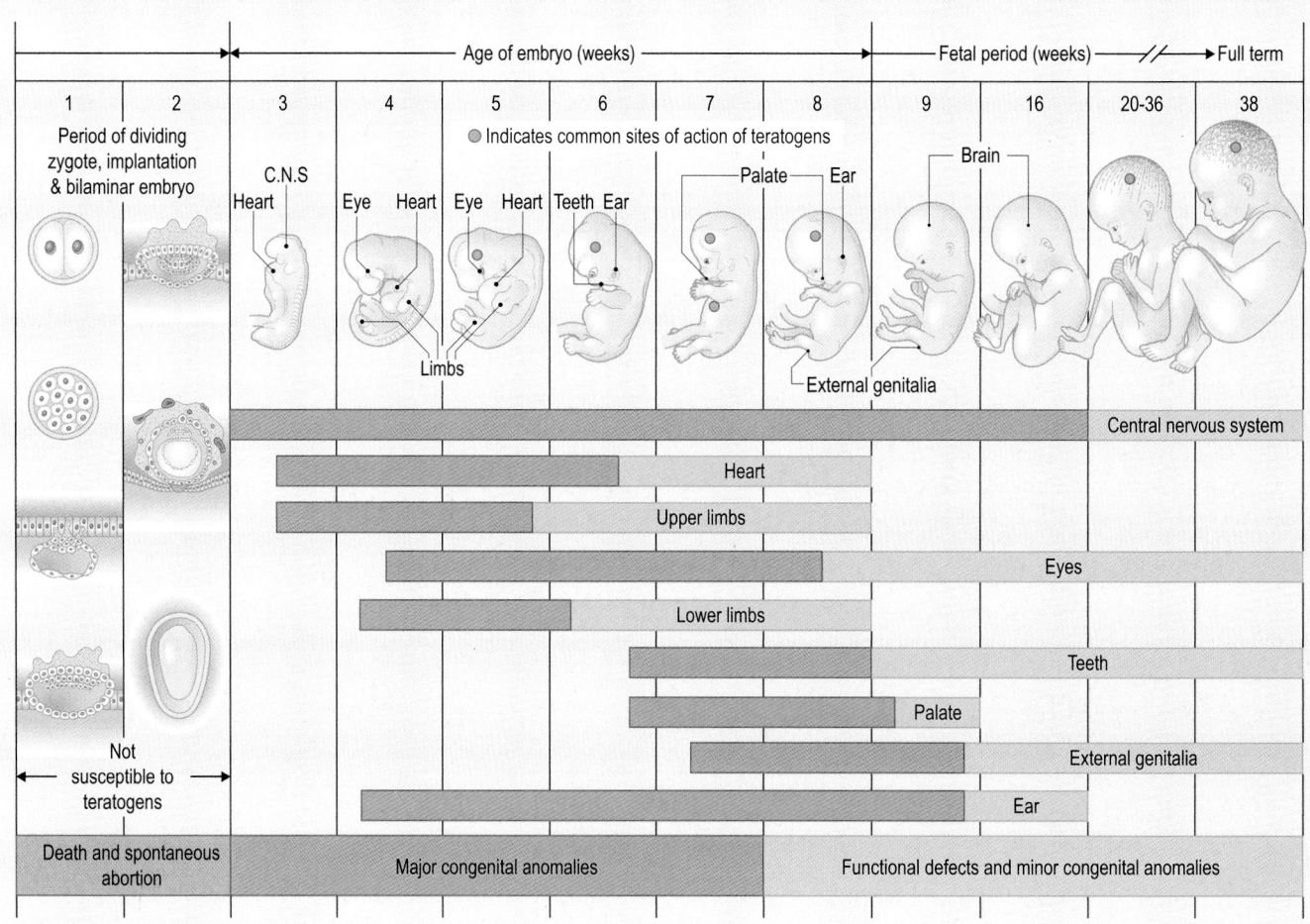

FIGURE 4.1.1 Critical periods in human development and the site of action of teratogens. Red denotes periods of maximum sensitivity to teratogens; yellow a lower risk of malformation upon exposure. (From Moore and Persaud 1993,[13] with permission.)

TABLE 4.1.2 THE SPECIFICITY OF ACTION OF SOME HUMAN TERATOGENS

Teratogen	Post fertilization age (days)	Malformation
Androgens (exogenous, tumors)	Before 90	Clitoral hypertrophy and labial fusion
	After 90	Clitoral hypertrophy
Diethylstilbestrol	After 14	50% vaginal adenosis
	After 98	30% vaginal adenosis
	After 126	10% vaginal adenosis
Goitrogens and iodine	After 180	Fetal goiter
Hyperthermia	18-30	Anencephaly
Radioiodine	After 65–70	Fetal thyroidectomy
Rubella virus	0–60	Cataracts or heat defects
	0–129+	Deafness
Tetracyclines	After 120	Enamel staining of primary teeth
	After 250	Staining of crowns of permanent teeth
Thalidomide	20–24	Eye and ear malformations
	24–33	Reduction defects upper extremities
	28–36	Reduction defects lower extremities
Warfarin (Coumadin)	Before 100	Nose hypoplasia, stippling of epiphyses
	After 100	Possible mental retardation

After Shephard 1986,[9] with permission.

nancy result in an adverse outcome. For instance, prenatal exposure to phenytoin causes congenital anomalies only in about 10% of exposed infants,[22] and prenatal exposure to thalidomide resulted in recognizable structural defects in fewer than 20% of exposed infants.[20] Studies in experimental animals as well as human epidemiologic studies have demonstrated that this sensitivity is largely dependent of the genetic constitution of the mother and the embryo or fetus.[16, 23–27]

While studies on experimental animals have greatly contributed to the understanding of the mechanism of action of many teratogenic agents,[28, 29] the results of studies to determine the teratogenicity of a given agent in laboratory animals must be interpreted with great care and cannot always be extrapolated to humans. Negative results do not guarantee that the drug or factor under study does not have the potential of adversely affecting human prenatal development. Conversely, a positive study does not mean that the agent is teratogenic in humans.[30]

Likewise, epidemiologic studies need to be interpreted cautiously. When a wide range of potentially teratogenic agents and outcomes are being studied, positive associations can be found by chance alone. Using the usual 5% level of significance, 5% of the statistically significant differences between exposed and non-exposed individuals may be spurious. On the other hand, negative studies may reflect a lack of sufficient statistical power to find differences between the risk of specific malformations among exposed and non-exposed individuals. This may be due to small sample size, especially when the investigators stratify by different teratogens and specific birth defects, etiologic heterogeneity, incomplete ascertainment of birth defects, and/or inadequate control of confounding factors.

The recognition of a teratogen is based on the following criteria:[31]

- Exposure produces an increase in occurrence of specific phenotypic effects, such as growth retardation and a recognizable pattern of major and minor anomalies.
- An animal model duplicates the effect in humans.
- A dose–response relationship has been demonstrated in either animals or humans so that the greater the exposure during pregnancy, the more severe is the phenotypic effect on the fetus.
- There is a plausible biologic explanation for the mechanism of action of the alleged fetal environmental agent.
- In exposed individuals, a group may be at increased risk owing to an underlying genetic susceptibility.

Unfortunately, all these criteria cannot always be established. Some agents have well recognized teratogenic effects while others are considered to be probably or possibly teratogenic. But for the vast majority of the drugs and chemicals to which the population is frequently exposed, substantive information about their potential teratogenic effects is lacking.[32–34]

Table 4.1.3 lists environmental disruptive events and their effects. Some agents are not established as teratogens and represent sporadic reports.

Physical agents

Radiation

The potential of producing adverse reproductive effects varies with the type of radiation and with the dose and timing of the exposure.[35] The most common types of radiation are ionizing radiation, ultrasound, low-frequency electromagnetic fields (EMF), and microwaves. Ultrasound and microwaves have been

TABLE 4.1.3 TERATOGENIC AGENTS

	Reported effects or associations	Comments
Radiation	Microcephaly, mental retardation, eye anomalies, intrauterine growth retardation (IUGR), visceral malformations depend on dose and state of exposure	Cell death and mitotic delay. No measurable risk with exposures of 5 rad or less of x-rays.
Hypoxia	Central nervous system (CNS) disruption, hypoxic ischemia encephalopathy, porencephaly	
Infectious agents		
Rubella	80% incidence of embryonic infection with exposure in first 12 weeks, 25% at end of second trimester, 100% at term. Defects include mental retardation, deafness, cardiovascular malformations, cataracts, glaucoma, microphthalmia	These infectious agents cause disruptions The cytotoxic effects and scarring or calcification during repair processes interfere with organogenesis and/or histogenesis. Characteristic syndromes are related to the specific tissue localization and pathologic characteristics of the infectious agent.
Cytomegalovirus	IUGR, risk of brain damage 50% after infection early in pregnancy	
Herpes simplex	Microcephaly, intracranial calcification, eye defects, vesicular rash	
Varicella-zoster	Skin and muscle defects, IUGR, limb reduction defects, eye anomalies, CNS abnormalities	
Venezuelan equine encephalitis	Hydranencephaly, microphthalmia, luxation of hip	
Toxoplasmosis	Hydrocephalus, microphthalmia, chorioretinitis	
Parvovirus	Stillbirth, abortion, hydrops, anemia, erythroblastosis, preductal coarctation. Increased maternal α-fetoprotein	
Syphilis	50% of offspring with defects after early exposure to primary or secondary syphilis and 10% after late exposures. Defects include maculopapular rash, hepatosplenomegaly, deformed nails, osteochondritis at joints of extremities, congenital neurosyphilis, abnormal epiphyses, chorioretinitis	
Thermodisruptions		
Hyperthermia	Microcephaly, CNS developmental defects, anencephaly, microphthalmia, distal limb deficiencies, cleft lip/palate, midface hypoplasia, neurogenic arthrogryposis, ear defects	Antimitotic teratogen
Heavy metals		
Lithium carbonate	Increased incidence of Ebstein anomaly, other heart and great vessel defects, neural tube defects	Mechanism has not been defined. Risk is estimated at 10%
Methylmercury	Minamata disease: cerebral palsy, microcephaly, mental retardation, blindness	Cell death due to inhibition of enzymes, especially sulfhydryl enzymes. Of liveborn exposed infants, 6% were affected; may be embryo lethal
Lead	Minor malformations, abortion, stillbirths	
Chemical agents		
Polychlorinated biphenyls	Cola-colored children: pigmentation of gums, nails, and groin; hypoplastic deformed nails; IUGR; abnormal skull calcification; growth retardation; stillbirth	Polychlorinated biphenyls are cytotoxic. Body residues in exposed women can affect subsequent offspring for up to 4 years after exposure
Gasoline	Mental retardation and neurologic abnormalities	Recreational inhalation during pregnancy has resulted in two infants affected

TABLE 4.1.3 TERATOGENIC AGENTS (*CONT'D*)

	Reported effects or associations	Comments
Methyl isocyanate	Cleft palate, hydronephrosis, diaphragmatic hernia, cardiac enlargement, meningomyelocele	Defects noted following Bhopal disaster in India
Maternal conditions		
Maternal starvation	CNS anomalies, IUGR, increased morbidity	High mitotic rate of fetus in general and CNS in particular is very sensitive to nutrient levels
Maternal diabetes mellitus	Caudal dysplasia or caudal regression syndrome, increased risk of several common defects	Insulin therapy protects fetus. Fetal growth retardation may result from vascular lesions in long-standing diabetics
Phenylketonuria	Mental retardation, microcephaly, IUGR	High levels of phenylketones interfere with cell metabolism
Systemic lupus erythematosus (SLE)	Cutaneous SLE lesions, congenital heart block, hematologic abnormalities	Transplacental transfer of IgG antibodies to fetus—anti-RO, anti-LA, anti-U, RNP
Myasthenia gravis	Congenital contractures	Effect of myasthenia on fetus causes contractures
Endocrinopathies	If condition is compatible with pregnancy, effects are similar to those following administration of hormone	Receptor-mediated exposures to high levels of sex hormones
Mechanical constraints		
Uterine malformations	Birth defects involving foot position, limb and skin development, head and ear shape, midline closure, jaw and muscle maldevelopment	Physical constraint can result in distortion and reduction in blood supply
Placental implantation abnormalities		
Oligohydramnios		
Drugs		
Acetazolamide	Sacrococcygeal teratoma, polyhydramnios	
Albuterol	Fetal tachycardia	
Alcohol	Fetal alcohol syndrome: IUGR, maxillary hypoplasia, reduction in width of palpebral fissures, microcephaly, mental retardation, heart defects	Usually exposure in utero of at least 4 oz (118 ml) pure alcohol daily, but variable
Amantadine	Single ventricle with pulmonary atresia	
Amitriptyline	Micrognathia	
Amobarbital	Anencephaly, congenital heart malformations, limb reduction, swelling of hands and feet, severe limb deformities, congenital hip dislocation, polydactyly, clubfoot, oral cleft, intersex, soft tissue deformity of neck	
Angiotensin-converting enzyme (ACE) inhibitors	Oligohydramnios, growth retardation, skull hypoplasia, renal tubular dysgenesis with neonatal anuria	Some affected infants have been exposed only during third trimester
Aspirin	Intracranial hemorrhage; heavy use may result in low birth weight but no increase in malformations	Doses toxic for mother are likely to be both maternal and embryo toxic
Azathioprine	Pulmonary valvular stenosis, goiter	
Bromides	Polydactyly, clubfoot, congenital dislocation of hip	
Caffeine	Caffeine is not likely to be a human teratogen; increased risk of fetal loss	Excess consumption is likely to be both maternal and embryo toxic
Captopril	Leg reduction, stillbirth	
Carbon monoxide	Cerebral atrophy, hydrocephalus	
Chlordiazepoxide	Microcephaly, congenital defects of heart, duodenal atresia	

TABLE 4.1.3 TERATOGENIC AGENTS (*CONT'D*)

	Reported effects or associations	Comments
Chloroquine	Up-slanting palpebral fissures, flat philtrum, microcephaly, thin upper lip, brachydactyly of fifth finger; auditory, vestibular, retinal, and other neurologic dysfunction	
Chlorpheniramine	Hydrocephalus, polydactyly, congenital dislocation of hip	
Clomiphene	Meningomyelocele, hydrocephalus, microcephaly, anencephaly, syndactyly, clubfoot, polydactyly, esophageal atresia	
Codeine	Hydrocephalus, congenital cardiac defects, musculoskeletal malformations, dislocated hip, pyloric stenosis, oral cleft, respiratory malformations	
Cortisone	Cleft lip/palate, congenital cardiac defects	
Coumadin (coumarin, dicumarol, warfarin)	Nasal hypoplasia; stippling of secondary epiphysis; IUGR; anomalies of eyes, hands, and neck; variable CNS effects	Metabolic inhibitor; bleeding is an unlikely explanation for effects. Risk from exposure 10–25% during weeks 8–14 of gestation (weeks 6–12 post conception)
Cytarabine	Anencephaly, tetralogy of Fallot, lobster claw of three digits, missing feet digits, syndactyly	
Dextroamphetamine	Exencephaly, more cardiac defects than controls, atrial septal defects	
Diazepam	Spina bifida, more cardiac defects than controls	
Diphenylhydantoin (phenytoin, hydantoin)	Hydantoin syndrome: hypoplastic nails and distal phalanges, cleft lip/palate, microcephaly, mental retardation	
Disulfiram	Vertebral fusion, clubfoot, radial aplasia, phocomelia, tracheoesophageal fistula	
Ethosuximide	Hydrocephalus, short neck, radial aplasia, absent thumbs, aplasia of esophagus and duodenum	
Fluphenazine	Poor ossification of frontal bone, limb deformities, bleeding	
Haloperidol	Limb deformities	
Heparin	Bleeding	
Imipramine	Exencephaly, limb reduction, cleft palate, renal cystic degeneration	
Indometacin*	Phocomelia	
Isoniazid	Meningomyelocele	
Lysergic acid diethylamide	Hydrocephalus, encephalocele, meningomyelocele, limb reduction defects, limb deficiencies	
Meclizine	Hypoplastic left heart	
Meprobamate	Congenital heart malformations, bilateral defects of limbs	
Metronidazole	Midline facial defects	
Nortriptyline	Limb reduction	
Nicotine, tobacco, smoking	Placental lesions and IUGR but no defined malformations; increased postnatal morbidity and mortality (including SIDS)	Maternal or placental complications can result in fetal death
Oral contraceptives	Meningomyelocele, hydrocephalus, anencephaly	

TABLE 4.1.3 TERATOGENIC AGENTS (*CONT'D*)

	Reported effects or associations	Comments
Oxazolidine-2,3-diones (trimethadione, paramethadione)	Fetal trimethadione syndrome: V-shaped eyebrows, low-set ears with anteriorly folded helix, high-arched palate, irregular teeth, CNS anomalies, developmental delay, microcephaly, malformed hands, congenital cardiac defects, esophageal atresia	Affects cell membrane permeability. Wide variation in reported risk. Associations documented only with chronic exposure
Paramethadione	Tetralogy of Fallot, pyloric stenosis, growth retardation	
Penicillamine	Ventricular septal defect, digital anomalies, cleft palate, ileal atresia, growth retardation, pulmonary hypoplasia	
Phenobarbital	Hydrocephalus, meningomyelocele	
Phenothiazines	Microcephaly, syndactyly, clubfoot, omphalocele, abdominal distention	
Phenylephrine	Eye and ear abnormalities, syndactyly, clubfoot, congenital dislocation of hip, umbilical hernia	
Phenylpropanolamine	Pectus excavatus, polydactyly, congenital dislocation of hip	
Phenytoin (Dilantin, hydantoin)	Hydantoin syndrome: microcephaly, mental retardation, wide fontanelles, congenital heart malformation, rib-sternal abnormalities, short nose, broad nasal bridge, broad alveolar ridge, short neck, hypertelorism, low-set ears, hypoplastic nails and distal phalanges, digital thumb, dislocated hip, cleft palate/lip, growth retardation	Direct effect on cell membranes and folate and vitamin K metabolism. Wide variation in reported risk. Association documented only with chronic exposure
Primidone	Goldenhar syndrome, anterior encephalocele, aqueductal stenosis	
Procarbazine	Cerebral hemorrhage	
Sympathomimetics	Limb reduction defects, gastroschisis	May be related to vascular disruption due to vasoconstriction
Spermicides	Limb reduction	
Sulfonamide	Hypoplasia of limb or part of it, foot defects, urethral obstructions	
Tetracycline	Hypoplastic tooth enamel, tooth and bone staining	Effects seen only if exposure is during second or third trimester
Thioguanine	Missing digits, growth retardation	
Tolbutamide	Finger-toe syndactyly, absent toes, accessory thumb	
Thalidomide	Bilateral limb reduction defects (preaxial preferential effects, phocomelia), facial hemangioma, esophageal or duodenal atresia; anomalies of external ears, kidneys, and heart	Multiple theories have been proposed, but primary mechanism is unknown
Thyroid: iodine deficiency, iodides, radioiodine, antithyroid drugs (propylthiouracil)	Hypothyroidism or goiter; neurologic and aural damage is variable	Fetopathic effect of endemic iodine occurs early in development. Fetopathic effect of iodides, antithyroid drugs, and radioiodine involves metabolic block, decreases thyroid hormone synthesis and gland development. Maternal intake of 12 mg iodide per day or more increases risk of fetal goiter.
Trifluoperazine	Transposition of great arteries, phocomelia	

TABLE 4.1.3 TERATOGENIC AGENTS (*CONT'D*)

	Reported effects or associations	Comments
Retinoic acid	Hydrocephalus; microcephaly; various congenital heart defects; malformations of cranium, ear, face, and ribs; limb deformities; stillbirth. Urogenital anomalies in humans have been associated with massive doses. Isotretinoin is a human teratogen; defects include ear malformations, open neural tube, cleft palate, facial abnormalities	Retinoic acid is cytotoxic; it may interact with DNA to delay differentiation and/or inhibit protein synthesis; *Hox* dysregulation
Valproic acid	Lumbosacral meningomyelocele, microcephaly, wide fontanel, tetralogy of Fallot, depressed nasal bridge, hypoplastic nose, low-set ears, small mandible, oral cleft, growth deficiency	
Zidovudine	Extra digits, ventricular septal defect, hydronephrosis, ureteral pelvic junction obstruction, single umbilical artery, hypoplastic left heart, mitral atresia	Antiretroviral therapy for HIV infection
Antineoplastic drugs		
Aminopterin, methotrexate	Hydrocephalus, cleft palate, meningomyelocele, IUGR, abnormal cranial ossification, reduction in derivatives of first branchial arch	Folic acid antagonists that inhibit dihydrofolate reductase, resulting in cell death
Busulfan	Growth failure, cleft palate, eye defects, cytomegaly of cells	
Cyclophosphamide	Growth retardation, ectrodactyly, syndactyly, cardiovascular anomalies, other minor anomalies. Magnitude of risk unknown	Requires cytochrome P-450 mono-oxidase activation; interacts with DNA, resulting in cell death
Tamoxifen	Goldenhar syndrome: defect involving 1st and 2nd branchial arches resulting in abnormalities of eyes, ears, vertebrae	Non-steroidal antiestrogenic drug used in treatment of breast carcinoma
Hormones		
Androgens (e.g. danazol)	Masculinization of female embryo: clitoromegaly with or without fusion of labia minora	Effects are dose dependent; stimulate growth and differentiation of receptor-containing tissue
Diethylstilbestrol	Masculinization of female embryo: vaginal adenocarcinogenesis, anomalies of cervix and uterus. The dosage that increases risk of genitourinary abnormalities in males is controversial	Stimulates estrogen receptor-containing tissue, may cause misplaced tissue. Vaginal adenosis from exposures before 9th week of pregnancy: 75% risk; risk of adenocarcinoma is low (1 in 10 000).
Progestins	Masculinization of female embryo exposed to high doses. Stimulates or interferes with growth and differentiation of receptor-containing tissue	
Vascular disruptions		
Cocaine	Placental abruption, cerebral hemorrhages, limb defects, bowel atresia	Vascular disruption
Vitamins		
Retinoic acid	Urogenital anomalies in humans have been associated with massive doses. Isotretinoin is a human teratogen; defects include ear malformations, open neural tube, cleft palate, facial abnormalities	Retinoic acid is cytotoxic; it may interact with DNA to delay differentiation and/or inhibit protein synthesis

TABLE 4.1.3 TERATOGENIC AGENTS (*CONT'D*)

	Reported effects or associations	Comments
Vitamin A	Excess causes absence or hypoplasia of ears, CNS anomalies, congenital heart disease, cortical blindness	Associated with high dosage >25,000 IU
Vitamin D	Large doses given in vitamin D prophylaxis are possibly involved in etiology of supravalvular aortic stenosis, elfin facies, and mental retardation (Williams-like syndrome)	Mechanism is likely to involve disruption of cell calcium regulation
Folic acid deficiency	Deficiency causes neural tube defects, aneuploidy, growth retardation	Accounts for 70% of neural tube defects; fortifying food with folic acid is recommended
Vitamin K deficiency	Stippled calcification along vertebral bodies	
Herbicides		
Agent Orange	No causal relationship between herbicide 2,4,5-T in Agent Orange and human malformations. Teratogenic exposures to toxic contaminant dioxin are not likely to be attainable in humans	The contaminant dioxin is cytotoxic

*Prostaglandin inhibitors (indomethacin and ibuprofen) given in the third trimester may cause oligohydramnios and closure of the ductus arteriosus.

shown to produce malformations in experimental animals by inducing hyperthermia; however, the capacity of low-frequency EMF for hyperthermia and cytotoxicity is insignificant. **No evidence at present indicates that radiowaves, shortwaves, or microwaves can cause non-thermal injury to the developing embryo.** Only the very high-frequency photons of ionizing radiation (mainly γ-rays and X-rays) can remove orbital electrons and produce ionization in tissues, resulting in cytotoxicity, chromosomal damage, and point mutations.[35]

Ionizing radiation

Before implantation, the mammalian embryo is insensitive to the teratogenic and growth-retarding effects of ionizing radiation, but sensitive to the lethal effects.[36–38] Permanent and sometimes severe growth retardation, however, results after midgestation radiation. Because of its extended periods of organogenesis and histogenesis the CNS has the greatest sensitivity of all organ systems to the detrimental effects of radiation through the later fetal stages.

The most likely mechanisms by which ionizing radiation adversely affects prenatal development are cell death, mitotic delay, inhibition of cell migration, communication and differentiation, and interference with histogenesis.[35]

Studies of the effects of in utero radiation exposure in the survivors of the atomic bombings of Hiroshima and Nagasaki indicate no statistically significant long-term effects on the frequencies of stillbirth, neonatal death, or chromosomal abnormalities.[39] However, **microcephaly** and **mental retardation** were frequently observed among the offspring of pregnant women exposed between the 8th and 15th weeks of gestation. No visceral or external malformations were present unless a child exhibited growth retardation at birth, was microcephalic, or had a readily apparent eye malformation. Thirty years after the event, survivors have shown increased frequency of hematopoietic malignancies, of which leukemia is a leading example. An in utero exposure dose of 156 rad is estimated to have doubled the frequencies of cancers of many types, including **leukemias and lymphomas**.[39–41] One cancer death occurs for each 990 prenatal radiation exposures.[42, 43]

In the atomic bomb exposure, microcephaly was common and its severity was related to the distance the mother was from the epicenter.[44] Mental retardation was found after 50-rad doses in Hiroshima but 200-rad doses in Nagasaki. Other significant defects were not found in survivors,[45, 46] but a 0.1% rate of subsequent leukemia was found in children who were within 1500 m of the epicenter.[46]

The rate of mental retardation among 1600 offspring exposed to the bomb was 2.4% at dose levels of 10–49 rad, and 17.6% at dose levels of 50–99 rad.[47] The most critical exposure period was 8–15 weeks after fertilization.[47]

The brain maintains its sensitivity to radiation throughout gestation and the neonatal period whereas other organs can be malformed only from the second to fourth weeks after conception.[48] Significant exposures between the second and fourth weeks are rare and usually result in abortion. Almost all studies of human fetal radiation exposures of less than 5 rad fail to show an increase in fetal malformations. Animal studies suggest that exposures of 50 rad or less should not produce malformations.[10]

The **brain and eyes** sustain the brunt of radiation injury during embryogenesis.[49] Dosages in excess of 25 rad are required for discernible damage. **Microcephaly, hydrocephalus, microphthalmia, cleft palate, micromelia, skull defects, optic atrophy, retinal dysplasia**, and **cataracts** are reported, usually after exposures of 100 rad or more.[49] Skeletal, visceral, and genital abnormalities are noted less commonly. Growth impairments always accompany those more specific abnormalities. Radiation and chemotherapy in Hodgkin disease may affect pregnancy outcome.[40, 50]

There is no evidence in humans that exposure to diagnostic levels of radiation is associated with an increase in the incidence of congenital malformations. A report from the National Council on Radiation Protection[51] stated that 'the risk of anomalies is considered negligible at 5 rad (0.05 Gy) or less if compared to the other risks of pregnancy, and the risk of malformations is substantially increased only at doses above 15 rad (0.15 Gy). However, the exposure of the fetus to radiation deriving from diagnostic procedures must rarely constitute a reason for the interruption of pregnancy.'

Cosmic radiation is composed of mostly high energy proton radiation from outer space, together with lower energy protons originating from the sun, which are much less significant except when given off in bursts during solar flares. At ground level, cosmic radiation is below doses that may be considered dangerous for the embryo or fetus. Similarly, the dose rate during high-altitude flights, though larger, has no impact on pregnancy for the casual traveler. However, airline crews and other frequent flyers may receive exposures that are above currently recommended limits.[52, 53] Epidemiologic studies investigating the relationship between exposure to cosmic radiation in flight attendants and other airline personnel and cancer have had conflicting results.[54, 55] No studies of its potential teratogenic effects are available in the literature.

Effects of testicular radiation for testicular carcinoma and prenatal ovarian radiation The least differentiated cells (spermatogonia) are the most radiosensitive, and the more mature cells (spermatozoa) are relatively radioresistant. Fertilization of an ovum by a radiation-damaged spermatozoon may result in lethal or serious non-lethal abnormalities in the fetus.[56] Li[57] reported the outcome of pregnancies in 99 women who had received abdominal radiation as children, when treated to ablate Wilms tumor. Among the 114 pregnancies that occurred in this population of previously irradiated patients, 34 (30%) had an adverse outcome: 17 perinatal deaths and 17 other low birth weight infants. The absence of adverse outcomes in the pregnancies fathered by irradiated male patients suggests that radiation-induced germinal mutation is an unlikely explanation for these findings.[57]

Isotopes

Iodine isotopes administered to a pregnant woman after 10 weeks of gestation can **ablate the fetal thyroid gland,** resulting in hypothyroidism.[58] Isotopes have been largely replaced by technetium pertechnetate, with which there is less total radiation and less concentration in the fetal thyroid gland. The incidence of fetal malformations is not increased after administration of radioactive isotopes.[59]

Iodine-123 (I-123), like the other radioactive iodine isotopes, crosses the placenta, concentrates in the fetal thyroid, and causes intrauterine hypothyroidism.[59] Since the fetal thyroid gland does not begin to function until the 12th to 14th week of gestation, administration during the first trimester is rarely associated with fetal hypothyroidism. However, among six cases with hypothyroidism following therapeutic doses of I-131, three had been exposed during the first trimester.[60]

I-123 is also excreted into breast milk. The amount of absorption from breast milk is uncertain; therefore, there is no consensus as to safe exposure by this route.[61]

I-125 rather than I-131 is used to label fibrinogen to scan for deep vein thrombosis because it has a longer half-life (60.2 days) and gives a smaller radiation dose. Use of this agent during pregnancy is contraindicated because unbound I-125 crosses the placental barrier to enter the fetal circulation and may accumulate in the fetal thyroid.[62] The risk of radiochemical thyroidectomy increases with the onset of the iodide-concentrating ability of the fetal thyroid gland around the 12th to 14th week of gestation.[63–65] No increased incidence of birth defects or chromosomal abnormalities has been documented in offspring of women who received high doses of radioactive iodine before becoming pregnant.[64]

Ultrasonography

Examinations using ultrasonography in microsecond pulses separated by 1–2 pauses have not been associated with any adverse effect on the fetus.[66] Continuous wave ultrasound can disrupt cellular structure when it increases core temperature, as demonstrated in experimental animals.[35] Growth impairment, microcephaly, sacral dysgenesis, and developmental impairment occurred in an infant born after therapeutic ultrasound examination of the psoas bursa of the mother at days 6–29 post ovulation.[67] No cause and effect relationship can be inferred from this single case.

Magnetic fields

Human exposures to magnetic fields, primarily from video display terminals and magnetic resonance imaging machines, have not been associated with fetal malformations, but the risk of pregnancy loss may be increased.[35, 68]

Thermodisruptions

Hyperthermia

Hyperthermia is defined as a body temperature of at least 102°F (38.9°C) and is an antimitotic teratogen when the exposure occurs between weeks 4 and 14 post conception.[69]

In a retrospective study, Smith and colleagues reported on 21 patients who had been exposed during pregnancy to hyperthermia caused by infections or by sauna bathing.[70] The most common abnormalities identified in these patients were severe **mental deficiency, seizures** in infancy, **microphthalmia, midface hypoplasia**, and **mild distal limb abnormalities**. Infants exposed to maternal hyperthermia at 7–16 weeks of gestation have hypotonia, neurogenic **arthrogryposis**, or CNS dysgenesis

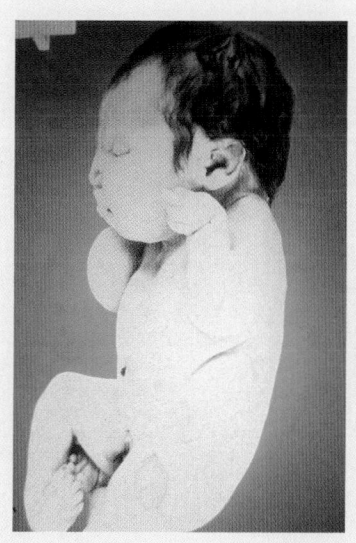

FIGURE 4.1.2 Neurogenic arthrogryposis due to hyperthermia. The mother had taken a sauna bath at the third to fourth week of gestation. She developed a high temperature and felt faint. The infant was born with neurological deficits and mental retardation.

(Fig. 4.1.2).[71] Shiota studied 100 embryos with CNS defects and found that 18% of mothers of anencephalic infants had experienced hyperthermia at the critical embryonic stage.[71] Occipital encephalocele has also been related to hyperthermia.[72] Embryonic studies in the guinea pig and rat have highlighted the extreme sensitivity of brain growth to elevated temperatures.[73–75]

The nature of the defects correlates with the timing and degree of the hyperthermia. In different studies most of the mothers had febrile illnesses with temperatures of 38.9°C or higher, commonly 40°C or above,[70, 76–79] frequently induced by sauna bathing. Retrospective human studies suggest that possibly 10% of neural tube defects (NTDs), including anencephaly, meningomyelocele, and occipital encephalocele, may be related to hyperthermia,[71] but this has not been corroborated by any epidemiologic study. Microcephaly, neuronal heterotopias, polymicrogyria, micrognathia, cleft lip and palate, defects in ear morphogenesis, and syndactyly have also been reported. Maternal hyperthermia has been noted in the pregnancy history of infants born with **Möbius sequence** (oromandibular limb hypogenesis sequence).[80, 81]

Hypothermia

Cardiopulmonary bypass in pregnant patients is associated with a fetal mortality rate of 16–33%. One infant with 'multiple congenital defects' has been described. Another infant had severe disruptive defects of the brain and distal spinal cord, suggesting hypoperfusion injuries possibly related to hypothermia.[82]

Infectious agents

The lethal or developmental effects of infectious agents are the result of mitotic inhibition, direct cytotoxic effects, or a vascular disruptive event on the embryo or fetus. However, a repair process may result in scarring or calcification, which causes further damage by interfering with histogenesis.[83]

Infections that do not result in congenital malformations but may cause fetal or **neonatal death** include enteroviruses (coxsackievirus, poliovirus and echovirus) and **hepatitis, variola, vaccinia,** and **mumps** viruses.[84] Non-radioactive in situ hybridization of formalin-fixed, paraffin-embedded placental and fetal tissue, using virus-specific DNA or RNA probes, is helpful for diagnosing fetal virus infections such as cytomegalovirus (CMV), parvovirus B-19, and varicella-zoster virus that cause fetal hydrops, placentitis, and abortion.[85]

Acquired immunodeficiency syndrome

An 'acquired immunodeficiency syndrome (AIDS) embryopathy' was suggested in the offspring of some women infected with human immunodeficiency virus (HIV). Reported features included growth deficiency, microcephaly, box-like cranial configuration, flat nasal bridge, ocular hypertelorism, up-slanting palpebral fissures, prominent eyes, frontal bossing, and a full upper lip.[86] However, many of the features represent normal racial variation in the population studied.[87] The existence of a distinct pattern of malformations has not been confirmed and further study is necessary to delineate the risks for HIV teratogenesis, if any.

Around 30–50% of infants born of untreated HIV-seropositive women develop AIDS or HIV-mediated disease.[88–92] Infected infants exhibit growth retardation, microcephaly, seborrheic dermatitis, adenopathy, and recurrent infections.[88–90]

Common cold viruses

A single retrospective case control study, in a relatively small population sample, found a 'modestly elevated risk of birth defects among women who reported having a cold in the first trimester of pregnancy'. However, these findings should be interpreted cautiously, as medications, which are frequently consumed simultaneously, could be an important confounding factor.[93]

Coxsackievirus

There has been serologic evidence for coxsackievirus infection in the etiology of congenital heart disease, in particular endocardial fibroelastosis, and fetal pericarditis, as well as meningoencephalitis.[94, 95]

Cytomegalovirus

CMV infection is a common and serious infection occurring in approximately 1–2% of live births in most populations.[96–98] About 1–5% of infants with congenital CMV infection have typical cytomegalic inclusion disease and another 5% have atypical illness. Clinically significant neurologic sequelae are present in almost half of these children.[98, 99] The remaining 90% are asymptomatic

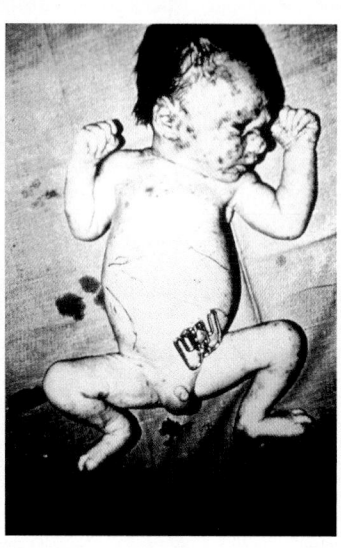

FIGURE 4.1.3
Hepatosplenomegaly and widespread petechial hemorrhages in an infant with cytomegalovirus embryopathy.

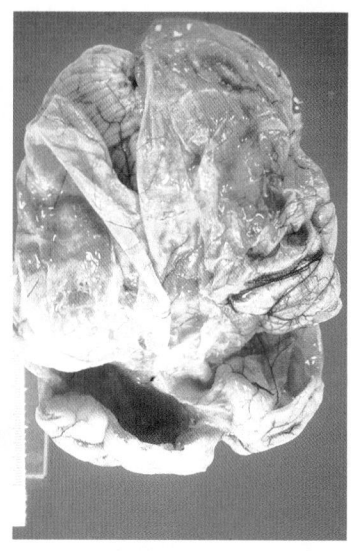

FIGURE 4.1.4 Herpes virus type 2 infection. Brain showing hydranencephaly with disruption of the cerebral cortices, leaving an empty sac.

at birth,[96] but 8–13% of them will eventually develop neurologic defects.[98]

Cellular necrosis is the principal mechanism by which CMV damages organs. Of every 10 000 infants born in the USA, 6–20 are brain damaged by CMV. If a woman is infected with CMV early in pregnancy, however, the incidence of brain damage in the newborn may reach up to 50%. Infections at any time in pregnancy will result in an approximately 65% incidence of some **eye anomaly, hearing loss**, and/or **learning disability**.[10] A review of a series of studies showed that 22–65% of children with symptomatic CMV had sensorineural hearing loss, in contrast with 6–23% of children with asymptomatic infection.[100]

CMV causes intrauterine growth retardation (IUGR), hepatitis, meningoencephalitis, and pneumonitis. Necrotizing meningoencephalitis results in microcephaly, periventricular calcification, mental retardation, seizures, deafness, and motor deficits. Uncommonly, obstructive hydrocephalus occurs. Optic atrophy and chorioretinitis can leave residual visual impairment. Other findings include hepatosplenomegaly, thrombocytopenia (Fig. 4.1.3), and hemolytic anemia.[96]

A recent non-randomized trial of CMV-specific hyperimmune globulin in the treatment of pregnant women with primary CMV infection was associated with a significantly lower risk of congenital CMV disease in the offspring of these women.[99] Though the study showed that the hyperimmune globulin was safe and effective, a controlled trial of this agent is needed to determine its effectiveness in the prevention and treatment of congenital CMV infection. In addition, several vaccines are currently being evaluated in clinical trials.[101, 102]

Herpes virus

Human herpes simplex virus (HSV) consists of two types. Type 1 is responsible for 98% of mouth and oral infections and approxi-

mately 100% of cases of encephalitis beyond the newborn period. Type 2 causes 90% of genital lesions and most cases of neonatal aseptic meningitis,[97] and represents 70–85% of cases of neonatal HSV infection. Neonatal HSV infection is a severe disease associated with significant morbidity and mortality. The estimated incidence is 1:5000–1:7500 live born infants.[103]

HSV infection of the newborn can be acquired in utero, intrapartum, or postnatally. In approximately 90% of cases, HSV is acquired at the time of delivery, through direct contact of the newborn with infected maternal genital secretions or, less frequently, from an ascending infection from the vaginal tract in cases of premature rupture of the membranes.[19, 104–108] Early postnatal acquisition of the virus has also been described. Finally, in 5% of the cases, HSV infection is acquired in utero.

The diagnostic criteria of intrauterine HSV infection include identification of infected infants in the first 48 h of life, virologic confirmation of infection, and exclusion of other congenital infections.[107, 108] The classic triad of findings associated with this syndrome consists of skin vesicles or scarring, lesions of the eye, and neurologic damage, frequently including **microcephaly** or **hydranencephaly** due to widespread **tissue necrosis of the brain** (Fig. 4.1.4). Other abnormalities caused by HSV infection include **intracranial calcifications, microphthalmia, retinal dysplasia**, and **liver necrosis**.[10] Short digits, and patent ductus arteriosus (PDA) have been reported.[105]

Maternal HSV infection has also been associated with an increased incidence of **spontaneous abortion and premature labor**.[106] The risk of neonatal infection is greater when the mother has a primary, rather than a recurrent, infection.

Influenza

Some studies have found a small increase in the prevalence of congenital malformations in general or of specific malformations following maternal influenza. However, it is possible that this is an effect of the fever rather than the viral infection.[109–111] There is no compelling evidence to incriminate influenza virus or infection during pregnancy as a cause of malformations.[19]

Lymphocytic choriomeningitis

Lymphocytic choriomeningitis virus (LCMV) is transmitted to humans by infected rodents (e.g. mice and hamsters) that excrete the virus in their urine. Human LCMV infection is usually mild and produces a flu-like episode with fever, headache, nausea, and myalgia. Occasionally, LCMV infection can result in meningitis and meningoencephalitis.

Infection during the first trimester of pregnancy is associated with spontaneous abortions.[112, 113] Fetal infection in the second and third trimesters may result in intrauterine or early neonatal death, as well as in hydrocephalus and chorioretinitis.[114, 115]

The Centers for Disease Control and Prevention (CDC) has issued the following recommendation for pregnant women or women who are considering pregnancy:[116]

- Avoid contact with wild rodents. Pregnant women who reside in a household with a wild rodent infestation should have the infestation addressed promptly by a professional pest control company or another member of the household.
- Keep pet rodents in a separate part of the home. Pregnant women should ask another family member or friend to clean the cage and care for the pet or arrange for temporary adoption of the pet by a responsible person. Pregnant women should avoid prolonged stays in any room where a rodent resides.

Mumps virus

Mumps virus during pregnancy does not cause malformations, but endocardial fibroelastosis has been noted in infants with a positive mumps antigen skin test; this relationship has not been consistent.[19]

Parvovirus

Human parvovirus B-19 is able to cross the placenta and results in fetal infection, which may occur whether the mother is symptomatic or asymptomatic. It is associated with a higher than average fetal loss and may lead to **spontaneous abortion** in the first trimester, **hydrops fetalis** (Fig. 4.1.5) in the second trimester, and **stillbirth** at term.[117, 118]

Generalized **myocarditis, myositis** of skeletal muscles, and **abnormalities of the eyes** have been reported.[119] Human parvovirus B-19 has an affinity for the erythropoietic tissue of the host and is therefore associated with **fetal anemia** leading to cardiac failure. Fetal toxicity and fetal demise have been reported in 10–38% of cases. **Elevations in maternal levels of α-fetoprotein** may be a sensitive marker for early fetal involvement in parvovirus infection and indicate an unfavorable prognosis. Malformations have not been described. The placenta shows changes of

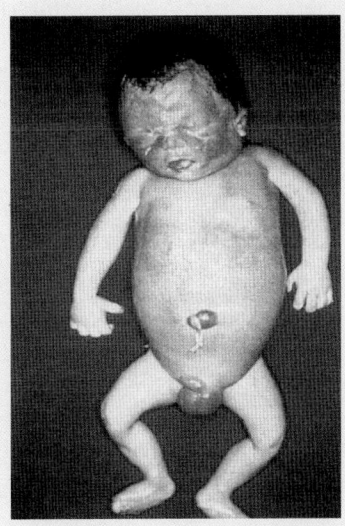

FIGURE 4.1.5 Infant with hydrops due to parvovirus B-19.

erythroblastosis with nucleated red blood cells in the fetal capillaries, some of which may contain intranuclear inclusions.[93] Parvovirus virions can be identified by electron microscopy from paraffin blocks in erythroid line cells in fatal hydrops fetalis,[120] but immunohistochemistry or PCR are more practical to demonstrate this infection.

Rubella virus

The frequency of embryonic rubella infection after maternal rubella with a rash is more than 80% during the first 12 weeks of pregnancy, 54% at 13–14 weeks, and 25% at the end of the second trimester.[121] Defects attributable to rubella result from infections occurring before the 16th week of gestation, however.[121] Rubella causes damage by means of several mechanisms: cell necrosis, obliterative angiitis that reduces blood flow to fetal tissues, and release of a mitotic inhibitor from infected cells. The permanent consequences are most probably due to mitotic inhibition, cell death, and interference with histogenesis by repair processes resulting in calcification and scarring.[122]

Rubella infection during the first trimester is accompanied by abortion (10%) and stillbirth (4%), with higher rates of fetal death during the first 2 months of gestation.[123]

In about of one-half of the cases, rubella embryopathy causes congenital rubella syndrome, (CRS) (Fig. 4.1.6) which includes unilateral or bilateral hearing loss, retinopathy, nuclear cataract, glaucoma, microphthalmia, myopia, and mental retardation (Fig. 4.1.7).

Cardiovascular defects include PDA and pulmonary artery stenosis, pulmonary valvular stenosis, aortic valvular stenosis, and ventricular septal defects (VSD).[19] Continuing infection impairs growth, interrupts bone growth and maturation, causes pancytopenia, and produces widespread visceral involvement.[19] Around 30% of adults who had CRS have developed diabetes mellitus.[19]

Rubella virus vaccine is a live, attenuated virus vaccine. Its administration is contraindicated during pregnancy because of

Other possible defects

Large fontanelle

Encephalitis

Petechiae

Dental enamal defects

Unusual dermatoglyphics

Interstitial pneumonia

Myocarditis

Hepatomegaly jaundice

Diabetes?

Splenomegaly

Abnormal bone trabeculations and growth plate

Skin dimples

Purpura

Immunologic defects

Hypotonia

Major defects

Microcephaly, mental retardation

Cataracts, glaucoma, retinitis, microphthalmia

Deafness

Congenital heart disease especially patent ductus arteriosus or pulmonic stenosis

Small for gestational age

Postnatal growth retardation

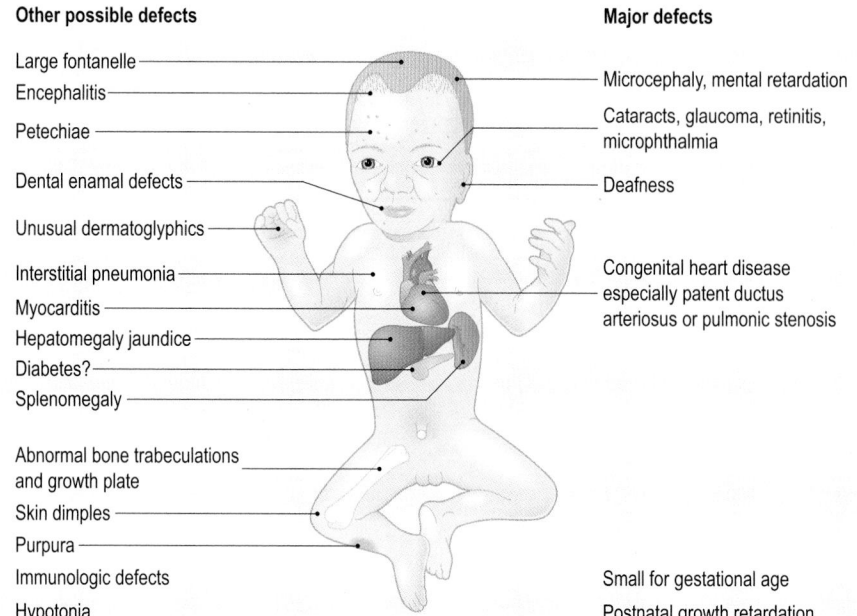

FIGURE 4.1.6 Malformations seen in rubella embryopathy.

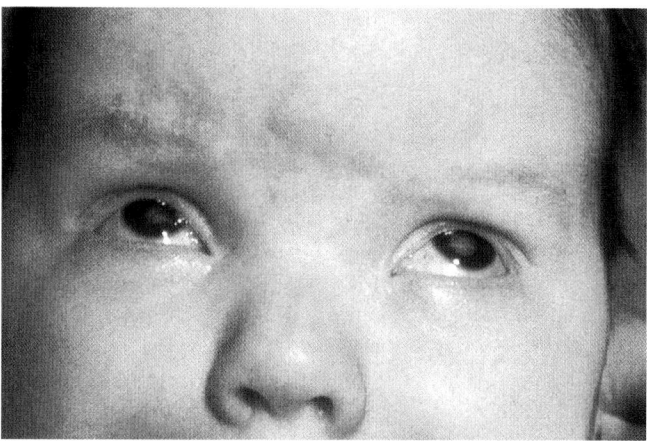

FIGURE 4.1.7 Rubella embryopathy. Bilateral congenital cataracts are evident.

theoretical risk to the fetus, since the vaccine strain may be transmitted transplacentally.[124] A report from the CDC states that the theoretical risk of CRS in infants born to women who received rubella vaccine within 3 months before or 3 months after conception is 0–1.6% (95% confidence intervals), substantially less than the greater than 20% risk of CRS associated with maternal infection with wild virus in the first trimester.[125] Since the licensure of the rubella vaccine in 1969, the CRS has practically disappeared from the USA and other industrialized countries.

Syphilis (see also Ch. 10)

It is believed that the fetus cannot be infected with syphilis early in pregnancy because a cytotrophoblastic layer of cells in the chorionic villi of the placenta prevents the spirochete from passing from maternal to fetal blood. This cell layer disappears at the 6th month. Since the spirochete usually does not reach the conceptus during the first trimester, it is not a cause of abortion or malformation.[126]

In untreated maternal syphilis of less than 2 years' duration, about half the infants are liveborn without infection. In untreated maternal syphilis in the primary or secondary stages, 50% are stillborn or die within 4 weeks after birth. In untreated maternal syphilis in the early part of the tertiary stage, 20–60% of the infants are normal, 40% have congenital syphilis, 20% are born prematurely, and 16% are stillborn or die within 4 weeks after birth. In untreated syphilis in the late part of the tertiary stage, 75% of babies are unaffected, 10% have congenital syphilis, 9% are born prematurely, 10% are stillborn, and 1% die within 4 weeks after birth.[127]

Adequate treatment during pregnancy can result in minimal effects in the infant; however, if the damage is severe, treatment might not prevent a miscarriage or stillbirth. In the absence of obvious signs of infection at birth, treatment of the infant can prevent the morbidity of congenital syphilis.[19]

Treponema pallidum is disseminated to every organ system, with a predilection for skin, mucous membranes, liver, CNS, and bones. Large bulky placenta, hydrops fetalis, and IUGR are frequent.[19]

The following are frequently found in infants with early congenital syphilis: copious nasal discharge (Fig. 4.1.8), hepatosplenomegaly, hepatitis, jaundice, anemia, thrombocytopenia, leukemoid reactions, rhinitis, maculopapular eruptions, bullous eruptions, condylomata lata, syphilitic nephrosis, fibrosing pneumonia (pneumonia alba), progressive hydrocephalus, chorioretinitis, uveitis, optic atrophy, and glaucoma. Later manifestations include interstitial keratitis, ocular pain, tearing, deafness,

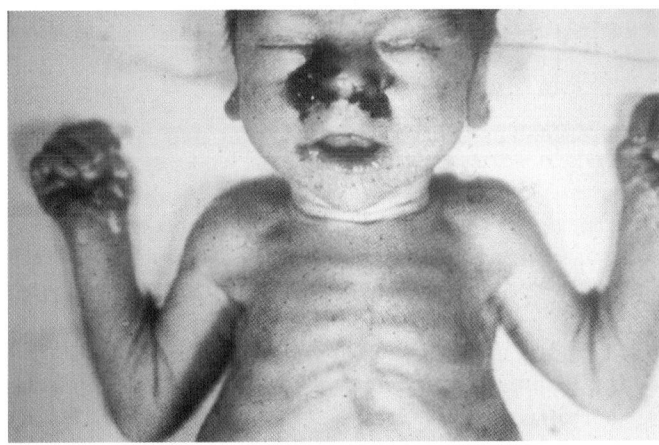

FIGURE 4.1.8 Newborn infant with congenital syphilis. Note the copious nasal discharge (snuffles).

Clutton joints, frontal bossing, saber shins, saddle-nose deformity, mental retardation, optic atrophy, and deep cutaneous scarring.[126] Abnormalities of the permanent teeth occur after the first trimester, including abnormal tapering of the incisors, and enamel-covered notching of the central incisors (**Hutchinson teeth**), and crowding of the cusps of the first molars (mulberry molars).[128]

Radiologic abnormalities include **periostitis** of the long bones.[129]

Toxoplasmosis

Primary maternal infection with *Toxoplasma gondii* occurs in 1 per 1000 pregnancies in the USA.[130] Infection is disseminated to the offspring in 40% of cases through placental infection. Malformations do not occur; however, hydrocephalus and microcephaly result from chronic destructive meningoencephalitis. Chorioretinitis may progress to scarring and loss of vision. Hydrocephalus and cerebral calcifications, hepatitis, and lymphadenopathy are the most common complications in infants infected prenatally.[130] Organisms have been recovered from the brain of a congenitally infected infant after 5 years.

Varicella-zoster virus

First-trimester **varicella** infection rarely causes fetal infection. However, it may result in cell necrosis with **meningoencephalitis, cutaneous lesions** (Fig. 4.1.9), and **diffuse visceral involvement**.[131, 132] Such infections are usually fatal; those who survive may have residual optic atrophy, microphthalmia, chorioretinitis, cortical atrophy, seizures, or motor disabilities. Infection with varicella late in pregnancy may cause fetal infection, manifested by cutaneous vesicles at birth.[129] Infection acquired during pregnancy causes fetal damage in 5–10% of cases.

A pattern of congenital anomalies, the 'congenital varicella syndrome', associated with varicella infection during the first

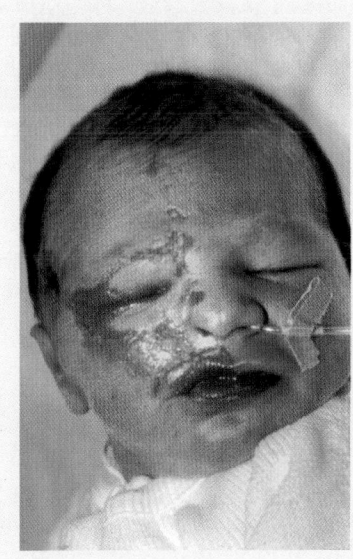

FIGURE 4.1.9 Varicella embryopathy. Note extensive cutaneous facial scarring. Infant still is unable to swallow.

TABLE 4.1.4 FETAL VARICELLA SYNDROME: COMMON ANOMALIES

Anomaly	Percentage
Cicatricial cutaneous defects in dermatomal distribution	100
Limb atrophy	80
Eye anomalies (chorioretinitis, microphthalmia, cataracts, anisocoria, nystagmus, corneal opacity, heterochromia)	68
Central nervous system abnormalities	77
Limb paresis	65
Hydrocephalus/cortical atrophy	35
Seizures	24
Horner syndrome	24
Mental retardation	18

After Alkalay et al 1987,[131] with permission.

trimester, consists of limb hypoplasia, cortical atrophy, skin scarring, eye defects, mental deficiency, and retarded growth (Table 4.1.4).[64]

In 52 infants with adverse effects after their mothers contracted varicella infection during pregnancy, 27 had congenital malformations and another 25 developed neonatal herpes zoster.[133] Varicella-related birth defects may be due to herpes zoster that is a reactivation of the latent varicella virus.[133]

Venezuelan equine encephalitis virus

Venezuelan equine encephalomyelitis (VEE) is recognized as an important human and equine disease in northern South America.

The etiologic agent, VEE virus, is a mosquito-borne alphavirus in the family Togaviridae, first isolated and characterized serologically in 1938. Subsequently, many antigenically related VEE viruses have been discovered in South, Central, and North America. It occurs in outbreaks and affected individuals present with either mild flu-like symptoms of fever, chills, severe headache, and myalgia, to encephalitis and death. Abortions and delivery of stillborn infants may occur among acutely ill pregnant women, although the full extent of fetal loss associated with each outbreak is unknown. VEE virus has been recovered from the brains of the aborted or stillborn term fetuses studied in some of the outbreaks.[134-136]

West Nile virus

West Nile virus (WNV), a mosquito-born flavivirus epidemic in the USA, is a human neuropathogen that causes disease in man, including encephalitis, paralysis, and death.[137] The virus may also be transmitted by blood and organ transplantation in human patients, as well as by accidental laboratory infection.[138, 139] Intrauterine infection of fetuses with WNV has been implicated in cases of women infected during pregnancy.[140] A woman infected with WNV during pregnancy gave birth to a seropositive baby with chorioretinal scarring and brain abnormalities.[140, 141] Other reports of maternal infection with WNV during pregnancy, however, have shown no evidence for morbidity of the fetus.[142] The CDC has issued recommendations for the evaluation of the fetuses of pregnant women with WNV infection and for the evaluation of infants born to mothers infected with WNV during pregnancy.[143]

Other viral infections

Other viruses have not resulted in congenital anomalies but have caused significant fetal pathology. **Poliovirus** has been associated with abortion, stillbirth, and meningomyelitis;[144] **echovirus** with disseminated viremia;[145] **variola and vaccinia** with necrotizing cutaneous and visceral infection; and **hepatitis virus** with neonatal hepatitis.[146]

Although premature rupture of membranes and perinatal mortality may result from *Ureaplasma (Mycoplasma)*, bacteria, *Candida* infection, Lyme disease,[147] and leptospirosis, no association with congenital defects has been documented.

Potentially teratogenic drugs and chemicals

The teratogenic effects of common drugs and chemicals including chemotherapeutic and immunosuppressive drugs are shown in Table 4.1.3.

Accutane™ (isotretinoin)

Accutane™ (isotretinoin or 13-cis-retinoic acid) is a prescription oral medication approved to treat severe, recalcitrant nodular acne. The drug, recognized as an animal teratogen before it was first marketed in 1982,[148] was identified less than a year later to be associated with spontaneous abortions and congenital malformations. Subsequent reports have documented the association between exposure to Accutane™ during the first weeks of pregnancy and a characteristic pattern of malformation (Fig. 4.1.10) that includes **microtia** or **absent external ears, cleft palate, CNS defects (hydrocephalus, microcephaly, cerebellar micro/macro dysgenesis), cardiovascular defects** [aortic arch anomalies, VSD, atrial septal defect (ASD), tetralogy of Fallot], and **hypoplastic adrenal cortex**.[149-152] The spectrum of malformations observed among these infants resembles that found in the animal studies. Table 4.1.5[153] lists the abnormalities related to isotretinoin exposure. A pregnancy prevention program in women of child-bearing age receiving isotretinoin has been established (Fig. 4.1.11).[154]

An extensive review of retinoid regulated gene expression has been published.[155] Many of the effects of retinoids on cell differentiation and proliferation are due to their induction or repression of *HOX* genes, of growth factors including epidermal growth factors, transforming growth factor-β, heparin-binding growth factors, insulin and insulin-like growth factors I and II, interleukins, interferons, colony stimulating factors, leukemia inhibitory factor, and nerve growth factor.

Isotretinoin is one of the most potent human teratogens known. It appears to interfere with the migration of neural crest cells.[156] Accutane™ is not absorbed through the dermis, and therefore no systemic toxicity has been reported. Topical application during the first trimester of pregnancy has not been associated with birth defects.[157]

Like its congener isotretinoin, **etretinate** can cause **CNS, cardiovascular**, and **skeletal malformations**. In contrast to isotretinoin, etretinate is bound to lipoproteins and persists in the circulation for years after use. Measurable concentrations of this drug in the serum have been identified more than 2 years after discontinuation of therapy.[158] **Unilateral limb defects** have been observed in a fetus conceived 4 months after the mother's last dose of etretinate. **Acitretin**, the acid analog of etretinate, has similar characteristics and is also a potent teratogen.[159, 160]

Alcohol

The effects of alcohol on the developing embryo and fetus as well as the basic diagnostic features of the fetal alcohol syndrome (FAS) were first described in 1973.[161, 162] The lifelong physical and cognitive deficits resulting from exposure to alcohol during prenatal development constitute the leading preventable cause of birth defects and developmental disabilities. The prevalence of FAS in the USA ranges between 0.2 and 1.5 cases per 1000 live births.[163-165]

The phenotypic variability of the embryo–fetotoxicity (Fig. 4.1.12) associated with maternal alcohol consumption

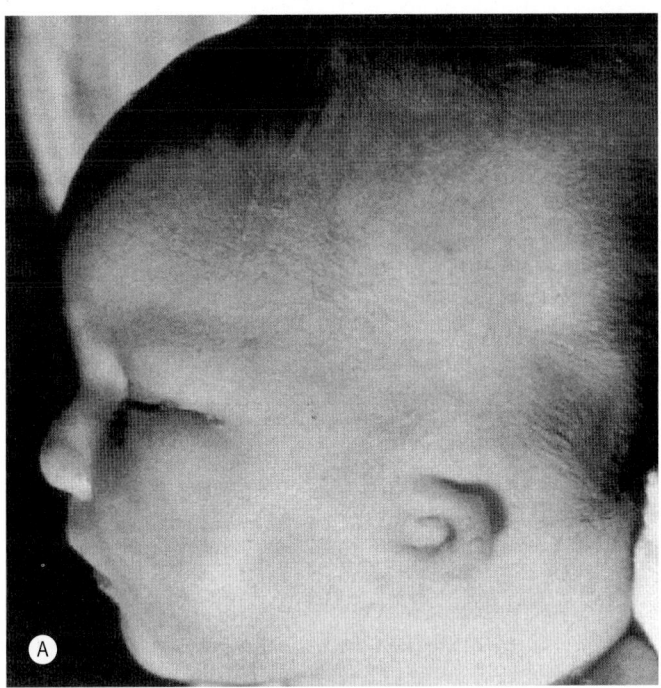

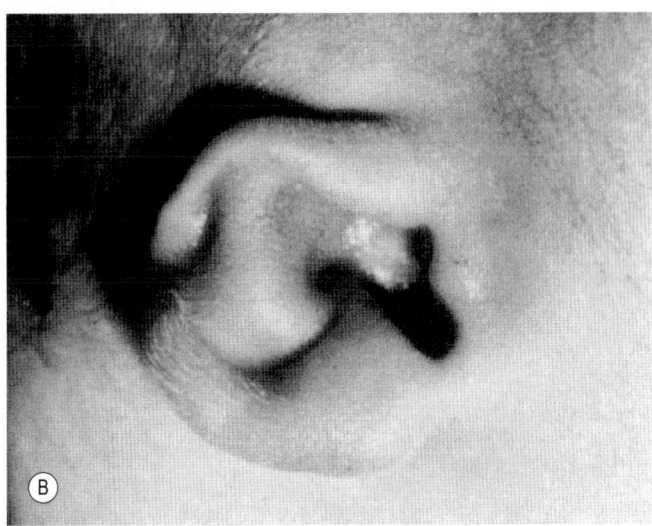

FIGURE 4.1.10 Ear anomalies in Accutane embryopathy. (Courtesy of Dr Robert Gorlin.)

TABLE 4.1.5 MANIFESTATIONS IN ISOTRETINOIN EMBRYOPATHY

Abnormality	Manifestations
Brain	Hydrocephalus, leptomeningeal heterotopias, vermis hypoplasia, Dandy-Walker malformation, corticospinal tract malformations
Brain (occasional)	Gyral defects including grade 3 lissencephaly, regional pachygyria, subcortical heterotopias
Brain function	Severe or profound mental retardation, hypotonia, diminished deep tendon reflexes, absent or abnormal primitive reflexes, hypoactive
Craniofacial	Low-set, small or atretic, malformed ears; small or atretic external auditory meatus; microphthalmia; telecanthus; epicanthal folds; low nasal bridge; small jaw, sometimes with U-shaped cleft palate (Robin sequence)
Heart	Ventricular septal defect, truncus arteriosus, double-outlet right ventricle, interrupted aortic arch, patent ductus arteriosus
Chromosomes	Normal
Other	Exposure at 2–8 weeks' gestation

After Dobyns 1987,[153] with permission.

during pregnancy has led to the use of numerous terms, in addition to FAS. These include fetal alcohol effects (FAE), alcohol-related birth defect (ARBD), and alcohol-related neurodevelopmental defects (ARND).[166] A new term, fetal alcohol spectrum disorders (FASD), has been recently proposed[167] to replace previous terms and encompass all different shades of expression of the effects of prenatal alcohol exposure. FASD is defined as the range of effects that can occur in a person whose mother drank alcohol during pregnancy, including physical, mental, behavioral, and learning disabilities, with possible lifelong implications.[167]

Structural and functional impairments occur in up to one-half of infants born to alcoholic women who drink heavily (2 oz, ie 59.4 ml, or more of absolute alcohol daily). Functional and growth disturbances without other morphologic changes can occur in infants whose mothers drink moderately (1–2 oz, ie 29.7–59.4 ml, of absolute alcohol daily). No malformations have been documented in infants of mothers who drink less than 1 oz (29.7 ml) of absolute alcohol daily. However, the risk of spontaneous abortion is twice the normal rate in women who drink 1 oz (29.7 ml) of absolute alcohol twice a week.[60] 'Binge' drinking in the first trimester may be a cause of fetotoxicity.[168] In view of the limited understanding of the effects of prenatal exposure to alcohol, total abstinence from alcohol during pregnancy is a wise precaution.

The patient with FAS must have three main characteristics: **prenatal and postnatal growth retardation** (>2 standard deviations for length and weight), **facial anomalies**, and **CNS dysfunc-**

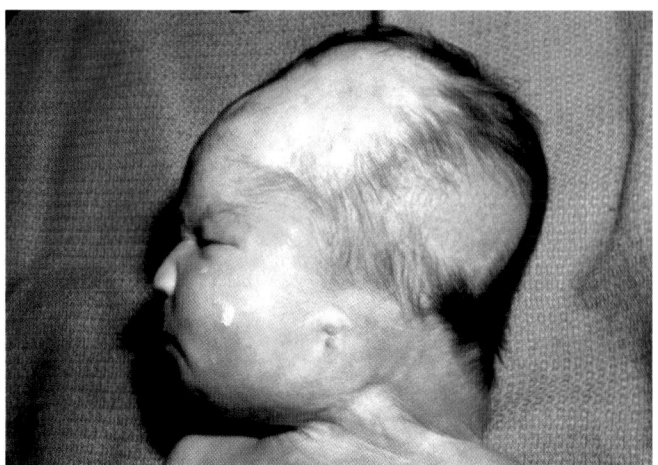

FIGURE 4.1.11 Vitamin A congener embryopathy. Extreme microtia is evident.

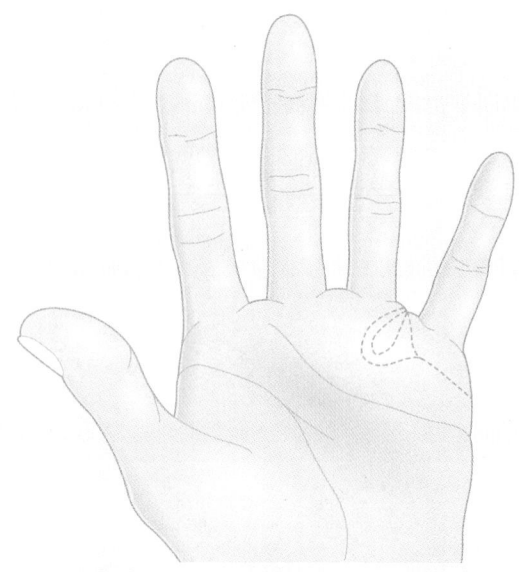

FIGURE 4.1.13 Palmar dermatoglyphics in fetal alcohol syndrome. Note prominent thenar crease, nearly absent transverse palmar crease, abrupt turning of the distal transverse crease into the second interdigital space, and fourth interdigital loop.

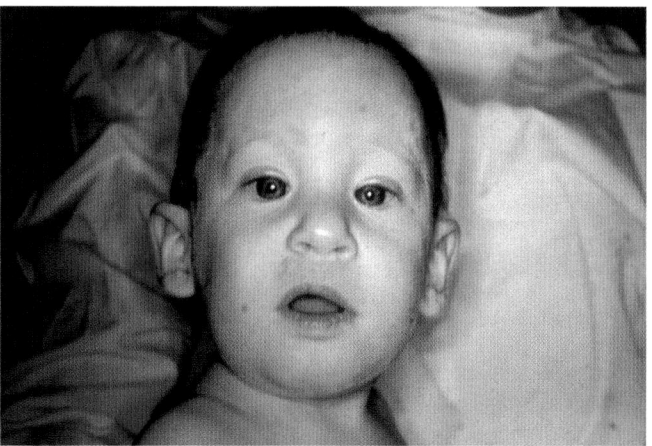

FIGURE 4.1.12 Infant with fetal alcohol syndrome. Note short palpebral fissures, mild ptosis, nostrils, smooth philtral area and narrow vermillion of the upper lip.

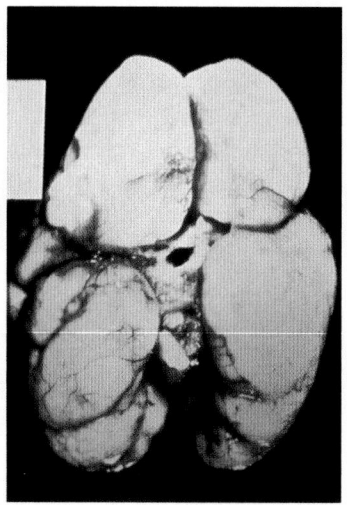

FIGURE 4.1.14 Brain in fetal alcohol syndrome. Abnormal gyration with lissencephaly.

tion (Table 4.1.6).[169] Patients with the syndrome usually weigh less than 2500 g at birth. Among the distinctive facial anomalies are absent or indistinct philtrum; epicanthal folds; short palpebral fissures; thin vermilion border of the upper lip; and short, upturned nose (see Fig. 2.18) Joint, limb, and cardiac anomalies are often present. CNS dysfunction includes mental retardation, hyperactivity, sleep disorders, spastic tetraplegia, seizures, and miscellaneous behavior difficulties. ASD and VSD are the most common cardiac defects. Radioulnar and cervical vertebral fusions, camptodactyly, hip dislocation, deformations of the feet, hypoplastic distal phalanges and nails, and altered palmar creases (Fig. 4.1.13) are skeletal components of the full syndrome. Less common defects include protuberant ears, cleft lip and palate, urogenital abnormalities, hemangiomas, and radial ray deficiencies.[170] The unusual **hirsutism** that is present at birth usually disappears with age, but it may be retained in Native Americans. Brain malformations include **hydrocephalus, lissencephaly**

(Fig. 4.1.14), and *NTDs*.[171] The occasional presence of **cystic hydrops** requires the consideration of FAS in the differential diagnosis of patients with this malformation. FAS has been reported in dizygotic twins.[172] Acetaldehyde is also a carcinogen and may cause tumors virtually identical to those seen in the fetal hydantoin syndrome. An association between paternal alcohol consumption and low birth weight has been reported.[173] Despite small head circumference and initially slow psychomotor maturation, some infants with FAS may progress and develop intelligence

TABLE 4.1.6 CHARACTERISTICS OF FETAL ALCOHOL SYNDROME

Affected system	Frequent anomalies	Occasional anomalies
Growth Deficiency		
Prenatal	2 SD for length and weight*	
Postnatal	2 SD for length and weight*	
	Disproportionately diminished adipose tissue	
Central Nervous System		
Dysfunction	Mild to moderate mental retardation	
Intellectual	Microcephaly*	
Neurologic	Poor coordination, hypotonia	
Behavioral	Irritability in infancy*, hyperactivity in childhood	
Dermatoglyphics		
Prominent thenar crease		
Nearly absent proximal transverse crease		
Abrupt turning of distal transverse crease		
into second interdigital space		
Fourth interdigital loop		
Facial Characteristics		
Eyes	Short palpebral fissures*	
Nose	Short, upturned[†]	
Maxilla	Hypoplastic philtrum*	
Mouth	Hypoplastic[†]	
	Thin upper vermilion*	
	Retrognathia in infancy	
	Micrognathia or relative prognathia in adolescence[†]	
Associated Anomalies		
Eyes	Ptosis, strabismus, epicanthal folds	Myopia, clinical microphthalmia, blepharophimosis
Ears	Posterior rotation	Poorly formed concha
Mouth	Prominent lateral palatine ridges	Cleft lip or cleft palate, small teeth with faulty enamel
Cardiac system	Murmurs, especially in early childhood, often atrial septal defect	Ventricular septal defects, great vessel anomalies, tetralogy of Fallot
Urogenital system	Labial hypoplasia	Hypospadias, small rotated kidneys, hydronephrosis
Cutaneous system	Hemangiomas	Hirsutism in infancy
Skeletal system	Aberrant palmar crease, pectus excavatum	Limited joint movements (especially fingers and elbows), nail hypoplasia, synostosis, pectus carinatum, bifid xiphoid, Klippel-Feil anomaly, scoliosis
Muscular system		Hernias of diaphragm, umbilicus, or groin, diastasis recti
Central nervous system	Errors in neuronal migration	Cortical nuclear and white matter dysplasia, rudimentary cerebellum, dysplastic brainstem, hydrophobia, lissencephaly

After Potter and Hetzel 1981,[169] with permission.
*Reported in 26–50% of patients.
[†]Reported in 1–25% of patients.
SD, Standard deviation.

within the normal range. Endocrine investigations reveal normal levels of growth hormone, cortisol, and gonadotropins.[174]

Acetaldehyde is implicated as the cause of FAS through its inhibiting effects on DNA synthesis, placental amino acid transport, and development of the fetal brain.[175] The biologic basis for

FAS is related to genetic polymorphisms identified for alcohol dehydrogenase (ADH), which converts alcohol to acetaldehyde, and for acetaldehyde dehydrogenase (ALDH$_2$), which converts acetaldehyde to acetate. Genetic differences in ADH alleles make some infants exposed to the same level of alcohol in utero more likely to have longer or higher levels of exposure to acetaldehyde.[26] This may explain the greater frequency of FASD in American blacks and Native Americans.

Amphetamines

Newborns of mothers who used methamphetamine during pregnancy have sometimes shown growth retardation at birth and have abnormal sleep patterns, poor feeding, tremors, and hypertonia in the neonatal period.[34] **Congenital cardiac defects** have been reported.[176]

Androgens

Masculinization of the external genitalia of female infants has been reported after in utero exposure to large doses of exogenous testosterone,[177] methyltestosterone,[178] and testosterone xanthate.[179] Congenital adrenal hyperplasia (CAH), most commonly due to 21-hydroxylase (CYP21) deficiency, is the leading endogenous cause of fetal masculinization.[180] In addition, any maternal source of elevated androgens can induce virilization of the female fetus. Most common among these disorders is the luteoma of pregnancy, a benign chorionic gonadotropin-dependent ovarian tumor which causes masculinization in 65% of females born to affected women.[181, 182] Other potentially virilizing ovarian tumors include the arrhenoblastomas, hilar-cell tumors, masculinizing ovarian stromal cell tumors, and the Krukenberg tumor. Maternal adrenal causes, other than untreated maternal virilizing CAH, are rare.[183, 184]

The masculinization is characterized by **clitoromegaly** with or without **fusion of the labia minora,** enlargement of the labia majora, and persistence of the urogenital sinus.

Either an excess or a deficiency in androgens affects only those tissues with androgen receptors. **Masculinization of the urogenital sinus** and its derivatives and of the external genitalia results, although there is little effect on the müllerian derivatives.

Angiotensin-converting enzyme inhibitors

Angiotensin-converting enzyme inhibitors (ACEIs), such as captopril, enalapril and lisinopril, are effective antihypertensive drugs, but their use during the second and third trimesters of pregnancy has been associated with a pattern of defects resulting from fetal renal tubular dysplasia. Associated anomalies include **neonatal respiratory distress, IUGR, limb and CNS defects, PDA, oligohydramnios,** and **calvarial hypoplasia.**[185] These features may be secondary to decreases in fetal angiotensin or increased bradykinin.[186, 187] The fetal effects of ACEIs during the first trimester of pregnancy have not been systematically studied and the existing reports are controversial. A recent case-control study of 209 infants with only first-trimester exposure to ACE inhibitors showed an increased risk of major congenital malformations (OR 2.71; 95% CI 1.72–4.27). More specifically, these

infants were at increased risk for malformations of the cardiovascular system (OR 3.72; 95% CI 1.89–7.30) and the CNS (OR 4.39; 95% CI 1.37–14.02).[187a]

Antabuse™

Antabuse™ (disulfiram) is a thorium derivative used as an adjunct in the management of selected cases of alcohol dependence. Only one prospective series has been reported, and no malformations were observed in the children whose mothers did not drink.[188] Several small series and case reports of infants exposed in the first trimester mention congenital malformations, but no specific pattern emerges from them. **Pierre Robin sequence with coronary defects, phocomelia of the lower extremities,** multiple abnormalities, microcephaly, and mental retardation, and talipes equinovarus have been reported.[189, 190] One of the pregnancies resulted in a spontaneous abortion.[190] None of these cases was reported to involve prenatal alcohol abuse. Other authors have found no congenital malformation among prenatally exposed children.[191, 192]

Antibiotic drugs

Streptomycin therapy during pregnancy may be associated with ototoxicity in the offspring. The risk to the fetus of eighth cranial nerve damage has been estimated at 1:12 based on a total of 49 cases in 587 exposures.[64] **Isoniazid,** in the absence of supplementary vitamin B_6, can damage the fetal brain.[193] The use of **tetracycline** during the second and third trimesters has been associated with a characteristic **dental defect** caused by the potent chelating ability of the drug. Tetracycline forms a complex with calcium orthophosphates and becomes incorporated into bones and teeth undergoing calcification. In teeth, this causes permanent discoloration (Fig. 4.1.15). Since deciduous teeth begin to calcify around 5 to 6 months in utero, use of tetracycline after this time results in staining and dentine defects.[193] The use of **aminoglycosides** during pregnancy may result in profound non-syndromic hearing loss if the fetus has a mitochondrial 12S rRNA mutation.[194, 195]

Anticonvulsants

Maternal epilepsy treatment with anticonvulsant drugs increases the risk of congenital anomalies in the exposed infant by two- to three-fold, as compared to non-exposed infants.[34, 196] All the 'classic' anticonvulsants have been proved to be teratogenic, although to different degrees, and phenytoin, phenobarbital, and carbimazole exposure in utero may result in similar phenotypic features.

No data are available on the potential teratogenicity of anticonvulsants marketed in the last decade or so, such as gabapentin, tiagabine, topiramate, zonisamide, lamotrigine, and others.

Since the teratogenic risk when the mother is receiving more than one anticonvulsant is higher than when receiving a single

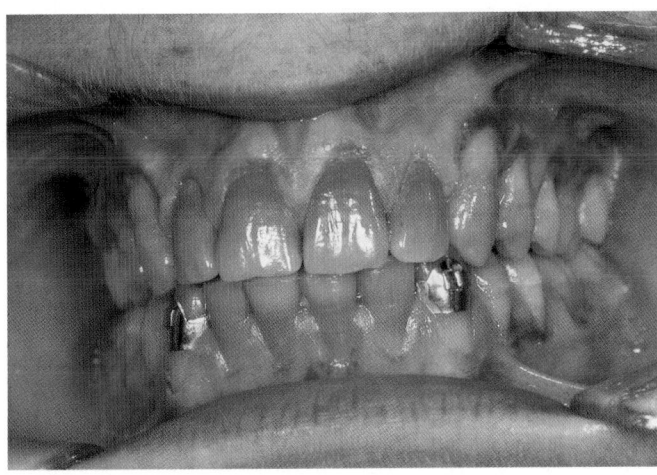

FIGURE 4.1.15 Tetracycline embryopathy. Long-term tetracycline therapy results in a yellow pigmentation of the teeth that darkens with age.

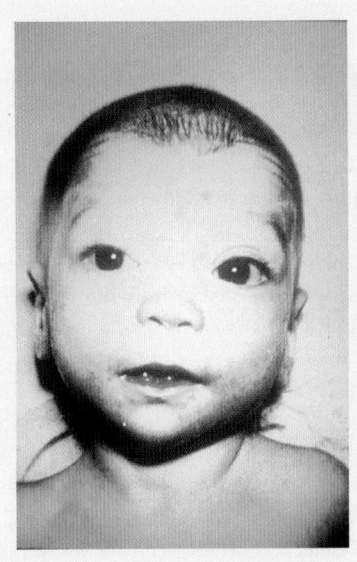

FIGURE 4.1.16 Phenytoin (Dilantin) embryopathy: hypertelorism, prominent eyes, depressed nasal bridge, macrognathia, and microcephaly.

the microsomal enzyme epoxy hydrolase.[133] There appears to be genetic susceptibility to phenytoin fetal toxicity. Twins have been discordant for manifestations of the hydantoin syndrome.[133]

Dilantin, phenobarbital and carbimazole anticonvulsant exposure in utero may result in similar phenotypic features. The so-called anticonvulsant face is characterized by a depressed and/or broad nasal bridge, anteverted nostrils, and a long philtrum.[199]

The risk of developmental disturbance in phenytoin-exposed children ranges from 1 to 11%.[133] Chronic exposure presents a maximum of 10% risk for the full syndrome and a maximum of 30% risk for some anomalies.[22, 197, 200, 201]

Craniofacial and limb abnormalities appear to be the most constant features of the syndrome.[202–205] These include microcephaly, hypertelorism, depressed nasal bridge, ptosis, and wide mouth. Other features include: cleft lip and palate; cardiac defects; colobomas, glaucoma, and other ocular abnormalities; and diaphragmatic, umbilical, and inguinal hernias. The use of phenytoin (frequently in combination with a barbiturate) during pregnancy has been associated with an **increased risk of neuroectodermal tumors**, including **ependymoma, mesenchymoma, neuroblastoma, ganglioneuroblastoma, melanotic ectodermal tumor**, and **Wilms tumor**, later in childhood.[198] A distinctive malformation is stiffness of the interphalangeal joints (symphalangism) with tapering of the fingers and severe nail hypoplasia. Many of the features of the syndrome may be genetically linked to epilepsy itself rather than to the drugs used to treat the disorder. The current view is that only hypertelorism and digital hypoplasia are clearly linked to phenytoin exposure.[206] The teratogenicity is related to oxidative metabolites that are normally eliminated by the enzyme epoxide hydrolase. Low levels of epoxide hydrolase in the amniotic fluid appear to correlate with the risk of a fetus developing features of the syndrome.[204]

Carbamazepine (Tegretol™)

Carbamazepine is an anticonvulsant frequently used in combination with other drugs in the prevention of grand mal, psychomotor, and petit mal seizures. In utero exposure to this agent, particularly if taken in combination with valproic acid, is associated with a phenotype consisting of **round facies, up-slanting palpebral fissures, hypertelorism, hypoplastic nasal bridge, short upturned nose, nevus flammeus, large anterior fontanelle**, and variable nail hypoplasia.[197, 206] There is a risk of 0.5–1.7% of spina bifida in the offspring of women treated with carbamazepine during pregnancy, alone or in combination with other antiepileptic drugs.[207–209]

Similar to phenytoin and phenobarbital, carbamazepine is biotransformed to oxidative metabolites such as epoxides, which are highly reactive compounds capable of binding covalently to nucleic acids. The microsomal enzyme epoxide hydrolase detoxifies the epoxides by converting them to dihydrodiols, which are easily eliminated. Fetuses with low levels of epoxide hydrolase who are exposed to carbamazepine are at a higher risk of having congenital abnormalities.[210]

drug, monotherapy is recommended in women with epilepsy who are contemplating pregnancy. The drug should be given at the lowest effective dose. In addition, because of the known folic antagonism of several anticonvulsant drugs, supplementation with folic acid at doses of 4 mg/day, starting at least one month before conception and continuing throughout the first trimester, is warranted.

Dilantin™ (hydantoin, phenytoin)

A pattern of anomalies, termed the **fetal hydantoin syndrome** (Fig. 4.1.16), consists of developmental delay or frank **mental deficiency, dysmorphic craniofacial features**, and **hypoplasia of the distal phalanges**.[197, 198] The presence of major phenytoin-associated birth defects in a child correlates with a deficiency of

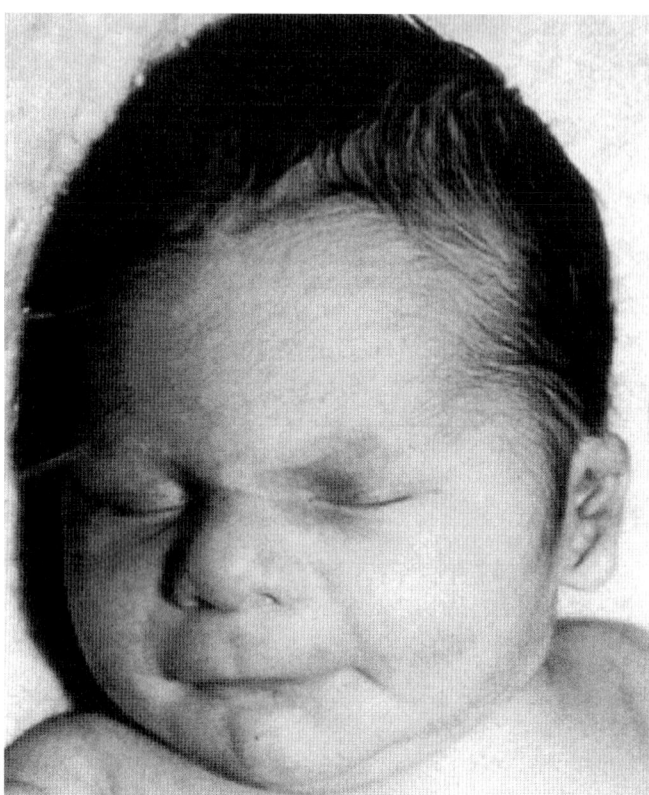

FIGURE 4.1.17 Facial dysmorphism and ear anomalies due to the effects of trimethadione exposure. (Courtesy of Dr Robert Gorlin.)

Phenobarbital

No increase in malformations was found in the Collaborative Perinatal Project.[211] Other studies, however, have reported increased frequencies of mild mental deficiency, cleft lip, cleft palate, and congenital heart disease after prenatal **phenobarbital exposure**.[212–214]

Trimethadione, paramethadione

Maternal use of these drugs results in **spontaneous abortion** in 25% of pregnancies. Most liveborn infants have **prenatal and postnatal growth deficiency, developmental delay, malformations, and distinctive facies**, including brachycephaly with midfacial hypoplasia, V-shaped eyebrows with or without synophrys, broad nasal bridge, arched or cleft palate, and malpositioned ears, with anterior cupping and/or excessive folding of the superior helices (Fig. 4.1.17).[199] **Cardiovascular defects,** particularly septal defects and tetralogy of Fallot; renal malformations, **tracheoesophageal anomalies,** hernias, and hypospadias are most common. Survivors often have mild to moderate mental retardation and speech impairment.[199]

Valproic acid (Depakene™)

Valproic acid and related compounds (valproate sodium, divalproex sodium) are used to treat grand mal, temporal lobe, and petit mal seizures, either as a single agent or in combination with other antiepileptic agents.

Valproic acid readily crosses the placenta and is found in fetal serum at levels equal to or greater than maternal serum levels.[193] A risk of fetal liver damage has been suggested.[133] Maternal valproic acid administration is associated with a pattern of minor anomalies known as the **fetal valproate syndrome**, which has features similar to those seen in fetal hydantoin syndrome, including **craniofacial anomalies, epicanthal folds** (inferior), **small anteverted nose, thin vermilion border, hyperconvex nails, long thin overlapping fingers and toes, hypospadias** and **IUGR.**[215–217] In addition, there is an increased risk of **lumbosacral spina bifida**[218] that may be associated with hydrocephalus and other **midline defects** within or outside the CNS.[219] The absolute risk of spina bifida has been estimated to be 1–2%.[64, 200, 220, 221] Women taking high daily doses of valproic acid (more than 1000 mg) or multiple anticonvulsant drugs are at a higher risk than those taking lower doses or monotherapy.[200, 219]

Neonatal afibrinogenemia and fatal hemorrhage after prenatal valproate exposure has been reported in one case.[133]

Mysoline™ (primidone)

Primidone, a derivative of phenobarbital, is used as an anticonvulsant medication. Since primidone is largely converted to phenobarbital, it is thought to have a similar teratogenic effect.[222]

Primidone freely crosses the placenta and is a possible cause of congenital anomalies.[193a] The most common human fetal anomalies attributed to primidone are cardiac malformations, craniofacial abnormalities, IUGR, and developmental delay.[193] Several women who took only primidone had children born with features similar to those of fetal hydantoin syndrome.[220] Twenty-four infants of 147 pregnant women who took primidone in combination with other anticonvulsant medications had abnormalities. Congenital defects included meningocele, cleft lip, cleft lip and palate, cardiac defects, and reduced head circumference. Only the incidence of cleft lip and palate was significantly increased over the expected rate in the population.[117] No controlled data permit a prediction of the frequency with which primidone therapy in the mother might lead to abnormalities.

Chloroquine

Minimal knowledge is available of the effects of chloroquine malarial prophylaxis used during pregnancy. Van Allen and colleagues[223] studied the effects of chloroquine on women in Tanzania who were taking 500 mg/week from the time they became pregnant. Malformations observed in three half-siblings included up-slanting palpebral fissures, flat philtrum, thin upper lip, and brachydactyly of the fifth finger. Maternal chloroquine use during pregnancy may be associated with auditory, vestibular, retinal, and other neurologic dysfunction in children.

Cigarette smoking

Since first reported by Simpson in 1957,[224] the association between cigarette smoking during pregnancy and IUGR has been corroborated by numerous studies. Maternal cigarette smoking is recognized as the largest preventable risk factor for IUGR in higher-income countries.[225] Smoking 10–20 cigarettes per day during pregnancy reduces birth weight by an average of 200 g. The magnitude of this association appears to be modified by maternal genetic polymorphisms.[226]

The effect of smoking on the risk of birth defects is controversial. Some reports indicate an association between smoking and congenital heart defects and other cardiovascular problems, urogenital defects, inguinal hernias, strabismus, anencephaly, cleft lip and palate, and clubfoot; other studies, including the Collaborative Perinatal Project, indicate no increase in incidence of congenital defects.[227] However, several studies have found an increased risk of orofacial clefts in the offspring of women who smoke during pregnancy.[228-233] A gene–environment interaction between maternal smoking, transforming growth factor-α, and clefting has been reported but not fully confirmed.[25, 234, 235]

Tobacco smoke contains approximately 4000 chemical compounds including nicotine, polycyclic aromatic hydrocarbons, tar, carbon particles, and carbon monoxide. Nicotine, a cholinergic agonist, is a vasoconstrictor that results in uterine vascular constriction and may be an important factor in IUGR through decreased perfusion of fetal tissues.[236]

Cigarette smoking during pregnancy raises the risk of perinatal mortality and morbidity.[237] The increased mortality is attributed to abruptio placentae, placenta previa, spontaneous abortion, prematurity, and IUGR.[227a] A mother who smokes is 80% more likely than a non-smoker to have a spontaneous abortion, and there is a higher prevalence of sudden infant death in babies born to smokers.[227a]

Carbon monoxide from cigarette smoke also crosses the placenta and produces an increase in carboxyhemoglobin (HbCO) levels; there is a longer half-life of HbCO in fetal blood than in maternal blood.[238] With maternal smoking, there are increased levels of biocyanate that deplete vitamin B_{12} and sulfur-containing amino acids, as well as depleted serum and red blood cell folic acid levels. A depleted supply of these vitamins and/or amino acids may inhibit protein synthesis. Nutritional deficits are not uncommon in women who smoke. All these factors may contribute to IUGR.[239-241]

Although a biologic causal mechanism has not been clearly identified, a robust body of evidence indicates that the chemicals in tobacco smoke are capable of producing deleterious changes in the placenta and the fetus.[242]

Cocaine

Cocaine is metabolized very slowly in the fetus because the fetus has low plasma levels of cholinesterase.[243] Cocaine acts by blocking the presynaptic reuptake of neurotransmitters at the nerve terminals, which results in increased levels of norepinephrine and

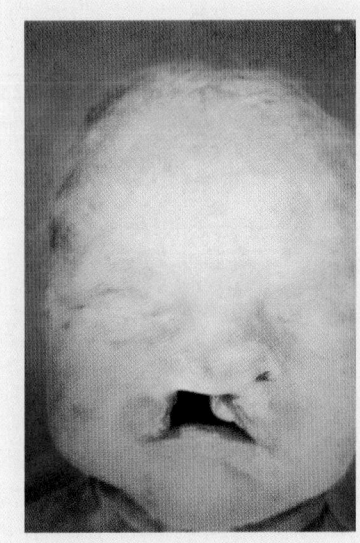

FIGURE 4.1.18 Cleft lip and cleft palate in a newborn after maternal ingestion of large doses of prednisone during pregnancy. The infant also had an endocardial cushion defect of the heart.

dopamine.[244] It may alter the availability and utilization of calcium, and reduces blood flow from the uterus to the placenta.

Available information on the teratogenic effects of cocaine is controversial. Case reports and small series show an increase in **abruptio placentae, cerebral hemorrhage, IUGR, limb defects, bowel atresias,** and other congenital anomalies, which appear to be related to vascular disruption.[245] Prospective studies, on the other hand, have found a relatively low incidence of vascular disruptions and a high frequency of growth problems.[246] Cocaine-exposed children also have an increased incidence of prematurity and sudden infant death syndrome (SIDS).[247] Newborns exposed to a high level of cocaine in utero exhibit asymmetric IUGR and microcephaly (see Part 2 of this chapter).[248]

Corticosteroids

There has been long-standing concern over the potential prenatal effects of exogenous corticoids, such as cleft palate, adrenal atrophy, and congenital cardiac defects.[249] We observed cleft lip and palate after maternal prednisone medication during pregnancy for severe asthma (Fig. 4.1.18). Cysts and impaired sperm production have been reported.

Cytotoxic and chemotherapeutic agents

Antineoplastic drugs inhibit cell growth or kill rapidly growing cells. The cytotoxic agents that produce malformations are shown in Table 4.1.3 and include the alkylating agents **busulfan** and **cyclophosphamide** and the antimetabolites **aminopterin** and **methotrexate**.[250] The risk of malformations with these agents is substantial, between 10 and 20% with both busulfan and aminopterin.[251] **Cleft palate, eye defects,** and generalized **cytomegaly** are related to maternal administration of busulfan.[251]

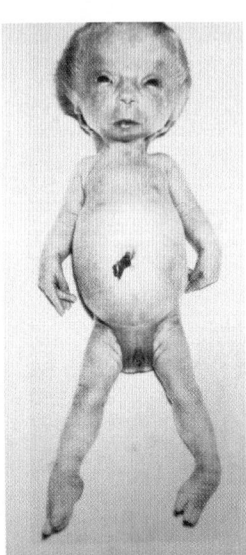

FIGURE 4.1.19 Aminopterin embryopathy in a newborn infant weighing 1280 g after a gestation of 42 weeks. The mother had taken aminopterin tablets in early pregnancy.

Cytoxan (cyclophosphamide) is an alkylating agent used in cancer chemotherapy and as an immunosuppressant. Cytoxan increases teratogenic risk. Cytochrome P-450 monooxygenase converts cyclophosphamide to 4-hydroxycyclophosphamide, which in turn breaks down to phosphoramide mustard and acrolein.[252] It interferes with DNA replication in dividing cells. Cytoxan is teratogenic in all animal species tested.[104] Observed defects include **facial clefts and limb reduction anomalies**.[104] Exposures of primates during early gestation result in cleft lip/palate; later exposures result in craniofacial dysmorphisms.[104]

In human pregnancies, Cytoxan exposures that occur during the first trimester have been associated with **IUGR, ectrodactyly, syndactyly, cardiovascular anomalies,** and other **minor anomalies**,[253, 254] such as **skeletal and palate defects** and **malformations of the limbs and eyes**.[104] Seven malformed infants resulted from first-trimester exposure when radiation therapy was also given to the mothers; at least one of these patients was also treated with antibiotics.[170] The use of Cytoxan therapy during the **second and third trimesters** is associated with a much smaller risk of congenital malformations, but it may induce **pancytopenia** and **impaired fetal growth**.[170]

Absence of digits was reported in two infants exposed to Cytoxan after the period of organogenesis.[253, 255]

Aminopterin has been used to induce therapeutic abortions during the first trimester of pregnancy. Malformations (hydrocephalus, cleft palate, meningomyelocele) and severe IUGR have been reported in the abortuses and in the offspring, when the abortion failed.[256] A recognizable fetal aminopterin/methotrexate syndrome has been described. It includes growth deficiency of prenatal onset, microcephaly, hypoplasia and delayed ossification of the calvarial bones, hypertelorism, wide nasal bridge, upsweep of frontal scalp hair, micrognathia, low set ears, and mesomelic shortening of the extremities (Fig. 4.1.19).

Methotrexate (methylaminopterin) ingestion during the first 2 months[257] or for 5 days between the eighth and tenth weeks of gestation[258] has resulted in the absence of digits. Both aminopterin and methotrexate are **folic acid antagonists** that inhibit dihydrofolate reductase. Bony malformations of the skull include absent or defective ossification, misshapen bones, sutural synostosis, and **anencephaly**. The **globular head**, wide-spaced and **prominent eyes, micrognathia, malformed ears** and **underdeveloped supraorbital ridges** compose a characteristic face. **Cleft lip and/or palate, dislocated hips and elbows**, clubfoot, and delayed bone maturation have been reported.

Diethylstilbestrol

There is a 75% risk of **vaginal adenosis** in exposures occurring before the ninth week of pregnancy; however, the risk of developing adenocarcinoma is extremely low, 1:10 000.[178]

Over half of women exposed prenatally to diethylstilbestrol (DES) have vaginal adenosis with persistence of müllerian mucosa over the cervix and upper vagina. The **uterus may be hypoplastic** and the **fallopian tubes are short and narrow**, with short ostia and absent fimbriae. Vaginal müllerian **adenocarcinoma** has been rarely reported in young women whose mothers had received DES.

The critical perinatal exposure period for this neoplasm seems to be between the 4th and 12th weeks of gestation. Early timing, long exposure, and high dosage are important determinants of risk of vaginal epithelial changes.[257] In all patients with vaginal and cervical carcinoma, maternal ingestion of the hormone occurred before the 18th week; in 80%, DES ingestion was before the 12th week.[64, 259] It has been hypothesized that women with DES induced genital changes have more metaplastic squamocolumnar epithelial cells, and therefore may be at greater risk for squamous neoplasia of the genital tract. **Malformations**, including virilization of the external genitalia, have been described **in the vagina and uterus** of exposed women; it has been reported in female fetuses after maternal treatment with high doses of **norethindrone**.[260]

Approximately one-third of males exposed prenatally to DES have some abnormalities, including **small penis with hypospadias or meatal stenosis, cryptorchidism, small testes** with induration of capsule, **epididymal cysts, testicular tumors**, and **impaired sperm production**.

Ergotamine

Ergotamine is a natural alkaloid of ergot that causes smooth muscle contraction. The constrictive effects of ergotamine on fetal blood vessels may be responsible for IUGR and jejunal atresia.[261] The Collaborative Perinatal Project did not find an association between the use of this drug during pregnancy and congenital abnormalities.[64]

No adverse effect on pregnancy was found in one study of women who took ergotamine for the treatment of migraine.[68, 262] A report from the database of the Hungarian Case-Control Surveillance of Congenital Anomalies (1980–1986) showed that amongst the mothers of 726 children born with NTDs, three had been exposed to ergotamine in the first 3 months of pregnancy while none of the mothers of the 726 controls had been exposed (p = 0.01).[263] Larger controlled studies on ergotamine use during pregnancy are needed to validate this observation.

Estrogen and progesterone

Estrogen and progesterone preparations have been used in the past to treat threatened abortion. It is possible that bleeding in early pregnancy is a sign of an abnormal embryo; therefore, medications used to treat such bleeding might, in these instances, be associated with an abnormal pregnancy outcome that was inevitable before the medication was given.[264]

Early studies concluded that estrogen/progesterone compounds or progesterone alone was associated with a variety of congenital anomalies, including limb reduction defects, esophageal atresia, defects of the cardiovascular system and CNS, and the VACTERL association.[265–271] Other reports have found no association between use of these compounds and any congenital defect.[272–276] A reanalysis of previously published data showed no association between the use of progestogens during pregnancy and congenital malformations.[277]

Genital abnormalities appear to be associated with the use of **progestogens** in pregnancy. **Masculinization is observed in approximately 1% of female fetuses** when exposure occurs during the eighth to tenth week of development. An increased risk of hypospadias has been reported in male fetuses exposed during early pregnancy, possibly resulting from interference with the production or action of fetal androgens, which are critical in the normal closure of the urethra.[278, 279]

Maternal progesterone and estrogen may stimulate fetal breast engorgement, neonatal vaginal bleeding, and gestational herpes. These effects, however, are transient.

Folic acid deficiency and folic acid antagonists

Folic acid deficiency has been observed in a high percentage of women who have had infants with an NTD; **folic acid antagonists** also may increase the risk of NTD affected pregnancies.

In 1976, Smithells and collaborators observed that women who gave birth to infants with NTD had low serum levels of micronutrients, including some vitamins.[280] Subsequent randomized and non-randomized clinical trials have conclusively demonstrated that women with higher dietary intakes of folate and those who have taken multivitamin or folic acid supplements periconceptionally have decreased their risk of NTD by at least 70%.[281–286] Folic acid, or pteroylmonoglutamic acid, is a water-soluble vitamin of the B complex. It is the synthetic form present in pharmaceutical preparations and fortified food. Dietary folic acid is a mixture of folates (polyglutamates) and it is easily denatured by cooking, processing, and prolonged storage. Folates are initially deconjugated in the cells of the intestinal wall to the monoglutamate form.[287, 288]

The underlying biologic mechanism by which periconceptional folic acid use protects against NTDs is unknown. Folic acid participates in DNA synthesis and is, therefore, essential for rapid cell division and organ/tissue formation in early development. Folates function as carbon donors in the synthesis of serine. In addition, they play an important role in the synthesis of purines and pyrimidine bases, in the synthesis of transfer RNA, and as methyl donors to create methylcobalamin, which is used for remethylation of homocysteine to methionine.[289]

It has been shown that 5–15% of normal Western populations is homozygous for a point mutation (C677T) in the 5,10-methylenetetrahydrofolate reductase (MTHFR) gene, which maps to 1p36.3. This mutation is associated with a moderate increase of NTDs, with mild hyperhomocysteinemia and probably with increased risk of cardiovascular disease in adults.[290]

In September 1992, the USPHS recommended that 'all women of childbearing age in the United States who are capable of becoming pregnant consume 0.4 mg folic acid per day for the purpose of reducing their risk of having a pregnancy affected with spina bifida or other NTDs'.[291] Subsequently, the Food and Drug Administration issued a regulation requiring all enriched grain products to be fortified with 140 μg folic acid per 100 g as of January of 1998. These efforts have resulted in approximately a 30% decrease in the prevalence of NTDs in the USA.[292]

Lithium

Cardiovascular malformations, in particular **Ebstein anomaly** and **tricuspid atresia**, have been related to lithium exposure.[193, 259, 293–295] Infants exposed in utero to lithium may experience transient lethargy, hypotonia, cyanosis, poor feeding, and poor respiratory efforts during the early neonatal period.[293] Other defects that have been noted in infants exposed to lithium in utero include malformations of the CNS, ear, and ureter; altered thyroid and cardiac function; and congenital goiter.[259] It was initially reported that 6–10% of newborn infants of mothers exposed to lithium during the first trimester could be so affected.[259] Prospective studies of women on lithium treatment have shown that the risk is much lower, possibly a risk of about 1% for congenital heart defects.[296]

Lysergic acid diethylamide

Case reports have shown that children born to mothers who used lysergic acid diethylamide (LSD) before or during pregnancy have had a variety of anomalies. Defects of the limbs, eyes, CNS and arthrogryposis (Fig. 4.1.20) may be present.[297] However, no consistent pattern of anomalies has been observed in these children. The assessment of the effects of LSD use during pregnancy has been difficult, since the woman's lifestyle may also include use of alcohol and other drugs, poor medical care and nutrition, and exposure to illness. There is no indication that the risk of congenital anomalies is great.[298] LSD-induced chromosomal damage may last up to 2 years but is usually transient.[299, 300]

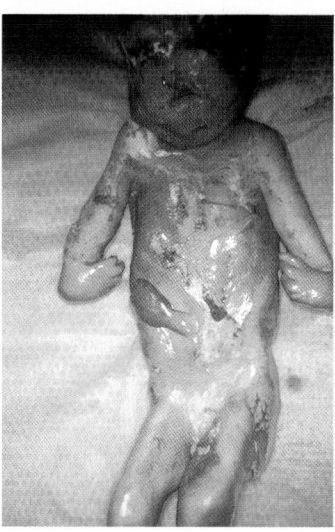

FIGURE 4.1.20 Skeletal defects, including radial aplasia and microcephaly, after lysergic acid diethylamide (LSD) exposure.

There is no evidence that paternal exposure to LSD in small doses before conception is associated with an increased rate of spontaneous abortion, premature birth, or birth defects.[301]

Marijuana

The active ingredient in marijuana is **8,9-tetrahydrocannabinol,** which is fat soluble, crosses the placenta easily, and may persist in the fetus for as long as 30 days.[302–304] **Growth retardation** and malformations are reported after maternal marijuana use during pregnancy. However, other potentially teratogenic drugs are probably used by women who smoke marijuana. An increased risk of **non-lymphoblastic leukemia** has been reported.[305]

Mercury

Mercury (Hg) is ubiquitous in the environment as a result of its natural sources, its widespread use in industrial and commercial products, and its emission from combustion processes.[306, 307] Thus, the population can be exposed to elemental (broken thermometers, dental amalgams), inorganic (Hg salts), and organic Hg [predominantly methylmercury (MeHg)]. Organic forms of mercury are more toxic than the inorganic forms. MeHg is formed by biotransformation of inorganic Hg that has contaminated lakes and oceans. It accumulates up the food chain in aquatic systems and leads to high concentrations of MeHg in predatory fish (e.g. tuna, swordfish, shark, and whale) and shellfish, which, when consumed by humans, can result in toxic effects. It is rapidly absorbed from the gastrointestinal tract, crosses the blood–brain barrier, and accumulates in the brain, where it is gradually converted to inorganic Hg.[307]

MeHg poisoning produces permanent atrophy of the granular layer of the cerebellum and spongious softening in the visual cortex and other cortical areas of the brain;[308] polyneuritis can also occur. The mechanisms by which MeHg causes neurotoxicity are not known.

The adverse effects of MeHg on the developing brain have been corroborated both in humans and animals.[309] Consumption of contaminated fish by pregnant women (and cats) in the island of Minimata, Japan resulted in severe effects of epidemic proportion in their offspring, which included mental retardation, cerebral palsy, deafness, and blindness (**Minamata disease**).[310, 311] A similar exposure occurred in Iraq after the ingestion of bread prepared from wheat treated with MeHg that had been used as a fungicide.[308]

Chronic, low-dose prenatal MeHg exposure from maternal consumption of fish has been associated with more subtle signs of neurotoxicity in children.[307, 312–315]

Elemental and inorganic mercury do not cross the placenta well and have not been proved to be human teratogens.[132]

Metronidazole (Flagyl™)

Metronidazole is an antibiotic and antiprotozoal agent commonly used in the treatment of gynecologic infections. It has been associated with birth defects in isolated cases.[316] However, case-control studies and other epidemiologic data indicate that use of this drug during pregnancy is not associated with an increased incidence of teratogenicity, spontaneous abortions, stillbirths, or prematurity.[317–320]

Misoprostol™

Misoprostol™ is a synthetic analog of prostaglandin E1 that has been used in combination with methotrexate to induce abortion.[321] Epidemiologic studies and case reports have shown an association between unsuccessful elective terminations of pregnancy using misoprostol and congenital defects. These are mostly vascular disruptions and include, among others, Möbius sequence, terminal transverse limb reduction defects, arthrogryposis with amyoplasia congenita, and gastroschisis.[322–325]

Penicillamine

Penicillamine is a chelating agent used to treat Wilson disease, cystinuria, and rheumatoid arthritis. Collagen tissue abnormalities, particularly cutis laxa and hyperextensibility disorders, associated with **low blood copper levels** may induce both elastic and collagen tissue anomalies.[326] Several cases of cutis laxa, hyperextensible joints, and occasionally other anomalies have been reported after penicillamine exposure in utero. Cutis laxa disappeared after a time in two survivors, suggesting that once the drug has been cleared from the body, normal collagen production can resume.[327] As a chelating agent, penicillamine can chelate zinc as well as copper, and the **low serum zinc level** may cause congenital defects.[327]

Phenothiazines

Phenothiazines are tranquilizers used as antipsychotics and as antiemetics. Some reports have found no association between maternal use of phenothiazines and the occurrence of congenital malformations.[328] Other case reports[329, 330] have documented neurologic abnormalities as well as hydronephrosis[328] and ureteropelvic junction obstruction attributed to in utero exposure to **fluphenazine**, but no causal relation can be established from these anecdotal reports.

Polychlorinated and polybrominated biphenyls

Polychlorinated and polybrominated biphenyls (PCBs) are synthetic hydrocarbon compounds once used as insulating and hydraulic fluids, lubricants in electric transformers, plasticizers, and chemical additives. They were banned in most industrialized nations in the 1970s, but residues persist in the soil and water worldwide. They have been found in game fish caught in PCB-contaminated bodies of water.[331]

Transplacental transfer of PCBs occurs in humans,[332] but only small amounts reach the fetus. However, as these compounds are highly lipophilic, much larger amounts are transferred via the mother's milk.

Accidental cooking oil contamination occurred in Japan and Taiwan in 1968 and 1979, respectively. Adults who consumed the contaminated oil develop chloracne, dark brown pigmentation of the skin and lips, swollen eyelids, and swelling and pain in the joints.[333] The offspring of women who had ingested the oil during pregnancy had deeply pigmented skin ('**cola baby**'); low birth weight; enlarged sebaceous glands in the eyelids; hypoplastic deformed nails; natal teeth; and abnormal pigmentation of the gums, nails, and groin.[331, 334] Neonatal mortality occurred in 20% of the affected infants in Taiwan.[335]

Children born to mothers with chronic exposure to PCB from environmental sources, as has occurred with consumption of contaminated fish in Lake Michigan, have shown moderately low birth weight and developmental deficits that persist at least through school age.[333] Higher levels of exposure are associated with more severe reduction of birth weight, small head size and hypotonicity and hyporeflexia.[334]

There is no evidence of reproductive risk to humans as long as occupational exposures to PCBs are kept at or below the recommended airborne levels of 0.001 mg/m³.[293] PCBs may interfere with male reproductive function by exerting estrogenic agonist/antagonist activity.[336]

Prostaglandin inhibitors

Aspirin, indometacin, and **naproxen** act by inhibiting the synthesis of prostaglandins from arachidonic acid. They readily cross the placenta and have been shown to cause severe constriction and occasionally **closure of the ductus arteriosus** in the fetus in the third trimester.[337] This increases pulmonary arterial pressure in the fetus. When used chronically, these drugs can lead to an increase in the mass of muscle in the small pulmonary arteries, resulting in **persistent pulmonary arterial hypertension** in the newborn.[338] Fetal indometacin exposure is related to **renal tubular dysgenesis,** resulting in anuria and oligohydramnios.[338a]

Human studies are contradictory. While some have failed to find an association between aspirin and birth defects,[211, 339] others have found positive associations with cleft palate, truncus arteriosus, gastroschisis and other vascular disruptions, and an increase in stillbirth rate and reduced birth weight.[340–343]

Sympathomimetics

Pseudoephedrine is a sympathomimetic agent. The Collaborative Perinatal Project found an association between first trimester sympathomimetic use and certain minor malformations, inguinal hernia, and clubfoot. Werler and associates reported an association between use of pseudoephedrine and **gastroschisis**.[342, 344]

We observed two cases of severe limb defects in infants after the use of sympathomimetic drugs during pregnancy. The mother of one had taken large doses of Primatene™ (ephedrine, theophylline, phenobarbital) as tablets and mist throughout pregnancy.[345] The infant was born with oligoectrosyndactyly (Fig. 4.1.21). In the other infant, maternal ingestion of sympathomimetic drugs, with Triaminic, pseudoephedrine, phenylephrine, and phenylpropanolamine, was associated with distal limb defects (Fig. 4.1.22). Sympathomimetic agents can produce cardiac defects[346] and limb malformations[347] in the chick embryo.

Sedatives

Data on the potential teratogenic effects of **benzodiazepine**-containing drugs are inconsistent. While several large case-control studies have shown no increased risk of birth defects in the children of mothers who took benzodiazepines during pregnancy,[348, 349] others have found elevated risks, especially for oral clefts.[350, 351] Taken in large amounts during the first trimester of pregnancy, benzodiazepines have been reported to produce IUGR, cleft lip, and facial features that resemble the characteristic findings of FAS.[350]

Thalidomide

Thalidomide is a proved teratogen. It was used to prevent nausea during pregnancy in several European countries, Australia, Canada, Japan, and Brazil in the 1960s but not in the USA. It causes **limb reduction defects; facial hemangiomas; esophageal and duodenal atresia; cardiac defects, particularly tetralogy of Fallot; renal agenesis; anomalies of the external ear; facial palsy; external ophthalmoplegia; anophthalmia or microphthalmia; and coloboma** (see Box 4.1.1).[352–354] Cleft palate is a rare complication; the CNS is not affected. The children are of normal

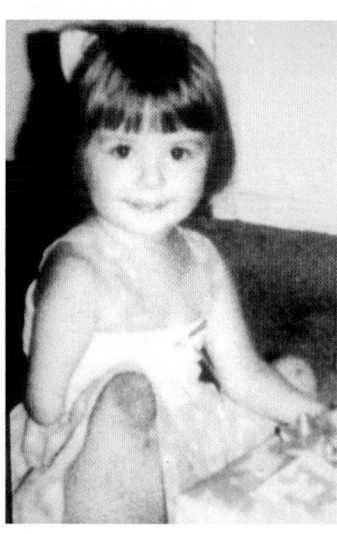

FIGURE 4.1.21 Limb reduction defects involving all extremities in a child whose mother took high doses of sympathomimetic drugs throughout pregnancy.

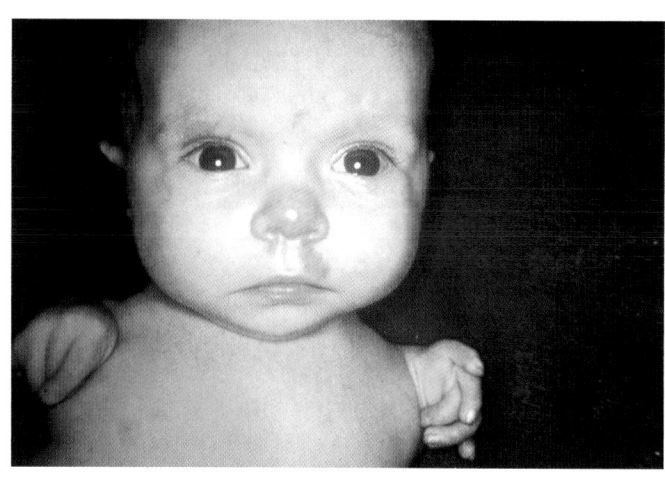

FIGURE 4.1.23 Phocomelia of upper extremities in thalidomide embryopathy.

intelligence. The critical period during which thalidomide produces human malformations spans about 2 weeks, between days 20 and 38 post conception. About 50% of pregnancies exposed during this period resulted in infants with anomalies, the most notable of which are limb defects ranging from triphalangeal thumb to tetra-amelia or phocomelia of the upper and lower limbs (Fig. 4.1.23), at times with preaxial polydactyly of six or seven toes per foot. Congenital heart defects, urinary tract anomalies, genital defects, gastrointestinal anomalies, eye defects, ear malformations, and dental anomalies have been observed.

McCredie postulated an interference with neural crest-based sclerotomal organization as the pathogenetic basis of the limb malformations.[355–357] North and McCredie expanded their retrospective studies of the visceral anomalies in infants who died with multiple congenital anomalies with longitudinal limb defects by attempting to determine whether neural crest injury would impair development of structures supplied by the sensory autonomic nerves derived from the injured zone of the neural crest.[358] Application of sclerotomal and viscerotomal maps to the autopsy data showed a neuroanatomic correlation in 89% of cases. The authors proposed a developmental correlation within a multiple congenital anomaly syndrome on the basis of neurotomes or embryonic developmental fields with common regional innervation. Some authors have postulated that thalidomide is an inhibitor of angiogenesis and that the antiangiogenic activity correlates with its teratogenicity and mechanism of action.[21, 359]

However, the molecular mechanisms are not known. A large number of hypotheses have been put forth, but there is no

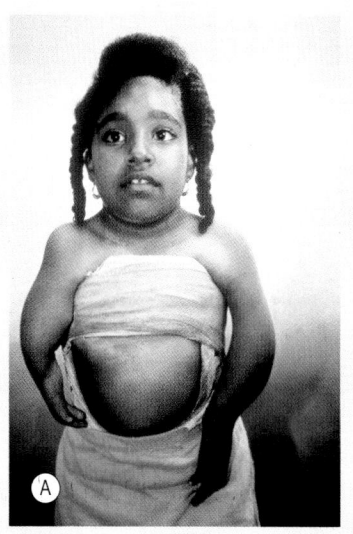

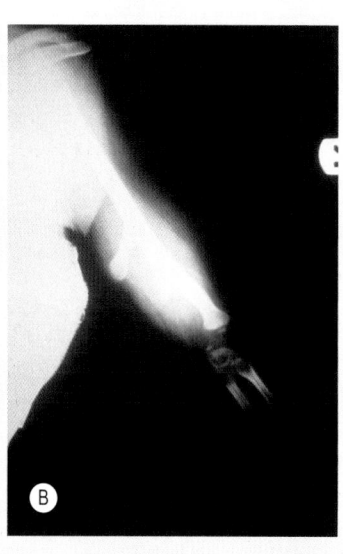

FIGURE 4.1.22 Oligoectrosyndactyly.
(A) Limb defects of upper extremities. The mother was exposed to high doses of Primatene (ephedrine, theophylline, phenobarbital) throughout pregnancy. (B) Radiograph of upper limb showing fusion of humerus and ulna and spur formation.

BOX 4.1.1 ABNORMALITIES REPORTED IN THALIDOMIDE EMBRYOPATHY

Skeletal defects
  Absent radii
  Hand
    Limited extension
    Club hand
    Hypoplastic or fused phalanges
    Finger syndactyly
    Carpal hypoplasia or fusion
    Radial deviation
  Ulna
    Short and malformed
    Unilaterally absent
    Bilaterally absent
  Humerus
    Hypoplastic
    Absent
  Shoulder girdle
    Abnormally formed with absent glenoid
    Fossa and acromion process
    Hypoplastic scapula and clavicle
  Hips
    Unilaterally or bilaterally dislocated
  Legs
    Coxa valga
    Femoral torsion
    Tibial torsion
      Bilateral
      Unilateral
    Stiff knee

    Abnormal tibiofibular joint
    Dislocated patella(e)
  Feet
    Over-riding fifth toe
    Calcaneovalgus deformity
    Other foot deformity
  Ribs
    Asymmetric first rib
    Cervical rib
  Spine
    Cervical spina bifida
    Fused cervical spine
Cardiac anomalies
  Tetralogy of Fallot
  Atrial septal defect
  Patent foramen ovale
  Dextrocardia
  Congestive heart failure leading to death
  Systolic murmur
  Cardiomegaly
  Suspected congenital heart disease
Other abnormalities
  Apparently low-set ears and malformations extending to microtia
  Urogenital anomalies
  Micrognathia
  Mandibular hypoplasia
  Maxillary hypoplasia
  Meckel diverticulum
  Uterine anomalies

From Gilbert-Barness and Opitz 1991,[354] with permission.

consensus regarding their validity. These include, in addition to the inhibition of angiogenesis;[359] down-regulation of integrins,[360] anti-tumor necrosis factor-α activity,[361] oxidative DNA damage,[362] and reverse of the stimulatory effect of insulin-like growth factor 1 and fibroblast growth factor 2 on the vascularization of the limb bud and other embryonic structures.[363]

Over 10 000 infants are known to have been injured by prenatal exposure.[64] During the critical period of 24–33 days after fertilization the upper limbs are more severely involved than the lower limbs. Any of the long bones can be defective or, in severe cases, totally absent. The hands in some cases are normal or lack thumbs or other fingers when oligodactyly, syndactyly, and polydactyly occur.

Thyroid medications

Transient hypothyroidism in the newborn infant may occur when the fetal thyroid gland has been suppressed by antithyroid drugs, iodine, radioactive iodine,[373] or, possibly, maternal antibodies.[374]

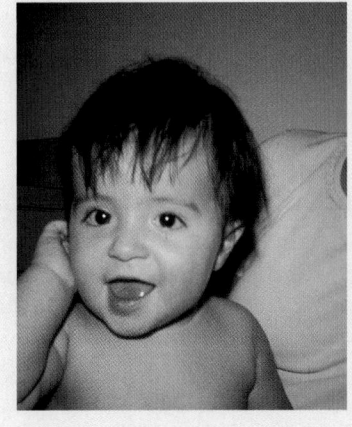

FIGURE 4.1.24 Toluene embryopathy. Note characteristics of face that are similar to those caused by alcohol embryopathy; including mid-face hypoplasia, short palpebral fissures, mild ptosis, smooth philtral area and narrow vermillion border of the upper lip. (From Arnold et al 1994,[364] with permission.)

Thyroid function returns to the euthyroid state during the first days or weeks of life.

Antithyroid drugs interfere with thyroid hormone synthesis by inhibiting iodine organification and coupling of the iodotyrosines to form T_3 and T_4 in the thyroid. The most commonly used antithyroid drugs are the thionamides (propylthiouracil, methimazole, and carbimazole). These drugs cross the placenta, though in small amounts, and may alter thyroid function in the fetus, resulting in hypothyroidism and goiter if administered after week 10 of gestation, as the pituitary–thyroid axis starts functioning between week 12 and 14 post fertilization.[168, 332, 375]

Propylthiouracil has not been found to be associated with an increased risk of congenital anomalies.[376, 377] However, ulcer-like midline scalp defects (aplasia cutis) have been described after maternal methimazole (Tapazole®) or carbimazole (a carboxy derivative of methimazole) medication during pregnancy.[375] Two infants have also had umbilical defects (patent urachus, persistent vitelline duct).[378] Other authors have reported additional malformations in children receiving methimazole or carbimazole that may constitute a recognizable syndrome. The observed structural abnormalities include, in addition to scalp defects, choanal atresia, hypoplastic nipples, and tracheoesophageal fistula.[379]

Amiodarone, an iodine-rich drug widely used for the treatment of cardiac tachyarrhythmias, may also induce hypothyroidism in the offspring of mothers treated during pregnancy. Due to its long half-life, the drug may affect thyroid function even if taken before the 10th week of development. The therapeutic dose (400 mg/day) is equivalent to 12 mg of iodine.[380]

Toluene

Toluene embryopathy (Fig. 4.1.24)[364] includes prenatal and postnatal **growth deficiency, microcephaly, anencephaly, developmental delay, cardiac and limb defects,** and **craniofacial anomalies** similar to FAS (see earlier in this chapter).[332, 365–372] Toluene is also teratogenic to animals.[332]

Phenotypic facial abnormalities similar to those of FAS suggest a common mechanism of craniofacial teratogenesis for toluene and alcohol due to deficiency of craniofacial neuroepithelium and mesodermal components due to increased embryonic cell death.[372]

The greatest risk of accidental exposure is likely to occur among workers in the paint, dye, chemical, and petrochemical industries.[368] One case of toluene in the serum of a newborn has been reported.[369] Toluene embryopathy, to date, has been found only in infants of maternal paint sniffers or others who abuse toluene for its euphoric effect.

Of 18 infants with a history of in utero toluene exposure who were examined at birth, 39% were born prematurely and 9% died during the perinatal period. Also 54% were small for gestational age, 52% exhibited continued postnatal growth deficiency, 33% had prenatal microcephaly, 67% had postnatal microcephaly, and 80% showed developmental delay. A total of 83% of the patients had craniofacial features similar to FAS, and 89% of these children had other minor anomalies.[372]

Vitamin A

No increased risk of malformations was observed in two large studies in which mothers had consumed more than 6000 IU of vitamin A.[381, 382] Another study with an intake of more than 10 000 IU of preformed vitamin A showed that 1 infant in 57 had a malformation.[383] Malformations have been reported in association with **vitamin A toxicity** and include **absence or hypoplasia of the external ears, CNS anomalies, cortical blindness, and severe congenital heart disease.**[384] This occurs with doses of vitamin A greater than 25 000 IU. It is recommended that the maximum vitamin A supplement before or during pregnancy be 8000 IU/day.

Consumption of high doses of naturally occurring vitamin A (β-carotenes) does not lead to toxicity or have teratogenic effects.

Vitamin D

Excessive maternal vitamin D intake was once linked to the so-called idiopathic hypercalcemia syndrome (**Williams-like syndrome**).[385] Williams syndrome in both familial and sporadic cases is due to a submicroscopic deletion within chromosomal subunit 7q11-23, including the elastin gene. The elastin gene deletion can explain the vascular and connective tissue abnormalities but not the hypercalcemia. The relationship of the syndrome to vitamin D metabolism is unknown, although hypercalcemia due to hypervitaminosis D appears to be a phenocopy. **Intrauterine and postnatal growth retardation, mental retardation,** and multiple system involvement with facial dysmorphism are characterized as the elfin facies with broad forehead, prominent and widely spaced eyes, reticular pattern to the stroma of the iris, strabismus, depressed nasal bridge with anteverted nostrils, rounded cheeks, and prominent lips. The **corneas** may contain **calcium deposits**. **Cardiovascular abnormalities** include supravalvular aortic stenosis and coarctation.

Vitamin K

Vitamin K deficiency during the first trimester of pregnancy resulting from vitamin K epoxide reductase deficiency appears to be the cause of vitamin K-related chondrodysplasia punctata[386] similar to that seen in warfarin embryopathy. An additional mechanism – maternal malabsorption of vitamin K – was postulated by Menger et al[386] in three cases with a similar constellation of anomalies. Disturbed vitamin K effects in the embryonic period are listed in Table 4.1.7.

Warfarin (dicumarol, coumarin derivatives)

Women with a history of thromboembolic disease or artificial heart valves often require long-term anticoagulant therapy common derivatives.

TABLE 4.1.7 DISTURBED VITAMIN K EFFECTS IN THE EMBRYONIC PERIOD*

Mechanism	Disorder
Malabsorption/malnutrition in maternal celiac disease	Vitamin K deficiency – embryopathy
Embryonic enzyme deficiency of vitamin K epoxide reductase	Pseudo warfarin embryopathy
Pharmacologic inhibition by coumarin derivates	Warfarin embryopathy

*Courtesy of Professor J Spranger.

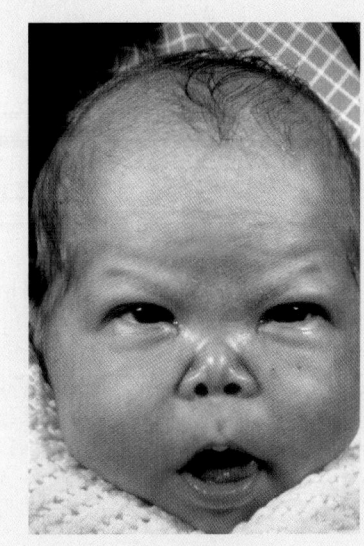

FIGURE 4.1.25 Warfarin embryopathy. Note the nasal hypoplasia. (Courtesy of Dr Renata Laxova.)

Warfarin inhibits the formation of carboxyglutamyl from glutamyl residues, decreasing the ability of proteins to bind calcium.[387] There is an estimated 25% risk for affected infants after exposure during 8–14 weeks of pregnancy. **Choanal stenosis** may occur. **Calcific stippling** occurs primarily in the tarsals, proximal femurs, and paravertebral processes. **Brachydactyly and small nails**, with greater severity in the upper limbs, has been present in about half of affected infants. **Optic atrophy,** microphthalmia, and blindness can result from exposure during the first or second trimester. **Brain anomalies** include microcephaly, optic atrophy, visual impairment, seizures, hypotonia, and mental retardation. **Midtrimester exposure** can result in optic atrophy, brain anomalies, and mental impairment. The inhibition of calcium binding by proteins during a critical period of ossification may explain **the nasal hypoplasia, stippled calcification, and skeletal abnormalities of warfarin embryopathy** (Fig. 4.1.25).[387]

A review of the outcome of 418 pregnancies in which coumarin derivatives were used showed that one-sixth of the liveborn infants were abnormal, one-sixth of the pregnancies resulted in abortion or stillbirth, and two-thirds of the pregnancies resulted in normal infants.[64] The risk of fetal malformation when coumarin derivatives are used is thought to be 1:5.[64] In 22 coumarin-exposed children with a mean age of 4 years, mental and physical development was found to be comparable with matched controls.[387]

Third-trimester exposure can anticoagulate the fetus, predisposing to perinatal hemorrhage.

Drugs and chemicals apparently not teratogenic in humans

Agent orange

Agent Orange exposure, particularly that which occurred in Vietnam, has stimulated extensive study of health and reproductive effects. The three largest studies have found no significant increase in congenital anomalies among the offspring of Vietnam veterans.[388–391] In one study an analysis of the data from sprayed areas in Vietnam found an increase in spontaneous abortions, stillbirths, cleft palate, and spina bifida in surviving infants after maternal exposure.[389] No conclusion is warranted at this time.

Bendectin

This compound originally contained pyridoxine, doxylamine, and dicyclomine; later, pyridoxine was eliminated. At least 10 large epidemiologic studies involving over 17 000 pregnant women have failed to find an association between the use of this compound and the occurrence of birth defects in the offspring.[392]

Caffeine

There is no evidence that caffeine is teratogenic in humans.[392a] A dose response has been reported between the consumption of caffeinated beverages and the time it takes to become pregnant. Failed ovulation has been excluded as the responsible factor, so a failure of implantation and an excess of early embryo losses are mechanisms that should be explored.[393]

Maternal conditions
Assisted reproductive techniques

Several studies have consistently documented an association between assisted reproductive techniques (ART) and low birth weight and preterm delivery.[394–396] In addition, over the past few years, evidence has begun to accumulate suggesting that the use of ART may also be associated with increased risks of neurodevelopmental abnormalities, birth defects including chromosomal aneuploids and syndromes resulting from genetic imprinting disorders, and possibly some types of cancer.[397–401] Data are still considered by some to be controversial, and this is a very active area of investigation.

Diabetes mellitus

Although hyperglycemia may be key in the pathogenesis of diabetic embryopathy, other circulating factors contained in diabetic serum may also be of importance in the pathogenetic mechanism altering embryonic development.[402] **Hyperglycemia** leads to inhibition of myoinositol uptake that is essential for embryonic development during the gastrulation and neurulation stages of embryogenesis.[403, 404] Deficiency of myoinositol appears to cause perturbations in the phosphoinositide system that lead to abnormalities in the arachidonic acid-prostaglandin pathway. The gastrulation and neurulation stages of development are particularly sensitive to **hypoglycemia** and result in growth retardation as well as cranial and caudal NTDs. Obesity associated with a number of metabolic abnormalities, including abnormal glucose metabolism, is associated with a higher risk of malformations.[405] A possible role of free oxygen radicals in diabetic teratogenicity has been suggested. The pathogenesis of diabetic embryopathy is heterogeneous;[402, 402a, 403] the maintenance of glucose homeostasis is important for the prevention of diabetic embryopathy.

Infants born of mothers with diabetes mellitus classes A, B, and C grow excessively before birth, presumably because of excessive glucose availability and fetal hyperinsulinism.[406] Infants of diabetic mothers (IDMs) with vascular complications can be growth impaired during fetal life.

Hyperinsulinemia in utero affects major organ systems, including the placenta. Insulin acts as the primary anabolic hormone of fetal growth and development, resulting in **macrosomia** and **visceromegaly**, especially affecting the heart and liver. In the presence of excess glucose, increased fat synthesis and deposition occur during the third trimester. Fetal macrosomia is reflected by increased body fat and muscle mass and organomegaly, but not in increased size of the brain or kidneys.[407, 408] After delivery there is a rapid fall in plasma glucose and persistently low concentrations of plasma free fatty acids (FFAs), glycerol, and β-hydroxybutyrate. Severe hypoglycemia at birth may be life threatening and require intravenous glucose infusions.

There is a correlation between elevated *hemoglobin* A_{1c} (HbA_{1c}) and the incidence of major congenital anomalies in IDMs.[409] HbA_{1c} is a normal, minor hemoglobin that is distinguished from HbA by the addition of a glucose moiety to the amino-terminal valine of the β chain. Glycosylation of hemoglobin A occurs during circulation of the red cell and depends on the average concentration of glucose to which the red cell has been exposed during its life cycle.[410] Measurement of HbA_{1c} provides an index of chronic glucose elevation, and therefore of diabetes control.[411] HbA_{1c} levels during pregnancy that exceeded 11.5% were associated with congenital abnormalities in 66% of the offspring, but levels below 9.5% were not associated with an increased frequency of anomalies in the infants.[412]

The overall incidence of major malformations is 6–9% in large series of women with uncontrolled diabetes, representing a threefold increase in IDMs. **Defects of the heart, CNS, kidneys**, and **skeleton** predominate. Transposition of the great vessels, VSD, and dextrocardia occur with greatest frequency. Anencephaly, spina bifida, hydrocephaly, and holoprosencephaly are the major CNS malformations. Other rare malformations include

situs inversus and **caudal dysplasia**, vertebral and renal anomalies, imperforate anus, radius aplasia, renal abnormalities including agenesis and dysplasia, and other multiple defects. Brain development is often impaired. Frequently the anomalies include those observed in the VATER association. Minor physical abnormalities include anteverted nares, flattened nasal bridge, excess skin folds on the neck, and tapered fingers with hyperconvex nails. Other complications include hyperbilirubinemia, hypocalcemia, vascular thromboses (particularly renal vein thrombosis), and respiratory distress syndrome.

Hyperglycemia during the embryonic period can cause malformations (disruptions) in virtually every organ and tissue. The molecular pathogenesis of these defects is an active area of research, but it is known that in maternal (and thus embryonic) hyperglycemia, excess glucose metabolism by embryos disturbs a complex network of biochemical pathways, leading to oxidative stress, which in turn results in impaired embryonic gene expression leading to **enchanced apoptosis**, disturbed cell signalling and abnormal organogenesis.[402a, 412a, 412b, 412c]

No increase in the rate of spontaneous abortion was found in diabetics with reasonable control; however, high HbA_{1c} levels have been associated with an increased incidence of spontaneous abortion.

In **caudal dysplasia** (Fig. 4.1.26) the spine has faulty segmentation or may terminate in the lumbar or sacral region. Anal and urethral sphincters may be incompetent and motor function of the lower extremities impaired. **Sirenomelia** occurs as a part of this spectrum. Malformations of the lower and upper extremities can occur independently of caudal regression. Holoprosencephaly and caudal dysplasia occur with a several hundredfold increase in these infants.

Caudal dysplasia syndrome, with varying degrees of sacral agenesis, is sometimes associated with defects of the palate and branchial arches and occurs in 1% of diabetic offspring.[413, 414] A 10-fold increase in NTDs among over 400 pregnancies has been reported.[414] The relative risk of major malformations among infants of women with insulin-dependent diabetes mellitus is 8 compared with infants of non-diabetic mothers. Infants of women with gestational diabetes mellitus who required insulin during the third trimester of pregnancy have been found to be up to 20 times more likely to have major cardiovascular system defects than infants of non-diabetic women.[114a] All these anomalies are explained by the apoptotic effect of hyperglycemia.[402a, 412a, 412c]

In one study the incidence of malformations in IDMs reported was apparently not related to the control of glycemia during organogenesis.[415] This is in disagreement with numerous studies that demonstrate that timely institution of intensive therapy is associated with rates of spontaneous abortion and congenital malformation similar to those observed in the nondiabetic population.[416]

A possible association of gestational diabetes mellitus (GDM) and congenital malformations has been reported. The defects observed in positive studies are similar to those found in the infants of women with diabetes type 1 or 2, though less frequent.[417, 418] The malformations may be related to the fact that many of the women diagnosed as having GDM have instead previously undiagnosed pregestational diabetes.[419]

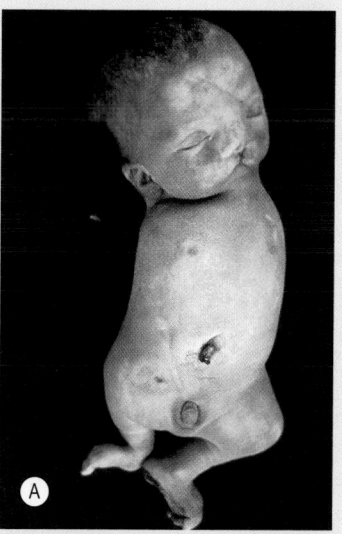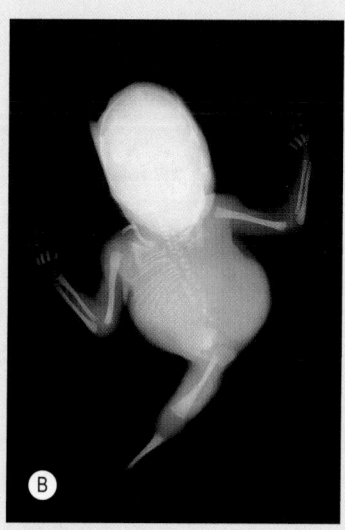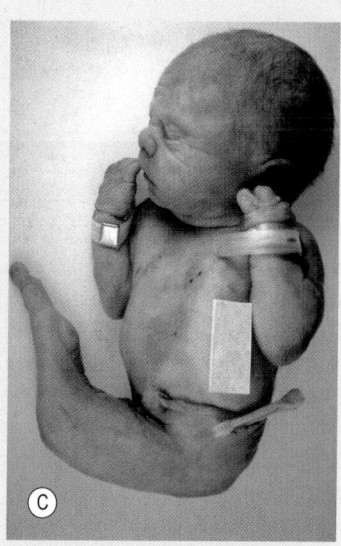

FIGURE 4.1.26 Diabetic embryopathy. (A) Infant with amelia, cleft lip, micrognathia, and caudal dysplasia. (B) Radiograph showing amelia and caudal dysplasia. (C) Sirenomelia.

The frequency of defects appears to be higher in women with GDM and obesity.[420]

Homocystinuria, Hartnup disease

Hydrocephalus has been reported in one each of infants born of mothers with *homocystinuria* and **Hartnup aminoaciduria**.[421] These are probably chance occurrences.

Hyperparathyroidism

Infants of mothers with untreated hypoparathyroidism may have transient **hyperparathyroidism** during the fetal and neonatal periods.[422] The fetal parathyroid hyperplasia that occurs in response to low maternal and fetal serum calcium concentrations is mediated by the maternal parathyroid dysfunction. **Bone demineralization** and subperiosteal reabsorption occurs in the long bones. **IUGR, pulmonary artery stenosis, VSD**, and **muscle hypotonia** have been reported.

Hyperparathyroidism in the mother results in excessive production of parathyroid hormone and hypercalcemia reflected in **fetal hypercalcemia,** which in turn depresses the fetal parathyroid gland and results in fetal **hypoparathyroidism**. It is usually due to a parathyroid adenoma in the mother. Maternal hyperparathyroidism results in an increase in abortion and stillbirth, and because of suppression of the fetal parathyroid, the newborn is at risk for hypocalcemia and tetany.

Immunologic disruption sequences

Fetal graft-versus-host (GVH) disease is mediated through an immunologic response of the fetus against the mother, and results in GVH response.

Paternal leukocyte injections received by the mother for multiple abortions cause IUGR in 50% of fetuses; also, these infants may have a brainstem defect with choreoathetoid movements in a syndrome reminiscent of animals with maternally induced runt disease of GVH reaction.[423]

Myotonic dystrophy

Myotonic dystrophy is one of the most common muscular dystrophies in adults. The disorder follows an autosomal dominant mode of inheritance and the mutated gene contains a segment of CTG repeats that tends to amplify in each generation (anticipation).[424, 425] Severity of the disease correlates with the number of triplet repeats. Infants born of women with myotonic dystrophy may show arthrogryposis resulting from fetal hypokinesia, and may experience difficulty in respiration and feeding. The facies characteristically shows **tenting of the upper lip,** ptosis, absence of movement, and **anterior cupping of the pinnas. Clubfoot** is often present. Postnatal growth is slow.[426]

Obesity

The current obesity epidemic in the USA and other countries[427] has prompted the study of the risk of congenital defects and prepregnancy obesity, defined as body mass index (BMI) $\geq$ $\geq 30\,\mathrm{kg/m^2}$. Different epidemiologic studies have found an increase in the risk of NTDs[428, 429] as well as omphalocele, heart defects, and multiple anomalies among infants of obese women has also been reported.[430–432a]

Although the mechanism is not known, depletion of folic acid levels and the possibility of undiagnosed pregestational or gestational diabetes have been suspected.

Phenylketonuria

Phenylketonuria (PKU) in women who do not adhere to their phenylalanine-restricted diets leads to a well-recognized pattern of congenital defects, the maternal PKU syndrome (MPKU), characterized by **intrauterine and postnatal growth restriction, microcephaly and mental retardation, cardiovascular defects, dislocated hips**, and other anomalies.[433] These effects are directly related to the maternal phenylalanine level: when the level exceeds 20 mg/dL, 92% of infants have mental retardation, 73%, microcephaly, 40%, IUGR, and 12%, cardiac malformations. A quarter of pregnancies are spontaneously aborted.

The effectiveness of a phenylalanine-restricted diet to prevent the MPKU syndrome has been well established. However many affected women do not adhere to it because of lack of appropriate access to care, insufficient economic resources, and psychological and social issues.[434]

Thyroid disorders (see also Ch. 31)

Congenital hypothyroidism associated with deafness and mental retardation is found in the offspring of hypothyroid mothers. Deafness persists in spite of thyroid replacement therapy. Developmental changes in the brain and cerebellum have been described.[435] Children of women with mild or subclinical maternal hypothyroidism have been reported to perform poorly on neuropsychological tests.[436]

Fetal iodine deficiency results in **cretinism** characterized by mental retardation, spastic diplegia, deafness, and strabismus.[437, 438] It requires severe maternal iodine deficiency (< 20 μg/day) during the first half of gestation, which occurs primarily in Northern Italy and in some mountainous areas of New Guinea, the Himalayas, and the Andes.

Hypothyroidism in infants occurs when the fetal thyroid gland has been suppressed by antithyroid drugs (propylthiouracil, carbimazole, iodides), radioactive iodine,[373] or possibly maternal antibodies.[374]

Iodine is a disinfectant for drinking water; iodide salts (potassium iodide) are expectorants and topical antiseptics. Excess iodine intake is thought to interfere with the development of the fetal thyroid gland when the gland becomes functional, at about 10 weeks' gestation. Iodide preparations implicated in conjunction with fetal goiter include ammonium, potassium, and sodium iodides.

Transfer of maternal thyroxin to the fetus is negligible during early pregnancy. During the final weeks of pregnancy, thyroid-binding globulin (TBG) may compete for thyroxin. Triiodothyronine is less bound by TBG and can more freely cross the placenta. Thyroid-stimulating hormone does not cross the placenta, but immunoglobulins that stimulate the thyroid gland do stimulate the fetal thyroid gland.[439]

Hyperthyroidism during pregnancy is usually due to Graves disease. The presence of thyroid-stimulating globulins may result in thyrotoxicity in the fetus and newborn regardless of the treatment of the maternal disease. **Neonatal thyrotoxicosis** is usually a transient phenomenon commonly lasting several months.[440, 441] Affected infants have goiter, exophthalmos, restlessness and tachycardia, periorbital edema, ravenous appetite, temperature elevations, cardiomegaly, cardiac failure, and hepatosplenomegaly. Craniosynostosis has been reported.[441a]

Systemic lupus erythematosus

Three forms of neonatal lupus erythematosus (NLE) consist of:
- skin lesions only;
- skin lesions associated with systemic manifestations; and
- heart involvement with or without skin manifestations.

NLE is believed to be caused by transplacental transfer of a **maternal IgG antibody to the fetus**. The antibody usually incriminated is **anti-Ro**, but **anti-La** and **anti-U$_1$RNP** have also been implicated.[442] The full clinical expression of NLE is characterized by **cutaneous SLE lesions, congenital heart block, and hematologic abnormalities**.

Uterine and placental implantation abnormalities

Abnormalities of the uterus, including bicornuate uterus and uterus didelphys, uterine fibroids, abnormal placental implantation, and oligohydramnios, may cause fetal compression and constraint, resulting in deformations of the fetus.[205] In addition, uterine malformations predispose to abnormalities of body stalk formation, late fetal cord compression or torsion, and increased risk of stillbirth.[443]

References

Teratogenic disruptions

1. Brent RL, Beckman DA, Landel CP. Clinical teratology. Curr Opin Pediatr 1993; 5:201–211.
2. De Santis M, Carducci B, Cavaliere AF, et al. Drug-induced congenital defects: strategies to reduce the incidence. Drug Saf 2001; 24:889–901.
3. Prolifka JE, Friedman JM. Clinical teratology: identifying teratogenic risks in humans. Clin Genet 1999; 56:409–420.
4. Robert CJ, Lowe CR. Where have all the conceptions gone? Lancet 1975; 1:498–499.
5. Holmes LB. The malformed newborn: practical perspectives. Boston: Developmental Disabilities Council; 1976.
6. Wilson JG. Environmental and birth defects. New York: Academic Press; 1973.
7. Fraser FC. Relation of animal studies to the problem of man. In: Wilson JC, Fraser FC, eds. Handbook of teratology. New York: Plenum Press; 1977:75–96.
8. Kalter H, Warkany J. Medical progress. Congenital malformations etiologic factors and their role in prevention. N Engl J Med 1983; 308:424–431.
9. Shephard TH. Human teratogenicity. Adv Pediatr 1986; 33:225–268.
10. Brent RL, Beckman DA. Etiology of human birth defects, with comments on the role of placental transport of human teratogens. In: Brent RL, Beckman DA, eds. Transplacental disorders, perinatal detection, treatment and management. New York: Alan R Liss; 1990:17–36.
11. Brent RL, Jensh RP. Intrauterine growth retardation. Adv Teratol 1967; 2:139–227.

12. Brent RL. Environmental causes of human congenital malformations: the pediatrician's role in dealing with these complex clinical problems caused by a multiplicity of environmental and genetic factors. Pediatrics 2004; 113: 957–968.

13. Moore KL, Persaud TVN. The developing human: clinically oriented embryology. 5th edn. Philadelphia: WB Saunders; 1993.

14. Bándihi F, Lowry RB, Czeizel AE. Risk and benefit of drug use during pregnancy. Int J Med Sci 200; 2:100–106.

15. Opitz JM. Blastogenesis and the 'primary field' in human development. Birth Defects OAS 1993; 29:3–37.

16. Finnell HF, Gelineau-van Waes J, Eudy JD, et al. Molecular basis of environmentally induced birth defects. Annu Rev Pharmacol Toxicol 2002; 42: 181–208.

17. Frías JL, Thomas IT. Teratogens and teratogenesis: General principles of teratology. Ann Clin Lab Sci 1988; 18:174–179.

18. Prolifka JE, Friedman JM. Medical genetics: 1. Clinical teratology in the age of genomics. CMAJ 2002; 167:265–273.

19. Stevenson RE. Environment causes of malformation. In: Stevenson RE, Hall JG eds. Human malformations and related anomalies. New York: Oxford University Press; 2006:35–58.

20. Newman CGH. Clinical aspects of thalidomide embryopathy – a continuing preoccupation. In: Sever JL, Brent RL, eds. Teratogen update: environmentally induced birth defects risk. New York: Alan R Liss; 1986:1–12.

21. McCredie J, Willert HG. Longitudinal limb deficiencies and the sclerotomes. J Bone Joint Surg (Br) 1999; 81-B:9–23.

22. Holmes LB, Harvey EA, Coull BA, et al. The teratogenicity of anticonvulsant drugs. N Engl J Med 2001; 344:1132–1138.

23. Botto LD, Mastroiacovo P. Exploring gene–gene interactions in the etiology of neural tube defects. Clin Genet 1998; 53:456–459.

24. Diehl RS, Erickson RP. Genome scan for teratogen-induced clefting susceptibility loci in the mouse: evidence of both allelic and locus heterogeneity distinguishing cleft lip and cleft palate. Proc Natl Acad Sci 1997; 94:5231–5236.

25. Hwang SJ, Beaty TH, Panny SR, et al. Association study of transforming growth factor α (TGF α) TaqI polymorphism and oral clefts: indication of gene–environment interaction in a population-based sample of infants with birth defects. Am J Epidemiol 1995; 141:629–636.

26. Stoler JM, Ryan LM, Holmes LB. Alcohol dehydrogenase 2 genotypes, maternal alcohol use, and infant outcome. J Pediatr 2002; 141:780–785.

27. Vieira AR, Avila JR, Daack-Hirsch S, et al. Medical sequencing of candidate genes for nonsyndromic cleft lip and palate. PLoS Genet 2005; 1:e64.

28. Kapron CM, Trasler DG. Genetic determinants of teratogen-induced abnormal development in mouse and rat embryos in vitro. Int J Dev Biol 1997; 41:337–344.

29. Newman LM, Johnson EM, Staples RE. Assessment of the effectiveness of animal developmental toxicity testing for human safety. Reprod Toxicol 1993; 7:359–390.

30. Brent RL. Utilization of animal studies to determine the effects and human risks of environmental toxicants (drugs, chemicals, and physical agents). Pediatrics 2004; 113: 984–995.

31. Larsen JW Jr, Greendale K. Letter to the editor: ACOG Technical Bulletin Number 84, February 1985: Teratology. Teratology 1985; 32:493–496.

32. Brent RL. The cause and prevention of human birth defects: What have we learned in the past 50 years? Cong Anom 2001; 41:9–21.

33. Lo WY, Friedman JM. Teratogenicity of recently introduced medications in human pregnancy. Obstet Gynecol 2002; 100:465–473.

34. Schardein JL.Chemically induced birth defects. 3rd edn. New York: Marcel Dekker; 2000.

Physical agents

35. Brent RL. Utilization of developmental basic science principles in the evaluation of reproductive risks from pre- and post-conception environmental radiation exposures. Teratology 1999; 59:182–204.

36. Brent RL, Bolden BT. The indirect effect of irradiation on embryonic development. IV. The lethal effects of maternal irradiation on the first day of gestation in the rat. Proc Soc Exp Biol Med 1967; 125:709–712.

37. Russell LB. Russell WL. Radiation hazards to the embryo and fetus. Radiology 1952; 58:369–377.

38. Russell LB, Russel WL. An analysis of the changing radiation response of the developing mouse embryo. J Cell Physiol 1954; 43(Suppl 1):103–149.

39. Schull WJ, Otake M, Neel JV. Genetic effects of the atomic bombs, a reappraisal. Science 1981; 213:1220–1227.

40. Brent RL. Radiation teratogenesis. Teratology 1980; 21:281–298.

41. Yoshimoto Y, Kato H, Schull WJ. Risk of cancer among children exposed in utero to A-bomb radiations, 1950–84. Lancet 1988; 2:665–669.

42. Gilman EA, Kneale GW, Knox EG, et al. Pregnancy, x-rays and childhood cancers: effects of exposure age and radiation dose. J Soc Radiol Protection 1987; 8:3–8.

43. Knox EG, Stewart AM, Kneale GW, et al. Prenatal irradiation and childhood cancer. J Soc Radiol Protection 1987; 7:177–189.

44. Plummer G. Anomalies occurring in children exposed in utero to the atomic bomb in Hiroshima. Pediatrics 1952; 10:687.

45. Neel JV, Schull WJ. The effect of exposure to the atomic bombs on pregnancy termination in Hiroshima and Nagasaki. National Academy of Science. Washington: National Research Council publication; 1956.

46. Miller RW. Delayed effects occurring within the first decade after exposure of young individuals to the Hiroshima atomic bomb. Pediatrics 1956; 18:1–18.

47. Otake M, Schull WJ. In utero exposure to A-bomb radiation and mental retardation: a reassessment. Br J Radiol 1984; 57:409–414.

48. Brent RL. The effect of embryonic and fetal exposure to x-ray, microwaves and ultrasound: counseling the pregnant and non-pregnant patient about these risks. Semin Oncol 1989; 16:347.

49. Dekaban A. Abnormalities in children exposed to x-radiation injury to the human fetus. Part 1. J Nucl Med 1968; 9:471–477.

50. McKeen EA, Mulvihil JJ, Rosner F, et al. Pregnancy outcome in Hodgkin's disease. Lancet 1979; 2:590.

51. National Council on Radiation Protection. Medical radiation exposure of pregnant and potentially pregnant women. Report No. 54. Washington: NCRP; 1977.

52. Barish RJ. In-flight radiation exposure during pregnancy. Obstet Gynecol 2004; 103:1326–1330.

53. Fattibene P, Mazzei F, Nuccetelli C, et al. Prenatal exposure to ionizing radiation. Sources, effects, and regulatory aspects. Acta Pediatr 1999; 88:693–702.

54. Kojo K, Pukkala E, Auvinen A. Breast cancer risk among Finnish cabin attendants: a nested case-control study. Occup Environ Med 2005; 62:488–493.

55. Sigurdson AJ, Ron E. Cosmic radiation exposure and cancer risk among flight crew. Cancer Invest 2004; 22:743–761.

56. Orecklin JR. Fertility in patients treated for malignant testicular tumors. J Urol 1973; 109:293–295.

57. Li FP. Outcome of pregnancy in survivors of Wilms' tumor. JAMA 1987; 257:216–219.

58. Fisher WD, Voorhess MI, Gardner LI. Congenital hypothyroidism in infant following maternal I-131 therapy. J Pediatr 1963; 62:132–146.

59. Cooper DS, Ridgway ED. Clinical management of patients with hyperthyroidism. Med Clin North Am 1985; 69:953–971.

60. Hollingsworth DR. Graves disease. Clin Obstet Gynecol 1983; 26:615–634.

61. Romney BM. Radionuclide administration to nursing mothers; mathematically derived guidelines. Radiology 1986; 160:549–554.

62. Rutherford SE, Phelan JP. Thromboembolic disease in pregnancy. Clin Perinatol 1986; 13:719–739.

63. Schardein JL. Chemically induced birth defects. 2nd en. New York: Marcel Dekker; 1993.

64. Kelly-Buchanan C. Peace of mind during pregnancy. New York: Facts on File Publication; 1988.

65. Shepard TH. Catalog of teratogenic agents. 7th edn. Baltimore: Johns Hopkins University Press; 1992.

66. Carstensen EL, Gates AH. The effects of pulsed ultrasound on the fetus. J Ultrasound Med 1984; 3:145–147.

67. McLeod DR, Fowlow SB. Multiple malformations and exposure to therapeutic ultrasound during embryogenesis. Am J Med Genet 1989; 34:317–319.

68. Goldhaber MK, Polen MR, Hiatt RA. The risk of miscarriage and birth defects among women who use video display terminals during pregnancy. Am J Ind Med 1988; 13:695–706.

69. Plect H, Graham JM, Smith DW. Central nervous system and facial defects associated with maternal hyperthermia at 4 to 14 weeks' gestation. Pediatrics 1981; 67:785–789.

70. Smith DW, Clarren SK, Harvey MAS. Hyperthermia as a possible teratogenic agent. J Pediatr 1978; 92:878–883.

71. Shiota K. Neural tube defects and maternal hyperthermia in early pregnancy: epidemiology in a human embryonic population. Am J Med Genet 1982; 12:281–288.

72. Fisher NL, Smith DW. Hyperthermia as a possible cause of occipital encephalocoele. Clin Res 1980; 28:116A.

73. Edwards MJ. Congenital defects in guinea pigs: fetal resorptions, abortions and malformations following induced hyperthermia during gestation. Teratology 1969; 2:313.

74. Edwards MJ. Congenital defects in guinea pigs following induced hyperthermia during gestation. Arch Pathol 1967; 84:42.

75. Edwards MJ. The experimental production of clubfoot in guinea pigs by maternal hyperthermia during gestation. J Pathol 1971; 103:49.

76. Clarren SK, Smith DW, Harvey MAS, et al. Hyperthermia – a prospective evaluation of a possible teratogenic agent in man. J Pediatr 1979; 95:81–83.

77. Fisher NI, Smith DW. Occipital encephalocele and early gestational hyperthermia. Pediatrics 1981; 68:480–483.

78. Miller P, Smith DW, Shepard T. Maternal hyperthermia as a possible cause of anencephaly. Lancet 1978; 1:519–521.

79. Jones KL. Smith's. Recognizable patterns of human malformations 6th ed. Philadelphia: Elsevier Saunders; 2006.

80. Supernau DW, Wertelecki W. Brief clinical report: similarity of effects – experimental hyperthermia as a teratogen and maternal febrile illness associated with oromandibular and limb defects. Am J Med Genet 1985; 21: 575–580.

81. Lipson AH, Webster WS, Brown-Woodman PDC, et al. Möbius syndrome: animal model – human correlations and evidence for a brainstem vascular etiology. Teratology 1989; 40:339.

82. Jones MC, Kosaki K, Bird LM. Disruptive defects of the brain and spinal cord as a consequence of cardiopulmonary bypass and hypothermia at 18 weeks gestation. Proc Greenwood Genet Ctr 1995; 14:58.

Infectious agents

83. Sever JL, Larsen JW, Grossman JH. Handbook of perinatal infections. Boston: Little, Brown; 1979.

84. Beckman DA, Brent RL. Mechanism of known environmental teratogens: drugs and chemicals. Clin Perinatol 1986; 13:649–687.

85. Mehraein Y, Rehder H, Draeger HG, et al. Diagnosis of fetal virus infections by in situ hybridization. Geburtshilfe Frauenheilkd 1991; 51:984–989.

86. Marion RW, Wiznia AA, Hutcheon RC, et al. Human T-cell lymphotropic virus type II (tiv-III) embryopathy. Am J Dis Child 1986; 140:638–640.

87. Cordero JF. Issues concerning AIDS embryopathy. Am J Dis Child 1988; 142:9.

88. Oleske J, Minnefor A, Cooper RJ, et al. Immune deficiency syndrome in children. JAMA 1983; 249:3245–2349.

89. Rubinstein A, Sicklick M, Gupta A, et al. Acquired immunodeficiency with reversed T4-T8 ratios in infants born to promiscuous and drug-addicted mothers. JAMA 1983; 249:2350–2356.

90. Scott GB, Bucke BE, Letterman JG, et al. Acquired immunodeficiency syndrome in infants. N Engl J Med 1984; 310:76–81.

91. Peterman TA, Drotman DP, Curran JW. Epidemiology of acquired immunodeficiency syndrome (AIDS). Epidemiol Rev 1985; 7:1–21.

92. Iosub S, Bamji M, Stone RK, et al. More on human immunodeficiency virus embryopathy. Pediatrics 1987; 80:512–516.

93. Zhang J, Wen-wei C. Association of the common cold in the first trimester of pregnancy with birth defects. Pediatrics 1993; 92:559–563.

94. Brown GC, Evans TN. Serologic evidence of coxsackievirus etiology of congenital heart disease. JAMA 1967; 199:183–187.

95. Gauntt CG, Gudvangen RJ, Brans YW, et al. Coxsackievirus group B antibodies in the ventricular fluid of infants with severe anatomic defects in the central nervous system. Pediatrics 1985; 76:64–68.

96. Avery ME, Taeusch HW Jr. Schaffer's diseases of the newborn. 5th edn. Philadelphia: WB Saunders; 1984.

97. Nahmias AJ, Josey WE, Naib ZM, et al. Antibodies to herpesvirus hominis types 1 and 2 in humans. In. Patients with genital herpes infection. Am J Epidemiol 1970; 91:539–546.

98. Stagno S. Cytomegalovirus. In: Remington JS, Klein JO, eds. Infectious diseases of the fetus and newborn infant. 5th edn. Philadelphia: WB Saunders; 2001:389–424.

99. Nigro G, Adler SP, La Torre R, et al. Passive immunization during pregnancy for congenital cytomegalovirus infection. N Engl J Med 2005; 353:1350–1362.

100. Fowler KB, Boppana SB. Congenital cytomegalovirus (CMV) infection and hearing deficit. J Clin Virol 2006; 35:226–231.

101. Adler SP, Hempfling SH, Starr SE, et al. Safety and immunogenicity of the Towne strain cytomegalovirus vaccine. Pediatr Infect Dis J 1998; 17:200–206.

102. Pass RF, Duliege AM, Boppana S, et al. A subunit cytomegalovirus vaccine based on recombinant envelope glycoprotein b and a new adjuvant. J Infect Dis 1999; 180:970–975.

103. Hutto C, Arvin A, Jacobs R, et al. Intrauterine herpes simplex virus infections. J Pediatr 1987; 110:97–101.

104. Vasileiadis GT, Roukema HW, Romano W, et al. Intrauterine herpes simplex infection. Am J Perinatol 2003; 20:55–58.

105. Montgomery J, Flanders RW, Tow MD. Congenital anomalies and herpesvirus infection. Am J Dis Child 1973; 126:364–366.

106. Sullender WM, Arvin AM, Diaz PS, et al. Type-specific antibodies to herpes simplex virus type 2 (HSV-2) glycoprotein G in pregnant women, infants exposed to maternal HSV-2 infection at delivery, and infants with neonatal herpes. J Infect Dis 1988; 157:164–171.

107. Whitley RJ. Herpes simplex virus. In: Fields B, Knippe D, Howley P, eds. Fields virology. 3rd edn. Philadelphia: Lippincott-Raven; 1995:2297–2333.

108. Arvin A, Whitley RJ. Herpes simplex virus infections. In: Remington JS, Klein JO, eds. Infectious diseases of the fetus and newborn infant. 5th edn. Philadelphia: WB Saunders; 2001:425–446.

109. Botto LD, Lynberg MC, Erickson JD. Congenital heart defects, maternal febrile illness, and multivitamin use: a population-based study. Epidemiology 2001; 12: 485–490.

110. Martínez-Frías ML, Garcia Mazario MJ, Caldas CT, et al. High maternal fever during gestation and severe congenital limb disruption. Am J Med Genet 2001; 98: 201–203.

111. Acs N, Bánhidy F, Puhó E, et al. Maternal influenza during pregnancy and risk of congenital abnormalities in offspring. Birth Defects Res A: Clin Mol Teratol 2005; 73:989–996.

112. Ackermann R, Stammler A, Armbruster B. Isolation of the lymphocytic choriomeningitis virus from curettage material after contact of the pregnant woman with a Syrian gold hamster (Mesocricetus auratus). Infection 1975; 3:47–49.

113. Barton LL, Mets MB, Beauchamp CL. Lymphocytic choriomeningitis virus: emerging fetal teratogen. Am J Obstet Gynecol 2002; 187:1715–1716.

114. Wright R, Johson D, Neumann D, et al. Congenital lymphocytic choriomoningitis virus syndrome: a disease that mimics congenital toxoplasmosis or Cytomegalovirus infection. Pediatrics 1997; 100:e9.

115. Enders G, Varho-Göbel M, Löhler J, et al. Congenital lymphocytic choriomeningitis virus infection: an underdiagnosed disease. Ped Infect Dis J 1999; 18:652–655.

116. CDC. Interim guidance for minimizing risk for human lymphocytic choriomeningitis virus infection associated with rodents. Morb Mortal Wkly Rep 2005; 54:747–749.

117. Carrington D. Maternal serum α-fetoprotein – a marker of fetal aplastic crisis during intrauterine human parvovirus infection. Lancet 1987; 1:433–435.

118. Schwarz TF, Nerlich A, Hottenrager B, et al. Parvovirus B19 infection of the fetus. Histology and in situ hybridization. Am J Clin Pathol 1991; 96:121–126.

119. Weiland HT, Vermey-Keers C, Salimans MM, et al. Parvovirus B19 associated with fetal abnormality. Lancet 1987; 1:682–683.

120. Knisely AS, O'Shea PA, McMillan P, et al. Electron microscopic identification of parvovirus virions in erythroid-line cells in fatal hydrops fetalis. Pediatr Pathol 1988; 8:163–170.

121. Miller RK, Cradock-Watson JE, Pollock TM. Consequences of confirmed rubella at successive stages of pregnancy. Lancet 1982; 2:781–784.

122. Naeye RI, Blanc WA. Pathogenesis of congenital rubella. JAMA 1965; 94: 1277–1283.

123. Menser MA, Forrest JM, Bransby RD. Rubella infection and diabetes mellitus. Lancet 1978; 1:57–60.

124. Best JM. Rubella vaccines: past, present and future. Epidemiol Infect 1991; 107:17–30.

125. Rubella prevention recommendations of the Immunization Practices Advisory Committee (ACIP). MMWR Recomm Rep 1990; 39(RR-15):1–18.

126. Ingall D, Sánchez PJ. Syphilis. In: Remington JS, Klein JO, eds. Infectious diseases of the fetus and newborn infant 5th ed. Philadelphia: WB Saunders; 2006:643–681.

127. Harter CA, Benirschke K. Fetal syphilis in the first trimester. Am J Obstet Gynecol 1976; 124:705–711.

128. Putkonen T. Does early treatment prevent dental changes in congenital syphilis? Acta Derm Venereol 1963; 43:240–249.

129. Abler C. Neonatal varicella. Am J Dis Child 1964; 107:492–494.

130. Sever JL, Ellenberg JH, Ley AC, et al. Toxoplasmosis: maternal and pediatric findings in 23,000 pregnancies. Pediatrics 1988; 82:181–192.

131. Alkalay AL, Pomerance JJ, Rimoin DL. Fetal varicella syndrome. J Pediatr 1987; 111:320–323.

132. Paryani SG, Arvin AM. Intrauterine infection with varicella-zoster virus after maternal varicella. N Engl J Med 1986; 314:1542–1546.

133. Reprotox database. Washington: Reproductive Toxicology Center; 1990.

134. Rico-Hesse R, Weaver SC, de Siger J, et al. Emergence of a new epidemic/epizootic Venezuelan equine encephalitis virus in South America. Proc Natl Acad Sci 1995; 92:5278–5281.

135. Wang E, Bowen RA, Medina G, et al. Cysticercosis Working Group in Peru: Virulence and viremia characteristics of 1992 epizootic subtype IC Venezuelan equine encephalitis viruses and closely related enzootic subtype ID strains. Am J Trop Med Hyg 2001; 65:64–69.

136. Weaver SC, Salas R, Rico-Hesse R, et al. Re-emergence of epidemic Venezuelan equine encephalomyelitis in South America. VEE Study Group. Lancet 1996; 348:436–440.

137. Andersonn RC, Horn KB, Hoang MP, et al. Punctate exanthem of West Nile Virus infection: report of 3 cases. J Am Acad Dermatol 2004; 51:820–823.

138. Macedo de Oliveira A, Beecham BD, Montgomery SP, et al. West Nile virus blood transfusion-related infection despite nucleic acid testing. Transfusion 2004; 44:1695–1699.

139. Wadei H, Alangaden GJ, Sillix DH, et al. West Nile virus encephalitis: an emerging disease in renal transplant recipients. Clin Transplant 2004; 18:753–758.

140. CDC. Intrauterine West Nile virus infection – New York, 2002. Morb Mortal Wkly Rep 2002; 51:1135–1136.

141. Alpert SG, Fergerson J, Noel LP. Intrauterine West Nile virus: ocular and systemic findings. Am J Ophthalmol 2003; 136:733–735.

142. Bruno J, Rabito FJ, Dildy GA. West Nile virus meningoencephalitis during pregnancy. J La State Med Soc 2004; 156:204–205.

143. CDC. Interim guidelines for the evaluation of infants born to mothers infected with West Nile virus during pregnancy. Morb Mortal Wkly Rep 2004; 53:154–157.

144. Siegel M, Greenberg M. Poliomyelitis in pregnancy. Effect on fetus and newborn infant. J Pediatr 1956; 49:280–288.

145. Moss PD, Heffernan CK, Thurston JG. Enteroviruses and congenital abnormalities. Br Med J 1967; 1:110–111.

146. Lin HH, Lee TY, Chen DS, et al. Transplacental leakage of HBeAg-positive maternal blood as the most likely route in causing intrauterine infection with hepatitis B virus. J Pediatr 1987; 111:877–881.

147. MacDonald AB. Gestational Lyme borreliosis. Implication for the fetus. Rheum Dis Clin North Am 1989; potentially 15:657–677.

Potentially teratogenic drugs and chemicals

148. CDC. Epidemiologic notes and reports. Isotretinoin – A newly recognized human tetratogen. Morb Mortal Wkly Rep 1984; 33:171–173.

149. Wilhite CC, Hill RM, Irving DW. Isotretinoin-induced craniofacial malformations in humans and hamsters. J Craniofac Genet Dev Biol Suppl. 1986; 2:193–209.

150. The Teratology Society. Recommendations for vitamin A use during pregnancy. Teratology 1987; 35:269–275.

151. Lammer EJ, Chen DT, Hoar RM, et al. Retinoic acid embryopathy. N Engl J Med 1985; 313:837–841.

152. Coberly S, Lammer E, Alashari M. Retinoic acid embryopathy: case report and review of the literature. Pediatr Pathol Lab Med 1996; 16:823–836.

153. Dobyns NB. Developmental aspects of lissencephaly and the lissencephaly syndrome. Birth Defects 1987; 23:225–241.

154. Mitchell AA, van Pennekon CM, Louik C. A pregnancy-prevention program in women of child-bearing age receiving isotretinoin. N Engl J Med 1995; 333:101–106.

155. Sporn M, Roberts A, Goodman D. Cellular biology and biochemistry of retinoids. New York: Raven Press; 1994.

156. Holmes LB. Fetal environmental toxins. Pediatr Rev 1992; 13:364–369.

157. Jick SS, Terris BZ, Jick H. First trimester tropical tretinoin and congenital disorders. Lancet 1993; 341:1181–1182.

158. Di Giovanna JJ, Zech LA, Ruddel ME, et al. Etretinate. Persistent serum levels after long-term therapy. Arch Dermatol 1989; 125:246–251.

159. Barbero P, Lotersztein V, Bronberg R, et al. Acitretin embryopathy: A case report. Birth Defects Res A: Clin Mol Terat 2004; 70:831–833.

160. de Die-Smulders CEM, Sturkenboom MCJM, Veraart J, et al. Severe limb defects and craniofacial abnormalities in a fetus conceived during acitretin therapy. Teratology 1995; 52: 215–219.

161. Jones and Smith 1973. Recognition of the fetal alcohol syndrome in early infancy. Lancet 1973; 2:999–1001.

162. Jones KL, Smith DW, Ulleland CN, et al. Pattern of malformation in offspring of chronic alcoholic mothers. Lancet 1973; 1:1267–1271.

163. CDC. Update: trends in fetal alcohol syndrome – United States, 1979–1993. Morb Mortal Wkly Rep 1995; 44:249–251.

164. CDC. Surveillance for fetal alcohol syndrome using multiple sources – Atlanta, Georgia, 1981–1989. Morb Mortal Wkly Rep 1997; 46:1118–1120.

165. CDC. Fetal alcohol syndrome – Alaska, Arizona, Colorado, and New York, 1995–1997. Morb Mortal Wkly Rep 2002; 51:433–435.

166. Stratton K, Howe C, Battaglia F. Fetal alcohol syndrome: diagnosis, epidemiology, prevention, and treatment. Washington: Institute of Medicine, National Academy Press; 1996.

167. Bertrand J, Floyd RL, Weber MK. Guidelines for identifying and referring persons with fetal alcohol syndrome. Morb Mortal Wkly Rep 2005; 54:1–10.

168. Briggs GG. Drugs in pregnancy and lactation. 3rd edn. Baltimore: Williams & Wilkins; 1990.

169. Potter BJ, Hetzel BS. Fetal alcohol syndrome. In: Hetzel BS, Smith RM, eds. Fetal brain disorders – recent approaches to the problem of mental deficiency. New York: Elsevier/North-Holland; 1981.

170. Jones KL. Fetal alcohol syndrome. Pediatr Rev 1986; 8:122–126.

171. Clarren SK, Alvord EC, Sumi SM, et al. Brain malformations related to prenatal exposure to ethanol. J Pediatr 1978; 92:64–67.

171a. Romero R, Pilu G, Jeanty P. Prenatal diagnosis of congenital anomalies. New York: Appleton and Lange 1988:115.

172. Christoffel KK, Salafsy I. Fetal alcohol syndrome in dizygotic twins. J Pediatr 1975; 87:963–967.

173. Little RE, Sing CF. Fathers' drinking and infant birth weight: report of an association. Teratology 1987; 26:59–65.

174. Tze WJ, Friesen HG, MacLeod PM. Growth hormone response in fetal alcohol syndrome. Arch Dis Child 1976; 51:703–706.

175. Kumar SP. Fetal alcohol syndrome, mechanisms of teratogenesis. Ann Clin Lab Sci 1982; 12:254–257.

176. Gilbert EF, Khoury GH. Dextroamphetamine and congenital cardiac malformations (Letter to the Editor). J Pediatr 1970; 76:638.

177. Grumbach MM, Hughes LA, Conte FA. Disorders of sex differentiation. In: Williams Textbook of Endocrinology 10th ed. Larsen PR, Kronenberg HM, Melmod S, Polonsky KS, eds. Philadelphia: WB Saunders 2003:842–1002.

178. O'Brien PC, Noller KL, Robboy SJ, et al. Vaginal epithelial changes in young women enrolled in the National Cooperation Diethylstilbestrol Adenosis (DESAD) Project. Obstet Gynecol 1979; 53:300–308.

179. Grunwaldt E, Bates T. Nonadrenal female pseudohermaphroditism after administration of testosterone to mother during pregnancy. Report of a case. Pediatrics 1957; 20:503–505.

180. Merke D, Bornstein S. Congenital adrenal hyperplasia. Lancet 2005; 365: 2125–2136.

181. Manganiello PD, Adams LV, Harris RD, et al. Virilization during pregnancy with spontaneous resolution postpartum a case report and review of the English literature. Obstet Gynecol Surv 1995; 50:404–410.

182. Wang YC, Su HY, Liu JY, et al. Maternal and female fetal virilization caused by pregnancy luteomas. Fertil Steril 2005; 84:509e15–509e17.

183. Forest MG. Ambiguous genitalia/intersex: endocrine aspects. In: Gearhart JP, Rink RC, Mouriquand PDE, eds. Pediatric urology. Philadelphia: WB

Saunders; 2001, vol I:623–658.

184. Forest MG, Nicolino M, David M, et al. The virilized female: endocrine background. BJU Int 2004; 93 (suppl 3):35–43.

185. Brent RL, Beckman DA. Angiotensin-converting enzyme inhibitors, an embryopathic class of drugs with unique properties: information for clinical teratology counselors. Teratology 1991; 43:543–546.

186. Barr M. Teratogen update: angiotensin-converting enzyme inhibitors. Teratology 1994; 50:399–409.

187. Shotan A, Widerhorn J, Hurst A, et al. Risks of angiotensin-converting enzyme inhibition during pregnancy: experimental and clinical evidence, potential mechanisms, and recommendations for use. Am J Med 1994; 96:451–446.

187a. Cooper WO, Hernandez-Diaz S, Arbogast PG, et al. Major congenital malformations after first-trimester exposure to ACE inhibitors. N Engl J Med 2006; 354:2443–2451.

188. Jones KL, Chambers CC, Johnson KA. The effect of disulfiram on the unborn baby. Teratology 1991; 43:438.

189. Nora AH. Limb reduction in infants born to disulfiram-treated alcoholic mothers. Lancet 1977; 2:664.

190. Koren G. Maternal-fetal toxicology: a clinician's guide. 2nd edn. New York: Marcel Dekker; 1994.

191. Helmbrecht G, Iffath A. First trimester disulfiram exposure: report of two cases. Am J Perinatol 1993; 10:5–7.

192. Wilson JG, Fraser FC. Handbook of teratology. Vol 1. New York: Plenum Press; 1977.

193. Berkowitz RL. Handbook for prescribing medications during pregnancy. 2nd edn. Boston: Little, Brown; 1986.

193a. Ornoy A. Neuroteratogens in man: an overview with special emphasis on the teratogenicity of antiepileptic drugs in pregnancy. Reprod Toxicol 2006; 22:214–226.

194. Fischel-Ghodsian N, Prezant TR, Fournier P, et al. Mitochondrial mutation associated with nonsyndromic deafness. Am J Otolaryngol 1995; 16:403–408.

195. Guan MX. Molecular pathogenetic mechanism of maternally inherited deafness. Ann NY Acad Sci 2004; 1011: 259–271.

196. Kallen B. Epidemiology of human reproduction. London: CRC Press; 1988.

197. Jones KL. Pattern of malformations in the children of women treated with carbamazepine during pregnancy. N Engl J Med 1989; 320:1061–1066.

198. Hanson JW, Smith DW. The fetal hydontion syndrome. J Pediatr 1975; 87:285–290.

199. Friedman JM. Effects of drugs and other chemicals on fetal growth. Growth Genet 1992; 8:1–5.

200. Killpatrick CJ, Moulds RF. Anticonvulsants in pregnancy. Med J Aust 1991; 154:199–202.

201. Speidel BD, Meadow SR. Maternal epilepsy and abnormalities of the fetus and newborn. Lancet 1972; 2:839–843.

202. Hanson JW. Fetal hydantoin effects. In: Severe JL, Brent RI, eds. Teratogen update: environmentally induced birth defect risks. New York: Alan R Liss; 1986:29–33.

203. Gaily E, Granstrom ML, Hiilesmaa V. Minor anomalies in offspring of epileptic mothers. J Pediatr 1988; 112:520–529.

204. Buehler BA, Delimont D, Van Waes M, et al. Prenatal prediction of risk of the fetal hydantoin syndrome. N Engl J Med 1990; 322:1567–1571.

205. Gilbert EF, Optiz JM. Congenital anomalies and malformation syndromes. In: Stocker JT, Dehner L, eds. Pediatric pathology. Philadelphia: JB Lippincott; 1992.

206. Van Allen MI. Increased major and minor malformations in infants of epileptic mothers: preliminary results of the pregnancy and epilepsy study. Am J Hum Genet 1988; 43:A73.

207. Hernández-Díaz S, Werler MM, Walker AM, et al. Neural tube defects in relation to use of folic acid antagonists during pregnancy. Am J Epidemiol 2001; 153:961–968.

208. Matalon S, Schechtman S, Goldzweig G, et al. The teratogenic effect of carbamazepine: a meta-analysis of 1255 exposures. Reprod Toxicol 2002; 16:9–17.

209. Samren EB, van Duijn CM, Cristianes GC, et al. Antiepileptic drug regimens and major congenital abnormalities in the offspring. Ann Neurol 1999; 46:739–746.

210. Finnell RH. Teratology: general considerations and principles. J Allergy Clin Immunol 1999; 103:S337–S342.

211. Heinonen OP. Birth defects and drugs in pregnancy, Littleton: Publishing Sciences Group; 1977.

212. Rothman KJ, Fyler DC, GoldblattbA, et al. Exogenous hormones and other drug exposures of children with congenital heart disease. Am J Epidemiol 1979; 109:433–439.

213. Dansky LV, Finnell RH. Parental epilepsy, anticonvulsant drugs, and reproductive outcome. Epidemiologic and experimental findings spanning 3 decades; 2: Human studies. Reprod Toxicol 1991; 5:301–335.

214. Reinisch JM, Sanders SA, Rubin DB. In utero exposure to phenobarbital and intelligence deficits in adult men. JAMA 1995; 724:1518–1525.

215. Cotariu D, Zaidman JL. Developmental toxicity of valproic acid. Life Sci 1991; 48:1341–1350.

216. Yerby MS, Leavitt A, Erickson DM. Antiepileptics and the development of congenital anomalies. Neurology 1992; 42(suppl 5):132–140.

217. DiLiberti JH, Farrndon PA, Dennis NR, et al. The fetal valproate syndrome. Am J Med Genet 1984; 19:473–481.

218. Robert E, Guibaud P. Maternal valproic acid and congenital neural tube defects. Lancet 1982; 2:937.

219. Lindhout D, Omtzigt JG, Cornel MC. Spectrum of neural-tube defects in 34 infants prenatally exposed to antiepileptic drugs. Neurology 1992; 42(suppl 5):111–118.

220. Omtzigt JG, Los FJ, Grobbee DE, et al. The risk of spina bifida aperta in first-trimester exposure to valproate in a prenatal cohort. Neurology 1992; 42(suppl 5):119–125.

221. Finnell RH. Genetic differences in susceptibility to anticonvulsant drug-induced developmental defects. Pharmacol Toxicol 1991; 69:223–227.

222. Smithells RW. Environmental teratogens of man. Br Med Bull 1976; 32:27–33.

223. Van Allen M, Jilek-Aall, Rwiza HT, et al. Possible fetal chloroquine syndrome. Proc Greenwood Genet Ctr 1995; 14:15.

224. Simpson WJ. A preliminary report of cigarette smoking and the incidence of prematurity. Am J Obstet Gynecol 1957; 73:808–815.

225. Kramer MS. Socioeconomic determinants of intrauterine growth retardation. Eur J Clin Nutr 1998; 52(suppl 1):529–533.

226. Wang X, Zuckerman B, Pearson C, et al. Maternal cigarette smoking, metabolic gene polymorphism, and infant birth weight. JAMA 2002; 287:195–202.

227. Naeye RL. Environmental influences on the embryo and early fetus. In: Naeye RL, ed. Disorders of the placenta, fetus, and neonate: diagnosis and clinical significance. St Louis: Mosby-Year Book; 1989.

228. Chung KC, Kowalski CP, Kim HM, et al. Maternal cigarette smoking during pregnancy and the risk of having a child with cleft lip/palate. Plast Reconstr Surg 2000; 105:485–491.

229. Ericson A, Kallen B, Westerholm P. Cigarette smoking as an etiologic factor in cleft lip and palate. Am J Obstet Gynecol 1979; 135:348–351.

230. Khoury MJ, Weinstein A, Panny S, et al. Maternal cigarette smoking and oral clefts: a population-based study. Am J Public Health 1987; 77:623–625.

231. Khoury MJ, Gomez-Farias M, Mulinare J. Does maternal cigarette smoking during pregnancy cause cleft lip and palate in offspring? Am J Dis Child 1989; 143:333–337.

232. Meyer KA, Williams P, Hernandez-Diaz S, et al. Smoking and the risk of oral clefts: exploring the impact of study designs. Epidemiology 2004; 15:671–678.

233. Wysyzynski DF, Duffy DL, Beaty TH. Maternal cigarette smoking and oral clefts: a meta-analysis. Cleft Palate Craniofac J 1997; 34:206–210.

234. Shaw GM, Velie EM, Schaffer D. Risk of neural tube defect-affected pregnancies among obese women. JAMA 1996; 275:1093–1096.

235. van Rooij IALM, Wegerif MJM, Roelofs HMJ, et al. Smoking, genetic polymorphisms in biotransformation enzymes, and nonsyndromic oral clefting: a gene–environment interaction. Epidemiology 2001; 12:502–507.

236. Trease GE, Evans WC. The pharmacological action of plant drugs. In: Trease GE, Evans WC, eds. Pharmacognosy. 12th edn. London: Bailliere Tindall; 1983:147–154.

237. Landesman-Dwyer S, Landesman-Dwyer IE, Emmanuel I. Smoking during pregnancy. Teratology 1979; 19:119–125.

238. Bureau MA, Monette J, Shapcott D, et al. Carboxyhemoglobin concentration in fetal cord blood and in blood of mothers who smoked during labor. Pediatrics 1982; 69:371–373.

239. Bottoms SF, Kuhnert DD, Kuhnert PM, et al. Maternal passive smoking and fetal serum thiocyanate levels. Am J Obstet Gynecol 1982; 144:787–791.

240. Curet LB, Rao AV, Zachman RD, et al. Maternal smoking and respiratory distress syndrome. Am J Obstet Gynecol 1983; 147:446–450.

241. Gluck L, Kulovich MV. Lecithin/sphingomyelin ratios in amniotic fluid in normal and abnormal pregnancy. Am J Obstet Gynecol 1973; 115:539–546.

242. Walsh RA. Effects of maternal smoking on adverse pregnancy outcomes: examination of the criteria of causation. Hum Biol 1994; 66:1059–1092.

243. Cregler LL, Mark H. Medical complications of cocaine abuse. N Engl J Med 1986; 315:1495–1500.

244. Hodach RJ, Hodach AE, Fallon JF, et al. The role of β-adrenergic activity in the production of cardiac and aortic arch anomalies in the chick embryo. Teratology 1975; 12:33–45.

245. Little BB, Snell LM, Klein VR, et al. Cocaine abuse during pregnancy: maternal and fetal implications. Obstet Gynecol 1989; 73:157–160.

246. Behnke M, Eyler FD, Garvan CW, et al. The search for congenital malformations in newborns with fetal cocaine exposure. Pediatrics 2001; 107:e74.

247. Volpe JJ. Mechanisms of disease: effect of cocaine use on the fetus. N Engl J Med 1992; 327:399–407.

248. Bateman DA, Chiriboga CA. Dose-response effect of cocaine on newborn head circumference. Pediatrics 2000; 106:e33.

249. Pexider T. Teratogens. In: Pierpont ME, Moller JH, eds. Genetics of cardiovascular disease. Boston: Martinus Nijhoff; 1986:25–68.

250. Doll DC, Ringenberg S, Yarbro JW. Antineoplastic agents and pregnancy. Semin Oncol 1989; 16:337–346.

251. Nicholson HO. Cytotoxic drugs in pregnancy. J Obstet Gynaecol Br Commonw 1968; 75:307–312.

252. Mirkes PE. Cyclophosphamide teratogenesis: a review. Teratog Carcinog Mutagen 1985; 5:75–88.

253. Greenberg LH, Tanaka KR. Congenital anomalies probably induced by cyclophosphamide. JAMA 1964; 188:423–426.

254. Toledo TM, Harper RC, Moser RH. Fetal effects during cyclophosphamide and irradiation therapy. Ann Intern Med 1971; 74:87–91.

255. Shepard TH, Fantel AG. Teratology of therapeutic agents. In: Iffy L, Kaminetzky HA, eds. Principles and practice of obstetrics and perinatology. New York: John Wiley; 1981:461–481.

256. Goetsch C. An evaluation of aminopterin as an abortifacient. Am J Obstet Gynecol 1962; 83:1474–1477.

257. Powell HR, Ekert H. Methotrexate-induced congenital malformations. Med J Aust 1971; 2:1076–1077.

258. Milunsky A, Graef JW, Gaynor MF. Methotrexate-induced congenital malformations with a review of the literature. J Pediatr 1968; 72:790–795.

259. Schou M, Amdisen A, Steenstroup OR. Lithium and pregnancy II. Hazards to women given lithium during pregnancy and delivery. Br Med J 1973; 21:137–138.

260. Schardein JL. Congenital abnormalities and hormones during pregnancy: a clinical review. Teratology 1980; 22:251–270.

261. Graham JM Jr, Marin-Padilla M, Hoefnagel D. Jejunal atresia associated with Cafergot ingestion during pregnancy. Clin Pediatr 1983; 22:226–228.

262. Raymond GV. Tertogen update: ergot and ergotamine. Teratology 1995; 51:344–347.

263. Czeizel A. Teratogenicity of ergotamine. J Med Genet 1989; 26:69–70.

264. Kullander S, Kallen B. A prospective study of drugs and pregnancy. 3. Hormones. Acta Obstet Gynecol Scand 1976; 55:221–224.

265. Hoffman F, Overzier C, Uhde G. Zur Frage der hormonalen Erzeugung fötaler Zwittenbildungen beim Menschen. Geburtshilfe Frauenheipkd 1955; 15:1061–1070.

266. Janerich DT, Piper JM, Glebatis DM. Oral contraceptives and congenital limb-reduction defects. N Engl J Med 1974; 291:697–700.

267. Levy EP, Cohen A, Frase FC. Hormone treatment during pregnancy and congenital heart defects. Lancet 1973; 1:611.

268. Nora JJ, Nora AH, Blu J, et al. Exogenous progestogen and estrogen implicated in birth defects. JAMA 1978; 240:837.

269. Nora JJ, Nora HA. Birth defects and oral contraceptives. Lancet 1973; 1:941.

270. Janerich DT, Piper JM, Glebatis DM. Oral contraceptives and congenital limb-reduction defects. N Engl J Med 1974; 291:697–700.

271. Heinonen OP, Stone D, Monson RR, et al. Cardiovascular birth defects and antenatal exposure to female sex hormones. N Engl J Med 1977; 296:67–70.

272. Gal I, Kirman B, Stern J. Hormonal pregnancy tests and congenital malformations. Nature 1967; 216:83.

273. Wilson JG. Teratogenic effects of environmental chemicals. Fed Proc1977; 36:1698.

274. Yasuda M, Miller JR. Prenatal exposure to oral contraceptives and transposition of the great vessels in man. Teratology 1975; 12:239–243.

275. Lammer EJ, Cordero JF. Exogenous sex hormone exposure and the risk for major malformations. JAMA 1986; 255:3128–3132.

276. Yovich JL, Turner SR, Draper R. Medroxyprogesterone acetate therapy in early pregnancy has no apparent fetal effects. Teratology 1988; 38:135–144.

277. Wiseman RA, Dodds-Smith IC. Cardiovascular birth defects and antenatal exposure to female sex hormones: a reevaluation of some base data. Teratology 1984; 30:359–370.

278. Sharpe RM, Skakkebaek NE. Are oestrogens involved in falling sperm counts and disorders of the male reproductive tract? Lancet 1993; 341:1392–1395.

279. Carmichael SL, Shaw GM, Laurent C, et al. Maternal progestin intake and risk of hypospadias. Arch Pediatr Adolesc Med 2005; 159:957–962.

280. Smithells RW, Sheppard S, Schorah CJ. Vitamin deficiencies and neural tube defects. Arch Dis Child 1976; 51:944–950.

281. Mulinare J, Cordero JF, Erickson JD, et al. Periconceptional use of multivitamins and the occurrence of neural tube defects. JAMA 1988; 260:3141–3145.

282. Bower C, Stanley FJ. Dietary folate as a risk for the neural-tube defects: evidence from a case-control study in Western Australia. Med J Aust 1989; 150:613–619.

283. Shaw GM, Schaffer D, Velie EM, et al. Periconceptional vitamin use, dietary folate, and the occurrence of neural tube defects. Epidemiology 1995; 6:219–226.

284. Milunsky A, Jick H, Jick SS, et al. Multivitamin/folic acid supplementation in early pregnancy reduces the prevalence of neural tube defects. JAMA 1989; 262:2847–2852.

285. Berry RJ, Li Z, Erickson JD, et al. Prevention of neural tube defects with folic acid in China. N Engl J Med 1999; 341:1485–1490.

286. Werler MM, Shapiro S, Mitchell AA. Periconceptional folic acid exposure and risk of occurrent neural tube defects. JAMA 1993; 269:1257–1261.

287. Hall JG, Solhedin F. Folate and its various ramifications. Adv Pediat 1998; 45:1–35.

288. Johnston RB. Folic acid: new dimensions of an old friendship. Adv Pediat 1997; 44:231–261.

289. Rosenblatt DS, Fenton WA. Inherited disorders of folate and cobalamin transport and metabolism. In: Scriver CR, Beaudet AL, Valle D, et al, eds. The metabolic and molecular bases of inherited disease. 8th edn. Vol 3. New York: McGraw-Hill; 2001:3897–3933.

290. Botto LD, Moore CA, Khoury MJ, et al. Neural-tube defects. N Engl J Med 1999; 341: 1509–1519.

291. CDC. Recommendation for the use of folic acid to reduce the number of cases of spina bifida and other neural tube defects. Morb Mortal Wkly Rep1992; 41(RR-14):001.

292. CDC. Spina bifida and anencephaly before and after folic acid mandate – United States, 1995–1996 and 1999–2000. Morb Mortal Wkly Rep 2004; 53:362–365.

293. Warkany J. Teratogen update: lithium. Teratology 1988; 38:593–597.

294. Cohen LS, Friedman JM, Jefferson JW, et al. A reevaluation of risk of in utero exposure to lithium. JAMA 1994; 271:146–150.

295. Jacobson SJ. Prospective multicentre study of pregnancy outcome after lithium exposure during first trimester. Lancet 1992; 339:530–533.

296. Shepard TH, Brent RL, Friedman JM, et al. Update on new developments in the study of human teratogens. Teratology 2002; 65:153–161.

297. Zellweger H, Mc Donald IS, Abbo G. Is lysergic-acid-diethylamide a teratogen? Lancet 1967; 2:1066–1068.

298. TERIS on-line database: the teratogen information system. Seattle: University of Washington; 1987.

299. Irwin S, Egozcue J. Chromosomal abnormalities in leukocytes from LSD-25 users. Science 1967; 157:313–314.

300. Hungerford DA, Taylor KM, Shagass C, et al. Cytogenic effects of LSD-25 therapy in man. JAMA 1968; 206:2287–2291.

301. Hecht F, Beals RK, Lees MH, et al. Lysergic-acid-diethylamide and cannabis as possible teratogens in man. Lancet 1968; 2:1087.

302. Idanpaan-Heikkila J, Fritchie GE, Englert LF, et al. Placental transfer of tritiated-1-tetrahydrocannabinol. N Engl J Med 1969; 281:330.

303. Klausner HA, Dingell JV. The metabolism and excretion of δ-9-tetrahydrocannabinol in the rat. Life Sci 1971; 10:49–59.

304. Kreuz DS, Axelrod J. δ-9-tetrahydrocannabinol: localization in body fat. Science 1973; 179:391–393.

305. Robinson LL, Buckley JD, Daigle AE, et al. Maternal drug use and risk of childhood non-lymphoblastic leukemia among offspring. Cancer 1989; 63:1904–1911.

306. National Academy of Sciences. Toxicological effects of methylmercury. Washington: National Research Council; 2000.

307. Schober SE, Sinks TH, Jones RL, et al. Blood mercury levels in US children and women of childbearing age, 1999–2000. JAMA 2003; 289:1667–1674.

308. Amin-zaki L, Majeed MA, Elhassani SB, et al. Prenatal methylmercury poisoning: clinical observations over five years. Am J Dis Child 1979; 133:172–177.

309. Friberg L. Methylmercury in fish: a toxicological-epidemiologic evaluation of risks report from an expert group. Nord Hyg Tidskr 1971; 4(suppl):19–364.

310. Murakami U. The effect of organic mercury on intrauterine life. Adv Exp Med Biol 1971; 27:301–306.

311. Harada M. Minamata disease: methylmercury poisoning in Japan caused by environmental pollution. Crit Rev Toxicol 1995; 25:1–24.

312. Kjellström T, Kennedy P, Wallis S, et al. Physical and mental development of children with prenatal exposure to mercury from fish. Stage I: Preliminary tests at age 4. Report 3080, Solna, Sweden. National Swedish Environmental Protection Board 1986.

313. Kjellström T, Kennedy P, Wallis S, et al. Physical and mental development of children with prenatal exposure to mercury from fish. Stage II: Interviews and psychological tests at age 6. Report 3642, Solna, Sweden. National Swedish Environmental Protection Board 1989.

314. Lebel J, Mergler D, Lucotte M, et al. Evidence of early nervous system dysfunction in Amazonian populations exposed to low-levels of methylmercury. Neurotoxicology 1996; 17:157–168.

315. Grandjean P, Weihe P, White RF, et al. Cognitive deficit in 7-year-old children with prenatal exposure to methylmercury. Neurotoxicol Teratol 1997; 19:417–428.

316. Greenberg F. Letter to the editor: Possible metronidazole teratogenicity and clefting. Am J Med Genet 1985; 22:825.

317. Morgan I. Metronidazole treatment in pregnancy. Int J Gynaecol Obstet 1978; 15:501–502.

318. Rosa FW, Baum C, Shaw M. Pregnancy outcomes after first trimester vaginitis drug therapy. Obstet Gynecol 1987; 69:751–755.

319. Burtin P, Taddio A, Ariburnu O, et al. Safety of metronidazole in pregnancy: a meta-analysis. Am J Obstet Gynecol 1995; 172:525–529.

320. Caro-Paton T, Carvajal A, Martin de Diego I, et al. Is metronidazole teratogenic? A meta-analysis. Br J Clin Pharmacol 1997; 44:179–182.

321. Hausknecht RU. Methotrexate and misoprostol to terminate early pregnancy. N Engl J Med 1995; 333:537–540.

322. Costa SH, Vessey MP. Misoprostol and illegal abortion in Rio de Janeiro, Brazil. Lancet 1993; 341:1258–1261. [Erratum, Lancet 1993; 341:1486.]

323. Schuler L, Pastuszak A, Sanseverino TV, et al. Pregnancy outcome after exposure to misoprostol in Brazil: a prospective, controlled study. Reprod Toxicol 1999; 13:147–151.

324. Coelho KE, Sarmento MF, Veiga CM, et al. Misoprostol embryotoxicity: clinical evaluation of fifteen patients with arthrogryposis. Am J Med Genet 2000; 95:297–301.

325. Adam MP, Manning MA, Beck AE, et al. Methotrexate/misoprostol embryopathy: report of four cases resulting from failed medical abortion. Am J Med Genet 2003; 123:72–78.

326. Linares A. Reversible cutis laxa due to maternal D-penicillamine treatment. Lancet 1979; 2:43.

327. Harpey JP, Jaudon MC, Clavel JP, et al. Cutis laxa and low serum zinc after antenatal exposure to penicillamine. Lancet 1983; 2:858.

328. Merlob P, Stahl B, Maltz E. Is fluphenazine a teratogen? Am J Med Genet 1994; 52:231–232.

329. Donalson GL, Bury RG. Multiple congenital abnormalities in a newborn boy associated with maternal use of fluphenazine enanthate and other drugs during pregnancy. Acta Paediatr Scand 1982; 71:335–338.

330. Slone D, Siskind V, Heinonen OP, et al. Antenatal exposure to phenothiazine in relation to congenital malformations, perinatal mortality rate, birth weight and intelligence quotient score. Am J Obstet Gynecol 1977; 128:486.

331. Longo LD. Environmental pollution and pregnancy; risks and uncertainties for the fetus and infant. Am J Obstet Gynecol 1980; 137:162–173.

332. daSilva VA, Malheiros LR, Paumgartten FL, et al. Developmental toxicity of in utero exposure to toluene on malnourished and well nourished rats. Toxicology 1990; 64:155–168.

333. Jacobson JL, Jacobson SW. Teratogen update: polychlorinated biphenyls. Teratology 1997; 55:338–347.

334. Rogan WJ. PCBs and cola-colored babies: Japan, 1968, and Taiwan, 1979. In: Sever JL, Brent RL, eds. Teratogen update: environmentally induced birth defects risks. New York: Alan R Liss; 1986:127–130.

335. Hsu S, Ma C, Hsu SK, et al. Discovery and epidemiology of PCB poisoning in Taiwan. Environ Health Persp 1985; 59:5–10.

336. Paul M. Occupational and environmental reproductive hazards. Baltimore: Williams & Wilkins; 1993.

337. Rudolph AM. The effects of nonsteroidal anti-inflammatory compounds on fetal circulation and pulmonary function. Obstet Gynecol 1981 58(Suppl 1): 63S–67S.

338. Danforth DN. Obstetrics and gynecology. Philadelphia: Harper & Row; 1982.

339. Werler MM, Mitchell AA, Shapiro S. The relation of aspirin use during the first trimester of pregnancy to congenital cardiac defects. N Engl J Med 1989; 321:1639–1642.

340. Turner G, Collins E. Fetal aspects of regular salicylate ingestion in pregnancy. Lancet 1975; 2:338–339.

341. Torfs CP, Katz EA, Bateson TF, et al. Maternal medications and environmental exposures as risk factors for gastroschisis. Teratology 1996; 54:84–92.

342. Werler MM, Sheehan JE, Mitchell AA. Maternal medication use and risks of gastroschisis and small intestinal atresia. Am J Epidemiol 2002; 155:26–31.

343. Werler MM, Bower C, Payne J, et al. Findings on potential teratogens from a case-control study in Western Australia. Aust N Z J Obstet Gynaecol 2003; 43:443–447.

344. Werler MM, Mitchell AA, Shapiro S. First trimester maternal medication use in relation to gastroschisis. Teratology 1992; 45:361–367.

345. Gilbert-Barness E, Telleli J, Drut RM, et al. Teratogenicity of an over-the-counter oral sympathomimetic/methyl xanthine/barbiturate combination in rabbits. Vet Hum Toxicol (in press).

346. Gilbert EF, Bruyere HJ Jr, Ishikawa S, et al. The role of catecholamines and other cardiac stimulants in cardiovascular teratogenesis. Recent observations and proposed mechanisms. In: Pexieder T, ed. Perspectives in cardiovascular research Vol. 5. Mechanisms of cardiac morphogenesis and teratogenesis. New York: Raven Press; 1980:473–484.

347. Bruyere HJ Jr, Fallon JF, Gilbert EF. External malformations in chick embryos following concomitant administration of methylxanthine and β-adrenomimetic agents: 1. Gross pathologic features. Teratology 1983; 28:257–269.

348. Aselton P, Jick H, Milunsky A, et al. First-trimester drug use and congenital disorders. Obstet Gynecol 1985; 65:451–455.

349. Czeizel AE, Mosonyi A. Monitoring of early human fetal development in women exposed to large doses of chemicals. Environ Mol Mutagen 1997; 30:240–244.

350. Laegreid L, Olegard R, Walstrom J. Teratogenic effects of benzodiazepine use during pregnancy. J Pediatr 1989; 114:126–131.

351. Bracken MB, Holford TR. Exposure to prescribed drugs in pregnancy and association with congenital malformations. Obstet Gynecol 1981; 58:336–344.

352. Lenz W, Knapp K. Thalidomide embryopathy. Arch Environ Health 1962; 5:100–105.

353. Henkel L, Willert HE. Dysmelia: a classification and pattern of malformation in a group of congenital defects of the limbs. J Bone Joint Surg 1969; 51B:399–414.

354. Gilbert-Barness EF, Opitz JM. Congenital anomalies and malformation syndromes. In: Wigglesworth JS, Singer DB, eds. Textbook of fetal and perinatal pathology. Oxford: Blackwell Scientific; 1991:388.

355. McCredie J. Embryonic neuropathy: a hypothesis of neural crest injury as the pathogenesis of congenital malformations. Med J Aust 1974; 1:159–163.

356. McCredie J. Neural crest defects: a neuroanatomic basis for classification of multiple malformations related to phocomelia. J Neurol Sci 1976; 28:373–387.

357. McCredie JM. Comments on 'Proposed mechanisms of action in thalidomide embryopathy,' Letter to the Editor. Teratology 1990; 41:239–242.

358. North K, McCredie J. Neurotomes and birth defects: a neuroanatomic method of interpretation of multiple congenital malformations. Enid Gilbert-Barness Festschrift. Am J Med Genet 1987; 3(suppl):29–42.

359. D'Amato RJ, Loughnan MS, Flynn E, et al. Thalidomide is an inhibitor of angiogenesis. Proc Natl Acad Sci 1994; 91:4082–4085.

360. Neubert R, Hinz N, Thel R, et al. Downregulation of adhesion receptors on cells of primate embryos as a probable mechanism of the teratogenic action of thalidomide. Life Sci 1996; 58:295–316.

361. Argiles JM, Carbo N, Lopez-Soriano FJ. Was tumor necrosis factor – a responsible for the fetal malformations associated with thalidomide in the early 1960s? Med Hypotheses 1998; 50:313–318.

362. Parman T, Wiley MJ, Wells PG. Free radical-mediated oxidative DNA damage in the mechanism of thalidomide teratogenesis. Nat Med 1999; 5:582–585.

363. Stephens TD, Fillmore BJ. Hypothesis: thalidomide embryopathy - proposed mechanism of action. Teratology 2000; 61:189–195.

364. Arnold GL, Kirby RS, Langendoerfer S, et al. Toluene embryopathy: clinical delineation and developmental follow-up. Pediatrics 1994; 93:216–220.

365. Toutant C, Lippmann S. Fetal solvents syndrome. Lancet 1979; 1:1356.

366. Arnold GL, Wilkens-Haug L. Toluene-embryopathy syndrome. Am J Hum Genet 1990; 47:A46.

367. Hersh JH, Podruch PE, Rogers G, et al. Toluene embryopathy. J Pediatr 1985; 106:922–927.

368. Donald JM, Hooper K, Hopenhayn-Rich C, et al. Reproductive and developmental toxicity of toluene: a review. Environ Health Perspect 1991; 94:237–244.

369. Utidjian HM. Excerpts from criteria for a recommended standard – occupational exposure to toluene. J Occup Med 1974; 16:107–109.

370. McDonald JC. Chemical exposures at work in early pregnancy and congenital defect: a case reference study. Br J Ind Med 1987; 44:527–533.

371. Hersh JH. A Toluene embryopathy: two new cases. J Med Genet 1989; 26:233–237.

372. Pearson MA, Hoyme HE, Seaver LH, et al. Toluene embryopathy: delineation of the phenotype and comparison with fetal alcohol syndrome. Pediatrics 1994; 93:211–215.

373. Burrow GN, Bartsocas C, Klatskin EH, et al. Children exposed in utero to propylthiouracil: subsequent intellectual and physical development. Am J Dis Child 1968; 116:161–165.

374. Sutherland JM, Esselborn VM, Burket RL, et al. Familial nongoitrous cretinism apparently due to maternal antithyroid antibody. N Engl J Med 1960; 263:336–341.

375. Milham S, Elledge W. Maternal methimazole and congenital defects in children (letter). Teratology 1972; 5:125.

376. Momotani N, Ito K. Treatment of pregnant patients with Basedow's disease. Exp Clin Endocrinol 1991; 97:268–274.

377. Ganheim A, Atkins P. Management of thyrotoxicosis in pregnancy. Int J Clin Pract 1998; 52:36–38.

378. Milham S. Scalp defects in infants of mothers treated for hyperthyroidism with methimazole or carbimazole during pregnancy. Teratology 1985; 32:321.

379. Ornoy A, Diav-Citrin O. Teratogen update: antithyroid drugs. Methimazole and propylthiouracil. Teratology 2002; 65:38–44.

380. Lomenick JP, Jackson WA, Backeljauw PF. Amiodarone-induced neonatal hypothyroidism: a unique form of transient early-onset hypothyroidism. J Perinatol 2004; 24:397–399.

381. Martínez-Frías ML, Salvador J. Epidemiological aspects of prenatal exposure to high doses of Vitamin A in Spain. Eur J Epidermiol 1990; 6:118–123.

382. Dudas I, Czeizel AE. Use of 6,000 Iu Vitamin A during early pregnancy without teratogenic effect. Teratology 1992; 45:335–336.

383. Rothman KJ, Moore LL, Singer MR, et al. Teratogenicity of high vitamin A intake. N Engl J Med 1995; 333:1369–1373.

384. Strange L. Hypervitaminosis A in early human infancy and malformations of the central nervous system. Acta Obstet Gynecol Scand 1978; 57:289–291.

385. Culler FL, Jones KL, Deftos LJ. Impaired calcitonin secretion in patients with Williams syndrome. J Pediatr 1985; 107:720–723.

386. Menger H, Lin AE, Toriello HV, et al. Vitamin K deficiency embryopathy: a phenocopy of the warfarin embryopathy due to a disorder of embryonic Vitamin K metabolism. Am J Med Genet 1997; 72:129–134.

387. Pauli RM. Mechanisms of bone and cartilage maldevelopment in the warfarin embryopathy. Pathol Immunopathol Res 1988; 7:107–112.

Drugs and chemicals apparently not teratogenic in humans

388. Steele EJ. Reappraisal of the findings on Agent Orange by the Australian Royal Commission. Toxicol Lett 1990; 51:261–268.

389. Erickson JD, Mulinare J, McClain PW, et al. Vietnam veterans' risk for fathering babies with birth defects. JAMA 1984; 252:903–912.

390. Hatch MC, Stein ZA. Agent Orange and risks to reproduction: the limits of epidemiology. Teratog Carcinog Mutagen 1986; 6:185–202.

391. Stellman SD, Stellman JM, Sommer JF Jr. Health and reproductive outcomes among American legionnaires in relation to combat and herbicide exposure in Vietnam. Environ Res 1988; 47:150–174.

392. Holmes LB, Bendectin. In: Sever JL, Brent RL, eds. Teratogen update: environmentally induced birth defect risks. New York: Alan R Liss; 1986:53–59.

392a. Browne ML. Maternal exposure to caffeine and risk of congenital anomalies: a systematic review. Epidemiology 2006; 17:324–331.

393. Infante-Rivard C, Fernandez A, Gauthier R, et al. Fetal loss associated with caffeine intake before and during pregnancy. JAMA 1993; 270:2940–2943.

Maternal conditions

394. Helmerhorst FM, Perquin D, Donker DAM, et al. Perinatal outcome of singletons and twins after assisted conception a systematic review of controlled studies. BMJ 2004; 328:261–265.

395. Jackson RA, Gibson KA, Wu YW, et al. Perinatal outcomes in singletons following in vitro fertilization a meta-analysis. Obstet Gynecol 2004; 103:551–563.

396. Schieve LA, Ferre C, Peterson HB, et al. Perinatal outcome among singleton infants conceived through assisted reproductive technology in the United States. Obstet Gynecol 2004; 103:1144–1153.

397. Ohtani-Fujita N, Fujita T, Aoike A, et al. CpG methylation inactivates the promoter activity of the human retinoblastoma tumor-suppressor gene. Oncogene 1993; 8:1063–1067.

398. Bergh T, Ericson A, Hillensjö T, et al. Deliveries and children born after invitro fertilisation in Sweden 1982-95: a retrospective cohort study. Lancet 1999; 354:1579–1585.

399. Anthony S, Buitendijk SE, Dorrepaal CA, et al. Congenital malformations in 4224 children conceived after IVF. Hum Reprod 2002; 17:2089–2095.

400. DeBaun MR, Niemitz EL, Feinberg AP. Association of in vitro fertilization with Beckwith-Wiedemann syndrome and epigenetic alterations of LIT1 and H19. Am J Hum Genet 2003; 72:156–160.

400a. Sutcliffe AG, Peters CJ, Bowdin S, et al. Assisted reproductive therapies and imprinting disorders – a preliminary British survey. Hum Reprod 2006; 21:1009–1011.

401. Klemetti R, Gissler M, Sévon T, et al. Children born after assisted fertilization have an increased rate of major congenital anomalies. Fertil Steril 2005; 84:1300–1307.

402. Sadler TW, Hunter ES III, Wynn RE, et al. Evidence for multifactorial origin of diabetes-induced embryopathies. Diabetics 1989; 38:70–74.

402a. Zhao Z, Reece EA. Experimental mechanisms of diabetic embryopathy and strategies for developing therapeutic interventions. J Soc Gynecol Investig 2005; 12:549–557.

403. Sadler TW, Denno KM, Hunter ES III. Effects of altered maternal metabolism during gastrulation and neurulation stages of embryogenesis. Ann N Y Acad Sci 1993; 678:48–61.

404. Baker L, Piddington R. Diabetic embryopathy: a selective review of recent trends. Diabetes Complications 1993; 7:204–212.

405. Waller DK, Mills JL, Simpson JL, et al. Are obese women at higher risk for producing malformed offspring? Am J Obstet Gynecol 1994; 170:541–548.

406. North AFJ, Mazumdar S, Logrillo VM. Birthweight, gestational age, and perinatal deaths in 5,471 infants of diabetic mothers. J Pediatr 1977; 90:444–447.

407. Naeye RL. Infants of diabetic mothers: a quantitative morphologic study. Pediatrics 1965; 35:980–988.

408. Susa JB, McCormick KL, Widness JA, et al. Chronic hyperinsulinemia in the fetal rhesus monkey. Effects on fetal growth and composition. Diabetes 1979; 28:1058–1063.

409. Miller E, Hare JW. Elevated maternal hemoglobin A_{1c} in early pregnancy and major congenital anomalies in infants of diabetic mothers. N Engl J Med 1981; 304:1331–1334.

410. Bunn HF, Haney DN, Kamin S, et al. The biosynthesis of human hemoglobin A_{1c}: slow glycosylation of hemoglobin in vivo. J Clin Invest 1976; 57:1652–1659.

411. Dunn PJ, Cole RA, Soeldner JS, et al. Temporal relationships of glycosylated hemoglobin concentrations to glucose control in diabetics. Diabetologia 1979; 17:213.

412. Key TC, Giuffrida RG, Moore TR, et al. Predictive value of early pregnancy glycohemoglobin in the insulin-treated diabetic patient. Am J Obstet Gynecol 1987; 156:1096–1100.

412a. Loeken MR. Advances in understanding the molecular causes of diabetes-induced birth defects. J Soc Gynecol Investig 2006; 13:2–10.

412b. Reece EA, Ji I, Wu YK, et al. Characterization of differential gene expression profiles in diabetic embryopathy using DNA microarray analysis. Am J Obstet Gynecol 2006; 195:1075–1080.

412c. Gareskog M, Cederberg J, Eriksson UJ, et al. Maternal diabetes in vivo and high glucose concentration in vitro increases apoptosis in rat embryos. Reprod Toxicol 2006 Sep 1; [Epub ahead of print].

413. Kucera J. Rate and type of congenital anomalies among offspring of diabetic women. J Reprod Med 1971; 7:73–82.

414. Passarge E. Congenital malformation and maternal diabetes. Lancet 1965; 1:324–325.

414a. de Vigan, Vérité V, Vodovar V, et al. Diabetes and congenital anomalies: data from Paris registry of congenital anomalies, 1985–1997. Reprod Toxicol 2000; 14:76.

415. Mills JL, Knopp TH, Simpson JL, et al. Lack of relation of increased malformation rates in infants of diabetic mothers to glycemic control during organogenesis. N Engl J Med 1988; 318:671–672.

416. Greene MF. Spontaneous abortions and major malformations in women with diabetes mellitus. Semin Reprod Endocrinol 1999; 17:127–136.

417. Martínez-Frías ML, Bermejo E, Rodríguez-Pinilla E, et al. Epidemiologic analysis of outcomes of pregnancy in gestational diabetes. Am J Med Genet 1998; 78:140–145.

418. Schaefer-Graf UM, Buchanan TA, Xiang A, et al. Patterns of congenital anomalies and relationship to initial maternal fasting glucose levels in pregnancies complicated by type 2 and gestational diabetes. Am J Obstet Gynecol 2000; 182:313–320.

419. Feig DS, Palda VA. Type 2 diabetes: a growing concern. Lancet 2002; 359: 1690–1692.

420. Martínez-Frías ML, Frías JP, Bermejo E, et al. Pregestational maternal body mass index predicts an increased risk of congenital malformations in infants of mothers with gestational diabetes. Diabetes Care 2005; 22:775–781.

421. MacCarthy JMT, Carey BC. Bone changes in homocystinuria. Clin Radiol 1968; 19:128–134.

422. Landing BH, Kamoshita S. Congenital hyperparathyroidism secondary to maternal hypoparathyroidism. J Pediatr 1970; 77:842–847.

423. Scott JR, Rote NS, Branch PW. Immunologic aspects of recurrent abortion and fetal death. Obstet Gynecst 1987; 70:645–656.

424. Brook JD, McCurrach ME, Harley HG, et al. Molecular basis of myotonic dystrophy: expansion of a trinucleotide (CTG) repeat at the 3′ end of a transcript encoding a protein kinase family member. Cell 1992; 68:799–808.

425. Hall JG. Genomic imprinting. Arch Dis Child 1990; 65:1013–1015.

426. Upadhyay K, Thomson A, Luckas MJ. Congenital myotonic dystrophy. Fetal Diagn Ther 2005; 20:512–514.

427. Mokdad AH, Bowman BA, Ford ES, et al. The continuing epidemics of obesity and diabetes in the United States. JAMA 2001; 86:1195–1200.

428. Prentice A, Goldberg G. Maternal obesity increases congenital malformations. Nutr Rev 1996; 54:146–150.

429. Werler MM, Louik C, Shapiro S, et al. Prepregnant weight in relation to risk of neural tube defects. JAMA 1996; 275:1089–1092.

430. Shaw GM, Todoroff K, Schaffer DM, et al. Maternal height and prepregnancy body mass index as risk factors for selected congenital anomalies. Paediatr Perinat Epidemiol 2000; 14:234–239.

431. Shaw GM, Nelson V, Moore CA. Prepregnancy body mass index and risk of multiple congenital anomalies. Am J Med Genet 2002; 107:253–255.

432. Watkins ML, Rasmussen SA, Honein MA, et al. Maternal obesity and risk for birth defects. Pediatrics 2003; 111: 1152–1158.

432a. Scialli AR. ACE inhibitors and major congenital malformations. N Engl J Med 2006; 355:12.

433. Yu JS, O'Halloran MT. Children of mothers with phenylketonuria. Lancet 1970; 1:210–212.

434. National Institutes of Health Consensus Development Conference Statement. Phenylketonuria: screening and management, October 16–18, 2000. Pediatrics 2001; 108:972–982.

435. Reteoff SS, Dumont JE, Vassant G, Reteoff S. Thyroid disorders. In: Scriver CR, Beaudet AL, Valle D, et al, eds. The metabolic and molecular bases of inherited disease 8th ed. New York: McGraw-Hill; 2001:4029–4075.

436. Haddow JE, Palomaki GE, Allan WC, et al. Maternal thyroid deficiency during pregnancy and subsequent neuropsychological development of the child. N Engl J Med 1999; 341:549–555.

437. Connolly KJ, Pharoah POD, Hetzel BS. Fetal iodine deficiency and motor performance during childhood. Lancet 1979; 2:1149–1151.

438. Hetzel BS, Hay ID. Thyroid function, iodine nutrition, and fetal brain development. Clin Endocrinol 1979; 11:445–460.

439. Davis LE, Lucas MJ, Hankins GDV, et al. Thyrotoxicosis complicating pregnancy. Am J Obstet Gynecol 1989; 160:63–70.

440. Nutt J, Clark F, Welch RG, et al. Neonatal hyperthyroidism and long-acting thyroid stimulator protector. Br Med J 1974; 2:695–696.

441. Gilbert EF. The effects of metabolic diseases on the cardiovascular system. Symposium on cardiovascular diseases of infancy and childhood. Am J Cardiovasc Pathol 1987; 1:189–213.

441a. Zimmerman D. Fetal and Neonatal hyperthyroidism. Thyroid 1999; 9:72–73.

442. Scott JS, Maddison PJ. Connective tissue disease, antibodies to ribonucleoprotein, and congenital heart block. N Engl J Med 1983; 309:209–212.

443. Gilbert EF, Opitz JM. Congenital anomalies and malformation syndromes. In: Stocker T, Dehner L, eds. Pediatric pathology. Philadelphia; JB Lippincott; 1992.

444. Martinez-Frías ML, Bermejo E, Rodriguez-Pinilla E, et al. Congenital anomalies in the offspring of mothers with a bicornuate uterus. Pediatrics 1998; 101:E10.

PART 2   *Enid Gilbert-Barness and Margot I. Van Allen*

Vascular disruptions

'It is not birth, marriage or death that is the most important time in your life but gastrulation.'

Wolpert

Embryology of human blood vessels and mechanisms of vascular disruption 178	Isolated structural anomalies and disruption sequences due to vascular disruption 186
Evidence for structural anomalies from vascular disruption 184	Short umbilical cord 199
	Amnion disruption sequence 200

Disruption of embryonic and fetal vasculature is a common cause of structural anomalies. Disruption is defined as a structural anomaly of an organ, part of an organ, or a larger region of the body resulting from the extrinsic breakdown of, or an interference with, an originally normal conceptus.[1,2] A variety of agents and events can result in disruption of the embryo and fetus, summarized in part 1 of this chapter and in Box 4.2.1.

The overall **incidence** of structural anomalies resulting from all types of disruption is not known. The Metropolitan Atlanta Congenital Defects program found an incidence of 0.13/1000 of newborns with more than one structural anomaly considered to be due to vascular disruption.[5a]

Vascular disruption refers specifically to structural anomalies resulting from damage to, or interruption of, normal embryonic or fetal development of the arteries, veins, and capillaries.[3] The resultant types of structural anomalies depend on the timing in embryogenesis and the severity of the disruptive event, as well as the location of the damaged tissue and whether there are secondary adhesions of necrotic tissue between contiguous organs (e.g. splenogonadal fusion and amnion adhesions).[3, 4]

The prevalence in live-borns of structural anomalies caused by vascular disruption is not known. In fetuses identified as having structural anomalies by ultrasound examination, 9.2% result from vascular disruption.[5] Luebke and colleagues[6] determined that 3.6% of stillbirths had structural anomalies due to vascular disruption.

Structural anomalies from vascular disruption are usually distinctive in appearance. There is loss of tissue, aberrant differentiation as well as incomplete development of adjacent tissues, and adhesions of damaged tissues to surrounding tissues or to amnion. A structural anomaly from disruption contrasts with a primary malformation, such as duodenal atresia or persistent cloaca, which represent errors in morphogenesis, and the pathogenesis is understandable within the context of errors in normal morphogenesis.[1, 2]

During embryogenesis, disruptive events that damage blood vessels result in hemorrhagic necrosis of tissues from hypoxia and from compression by the enlarging hematoma. There is resultant loss of developing tissues, distortion and aberrant differentiation of contiguous tissues, and incomplete development of structures within the same or secondarily affected developmental fields (Fig. 4.2.1).

Anomalies from vascular disruption occurring during the fetal period result from occlusion of blood vessels due to emboli, thrombi, or external compression; and from hypoperfusion.[3, 4, 7, 8, 9] Anomalies due to occlusion are usually limited to the tissues supplied by the occluded vessel(s) (e.g. porencephalic cyst secondary to obstruction of the middle cerebral artery). When there is acute vascular insufficiency, the anomalies are typically found in areas of watershed blood supply. When there is chronic vascular insufficiency, there can be hypoplasia of a structure, with possible loss of the tissue that is the least perfused (Fig. 4.2.2)

Temporal dating of structural anomalies from vascular disruption can be difficult. Unlike errors in morphogenesis where discrete timing based on normal embryogenesis is possible, with vascular disruption an event occurring after a tissue is formed can result in a structural anomaly, for example, anencephaly caused by failure of neural tube closure occurs prior to 28 days' gestation. Anencephaly from amnion disruption sequence can result from damage to cranial tissue after 28 days.[10] The gestational timing of an anomaly resulting from disruption can only be inferred by

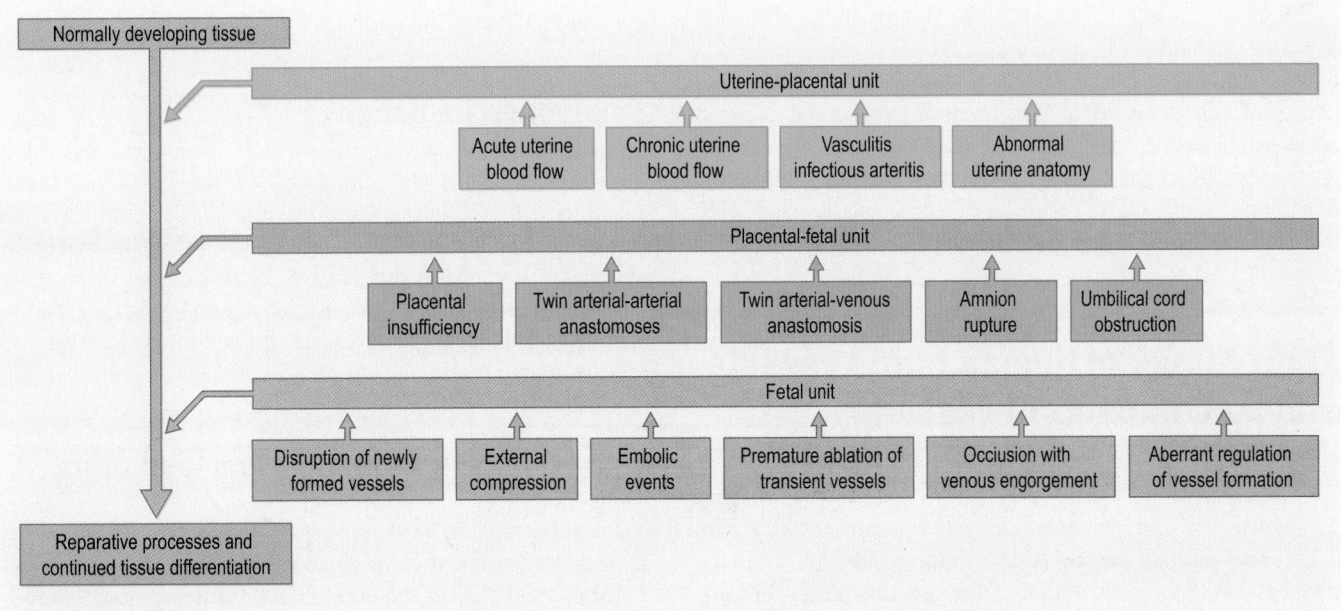

FIGURE 4.2.1 Summary of vascular disruption in the developing embryo and fetus. (From Van Allen 1981,[3] with permission.)

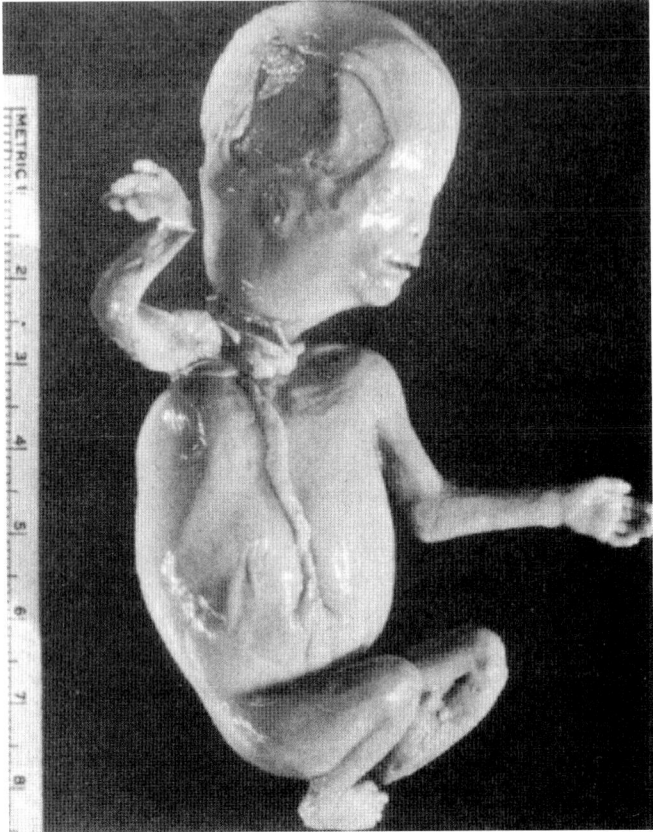

FIGURE 4.2.2 Hypoplasia of the right arm due to decreased perfusion from constriction by the umbilical cord. Subsequent obstruction of umbilical flow resulted in fetal death and maceration.

TABLE 4.2.1 MECHANISMS OF VASCULAR DISRUPTION IN THE EMBRYO AND FETUS

Mechanism	Examples of resultant structural anomalies
Disruption of embryonic capillary plexus	Early amnion disruption sequence Limb body wall complex Oromandibular hypogenesis syndrome
Persistence of embryonic vessels	Structural anomalies of limbs, e.g. radial aplasia, tibial aplasia, clubfoot, fibular aplasia
Premature ablation of embryonic vessels	Subclavian artery supply disruption sequence (Poland, Möbius, Klippel-Feil sequences) Horseshoe kidney
Failure of maturation of vessels	Capillary hemangiomas Arteriovenous fistulas Berry aneurysms
Occlusion (external compression) of vessels	Amniotic band syndrome Anomalies associated with fibroids, tubal pregnancies, and bicornuate uterus
Occlusion (emboli, thrombosis) of vessels	See Box 4.2.3 for twin anomalies, comparable anomalies in singletons
Altered hemodynamics	Anomalies associated with maternal cocaine use

associated structural anomalies, by documentation by sonogram,[11] or if the date of the disruptive event is known [e.g. the date of abdominal trauma or intrauterine device (IUD) removal].[5, 12]

There is etiologic heterogeneity for many of the structural anomalies attributable to vascular disruption, so care is needed in making this diagnosis. Familial predisposition to abnormal embryonic development of blood vessels can be the cause of apparent autosomal dominant or recessive inheritance of anomalies appearing similar to those of sporadic vascular disruption, including Adams-Oliver syndrome, cutis aplasia, and split hand/split foot syndrome.

Embryology of human blood vessels and mechanisms of vascular disruption

Mechanisms of vascular disruption are summarized in Figure 4.2.1. The vascular supply to the embryo and fetus can be divided into three units. The first, the **uterine–placental unit,** refers to blood supply to the uterus, uterine spiral arteries, and placental implantation and function. The second, the **placental–fetal unit,** refers to embryonic vessels in the placenta and the umbilical cord vessels. The third, the **fetal unit,** refers to the blood vessels in the embryo and fetus proper, the yolk sac and the allantois. The embryonic development of the blood vessels in the context of the mechanisms of damage and the resultant structural anomalies are reviewed in Table 4.2.1.

Embryonic circulation

The embryo has a rich blood supply, the circulation being established by 21 days post conception (Fig. 4.2.3).[13, 14] The cardiovascular system is described by Moore[15] as the first organ system to function in the embryo. Establishment of placental circulation is necessary for nutrient supply and removal of waste material, owing to a relatively limited function of the yolk sac (compared with avian embryos).

Capillary plexus formation and disruption[15–18]

The first blood vessels arise on day 13–15 post conception (pc), in the extraembryonic mesenchyme covering the yolk sac, connecting stalk, and wall of the chorionic sac. Angiogenesis of blood vessels begins as lacunae that coalesce to form a fine capillary

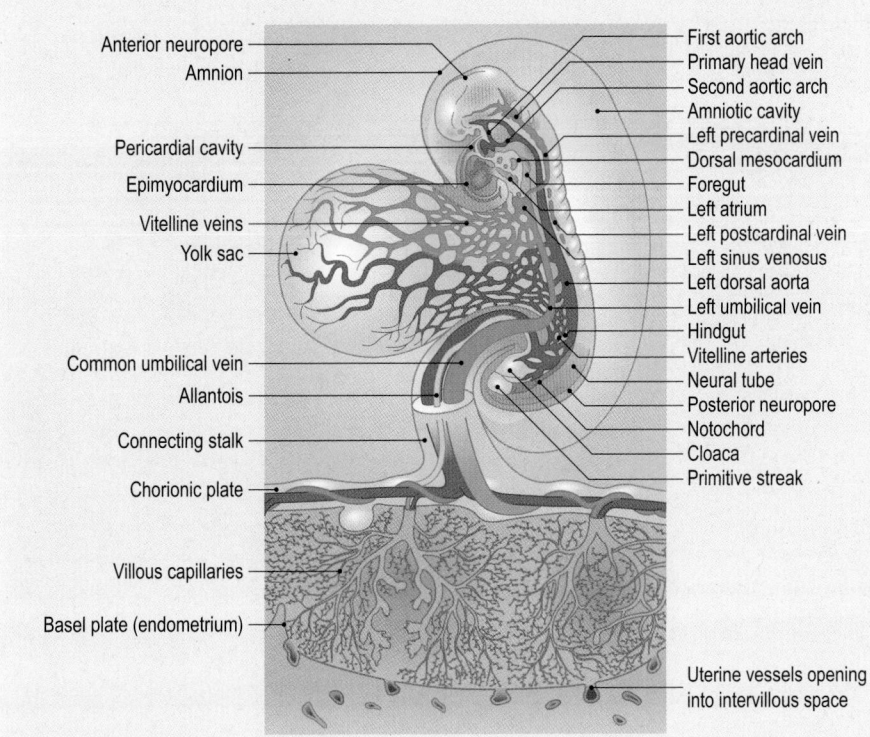

Anterior neuropore
Amnion

Pericardial cavity
Epimyocardium
Vitelline veins
Yolk sac

Common umbilical vein
Allantois
Connecting stalk
Chorionic plate

Villous capillaries
Basel plate (endometrium)

First aortic arch
Primary head vein
Second aortic arch
Amniotic cavity
Left precardinal vein
Dorsal mesocardium
Foregut
Left atrium
Left postcardinal vein
Left sinus venosus
Left dorsal aorta
Left umbilical vein
Hindgut
Vitelline arteries
Neural tube
Posterior neuropore
Notochord
Cloaca
Primitive streak

Uterine vessels opening
into intervillous space

FIGURE 4.2.3 Cardiovascular system of a dissected human embryo at stage 11; 2.4–2.5 mm; 24 days; 13–20 pairs of somites. The yolk sac is intact and the amnion is cut in the sagittal plane. (From Stephen 1989,[13] with permission. Redrawn from illustration by Didusch 1930,[14] with permission.)

plexus. Intraembryonic vessels arise on day 15–17 pc, with formation of a pulsatile primitive cardiac tube on day 21. As the blood flow increases, the capillaries form primitive vessels, which segmentally branch from the paired embryonic aortic arteries and cardinal veins. The vessels of the capillary plexus easily rupture after changes in blood pressure, compression, occlusion, or vasoactive teratogenic agents. Rupture of vessels, subcutaneous blisters, and local hemorrhage have been observed in animal studies after a number of teratogenic agents[3]; amnion puncture;[19, 20] occlusion of uterine, placental, and embryonic blood vessels;[21, 22] and maternal hypotension[23] and hyperthermia.[24] In humans, structural anomalies most likely due to disruption of the capillary plexus have been reported after uterine and embryonic trauma from IUD removal or attempted abortion,[3, 5, 12, 25] vasoactive teratogenic agents (e.g. cocaine),[26, 27] placental chorionic villus sampling (CVS) before 9 weeks' gestational age,[28–31] and maternal hypotension.[3, 32] Although limb reduction anomalies and club feet have been reported after amniocentesis particularly when done between 12–15 weeks of gestation, it is not clear that they are causally related.[33, 34]

Vitelline and placental circulations

The vitelline artery and vein supply the embryonic yolk sac an important source of nutrients and blood cells during the first weeks of pregnancy. In **sirenomelia,** there is frequently persistence of a large vitelline artery, which has apparently remained the predominant fetal blood vessel in the body stalk, replacing the umbilical artery in the placenta circulation. It has been

hypothesized that the vitelline artery causes a vascular steal, shunting blood from the caudal end of the embryo (Fig. 4.2.4).[35] Inadequate delivery of nutrients and oxygen in the caudal embryo may cause loss of tissue and failure of lateralization of the hind limbs, resulting in the common lower limb that typifies sirenomelia (Fig. 4.2.5).[35]

The placental circulation is normally established by 18–21 days when the umbilical-allantoic vessels of the embryo connect with those of the placenta via the body stalk. In monozygotic twins with a common placenta, random coalescence of lacunae results in vascular anastomoses between twins.[36, 37] When there are vascular placental anastomoses, combined with an abnormal cardiac function in one of the pair (e.g. an acardiac twin), the **twin reversed arterial perfusion (TRAP) sequence** can develop (Figs 4.2.6 –4.2.9).[36]

Development of vascular anastomoses in normal monozygotic twins results in a **twin to twin transfusion** sequence (see Ch. 9), with a risk of discordant placental blood flow to twins and embolic occlusion of vessels, with resultant tissue infarction.[37] Another concern for monoamnionic, monochorionic twins is entanglement of the umbilical cords and vascular insufficiency (see Fig. 9.21B).

Embryonic arteries and veins

During organogenesis, the embryonic vessels are formed at the same time as the tissue and organs they supply. As the tissue differentiates transient embryonic arteries and veins form that are important in supplying embryonic structures but have

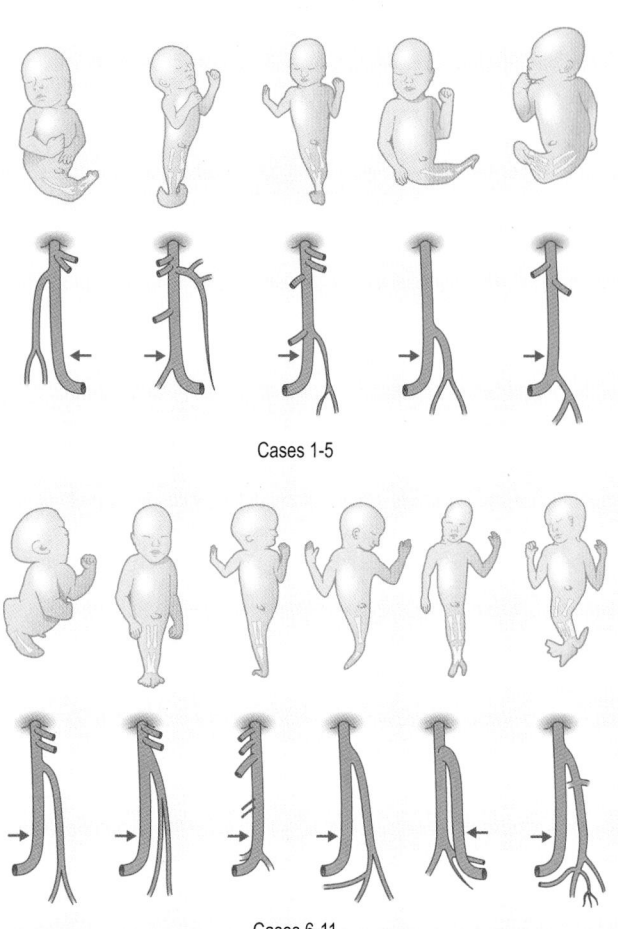

Cases 1-5

Cases 6-11

FIGURE 4.2.4 Lower limb configuration and long bones in 11 cases of sirenomelia, with respective configuration of major abdominal arteries. The vitelline artery is noted by the arrowheads. (From Stevenson et al 1986,[35] with permission.)

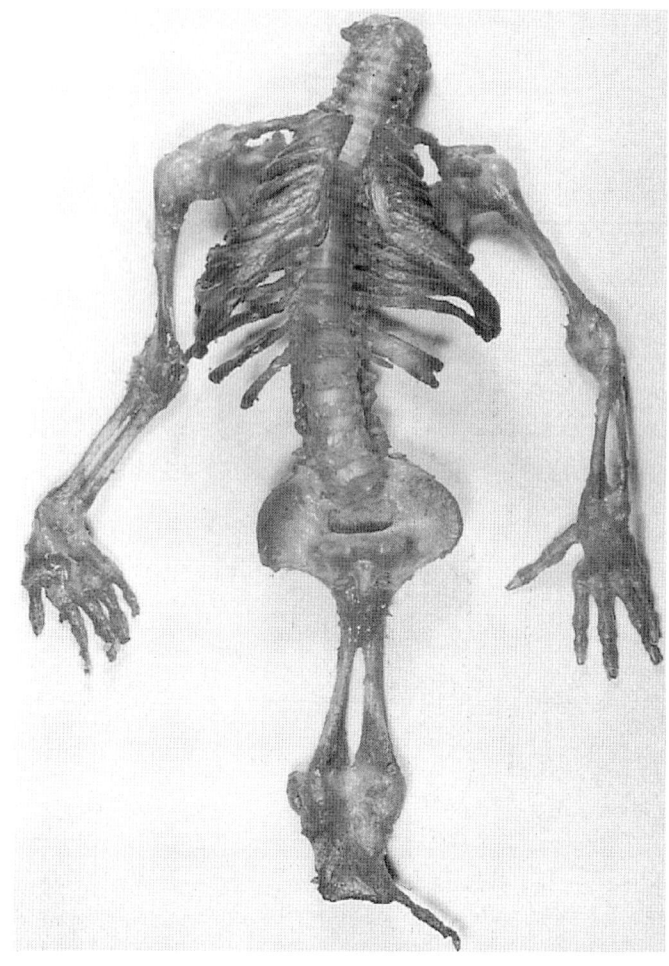

FIGURE 4.2.5 Skeleton of an infant with sirenomelia, showing abnormal sacrum and pelvis with partial fusion of the femurs and fused upper portion of the tibias. The remainder of the lower extremities are absent.

regressed by the fetal period. Embryonic blood vessels regress and are replaced by definitive vessels histologically similar to adult vessels. Premature ablation of embryonic blood vessels has been hypothesized to cause structural anomalies. Damage to the transient aortic arches and altered embryonic blood pressure are frequently associated with congenital heart defects (e.g. **DiGeorge sequence**.)[38] Damage to the transient stapedial artery that supplies the embryonic face from 32 to 54 days pc results in **oculoauriculovertebral spectrum** (also called facioauriculovertebral spectrum, hemifacial microsomia).[3, 39, 40] **Poland sequence** (absent pectoral muscle, syndactyly,[39a] or transverse limb reduction defect), **Klippel-Feil anomaly** (fused cervical vertebrae and other anomalies), and **Möbius sequence** (cranial nerve palsies and transverse limb reduction anomalies) all appear to result from disruption of the embryonic subclavian artery and its branches during the sixth week pc.[41] **Gastroschisis** has been attributed to premature ablation or occlusion of the omphalomesenteric

artery.[42] **Horseshoe kidney** is hypothesized to result from premature ablation of the segmental renal arteries that supply the kidneys as they migrate from the pelvis to their position in the retroperitoneum.[43] **Hypoplastic left heart syndrome** and **coarctation of the aorta** are associated with an increase in structural anomalies identified on autopsy, particularly in the lower half of the body ($p = 0.002$) most likely due to hypoperfusion of the caudal embryo.[38a]

The anatomic relationships and pattern of change of the embryonic vessels have been studied in human embryos.[39, 44–48] Embryonic vessels can be identified on anatomic dissections by their anatomic relationships to muscles and nerves. Limb abnormalities, including **radial aplasia and hypoplasia** (Fig. 4.2.10),[44] **tibial aplasia, fibular aplasia, clubfoot,**[44] **sirenomelia** (see Fig. 4.2.4),[35] and other disorders, have been reported to show persistence of embryonic vessels and failure of formation of adult vessels. Absence of segmental branches of the vertebral artery has been observed in **meningomyelocele** (Fig. 4.2.11),[48] but it is not

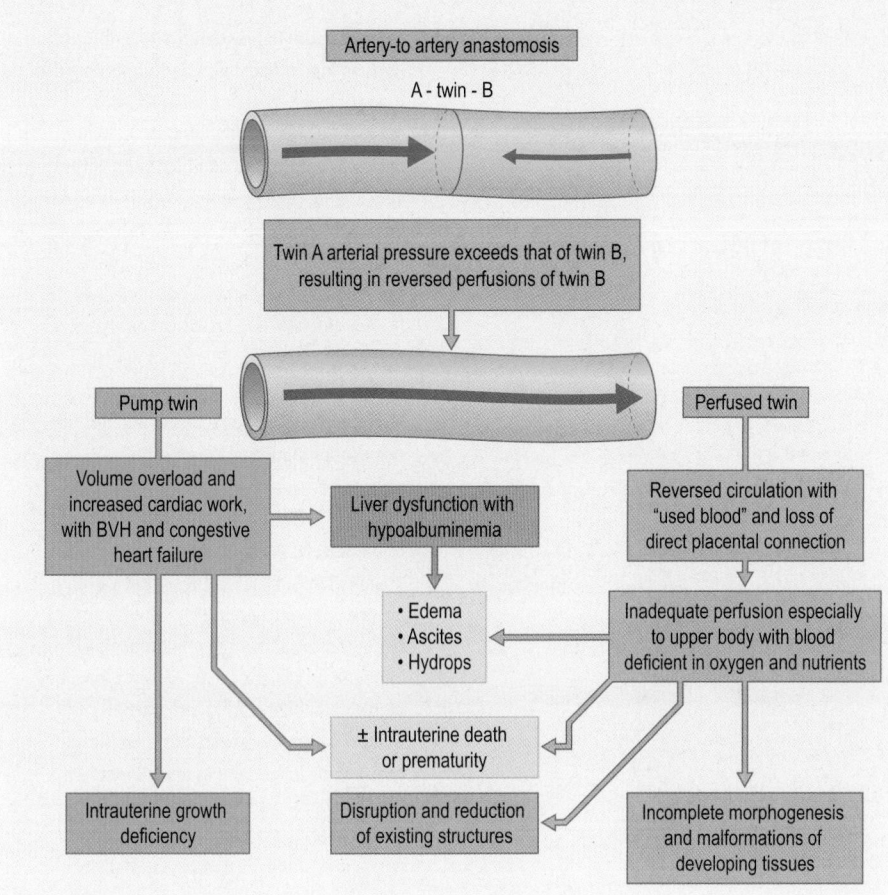

FIGURE 4.2.6 Development of the twin reversed arterial perfusion (TRAP) sequence. Anastomoses between major vessels of the developing arteries lead to reversed arterial blood flow and disruption of normal development in the recipient. BVH, biventricular hypertrophy. (From Van Allen et al 1983,[36] with permission.)

clear if this is causally related to the neural tube defect or is secondary to a mesenchymal tissue abnormality. Persistence of embryonic vessels can result in vascular insufficiency from inadequate caliber or in surgical complications due to the unanticipated anatomic locations.

Regulation of angiogenesis and blood vessel maturation

Embryonic control of angiogenesis and maturation of blood vessels are not completely understood. Abnormal histogenesis of major blood vessels resulting in coarctation of the aorta, renal artery stenosis, and essential hypertension is found in a number of disorders. Among the most common genetic and multiple congenital anomaly disorders with errors in histogenesis of blood vessels are **Turner syndrome, Williams syndrome, vascular neurofibromatosis, Klippel-Trenaunay-Weber syndrome, congenital rubella syndrome, arteriohepatic dysplasia syndrome**, and others, many of which present in adulthood.[38]

Dysplasia of blood vessels is seen in **Klippel-Trenaunay-Weber** syndrome, Sturge-Weber syndrome, arteriovenous fistulas, lethal multiple pterygium syndrome, hemangiomas, neurofibromatosis, Maffucci syndrome, and related disorders.[38, 49] In these disorders, there appears to be abnormal control of blood vessel formation and structure. In animal studies, sympathetic denervation is associated with an increase in blood flow and in formation of arterial-to-venous fistulas in the rabbit ear.[50]

Occlusion of blood vessels

External compression

The type of structural anomaly that results from external compression of vessels depends on the location, amount, and duration of the external pressure, as well as the timing during gestation.[3] **Pressure necrosis** is caused by **occlusion of vessels, local tissue damage from stasis, anoxia, accumulation of metabolites,** and **extravasation of fluid.**[3, 51, 52] **External compression** can result from **amniotic entanglement** (ring constrictions, amniotic band syndrome) (Fig. 4.2.12),[10, 11, 53] **strangulation** of an extremity (Fig. 4.2.2) or neck with the umbilical cord, in utero constraint from a fallopian tube pregnancy, bicornuate uterus, or uterine fibroma.[54–56]

Matsunaga and Shiota[54] studied 3614 specimens from elective first-trimester abortions and demonstrated a non-random excess of unilateral limb defects in 43 tubal pregnancies,

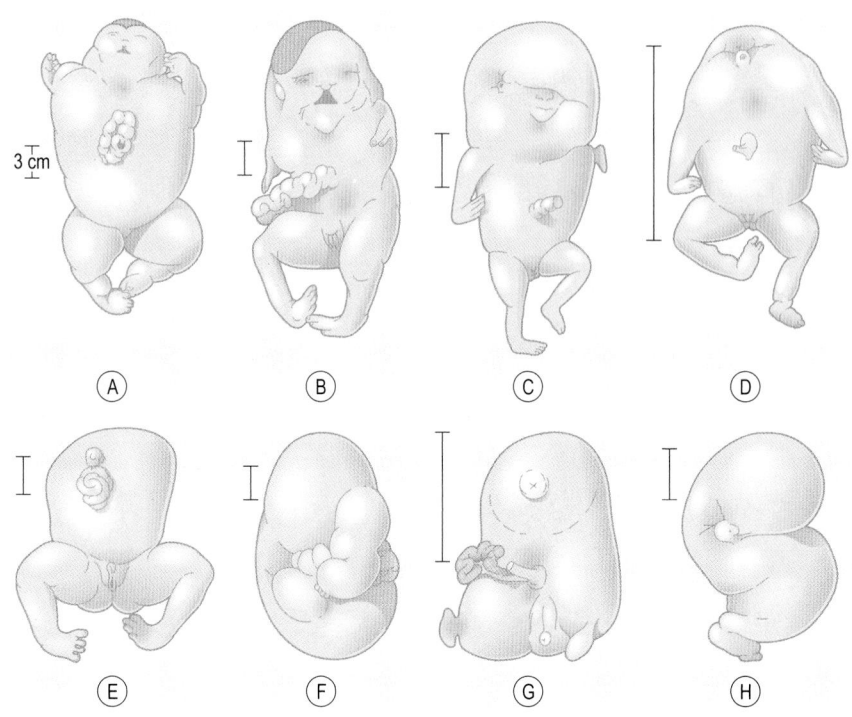

3 cm

(A)   (B)   (C)   (D)

(E)   (F)   (G)   (H)

FIGURE 4.2.7 Representative examples of perfused (acardiac) twins demonstrating the gradation of loss of normal form, with relative sparing of the lower body. Unique external features are demonstrated in these specimens. (A) An edematous 1.21 kg female twin with anencephaly, midline cleft lip and palate, micro-ophthalmia, radial aplasia, limb reductions, oligodactyly, and syndactyly. (B) A 3.1 kg twin female with anencephaly, micro-ophthalmia, midline cleft lip and palate, gastroschisis, phocomelia, and oligodactyly. (C) A 700 g triplet female with micro-ophthalmia, radial aplasia, phocomelia, and oligodactyly. (D) A 100 g female twin having cyclopia with a proboscis, omphalocele, radial aplasia, oligodactyly, absent cranial vault, clubfeet, and marked edema. (E) A 530 g female twin with absent head, thorax, and arms; omphalocele; clubfeet; and oligodactyly. (F) A 3.2 kg male twin with absent cranial end, partial abdominal cavity, omphalocele, reduced lower limbs, oligodactyly, and syndactyly. (G) A 770 g twin with absent cranium, minimal thoracic cavity, omphalocele, herniation of the gut from the umbilicus, cloacal extrophy, and skin tags suggestive of limbs. (H) A 500 g female triplet with hemipelvis, a single leg with a single toe, having a small omphalocele with complete absence of thoracic and cranial structures.

and caudal dysplasia in 97 pregnancies from myomatous uteri. Isolated limb reduction anomalies have been reported in association with bicornuate uteri and with large uterine fibroids.[3, 55, 56] These studies are consistent with external constraint and inadequate blood supply to the developing embryo being teratogenic.

Emboli and thrombosis

Studies of twins have provided considerable evidence of embolic occlusion of embryonic or fetal vessels causing structural anomalies. **Limb reduction anomalies** in singletons have been reported associated with **segmental infarction of the placenta,** with tissue infarction from either emboli of necrotic tissue or **transient hypotension** (Fig. 4.2.13).[8] In utero artery and vein thrombosis due to hypercoagulable states, such as occurs in infants of diabetic mothers (IDMs), can cause gangrene and subsequent tissue loss (Fig. 4.2.14).[7] Cutis aplasia can result

from focal abnormal blood supply, can develop after embolic events, or can be due to external pressure occluding terminal blood vessels.

Altered hemodynamics

Alteration in blood flow to the uterine-placental unit, from either chronic or acute reduction of uterine blood supply, affects the developing embryo and fetus (Table 4.2.2).[3,4] Acute reduction in blood flow has been studied after maternal trauma, hypotension, sympathetic nerve stimulation,[56] and clamping of uterine vessels.[21, 22] The clinical implications of these studies are striking with reference to maternal use of **cocaine**[26, 58, 59] and other vaso-active agents.[3] Control of uterine blood flow is achieved by sympathetic adrenergic vasoconstrictors. The resting tonus of these fibers is minimal, a widely dilated vascular bed being the usual state.[57] Agents such as cocaine that stimulate sympathetic nervous activity would reduce the uterine blood flow.[26] Although

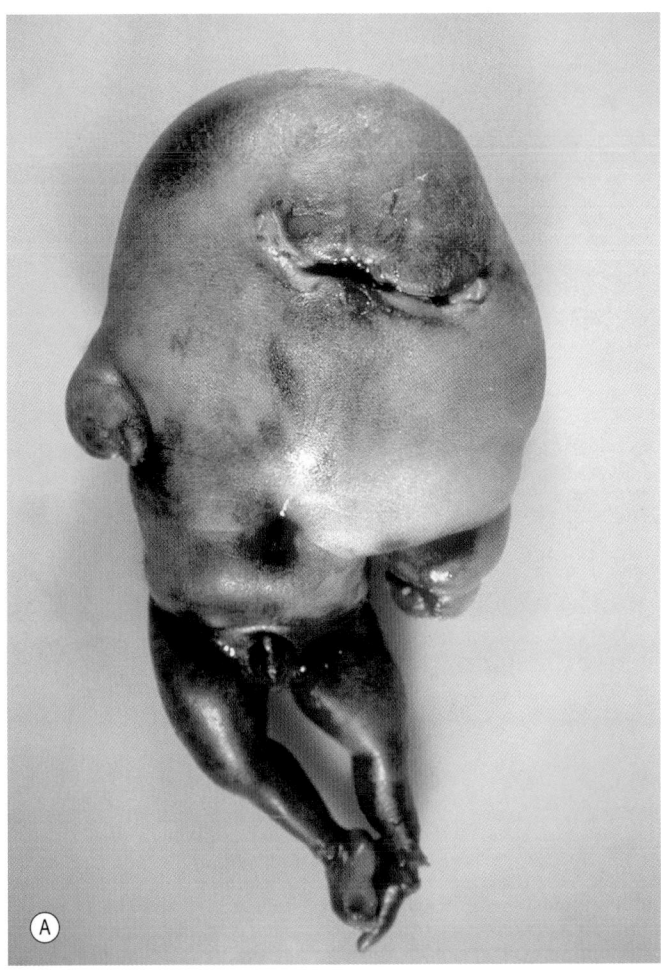

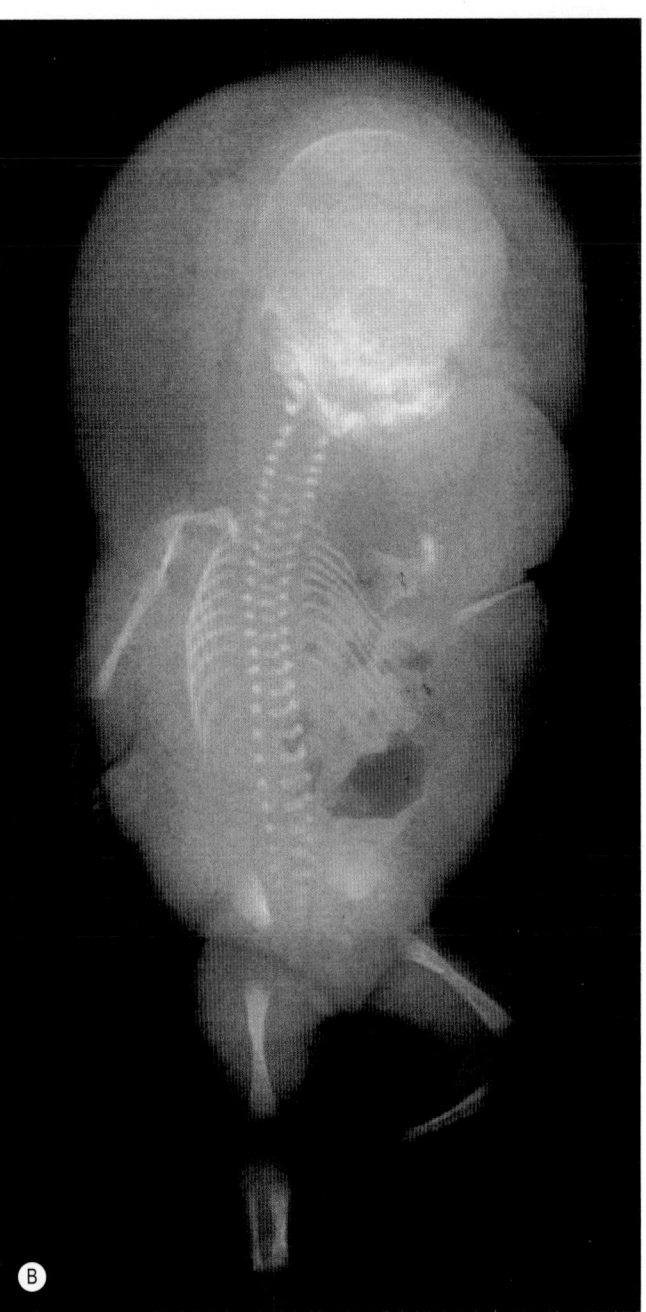

FIGURE 4.2.8 (A) The perfused twin illustrated in Figure 4.2.7C demonstrating the abundance of myxedematous tissue. (B) Relative preservation of the skeleton, which has differentiated even in the presence of low oxygen tension.

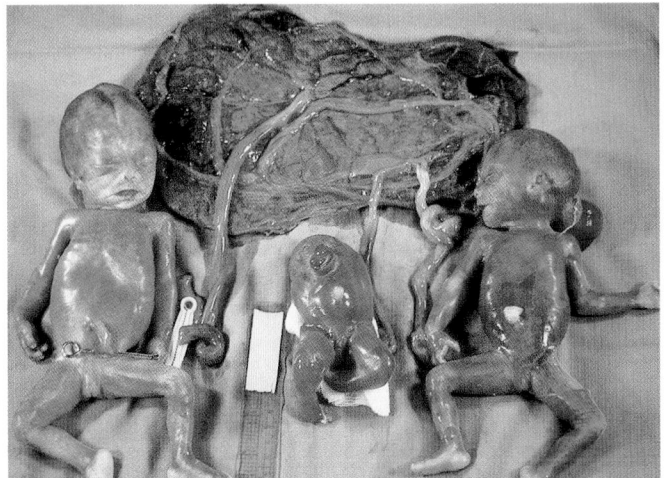

FIGURE 4.2.9 Triplet monochorionic fetuses, with normal triplet (left) having a separate amniotic sac from its co-triplets, one with acephalus acranium and the other with an occipital encephalocele. Note the umbilical artery anastomoses between the two abnormal twins on the surface of the chorion.

TABLE 4.2.2 DRUGS AND EFFECTS THAT INDUCE HEMORRHAGE IN EXPERIMENTAL ANIMAL MODELS

Drugs	Effects
Epinephrine	Hypotension
Norepinephrine	Uterine artery occlusion
Vasopressin	Sympathetic nerve stimulation
Trypan blue	Hypertension
Cocaine	Fetal hypoxia
Salicylates	Acute amnion rupture
Anticoagulants	Placental manipulation
Triazene	
Thalidomide	

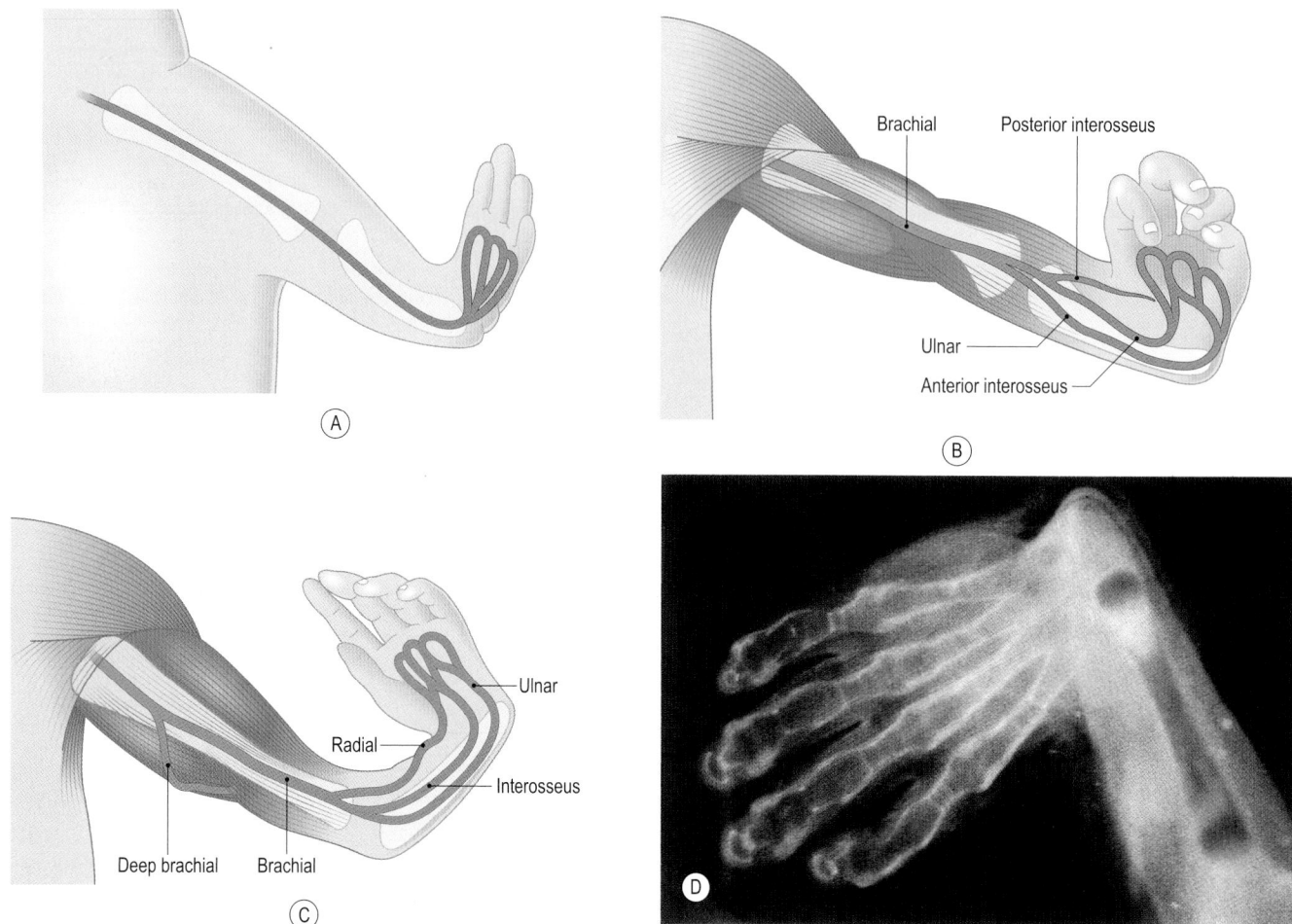

FIGURE 4.2.10 Vascular patterns in radial aplasia. (A) Type I. The limb is supplied by a single superficial midline artery, a persistent embryonic axial artery that arborized in the hand to form a circular arcade. (B) Type II. The radial artery is absent, with or without persistence of the embryonic medial artery, and the ulnar and interosseous arteries have their usual course. (C) Type III. The radial artery is present with an aberrant course to the posterior surface of the hand. (D) Absence of radius and thumb. Alcian red preparation. (From Van Allen et al 1982,[44] with permission.)

the maternal intervillous and fetal villous blood are not interconnected, the placental blood flow is dependent on maternal blood pressure rather than the activity of the embryonic heart. **Stasis of placental blood flow** can result in **circulatory failure in the embryo** (Fig. 4.2.15).

Whether or not the anoxia or vascular disruption results from altered placental–embryonic/fetal hemodynamics depends on the duration and severity of the **reduced uterine blood flow.** The embryonic and fetal tissues that are most sensitive to hyper- or hypoperfusion are tissues that are actively differentiating, tissues with high oxygen and nutrient requirements (e.g. brain, liver), tissues with a high circulatory-flow rate, newly formed vessels (the capillary plexus), distal vasculature, and tissues with a watershed blood supply. Changes observed in blood vessels of laboratory animals after uterine-artery ligation are initial loss of integrity of the vessel wall, plasma leakage and subcutaneous bleb formation, followed by vessel rupture, hemorrhagic necrosis, and tissue loss.[21, 38] If the fetus survives acute reduction of uterine blood flow, reparative processes

begin; damaged tissues are resorbed without reformation of previously existing structures, and morphogenesis of developing tissues is abnormal or incomplete.

Evidence for structural anomalies from vascular disruption

Evidence for vascular disruption causing structural anomalies comes from studies of discordant monozygotic (MZ) twins, singletons with amniotic entanglement, dissection of vasculature, fetal and maternal trauma, prospective ultrasound observations, Doppler flow studies, exposure to vasoactive teratogens (e.g. cocaine), the epidemiology of at-risk populations, and experimental animal models. The most common structural anomalies resulting from vascular disruption are discussed below.

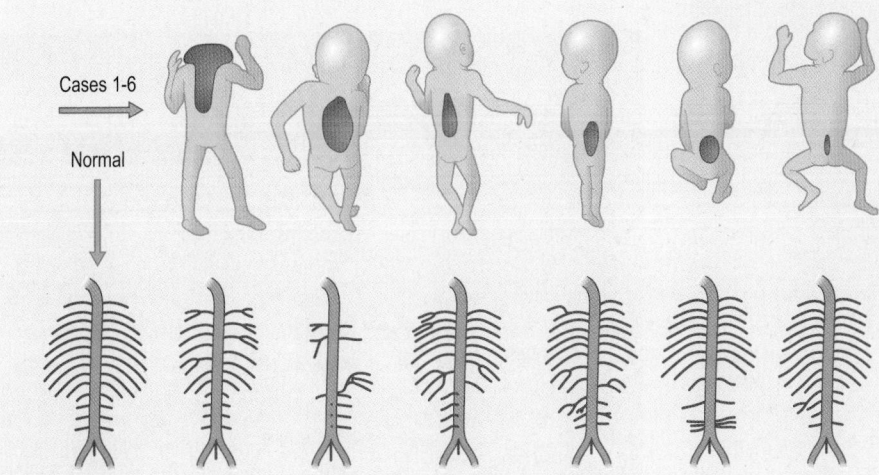

FIGURE 4.2.11 Artery dissections of five fetuses with meningomyelocele and one fetus with craniorachischisis. Top, Location and size of spinal defects in fetuses from the study. Bottom, Aorta and dorsal intersegmental arteries in the control fetus and in six fetuses with abnormalities of spinal closure.

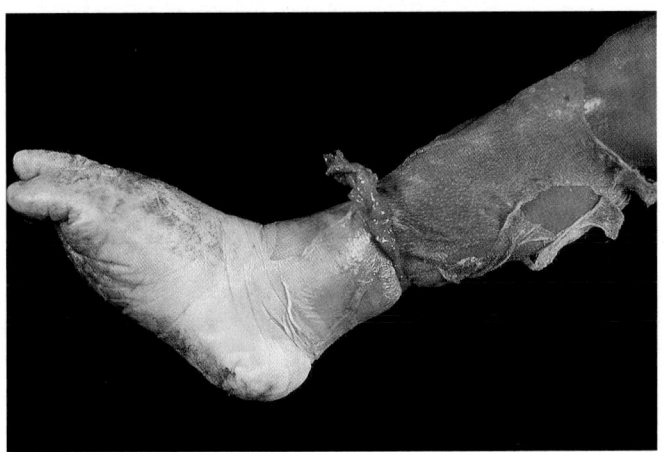

FIGURE 4.2.12 Ring constriction from amniotic entanglement resulting in occlusion of venous supply and engorgement of the distal limb.

Twin studies and placental arterial-to-venous anastomoses

Structural anomalies are 50% more frequent in twins than in singletons.[60] This increased risk is attributable to an excess of anomalies in MZ twins.[61] Many of these anomalies may be caused by vascular disruption from arterial-to-venous anastomoses between twins because of a shared placenta. Injection studies of monochorionic placentas demonstrate that **anastomoses are present in 94–98% of MZ twins.**[62,63] In dizygotic (DZ) twins, **vascular anastomoses** can occur if the dichorionic placentas have fused, and are present in 1.5% of fetuses studied.[62] As expected from the placental studies, structural anomalies from vascular disruption are more common in MZ than in DZ twins.

Events leading to **vascular disruption in twins** are hypothesized to result from:

- **emboli** from the placenta to both MZ twins, causing death of one twin and structural anomalies from embolic infarction in the surviving twin (either after a single embolic episode or after showers of emboli at different times on the basis of histologic examination);[64]
- **thromboplastin** from the demised co-twin causing disseminated intravascular coagulation and structural anomalies in the surviving twin;
- **altered fetal hemodynamics** with transient hypotension or hypertension;
- **altered growth and anomalies from embryonic hypoperfusion;** or
- **disparate placental blood flow** (maternal–placental unit) resulting in altered growth and anomalies from hypo- or hyperperfusion.

Structural anomalies reported in twins after in utero demise of the co-twin attributed to vascular disruption are summarized in Box 4.2.2. In surviving twins the most common structural anomalies identified after death of a co-twin are **central nervous system (CNS) anomalies** in 72%; **gastrointestinal anomalies (intestinal atresias, hepatic and splenic infarcts)** in 19%; **kidney anomalies** in 15%; and **lung anomalies** (usually infarcts) in 8%.[64] Other anomalies have also been reported in MZ twins at a frequency greater than expected as based on the incidence in singletons.[65,66]

Serial ultrasound examinations have provided evidence that supports vascular disruption occurring after death of a co-twin by observing the appearance of structural anomalies in previously normal fetuses. Serial fetal ultrasound examinations have documented the appearance of CNS damage and other anomalies in fetuses after the demise of a co-twin.[65–70] **Acrosyndactyly, ring constrictions without amniotic entanglement,** and **cleft lip and palate** were present in a newborn, with ultrasound documentation of death of a co-twin in the first trimester (Fig. 4.2.16).[11] Had the ultrasound not documented the twin pregnancy and the absence of an abnormal amnion, the cause of the anomalies would have been unclear.

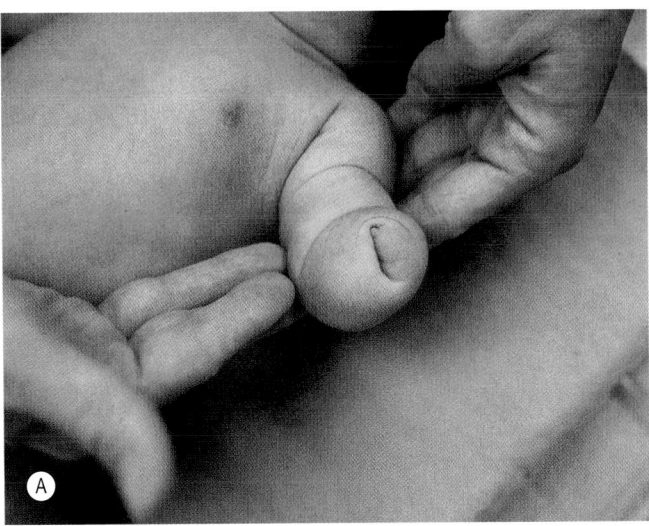

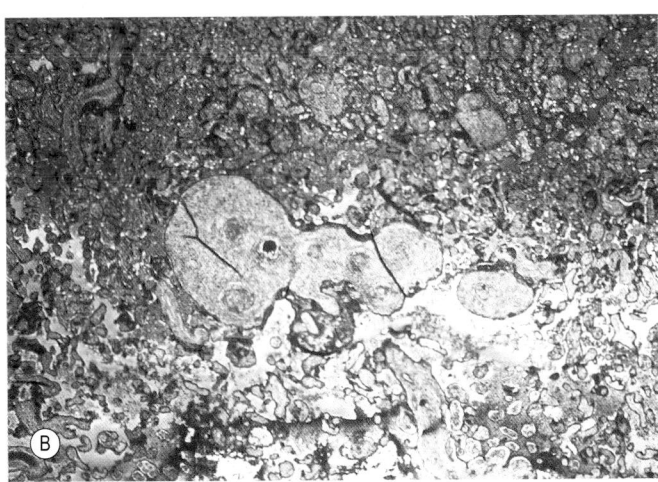

FIGURE 4.2.13 (A) Limb reduction anomalies. (B) Infarct of placenta. (From Hoyme et al 1982,[8] with permission.)

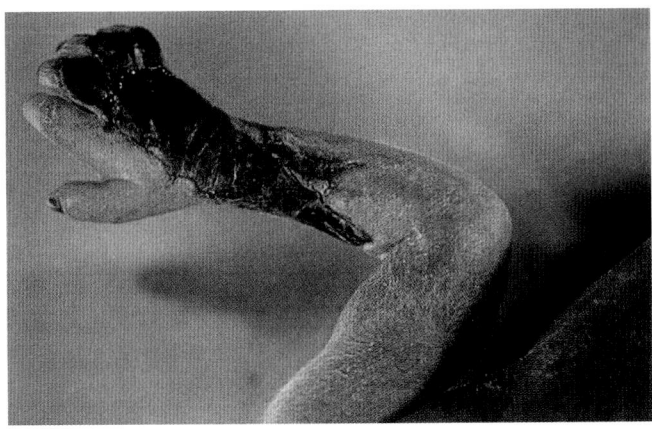

FIGURE 4.2.14 In utero thrombosis of the subclavian artery of an infant of an insulin-dependent diabetic mother resulting in neonatal gangrene in a 32-week gestation pregnancy. Postnatally, there was development of collaterals with progression of non-bacterial gangrene. The infant died at 23 days of age of complications resulting from thrombosis of the renal, superior, and inferior mesenteric arteries. (From Van Allen et al 1989,[7] with permission.)

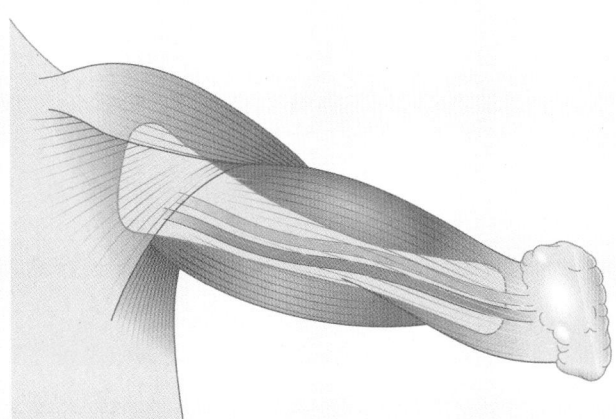

FIGURE 4.2.15 Brachial artery thrombosis after maternal blood loss from abruptio placentae, hypotension, and severe secondary anemia. Distal necrosis of the limb occurred with autoamputation in utero, followed by spontaneous abortion. (From Hoyme et al 1982,[8] with permission.)

Isolated structural anomalies and disruption sequences due to vascular disruption

Structural anomalies due to vascular disruption are common in singletons. It is usually difficult to determine the specific etiologic factor that caused the disruption. The pregnancy history, with respect to a known mechanism of disruption, is usually negative. Epidemiologic studies suggest that young and/or primiparous mothers are more at risk for having offspring with structural anomalies from vascular disruption in some disorders, including gastroschisis and hydranencephaly.[71–73] Age was not found to be a contributing factor in limb–body wall complex (LBWC) in a study performed in Japan.[74]

Congenital encephaloclastic porencephaly

Congenital encephaloclastic porencephaly consists of a cavity in the brain resulting from destruction of normal brain tissue.[75, 76] The lesion can be single or multiple, unilateral or bilateral. It has a variety of causes, including vascular accidents, trauma, and toxic

Central nervous system
Parietal, occipital infarcts
Cerebellar infarcts
Porencephaly
Hydranencephaly
Hydrocephalus
Multicystic encephalomalacia
Microcephaly
Transverse myelia

Gastrointestinal
Hepatic infarct
Subhepatic cyst
Splenic infarct
Gallbladder atresia
Small bowel atresia
Colonic atresia
Appendiceal atresia
Gastroschisis

Limbs
Transverse limb reduction
Constriction bands
Digital amputations
Gangrene, arterial thrombosis
Craniofacial
Cleft lip/palate
Facial clefts
Hemifacial microsomia

Lung
Arterial thrombi
Pulmonary infarcts

Kidney
Renocortical infarction
Renomedullary infarction
Unilateral renal atresia
Horseshoe kidney
Splenogonadal fusion
Bilateral anorchia

Other disorders
Cutis aplasia
Oromandibular limb hypogenesis
Poland disruption sequence
Limb body wall disruption sequence
Twin reversed arterial perfusion (TRAP) sequence

softening and destruction of the brain. They usually communicate with the ventricular or subarachnoid space, or both. Microscopic examination demonstrates proliferation of astrocytes and blood vessels around the edge of the defect. Hydrocephalus is a common associated finding.

Multicystic encephalomalacia

Multicystic encephalomalacia has been reported in twins and is thought to result from multiple emboli occluding cerebral vessels.[66,75] (Fig. 4.2.16B) Multicystic encephalomalacia is also seen in **Aicardi syndrome,** a sporadic disorder of unknown etiology.

Hydranencephaly

In hydranencephaly, all or nearly all of the telencephalon is absent. This is thought to result from destruction of a previously formed brain. Within the skull there is a fluid-filled cavity surrounded by leptomeninges, usually with a gliotic molecular layer and sometimes small islands of partly preserved cerebral cortex.[75–77] There may be relative sparing of the interior temporal and occipital regions of the brain.

Clinical and experimental evidence supports vascular disruption in the pathogenesis of hydranencephaly. Death of an MZ co-twin,[37,64,66,66a] hemorrhagic states such as **factor XIII deficiency,**[78] serial ultrasound examinations after an in utero stroke,[67–70] prenatal infections with **toxoplasmosis**[79] and **herpes simplex,**[80] and **maternal hypoxemia**[81] are all associated with hydranencephaly, supporting vascular occlusion or necrosis in the etiology of this disorder. Carotid occlusion using paraffin balls in puppies, and ligation of the carotid arteries and jugular veins in monkeys, produce massive liquefaction necrosis of the brain and a condition equivalent to hydrancephaly.[82,83] Hydranencephaly has been reported in association with congenital vascular malformations (port wine stains, generalized nevus flammeus, anomalous retinal vessels and internal carotid flow), as well as with malformations of larger vessels (e.g. webbing of the carotid alteries and an absent internal carotid artery system).[83a] Collapse of the cranium, microcephaly, and cutis verticis gyrata result in a clinical situation that resembles fetal brain disruption sequence (Fig. 4.2.17).[84] The usual pattern of destruction suggests bilateral carotid artery insufficiency with preservation of the vertebrobasilar circulation.[75–77]

Oculoauriculovertebral spectrum

Oculoauriculovertebral spectrum (OAV, hemifacial microsoma, Goldenhar syndrome)[85–87] is characterized by uni- or bilateral microtia, mandibular hypoplasia, and anomalies of the cervical spine and/or epibulbar dermoids or lipodermoids (Fig. 4.2.18). There is facial asymmetry with mandibular as well as maxillary, temporal, and malar bone hypoplasia, with occasional bilateral

and infectious agents. The disruptive vascular etiology of porencephaly has been well documented.[75,76] In most cases the cerebral destruction is restricted to the distribution of the middle cerebral artery.

Encephaloclastic lesions can result from insults during the fetal period, at birth, or postnatally. They result from necrotic

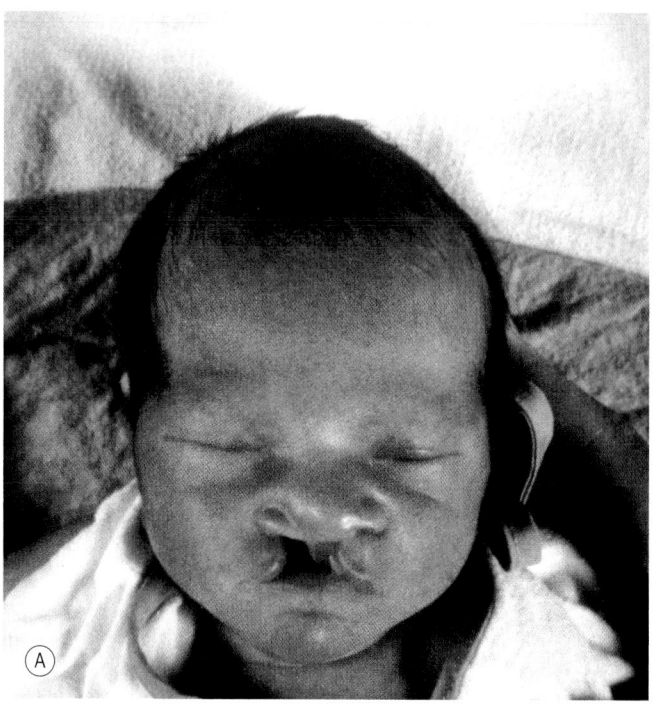

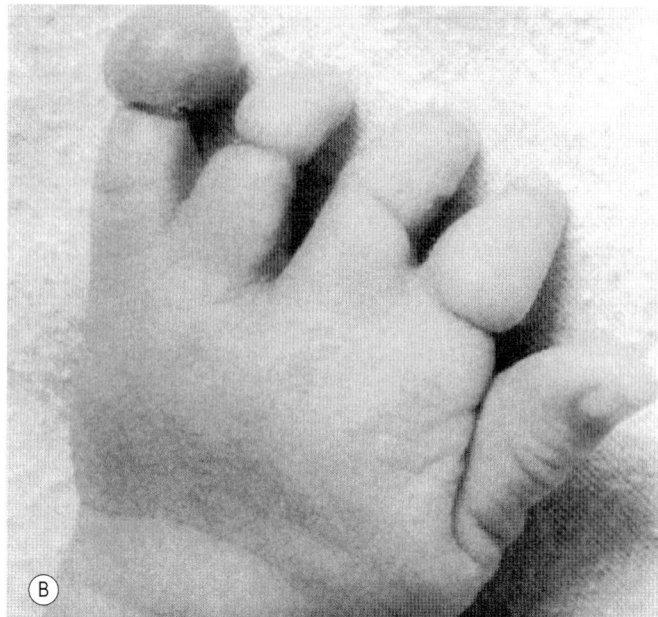

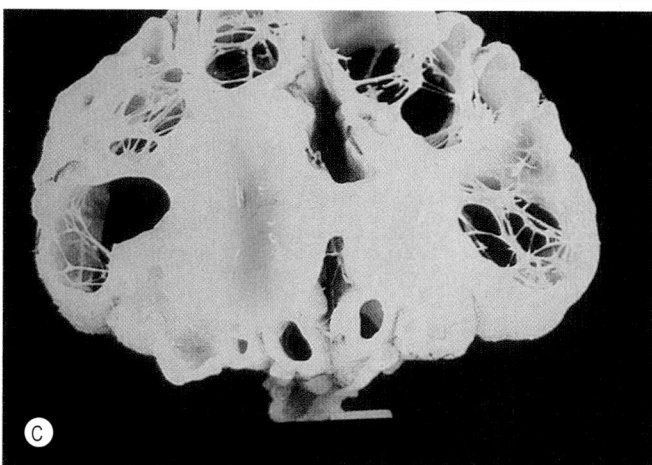

FIGURE 4.2.16 First-trimester ultrasound examination demonstrated a monochorionic, diamniotic twin pregnancy and a smaller, nonviable co-twin. There was no evidence of amniotic strands or persistence of the extraembryonic coelom. At birth the following anomalies were present in the surviving twin. (A) Left cleft lip and cleft palate. (B) Acrosyndactyly of left hand with ring constrictions and reduction of digits 2–5 with proximal syndactyly. The constriction pattern found on the digits strongly suggests that this malformation (and thus the cleft lip and palate of the same child) likely results from amniotic bands, even though such bands could not be identified after careful examination of the placenta. (C) Encephaloclastic porencephaly. Multiple porencephalic cysts are present in the brain, caused by either emboli from necrotic tissue or absorption of toxic substances from a dead twin, resulting in cerebral vascular disruption. (A and B from Van Allen et al 1992,[11] with permission.)

involvement. The ipsilateral ear is dysplastic, with nubbins of tissue (undifferentiated hillocks of His), anotia, and canal atresia. The contralateral ear can also be abnormal. Supernumerary ear tags can occur anywhere from the tragus to the angle of the mouth. Eye involvement is present in 35% with epibulbar dermoids (white solid masses), lipodermoids (yellow, movable, conjunctival), or dermis-like or complex dermoids (mesoectodermal). Other eye anomalies can occur, including microphthalmia and microcornea, as can bilateral involvement.

Common associated anomalies[85–87] include **CNS defects** in 5–15%, including **frontal and occipital encephaloceles, hydrocephaly, lipoma,** and others. **Cranial nerve involvement** is frequent, with lower facial muscle weakness in 10–20% (CN VII) as well as other cranial nerves (CN III, IV, VI, IX). Congenital **heart anomalies** are common (5–58%, depending on the series). In particular, ventricular septal defect (VSD) and tetralogy of Fallot account for at least half the anomalies. **Vertebral defects,**

especially in the cervical region, occur in 20–30%. Further anomalies include talipes equinovarus in 20%, radial limb anomalies in 10%, and other anomalies of the **VACTERL** association (vertebral, anal, cardiac, tracheoesophageal, renal, and limb abnormalities).

Differential diagnosis[87] includes **Townes-Brocks syndrome,** an autosomal dominant disorder with similar facial anomalies, hearing loss, anal defects, and renal anomalies; and **branchio-otorenal (BOR) syndrome,** an autosomal dominant disorder with hearing loss, preauricular pits, branchial fistulas or cysts, abnormal pinna, and/or renal dysplasia. Characteristic features of OAV spectrum are distinguishable from **mandibulofacial dysostosis** and **Nager acrofacial dysostosis,** which have bilateral involvement, and other anomalies.

Poswillo[88–90] demonstrated with an animal model that disruption of the **embryonic stapedial artery** resulted in an

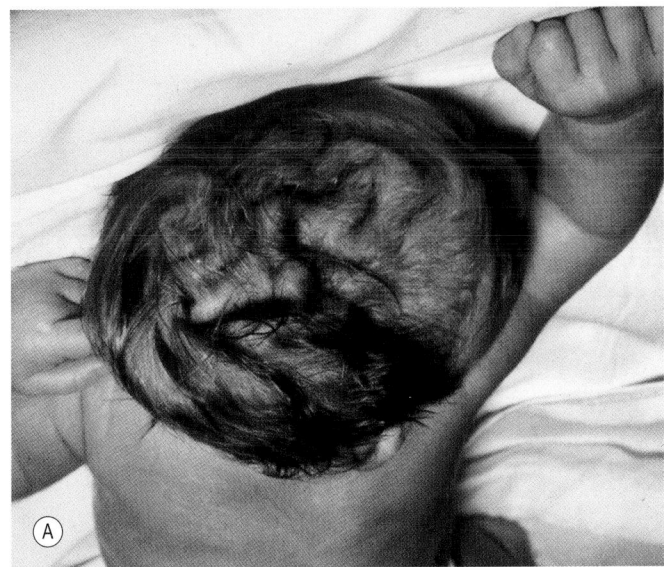 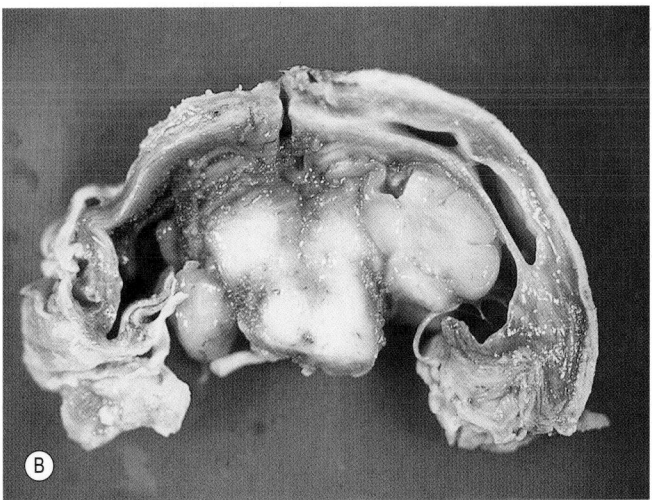

FIGURE 4.2.17 Cutis verticis gyrata. Third trimester in utero thrombosis of the sinus venosis with necrosis of the cerebral cortex and collapse of the skull resulting in cutis verticis gyrata congenita and severe microcephaly.

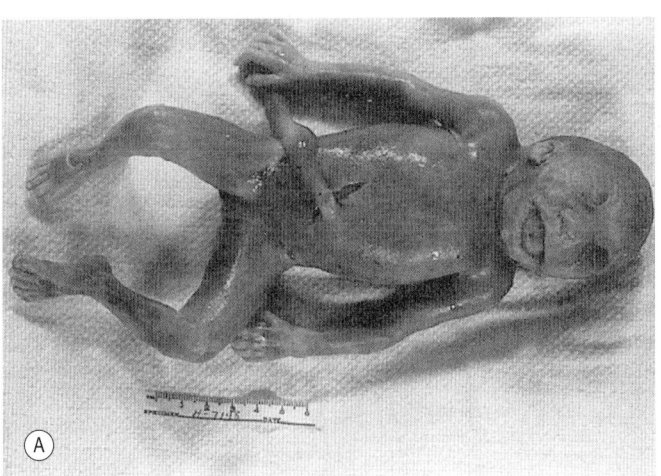 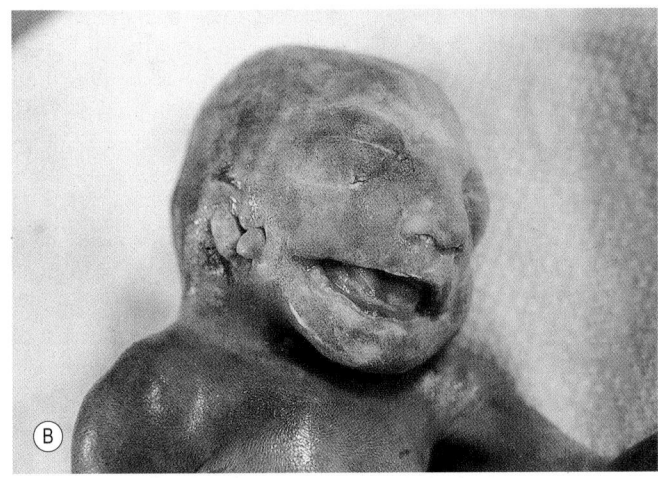

FIGURE 4.2.18 (A) A 430 g, 19-week female fetus with oculoauriculovertebral syndrome. Anomalies include occipital encephalocele and bilateral facial microsomia, with the left side more severely reduced than the right and macrosomia. (B) There is macrostomia and abnormal left auricle development with ear tags and absent ear canal. The right ear has a normally formed auricle plus five preauricular ear tabs. Additionally there are cleft palate, cervical vertebral defects, ventricular septal defect, and no eye anomalies.

expanding hematoma with destruction of differentiating tissues in the region of the ear and jaw.

During embryogenesis, the stapedial artery courses next to the facial nerve, with two branches – the ventral stem, which branches into the maxillary (infraorbital) and mandibular arteries, and the dorsal or supraorbital division, which supplies the primitive orbit and the gasserian ganglion.[91] The severity of tissue destruction determines the degree of resultant damage. Similar observations have been made in humans.[92, 93] The constellation of anomalies suggests that disruption occurs between 30 and 45 days pc in humans. Another possible mechanism consists of disturbances in the branchial arches or various populations of neural crest cells that may inhibit development of adjacent medial or frontonasal processes. These could have a variety of causes.[84–87]

Other causes of OAV are teratogens (e.g. retinoic acid, maternal diabetes, thalidomide, primidone) and chromosomal disorders [(del(5p), del(6q), trisomy 7 mosaicism, del(8q), trisomy 9 mosaicism, trisomy 18, recombinant chromosome 18, del(18q), ring 21 chromosome, del(22q), 49,XXXXY, 47,XXY].[85–87, 94]

Most cases of OAV are sporadic, but familial cases have been reported.[87, 94] Discordance for OAV in MZ twins has been reported. Rarely, concordance with variable expression has been documented in MZ twins.

Gastroschisis

Gastroschisis is an abdominal wall defect lateral to the umbilical cord (more commonly on the left; see also Ch. 21). It is distinguished from an omphalocele by the absence of a membranous sac. There is usually extrusion of abdominal organs into the amniotic cavity rather than the extracoelomic space, as occurs in a lateral body wall defect (e.g. LBWC). There is good evidence to support the hypothesis of Hoyme and colleagues[42] that gastroschisis results from **premature ablation and/or disruption of the embryonic omphalomesenteric artery.**

The paired omphalomesenteric arteries are among the first arteries to form in the embryo, connecting the aorta with the yolk sac by 23 days' gestation (Fig. 4.2.19).[42, 95] The superior mesenteric artery (SMA), which supplies the small intestines, is derived from this embryonic artery. By a process of a controlled cell death and formation of new vascular connections, the left omphalomesenteric artery is ablated. The right omphalomesenteric artery continues to supply the omphalocele sac and the skin at the base of the umbilical cord after the intestine returns to the peritoneal cavity by 10 weeks' pc. Premature ablation of the left or disruption of the right omphalomesenteric artery will result in local necrosis and tissue loss. The resultant abdominal wall defect leads to extrusion of abdominal contents into the amniotic cavity.

Associated structural anomalies, in particular in the gastrointestinal tract, are present in 40–50% of cases with gastroschisis.[42, 96] Frequent associated anomalies include non-duodenal intestinal atresia or stenosis, atresia of the appendix, 'apple-peel' bowel (see below), atresia of the gallbladder, absence of one kidney, hydronephrosis and hydroureters, and porencephaly.

Decongestant use, particularly ephedrine, pseudoephedrine, methylenedioxymethamphetamine and phenylpropanolamine in the first trimester has been associated with an increased risk of gastroschisis, small intestinal abrasion, atresia of the appendix, and hemifacial microsomia; all thought to arise from vascular disruption.[96a] This risk appears to be enhanced by the vasoconstrictive effects of cigarette smoking and alcohol intake.[96a]

Intestinal atresia

It is well accepted that segmental intestinal atresia, with or without a fibrous cord, and 'apple-peel' bowel are secondary to disruption of the SMA. Associated structural anomalies include **gastroschisis, gallbladder abnormalities, abnormal cystic artery and duct, biliary duct anomalies, and hypospadias.** All of these have been associated with disruptions, but there are other causes.

'Apple-peel' bowel is a descriptive term referring to the configuration of the distal small bowel in some cases of jejunal atresia.[97] This defect has been shown by arteriographic studies to be secondary to in utero interruption of the SMA.[42, 98, 99]

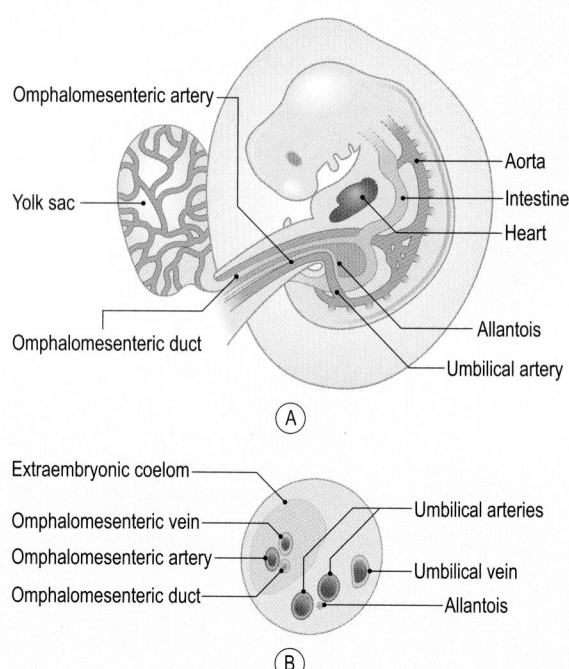

FIGURE 4.2.19 Gastroschisis results from premature ablation or disruption of the omphalomesenteric artery. (A) Diagrammatic representation of a sagittal view of a 5-mm crown-rump length (32-day) human embryo. Arteries are represented in red; the extraembryonic coelom and peritoneal cavity are shown in darker brown; veins are not shown. (B) Cross-section of the base of the umbilical cord. Note the position of the omphalomesenteric duct and vessels at the right portion of the cord. (From Hoyme et al 1981,[42] with permission.)

Non-duodenal intestinal atresia has been produced experimentally[100] by in utero ligation of branches of the SMA of fetal puppies. Complete ligation resulted in intestinal infarction, resorption, and atresia; partial occlusion of blood supply resulted in intestinal stenosis.

Limb reduction defects

Limb reduction defects are multifactorial in nature. Isolated limb anomalies, especially terminal transverse defects that are sporadic, may be due to vascular disruption. **Terminal transverse defects** have an incidence of 1.8 per 10 000 in British Columbia, being the second most common type of limb abnormalities after terminal longitudinal defects (3.3 per 10 000).[101] Evidence of amniotic entanglement (amniotic band syndrome), placental infarctions, deceased blood flow to co-twins, and maternal factors that place the conceptus at risk for vascular disruption provide support for the theory that this is the cause of the limb anomaly. Monogenic or chromosomal disorders should be excluded.

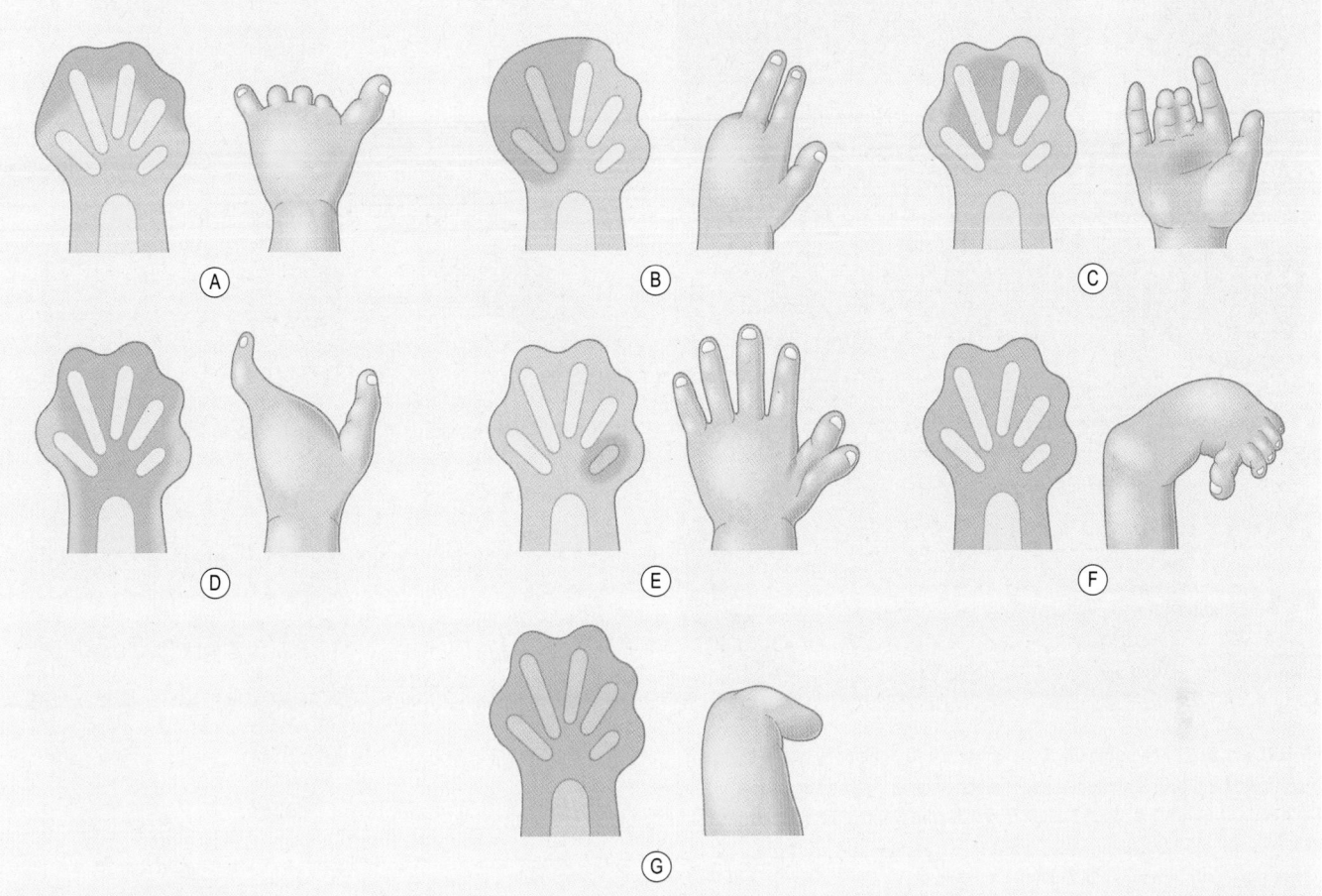

FIGURE 4.2.20 Various types of limb reduction anomalies resulting from vascular disruption. Stippling indicates areas of hemorrhagic necrosis affecting the embryonic limb. See text for discussion. (From Van Allen et al 1987,[106] with permission.)

There is an intimate relationship between vascular development and normal limb morphogenesis in humans and experimental animals. A direct interrelationship between the development of the apical ectodermal ridge (AER) and the marginal vessels (the marginal vein and the capillary plexus) of the limb bud has been found. Damage to the AER leads to disruption of the vascular pattern, with failure of normal development of embryonic vessels and of the limb.[102] Conversely, damage to the marginal vein or terminal capillary plexus may result in damage to the contiguous AER and abnormal limb development.

The AER controls normal limb development through its interaction with the underlying mesoderm.[103–105] The AER is located at the distal rim of the developing limb bud. Excision of part of the AER results in failure of the corresponding terminal parts of the limb bud to develop. Excision and transplantation of the AER to another location on the embryo leads to continued growth and differentiation of the limb tissue. If the AER is removed from the limb bud (after stage 18 of the chick), ectodermal healing takes place, but the ridge does not regenerate and a truncated limb is formed. The earlier the

ablation is performed, the greater will be the ensuing limb defect.[105]

Figure 4.2.20 illustrates various types of limb reduction anomalies resulting from vascular disruption.[106] The stippling indicates the hypothesized area of the limb in which hemorrhagic necrosis affected the embryonic limb. This illustration is based on experimental studies of normal and abnormal limb development[20, 102, 104, 105] and on human studies of radial aplasia and LBWC.[12, 44, 106] Damage to the AER due to rupture of the marginal vein leads to oligodactyly (Fig. 4.2.20A and B) and transverse limb defects. The extent of limb deficiency depends on the size of the hematoma and the timing in gestation when disruption occurred. Transverse limb defects, absent limbs, and limb girdles result from extensive involvement by the hematoma or disruption during early limb bud formation (Fig. 4.2.20G). Hematomas in the middle of the developing hand area of the limb bud lead to split hand or foot with or without oligodactyly, depending on the extent of tissue damage (Fig. 4.2.20D). Hemorrhages in the interdigital spaces lead to syndactyly and acrosyndactyly (pseudosyndactyly) (Fig. 4.2.20C). The interdigital areas of necrosis heal with adhesions between the digits, the undamaged distal tissue

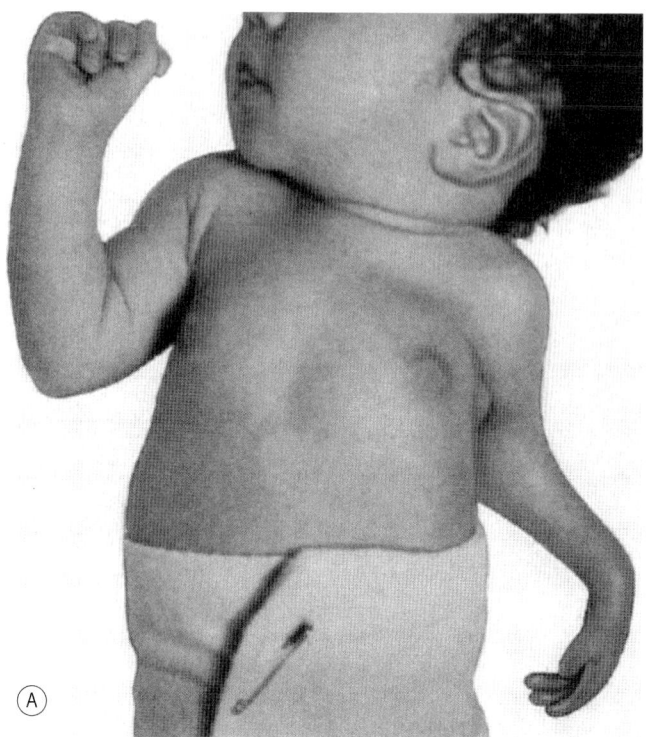

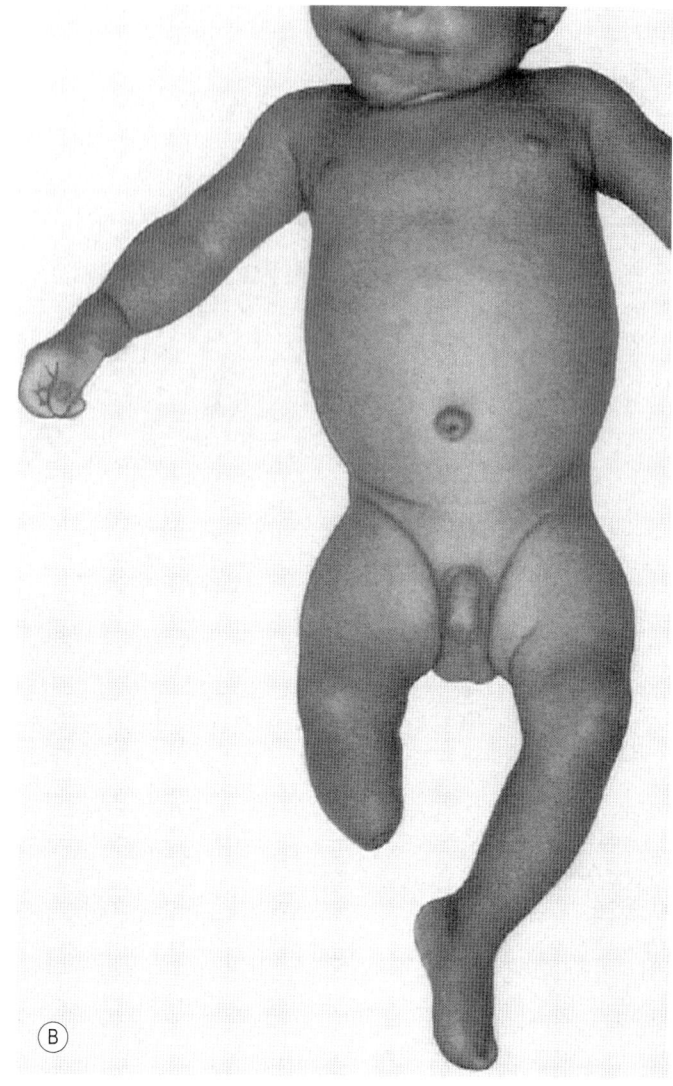

FIGURE 4.2.21 (A) Hypoplasia of the left arm and deficiency of the superior insertion of the pectoral muscle; anomalies seen in Poland sequence. (B) Amniotic bands causing midcalf terminal transverse limb reduction defect, with ring constriction and scarring of right forearm and amputation of left toes.

primordia forming fingers. Syndactyly and acrosyndactyly (pseudosyndactyly) most likely occur in the limb bud that has begun to develop fingers and have a relatively small area of hemorrhagic necrosis. Splitting of a digit by a small hematoma may result in polydactyly (Fig. 4.2.20E). Damage by a hematoma in the soft tissue of the foot may lead to clubfoot (Fig. 4.2.20F), with abnormal tendon insertions and persistence of embryonic vessels.[47]

Figures 4.2.21–4.2.24 illustrate typical limb anomalies resulting from vascular disruption.

Microgastria with limb anomalies

Congenital microgastria is a rare anomaly in which patients suffer from feeding dysfunction, dumping syndrome, reflux, and failure to thrive.[107] Many of the reported structural anomalies associated with microgastria are typical of anomalies resulting from vascular disruption. These include splenogonadal fusion,[108,109] congenital megacolon,[110] abnormal lung lobation,[107,108,110,111] anophthalmia and porencephalic cyst,[112] bicornuate uterus,[111] absence of the kidney,[113] horseshoe kidney, hemifacial microsomia with ipsilateral seventh nerve palsy,[107] and congenital cardiac defects.[108] Shackelford and colleagues[110] described a patient in whom microgastria was associated with components of the VACTERL association with esophageal atresia, lumbosacral vertebral anomalies, and imperforate anus.

Limb anomalies associated with microgastria include predominantly distal ray anomalies, in particular hypoplastic forearm bones, hand, and wrist; radial ray hypoplasia and absent thumb; and peromelia.[107,109,114]

Microgastria associated with specific limb anomalies is not known for certain to be related to vascular disruption. Microgastria is a sporadic disorder. Anomalies of the limb are unilateral. The forearm and hand develop simultaneously with the stomach and spleen, which arise from the dorsal mesogastrium during the fifth embryonic week. The gonad at that time in gestation is in close proximity to the spleen. Hemorrhagic

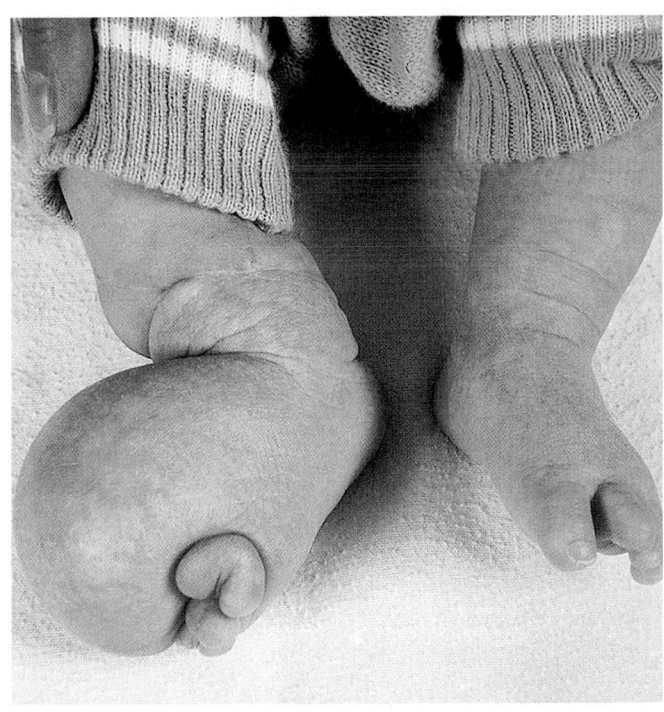

FIGURE 4.2.22 Hypoplasia of the toes and foot seen in a number of disorders associated with vascular disruption. It is most likely due to hypoperfusion during embryogenesis of the foot.

necrosis of tissues may result in adhesion of the gonad to the spleen, preventing descent of the gonads in the peritoneal cavity to the perineum. Previous investigations of the vascular anomalies of radial aplasia suggest that many, though not all, sporadic disorders with these anomalies are the result of abnormal artery development or disruption of embryonic arteries.[3,4] Lueder and associates[107] report a half sib pair, one with microgastria, radial ray anomalies, hemifacial microsomia, and other anomalies. The other child had Klippel-Feil sequence, Sprengel deformity of the right scapula, and congenital fusion of the fourth to sixth cervical vertebrae, which fits into the spectrum of anomalies of subclavian artery supply disruption sequence (SASDS) (see later).[41] The authors suggest a possible monogenic etiology. This may well be the case with an underlying disorder of embryonic vessel development resulting in an increased risk of structural anomalies from vascular disruption.

Adams-Oliver syndrome

Adams-Oliver syndrome is an autosomal dominant disorder associated with **vertex cranial cutis aplasia and terminal transverse limb reduction anomalies.**[115–117] Cutis marmorata and tortuous, dilated scalp veins have been reported in families.[118] Despite large cranial scalp defects, CNS abnormalities are not a feature of this disorder; if they are present, alternative diagnoses need to be considered.[116] There is variable expression, so that

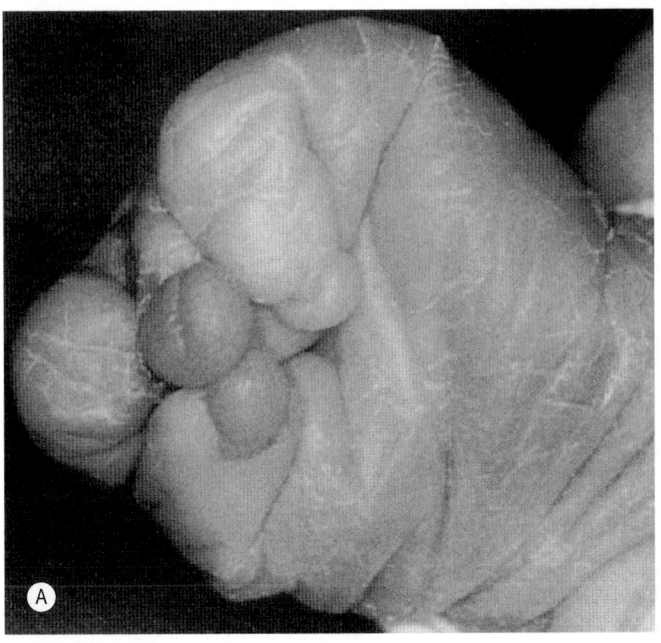
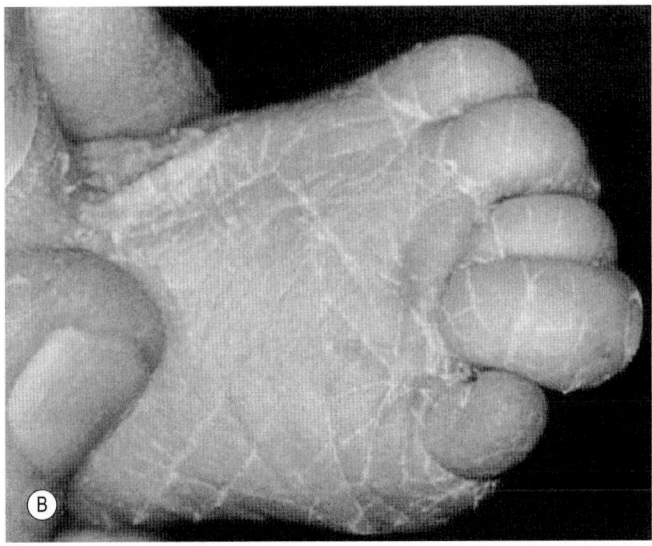

FIGURE 4.2.23 (A) Left hand of a newborn with acrosyndactyly. There is syndactyly of the second and third digits proximally, distal digital fusion of the thumb to the first to third digits, with a ring constriction and a fibrous band ending in a common pedunculated digit. There was no evidence of abnormal amnion or amniotic entanglement. (B) Left foot of a newborn with a shortened big toe of narrow caliber. (From Van Allen et al 1992,[11] with permission.)

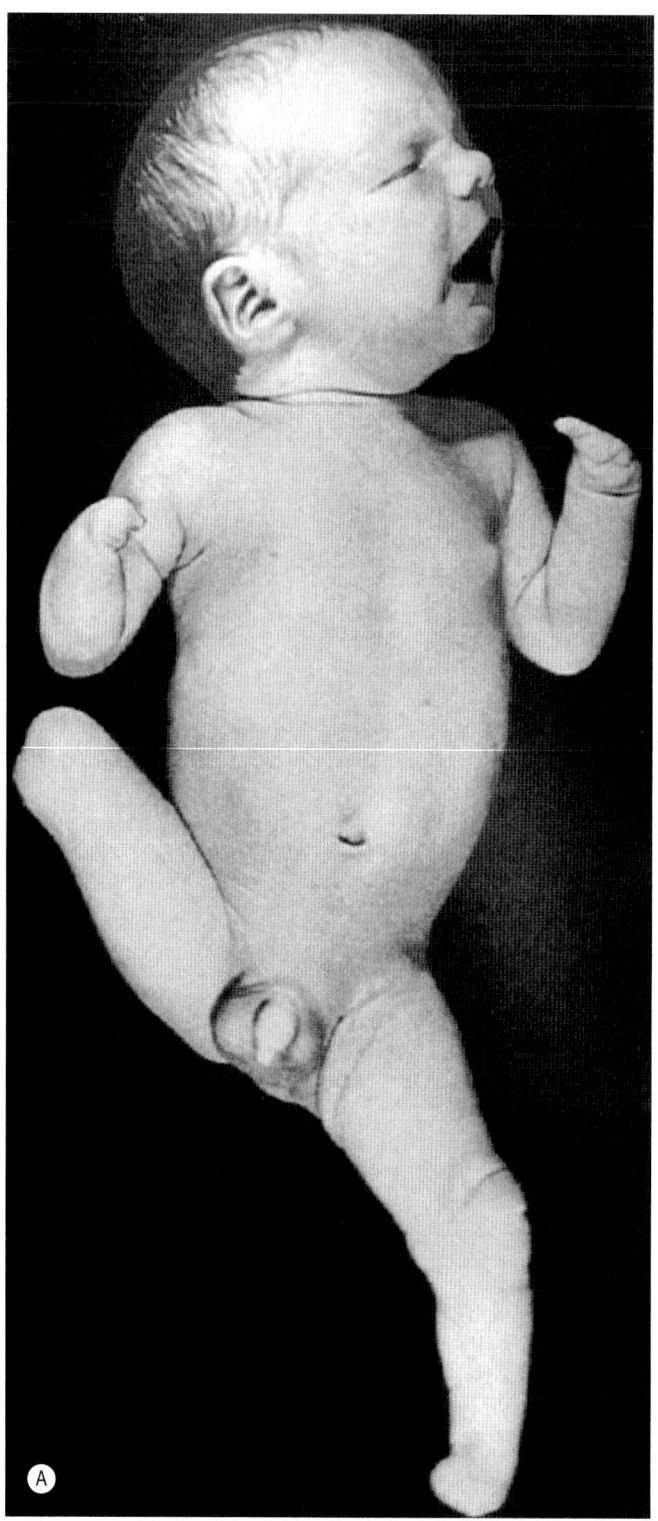

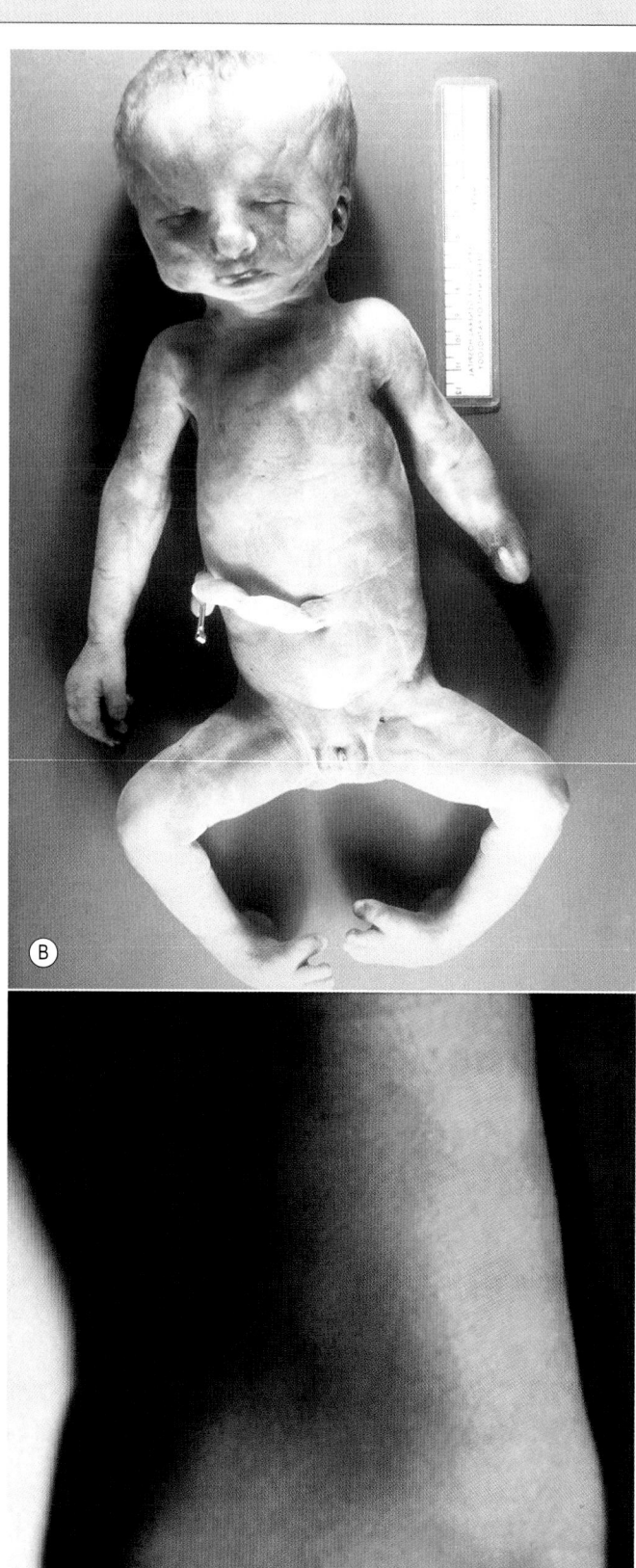

FIGURE 4.2.24 Newborns with oromandibular limb hypogenesis (OMLH) syndrome. Similar structural anomalies have been reported after chorionic villus sampling performed before 10 weeks' gestation (8 weeks' embryonic age). (A) Terminal transverse limb anomalies without involvement of the tongue and mandible. (B) OMLH with mandibular hypoplasia, ankyloglossia, and Möbius syndrome (cranial nerves VI and VII affected), and terminal limb reduction anomalies. (C) Transverse digital reduction defects. (Courtesy of Dr P.J.M. MacLeod.)

minimal clinical findings can be a small bald area at the vertex cranium.[119] Although most families have autosomal dominant inheritance.[115–117] Autosomal recessive inheritance has been reported.[120]

The scalp lesions have been described as areas of thin, atrophic skin or deeper lesions that extend from the skin through the skull to the dura, ranging from 0.5 to 10 cm in diameter.[115, 117, 121] Cutis marmorata is a common associated cutaneous finding.[118]

In the scalp lesion, histologically normal skin abuts a well-demarcated 'membrane' of atrophic epidermis that is thin and gradually fades out entirely.[115–117, 119] In the area of the membrane, there is compact collagen, minimal adipose tissue, and no sebaceous or sweat glands. In the atrophic portion of the scalp, hair follicles are calcified. Some lesions appear to be highly vascular. Deep lesions rarely involve the sagittal sinus, predisposing to episodes of spontaneous hemorrhage, surgical complications, and (in rare cases) death. With open scalp lesions, there is a risk of sepsis and/or meningitis.

Limb defects are typically asymmetric, being more severe in one arm or leg, often with one or more limbs unaffected.[115, 116] The full spectrum of observed defects ranges from **hypoplastic nails, cutaneous syndactyly, bony syndactyly, transverse reduction defects, zygodactyly, ectrodactyly, polydactyly, and brachydactyly.**[119] More severe defects include complete absence of a hand or foot, or virtual absence of a limb (hemiamelia) as in the original proband.[115] Radiographic findings correspond to the structural limb anomaly.

Chorionic Villus Sampling (CVS)

Chorionic villi sampling for prenatal testing uses suction to shear off villi using a catheter. This procedure is associated with an increased risk over the background risk for anomalies resulting from vascular disruption and for miscarriages. If **CVS is performed prior to 10 weeks** (70 days) of gestation (8 weeks post conception) **transverse limb reduction defects, ring constrictions** and **oromandibular hypogenesis spectrum** have been reported (Fig. 4.24).[115a] These anomalies most likely result from vascular disruption but amnion rupture may occur in some cases. The **frequencies of gastroschisis, intestinal atresias and club feet have also been increased with CVS.**[115b] Terminal transverse limb defects have been more likely to affect one or two middle fingers and the absence of the distal portion of the third finger with tapering and stiff joints appears to be a distinctive effect of CVS.[115c]

Teratogenic exposures

Misoprostil is a highly effective abortifactant when taken during the first trimester. In surviving pregnancies, there is a risk for **athrogyposis of the amyoplasia congenital type; terminal transverse limb reduction defects; moebius syn-** drome including cranial nerve palsies plus limb reduction anomalies.

Limb-body wall disruption sequence

In LBWC, a disorder sometimes included in early amnion rupture sequence, evidence has been published in support of the hypothesis of vascular disruption as the cause.[12, 106] This hypothesis has been substantiated by other studies and is believed to be generalizable to other disorders within the early amnion disruption sequence.

Diagnosis of LBWC is based on the presence of two of three of the following characteristics: exencephaly or encephalocele with facial clefts; **thoracoschisis** (upper body wall deficiency) (Fig. 4.2.25), **abdominoschisis** (lower body wall deficiency) (Fig. 4.2.26), or **thoracoabdominoschisis** (Fig. 4.2.27); and limb defects.[12, 106] Classically, **pleurosomas** refers to body wall and upper limb defects, and **cyllosomas** to body wall deficiency and lower limb defects. Structural anomalies of all organ systems are present.

The pathogenesis of LBWC is summarized in Figure 4.2.28[12] and discussed further in Chapter 21. In a study that evaluated vascular disruption as the cause of LBWC, 95% (24/25) of the fetuses with LBWC had associated internal structural anomalies. In 72% of these fetuses (18/25), the internal anomalies are recognized to be secondary to vascular disruption as defined by twin studies (see Box 4.2.2).

Concordances were not found between the side and location of the body wall defect with respect to the location of the limb, internal, and cranial defects.[12, 106] This is consistent with a systemic event, such as circulatory failure, rather than external compression or anomalies resulting from damage to contiguous developmental fields. In 85% of the fetuses, evidence of persistence of the extraembryonic coelom associated with persistence of the ectodermal–amnion margin was found by examination of the placenta, the amnion being continuous with the skin of the body wall defect. In 40% (10/25), there were tags and amniotic adhesions at other sites, suggesting secondary amniotic adhesions and entanglements. There was no difference in the types or incidence of internal structural anomalies among fetuses with, and those without, amniotic adhesions, suggesting that this was a secondary rather than a primary cause of the anomalies.

Urethral obstruction sequence and lower limb deficiency

Over 28 reported examples of urethral obstruction sequence (UOS) with associated lower limb deficiency can be found in the medical literature.[124] UOS is found predominantly in boys and consists of bilateral obstructive changes of the urinary tract most commonly due to urethral valves or atresia, undescended testes, and hypoplasia of the abdominal muscles, giving rise to the wrinkled, **'prune-belly'** appearance in which loops of bowel

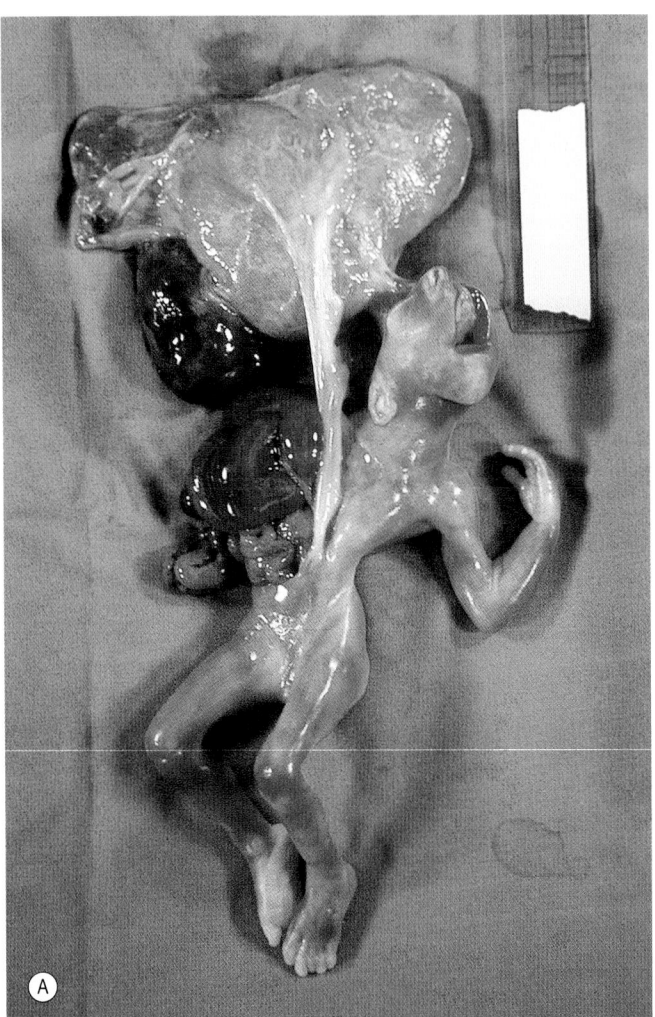
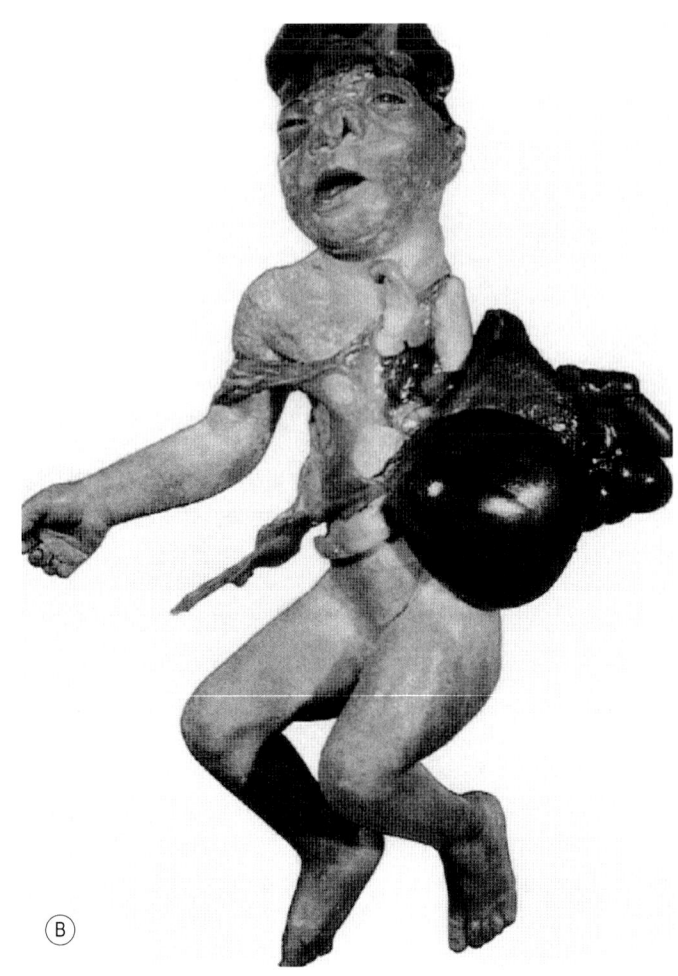

FIGURE 4.2.25 Limb body wall complex with thoracoschisis. (A) Fetus with thoracoschisis and facial cleft. The amnion is continuous with the skin of the cranium, forming a pseudoencephalocele. There is severe scoliosis, absent right arm, and internal structural anomalies. Note the short umbilical cord. (From Van Allen et al 1987,[12] with permission.) (B) Thoracoschisis, absent left arm with a pedicle of tissue forming a rudimentary finger, exencephaly, hypertelorism, and entanglement in the amnion.

are visible through the thin body wall (Fig. 4.2.29). The condition is also known as the **prune-belly syndrome, triad syndrome,** or **Eagle-Barrett syndrome,** but the acceptable term now, based on the pathogenesis, is UOS.[125] Other anomalies are frequently associated with UOS, in particular lower limb deficiency, which is estimated to occur in about 3–5.5% of reported cases.[124, 126, 127]

One proposed etiology for limb reduction defects associated with UOS is vascular compromise by the distended bladder of the iliofemoral vessels, leading to a reduction of vascular supply to the lower limb. Hypoplasia, distal hypoxia with reabsorption of tissue, and/or gangrene would result from the insufficient blood supply. This is supported by the observation of gangrene of the leg at birth.[124]

In other cases the primary event appears to result from damage to the intermediate mesoderm that gives rise to the urinary tract system, and to the lateral mesoderm that gives rise to the lower limbs. An example is teratogenesis from cocaine, which results in an increased risk for UOS as well as limb reduction anomalies.[124, 128, 129] Emboli from the placenta have been associated with two cases of UOS and limb reduction defects.[130]

Cocaine embryopathy and fetopathy

Cocaine has been hypothesized to cause disruption of embryonic and fetal vasculature, **especially in the second and third trimesters.**[26, 131, 132] Structural anomalies reported in infants exposed in utero to cocaine that are consistent with vascular disruption are **non-duodenal intestinal atresia or infarction, unilateral terminal transverse limb reduction defects, atypical ectrodactyly, asymmetric radial ray anomalies, single forearm bone and digit, aplasia cutis congenita, unilateral renal agenesis, UOS, cerebral infarctions and hemorrhage, and placental infarctions and abruptions.**[26, 27, 132–134]

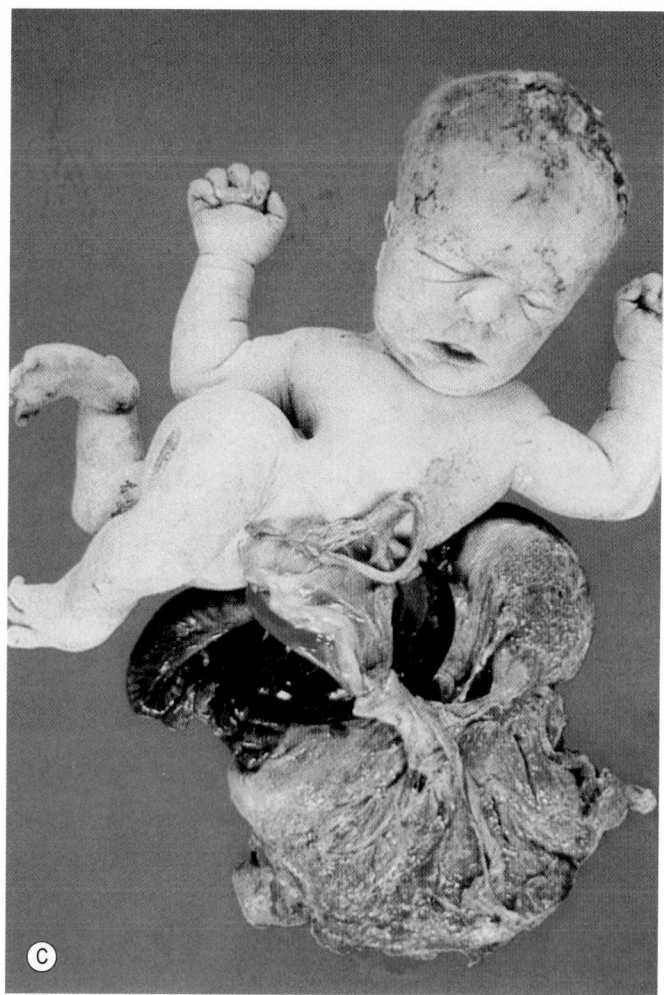

FIGURE 4.2.25 *(cont'd)* (C) Short umbilical cord with placenta adherent to the viscera and marked deformation of the fetus.

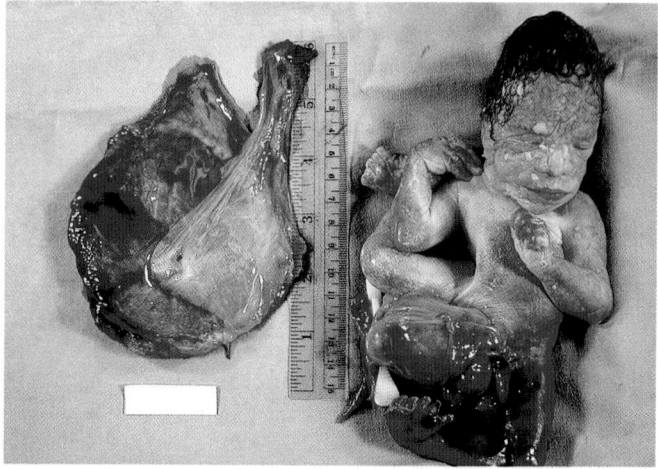

FIGURE 4.2.26 Abdominoschisis with extrophy of the bladder and abdominal organs, absent external genitalia, and foot and lower limb anomalies. Note the short umbilical cord and how the amnion is non-adherent to the placenta. The visceral organs extruded into the extraembryonic coelom, and the amnion margin is continuous with the skin of the abdominal defect. (From Van Allen et al 1987,[12] with permission.)

The most likely mechanism for cocaine causing vascular disruption is alteration of blood flow at the uterine–placental unit, by a direct effect on the embryonic–fetal vasculature and blood pressure, and/or the effects of toxic oxygen free-radicals.[26, 135, 136] Cocaine prevents uptake of neurotransmitters at the nerve terminals, increasing levels of the vasoactive amines serotonin, epinephrine, and norepinephrine. Sympathetic nerve stimulation decreases uterine blood flow to the placenta and causes fetal hypertension and vasoconstriction. Secondary stasis of placental blood flow and circulatory failure, anoxia, placental infarction with subsequent embolic infarction, maternal hyperthermia, and a direct effect on embryonic–fetal hemodynamics are all mechanisms that would explain structural anomalies occurring in cocaine-exposed pregnancies.

How frequently cocaine causes structural anomalies from vascular disruption, and whether this risk is increased over the background risk of non-cocaine users, have not been determined with certainty. Meta-analysis of published studies of pregnancy outcome in women using cocaine during pregnancy compared with drug-free controls has demonstrated a **decrease in mean size for head circumference, gestational age, birth weight, and birth length.**[137] This effect is no longer apparent when cocaine-exposed infants are compared with infants of mothers who are polydrug users without cocaine. Meta-analysis of congenital anomalies supports an association of congenital **genitourinary malformations with cocaine use during pregnancy.** This study was not able to assess the risk of specific structural anomalies associated with vascular disruption, including in utero stroke, gastroschisis, and limb reduction defects, because of the sample size.

Neonatal gangrene

Neonatal gangrene of a limb at the time of birth is rare; most arterial thromboses in infants occur postnatally as a complication of umbilical artery catheters. At least 32 infants with upper and/or lower limb gangrene at birth have been reported in the literature.[7] In utero thrombosis is associated with necrosis and loss of tissue dependent on the occluded artery (see Fig. 4.2.14). Recanalization and development of collateral blood supply is evident in infants who survive. Extensive necrosis or overwhelming infection may require operative therapy, including thrombectomy and amputation of the limb.

Of these newborns, 22% were infants of insulin-dependent or gestationally diabetic mothers. Venous thrombosis and thromboembolism is far more common in IDMs than arterial thrombosis and may contribute to embolic occlusion of the femoral or brachial artery. **The most likely cause of arterial as well as venous thrombosis in IDMs is a hypercoagulable state associated with poorly controlled maternal diabetes.**[138, 139] Other contributing factors for in utero arterial thrombosis include macrosomia with in utero constraint, neonatal asphyxia or dehydration, limb compression, polycythemia, and embolic thrombi from venous thrombosis.

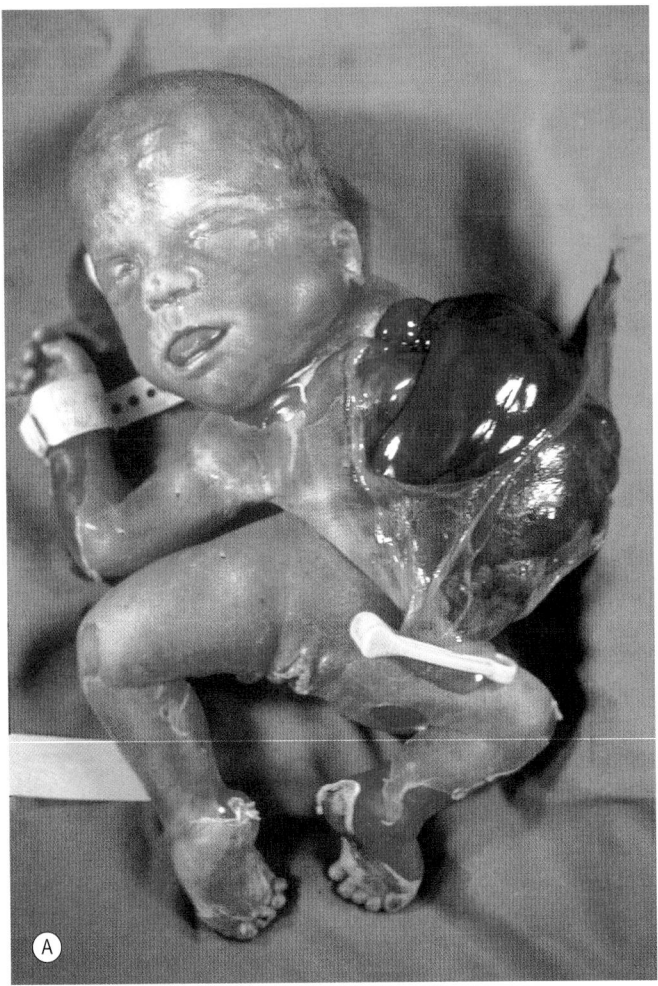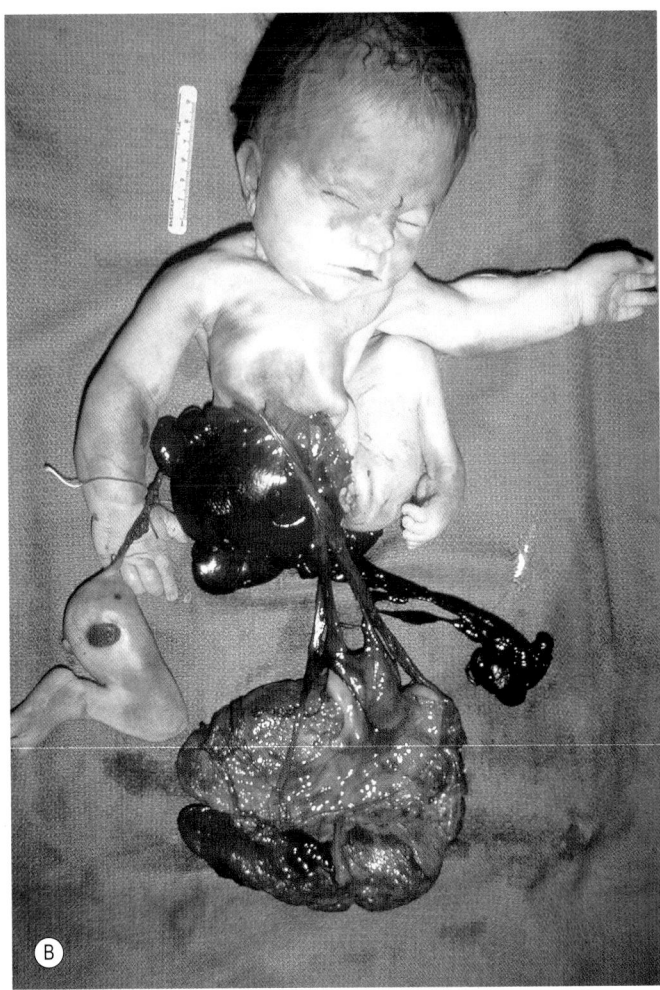

FIGURE 4.2.27 Two fetuses with thoracoabdominoschisis with absent (A) or rudimentary (B) left arm, severe scoliosis, abnormal rotation of the foot, and [in (A)] bilateral clubfeet; other visceral anomalies are present. In (B) there is a very short umbilical cord with placenta adherent to the eviscerated organs. [(A) from Van Allen et al 1987,[12] with permission.]

Cleft lip and cleft palate with limb reduction anomalies

The usual cleft lip, either unilateral or bilateral, can be associated with constriction bands and distal limb reduction (see Fig. 4.2.16). Occasional anomalies include unilateral renal agenesis, porencephaly, and congenital heart anomalies, in particular ventricular septal defect.[11]

Subclavian artery supply disruption sequence

A unifying hypothesis for the overlapping clinical presentation of **Poland, Klippel-Feil,** and **Möbius sequences** has been proposed.[41] The overlapping anomalies of absence of the pectoralis major muscle with breast hypoplasia, terminal transverse limb defects, cranial nerve palsies, and Sprengel anomaly have been grouped together as **SASDS.**[41]

Bavinck and Weaver proposed and provided evidence for interruption of the early embryonic blood supply in the subclavian arteries, the vertebral arteries, and/or their branches during the sixth week of embryonic development, resulting in these constellations of anomalies.[41] See also Chapter 21.

Poland sequence

Poland sequence consists of **congenital unilateral absence of the sternocostal head of the pectoralis major muscle combined with variable defects of other pectoral and chest wall muscles,** along with ipsilateral symbrachydactyly or other anomalies of the hand and arm. Other associated ipsilateral anomalies include hypoplasia or absence of the nipple and breast, defects of the ribs and vertebrae, and genitourinary anomalies.[140–142]

Less frequently, the findings of Poland sequence overlap in anomalies with Adams-Oliver syndrome, specifically cutis aplasia; limb anomalies in the two disorders are quite similar in

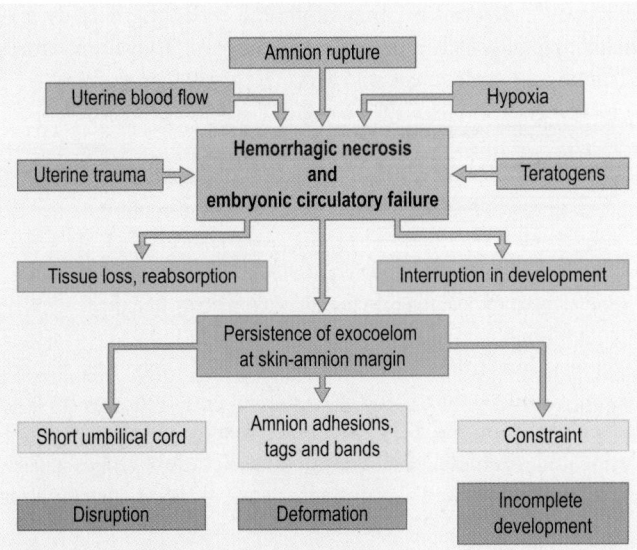

FIGURE 4.2.28 Schemata of the multiplicity of events resulting in structural anomalies from vascular disruption as illustrated by the pathogenesis of limb body wall complex. (From Van Allen et al 1987,[12] with permission.)

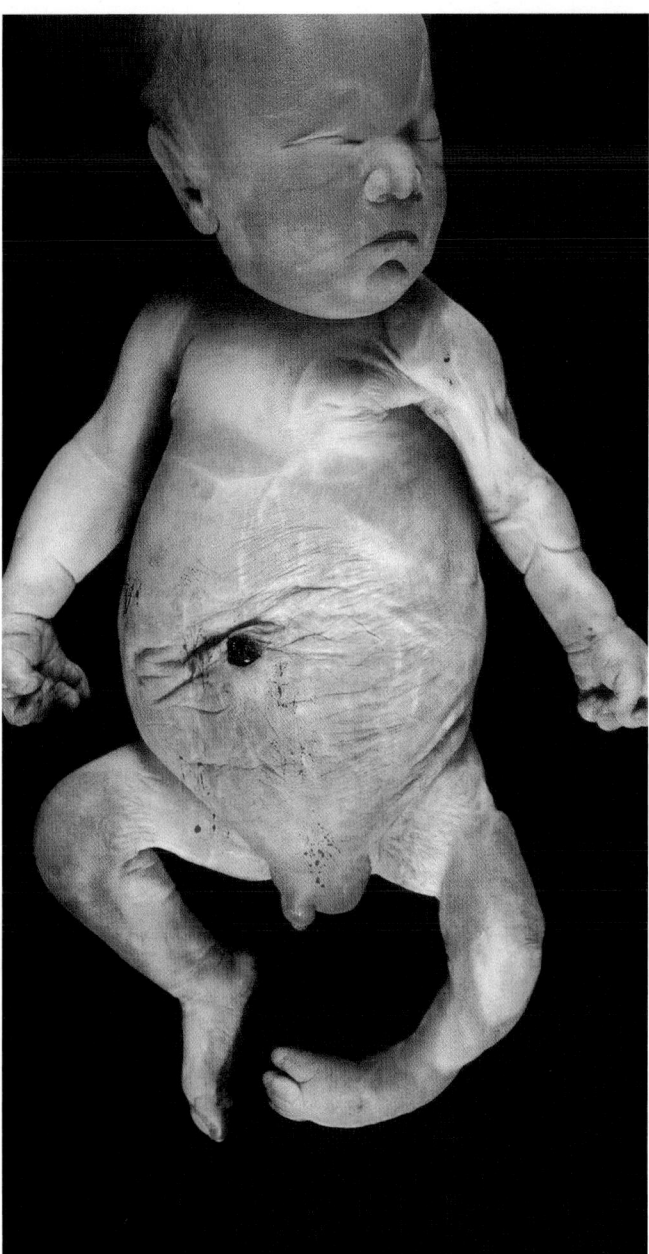

FIGURE 4.2.29 Prune-belly sequence in a fetus with bladder outlet obstruction, an urachal cyst, and hypoplasia of the kidneys.

appearance.[143] Adams-Oliver syndrome has also been associated with pulmonary arterio-venous malformation further supporting a vascular hypotheses.[143a] The additional findings of cranial nerve palsies and Klippel-Feil and Sprengel anomalies are suggestive of the more extended spectrum of anomalies of SASDS.[41] Isolated absence of the nipple and mammary gland with a normal pectoral muscle and normal limbs most likely represents a separate entity.

Poland sequence more frequently involves the right side of the body than the left, in a ratio of 1.7:1, and is more common in males than in females (3:1).[41, 144–147] The estimated population incidence is 1 in 30 000 to 1 in 50 000.[145–147]

The cause of Poland sequence is unknown. Disruption of the branchial artery and its branch that supplies the pectoral muscle is a likely pathogenesis for Poland sequence. The primary defect may be the development of the proximal subclavian artery with early deficit of blood flow to the distal limb and the pectoral region resulting in partial loss of tissue in these regions.[148a] Subclavian artery **disruption sequence at around 6 weeks gestation may cause various combinations of Poland, Klippel-Feil and Möbius anomalies.**[148b] Furthermore the **association of Poland-Möbius syndrome and cocaine abuse** has been reported.[148c] Most reported cases are sporadic, but familial cases have been described.[140, 142, 143, 148]

Sprengel anomaly

In Sprengel anomaly, one or both scapulae are hypoplastic, or in a congenitally high position with the lower angle turned toward the spine. This anomaly can be an isolated condition but is frequently seen as part of Poland sequence and Klippel-Feil

defects. Complete or partial obstruction of blood flow in the subclavian, internal thoracic, and/or suprascapular arteries is hypothesized in the pathogenesis of this disorder.[41]

Short umbilical cord

The normal umbilical cord has an average length of about 55 cm, with a range of 32–120 cm in normal full term fetuses.[149–152] Standard curves for umbilical cord length have been developed.[151]

TABLE 4.2.3 SHORT UMBILICAL CORD (SUC) SYNDROME AND SIMILAR ANOMALY CONSTELLATIONS

Group	Anomalies
Group I: SUC + amnion bands	ADAM sequence
	Variable clefts
	Variable amputations
Group II: SUC + abdominal wall defect	Severe SUC (< 10 cm)
	Abdominal wall defect
	Bent fetal body axis (pleurosomus, cyllosomus)
	Missing extremity
Group III: SUC + severe midline field schisis defect	Midline developmental field schisis defect with omphalocele, CL/CP, ectopia cordis, bladder exstrophy, neural tube defect
Group IV: SUC + acephalus-acardia	Abnormal twinning
Group V: SUC + fetal hypokinesia	Neuromuscular disorder
	Arthrogryposis
	Extremity defect
Group VI: SUC primary defect	Abdominal wall defect
	Omphalocele

Data from Gilbert-Barness et al 1993,[150] Grange et al 1986,[160] and Blackburn and Cooley 1993,[149] with permission.

ADAM, Amniotic deformity adhesions and mutilation; CL/CP, cleft lip and/or palate

At term,[151] males have longer cords than females: 38–90 cm with a mean of 60 cm. Females have cords of 36–86 cm with a mean of 57 cm. These gender differences may be related to the average body weight and length, rather than sex.[150]

An umbilical cord shorter than 32 cm is defined to be abnormally short[149, 150, 154] and is frequently associated with underlying major structural anomalies in the fetus.[150] It is estimated that an umbilical cord must be at least 32 cm long to allow for normal labor and delivery, so that shorter cords carry an increased risk of complications.[152, 155–157] Studies indicate that the human umbilical cord grows almost linearly during the whole period of gestation.[158, 159]

Multiple congenital anomalies are frequently associated with a short umbilical cord (SUC), in particular if there are a lateral body wall defect, severe CNS abnormalities, or amniotic bands (see Figs 4.2.25A-C and 4.2.27B). Gilbert-Barness and colleagues[150] divided cases of SUC into seven groups based on similarities in the constellation of anomalies and the proposed pathogenesis (Table 4.2.3).

Previous studies had hypothesized that the length of the umbilical cord is determined by fetal activity and the tension placed on the cord during growth.[160, 161] The observation that fetuses with structural malformations that limit movement are more likely to have a SUC has been supported by experimental animal studies. In a study of pregnant rats, Moessinger and associates[162] determined that umbilical cord length is directly related to fetal activity and tension on the cord. They found that:

- chronic oligohydramnios at 15 days of rat gestation (6 weeks of human gestation) resulted in umbilical cords 65% of control length;
- paralysis of embryos with tubocurarine during the last few days of rat gestation resulted in umbilical cords 85% of control length; and
- rat fetuses removed from the uterus in the last few days of gestation and allowed to float freely in the abdominal cavity had cords 144% of control length.

In another study by Moessinger,[163] paralysis was experimentally induced during the last 3 days of gestation. The rat pups had polyhydramnios, SUC, low body weight, pulmonary hypoplasia, and multiple joint contractures. These changes closely resemble the human equivalent, fetal akinesia deformation sequence, also called Pena-Shokeir syndrome.

Amnion disruption sequence

Amnion disruption sequence (ADS) encompasses a heterogeneous group of disorders of varying severity with distinctive structural anomalies and abnormal amnion attachments, amniotic strands, or amniotic entanglement. Synonyms for this spectrum of disorders include amniotic band disruption sequence, amniotic band syndrome, amniotic band sequence, amniotic deformity adhesions and mutilation (ADAM) complex, LBWC (pleurosomas, cylosomas), and congenital annular constriction bands. The amniotic band syndrome is further discussed in Chapter 21.

A spectrum of structural anomalies is seen in ADS. The type of anomalies depends on the stage of embryonic development and the severity of the disruptive event. Classification of patients with ADS into four main groups is based on the type of structural anomalies, the associated anomalies, and the type of amnion abnormalities (Table 4.2.4).

The prevalence of ADS in liveborn infants has been estimated to be 0.7 to 8.1 per 10 000.[6, 53, 165–169] These figures are based on studies from birth defect registries and retrospective hospital record reviews, all of which are subject to limitations of study design.

A much higher prevalence of ADS has been found in previable fetuses and stillbirths than in liveborn infants. The Wisconsin Stillbirth Service Project (WiSSP) found a prevalence of 140 per 10 000 (1.4%) for the more severe disruptions classified as 'early' ADS (group I).[6] When corrected for referral bias within their catchment area, a minimal estimate of 60 per 10 000 (0.6%) was made. In fetuses with structural anomalies identified by ultrasound examination, 3.6% have structural anomalies due to ADS.[5]

Studies of previable fetuses consecutively referred to embryopathology laboratories have found an ADS prevalence of 11.4 per 10 000 previable fetuses of less than 28 weeks' gestation,[170] and 178.2 per 10 000 (1.7%) in fetuses from spontaneous miscarriages and induced abortions of 9–18 weeks.[171] In utero death and

TABLE 4.2.4 CLASSIFICATION OF DISORDERS WITHIN AMNION DISRUPTION SEQUENCE

Group	Disruption complex	Prognosis
Group I: Early embryonic period 1. Before 4 weeks' pc 2. 3-6 weeks' pc	i. Anencephaly with amniotic bands ii. Craniofacial clefts with ectopia cordis iii. Limb body wall complex iv. Unusual facial clefting v. Encephalocele/pseudoencephalocele	Neonatal lethal Almost always lethal Usually neonatal lethal Variable; amenable to plastic surgery Variable intellectual impairment; dependent on degree of brain malformation
Group II: Midembryonic period (4–7 weeks pc)	i. CL/CP ± limb defect ± CHD ± associated internal anomalies ii. Limb reduction defect ± associated anomalies ± constriction bands	Usually good but dependent on associated anomalies Good but dependent on associated anomalies
Group III: Late embryonic to early fetal period (7–12 weeks pc)	i. Pierre Robin sequence secondary to transient oligohydramnios ii. Oligohydramnios sequence from persistent oligohydramnios	Good Dependent on degree of pulmonary hypoplasia
Group IV: Late embryonic to fetal period (after 9 weeks pc)	i. Limb entanglement in amnion Limb amputation Constriction bands Distal lymphedema	Good

CL/CP, Cleft lip and/or palate; CHD, congenital heart defect.

spontaneous miscarriages were not necessarily related to the severity of the structural anomalies, 11/18 fetuses having defects limited to limbs or digits. Umbilical cord constriction by amniotic bands was the attributable cause of death in 6/11 with placentas available for evaluation.

An identifiable cause or causes for amnion rupture or vascular disruption with amniotic adhesions cannot be determined in most pregnancies. The frequency of amniotic entanglement in previable fetuses[171] suggests that this is a common error of morphogenesis that occurs spontaneously rather than being the result of a specific etiologic agent.

Individual case reports have suggested the following postulated etiologies documented to have occurred at the appropriate time during embryogenesis: abdominal trauma,[170] chorioamnionitis, removal of an IUD,[12, 25] maternal oophorectomy,[172] and busulfan (an antimitotic drug) treatment for idiopathic thrombocytopenia purpura.[171]

Oligohydramnios disruption sequence is a well-documented complication of amniocentesis[173] and CVS.[174] Although limb reduction defects and amniotic bands have been reported after amniocentesis, the occurrence may not be increased over the background risk for these types of anomalies.[33, 34, 175, 176] After CVS, especially when performed earlier than 10 weeks of pregnancy (8 weeks post conception), transverse limb reduction defects, ring constrictions, and oromandibular hypogenesis spectrum have been reported.[28, 177, 178] These anomalies most likely result from vascular disruption, but amnion rupture may also occur in some cases.[4] Table 4.2.5 summarizes the anomalies resulting from amniotic bands which may simulate genetic disorders.[179–187]

Connective tissue disorders resulting in an abnormality of amnion collagen formation have been reported in osteogenesis imperfecta and in Ehlers-Danlos syndrome type IV.[181–184] Amniotic bands have also been reported in association with epidermolysis bullosa.[185]

Amniotic bands that may or may not be causally associated with the underlying disorder have also been reported in the pump twin of TRAP sequence[186] and in a fetus with 47,XYY.[187]

It has been controversial whether the disorders of ADS result from mechanical trauma by collapse of the amnion and subsequent entanglement, as supported by Torpin,[165, 188] Miller and colleagues,[53] and Higginbottom and colleagues,[10] or from a mesodermal defect, as supported by Streeter.[189] More recently, disruption of embryonic vasculature from either amnion rupture or other teratogenic events has been proposed as the primary mechanism of damage based on clinical studies and experimental animal models of amnion puncture. Amnion entanglement appears to be a secondary phenomenon, or, to be more important in the pathogenesis of isolated limb reduction anomalies that can occur during the fetal period.

Experimental animal studies have provided evidence that amnion puncture or rupture results in disruption of developing embryonic vasculature, with resultant structural anomalies similar to those seen in humans. The following observations were made in rat embryos[190–192] after artificial rupture of the amnion with or without withdrawal of fluid in 15-day-gestation pregnancies during limb development. Immediately after amnion puncture, rupture of the marginal vein of the limb buds was observed followed by hemorrhage into the interdigital spaces and disruption of the capillary plexus of the limb buds.[19, 52, 193]

TABLE 4.2.5 DISORDERS INCLUDED IN THE AMNION DISRUPTION SEQUENCE

Disorder	Characteristic features	Associated anomalies
Anencephaly with amniotic bands	Anencephaly with amnion continuous with skin–amnion margin	Frequent
Craniofacial clefts with ectopia cordis	Ectopia cordis, midline sternal cleft, exencephaly or anencephaly, frontonasal dysgenesis, facial clefts, congenital heart defect, fibrous amniotic strands attached to face and head	Absent pericardium, absent ventral diaphragm, supraumbilical omphalocele, anophthalmia; no limb defects
Limb body wall complex	Lateral body wall defect (thoracoabdominoschisis, abdominoschisis), limb reduction defect, neural tube defects, facial clefts	Frequent; 95% with internal structural anomalies involving all organs
Unusual facial clefting	Bizarre facial clefting, CL/CP; microcephaly, anophthalmia, coloboma, other eye anomalies; amnion adherent to face, swallowed amnion	Frequently associated brain malformations, microcephaly, deficiency of anterior calvaria or unusually placed encephaloceles
Encephalocele/ pseudoencephalocele	Encephalocele(s) that are asymmetric, are usually anteriorly placed, and can be multiple; amnion adherent to skin with exencephaly gives appearance of encephalocele (pseudoencephalocele); cranium adherent to placenta	Frequently associated with facial clefting, brain anomalies, digital and limb anomalies
CL/CP ± limb defects	Usual CL/CP with limb reduction anomalies	Occasional; unilateral renal agenesis, porencephaly, congenital heart anomalies
Limb reduction defects	Ring constrictions, syndactyly, acrosyndactyly, ectrodactyly, preaxial polydactyly, transverse amputations, oligodactyly, clubfeet; distal lymphedema, neurapraxias	Usually absent; rule out renal and brain disruptions
Robin sequence secondary to transient oligohydramnios	U-shaped CP, micro- and retrognathia, glossoptosis; ear anomalies; anomalies of oligohydramnios sequence	Occasional; congenital heart defects; limb anomalies, clubfoot, ring constrictions, syndactyly, hypoplastic digits, Poland anomaly, transverse limb reduction defects; congenital dislocated hip; exclude other causes
Oligohydramnios sequence	Compression deformities of face and limbs; pulmonary hypoplasia, redundant skin	With chronic leakage of amniotic fluid there are usually no internal structural anomalies, except for pulmonary hypoplasia

CL/CP, Cleft lip and/or palate.

Examination of the limbs 30 min after amniocentesis demonstrated extension of the hemorrhage, hemorrhagic necrosis with perivascular edema, subectodermal blebs, and vascular congestion. There was reabsorption of the damaged tissues and continued differentiation during the next 24 h of observation. Hemorrhages were seen in up to 77% of the limb buds of observed embryos.[193] Limb deficiency defects were noted, including terminal transverse limb reduction anomalies, preaxial and postaxial polydactyly, bifid distal phalanges syndactyly, oligodactyly, and ring constrictions.

After amnion puncture in rats, there was a delayed systemic effect characterized by embryonic hypotension, bradycardia, decreased peripheral blood flow, rupture of vessels, and hemorrhages.[19, 52, 193] Kino[19] found no association between the amount of amniotic fluid removed and the severity of damage to the embryo. He hypothesized that amnion puncture leads to uterine contractions, decreasing blood supply to the placenta and circulatory collapse in the embryo.

In ADS, structural anomalies result from:
- disruption of existing and developing tissues due to damage of developing vasculature, or mechanical disruption of the embryo and fetus;

- deformations secondary to in utero constraint if there is persistent oligohydramnios from fluid leakage; and
- the fetus becoming entangled in the amnion either at the time of the initial amnion rupture or with subsequent activity.

Persistence of the extraembryonic coelom so that the amnion is not adherent to the chorion may predispose to amniotic entanglement by an active fetus.

Not all structural anomalies in ADS result from disruption during the embryonic period. Fetal entanglement in the amnion without resultant constriction and distal limb ischemia, with or without limb amputation, is a common cause of structural anomalies. Reports of infants with transverse reduction anomalies and abnormal amniotic entanglement, with the amputated limb recovered at delivery, suggest the amputation occurred in the second or third trimester.[165, 194] A report by Yang and associates[194] of a foot measuring 19 mm in length in the presence of a fibrotic amnion that was partially stripped off the underlying chorion suggests that the amputation occurred at 14–16 weeks' gestation.

Management and treatment depend on the severity of structural anomalies and parental preferences. Postnatal survival after a live birth of a child with ADS is related to the embryonic timing

TABLE 4.2.6 DISORDERS PHENOTYPICALLY SIMILAR OR WITH AN INCREASED RISK FOR AMNION DISRUPTION SEQUENCE

Disorder	Clinical features
Adams-Oliver syndrome (AD)	Vertex cranial cutis aplasia congenita, terminal limb reduction defects, syndactyly, constriction bands
Disorganization gene (mouse mutant Ds; semidominant)	Cranioschisis and exencephaly (53%), hamartomas (40%), limb abnormalities (33%), eye defects (21%), craniopharyngeal defects (18%), thoraco/gastroschisis (16%), other (< 15%)
Ehler-Danlos type IV (AD, AR)	Collagen type III defect with joint laxity, premature rupture of amnion in disorder with rupture of visceral organs, blood vessels, and amnion; ring constrictions, lymphedema
Epidermolysis bullosa	Blisters in upper layers of dermis, with typical histopathology and electron microscopy with interruption of basement membrane and decreased anchoring fibrils; pyloric atresia; constriction bands, limb reduction defects, oligodactyly, cutis aplasia
Osteogenesis imperfecta	Blue sclera, minimal calvarial mineralization, wormian bones, long and short bones bowed with multiple fractures; other skeletal anomalies; type I collagen defect, fragility and premature rupture of membranes
Twin reversed arterial perfusion sequence (TRAP)	Placental vascular anastomoses in large vessels of MZ twins; perfused twin (acardiac) with severe reduction and anomalies of all organs; amniotic entanglement unusual
Twins	Monochorionic twins (both MA and DA), twins discordant for amnion rupture sequence, including anencephaly, facial clefts, limb body wall complex, ring constrictions, limb amputations and anomalies
Vascular disruption during embryogenesis	Structural anomalies typical of vascular disruption, including limb reduction anomalies, ring constrictions, and other anomalies from secondary amniotic adhesions in areas of tissue necrosis

AD, Autosomal dominant; AR, autosomal recessive; DA, diamnionic; MA, monoamnionic; MZ, monozygotic.

and severity of the initial disruption (see Table 4.2.4). Despite the most aggressive medical treatment, newborns with early ADS who have severe neural tube and body wall defects rarely survive. Similarly, if there has been prolonged oligohydramnios, severe pulmonary hypoplasia limits survival independent of the associated structural anomalies. Infants with limb reduction defects and ring constrictions with or without cleft lip and palate have the best long-term outcome.

ADS is usually sporadic with a low risk of recurrence in subsequent pregnancies. Caution is required in counseling couples regarding recurrence risks because of a limited number of families with more than one affected individual.[195–197] Incorrect diagnosis of ADS in the presence of disorders with a similar phenotype, including Adams-Oliver syndrome, connective tissue disorders, teratogenic agents causing vascular disruption, and familial disorders of limb malformations, could falsely underestimate the risk of a subsequent affected child (Table 4.2.6). The corollary is overestimation of the recurrence risk when an anomaly for ADS is incorrectly diagnosed as a multifactorial disorder such as a neural tube defect or omphalocele.

Early amnion rupture sequence is probably more frequent than generally presumed because of the early abortion risk and it may be impossible to find remnants of the amniotic bands.[196a] Some cases of amniotic band like anomalies associated with cleft lip and palate may represent mutations on the genes disorganization, p63 or IRF6.[196b] Amniotic disruption with loss of amniotic fluid, causing fetal compression and localized fetal ischemia may result in extremely variable abnormalities.[196c]

Prenatal diagnosis of amniotic bands and disorders included in ADS is possible with fetal ultrasound.[197–203] Not all abnormal amniotic strands necessarily result in entanglement by the fetus.

Anencephaly with amniotic bands

An estimated 5% of fetuses and newborns with anencephaly have associated attachment of amniotic bands.[204, 205] Amnion-arachnoid adhesions, facial clefts, and SUC are frequently associated (Fig. 4.2.30).[10, 11, 122, 206–208] Disruption is most likely around the time of neural tube closure at 26–28 days' gestation. Amniotic entanglement of limbs can occur but is most likely after the initial disruptive event. When anencephaly is associated with body wall defects and herniation of thoracic and abdominal contents, it is diagnosed as LBWC.[11, 106, 207]

Craniofacial clefts with ectopia cordis

Disruption of the amnion during the third week of gestation (21–25 days post conception) can result in ectopia cordis with amniotic bands. The usual **structural anomalies include ectopia cordis, congenital heart defects, supraumbilical omphalocele, ventral diaphragmatic defect, SUC, and frequently anencephaly with midfacial clefts.** Fibrous amniotic strands are usually attached to the face, head, and the body wall (Fig. 4.2.31).[205, 209] Limb defects are unusual. **Placental changes consistent with amnion disruption, anencephaly, facial clefts, and the presence of amniotic attachments distinguish this disorder from the usual case of ectopia cordis and Cantrell**

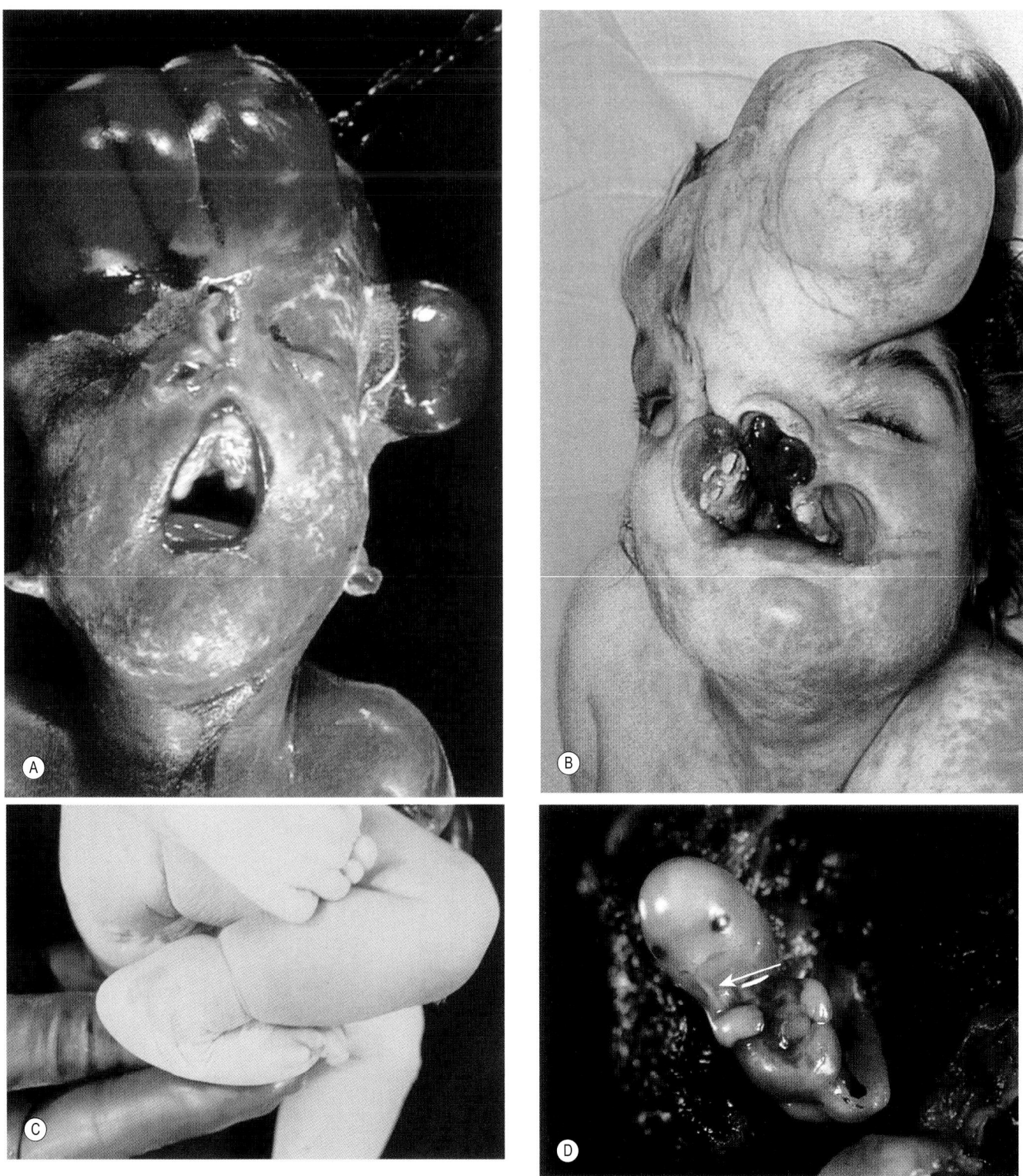

FIGURE 4.2.30 (A) Amnion disruption sequence. Two encephaloceles, cleft palate, and distorted nostrils with multiple adherent amniotic bands. (B) Amnion disruption sequence. There is a large frontal encephalocele and clefting of the mouth, premaxilla, and palate caused by swallowing amniotic membranes. This girl was 27 years old at the time of death and had been fed by a gastrostomy tube. (C) Constriction ring (Streeter band) around ankle—the least severe form of amniotic band disruption. (D) Embryo at 10 week's gestation with an amniotic band attached to the lip (arrow).

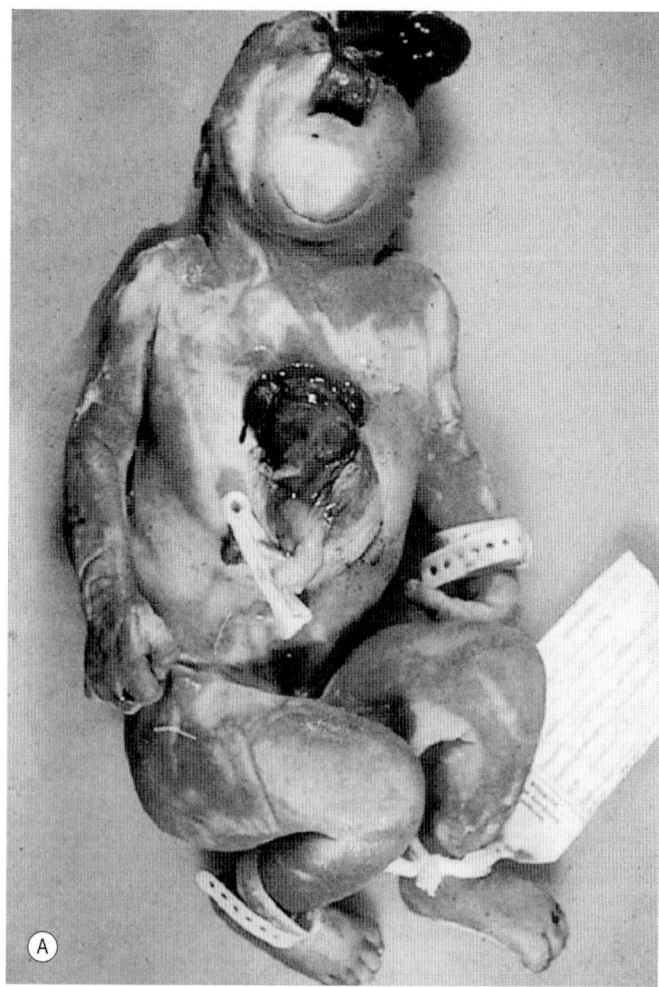

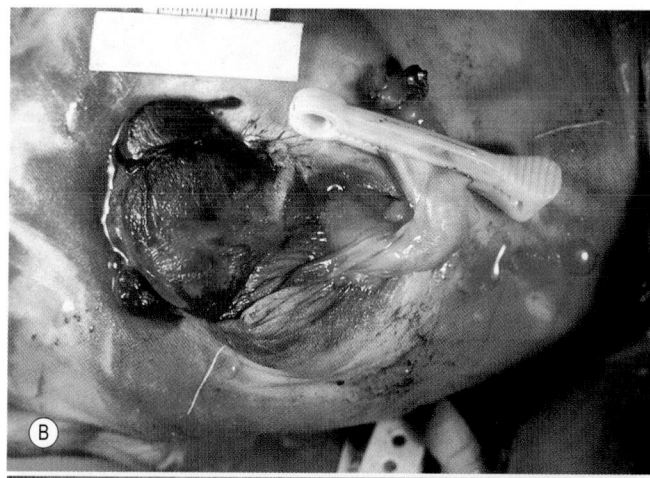

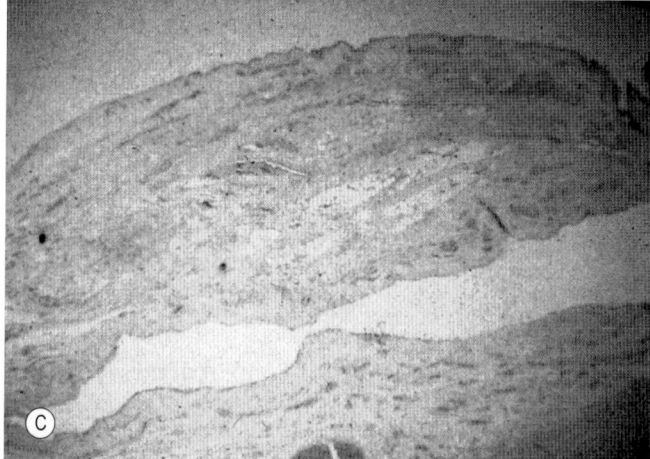

FIGURE 4.2.31 (A) A 33-week gestation female fetus with exencephaly, midline facial cleft, bilateral cleft lip, ectopia cordis thoracalis, supraumbilical omphalocele, and amnion attached to the cranium and cardiac apex. (B) Ectopia cordis thoracalis with midline sternal cleft and fused manubrium. A fibrous band is attached to the apex of the heart. A supraumbilical omphalocele is continuous with the thoracic defect, and the umbilicus is superiorly displaced in the midepigastrium. (C) Histologically, the band from the apex of the heart is composed of fibrous connective tissue. There are numerous vascular spaces and a suggestion of amniotic columnar epithelium along its surface. The bands attached to the head are typical of amnion. (From Van Allen and Myhre 1985,[209] with permission.)

pentalogy. The pathogenesis of ectopia cordis with anencephaly and facial clefts is summarized in Figure 4.2.32.

Encephalocele/pseudoencephalocele

Encephaloceles caused by early amnion rupture are usually asymmetric and anteriorly placed; the amnion is continuous with the skin margin.[10, 11, 122, 207] They can be multiple. Amnion is adherent to the skin with exencephaly, giving the appearance of an encephalocele (pseudoencephalocele; see Fig. 4.2.30A). Arachnoid-to-amnion adhesions, SUC, and the cranium can be adherent to the placenta. Frequently associated anomalies include facial clefts, brain anomalies, exencephaly, and digital and limb anomalies.

Limb reduction defects

Characteristic limb anomalies resulting from vascular disruption with or without amniotic entanglement include ring constrictions, syndactyly, acrosyndactyly, ectrodactyly, preaxial polydactyly, transverse amputations, oligodactyly, and clubfeet (Fig. 4.2.33; see also Fig. 4.24). Constrictions can be tight enough to result in distal lymphedema, vascular insufficiency, and neuropraxis.[19, 106, 165, 199, 210] Associated structural anomalies are not common. Structural anomalies due to disruption should be excluded in the kidneys and brain. Organ infarctions are common on autopsy but are usually asymptomatic unless they involve the brain. Limb reduction defects appear to be due to vascular disruption in 35% of cases.[210a]

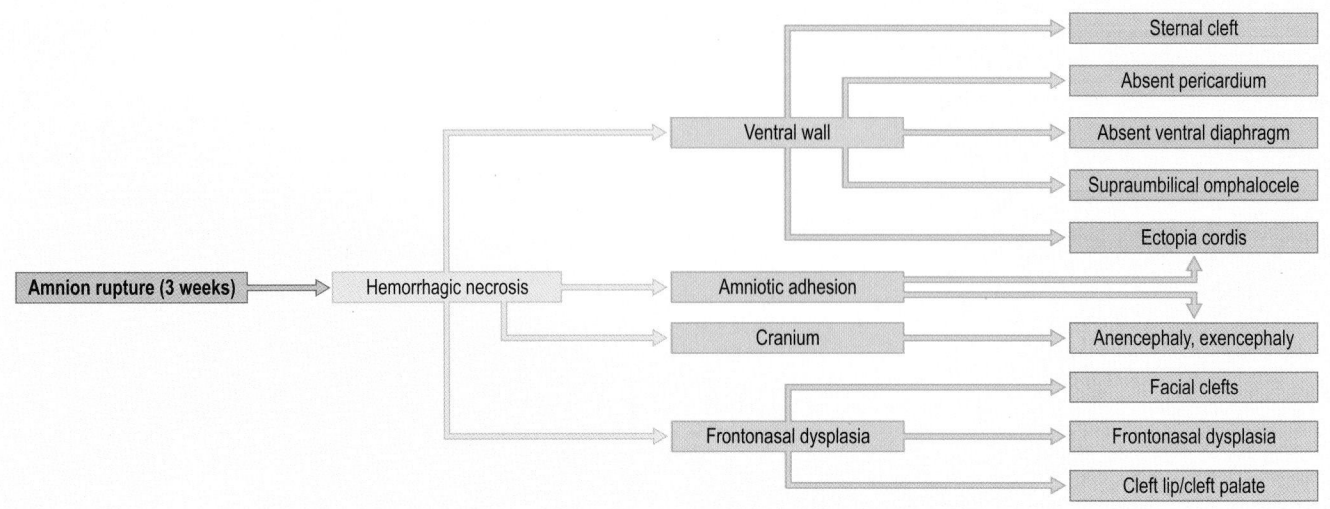

FIGURE 4.2.32 Schematic representation of the pathogenesis of ectopia cordis with craniofacial disruptions and amniotic adhesion resulting from early amnion rupture. (From Van Allen and Myhre 1985,[209] with permission.)

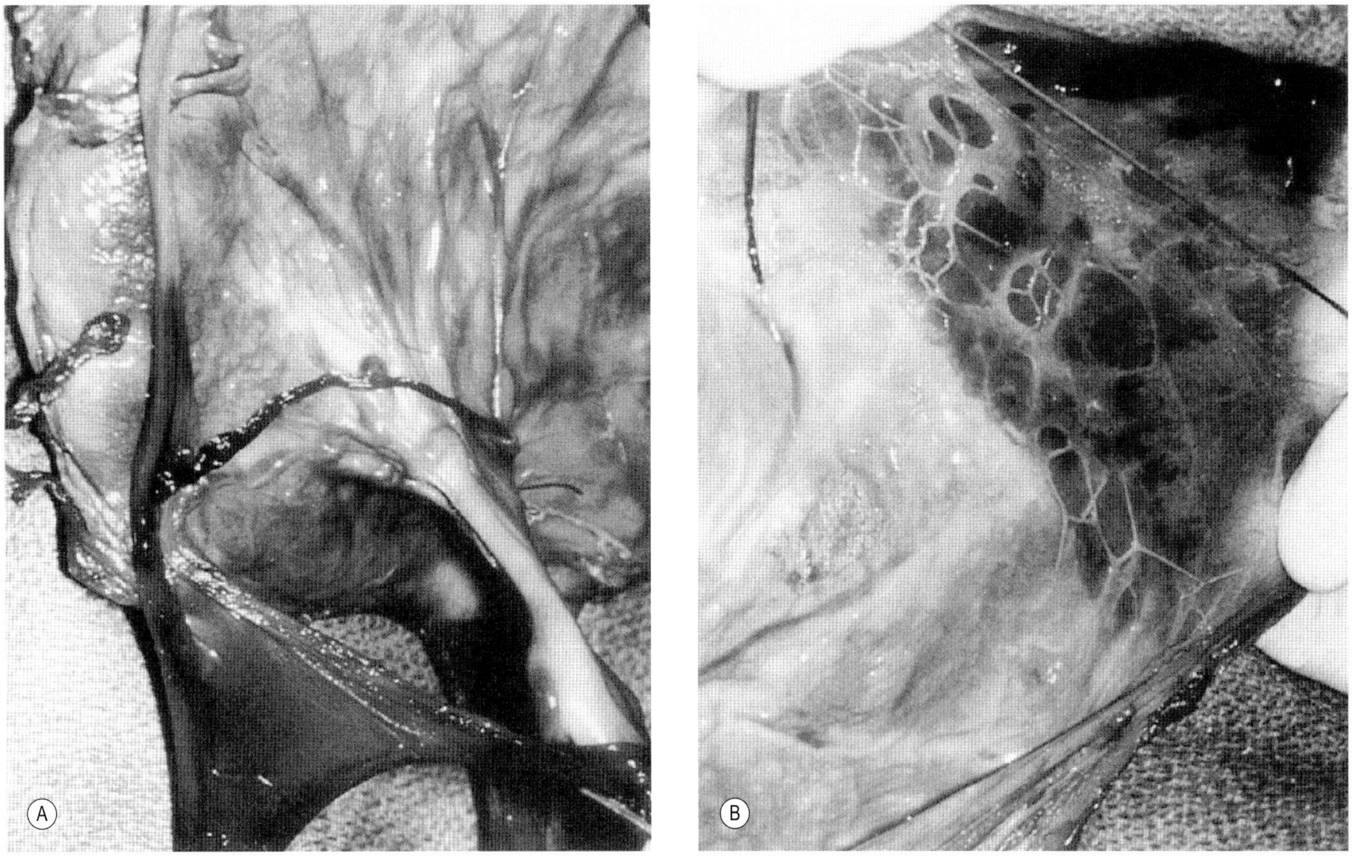

FIGURE 4.2.33 Placenta from a newborn with amniotic band syndrome. (A) Amnion stripped from chorion with abnormal insertion into the umbilical cord. (B) Friable amnion and amnion nodosum.

Pierre Robin sequence

Pierre Robin sequence results from transient oligohydramnios during early embryogenesis during palate closure and is characterized by a U-shaped cleft palate, micro- and retrognathia, and glossoptosis; ear anomalies; and anomalies of the oligohydramnios sequence.[56, 211, 212] Occasional findings include congenital heart defects (flow lesions), limb anomalies, clubfoot, ring constrictions, syndactyly, hypoplastic digits, Poland anomaly, transverse limb reduction defects, and congenital dislocated hip. Other disorders should be excluded, in particular Stickler syndrome and chromosomal aneuploidy.[212]

Potter sequence (oligohydramnios deformation sequence)

In utero constraint during the second and third trimesters due to lack of amniotic fluid from either renal agenesis/dysgenesis or chronic leakage of amniotic fluid results in a distinctive clinical phenotype.[213–215] Characteristic features include compression deformities of the face and limbs, pulmonary hypoplasia, redundant skin, and clubfeet.

References

Vascular disruptions

1. Aase JM. Diagnostic dysmorphology, New York: Plenum Press; 1990.
2. Spranger J, Benirschke K, Hall JG, et al. Errors in morphogenesis: concepts and terms. J Pediatr 1982; 100:160–165.
3. Van Allen MI. Fetal vascular disruptions: mechanisms and some resulting birth defects. Pediatr Ann 1981; 10:219–233.
4. Van Allen MI. Structural anomalies resulting from vascular disruption. Pediatr Clin North Am 1992; 39:255–277.
5. Van Allen MI, Johnson JM, Toi A, et al. Occurrence of vascular disruption in 250 fetuses with structural anomalies identified by ultrasound. Proc Greenwood Genetics Center 1992; 11:70.
5a. Martin ML, Khoury MJ, Cordero JF, Waters GD. Trends in rates of multiple vascular disruption defects, Atlanta 1968–1989: is there evidence of a cocaine teratogenic epidemic? Teratology 1992; 45(6):647–653.
6. Luebke HJ, Reiser CA, Pauli RM. Fetal disruptions: assessment of frequency, heterogeneity, and embryologic mechanisms in a population referred to a community-based stillbirth assessment program. Am J Med Genet 1991; 39:239–240.
7. Van Allen MI, Jackson JC, Knopp RH, et al. In utero thrombosis and neonatal gangrene in an infant of a diabetic mother. Am J Med Genet 1989; 33:323–327.
8. Hoyme HE, Jones KL, Van Allen MI, et al. Vascular pathogenesis of transverse limb reduction defects. J Pediatr 1982; 101:839–843.
9. Hrynchak M, Van Allen MI. Monozygotic twins with dyserythropoietic anaemia type I and limb abnormalities – are they related? Clin Res 1994; 42:51A.
10. Higginbottom MC, Jones KL, Hall BS, et al. The amniotic band disruption complex: timing of amniotic rupture and variable spectra of consequent defects. J Pediatr 1979; 95:544–549.
11. Van Allen MI, Siegel-Bartelt J, Dixon J, et al. Constriction bands and limb reduction defects in two newborns with fetal ultrasound evidence for vascular disruption. Am J Med Genet 1992; 44:598–604.
12. Van Allen MI, Curry C, Gallagher L. Limb body wall complex: I. Pathogenesis. Am J Med Genet 1987; 28:529–548.

Embryonic circulation

13. Stephen SG. Pictorial human embryology. Seattle: University of Washington Press; 1989.
14. Didusch J. In: Heuser CH, ed. A human embryo with 14 pairs of somites. Carnegie Contrib Embryol 1930; 22:135.

Capillary plexus formation and disruption

15. Moore KL. Before we are born: basic embryology and birth defects. 3rd edn. Philadelphia: WB Saunders; 1989.
16. Gilbert SG. Pictorial human embryology. Seattle: University of Washington Press; 1989.
17. O'Rahilly F, Muller F. Human embryology and teratology. New York: Wiley-Liss; 1992.
18. Congdon ED. Transformation of the aortic-arch system during the development of the human embryo. Contrib Embryol Carnegie Inst 1922; 14:47.
19. Kino Y. Clinical and experimental studies of the congenital constriction band syndrome, with an emphasis on its etiology. J Bone Joint Surg 1975; 57A:636–643.
20. Houben JJ. Immediate and delayed affects of oligohydramnios on limb development in the rat. Teratology 1984; 30:403–411.
21. Millicovsky G, DeSesso JM. Differential embryonic cardiovascular responses to acute maternal uterine ischemia: an in vivo microscopic study of rabbit embryos with either intact or clamped umbilical cords. Teratology 1980; 22:335–343.
22. Brent RL, Franklin JB. Uterine vascular clamping: new procedure for the study of congenital malformations. Science 1960; 132:89.
23. Danielsson BRG, Reiland S, Rundqvist E, et al. Digital defects induced by vasodilating: relationship to reduction in uteroplacental blood flow. Teratology 1989; 40:351–358.
24. Nilsen NO. Vascular abnormalities due to hyperthermia in chick embryos. Teratology 1984; 30:237–251.
25. Csecsei K, Szeifert GT, Papp Z. Amniotic bands associated with early rupture of amnion due to an intrauterine device. Zentralbl Gynakol 1987; 109:738–741.
26. Hoyme HE, Jones KL, Dixon SD, et al. Prenatal cocaine exposure and fetal vascular disruption. Pediatrics 1990; 85:743–747.
27. Kapur RP, Shaw CM, Shepard TH. Brain hemorrhages in cocaine-exposed human fetuses. Teratology 1991; 33:11–18.
28. Christiaens GC, Van Baarlen J, Huber J, et al. Fetal limb constriction: a possible complication of CVS. Prenat Diagn 1989; 9:67–71.
29. Firth HV, Boyd PA, Chamberlain P, et al. Severe limb abnormalities after chorion villus sampling at 56–66 days' gestation. Lancet 1991; 337:762–763.
30. Mastroiacovo P, Cavalcanti DP. Limb reduction defects and chorion villus sampling. Lancet 1991; 337:1091.
31. Olney RS, Khoury MJ, Alo CJ, et al. Increased risk for transverse digital deficiency after chorionic villus sampling: results of United States multistate case-control study, 1988–1992. Teratology 1995; 51:20–29.
32. Leist KH, Grauwiler J. Fetal pathology in rats following uterine-vessel clamping on day 14 of gestation. Teratology 1974; 10:55–67.
33. Kohn G. The amniotic band syndrome: a possible complication of amniocentesis. Prenat Diagn 1987; 7:303–305.
34. Lage JM, VanMarter LJ, Bieber FR. Questionable role of amniocentesis in the etiology of amniotic band formation: a case report. J Reprod Med 1988; 33:71–73.

Vitelline and placental circulations

35. Stevenson RE, Jones KL, Phelan MC, et al. Vascular steal: the pathogenetic mechanism producing sirenomelia and associated defects of the viscera and soft tissues. Pediatrics 1986; 78:451–457.
36. Van Allen MI, Smith DW, Shepard TH. Twin reversed arterial perfusion (TRAP) sequence: a study of 14 twin pregnancies with acardius. Semin Perinatol 1983; 7:285–293.

37. Schinzel AGL, Smith DW, Miller JR. Monozygotic twinning and structural defects. J Pediatr 1979; 95:921–930.

Embryonic arteries and veins

38. Blackburn WR, Cooley NR Jr. Vascular pathology in hypertensive children. In: Logie JMH, ed. Pediatric hypertension. Boston: Blackwell Scientific Publications; 1992.

38a. Davies BR, Rizo T, Arroyo-Valerio A. Congenital heart disease and its association with other congenital malformations found at autopsy. Pediatr Pathol Mod Med 2002; 21:541–549.

39. Padget DH. The development of the cranial arteries in the human embryo. Carnegie Contrib Embryol 1948; 32:207.

39a. Abramson DL, Cohen MM Jr, Mulliken JB. Mobius syndrome: classification and grading system. Plast Reconstructr Surg 1998; 102: 961–967.

40. Poswillo D. Experimental first-trimester amniocentesis in nonhuman primates. Teratology 1972; 6:227–234.

41. Bavinck JNB, Weaver D. Subclavian artery supply disruption sequence: hypothesis of a vascular etiology for Poland, Klippel-Feil, and Moebius anomalies. Am J Med Genet 1986; 23:903–918.

42. Hoyme HE, Higginbottom MC, Jones KL. The vascular pathogenesis of gastroschisis: intrauterine interruption of the omphalomesenteric artery. J Pediatr 1981; 98:228–231.

43. Gray SW, Skandalakis JE. Embryology for surgeons, the embryological basis for the treatment of congenital defects. Philadelphia: WB Saunders; 1972.

44. Van Allen MI, Hoyme HE, Jones KL. Vascular pathogenesis of limb defects. I. Radial artery anatomy in radial aplasia. J Pediatr 1982; 101:832–838.

45. Hootnick DR, Packard DS Jr, Levinsohn EM. Congenital tibial aplasia with preaxial polydactyly: soft tissue anatomy as a clue to teratogenesis. Teratology 1983; 27:169–179.

46. Hootnick DR, Levinsohn EM, Randall PA, et al. Vascular dysgenesis associated with skeletal dysplasia of the lower limb. J Bone Joint Surg 1980; 62A:1123–1129.

47. Hootnick DR, Levinsohn EM, Crider RJ, et al. Congenital arterial malformations associated with club foot. Clin Orthop 1982; 167:160–163.

48. Stevenson RE, Kelly JC, Aylsworth AS, et al. Vascular basis for neural tube defects: a hypothesis. Pediatrics 1987; 80:102–106.

Regulation of angiogenesis and blood vessel maturation

49. Fitch N, Rochon L, Srolovitz H, et al. Vascular abnormalities in a fetus with multiple pterygia. Am J Med Genet 1985; 21:755–760.

50. Morris JL, Bevan RD. Proliferation of arteriovenous anastomoses in the developing rabbit ear is enhanced after denervation. Am J Anat 1986; 176:497–509.

Occlusion of blood vessels

51. Grabowski CT, Tsai ENC, Toben HR. The effects of teratogenic doses of hypoxia on the blood pressure of chick embryos. Teratology 1969; 2:67.

52. Kennedy LA, Persaud TVN. Pathogenesis of developmental defects induced in the rat by amniotic sac puncture. Acta Anat 1977; 97:23–35.

53. Miller ME, Graham JM Jr, Higginbottom MC, et al. Compression related defects from early amnion rupture: evidence for mechanical teratogenesis. J Pediatr 1981; 98:292–297.

54. Matsunaga E, Shiota K. Ectopic pregnancy and myomata uteri: teratogenic effects and maternal characteristics. Teratology 1980; 21:61–69.

55. Graham JM Jr, Miller ME, Stephan MJ, et al. Limb reduction anomalies and early in utero limb compression. J Pediatr 1980; 96:1052–1056.

Altered hemodynamics

56. Graham JM Jr. Smith's recognizable patterns of human deformation. 2nd edn. Philadelphia: WB Saunders; 1988.

57. Greiss FC, Gobble FL. Effect of parasympathetic nerve stimulation on the uterine vascular bed. Am J Obstet Gynecol 1967; 199:1067–1072.

58. Moore T, Sorg J, Miller L, et al. Hemodynamic effects of intravenous cocaine on the pregnant ewe and fetus. Am J Obstet Gynecol 1986; 155:883–888.

59. Woods J, Plessinger M, Clark KE. Effects of cocaine on uterine blood flow and fetal oxygenation. JAMA 1987; 257:957–961.

Twin studies and placental arterial-to-venous anastomoses

60. Layde PM, Ericson JD, Falek A, et al. Congenital malformations in twins. Am J Hum Genet 1980; 32:69–78.

61. Myrianthopoulis NC. Congenital malformations in twins. Acta Genet Med Gemellol (Roma) 1976; 25:331.

62. Robertson EG, Neer KJ. Placental injection studies in twin gestations. Am J Obstet Gynecol 1979; 147:170.

63. Bleisch VR. Placental circulation of human twins. Am J Obstet Gynecol 1965; 91:862–869.

64. Szymonowicz W, Preston H, Yu VYH. The surviving monozygotic twin. Arch Dis Child 1986; 61:454–458.

65. Schinzel AGL, Smith DW, Miller JR. Monozygotic twinning and structural defects. J Pediatr 1979; 95:921–930.

66. Hoyme HE, Higginbottom MC, Jones KL. Vascular etiology of disruptive structural defects in monozygotic twins. Pediatrics 1981; 67:288–291.

66a. Hahn JS, Lewis AJ, Barnes P. Hydranencephaly wing to twin-twin transfusion: serial fetal ultrasonography and magnetic resonance imaging findings. J Child Neurol 2003; 18:367–370.

67. Anderson RL, Gobus MS, Curry CJR, et al. Central nervous system damage and other anomalies in surviving fetus following second trimester antenatal death of co-twin. Prenat Diagn 1990; 10:513–518.

68. Hughes HE, Miskin M. Congenital microcephaly due to vascular disruption: in utero documentation. Pediatrics 1985; 78:85.

69. Greene MF, Benacerraf B, Crawford JM. Hydranencephaly: US appearance during in utero evolution. Radiology 1985; 156:779–780.

70. Haid HA, Mashini IS, Devoe LD, et al. Ultrasonographic prenatal diagnosis of hydrancencephaly: a case report. J Reprod Med 1986; 31:254–256.

Isolated structural anomalies and disruption sequences

71. Lubinski M. Prenatal vascular disruptions associated with decreased maternal age. Proc Greenwood Genetics Center 1994; 14:74.

72. Mastroiacovo P, Kallen B, Knudsen LB, et al. Absence of limbs and gross body wall defects: an epidemiological study of related rare malformation conditions. Teratology 1992; 46:455–464.

73. Goldbaum G, Daling J, Milham S. Risk factors for gastroschisis. Teratology 1990; 42:397–403.

74. Kurosawa K, Imaizumi K, Masuno M, et al. Epidemiology of limb-body wall complex in Japan. Am J Med Genet 1994; 51:143–146.

Congenital encephaloclastic porencephaly

75. Hunter AGW. Brain. In: Stevenson RE, Hall JG, Goodman RM, eds. Human malformations and related anomalies. Vol II. New York: Oxford University Press; 1993:74.

76. Lemire RJ, Loeser JD, Leech RW, et al. Normal and abnormal development of the human nervous system. New York: Harper & Row; 1975.

Hydranencephaly

77. Crome L. Hydranencephaly. Dev Med Child Neurol 1972; 14:224–226.

78. Takada K, Shiota M, Ando M, et al. Porencephaly and hydranencephaly: a neuropathological study of four autopsy cases. Brain Dev 1989; 1:51–56.

79. Plantaz D, Joannard A, Pasquier B, et al. Hydranencephalie et toxoplasmose congenitale: à propos de quatre observations. Pediatrie 1987; 42:161–165.

80. Christie JD, Rkusan TA, Martinez MS, et al. Hydranencephaly caused by congenital infection with herpes simplex virus. Pediatr Infect Dis 1986; 5:473–478.

81. Fernandez F, Perez-Higuerez A, Hernandez R. Hydranencephaly after maternal butane-gas intoxication during pregnancy. Dev Med Child Neurol 1986; 28:361–363.

82. Becker H. Uber Hirnefassausschaltungen. II. Intrakranielle Gefassverschlusse. Über experimentalle Hydranencephalie (Blasenhirn). Dtsch Z Nervenheilkd 1949; 161:446.

83. Meyers RE. Brain pathology following fetal vascular occlusion: an experimental study. Invest Ophthalmol 1969; 8:41.

83a. Steveson DA, Hart BL, Clericuzio CL. Hydraencephaly in an infant with vascular malformations. Am J Med Genet 2001; 104:295–298.

84. Moore CA, Weaver DD, Bull MJ. Fetal brain disruption sequence. J Pediatr 1990; 116:383–386.

Oculoauriculovertebral spectrum

85. Rollnick BR, Kaye CI, Nagatoshi K, et al. Oculoauriculovertebral dysplasia and variants: phenotypic characteristics of 294 patients. Am J Med Genet 1987; 26:361–375.

86. Rollnick BR. Oculoauriculovertebral anomaly: variability and causal heterogeneity. Am J Med Genet 1988; (suppl) 4:41–53.

87. Gorlin RJ, Cohen MM Jr, Levin LS. Branchial arch and oroacral disorders. In: Gorlin RJ, Cohen MM Jr, Levin LS, eds. Syndromes of the head and neck. 3rd edn. New York: Oxford University Press; 1990.

88. Poswillo D. Experimental first-trimester amniocentesis in nonhuman primates. Teratology 1972; 6:227–234.

89. Poswillo D. The pathogenesis of the first and second branchial arch syndrome. Oral Surg 1974; 35:302.

90. Poswilo D. Hemorrhage in development of the face. Birth Defects 1975; 11:61.

91. Padget DH. The development of the cranial arteries in the human embryo. Carnegie Contrib Embryol 1948; 32:207.

92. Robinson L, Hoyme HE, Edwards DK, et al. Vascular pathogenesis of unilateral craniofacial defects. J Pediatr 1987; 11:236–239.

93. Gorlin RJ, Jue KL, Jacobsen U, et al. Oculoauriculovertebral dysplasia. J Pediatr 1963; 63:991.

94. Rollnick BR, Kaye CI. Hemifacial microsomia and variants: pedigree data. Am J Med Genet 1983; 15:233–253.

Gastroschisis

95. Blackburn W, Cooley NR Jr. The umbilical cord. In: Stevenson RE, Hall JG, Goodman RM, eds. Human malformations and related anomalies. Vol II. New York: Oxford University Press; 1993.

96. Sermer M, Benzie RJ, Pitson L, et al. Prenatal diagnosis and management of congenital defects of the anterior abdominal wall. Am J Obstet Gynecol 1987; 156:308–312.

96a. Werler MM, Shehan JE, Mitchell AA. Association of vasoconstrictive exposures with risks of gastroschisis and small intestinal atresia. Epidemiology 2003; 14:349–354.

96b. Werler MM. Teratogen update: Pseudoephedrine. 2006; 76:445–452.

97. Louw JH. Jejeunoileal atresia and stenosis. J Pediatr Surg 1966; 1:8.

Intestinal atresia

98. Wetzman JJ, Vanderhoof RS. Jejunal atresia with agenesis of the dorsal mesentery with 'Christmas tree' deformity of the small intestine. Am J Surg 1966; 11:443–449.

99. Jemnez FA, Reiner L. Arteriographic findings in congenital abnormalities of the mesentery and intestines. Am J Gynecol Obstet 1961; 113: 346–352.

100. Louw JH, Barnard CN. Congenital intestinal atresia: observation on its origin. Lancet 1955; 2:1065_1067.

Limb reduction defects

101. Froster-Iskenius U, Baird PA. Limb reduction defects in over one million consecutive livebirths. Teratology 1989; 39:127–135.

102. Freinberg RN, Saunders MW Jr. Effects of excising the apical ectodermal ridge on the development of the marginal vasculature of the wing bud in the chick embryo. J Exp Zool 1982; 219:345.

103. Goetnick PF. Genetic aspects of skin and limb development. In:Monroy A, Moscona AA, eds. Current topics in developmental biology. New York: Academic Press; 1966:253.

104. Saunders JW Jr. Developmental control of three-dimensional polarity in the avian limb. Ann N Y Acad Sci 1972; 193:29–42.

105. Saunders JW Jr. The experimental analysis of chick limb development. In: Ede DA, Hichliffe JR, Balls M, eds. Vertebrate limb and somite morphogenesis. Cambridge: Cambridge University Press; 1977.

106. Van Allen MI, Curry C, Walden CE, et al. Limb-body wall complex: II. Limb and spine defects. Am J Med Genet 1987; 28:549–565.

Microgastria with limb anomalies

107. Lueder GT, Fitz-James A, Dowton SB. Congenital microgastria and hypoplastic upper limb anomalies. Am J Med Genet 1989; 32:368–370.

108. Putschar WGJ, Manion WC. Congenital absence of the spleen and associated anomalies. Am J Clin Pathol 1956; 26:429–470.

109. Mandell GA, Heyman S, Alavi A, et al. A case of microgastria in association with splenic-gonadal fusion. Pediatr Radiol 1983; 13:95–98.

110. Shackelford GD, McAlister WH, Brodeur AE, et al. Congenital microgastria. AJR Am J Roentgenol 1973; 118:72–76.

111. Kessler H, Smulewicz JJ. Microgastria associated with agenesis of the spleen. Radiology 1973; 107:393–396.

112. Anderson KD, Guzzetta PC. Treatment of congenital microgastria and dumping syndrome. J Pediatr Surg 1983; 18:747–750.

113. Peterman MG. Congenital absence of spleen and left kidney. JAMA 1932; 99:1252.

114. Aintablian NH, Slim MS, Antoun BW. Congenital microgastria: case report and review of the literature. Pediatr Surg Int 1987; 2:307.

Adams-Oliver syndrome

115. Adams FH, Oliver CP. Hereditary deformities in man due to arrested development. J Hered 1945; 36:2.

115a. Gilbert-Barness E, Spicer DB. Embryo and fetal pathology color atlas with ultrasound correlation. Cambridge: Cambridge University Press; 2004; 304.

115b. Stoler JM, McGuirk CK, Lieberman E, et al. Malformations reported in chorionic villus sampling exposed children: a review and analytic synthesis of the literature. Genet Med 1999; 1:315–322.

115c. Golden CM, Ryan LM, Holmes LB. Chorionic villus sampling: a distinctive teratogenic effect on fingers? Birth Defects Res A Clin Mol Teratol 2003; 67:557–562.

116. Whitley CB, Gorlin RJ. Adams-Oliver syndrome revisited. Am J Med Genet 1991; 40:319–326.

117. Küster W, Lenz W, Kääriäinen H, et al. Congenital scalp defects with distal limb anomalies (Adams-Oliver syndrome): report of ten cases and review of the literature. Am J Med Genet 1988; 31:99–115.

118. Toriello HV, Graff RG, Florentine MF, et al. Scalp and limb defects with cutis marmorata telangiectatica congenita: Adams-Oliver syndrome? Am J Med Genet 1988; 29:269–276.

119. Sybert VP. Aplasia cutis congenita: a report of 12 new families and review of the literature. Pediatr Dermatol 1985; 3:1–14.

120. Koiffman CP, Wajntal A, Huyke BJ, et al. Congenital scalp skull defects with distal limb anomalies (Adams-Oliver syndrome – McKusick 10030): further evidence of autosomal recessive inheritance. Am J Med Genet 1988; 29:263–268.

121. Irons GB, Olson RM. Aplasia cutis congenita. Plast Reconstr Surg 1980; 66:199–203.

122. Moerman P, Fryns J-P, Vandenberghe K, et al. Constrictive amniotic bands, amniotic adhesions and limb-body wall complex: discrete disruption sequences with etiopathogenetic overlap. Am J Med Genet 1992; 42: 470–479.

123. Lockwood C, Ghidini A, Romero R. Amniotic band syndrome in monozygous twins. Prenatal diagnosis and pathogenesis. Obstet Gynecol 1988; 71:1012–1016.

Urethral obstruction sequence and lower limb deficiency

124. Perez-Aytes A, Graham JM, Hersh JH, et al. Urethral obstruction sequence and lower limb deficiency: evidence for the vascular disruption hypothesis. J Pediatr 1993; 123:398–405.

125. Pagon R, Smith DW, Shepard TH. Urethral obstruction malformation complex: a cause of abdominal muscle deficiency and the 'prune belly'. J Pediatr 1979; 94:900–906.

126. Carey JC, Eggert L, Curry C. Lower limb deficiency and the urethral obstruction sequence. Birth Defects 1982; 18:19–28.

127. Gilbert EF, Hogan GR, Stevenson MM, et al. Gangrene of an extremity in the newborn. Pediatrics 1970; 45:469–472.

128. Chavez GF, Mulinare J, Cordero JF. Maternal cocaine use during early pregnancy as a risk factor for congenital urogenital anomalies. JAMA 1989; 262:795–798.

129. Mahalik MP, Gautieri RF, Mann DE. Teratogenic potential of cocaine hydrochloride in CF-1 mice. J Pharm Sci 1980; 69:703–706.

130. Genest DR, Driscoll SG, Bieber FR. Complexities of limb anomalies: the lower extremity in the 'prune belly' phenotype. Teratology 1991; 44: 365–371.

Cocaine embryopathy and fetopathy

131. Chasnoff IJ, Bussey ME, Savich R, et al. Perinatal cerebral infarction and maternal cocaine use. J Pediatr 1986; 108:456–459.

132. Chasnoff IJ, Chisum GM, Kaplan WE. Maternal cocaine use and genitourinary tract malformations. Teratology 1988; 37:201–204.

133. Bingol N, Fuchs M, Diaz V, et al. Teratogenicity of cocaine in humans. J Pediatr 1986; 23:903.

134. Dixon SD, Bejar R. Echoencephalographic findings in neonates associated with maternal cocaine and methamphetamine use: incidence and clinical correlates. J Pediatr 1989; 115:770–778.

135. Danielsson BR. Malformations and hypoxia induced by pharmacological action. Teratology 1994; 49:238.

136. Zimmerman EF, Potturi RB, Resnick E, et al. Role of oxygen free radicals in cocaine-induced vascular disruption in mice. Teratology 1994; 49: 192–201.

137. Lutiger B, Graham K, Einarson TR, et al. Relationship between gestational cocaine use and pregnancy outcome: a meta-analysis. Teratology 1990; 44:405.

Neonatal gangrene

138. Stuart MJ, Sunderji SG, Allen JB. Decreased prostacyclin production in the infant of the diabetic mother. J Lab Clin Med 1981; 98:412–416.

139. Ambrus CM, Ambrus JL, Courey N, et al. Inhibitors of fibrinolysis in diabetic children, mothers and their infants. Am J Hematol 1979; 7:245–254.

Poland sequence

140. Fuhrmann W, Mösseler U, Neuz H. Zur Klinik und Genetik des Poland-Syndroms. Dtsch Med Wochenschr 1971; 96:1076.

141. Freire-Maia N, Chautard EA, Opitz JM, et al. The Poland syndrome – clinical and genealogical data, dermatoglyphic analysis, and incidence. Hum Hered 1973; 23:97–104.

142. Fraser FC, Ronen GM, O'Leary E. Pectoralis major defect and Poland sequence in second cousins: extension of the Poland sequence spectrum. Am J Med Genet 1989; 33:468–470.

143. Der Kaloustian VM, Hoyme HE, Hogg H, et al. Possible common pathogenetic mechanisms for Poland sequence and Adams-Oliver syndrome. Am J Med Genet 1991; 38:69–73.

143a. Maniscalco M, Zedda A, Faraone S, et al. Association of Adams-Oliver syndrome with pulmonary arteriovenous malformation in the same family: a further support to the vascular hypothesis. Am J Med Genet 2005; 136:269–274.

144. Ireland DC, Takayama N, Platt AE. Poland's syndrome. A review of forty-three cases. J Bone Joint Surg 1976; 58A:52–58.

145. McGillivray BC, Lowry RB. Poland syndrome in British Columbia: incidence and reproductive experience of affected persons. Am J Med Genet 1977; 1:65–74.

146. Castilla EE, Paz JE, Orioli IM. Pectoralis major muscle defect and Poland complex. Am J Med Genet 1982; 4:263.

147. Lowry RB, Bovet JP. Familial Poland anomaly. J Med Genet 1983; 20:152.

148. Sujansky E, Riccardi VM, Matthew AM. The familial occurrence of Poland syndrome. Birth Defects 1977; 13:117–121.

148a. Riyaz N, Riyaz A. Poland syndrome (anomaly) with congenital hemangioma: a new association. Indian J Dermatol Venereol Leprol 2006; 72: 222–223.

148b. Issaivanan M, Virdi A, Parmar VR. Subclavian artery supply disruption sequence-Klippel-Feil and Mobius anomalies. Indian J Pediatr 2002; 69:441–442.

Short umbilical cord

149. Gardiner JP. The umbilical cord: normal length; length in cord complications; etiology and frequency of coiling. Surg Gynecol Obstet 1922; 34:252.

150. Gilbert-Barness E, Drut RM, Drut R, et al. Developmental abnormalities resulting in short umbilical cord. Birth Defects1993; 29:113–140.

151. Blackburn W, Cooley NR Jr. The umbilical cord. In: Stevenson RE, Hall JG, Goodman RM, eds. Human malformations and related anomalies. New York: Oxford University Press; 1993:1097.

152. Benirschke K. The pathology of the human placenta. New York: Springer-Verlag; 1990.

153. Mills JL, Fishe R, Knopp RH, et al. Malformations in infants of diabetic mothers: problems of study design. Prev Med 1983; 12:274–286.

154. Miller ME, Higginbottom M, Smith DW. Short umbilical cord: its origin and relevance. Pediatrics 1981; 67:618–621.

155. Pal SK, Bhattacharya B. Absolute short umbilical cord (a case report). J Obstet Gynecol India 1977; 27:442.

156. Pal SK. Absolute short cord dystocia. J Indian Med Assoc 1980; 74:134–136.

157. Rayburn WF, Beynen A, Brinkman DL. Umbilical cord length and intrapartum complications. Obstet Gynecol 1981; 57:450–452.

158. Funinaga M, Chinn A, Shepard TH. Umbilical cord growth in human and rat fetuses: evidence against the 'stretch hypothesis'. Teratology 1990; 41:33–339.

159. Naeye RL, Tafari N. Noninfectious disorders of the placenta, fetal membranes and umbilical cord. In: Risk factors in pregnancy and disease of the fetus and newborn. Baltimore: 1983, Williams & Wilkins; 1983: 145.

160. Grange DK, Arya S, Opitz J, et al. The short cord syndrome. Pediatr Pathol 1986; 5:96.

161. Miller ME, Jones MC, Smith DW. Tension: the basis of umbilical cord length. J Pediatr 1982; 101:844.

162. Moessinger AC, Blanc WA, Marone PA, et al. Umbilical cord length as an index of fetal activity: experimental study and clinical implications. Pediatr Res 1982; 16:109–112.

163. Moessinger AC. Fetal akinesia deformation sequence: an animal model. Pediatrics 1983; 72:857–863.

164. Mastroiacova P, Calabro A. Amniotic-adhesion malformations in Italy. Lancet 1980; 2:801.

Amnion disruption sequence

165. Torpin R. Fetal malformations caused by amnion rupture during gestation. Springfield: Charles C Thomas; 1968.

166. Garza A, Cordero JF, Mulinare J. Epidemiology of the early amnion rupture spectrum of defects. Am J Dis Child 1988; 142:541–544.

167. Ossipof V, Hall BD. Etiologic factors in the amniotic band syndrome: a study of 24 patients. Birth Defects 1977; 13:117–132.

168. Salvador J, Prieto L, Cereijo A, et al. An epidemiologic study of the amniotic band disruption sequence. Proc Greenwood Genet Center 1986; 5:182.

169. Baker CJ, Rudolph AJ. Congenital constrictions and intrauterine amputations. Am J Dis Child 1971; 121:393.

170. Byrne J, Blanc WA, Baker D. Amniotic band syndrome in early fetal life. Birth Defects 1982; 18:43.

171. Kalousek DK, Bamforth S. Amnion rupture sequence in previable fetuses. Am J Med Genet 1988; 31:63–73.

172. Tanaka O, Toshikiyo K, Otani H. Amniogenetic band anomalies in a fifth-month fetus and in a newborn from maternal oophorectomy during early pregnancy. Teratology 1986; 33:187–193.

173. Jackson LG, Wapner RA, Barr MA. Safety of chorionic villus biopsy. Lancet 1986; 1:674–675.

174. Turnpenny PD, Hakim MM, Thwaites RJ, et al. Oligohydramnios sequence in a live-born infant following chorionic villus sampling. Prenat Diagn 1990; 10:675.

175. Moessinger AC, Blanc WA, Byrne J, et al. Amniotic band syndrome associated with amniocentesis. Am J Obstet Gynecol 1981; 141:588.

176. Rehder H, Weitzel H. Intrauterine amputations after amniocentesis. Lancet 1978; 1:382.

177. Planteydt HT, VanDer Vooren MJ, Verweij H. Amniotic bands and malformations in child born after pregnancy screened by chorionic villus biopsy. Lancet 1986; 2:756–757.

178. Boyd PA, Keeling JW, Selinger M, et al. Limb reduction and chorion villus sampling. Prenat Diagn 1990; 10:437.

179. Donnai D, Winter RM. Disorganisation: a model for 'early amnion rupture'? J Med Genet 1989; 26:421–425.

180. Winter RM, Donnai D. A possible human homologue for the mouse mutant disorganization. J Med Genet 1989; 26:417–420.

181. Young ID, Lindenbaum RH, Thompson EM, et al. Amniotic bands in connective tissue disorders. Arch Dis Child 1985; 60:1061–1063.

182. Van Der Rest M, Hayes A, Marie P, et al. Lethal osteogenesis imperfecta with amniotic band lesions: collagen studies. Am J Med Genet 1986; 24:433–446.

183. Barabas AP. Ehlers-Danlos syndrome: associated with prematurity and premature rupture of foetal membranes; possible increase in incidence. Br Med J 1966; 2:682.

184. Rudd NL, Nimrod C, Holbrook KA, et al. Pregnancy complications in type IV Ehlers-Danlos syndrome. Lancet 1983; 1:50–53.

185. Marras A, Dessi C, Macciotta A. Epidermolysis bullosa and amniotic bands. Am J Med Genet 1984; 19:815–817.

186. Draeger A, Nerlich A. Syndrome des bandes amniotiques associé à une malformation acardiaque observé dans une grossesse gemellaire: à propos d'un cas. Ann Pathol 1988; 8:317.

187. Hernando I, Plasencia A, Pena E, et al. Sindrome de bandas amnioticas y cariotipo 47,XYY. An Exp Pediatr 1987; 27:75.

188. Torpin R. Amniochorionic mesoblastic fibrous strings and amniotic bands: associated constricting fetal malformations or fetal death. Am J Obstet Gynecol 1965; 91:65–75.

189. Streeter GL. Focal deficiencies in fetal tissues and their relation to intrauterine amputation. Contrib Embryol 1930; 22:1.

190. DeMyer W, Baird O. Mortality and skeletal malformations from amniocentesis and oligohydramnos in rats: cleft palate, club foot, microstomia and adactyly. Teratology 1971; 2:33.

191. Trasler DG, Wlker BE, Fraser FC. Congenital malformations produced by amniotic-sac puncture. Science 1956; 124:439.

192. Poswillo D. Observations of fetal posture and causal mechanisms of congenital deformity of palate, mandible, and limbs. J Ent Res 1966; 45 (suppl 3):584.

193. Houben JJ. Immediate and delayed effects of oligohydramnios on limb development in the rat: chronology and specificity. Teratology 1984; 30:403–411.

194. Yang SS, Sanborn JR, Levine AJ, et al. Amniotic rupture, extraamniotic pregnancy, and vernix granulomata. Am J Surg Pathol 1984; 8:117–122.

195. Etches PC, Stewardt AR, Ives EJ. Familial congenital amputations. J Pediatr 1982; 101:448–449.

196. Lubinsky M, Sujansky E, Sanger W, et al. Familial amniotic bands. Am J Med Genet 1983; 14:81.

196a. Czichos E, Lukaszek S, Krekora M, et al. Early amnion rupture and fetal and newborn defects as an obstetrical and pathomorphological problem. Ginekol Pol 2005; 76:448–456.

196b. Robin NH, Franklin J, Prucka S, et al. Clefting, amniotic bands, and polydactyly: a distinct phenotype that supports an intrinsic mechanism for amniotic band sequence. Am J Med Genet 2005; 137:298–301.

196c. Morovic CG, Berwart F, Varas J. Craniofacial anomalies of the amniotic band syndrome in serial clinical cases. Plast Reconstr Surg 2004; 113:1556–1562.

197. Brown DL, Felker RE, Emerson DS. Intrauterine shelves in pregnancy: sonographic observations. AJR Am J Roentgenol 1989; 153:821–824.

198. Herbert WNP, Seeds JW, Cefalo RC, et al. Prenatal detection of intraamniotic bands: implications and management. Obstet Gynecol 1985; 65(3 suppl):35S–38S.

199. Hill LM, Kislak S, Jones N. Prenatal ultrasound diagnosis of a forearm constriction band. J Ultrasound Med 1988; 7:293–295.

200. Mahony BS, Filly FA, Callen PW, et al. The amniotic band syndrome: antenatal sonographic diagnosis and potential pitfalls. Am J Obstet Gynecol 1985; 152:63–68.

201. Patten RM, Van Allen MI, Mack LA, et al. Limb-body wall complex: in utero sonographic diagnosis of a complicated fetal malformation. AJR Am J Roentgenol 1986; 146:1019–1024.

202. Papp Z, Tough Z, Csecei K, et al. Letter to the Editor. Are there 'innocent' amniotic bands? Am J Med Genet 1986; 24:207–209.

203. Yamaguchi M, Yasuda H, Kuroki T, et al. Early prenatal diagnosis of amniotic band syndrome. Am J Perinatol 1988; 5:5.

Anencephaly with amniotic bands

204. Holmes LB, Driscoll SG, Atkins L. Etiologic heterogeneity of neural-tube defects. N Engl J Med 1976; 294:365.

205. Lemire RJ, Beckwith JB, Warkany J. Anencephaly. New York: Raven Press; 1978.

206. Keller H, Neuhauser G, Durkin-Stamm MN, et al. 'ADAM complex' (amniotic deformity, adhesions, mutilations) – a pattern of craniofacial and limb defects. Am J Med Genet 1978; 2:81.

207. Pagon RA, Stephens TD, McGillivary BC, et al. Body wall defects with reduction limb anomalies: a report of fifteen cases. Birth Defects 1979; 15:171–185.

208. Yang SS. ADAM sequence and innocent amniotic band: manifestations of early amnion rupture. Am J Med Genet 1990; 37:562–568.

Craniofacial clefts with ectopia cordis

209. Van Allen MI, Myhre S. Ectopia cordis thoracalis with craniofacial defects resulting from early amnion rupture. Teratology 1985; 32:19–24.

Limb reduction defects

210. Barenberg LM, Greenberg B. Intrauterine amputations and constriction bands: report of a case with anesthesia below the constriction. Am J Dis Child 1942; 64:87.

210a. McGuirk CK, Westgate MN, Homes LB. Limb deficiencies in newborn infants 2001; 108:E64.

Pierre Robin sequence

211. Hanson J, Smith DW. U-shaped palatal defect in the Robin anomaly: developmental and clinical relevance. J Pediatr 1975; 87:30–33.
212. Gorlin RJ, Cohen MM, Levin LS. Robin sequence. In: Gorlin RJ, Cohen MM Jr, Hennekam RCM, eds. Syndromes of the head and neck. 4th edn. New York: Oxford University Press; 2001.

Potter sequence

213. Potter EL. Bilateral renal agenesis. J Pediatr 1946; 29:68.
214. Curry CJR, Jensen K, Holland J, et al. The Potter sequence: a clinical analysis of 80 cases. Am J Med Genet 1984; 19:679–702.
215. Evans JR. Renal agenesis. In: Stevenson RG, Hall JG, Goodman RM, eds. Human malformations and related anomalies. New York: Oxford University Press; 2006:1184–1190.

Chromosomal abnormalities

5

Enid Gilbert-Barness   Luc L. Oligny

'Man is an instrument designed by DNA for the purpose of understanding itself.'

Anonymous

Terminology and techniques

General considerations of chromosomal abnormalities

Chromosomal abnormalities represent the largest category of causes of conceptual loss. Abortuses that have reached a 2 week stage of development have a 78% rate of chromosomal abnormalities.[1,2] For abortions occurring after the first missed period but before week 20, the rate declines to 62%.[1,2] The rate further declines to 6% for stillborn infants, and in liveborn infants the rate is 0.5%.[3] Chromosomal imbalance may be the major cause of failure of development of 31% of ova lost before implantation. From the time of conception, it is estimated that at least half of all human ova have a chromosomal abnormality.[4,5] The incidence of the types of chromosomal abnormalities in spontaneous abortions is shown in Table 5.1. Advanced maternal age has long been known as a predisposing factor for chromosomal abnormalities, and advanced paternal age has recently been shown to also constitute a risk. Amniocentesis is offered when maternal age, ultrasonographic findings, and/or other screening techniques such as the triple screen suggest an elevated risk of fetal aneuploidy.

Approximately 99% of all conceptuses with chromosomal abnormalities die prenatally, including monosomy X and autosomal

TABLE 5.1 INCIDENCE OF THE TYPES OF CHROMOSOMAL ABNORMALITIES IN 1500 SPONTANEOUS ABORTIONS

Abnormalities	Rate of occurrence (%)
Autosomal trisomies	52.00
Triploidy	19.86
45,X	15.30
Tetraploidy	6.18
Double trisomy	1.73
Translocations	3.80
Mosaicism	1.08

After Boué et al 1975,[4] with permission.

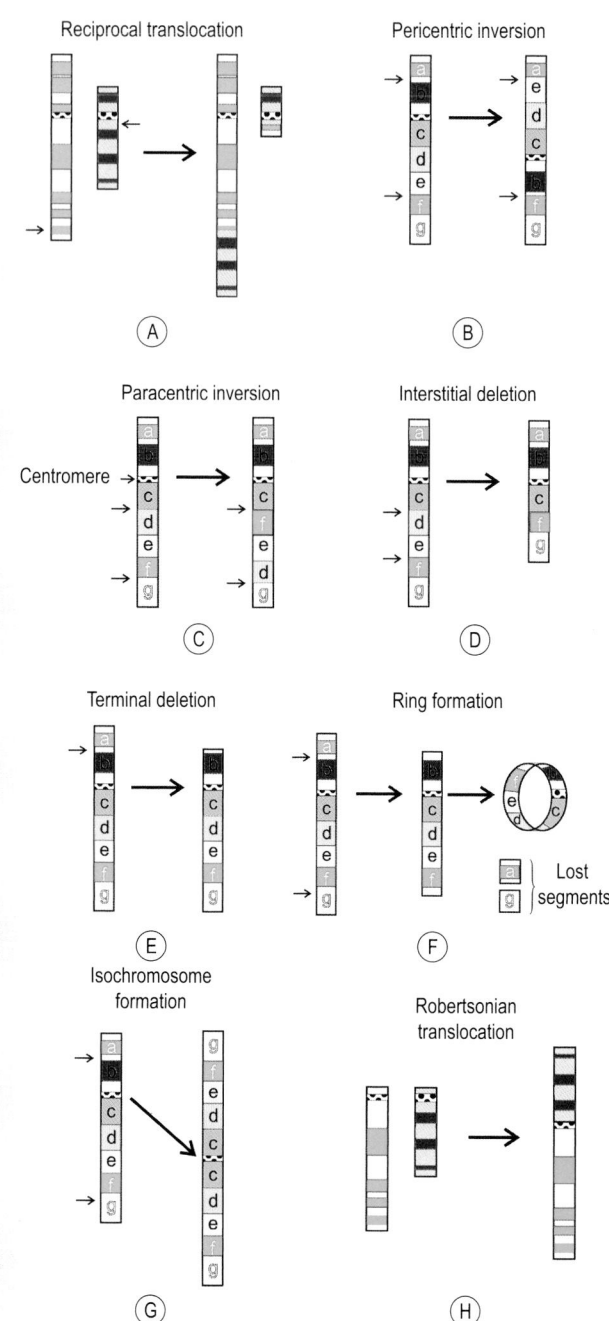

FIGURE 5.1 Diagrammatic view of the most common structural chromosomal rearrangements (see Box 5.1).

trisomy; more than half of fetuses with trisomy 21 die prenatally.[6] Survival of triploid fetuses to term are exceptional. Around 40% of liveborn children with Down syndrome (DS) have died by the end of the first year of life.[7,8] Machin and Crolla[9] found a chromosomal abnormality in 13.4% of infants and fetuses with lethal malformations. **Meiotic non-disjunction,** which causes numerical abnormalities, appears to be non-random because women who have had an aneuploid fetus are more likely to have another aneuploid fetus if they miscarry again than women whose first miscarried fetus was chromosomally normal.

An extra sex chromosome (e.g. 47,XXX; 47,XYY) can be found in more than one-third of cytogenetically abnormal liveborn infants and does not seem to produce excessive prenatal mortality. Approximately 25% of liveborn infants with chromosomal abnormalities have autosomal trisomy, and approximately 40% have a structural chromosomal defect. Those with inherited balanced chromosomal translocations are phenotypically normal, but have about 15% fewer liveborn offspring than their chromosomally normal siblings.[10] Patients with de novo balanced translocations have an increased risk of maldevelopment.

Terminology for normal human chromosomes and for structural and numerical chromosomal abnormalities has been established by the International Standing Committee on Human Cytogenetic Nomenclature.[11] Box 5.1 defines some of these terms (see also Fig. 5.1). High-resolution methods have increased the number of recognizable human chromosomal regions and bands to more than 1200, enabling more precise determinations of chromosomal abnormalities.[12,13] However, the routine cytogenetic analysis is based on 550 bands per haploid set, but extended or prometaphase banding analyzes chromosomes at the 800 band level. Fluorescence in situ hybridization (**FISH**) is more sensitive than conventional karyotyping in the diagnosis of very small deletions (**microdeletions or cryptic deletions**).

Although the common chromosomal syndromes are discussed in this chapter, more extensive and detailed reviews of chromosomal abnormalities can be found in publications by Yunis,[14] Zellweger and Simpson,[15] de Grouchy and Turleau,[16] Schinzel,[17] McKinlay Gardner and Sutherland,[18] Borgaonkar,[19,20] Gilbert and Opitz,[21] Gilbert and colleagues,[22] and the many monographs on new chromosomal syndromes from the Annual Birth Defects Meetings, published in the Birth Defects Original Articles Series

and the Proceedings of the International Congress of Human Genetics.[23]

Numerical chromosome abnormalities may involve an individual chromosome (**aneuploidy**) resulting in monosomy, trisomy, higher degrees of aneuploidy, or double trisomies; or haploid sets resulting in triploidy (69 chromosomes) or tetraploidy (92 chromosomes).

BOX 5.1 CYTOGENETIC TERMINOLOGY

Aneuploid. An unbalanced state that arises through loss or addition of whole or pieces of chromosomes; always considered deleterious.

Chromosome. The location of hereditary (genetic) material within the cell. This hereditary material is packaged in the form of a very long, double-stranded molecule of DNA surrounded by and complexed with several different forms of protein. Genes are found arranged in a linear sequence along chromosomes, in addition to a large amount of DNA of unknown function.

Confined placental mosaicism. A viable mutation in trophoblast or extraembryonic progenitor cells of the inner cell mass resulting in dichotomy between the chromosomal constitution of the placenta and the embryo or fetus (Fig. 5.1B and C).

Deletion. Missing segments of, or whole chromosomes (Fig. 5.1D, E and F).

Diploid (2n). The whole set of 46 chromosomes in a somatic cell, comprised two haploid sets.

Duplication. Presence of two copies of a segment of chromosome contiguous with one another, within the chromosome normally carrying that segment.

Endomitosis. Duplication of the chromosomes without accompanying spindle formation or cytokinesis resulting in a polyploid nucleus.

Fluorescence in situ hybridization (FISH). This technique can use non-dividing cells from smears or sections, or cells in metaphase. By use of commercially available or in-house, chromosome-specific fluorescent probes that can hybridize to complementary DNA sequences, the number of fluorescent signals in interphase cells can be counted to determine the number of copies of the target chromosomes present in those cells. The use of different colored probes recognizing contiguous chromosomal segments can identify translocations and other rearrangements within that segment.

Fragile X. The most frequent mental retardation syndrome caused by a mutant gene. The syndrome is due to an altered gene on the X chromosome characterized by too many copies of a CGG repeat that compromises the function of the gene FMR1 involved in brain development. Since it is X-linked, it is more frequent in males, but it also occurs in heterozygous females who have extensive amplification of the CGG trinucleotide.

Genotype. The total of the genetic information contained in the chromosomes of an organism; the genetic make-up of an organism.

Haploid (n). Refers to the set of 23 chromosomes present in a normal gamete.

Homologue. The individual members of a pair of chromosomes.

Inversion. Inversions require two chromosomal breaks. Both breaks on one side of the centromere produce a paracentric inversion (Fig. 5.1C); breaks in both arms produce a pericentric inversion (Fig. 5.1B).

Isochromosome. Chromosomes that arise from several different mechanisms, principally transverse rather than longitudinal division of the centromere during mitosis or meiosis. Isochromosomes have either two long or two short arms (Fig. 5.1G), resulting in a trisomy of the duplicated arm, and a monosomy of the other arm.

Monosomy. Lack of one whole chromosome.

Mosaicism. Two or more chromosomally different cell lines derived from a single zygote in one individual.

Non-disjunction. Failure of paired chromosomes or sister chromatids to disjoin at anaphase during mitotic division or in the first or second meiotic division.

Oncogenes. Normal growth-related genes that become activated and/or amplified in somatic cells, thereby causing increased cell proliferation and abnormal growth.

Phenotype. The observable properties of an organism resulting from the interaction between its genotype and the environment.

Polymorphisms. Chromosomes or chromosome regions that may vary in size without phenotypic effect, because they are composed of heterochromatin (non-transcribed DNA). The most common human chromosomal polymorphisms involve 1q, 9q, 13p, 14p, 15p, 16q, 21p, 22p, and Yq. Polymorphisms can also refer to molecular differences observed between alleles, when they do not have any phenotypic effect.

Polyploidy. More than two haploid sets of chromosomes (i.e. 69 is triploidy, 92 is tetraploidy).

Ring chromosomes. Formed when two chromosomal breaks occur within both the short and long arms of a chromosome (Fig. 5.1F). Ring chromosomes are meiotically and mitotically unstable; gonocytes harboring them rarely survive meiosis to be transmitted to the next generation.

Southern blotting. Molecular technique where DNA is cut by restriction enzymes and restriction fragments are separated through gel electrophoresis prior to being blotted onto a membrane and visualized through hybridization with labeled probes. It can be used to assess allelic polymorphisms and gene copy number.

Tetraploidy. Four copies of haploid set (92,XXXX, or 92,XXXY, or 92,XXYY). This occurs in many tumors and also occurs at conception or shortly thereafter, resulting in spontaneous abortion, or (exceptionally) in term delivery of a malformed infant.

Tetrasomy. Two extra chromosomes of one pair; if they belong to two different pairs, the state is called double trisomy.

Translocation. Exchange of material between two chromosomes in which the unbalanced state of one or the other altered chromosome in offspring represents a duplication or deletion (Fig. 5.1A). Robertsonian translocation involves only acrocentric chromosomes (Fig. 5.1H); the breakpoints are in the short arms, and the translocation arises from end-to-end pairing, resulting in a chromosome with two long arms and no short arm.

Triploidy. Three copies of haploid set (69,XXX, or 69,XXY, or 69,XYY) due to an accident at fertilization (dispermy), or from a meiotic error of sperm or oocyte. Triploidy is not viable and results in spontaneous abortion or premature delivery of a nonviable infant with multiple malformations.

Trisomy. One whole extra chromosome.

After Behrman and Vaughan 1992,[150] and Kalousek and Gilbert-Barness 1997,[100] with permission.

A prerequisite to routine chromosome analysis is the presence of dividing cells obtained through tissue culture. **Tissue culture** includes short-term peripheral blood culture, culture of chorionic villi, amniotic fluid cell culture, culture of skin biopsy or other tissue, and direct (1–3 h incubation) or cultured bone marrow specimens. Lung or cartilage cells can be grown from macerated fetuses with some success. The tissue is grown in culture medium until there are sufficient dividing cells, at which time Colcemid is added to the cultures to disrupt spindle formation and arrest the cells in prometaphase or metaphase, when chromosomes are sufficiently contracted to be visible. The metaphase cells are then harvested, placed on slides, stained and examined under the microscope. The most common banding technique, called G-banding, involves treating slides with trypsin or other proteases, followed by staining with Giemsa. The typical cytogenetic analysis is based on a resolution of 550 bands per haploid set, but prometaphase banding analyzes chromosomes at the 800 band level.

The mechanisms yielding chromosome banding are poorly understood. During **G-banding,** trypsin cannot access and digest the histone and other chromatin proteins within the tightly condensed chromatin; thus, only loosely condensed chromatin is digested, accounting for the dark (protein-rich) and light bands, respectively. Likewise, transcription factors and other components of the transcription machinery cannot access heterochromatin, providing a mechanism for its lack of transcription.

Fluorescence in situ hybridization

Cytogenetic analysis with FISH using chromosome- and locus-specific DNA **probes** can identify chromosome rearrangements and aneuploidy in interphase cells such as leukocytes, amniocytes, and chorionic villus samples. Hundreds of commercial and in-house probes are currently available, allowing the specific identification and characterization of virtually all chromosomal rearrangements. This makes FISH a valuable tool in clinical cytogenetics for the confirmation of G-banded karyotypes (Fig. 5.2),[24] or as a primary diagnostic modality for metaphase and interphase cells, in the investigation of syndromic malformations and of tumor-specific chromosomal anomalies.

This technique can use non-dividing (interphase) cells from smears or sections. Chromosome-specific fluorescent probes hybridize to complementary DNA sequences, and the number of fluorescent signals in interphase cells can be counted to determine the number of copies of the target chromosomes present in those cells. Aneuploidy involving chromosomes 13, 18, 21, X and Y account for more than 80% of chromosomal abnormalities detected in prenatal diagnosis.[25] Multicolor probe 'cocktails' can be used to identify the most common aneuploidy in amniotic fluid and autopsy cells in interphase, which is more rapid than karyotyping, but not as sensitive, as only the anomalies recognized by the probes can be found.[26, 27]

To identify **microdeletions,** i.e. deletions too small to be reliably identified through conventional high-resolution karyotyping, FISH probes are used on metaphases to heighten the technique's resolution (Fig. 5.3). Multicolor probe cocktails are now routinely used in oncology (Figs 5.4 and 5.5) to identify chromosomal rearrangements, such as the t(9;22) of chronic myelogenous leukemia and acute lymphoblastic leukemia (ALL), rearrangements of the MLL gene on 11q23 in acute leukemias (Fig. 5.6), or the t(8;21), t(15;17) and inv(16) characteristic of acute myelocytic leukemia (AML).

A variant of the FISH technique is **primed in situ (PRINS)** labeling, whereby the fluorescent probe is constructed onto slides with interphase nuclei or metaphase spreads, through polymerase chain reaction (PCR) amplification. This technique allows color-specific identification of chromosomes (Fig. 5.7).[28–30] PRINS is rapid and cheaper than FISH, but for now is limited to the identification of repetitive DNA sequences.

FISH using **subtelomeric probes** (which recognize the subtelomeric regions of the long and short arms of each chromosome, Fig. 5.8) has been the subject of recent studies in patients with either minor malformations and/or mental retardation of unknown origin. This technique shows subtelomeric rearrangements which cannot be identified with routine and high-resolution karyotypes. Some centers advocate systematic screening of patients fulfilling a set of stringent criteria, as this technique is positive in approximately 10% of such patients.[31–33] Systematic population screens are not practical with current technology, and alternatives are sought.[34]

Cocktails of probes are available to identify specifically each of the 24 human chromosomes, which are thus color-coded. This **spectral karyotyping** (or **SKY**) allows the study of complex chromosomal rearrangements, and has proven particularly helpful in oncology (Fig. 5.9);[35–38] nevertheless, SKY cannot detect chromosomal inversions.

In comparative genomic hybridization **(CGH)**,[39] tumoral DNA is labeled with a green fluorescent dye. Red-labeled normal genomic DNA is added in equimolar amounts to the tumoral DNA. The mixture is hybridized onto normal metaphase spreads. Segments of chromosomes deleted in the tumor are red, whereas duplicated (amplified) segments are green; unaltered segments are yellow (Fig. 5.10A). Multiple metaphases are analyzed digitally to improve sensitivity and specificity, and an idiogram of the results is generated (Fig. 5.10B). This technique cannot recognize rearrangements if there is no loss or gain of chromosomal material (e.g. balanced translocations). A registry of tumor-type specific karyotypic, CGH and SKY correlations is operated by the National Institute of Health (USA).[37, 38]

DNA microarray technology is an offshoot of CGH: up to several thousand small segments of DNA or genes from normal individuals (e.g. cDNA, DNA cloned in yeast artificial chromosomes, bacterial artificial chromosomes, or other sources) are spotted (fixed) onto a microscope slide, each in a specific spot within rows and lines of such spots (arrays). The slide is hybridized with an equimolar mixture of tumoral and normal DNA, respectively fluorescent-labeled in green and red. If no genetic material has been lost or gained in the test sample, the dot will be yellow; color shifts indicate loss or gain.[40] This technology holds great promise in the study, characterization, and treatment of cancer.[41–43] Modifications of the technique allow the study of gene expression, through the quantification of mRNA which is

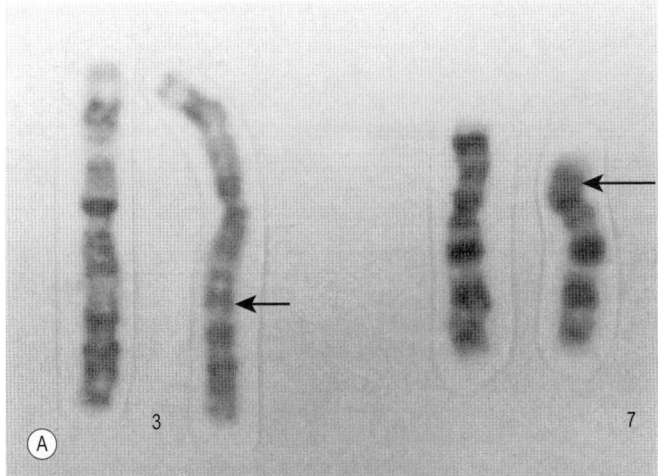

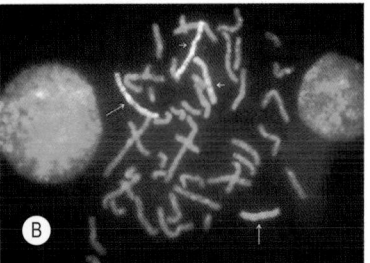

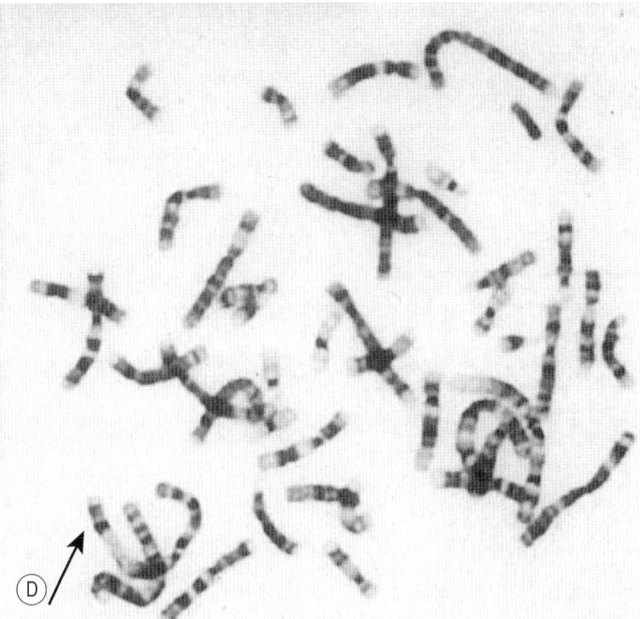

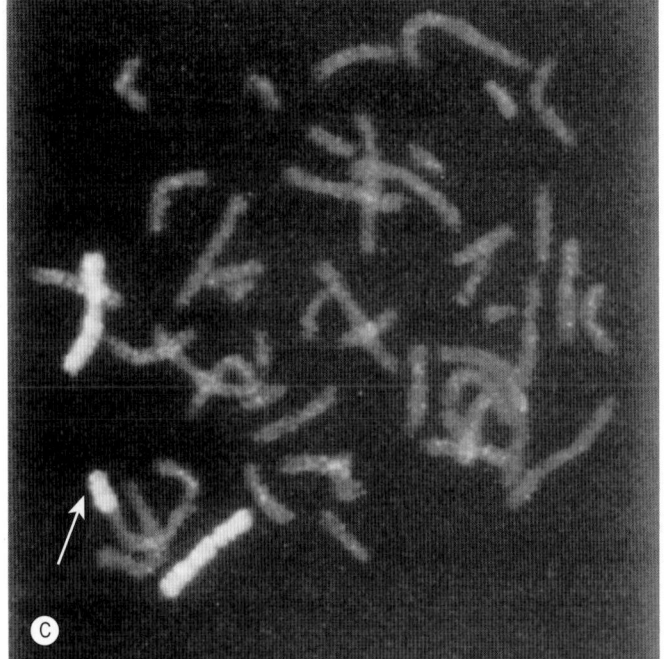

FIGURE 5.2 (A) Partial karyotype using trypsin-Giemsa banding (G-banding) suggests an interchromosomal insertion: a small segment from the short arm of one chromosome 7 (long arrow) has been transposed into the long arm of one chromosome 3 (short arrow). (B) Fluorescent in situ hybridization (FISH) technology. Chromosome painting probes for chromosome 3 (spectrum orange) and chromosome 7 (spectrum green) confirm an insertional translocation of chromosome 7 material into the chromosome 3 long arm. Normal and abnormal chromosomes 3 and 7 are shown with short and long yellow arrows, and short and long white arrows respectively. (C) and (D): Translocation between chromosomes 1 and 7. (C) A GTL-banded metaphase from an amniotic fluid culture processed with a chromosome 7 painting. (D) This combination method helped establish that chromosome 7 was involved and that the break and fusion point on chromosome 1 was 1p36.3. [(A) and (B) courtesy Karen David and Archives of Pediatric and Adolescent Medicine; (C) and (D) courtesy Dr Jalal and American Journal of Medical Genetics.]

hybridized to the array. DNA microarrays should not be confused with **tissue microarrays,** where tissues of interest from paraffin-embedded blocks are core-sampled, and transferred along with 100 other such specimens to a paraffin block, enabling all these specimens to be immunostained together on one slide.

Molecular techniques in DNA diagnosis

There is increasing overlap between cytogenetics and molecular biology, so that the boundary between these two diagnostic modalities is becoming blurred.[44] Only a brief overview of DNA-based molecular techniques will be given here. For a detailed discussion, the reader is referred to a standard textbook of molecular biology[45, 46] or a web-based primer.[47, 48] A knowledge of molecular-based DNA diagnosis is now considered essential to the practice of pathology. Since the human genome has been essentially totally sequenced, we can only expect that molecular diagnosis will take an ever-growing place in medicine. As such, today's molecular techniques may become obsolete in the near future, and diagnostic methods may change rapidly.[49]

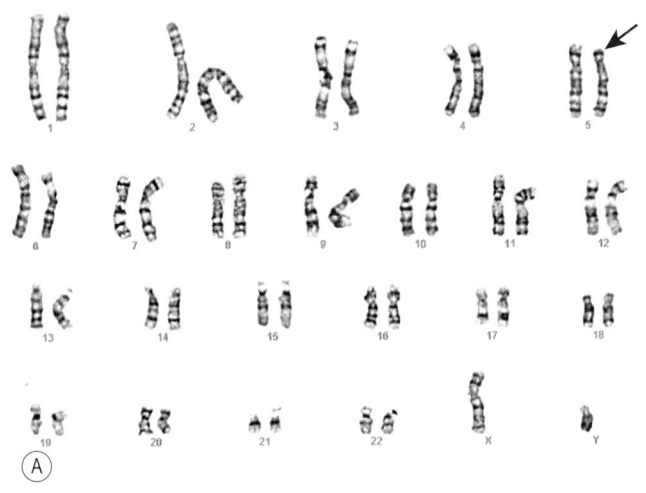

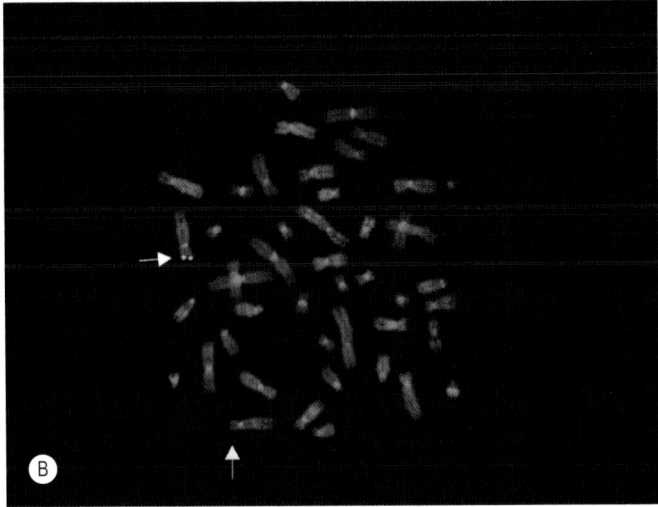

FIGURE 5.3 (A) Karyotype of male patient with cri du chat (del 5p) syndrome. The deletion is shown with an arrow. (B) FISH, same patient. Chromosomes 5 are identified with a red probe (arrows), and the telomeric portion of the short arms are labeled with a green probe, demonstrating the deletion of the short arm of one chromosome 5 (yellow arrow). (Courtesy of Drs Raouf Fetni and Nicole Lemieux.)

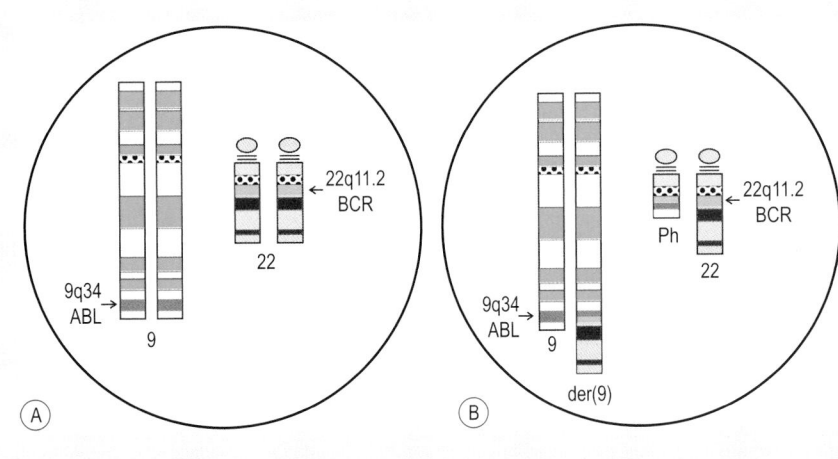

FIGURE 5.4 Identification of the t(9;22) translocation using dual color, dual fusion translocation probes. (A) Normal nucleus labeled with an orange probe spanning the ABL breakpoint, and a green probe spanning the breakpoint cluster region breakpoint. Chromosomes 9 are shown in blue, 22s in red. In interphase and metaphase, each nucleus shows two orange dots and two green dots. (B) Nucleus with a t(9;22), labeled with same probes. The two normal chromosomes yield an orange and a green spot, while the two rearranged chromosomes (derivative 9 and Philadelphia chromosome) each give a yellow signal, as the combined green and orange fluorescence signals merge to appear as a single yellow dot.

Southern blotting can be used to assess gene or **DNA sequence copy number** by employing specific endonucleases to cut the DNA into fragments. By means of gel electrophoresis to separate the fragments on the basis of size, followed by use of specific radioactive isotope- or fluorescent-labeled DNA probes that hybridize to the target sequence, the presence of normal and abnormal DNA sequences can be detected. This is the basis of molecular testing for the fragile X, for example, in which the band hybridizing to the probe can be demonstrated by autoradiography (see discussion of fragile X, below). The study of restriction fragment length polymorphism is based on the Southern blot technique; the power of the Southern blot has been greatly increased through the use of **allele-specific oligonucleotide (ASO)** probes, which allow the detection of known mutations.

PCR is much more rapid than Southern blots, and requires minute amounts of DNA (often the DNA of a single cell is sufficient). **ASO primers** can be used to identify different alleles of a gene, both normal and mutant.

Northern blots and **reverse transcriptase-polymerase chain reaction** (RT-PCR) identify the presence of mRNA, i.e. of transcribed (active) genes. **Microdissecting** cells from a slide, using a laser, can sample a homogeneous cell population (e.g. tumor cells free of stromal cells, or subpopulations of phenotypically different tumor cells). Isolated cells can be analyzed through PCR for the presence of abnormal genes, or through RT-PCR for the analysis of actively transcribed genes.

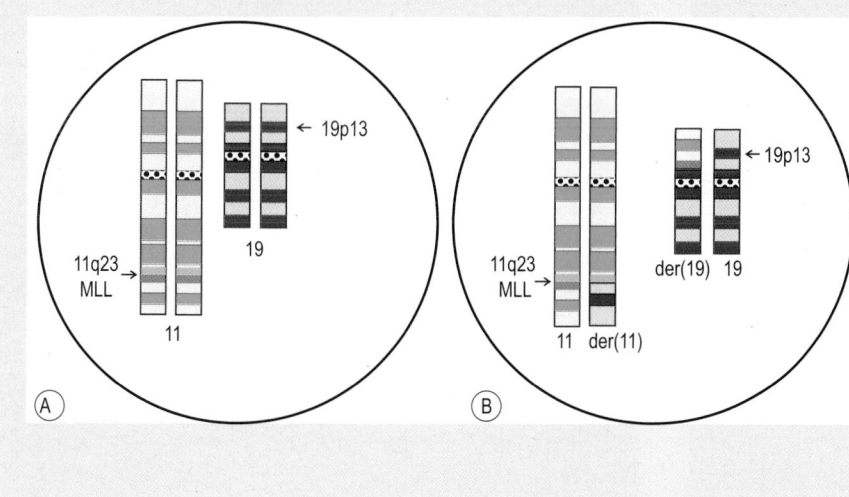

FIGURE 5.5 Identification of a rearrangement at 11q23 using a dual color, break-apart rearrangement probe. (A) Normal nucleus labeled with two probes, one green, centromeric to the breakpoint cluster region (BCR) of the translocations involving the MLL gene, and one orange distal to the BCR. Each nucleus yields two yellow signals. (B) Nucleus with a translocation at the level of the MLL BCR. The normal chromosome 11 yields one yellow signal, the derivative 11 one green signal, and the other derivative (in this case, chromosome 19) one orange signal. Dual color, break-apart probes are useful to identify translocations involving one constant breakpoint (11q23) with a multitude of other chromosomes [e.g. t(4;11)(q21;q23), t(9;11)(p22;q23), and the t(11;19)(q23;p13) shown here].

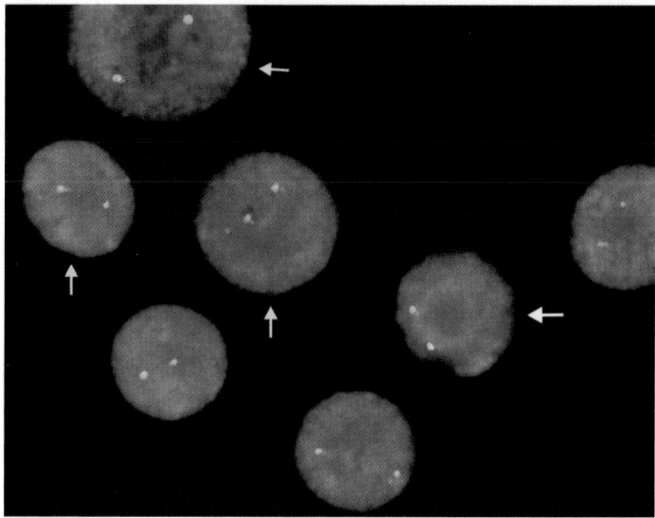

FIGURE 5.6 FISH using the MLL dual color, break apart rearrangement probe. A normal nucleus is shown by a white arrow, with two fusion signals; abnormal nuclei (yellow arrows) show a translocation at 11q23 with two abnormal signals (one red and one green) in addition to the normal fusion signal (adjacent red and green signals). (Courtesy of Dr Raouf Fetni.)

Minor anomalies and mild malformations

In live births, most congenital anomalies in chromosomal disorders are minor anomalies or mild malformations. **Minor anomalies** should be regarded as **defects of phenogenesis** and **mild malformations** as **defects of organogenesis.** Minor anomalies comprise all those human developmental variants and dysmorphisms commonly seen in normal populations, including epicanthal folds, mongolian spots, variants of scalp hair patterns, ear configuration, height of bridge of nose, variant dermatoglyphics, broad thumbs, clinodactyly, 'trigger' thumbs, synophrys, vertebral segmentation defects, and others.

A mild malformation is a morphologic anomaly that should be interpreted as a reduced expressivity (severity) of a major anomaly under the following circumstances:

- Anomalies in laterally paired organs are of unequal severity.
- Anomalies are known to be associated with the defect as part of a developmental field defect (e.g. single umbilical artery with unilateral renal agenesis).
- The defect occurs in a more severe form in a twin or other first-degree relative.
- Associated functional or structural defects indicate **pleiotropy** (i.e. the production of apparently multiple effects at the clinical or phenotypic level, by a single genetic anomaly, such as the hydrops, cardiac and aortic malformations, horseshoe kidneys and slightly short fourth metacarpals characteristic of Turner syndrome).

Mild malformations frequently seen in chromosomal syndromes are listed in Box 5.2.

Atavisms, such as the retention of a coccygeal tail and the presence of the pectoralis minimus and latissimocondyloideus muscles in the trisomy 18 syndrome, are due to the expression of normally-repressed genes that code for phylogenetically older structures.[50]

Chromosomal anomalies

It must be realized that the vast majority of zygotes with a chromosomal anomaly, be it a triploidy, a trisomy, a monosomy, an interstitial duplication or deletion, or an unbalanced translocation, are spontaneously aborted very early in the pregnancy.

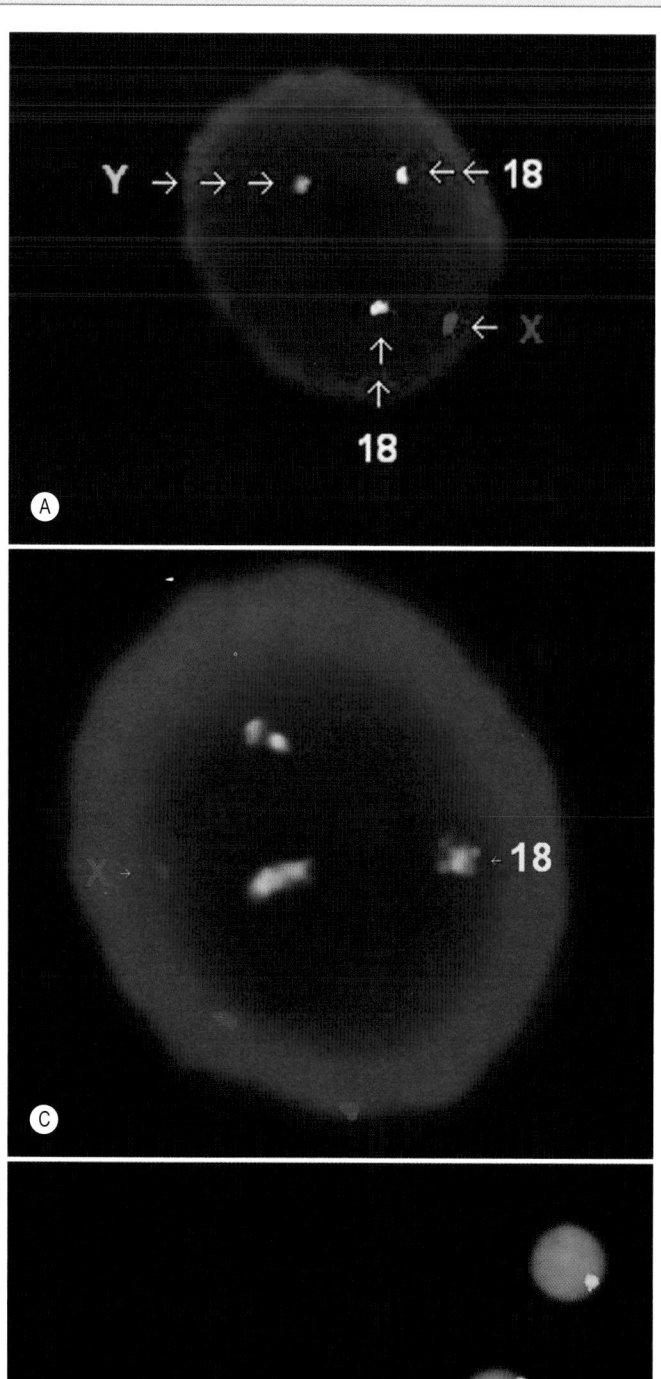

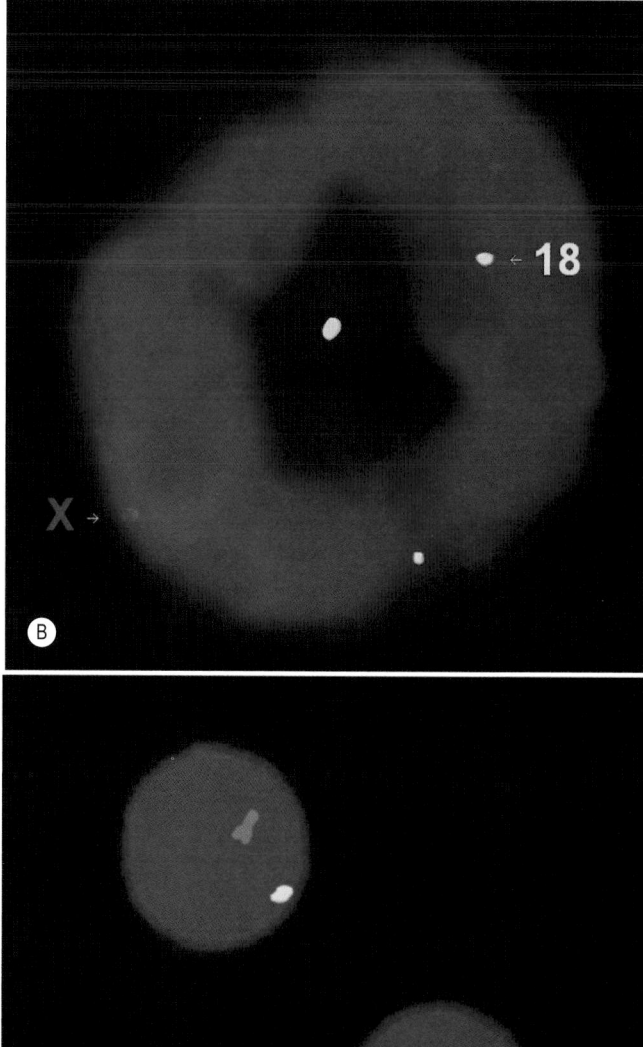

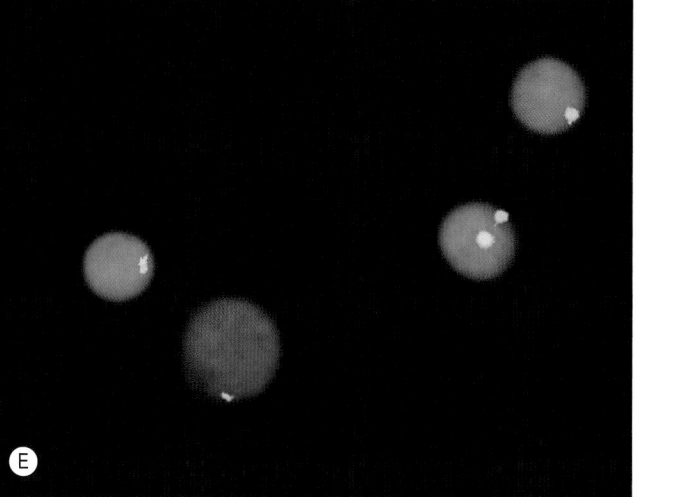

FIGURE 5.7 (A) Normal amniocyte nucleus, stained with a tricolor PRINS technique to identify chromosomes 18, X and Y. (B) and (C) Same technique (prenatal diagnosis) showing a trisomy 18 in a female fetus, and triploidy in a female fetus, respectively. (D) Bone marrow transplantation with sex mismatch; circulating lymphocytes demonstrate the chimeric state (chromosomes X and Y giving red and green signals, respectively). (E) PRINS for chromosome 7 in a patient with a myelodysplastic syndrome, demonstrating a monosomy 7 in three of the four nuclei.
[Figs (A)–(D) courtesy of Dr Régen Drouin, Fig. (E) courtesy of Dr Stéphane Barrette.]

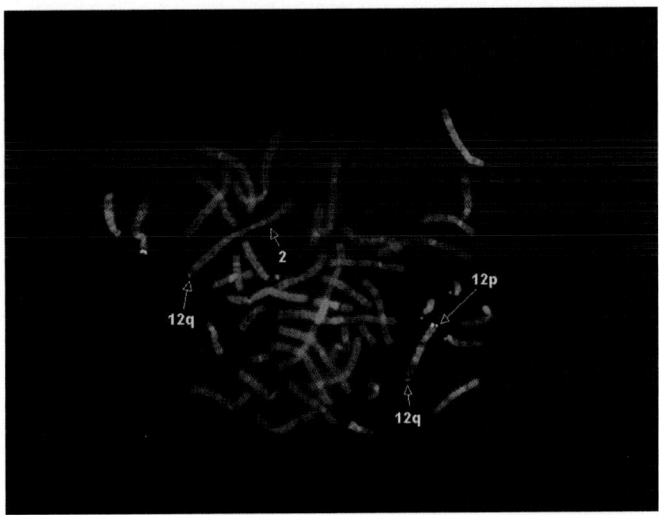

FIGURE 5.8 The subtelomeric regions of the short and long arms of chromosomes 12 are respectively recognized by green and red probes, through a FISH technique. Subtelomeric probes can be used to identify cryptic chromosomal deletions. Here, the technique demonstrates no such deletion, but rather that one chromosome 12 is rearranged (in a 2;12 translocation); the normal chromosome 12 is seen on the right. Subtelomeric probes do not allow characterization of the breakpoints. (Courtesy of Drs Raouf Fetni and Nicole Lemieux.)

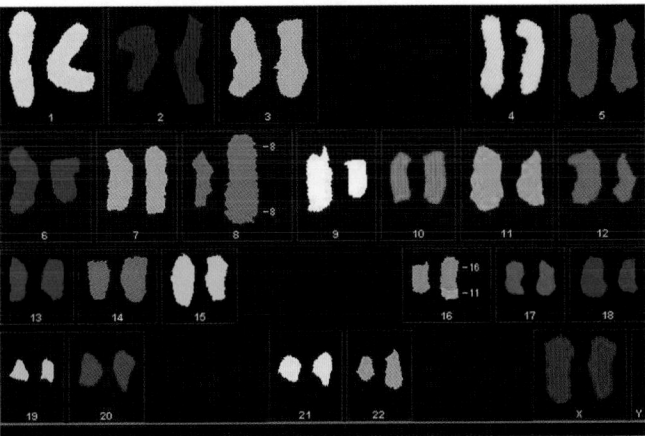

FIGURE 5.9 SKY labeling of a metaphase spread. Each chromosome appears with a specific color, enabling an accurate identification of translocations which could be cryptic or difficult to characterize. Prolymphocytic T-cell leukemia with an unbalanced translocation between chromosomes 11 and 16, and an isochromosome 8 [i(8)(q10)]. (Courtesy of Drs Josée Hébert and Raouf Fetni.)

BOX 5.2 MINOR MALFORMATIONS ASSOCIATED WITH CHROMOSOME DISORDERS

Single umbilical artery

Bipartite uvula

Intrahepatic gallbladder

Abnormal branching of bile ducts

Abnormal lobation of lungs, spleen, or liver

Malrotation of gut

Meckel diverticulum

Annular pancreas

Urogenital malformations

Kinked ureters

Megapelvis

Renal microcysts

Mingling of different organ tissues (developmental dysplasias)

Accessory spleens

Costal and sternal defects

Hence, the malformed fetuses which come to attention are those whose anomaly was 'less severe' genetically. For example, embryonal trisomy 1 has never been found in a non-mosaic state, presumably because it is highly lethal in very early embryos. Early spontaneous abortion is a very common occurrence in humans, with approximately half of all conceptuses lost (see Ch. 1). A significant proportion of these abortions are secondary to meiotic non-disjunction of the oocyte, which occurs in approximately 20% of all oocytes (range of 1.3–57.7%, in a review of 59 studies).[51]

The risk of live birth and the severity of malformations for numerical chromosomal anomalies is well known, but is much more difficult to predict in cases of interstitial duplications and/or deletions (except for well characterized alterations, such as Cri du chat syndrome, Miller-Dieker syndrome, or Wolf-Hirschhorn syndrome). It depends on the amount of altered genetic material, and of the genes present in these segments. As a general rule, the more is altered, the greater the risk of non-viability, and deletions of chromosomal segments tend to be more lethal than are trisomies of the same segment. For specific cases, the reader is referred to catalogues.[18, 19, 52] The preimplantation embryos of known carriers of balanced translocations and of carriers of diseases amenable to genetic testing can be grown in vitro and screened, so as to implant only normal conceptuses.[53]

Autosomal trisomy is associated with increased maternal age; young mothers and older fathers are at increased risk of conceiving a child with monosomy X. Radiation and other environmental factors such as drugs and viruses can increase the risk of non-disjunction.[54]

Chromosomal abnormalities may be manifestations of underlying **defects of DNA repair,** as seen in **Bloom syndrome, ataxia telangiectasia, xeroderma pigmentosum,** and **Fanconi aplastic anemia.** In these disorders, the chromosomal abnormalities, including breaks, are a result, not a cause, of the condition.

Aneuploidy is usually associated with disturbances of growth manifesting as an intrauterine growth retardation or restriction **(IUGR).** All unbalanced chromosomal abnormalities are associated with multiple congenital anomaly syndromes consisting of various combinations of minor and major anomalies. Most cases

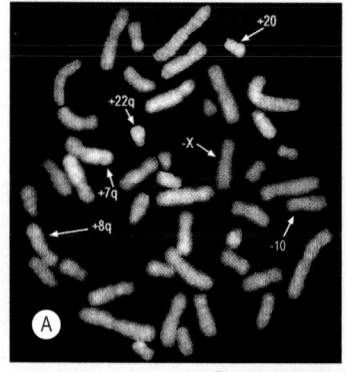

FIGURE 5.10 (A) Metaphase spread labeled with the CGH technique, in a case of medulloblastoma. Arrows show the most important gains and deletions. (B) Ten metaphases were scanned (a total of 20 autosomes, 10 chromosomes X, and 10 chromosomes Y are analyzed); the mean fluorescence ratios are shown as a blue line for each chromosome. Idiograms allow precise determination of chromosomal segments gained (in green, to the right) and lost (in red, to the left). (Courtesy of Sophie Dubé and Dr Nicole Lemieux.)

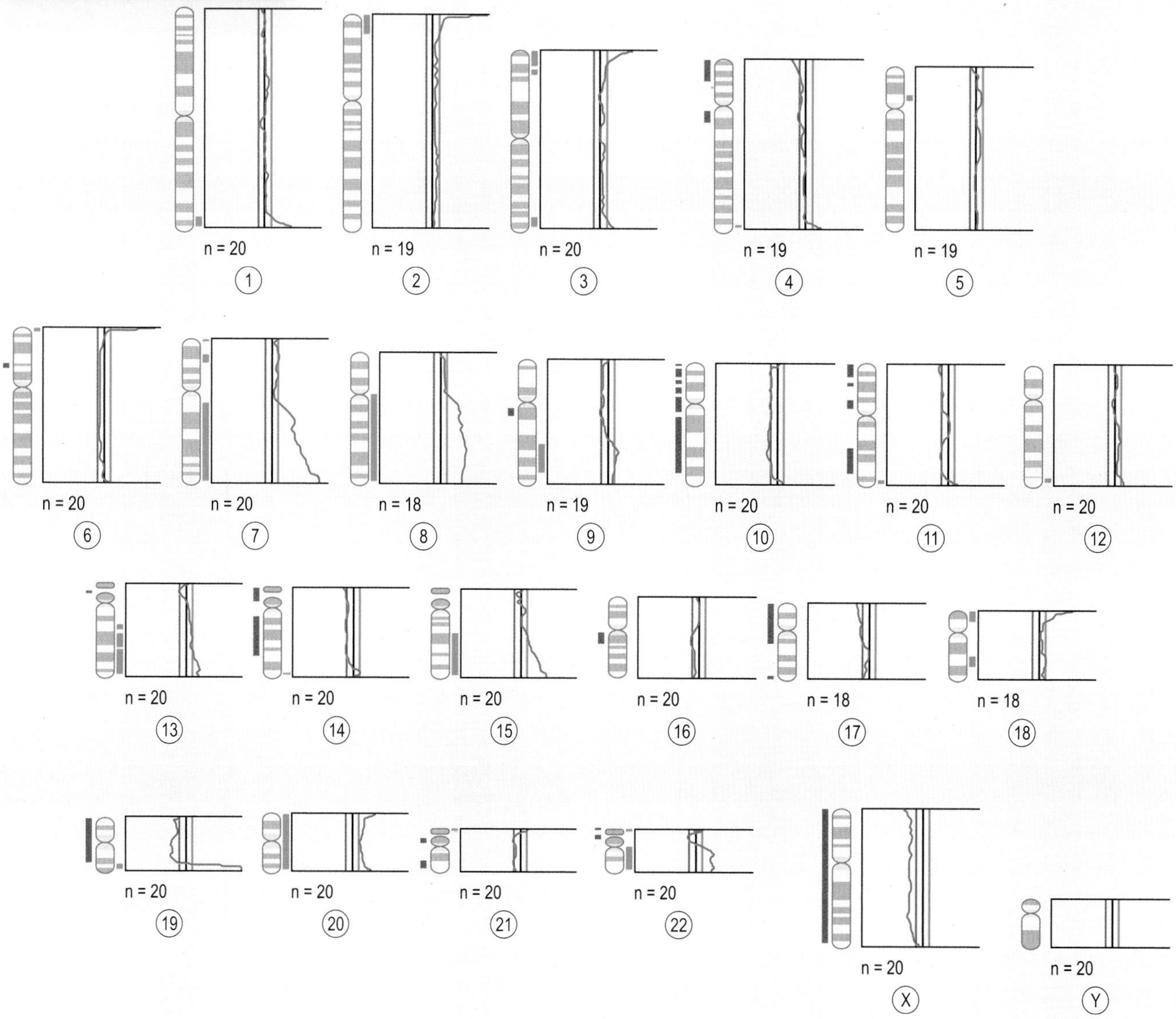

n = 20 (1) n = 19 (2) n = 20 (3) n = 19 (4) n = 19 (5)

n = 20 (6) n = 20 (7) n = 18 (8) n = 19 (9) n = 20 (10) n = 20 (11) n = 20 (12)

n = 20 (13) n = 20 (14) n = 20 (15) n = 20 (16) n = 18 (17) n = 18 (18)

n = 20 (19) n = 20 (20) n = 20 (21) n = 20 (22) n = 20 (X) n = 20 (Y)

of chromosomal imbalance affect central nervous system (CNS) function, manifesting as mental retardation.

All gross aneuploidy has unfavorable developmental effects on gonads. For example, Turner syndrome is associated with gonadal dysgenesis or late fetal ovarian degeneration, and patients with Klinefelter syndrome have congenital micro-orchidism and despite undergoing puberty, remain azoospermic.

Many chromosomal aberration syndromes pose an increased risk of cancer.[55] Some examples are the association of del(13q) with retinoblastoma; del(11p) and trisomy 18 with Wilms tumor;

trisomy 21 with leukemia, retinoblastoma, and probably CNS and testicular tumors; Klinefelter syndrome with breast cancer; and trisomy 13 with retinoblastoma and leukemia.

Structural chromosomal abnormalities

Structural chromosomal abnormalities include reciprocal translocations, inversions, deletions, ring chromosomes, isochromosomes, chromosomal insertions, intrachromosomal duplications, dicentric chromosomes, isochromosome formation, and Robertsonian translocation (Fig. 5.1). The nomenclature used in describing cytogenetic alterations in patients and their tumors has been the subject of an international consensus.[56]

Reciprocal translocations (Fig. 5.1A) occur when there is an exchange of chromosomal material between chromosomes. Translocations can be **balanced or unbalanced.** Balanced translocation represents no loss or gain of genetic material; the individual has a normal chromosomal complement and is usually phenotypically normal. Meiosis in a balanced translocation carrier may produce gametes with a normal chromosomal complement or a complement with the balanced translocation, or may harbor a segmental trisomy (duplication) and/or monosomy (deletion). In unbalanced translocation, there is either some gain and/or loss (duplication or deletion) of chromosomal material. A reciprocal translocation between chromosomes 11 and 22 with breakpoints at 11q23 and 22q11 is common.[57] Rarely breaks occur between genes, preventing transcription. This may occur in Duchenne muscular dystrophy associated with reciprocal translocation between X chromosomes and autosomes.[58]

Inversions involve two breaks within a single chromosome with an inversion of the intervening segment. The inversions can be pericentric when the breaks occur on both sides of the centromere (Fig. 5.1B), or paracentric when both breaks occur in either the long or short arm of the chromosome (Fig. 5.1C). During meiosis, the pairing of one normal chromosome with its inverted homologue can produce terminal deletions and/or duplications, resulting in the production of very abnormal chromosomes when cross-overs occur within the abnormal segment.[17]

Deletions can either be the result of two internal breaks on the chromosome (leading to an **interstitial deletion,** Fig. 5.1D), or of a distal break (leading to a **terminal deletion,** Fig. 5.1E). Deletions result in lost portions of chromosomal material.

Ring chromosomes are formed when breaks occurring on the short and long arms of a chromosome fuse (Fig. 5.1F). Ring chromosomes are unstable during meiosis.

Isochromosomes are mirror image chromosomes that result from single breaks close to the centromere, eliminating the whole of a long or short arm, followed by the duplication of the remaining arm (Fig. 5.1G).

Chromosomal insertions are characterized by a segment of a chromosome inserted into another part of the chromosome or into a different chromosome.

Intrachromosomal duplications occur when a segment of chromosome is duplicated and inserted next to the normal segment. They result in a segmental trisomy.

Dicentric chromosomes are chromosomes with two contiguous centromeres. They result from unbalanced translocations involving one chromosomal pair [e.g. i(15p) which often have two centromeres, with a minuscule segment of the long arm between them] or different chromosomes [e.g. der(14;21) which can have a very small segment of the short arm of either chromosome 14 or 21 between the two centromeres].

In **Robertsonian translocations** (Fig. 5.1H), the short arms of two acrocentric chromosomes (comprising chromosomes 13, 14, 15, 21, and 22) are lost and a dicentric fused chromosome is formed, containing the long arms of the involved chromosomes.[59]

For a more detailed description of structural chromosomal abnormalities, the reader is referred to the Schinzel catalogue of unbalanced chromosome aberrations in man.[17] The clinical implications of chromosomal anomalies are reviewed by McKinlay et al.[18]

Chromosomal mosaicism

When a chromosomal abnormality arises after zygote formation, the conceptus may be comprised of two or more cell lines. The resultant mosaic pattern may be generalized in the conceptus and placenta or confined within the placenta or fetus (Fig. 5.11 A, B and C respectively).

Generalized chromosomal mosaicism is the result of a very early mutational event, and all tissues of the conceptus and placenta are affected. It may occur in liveborn autosomal trisomies, sex chromosome aneuploidy, polyploidy and other chromosomal rearrangements such as ring chromosomes and dicentric chromosomes. The phenotype depends on the percentage of the abnormal cell line and its tissue distribution.

Confined placental mosaicism (CPM) (Fig. 5.11B) results from mutations occurring in the trophoblast or extraembryonic progenitor cells of the inner cell mass. It is found in 1–2% of pregnancies in which chorionic villus sampling has been performed at 9–12 weeks' gestation.[60] Although some pregnancies with CPM progress uneventfully to term, CPM may be associated with intrauterine fetal death and intrauterine growth retardation and prenatal mortality. It appears that mosaic aneuploidy interferes with normal placental function and the survival of a chromosomally normal fetus.[60] Three types of CPM have been defined by Tyson and Kalousek and are listed below.[61]

- **Type 1: abnormal cell line in cytotrophoblast** associated with chromosomally normal placental stroma; the most common type.
- **Type 2: abnormal cell line in placental stroma** associated with diploidy in cytotrophoblast and embryo/fetus.
- **Type 3: diploidy in fetus** associated with mosaic or non-mosaic cell line in placental stroma and cytotrophoblast.

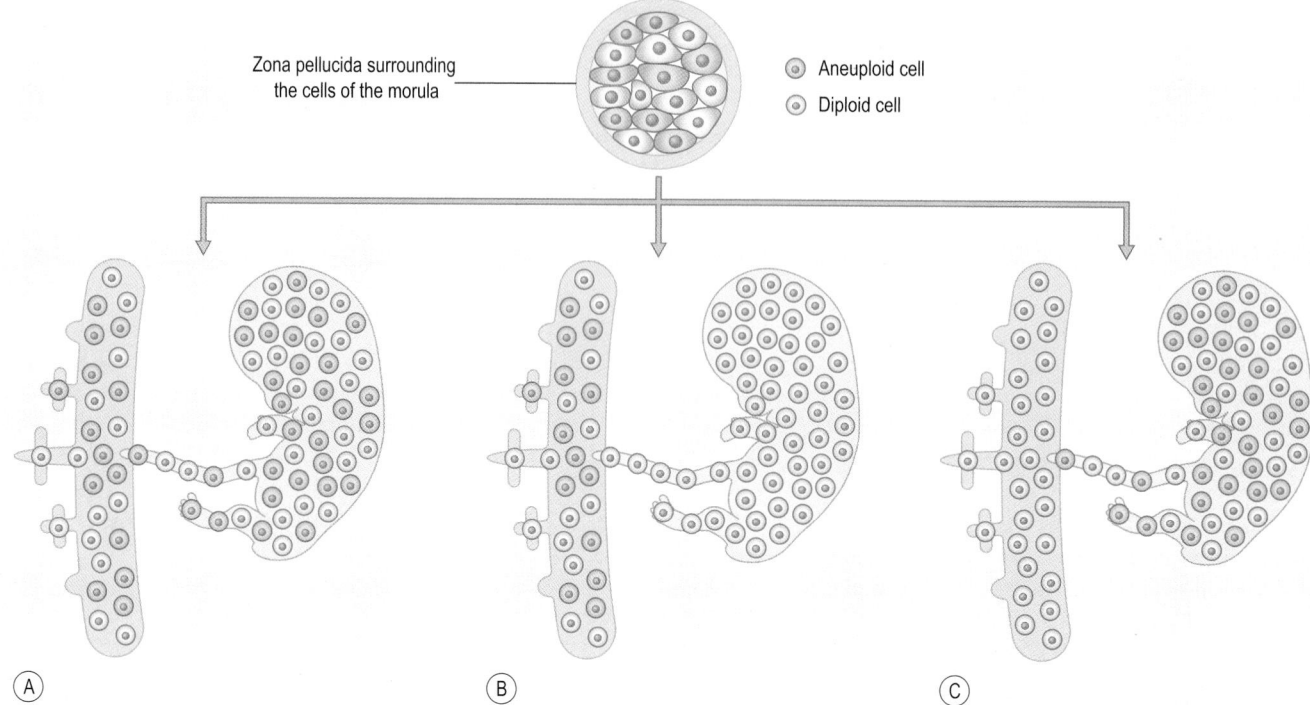

FIGURE 5.11 Diagrammatic representation of chromosomal mosaicisms. (A) Generalized chromosomal mosaicism occurring as a result of a very early mutational event. (B) Mosaic placenta, with normal embryo (confined placental mosaicism), resulting from unequal distribution of embryonic and progenitor cells during compaction and inner cell mass formation during the early blastocyst stage. (C) Confined fetal chromosomal mosaicism caused by mutation in early embryonic progenitors. (After Dimmick and Kalousek 1992,[281] with permission.)

Abnormalities of chromosome 21

Trisomy 21: Down syndrome

Approximately 95% of all cases of Down syndrome (**DS**) represent trisomy 21 due to **non-disjunction;** almost 4% have a **translocation,** and half of these have a balanced translocation carrier parent. The most frequent translocation is a Robertsonian t(14;21)(q10;q10). More than 50% of the t(14;21) and 90% of the t(21;21) occur de novo, with both parents having normal karyotypes. The remaining cases with t(14;21) and t(21;21) have a parent with the same translocation in a balanced form, warranting a cytogenetic screen in these families. The risk of DS to offspring of t(14;21) translocation in the mother is 11% and 2.4% in the father. In the very rare instances of parental balanced t(21q;21q), the risk to offspring is essentially 100%.[62] Most of the phenotypic manifestations of DS result from the additional genetic material contained in band 21q22.

Mosaicism for the extra chromosome 21 is found in 1% of patients with DS. In such cases, as in all patients with a chromosomal mosaicism, the severity of the phenotype depends on the percentage of trisomic cells in the various tissues during development (e.g. brain, heart, marrow). Hence, the phenotype cannot be predicted by a determination of the proportion of abnormal cells in blood or amniotic fluid. In such cases, genetic counseling is very difficult.

Risk for offspring with DS increases exponentially with increasing maternal age. In mothers 15–19 years of age, it is 1/2500, and rises to 1/25 in mothers older than 40 years of age (Table 5.2).[63] However, due to extensive screening of **mothers of advanced age,** 75% of babies with DS are currently born to women under 35. There is also an increased risk with maternal age under

TABLE 5.2 DOWN SYNDROME AND MATERNAL AGE

Age of mother (Year)	Risk of Down syndrome
20	1/1000
25	1/1524
30	1/1163
32	1/610
35	1/324
38	1/322
40	1/95
43	1/64
45	1/30

From Trimble and Baird 1978,[62] with permission.

TABLE 5.3 CLINICAL FEATURES OF TRISOMY 21 IN THE NEWBORN

Sign	Frequency of occurrence in Down syndrome (%)
Flat face (hypoplastic maxilla)	90
Slanting palpebral fissures	80
Abundant nuchal skin	80
Hyperextensibility of joints	80
Muscular hypotonia	80
Absent Moro reflex	80
Dysplastic pelvis	70
Dysplastic ears	60
Dysplastic middle phalanx of fifth finger	60
Single palmar crease (of at least one hand)	50

After Hall 1966,[71] with permission.

17 years, and a slightly increased risk with a paternal age greater than 55 years.[64–66] The chromosomal aberration corresponding to trisomy 21 is also found in non-human primates, including the chimpanzee, gorilla, and orangutan.[67–69]

For mothers of a child with trisomy 21, the risk of having a subsequent child with a chromosome variation has been empirically determined to be approximately 1%. For parents of a child with translocation, the recurrence risk varies depending on the type of translocation. In cases of translocations between chromosome 21 and other acrocentric chromosomes, the risk of recurrence is about 16% if the mother is a carrier and about 5% if the father is a carrier.[70] Although fertility is rare in males with DS, pregnancy among women with DS is possible, and there is a 50% chance of DS occurring in the infant.[71]

IUGR is a consistent finding in infants with DS. They are hypotonic with hyperextensibility of joints and have diminished sucking and swallowing reflexes. Certain cardinal signs of trisomy 21 are present in the newborn (Table 5.3).[72] The phenotype of DS is generally easily recognized at birth (Fig. 5.12). Clinodactyly of the fifth finger is present in 83% of cases, and after the 16th week of gestation, an absent or hypoplastic phalanx of the fifth finger is observed in 78%. The **dermatoglyphic patterns** include an increased number of ulnar loops, third interdigital distal loops, radial loops on digits 4 and 5, a decreased number of whorls and arches, a single palmar transverse crease or an extended proximal transverse crease (Sydney line), and a distal axial triradius (Fig. 5.12).[73–76]

The most consistent manifestation of DS is **mental retardation,** with an IQ score usually in the range of 35 to 55.[15] The common anomalies, in descending order of frequency, are **cardiovascular malformations, duodenal obstruction, talipes equinovarus, cataract, imperforate anus, cleft lip or palate, congenital megacolon (Hirschsprung disease), and meningomyelocele.**[21] The incidence of congenital cardiovascular malformations is about 70% (atrioventricular canal, atrial or ventricular septal defects, tetralogy of Fallot, persistent left vena cava, retroesophageal right subclavian artery, aortic coarctation, and pulmonary stenosis);

trisomy 21 accounts for more than 5% of all cases of congenital malformations of the heart.[77] Pulmonary hypertension and pulmonary vascular sclerosis occur more often in DS than in the general population.[78] **Polyarteritis nodosa** involving the coronary vessels in DS has been recognized.[21] Calcified and cystically dilated Hassall corpuscles are fairly consistent findings (Fig. 5.13).

Renal anomalies, although uncommon, may be present. **Hematologic abnormalities** are common. DS increases the risk of **leukemia** 10–20 fold in early childhood, and decreases with age; 1% of patients with DS develop leukemia.[79–81] In DS, the three most frequent types of leukemia are:

- ALL with blasts that are TdT-positive B-cell precursors;
- cytochemically positive AML with blasts positive for myeloperoxidase (MPO)[82]; and
- the largest group, AML, negative for MPO with marked leukocytosis and atypical megakaryocytes and blasts in the bone marrow – this type has been classified as megakaryoblastic leukemia (AML-M7).[83]

The latter may undergo spontaneous remission. The regressing condition is then termed **transient myeloproliferative disorder (TMD)** of DS, and occurs in 10% of DS.[80, 84] This is generally seen in newborns and infants under 6 months of age, and regresses within 4–7 weeks, but re-emerges as an irreversible acute megakaryoblastic leukemia in up to 33% of these patients.[80, 85] Hepatic fibrosis may accompany TMD.[86]

DS with TMD and with AML-M7 characteristically have a mutation of the GATA1 gene (located on Xp11.23), an essential transcriptional regulator of normal megakaryocyte differentiation.[80] DS is associated with an increased risk of retinoblastoma, germ cell tumors, and perhaps lymphoma, but with a lower risk of chronic myeloid leukemia, chronic lymphocytic leukemia, and solid tumors.[81, 87] Breast cancer is exceptional, and the risk of development of a second malignancy after treatment for leukemia is decreased.[81] It is postulated that the increased susceptibility to apoptosis in DS may result in cell death rather than malignant transformation.[81]

The morphology of the brain varies. The weight of the brain in DS is usually less than normal; the brain is delayed in maturity for gestational age, and the convolutions are small. Myelination is retarded, the cerebral convolutions are flat, and the frontal and temporal poles are compressed. The gyri, particularly of the frontal poles, are flattened. A **brachycephalic brain** with an **open operculum** and hypoplastic superior temporal gyrus are characteristic features (Fig. 5.14A). A short corpus callosum, hypoplasia of the brainstem and medulla, and hypoplasia of the cerebellar hemispheres are frequently reported. The cerebellum shows the frequent presence of **tuber flocculus** (Fig. 5.14B), which consists of undifferentiated piles of cells found in the earliest differentiation of the cerebellum at about 5 weeks' gestation, and persisting in more than 60% of the brains of patients with DS. Tuber flocculus is rarely seen in other developmental disorders of the brain.

Spinal cord changes include enlargement of the central canal with irregular ependymal proliferation, hypoplasia of the gray matter, and lack of separation of Clarke columns.[88] Atlantooccipital or atlantoaxial instability is common in DS and may potentiate spinal cord injury as well as being implicated in sudden infant death.

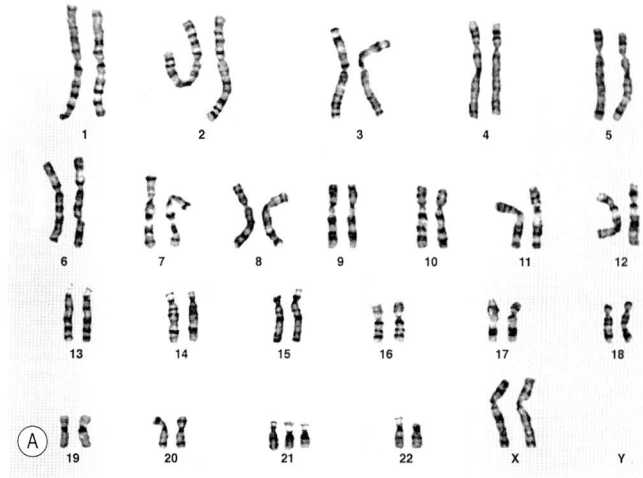

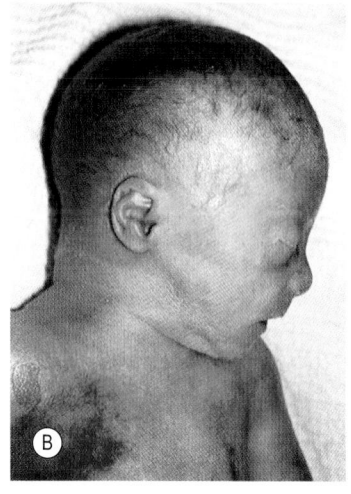

FIGURE 5.12 Characteristic features of trisomy 21. (A) Karyotype of trisomy 21, 47,XX,+21. (B) Fetus of trisomy 21 at 22 weeks' gestation with typical facial features. (C) Dermatoglyphics of Down syndrome compared with the normal. [(A) Courtesy Dr Nicole Lemieux. (B) From Gilbert and Opitz 1982,[21] with permission. (C) From Jones 1988,[75] with permission.]

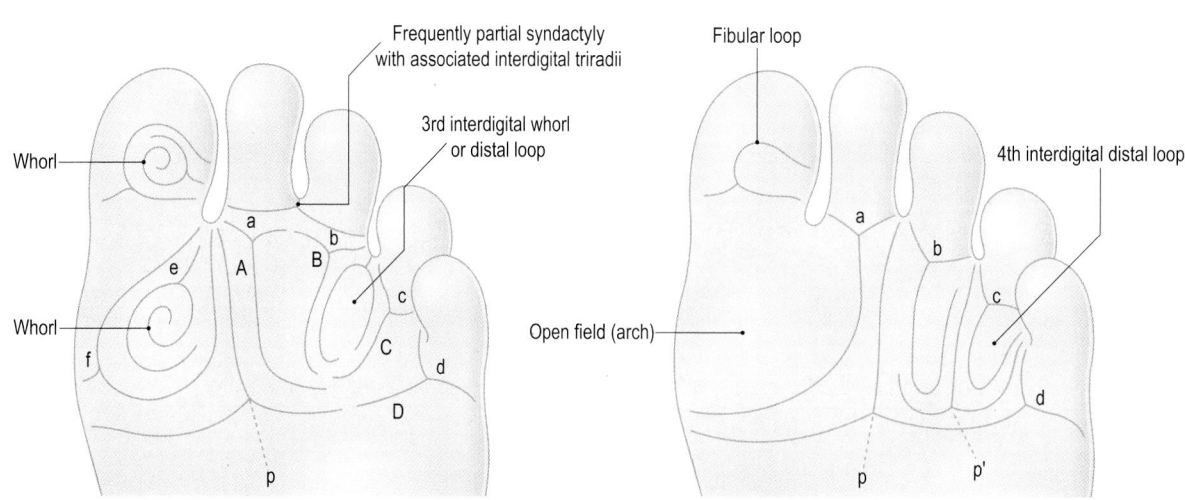

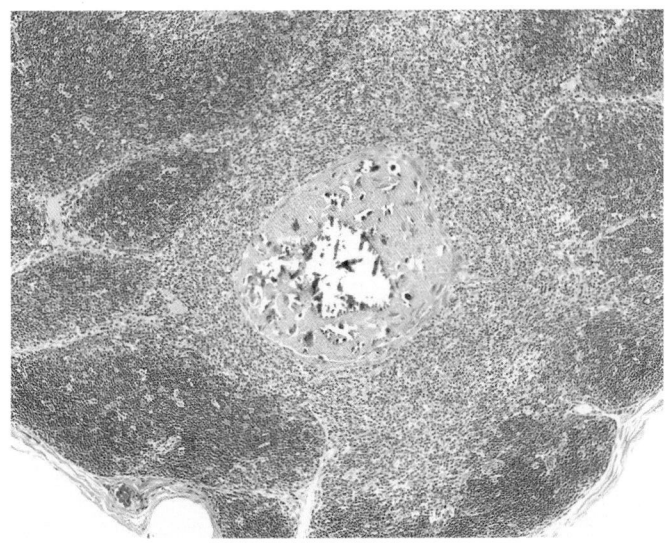

FIGURE 5.13 Microscopic section of the thymus in a patient with Down syndrome. Hassall corpuscles are large, cystic, and calcified. (HPS; original magnification × 100.)

The architecture of the cortex of the cerebrum and cerebellum is irregular, with alternating zones of dense and scanty neurons. Colon found a paucity of neuronal elements, although the existing neurons had increased nucleoplasm.[89]

Alzheimer disease and chromosome 21

Typical Alzheimer changes with senile plaques and neurofibrillary tangles can be found in the brain of adolescents and young adults with trisomy 21 (Fig. 5.14C). Granulovacuolar degeneration of neurons may occur by 30 years of age, and by 50 years of age, more than half of DS patients develop Alzheimer disease.[90] Up to 84% of demented DS patients develop seizures, while early-onset epilepsy is associated with an absence of dementia.[90] Factors which influence β-amyloid levels, rather than overexpression of amyloid precursor protein, may account for differences in age at onset of dementia in DS.[91]

The gene for the **amyloid β-protein** is found on chromosome 21. The accumulation of amyloid in Alzheimer disease is sometimes caused by the overexpression of a mutant β-*protein* gene that resides on chromosome 21 and that mimics the gene-dosage effect of DS. Some families in which Alzheimer disease is inherited as an autosomal dominant mutation produce a significantly higher-than-normal number of DS children.[92–94]

Other systems

Other abnormalities, including endocrine, immunologic and reproductive organ disorders as well as morphologic changes in the CNS, spinal cord, and liver, are listed in Box 5.3.

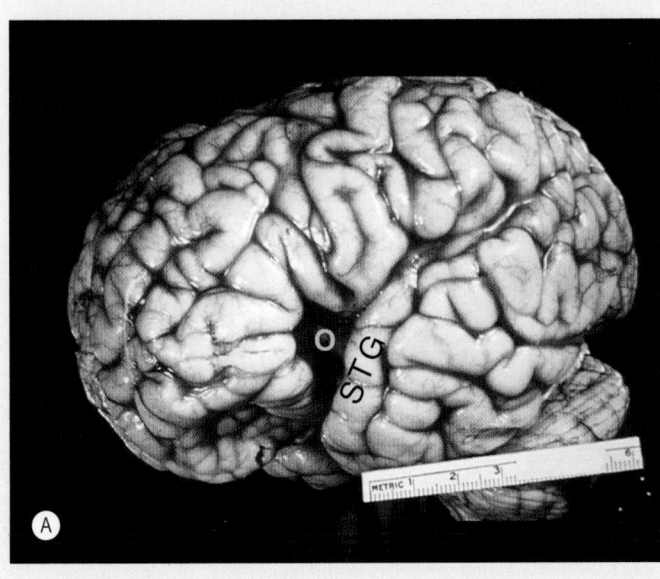

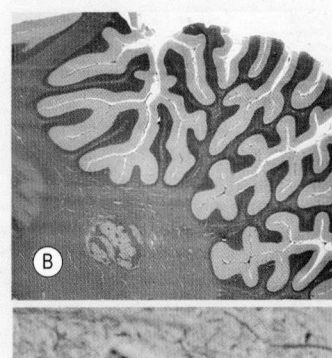

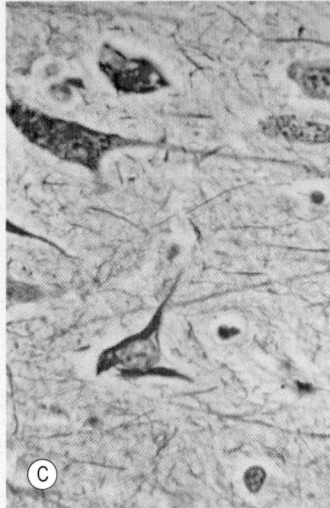

FIGURE 5.14 (A) Brain in Down syndrome (DS). There is a short anteroposterior diameter, an open operculum (O), and a hypoplastic superior temporal gyrus (STG). (B) Brain in DS showing a tuber flocculus within the cerebellum (× 10). (C) Microscopic section of the brain in trisomy 21 showing neurofibrillary tangles as seen in an Alzheimer brain. (H&E × 100) (From Gilbert and Opitz 1982,[21] with permission.)

BOX 5.3 SYSTEM ABNORMALITIES IN TRISOMY 21

General disturbances of growth and development
Intrauterine growth retardation
Diminished sucking and swallowing reflexes
Mental retardation
Dermatoglyphics (Fig. 5.12C)
Palmar
Ulnar loops increased
Third interdigital distal loops
Radial loops on digits 4 and 5
Decreased numbers of whorls and arches
Single palmar crease
Extended proximal transverse crease (Sydney line)
Distal axial triradius
Plantar
Fibular loops
Fourth interdigital distal loop
Subhalucal open field

Cardiac defects
Endocardial cushion defects
Tetralogy of Fallot
Ventricular septal defect
Double-outlet right ventricle
Pulmonary hypertension
Pulmonary vascular sclerosis

Hepatic defects
Liver enlargement
Moderate to severe steatosis

Gastrointestinal
Esophageal atresia 1%
Duodenal atresia 30%
Annular pancreas
Congenital intestinal agangliosis (Hirschsprung disease) 2%
Anorectal malformations 2%
Diastases recti
Umbilical hernia

Renal
Stricture at ureteropelvic junction
Hydronephrosis
Focal cystic malformation
Collecting tubules
Immature glomeruli
Renal cystic dysplasia
Nephrogenic rests
Kidneys small
Hemangiomas of kidney

Endocrine
Hypothyroidism
Precocious puberty
Diabetes mellitus
Hyperthyroidism

Adrenal hyperplasia
Hypogenitalism
Penis and testes small
Cryptorchidism
Macrogenitosomia precox
Testes: interstitial fibrosis, hypoplasia of seminiferous tubules
Ovaries usually small
Hypoplasia with persistence of atretic corpora lutea
Development of axillary and pubic hair, and breasts deficient

Immune system
T-cell immunodeficiency
Thymus usually small
Large Hassall corpuscles
Calcification and cystic changes of Hassall corpuscles
Spleen: lymphocyte depletion
Lymph nodes: depleted T-dependent zones
Hepatitis B surface antigenemia

Hematologic
Polycythemia
Leukemia (1%)
Congenital acute myeloblastic leukemia
Acute lymphoblastic leukemia in childhood
Acute megakaryocytic leukemia
Myeloproliferative disorder (transient early in infancy)

Central nervous system
Brain
Weight usually less than normal
Delayed maturity
Convolutions small
Myelination retarded
Cerebral convolutions: flat frontal and temporal poles compressed
Gyri: frontal poles flattened
Hypoplastic brachycephalic brain
Hypoplasia of superior temporal gyrus
Open operculum
Short corpus callosum
Hypoplasia of brainstem and medulla
Hypoplasia of cerebellar hemispheres
Tuber flocculus

Spinal cord
Enlargement of central canal
Irregular ependymal proliferations
Hypoplasia of gray matter
Lack of separation of Clarke columns
Atlanto-occipital or atlantoaxial instability
Paucity of neuronal elements
Alzheimer changes
Senile plaques
Neurofibrillary tangles
Tuber flocculus

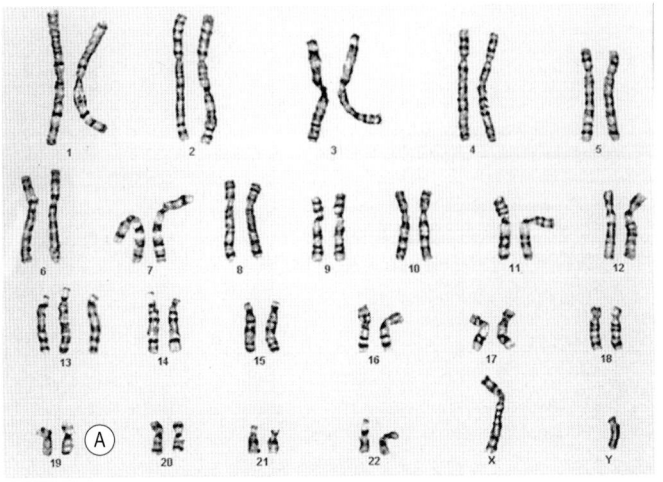

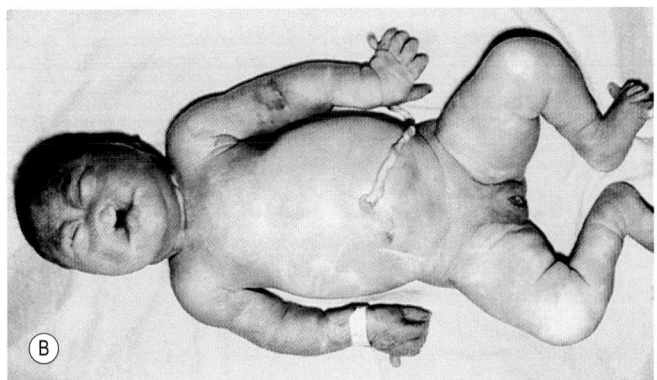

FIGURE 5.15 (A) Karyotype of boy with trisomy 13. (B) Trisomy 13: midline facial defect, hypotelorism, and polydactyly. [(A) Courtesy of Dr Nicole Lemieux. (B) From Gilbert and Opitz 1982,[21] with permission.]

Placenta

Third trimester fetuses with trisomies, particularly 21, 13, and 18, have placentas with high vascular resistance owing to the small size, reduced number, and sclerotic obliteration of arteries in the stem and peripheral villi. In addition, villous maturational arrest with resultant villous immaturity and large atypical Hofbauer or trophoblastic cells is often present in trisomic chromosomal abnormalities and there is a high incidence of single umbilical artery.

Monosomy 21

Monosomy 21 is only very rarely seen in live births and most if not all cases are mosaics. Abnormalities include intrauterine growth retardation, failure to thrive, craniofacial dysmorphism, down-slanting palpebral fissures, micrognathia, low-set large ears, flexion contractures, and neuropathologic and cardiac abnormalities.[95, 96]

Abnormalities of chromosome 13

Trisomy 13

Patau and colleagues first cytogenetically defined trisomy 13,[97] and the clinical phenotype was described by Smith.[98] Trisomy 13 caused by **non-disjunction** is found in most cases. **Translocation** of chromosomes 13 and 14 [46,XX or XY,der(13;14)(q10;q10),+13] is present in approximately 20% of cases. Half of these translocation cases have a carrier parent with a balanced Robertsonian translocation [45,XX or XY, der(13;14)(q10;q10)]. **Trisomy 13 mosaicism** is found in less than 10%.[15] Phenotypic abnormalities that may be found in trisomy 13 are listed in Box 5.4.

Trisomy 13 is estimated to occur in 1 in 5000 live births, and increased risk is associated with **advanced maternal age.**[99] Prenatal wastage is high: 97% of trisomy 13 conceptuses are spontaneously aborted. At least 85% of translocations involve two D chromosomes (chromosomes 13, 14 and 15).

Survival beyond 10 years of age in patients with this disorder is extremely rare. Two cases of patients reaching 11 and 19 years of age are reported.[100, 101] In a large series of 200 liveborn infants with trisomy 13, 28% died within the first week, 44% within the first month, and 73% within the first 4 months of life.[102]

The phenotype of trisomy 13 (Fig. 5.15) is that of a small-for-gestational-age infant with a spectrum of **midline facial defects** that include premaxillary agenesis, cebocephaly, ethmocephaly, and cyclopia (Fig. 5.16). Other classic external phenotypic abnormalities include micrognathia, malformed ears, and polydactyly. About one-third have a **scalp defect** (Fig. 5.17A) in the region of the vertex, and two-thirds have capillary hemangiomas. Omphalocele, large umbilical hernia, retroflexed thumb, hyperconvex nails, and anomalies of the feet (e.g. talipes equinovarus and talipes calcaneovalgus) are frequent. **Rocker-bottom feet** (with prominence of the calcaneus) and abnormal lobation of the lungs, liver, and spleen are common, although with less frequency than in trisomy 18.

Dermatoglyphic patterns include a high incidence of a single palmar crease and distal axial triradius. An S-shaped fibular arch pattern in the hallucal areas of the soles is a valuable diagnostic sign of trisomy 13.[21]

The persistence of **atavistic muscle groups** has been observed.[103] The six most frequent and consistent muscle variations are absence of the palmaris longus, peroneus tertius, palmaris brevis, plantaris, pectorodorsalis, and extensor indicis muscles.

Congenital **cardiovascular malformations** are found in 80% of cases.[102] Respiratory tract defects include abnormal lobation of the lungs, tracheoesophageal fistula, and bifid uvula. Abdominal malformations include, in addition to omphalocele, malrotation of the gut, and (less often) Meckel diverticulum, heterotopias of

BOX 5.4 ABNORMALITIES OBSERVED IN TRISOMY 13

External malformations
Intrauterine growth retardation
Microcephaly
Receding forehead
Epicanthal folds
Deep-set eyes
Absent philtrum
Sparse, curled eyelashes
Midline scalp defect at vertex of head
Horizontal palpebral fissures
Proboscis
Broad, flat nose
Low-set, flat, poorly defined ears
Midline facial defect, cleft lip palate
Dysmorphic ears
Preauricular tag
Incisor teeth present at birth
Cranial line defect
Hypotelorism
Micrognathia
Prominent calcaneus
Rocker-bottom feet
Talipes equinovarus
Talipes calcaneovalgus
Flexion contracture
Hexadactyly of hands and feet
Flexed fingers, retroflexed thumbs
Clinodactyly of little fingers
Camptodactyly
Abnormal flexion creases
Cleft hands with four digits
Narrow, hyperconvex nails 'hammer' toes
Hemangiomas on face, forehead, nape of neck
Hypoplastic or absent 12th ribs
Hypoplastic pelvis with flattened acetabular angle
Kyphoscoliosis

Placenta
Single umbilical artery
Polyhydramnios
Oligohydramnios

Cardiovascular malformations
Ventricular septal defects
Patent ductus arteriosus
Atrial septal defect
Dextrocardia/dextroposition
Patent foramen ovale
Pulmonic valvular stenosis
Pulmonic valvular atresia
Bicuspid aortic valve
Transposition of great vessels
Truncus arteriosus
Double-outlet right ventricle

Aortic coarctation
Left superior vena cava
Polyvalvular dysplasia

Hematologic abnormalities
Multiple projections in neutrophil nuclei
Increased fetal and Gower-2 hemoglobin
Extramedullary hematopoiesis

Dermatoglyphics
Distal axial triradius
Single palmar crease
Arch fibular or arch fibular S pattern

Visceral malformations
Abnormal lobation of lungs
Pulmonary hypoplasia
Abnormal lobation of liver
Malrotation of intestines
Elongated, hypoplastic, or malrotated or hydropic gallbladder
Cholestasis
Focal hepatic calcification
Ectopic pancreas in spleen
Abnormally large fetal cortex of adrenals
Omphalocele
Gastroschisis
Accessory spleens
Ectopic spleen
Meckel diverticulum
Absent mesentery
Inguinal and/or umbilical hernia
Adrenal hypoplasia
Ectopic adrenal tissue

Genitourinary malformations
Micromulticystic kidneys
Double kidney
Double ureter
Hydronephrosis and hydroureter
Renal dysplasia
Horseshoe kidney
Renal hypoplasia
Males
Cryptorchidism
Anomalies of scrotum
Small micropenis
Hyperplasia of Leydig cells
Agenesis of testes
Hypospadias
Females
Bicornuate uterus
Hypertrophy of clitoris
Double separate vagina
Uterus didelphys

BOX 5.4 ABNORMALITIES OBSERVED IN TRISOMY 13 (*cont'd*)

Ocular malformations

Microphthalmia, anophthalmia
Cataracts
Corneal opacities
Retinoschisis
Hypoplasia of optic nerve
Coloboma of iris or retina
Aniridia
Retinal dysplasia
Retinoblastoma
Abnormal central gyration

Central nervous system malformations

Arrhinencephaly-holoprosencephaly
Cerebellar anomalies
Corpus callosum defects
Heterotopias
Arnold-Chiari malformation
Vascular malformations
Anencephaly
Migration defects
Dandy-Walker malformation

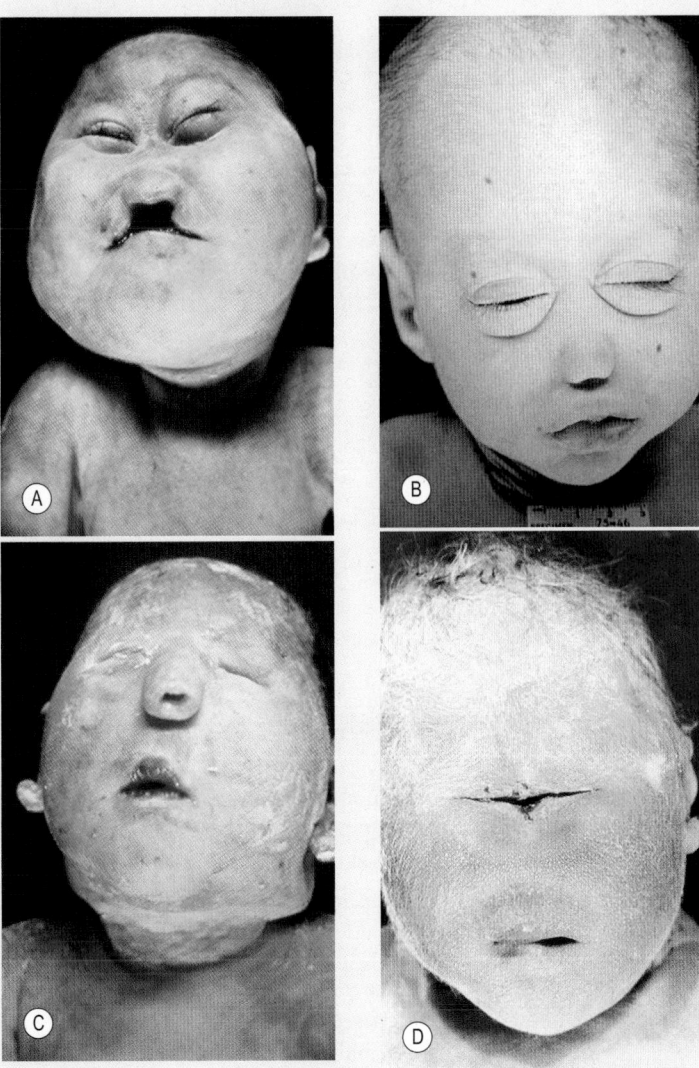

FIGURE 5.16 Midline facial defects in trisomy 13. (A) Bilateral cleft lip, premaxillary aplasia, and hypotelorism. (B) Cebocephaly. (C) Ethmocephaly. (D) Cyclopia. (From Gilbert and Opitz 1982,[21] with permission.)

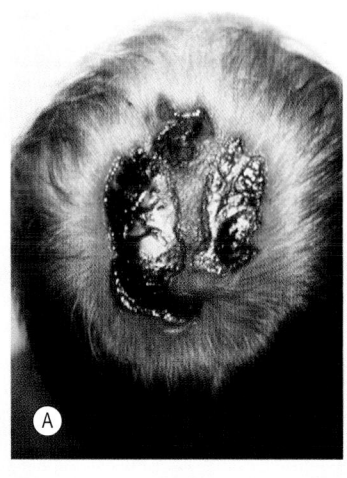

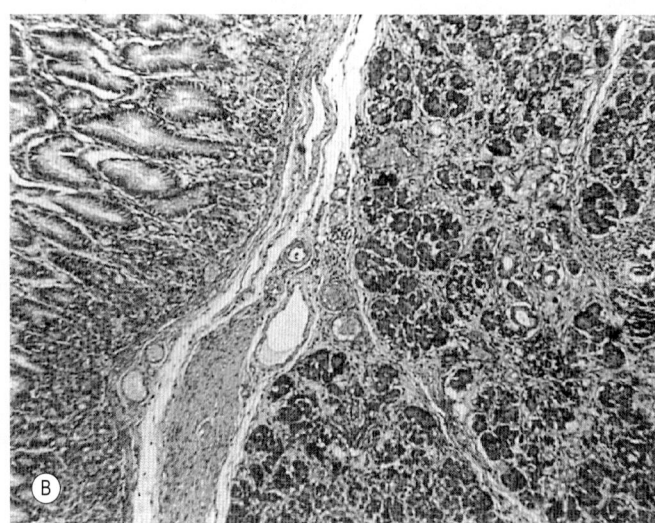

FIGURE 5.17 (A) Trisomy 13: midline defect over the vertex of the scalp. (B) Heterotopic pancreas in the wall of the duodenum. (From Gilbert and Opitz 1982,[21] with permission.)

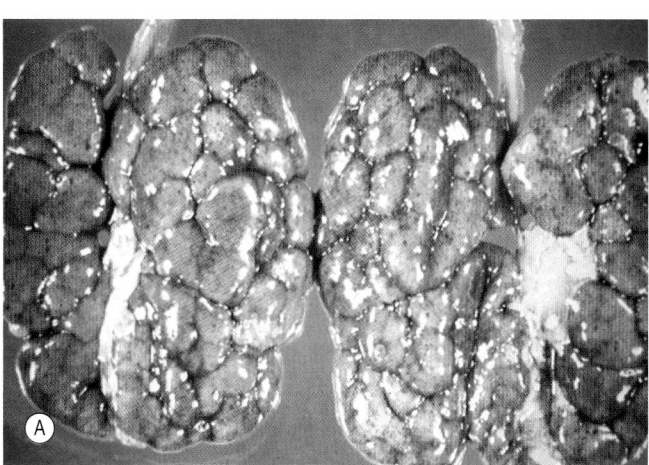

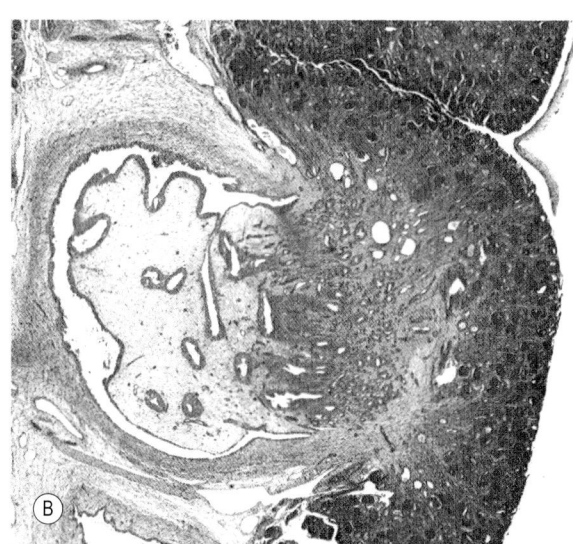

FIGURE 5.18 Trisomy 13. (A) Kidney with excessive fetal lobulation and multiple cortical cysts. (B) Micromulticystic kidney. (HPS × 25) (5.18A from Gilbert and Opitz 1982,[21] with permission.)

the pancreas (Fig. 5.17B), and accessory spleens. The appendix may show multiple diverticula along the serosal surface, commonly referred to as a dinosaur tail. The adrenal glands may be enlarged, and the association of adrenocortical carcinoma and neuroblastoma has been described.[104, 105]

Genital abnormalities in the female include bicornuate uterus (in 80% of cases) and biseptate uterus or uterus duplex; the fallopian tubes may insert abnormally. Anomalies of the external genitalia, such as clitoral hypertrophy and duplication of the labia, are rare; ovaries may be absent, normal, hypoplastic, or enlarged.[104, 106] In the male, cryptorchidism and hypoplasia of the external genitalia are common.

Urologic abnormalities include lobulated kidneys (Fig. 5.18A) and micromulticystic kidneys, a very frequent finding (Fig.

5.18B), as well as hydroureter, duplication of kidneys and ureters, dysplastic kidneys, unilateral renal agenesis, and nephrogenic rests.[107–110] Kidneys tend to be heavier than normal. Horseshoe kidneys are less common than in trisomy 18 and Turner syndrome. Megacystis and persistent urachus are infrequent.

Cryptorchidism is an almost constant finding. The penis and scrotum are small, hypospadias is sometimes present, and scrotal skin may extend to the penis. Urogenital anomalies are much more frequent in trisomy 13 than in other chromosomal defects, suggesting that the extra 13 chromosome affects fusion at the caudal end of the Müllerian duct.

Hematologic abnormalities include a decreased rate of replacement of fetal hemoglobin with adult hemoglobin, neutrophilic nuclear projections, and persistence of hemoglobin Gower

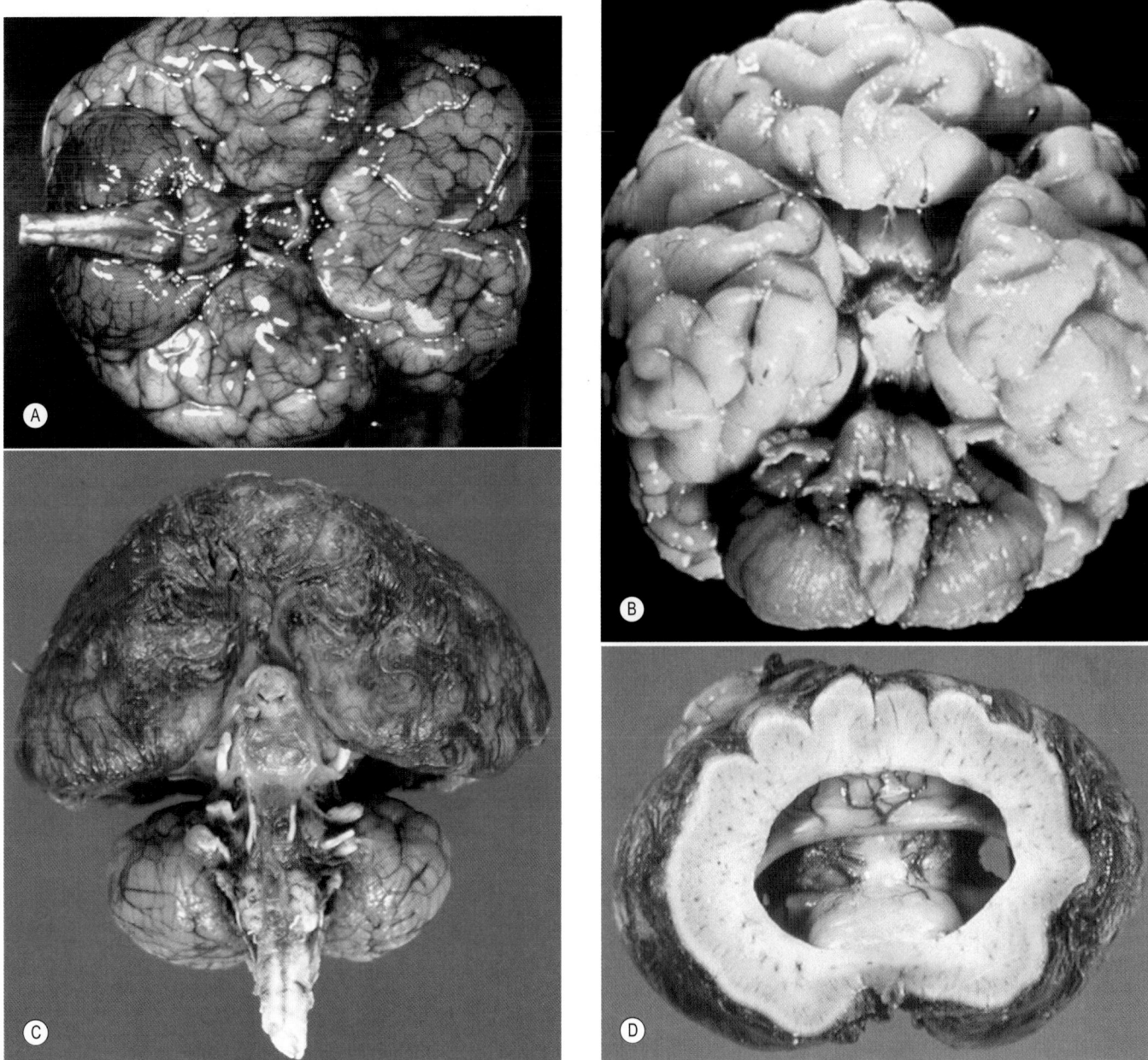

FIGURE 5.19 Brain in trisomy 13. (A) Arrhinencephaly: absence of olfactory bulbs and tracts. (B) Lobar holoprosencephaly. (C) Alobar holoprosencephaly. (D) Coronal section of (C): single central ventricle with absent corpus callosum. (From Gilbert and Opitz 1982,[21] with permission.)

2 throughout the gestational period and into the early neonatal period.[111–113] Acute myeloblastic leukemia has been reported in trisomy 13.[114, 115]

CNS abnormalities in trisomy 13 encompass the spectrum of arrhinencephaly–holoprosencephaly (Fig. 5.19).[116, 117] DeMyer and colleagues correlated the severity of the facial defects to the degree of malformation of the brain, albeit not in all cases.[118] Mesoderm normally migrates anterior to the notochord and is responsible for the induction of differentiation of the forebrain and midline facial structures. Failure of this migration produces a defect encompassing this developmental field. The holopros-

encephaly complex is genetically heterogeneous and includes cyclopia, ethmocephaly, cebocephaly medial clefts, and normocephaly (Box 5.5).

Arnold-Chiari and Dandy-Walker malformations and myelomeningocele may coexist. The optic chiasm and optic nerves are usually hypoplastic, and are typically associated with hypertelorism. **Heterotopias** occur frequently within the cortex and especially in the dentate nucleus of the cerebellum. Herniation of the cochlear nuclei into the eighth cranial nerve (Fig. 5.20), the presence of gray matter in the 11th cranial nerve, arteriovenous malformations of leptomeningeal and intracerebral vessels,

Genetics (eight genes involved: SHH, PTCH, TGIF, TDGF1, ZIC2, SIX3, GLI2, FAST1)[116, 117]

1. Sporadic

2. Autosomal recessive

3. Autosomal dominant

4. Component part of malformation complex (aneuploidy in 40% of cases, half with trisomy 13)

Cyclopia

Single or partially divided eye in single midline orbit

Absence of nose or supraorbital proboscis

Fusion of anterior lobes of brain

Ethmocephaly

Severe hypotelorism with two separate orbits; synophthalmia possible

May have absence of nose or an infraorbital proboscis, fusion of forebrain

Cebocephaly

Hypotelorism with separate orbits

Proboscis-like nose

Fusion of forebrain

Median cleft lip (absence of primary palate)

Hypotelorism with separate orbits

Hypoplastic nose

Absence of median portion of upper lip

Lobar or semilobar holoprosencephaly

Others

Mild dysmorphic changes

Single central maxillary incisor

Normocephaly

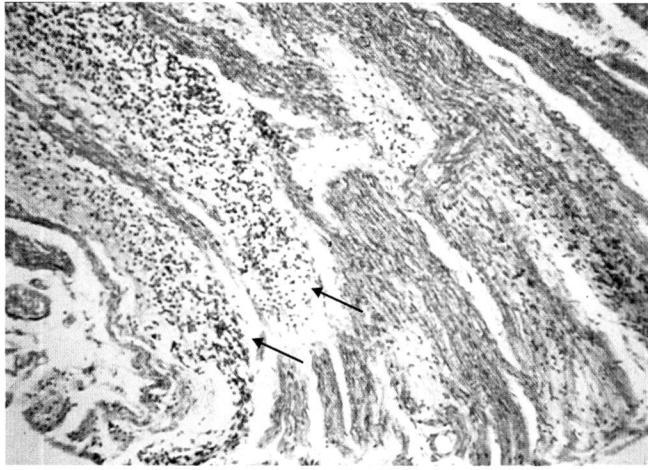

FIGURE 5.20 Trisomy 13. Microscopic section of brain showing heterotopic glial cells in the eighth cranial nerve (arrows). (Kluver stain × 100)

arachnoid cyst of the cauda equina, and retinal pigment epithelium within the optic nerve have been observed.[7] Heterotopic neuroblasts may exist within the external granular layer of the cerebellum. The corticospinal tracts of the spinal cord may lack myelination.

As a result of defective formation of the ocular vesicle, **ocular malformations** may occur, including colobomas, anophthalmia, microphthalmia, and cyclopia.[107, 119] Dysplastic changes of the cornea, iris, and anterior chamber can lead to corneal opacity, hypoplasia of iris stroma, and immature chamber angle. Retinoblastoma,[120] partial absence of Descemet membrane and corneal epithelium, may occur. **Retinal dysplasia** is a constant feature.

Other abnormalities of chromosome 13

The effects of duplications of specific segments of chromosome 13 are shown in Fig. 5.21. With banding techniques, duplications are categorized into two groups: those trisomic for the proximal one-third to one-half and those trisomic for the distal two-thirds to one-half of the long arm of chromosome 13.[121] Excess of the distal or of the proximal segment is associated with specific malformations.[122–124]

Duplication of the proximal segment of the long arm of chromosome 13 is associated with non-specific clinical features such as psychomotor retardation, microcephaly, low-set ears, microstomia, micrognathia, distal triradius, and incurved fifth fingers. A few patients also exhibit microphthalmia, hemangioma, cleft palate, and epicanthal folds.

Duplication of the distal two-thirds to one-half of the long arm of chromosome 13 is associated with features not very different from those of the complete trisomy 13 syndrome, although deafness, eye malformations, cleft palate, cleft lip, and cardiac defects are observed less frequently. However, duplication of the distal one-third to one-half of the long arm of chromosome 13 seems to be critical for polydactyly, hemangioma, frontal bossing, and narrow temples.[122] Midbrain defects with receding forehead, cleft lip, eye malformations, and an increased number of nuclear projections of neutrophils probably depend on trisomy of most of the long arm. Fetal hemoglobin concentration was normal in patients with trisomy for the distal one-third of the long arm. Two patients trisomic for the distal portion had a hallucal fibular arch. Simple arches on all 10 fingers, a finding more characteristic of trisomy 18, may be observed.[121]

Mosaicism and chromosome 13 deletion syndromes

Approximately 60% of chromosome 13 deletions are associated with a ring chromosome formation. About 25% of patients with a del(13q) chromosome constitution have a terminal or interstitial deletion. A prosencephalic brain defect may be observed in del(13q). Ventricular and atrial septal defects, aplasia of the gallbladder, and hypoplastic kidneys occur frequently. Unilateral

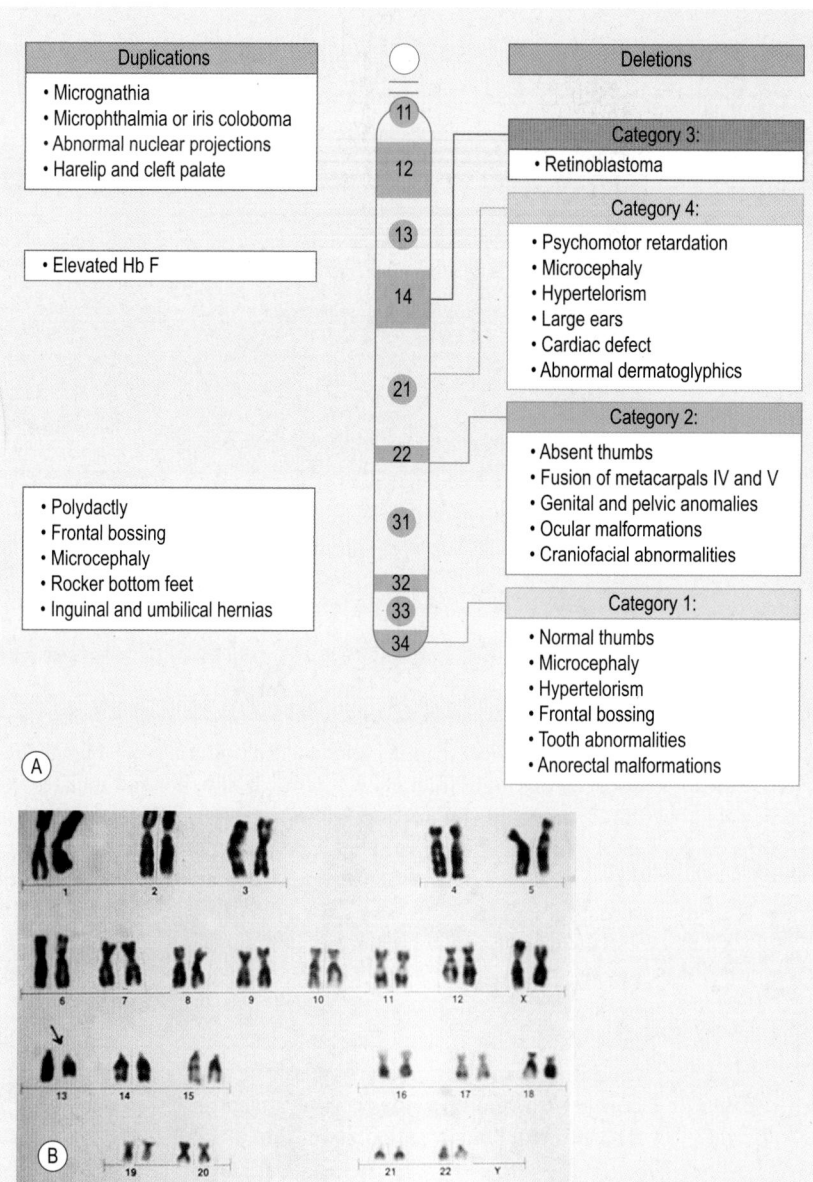

Duplications
- Micrognathia
- Microphthalmia or iris coloboma
- Abnormal nuclear projections
- Harelip and cleft palate

- Elevated Hb F

- Polydactly
- Frontal bossing
- Microcephaly
- Rocker bottom feet
- Inguinal and umbilical hernias

Deletions

Category 3:
- Retinoblastoma

Category 4:
- Psychomotor retardation
- Microcephaly
- Hypertelorism
- Large ears
- Cardiac defect
- Abnormal dermatoglyphics

Category 2:
- Absent thumbs
- Fusion of metacarpals IV and V
- Genital and pelvic anomalies
- Ocular malformations
- Craniofacial abnormalities

Category 1:
- Normal thumbs
- Microcephaly
- Hypertelorism
- Frontal bossing
- Tooth abnormalities
- Anorectal malformations

FIGURE 5.21 Chromosome 13. (A) Diagrammatic representation of chromosome 13 showing the effects of deletions and duplications of specific segments. Hb F, Fetal hemoglobin. (B) Deletion of 13q14 in retinoblastoma. [(A) From Gilbert and Opitz 1982,[21] with permission.]

renal agenesis and hydronephrosis are sometimes present. Prominent nasofrontal bones; large ears with deep sulci and large, overdeveloped lobules; hypoplasia or agenesis of the thumbs; and imperforate anus are conspicuous features.

Category 1 may reflect a peculiar behavior of the ring chromosome in early embryonic life. Loss of the telomere and the most distal band of 13q34 are essential for the development of these abnormalities. Microcephaly with hypertelorism; ears with large, deep sulci and overdeveloped lobules; ocular abnormalities; and anogenital malformations are occasional features.

Category 2 patients have absent or hypoplastic thumbs. Craniofacial abnormalities include a triangular shape of the calvaria, frontal bossing, hypertelorism, epicanthal folds, and a protruding maxilla. Microphthalmia, colobomas, and genital malformations are frequent. Thumb defects range from a unilateral, boneless, rudimentary fold to bilateral absence of the thumbs without rudiments. Bilateral fusion of the fourth and fifth toes, and missing fifth toes with only four metatarsals, occur. Only mild psychomotor retardation associated with very few congenital malformations is reported. Deletion of the 13q31 segment is necessary for the development of category 2 features.[121]

Category 3 is linked to a deletion of 13q14 and is associated with the development of retinoblastoma.[125–127]

Category 4 is associated with deletion of 13q21.[121] Microcephaly, hypertelorism, large but well-formed ears, psychomotor

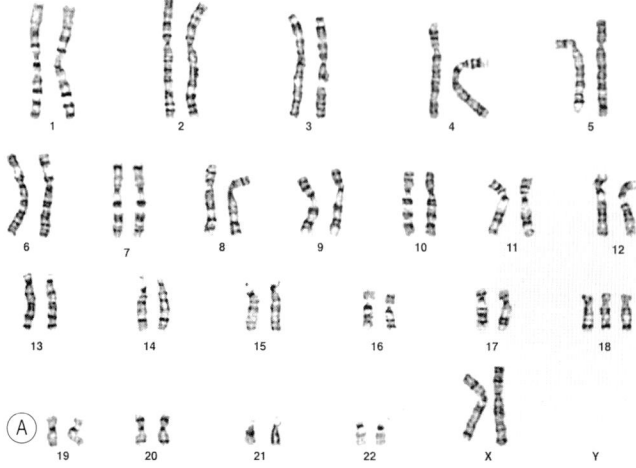
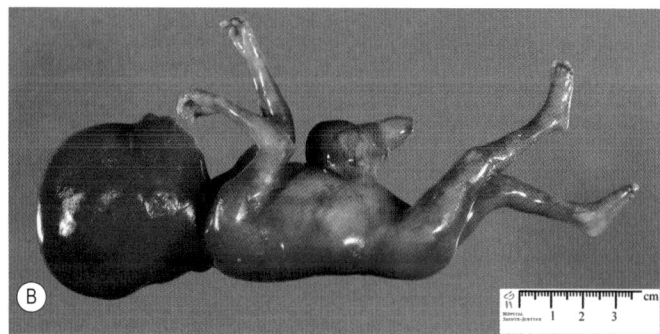

FIGURE 5.22 Trisomy 18. (A) Karyotype 47,XX,+18. (B) Nineteen weeks' gestation fetus showing the typical phenotype of trisomy 18 including micrognathia, low-set ears, slender bridge of the nose, clenched fists with overlapping second and fifth fingers, in addition to an omphalocele. [(A) Courtesy Dr Nicole Lemieux.]

retardation, and cardiac defects characterize this condition. The thumbs are normal, and retinoblastoma does not occur. Microstomia and mongoloid slant of the palpebral fissures are sometimes seen.

Trisomy 13 mosaicism has recognizable trisomy 13 features; however, with relatively fewer trisomic cells, the phenotype is less diagnostic.

Abnormalities of chromosome 18

Trisomy 18

The incidence of trisomy 18 is estimated to be between 1 in 3500 to 1 in 8000 live births; most are spontaneously aborted. Of those born, more than half die by 2 months of age, and survival beyond 1 year is rare. The female-to-male ratio is approximately 3:1.[128] As in other trisomic states, there is a correlation with **advanced maternal age.** Trisomy 18 is due to non-disjunction in approximately 80% of cases, mosaicism in 10%, translocation in 5%, and trisomy 18 plus sex chromosomal aneuploidy in 5%.[15]

The spectrum of clinical and autopsy findings in trisomy 18 syndrome[129] includes a consolidated list of the abnormalities shown in Box 5.6. The typical phenotype of trisomy 18 can generally be recognized in the fetus by the second trimester.

More than half of the cases are associated with **polyhydramnios**; this may be related to defective sucking and swallowing reflexes in utero. The placenta is often disproportionately small and may have a single umbilical artery. Some anomalies occur with equal frequency in trisomy 13 and trisomy 18. Delayed psychomotor development and severe mental retardation are constant findings. The classic phenotype is that of an infant with prenatal growth failure, hypertonia, limited hip abduction, and flexion deformities (Fig. 5.22). A dolichocephalic head with a prominent occiput, low-set ears with a pointed upper helix, small palpebral fissures, small mouth, micrognathia, barrel chest with short sternum and small pelvis, camptodactyly with the index finger overlapping the middle and ring fingers (Fig. 5.23A), short thumb and short hallux, and rocker-bottom feet (Fig. 5.23B) occur with high frequency. Clefts of the lip and palate and abnormal retina are not as common as in trisomy 13.[130] Diastasis recti, umbilical hernia, omphalocele, short and dorsiflexed hallux, and partial syndactyly between the second and third toes are sometimes seen.

Dermatoglyphics include a high number of arches in the fingers. In extensive anatomic dissections of the head and neck, Ramirez-Castro and Bersu described hypoplasia of the muscles of facial expression, fusion of the muscles around the corners of the mouth, and a supernumerary muscle band that extends from the corner of the mouth to the occipital attachment of the trapezius.[131] The otomandibular region manifests a spectrum of muscular, skeletal, arterial, and salivary gland variations.

A **congenital cardiac defect,** most frequently ventricular septal defect, is present in more than 95% of trisomy 18.[132] The atrioventricular and semilunar valves of the heart are dysplastic, with valvular and lacunar degeneration of the spongiosa and a lack of elastic tissue in the proximalis and spongiosa layers. In more than 60% of trisomy 18, the valves have a gelatinous, nodular appearance, with obliterated interchordal spaces and hyperplastic papillary muscles, described as polyvalvular disease (Fig. 5.24).[133] These valvular lesions are reminiscent of the normal fetal appearance of valves during the fourth month of gestation, suggesting failure of maturation of the loose myxoid mesenchyme of the valvular anlagen. Endocardial fibroelastosis and diffuse myocardial fibrosis occur.[134, 135] Coarctation of the aorta, atrial or ventricular septal defect and a persistent left superior vena cava are each present in 15–20% of cases.

CNS abnormalities may include abnormal gyri, parietal lobe defects, absent corpus callosum, cerebellar abnormalities, hydrocephalus, and meningomyelocele.[3] Holoprosencephaly and anencephaly are less common than in trisomy 13.[136]

BOX 5.6 ABNORMALITIES OBSERVED IN TRISOMY 18

Craniofacial dysmorphism
Dolichocephaly
Protuberant occiput
Small bitemporal diameter
Microencephaly
Wide fontanelles
Slender bridge of nose
Nares upturned
Horizontal palpebral fissures
Epicanthal folds
Hypertelorism
Microstomia
Micrognathia
Cleft lip/cleft palate (rare)
Low-set, 'fawn-like' ears with flat pinna and pointed upper portions
Atresia of external auditory canal (rare)
Patent metopic suture
Choanal atresia
Small face
Small mouth
Preauricular tag
High-arched palate
Low hairline
Holoprosencephaly (in 70% of cases)

Thorax and abdomen
Short webbed neck
Short sternum
Small nipples
Umbilical and inguinal hernia
Diastasis recti
Narrow pelvis
Marked lanugo at birth
Pilonidal sinus

Skeletal and limb
Hyperflexed position
Clenched fists
Index finger and fifth finger overlap third and fourth fingers
Camptodactyly
Clinodactyly
Hypoplastic, hyperconvex nails
Limitation of thigh abduction
Congenital dislocation of hips
Radial hypoplasia or aplasia
Thumb aplasia
Thumb duplication
Rocker-bottom feet
Short and dorsiflexed great toe
Absent twelfth ribs
Syndactyly of second and third digits
Postaxial hexadactyly
Medial aplasia
Lobster-claw anomaly

Phocomelia
Partial cutaneous syndactyly of toes
Arthrogryposis
Talipes equinovarus
Single palmar crease
Digital arches
Ulnar deviation of hands
Cleft in hand

Cardiovascular
Ventricular septal defect with or without overriding aorta
Patent ductus arteriosus
Pulmonic stenosis/bicuspid valve
Bicuspid aortic valve
Atrial septal defect
Dysplastic valve
Coarctation of aorta
Double-outlet right ventricle
Hypoplastic left heart
Abnormal coronary artery
Persistent left superior vena cava
Absent right superior vena cava
Transposition of great vessels
Tetralogy of Fallot
Eisenmenger complex
Dextrocardia
Dextroversion
Hypoplastic left atrium
Parachute mitral valve
Abnormal coronary arteries
Diffuse myocardial fibrosis
Endocardial fibroelastosis
Double inferior vena cava
Polyvalvular dysplasia
Endocardial cushion defect
Mitral atresia
Malrotation of great vessels
Esophageal subclavian veins
Common atrium
Anomalous pulmonary venous return
Single coronary ostium

Genitourinary
Horseshoe kidney
Ectopic kidney
Hydronephrosis
Megaloureter or double ureter
Micromulticystic kidneys
Severe hypoplasia of kidneys
Bilateral duplication of ureters and pelvis
Urethral atresia
Megacystis
Patent urachus
Hydroureter

Renal cystic dysplasia
Bladder diverticulum
Bladder outlet obstruction
Male
Cryptorchidism
Hypospadias
Female
Vaginal agenesis (rare)
Hypoplasia of clitoris
Hypoplasia of labia majora
Bifid uterus
Septate uterus
Abdominal external genitalia
Ovarian hypoplasia, dysplasia
Streak ovaries (rare)

Visceral
Thymic hypoplasia
Thyroid hypoplasia
Tracheoesophageal fistula
Pulmonary hypoplasia
Abnormal lobation of lung
Adrenal hypoplasia
Diaphragmatic eventration
Accessory spleens
Umbilical and inguinal herniae
Prominent extramedullary hematopoiesis

Gastrointestinal
Esophageal atresia
Absent gallbladder
Meckel diverticulum
Heterotopic pancreas in spleen
Pyloric stenosis
Omphalocele
Malrotation of intestine
Hypoplasia of intestine
Exstrophy of cloaca

Ectopic pancreas in duodenal wall
Anomalies of pancreas
Dysplastic development of pancreas
Ileal atresia
Absent appendix
Imperforate anus

Central nervous system
Large anterior fontanelle, thick fontanelle
Meningomyelocele
Cerebellar anomalies
Abnormal gyri
Hydrocephalus
Arnold-Chiari malformation
Corpus callosum defects
Holoprosencephaly
Frontal lobe defect
Migration defect
Anencephaly
Microcephaly
Heterotopias
Abnormal olivary nuclei
Osteoma of skull
Arachnoid cyst
Hypoplastic cerebellar vermis

Ocular (rare)
Abnormal retinal pigmentation
Cataract
Coloboma
Clouding of cornea
Microphthalmia
Placenta
Two-vessel umbilical cord
Polyhydramnios
Villitis
Chorioamnionitis
Trophoblast inclusions

Malformations of the **genitourinary tract** are found in approximately 75% of cases, and horseshoe kidneys in 25%. Also found are duplication of ureters or kidneys, hydroureter, hydronephrosis, cystic dysplastic kidneys, renal hypoplasia, unilateral aplasia or agenesis, cryptorchidism and hypospadias, nests of undifferentiated metanephric blastema resembling minute foci of Wilms tumor, and overt Wilms tumor.[137]

Iso(18p) syndrome

The presence of a supernumerary isochromosome comprising two short arms of chromosome 18 results in a tetrasomy 18p

[47,XX or XY,+i(18p)]. It is often present in a mosaic form, and gonadal mosaicism has been reported (a phenotypically normal parent harboring germ cells carrying the +i(18p)).

Del(18p) syndrome

Deletion of the short arm of chromosome 18 has a 2:1 male-to-female ratio and is associated with variable degrees of mental retardation. Birth weight is low, somatic growth is retarded, and the ears are low-set, large, floppy, and poorly formed. The phenotype includes hypotonia, hypertelorism, short neck, ptosis, micrognathia, epicanthal folds, pterygium colli, and microcephaly

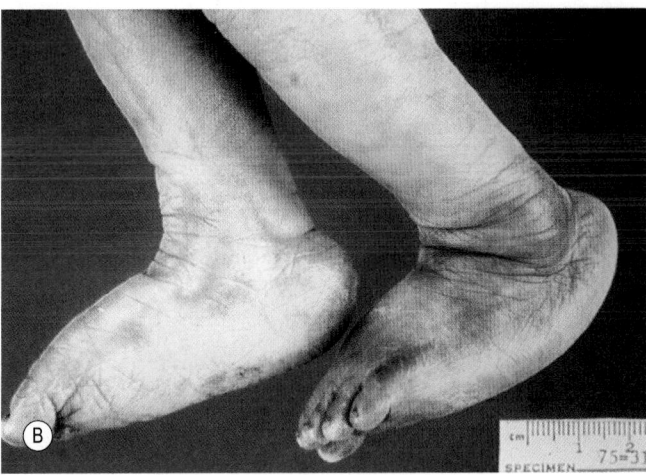

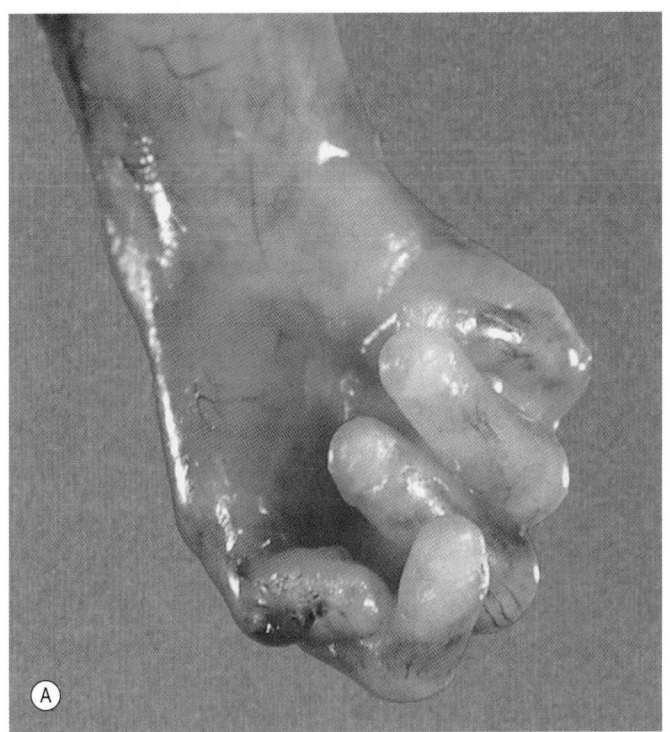

FIGURE 5.23 Trisomy 18. (A) Overlapping of the index finger over the middle finger. (B) Rocker-bottom feet. [(B) From Gilbert and Opitz 1982,[21] with permission.]

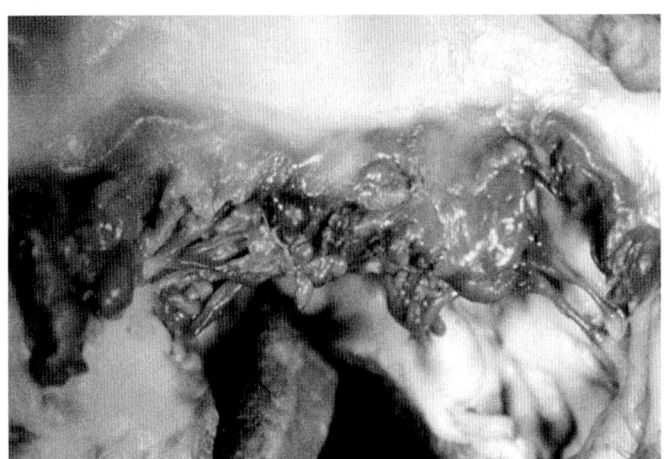

FIGURE 5.24 Multivalvular heart anomalies in trisomy 18. The tricuspid valve leaflets are thickened, rolled, and distorted. (From Gilbert and Opitz 1982,[21] with permission.)

with striking resemblances to the Turner and Noonan syndromes.[15] Short fingers and alopecia are less frequently observed, as are various degrees of holoprosencephaly, including cyclopia and agenesis of the corpus callosum.[138–141] Extremely severe rheumatoid arthritis of early onset was observed in one patient.[140]

Del(18q) syndrome

Deletion of the long arm of chromosome 18 is associated with severe mental and somatic growth retardation. Hypotonia and seizures are frequent. **Skin dimples** may be present over the subacromial and epitrochlear areas, lateral to the patellae, and over the metacarpophalangeal joints. **Subcutaneous nodules** may develop on the cheeks at the usual site of the dimples, the fingers are long and tapered, and supernumerary ribs may be present. **Cardiovascular anomalies,** usually a ventricular septal defect and **hypogenitalism** in both sexes are frequent. Cryptorchidism and hypospadias may be present, as are horseshoe kidney and bilateral cortical nephroblastomatosis.[21, 142] This renal aberration has also been seen in partial dup(20p).[143, 144] Craniofacial dysmorphism includes midfacial hypoplasia and microcephaly with recessed orbits, often with eye defects, carp-shaped mouth, short nose, and abnormalities of the ears, especially atresia of the external auditory canals. Cleft lip or cleft palate is present in 40% of cases. Serum levels of immunoglobulin A are low.[142] **Dermatoglyphic characteristics** include fingerprint whorls exceeding five and a high frequency of large, composite patterns.[145]

Additional features include intrauterine growth retardation, micrognathia, depressed nasal bridge, macrostomia, highly arched palate, puffy lower eyelids with semilunar-shaped and minimal mongoloid slant of the palpebral fissures, extremely well developed dermal ridges, rocker-bottom feet, umbilical hernia, and a very short perineal body.[21] Papillary thyroid carcinoma with lymph node metastases was reported in one patient at 9 years of age.[21]

Dup(18q) syndrome

Most cases of duplications of the long arm of chromosome 18 have a specific duplicated chromosomal segment, 18q21, and

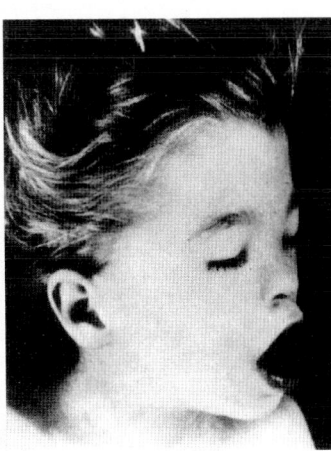

FIGURE 5.25 Patient with carp-shaped mouth, sloping forehead, and maxillary hypoplasia of dup(18q). (From Gilbert and Opitz 1982,[21] with permission.)

most of these cases have the major features of full trisomy 18. This suggests that the 18q21 segment is responsible for the major characteristics of the trisomy 18 phenotype.

A carp-shaped mouth, maxillary hypoplasia, hypoplastic ears, upper epicanthal folds, short palpebral fissures (Fig. 5.25), congenital cataracts, maleruption and malocclusion of the teeth, micrognathia, camptodactyly (Fig. 5.26A), abnormal dermatoglyphics, rocker-bottom feet, crowding of toes, and congenital cardiac defects, including double-outlet right ventricle, ventricular septal defect, patent foramen ovale, and pulmonary artery stenosis, characterize this syndrome. The neuropathologic findings in the brain may strongly resemble those seen in DS (Fig. 5.26B).[21]

Wolf-Hirschhorn syndrome [del(4p)]

One-third of patients with a deletion of the short arm of chromosome 4 comprising band 4p16.3 (Wolf-Hirschhorn syndrome, MIM 194190) die during the first year of life.[17] Survival beyond 20 years of age is rare.[146–148] The clinical features include severe psychomotor and growth retardation, low birth weight, diminished fetal activity, hypotonia, seizures, microcephaly, midline scalp defects, cleft lip or cleft palate, and micrognathia (Fig. 5.27).[146–154] A more comprehensive and consolidated list of the clinical features of Wolf-Hirschhorn syndrome is given in Box 5.7. **Hemangioma** on the brow, prominent glabella, and **ocular abnormalities,** including hypertelorism, divergent strabismus, eyelid ptosis, down-slanting palpebral fissures, and iris colobomas, are occasionally seen. **Congenital cardiac defects** are frequent.[155] Cryptorchidism and hypospadias may occur in males, and absent uterus and streak gonads in females.[156] **Abnormal dermatoglyphic patterns** include transverse palmar creases, dermal ridges, and hypoplastic fingers. The phenotype is inconsistent, as breakpoints, and thus the length of the deleted segment, are variable, and may include a concomitant duplication of a more proximal segment of 4p or the formation of ring chromosomes.[157] **Advanced parental age** correlates with this chromosomal defect.[115]

Cri-du-chat (Cat cry) syndrome [del(5p)]

The deletion of the short arm of chromosome 5 (Cri-du-chat or cat cry syndrome, MIM 123450) is the most frequent autosomal

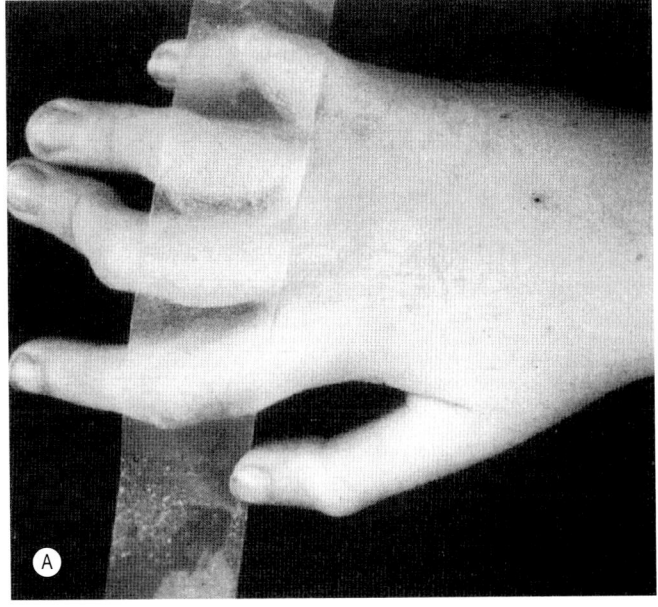

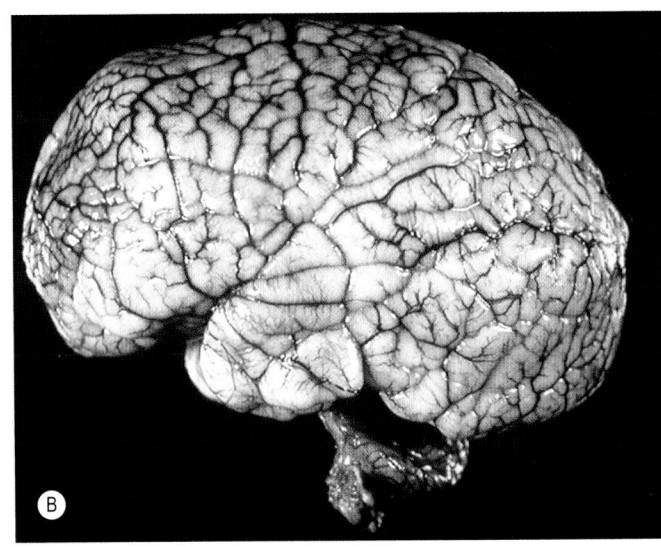

FIGURE 5.26 Dup(18q) (A) Camptodactyly of the fingers. (B) Brain. Notice the similarity to the appearance of DS: brachycephaly with open operculum and hypoplastic superior temporal gyrus. (From Gilbert and Opitz 1982,[21] with permission.)

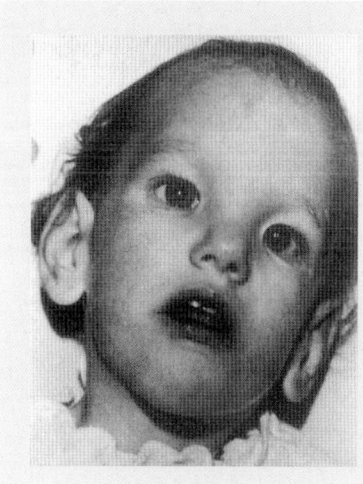

FIGURE 5.27 Del(4p) – Wolff-Hirschhorn syndrome: hypertelorism, microcephaly, and large ears.

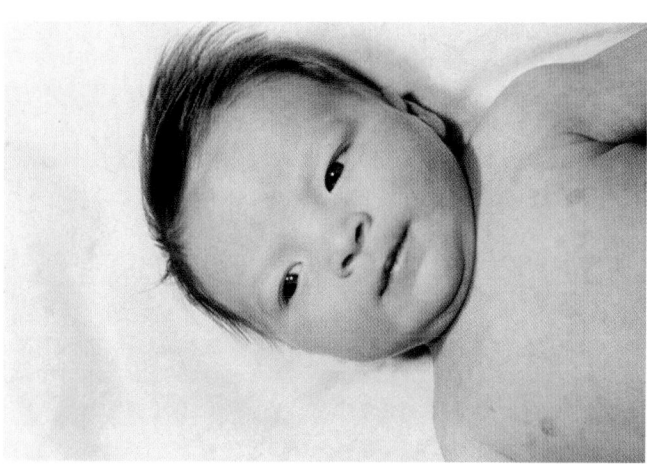

FIGURE 5.28 Cri-du-chat syndrome: hypertelorism, oval face, antimongoloid slant of the eyes and large ears. (From Gilbert and Opitz 1982,[21] with permission.)

and the face becomes thin and the philtrum short. Premature graying of the hair occurs in about 30% of cases. Oligosyndactyly, bowel malrotation, and thymic dysplasia are noted in more severe cases.[162] None are known to have reproduced, although females menstruate and develop normal secondary sex characteristics. Dental malocclusion is common.

Musculoskeletal anomalies include flat feet, mild scoliosis, large frontal sinuses, small ilia, syndactyly, and short metacarpals and metatarsals.[163, 164] **Dermatoglyphic abnormalities** include palmar creases in 35%; 50% have thenar patterns, distal axial triradii, and deficiency of ulnar loops.[165]

Trisomy 7

Conceptions with this condition rarely survive into the second trimester.[166] A report of a single fetus with trisomy 7[167] described IUGR, imperforate anus, and abnormal external genitalia. Internal anomalies were hemivertebrae, pulmonary hypoplasia, renal agenesis and dysplasia, urethral agenesis, and a blind-ending vagina. The urinary malformation resulted in a Potter sequence, with characteristic facies and distal contractures. Most trisomy 7 conceptuses abort early.

Del(7q) syndrome

Approximately 30 cases of a terminal deletion of 7q have been reported. Most of these *de novo* deletions involved a break at q32.[168]

Clinical findings[169, 170] include growth retardation, prominent forehead, developmental delay, single transverse palmar crease, male genital malformations, ocular anomalies, hypotonia, broad nasal bridge, and microcephaly. Other findings include feeding problems, micrognathia, hypotelorism, and chest abnormalities,[171] holoprosencephaly,[168] absence of the adrenal glands,[172] elements of the caudal deficiency sequence[173] and third and fourth branchial arch defects, including right aortic arch, a high ventricular septal defect, and truncus arteriosus.

Williams-Beuren syndrome [del(7)(q11.2)]

Williams-Beuren syndrome (WBS, MIM 194050) results from a mutation or a deletion of the ELASTIN gene located on 7q11.2. Most cases have cryptic deletions, detected only through FISH (Fig. 5.29). It is a contiguous gene syndrome, with deletions of the genes LIMK1, RFC2 and CYLN2 also probably having an impact on the phenotype. WBS is characterized by supravalvular aortic stenosis, multiple peripheral pulmonary arterial stenoses, elfin facies, characteristic dental malformation, and infantile hypercalcemia. IQ is reduced (range 20–106, mean 58), with cognitive

deletion syndrome detected by standard cytogenetic testing. It has an estimated incidence of 1 in 50 000 live births. There is no maternal age effect, and its prevalence among the mentally retarded is 1.5 per 1000. Karyotype is 46,XX or XY,del(5)(p13 or 15.1-pter), but band 5p15.2 is involved by definition[17, 152, 158–160] (Fig. 5.3; Box 5.8).

Balanced translocation in a parent accounts for 10–15% of cases.[161] The Cri-du-chat syndrome is characterized by a **weak, shrill, catlike cry** of the affected infant, caused by hypoplasia of the larynx. The characteristic cry usually disappears with time, sometimes only a few weeks after birth. Growth and mental retardation are severe (IQ less than 35), with failure to thrive, and hypotonia in infancy. The head is microcephalic and the face round; hypertelorism, down-slanting palpebral fissures, epicanthal folds, bilateral alternating strabismus, broad nasal bones, and low-set ears with high-pitched cry in the neonatal period constitute the typical phenotype (Fig. 5.28).

Preauricular tags and mild micrognathia may be seen. In time the **roundness of the face** and the ocular hypertelorism disappear,

BOX 5.7 ABNORMALITIES OBSERVED IN WOLF-HIRSCHHORN SYNDROME

Craniofacial dysmorphism
  Frontal bossing
  High frontal hairline
  Hemangioma over forehead or glabella
  Proptosis due to hypoplasia of orbital ridges
  Hypertelorism
  Up-slanting palpebral fissures
  Ptosis
  Exotropia and ectopic pupils
  Broad and beaked nose
  Prominent bridge of nose and shallow septum
  Stenosis or atresia of nasolacrimal ducts
  Short prominent philtrum
  Down-turned corners of mouth
  Small mandible
  Large, floppy, mis-shapen ears
  Scalp defect with or without underlying bony defect

Trunk and skeletal malformations
  Long slender fingers with additional flexion creases
  Long, narrow chest
  Hypoplastic, widely spaced nipples
  Diastasis recti
  Sacral sinus
  Umbilical or inguinal hernias
  Hypoplasia or duplication of thumbs
  Hypoplasia or duplication of great toes
  Hypoplasia of pubic bones
  Abnormalities of vertebrae and ribs
  Defective calcification of calvarian bones
  Osteoporosis
  Delay in bone maturation

Internal malformations
  Accessory spleens
  Abnormal shape of pancreas
  Absence of gallbladder
  Abnormal lung lobation

Cardiovascular malformations
  Persistent left superior vena cava
  Abnormalities of valves
  Complex cardiac defects

Genitourinary malformations
  Hypoplastic kidneys
  Cystic dysplastic kidneys
  Unilateral renal agenesis
  Hydronephrosis
  Exstrophy of bladder
  Male
  Hypoplastic external genitalia
  Cryptorchidism and hypospadias
  Female
  Large clitoris
  Uterine hypoplasia
  Bicornuate or unicornuate uterus
  Agenesis of vagina, cervix, or uterus
  Ovarian streaks

Central nervous system malformations
  Hypoplasia of cerebellum
  Cavum septum pellucidum
  Hypoplasia or aplasia of corpus callosum
  Hypoplasia or absence of olfactory bulbs and tracts
  Microgyria
  Migration defects
  Hydrocephalus

Ocular malformations
  Colobomas
  Microphthalmia
  Megalo- or sclerocornea
  Cataract
  Hypoplastic anterior chamber
  Hypoplastic ciliary body of iris
  Persistence of lenticular membrane
  Hypoplastic retina with formation of rosettes
  Cup-shaped optic discs
  Congenital nystagmus
  Rieger anomaly

Dermatoglyphics
  Hypoplastic dermal ridges ('laundress hands')

deficits including poor visual-motor integration, often masked by relatively spared language skills.

Abnormalities of chromosome 8

Trisomy 8

Trisomy 8 mosaicism (Fig. 5.30A) is more common than complete trisomy 8, which is usually lethal. The phenotype of trisomy 8 mosaicism is highly variable, ranging from a phenotypically normal individual to a polymalformation syndrome (Warkany syndrome). Mental retardation varies from mild to severe, although some patients have normal intelligence,[174–178] as mosaicism may spare the brain cells. Box 5.9 lists the abnormalities throughout the range of severity of the syndrome. The most common abnormalities include an abnormally shaped skull, reduced joint mobility, various vertebral anomalies, supernumerary ribs, strabismus, absent patellae, short neck, long slender trunk, cleft palate, and deep palmar and plantar creases. **Deep plantar creases** are highly characteristic of the syndrome;

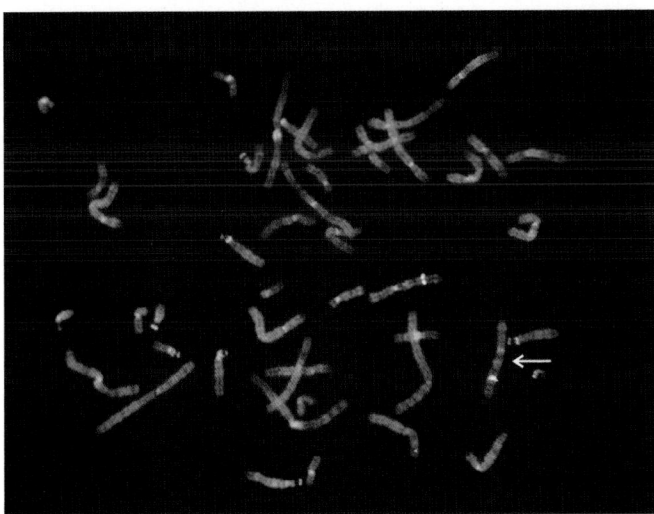

FIGURE 5.29 Williams-Beuren syndrome (FISH): chromosomes 7 are identified by a green spot, and labeling band 7q11.2 in red shows it to be deleted on the chromosome on the right (arrow).

BOX 5.8 ABNORMALITIES OBSERVED IN CRI DU CHAT (CAT CRY) SYNDROME

At birth

Growth retardation
Microcephaly
Mewing cry
Full cheeks, round face
Depressed nasal bridge
Inner epicanthal folds
Downward slant of palpebral fissures
Short fingers
Clinodactyly of little fingers
Talipes equinovarus
Cleft palate
Preauricular fistulas
Hypospadias
Cryptorchidism
Syndactyly of second and third toes and fingers
Oligosyndactyly
Thymic dysplasia
Malrotation of gut

Childhood

Small, narrow, often asymmetric face
Malocclusion
Scoliosis
Muscle tone normal or increased
Shortening of metacarpals three through five
Premature graying of hair

---

however, they were also seen in a patient with del(6p) syndrome and in two patients with partial trisomy for the long arm of chromosome 10.[179, 180] Camptodactyly is common and digital abnormalities of both feet have been observed.[21] A few patients exhibited agenesis of the corpus callosum.

Cardiac defects include ventricular septal defect, patent ductus arteriosus, and cor triatriatum. In 75% of cases, severe **ureteral and renal anomalies** occur, predominantly obstructive uropathy with hydronephrosis and secondary chronic pyelonephritis.[181, 182]

Dermatoglyphic patterns include a low total ridge count and increased number of arches, distal palmar triradius, and a single palmar crease. Partial factor VII deficiency has been reported.[183] **Skeletal malformations** may include supernumerary skeletal and lumbar vertebrae, supernumerary ribs, small pelvic bones, absent patellae, vertebral dysplasia, locked vertebrae, hemivertebrae, and spina bifida.

Localization of the *glutathione reductase* gene on chromosome 8 bears diagnostic importance in patients with trisomy 8, in whom high levels of the enzyme are detected.[184]

We have observed an infant with **complete trisomy 8.** Such infants may represent cases in which somatic mosaicism was not excluded, although in trisomy 8 there is rarely survival to the second trimester. Abnormalities include generalized lymphedema, brachycephalic skull, down-slanting palpebral fissures, flat nasal bridge, ankylosis of the tongue, hypertelorism, epicanthal folds, cleft palate, micrognathia (Fig. 5.30B), abnormally shaped ears (Fig. 5.30C), bilateral short broad fingers with camptodactyly (Fig. 5.30D), shield chest, shortened neck, sacral dimple, hypospadias, deep furrows on the soles of the feet (Fig. 5.30E), truncus arteriosus with a supracristal ventricular septal defect, aplasia of the left diaphragm, hypoplasia of the left lung, and posterior urethral valves causing urinary obstruction with bilateral hydronephrosis and hydroureter, and absent patellae (Fig. 5.30F).

Recombinant chromosome 8 syndrome

The recombinant chromosome 8 syndrome is an inherited chromosomal abnormality associated with multiple congenital anomalies described in 33 large kindreds in the western USA.[185] The abnormal chromosome results from the unequal meiotic recombination in the gamete cells of a parent who is heterozygous for a specific pericentric inversion of chromosome 8, inv(8)(p23q22). All the kindreds have been of Hispanic origin.[186] The partial trisomy is caused by a derivative chromosome 8 due to unequal crossover during meiosis, leading to a duplication of the long arm and, probably, a deletion of a very small portion of the distal end of the short arm of that chromosome.

Developmental delay and mental retardation become evident soon after birth. **External malformations** include hypertelorism; short but prominent philtrum; hirsutism; a broad, square face; low frontal hairline; brachycephaly; a short, thick neck; long palpebral fissures; anteverted nostrils; high nasal bridge; square ear lobules; camptodactyly of the fifth fingers; dermal arch pattern on five or more digits; and deep plantar furrows.[186] Internal malformations include a high incidence of **congenital cardiac and genitourinary**

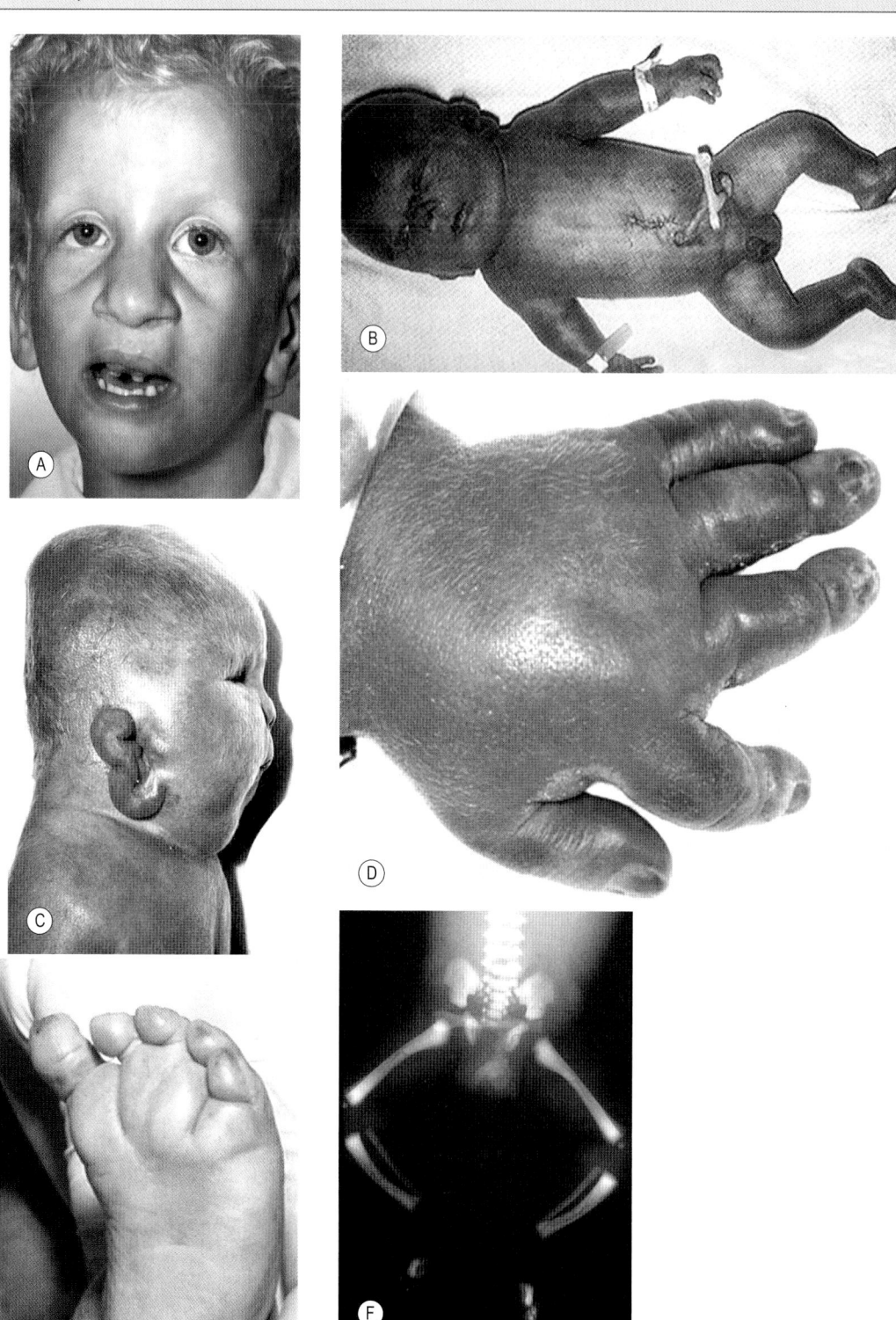

FIGURE 5.30 (A) Trisomy 8 mosaicism: flat nasal bridge and widely spaced central incisor teeth. (B) Complete trisomy 8 in an infant who died shortly after birth with lymphedema and multiple anomalies. (C) The ears are malformed and edematous. (D) The hands are broad and the fingers short and malformed. (E) Deep plantar furrows and malpositioned toes (four on the left foot). (F) Radiograph of the lower limbs showing absent patellae. [(A) Courtesy Dr Robert Gorlin. (B)– (F) From Gilbert and Opitz 1982,[21] with permission.]

BOX 5.9 ABNORMALITIES OBSERVED IN TRISOMY 8 MOSAICISM

Craniofacial dysmorphism
  Scaphocephaly
  Dysmorphic ears
  Hypertelorism
  Strabismus
  Broad-bridged, upturned nose
  Thick, everted lower lip
  Micrognathia
  High-arched palate
  Coarse, pear-shaped nose
  Down-slanting palpebral fissures

Limb and trunk malformations
  Clinodactyly
  Deep skin furrows on soles and/or palms
  Camptodactyly
  Syndactyly of toes
  Narrow pelvis
  Long, slender trunk

Skeletal malformations
  Hemivertebrae
  Extra vertebrae
  Butterfly vertebrae
  Spina bifida occulta
  Broad dorsal ribs
  Narrow and hypoplastic iliac wings
  Absent patellae
  Kyphoscoliosis
  Pectus carinatum

  Radioulnar synostosis
  Normal or advanced growth

Genitourinary malformations
  Hydronephrosis
  Ureteral obstruction
  Horseshoe kidney
  Unilateral agenesis of kidney
  Male
  Cryptorchidism
  Testicular hypoplasia
  Hypospadias

Cardiovascular malformations
  Interrupted aortic arch

Gastrointestinal malformations
  Diaphragmatic hernia
  Esophageal atresia
  Malrotation or absence of gallbladder

Ocular malformations
  Microphthalmia
  Iridal coloboma
  Glaucoma
  Corneal or lenticular opacities

Central nervous system malformations
  Hydrocephalus
  Agenesis of corpus callosum
  Large sella turcica

defects. Cardiac anomalies include ventricular septal defect, atrial septal defect, patent ductus arteriosus, tetralogy of Fallot, pulmonary atresia and stenosis, and persistent left superior vena cava. Genitourinary abnormalities include bilateral ureterovesical obstruction, double collecting system, cystic kidneys, hypoplastic ureters, hydronephrosis, dysplastic kidneys, and cryptorchidism.

CHARGE syndrome [del(8)(q12.1)]

CHARGE (MIM 214800) is an acronym for *C*oloboma, *H*eart anomaly (atrial and ventricular septal defects), *A*tresia choanae, *R*etardation of mental and physical development, including microcephaly, *G*enital hypoplasia and *E*ar anomalies/deafness. More than half have a CNS malformation, predominantly involving the forebrain – particularly arrhinencephaly and holoprosencephaly. Cleft palate and esophageal atresia are commonly associated. Most affected individuals have mutations of the *chromodomain helicase DNA-binding protein 7* (*CHD7*) gene

located on 8q12.1, sometimes manifesting as a deletion of that region, either cytogenetically or, more commonly, by FISH.

Abnormalities of chromosome 9

Trisomy 9

Full trisomy 9 is characterized by **craniofacial anomalies,** microcephaly, flat nasal bridge, epicanthal folds, micrognathia, low-set ears, cleft palate, and limb contractures (Fig. 5.31). Bilateral cystic dysplastic kidneys with atresia of the proximal ureters and a rudimentary atretic urinary bladder and hepatic and pancreatic dysplasia[187–195] are included in the complete range of abnormalities listed in Box 5.10. Complex **congenital cardiac defects** occur in two-thirds of cases, renal malformations in about one-half, and brain defects, particularly cystic dilation of the fourth ventricle with lack of midline fusion of the cerebellum, in two-thirds. Less frequent anomalies include microphthalmia, corneal opacities, coloboma of the iris, absence of the corpus

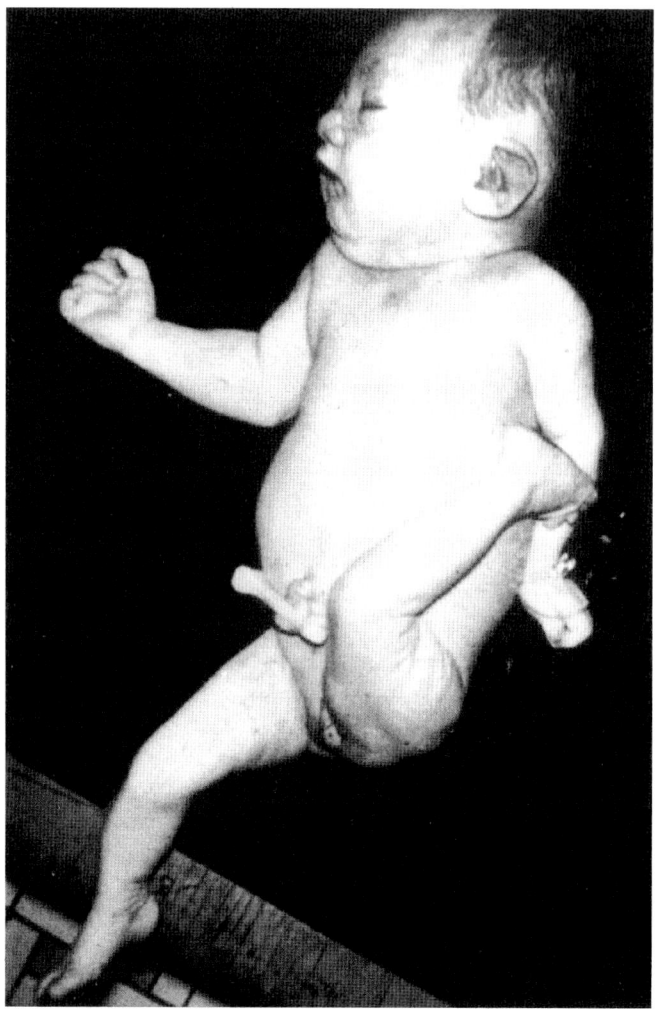

FIGURE 5.31 Trisomy 9: arthrogryposis; the head is brachycephalic and the ears are large and malformed. (From Gilbert and Opitz 1982,[21] with permission.)

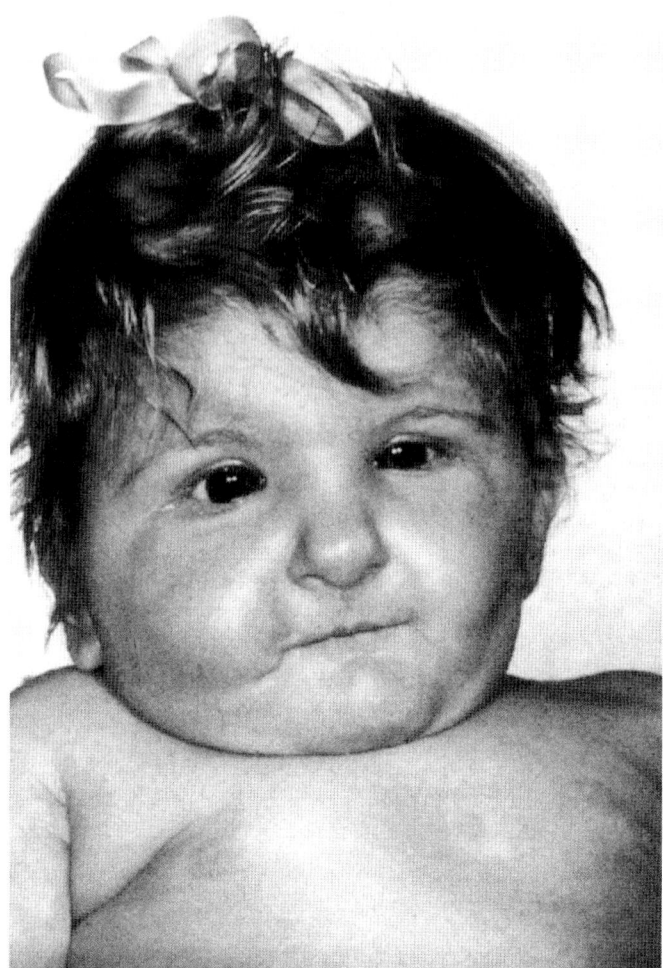

FIGURE 5.32 Trisomy 9 mosaicism: sloping forehead, deep-set eyes, and micrognathia. (Courtesy Dr Robert Gorlin.)

callosum, cleft lip or palate, abnormal lobation of lungs, malrotation of the large bowel, imperforate anus, and vertebral anomalies.

Trisomy 9 mosaicism syndrome

The trisomy 9 mosaicism syndrome was first reported by Haslam and colleagues.[194] It is associated with joint contractures, congenital cardiac defects, apparently low-set, malformed ears, sloping forehead, deep-set eyes and micrognathia (Fig. 5.32). Genitourinary abnormalities include micropenis, cryptorchidism, bladder diverticulum, double ureters, and microscopic renal cysts.[195] A phenotype of **tetrasomy 9p** has also been reported, resulting from the presence of an isochromosome 9p [47,XX or XY,+i(9p)]. Characteristic sonographic features include IUGR, ventriculomegaly, Dandy-Walker malformation, cleft lip and/or palate and renal anomalies. At birth, facial features include ear anomalies, hypertelorism, broad nasal bridge/bulbous or beaked nose, and micrognathia.[196–198] Most cases of tetrasomy 9p are mosaic, and non-mosaic patients are more severely malformed.[199]

We have seen one case of triplication of the long arm of chromosome 9, resulting in a **tetrasomy 9q**, in a patient investigated to rule out Down syndrome.

WAGR syndrome [del(p11-p13)]

The **association of Wilms tumor, Aniridia, ambiguous Genitalia, and mental Retardation (WAGR** syndrome, MIM 194072) comprises the characteristic clinical features of an interstitial short arm deletion of chromosome 11p13 (Fig. 5.33).[200, 201] Facial characteristics include a prominent nasal bridge, eversion of the lower lip, prominent forehead, cranial asymmetry, highly arched narrow palate, short neck, simplified pinna, and ptosis. **Ocular abnormalities** include poor vision, nystagmus, glaucoma, pale fundus or optic disc, and cataracts. **Dermatoglyphic findings** include helical open field patterns and digital radial loops. Wilms

BOX 5.10 ABNORMALITIES OBSERVED IN TRISOMY 9

Frequent malformations

Microcephaly or dolichocephaly
Low-set, malformed ears
Micrognathia
Broad nose with bulbous tip
Abnormal brain
Congenital heart defects
Abnormal hands/feet
Dislocation of joints: elbow/knee/hip
Cryptorchidism
Micropenis
Growth failure, psychomotor retardation, and/or early death
Third fontanel
Narrow temples
Occipital bossing
Facial asymmetry
Anophthalmos
Small palpebral fissure
Hypotonia
Epicanthal folds
Mongoloid slant
Hypertelorism
Hypotelorism
High-arched palate
Cleft lip/palate
Small mouth
Thin upper lip
Prominent maxilla
Low hairline
Loose, webbed, or short neck
Shield chest
Widely spaced nipples
Umbilical hernia
Kyphosis/scoliosis
Renal cysts
Hydronephrosis
Absent pubic bone
Absent/hypoplastic tibia/fibula
Abnormal/absent toes
Hypoplastic scrotum

Rare malformations

Malformed or overlapping fingers
Deeply furrowed palms
Hypoplastic or hyperconvex nails
Hypoplastic or absent phalanges or metacarpal bones
Rocker-bottom feet

Talipes calcaneovalgus
Longitudinal sole crease
Short humerus and femur
Folded helix, prominent antihelix, posterior rotation
Brachycephaly
Hydrocephalus
Pouched cheeks
Low-pitched cry
Long philtrum
Long trunk
Narrow chest
13 ribs
Abnormal vertebrae
S-shaped upper lip
Short xiphoid
Hyposegmented lungs
Malrotation of large bowel
Adrenal hypoplasia
Posterior urethral valves
Cholestasis
Absent fifth sacral segment
Absent tarsal/calcaneal bone
Inguinal hernia
Ectopic adrenal tissue on testis
Single umbilical artery
Renal hypoplasia
Renal ectopia
Horseshoe kidney
Hydronephrosis
Renal microcysts

Central nervous system malformations

Large fourth ventricle
Non-fusion of cerebellum
Hypoplastic temporal lobes
Wide cranial sutures
Leukomalacia

Cardiovascular malformations

Dextroposition of aorta
Aorta originating from right ventricle
Persistent left superior vena cava
Ventricular septal defect
Atrial septal defect
Patent ductus arteriosus
Coarctation of the aorta
Pulmonic/tricuspid valve dysplasia or atresia
Pulmonary stenosis

tumor develops in one-third of patients, with an average age of appearance of 18 months (range up to 5 years of age).

In the UK, aniridia was found in approximately 2% of patients with Wilms tumor; bilateral tumors were present in 36% (in Wilms tumor without aniridia, only one had bilateral tumors).

WAGR syndrome is a **contiguous gene syndrome,** Wilms tumors resulting from a **deletion** of the **WT1 gene,** and aniridia from a deletion of the **AN2 gene.** Riccardi and colleagues reported Wilms tumor with sporadic aniridia and normal chromosomes,[202] but the possibility of a cryptic translocation of 11p13 was not assessed

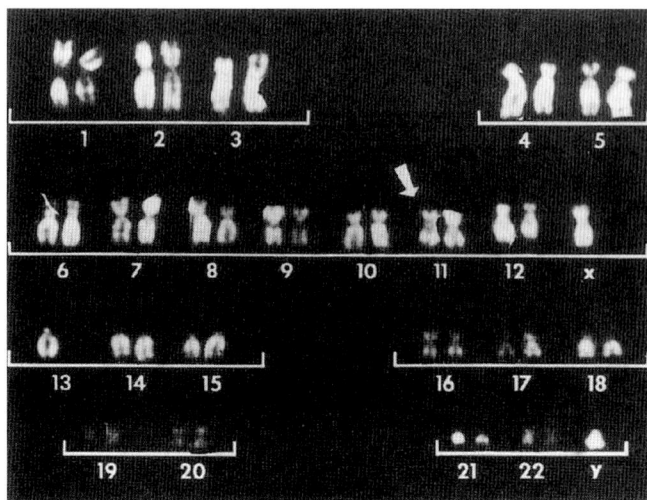

FIGURE 5.33 Karyotype of del(11p) in WAGR (Wilms tumor, Aniridia, ambiguous Genitalia, and mental Retardation).

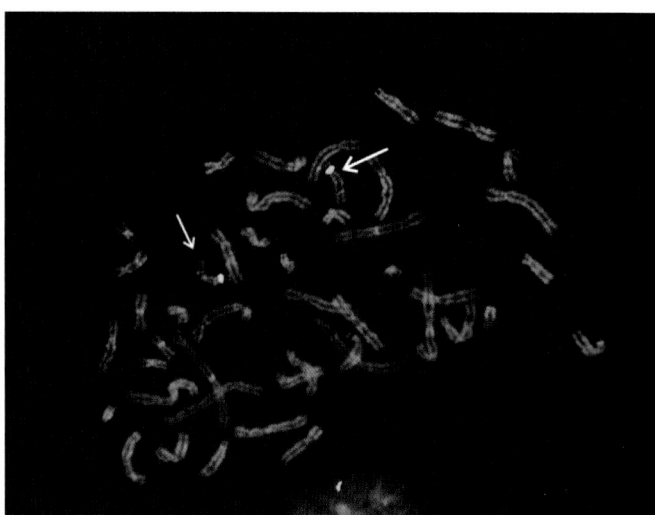

FIGURE 5.34 Prader-Will and Angelman syndrome determination through FISH. Chromosomes 15 are hybridized to a centromeric (green) and a telomeric (red) probe, making them readily identified (arrows). The PWS-AS probe hybridizing just below the centromere (in 15q11-q13) reveals a deletion of the chromosome 15 to the right (long arrow), the other being normal. (Courtesy Drs Raouf Fetni and Nicole Lemieux.)

by FISH. The WT1 gene (Wilms tumor 1) maps to 11p13 and functions as a tumor suppressor. It encodes a zinc finger DNA-binding protein; this master switch gene acts as a transcriptional activator or repressor, and is required for normal development of the genitourinary system and mesothelial tissues. The Denys-Drash syndrome (MIM 194080) generally results from a point mutation of the WT1 gene.

In one study[203] a woman had a balanced translocation from the short arm of chromosome 11 to the long arm of chromosome 2; familial Wilms tumor with aniridia syndrome occurred in three first-degree relatives.

Two patients with Wilms tumor and iris dysplasia, with normal chromosomes and no gene loss demonstrable by enzyme markers and direct DNA analyses, suggesting that aniridia defines a risk for Wilms tumor even in the absence of del(11)(p13).[203] It has not yet been determined whether patients with Wilms tumor and aniridia exhibit the subcapsular nephroblastomatosis found in children with the hereditary form of Wilms tumor.[204]

Disorganization of the renal parenchyma was noted in the del(11p) syndrome with a Wilms tumor that occupied the medulla of the kidney rather than its usual location in the cortex.[205]

Pallister-Killian syndrome [47,+i(12p)]

Pallister-Killian syndrome (MIM 601803) is characterized by the presence of a supernumerary isochromosome 12p, which results in patients having four copies of the short arm of chromosome 12 per cell **(tetrasomy 12p).** It is frequently present in mosaic form, which impacts on the phenotypic

manifestations. At birth, infants are of normal or of increased weight and size, but postnatal deceleration of length and head circumference develops, often with obesity. Profound mental deficiency is characteristic, often with seizures. Dysmorphisms and malformations are numerous. Streaks of hyper- and hypopigmentation may occur, and these areas should be individually sampled for karyotyping, as they are often the manifestation of mosaicism.

Prader-Willi and Angelman syndromes [del(15)(q11-q13)]

Prader-Willi (PWS, MIM 176270) and **Angelman** (AS, MIM 105830) syndromes are non-Mendelian disorders which can result from a deletion of the paternal and maternal chromosomal region 15q11-q13, respectively, or from a maternal uniparental disomy (UPD, i.e. with both chromosomes derived from a single parent; see Ch. 1) and a paternal UPD for chromosome 15, respectively.

The incidence of **PWS** is approximately 1/25 000 to 1/50 000 births; it is usually sporadic with no maternal age effect. A deletion can be demonstrated by FISH in 70% of PWS (Fig. 5.34), whereas 25% of cases result from maternal uniparental disomy. The infant is extremely hypotonic at birth, with hypogonadism, hypopigmentation, and short stature with small hands and feet (Fig. 5.35). In the second year of life, hyperphagia and obesity develop. Mental retardation is moderate, and obesity progresses with age. They are at risk for

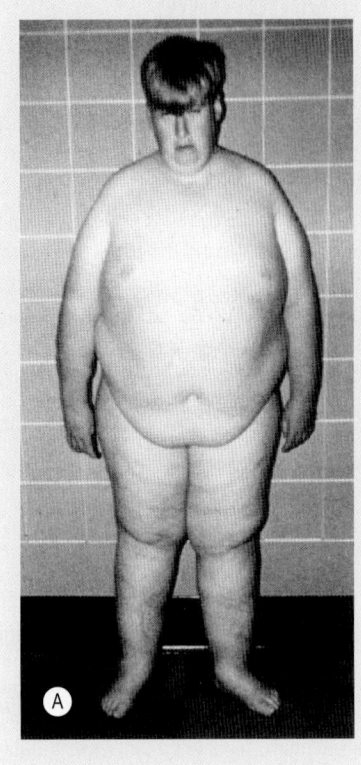
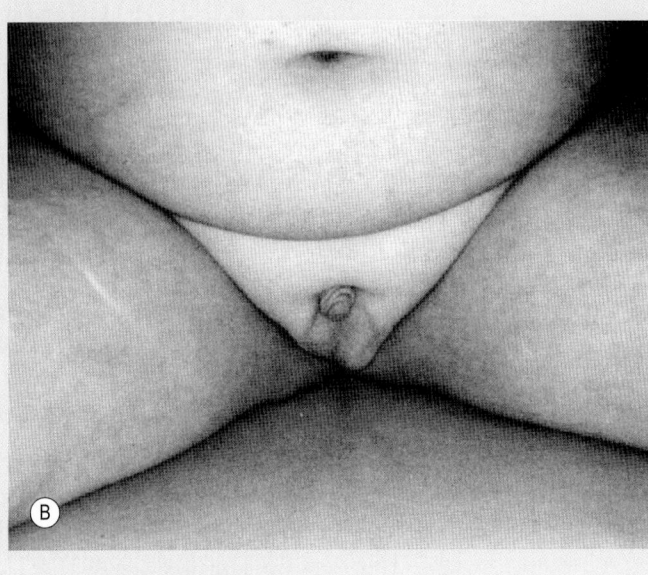

FIGURE 5.35 Prader-Willi syndrome.
(A) Characteristic: marked obesity.
(B) Hypogenitalism: small penis and cryptorchidism.
(Courtesy Dr Robert Gorlin.)

sudden death, and growth hormone therapy may be a risk factor.[206] PWS is a contiguous gene syndrome, and results from a deletion of the paternal allele [46,XX or XY,del (15)(q11.2-q13.1)pat] or from maternal UPD of chromosomes 15 which results in a lack of expression of the SNRPN and NECDIN genes,[207, 208] and possibly of other imprinted genes located in the 15q11-q13 region. These two genes are maternally imprinted (only the paternal allele is expressed), which explains the fact that PWS can result from a maternal UPD for chromosome 15, as well as from a deletion of the 15q11-q13 region of the paternal chromosome 15.

AS **(happy puppet syndrome)**[209] is characterized by severe mental retardation and seizures, abnormal puppet-like gait with ataxia and jerky arm movements, characteristic facies, and frequent paroxysms of laughter and absent speech. Microbrachycephaly, ocular anomalies, maxillary hypoplasia, large mouth and tongue, and widely spaced teeth are seen. Some cases have a familial incidence where no deletion has been identified. It is therefore likely that only one or very few genes are responsible for the AS phenotype. The cause of the syndrome resides in the *E6-associated protein ubiquitin-protein ligase* gene (*UBE3A*).[210] This gene is paternally imprinted (only the maternal allele is expressed), accounting for the fact that AS can result from unipaternal disomy for chromosome 15 and from a deletion of 15q11.2-q13mat. One must keep in mind that **FISH** studies will identify the AS and PWS patients harboring a deletion, but **molecular studies** are required to make the diagnosis of patients with *UPDs*[211] or with a mutation. A deletion can be demonstrated

by FISH in ~ 70% of AS, a paternal UPD is found in ~ 7% of cases and a mutation of UBE3A is found in ~ 10% of cases.

Other abnormalities of chromosome 15

+i(15p)

The isochromosome 15p accounts for approximately half of all marker chromosomes seen in constitutional karyotypes. It does not have any phenotypic manifestations, such patients and their offspring receiving the supernumerary chromosome being normal. The nature of such markers can be confirmed by FISH.

Del(15q)

Del(15q) is associated with different syndromes, depending on the exact segment missing and whether maternal or paternal genes are lost when the 15q11-q13 region is involved. See Prader-Willi/Angelman syndromes.

Trisomy 15

Approximately 1/1000 conceptions is trisomic for chromosome 15, which is about the same incidence as for trisomy 13. However, unlike trisomy 13, survival into the fetal period and live birth is very rare as most abort early. Only one case of

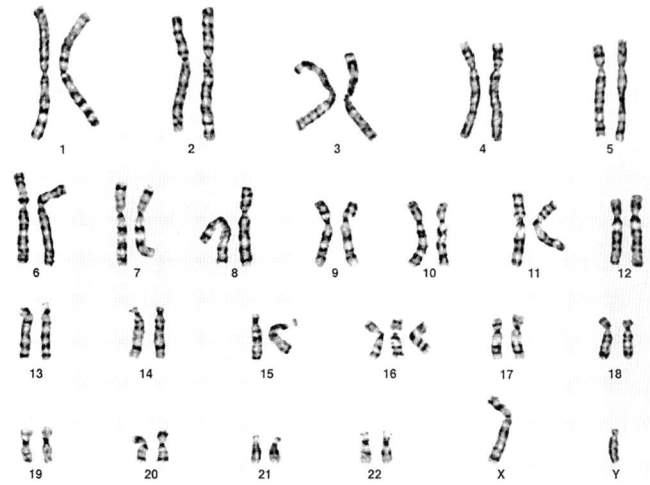

FIGURE 5.36 Karyotype of trisomy 16 (47,XY,+16). (Courtesy Dr Nicole Lemieux.)

liveborn non-mosaic trisomy 15 is reported.[212] This term-gestation, growth-retarded, hypotonic female infant had facial dysmorphic features consisting of small palpebral fissures, epicanthic folds, broad nasal bridge, small mouth, and abnormal ears. Positional deformities of the extremities and bony abnormalities were noted on X-ray films. Pulmonary hypoplasia and cardiac defects consisted of a small left atrium, ventricular dilation, muscular ventricular septal defect, and coarctation of the aorta.

Trisomy 16

Trisomy 16 is common in embryos and fetuses that abort early during development (Fig. 5.36). **Mosaicism** for trisomy 16 is sometimes encountered during prenatal diagnosis, particularly with chorionic villous biopsy specimens, and until recently was thought to be confined to the placenta. However, several liveborn infants with trisomy 16 mosaicism have been described. The extra chromosome 16 in the infant appears maternal in origin and suggests that the non-disjunction is a first meiotic division error. Investigation of multiple tissues is required before it can be concluded that mosaicism is confined to the placenta. Trisomy 16 mosaicism at prenatal diagnosis may be associated with a highly variable phenotype that may occasionally be compatible with extrauterine life.[213]

Trisomy 16 is the most common trisomy encountered in first-trimester spontaneous abortions. A single term-gestation infant boy with trisomy 16 who died shortly after birth had microcephaly with a flattened occiput, hypertelorism, microphthalmos, cleft lip and palate, and abnormally shaped ears; a ventricular septal defect, intestinal malrotation, and a germ cell tumor replacing one of the undescended testes were identified, with the other gonad dysgenetic.[213]

Rubinstein-Taybi syndrome [del(16)(p13.3)]

Rubinstein-Taybi syndrome (RSTS, MIM 180849) can be caused by a mutation of the gene CREBBP located on 16p13.3, or its deletion. Genetic heterogeneity exists (it can be caused by mutations of other genes, such as EP300, located on 22q13). It is characterized by mental retardation, broad thumbs and toes, facial anomalies, shawl scrotum and a propensity for fractures. One-third of patients have a cardiac anomaly. RSTS patients are at risk of developing neoplasias, both benign and malignant. Microdeletions of the 16p13.3 region can be demonstrated by FISH in approximately 10% of RSTS patients.[214, 215]

Smith-Magenis syndrome [del(17)(p11.2)]

Smith-Magenis syndrome (SMS, MIM 182290) results from a deletion of 17p11.2, possibly due to a disruption of the RAI1 gene. It is characterized by brachycephaly, midface hypoplasia with broad nasal bridge, prognathism, hoarse voice, speech delay, and psychomotor and growth retardation. In older patients, the phenotype is said to be characteristic, but cytogenetic/FISH confirmation is necessary.

Miller-Dieker lissencephaly syndrome [del(17)(p13.3)]

Miller-Dieker lissencephaly syndrome (MDLS, MIM 247200) is a contiguous gene syndrome resulting from the micro-deletion of 17p13.3. It is characterized by growth retardation, failure to thrive, minor facial anomalies, occasional hirsutism, clouding of corneas, polydactyly, variable malformations of other organs, and microcephaly with severe brain anomalies, including an absence of convolutions and gyri (lissencephaly) and only four instead of six cortical layers.[216–227] More than 50 genes have been mapped within the MDLS deletion region, but only the *LIS1* gene has been associated with a specific phenotypic feature of MDLS. *LIS1* hydrolyzes platelet activating factor, an inhibitor of neuronal migration.

Congenital heart disease, unilateral renal agenesis, fetal lobulation, and **cystic kidneys,**[106, 216, 222] and, in two of four cases, renal abnormalities included bilateral double-collecting systems, hydronephrosis, and abnormal calyceal patterns.

By high-resolution chromosome analyses, Dobyns and collea-gues found abnormalities of chromosome 17 in two of three unrelated patients with MDLS, one with a ring chromosome 17 and the other with an unbalanced translocation that resulted in partial monosomy of 17p13.[228] Abnormalities of chromosome 17 were found in all previously reported families in which two or

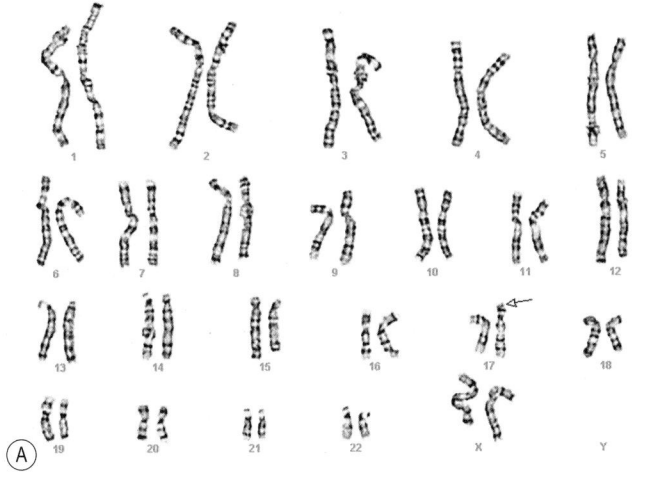
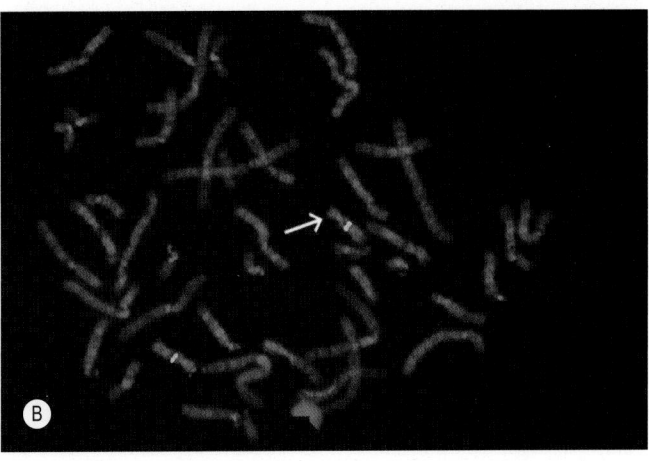

FIGURE 5.37 Miller-Dieker lissencephaly syndrome. (A) Karyotype shows an asymmetry in the length of the short arms of chromosomes 17, the one highlighted by an arrow having suffered a deletion. (B) Both chromosomes 17 are marked in green by this two-color FISH technique, which demonstrates the deletion of band 17p13.3 (red probe) on one of these two chromosomes (arrow). (Both figures courtesy of Drs Raouf Fetni and Nicole Lemieux.)

more children had MDLS. Two patients had normal chromosomes; submicroscopic deletions of 17p are suspected in these cases.[218]

A de novo microdeletion occurs in 80% of MDLS patients; the other patients inherit the deletion from a parent with a balanced chromosomal translocation. Hence, parental chromosomes should be investigated for this deletion through conventional karyotyping and FISH analysis (Fig. 5.37).

Trisomy 20

A few documented cases have survived into the second trimester[229] with failure to thrive, hypertelorism, micrognathia, cleft palate, low-set ears, positional deformities of the feet, and spinal abnormalities. Heart defects and intestinal malrotation and duplications have been observed. Persistent renal blastema and confined placental mosaicism for trisomy 20 are common and are associated with fetal anomalies only if the percentage of amniotic cells trisomic for chromosome 20 is more than 50%.[230]

Alagille syndrome [del(20)(p12)]

Alagille syndrome (AGS, MIM 118450) is caused by a mutation of the *Jagged-1* gene (*JAG1*) located on 20p12; it has reduced penetrance and variable expressivity. It is characterized by intrahepatic bile duct paucity manifesting as neonatal jaundice, arteriohepatic dysplasia, ocular anomalies, pulmonic valvular and peripheral arterial stenoses, butterfly vertebrae and other spinal defects, a broad forehead, a pointed mandible, a bulbous nose and short fingers. Approximately 5% of patients have a deletion of 20p12.[231]

Monosomy 22

Monosomy 22 is rarely identified in a non-mosaic state. Malformations in monosomy 22 include IUGR; microcephaly; hypertelorism; and skeletal, brain, cardiac, and gastrointestinal abnormalities, as well as humoral immunodeficiency.[232]

DiGeorge syndrome/velocardiofacial syndrome [del(22)(q11.2)]

DiGeorge syndrome (DGS, MIM 188400) results from deletion in 22q11.2, which leads to a deletion of the *TBX1* gene (among others; it is probably also a contiguous gene deletion syndrome). It appears that the velocardiofacial syndrome (MIM 192430) belongs to the DGS spectrum, as it too is characterized by the deletion of the *TBX1* gene. This deletion is best diagnosed by FISH (Fig. 5.38). DGS is characterized by hypocalcemia arising from parathyroid hypoplasia/aplasia, thymic hypoplasia, outflow tract defects of the heart, and anomalies of the lower face (discussed in Ch. 1).

Del(22q) syndrome

The features produced by the deletion of the long arm of chromosome 22 include severe mental retardation, muscular hypotonia, microcephaly, epicanthal folds, ptosis, flat nasal bridge, large and apparently low-set ears, high-arched palate, syndactyly of toes, and bifid uvula. Dermatoglyphic analyses

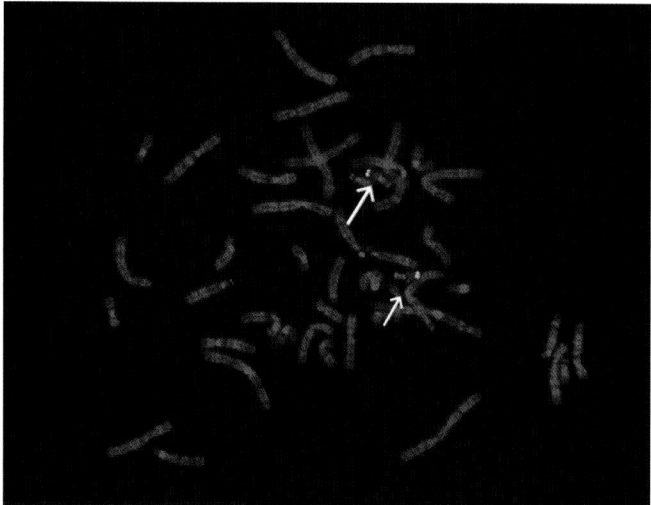

FIGURE 5.38 Evaluation of the 22q11.2 region through FISH. Chromosomes 22 are identified through a telomeric green probe (arrows); the region of interest, hybridized to a red probe, is seen to be deleted on the top chromosome (long arrow), confirming the diagnosis of DiGeorge syndrome. (Courtesy of Drs Raouf Fetni and Nicole Lemieux.)

indicate a marked increase in furrows, a decrease in ulnar and radial loops, a distal axial triradius, and hypothenar patterns. Leukocyte alkaline phosphatase is increased.[228]

Cat-eye syndrome [+(22)(pter-q11)]

Trisomy 22p/tetrasomy 22p

Cat-eye syndrome (MIM 115470) is characterized by an extra **isodicentric chromosome 22** with an inversion-duplication involving 22pter-q11,[233] which results in a tetrasomy of the short arm and of a pericentromeric segment of the long arm of chromosome 22.[234, 235] Trisomy of band 22q11.2 is sufficient to cause the phenotype.[233, 236]

Clinical features vary greatly, and a condensed list is given in Box 5.11. Patients with partial trisomy 22 (excluding band 22q11.2) may have near-normal intelligence. Familial occurrence is more frequent in trisomy 22p than in other trisomies. In milder forms of this disorder, reproduction has occurred, allowing for a dominant mode of inheritance.[98]

Characteristic features (Fig. 5.39) include **down-slanting palpebral features; ocular coloboma,** which can involve the iris, choroid, and optic nerve; **preauricular skin tags or pits,** which are probably the most consistent features; **congenital heart defects; anal atresia** with a fistula; and **renal malformations,** such as unilateral absence, uni- or bilateral hypoplasia, and cystic dysplasia. Intelligence is usually low to normal, although moderate retardation is also reported.

Less frequent, but also characteristic, findings are microphthalmia, microtia with atresia of the external auditory canal, intra- or extrahepatic biliary atresia, and malrotation of the gut.

Other rare autosomal trisomies and monosomies

Full non-mosaic fetuses with **trisomies of autosomes** other than chromosomes 13, 18, or 21 rarely survive into the second or third trimester.

Autosomal monosomies at term have been reported only for sex chromosomes and chromosomes 21 and 22. Rare mosaic monosomies for chromosomes 16, 18, and 20 have been recorded in the fetus.[19]

Triploidy

The extra haploid set of chromosomes in triploidy (Fig. 5.40A) is the result of double fertilization of the ovum (diandry) or failure of the ovum to extrude a polar body (digyny). Study of fetal and parental heteromorphisms shows that 66% of triploids are the result of **dispermy,** 24% are the result of **fertilization of a haploid ovum by a diploid sperm** caused by failure of the first meiotic division in the male, and 10% are the result of

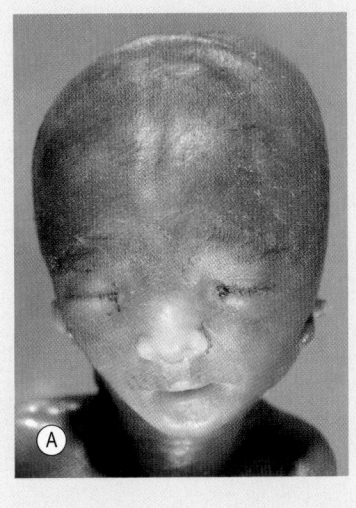

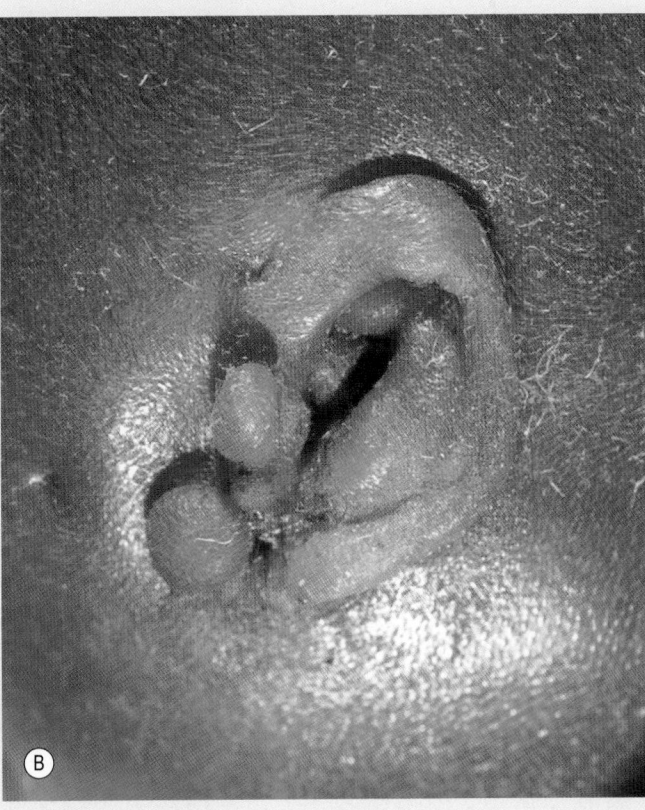

FIGURE 5.39 Trisomy 22p (cat-eye syndrome). (A) Down-slanting palpebral fissures and hypertelorism. (B) Malformed ear with preauricular tag.

either a **diploid meiotic division in the male or a diploid egg** from failure of the first maternal meiotic division.[237, 238]

Triploidy is the most frequent chromosomal aberration in first-trimester abortions and occurs in approximately 1% of all recognized human pregnancies.[239] Rarely do triploid gestations reach term;[237, 240–242] if the infant is liveborn, death occurs within a few hours after birth, although one XXX triploidy infant lived for 26 days.[243] About two-thirds of cases of triploidy have been XXY and about one-third XXX; they are rarely XYY.[243] We have observed one triploidy with one extra sex chromosome (70,XXYY). The external and internal genital development of triploid fetuses is controlled by the Y chromosome; in females, the ovaries are hypoplastic with poorly developed primordial folicles.[244] We have observed testicular Leydig cell hyperplasia in the majority of male molar triploidies.

McFadden and Kalousek divide triploid fetuses into two types.[245] Both types show the classical malformations. **Type I (or molar triploidy),** with the extra haploid set of chromosomes of **paternal origin (diandry),** shows a mild symmetrical IUGR with a partial hydatidiform molar placenta. **Type 2,** with the extra haploid set of **maternal origin (digyny, or non-molar triploidy),** shows a severe asymmetrical IUGR (with relative macrocephaly) with extreme placental hypoplasia (Fig. 5.40B) characterized by markedly hypermature and fibrotic villi, devoid of molar changes (Fig. 50.40F). Non-molar triploidy has a longer survival in utero and commonly results from an error in meiosis I division of oocytes.

In both molar and non-molar triploidies, microphthalmia, coloboma, ovoid cornea, hypertelorism, and dysmorphic ears and syndactyly of the third and fourth fingers and toes are frequent features; more severe malformations of fingers and toes, and talipes equinovarus may be present (Fig. 5.40C and D).[21] Congenital cardiac lesions occur in two-thirds of cases and include atrial and ventricular septal defects, endocardial cushion defects, pulmonary valvular stenosis, and valvular anomalies. Most show renal cysts, histologically of the dysplastic type. Sacrococcygeal rachischisis is frequent, and meningomyelocele has been described. The adrenal glands are extremely hypoplastic. Transverse creases are not infrequent. Rarer anomalies include: Dandy-Walker malformation; eccentric pupils; colobomas; hypoplasia of the iris or retina; choanal atresia; hypoplasia of the thyroid, thymus, and pancreas; tracheoesophageal fistula; omphalocele; diaphragmatic hernia; chondrodysplasia punctata; and thumb duplication.[244, 246, 247] We observed large hyperchromatic cells in the islets of Langerhans in the pancreas that were immunoperoxidase positive for somatostatin (Fig. 5.40E), and nodular Leydig cell hyperplasia. Box 5.12 presents a more comprehensive list of abnormalities observed in triploidy. Triploid pregnancy is associated with polyhydramnios and maternal proteinuria, hypertension, edema, and midtrimester pre-eclampsia.[248]

Triploid placentas with an extra set of paternal chromosomes form **partial hydatidiform moles** (Fig. 5.41). In 85% of cases of

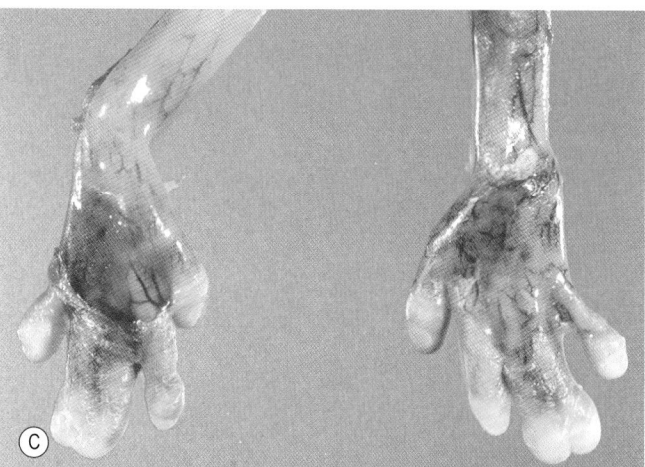

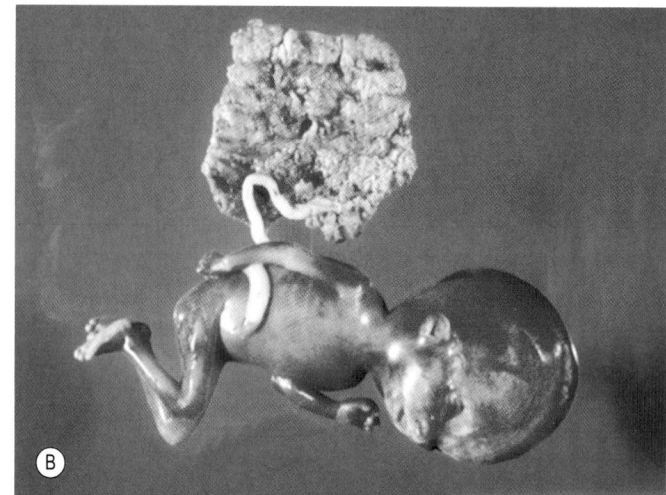

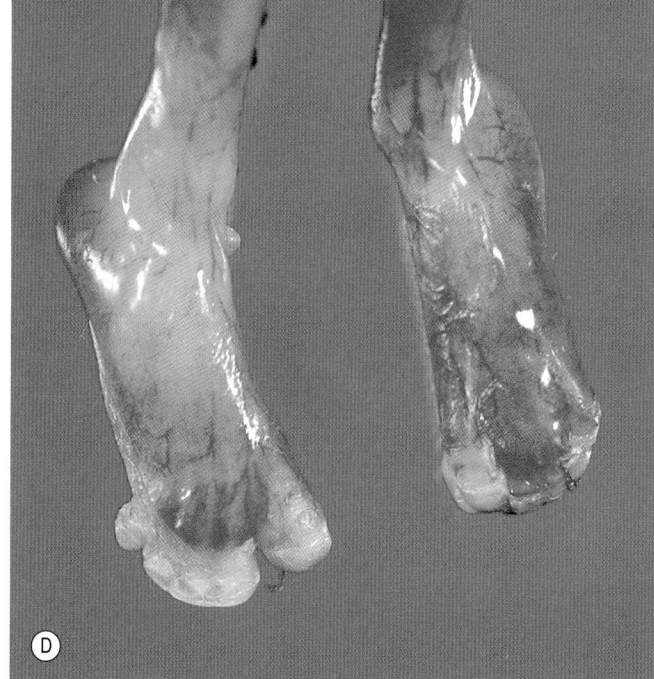

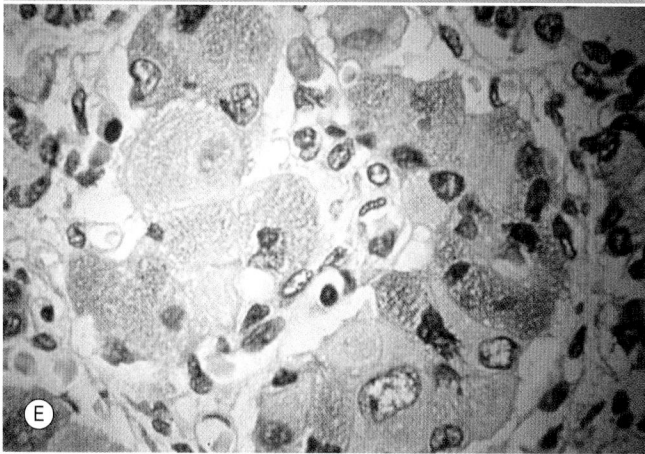

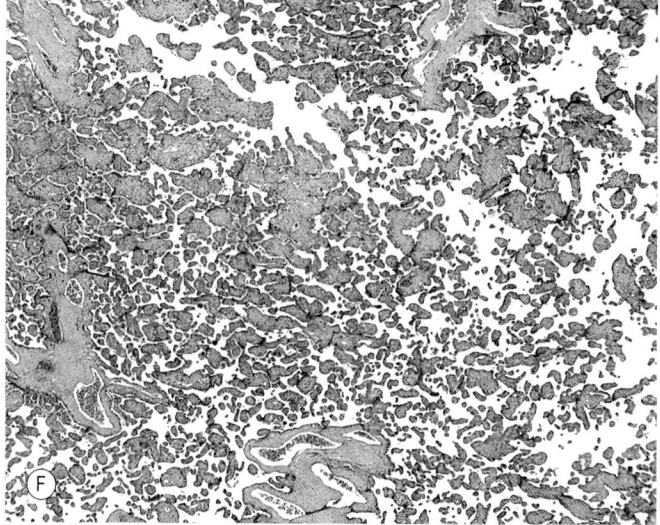

FIGURE 5.40 Triploidy. (A) Karyotype 69,XXY. (B) Triploid fetus (non-molar triploidy): hypertelorism, bulbous nose, sloping forehead, small mouth and extreme placental hypoplasia. (C) The hands with syndactyly of the third and fourth fingers, and camptodactyly. (D) Bizarre appearance of toes, with bilateral syndactyly of the second, third and fourth toes. (E) Microscopic appearance of the pancreatic islet in a molar triploidy: cytomegaly of the cells that are somatostatin positive. (Immunoperoxidase stain for somatostatin × 400) (F) Microscopic section of a non-molar triploidy. The villi are hypoplastic, fibrous and hypovascular. (HPS stain, original magnification × 25) [(A) Courtesy Diane Lachance and Dr Nicole Lemieux. (E) From Gilbert and Opitz 1982,[21] with permission.]

BOX 5.12 ABNORMALITIES OBSERVED IN TRIPLOIDY

Maternal features

- Midtrimester pre-eclampsia
- Polyhydramnios
- Proteinuria, hypertension

Fetal malformations at birth

- Fetal growth failure

Extremities and skeletal malformations

- Transverse crease
- Large posterior fontanelle
- Incomplete ossification of calvarium
- Syndactyly between third and fourth fingers/toes
- Talipes equinovarus
- Proximal displacement of thumbs
- Lumbosacral myelomeningocele

Central nervous system malformations

- Hydrocephalus
- Arnold-Chiari syndrome
- Meningomyelocele
- Holoprosencephaly
- Hypoplasia of basal ganglia, cerebellum, and occipital lobe
- Aplasia of corpus callosum

Ocular malformations

- Iris coloboma
- Microphthalmia

Craniofacial malformations

- Malformed ears
- Large, bulbous nose
- Cleft lip and palate

Genitourinary malformations

- Renal hypoplasia and cysts
- Hypospadias
- Cryptorchidism
- Leydig cell hyperplasia of testes in molar triploidies
- Hydronephrosis
- Micropenis
- Bifid scrotum
- Hypoplasia of ovaries

Cardiopulmonary malformations

- Ventricular septal defect
- Retroesophageal right subclavian artery
- Tetralogy of Fallot
- Atrial septal defect, secundum type
- Persistent left superior vena cava

Gastrointestinal malformations

- Malrotation of colon
- Aplasia of gallbladder

Endocrine malformation

- Adrenal hypoplasia

Placental abnormalities in molar triploidies

- Partial hydatidiform mole
- Mild trophoblastic proliferation
- Hydropic villi with scalloping
- Large cisternae within villi
- Trophoblastic inclusions

Placental abnormalities in non-molar triploidies

- Extreme hypoplasia
- Marked villous fibrosis

triploidy, the extra haploid set is of paternal origin.[249–252] The placenta of triploidy of maternal origin is usually non-hydropic. The presence of distinct phenotypes confirms the role of genomic imprinting in the development of human triploid conceptions, including their placentas.

Histologically, the partial mole of triploidy is characterized by molar changes interdigitating with seemingly unaffected placental villi.[250, 251, 253] Hydatidiform changes include large villi with scalloping of their margins and mild trophoblastic hyperplasia with vacuolization, similar to that seen in young placentas up to weeks 6 or 7 of gestation (Fig. 5.41B and C). Large cisternae are present within the edematous villi. Trophoblastic inclusions, seen as deep and narrow invaginations of trophoblast into the villous stroma, are seen in 70% of cases.[254–256]

We observed a triploid infant with elevated maternal serum and borderline elevated amniotic α-fetoprotein levels. This may be related to the partial hydatidiform molar placenta that may pass more α-fetoprotein back from the amniotic fluid to the maternal serum.[257]

Sex chromosome abnormalities

Klinefelter syndrome

Klinefelter syndrome has an incidence of 1 in 850 live male births and includes 47,XXY (Fig. 5.42A), 48,XXYY, 46,XY mosaicism, and other, rarer forms such as 48,XXXY, 49,XXXYY, and 49,XXXXY. Around 80% are XXY, 10% are mosaic, and the remainder is XXYY or a less frequently occurring type 47,XXY. Klinefelter syndrome is characterized by a hypogonad male with azoospermia, gynecomastia, increased length of extremities, and an increased incidence of mental deficiency, which increases with the number of X chromosomes. About 10% of cases of male sterility are due to Klinefelter syndrome.[258] Some cases have associated trisomy 21. Tall stature (Fig. 5.42B), borderline intelligence, and aggressive behavioral problems occur in some cases, especially in examples of 48,XXYY. The testes are atrophic and show hyalinization of the tubules with clusters of Leydig cells (Fig. 5.42C).

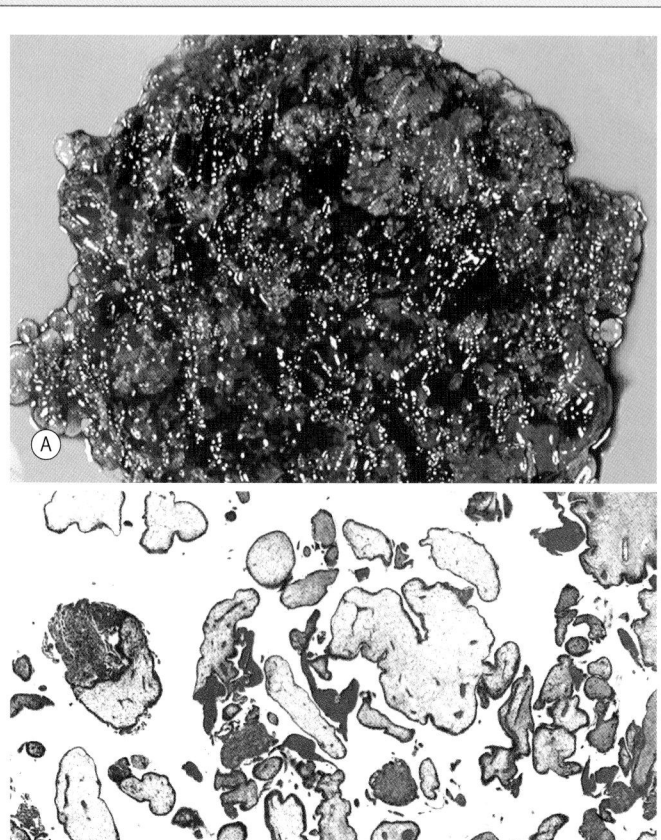

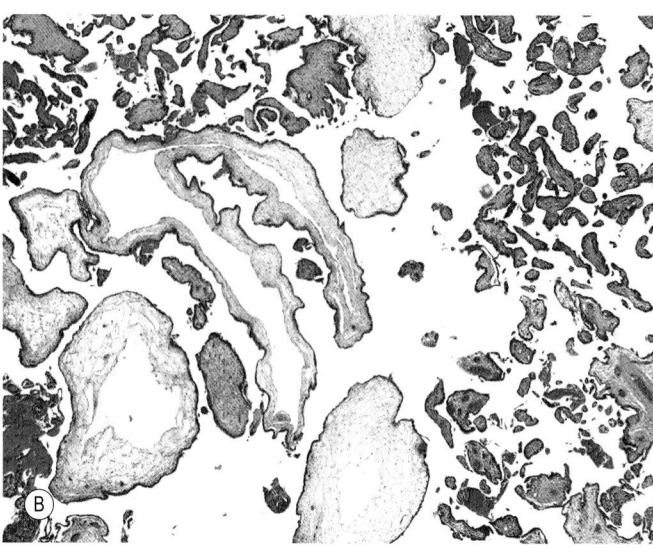

FIGURE 5.41 Triploidy. (A) Placenta in triploidy with partial hydatidiform mole. (B) and (C) Microscopic section of the placenta. The chorionic villi are large, with scalloping at the margins, trophoblastic inclusion, and an edematous stroma. (HPS stain, original magnification × 25) [(A) From Gilbert and Opitz 1982,[21] with permission.]

Before puberty the testis may be normal in size and microscopic appearance. However, during adolescence the testes fail to enlarge and the seminiferous tubules become atrophic, hyalinized, irregularly arranged and are lined only by Sertoli cells; elastic fibers are absent around the tunica propria of the tubules, Leydig cells are clumped, and spermatogonia and spermatogenesis are inconspicuous or absent. The penis is usually of normal circumference but can be shorter than normal. The size of the penis is inversely proportional to the number of Xs; in those with XXXXY it is minuscule.

Renal cysts, hydronephrosis, hydroureter, and ureterocele have been reported.[107] These kidneys have been described as symmetrically enlarged, with small cysts 0.1–0.8 cm in diameter throughout the parenchyma.[259] The ureters may be very thin but not atretic; the bladder is small and cylindric. Calyces and papillae may not be recognized.

Gynecomastia develops after puberty in about 50% of these patients (Fig. 5.42B); facial hair is sparse, axillary hair may be deficient, and 50% have a female pubic escutcheon. Mosaic individuals may be less severely affected. An increased incidence of diabetes mellitus, chronic pulmonary diseases, chronic bronchitis, bronchiectasis, asthma, and emphysema is common.[260–262] Low

concentration of plasma testosterone and elevated plasma concentrations of luteinizing and follicle-stimulating hormones are found, accounting for the gynecomastia.[263] Patients with Klinefelter syndrome have decreased radioactive iodine uptake and diminished response to thyroid-stimulating hormone; however, growth hormone and glucocorticoid secretion are normal.

Monosomy X (Turner syndrome and variants)

Depending on the studies, approximately 45% of patients with Turner syndrome are 45,X (Fig. 5.43A), 7% have an isochromosome X [46,X,i(Xq)] which results in trisomy Xq and monosomy Xp, 8% show 45,X/46,X,i(Xq), 16% have a ring X chromosome [45,X/46,X,r(X)] and 13% are mosaic (45,X/46,XX); all show the same phenotype. The remainder of cases comprise various anomalies of the Y chromosome (6%), 45,X/46,XX/47,XXX and other sex-chromosome mosaics, and other sex chromosome anomalies.[18, 264] 45,X/46,XX mosaicisms have a variable phenotype. Those who come to clinical attention usually have typical monosomy-X phenotype.

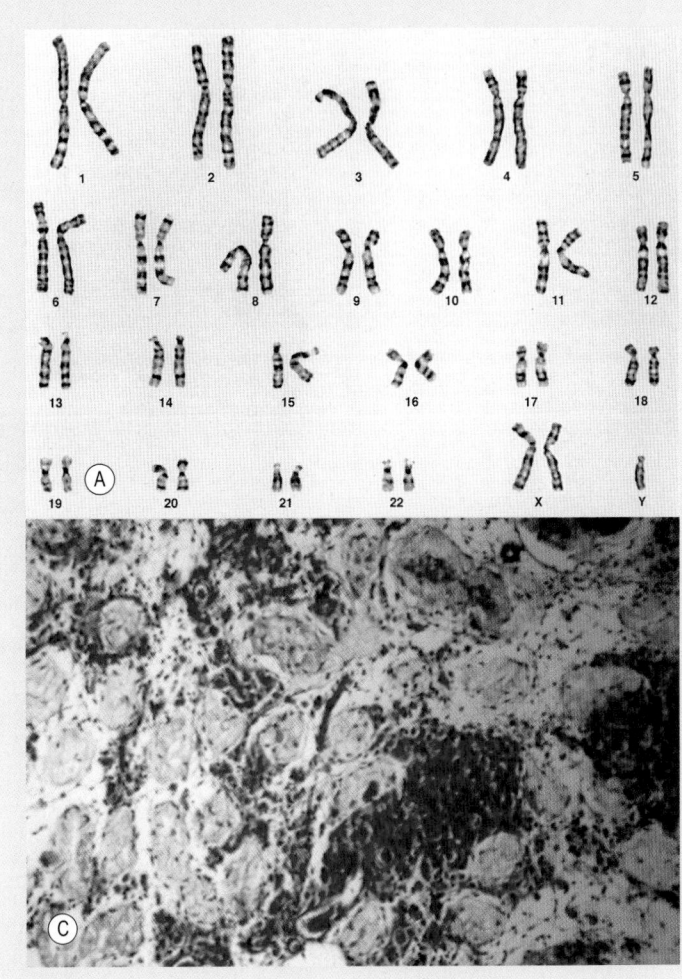

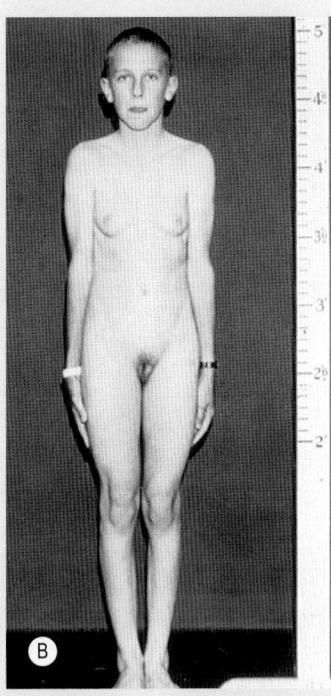

FIGURE 5.42 (A) Karyotype 47,XXY. (B) Phenotype: tallness with arachnodactyly and gynecomastia. (C) Microscopic section of testis in Klinefelter syndrome. The tubules are atrophic and there are hyperplastic clusters of Leydig cells. (H&E × 250) [(A) Courtesy Dr Nicloe Lemieux. (B) Courtesy Dr Robert Gorlin.]

A deletion of the short arm of the X chromosome is also associated with the typical phenotype.[264] Terminal deletions of the short arm of the X chromosome are associated with infertility, but somatic stigma vary, depending on the extent of the deletion. Deletions of the whole short arm of the X chromosome generally results in the full phenotype. Loss of an interstitial or terminal segment of Xq can result in short stature and primary or secondary ovarian failure. Deletions distal to Xq21 appear to have no effect on stature.

Turner syndrome has been estimated to occur in 1/2500–1/3000 live female births.[98, 264] Embryonal and fetal mortality is high, with 95–98% of all conceptions spontaneously aborted.

In nearly 85% of 45,X Turner patients, the X chromosome is of maternal origin (resulting from a loss of the sex chromosome in the fertilizing sperm),[265] except in the conceptions of very young mothers, in which case the remaining X chromosome is more commonly of paternal origin (due to a loss of an X during meiosis of the oocyte).[266] PCR-based diagnosis has been reported to establish the parental origin of the X chromosome and the presence of mosaicism.[265]

Phenotypic features of Turner syndrome include short stature, broad chest with widely-spaced nipples, ovarian dysgenesis with hypoplasia or absence of oogonia, primary amenorrhea, sexual infantilism, and sterility.[21] Congenital lymphedema with residual puffiness of the dorsum of the feet and of the fingers and toes (80%), anomalous ears, webbed posterior neck (50%), excessive numbers of pigmented nevi (50%), and cardiac defects (20%) are common (Box 5.13).

Developmental and behavioral concerns: most patients with Turner syndrome have normal intelligence; approximately 10% have substantial developmental delays, irrespective of karyotype. Nevertheless, approximately 70% have learning disabilities affecting non-verbal perceptual motor and visuospatial skills, more commonly in 45,X than in 45,X/46,XX.[264] **Imprinted genes on the X chromosome are postulated** to explain the **cognitive development** of Turner patients; if this were the case, the phenotype would depend on the **parental origin of the X chromosome.**[267–271] Loss of the Xp22.3 region appears to be associated with the neurocognitive anomalies of Turner syndrome.[264]

Skeletal anomalies include skeletal dysplasia with short stature, mild epiphyseal dysplasia, and typical bony alterations:

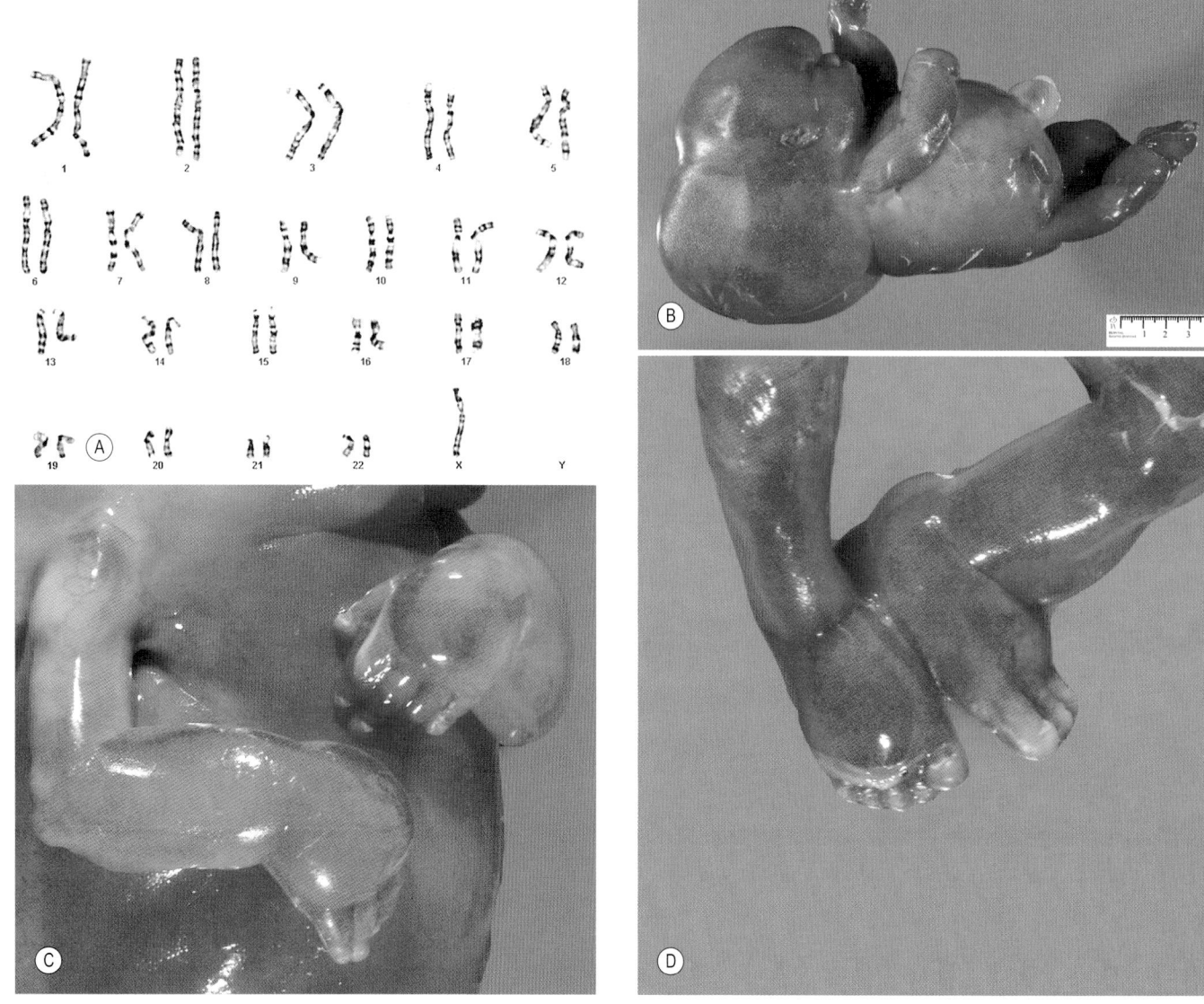

FIGURE 5.43 Monosomy X. (A) Turner patient with 45,X karyotype. (B) Fetus with Turner syndrome showing cystic hygroma of the neck. (C) and (D) In limbs, edema is characteristically most prominent on the dorsum of the hands and feet. [(A) Courtesy Dr Nicole Lemieux.]

malformation of the ulnar head leading to cubitus valgus (the typical increased 'carrying angle' of the arm) which may cause a limited range of motion, short fourth metacarpals, deformity of the medial tibial condyle, chondrodysplasia of the distal radial epiphysis (Madelung's deformity), osteoporosis with hypoplasia of the first cervical vertebra, and small carpal angle.[264, 272–274]

Congenital lymphedema is most likely to occur in **45,X. Cystic hygroma** (Fig. 5.43B) is common prenatally, and manifests postnatally as a **webbed neck**.[275] It has been suggested that the lymphedema results from the generalized hypoplasia and partial agenesis of the lymphatic system that ceases to extend peripherally at an early embryonic stage.[276] The **fetal hydrops** also explains the **widely spaced nipples** and **shield-chest. Edema of the hands and feet** (Figs 5.43C and D) due to lymphatic and venous malformations is present in the newborn, and may take years to resolve.[264, 277] Intestinal hemorrhage due to congenital

hemangiomas, venous ectasia, or telangiectasia has been reported.[278] Multiple telangiectasias of the intestinal wall may lead to anemia as a result of repeated gastrointestinal bleeding.[279]

Renal anomalies occur in 40–75% of cases; horseshoe kidney, double or clubbed renal pelvis, hypoplasia or hydronephrosis and bifid ureters, duplication of kidneys or ureters, unilateral renal agenesis with abnormalities of the contralateral kidney, and renal hypoplasia are most common.[280–286] Silent hydronephrosis resulting from obstruction of a duplicated segment occurs in 10%.[264] Micromulticystic renal disease is observed.[21]

Cardiovascular malformations are found in approximately 40% of Turner cases, with no clear genotype–phenotype correlation.[264, 287, 288] Congenital aortic valvular stenosis, partial anomalous pulmonary venous return,[287] dilation of the proximal aorta, and cystic medial necrosis of the aortic wall may occur with aortic rupture.[289] There are more than 80 reports of aortic

BOX 5.13 ABNORMALITIES OBSERVED IN TURNER SYNDROME

Infant
  Small for gestational age
  Lymphedema of dorsum of hands and feet
  Deep-set nails
  Excess skin on nape of neck (becomes pterygium colli later in life)
  Cystic hygroma

In childhood and adolescence
  Small stature
  Short, webbed neck
  Low posterior hairline
  Cubitus valgus
  Short fourth and fifth metacarpals (brachymetacarpia)
  Multiple nevi
  Hypoplastic, hyperconvex nails
  Tendency to keloid formation

Craniofacial dysmorphism
  Triangular face
  Antimongoloid slant of palpebral fissures
  Epicanthal folds
  Ptosis
  High-arched palate
  Hypoplasia of mandible, retrognathia
  Low-set ears

Thorax malformations
  Broad, shield-shaped chest
  Widely spaced, hypoplastic nipples

Gastrointestinal malformations
  Intestinal hemorrhage due to hemangiomas or telangiectasia

Genitourinary malformations
  Infantile female external genitalia
  Pubic hair scanty or absent
  Axillary hair absent
  Clitoral hypertrophy
  Streak gonads
  Hypoplastic, sometimes bifid uterus
  Failure of development of secondary sex characteristics
  Horseshoe kidney
  Double or clubbed renal pelvis
  Anomalies of renal rotation
  Hypoplasia or renal agenesis
  Hydronephrosis
  Bifid ureters
  Micromulticystic kidneys

  Membranoproliferative glomerulonephritis
  Gonadal malignancy if Y chromosomal component present

Cardiovascular malformations
  Coarctation of aorta
  Cystic medial necrosis of aorta
  Dissecting aneurysm
  Floppy mitral or aortic valves (myxoid degeneration)
  Aortic valvular stenosis

Central nervous system malformations
  Slight cortical dysplasia
  Gray matter heterotopia
  Hydrocephalus

Ocular malformations
  Severe myopia
  Congenital cataracts
  Congenital deafness

Skeletal malformations
  Low inner tibial plate, slightly slanted downward and inward and projecting beyond metaphysis (Kosowicz sign)
  Shortness of fourth and fifth metacarpals
  Raised semilunar carpal bones

Endocrine abnormalities
  Low serum levels of estrogens and pregnanediol; increased follicle stimulating hormone
  Low urine levels of 17-ketosteroids
  Hashimoto thyroiditis (autoimmune)

Non-gonadal neoplasms
  Ganglioneuroblastoma of adrenal
  Carcinoid tumor of cecum and appendix
  Multiple granular cell myoblastomas
  Medulloblastoma
  Cerebellar glioma
  Meningioma
  Melanoma
  Pituitary chromophobe adenoma
  Retroperitoneal mesenchymoma
  Thyroid carcinoma
  Anaplastic lung tumor
  Hibernoma
  Adenocarcinoma of endometrium
  Gastrointestinal adenocarcinoma (stomach and large bowel)
  Squamous cell carcinoma of vulva
  Acute myelogenous leukemia

dissection in Turner patients.[264] Some degree of coarctation of the aorta is an almost constant feature that can be identified in the fetus; other cardiovascular malformations include atrial septal defect, patent ductus arteriosus, transposition of the great arteries, and retroesophageal subclavian artery.[289, 290]

Gonadal dysgenesis is a cardinal feature of Turner syndrome. The gonads consist of long streaks of white, wavy, connective tissue stroma, generally without follicles, although follicles may be present in fetal and infantile ovaries.[290] **Hormone replacement** therapy is required in 90% of Turner patients to initiate puberty and complete growth.[264] Normal **gonadotropin levels** in the first 3–6 months of life suggests a residual ovarian function, but does not ensure that the initiation and progression of puberty will be normal. Spontaneous fertility is rare. **Gonadoblastomas** occur in the streak gonads of 7–30% of Turner patients with a cell population exhibiting a **mosaicism for the Y chromosome.** FISH analysis for a Y chromosome has been advocated for all girls with a 45,X karyotype, but clinical evidence indicates that such an approach is merited only in those with masculinization or a mosaicism for an unidentified marker chromosome.[264] **Prophylactic gonadectomy** is indicated if a Y chromosome is present.[264] PCR screening for Y-chromosome sequences is not recommended, as it yields a high false-positive rate.[264] The relative **risk of other cancers is not increased** in Turner syndrome.

Hypothyroidism occurs in 15–30% of patients; its onset is generally during adulthood, but 10–15% of cases occur prior to adolescence.[264] The majority of patients with Turner syndrome and **diabetes mellitus** develop the adult-onset type, and most are overweight.[264]

Clinically significant **strabismus** is found in 18%, **ptosis** in 13%, and the risk of **cataracts** and **nystagmus** is also increased.[264] The majority of children with Turner syndrome have **recurrent otitis media,** probably as a result of small dysfunctional eustachian tubes and palatal dysfunction.[264] **Sensorineural hearing loss** develops in 90% of adults.[264]

Gastrointestinal manifestations include feeding problems, gastroesophageal reflux, failure to thrive and celiac disease. In adults, Crohn disease, ulcerative colitis, and chronic diarrhea of unknown cause are increased, more commonly in association with an *i(Xq)* cell lineage.[264]

The placenta of monosomy X shows variable cellularity and stromal fibrosis of the chorionic villi with trophoblastic hypoplasia and deficient syncytial budding.

Other sex chromosome abnormalities

There are no consistent abnormalities in fetuses or newborns with **47,XXX** or **47,XXY** reported so far. The phenotype of **47,XYY** fetuses is normal, and these males eventually become normally fertile as the supernumerary Y is lost during meiosis.

47,XXX, 48,XXXX, and 49,XXXXX are associated with early puberty, premature menopause, and some decrease in IQ. In males and females, the severity of the mental retardation is proportional to the number of supernumerary X chromosomes.

Fragile X syndrome

Comprehensive and detailed collections of papers on fragile X syndrome have been published as special issues in the *American Journal of Medical Genetics.*[291, 292] Clinical and molecular aspects of this syndrome have also been reviewed. [293–295]

Fragile X syndrome (MIM 309550) is the most common form of inherited mental retardation in humans, with an estimated frequency of 1/4500 males,[295] and 1/9000 in females, who tend to exhibit a milder form of mental retardation. Fragile X syndrome segregates as an **X-linked dominant condition** with incomplete penetrance, since patients of either sex, when carrying the fragile X mutation, may exhibit mental deficiency to variable extent. Approximately 30% of carrier females are affected, and 20% of males carrying the fragile X chromosome are phenotypically normal but may transmit the disorder through their daughters. The sons of these daughters may develop fragile X syndrome, and the daughters of these daughters may have mental retardation.[296, 297] This transmission has been explained through the elucidation of the trinucleotide expansion which occurs in the meiosis of oogonia (reviewed in Ch. 1).

Fragile X syndrome typically presents with a combination of mental retardation with developmental and speech delay. Hyperactivity, short attention span, hand flapping, poor eye contact, and poor gross motor coordination are features that suggest autism. Hyperextensibility of joints, pes planus, mitral valve prolapse and mild aortic dilation suggest a mild connective tissue dysplasia. **Abnormal facial features** (Fig. 5.44A) include large, cupped, or protruding ears; head circumference greater than the 75th percentile; prominent jaw; long and narrow face; high-arched palate; flattened nasal bridge; hypertelorism; and epicanthal folds.[298] Large testes **(macroorchidism)** are common in young patients (Fig. 5.44B).

A characteristic dermatoglyphic pattern with an increased frequency of radial loops, whorls, and arches on the fingertips; a pronounced transverse course of the palmar ridges; a lower a-bridge count; and the absence of c-triradii, have been described.[299, 300]

Fragile X syndrome, as implied by the name, is associated with a fragile site (Fig. 5.45). This in vitro phenomenon appears as a break, a fraying or a gap in X chromosomes at position Xq27.3.[173] Verkerk and associates[296] reported the isolation of a cDNA from the region of the fragile X mutation. It was derived from a **gene denoted FMR-1** (*fragile X mental retardation-1*). This gene has been cloned and found to include a repeated sequence of cytosine-guanine-guanine (the **CGG trinucleotide repeat**) that causes the X chromosome to break in vitro when the expansion is greater than 200 repetitions.[301, 302] A 4.8 kb mRNA transcript from this gene was found in a variety of tissues, with brain tissue showing the highest level of expression. Additional results indicate that testis, uterus, and placenta all have similar high levels of the transcript. It has recently become apparent that patients with a **premutation** (between 55 and 200 CGG repeats) are at risk for developing mild **cognitive and/or behavioral deficits, premature ovarian failure,** and a neurodegenerative disorder, the **fragile-X-associated tremor/ataxia syndrome** (FXTAS).[303]

Cytogenetic diagnosis relies on the presence of the fragile site and depends on folic acid-deficient tissue culture medium. The development of this technique was historically important for three reasons: it allowed a specific diagnosis to be made in a mentally retarded male; chromosome studies of female relatives of the proband allowed detection of carriers of the fragile X chromosome who were at risk for a son with mental retardation; and chromosome studies of amniotic cells from pregnant carriers of

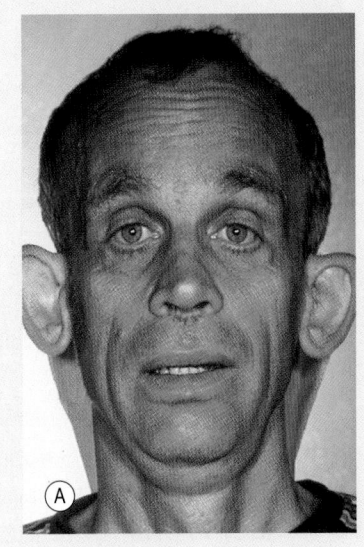

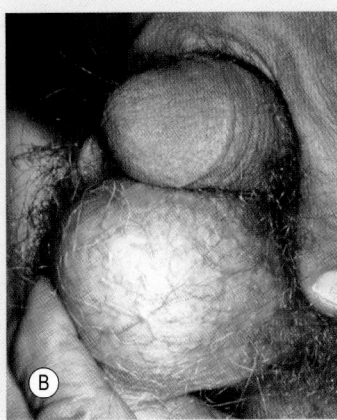

FIGURE 5.44 Fragile X. (A) Phenotype: large, floppy ears. (B) Macroorchidism. (Courtesy Dr Robert Gorlin.)

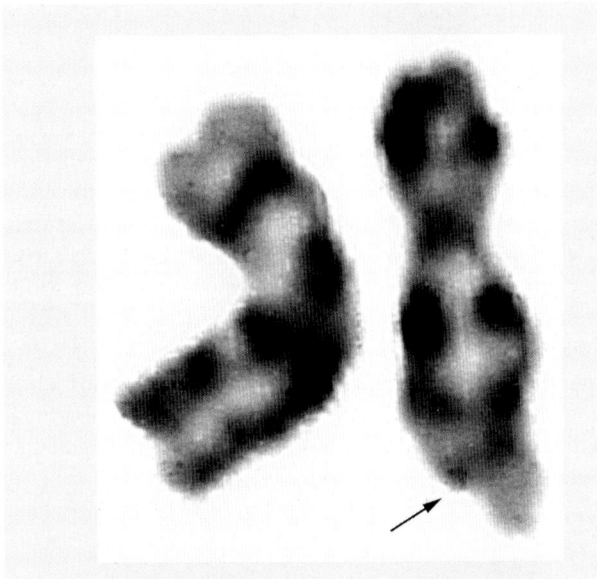

FIGURE 5.45 Fragile X with partial karyotype of the X chromosomes. The break at Xq27.3 is shown with an arrow. (Courtesy of Dr Nicole Lemieux.)

the fragile X could identify whether or not a male fetus carried the X chromosome bearing the mutation.[304] This test has proved unreliable, as it detects only about half of obligate carriers. Direct DNA analysis using PCR and/or Southern blotting is the gold standard, and has proven to be an extremely reliable method of diagnosis.[305] Fragile X testing should be considered for all children with developmental delay of unknown cause.[306, 307]

DNA methylation occurs through the attachment of a methyl group, -CH$_3$, to cytosines which are followed immediately by a guanine (CpG). This produces 5-methyl deoxycytidine, an alteration in DNA that plays a major role in the inhibition of gene expression, including X inactivation (see Ch. 1 for a review of epigenetic control of transcription). Thus, CpG islands can be perceived as on/off switches (depending on their methylation status) that control genes in their vicinity,[301, 302] and their methylation status can be detected through methyl-sensitive restriction enzymes. When CpG islands are not methylated, the CG sequences within them can be cleaved by these methyl-sensitive restriction enzymes (e.g. Eag1). When methylation of these sequences occurs, these methyl-sensitive restriction enzymes fail to recognize the methylated restriction site, and the DNA is thus not cleaved.

DNA-based analyses are considerably more accurate than cytogenetic screens for the diagnosis of the fragile X syndrome. Nevertheless, in the initial screening of patients with a phenotype suggestive of fragile X, cytogenetic analysis is indicated since as many patients will have the FMR1 mutation as will have a non-related cytogenetic anomaly. Southern blot and PCR-based assays are both routinely used to detect the FMR1 trinucleotide repeat mutation.[298] The **PCR** assay uses two primers which flank the repeating sequence (Figs 5.46 and 5.47). The molecular weight of the amplification product thus exactly reflects the number of times the CGG is repeated. Women have two alleles of the FMR1 gene; when these two alleles are of similar weight, they appear as a single band on the PCR assay. Women with a full mutation also often show only a single band, as the allele with more than 200 repetitions fails to amplify through the PCR technique. **Southern blotting** resolves this issue. DNA is cleaved with two restriction enzymes, with *Eco*R1 which yields a normal fragment of 5.2 kb containing the gene FMR1, and with the methyl-sensitive Eag1 which cleaves the unmethylated 5.2 kb fragment into a 2.8 kb segment containing FMR1 (Figs 5.48 and 5.49). Hence, normal men show a band of 2.8 kb, while normal women show two bands,

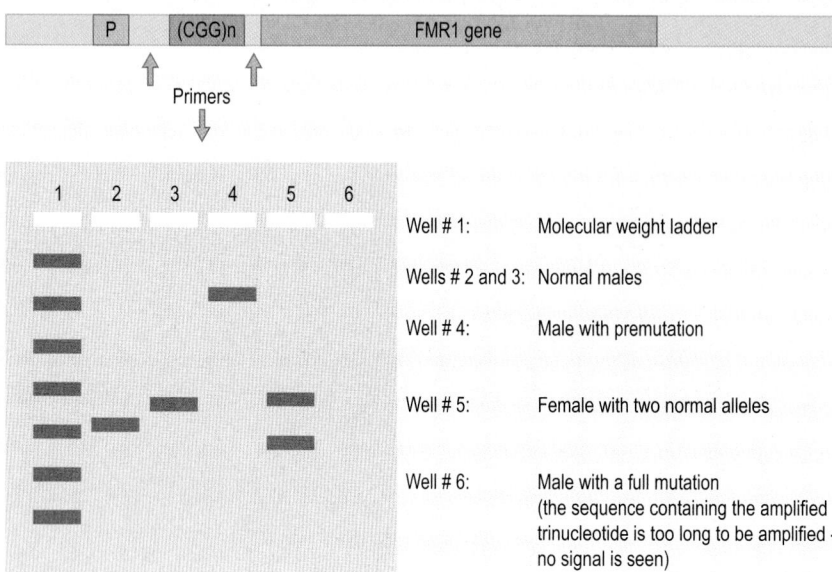

FIGURE 5.46 Diagrammatic representation of FMR1 gene, with its promoter and the intervening CGG trinucleotide repeated n times. The gene is amplified by PCR using primers flanking the trinucleotide repeat, and the length of the amplified segment is evaluated by gel electrophoresis, to calculate 'n'. Note that longer segments of DNA migrate shorter distances.

Well # 1:   Molecular weight ladder

Wells # 2 and 3: Normal males

Well # 4:   Male with premutation

Well # 5:   Female with two normal alleles

Well # 6:   Male with a full mutation
(the sequence containing the amplified trinucleotide is too long to be amplified – no signal is seen)

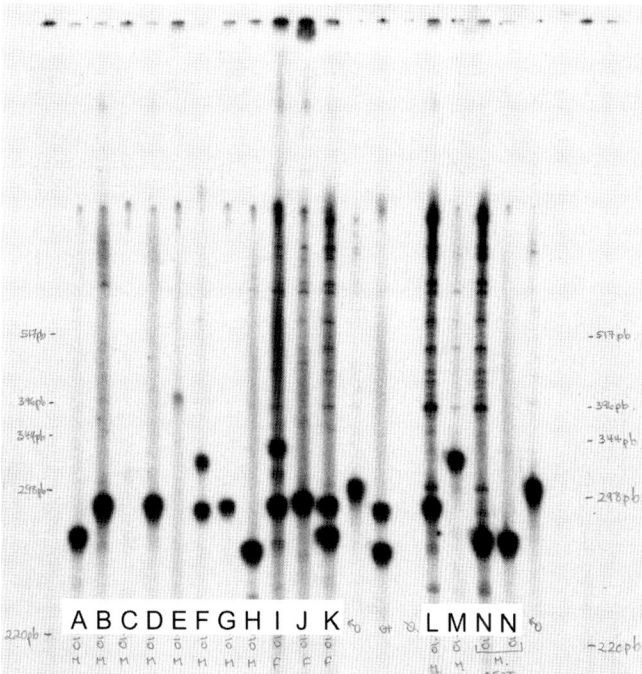

FIGURE 5.47 PCR determination of the number of CGG trinucleotide repeats. Patients A and B are normal males. Patient E (male) shows a premutation (which amplifies poorly). Patient F is phenotypically male, yet shows two bands; this finding was explained when his karyotype revealed that he has Klinefelter syndrome (47,XXY). Patients C (male) and J (female) show full mutations, the latter appearing as a thick band at the origin. Patient N, a normal male, was evaluated twice on the same gel.

of 2.8 kb and 5.2 kb corresponding respectively to the alleles on their active and inactive X chromosomes (respectively cleaved and non-cleaved by Eag1). Men with a premutation (i.e. with their CGG repeated more than 55 times but less than 200 times, and thus with essentially unmethylated CGGs) have a band larger than 2.8 kb, whereas men with a full mutation show a band larger than 5.2 kb. Women with a premutation can show up to four bands (2.8 kb and 5.2 kb corresponding to the normal alleles on the active and inactive Xs, and slightly larger than 2.8 kb and 5.2 kb corresponding to the premutated alleles). Women with a full mutation show three bands, of 2.8 kb, 5.2 kb and an abnormal band larger than 5.8 kb (i.e., with more than 600 nucleotides, or 200 trinucleotides, added to the mutated allele).

Imprinted chromosomes

Imprinting has been discussed in Chapter 1. **Imprinted domains** have been identified on chromosomes 1, 6, 7, 11, 14, 15, 18, 19, 20, and possibly also on chromosomes 13 and X. The chromosomal regions, along with the genes involved, are shown in Table 5.4.[308–310]

Neoplasia associated with chromosomal aberrations

Research originating in the 1980s has uncovered many of the molecular origins of neoplasia (see Chs 29 and 32). Of the

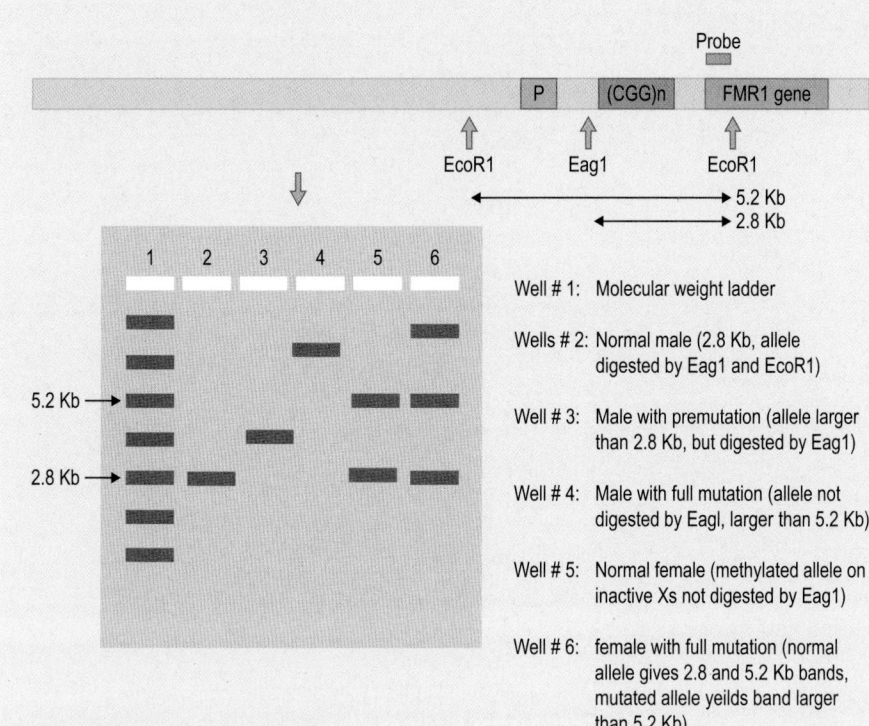

Well # 1: Molecular weight ladder

Wells # 2: Normal male (2.8 Kb, allele digested by Eag1 and EcoR1)

Well # 3: Male with premutation (allele larger than 2.8 Kb, but digested by Eag1)

Well # 4: Male with full mutation (allele not digested by EagI, larger than 5.2 Kb)

Well # 5: Normal female (methylated allele on inactive Xs not digested by Eag1)

Well # 6: female with full mutation (normal allele gives 2.8 and 5.2 Kb bands, mutated allele yeilds band larger than 5.2 Kb)

FIGURE 5.48 Diagrammatic representation of the Southern technique used in the diagnosis of fragile X. The DNA is digested by the restriction enzymes EcoR1 and Eag1. Normal males show a single band of 2.8 kb (lane 2). Males with a premutation do not methylate their gene, and thus show a band between 2.8 and 5.2 kb. Normal women have two X chromosomes, one active (cut by Eag1, giving rise to a 2.8 kb band), one inactive (methylated, and thus not cut by the methylation-sensitive Eag1, giving rise to a 5.2 kb band). Women with full mutations have half of their normal Xs active and half inactive (giving rise to the 2.8 and 5.2 kb bands, respectively), while all their mutated Xs are methylated, giving a band heavier than 5.2 kb.

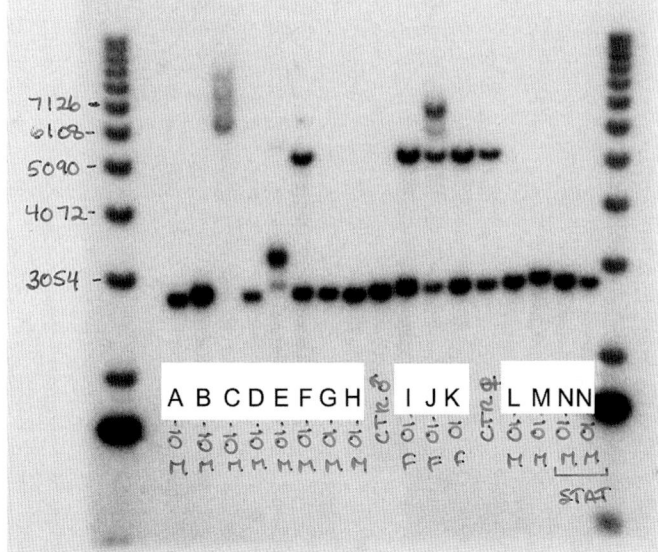

FIGURE 5.49 Evaluation of the FMR1 gene through Southern blotting (same patients as shown in Fig. 5.47). Patients A and B are examples of normal males, with a 2.8 kb allele. Patient C is a male with a full mutation; his band shows as a smear, ranging from 6.5 to more than 9 kb, as the CCG trinucleotide is unstable in mitosis, leading to the expansion of 'n' (from ~1200 to ~3000 repeats). Patient E has a premutation, with a light band of near-normal size corresponding to a portion of his cells having truncated the mutated CGG trinucleotide. Patient F (47,XXY) shows two bands, due to Lyonization. Patients I and K are normal females, with the 2.8 and 5.2 kb bands, while patient J is a female with a full mutation.

20 000–25 000 genes in the human genome, only about 50 can act as oncogenes/tumor suppressor genes.[311]

Cytogenetic studies have identified specific chromosomal changes as diagnostic and prognostic factors in hematologic malignancies and in solid tumors. Cytogenetic alterations identified in various neoplasias have been extensively cataloged.[312–317] Chromosomal changes in some pediatric hematologic malignancies and solid tumors are shown in Tables 5.5 and 5.6, and are of marked diagnostic and therapeutic importance.[315, 317–322] The fact that many chromosomal alterations found in pediatric tumors are tumor-specific has allowed the development of molecular-based diagnostic techniques, which are much more rapid and sensitive than their karyotype-based counterparts. For example, RT-PCR in conjunction with FISH is now routinely used in the diagnosis of rhabdomyosarcoma, Ewing sarcoma/peripheral primitive neuroectodermal tumor, Burkitt lymphoma, synovial sarcoma, gastrointestinal stromal tumor, desmoplastic small round blue cell tumor, myxoid liposarcoma, etc. Other tumor-specific translocations are more efficiently evaluated using FISH, especially when variant translocation partners exist; the FISH panels used at the CHU Sainte-Justine in the investigation of leukemias and lymphomas are shown in Tables 5.7 and 5.8. The quantification of N-MYC amplification in neuroblastoma is also efficiently assessed by FISH (Fig. 5.50).

Chromosomal abnormalities are very frequent in pediatric neoplasias, and lead to the activation of proto-oncogenes, or to the

TABLE 5.4 IMPRINTED CHROMOSOMAL REGIONS AND CORRESPONDING GENES

Chromosome band	Gene	Allele expressed	Name of protein or function
1p36	TP73	M	Tumor related protein
11p31	ARHI	P	Ras homolog
6q24	HYMAI	P	NT-RNA
6q24	PLAGL1	P	Zinc finger protein
7p12	GRB10	P/M (isoform dependent)	Growth factor receptor-bound protein
7q21	CALCR	M	Calcitonin receptor
7q21	SGCE	P	Sarcoglycan, epsilon
7q21	PEG10	P	Retroviral gag pol homologue
7q21	PPP1R9A	M	Protein phosphatase inhibitor
7q21	PON-1	P	Paraoxonase 1
7q21	PON2	M	Paraoxonase 2
7q21	PON3	M	Paraoxonase 3
7q21	ASB4	M	Ankyrin repeat and SOCS box
7q21	DLX5	M	Homeo box
7q32	CPA4	M	Carboxypeptidase
7q32	MEST	P	α/β hydrofold family
7q32	MESTIT1	P	MEST AS RNA, NT
7q32	COPG2IT1	P	COPG2 AS RNA, NT
7q32	COPG2	P	Coatomer protein complex subunit
11p15.5	H19	M	H19 RNA, NT
11p15.5	IGF2	P	Insulin-like growth factor 2
11p15.5	IGF2AS	P	IGF2 AS RNA, NT
11p15.5	INS2	P	Insulin
11p15.5	ASCL2?	P	HLH-type transcription factor
11p15.5	TRPM5?	P	Ca^{2+}-acivated cation channel
11p15.5	KCNQ1	M	Voltage-gated potassium channel
11p15.5	KCNQ1OT1	P	KCNQ1 AS RNA, NT
11p15.5	KCNQ1DN	M	BWRT protein
11p15.5	CDKN1C	M	Cyclin-dependent kinase inhibitor
11p15.5	SLC22A1LS?	M	SLC22A1LS putative protein
11p15.5	SLC22A18	M	Organic cation transporter
11p15.5	PHLDA2	M	Pleckstrin homology-like domain
11p15.5	OSBPL5	M	Oxysterol binding protein-like 5
11p15.5	ZNF215?	M	Zinc finger protein 215
11p13	WT1-ALT transcript	P	Wilms tumor 1 protein
11p13	WT1AS	P	WT1 AS RNA, NT
13q14	HTR2A	?M	Serotonin receptor
14q32	DLK1	P	RNA-UF
14q32	MEG3	M	RNA-UF
15q11	MKRN3	P	Makorin 3, a ring finger protein
15q11	MAGEL2	P	MAGE-like protein
15q11	NDN	P	Necdin, neuronal growth suppressor
15q11	SNURF	P	SNRPN upstream reading frame
15q11	SNRPN	P	Small nuclear ribonuclear protein
15q11	HBII-436	P	RNA-UF
15q11	HBII-13	P	RNA-UF
15q11	HBII-437	P	RNA-UF
15q11	HBII-438A	P	RNA-UF
15q11	HBII-438B	P	RNA-UF
15q11	HBII	P	RNA-UF
15q11	PWCR1	P	RNA-UF
15q11	UBE3A-AS	P	UBE3A, AS-RNA

TABLE 5.4 IMPRINTED CHROMOSOMAL REGIONS AND CORRESPONDING GENES (*CONT'D*)

Chromosome band	Gene	Allele expressed	Name of protein or function
15q11	UBE3A	M	Ubiquitin protein ligase
15q11	ATP10A	M	ATPase, class V
15q11	GABRB3	P	γ-aminobutyric acid receptor
15q11	GABRA5	P	γ-aminobutyric acid receptor
15q11	GABRG3	P	γ-aminobutyric acid receptor
18q21	x	M	Transcription elongation factor
19q13	PEG3	P	Zinc finger protein
19q13	ZIM2	P	Zinc finger protein
20q11	NNAT	P	Neurontin
20q13	L3MBTL	P	Polycomb group protein
20q13	GNAS / NESP55	M	Neuroendocrine secretory protein 55
20q13	GNAS / GNASXL	P	Large isoform of GS-α
20q13	GNAS / Exon-1A	P	RNA-UF
20q13	*GNAS /GS-α*	M	Stimulatory G-protein
20q13	*SANG*	P	GNAS AS RNA

Chromosome X neurocognitive genes postulated to exist

P, Paternal expression (maternal imprinting); M, maternal expression; ?P/?M, preferential paternal / maternal expression postulated, provisional data; NT-RNA, non-translated RNA; RNA-UF, RNA of unknown function; AS RNA, antisense RNA; NT, not translated.

After Morison et al 2005,[308] and other sources.[309, 310]

Updated information is available through internet sites dedicated to human imprinting.[309, 310]

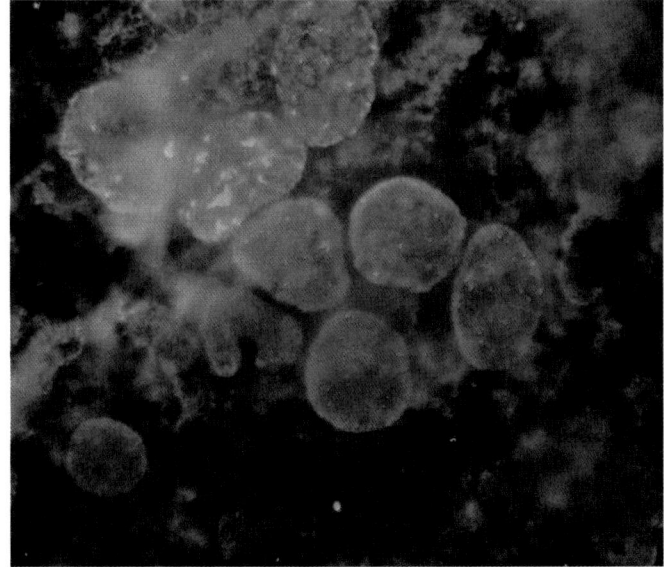

FIGURE 5.50 Determination of N-MYC status through FISH. Normal cells should have only two copies of the N-MYC gene. Each nuclei (blue spheres) from this neuroblastoma show multiple signals (in red), indicating that the N-MYC gene is amplified.

inactivation of tumor suppressor genes;[322–329] many chromosomal anomalies are consistently associated with specific types of human cancer (Tables 5.5 and 5.6).[324] Nevertheless, it is now appreciated that many cancers activate oncogenes and inhibit tumor sup-

pressor genes through epigenetic alterations.[330–333] A detailed discussion of tumor-specific cytogenetic alterations is beyond the scope of this chapter, and has been the topic of excellent reviews.[312–314, 321, 322, 325, 326]

The majority of lymphomas, AML and ALL are associated with chromosomal anomalies, many of which are tumor-specific.[312, 313, 315, 323] For example, inversion of chromosome 16 [inv(16)(p13q22)] is characteristic of **acute myelomonocytic leukemia** (AML-M4). Such specific chromosomal anomalies can be rapidly investigated with FISH analyses. Cytogenetic findings constitute the single most important prognostic factor of AML.[315]

In **Burkitt lymphoma** the human cellular c-myc oncogene, located on chromosome 8, becomes activated when rearranged with the normally-active promoter of the immunoglobulin heavy-chain gene of chromosome 14 or the immunoglobulin light-chain genes of chromosomes 2 and 22.[334–337] A translocation of chromosomes 8 and 14 or a variant form of this defect is present in 100% of cases of Burkitt lymphoma.[107, 327, 338]

In cells from **Ewing sarcoma,** two- and three-way reciprocal translocations always involve a break at band 22q12, most commonly resulting in the exchange of material between chromosomes 11 and 22 [t(11;22)(q24;q12)].[339, 340] This translocation is found in osseous, extraosseous Ewing and peripheral primitive neuroectodermal tumors. The karyotypes of **alveolar rhabdomyosarcomas** show a t(2,13)(q35;q14)[341, 342] or a t(1;13) (p36;q14).[342]

Cytogenetic analysis of **retinoblastomas** demonstrates deletions and rearrangements resulting in the loss of structural

TABLE 5.5 HEMATOLOGIC MALIGNANCIES ASSOCIATED WITH CHROMOSOMAL DEFECTS

Disease	Defects	Disease	Defects
Leukemias		B-cell non-Hodgkin lymphoma	t(3;11)(q27;q23.1)
Acute myeloid leukemias		Pre-B-cell ALL (L1)	*t(1;19)(q23;q12), [8][+4,+10,+17],
M1 (undifferentiated)	t(1;3)(p36;q21), t(3;v)(q26;v),		*t(1;4)(q23;q21), del(6q),
	t(1;6)(q23;q21), t(9;22)(q34;q11),		dic(7;9)(p11~13;p11), del(9p),
	+11, t(16;21)(p11;q22)		t(9;22)(q34;q11), t(11;19)(q23;p13),
M2 (with maturation)	t(1;17)(q23;q25) , +4,		der(12p), t(12;17)(p13;q21),
	t(6;9)(p21;q34), t(7;11)(p15;p15),		[8]t(12;21)(p12;q22),
	+8, †t(8;21)(q22;q22), +9,		t(14;22)(q32;q11), t(17;19)(q22;p13),
	t(9;22)(q34;q11), +11		−20, +21
M3 (promyelocytic)	t(11;17)(q23;q21),	Pro-B-cell ALL (L2)	dup(1)(q12~21q31~32),
	‡t(15;17)(q21;q1-q21)		*t(4;11)(q21;q23), del(6q), del(9p),
M4 (myelomonocytic)	t(1;3)p36;q21), t(1;7)(q10;p10),		i(9q), t (9;12)(p11~12;p11~13),
	t(1;17)(q23;q25), t(3;v)(q26;v),		t(9;22)(q34;q11), t(11;19)(q23;p13),
	+4, del(5q), t(6;9)(p21;q34),		t(17;19)(q22;p13), t(14;18)(q32;q21),
	t(6;11)(q27;q23), del(7q),		t(14;22)(q32;q11), +21
	+8, +9, +11, *11q23 anomalies,	B-cell ALL (L3)	dup(1)(q12~21q31~32),
	t(11;19)(q23;p13), +22		t(2;8)(p12;q24), t(8;14)(q24;q32),
M4Eo (M4 with eosinophilia)	t(1;12)(q25;p13), inv(16)(p13;q22),		t(8;22)(q24;q11),
	t(16;16)(p13;q22), del(16)(q22)		t(9;12)(p11~12;p11~13),
M5 (monocytic)	t(1;17)(q23;q25), t(6;11)(q27;q23),		t(14;18)(q32;q21)
	+8, t(8;16)(p11;p13), t(8;22)	B-cell ALL, any type	+8
	(p11;q13), +9, *t(9;11)(p21~22;q23),	T-cell ALL	t(1;11)(p32;q23), t(1;7)(p32;q34),
	t(10;11)(p11~15;q23), 11q23		t(1;7)(p34;q34),
	anomalies, t(11;19)(q23;p13)		t(1;14)(p32~34;q11), del(6q),
M6 (erythroleukemia)	t(3;5)(q21~25;q31~35),		t(7;9)(q34~36;q34),
	t(3;v)(q26;v), del(5q), del(7q)		t(7;9)(q34;q32),
M7 (megakaryoblastic)	t(1;22)(p13;q13),		t(7;10)(q34~36;q24),
AML, no FAB preference	t(1;11)(q23;p15), t(2;11)(q31;p15),		t(7;11)(q34~36;p13),
	t(3;21)(q26;q22), −5/del(5q),		t(7;19)(q35;p13), +8,
	t(5;14)(q33;q32) , −7/del(7q),		t(8;14)(q24;q11), del(9p),
	del(9q), del(12p), +13,		t(10;11)(p13~14;q14~21),
	t(16;21)(p11;q22), i(17)(q10),		t(10;14)(q24;q11), t(11;14)(p15;q11),
	del(20q), +21, −Y		t(11;14)(p13;q11), der(12p)
Other myeloid dysplasias and leukemias		CLL	del(6q), del(8q), del(11q), +12,
Myelodysplasia	t(3;21)(q26;q22), −7		del(13q), del(17p)
Refractory anemia with excess blasts	−7	**Pediatric non-Hodgkin lymphomas (excluding lymphoblastic lymphomas)**	
Chronic myelogenous leukemia, blast crisis	t(3;21)(q26;q22)	Diffuse large cell	t(2;3)(p12;q27), t(3;14)(q27;q32),
Chronic myelomonocytic leukemia	t(5;12)(q33;p13), t(1;7)(p15;p15),		t(3;22)(q27;q11)
Chronic myelogenous leukemia, adult type	t(9;22)(q34;q11)	Ki-1 (anaplastic large cell)	t(2;5)(p23;q35)
Chronic myelogenous leukemia, juvenile type	Normal, −7		
Acute lymphoblastic leukemias (ALL)			
B-cell ALL / Burkitt lymphoma	t(8;14)(q24;q32), t(2;8)(p12;q24), t(8;22)(q24;q11)		

Table prepared from multiple sources including Sandberg 1994,[318] Kalwinsky et al 1990,[319] Schneider 1993,[320] Ravindranath et al 2005,[315] Chessells et al 2002,[316] Heim and Mitelman 2004,[313] Pizzo and Poplack 2004.[321]

* Indicates variable translocation partners; † indicates poor prognostic factor;
‡ indicates favorable prognostic factor.
CML, Chronic myelocytic leukemia; CLL, Chronic lymphocytic leukemia.

TABLE 5.6 CHROMOSOMAL ABNORMALITIES FOUND IN SOLID TUMORS

Solid tumors	Chromosomal abnormality	Affected gene(s)
Medulloblastoma	del(10q), −11, del(17p)/i(17)(q10)	
Retinoblastoma	del(13)(q14)	RB
Neuroblastoma	del(1p)(p32;p36)*	N-MYC amplification*
Malignant rhabdoid tumor (kidney, CNS and extrarenal sites)	der(22)(q11.2)	SNF5/INI1
Brain	Monosomy 22	
Liver	del(3)(q21)	
Extrarenal	t(8;15)(q12;p11)	
Renal	del(13)(q14)	
Testicular germ cell tumor	i(12p)	
Wilms tumor	del(11)(p13)	WT1
	der(11)(p15)	IGF2 and others
Malignant melanoma of soft parts	t(12;22)(q13;q12)	EWS-ATF1
	DSRCT	t(11;22)(p13;q12)
	EWS-WT1	
Small round cell sarcoma	inv(22q)	EWS-ZSG
Ewing sarcoma/PPNET	t(11;22)(q24;q12)	EWS-FLI1
	t(21;22)(q22;q12)	EWS-ERG
	t(7;22)(p22;q12)	EWS-ETV1
	t(17;22)(q12;q12)	EWS-E1AF
	t(2;22)(q33;q12)	EWS-FEV1
Congenital fibrosarcoma/ mesoblastic nephroma	t(12;15)(p13;q25)	ETV6-NTRK3
	DFSP t(17;22)(q22;q13)	COL1A1-PDGFB
Alveolar rhabdomyosarcoma	t(1;13)(p36;q14)	PAX7-FKHR
	t(2;13)(q35;q14)	PAX3-FKHR
Synovial sarcoma	t(X;18)(p11;q11)	SYT-SSX1
	t(X;18)(p11;q11)	SYT-SSX2
Extraskeletal myxoid chondrosarcoma	t(9;22)(q22;q12)	EWS-CHN
Myxoid liposarcoma	t(12;16)(q13;p11)	TLS/FUS-CHOP
	t(12;22)(q13;q12)	EWS-CHOP
Liposarcoma	t(12;16)(q13;p11)	

DSRCT, Desmoplastic small round cell tumor; DFSP, dermatofibrosarcoma protuberans; *indicates a poor prognostic factor.

material from band 13q14, involving the gene Rb.[343, 344] This has been reported in cases of unilateral and bilateral tumors; the former is usually sporadic, and the latter is always heritable. It has also been reported in patients who carry deletions of 13q14 in somatic and tumor cells (constitutional 13q deletion syndrome).

Wilms tumor has been seen in association with aniridia (**WAGR syndrome,** MIM 194072, comprising Wilms tumor, Aniridia, Genitourinary anomalies, mental Retardation) in patients who carry constitutional deletions of 11p11-p13.[344]

Cytogenetic studies of *meningiomas* show the loss of one chromosome 22 in 70% of cases. In almost half of these cases with monosomy 22, other chromosomes are also missing.[345] The cytogenetic findings of 109 pediatric central nervous system tumors of various types have been reviewed.[346]

Dedication

Dr Oligny wishes to dedicate this chapter to Caroline Mangerel.

Acknowledgements

Dr Oligny wishes to thank Drs Nicole Lemieux and Raouf Fetni, as well as Fléchère Fortin, Sophie Dubé, and Mélanie Beaulieu for their insightful review of this manuscript, and Diane Lachance for assistance with the obtention karyotypes. The outstanding assistance of Mr Stéphane Dedelis, medical photographer at CHU Sainte-Justine, is gratefully acknowledged.

TABLE 5.7 FISH PANELS FOR THE INVESTIGATION OF LEUKEMIAS

Acute lymphoblastic leukemia

t(12;21)(p13;q22)	TEL/AML1	12p13/21q22
t(9;22)(q34;q11.2)	BCR/ABL	22q11.2/9q34
t(11q23)	MLL	11q23
+4	D4	4p11.1-q11.1
+10	D10	10p11.1-q11.1
+17	D17Z1	17p11.1-q11.1

Acute myeloid leukemia

M2 t(8;21)(q22;q22)	ETO/AML1	8q22 /21q22
M3 t(15;17)(q22;q21)	PML/RARA	15q22 /17q21.1
t(17q21.1)	RARA	17q21.1
M4 inv(16)(p13q22)	CBFB	16q22
t(11q23) MLL 11q23		
+ 8 D8Z2 8p11.1-q11.1		

Chronic lymphocytic leukemia panel

+12	D12Z3	12p11.1-q11.1
del(13q14)	D13S319	13q14.3
del(11q22.3)	ATM	11q22.3
del(17p13)	P5317	p13.1

Chronic myeloid leukemia

t(9;22)(q34;q11.2)	BCR/ABL	22q11.2/9q34

Multiple myeloma

del(13q14)	D13S319	13q14.3
t(14q32)	IGH	14q32
t(11;14)(q13;q32)	CCND1 / IGH	11q13/14q32

Myelodysplastic syndromes

−7/7q	D7Z1	7p11.1-q11.1
	D7S486	7q31
−5/5q-	D5S721/D5S23	5p15.2
	EGR1	5q31
20q-	D20S109	20q12

Table courtesy of Dr Raouf Fetni

TABLE 5.8 FISH PANELS FOR THE INVESTIGATION OF LYMPHOMAS

Anaplastic large cell lymphoma

t(2p23)	ALK	2p23

Burkitt lymphoma

t(8q24)	CMYC	8q24

Diffuse large cell lymphoma

t(3q27)	BCL6	3q27

Follicular lymphoma

t(14;18)(q32;q21)	IGH/BCL2	14q32/18q21

MALT lymphoma

t(11;18)	MALT1	18q21

Mantle cell lymphoma

t(11;14)(q13;q32)	CCND1 / IGH	11q13/14q32

Non-Hodgkin lymphoma

t(14q32)	IGH	14q32

Table courtesy of Dr Raouf Fetni

References

Terminology and techniques

1. Boué A, Thibault CD, eds. Les accidents chromosomiques de la reproduction. Paris: Inserm1973; 29.
2. Boué J, Philippe E, Giroud A, et al. Phenotypic expression of lethal chromosome anomalies in human abortuses. Teratology 1976; 14:3–19.
3. Jacobs PA. Epidemiology of chromosome abnormalities in man. Am J Epidemiol 1977; 105:180–191.
4. Boué J, Boué A, Lazar P. Retrospective and prospective epidemiological studies of 1500 karyotyped spontaneous human abortions. Teratology 1975; 12:11–26.
5. Witschi E. Teratogenic effects from overripeness of the egg. In: Fraser FC, McKusick VA, eds. Congenital malformations. New York: Excerpta Medica; 1970; 157–169.
6. Creasy MR, Crolla JA. Prenatal mortality of trisomy 21 (Down syndrome). Lancet 1974; 1:473–474.
7. Gustavson KH, Hagberg B, Hagberg G, et al. Severe mental retardation in a Swedish county. I. Epidemiology, gestational age, birth weight, and associated CNS handicaps in children born 1959-1970. Acta Pediatr Scand 1977; 66:373–379.
8. Gustavson KH, Hagberg B, Hagberg G. Severe mental retardation in a Swedish County. II. Etiologic and pathogenetic aspects of children born 1959–1970. Neuropaediatrie 1977; 8:293–304.
9. Machin GA, Crolla JA. Chromosome constitution of 500 infants dying during the perinatal period. Hum Genet 1974; 23:183–198.
10. Jacobs PA, Aitken J, Frackiewicz A, et al. The inheritance of translocations in man: data from families ascertained through a balanced heterozygote. Ann Hum Genet 1970; 34:119–136.
11. ISCN. An international system for human cytogenetic nomenclature. Cytogenet Cell Genet 1978; 21:309–409.
12. Francke U, Oliver N. Quantitative analysis of high resolution Trypsin-Giemsa bands of human prometaphase chromosomes. Hum Genet 1978; 45:137–165.
13. Yunis JJ. Nomenclature for high resolution human chromosomes. Cancer Genet Cytogenet 1980; 2:221.
14. Yunis JJ. New chromosomal syndromes. New York: Academic Press; 1977.
15. Zellweger H, Simpson J. Chromosomes of man. Philadelphia: JB Lippincott; 1977.
16. de Grouchy JD, Turleau C. Clinical atlas of human chromosomes. New York: John Wiley; 1984.
17. Schinzel A. Catalogue of unbalanced chromosome aberrations in man. 2nd edn. New York: Walter de Gruyter; 2001.
18. McKinlay Gardner RJ, Sutherland GR. Chromosome abnormalities and genetic counseling. 3rd edn. Oxford: Oxford University Press; 2004.
19. Borgaonkar DS. Chromosomal variation in man. A catalog of chromosomal variants and anomalies. 8th edn. New York: Alan R Liss; 1997.
20. Pai GS, Lewandowski RC, Borgaonkar DS. Handbook of chromosomal syndromes. New York: John Wiley; 2003.
21. Gilbert EF, Opitz JM. Developmental and other pathologic changes in syndromes caused by chromosome abnormalities. Perspect Pediatr Pathol 1982; 7:1–63.
22. Gilbert LA, Dudley AW, Meisner L, et al. New neuropathological findings in trisomy 13. Arch Pathol Lab Med 1977; 101:540–544.
23. Opitz JM, Ceizel A, Fraus JA. Nosologic grouping in birth defects. In: Vogel F, Sperling V, eds. Proceedings of the VII International Congress on Human Genetics, Berlin, 1988. Springer-Verlag; 1988; 382–385.
24. Sullivan BA, Leana-Cox J, Schwartz S. Clarification of subtle reciprocal rearrangements using fluorescence in situ hybridization. Am J Med Genet 1993; 47:223–230.
25. Luquet I, Mugneret F, Athis PD, et al. French multi-centric study of 2000 amniotic fluid interphase FISH analyses from high-risk pregnancies and review of the literature. Ann Genet 2002; 45:77–88.
26. Baart EB, Martini E, Van Opstal D. Screening for aneuploidies of ten different chromosomes in two rounds of FISH: a short and reliable protocol. Prenat Diagn 2004; 24:955–961.

27. Locatelli A, Mariani S, Ciriello E, et al. Role of FISH on uncultured amniocytes for the diagnosis of aneuploidies in the presence of fetal anomalies. Fetal Diagn Ther 2005; 20:1–4.

28. Gadji M, Krabchi K, Drouin R. Simultaneous identification of chromosomes 18, X and Y in uncultured amniocytes by using multi-primed in situ labelling technique. Clin Genet 2005; 68:15–22.

29. Coullin P, Roy L, Pellestor F, et al. PRINS, the other in situ DNA labelling method useful in cellular biology. Am J Med Genet 2002; 107:127–135.

30. Mennicke K, Yang J, Hinrichs F, et al. Validation of primed in situ labelling for interphase analysis of chromosomes 18, X, and Y in uncultured amniocytes. Fetal Diagn Ther 2003; 18:114–121.

31. Roberts AE, Cox GF, Kimonis V, et al. Clinical presentation of 13 patients with subtelomeric rearrangements and a review of the literature. Am J Med Genet A 2004; 128:352–363.

32. Walter S, Sandig K, Hinkel GK, et al. Subtelomere FISH in 50 children with mental retardation and minor anomalies, identified by a checklist, detects rearrangements including a de novo balanced translocation of chromosomes 17p13.3 and 20q13.33. Am J Med Genet A 2004; 128:364–373.

33. Sogaard M, Tumer Z, Hjalgrim H, et al. Subtelomeric study of 132 patients with mental retardation reveals 9 chromosomal anomalies and contributes to the delineation of submicroscopic deletions of 1pter, 2qter, 4pter, 5qter and 9qter. BMC Med Genet 2005; 6:21–31.

34. Rooms L, Reyniers E, Kooy RF. Subtelomeric rearrangements in the mentally retarded: a comparison of detection methods. Hum Mutat 2005; 25:513–524.

35. Belaud-Rotureau MA, Elghezal H, Bernardin C, et al. Le caryotype spectral (SKY): principe, avantages et limites en cytogénétique constitutionnelle et tumorale. Ann Biol Clin (Paris) 2003; 61:139–146.

36. Bayani JM, Squire JA. Application of SKY in cancer cytogenetics. Cancer Invest 2002; 20:373–386.

37. Knutsen T, Gobu V, Knaus R, et al. The interactive Online SKY/M-FISH & CGH database and the Entrez cancer chromosomes search database: linkage of chromosomal aberrations with the genome sequence. Genes Chromosomes Cancer 2005; 44:52–64.

38. http://www.ncbi.nlm.nih.gov/entrez/query.fcgi?CMD=search&DB=cancerchromosomes

39. Gebhart E. Comparative genomic hybridization (CGH): ten years of substantial progress in human solid tumor molecular cytogenetics. Cytogenet Genome Res 2004; 104:352–358.

40. Pinkel D, Albertson DG. Array comparative genomic hybridization and its application in cancer. Nat Genet 2005; 37 (suppl):S11–S17.

41. van Steensel B. Mapping of genetic and epigenetic regulatory networks using microarrays. Nat Genet 37 2005; (suppl):S18–S24.

42. Wheeler DB, Carpenter AE, Sabatini DM. Cell microarrays and RNA interference chip away at gene function. Nat Genet 2005; 37 (suppl): S25–S30.

43. Segal E, Friedman N, Kaminski N, et al. From signatures to models: understanding cancer using microarrays. Nat Genet 2005; 37 (suppl): S38–S45.

44. Speicher MR, Carter NP. The new cytogenetics: blurring the boundaries with molecular biology. Nat Rev Genet 2005; 6:782–792.

45. Nussbaum R, McInnes R, Willard H, eds.Thompson & Thompson's Genetics in Medicine Revised reprint, 6th edn. Philadelphia: Saunders; 2004.

46. Pasternak JJ. An introduction to human molecular genetics: mechanisms of inherited diseases. 2nd edn. New York: John Wiley; 2005.

47. http://web.indstate.edu/thcme/mwking/molecular-medicine.html

48. http://www.uni-koeln.de/math-nat-fak/biochemie/klein/material/MolBio.pdf

49. Dudarewicz L, Holzgreve W, Jeziorowska A, et al. Molecular methods for rapid detection of aneuploidy. J Appl Genet 2005; 46:207–215.

Minor anomalies and mild malformations

50. Barash BA, Freedman L, Opitz JM. Anatomic studies in the 18-trisomy syndrome. Birth Defects 1970; 6:3–15.

Chromosomal anomalies

51. Rosenbusch B. The incidence of aneuploidy in human oocytes assessed by conventional cytogenetic analysis. Hereditas 2004; 41:97–105.

52. Stene J, Stengel-Rutkowski S. Genetic risks of familial reciprocal and robertsonian translocation carriers. In: The cytogenetics of mammalian autosomal rearrangements. A Daniel, ed. New York: Alan R Liss; 1988:3–72.

53. Sampson JE, Ouhibi N, Lawce H, et al. The role for preimplantation genetic diagnosis in balanced translocation carriers. Am J Obst Gynecol 2004; 190:1707–1711.

54. Shaw EB, Steinback HL. Aminopterin-induced fetal malformation. Survival of infant after attempted abortion. Am J Dis Child 1968; 115:477–482.

55. Bersu ET. Anatomical analysis of the developmental effects of aneuploidy in man: the Down syndrome. Am J Med Genet 1980; 5:399–420.

Structural chromosomal abnormalities

56. Shaffer LG, Tommerup N. ISCN 2005 – An international system for human cytogenetic nomenclature (1995). Basel: S. Karger; 2005.

57. Zackai EH, Emmanuel BS. Site-specific reciprocal translocation, t(11;22) (q23;q11), in several unrelated families with 3:1 meiotic disjunction. Am J Med Genet 1980; 7:507–521.

58. Zatz M, Vianna-Morgenta AM, Campos P, et al. Translocation (X;6) in a female with Duchenne muscular dystrophy; implications for the localization of the DMD locus. J Med Genet 1981; 18:442–447.

59. Machin GA. The causes of malformations. In: Wigglesworth JS, Singer DB, eds. Textbook of fetal and perinatal pathology. Vol I. Oxford: Blackwell Scientific; 1991:307–338.

Chromosomal mosaicism

60. Kalousek DK, Dill FJ. Chromosomal mosaicism confined to the placenta in human conceptions. Science 1983; 221:665–667.

61. Tyson RW, Kalousek DK. Chromosomal abnormalities in stillbirth and neonatal death. In: Dimmick JE, Kalousek DK, eds. Developmental pathology of the embryo and fetus. Philadelphia: JB Lippincott; 1992:83–110.

Abnormalities of chromosome 21

62. Hamerton JL. Fetal sex. Lancet 1970; 1:516–517.

63. Trimble BK, Baird PA. Maternal age and Down syndrome: age-specified incidence rates by single-year intervals. Am J Med Genet 1978; 2:1–5.

64. Erickson JD, Bjerkedal T. Down syndrome associated with father's age in Norway. J Med Genet 1981; 18:22–28.

65. Hook EB. Unbalanced robertsonian translocations associated with Down's syndrome or Patau's syndrome: chromosome subtype, proportion inherited, mutation rates, and sex ratio. Hum Genet 1981; 59:235–239.

66. Stene J, Stene E, Stengen-Rutkowski S, et al. Paternal age and Down's syndrome. Data from prenatal diagnoses (DFG). Hum Genet 1981; 59:119–124.

67. Andrle M, Fiedler W, Rett A, et al. A case of trisomy 22 in *Pongo pygmaeus*. Cytogenet Cell Genet 1979; 24:1-6.

68. McClure HM. Features of Down's-like syndrome in a chimpanzee. Am J Pathol 1972; 67:413–417.

69. Turleau C, DeGrouchy J, Klein M. Phylogenie chromosomique de l'homme et des primates hominiens (*Pan troglodytes, Gorilla gorilla*, et *Pongo pygmaeus*): essai de reconstitution du caryotype de l'ancêtre commun. Ann Genet 1972; 15:225–240.

70. Lister TJ, Frota-Pessoa O. Recurrence risk for Down syndrome. Hum Genet 1980; 55:203–208.

71. Sheridan R, Llerena J, Matkins SS, et al. Fertility in a male with trisomy 21. J Med Genet 1989; 55:294–298.

72. Hall B. Mongolism in newborn infants. An examination of the criteria for recognition and some speculations on the pathogenetic activity of the chromosomal abnormality. Clin Pediatr 1966; 5:4–12.

73. Penrosel S. Memorandum on dermatoglyphic nomenclature. Birth Defects 1968; 4:1–13.

74. Reed T, Christian JC. A comparison of the dermatogram with other indices for the diagnosis of Down's syndrome. Clin Genet 1976; 10:139–144.

75. Zellweger H, Schochet S Jr, et al. Handbook of clinical neurology. Amsterdam: Elsevier/North Holland; 1977.

76. Jones KL. Smith's recognizable patterns of malformation syndromes. Philadelphia: WB Saunders; 1988:673.

77. Greenwood RD, Nadas AS. The clinical course of cardiac disease in Down's syndrome. Pediatrics 1976; 58:893–897.

78. Chi TPL, Krovetz LJ. The pulmonary vascular bed in children with Down syndrome. J Pediatr 1975; 86:533–538.

79. Kojima S, Matsuyama T, Sato T, et al. Down's syndrome and acute leukemia in children: an analysis of phenotype by use of monoclonal antibodies and electron microscopic platelet peroxidase reaction. Blood 1990; 76:2348–2353.

80. Hitzler JK, Zipursky A. Origins of leukemia in children with Down syndrome. Nat Rev Cancer 2005; 5:11–20.

81. Hasle H. Pattern of malignant disorders in individuals with Down's syndrome. Lancet Oncol 2001; 2:429–436.

82. de Alarcon PA, Patil S, Golberg J, et al. Infants with Down's syndrome: use of cytogenetic studies and in vitro colony assay for granulocyte progenitor to distinguish acute nonlymphocytic leukemia from a transient myeloproliferative disorder. Cancer 1987; 60:987–993.

83. Zipursky A, Peeters M, Poon A. Megakaryoblastic leukemia and Down's syndrome – a review. In: Oncology and immunology of Down syndrome. New York: Alan R Liss; 1987:33–56.

84. Litz CE, Davies S, Brunning RD. Morphologic and biologic features of the transient myeloproliferative syndrome in Down's syndrome. Mod Pathol 1993; 6:545A.

85. Massey GV. Transient leukemia in newborns with Down syndrome. Pediatr Blood Cancer 2005; 44:29–32.

86. Miyauchi J, Ito Y, Kawano T, et al. Unusual diffuse liver fibrosis accompanying transient myeloproliferative disorder in Down's syndrome: a report of four autopsy cases and proposal of a hypothesis. Blood 1992; 80:1521–1527.

87. Brichard B, Vermylen C, De Potter P, et al. Down syndrome: possible predisposition to retinoblastoma. Med Pediatr Oncol 2003; 41:73–74.

88. Solitaire GB. The spinal cord of the mongol. J Ment Defic Res 1969; 13:1–7.

89. Colon EJ. The structure of the cerebral cortex in Down syndrome. Neuropaediatrie 1972; 3:362–376.

90. Menéndez M. Down syndrome, Alzheimer's disease and seizures. Brain Dev 2005; 27:246–252.

91. Schupf N. Genetic and host factors for dementia in Down's syndrome. Br J Psychiatry 2002; 180:405–410.

92. Heston LL, Mastri AR. The genetics of Alzheimer's disease: associations with hematologic malignancy and Down's syndrome. Arch Gen Psychiatry 1977; 34:976–981.

93. Heston LL, Mastri AR, Anderson VE, et al. Dementia of the Alzheimer type: clinical genetics, natural history, and associated conditions. Arch Gen Psychiatry 1981; 38:1085–1090.

94. Heyman A, Wilkinson W, Hurwitz B, et al. Alzheimer's disease: genetic aspects and associated clinical disorders. Ann Neurol 1983; 14:507–515.

95. Wisniewski K, Dambska M, Jenkins EC, et al. Monosomy 21 syndrome: further delineation, including clinical, neuropathological, cytogenetic and biochemical studies. Clin Genet 1983; 23:102–110.

96. Pellissier MC, Phillip N, Voelckel-Baeteman MA, et al. Monosomy 21: a new case confirmed by in situ hybridization. Hum Genet 1987; 75:95–96.

Abnormalities of chromosome 13

97. Patau K, Smith DW, Therman E, et al. Multiple congenital anomaly caused by an extra chromosome. Lancet 1960; 1:790–793.

98. Jones KL, Smith DW. Smith's recognizable patterns of human malformation. 6th edn. Philadelphia: Elsevier; 2005.

99. Nielsen J, Sillesen J. Incidence of chromosome aberrations among 11148 newborn children. Hum Genet 1975; 30:1–12.

100. Marden PM, Yunis JJ. Trisomy D1 in a 10-year-old girl: normal neutrophils and fetal hemoglobin. Am J Dis Child 1967; 114:662–664.

101. Redheendran R, Neu RL, Bannerman RM. Long survival in trisomy-13 syndrome: 21 cases including prolonged survival in two patients 11 and 19 years old. Am J Med Genet 1981; 8:167–172.

102. Warkany J, Passarge E, Smith LD. Congenital malformations in autosomal trisomy syndromes. Am J Dis Child 1966; 112:502–517.

103. Pettersen JC, Koltis GG, White MF. An examination of the spectrum of anatomic defects and variations found in eight cases of trisomy 13. Am J Med Genet 1979; 3:183–210.

104. Marin-Padilla M, Hoefnagel D, Benirschke K. Anatomic and histopathologic study of two cases of D1(13-15) trisomy. Cytogenetics 1964; 48:258–284.

105. Nevin NC, Dodge JA, Allen IV. Two cases of trisomy D associated with adrenal tumors. J Med Genet 1972; 9:119–122.

106. Toews H, Jones HW. Cyclopia in association with D trisomy and gonadal agenesis. Am J Obstet Gynecol 1968; 102:53–56.

107. Egli F, Stalder G. Malformations of kidney and urinary tract in common chromosomal aberrations. Hum Genet 1973; 18:1–15.

108. Gilbert E, Opitz J. Renal involvement in genetic-hereditary malformation syndromes. In: Hamburger J, Crosnier J, Grunfeld JP, eds. Nephrology. New York: John Wiley; 1979:909–944.

109. Keshgegian AA, Chatten J. Nodular renal blastema in trisomy 13. Arch Pathol Lab Med 1979; 103:73–75.

110. Townes PL, Dehart GK Jr, Hecht F, et al. Trisomy 13-15 in a male infant. J Pediatr 1962; 60:528–532.

111. Huehns ER, Lutzner M, Hecht F. Nuclear abnormalities of the neutrophils in D1(13-15) trisomy syndrome. Lancet 1964; 13:589–590.

112. Powars D, Rohde R, Graves D. Foetal hemoglobin and neutrophil anomaly in the D1 trisomy syndrome. Lancet 1964; 18:1363–1364.

113. Walzer S, Gerald PS, Breau G, et al. Hematologic changes in the D1 trisomy syndrome. Pediatrics 1966; 38:419–429.

114. Schade H, Scheller L, Schultze KW. D-Trisomie (Patau-Syndrom) mit kongenitaler myeloider Leukaemie. Med Welt 1962; 50:2690–2692.

115. Zuelzer WW, Thompson RI, Mastrangelo R. Evidence for a genetic factor related to leukemogenesis and congenital anomalies: chromosomal aberrations in pedigree of an infant with partial D trisomy and leukemia. J Pediatr 1968; 72:367–376.

116. Hahn JS, Plawner LL. Evaluation and management of children with holoprosencephaly (Review). Pediatr Neurol 2004; 31:79–88.

117. Cohen MM. SHH and holoprosencephaly. In: Inborn errors of development – the molecular basis of clinical disorders of morphogenesis. Epstein CJ, Erickson RP, Wynshaw-Boris A, eds. Oxford Monographs of Medical Genetics No. 49. Oxford: Oxford University Press; 2004:240–248.

118. De Myer W, Zeman W, Palmer CG. The face predicts the brain: diagnostic significance of median facial anomalies for holoprosencephaly (arrhinencephaly). Pediatrics 1964; 34:256–263.

119. Taysi K, Tinaztepe K. Trisomy D and the cyclops malformation. Am J Dis Child 1972; 124:710–713.

120. Hoepner J, Yanoff M. Ocular anomalies in trisomy 13-15. Am J Ophthalmol 1972; 74:729–737.

121. Niebuhr E. Partial trisomies and deletions of chromosome 13. In: Yunis JJ, ed. New chromosomal syndromes. New York: Academic Press; 1977: 273–299.

122. Escobar JI, Sanchez O, Yunis JJ. Trisomy for the distal segment of chromosome 13. Am J Dis Child 1974; 128:217–220.

123. Escobar JI, Yunis JJ. Trisomy for the proximal segment of the long arm of chromosome 13. A new entity? Am J Dis Child 1974; 128:221–222.

124. Pettersen JC. Anatomical studies of a boy trisomic for the distal portion of 13q. Am J Med Genet 1979; 4:383–400.

125. Knudson AG, Meadows AT, et al. Chromosomal deletion and retinoblastoma. N Engl J Med 1976; 295:1120–1123.

126. Orye E, Delbeke MH, Vandenabeele B. Retinoblastoma and long arm deletion of chromosome 13. Attempts to define the deleted segment. Clin Genet 1974; 5:457–464.

127. Wilson MG, Melnyk J, Towner JW. Retinoblastoma and deletion D (14) syndrome. J Med Genet 1969; 6:322–327.

Abnormalities of chromosome 18

128. LeMarec B, Senecal J. Sex ratio et âge maternal dans la trisomie 18. J Genet Hum 1975; 23(suppl):119–120.

129. Moerman P, Fryns JP, Goddeeris P, et al. Spectrum of clinical and autopsy findings in trisomy 18 syndrome. J Genet Hum 1982; 30:17–38.

130. Rodriguez MM, Punnet HH, et al. Retinal pigment epithelium in a case of trisomy 18. Am J Ophthalmol 1973; 76:265–268.

131. Ramirez-Castro JL, Bersu ET, Valdes-Dapena M. Anatomical analysis of the developmental effects of aneuploidy in man – the trisomy 18 syndrome: II. Anomalies of the upper and lower limbs. Am J Med Genet 1978; 2:285–306.

132. Schinzel A. Cardiovascular defects associated with chromosome aberrations and malformation syndromes. Prog Med Genet 1983; 5:303–379.

133. Matsuoka R, Matsuyama S, Yamamoto Y, et al. Trisomy 18q: a case report and review on karyotype-phenotype correlations. Hum Genet 1981; 57:78–82.

134. Kurien VA, Duke M. Trisomy 17-18 syndrome: report of a case with diffuse myocardial fibrosis and review of cardiovascular abnormalities. Am J Cardiol 1968; 21:431–435.

135. Lewis AJ. The pathology of trisomy 18. J Pediatr 1964; 65:92–101.

136. Merrild U, Schioler V, Christensen F, et al. Anencephaly in trisomy 18 associated with elevated α-1-fetoprotein in amniotic fluid. Hum Genet 1978; 45:85–88.

137. Karayalcin G, Shanske A, Honigman R. Wilms' tumor in a 13-year-old girl with trisomy 18. Am J Dis Child 1981; 135:665–666.

138. Gorlin RJ, Yunis J, Anderson VED. Short arm deletion of chromosome 18 in cebocephaly. Am J Dis Child 1968; 115:473–476.

139. Nitowsky HM, Sindhavananda N, Konigsberg UR, et al. Partial 18 monosomy in the cyclops malformation. Pediatrics 1966; 37:260–269.

140. Sabater J, Antich J, et al. Deletion of short arm of chromosome 18 with normal levels of IgA. J Ment Defic Res 1972; 16:103.

141. Uchida IA, McRae KN, Ray M, et al. Familial short arm deficiency of chromosome 18 concomitant with arrhinencephaly and alopecia congenitalis. Am J Hum Genet 1965; 17:410–419.

142. Wertelecki W, Gerald PS. Clinical and chromosomal studies of the 18q-syndrome. J Pediatr 1971; 78:44–52.

143. Francke U. Partial duplication 20p. In: Yunis J, ed. New chromosomal syndromes. New York: Academic Press; 1977.

144. Schinzel A. Trisomy 20pter-q11 in a malformed boy from a t(13;20) (p11;q11) translocation-carrier mother. Hum Genet 1980; 53:169–172.

145. Mavalwala J, Wilson MG, Parker CD. The dermatoglyphics of the 18q-syndromes. Am J Phys Anthropol 1970; 32:443–449.

Wolf-Hirschhorn syndrome [del(4p)]

146. Fryns JP, DeMeulenaere A, van den Berghe H. The 4p- syndrome in a 24-year-old female. Ann Genet 1981; 24:110–111.

147. Wilson MG, Towner JW, Coffin GS, et al. Genetic and clinical studies in 13 patients with the Wolf-Hirschhorn syndrome [del(4p)]. Hum Genet 1981; 59:297–307.

148. Opitz JM. Editorial comment: twenty-seven year follow-up in the Wolf-Hirschhorn syndrome. Am J Med Genet 1995; 55:459–461.

149. Arias D, Passarge E, Engle MA, et al. Human chromosomal deletion – two patients with the 4p syndrome. J Pediatr 1970; 76:82–88.

150. Magill HL, Shackelford GD, McAlister WH, et al. 4p- (Wolf-Hirschhorn) syndrome. AJR Am J Roentgenol 1980; 135(2):283–288.

151. Miller OJ, Breg WR, Warburton D, et al. Partial deletion of the short arm of chromosome No. 4(4p-). Clinical studies in five unrelated patients. J Pediatr 1970; 77:792–801.

152. Schinzel A. Autosomal chromosomen aberrationen. Arch Genet (Zur) 1979; 52:1–204.

153. Taillemite JL, Tufferaud G, Hazael-Massieux P, et al. Délétion partielle du bras court du chromosome 4. À propos de trois observations. Ann Genet 1977; 20:93–100.

154. Wilcox LM, Bercovitch L, Howard RO. Ophthalmic features of chromosome deletion 4p- (Wolf-Hirschhorn syndrome). Am J Ophthalmol 1978; 86:834–839.

155. Schinzel A. Cardiovascular defects associated with chromosome aberrations and malformation syndromes. Prog Med Genet 1983; 5:303–379.

156. Judge CG, Garson OM, Pitt DB, et al. A girl with Wolf-Hirschhorn syndrome and mosaicism 46,XX/46,XX,4p-. J Ment Defic Res 1974; 18:79–85.

157. Beaujard MP, Jouannic JM, Bessieres B, et al. Prenatal detection of a de novo terminal inverted duplication 4p in a fetus with the Wolf-Hirschhorn syndrome phenotype. Prenat Diagn 2005; 25:451–455.

Cri-du-chat (cat cry) syndrome [del(5p)]

158. Niebuhr E. Anthropometry in the cri du chat syndrome. Clin Genet 1979; 16:82–95.

159. Niebuhr E. Cytologic observations in 35 individuals with a 5p- karyotype. Hum Genet 1978; 42:143–156.

160. Niebuhr E. The cri du chat syndrome. Epidemiology, cytogenetics, and clinical features. Hum Genet 1978; 44:227–275.

161. de Capoa A, Warburton D, Breg WR, et al. Translocation heterozygosis: a cause of five cases of the cri du chat syndrome and two cases with a duplication of chromosome number five in three families. Am J Hum Genet 1967; 19:586–603.

162. Taylor MJ, Josifek K. Multiple congenital anomalies, thymic dysplasia, severe congenital heart disease, and oligosyndactyly with a deletion of the short arm of chromosome 5. Am J Med Genet 1981; 9:5–11.

163. Mennicken U, Pfeiffer RA, Puyn U. Klinische and cytogenetische Befunde von 7 Patienten mit Cri-du-Chat Syndrom. Z Kinderheilkd 1968; 104:230–256.

164. Neuhauser G, Lother K. Das Katzenschrei Syndrom. Monatsschr Kinderheilkd 1966; 114:278–281.

165. Warburton D, Miller OJ. Dermatoglyphic features of patients with a partial short arm deletion of a B-group chromosome. Ann Hum Genet 1967; 31:189–207.

166. Del Mazo J, Abrisqueta JA. Maternal origin of a trisomy 7 in a spontaneous abortus. Obstet Gynecol 1979; 53(suppl):18S–20S.

167. Yunis E, Ramirez E, Uribe JG. Full trisomy 7 and Potter syndrome. Hum Genet 1980; 54:13–18.

168. Bogart MH, Cunniff C, Bradshaw C, et al. Terminal deletions of the long arm of chromosome 7: five new cases. Am J Med Genet 1990; 36:53–55.

169. Harris EL, Wappner RS, Palmer CG, et al. 7q deletion syndrome (7q32-qter). Clin Genet 1977; 12:233–238.

170. Bernstein R, Dawson B, Morcom G, et al. Two unrelated children with distal long arm deletion of chromosome 7: clinical features, cytogenetic and gene marker studies. Clin Genet 1980; 17:228–237.

171. Young RS, Weaver DD, Kukolich MK, et al. Terminal and interstitial deletions of the long arm of chromosome 7: a review with five cases. Am J Med Genet 1984; 17:437–450.

172. McMorrow LE, Toth IR, Gluckson MM, et al. A lethal presentation of de novo deletion 7q. J Med Genet 1987; 24:629–631.

173. Schrander-Stumpel C, Schrander J, Fryns JP, et al. Caudal deficiency sequence in 7q terminal deletion. Am J Med Genet 1988; 30:757.

Abnormalities of chromosome 8

174. Bishun NP. Normal trisomy C mosaicism in the mother of a 'mongoloid' child. Acta Paediatr Scand 1958; 57:243–244.

175. Caspersson T, Lindsten J, Zech L, et al. Four patients with trisomy 8 identified by the fluorescence and Giemsa banding techniques. J Med Genet 1972; 9:1–7.

176. Giraud F, Mattei JF, Blanc-Pardigon M, et al. Trisomie 8 en mosaïque. Arch Fr Pediatr 1975; 32:177–183.

177. Stenbjerg S, Husted S, Bernsen A, et al. Coagulation studies in patients with trisomy 8 syndrome. Ann Genet 1975; 18:241–242.

178. Stolte L, Evers J, Blankenborg G. Possible trisomy in chromosome 6-12 in a normal woman. Lancet 1964; 284:480–481.

179. de Grouchy J, Veslot J, Bonnette J, et al. A case of ?6p-chromosomal aberration. Am J Dis Child 1968; 115:93–99.

180. Yunis J, Sanchez O. A new syndrome resulting from partial trisomy for the distal third of the long arm of chromosome 10. J Pediatr 1974; 84:567–570.

181. Kosztolanyi G, Buhler EM, Elmiger P, et al. Trisomy 8 mosaicism. A case report and a proposed list of clinical features. Eur J Pediatr 1976; 123:293–300.

182. Riccardi V, Atkins L, Holmes LB. Absent patellae, mild mental retardation, skeletal and genitourinary anomalies, and C group autosomal mosaicism. J Pediatr 1970; 77:664–672.

183. de Grouchy J, Josso F, Beguin S, et al. Deficite en facteur VII de la coagulation chez trois subjects trisomiques 8. Ann Genet 1974; 17:105–108.

184. de la Chapelle A, Vuopio P, Icen A. Trisomy 8 in the bone marrow associated with high red cell glutathione reductase activity. Blood 1976; 47:815–826.

185. Williams TM, McConnell TS, Martinez F Jr, et al. Clinicopathologic and dysmorphic findings in recombinant chromosome 8 syndrome. Hum Pathol 1984; 15:1080–1084.

186. Lovell M, Herrera J, Coco R. A child with recombinant of chromosome 8 inherited from a carrier mother with a pericentric inversion. Medicina (Buenos Aires) 1982; 42:359–362.

187. Anneren G, Sedin G. Case report of trisomy 9 syndrome. Acta Pediatr Scand 1981; 70:125–128.

188. Juberg RC, Gilbert EF, Salisbury RS. Trisomy C in an infant with polycystic kidneys and other malformations. J Pediatr 1970; 76:598–603.

189. Blair JD. Trisomy C and dysplasia of kidneys, liver and pancreas. Birth Defects Orig Artic Ser 1976; 12:139–149.

190. Feingold M, Atkins L. A case of trisomy 9. J Med Genet 1973; 10:184–187.

191. Francke U, Benirschke K, Jones OW. Prenatal diagnosis of trisomy 9. Hum Genet 1975; 29, 243–250.

192. Frohlich GS. Delineation of trisomy 9. J Med Genet 1982; 19:316–317.

193. Mantagos S, McReynolds JW, Sheashore MR, et al. Complete trisomy 9 in two liveborn infants. J Med Genet 1981; 18:377–382.

Abnormalities of chromosome 9

194. Haslam RHA, Broske SP, Moore CM, et al. Trisomy 9 mosaicism with multiple congenital anomalies. J Med Genet 1973; 10:180–184.

195. Bowen P, Ying KL, Chung GSH. Trisomy 9 mosaicism in a newborn infant with multiple malformations. J Pediatr 1974; 85:95–97.

196. Dhandha S, Hogge WA, Surti U, et al. Three cases of tetrasomy 9p. Am J Med Genet 2002; 113:375–380.

197. Deurloo KL, Cobben JM, Heins YM, et al. Prenatal diagnosis of tetrasomy 9p in a 9-week-old fetus with Dandy-Walker malformation: a case report. Prenat Diagn 2004; 24:796–798.

198. Hengstschlager M, Bettelheim M, Drahonsky R, et al. Prenatal diagnosis of tetrasomy 9p with Dandy-Walker malformation. Prenat Diagn 2004; 24: 623–626.

199. de Azevedo Moreira LM, Freitas LM, Gusmao FA, et al. New case of non-mosaic tetrasomy 9p in a severely polymalformed newborn girl. Birth Defects Res A Clin Mol Teratol 2003; 67:985–988.

WAGR syndrome [del(p11-p13)]

200. Riccardi VM, Hittner HM, Francke U, et al. The aniridia-Wilms' tumor association: the critical role of chromosome band 11p13. Cancer Genet Cytogenet 1980; 2:131–137.

201. Shannon RS, Mann JR, Harper E, et al. Wilms' tumor and aniridia: clinical and cytogenetic features. Arch Dis Child 1982; 57:685–690.

202. Riccardi VM, Hittner HM, Strong LC, et al. Wilms' tumor with aniridia/iris dysplasia and apparently normal chromosomes. J Pediatr 1982; 100:574–577.

203. Yunis JJ, Ramsay NK. Familial occurrence of the aniridia-Wilms' tumor syndrome with deletion 11p13.1. J Pediatr 1980; 96:1027–1030.

204. Bove KE, McAdams AJ. The nephroblastomatosis complex and its relationship to Wilms' tumor: a clinicopathological treatise. Perspect Pediatr Pathol 1976; 3:185.

205. Trigg ME, Padilla-Nash H, Saxe D, et al. Aniridia and Wilms' tumor in a child constitutionally mosaic for 11p-; 12q+: a new chromosome change

also present in Wilms' tumor cells of the blastema types. Hum Pathol 1986; 17:1074–1077.

Prader-Willi and Angelman syndromes [del(15)(q11-q13)]

206. Van Vliet G, Deal C, Crock PA, et al. Sudden death in growth hormone-treated children with Prader-Willi syndrome. J Pediatr 2004; 144:129–131.

207. Jay P, Rougeulle C, Massacrier A, et al. The human necdin gene, NDN, is maternally imprinted and located in the Prader-Willi syndrome chromosomal region. Nat Genet 1997; 17:357–361.

208. MacDonald HR, Wevrick R. The necdin gene is deleted in Prader-Willi syndrome and is imprinted in human and mouse. Hum Mol Genet 1997; 6:1873–1878.

209. Williams CA, Frias JL. The Angelman ('happy puppet') syndrome. Am J Med Genet 1982; 11:453–460.

210. Kishino T, Lalande M, Wagstaff J. UBE3A/E6-AP mutations cause Angelman syndrome. Nat Genet 1997; 15:70–73.

211. Borelina D, Engel N, Esperante S, et al. Combined cytogenetic and molecular analyses for the diagnosis of Prader-Willi/Angelman syndromes. J Biochem Mol Biol 2004; 37:522–526.

212. Coldwell S, Fitzgerald B, Semmens JM, et al. A case of trisomy of chromosome 15. J Med Genet 1981; 18:146–148.

Trisomy 16

213. Taylor AI. Trisomy of chromosome 16 in a neonate, 47,XY,?16+. J Med Genet 1971; 18:123–125.

Rubinstein-Taybi syndrome [del(16)(p13.3)]

214. Wallerstein R, Anderson CE, Hay B, et al. Submicroscopic deletions at 16p13.3 in Rubinstein-Taybi syndrome: frequency and clinical manifestations in a North American population. J Med Genet 1997; 34:203–206.

215. Petrij F, Dauwerse HG, Blough RI, et al. Diagnostic analysis of the Rubinstein-Taybi syndrome: five cosmids should be used for microdeletion detection and low number of protein truncating mutations. J Med Genet 2000; 37:168–176.

Miller-Dieker lissencephaly syndrome [del(17)(p13.3)]

216. Daube JR, Chou SM. Lissencephaly: two cases. Neurology 1966; 16:179–191.

217. Dieker H, Edwards RH, et al. The lissencephaly syndrome. Birth Defects 1969; 5:53–64.

218. Dobyns WB, Stratton RF, Greenberg F. Syndromes with lissencephaly: I. Miller-Dieker and Norman Roberts syndromes and isolated lissencephaly. Am J Med Genet 1984; 18:509–526.

219. Garcia CA, Dunn D, Trevor R. The lissencephaly (agyria) syndrome in siblings: computerized tomographic and neuropathologic findings. Arch Neurol 1978; 35:608–611.

220. Hanaway J, Lee SI, Netsky NG. Pachygyria: relation of findings to modern embryologic concepts. Neurology 1968; 18:791–799.

221. Jellinger K, Rett A. Agyria-pachygyria (lissencephaly syndrome). Neuropediatrie 1976; 7:66–91.

222. Jones KL, Gilbert EF, Kaveggia EG, et al. The Miller-Dieker syndrome. Pediatrics 1980; 66:277–281.

223. Miller JQ. Lissencephaly in 2 siblings. Neurology 1963; 13:841–850.

224. Norman MG, Roberts M, Sirois J, et al. Lissencephaly. Can J Neurol Sci 1976; 3:39.

225. Stewart RM, Richman DP, Caviness VS Jr. Lissencephaly and pachygyria: an architectonic and topographical analysis. Acta Neuropathol (Berl) 1975; 31:1.

226. Toro-Sola MA, Rivera-de-Quinones H, Miranda JL. Lissencephaly: a clinicopathologic study in a Puerto Rican female. Birth Defects Orig Artic Ser 1978; 14:307–313.

227. Van Allen M, Clarren SK. A spectrum of gyral anomalies in Miller-Dieker (lissencephaly) syndrome. J Pediatr 1983; 102:559–564.

228. Dobyns WB, Stratton RF, Parke JT, et al. Miller-Dieker syndrome: lissencephaly and monosomy 17p. J Pediatr 1983; 102:552–558.

Trisomy 20

229. Pan SF, Fatora SR, Hass JE, et al. Trisomy of chromosome 20. Clin Genet 1976; 9:449–453.

230. Djalali M, Steinbach P, Schinger E, et al. On the significance of true trisomy 20 mosaicism in amniotic fluid culture. Hum Genet 1985; 69:321–326.

Alagille syndrome [del(20)(p12)]

231. Li L, Krantz ID, Deng Y, et al. Alagille syndrome is caused by mutations in human Jagged1, which encodes a ligand for Notch1. Nat Genet 1997; 16: 243–251.

Monosomy 22

232. Garcia Miranda JL, Otero Gomez A, Varela Ansedes H, et al. Monosomy 22 with humoral immunodeficiency: is there an immunoglobulin chain deficit? J Med Genet 1983; 20:69–72.

Cat-eye syndrome [+(22)(pter-q11)]

233. Schinzel A, Schmid W, Fraccaro M, et al. The 'cat eye syndrome': dicentric small marker chromosome probably derived from a no. 22 (tetrasomy 22pter to q11) associated with a characteristic phenotype. Report of 11 patients and delineation of the clinical picture. Hum Genet 1981; 57:148–158.

234. Mears AJ, Duncan AMV, Budarf ML, et al. Molecular characterization of the marker chromosome associated with cat eye syndrome. Am J Hum Genet 1994; 55: 134–142.

235. Mears AJ, El-Shanti H, Murray JC, et al. Minute supernumerary ring chromosome 22 associated with cat eye syndrome: further delineation of the critical region. Am J Hum Genet 1995; 57: 667–673.

236. Meins M, Burfeind P, Motsch S, et al. Partial trisomy of chromosome 22 resulting from an interstitial duplication of 22q11.2 in a child with typical cat eye syndrome. J Med Genet 2003; 40: 62–65.

Triploidy

237. Jacobs PA, Angel RR, Buchanan IM, et al. The origin of human triploids. Ann Hum Genet 1978; 42:49–57.

238. Jacobs PA, Morton NE. Origin of human trisomics and polyploids. Hum Hered 1977; 27:59–72.

239. Boué JG, Boué A. Les aberrations chromosomiques dans les avortements spontanés humains. Presse Méd 1970; 78:635–641.

240. Beischer NA, Fortune DW, Fitzgeeral MG. Hydatidiform mole and coexistent foetus, both with triploid chromosome constitution. Br Med J 1967; 3:476–478.

241. Jones WB, Lauerson NH. Hydatidiform mole with coexistent fetus. Am J Obstet Gynecol 1975; 122:267–272.

242. Szulman AE, Philippe E, Boué JG, et al. Human triploidy: association with partial hydatidiform moles and nonmolar conceptuses. Hum Pathol 1981; 12:1016–1021.

243. Butler LJ, Chantler C, France NE, et al. A liveborn infant with complete triploidy (69,XXX). J Med Genet 1969; 6:413–421.

244. Niebuhr E. Triploidy in man. Cytogenetical and clinical aspects. Hum Genet 1974; 21:103–125.

245. McFadden DE, Kalousek DL. Two different phenotypes of fetuses with chromosomal triploidy: correlation with parental origin of the extra haploid set. Am J Med Genet 1991; 38:535–538.

246. Saad AA, Juliar JF, Harm J, et al. Triploidy syndrome. A report of two live-born (69,XXY) and one stillborn (69,XXX) infants. Clin Genet 1976; 9:43–50.

247. Prats J, Sarret E, Moragas A, et al. Triploid live full-term infant. Helv Paediatr Acta 1971; 26:164–172.

248. Toaff R, Toaff ME, Peyser MR. Mid-trimester pre-eclamptic toxemia in triploid pregnancies. Isr J Med Sci 1976; 12:234–239.

249. Philipp T, Grillenberger K, Separovic ER, et al. Effects of triploidy on early human development. Prenat Diagn 2004; 24:276–281.

250. Genest DR. Partial hydatidiform mole: clinicopathologic features, differential diagnosis, ploidy and molecular studies, and gold standards for diagnosis. Int J Gynecol Pathol 2001; 20:315–322.

251. Devriendt K. Hydatidiform mole and triploidy: the role of genomic imprinting in placental development. Hum Reprod Update 2005; 11:137–142.

252. Jacobs PA, Szulman AE, Funkhouser J, et al. Human triploidy: relationship between parental origin of the additional haploid complement and development of partial hydatidiform mole. Ann Hum Genet 1982; 46:223–231.

253. Szulman AE, Surti U. The syndromes of hydatidiform mole. II. Morphologic evolution of the complete and partial mole. Am J Obstet Gynecol 1978; 132:20–27.

254. Honore LH, Dill FJ, Poland BJ. Placental morphology in spontaneous human abortuses with normal and abnormal karyotypes. Teratology 1976; 14: 151–156.

255. Philippe E. Histopathologie placentaire. Paris: Masson; 1974.

256. Philippe E, Boué JG. Le placenta des aberrations chromosomiques létales. Ann Anat Pathol (Paris) 1969; 14:249–266.

257. Meisner L, Louie RR, Arya S, et al. Triploidy with an extra sex chromosome (70,XXYY) and elevated α-fetoprotein levels. In: Gilbert EF, Opitz JM, eds. Genetic aspects of developmental pathology. New York: Alan R Liss; 1987:333–339.

Sex chromosome abnormalities

258. Williams DL, Runyan JW Jr. Sex chromatin and chromosome analysis in the diagnosis of sex anomalies. Ann Intern Med 1966; 64:422–459.

259. Coté GB, Tsomi K, Papadakou-Lagoyanni S, et al. Oligohydramnios syndrome and XYY karyotype. Ann Genet 1978; 221:226–228.

260. Daly JJ, Hunter H, Rickards DF. Klinefelter syndrome and pulmonary disease. Am Rev Respir Dis 1968; 98:717–719.

261. Domm BM, Vassallo CL. Klinefelter's syndrome, obesity and respiratory failure. Am Rev Respir Dis 1973; 107:123–126.

262. Rimoin DL, Schimke RN. Genetic disorders of the endocrine glands. St Louis: CV Mosby; 1971.

263. Hsueh WA, Hsu TH, Federman DD. Endocrine features of Klinefelter's syndrome. Medicine (Baltimore) 1978; 57:447–461.

264. Sybert VP, McCauley E. Turner's syndrome. N Engl J Med 2004; 351:1227–1238.

265. Pelotti S, Bini C, Ceccardi S, et al. Sex chromosome analysis in Turner syndrome by a pentaplex PCR assay. Genet Test 2003; 7:245–247.

266. Lemli L, Smith DW. The XO syndrome. A study of the differential phenotype in 25 patients. J Pediatr 1963; 63:577–588.

267. Skuse DH, James RS, Bishop DVM, et al. Evidence from Turner's syndrome of an imprinted X-linked locus affecting cognitive function. Nature 1997; 387:705–708.

268. Skuse DH. X-linked genes and mental functioning. Hum Mol Genet 2005; 14 Spec No 1:R27–32.

269. Davies W, Isles AR, Wilkinson LS. Imprinted gene expression in the brain (Review). Neurosci Biobehav Rev 2005; 29:421–430.

270. Raefski AS, O'Neill MJ. Identification of a cluster of X-linked imprinted genes in mice. Nat Genet 2005; 37:620–624.

271. Davies W, Isles A, Smith R, et al. Xlr3b is a new imprinted candidate for X-linked parent-of-origin effects on cognitive function in mice. Nat Genet 2005; 37:625–629.

272. Kosowicz J. The roentgen appearance of the hand and wrist in gonadal dysgenesis. AJR Am J Roentgenol 1965; 93:354–361.

273. de la Chapelle A. Cytogenetical and clinical observations in female gonadal dysgenesis. Acta Endocrinol (Copenh) 1962; 40(suppl 65):1–122.

274. Finby N, Archibald RM. Skeletal abnormalities associated with gonadal dysgenesis. AJR Am J Roentgenol 1963; 89:1222–1235.

275. van der Putte SC. Lymphatic malformation in human fetuses. A study of fetuses with Turner's syndrome or status Bonnevie-Ullrich. Virchows Arch A Patho Ana Histol 1977; 376:233–246.

276. Carr RF, Ochs RH, Ritter DA, et al. Fetal cystic hygroma and Turner's syndrome. Am J Dis Child 1986; 140:580–583.

277. Weiss SW. Pedal hemangioma (venous malformation) occurring in Turner's syndrome: an additional manifestation of the syndrome. Hum Pathol 1988; 19:1015–1018.

278. Burge DM, Middleton AW, Kamath R. Intestinal haemorrhage in Turner's syndrome. Arch Dis Child 1981; 56:557–558.

279. Schultz LS, Assimacopoulos CA, Lillihei RC. Turner's syndrome with associated gastrointestinal hemorrhage: a case report. Surgery 1970; 68:485–488.

280. Gilbert-Barness E, Opitz J. Renal abnormalities in malformation syndromes. In: Edelman CM, Bernstein J, eds. Pediatric kidney disease. 2nd edn. Boston: Little, Brown; 1992:1067–1119.

281. Egli F, Stalder G. Malformations of kidney and urinary tract in common chromosomal aberrations. Hum Genet 1973; 18:1–15.

282. Dimmick JE, Kalousek DK. Developmental pathology of the embryo and fetus. Philadelphia: JB Lippincott; 1992.

283. Cleeve DM, Older RA, Cleeve LK, et al. Retrocaval ureter in Turner syndrome. Urology 1979; 13:544–545.

284. Bernstein J, Gilbert-Barness E. Congenital malformations of the kidney. In: Tisher CC, Brenner BM, eds. Renal pathology. 3rd edn. Philadelphia: JB Lippincott; 1994:1355–1369.

285. Bernstein J, Gilbert-Barness E. Developmental abnormalities of the kidney. In: Sternberg SS, ed. Diagnostic surgical pathology. 2nd edn. New York: Raven Press; 1994:1631–1644.

286. Gilbert-Barness EF, Opitz JM, Barness LA. Heritable malformations of the kidney and urinary tract. In: Spitzer A, Avener ED, eds. Inheritance of kidney and urinary tract diseases. Norwell: Kluwer Academic Publishers; 1990:327–400.

287. Engle MA, Ehlers KH. Cardiovascular malformations in the syndrome of Turner phenotype with normal karyotype. Birth Defects 1972; 8:104–109.

288. Siggers DC, Polani PE. Congenital heart disease in male and female subjects with somatic features of Turner's syndrome and normal sex chromosomes. Br Heart J 1972; 34:41–46.

289. Kostich ND, Opitz JM. Ullrich-Turner syndrome associated with cystic medial necrosis of the aorta and great vessels. Am J Med 1965; 38: 943–950.

290. Weiss L. Additional evidence of gradual loss of germ cells in the pathogenesis of streak ovaries in Turner's syndrome. J Med Genet 1971; 8:540–544.

Fragile X syndrome

291. Sutherland GR, Brown WT, Hagerman R, et al. X-linked mental retardation-6. Special issue. Sixth International Workshop. The fragile X and X-linked mental retardation. Am J Med Genet 1994; 51:281–293.

292. Fryns JP, Borghgraef M, Brown TW, et al. 9th international workshop on fragile X syndrome and X-linked mental retardation. Am J Med Genet 2000; 94: 345–360.

293. Willemsen R, Oostra BA, Bassell GH, et al. The fragile X syndrome: from molecular genetics to neurobiology. Ment Retard Dev Disabil Res Rev 2004; 10:60–67.

294. Mandel JL, Biancalana V. Fragile X mental retardation syndrome: from pathogenesis to diagnostic issues. Growth Horm IGF Res 2004; 14 (suppl A): S158–S165.

295. O'Donnell WT, Warren ST. A decade of molecular studies of fragile X syndrome. Annu Rev Neurosci 2002; 25:315–383.

296. Verkerk AJ, Pieretti M, Sutcliffe JS, et al. Identification of a gene (FMR-1) containing a CGG repeat coincident with a breakpoint cluster region exhibiting length variation in fragile X syndrome. Cell 1991; 65:905–914.

297. Yu S, Pritchard M, Kremer E, et al. Fragile X genotype characterized by an unstable region of DNA. Science 1991; 252:1179–1181.

298. Meryash DL, Cronk CE, Sachs B, et al. An anthropometric study of males with the fragile X syndrome. Am J Med Genet 1984; 17:159–174.

299. Chudley AE, Hagerman RJ. Fragile X syndrome. J Pediatr 1987; 110: 821–831.

300. Simpson EN, Newman BJ, Parlington MW. Fragile X syndrome. III: Dermatoglyphic studies in males. Am J Med Genet 1984; 17:195–207.

301. Vincent A, Heitz D, Petit C, et al. Abnormal pattern detected in fragile-X patients by pulsed field electrophoresis. Nature 1991; 349:624–626.

302. Bell MV, Hirst MC, Nakahori Y, et al. Physical mapping across the fragile X: hypermethylation and clinical expression of the fragile X syndrome. Cell 1991; 64:861–866.

303. Hagerman PJ, Hagerman RJ. The fragile-X premutation: a maturing perspective. Am J Hum Genet 2004; 74:805–816.

304. Laxova R. Fragile X syndrome. Adv Pediatr 1994; 41:305–342.

305. Rousseau F, Heitz D, Biancalana V, et al. Direct diagnosis by DNA analysis of the fragile X syndrome of mental retardation. N Engl J Med 1991; 325: 1673–1681.

306. Tarleton JC, Saul RA. Molecular genetic advances in fragile X syndrome. J Pediatr 1993; 122:169–185.

307. McConkie-Rosell A, Finucane B, Cronister A, et al. Genetic counseling for fragile X syndrome: updated recommendations of the national society of genetic counsellors. J Genet Couns 2005; 14:249–270.

Imprinted chromosomes

308. Morison IM, Ramsay JP, Spencer HG. A census of mammalian imprinting. Trends Genet 2005; 21:457–465.

309. http://igc.otago.ac.nz/home.html

310. http://www.geneimprint.com/

Neoplasia associated with chromosomal aberrations

311. Weinberg RA. Oncogenes and tumor suppressor genes. CA Cancer J Clin 1994:160–170.

312. Mitelman F, Johansson B, Mertens F. Catalogue of chromosome aberrations in cancer. 5th edn. New York: Wiley-Liss; 1994.

313. Heim S, Mitelman F. Cancer cytogenetics. 2nd edn. New York: Wiley-Liss; 1995.

314. http://www.ncbi.nlm.nih.gov/entrez/query.fcgi?CMD=search&DB=cancerchromosomes

315. Ravindranath Y, Chang M, Steuber CP, et al. Pediatric oncology group (POG) studies of acute myeloid leukemia (AML): a review of four consecutive childhood AML trials conducted between 1981 and 2000. Leukemia, advance online publication, leukemia 2005; 19:2101–2160.

316. Chessells JM, Harrison CJ, Hempski H, et al. Clinical features, cytogenetics and outcome in acute lymphoblastic and myeloid leukaemia of infancy: report from the MRC childhood leukaemia working party. Leukemia 2002; 16:776–784.

317. Ellison DA, Parham DM, Sawyer JR. Cytogenetic findings in pediatric T-lymphoblastic lymphomas: one institution's experience and a review of the literature. Pediatr Dev Pathol 2005; 8:550–556.

318. Sandberg AA. Cancer cytogenics for clinicians. CA Cancer J Clin 1994; 44: 136.

319. Kalwinsky DK, Raimondi SC, Schnell JM, et al. Prognostic importance of cytogenetic subgroups in de novo pediatric acute non-lymphocytic leukemia. J Clin Oncol 1990; 8:75.

320. Schneider NR. Cytogenetic evaluation of childhood neoplasms. Arch Pathol Lab Med 1993; 117:1220.

321. Pizzo PA, Poplack DG. Principles and practice of pediatric oncology. 4th edn. Philadelphia: Lippincott, Williams & Wilkins; 2002.

322. Reddy KS, Perkins SL. Advances in the diagnostic approach to childhood lymphoblastic malignant neoplasms. Am J Clin Pathol 2004; 122 (suppl):S3.

323. Yunis JJ. The chromosomal basis of human neoplasia. Science 1983; 221:227.

324. Sandberg AA. The chromosomes in human cancer and leukemia. Amsterdam: Elsevier/North Holland; 1990.

325. Sandberg AA, Bridge JA. The cytogenetics of bone and soft tissue tumors. Boca Raton: CRC Press; 1994.

326. Ravindranath Y, Chang M, Steuber CP, et al. Pediatric oncology group (POG) studies of acute myeloid leukemia (AML): a review of four consecutive childhood AML trials conducted between 1981 and 2000. Leukemia 2005; 19:2101–2116.

327. Yunis JJ. Chromosomes and cancer: new nomenclature and future directions. Hum Pathol 1981; 2:494.

328. Yunis JJ. New chromosome techniques in the study of human neoplasia. Hum Pathol 1981; 12:540.

329. Yunis JJ, Oken MM, Kaplan ME, et al. Distinctive chromosomal abnormalities in histologic subtypes of non-Hodgkin's lymphoma. N Engl J Med 1982; 307:1231.

330. Oligny LL. Cancer and epigenesis: a developmental perspective. Adv Pediatr 2003; 50: 59.

331. Feinberg AP. The epigenetics of cancer etiology. Semin Cancer Biol 2004; 14:427.

332. Lund AH, van Lohuizen M. Epigenetics and cancer. Genes Dev 2004; 18:2315.

333. Baylin SB. Reversal of gene silencing as a therapeutic target for cancer – roles for DNA methylation and its interdigitation with chromatin. Novartis Found Symp 2004; 259:226.

334. Dalla-Favera R, Bregni M, et al. Human c-myc oncogene is located on the region of chromosome 8 that is translocated in Burkitt lymphoma cells. Proc Natl Acad Sci U S A 1972; 68:6724.

335. Dalla-Favara R, Martinotti S, Gallo RC, et al. Translocation and rearrangements of the c-myc oncogene locus in human undifferentiated B-cell lymphoma. Science 1983; 219:963.

336. Marcu KB, Harris LJ, et al. Transcriptionally active c-myc oncogene is contained within NIARD, and DNA sequence associated with chromosome translocation in B-cell neoplasia. Proc Natl Acad Sci U S A 1983; 80:519.

337. Taub R, Kirsch I, et al. Translocation of the c-myc gene into the immunoglobulin heavy chain locus in human Burkitt lymphoma and murine plasmacytoma cells. Proc Natl Acad Sci U S A 1982; 79:7837.

338. Yunis JJ. Specific fine chromosomal defects in cancer: an overview. Hum Pathol 1981; 12:503.

339. Aurias A, Rimbaut C, Buffe D, et al. Chromosomal translocations in Ewing sarcoma. N Engl J Med 1983; 309:496.

340. Turc-Carel C, Philip I, Berger MP, et al. Chromosomal translocation in Ewing sarcoma. N Engl J Med 1983; 309:497.

341. Seidal T, Mark J, Hagman B, et al. Alveolar rhabdomyosarcoma. Acta Pathol Microbiol Immunol Scand 1982; 90:345.

342. Fitzgerald JC, Scherr AM, Barr FG. Structural analysis of PAX7 rearrangements in alveolar rhabdomyosarcoma. Cancer Genet Cytogenet 2000; 117: 37.

343. Rivera H, Turleau C, et al. Retinoblastoma del(13q14): report of two patients, one with a trisomy sib due to maternal insertion. Gene-dosage effect for esterase D. Hum Genet 1981; 59:211.

344. Junien C, Turleau C, et al. Regional assignment of catalase (CAT) gene to band 11p13. Associate with the aniridia-Wilms' tumor-gonadoblastoma (WAGR) complex. Ann Genet 1980; 23:165.

345. Zankl H, Zang KD. Correlations between clinical and cytogenetical data in 180 human meningiomas. Cancer Genet Cytogenet 1980; 1:351.

346. Neumann E, Kalousek DK, Norman MG, et al. Cytogenetic analysis of 109 pediatric central nervous system tumors. Cancer Genet Cytogenet 1993; 71:40.

Pathology of abortion: the embryo and the previable fetus

Dagmar K. Kalousek   Luc L. Oligny

'The more we learn, the more we know how we can help an embryo within a range of normalcy to grow to full term pregnancy'.

R. Ringer Kemble

Dedication

Dr Oligny: This chapter is dedicated to Nicolas, Marie-Anne, Alexandre, Jean François, Noëlla and Yves Oligny, for their ongoing and constant support.

Acknowledgement

Dr Oligny wishes to thank his colleagues at CHU Sainte-Justine for providing an environment conducive to investing so much time into this book, and for their constant *joie de vivre*.

Definitions of spontaneous abortion and purpose of its study

Spontaneous abortion is generally defined as the loss of the conception before the period of viability. It is a common event in human reproduction. It has been estimated that **up to 70% of all conceptions fail to complete their development**.[1–4] Approximately 30% of all zygotes abort before implantation, and another 30% abort after implantation but before the mother recognizes that she is pregnant (the subclinical or occult pregnancies). Such losses are detectable only by sensitive assays for human chorionic gonadotropin (hCG).[5–8] A final 10% of all conceptions are lost after the mother becomes aware of being pregnant; these clinical miscarriages represent the 'tip of the iceberg'.[3] Live twin pregnancies detected prior to 7 weeks gestation result in live twin neonates in only 71% of cases, and this fetal loss rate is similar for in vitro fertilization (IVF) and non-IVF pregnancies.[9]

Among clinically recognized pregnancies, 15–20% are lost spontaneously before fetal viability, with the highest loss rate in the first trimester.[10] When a woman has had two or more successive spontaneous abortions, this condition becomes known as **recurrent spontaneous abortions**. An induced abortion or termination of pregnancy is most often performed for a variety of social reasons or for removal of a defective fetus.

The basic terms used in the morphologic study of abortions include the following: conceptus and products of conception, both of which describe all the structures that develop from the zygote, the embryo, or the fetus, and the gestational sac or the placenta and its corresponding membranes. **The developing human is considered to be an embryo from conception until the end of the eighth week**, by which time all major organ systems have developed.[11, 12] **From the beginning of the ninth week until birth the developing human is called a fetus. Developmental age of an embryo or a fetus extends from the day of fertilization** to the death of the embryo or fetus within the uterus or to its live birth. In contrast, **gestational or menstrual age extends from the last day of the menstrual period** to the expulsion or removal of the conceptus. The intrauterine retention period is the time between the death of the embryo or fetus and its expulsion or removal. Since the pathologic and genetic findings in embryonic and previable fetal loss significantly differ, early and late spontaneous abortions are discussed separately. **Early spontaneous abortion describes pregnancy loss in the embryonic period (up to 8 weeks of development); late spontaneous abortion refers to fetal death between the ninth and the 18th weeks** of development.

TABLE 6.1 ETIOLOGY OF SPONTANEOUS ABORTION

Etiology	Frequency	Reference
Chromosomal abnormalities	> 50%	4, 11, 13
– Trisomy 16, 21, 18, 13	~ 1/2	
– Monosomy X	~ 1/4	
– Triploidy (maternal or paternal)	~ 1/5	16
Maternal age, independently of chromosomal abnormalities	2.1% in 30–32 years old	
	2.8% in 33 years old	
Increasing maternal age	Proportional to age	55
Paternal age (greater than 45 years of age)	Twofold increase	56
	20–40% in > 40 years old	16
Failure of implantation (see Table 6.2)	?	4
Poorly-controlled type 1 diabetes mellitus	Fourfold increase	96
Maternal alcohol intake (> 5 drinks/week) at the time of conception	Two- to fivefold increase	36, 37
Paternal alcohol intake (> 10 drinks/week) at the time of conception	Two- to fivefold increase	36
Maternal caffeine ingestion > 375 mg/day	Twofold increase	37
Chorioamnionitis	Up to 30%	

The pathologist's detailed examination of spontaneous abortion specimens not only provides important information relating to the developmental age and morphology of the conceptus, but is also the basis for reproductive genetic counseling of parents. The prognosis for future pregnancies is critically dependent on recognizing an accurate pathogenesis of pregnancy loss. Spontaneous abortion in today's society is no longer accepted as 'just a part of human reproduction', as many parents delay having offspring until their thirties and expect a live, healthy baby from each conception. When pregnancy fails, the parents want to know why the failure occurred, whether it is likely to happen again, and whether there is any increased chance of having an abnormal liveborn infant in a future pregnancy. Because pathologists receive all aborted tissues, they have the responsibility of ensuring that answers are obtained whenever possible and that the information is communicated to the patient's obstetrician and geneticist.

Etiology of spontaneous abortion

The factors contributing to the occurrence of any given abortion are either **genetic or environmental** (including the maternal environment). At different gestational ages, different factors are usually effective. An early spontaneous abortion often represents a mechanism of natural selection removing most abnormal conceptuses with chromosomal and gene(s) defects. On the other hand, abortion can also be viewed as the outcome of abnormal events in the process of implantation, morphogenesis, and development of a normal conceptus. The etiology of spontaneous abortion involves many factors, only some of which are listed in Table 6.1.

Chromosomal abnormalities

Over 50% of early spontaneous abortions are chromosomally abnormal, with 30–70% of all 2–3 day postconception embryos being aneuploid. At least 30% of morphologically normal embryos are chromosomally abnormal, and chromosomal mosaicism has been reported in 30% of human blastocysts (reviewed by Macklon et al [3]).

The four main classes of chromosomal abnormalities are trisomy (27%), polyploidy (10%), sex chromosome monosomy (9%), and structural rearrangements (2%). About half of the abnormal karyotypes that occur in first-trimester abortions are various forms of autosomal trisomy. Trisomy 16 is the most frequent and accounts for about one-third of all trisomies;[13, 14] trisomy 16 always results from a maternal meiosis I nondisjunction, whereas trisomy 18 predominantly results from a second meiotic division error. Cytogenetic analysis of 2434 *oocytes* has shown aneuploidy in 8–54%, with an average of 27% (reviewed by Macklon et al [3]): 13% were hypohaploid, 8% hyperhaploid, 2% had structural anomalies and 4% were diploid. For all chromosomes except the largest, the non-disjunction rate increases with age, whereas monosomy X shows an inverse maternal age effect. However, the effect of maternal age on fetal aneuploidy has not been conclusively demonstrated to be a consequence of an increased rate of aneuploidy in oocytes. Hence, the difference in age-related aneuploidy between oocytes and miscarried embryos could result from different rates of preimplantation and early postimplantation losses.

Fluorescent in situ hybridization (FISH) studies of sperm show an overall rate of aneuploidy of 7%, but rates differ between patients, and the percentage of aneuploidy is significantly increased in patients with abnormal spermograms. Sperm of non-obstructive azoospermic men have higher rates of aneuploidy, especially involving sex chromosomes (reviewed by Macklon et al [3]).

The reported frequency of chromosomal abnormalities in late spontaneous abortions is between 4 and 44%. Such wide variation is caused by the prolonged intrauterine retention of demised aneuploid embryos, which are then often classified as late spontaneous abortion. However, if developmental age is evaluated in aborted specimens, a low frequency of 4–7% of chromosomal defects is found in the previable fetal period.[15]

TABLE 6.2 FACTORS ASSOCIATED WITH IMPLANTATION AND EARLY PREGNANCY MAINTENANCE

Factor	Example	Suggested role
Hormonal	Estradiol-17β, progesterone, βhCG	Endometrial maturation Release of progesterone by corpus luteum
Changes in endometrial epithelium	Cell adhesion molecules; mucin production	Blastocyst adhesion, trophoblastic differentiation and invasion
Cytokines, growth factors	Leukemia inhibiting factor; heparin-binding epidermal growth factor; hepatocyte growth factor; interleukin; vascular endothelial growth factor	Facilitate signaling between blastocyst and uterus; regulate endometrial prostaglandin production; promote endometrial invasion, proliferation and differentiation; regulate vascular permeability and remodeling
Immunologic factors	Interleukin-10; Crry (complement regulator) HLA-G Indolamine 2,3-dioxygenase	Immunosuppression Prevents immune recognition and rejection of fetus Degrades tryptophan (essential for macrophage action)
Trophoblast proteases and protease	Matrix metalloproteases, tissue inhibitors of metalloproteases; cathepsin B and L; cadherins; integrins	Regulates trophoblast invasion; facilitate trophoblast vascular mimicry
Other factors	Cyclooxygenase-2 Oxygen tension	Regulates prostaglandin production Regulates the balance between trophoblast proliferation and differentiation

After Norwitz et al 2001,[4] with permission.

Infections

The major effects of infection on a previable conceptus are intrauterine death, developmental disruptions, intrauterine growth retardation, and premature expulsion from the uterus. Almost one-third of non-macerated fetuses are aborted with placentas showing chorioamnionitis, while first-trimester infections are generally not recorded. The specific organisms causing intrauterine infections are discussed in Chapter 15. The only infections clearly associated with miscarriage are listeriosis, syphilis (mainly during the second trimester), parvovirus B19, HIV and malaria.[16]

Implantation and maternal diseases

The diseases of pregnant women frequently affect the viability of the fetus. The maternal diseases most likely to result in spontaneous abortion are those that rapidly change homeostasis (**hypovolemic shock, fever**) or those inducing increased myometrial irritability (**retroplacental hemorrhage, chorioamnionitis**). Spontaneous abortion rates are no higher among mothers with **diabetes mellitus** than among controls, except in those with poorly controlled disease.[17] However, women with type 1 diabetes presenting at their first obstetric visit with a glycated hemoglobin concentration above 7.5% had a fourfold increase in spontaneous abortion, a ninefold increase in major congenital malformations and a fivefold increase in perinatal mortality, compared with non-diabetic women and women with a fair glycemic control (HbA_{1c} < 7.5%) at presentation.[18]

Early pregnancy losses resulting from **abnormal implantation** in an unsupportive endometrial environment are due either to inadequate endometrial progesterone receptor function or to low progesterone production by the corpus luteum. The condition is usually described as **luteal phase deficiency**, and it has been estimated that it occurs in **35% of patients experiencing recurrent losses**.[17]

Implantation is a very complex phenomenon (reviewed by Norwitz et al[4]). Adhesion of the blastocyst to the endometrium through cell adhesion molecules (CAMs) begins on the 6th day post conception (pc): microvilli on the apical surface of trophoblast interdigitate with pinopodes (microprotrusions of epithelial cells). The next stage results in a stable adhesion characterized by increased interaction between the trophoblast and epithelial cells. The syncytiotrophoblast invades the endometrium by the 7th day pc, with the embryonic pole of the blastocyst oriented toward the endometrium. Cross-talk between the embryo and endometrium must be subtly regulated for implantation to be successful; we are only starting to understand the cascades involved (Table 6.2).[3]

The function of the maternal blood vessels that communicate with the placental intervillous space is an important determinant of fetal mortality. After implantation, some cytotrophoblasts change their CAMs so as to enable the invasion and replacement of the endothelial cells of the uterine spiral arterioles, resulting in an increase in the diameter of the vessels. The absence of such invasion and dilatation causes the arterioles to remain of small caliber, and thus high resistance vessels, which can result in gestational **maternal hypertension**, including pre-eclampsia and eclampsia; this predisposes to late abortion.[3, 19, 20]

Maternal thrombophilia can either be of genetic origin, and/or acquired. There is growing evidence implicating thrombophilias in the pathophysiological processes underlying miscarriage, intrauterine growth retardation (IUGR) and pre-eclampsia; all these conditions are associated with thrombotic damage in the placental bed.[21] Around 5% of women have two or more successive spontaneous abortions, and 1–2% have three or more; it has become clear that prothrombotic changes are associated with a substantial proportion of these fetal losses.[21]

Collectively, **heritable thrombophilias** are present in at least 15% of Western populations; as pregnancy is a physiological hypercoagulable state, it is not surprising that thrombophilias often first manifest during pregnancy.[21] The major hereditary forms of thrombophilia include deficiencies of the endogenous anticoagulant proteins: antithrombin, protein C and protein S; abnormalities of procoagulant factors, particularly mutations involving factor V (e.g. **FV-Leiden**), methylenetetrahydrofolate reductase (e.g. **MTHFR** C677T and A1298C), prothrombin (e.g. **PRT** G20210A) and transcobalamin (e.g. **TC** C776G). Approximately half of the population carry at least one mutated allele of MTHFR, and the frequency of the 677T mutation in a homozygous state ranges from 1 to 20%, depending on the population.[21, 22] Maternal MTHFR and TC mutations, through maternal hyperhomocysteinemia (HHC), lead to recurrent embryo loss as well as first embryo loss; one or more MTHFR 677T and 1298C allele, versus the wild type combined genotype, is associated with an increased odds ratio of spontaneous abortion of 14.2; the prevalence of the mutated TC 776G allele was also significantly increased, while the wild-type allele in a homozygous state was much lower among spontaneously aborted embryos than controls. Furthermore, embryos with MTHFR and TC double-mutant alleles had greater rates of spontaneous abortion than embryos with only one mutated gene.[22] It is postulated that a combined maternal and fetal MTHFR and/or TC mutation(s) would further increase the risk of spontaneous abortion, and that in the face of maternal and/or fetal mutations, preconceptional folate and B-vitamin supplementation may prove beneficial.[22] The presence of lupus anticoagulants, anticardiolipin antibodies and high levels of homocysteine are associated with increased risk of pregnancy loss before 9 weeks' gestation.[23] FV-Leiden carriers have an odds ratio of spontaneous abortion of 1.8.[23] Women with homozygous FV-Leiden and women with HHC are at increased risk of first trimester spontaneous abortion, with odds ratios of 6.25 reported for each of these thrombophilias.[23, 24] The odds ratios of first trimester spontaneous abortion in women with anticardiolipin antibodies and lupus anticoagulants are 3.40 and 2.97, respectively.[23] The odds ratios of third trimester losses for maternal heterozygous FV-Leiden and PT G20210A mutations are respectively 2.8 and 2.66.

Acquired thrombophilias include antiphospholipid antibodies, which are found in 15% of women with recurrent miscarriages (both early and late), anticardiolipin antibodies, lupus anticoagulant and anti-β-2-glycoprotein 1 antibodies, all of which increase thrombin generation and thrombotic placental infarction.[21, 25] These autoantibodies may also directly affect trophoblast differentiation and invasion.[26] Furthermore, lupus anticoagulant increases placental apoptosis, attenuates trophoblast mitotic rates and reduces trophoblastic invasion, thus impairing placentation; these effects are attenuated by heparin.[27] Fetal loss related to antiphospholipid antibodies is reduced with antithrombotic therapy, particularly with combination therapy using heparin and low-dose aspirin (71% live birth rates compared to 42% when using aspirin alone – odds ratio of 3.37 – and 10% when no pharmacological treatment is used).[21] Krabbendam and Dekker studied women with two or more spontaneous abortions; those diagnosed to have a hereditary thrombophilia and treated with this combination therapy had a 75% rate of live births; likewise, the women in this group with either HHC or MTHFR were treated with folate/vitamin B6 and B12 and 77% of these conceptions resulted in a live birth.[28] Hence, screening for antiphospholipid antibodies and possibly for other forms of thrombophilias should be routinely offered to all women with recurrent miscarriage as such antibodies are present in half of these women; however, universal screening for FV-Leiden in pregnancy is not cost effective.[21] In women suffering from the chronic myeloproliferative disease **essential thrombocytemia**, treatment with low dose aspirin doubled the rates of live birth, compared to lack of pharmacologic treatment.[29]

Anomalies of uterine development are relatively frequent, with a reported incidence of 1/200 to 1/6000 women. Overall, about 20–25% of women with anomalies of uterine fusion have problems with reproduction, recurrent abortion being the most frequent and serious.[17, 30] **Cervical incompetence** is a major factor in late spontaneous abortion. It is characterized by an asymptomatic dilatation of the internal cervical os, leading to dilatation of the cervical canal and external os during the second trimester of pregnancy. The consequent lack of support from the fetal membranes leads to their spontaneous rupture, which is usually followed by expulsion of the fetus and placenta. The most common cause of cervical incompetence is a congenital defect in the cervical tissue, but **cone biopsies** constitute a risk factor, more so when performed during adolescence. **Uterine leiomyomas**, especially if submucosal, may also be associated with repetitive abortion. Iatrogenic lesions, the most common of which is caused by a **retained intrauterine contraceptive device (IUD)**, represent another category of increased risk of pregnancy loss.[31]

A history of miscarriage increases the risk of recurrent spontaneous abortion, with rates of 12, 29 and 36% after one, two and three previous spontaneous abortions.[16] The risk of spontaneous abortion following an induced abortion is increased, by a factor of 1.3–3.3 depending on the studies quoted, and by as much as eightfold in women with three or more induced abortions;[16] nevertheless, Zhou et al found an increased risk only when the interpregnancy interval was less than 3 months, irrespective of the abortion method and of the number of prior induced abortions.[32]

Effects of maternal nutrition and medication

Maternal malnutrition affects fetal growth and development. Its effect depends on its initiation relative to the development of the conceptus, its duration, and its type and severity. For example, **deficiency of maternal dietary zinc** decreases the antimicrobial activity of amniotic fluid[33] and therefore may play a role in late spontaneous abortions due to chorioamnionitis.

The effects of maternal medication are so vast that anyone involved in developmental pathology must have access to the latest edition of a compendium listing references to the known and alleged teratogenicity of specific drugs.[34] It should be remembered that **drugs teratogenic to some individuals may predispose to spontaneous abortions in others**. Non-prescription drugs are a particular problem since they are easy to obtain, are taken in an unscheduled way, and are easily forgotten. A single substance, perhaps teratogenic, may be an ingredient of many medications and be present in varying amounts. For example, it has been suggested that agenesis of the cloacal membrane may be related to maternal ingestion of doxylamine succinate; this substance is contained in at least 14 prescription and non-prescription drugs.[35]

It is now generally accepted that **alcohol consumption** during pregnancy is associated with developmental defects that can be diagnosed in the newborn. It has also been demonstrated that the use of alcohol in pregnancy predisposes to spontaneous abortions.[36, 37] The risk of abortion due to **smoking** is difficult to evaluate and appears less dose dependent than that of alcohol;[36] nicotine can produce vasculitis secondary to vascular spasms, resulting in placental pathology.[31, 37] Daily **caffeine consumption** of > 375 mg has been reported to increase the rate of spontaneous abortion twofold, and caffeine doses of > 200 mg (approximately two cups) have been shown to lower blood flow in the placenta.[16, 37] Neither lysergic acid diethylamide (LSD) nor cannabis have been shown unequivocally to increase the risk of spontaneous abortion, whereas **cocaine** and its derivatives have, at least in part due to their effects on placental vasoconstriction.[16, 38]

Immunologic factors

In mammalian reproduction, the role of **immunogenetic incompatibility** between parents has been widely discussed. The major histocompatibility complex (MHC) of mammalian species is known to play a crucial role, both in self-recognition and in the recognition and response to antigens presented by an allograft. The role of the MHC in pregnancy has been studied chiefly in humans, mice, and rats. These species all have a hemochorial placentation that allows intimate contact between the maternal and fetal circulations. Although the placenta was once regarded as an inert or immunosuppressive barrier between the maternal and fetal circulations, it is now clear that a specific maternal immune reactivity against the fetus can be measured, and this response seems to facilitate fetal survival. It is now argued that immunomodulation (e.g. immunotherapy by lymphocyte allo-immunization or intravenous immunoglobulin) to prevent recurrent spontaneous abortions should no longer be performed in an ad-hoc fashion, but rather, be used to specifically correct documented cellular defects, and as such, be tailored for the specific pathway whose disruption causes the abortion.[39, 40] The immunologic features of successful and unsuccessful pregnancies have been summarized as follows:[39–45]

- **Complex immunoregulation** during pregnancy leads to the production of a protective rather than a destructive maternal immune response, and to factors that interfere with the function of immune cytotoxic effector cells capable of destroying or damaging target tissue. For example, a deficient production of leukemia inhibitory factor (LIF) by endometrial stromal cells and defects

(mutations) of LIF molecules can lead to sterility, which can be treated with recombinant LIF substitution therapy.[39, 40]

- The **trophoblast**, the fetal tissue at the maternal interface that completely surrounds the fetus, expresses in a modified form the major and minor histocompatibility and the developmental (oncofetal) antigens that are essential for recognition by the local maternal immune system, and the subsequent elicitation and expression of a local and systemic non-cytotoxic immune response.

- **Maternal immunologic stimulation** must occur. Maternal T lymphocytes and natural killer (NK) cells, activated by placental antigens and probably also directly by the embryo and endometrium, produce lymphokines, such as interleukins; activation of the 'innate immune system' is a requirement of successful pregnancy; the ratio of T-helper cells type 1 (Th1) over Th2 is postulated to play a role in immunotolerance, but alterations of this ratio (the so-called Th1/Th2 paradigm) and their effects are very controversial.[39, 40] The cascades involved in preventing the immune rejection of the embryo and fetus are very complex indeed, and poorly understood at present. They involve **sperm-related immunoregulation, B and T lymphocytes, uterine NK cells** (also called uNKs, or uterine large granular lymphocytes; uNKs, which can represent up to 70% of the uterine stroma in a peri-implantation uterus, are phenotypically strikingly different from peripheral NK cells; uNKs can secrete the crucial vascular growth factor angiopoietin-2), the **MHC**, many colony-stimulating factors (**CSFs**, partly under progesterone regulation) including granulocyte macrophage-CSF, complement inhibitors such as **Crry, interleukins** and other **cytokines** [such as IL-2, **IL-11**, IL-15, **interferons** (maternal IFN-g which also plays a role in vascular bed remodeling, and embryonal IFN-t), tumor necrosis factor (**TNF**) and maternal **LIF**], **HLA-A, HLA-B** (neither of which are expressed by human trophoblast cells), **HLA-C,** and **HLA-G** (which can protect otherwise NK-sensitive cells from NK cell-mediated lysis). Furthermore, it must be stated that the systemic effects of maternal immunomodulation are quite different from those observed in the microenvironment of implantation. A detailed exposure of the immunologic alterations associated with pregnancy and spontaneous abortions are beyond the scope of this chapter.[39, 40, 42–45]

- If these processes are not initiated, the critical features for the immunoprotection of the trophoblast are not achieved and it fails to proliferate in a manner necessary to support the fetus, or it may be rejected by allo- or autoimmune reactivity initiated in the mother. Maternal allorecognition of the fetus and placenta has been demonstrated, and such recognition is of sufficient strength to potentially cause embryo rejection, as is the case in any other allograft.[45]

Homozygosity of major histocompatibility genes may be a cause of spontaneous abortion in humans. The increased sharing of histocompatibility locus antigen (HLA) in couples experiencing recurrent spontaneous abortions can occur at all loci and is not restricted to one specific HLA locus.[46–48]

Shared HLA antigen loci may encode for trophoblastic antigen, thus preventing maternal recognition of trophoblast as semiallogeneic and thus also preventing production of blocking antibodies that inhibit cell-mediated immunity. HLA antigen sharing may result in lethal homozygous gene combinations, permit entry of maternal lymphocytes into the fetal circulation with runting or severe combined immunodeficiency (**fetal graft-versus-host disease**), or cause defective maternal vascular response to placentation similar to that seen with pre-eclampsia.[49] It has been found that HLA-A, HLA-B, and HLA-DR expression has no significant effect on pregnancy outcome;[50] however, the non-classical class I antigen HLA-G expressed in human trophoblast has been found to be of great importance.[51] It is not expressed by all tissues, but is highly expressed at the fetomaternal interface; some HLA-G polymorphisms are thought to protect from spontaneous abortion, whereas others may be predisposing.[42]

Gill suggests that genetic defects critical in determining the fate of the embryo are located in the HLA region of the MHC. He postulates that the most severe defects in MHC-linked genes would lead to the death of the embryo (recurrent spontaneous abortions); less severe defects would result in congenital abnormalities, and the least severe would lead to a predisposition to cancer.[52]

Other factors (contraception, environment, parental age)

There is a twofold increase in the risk of first- and second-trimester spontaneous abortion when pregnancy occurs in the presence of an IUD. Oral contraception, when discontinued at least 1 month before the last menstrual period, has not been associated with an increased risk of abortion. However, in pregnancy resulting from oral contraceptive failure, there is an increased risk of first-trimester abortion. During pregnancy the use of the diaphragm appears to reduce the incidence of second-trimester pregnancy loss, whereas the condom or rhythm methods have no impact on the abortion rate.

Many chemical compounds in the environment of working pregnant mothers have been implicated in the genesis of abortion, but few have been proved. Although some studies have shown an increased risk of abortion among female anesthesiologists, other studies do not support this finding. Information concerning a possible abortifacient effect after increased exposure to various environmental toxins is even less clear. Vianna[53] reported that the entire population of women exposed to toxic chemical wastes in the Love Canal area had no significant excess of spontaneous abortions, although groups of women living in certain areas with a higher exposure may have had an increased risk of abortion.

Maternal age is clearly associated with spontaneous abortions, independently of chromosomal abnormalities, and this risk increases markedly in very young mothers with a history of previous pregnancies, and in mothers older than 35 years of age. The risk of spontaneous abortion is reported to be of 2.1% in women 30–32 years of age, and to rise above 2.8% after 33 years of age, reaching 20–40% after 40 years of age.[16, 54, 55] It has also been suggested that paternal age greater than 45–50 years almost doubles the risk of fetal loss, particularly of late fetal death.[56]

TABLE 6.3 FREQUENCY OF DIFFERENT SPECIMEN MORPHOLOGY IN EARLY SPONTANEOUS ABORTIONS

Specimen morphology	Frequency (%)
Complete specimens	50
Embryos with growth disorganization	24
Normal embryos	10
Embryos with localized defect(s)	8
Degenerated embryos	8
Incomplete specimens	50
Ruptured/fragmented sacs	38
Decidua only	12

After Kalousek 1987;[58] with permission.

Specimens of early spontaneous abortion

The frequency of different types of specimens in early spontaneous abortion is given in Table 6.3. The morphologic evaluation of early spontaneous abortion is hampered by the fact that approximately one-half of specimens from early spontaneous abortions are either incomplete, which means that they contain only fragmented chorionic sacs and no embryo, or insufficient for any evaluation of the conceptus. The insufficient specimens are those with only decidua and blood clots. Decidua is not a product of conception, and specimens consisting of decidua only cannot be used for definitive confirmation of pregnancy loss, because hormonal treatment, ectopic pregnancy, and the premenstrual endometrium may mimic decidual change.

The complete specimens consist of either an intact chorionic sac or ruptured sac with an embryo. Gross examination of complete specimens can yield three types of useful findings: **embryonic growth disorganization (GD)**, **an embryo with normal morphology**, or an **embryo with localized defect(s)**. Examination of more than 2000 complete specimens has shown that embryonic GD is found in 58–70% of early spontaneous abortions; morphologically normal embryos in 16–24%; and embryos with localized developmental defect(s) in 5–18%.[57, 58]

Four types of embryonic GD have been described. The morphologic subclassification of GD allows more accurate estimates of the frequency of the underlying cytogenetic defects for the specific type of growth disorganization (Table 6.4). **GD$_1$ specimens** represent complete or very early failure of development of the embryo proper (Fig. 6.1). The intact chorionic sacs usually contain mucoid fluid with **no evidence of an embryo** or body stalk. Amnion, if present, is structurally abnormal; instead of being separated from the chorion by extraembryonic coelom, it is closely attached to it. The chorionic villi of these sacs are usually sparse, clubbed, and cystic. Microscopically, they are avascular and hydropic and show attenuated trophoblast cells.

GD$_2$ specimens (Fig. 6.2) consist of a chorionic sac containing **solid embryonic tissue 1–4 mm in length with no recognizable external features and no retinal pigment**. This embryonic tissue

TABLE 6.4 CORRELATION BETWEEN EMBRYONIC MORPHOLOGY AND CYTOGENETIC FINDINGS

Embryonic morphology	Abnormal cytogenetics (%)
GD_1	60
GD_2	73
GD_3	52
GD_4	37
Normal	20
Focal defects	92

After Kalousek 1987;[58] with permission.
GD, Growth disorganization.

may be firmly attached to the internal aspect of the amnion or it may have an identifiable short body stalk. A yolk sac can be distinguished from the embryo proper by its position between the amnion and the chorionic plate. The chorionic villi and amnion show abnormalities similar to those in GD_1.

GD_3 specimens (Fig. 6.3) contain **elongated, smooth embryos up to 10 mm long without any morphologic hallmarks but with retinal pigment** identifying the cephalic pole. Sparse, hypoplastic villi showing microscopically focal hydropic degeneration and reduced vascularization of villous stroma are common in these conceptions.

GD_4 specimens (Fig. 6.4) contain an embryo with **recognizable head, trunk**, and **limb buds**, characterized by **severe developmental inconsistencies** such as a small head for developmental

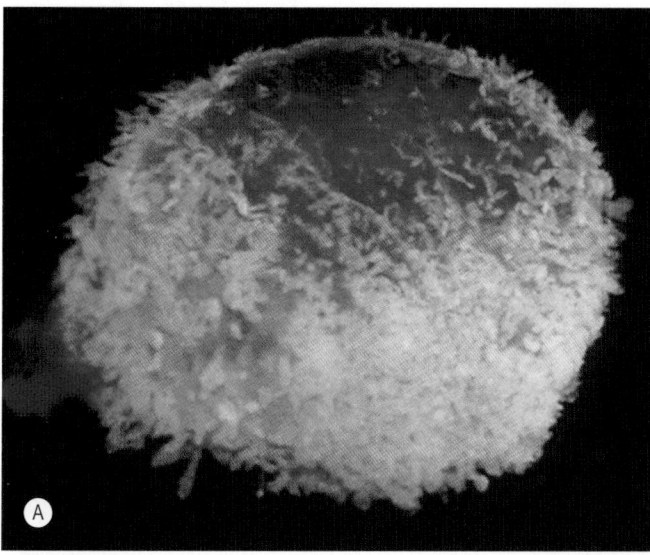
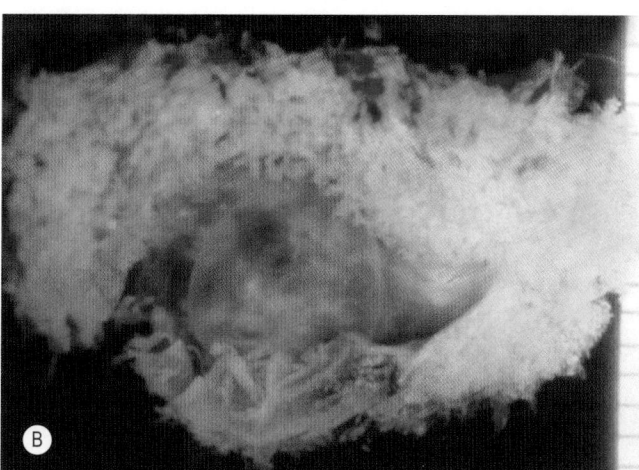

FIGURE 6.1 (A) Empty chorionic sac, 1 cm in diameter, showing inadequate development of villi. (B) Growth-disorganized (GD1) embryo with empty gestational sac.

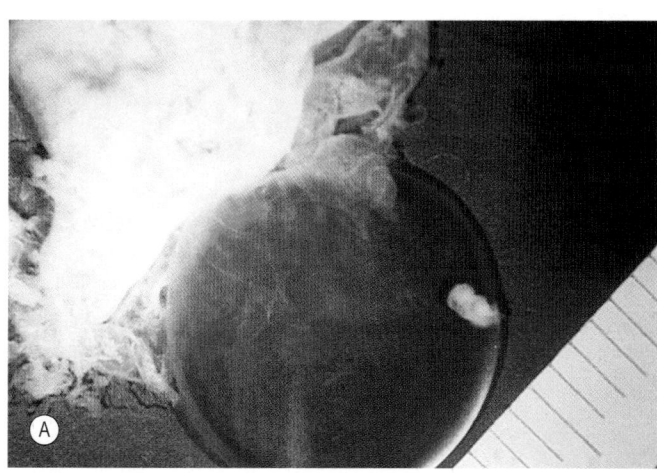
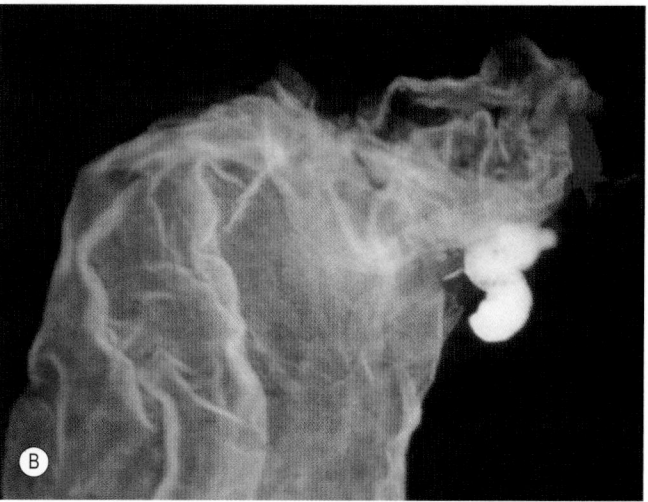

FIGURE 6.2 (A) Opened chorionic sac with amniotic sac. The embryo has failed to develop properly and is represented by a small white mass 2 mm in diameter inside the amniotic sac (GD2). (B) Close-up of embryonic disorganized tissue, 2 mm in length, firmly attached to the amnion (GD2).

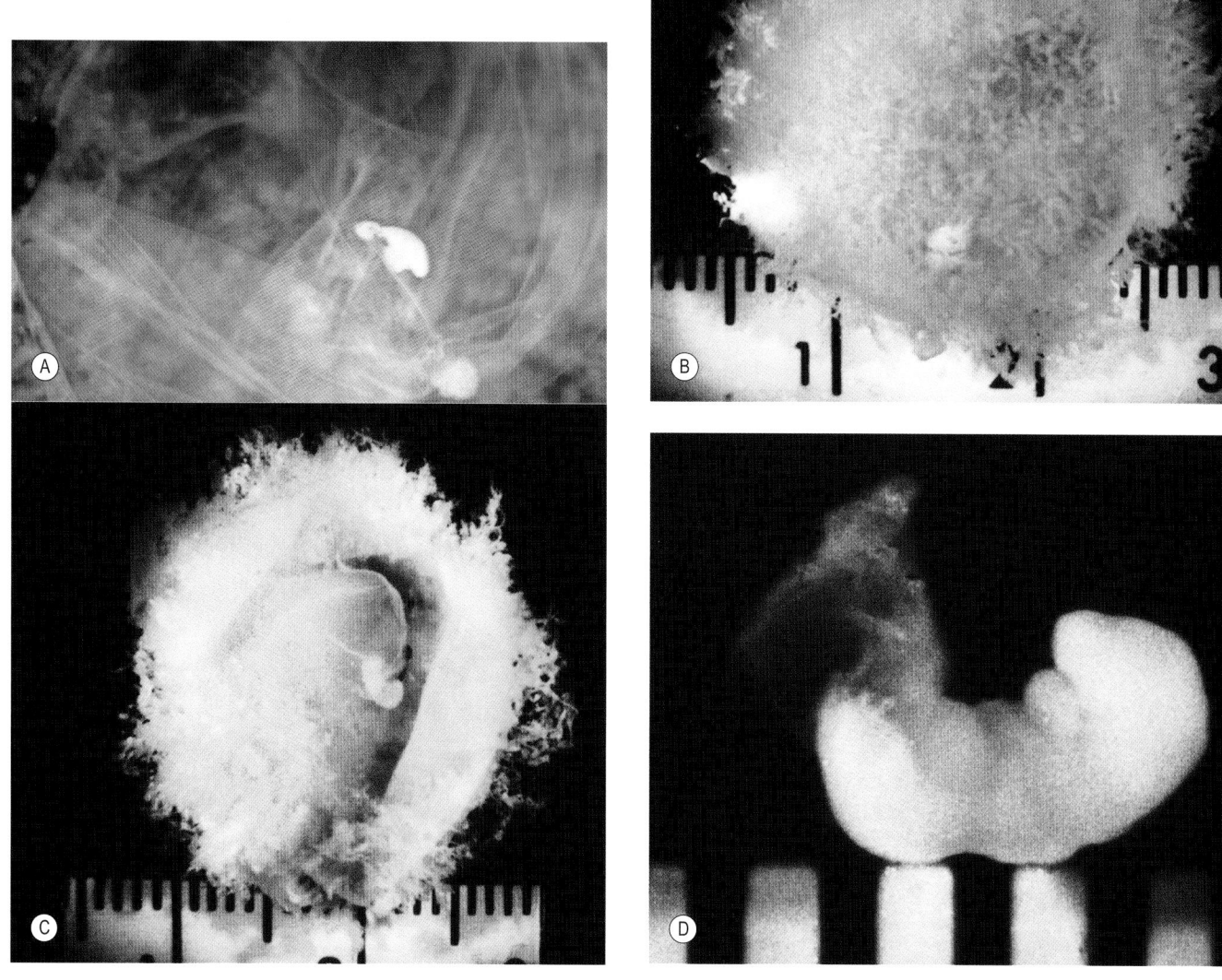

FIGURE 6.3 (A) GD3 embryo in an excessively large amniotic sac, which has become separated from the inverted chorionic sac. (B) Cystic enlargement and sparse development of villi in the chorionic sac, 2.8 cm in diameter, containing a GD3 embryo. (C and D) GD$_3$ embryo 3.5 mm in length with retinal pigment barely visible at the cephalic end. This embryo had a cytogenetic diagnosis of trisomy 16.

age (as established by embryonic length, usually 10–15 mm) or marked retardation in upper and lower limb development.

Embryos are classified as normal when orderly development of limbs, head, face, and trunk corresponds to that expected for an embryo of that specific measured crown-rump length (Fig. 6.5). **The normal development of human embryos is divided into 23 (Carnegie) stages.**[11] In the earlier stages the developmental stage of the embryo is determined by the number of somites, whereas in later stages the specific size of the embryo and its external features become important indicators for its staging. The main external features of each stage are summarized in Table 6.5.[11, 59–61] This staging allows an easy and accurate evaluation of normal

human embryos. A normal diploid chromosomal complement in a spontaneously aborted, morphologically normal embryo usually indicates implantation abnormality or maternal endocrine disorder.

Morphologically defective embryos may have single or multiple external defects (Fig. 6.6). Because morphogenesis is incomplete until the end of the embryonic period, the diagnosis of a specific defect in an embryo depends heavily on correct evaluation of its developmental stage.[62] For example, syndactyly cannot be diagnosed before stage 22. Most embryos with localized defect(s) show chromosomal abnormalities (Table 6.4), mainly various trisomies and triploidy.

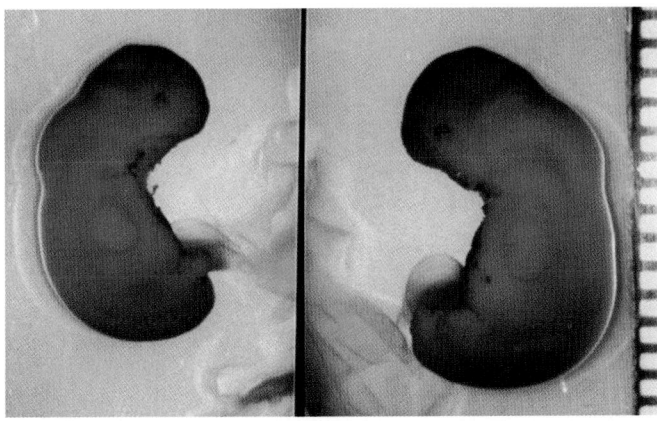

FIGURE 6.4 GD4 embryo 12 mm in length with a small head, dysplastic face, and growth-retarded limbs.

Histologic evaluation of placental tissue from early spontaneous abortions can be used for dating or descriptive classification. Its usefulness for correlation with cytogenetic findings is very limited. Szulman's dating of spontaneous abortion based on microscopic placental morphology is particularly useful in the evaluation of incomplete specimens of early spontaneous abortion.[63] He uses the chorionic villi vascularization and the presence of nucleated red blood cells as the main criteria for establishing

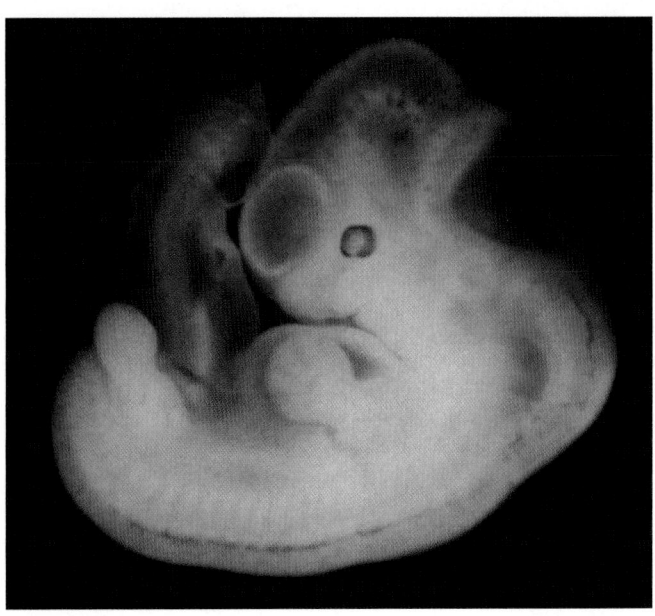

FIGURE 6.5 Normal embryo stage 16.

TABLE 6.5 SUMMARY OF EMBRYONIC DEVELOPMENT

Crown–rump length (mm)	Days after ovulation	Carnegie stage	Main external features
0.1	0–2	1	Fertilized oocyte
	2–4	2	Morula
	4–6	3	Blastocyst
		4	Bilaminar embryo
0.2–0.4	6–15	5	Bilaminar embryo with primary yolk sac
		6	Trilaminar embryo with primitive streak
0.4–1.0	15–17	7	Trilaminar embryo with notochordal process
1.0–1.5	18–20	8	Primitive pit and notochordal canal formed
1.5–2.0	20–22	9	Deep neural groove; first somites present; heart tubes begin to fuse
2.0–3.0	22–24	10	Neural folds begin to fuse; heart begins to beat; embryo straight; 4–12 pairs of somites
3.0–4.0	24–26	11	Rostral neuropore closing; embryo slightly curved; 13–20 pairs of somites
4.0–5.0	26–30	12	Upper limb buds appear; caudal neuropore closed; tail appearing; 21–29 pairs of somites
5.0–6.0	28–32	13	Four pairs of branchial arches; lower limb buds appear; tail present; 30 or more somites
6.0–7.0	31–35	14	Lens pits and nasal pits visible; optic cups present
7.0–10.0	35–38	15	Hand plates formed; lens vesicles and nasal pits prominent
10.0–12.0	37–42	16	Foot plates formed; nasal pits face ventrally; pigment visible in retina
12.0–14.0	42–44	17	Finger rays appear; auricular hillocks developed; upper lip formed
14.0–17.0	44–48	18	Toe rays and elbow region appear; eyelids are forming; ambiguous genital tubercle seen
16.0–20.0	48–51	19	Trunk elongating and straightening; midgut herniation to umbilical cord
20.0–22.0	51–53	20	Fingers distinct but webbed; scalp vascular plexus appears
22.0–24.0	53–54	21	Fingers free and longer; toes still webbed
24.0–28.0	54–56	22	Toes free and longer; eyelids and external ear more developed
28.0–30.0	56–60	23	Head more rounded; fusing eyelids

From Jirasek 1983,[59] Moore and Persaud 1993,[60] O'Rahilly and Muller 1987,[11] and Streeter 1951,[61] with permission.

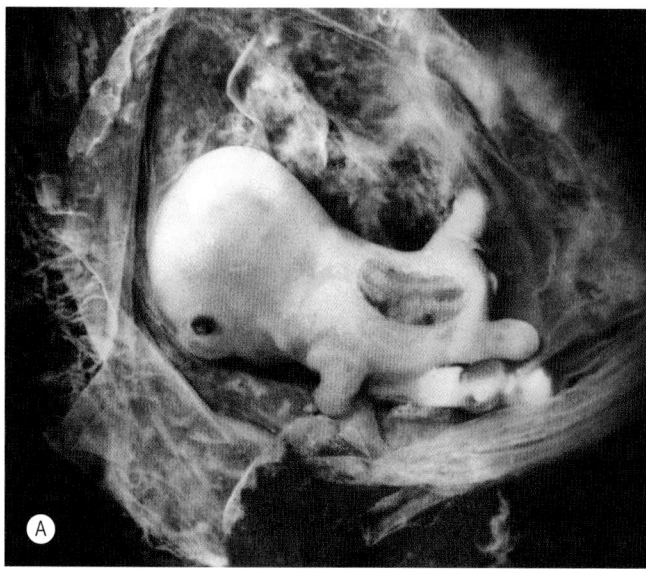
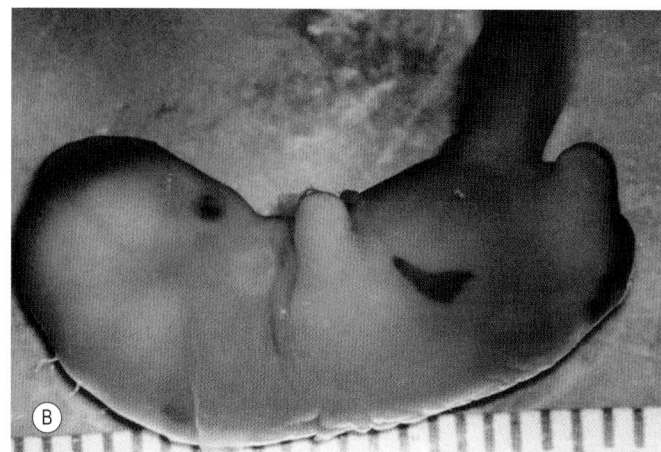

FIGURE 6.6 (A) Embryo, developmental age of 5½ weeks, with an open neural tube defect. (B) Embryo, developmental age of 5½ weeks, with multiple developmental defects including facial dysplasia, firm attachment of the chin to the chest, abnormal branchial arch development, and growth delay of limbs.

the embryonic age at the time of intrauterine demise. To classify incomplete specimens, Rushton[64] divides early conceptions (mean developmental age 9.4 weeks) into three main histologic categories:

- most villi showing microscopic hydropic change;
- most villi showing stromal fibrosis with vascular obliteration; and
- intermediate with about an equal proportion of those with hydropic villi and those with stromal fibrosis.

Several studies correlating morphologic and cytogenetic findings in placental tissue from early abortions have been performed, and all but the earliest ones[65, 66] concluded that there is no specificity in association of certain histologic villous alterations with chromosomal aberrations.[67–70] It appears that the placental villi may react similarly to chromosomal and non-chromosomal disturbances, and that villous morphology depends on the severity and the timing of the onset of the 'disorder' rather than on its type. The predictive value of the histologic appearance of chorionic villi for differentiating between chromosomally normal and abnormal abortions may be claimed in cases of the **partial hydatidiform mole**.[69, 71, 72] However, even this diagnosis is not absolutely specific for triploidy and may occasionally be associated with trisomic and with Beckwith-Wiedemann conceptions.[73]

Molecular techniques such as FISH, also known as interphase cytogenetic analysis, make the pathologist's job not only easier but also more affordable. Specific centromeric probes for the identification of various chromosomal aneuploidies and polyploidies can be utilized in specimens of early spontaneous abortion. **With probes for three different centromeres (X, Y, 16) accurate diagnosis of 60% of chromosomal defects can be made**.[74] The principle of hybridization in situ for the detection of chromosomal defect is simple.[75] Non-dividing interphase nuclei are exposed to a specific DNA centromere probe, such as D16Z1 (centromere probe for chromosome 16), which is fluorescent dye-labeled.

After the hybridization, numbers of positive signals are counted in 100–500 nuclei. Two signals in most nuclei mean that the specimen does not represent trisomy 16 conception. On the other hand, when three signals are found for D16Z1 and all the other probes show a normal number of signals, trisomy 16 can be diagnosed (Fig. 6.7). In the case of triploidy, three signals are seen for all the probes, including sex chromosomes. Tetraploidy is characterized by the presence of four signals for each probe tested and monosomy by the absence of one signal. Interphase cytogenetic analysis can be used for the detection of mosaicism[76] and archived material can be utilized.[77]

Clinical significance of pathologic evaluation of early spontaneous abortion

Examination of embryos is as important as the performance of perinatal autopsies. This is best illustrated by the example of embryonic localized developmental defects. Among embryos, frequent limb defects, cleft lip, and neural tube defects (Tables 6.6 and 6.7) have been recorded.[57, 78] The probability of recurrence of these defects in future pregnancies, and possibly in liveborn infants, depends on their cause. If the defects are multifactorial in origin, the recurrence is generally around 2–5%. It may be much higher for autosomal dominant and recessive mutant genes, or significantly lower if the defects are a part of a chromosomal syndrome, such as neural tube defect in triploidy. Therefore, detection of a specific defect and determination of its cause provide valuable information for genetic counseling and allow specific prenatal investigation in a future pregnancy. This would

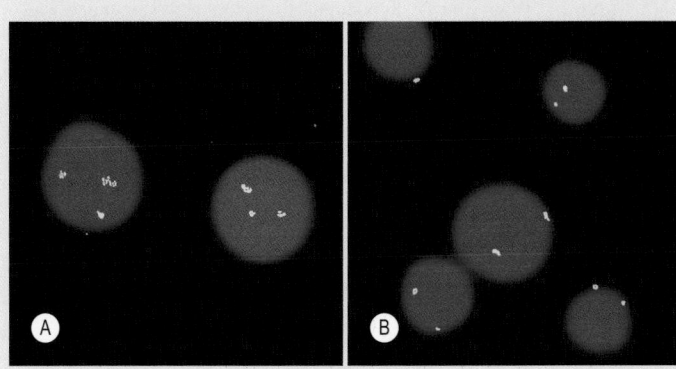

FIGURE 6.7 Fluorescence in situ hybridization using probe D16Z1. (A) Trisomy 16. (B) Disomy 16.

TABLE 6.6 PREVALENCE OF MAJOR DEVELOPMENTAL DEFECTS (PER 1000 EXAMINED)

System	Embryos	Previable fetuses	Stillborn fetuses	Newborns
CNS	23	12	49	1
CVS	16	96	15	7
Alimentary	12	76	10	5
Musculoskeletal	18	53	13	5

After Poland et al 1981,[57] with permission.
CNS, Central nervous system; CVS, cardiovascular system.

not be possible if pathologic investigation of early spontaneous abortion specimens had not been carried out and if a particular embryonic defect had remained undetected.

The identification of a well-developed, fresh embryo in an early spontaneous abortion specimen highly suggests abnormal hormonal function of the corpus luteum, endometrial insufficiency, or abnormal uterine structure. Some morphologically normal embryos may show an abnormal chromosomal complement, most commonly monosomy X and triploidy (Table 6.7). As the recurrence risk of pregnancy loss is higher if the abortus is cytogenetically normal than if the abortus is cytogenetically abnormal,[79] cytogenetic analysis of aborted morphologically normal embryos is clinically important.

The morphologic diagnosis of **embryonic GD is associated with chromosomal abnormalities in over 60% of specimens**, such as trisomy, monosomy, triploidy, and tetraploidy. Most of these chromosomal mutations are not hereditary and therefore carry no increased risk of recurrence for future pregnancies.[79] They originate de novo either in parental gametes (trisomy and monosomy) or are the result of failure of normal fertilization (triploidy and tetraploidy) and cleavage (tetraploidy). In couples with a history of habitual abortions, an understanding of the relationship between karyotype and phenotype of the conceptus is very important for the obstetrician. For example, the repeated finding of a normal karyotype in a specimen with embryonic GD suggests that a teratogenic effect may be interfering with normal embryogenesis or that submicroscopic lethal genetic defects may be preventing normal embryogenesis. The report of triploidy or tetraploidy indicates to the obstetrician an accidental and sporadic nature of the embryonic maldevelopment similar to that of trisomy and monosomy. Early pregnancy loss with chromosomal trisomy or monosomy explains the loss and does not place the couple at higher risk for repeated chromosomal trisomy and

TABLE 6.7 CORRELATION OF MORPHOLOGY AND KARYOTYPE IN 256 COMPLETE EARLY ABORTION SPECIMENS

Morphology	Normal karyotype	Trisomy*	Monosomy X	Triploidy	Tetraploidy	Structural rearrangement	Total
GD$_1$	15	13	2	1	3	3	37
GD$_2$	6	12		2	1		21
GD$_3$	10	11					21
GD$_4$	5	2	1				8
Normal embryos	32	4	5	3		1	45
Embryos with localized defects	10	29	18	25		7	89
Degenerated embryos	8	13	2	7	2	2	34
TOTAL	86	84	28	38	6	14	256

*Includes double trisomy.
Information from Registry of Handicapped Children and Adults in BC (1966–1973).
CNS, Central nervous system; CVS, cardiovascular system.

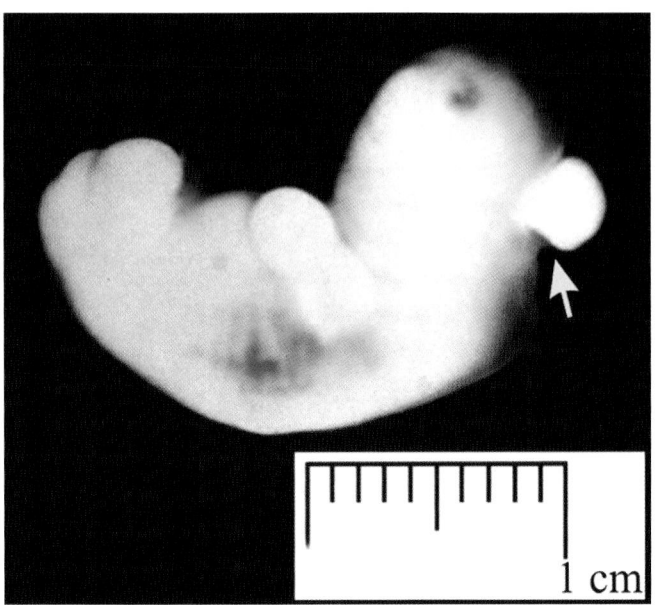

FIGURE 6.8 Embryo with monosomy X showing encephalocele (arrow).

pregnancy loss.[79] **Only the detection of chromosomal rearrangement indicates a high probability of one parent being a carrier of a balanced form of the rearrangement and a high risk of recurrence.**

Localized embryonic defects are common in **monosomy X,** triploidy, and trisomies 13 to 15. Embryos with monosomy X often show encephalocele (Fig. 6.8) and delayed limb development.[80] A typical embryonic **triploid phenotype** is characterized by advanced embryonic development with facial dysplasia, delayed upper and lower limb development, and symmetric or midline subectodermal hemorrhages. Facial clefting and neural tube defects, specifically a failure of the caudal neuropore to close, are common.[81, 82] Chromosomal triploidy is found in approximately 15% of chromosomally abnormal early spontaneous abortions. The gestational sac in triploidy may present with two different phenotypes, one characterized by cystic villi (Fig. 6.9), termed partial hydatidiform mole (Box 6.1), and the other being indistinguishable from any other chromosomally abnormal abortion.[71, 73] **Genomic imprinting** (discussed in Ch. 1) is the cause of these two specific placental phenotypes in triploidy (discussed in more detail below). **The partial hydatidiform** *mole* is characterized by the dominance of a paternal genome (fertilization of a single ovum by two spermatozoa or by a single diploid spermatozoon), whereas maternal triploidy (**i.e. non-molar triploidy, with two maternal chromosomal sets and only one paternal set**) is characterized by an **extreme placental hypoplasia with very severe fetal growth retardation; triploid fetuses, whether associated with molar or non-molar placentas, generally show malformations involving multiple systems** (see below).[83, 84] Among **trisomy 13** embryos, facial clefting, holoprosencephaly, and polydactyly are common findings. **Trisomy 14 and 15** embryos can also show facial clefting and growth retardation of limbs.

Before the introduction of ultrasound examination of early pregnancy, the incomplete early abortion specimens were most difficult to evaluate meaningfully on morphologic examination.[85–87] In the fragmented or ruptured chorionic sac with no embryo, the existence of an embryo proper and its level of development can now be established not only by histologic examination of villous vascularization,[53] but also by evaluation of the ultrasound images (Fig. 6.10). **Ultrasound examination** can document the presence of a well-developed embryo for its gestational age (Fig. 6.11) as well as a complete absence of an embryo or embryonic GD. Therefore the finding of avascular hydropic villi can be correlated with the ultrasound image (Fig. 6.12), and the specific diagnosis of an anembryonic sac with its high risk of *de novo* chromosomal error can be confidently made. The histologic evaluation of chorionic villi and a morphologic correlation with cytogenetic findings, by ploidy through flow-cytometry or through the expression of p57^{KIP2} (see complete hydatidiform moles, below) are usually successful in diagnosing chromosomal triploidy caused by **two paternal sets of chromosomes (diandric triploidy)**, as these conceptions have the specific morphology of a **partial hydatidiform mole** (Box 6.1). In any other chromosomal heteroploidy, the correlation between morphologic and cytogenetic findings is inconsistent, and in situ hybridization using chromosomal centromeric probes should be used to establish the presence or absence of numerical chromosomal defects to allow a more precise counseling of couples, especially those with a history of repeated pregnancy losses.

Specimens of late spontaneous abortion

Specimens of late spontaneous abortion consist of the fetus and the placenta. Examination of both is equally important for establishing the cause of the pregnancy loss. The principles of the examination are similar to those of perinatal autopsy.[12, 62] Placental abnormality is actually more common than fetal

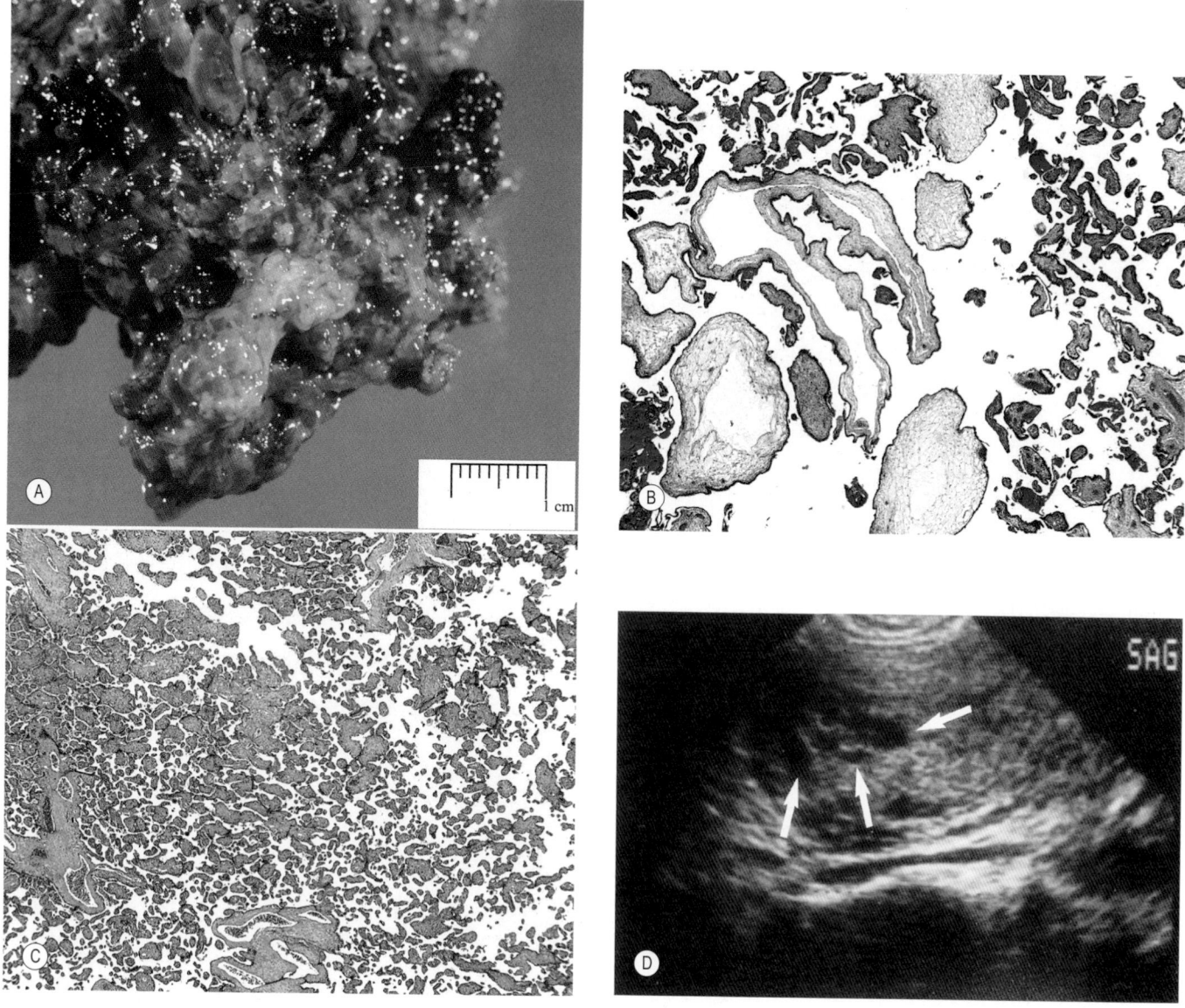

FIGURE 6.9 (A) Placenta with partial hydatidiform mole, showing large hydropic villi. (B) and (C) Histologic section of a partial hydatidiform mole and of a non-molar triploid placenta, respectively. (HPS stain; both magnified × 25) The villi of the partial mole are hydropic with cisternae, whereas those from the non-molar triploidy are hypoplastic and fibrous. (D) Ultrasound appearance of a partial mole with cystic dilatation of villi (arrows) on sagittal midline section through the placenta.

abnormalities during the previable fetal period.[88] In the analysis of **conceptions with a macerated fetus, over 50% of specimens showed a placental and related cause** of the loss compared with 25% unspecified causes and 25% fetal causes. Very similar findings were presented for specimens with fresh fetuses.[89]

In the natural history of a late spontaneous abortion it is common for the fetus to die before expulsion from the uterus. The interval between death and expulsion may be long, sometimes more than 8 weeks. Therefore, in evaluating the conceptus, it is important to distinguish those changes that occurred before fetal death from those that occurred after. The most obvious consequence of prolonged intrauterine retention is **maceration or autolysis** of the fetus, often diagnosed by ultrasound examination (Fig. 6.13).[90, 91] **No maceration occurs in the placenta** owing to its continuous nourishment from the maternal circulation. After fetal death the principal changes within the chorionic villi are **atrophy of the cytotrophoblast, clumping of nuclei in the syncytial trophoblast (syncytial knotting), fibrosis of the villous stroma,** and **collapse of the villous vessels** (Fig. 6.14). **Focal calcifications** in the villi are a common finding in retained second-trimester placentas. Secondary changes in the placenta after fetal death, apart from those described above, are **deposition of fibrin in the maternal placental compartment, subchorionic hemorrhage,** and **retroplacental hemorrhage**. Perivillous fibrin depositions are most marked close to the placental floor; when marked, this

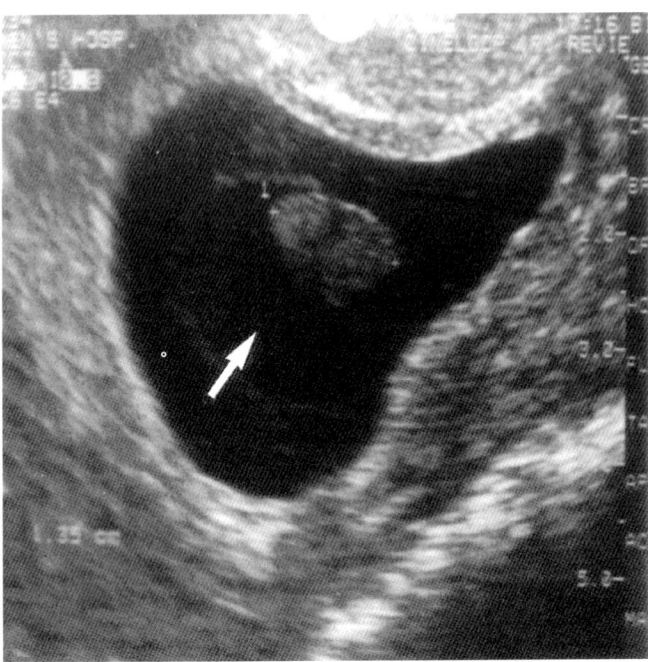

FIGURE 6.10 Endovaginal scan showing the uterine cavity with amniotic sac (arrow) and GD embryo measuring 1.35 cm in length. There was no heartbeat at the 10th gestational week.

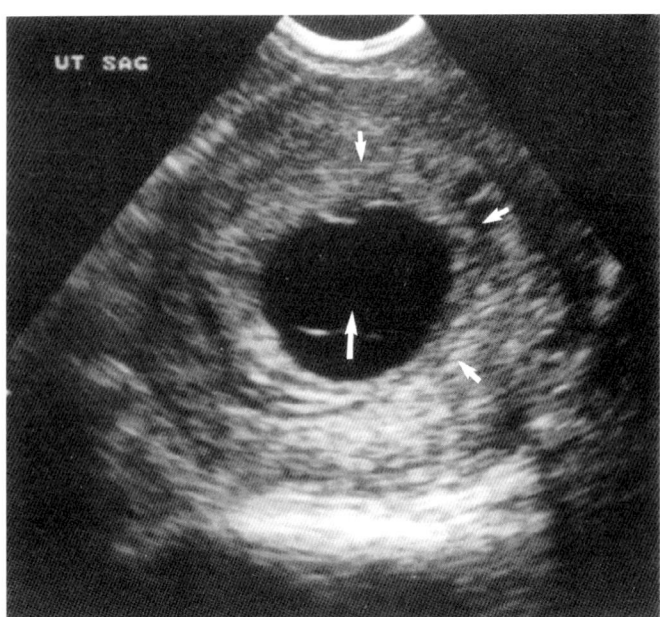

FIGURE 6.12 Endovaginal scan through the body of the uterus showing an anembryonic gestational sac with fluid (long arrow). Irregular villous tissue of the gestational sac is marked by several short arrows.

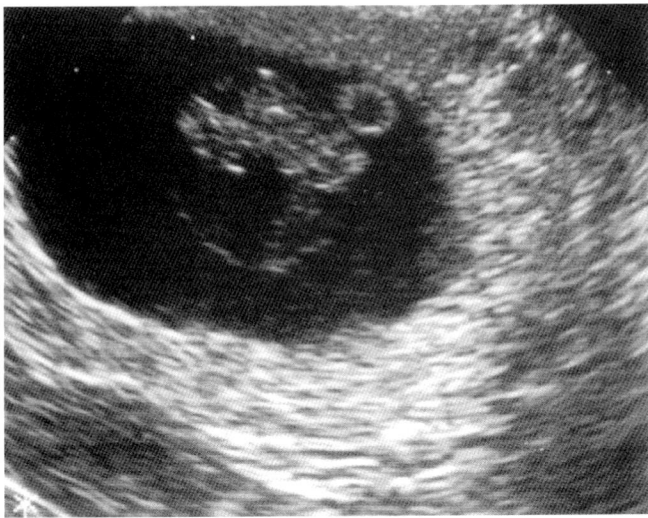

FIGURE 6.11 Ultrasound image of a normal gestational sac with an embryo.

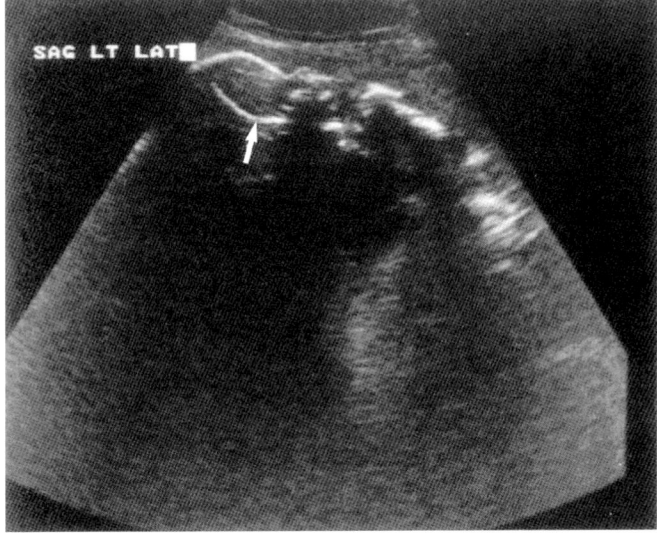

FIGURE 6.13 Ultrasound image of a macerated fetus with collapsed skull (arrow) and chest.

physiologic deposition must be differentiated from a **maternal floor infarct**. Subchorionic and retroplacental hemorrhages, referred to as **Breus moles**, are usually recent and extensive (Fig. 6.15).

Artifactual abnormalities are often present in spontaneously aborted fetuses.[92] Traumatic defects are commonly seen in the neck, thorax, and abdominal wall. Confusion with developmental defects can be avoided by careful microscopic examination of the margins of the defect. In traumatic defects the edges are irregular and show different layers of the area involved. Traumatic disruption can also mask developmental defects, such as an omphalocele

sac or an encephalocele. Vestiges of the ruptured sac are usually found around the circumference of the defect.

Autolyzed cerebral tissue in the retroperitoneal space can be confused with primitive neuroectodermal tumor in macerated fetuses. Brain tissue can also be found under pleura, in the neck area, and in inguinal areas (Fig. 6.16). This finding is common (one in four macerated fetuses) and is due to squeezing of autolyzed brain tissue into the spinal canal and along the spinal nerves into retroperitoneal and retropleural spaces or into the neck area. Detection of this artifact appears to be confined to a

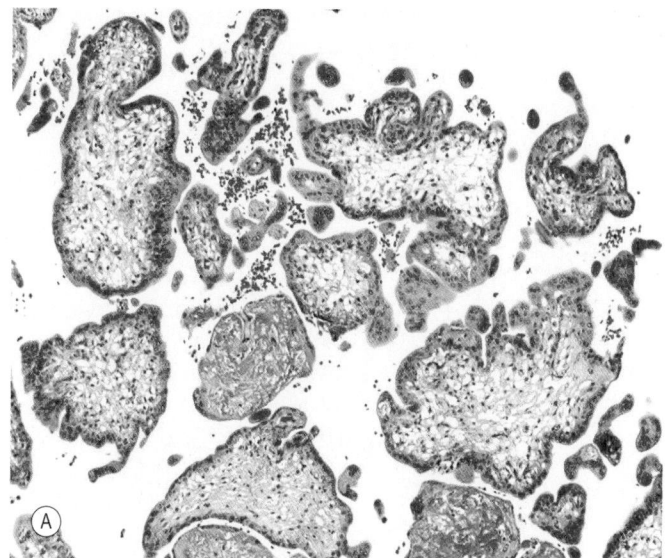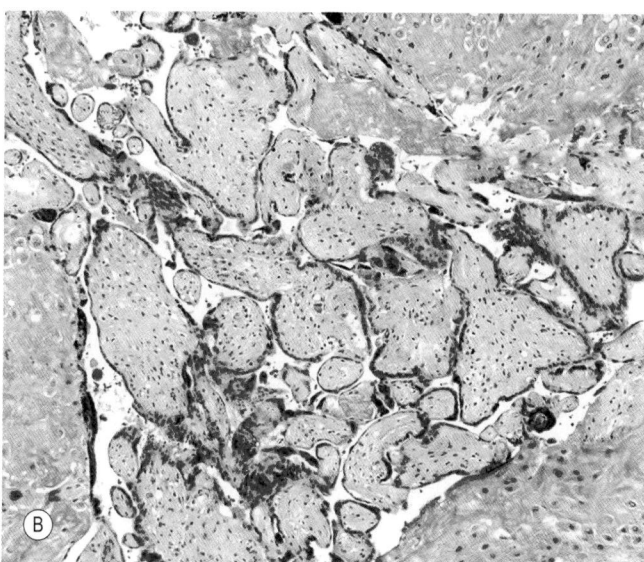

FIGURE 6.14 Histologic placental changes due to retention after intrauterine death of the fetus. (A) Villi with collapse of the blood vessels and partial condensation of the edematous stroma. (B) Villi showing hyalinization, clumping of syncytiotrophoblast nuclei, and collapse of the maternal vascular space.

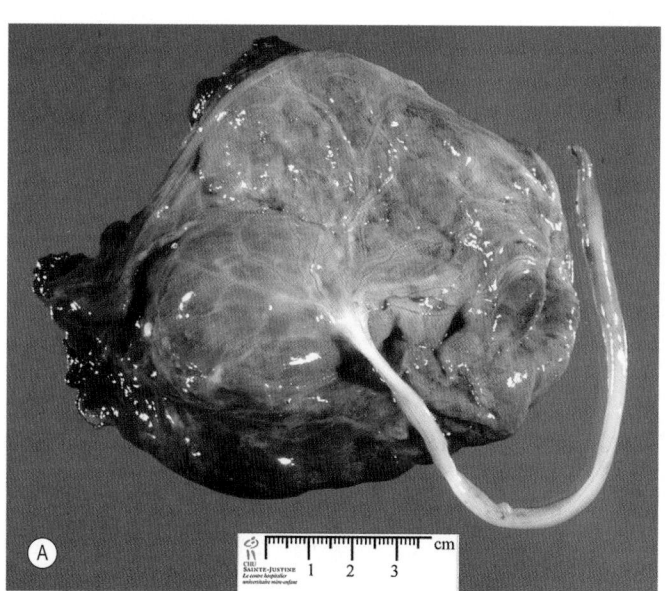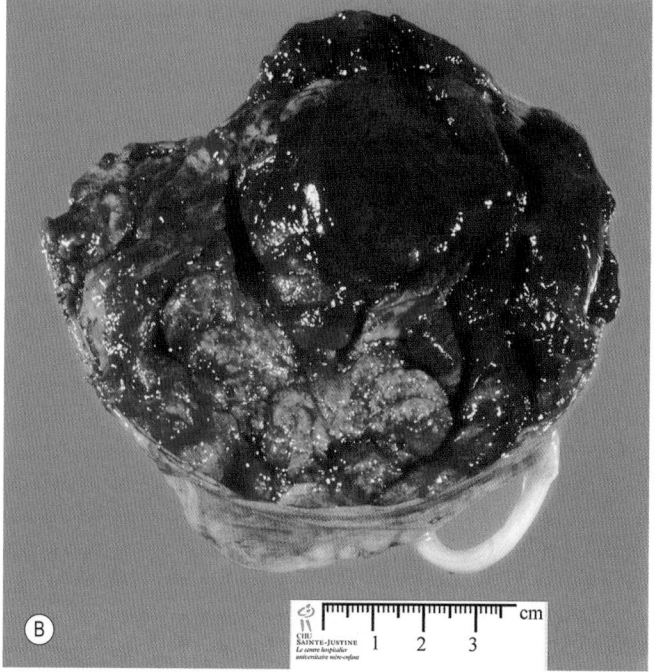

FIGURE 6.15 Subchorionic (A) and retroplacental (B) hemorrhage in the same patient.

developmental age between 9 and 16 weeks, which may signify certain developmental characteristics of this period.[93]

Autolysis and degeneration also interfere with evaluation of the normal development. In early fetuses, it is difficult to distinguish between opened eyes that are due to degeneration of eyelids and a primary defect in eyelid closure. Similar difficulty arises in evaluation of the lower lumbar and sacral areas in macerated fetuses of 9–11 weeks when the widening of the spinal canal may mimic an open neural tube defect.

Clinical significance of pathologic evaluation of late spontaneous abortion

Single malformations are more frequent among spontaneously aborted previable fetuses than among stillbirths or live births, as shown in Table 6.6. Their identification and accurate diagnosis

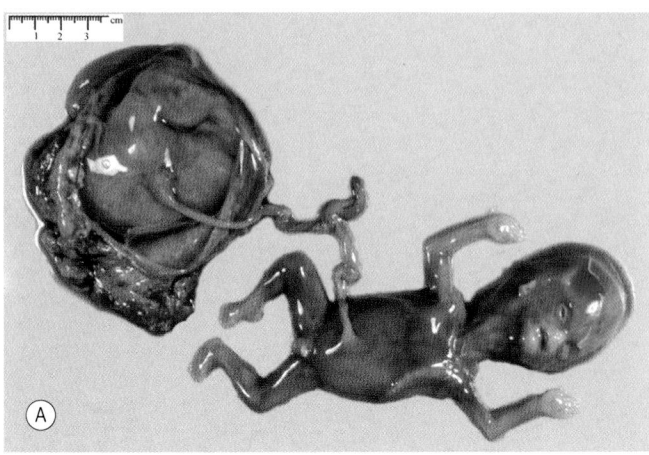

FIGURE 6.16 Autolyzed brain tissue in subcutaneous, subperitoneal, and lymphatic vessels areas.

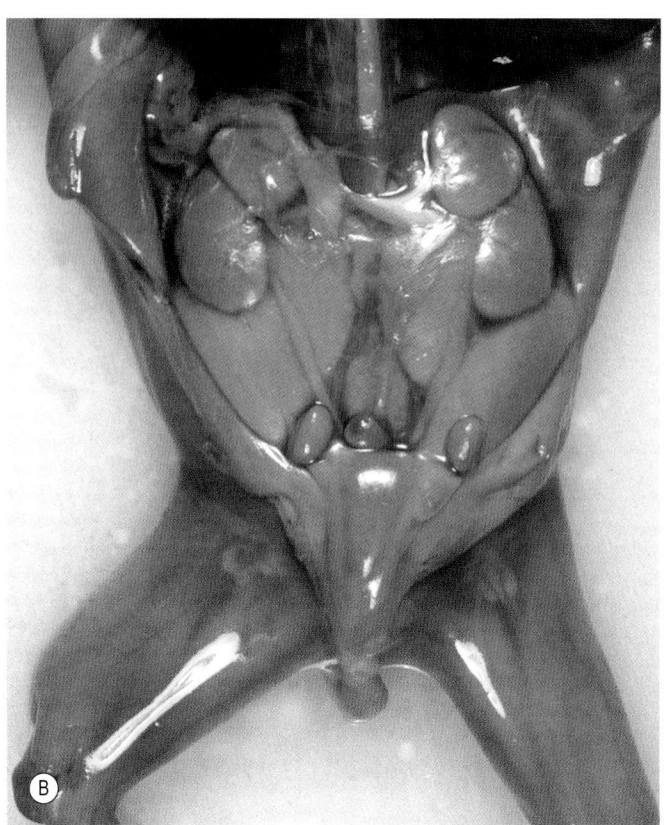

provide invaluable assistance in prenatal care of future pregnancies, as already illustrated in the example of embryonic defects.

A single lesion may have several pathogenetic mechanisms, and the distinction of a specific mechanism responsible for a defect provides guidance in the prevention effort for geneticists, obstetricians, and the family in future pregnancies. For example, congenital heart disease of multifactorial inheritance has a recurrence risk in future pregnancies of 2–5% (depending on the type of defect), whereas the recurrence risk for heart defect is not increased when associated with a chromosomal defect (e.g. trisomy 13). Neural tube defects are even more heterogeneous (Figs 6.17–6.19), as these can be of multifactorial origin, caused by

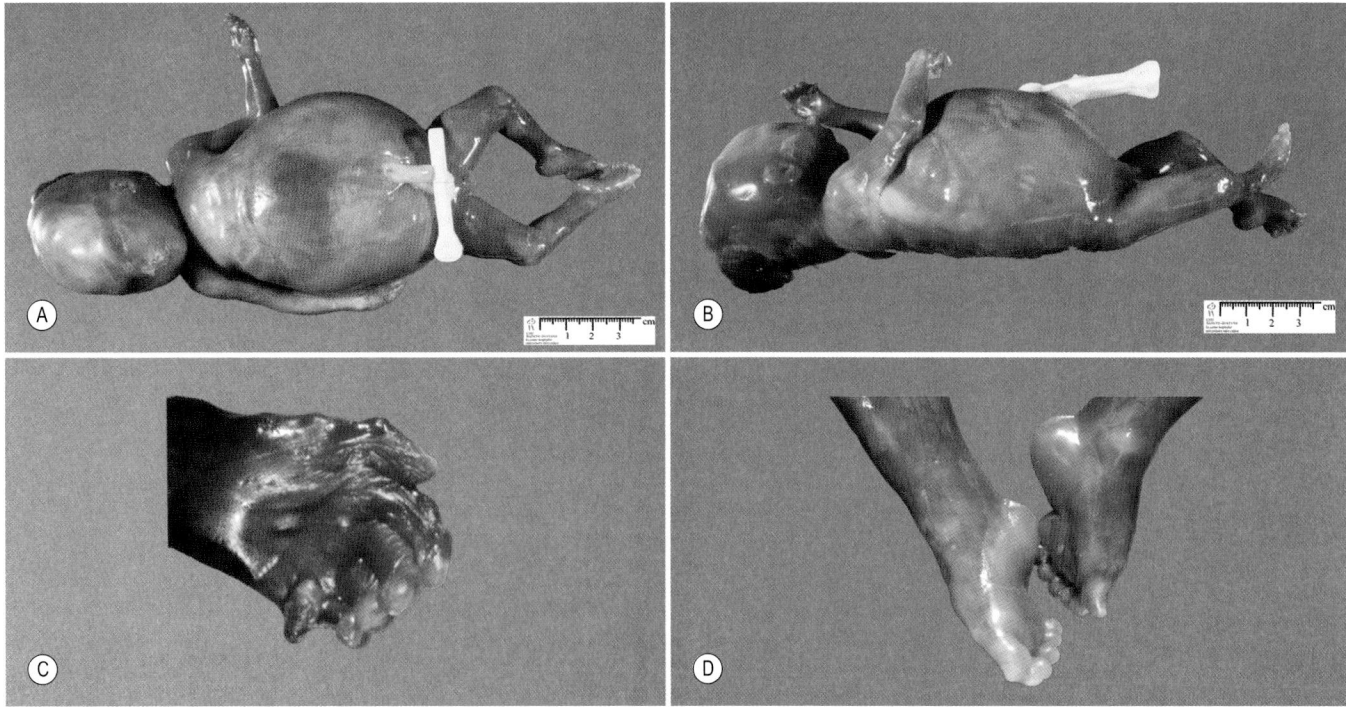

FIGURE 6.17 A fetus with Meckel-Gruber syndrome, exhibiting abdominal distension due to a severe renal multicystic dysplasia (a constant feature) (A), as well as an encephalocele (B) and polydactyly of hands and feet (C and D).

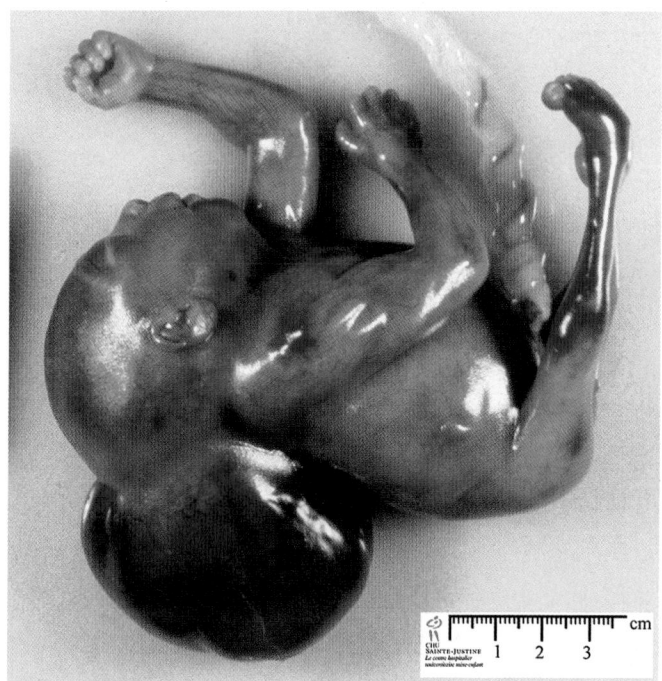

FIGURE 6.18 Neural tube defect (encephalocele) in a fetus with a normal chromosomal complement.

a single-gene defect (Meckel-Gruber syndrome type I, MIM 249000), chromosomal defect (trisomy 13, 18, triploidy), or a non-genetic mechanism (amniotic bands). The recurrence risk for each of these pathogenetic mechanisms differs substantially (Table 6.8). The common morphologic defects seen among spontaneously aborted or previable fetuses are described below.

Abortion of a morphologically normal previable fetus is usually related to uterine or placental abnormalities or an ascending infection. For future pregnancy management, clear identification of the normal development of such a fetus, and determination of the specific cause of late abortion, are important (Fig. 6.20).

The incidence of cytogenetic abnormalities among late abortions is substantially lower (5–10%) than among early abortions.[15]

The most frequently detected chromosomal abnormalities are specific autosomal trisomies (13, 18, 21), sex chromosome monosomy (45,X), and triploidy. Since these chromosomal defects are typically found among morphologically abnormal fetuses, chromosomal studies are indicated for all fetuses with developmental defects.

Most fetuses with chromosomal defects show a characteristic phenotype. A classic fetal phenotype for sex chromosomal monosomy (45, X) consists of generalized subcutaneous edema, posterior cervical cystic hygroma, and an aortic preductal coarctation (Fig. 6.21). This triad is found with high consistency among spontaneously aborted previable fetuses with sex chromosome monosomy.[94] Other developmental anomalies, such as abnormal bicuspid aortic valve, horseshoe kidney, ventricular septal defect and single umbilical artery are commonly, but not consistently, observed.[95] Isolated posterior cervical hygroma mandates a complete internal examination because it may be seen in a variety of conditions, such as Noonan syndrome, congenital heart disease, fetal alcohol syndrome, and autosomal chromosomal trisomies.[96] In fragmented or incomplete fetal specimens, a diagnosis of fetal 45,X can be supported by the presence of cutaneous edema with peripheral lymphatic hypoplasia.[97] The cytogenetic analysis of cultured fetal tissues or of interphasic nuclei remains essential for differential diagnosis of posterior cervical hygroma whenever aortic preductal coarctation is not identified.

The phenotype of **fetal triploidy** in spontaneous abortion depends on the parental origin of the extra haploid set of chromosomes. It is usually characterized by IUGR, **syndactyly of digits** (usually between the third and fourth fingers and toes), **abnormal development of brain** (hydrocephalus, neural tube defect), **cardiac malformations and severe adrenal hypoplasia**. In **non-molar triploidies** (resulting from an extra maternal haploid set), the **placenta is small and fibrosed**, the **fetus shows an extreme growth retardation with relative macrocephaly**[95] (Fig. 6.22). Triploidies of paternal origin are less frequent. Fetuses from these **molar triploidies** show a different phenotype characterized by **mild to moderate IUGR, microcephaly** and placental cystic changes typical for partial hydatidiform moles (Fig. 6.23).[98]

Only a few specific autosomal trisomies – 13, 18, 21 – are found among late abortions. Trisomies 13 and 18 are easily

TABLE 6.8 ETIOLOGY AND RECURRENT RISK OF NEURAL TUBE DEFECTS

Defect	Etiology	Recurrence risk (%)
Meningomyelocele	Triploidy	0
Meningomyelocele	Trisomy 13 (extra chromosome/translocation)	1–10
Meningomyelocele	Multifactorial inheritance	2
Encephalocele	Amnion rupture sequence	0
Encephalocele	Meckel-Gruber syndrome	25
Encephalocele	Multifactorial inheritance	2

After Kalousek 1991,[83] with permission.

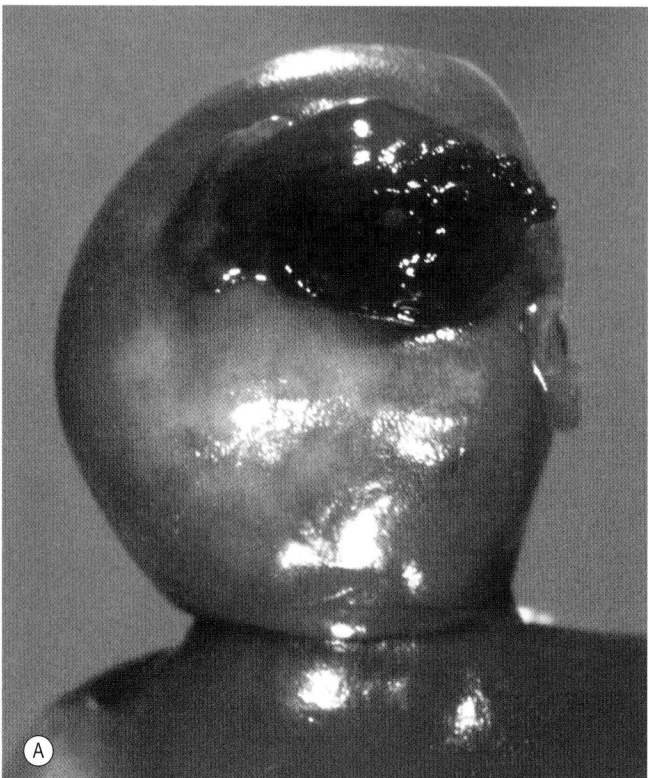

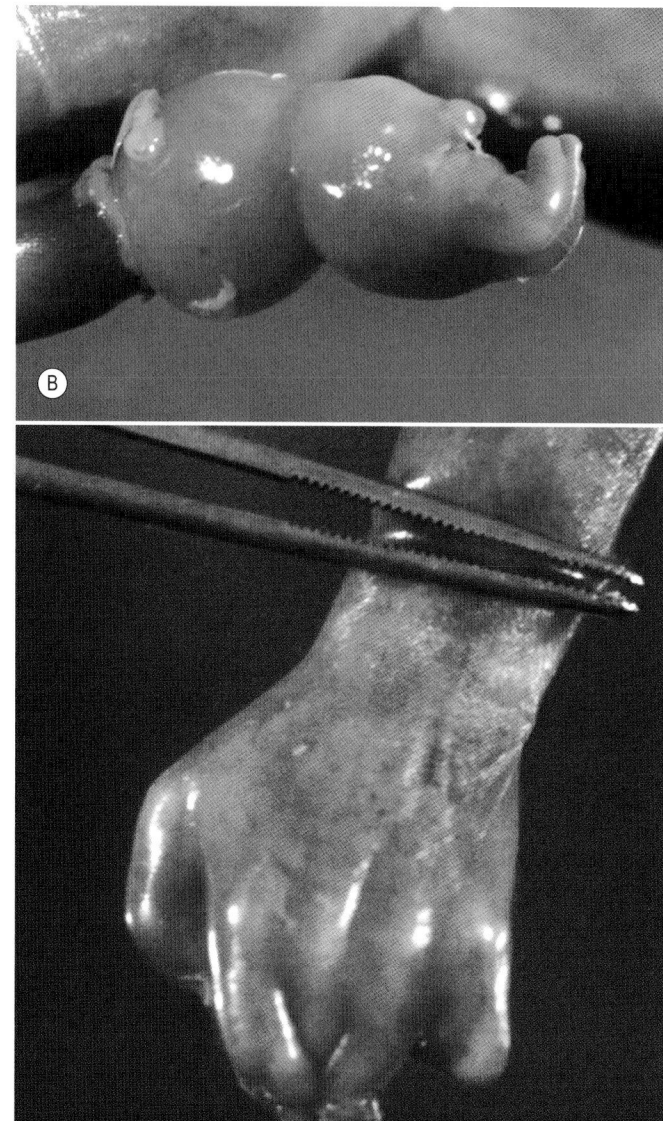

FIGURE 6.19 Amniotic bands producing deformation of the skull mimicking encephalocele (A); (B) the constriction of the forearm, amputations of fingers and (C) fusion of digits are also characteristic features.

diagnosed on the basis of morphologic examination alone, as they present characteristic phenotypes. Cardiac malformations, polydactyly, cleft lip and palate, and abnormal brain and eye development are the hallmarks of **trisomy 13** (Fig. 6.24). **Severe IUGR, abnormal positioning of second and fifth fingers overlapping the third and fourth fingers, congenital heart disease,** and **omphalocele** are commonly found in **trisomy 18** (Fig. 6.25). The phenotype of fetuses terminated after prenatal diagnosis of trisomy 21 is frequently normal; only a search for subtle features such as midphalangeal hypoplasia of the fifth finger, simian crease, flat occipital bone, and congenital heart disease (typically atrioventricular defect) may suggest trisomy 21. Spontaneously aborted fetuses with **trisomy 21** usually show **fetal hydrops** or at least cervical cystic hygroma (Fig. 6.26).

Common abnormal morphologic findings in late abortion specimens

Neural tube defects (see also Ch. 36)

Rachischisis is the most common neural tube defect seen among spontaneously aborted fetuses. It results from a failure of the spine to close and encircle the spinal cord, and may either be open (with the spinal cord bathing in amniotic fluid) or closed by skin and soft tissues, occasionally forming a cyst, the meningoceles and meningomyeloceles. **Triploidy and trisomies 13 and 18** must always be considered in spontaneously aborted fetuses showing

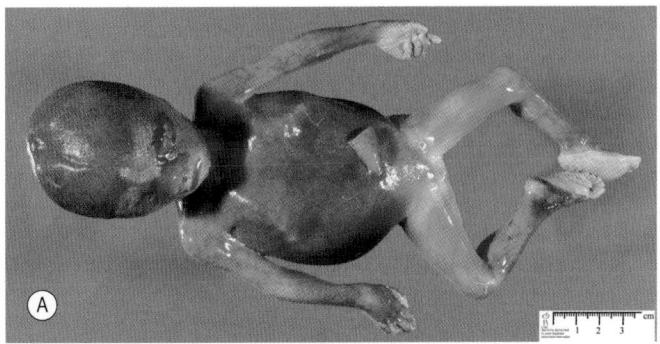

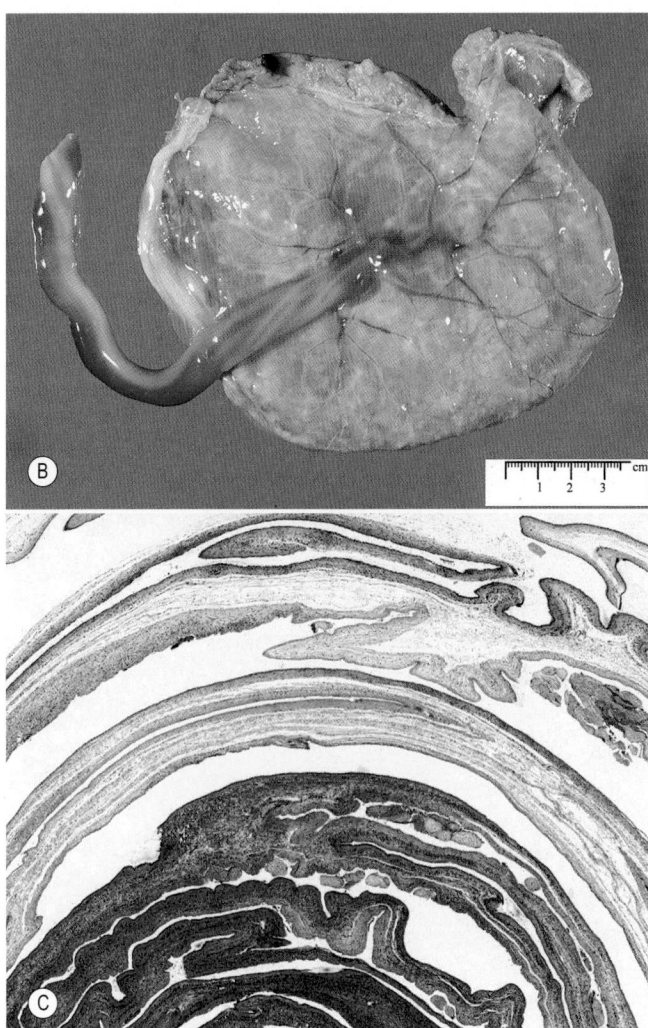

FIGURE 6.20 Spontaneously aborted, normally developed fetus at 16 weeks of gestational age, (A), with creamy membranes suggesting chorioamnionitis (B). Histologic examination of the amnion roll confirmed the diagnosis (C), and showed the causative organism to be Candida. (Stained with HPS; original magnification × 25)

such a defect, as there is a frequent association between thoracolumbar rachischisis and aneuploidy. Molecular cytogenetic examination of fetal or placental nuclei is particularly useful when fetal tissue cannot be karyotyped. Prenatally, meningomyelocele is usually diagnosed by a raised maternal α-fetoprotein concentration if open or by ultrasound examination when closed.

Other neural tube defects such as anencephaly and encephalocele are rare findings in late spontaneous abortion specimens (Fig. 6.27). They are usually diagnosed through ultrasound examination or by elevated maternal serum α-fetoprotein testing.

Hydrocephalus results from an increase in the amount of intraventricular cerebrospinal fluid. Although it is usually due to obstruction, the increase may also be due to an overproduction or defective absorption of cerebrospinal fluid. Hydrocephalus can develop as early as the second trimester of pregnancy. It may be associated with a variety of infections, mutant genes, and chromosomal triploidy.

Amnion rupture sequence

Amnion rupture sequence (ARS) is a disruption complex characterized by rupture of the amnion, with secondary effects on the fetus producing:

- **malformations** resulting from interruption of normal morphogenesis;
- **deformations** due to distortion of established structures; or
- **mutilations** of structures already formed.

Although ARS is an uncommon, sporadic condition among liveborn infants, its prevalence among previable fetuses is about 100 times higher than in the third trimester, and **constrictions of the umbilical cord by amniotic bands** (Fig. 6.28) **are a frequent cause of fetal intrauterine death and spontaneous abortion.**[99]

Posterior cervical cystic hygroma

Posterior cervical cystic hygroma, once considered diagnostic of fetal monosomy X, is now being recognized as a non-specific

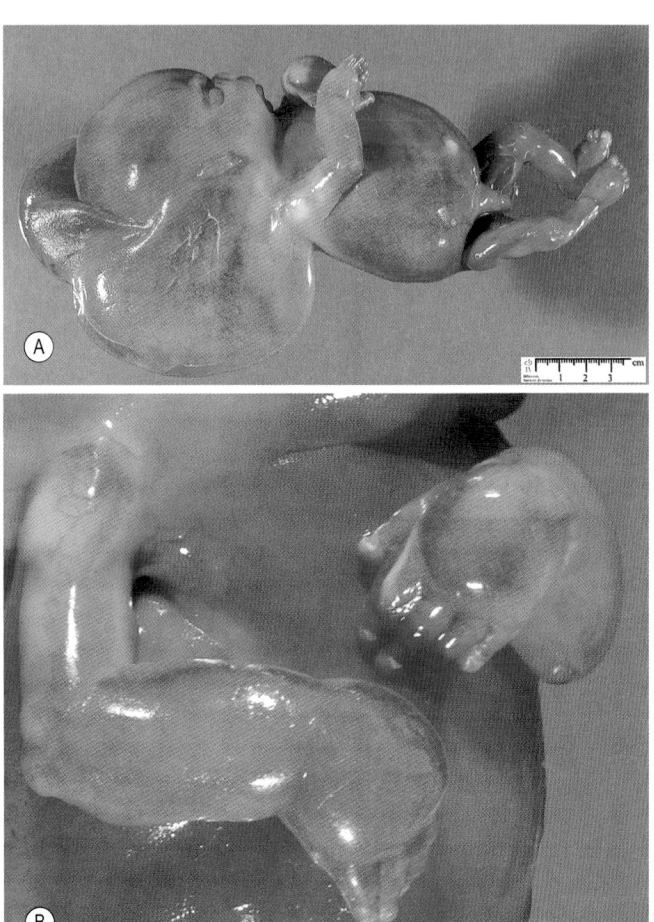

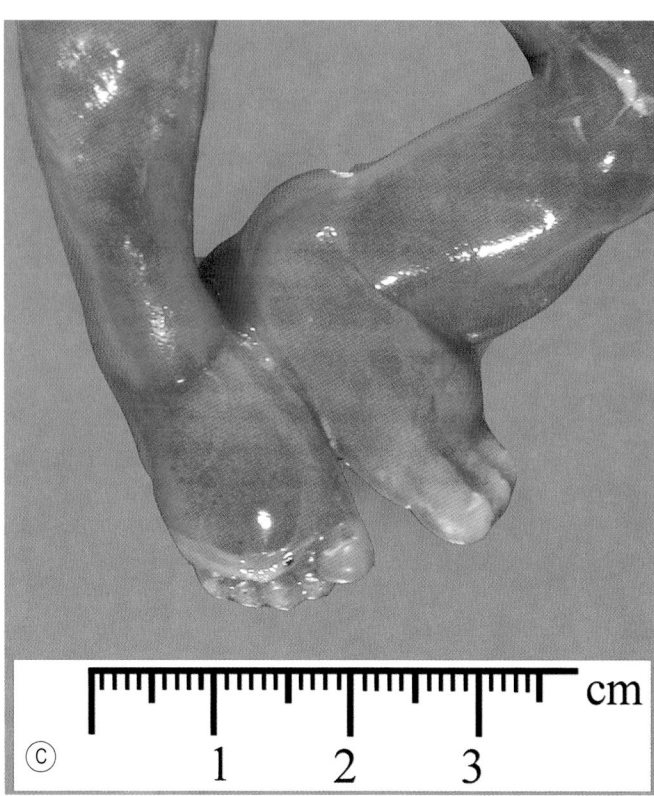

FIGURE 6.21 (A) Typical appearance of a fetus with monosomy X at 20 weeks' gestation. (B) and (C) Note the characteristic edema of the dorsum of the hands and feet.

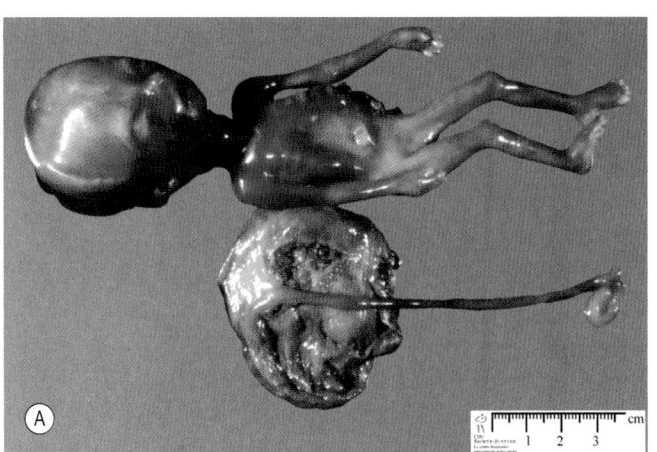

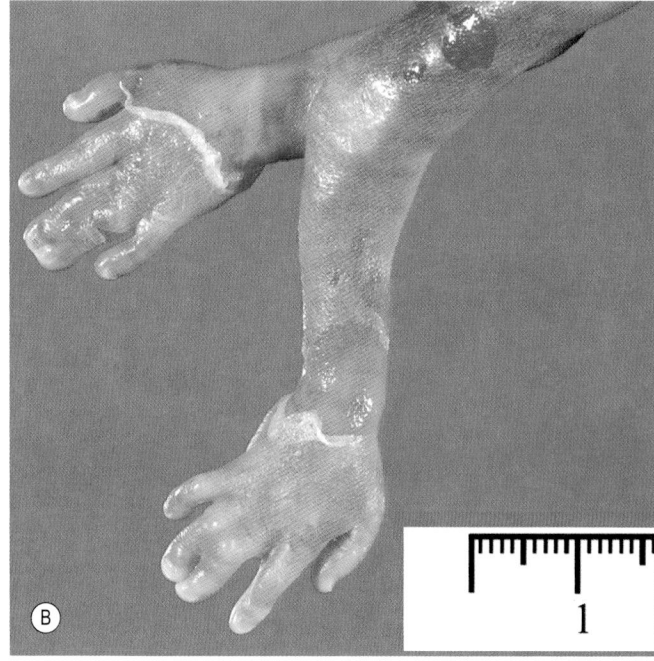

FIGURE 6.22 (A) Typical appearance of a fetus and placenta with non-molar triploidy due to an extra maternal haploid chromosomal complement. Note the macrocephaly and extreme placental hypoplasia. Syndactyly of the third and fourth digits, absent in this fetus, is not a constant feature. (B) Different triploid fetus, with characteristic 5–4 syndactyly.

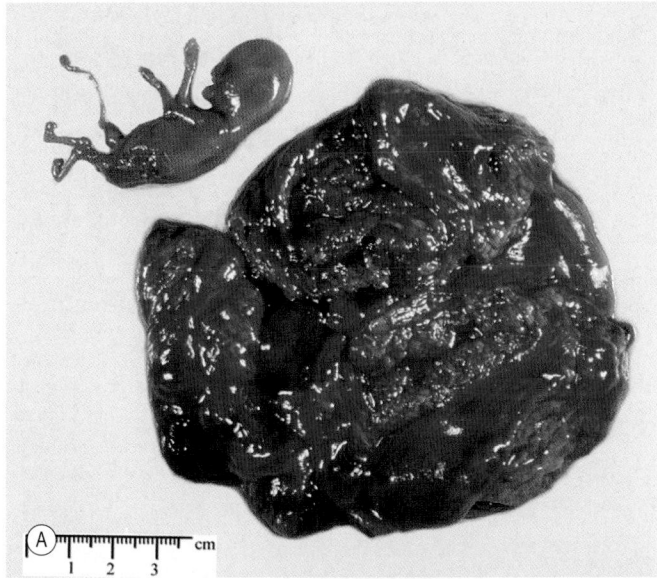

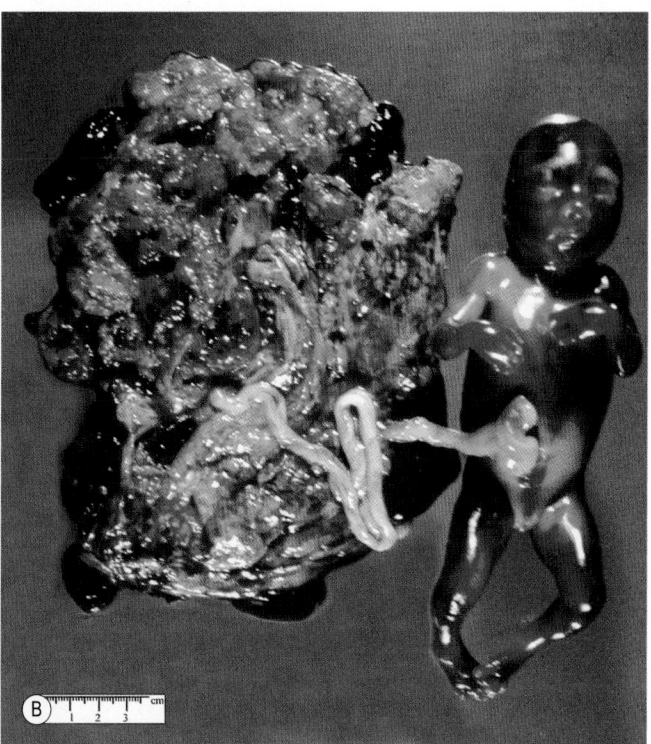

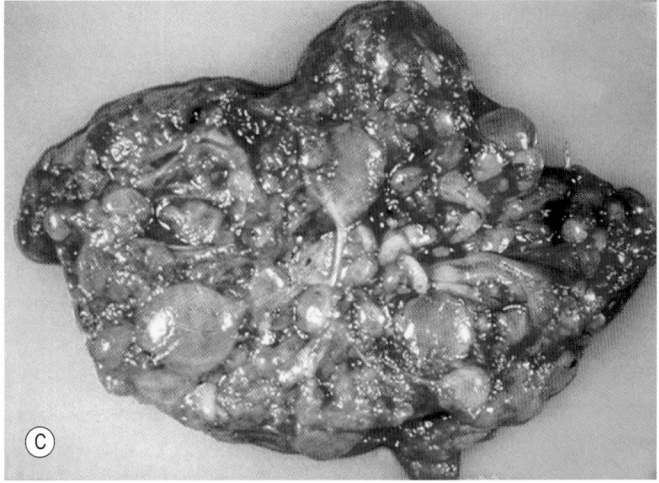

FIGURE 6.23 (A) and (B) Typical appearance of a fetus and placenta with molar triploidy due to an extra paternal haploid chromosomal complement. (C) Placenta of molar triploidy with large hydropic (cystic) cisternae.

abnormality found in several unrelated conditions, such as chromosomal trisomies, multiple lethal pterygium syndrome, Noonan syndrome, Roberts syndrome, congenital heart disease, infections (e.g. by parvovirus B19) and others.[96, 100] It consists of fluid accumulation in dilated lymphatic channels of the neck and surrounding connective tissue, and reflects failure or delay in development of the connection between the jugular lymph sac and the internal jugular vein.[101] Posterior cervical hygroma can easily be detected on ultrasound examination of midtrimester fetuses (Fig. 6.29). Among spontaneously aborted fetuses, posterior cervical hygroma is **usually associated with chromosomal trisomies, monosomy X**, and **multiple lethal pterygium syndrome** (MIM 253290). It is important that the correct fetal condition associated with the cervical hygroma be established, to allow accurate genetic counseling.

Abdominal wall defects (see also Ch. 21)

Omphalocele is commonly seen among spontaneously aborted fetuses. As a result of failure to correct the physiologic midgut

herniation (which should have closed by the end of the 11th week pc), omphalocele contents remain in a membranous sac composed of amnion and peritoneum (Fig. 6.30). Associated developmental anomalies are frequent.[62, 102] In two-thirds of the fetuses with prenatal diagnosis of omphalocele, chromosomal defects were found.[103] Omphalocele must be clearly distinguished from other abdominal wall defects, such as gastroschisis and body stalk defect, to allow accurate genetic counseling.

Facial clefts

Facial clefts (see also Ch. 20) are usually found at the fusion site of the frontonasal, maxillary, and mandibular prominences. Lateral or median cleft lip, with or without cleft palate, is the result of a fusion failure. Facial clefts are etiologically a heterogeneous group. They may occur as isolated abnormalities or as part of a syndrome. Isolated cleft lip, with or without cleft palate, is a different entity from cleft palate alone. Referral of the family to the clinical genetics service after diagnosis of cleft lip or palate in a

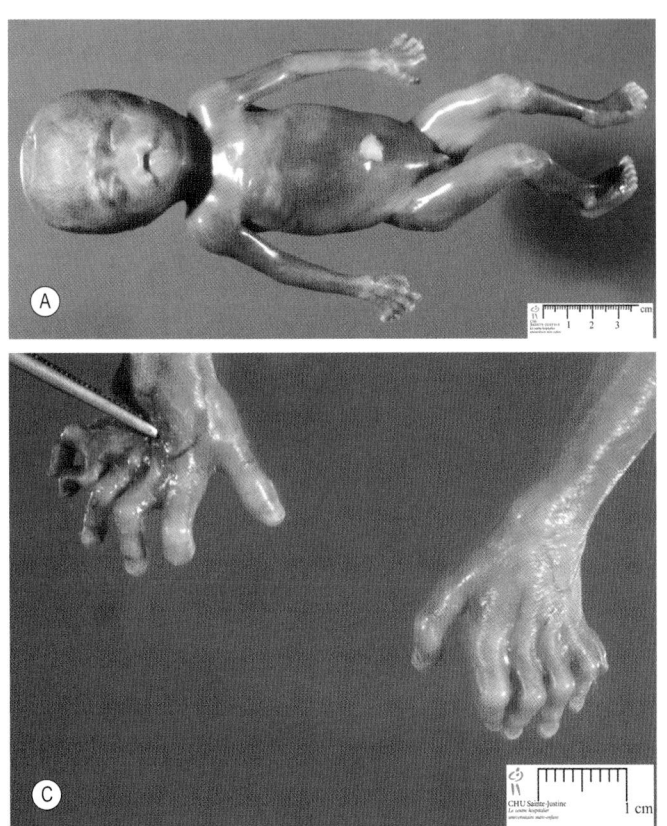

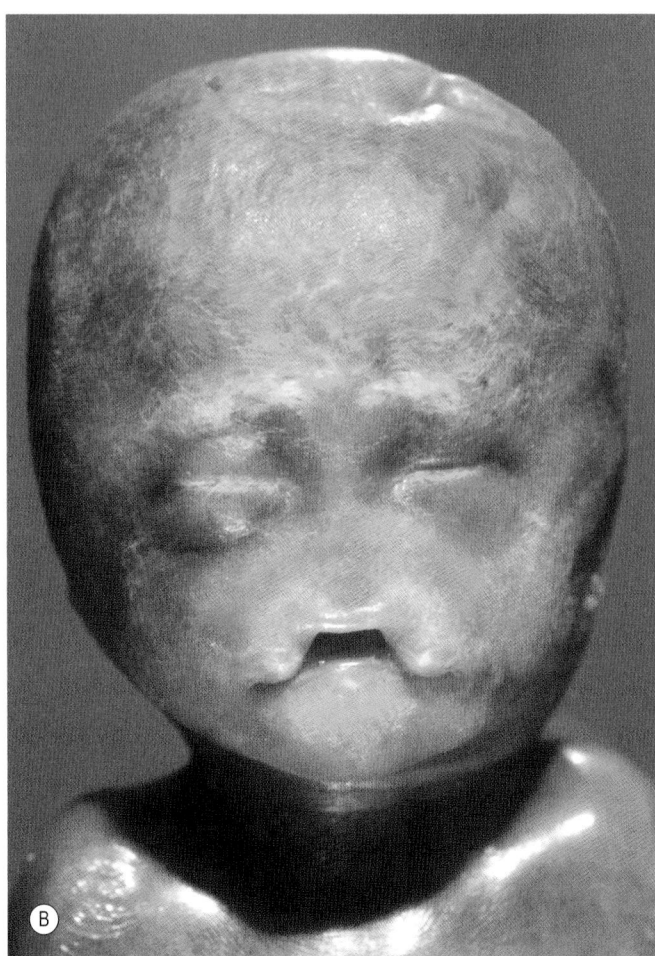

FIGURE 6.24 (A) Trisomy 13 fetus with microcephaly; (B) midline cleft lip and left-sided microphthalmia; and (C) polydactyly.

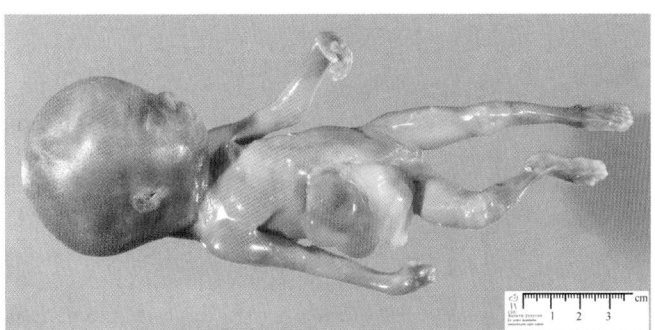

FIGURE 6.25 Trisomy 18 fetus with marked intrauterine growth retardation and omphalocele.

chromosomally normal conceptus is important for complete evaluation, as the inheritance may be dominant, X-linked, or multifactorial.

Cleft lip and palate are often found in fetuses with trisomy 18. In trisomy 13, over 50% of fetuses have facial clefts.[62] Other chromosomal abnormalities may also be associated with facial clefts. Irregular facial clefts or those occurring in areas other than physiologic raphes are usually produced by amniotic bands (Fig. 6.31).

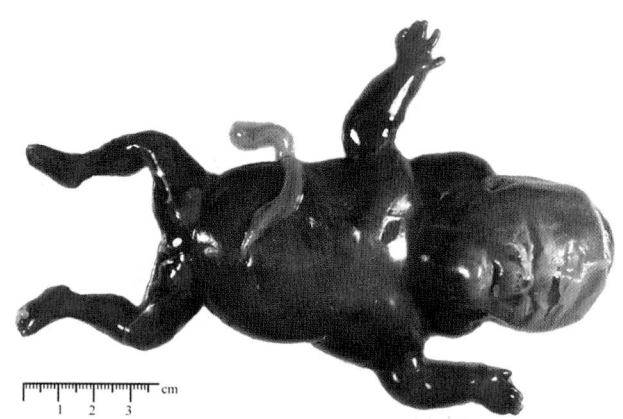

FIGURE 6.26 Trisomy 21 fetus with generalized hydrops and mild posterior cervical cystic hygroma, mimicking Turner syndrome.

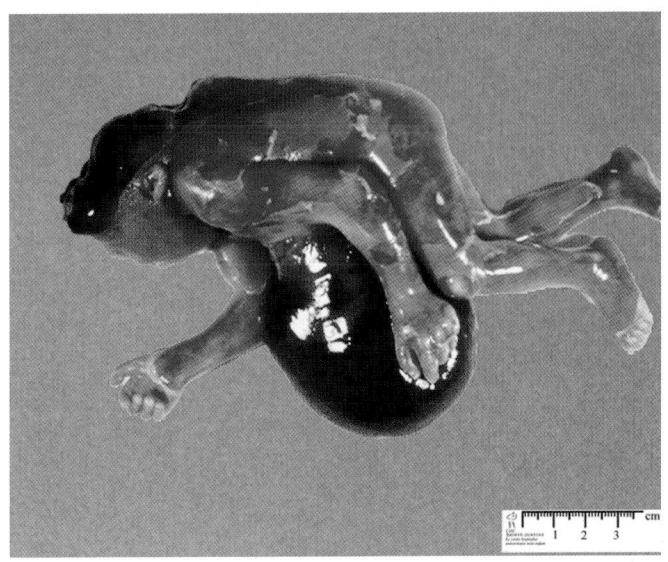

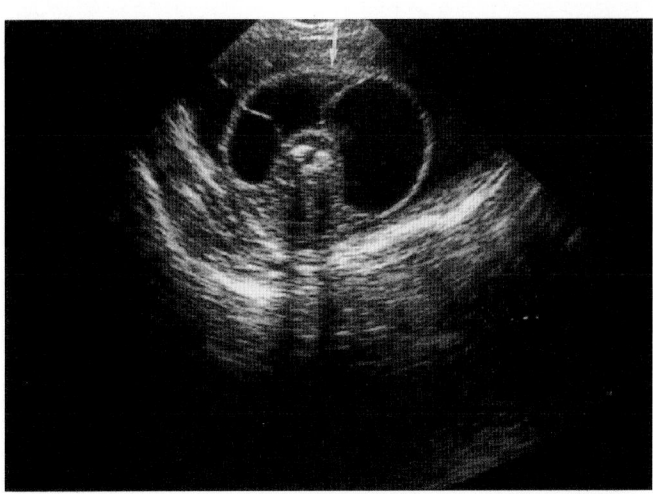

FIGURE 6.29 Ultrasound image of the fetal head with a large posterior cervical hygroma due to monosomy X. Arrows point to the septa within the hygroma.

FIGURE 6.27 Spontaneously aborted fetus with anencephalus, spina bifida, and omphalocele.

Renal anomalies and obstructive uropathies
(see also Ch. 27)

Oligohydramnios is the most common presenting symptom of significant renal anomalies. Lack of amniotic fluid interferes with normal lung development, even before 20 weeks' gestation,

causing **pulmonary hypoplasia**. The other components of the oligohydramnios sequence (i.e. the **Potter sequence**) seen at term (e.g. Potter facies, clubfeet, bowed legs and pterygia) are less frequently seen in previable fetuses. The renal anomalies which can cause early fetal oligohydramnios include bilateral renal agenesis (the **Potter syndrome**), cystic renal dysplasias, and infantile

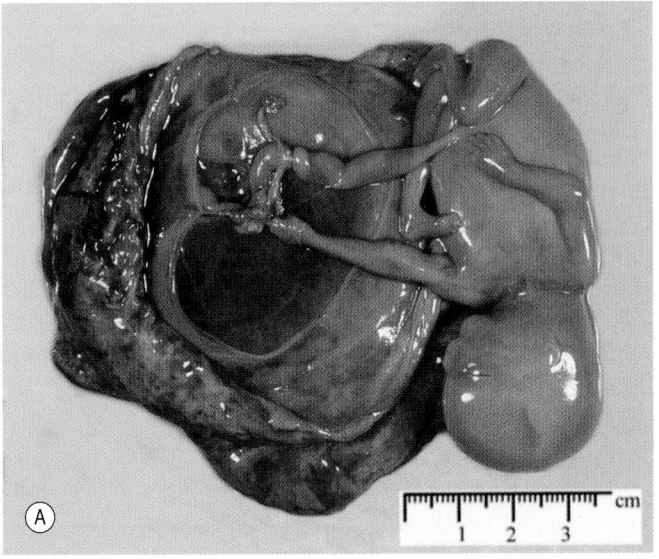

FIGURE 6.28 Macerated fetus with the umbilical cord strangulated by amniotic bands.

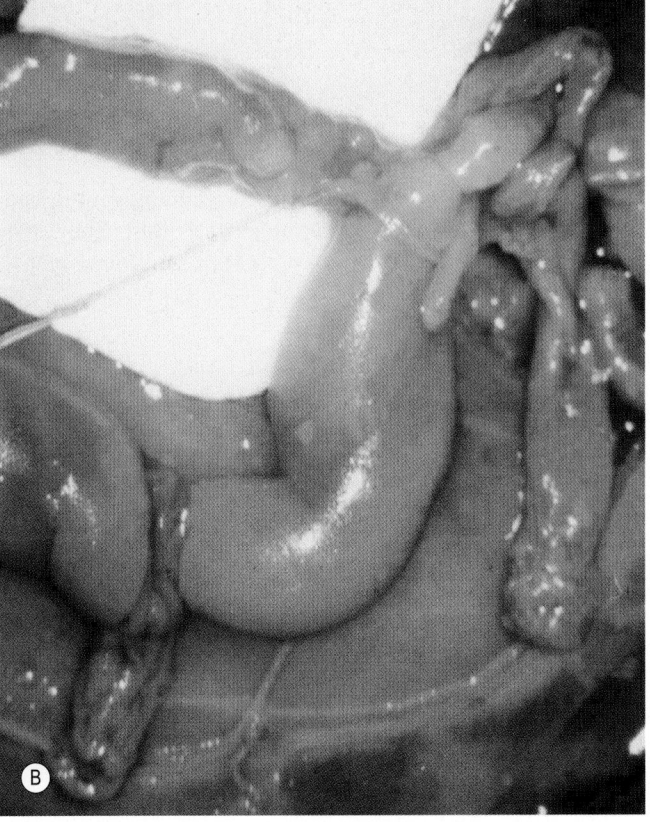

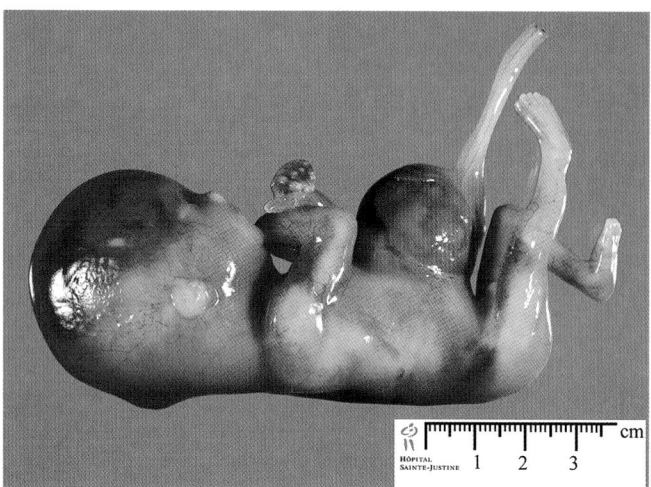

FIGURE 6.30 Fetus at 16 weeks of gestation with a large omphalocele containing liver and small bowel.

polycystic diseases. Pathologic examination helps distinguishing between the different types of renal disease so that accurate estimates of recurrence risks can be given to parents, and appropriate prenatal investigation initiated in subsequent pregnancies.[62, 104]

The **prune-belly syndrome** is characterized by a markedly enlarged bladder (megacystis), hydroureteronephrosis, renal cystic dysplasia and/or renal hypoplasia and/or isolated medullary hypoplasia. Although an abnormal primary mesenchymal defect of the abdominal wall has been postulated to explain this syndrome,[105] it probably results from a primary **urethral obstruction**.[106–108]

Heart defects

Heart defects (see Ch. 23) are a common finding among both spontaneously aborted and terminated fetuses. They may represent an isolated defect or be a part of a syndrome, such as chromosomal aneuploidies.[62]

Molar pregnancies

There are two types of molar pregnancies. **Complete hydatidiform mole (CHM)** is an abnormal pregnancy caused by proliferation of diploid cells containing only paternal chromosomes. **Partial hydatidiform moles (PHM)** are triploid conceptions with two paternal chromosomal sets and one maternal haploid set; their incidence is of 3/1000 pregnancies. Theses placentas may be associated with a triploid embryo or fetus, and rarely complicate an otherwise normal pregnancy (i.e. a twin pregnancy with one normal conceptus and one triploid molar twin). The risk of CHMs becoming malignant is stated to be 15%; PHMs proven to be triploid also have a non-negligible risk of

becoming malignant (defined as a plateau or a rise of hCG after pregnancy has been terminated), reported to be 0.5%.[109] Albeit considered a very rare event, PHMs can evolve into choriocarcinomas.[109] One study reported that in women who required medical treatment after evacuation of a PHM, the risk of evolution to choriocarcinoma was 20% (3 of 15 patients).[109]

Familial recurrent forms of hydatidiform moles exist; recurrences are generally CHMs, but rarely can be PHMs.[110]

Complete hydatidiform moles

The incidence of CHM in the USA is approximately 1 per 2000 pregnancies. It typically presents between the 11th and 25th weeks of pregnancy, with an average gestational age of approximately 16 weeks. Excessive uterine enlargement occurs and may be accompanied by severe vomiting and hypertension. The hCG level is markedly elevated. Ultrasonography often discloses a classic 'snowstorm' appearance. CHM is often voluminous, consisting of 300–500 mL or more of tissue. It is characterized by gross generalized villous edema. Enlarged villi form grape-like transparent vesicles measuring up to 2 cm. Only rarely is an embryo or fetus associated with CHM; in all instances, this finding represents a twin gestation.[111] Around 10–30% of cases of CHM result in persistent gestational trophoblastic disease.

CHM may show considerable cytologic atypia. Trophoblastic proliferation is highly variable; it may be exuberant or focal and minimal. It is often circumferential around the villi. The histologic grade of the trophoblast cells in CHM has no apparent effect on the overall prognosis. The villous stroma lacks the blood vessels that normally form when embryogenesis occurs. Cisterns within the stroma are usually present in some of the villi. Most complete moles have a 46,XX karyotype, resulting either from dispermy or from duplication of a haploid sperm in an anuclear ovum (diploid androgenesis).[112, 113] Undisputedly the result of dispermy, XY moles, which represent only some 4% of cases of CHM, originate from the fertilization of an anuclear ovum by two spermatozoa.[114] No significant difference has been noted between the gross and microscopic findings of the XY and XX forms of CHM.[112] Studies of invasive moles and choriocarcinomas have led to the suggestion that heterozygous CHM (caused by dispermy) may have a more malignant potential than their homozygous counterparts arising through diploid androgenesis.[115]

Partial hydatidiform moles

PHM is more common than CHM. Morphologically partial moles differ from complete moles in three respects:

- An embryo or fetus is usually present, and villi are often vascularized.
- The intravillous microcystic pattern may be diffuse or focal and is often not as prominent as in CHM.
- Trophoblastic hyperplasia is less prominent and sometimes strikingly focal. By definition, PHMs are triploid, with two paternal and one maternal haploid complements.[109, 116, 117]
  Placental PHM-like morphology has been described in trisomies, Beckwith-Wiedemann syndrome and other conditions.[118–120]

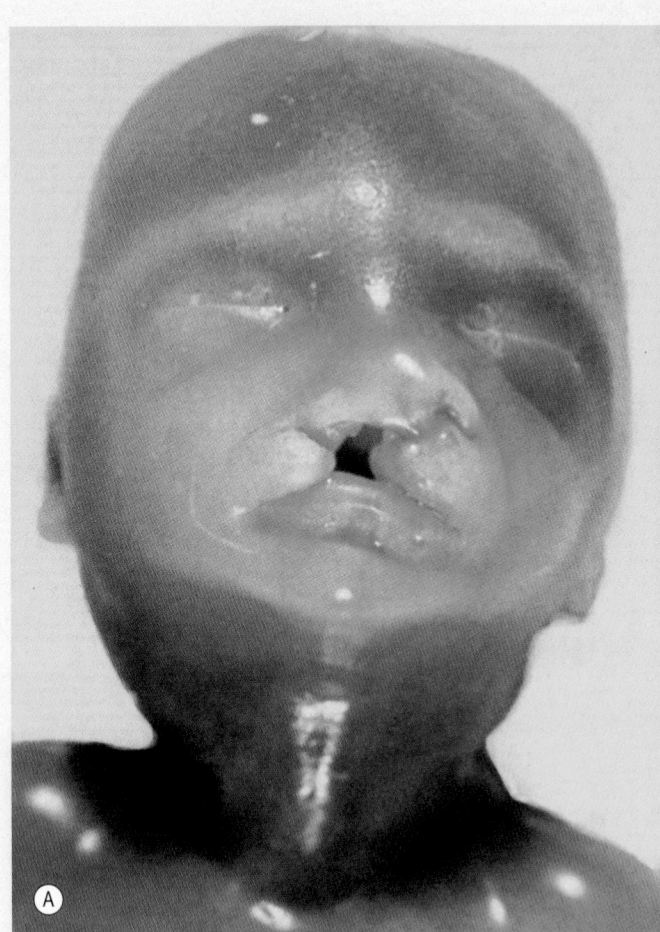

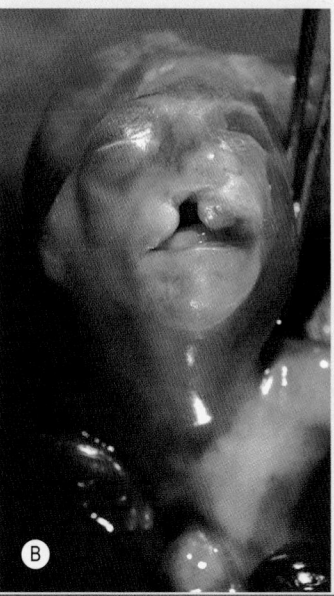

FIGURE 6.31 (A) Typical isolated lateral cleft lip, in physiological axis of closure. (B) and (C) Irregular facial clefting due to amniotic bands with associated disruptions of the face, skull and hands.

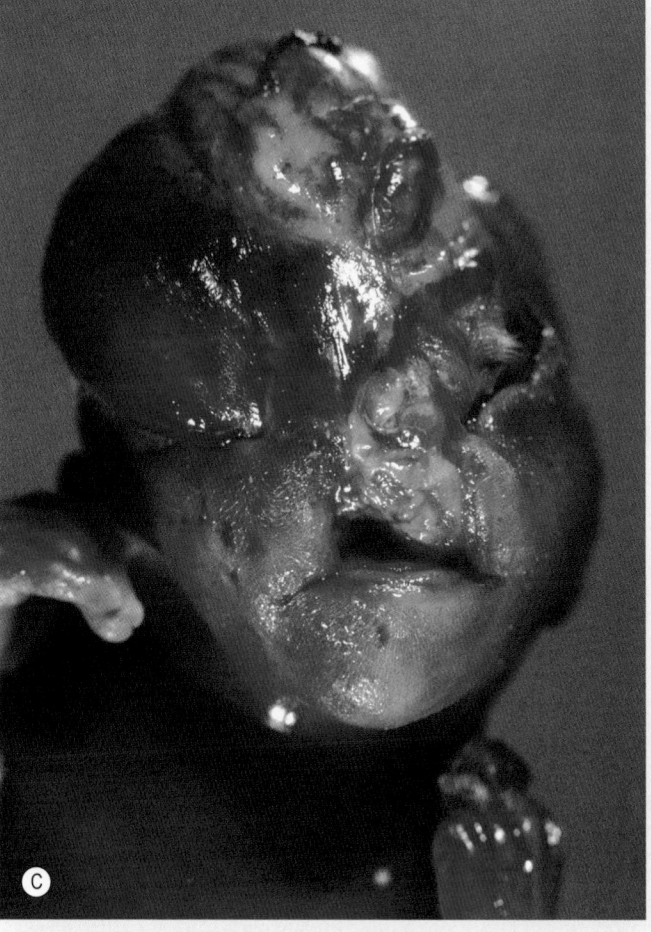

The gross specimen in PHM often shows hydropic villi like those seen in CHM mixed with histologically non-molar placental tissue. Microscopically, there tends to be a mixture of large, edematous villi and small, normal-sized villi without edema. Some of the hydropic villi show a central, acellular cistern similar to that seen in CHM. The small villi are often fibrotic. Trophoblastic hyperplasia is focal and often confined to the syncytiotrophoblasts. The villi often have irregular, scalloped outlines that

TABLE 6.9 DIFFERENTIAL FEATURES OF COMPLETE AND PARTIAL MOLES

Feature	Complete	Partial
Clinical presentation	Spontaneous abortion	Missed or spontaneous abortion
Gestational age	16–18 weeks	18–20 weeks
Uterine size	Often large for dates	Often small for dates
Serum βhCG	++++	+
Cytogenetics	Diploid, XX (over 90%) or XY (< 10%); all paternal	Triploid, XXY (58%), XXX (40%), XYY (2%); 2 ÷ 1 paternal ÷ maternal
Persistent gestational trophoblastic disease	10–30%	4–11%
Embryo/fetus	Absent	Often present
Histologic features		
• Villous outline	Round	Scalloped
• Hydropic swelling	Marked	Less pronounced
• Trophoblastic proliferation	Circumferential	Focal, minimal
• Trophoblastic atypia	Often present	Absent
• Immunocytochemistry		
– βhCG	++++	+
– αhCG	+	++++
– PLAP	++	++++
– PL	–	+++
• CDKN1C* (formerly p57[KIP2])		
Ploidy by flow cytometry*	Diploid	Triploid

After Silverberg and Kurman 1992,[121] Merchant et al 2005,[122] and Genest 2001,[123] with permission.
hCG, Human chorionic gonadotropin; PLAP, placental alkaline phosphatase; PL, placental lactogen.
* Denotes gold standard diagnostic modalities.

produce infoldings of trophoblastic cells into the villous stroma, resulting in villous inclusions. In fresh tissue, evidence of an embryo or of amnion is usually present; stromal vasculature and vessels may contain fetal nucleated erythrocytes; after longer postmortem intervals, the remnants of stromal vessels and fetal erythrocytes often disappear. Differential features between CHM and PHM are shown in Table 6.9.[98, 121]

Differential diagnosis

There is significant overlap between the histologic appearance of spontaneously aborted normal placentas (retained products of conception) and PHMs, as well as between PHMs and CHMs. However, the placentas from retained products of conception only seldom if ever show the same degree of hydropic changes and of syncytial hypertrophy as those seen in CHMs. Retention changes are typically accompanied by trophoblastic proliferation, and the immature villi have loose and edematous stroma. The trophoblastic proliferation in a non-molar hydropic abortus shows polarity characterized by column-like growth of the cells from only one pole of a villus, and the cells do not show cytologic atypia. Assessment of ploidy through flow cytometry studies of the placenta can be performed on paraffin blocks and is useful to distinguish between these conditions, as is the immuno-histochemical staining reaction directed toward the paternally imprinted (i.e. maternally-expressed) p57[KIP2] (now called CDKN1C).[122, 123]

Historically, immunohistochemistry for hCG, human placental lactogen (hPL), and placental alkaline phosphatase (PLAP) have been used to help in the distinction between complete and partial mole. The level of βhCG is much greater than that of PLAP in CHM; the opposite is found in PHM, which has greater staining with PLAP.[124, 125] Immuno-histochemical staining for PLAP is only focal in abortions with hydropic change, whereas it is diffuse in PHM. However, **the only conclusive means for resolving the differential diagnosis is the assessment of ploidy** through cytogenetics or flow cytometry, or assessment of p57[KIP2] expression, correlated with routine histologic assessment of placental tissues.[122, 123]

Acknowledgement

Drs Kalousek and Oligny wish to acknowledge the contribution of the files of the Embryopathology Laboratory at the Department of Pathology of BC Children's Hospital and of the Department of Pathology of the CHU Sainte-Justine. We are also grateful for Mr Stéphane Dedelis' photographic assistance.

References

Definitions of spontaneous abortion and purpose of this study

1. Opitz JM. Prenatal and perinatal death. The future of developmental pathology. Pediatr Pathol 1987; 7:363–394.
2. Simpson JL. Incidence and timing of pregnancy losses. Am J Med Genet 1990; 35:165–173.
3. Macklon NS, Geraedts JP, Fauser BC. Conception to ongoing pregnancy: the 'black box' of early pregnancy loss. Hum Reprod Update 2002; 8:333–343.
4. Norwitz ER, Schust DJ, Fisher SJ. Implantation and the survival of early pregnancy. N Engl J Med 2001; 345:1400–1408.
5. Miller JF, Williamson E, Glue J, et al. Fetal loss after implantation. A prospective study. Lancet 1980; 2:554–556.
6. Kline J, Stein Z. Very early pregnancy. In: Dixon RL, ed. Reproductive toxicology. New York: Raven Press; 1985:251–265.
7. Edmonds DR, Lindsay KS, Miller JR, et al. Early embryonic mortality in women. Fertil Steril 1982; 38:447–453.
8. Wilcox AJ, Weinberg CR, O'Conner JF, et al. Incidence of early loss of pregnancy. N Engl J Med 1988; 319:189–194.
9. Sampson A, de Crespigny L Ch. Vanishing twins: the frequency of spontaneous fetal reduction of a twin pregnancy. Ultrasound Obstet Gynecol 1992; 2:107–109.
10. Warburton D, Fraser CF. Spontaneous abortion risks in moms: data from reproductive histories collected in medical genetics unit. Am J Hum Genet 1964; 16:1–25.
11. O'Rahilly R, Muller F. Developmental stages in human embryos. Carnegie Institute of Embryology. Publication 637. Philadelphia: Washington; 1987.
12. Moore KL, Persaud TVN. The developing human: clinically oriented embryology. 7th edn. Philadelphia: WB Saunders; 2002.

Etiology of spontaneous abortion

13. Boué J, Boué A, Lazar P. Retrospective and prospective epidemiological studies of 1500 karyotypes from spontaneous human abortions. Teratology 1975; 12:11–26.
14. Jacobs PA, Hassold TJ. Chromosome abnormalities: origin and etiology in abortions and livebirths. In: Vogel F, Sperling K, eds. Human genetics. New York: Springer-Verlag; 1987:233–244.
15. Craver RD, Kalousek DK. Cytogenetic abnormalities among spontaneously aborted previable fetuses. Am J Med Genet 1987; 3(Suppl):113–119.
16. Garcia-Enguidanos A, Calle ME, Valero J, et al. Risk factors in miscarriage: a review. Eur J Obstet Gynecol Reprod Biol 2002; 102:111–119.
17. Simpson JL. Aetiology of pregnancy failure. In: Chapman M, Grudzinskas G, Chand T, eds. The embryo normal and abnormal development and growth. Berlin: Springer-Verlag; 1991:11–39.
18. Temple R, Aldridge V, Greenwood R, et al. Association between outcome of pregnancy and glycaemic control in early pregnancy in type 1 diabetes: population based study. BMJ 2002; 325(7375):1275–1276.
19. Robertson WB. Uteroplacental vasculature. J Clin Pathol 1976; (Suppl) 29:9–17.
20. Merviel P, Carbillon L, Challier JC, et al. Pathophysiology of preeclampsia: links with implantation disorders. Eur J Obstet Gynecol Reprod Biol 2004; 115:134–147.
21. Greer IA. Thrombophilia: implications for pregnancy outcome. Thromb Res 2003; 109:73–81.
22. Zetterberg H. Methylenetetrahydrofolate reductase and transcobalamin genetic polymorphisms in human spontaneous abortion: biological and clinical implications. Reprod Biol Endocrinol 2004; 2:7.
23. Robertson L, Wu O, Greer I. Thrombophilia and adverse pregnancy outcome. Curr Opin Obstet Gynecol 2004; 16:453–458.
24. Mtiraoui N, Borgi L, Gris JC, et al. Factor V Leiden, prothrombin G20210A and antibodies against phospholipids in recurrent spontaneous abortion. J Thromb Haemost 2004; 2:1482–1484.
25. Heilmann L, von Tempelhoff GF, Pollow K. Antiphospholipid syndrome in obstetrics. Clin Appl Thromb Hemost 2003; 9:143–150.
26. Tincani A, Balestrieri G, Danieli E, et al. Pregnancy complications of the antiphospholipid syndrome. Autoimmunity 2003; 36:27–32.
27. Bose P, Black S, Kadyrov M, et al. Adverse effects of lupus anticoagulant positive blood sera on placental viability can be prevented by heparin in vitro. Am J Obstet Gynecol 2004; 191:2125–2131.
28. Krabbendam I, Dekker GA. Pregnancy outcome in patients with a history of recurrent spontaneous miscarriages and documented thrombophilias. Gynecol Obstet Invest 2004; 57:127–131.
29. Candoni A, Fanin R, Michelutti T, et al. Pregnancy and abortion in women with essential thrombocythemia. Am J Hematol 2002; 69:233–234.
30. Glass RH, Golbus MS. Habitual abortion. Fertil Steril 1978; 29:257–265.
31. Rushton DI. Chromosomal abnormalities of the fetus. J Obstet Gynaecol Br Commonw 1968; 75:1225–1228.
32. Zhou JO. Risk of spontaneous abortion following induced abortion is only increased with short interpregnancy interval. J Obstet Gynaecol 2000; 20:49–54.
33. Naeye RL, Tafari N. Risk factors in pregnancy and diseases of the fetus and newborn. Baltimore, 1983, Williams & Wilkins; 1983:194.
34. Friedman JM, Polifka JE. Teratogenic effects of drugs: a resource for clinicians (TERIS). Baltimore: The Johns Hopkins University Press; 2000.
35. Robinson HB, Tross K. Agenesis of the cloacal membrane. A probable teratogenic anomaly. Perspect Pediatr Pathol 1984; 8:79–96.
36. Henriksen TB, Hjollund NH, Jensen TK, et al. Alcohol consumption at the time of conception and spontaneous abortion. Am J Epidemiol 2004; 160: 661–667.
37. Rasch V. Cigarette, alcohol, and caffeine consumption: risk factors for spontaneous abortion. Acta Obstet Gynecol Scand 2003; 82:182–188.
38. Chasnoff IJ, Burns WJ, Schnoll SH, et al. Cocaine use in pregnancy. N Engl J Med 1985; 313:667–669.
39. Chaouat G, Ledee-Bataille N, Dubanchet S, et al. TH1/TH2 paradigm in pregnancy: paradigm lost? Cytokines in pregnancy/early abortion: reexamining the TH1/TH2 paradigm. Int Arch Allergy Immunol 2004; 134:93–119.
40. Chaouat G, Ledee-bataill N, Dubanchet S. Is there a place for immunomodulation in assisted reproduction techniques? J Reprod Immunol 2004; 62:29–39.
41. Renard C. Effects of feto-maternal major histocompatibility differences on litter size in pigs. In: Beard RW, Sharp F, eds. Early pregnancy loss: mechanisms and treatment. London: Springer-Verlag; 1988:105.
42. Abbas A, Tripathi P, Naik S, et al. Analysis of human leukocyte antigen (HLA)-G polymorphism in normal women and in women with recurrent spontaneous abortions. Eur J Immunogenet 2004; 31:275–278.
43. Agrawal S, Pandey MK, Mandal S, et al. Humoral immune response to an allogenic foetus in normal fertile women and recurrent aborters. BMC Pregnancy Childbirth 2002; 2:6.
44. Clark DA, Coulam CB, Daya S, et al. Unexplained sporadic and recurrent miscarriage in the new millennium: a critical analysis of immune mechanisms and treatments. Hum Reprod Update 2001; 7:501–511.
45. Erlebacher A. Why isn't the fetus rejected? Curr Opin Immunol 2001; 13:590–593.
46. Thomas ML, Harger JH, Wagener DK, et al. HLA sharing and spontaneous abortion in humans. Am J Obstet Gynecol 1985; 151:1053–1058.
47. Weitkamp LR, Schachter BZ. Transferrin and HLA: Spontaneous abortion, neural tube defects and natural selection. N Engl J Med 1985; 313:925–932.
48. Ho MN, Gill TJ III, Hseih RP, et al. Sharing of human leukocyte antigens (HLA) in primary and secondary recurrent spontaneous abortions. Am J Obstet Gynecol 1990; 163:178–188.
49. Michel MZ, Khong TY, Clark DA, et al. A morphological and immunological study of human placental bed biopsies in miscarriage. Br J Obstet Gynaecol 1990; 97:984–988.
50. Eroglu G, Betz G, Torregano C. Impact of histocompatibility antigens on pregnancy outcome. Am J Obstet Gynecol 1992; 166:1364–1369.
51. Kovats S, Main EK, Librach C, et al. A class I antigen, HLA-G, expressed in human trophoblasts. Science 1990; 248:220–223.
52. Gill GT. Influence of MHC and MHC-linked genes in reproduction (invited editorial). Am J Hum Genet 1992; 50:1–5.

53. Vianna NJ. Adverse pregnancy outcomes – potential endpoints of human toxicity in the Love Canal. Preliminary results. In: Porter IH, Hook EB, eds. Human embryonic and fetal death. New York: Academic Press; 1980:165–168.

54. Roman E, Stevenson AC. Spontaneous abortion. In: Barron SL, Thompson AM, eds. Obstetrical epidemiology. London: Academic Press; 1983:61–87.

55. Heffner LJ. Advanced maternal age – How old is too old? N Engl J Med 2004; 351:1927–1929.

56. Nybo Andersen AM, Hansen KD, Andersen PK, et al. Advanced paternal age and risk of fetal death: a cohort study. Am J Epidemiol 2004; 160:1214–1222.

Specimens of early spontaneous abortion

57. Poland BJ, Miller JR, Harris M, et al. Spontaneous abortion: a study of 1961 women and their conceptuses. Acta Obstet Gynaecol Scand 1981; 102(Suppl):1–32.

58. Kalousek DK. Anatomic and chromosome anomalies in specimens of each spontaneous abortion: seven year experience. Birth Defects 1987; 23:153–168.

59. Jirasek JE. Atlas of human prenatal morphogenesis. Boston: Martinus Nijhoff; 1983.

60. Moore KL, Persaud TVN. The developing human: clinically oriented embryology. 5th edn. Philadelphia: WB Saunders; 1993.

61. Streeter GL. Developmental horizons in human embryos. Washington: Carnegie Institute of Embryology; 1951.

62. Kalousek DK, Fitch N, Paradice BA. Pathology of human embryo and previable fetus. New York: Springer-Verlag; 1990.

63. Szulman AE. Examination of the early conceptus. Arch Pathol Lab Med 1991; 115:696–700.

64. Rushton DI. The classification and mechanisms of spontaneous abortion. Perspect Pediatr Pathol 1984; 8:269–287.

65. Philippe E. Morphologie et morphométrie des placentas d'aberrations chromosomiques létale. Rev Fr Gynécol Obstét 1973; 6:655.

66. Honoré LH, Poland BJ. Placental morphology in spontaneous human abortions with normal and abnormal karyotypes. Teratology 1976; 14:151–166.

67. Novak R, Agamanolis D, Dasu S, et al. Histological analysis of placental tissue in first trimester abortions. Pediatr Pathol 1988; 8:477–482.

68. Minguillon C, Eiben B, Bahr-Porsch S, et al. The predictive value of chorionic villus histology for identifying chromosomally normal and abnormal spontaneous abortions. Hum Genet 1989; 82:373–376.

69. Rehder H, Coerdt W, Eggers R, et al. Is there a correlation between morphological and cytogenetic findings in placental tissue from early missed abortions? Hum Genet 1989; 82:377–385.

70. Van Lijnschsten G, Arends JW, de La Fuente AA, et al. Intra- and inter-observer variation in the interpretation of histological features suggesting chromosomal abnormality in early abortion specimens. Histopathology 1993; 22:25–29.

71. Szulman AE, Surti U. The clinicopathologic profile of the partial hydatidiform mode. Obstet Gynecol 1982; 59:597–602.

72. Van Lijnschsten G, Arends JW, Leffers P, et al. The value of histomorphological features of chorionic villi in early spontaneous abortion for the prediction of karyotype. Histopathology 1993; 22:557–563.

73. Jacobs P, Szulman A, Funkhouser J, et al. Human triploidy: relationship between paternal origin of the additional haploid complement and development of partial hydatidiform mole. Ann Hum Genet 1982; 46:223–231.

74. Philips C, Meadows L, Hebert M, et al. Screening for chromosomical abnormalities by fluorescent in situ technique: application to human spontaneous abortions. Am J Hum Genet 1992; 51:A11.

75. Nuovo GJ. PCR in situ hybridization. Protocols and applications. New York: Raven Press; 1992.

76. Lomax B, Kalousek DK, Kuchinka BD, et al. Utilization of interphase cytogenetic analysis for the detection of mosaicism. Hum Genet 1994; 93:243–247.

77. Kuchinka BD, Kalousek DK, Lomax BL, et al. Interphase cytogenetic analysis of single cell suspensions prepared from previously formalin fixed and paraffin embedded tissues. Mod Pathol 1995; 8:183–186.

Clinical significance of pathologic evaluation of early spontaneous abortion

78. Nishimura H. Prenatal versus postnatal malformations based on the Japanese evidence on induced abortions in human beings. In: Blandon RS, ed. Aging, gametes their biology and pathology. Basel: S Karger; 1975:349–368.

79. Warburton D, Kline J, Stein Z, et al. Does the karyotype of a spontaneous abortion predict the karyotype of a subsequent abortion? Evidence from 273 women with two karyotyped spontaneous abortions. Am J Hum Genet 1987; 41:465–483.

80. Warburton D, Byrne J, Canki N. Chromosome anomalies and prenatal development: an atlas, Oxford: Oxford University Press; 1991.

81. Harris MJ, Poland BJ, Dill FJ. Triploidy in 40 human spontaneous abortuses: assessment of phenotype in embryos. Obstet Gynecol 1981; 57:600–606.

82. Philipp T, Grillenberger K, Separovic ER, et al. Effects of triploidy on early human development. Prenat Diagn 2004; 24:276–281.

83. Kalousek DK. Pathology of abortion. Chromosomal and genetic correlations. In: Kraus FT, Damjanov I, eds. Pathology of reproductive failure. Baltimore: Williams & Wilkins; 1991: 228.

84. Hall J. Genomic imprinting – review and relevance to human diseases. Am J Hum Genet 1990; 46:857–873.

85. Robinson HP. The diagnosis of early pregnancy failure by sonar. Br J Obstet Gynaecol 1975; 82:849–857.

86. Stabile I, Campbell S, Grudzinskas JG. Ultrasonic assessment in complications of first trimester pregnancy. Lancet 1987; 2:1237–1240.

87. Stabile I. Anembryonic pregnancy. In: Chapman M, Grudzinskas G, Chard T, eds. The embryo: normal and abnormal development and growth. Berlin: Springer-Verlag; 1991:35–94.

Specimens of late spontaneous abortion

88. Benirschke K, Kaufmann P. Pathology of the human placenta. 2nd edn. New York: Springer-Verlag; 1990.

89. Ruston DI. Placental pathology in spontaneous miscarriage. In: Early pregnancy loss: mechanisms and treatment. Proceedings of the 18th Study Group of the Royal College of Obstetricians and Gynecologists, Lanes, UK. Ashton-under-Lyme: RCOG Publications, Peacock Press; 1988:149.

90. Saunders R, James AE, eds. The principles and practice of ultrasonography in obstetrics and gynaecology. New York: Appleton-Century-Crofts; 1980:454.

91. Deter RL, Harrist RB, Hadlock IP, et al. The use of ultrasound in the assessment of normal fetal growth: a review. J Clin Ultrasound 1981; 9:481–493.

92. Knowles SAS. Examination of products of conception terminated after prenatal investigation. J Clin Pathol 1986; 39:1049–1065.

Clincial significance of pathologic evaluations of late spontaneous abortion

93. Kalousek DK, Pantzar T, Craver R. So-called primitive neuroectodermal tumor in aborted previable fetuses. Pediatr Pathol 1988; 8:503–511.

94. Kalousek DK, Seller M. Differential diagnosis of posterior cervical hygroma in previable fetuses. Am J Med Genet 1987; 3(Suppl):83–92.

95. Byrne J, Blanc W, Warburton D, et al. The significance of cystic hygroma in fetuses. Hum Pathol 1984; 15:61–67.

96. Chervenak FA, Isaacson G, Blackemore K, et al. Fetal cystic hygroma. Cause and natural history. N Engl J Med 1983; 309:822–825.

97. Chitayat D, Kalousek D, Bamforth J. The lymphatic abnormalities in fetuses with posterior cervical cystic hygroma. Am J Med Genet 1989; 33:352–356.

98. McFadden DE, Kalousek DK. Two different phenotypes of fetuses with chromosomal triploidy: correlation with parental origin of the extra haploid set. Am J Med Genet 1991; 38:535–538.

Common abnormal morphologic findings in late abortion specimens

99. Kalousek DK, Bamforth S. Amniotic rupture sequence in previable fetuses. Am J Med Genet 1988; 31:63–73.

100. Azar G, Snijders RJM, Gosden CM, et al. Fetal nuchal cystic hygromata: associated malformations and chromosomal defects. Fetal Diagn Ther 1991; 6:46–57.

101. van der Putte SCJ, Van Limborgh J. The embryonic development of the main lymphatics in man. Acta Morphol Neerl Scand 1980; 18:323–335.

102. Gilbert W, Nicolaides KH. Fetal gastro-intestinal and abdominal wall defects: associated malformations and chromosomal abnormalities. Obstet Gynecol 1987; 70:633–635.

103. Nicolaides KH, Snijders RJM, Cheng M, et al. Fetal abdominal wall and gastrointestinal tract defects and associated malformations of gastrointestinal tract defects and chromosomal defects. Fetal Diagn Ther 1992; 7:102–115.

104. Nicolaides KM, Cheng M, Snijders RJM, et al. Fetal renal defects: associated malformations and chromosomal defects. Fetal Diagn Ther 1992; 7:1–11.

105. Popek EJ, Tyson RW, Miller GJ, et al. Prostate development in prune belly syndrome (PBS) and posterior urethral valves (PUV): etiology of PBS – lower urinary tract obstruction or primary mesenchymal defect? Pediatr Pathol 1991; 11:1–29.

106. Volmar KE, Fritsch MK, Perlman EJ, et al. Patterns of congenital lower urinary tract obstructive uropathy: relation to abnormal prostate and bladder development and the prune belly syndrome. Pediatr Dev Pathol 2001; 4:467–472.

107. Berry C. Patterns of congenital lower urinary tract obstructive uropathy: relation to abnormal prostate and bladder development and the prune belly syndrome (Letters to the editor). Pediatr Dev Pathol 2003; 6:202–203.

108. Volmar KE, Hutchins GM, Fritsch MK. Patterns of congenital lower urinary tract obstructive uropathy: relation to abnormal prostate and bladder development and the prune belly syndrome (Reply). Pediatr Dev Pathol 2003; 6:203.

Molar pregnancies

109. Seckl MJ, Fisher RA, Salerno G, et al. Choriocarcinoma and partial hydatidiform moles. Lancet 2000; 356:36–39.

110. Fisher RA, Hodges MD, Newlands ES. Familial recurrent hydatiform mole – a review. J Reprod Med 2004; 49:595–601.

111. Lage JM, Mark SD, Roberts DJ, et al. A flow cytometric study of 137 fresh hydropic placentas: correlation between types of hydatidiform moles and nuclear DNA ploidy. Obstet Gynecol 1992; 79:403–410.

112. Kajii T, Kurashige M, Ohama K, et al. XY and XX complete moles: clinical and morphological correlation. Am J Obstet Gynecol 1984; 150:57–64.

113. Kajii T, Ohama K. Androgenetic origin of hydatidiform mole. Nature 1977; 268:633–634

114. Ohama K, Kajii T, Okamoto E. Dispermic origin of XY hydatidiform moles. Nature 1981; 292:551–552.

115. Fisher AR, Lawler SD. Heterozygous complete hydatidiform moles: do they have a worse prognosis than homozygous complete moles? Lancet 1984; 2:51.

116. Lawler SD, Fisher A, Pickthall JV, et al. Genetic studies on hydatidiform moles. The origin of partial moles. Cancer Genet Cytogenet 1982; 5: 309–320.

117. Lawler SD, Povey S, Fisher FA, et al. Genetic studies on hydatidiform moles. II. The origin of complete moles. Ann Hum Genet 1982; 46:209–222.

118. Szulman AE, Surti U. The clinicopathologic profile of the partial hydatidiform mole. Obstet Gynecol 1982; 59:597–602.

119. Matsui H, Iitsuka Y, Yamazawa K, et al. Placental mesenchymal dysplasia initially diagnosed as partial mole. Pathol Int 2003; 53:810–813.

120. Paradinal JF, Sebire NJ, Fisher RA, et al. Pseudo-partial moles: placental stem vessel hydrops and the association with Beckwith-Wiedemann syndrome and complete moles. Histopathology 2001; 39:447–454.

121. Silverberg SG, Kurman RJ. Atlas of tumor pathology; tumors of the uterine corpus and gestational trophoblastic disease. Washington: Armed Forces Institute of Pathology; 1992.

122. Merchant SH, Amin MB, Viswanatha DS, et al. p57^{KIP2} immunohistochemistry in early molar pregnancies: emphasis on its complementary role in the differential diagnosis of hydropic abortuses. Hum Pathol 2005; 36: 180–186.

123. Genest DR. Partial hydatidiform mole: clinicopathological features, differential diagnosis, ploidy and molecular studies, and gold standards for diagnosis. Int J Gynecol Pathol 2001; 20:315–322.

124. Brescia RJ, Kurman RJ, Main C, et al. Immunocytochemical localization of chorionic gonadotropin, placental lactogen, and placental alkaline phosphatase in the diagnosis of complete and partial hydatidiform moles. Int J Gynecol Pathol 1987; 6:213–229.

125. Benkowitz R, Ozturk M, Goldstein D, et al. Human chorionic gonadotropin and free subunits of serum levels in patients with partial and complete hydatidiform moles. Obstet Gynecol 1989; 74:212–216.

Causes of fetal and neonatal death

7

M. Halit Pinar   Don B. Singer

'To the small part of ignorance that we arrange and classify we give the name knowledge.'

Ambrose Bierce 1842–1914?

Definitions of fetal and neonatal death

Fetal death occurs prior to the complete expulsion or extraction of the product of conception, irrespective of the duration of pregnancy, and is indicated by absent breathing, heartbeat, pulsating umbilical cord, or muscular movement. Intrauterine and intrapartum deaths are included. The **fetal mortality rate** (*FMR*) is the number of fetal deaths × 1000, divided by the sum of live births and fetal deaths in a population. **Stillbirth** or late fetal death occurs at gestations of at least 20 weeks, 23 weeks, 24 weeks, or 28 weeks depending on the country, jurisdiction, an investigator's, or a reporter's choice. In the USA, most jurisdictions require a death certificate at 20 weeks' gestation.[1, 2]

The fetal biophysical profile (fetal ultrasound for general appearance, serial evaluation of growth, fetal heart beat monitor, and/or Doppler study of umbilical blood flow), and the mother's report of fetal movement constitute signs of fetal status. Fetal death is apt to occur if the profile and the fetal movements deteriorate.[3] Absence of cardiac activity by ultrasonography confirms the diagnosis. Labor and delivery usually occur spontaneously within hours to 2 weeks; this interval is inversely related to the length of gestation. If the interval is longer than 8 h, the fetus will have autolysis of tissues (maceration).[4]

Infant death occurs when a liveborn infant of any gestational age dies within the first year after birth. The **infant mortality rate** (*IMR*) is the number of infant deaths per 1000 live births.

Neonatal death is that which occurs during the first 28 days of life. The **neonatal mortality rate** (*NMR*) is the number of neonatal deaths per 1000 live births. **Early neonatal death** occurs when a liveborn infant of any gestational age dies within the first 7 days of life; this is sometimes referred to as hebdomadal death, from the Greek *hebdomos*- seventh. **Perinatal deaths** include late fetal deaths at 28+ weeks' gestation and early neonatal deaths, <7 completed days of life. The **perinatal mortality rate** is the number of perinatal deaths × 1000 divided by the sum of live births and fetal deaths at 28+ weeks.

Low birth weight (*LBW*) is equal to or less than 2500 g, regardless of gestational age.[5] **Preterm birth** is birth of a fetus or baby before 37 completed weeks of gestation and usually corresponds to a weight of 2500 g. Unofficially, 'very preterm birth' describes a fetus or neonate before 32 completed weeks of gestation (~1500 g) and 'extremely preterm birth' occurs before 28 completed weeks (~1000 g).[5]

Vital statistics: fetal and neonatal death

The rates of fetal, perinatal, and neonatal death vary depending on statistical methods and on the country or jurisdiction. Since 1915 the IMR in the USA has declined steadily from 99.9 to only 6.9 per 1000 live births in 2002.[5] The socioeconomic status of the mothers and the quality of prenatal care affect the IMR.[5, 6]

The IMR is known for most countries in the world but fetal mortality rates are not readily available. To estimate FMR for industrialized countries, follow the rules-of-thumb in Box 7.1. In 2002, the USA had an IMR of 6.9 per 1000 live births and an NMR of 4.5 per 1000 live births. Using the rules-of-thumb, the perinatal mortality rate is about 3.1 per 1000 live births and fetal mortality rate is about 4.5 per 1000 live births + fetal deaths.[5]

Underlying causes of fetal and neonatal death

The only direct and immediate causes of death are failed circulation of blood or failed oxygenation of the tissues.[7] An **underlying** cause of death is 'the disease or injury which initiates the train of morbid events leading directly to death – or – the circumstances of the accident or violence which produces the fatal injury'.[5] Since embryos, fetuses, and neonates comprise a continuum, underlying causes include maternal disease, placental defects, embryonic and fetal genetic abnormality, metabolic defect, structural malformation, prematurity, multiple births, trauma, and perinatal infection.

The most current data for causes of infant mortality rates and the estimated neonatal, perinatal, and fetal death rates are shown in Table 7.1.

Fetal death before 24 weeks' gestation is often due to infection or congenital malformation. From 24 to 36 weeks asphyxia, hydrops, and anemia are predominant.[4,8] When the gestation is at least 36 weeks, the causes of fetal death are often unknown, (except for cord accident or extensive placental separation), even after thorough studies including autopsies.[4,9,10] Some unexplained late fetal deaths are associated with increased prepregnancy maternal weight, small for dates fetuses, primiparity, multiparity, few prenatal visits, low socioeconomic status, and maternal age more than 40 years.[11,12] Many unexplained fetal deaths are attributed to chronic hypoxia when elevated erythropoietin levels are found in the amniotic fluid.[13] Still, the true underlying causes of many late intrauterine deaths remain puzzling. The suggestion that fetal deaths of unknown cause are related to the sudden infant death syndrome (SIDS) gained some currency a few years ago but a side-by-side comparison of features shows no correlation in the large majority of cases.[14]

Fetal growth impairment (intrauterine growth restriction, IUGR) is prevalent in fetal and neonatal death.[15] Risk factors for IUGR are the same as the underlying causes of fetal death: malformation, infection, maternal undernutrition, smoking, drug use, hypoxia, or high altitude, preeclampsia, thrombophilia. The chances of fetal death are high if IUGR is detected prior to 26 weeks' gestation, especially with hydrops or impaired umbilical venous flow. Liveborn term infants (38–42 weeks) with IUGR have a perinatal morbidity and mortality 5–30 times that of infants with normal growth.[16] Fetuses in multiple births grow at the same rate as singletons until the sum of the fetal weights reaches 3000 g. From that point until delivery, multiple fetuses grow more slowly than singletons. Most other conditions that cause severe fetal growth restriction also operate in the latter half of pregnancy and result in an asymmetric small fetus i.e. the brain is near-normal while the body and organs are comparatively small (Fig. 7.1). The normal brain–liver weight ratio

TABLE 7.1 TEN LEADING CAUSES OF INFANT DEATH IN 2001* AND ESTIMATED RATES OF NEONATAL, PERINATAL, AND FETAL DEATHS

Cause of death	IMR	NMR	PMR	FMR
All causes	6.02	4.0	2.0	4.0
Congenital malformations, deformations and chromosomal abnormalities	1.36	0.89	0.45	0.89
Prematurity and low birth weight	1.09	0.72	0.36	0.72
Maternal complications during gestation	0.37	0.25	0.12	0.25
Placental and cord complications	0.25	0.17	0.09	0.17
Respiratory distress syndrome	0.25	0.17	0.09	NA
Bacterial sepsis	0.17	0.11	0.06	0.11
Disease of circulatory system	0.15	0.10	0.05	0.10
Intrauterine hypoxia or birth asphyxia	0.13	0.09	0.04	0.09
All other cause	2.25	1.49	0.74	1.49

IMR, Infant mortality rate; NMR, neonatal mortality rate, ≈ two-thirds of IMR; PMR, perinatal mortality rate, ≈one-third of IMR; FMR, fetal mortality rate ≈ NMR. IMR, NMR calculated as deaths per 1000 live births; PMR, FMR calculated as deaths per 1000 live births + fetal deaths.
After Arias et al 2003,[5] with permission.

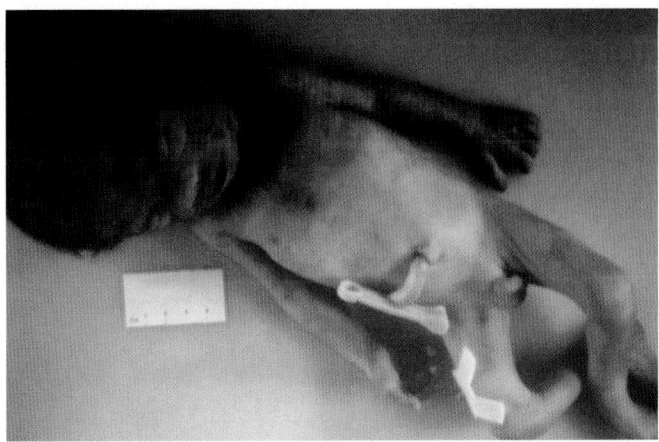

FIGURE 7.1 Asymmetric growth restriction. The head and brain have grown normally while the rest of the body is small for the gestation, 32 weeks. Note also the discolored left arm and head due to a shoulder presentation in the birth canal.

of 2.8:1 is changed to 5:1 or 6:1. Asymmetric growth restriction is caused by abnormal placental transfer of oxygen and nutrients. By contrast, symmetric growth restriction is usually due to a chromosomal or genetic abnormality or viral infection.[6]

Maternal factors in fetal and neonatal death

Maternal conditions associated with fetal death include very young or advanced age, hypertension, infections, thrombotic disorders, anemia, obesity, diabetes, incompetent cervix, premature rupture of membranes, and multiple pregnancy.[17, 18] Such conditions accounted for at least 12% of fetal deaths in a large Swedish study.[19]

Maternal age

Intrapartum death and IUGR are especially prevalent among teenage mothers.[5] When the mother is 35 years of age or older, chromosomal abnormalities and diabetes are increased but non-syndromic malformations are not increased.[11] With fathers 40 years or older and mothers 30 years or older, fetal deaths are only slightly increased.[20]

Maternal hypertensive disorders

The hypertensive disorders in pregnancy include mild to severe pregnancy induced hypertension (PIH), pre-eclampsia (PIH accompanied by proteinuria), HELLP syndrome (pre-eclampsia with intravascular *h*emolysis, *e*levated *l*iver enzymes and *l*ow

TABLE 7.2 HYPERTENSIVE DISORDERS IN 135 466 PREGNANCIES

	Incidence (%)	Relative risk for	
		SGA infants	Stillbirth
Mild PIH	7.7	1.3	1.1
Severe PIH	1.3	2.5	1.8
HELLP	0.2	3.8	2.5
Eclampsia	0.02	3.5	ND
Chronic hypertension	0.6	1.4	2.4
Chronic hypertension +PIH	0.4	2.2	4.4

SGA, Small for gestational age; mild PIH, pregnancy induced hypertension without proteinuria; severe PIH, pregnancy induced hypertension with proteinuria; HELLP, or eclampsia; HELLP syndrome, PIH with hemolysis, elevated liver enzymes, low platelets; ND, no data.
Overall rate of hypertensive disease in pregnancy = 10.1%
From Allen et al 2004,[21] with permission.

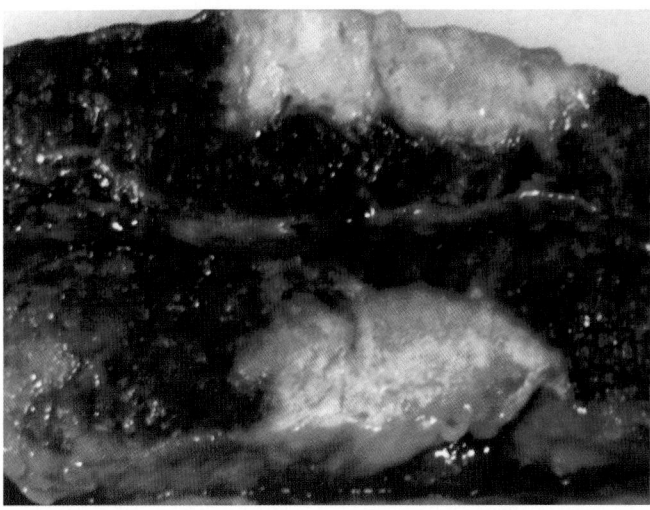

FIGURE 7.2 Placenta with multiple yellow infarcts due to pregnancy induced hypertension. Similar lesions develop with maternal thrombotic disorders.

*p*latelets), eclampsia (pre-eclampsia plus convulsions), and chronic hypertensive diseases (present before the pregnancy and continue after delivery). PIH can be superimposed on chronic hypertension.[21] The clinical onset of PIH is often in the first pregnancy and after 20 weeks' gestation but the initiating factor is failure of trophoblast to properly remodel endometrial arteries at implantation in the first week of gestation. Obesity, multiple gestations, and gestational diabetes predispose to PIH.[21] The effects of maternal hypertension on the placenta and fetal growth and stillbirth are listed in Table 7.2. Placental infarcts are common (Fig. 7.2).

Maternal infections

Infections are responsible for about 20–25% of fetal and perinatal mortality.[19] An infectious agent reaches the fetus by two main routes: blood-borne from the mother's circulation or

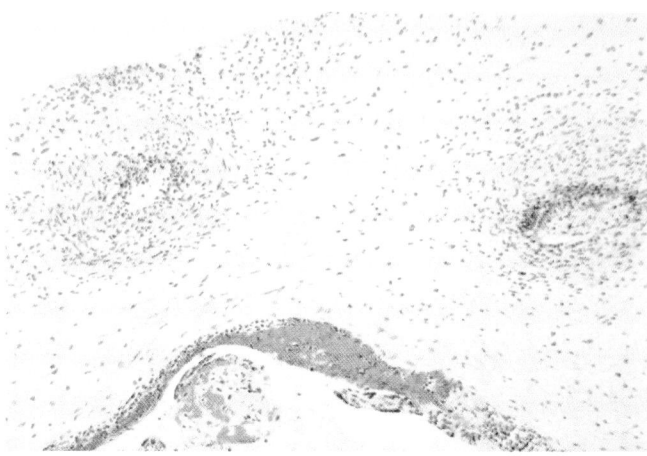

FIGURE 7.3 The amnion and fetal vessels are infiltrated with polymorphonuclear leukocytes. (Hematoxylin and eosin stain; 100 × original magnification.)

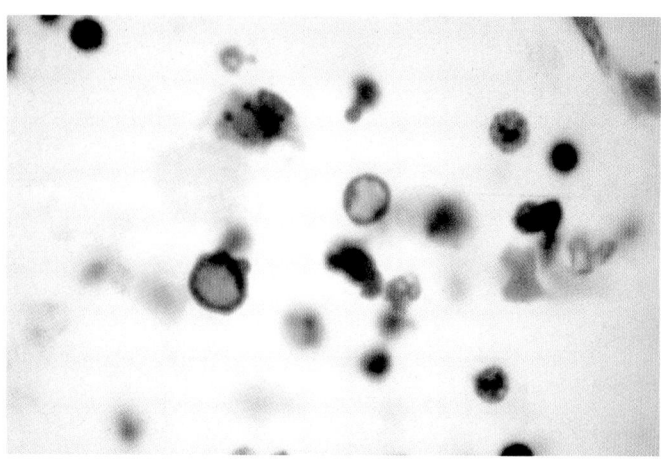

FIGURE 7.4 Parvovirus B19 inclusions in fetal erythroid precursors. The amphophilic inclusions displace chromatin to the margin of the nucleus in two enlarged cells at the center of the figure. (Hematoxylin and eosin stain; 400 × original magnification.)

ascending from the mother's genital tract. The placenta is an imperfect barrier to maternal blood-born bacteria, viruses, fungi, and protozoa. Ascending infections from colonized genitalia can invade prematurely ruptured placental membranes (PROM) or breach intact placental membranes to infect the amniotic sac. Choriodecidual colonization induces acute inflammation of the amnion and of the fetal vessels (Fig. 7.3). Endotoxins and exotoxins cause increases in prostaglandins and cytokines that tend to ripen the cervix and produce uterine contractions.[22] The fetus aspirates and swallows the organisms producing pneumonia, septicemia, and meningitis.[23]

Group B streptococcus (GBS) sepsis is one of the world's most prevalent causes of fetal and neonatal death.[24–28] Early onset GBS sepsis is that which begins in utero or within the first 96 h of life. Late onset sepsis is first noted after 96 h and is often heralded by meningitis. Screening and treatment protocols to reduce the morbidity and mortality from GBS infections call for treating women at risk with intravenous penicillin or a similar antibiotic at the onset of labor. The neonate is treated for several days after delivery.[29, 30] These protocols have reduced fatalities from 1.7 to 0.4 per 1000 live births.[31] Failures occur in about 7% of cases because of non-adherence to the protocols or lack of prenatal care.[32] Gram-negative organisms are not affected by the prescribed antibiotics. Furthermore, one-third of fatal GBS cases are fetuses infected before the onset of labor.[33, 34] Vaccinations with GBS capsular polysaccharide have been tried but results are inconclusive.[35]

Other bacterial species that mothers commonly pass to their fetuses and neonates include *Ureaplasma urealyticum, Mycoplasma hominis*, coagulase negative staphylococcus, non-typable *Hemophilus influenzae, Streptococcus viridans, Escherichia coli*, and *Aerobacter aerogenes*.[22] Mothers with human immunodeficiency virus (HIV) infections are especially prone to transmit *Mycobacterium tuberculosis* and *Treponema pallidum*.[36, 37]

Most perinatal viral diseases are from transplacental infections but HIV and herpes infections are usually acquired by exposure to maternal blood or an infected birth canal.[23] The most common lethal perinatal viral agent is parvovirus B19.[38–40] This virus causes more fetal deaths than HIV, cytomegalovirus, rubella, herpes, rubeola, and influenza combined.[23, 41–43] The virus infects fetal erythroid precursors producing characteristic intranuclear inclusions and profound anemia with fetal and placental hydrops[44] (Fig. 7.4). Intrauterine blood transfusions can be life-saving but almost half of the fetuses are dead by the time hydrops is noted on ultrasound.[38] Maternal HIV infection has few direct effects on the fetus until parturition.[45] Antiretroviral treatment (Zidovudine®) reduces vertical transmission to fetuses by 70%, but the prematurity rate (16%), LBW (18%) and stillbirth (0.6%) are essentially the same whether the mother is treated or not.[46, 47]

Candidiasis is an occasional yeast/fungal cause of fetal and neonatal infection. Diabetic women are especially at risk. The diagnosis can be suspected by examining the surface of the umbilical cord which is studded with small white colonies of candida organisms[48] (Fig. 7.5).

Malaria is the most common protozoan infection transmitted to the fetus. This is a major problem in malaria-endemic regions of the world with perinatal mortality rates up to 61 per 1000. It is especially prevalent with coexistent HIV infection.[49] Toxoplasmosis and trypanosomiasis are other notable protozoan maternal–fetal infections.[50–52]

Bacterial vaginosis, a polymicrobial infection with predominantly Gram-negative flora, mostly affects women of child-bearing age. Adverse effects are early fetal loss in the first and second trimesters, chorioamnionitis, preterm delivery, and IUGR in the last trimester.[53] Maternal urinary tract infection has a 2.4 fold risk for stillbirth and IUGR, and appendectomy during pregnancy, whether or not the appendix is inflamed, can result in fetal and neonatal complications.[54, 55] Lastly, maternal fever during labor (at least 38°C)

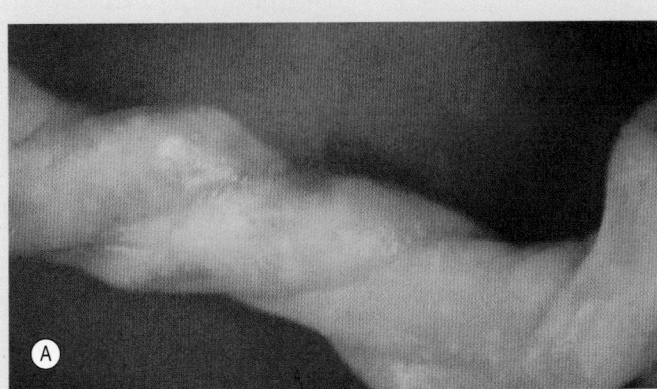

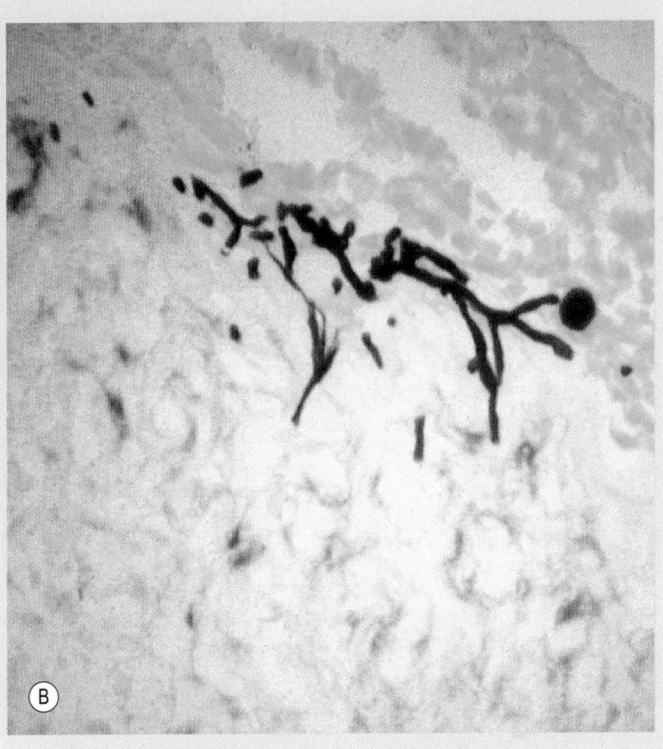

FIGURE 7.5 (A) *Candida albicans* infection of the umbilical cord produces rounded white spots measuring 1–2 mm. (B) *Candida albicans* hyphae in the surface of the umbilical cord. (Silver stain; 1000 × original magnification.)

is associated with increased prematurity and neonatal infections.[56]

Maternal thrombophilia

Pregnancy stresses the balance between procoagulant and anticoagulant pathways with progressive fall in protein S, an acquired resistance to activated protein C, and impaired fibrinolysis. The incidence of maternal thrombophilia may be as high as 65% in otherwise unexplained fetal deaths.[57] Specific thrombophilic disorders are factor V Leiden, prothrombin gene mutation, homocystinemia, especially that due to mutant methylenetetrahydrofolate reductase, marked deficiencies of protein S and protein C, and deficiency of antithrombin III. [57, 58] With any thrombophilia, the risk of fetal death is higher in the second and third trimesters than in the first. Thromboses and infarcts are found in the placentas of such cases but, in carefully controlled studies, fetal growth impairment, abruption, and pre-eclampsia are not increased[57] (Fig. 7.2) Recurrence in subsequent pregnancies can be reduced by immunosuppressive and anti-thrombotic therapies, such as low-molecular-weight heparins.[59, 60]

Lupus anticoagulants and antiphospholipid antibodies define two distinct but related conditions, each associated with thrombosis.[61] Lupus anticoagulant is a misnomer most often unassociated with lupus erythematosus and associated with thrombosis, not anticoagulants in vivo. These patients have increased early spontaneous abortions and fetal deaths in the second and third trimesters of gestation. The diagnosis is based on prolonged prothrombin time and partial thromboplastin time, confirmed by prolonged Russell snake venom clotting time and by specific antibody tests for phospholipids such as phosphatidylserine or cardiolipin.[61]

Maternal anemia

Maternal hemoglobinopathies are associated with excess prematurity, fetal growth impairment and stillbirth.[62] α thalassemia, when the fetus is homozygous for all four α chains, is uniformly fatal unless intrauterine transfusions are given; thereafter the infant will require life-long transfusions.[63, 64] With thalassemia minor, pregnancy and perinatal outcomes are favorable except for higher rates of IUGR.[65] Depending on the paternal contribution, homozygous thalassemia might affect the fetus.[66] The same would hold for sickle cell disease and other recessively inherited hemoglobinopathies. Spontaneous abortions occur in 36% of pregnancies if the mother is homozygous for the sickle cell gene and maternal death occurs in about 2% of these women.[67]

Maternal obesity and maternal diabetes

Maternal obesity is associated fetal macrosomia, shoulder dystocia, late fetal death, and congenital malformations, especially neural tube defects.[68] Maternal problems include pre-

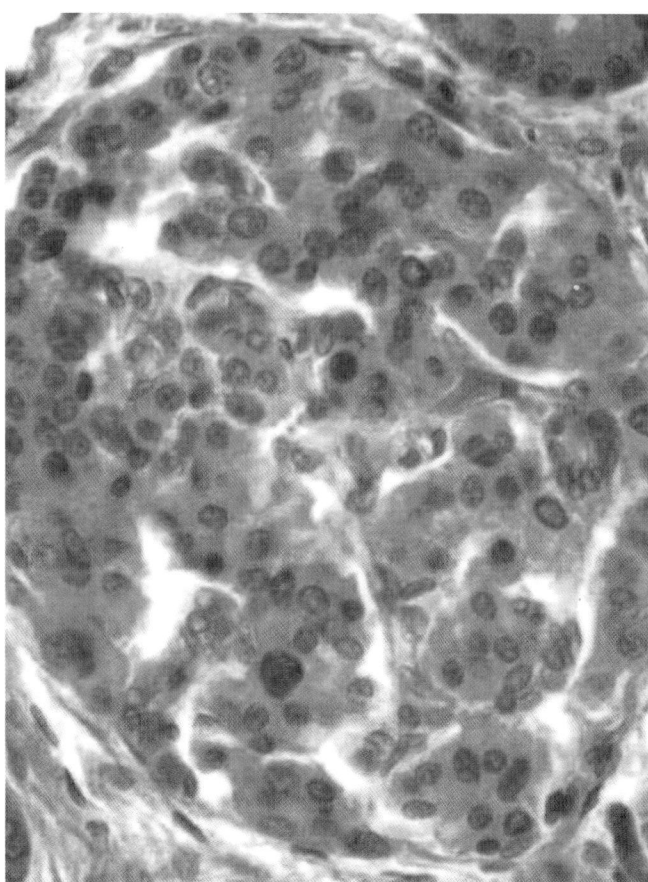

FIGURE 7.6 Pancreatic islets are enlarged and have large hyperchromatic β cells. (Hematoxylin and eosin stain; 200 × original magnification.)

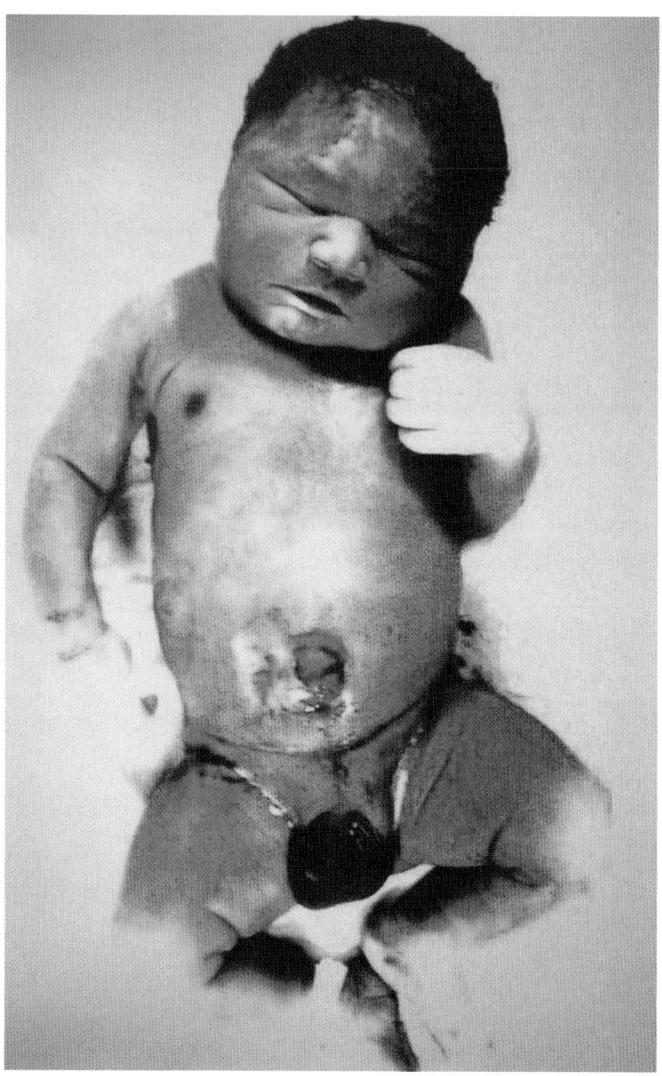

FIGURE 7.7 Macrosomic infant born to a diabetic mother with poor control of blood glucose. Abundant body fat is a feature along with overall excessive growth.

eclampsia, increased cesarean section rate, operative vaginal delivery, diabetes, and chorioamnionitis.[69]

Women with diabetic vascular disease have difficulty conceiving and when they do, fetuses have growth impairment, increased rates of stillbirth and preterm delivery. In offspring of women with type 1 and type 2 diabetes, malformations are increased. The skeleton, the cardiovascular system, central nervous system, urinary tract, and gastrointestinal tract are involved.[70–72] Transient myocardiopathy with left ventricular outlet obstruction has also been described.[73] Good preconceptional and early gestational control of maternal glucose markedly reduces congenital malformations but the incidence is still higher than in the general population.[74] Genetic etiology is not involved since paternal diabetes is not a factor.[70] Obesity increases risk of gestational diabetes which, though innocent of a role in congenital malformations, contributes to fetal and neonatal morbidity/mortality. Inflammatory cytokines generated by the placenta produce oxidative stress which in turn result in fetal brain injuries.[75, 76] The fetal pancreatic islets produce excess insulin, a potent growth factor for the fetus (Fig. 7.6). Macrosomia with cephalopelvic disproportion is a hazard[77] (Fig. 7.7). After separation from the mother, neonatal hyperinsulinemia may produce life-threatening hypoglycemia.[78] Fetal and neonatal

organs and physiologic processes are relatively immature. Near-term infants develop respiratory distress syndrome.[79] Fetuses and infants of diabetic mothers are at risk for thromboembolism because of high hematocrits, hyperviscosity, and protein C deficiency[80] (Fig. 7. 8).

Other maternal disorders that affect their offspring are listed in Table 7.3.

Maternal morbidity and mortality

Cardiac failure, hemorrhage, amniotic fluid embolus, pre-eclampsia–eclampsia, gestational diabetes, and postpartum hemorrhage, though rare, are causes of maternal disease and death.[81] Homicide must also be considered, particularly among teenagers and young women in the early stages of pregnancy.[82] Abruptio placenta, placenta previa, postpartum uterine atony, and placenta accreta can produce massive hemorrhage, the most common lethal event associated with pregnancy. In developing countries the maternal mortality rate is 7%. This is compared to a rate of 0.3% in the USA.[83]

Fetal and placental conditions associated with stillbirth

Since perinatal mortality includes both fetal and neonatal death, classification systems have addressed two populations with somewhat different disease processes. For example, conditions such as 'prematurity' and 'pulmonary hypoplasia' are not relevant causes for stillbirths. Attempts to collect uniform data on fetal death have been hampered by this lack of a separate classification. Such a classification must be practical, use standard terminology, be resistant to variable interpretation, easy to expand, and be based on clinical information and on placental and postmortem examinations. We present here a simple classification of fetal death based on underlying causes of the associated disorders. Causes are assigned when a fetal or placental lesion is deemed sufficient to result in or contribute significantly to the fetal death. The various causes are mutually exclusive (Table 7.4).

Infections

Deaths attributed to bacterial infections are divided into two groups:
- positive bacteriologic cultures and histologic evidence of inflammation;
- no positive bacteriologic cultures but with histologic criteria for amniotic fluid bacterial infection syndrome.

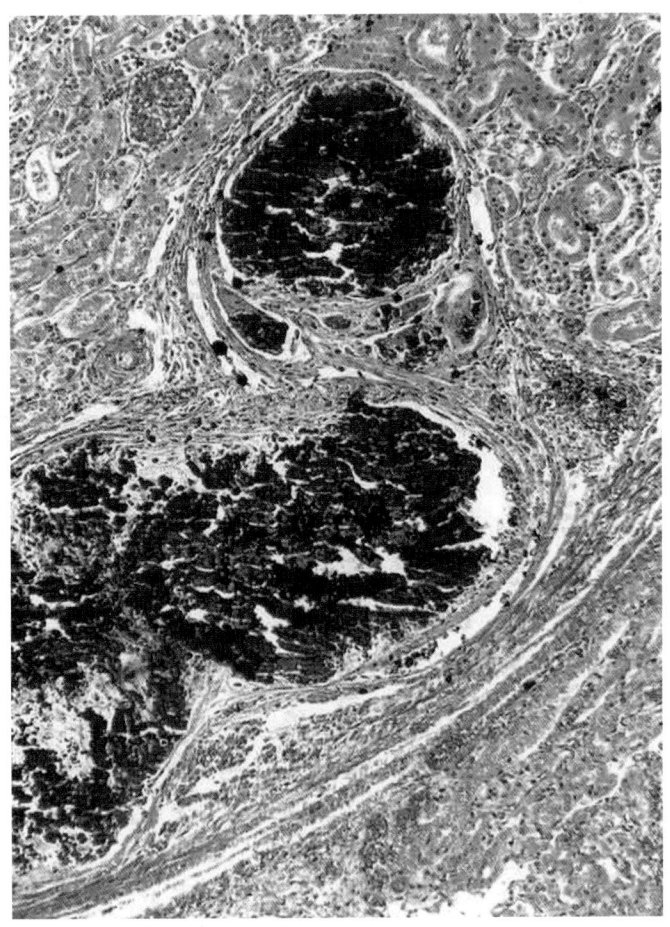

FIGURE 7.8 Calcified thrombi in renal veins in an infant of a diabetic mother. (Hematoxylin and eosin stain; 100 × original magnification.)

TABLE 7.3 OTHER MATERNAL CONDITIONS AFFECTING FETUSES AND NEONATES

Condition	Effect on fetus/neonate
Myasthenia gravis	Stillbirth uncommon; 10% neonates have myasthenia
Myotonic dystrophy	Mortality 15%; prematurity 20%; may inherit gene; mothers can not push during labor
Transplant recipients	Complications in 25%; stillbirth, IUGR; disturbed immune system
Liver disease	Prematurity; drug withdrawal; respiratory distress; IUGR; coagulopathy
Rheumatic diseases	Prematurity 20%
Systemic lupus erythematosus	Prematurity; premature rupture of membranes; IUGR
Autoimmune thyroid diseases	Little effect on the fetus if mother is adequately treated
Anti-SSA/Ro antibodies	Spontaneous abortion; prematurity; rare congenital heart block
Cardiovascular disease	Increased early abortion; stillbirth; respiratory distress; asphyxia; hyperacidemia in 30%; congenital heart disease risk is two to three times if mother has congenital lesion
Renal disease	Poor outcome twice normal; outcome good if mother has low creatinine; prematurity
Periodontal disease*	IUGR; premature rupture of membranes; premature delivery
Smoking and drug abuse	IUGR; prematurity; fetal and neonatal death, especially with cocaine
Diabetes	IUGR, LGA – outcome good with good maternal glycemic control
Chemotherapy	IUGR; prematurity; fetal and neonatal death

*Gingival inflammation, bleeding, and/or hypertrophy.
LGA, Large for gestational age; IUGR, intrauterine growth restriction.

TABLE 7.4 CAUSES OF FETAL DEATH IN 388 CASES WITH AUTOPSY*

	No	%
INFECTIOUS DISORDERS		
Acute		
Acute infections placentitis and amniotic fluid infection syndrome – bacterial		
Culture positive	35	
Culture negative	23	
Chronic		
Chronic infectious placentitis with morphologic evidence of fetal infection – viral	7	
	65	16.8
CONDITIONS CAUSING CIRCULATORY COMPROMISE		
Acute		
Umbilical cord/membranous fetal blood vessel avulsion or puncture		
Cord prolapse	1	
Nuchal cord with pathological evidence of circulatory compromise		
Abruptio placenta, acute	20	
Fetomaternal hemorrhage	1	
Acute and/or chronic		
True knot of the umbilical cord		
Cord sections lacking Wharton's jelly (includes furcate insertion)		
Velamentous cord insertion		
Circumvallate membrane insertion	1	
Fetal thrombotic vasculopathy	3	
Chronic		
Maternal and fetal conditions* resulting in intrauterine growth impairment of the fetoplacental unit and cause destructive, reparative and developmental placental lesions involving <50% of placental mass†	51	
	77	19.8
DEVELOPMENTAL DISORDERS		
Umbilical cord abnormalities		
Short umbilical cord	3	
Long umbilical cord	2	
Decreased coil index		
Increased coil index	1	
Multiple gestation		
Dichorionic diamnionic twining	8	
Monochorionic twining		
TTT syndrome‡	10	
TRAP sequence§	3	
Cord entanglement	3	
Monochorionic twining no obvious lesions	3	
Multifetation (number of fetuses > 2)	8	
Intrauterine growth restriction (IUGR)	23	
Overgrowth syndromes (placenta and fetus)	4	
Vascular malformations		
Mesenchymal dysplasia	3	
Early amnion rupture sequence	6	
Chromosomal disorders		
Aneuploidy syndromes		
Trisomy 21	7	
Trisomy 18	5	
Trisomy 13	3	
Monosomy X	3	
Triploidy	1	
Other	3	
Confined placental mosaicism		
Uniparental isodisomy		
Lethal or non-lethal malformations without overt chromosomal abnormalities (at 800 band resolution)		
Oligohydramnios sequence		
Renal agenesis	3	
Autosomal recessive polycystic kidney disease	2	
Autosomal dominant polycystic kidney disease	1	
Cystic dysplastic kidneys	2	
Cloacal dysgenesis	5	

	No	%
Neural tube defects and neuronal migrational disorders		
Anencephaly	9	
Craniorachischisis	4	
Holoprosencephaly	3	
Skeletal dysplasias	4	
Osteogenesis imperfecta		
Thanatophoric dysplasia	3	
Other	4	
Complex congenital heart malformations	14	
	154	39.7
IMMUNOLOGICAL DISORDERS		
Villitis of undetermined etiology (VUE)	1	
Isoimmunization		
Autoimmune diseases		
	1	0.3
HEMATOLOGICAL DISORDERS		
Hemoglobinopathies with hydrops	5	
Hemoglobinopathies without hydrops	3	
Hereditary thrombophilic disorders	4	
	12	3.1
METABOLIC DISORDERS		
Gestational diabetes	8	
Type I diabetes	2	
Type II diabetes		
	10	2.6
ENVIRONMENTAL DISORDERS – FACTORS		
Acute		
Homicide – suicide		
Substance overdose		
Motor-vehicle or other accidents		
Chronic		
Environmental toxin exposure	6	
Chronic substance abuse	6	
	6	1.5
NEOPLASTIC		
Placenta		
Chorangioma, solitary > 20% placental volume	2	
Chorangiomatosis involving > 20% placental volume	2	
Fetal		
Vascular		
Hemangioma, hemangioendothelioma	1	
Solid		
Rhabdomyoma		
Teratomas	1	
Neuroblastoma	1	
OTHER		
Hydrops fetalis – cause undetermined	6	
Congenital uterine malformations	3	
Evidence of CNS hypoxia – cause undetermined	6	
Preterm prolonged rupture of membranes – no other pathology	12	
	27	7
NO KNOWN ASSOCIATION	29	7.5
Grand total	388	

*Conditions associated with decreased placental perfusion are pre-eclampsia, chronic hypertension, HELLP syndrome, and chronic abruption.

†Placental lesions associated with decreased placental perfusion are: increased syncytial knots, villous agglutination, increased intervillous fibrin (fibrin-type fibrinoid), distal villous hypoplasia, acute atherosis, mural hypertrophy of membrane arterioles, muscularized basal plate arteries, increased placental site giant cells, proliferation of immature extravillous cytotrophoblast (evCTB) (intermediate trophoblast) and thin umbilical cord

‡Twin-twin transfusion syndrome

§Twin reversed arterial perfusion syndrome

From the autopsy files at Women and Infants' Hospital, Brown University School of Medicine, Providence, Rhode Island.

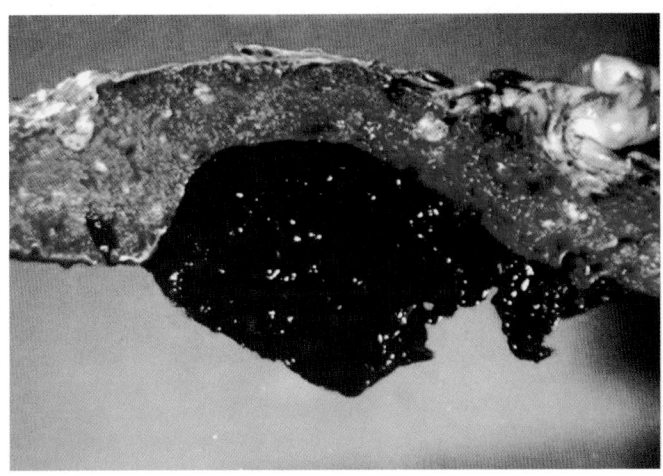

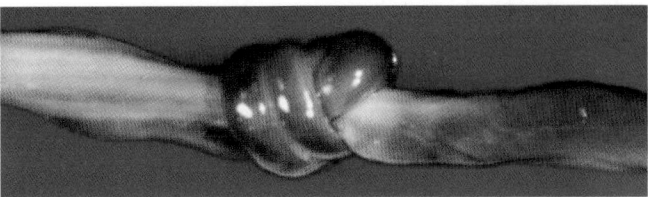

FIGURE 7.10 A true knot in the umbilical cord with distension of vessels within the knot.

FIGURE 7.9 A large hematoma separates the central portion of the placenta from its attachment to the uterus. Surrounding tissue is ischemic.

This consists of polymorphonuclear leukocytes in the lungs, upper gastrointestinal tract, or hepatic sinusoids and/or acute chorioamnionitis, funisitis or umbilical vasculitis (Fig. 7.3). In our series Group B streptococcus was isolated in 20 of 35 culture positive cases. In some cases with positive cultures, the fetuses have sparse or absent polymorphonuclear infiltrates. We assume death is related to cytokines induced by the infectious agent and that precede a neutrophilic response.[84] Infections can account for about 15–20% of fetal deaths, especially in mid gestation. The most common causative organisms are coagulase negative staphylococci, GBS, *S. viridans, E. coli,* and *A. aerogenes.*[85] The circumstances that lead to fetal infections are discussed in the previous section on maternal conditions. Recurrence in subsequent pregnancies is a distinct hazard.

Circulatory disorders

Acute circulatory disorders include abruptio placenta and compromise of umbilical circulation. Abruptio placenta accounts for about 10% of all fetal deaths.[86] To diagnose abruption requires evidence of a retroplacental hematoma and surrounding parenchymal necrosis (Fig. 7.9). Cord accidents (nuchal cord, true knots, and prolapse) require morphologic evidence such as thrombotic obstruction of the fetal blood vessels or color difference between the afferent and efferent segments of the obstructed cord (Figs 7.10 and 7.11). Either excessive or reduced coiling of the umbilical cord is associated with adverse perinatal outcome; about one-third of such fetuses are stillborn (Fig. 7.12). Growth impairment is also increased with both abnormal cord coil index values.[87]

A fetus can bleed excessively into the placenta or to a twin, triplet, etc. Fetomaternal hemorrhage (FMH) is common, occurring in approximately 75% of all pregnancies but is clinically important only when large. FMH may be a consequence of

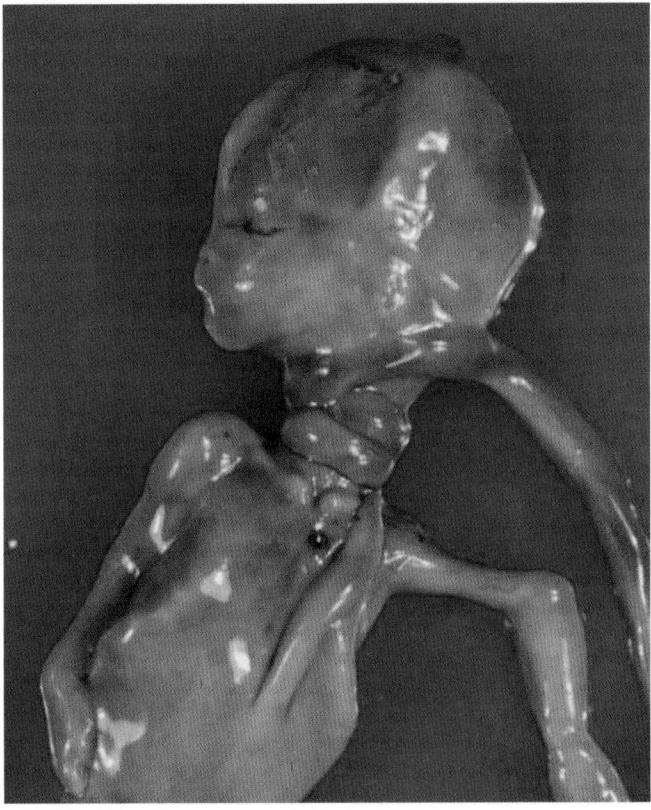

FIGURE 7.11 A nuchal cord with three loops around the neck. The fetus had been dead for at least a week, indicated by the brown discoloration and autolysis of tissues.

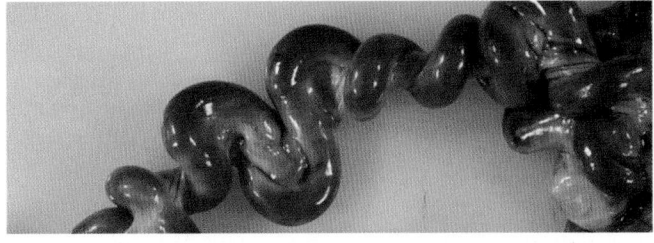

FIGURE 7.12 Excessive coiling and postmortem discoloration of the umbilical cord in a case of fetal death.

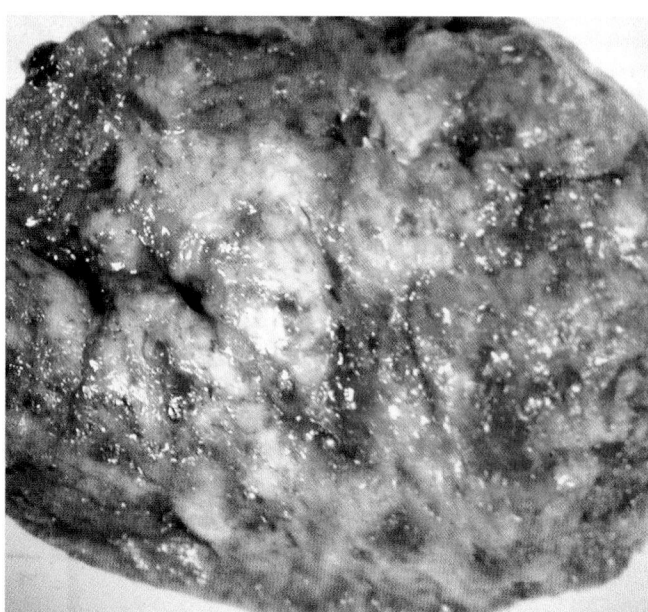

FIGURE 7.13 Maternal surface (floor) of the placenta with extensive fibrin deposits.

abdominal trauma with placental abruption or with complications such as anterior placenta or chorangioma. Massive FMH causes death with hypovolemic shock, pallor, cardiac failure, and hydrops.[88] If fetal cells are antigenically incompatible, the mother may have serious reactions including disseminated intravascular coagulation and renal failure. Blood group incompatibility, especially Rh sensitization, causes fetal and neonatal problems in subsequent pregnancies with fetal hydrops or neonatal hyperbilirubinemia.[64]

FMH and the quantity transfused is best detected by flow cytometry of maternal blood.[89] Immediate transfusion may save the life of the fetus or neonate. Since fetal cells can persist in the maternal circulation for days, perhaps weeks, flow cytometry (or the older Kleihauer-Betke stain) should be performed routinely in all cases of unexplained stillbirth, fetal distress, and neonatal anemia.[90]

Chronic circulatory compromise is due mostly to decreased placental perfusion and results in asymmetric IUGR.[91] Maternal hypertension is the most common disorder in this category (Table 7.2). Chronic abruption and some thrombophilic states affect maternal and fetal circulation with prominent placental syncytial knots, villous agglutination, increased intervillous fibrin, distal villous hypoplasia, acute atherosis, mural hypertrophy of membrane arterioles, muscularized basal plate arteries, increased decidual giant cells, proliferation of immature extravillous cytotrophoblast (intermediate trophoblast) and thin umbilical cord.[92] These lesions are the precursors of more easily recognized parenchymal lesions such as infarcts, fibrin deposits, thrombi, Breus' mole, or extensive maternal floor fibrin deposits (misnamed maternal floor infarcts) (Fig. 7.13). Any of these lesions can cause fetal death when they involve 50% of the placental mass.[86, 92]

In chronic abruption, oligohydramnios, hypoplastic lungs, and pulmonary hypertension complicate the course in survivors.[93] Twin-to-twin-transfusion (T^4 syndrome) of blood through anastomoses in monochorionic twin placentas can exsanguinate the donor and overload the circulation in the recipient with death in both. Techniques to ablate the feto–fetal anastomoses have improved the outcome in such cases.[94]

Fetal thrombosis

Conditions that reduce plasma volume and maintain or increase formed blood elements contribute to fetal and neonatal thromboembolism. These conditions include congenital nephrotic syndrome, septicemia, and necrotizing enterocolitis. Hypoxia and other sources of oxidative stress damage the endothelium allowing platelet aggregation and thrombus formation. Intravenous and intra-arterial probes and catheters promote thrombi. Infants of diabetic mothers are prone to thromboembolism, mainly on the basis of high hematocrits and hyperviscosity. In fetal life, small renal venules thrombose and propagate to larger veins and the vena cava (Fig. 7.8). Factor V Leiden and genetic deficiencies of protein C, protein S, antithrombin III are responsible for some cases of fetal thrombosis.[57] Fetal vascular obstructive diseases are reflected by avascular placental villi, endothelial karyorrhexis, thrombi in large placental vessels, and intimal fibrinous cushions, sometimes with calcification or fibrosis. Syncytial trophoblast has excessive karyorrhexis.[95] Fetal thromboemboli are associated not only with increased fetal and neonatal death but also increased cerebral palsy.[96]

Developmental disorders

The developmental disorders include several subcategories such as short and long umbilical cords, multiple gestations, symmetric IUGR, overgrowth syndromes, vascular malformations such as chorangioma, hemangioma, arteriovenous fistulae, chromosomal disorders, confined placental mosaicism, uniparental disomy, and structural malformations with and without chromosomal defects or known genetic defects.

Malformations in stillbirths

Malformations rarely directly cause intrauterine death. Exceptions are severe chromosomal defects or cardiac defects with congestive failure and hydrops. Nevertheless, the rate of malformations among stillborn fetuses (~20%) is higher than in the general population (~2–3%).[97] In a large Swedish study, 10% of the stillbirths were attributed to congenital malformations while in the USA the rate approaches 20%.[5, 19] In our series, the combined chromosomal anomalies and structural malformations accounted for 20% of fetal deaths (Table 7.4) Major anomalies mostly involved the central nervous system, renal, cardiac, and

and rocker-bottom feet provide clues to the diagnosis. Ventricular septal defects, nodular dysplasia of the valves, and hypoplastic lungs may be seen. In trisomy 13 (Patau syndrome) the anomalies are frequently severe and include cyclopia, polydactyly, neural tube defects, scalp defects and cleft lip and palate. Triploidy (69 chromosomes) causes early fetal loss with profound asymmetric IUGR, syndactyly, and multiple internal anomalies if the extra haploid set is contributed by the mother. Hydatid changes in the placenta (partial mole) are the main features of triploidy if the father contributes the extra chromosomes.[101]

Single gene disorders are important since recurrence in subsequent pregnancies is a risk. Those affecting stillborn fetuses are listed in Table 7.5.[102] Multifactorial inheritance, i.e. with isolated malformations, also contributes to stillbirth but one must carefully rule out multiple anomalies before invoking such a diagnosis.

Confined placental mosaicism (CPM) has been detected at all stages of gestation.[103] Chromosomal mosaicism is defined as two or more karyotypically different cell lines arising from a single zygote. The three types of CPM are shown in Table 7.6. CPM may persist in placentas with normal full-term neonates, but up to 20% of these gestations have complications (Fig. 7.15). The most common chromosomes involved are trisomies of 2, 7, 9, 15, and 16.[104] Recent studies show that CPM is not as prevalent as previously thought.[105]

The contributions of gene mutations or confined placental mosaicism to stillbirth remain largely unexplored since they often go undiscovered within records of other causes, such as asphyxia and IUGR.

Uniparental disomy occurs when homologous chromosomes in a pair originate from one parent. Through imprinting, maternally derived genes may function differently than paternally derived ones (see Ch. 1).[106] Known cases have produced viable neonates and children, but it seems reasonable to assume that uniparental disomy will cause stillbirth as well.

Multiple gestations

The stillbirth rate among twins is much higher than among singletons and is higher still among triplets, quadruplets, etc. When the placentas are monochorionic, twin-to-twin transfusions (T^4 syndrome) can exsanguinate the donor and overload the circulation of the recipient, resulting in two fetal deaths. If one fetus dies and the other(s) survive, the dead twin syndrome may develop. The surviving fetuses develop massive infarcts of the kidneys, spleen, brain, etc. Once thought to represent bleeding into the dead twin's stagnant circulation, these lesions are now considered a sublethal insult caused by the same condition that produced the stillbirth.[4]

Intrauterine growth restriction

The incidence of IUGR is higher among stillborn fetuses than the general population. Most of the maternal conditions already

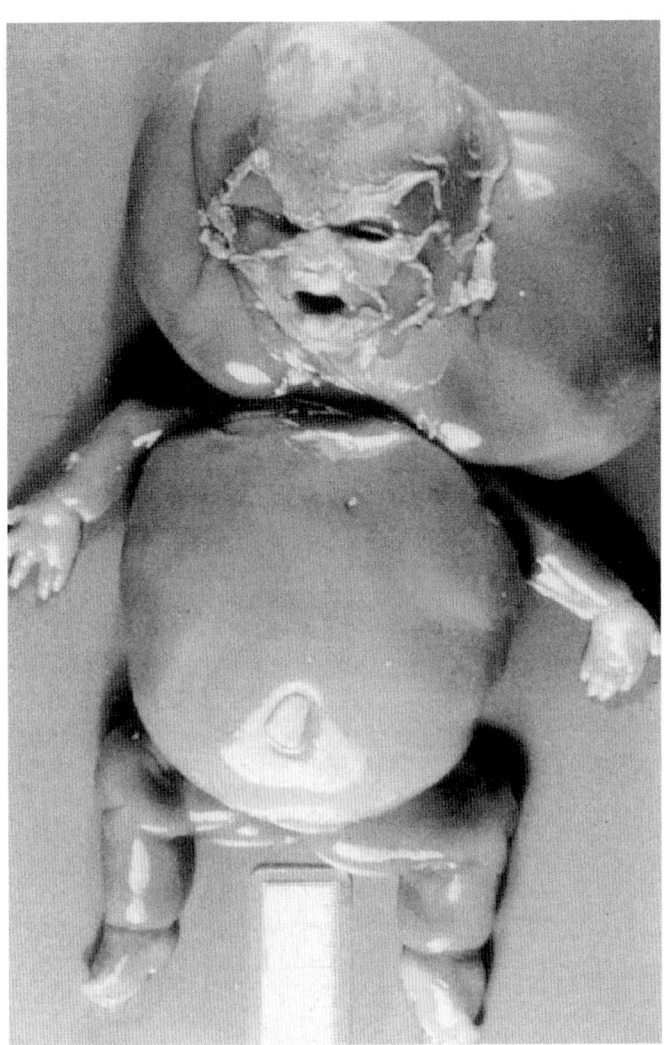

FIGURE 7.14 Fetus with monosomy X and pronounced edema. A large nuchal hygroma is characteristic of this chromosomal defect. (From Kalousek and Gilbert-Barness 1997,[100] with permission.)

skeletal system. Minor anomalies are also increased in stillborn fetuses compared with the general population. For example, a single umbilical artery occurs three times more frequently in stillborn fetuses than in the general population.[98]

Chromosomal abnormalities are found in up to 10% of stillborn fetuses.[99] The most common of these is monosomy X with nuchal cystic hygromas in early fetal life and characteristic webbed neck, broad chest, and increased carrying angle of arms in near-term fetuses (Fig. 7.14).[100] Trisomies 21, 18, and 13 together make up a significant proportion of the genetic conditions causing stillbirth. Phenotypic features may be subtle in trisomy 21 (Down syndrome) until the third trimester. Careful examination may show single palmar creases, clinodactyly of the fifth finger with a hypoplastic middle phalanx, and increased acetabular angle in radiographs of the pelvis and hips. Half of Down fetuses have congenital heart anomalies and half of these are endocardial cushion defects (atrioventricular canal, cleft mitral valve, septum primum defects). In trisomy 18 (Edward syndrome) marked IUGR with abnormal clenching of the hands

TABLE 7.5 COMMON MENDELIAN DISORDERS IN STILLBIRTH

McKusick* no.	Condition	Inheritance
200600	Achondrogenesis type 1 (Parenti-Fraccaro)	AR
200610	Achondrogenesis type 2 (Langer-Saldino)	AR
208500	Asphyxiating thoracic dystrophy	AR
211180	Bowen-Conradi syndrome	AR
211990	Camptomelic dysplasia	AR
302950	Chondrodysplasia punctata (severe form)	AR
219000	Cryptophthalmos syndrome (Fraser)	AR
219150	Cutis laxa	AR
256050	De la Chapelle neonatal osseous dysplasia	AR
200995	Elejalde acrocephalopolydactyly syndrome	AR
228520	Fibrochondrogenesis	AR
305600	Focal dermal hypoplasia (Goltz syndrome)	XD
229850	Fryns syndrome	AR
231680	Glutaric aciduria type II	XR
230500	GM$_1$ (generalized gangliosidosis type 1)	AR
236680	Hydrolethalus	AR
146000	Hypochondroplasia	AR
171760	Hypophosphatasia (severe form)	AR
252500	I-cell (mucolipidosis type 2)	AR
208530	Ivemark syndrome (asplenia or polysplenia)	AR
277300	Jarcho-Levin syndrome	AR
246620	Leprechaunism	AR
275000	Lethal multiple pterygium syndrome: type Chen	AR
249000	Meckel-Gruber syndrome	AR
249210	Megacystic microcolon–intestinal hypoperistalsis syndrome	AR
249420	Melnick-Needles syndrome	XD
256520	Neu-Laxova syndrome	AR
257350	Nuchal blebs–lethal dysplasia	AR
120150	Osteogenesis imperfecta (OI) congenita type II	AD
265000	Popliteal pterygium (severe lethal), Bartsocas-Papas type	AR
264090	Progeria, neonatal form	AR
268300	Roberts syndrome (pseudothalidomide syndrome)	AR
269250	Schneckenbecken dysplasia	AR
263530	Short rib polydactyly type 1 (Saldino-Noonan) and type 3 (Naumoff)	AR
263520	Short rib polydactyly type 2 (Majewski)	AR
236670	Walker-Warburg (Hard E syndrome)	AR
214100	Zellweger (cerebrohepatorenal) syndrome	AR

AD, Autosomal dominant; AR, autosomal recessive; XD, X-linked dominant; XR, X-linked recessive.

From Kalousek and Gilbert-Barness 1997,[100] with permission.

*McKusick 1994,[102] modified according to Online Mendelian Inheritance in Man™ 2004.

TABLE 7.6 CONFINED PLACENTAL MOSAICISM

	Type I	Type II	Type III
Cytotrophoblast	N A	N	N A
Chorionic stroma	N/A	N A	N A
Fetus	N/A	N	N

N A, Both normal and abnormal cell lines are present; N/A, only normal or only abnormal cell lines are found in the chorionic stroma and the fetus; N, only a normal cell line is present.

From Kalousek and Gilbert-Barness 1997,[100] with permission.

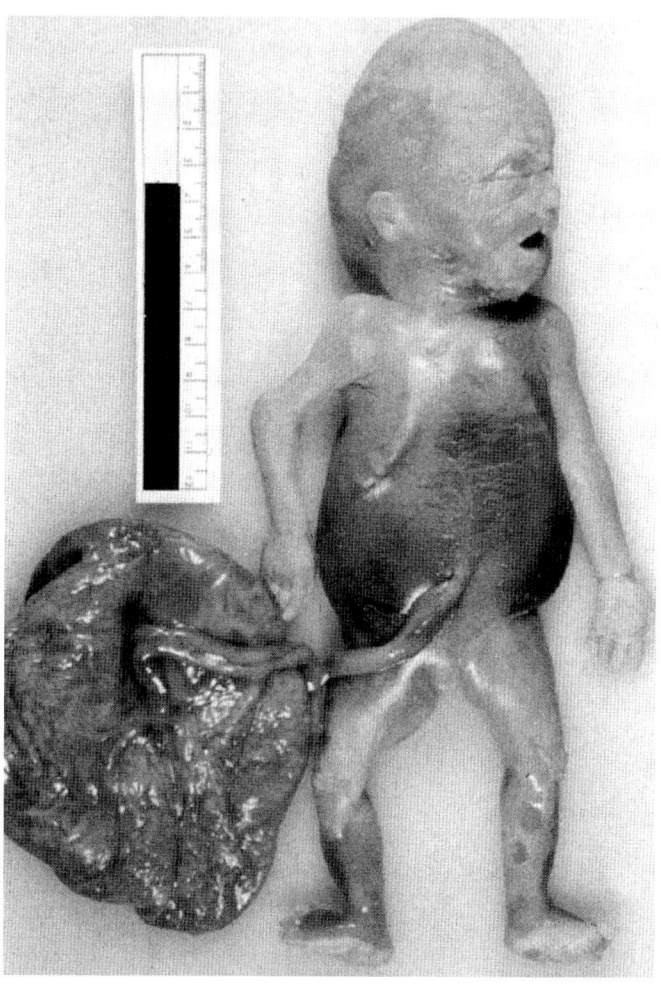

FIGURE 7.15 Confined placental mosaicism results in trisomic zygote rescue. (From Kalousek and Gilbert-Barness 1997,[100] with permission.)

described contribute to asymmetric IUGR. Impaired fetal growth is most commonly due to poor placental perfusion but viral infections, thrombotic disorders, and developmental defects contribute a sizeable share. Symmetric IUGR is usually due to genetic or chromosomal defects or structural malformations.

Large for gestational age

Large fetuses, aside from those with diabetic mothers and those with cephalopelvic disproportion, are rarely stillborn. The normal fetal:placental weight ratio ranges from 3–4:1 at 20 weeks' gestation to 6–7:1 at 40 weeks. When the fetal:placental weight ratio is 8:1 at term, fetal death can occur, presumably on the basis of failed placental growth (hypoplasia or true placental insufficiency). As yet no controlled studies on this condition have been reported.

Amniotic deformities adhesions mutilations complex

Random amputations of digits or extremities, irregular abdominal wall defects and facial clefts, open cerebral and spinal defects, placentas adherent to the scalp and similar bizarre lesions are the features of amniotic deformities adhesions mutilations (ADAM) complexes. The initiating event is rupture of the amniotic membrane. Threads and cords of amnion attach to embryonic or fetal surfaces, encircle limbs, or are swallowed. The raw surfaces of the torn membranes may heal by attaching the placenta to a body part, often the scalp. The amniotic bands become fibrotic and, as the fetus grows, the bands increasingly constrict resulting in sterile gangrene, mummification, or outright amputation or if swallowed, the tethered bands cut into the face producing irregular clefts in the developing mouth, palate, nose, and eyes. Bands may slice into the brain.[107] Though often fatal in utero, ADAM lesions are compatible with live birth, without any impact on long term survival.

Mesenchymal dysplasia

Mesenchymal dysplasia is a rare defect of the placental vasculature that macroscopically resembles hydatidiform mole. Villi are edematous and stem villi contain peripherally placed, dilated vessels. Growth of the fetus is usually normal or they are large. Stillbirth rarely results.[108]

Immunologic disorders

Villitis of unknown etiology consists of infiltrates of maternal leukocytes, including macrophages, into the placental villi (Fig. 7.16). The fetus may be growth impaired or stillborn. Recurrence in later pregnancies is a significant risk. This is apparently an immunologic response of the mother to a fetal or placental product.[95] Alloimmune thrombocytopenia does not usually result in fetal death, but hemorrhages are a risk in postnatal life.[109] Fetal maternal blood group incompatibility can result in profound anemia in the fetus. Most such cases are the result of Rh factor on the surfaces of fetal red blood cells that immunize an Rh negative mother. Infants are usually liveborn,

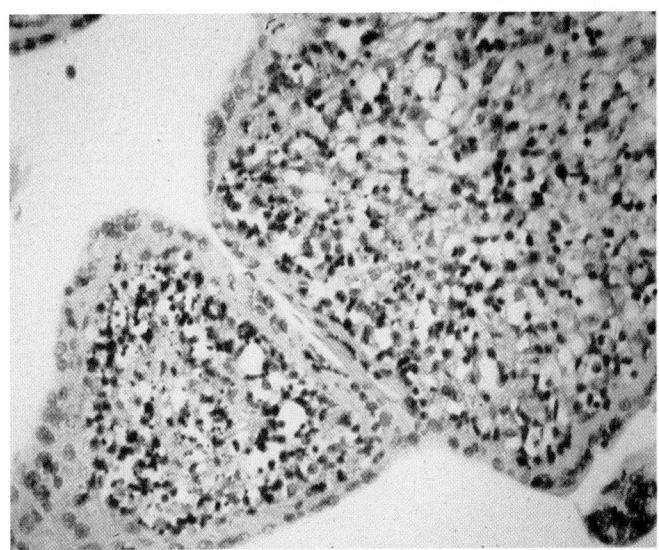

FIGURE 7.16 Villitis of unknown etiology. Maternal leukocytes, including macrophages infiltrate the placental villi. (Hematoxylin and eosin stain; 100 × original magnification.)

but fetal death with profound anemia and hydrops was once common. The use of Rh-immune globulin has almost eliminated this disorder in industrialized countries but other red cell antigens can produce similar disease.[110]

Hematologic disorders

α thalassemia is uniformly fatal when the fetus is homozygous for all four α chains. β thalassemia and sickle cell disease do not adversely affect the fetus since the β chains of hemoglobin are sparse in fetal red blood cells. Thrombotic disorders include factor V Leiden, deficiencies of protein C, protein S, and antithrombin III (see the section on maternal conditions).

Metabolic disorders

The metabolic disorders that cause fetal death are rare. An exception is the fetus of a diabetic mother. This is described in the section on maternal conditions. Metabolic disorders affecting the liveborn neonate are addressed below.

Environmental disorders

Homicide usually involves fetuses as incidental victims. Maternal use of drugs, including those prescribed for medical conditions, can adversely affect fetal development. Fetal deaths are recorded in instances of low maternal folate levels and malformations in mothers who receive antiepileptic medication, especially valproic acid.[111]

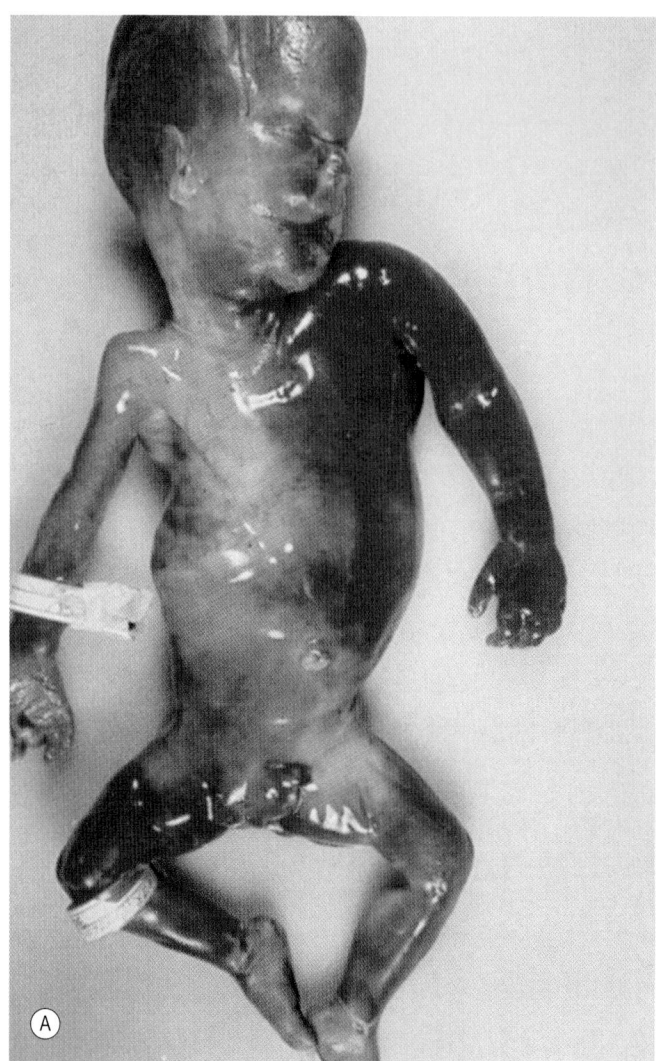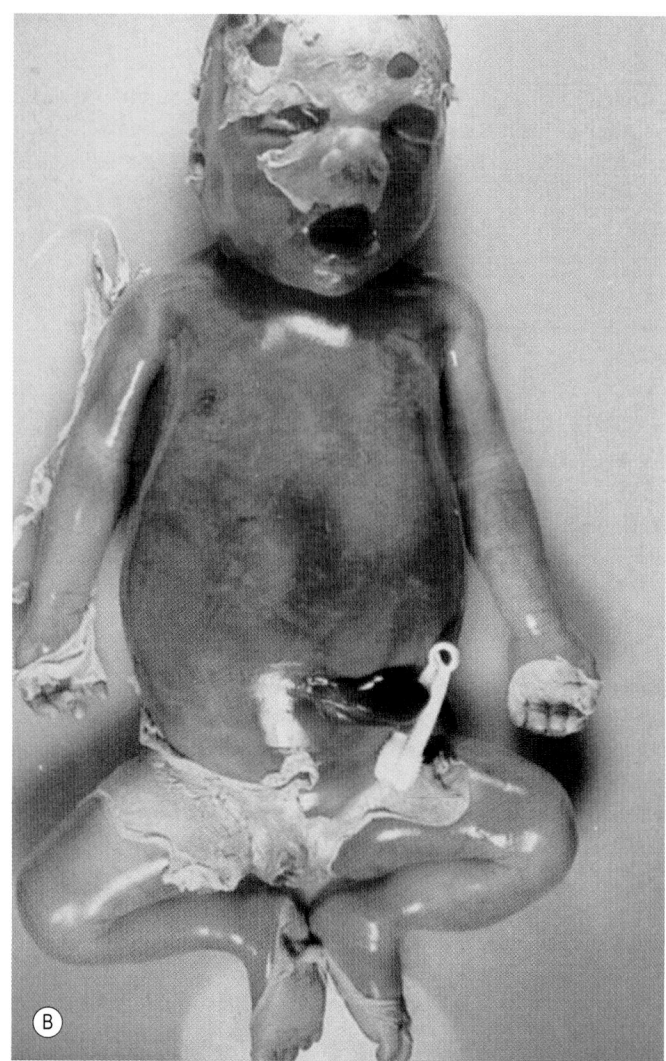

FIGURE 7.17 Maceration. (A) Fetus retained in utero for up to 8 h. The skin is red and early skin slippage is noted on the ankles. (B) Fetus retained in utero for ≥ 2 days. Extensive skin slippage and heme-staining of the skin. The umbilical cord is dark red and the mouth is open due to relaxation of autolyzed muscles.

Effects of intrauterine retention after fetal death

Depending on the duration of intrauterine retention between fetal death and delivery, the degree of maceration may vary from none to slight to severe. The best estimates of duration of postmortem retention in the uterus have been established by Genest et al.[112–114] In 6 or 8 h small areas of desquamation develop and the umbilical cord turns brown–red. Skin begins to desquamate from the face, abdomen, or back in 12 h; desquamation involves 5% or more of the body surface in ≥ 18 h; brown skin discoloration develops in ≥ 24 h; and a moderate or severe extent of desquamation is found in ≥ 24 h. The only late change that correlates with a specific duration of intrauterine retention is mummification (≥2 weeks) wherein most of the interstitial, intravascular, and cavity fluids have

exuded into the amniotic sac. These changes may be helpful to establish the time of death when a complete autopsy and histologic examinations cannot be performed (Fig. 7.17).[115]

The placental changes after fetal death seem to be more constant than those in the fetus and include:

- villous intravascular karyorrhexis (≥ 6 h);
- vascular lumen abnormalities of stem villi, including fibroblast 'septation' and total luminal obliteration (multifocal, ≥ 2 days; extensive, ≥2 weeks); and
- extensive fibrosis of terminal villi (≥ 2 weeks).

In the histologic examination of fetal tissues, the 10 most consistent histologic features and their predicted death-to-delivery intervals are: loss of nuclear basophilia in individual cells in renal cortical tubules (4 h), liver (24 h), inner half of the myocardium (24 h), outer half of the myocardium (48 h), bronchial epithelium (96 h), and tracheal cartilage (1 week); and loss of nuclear basophilia of all cells in the liver (96 h),

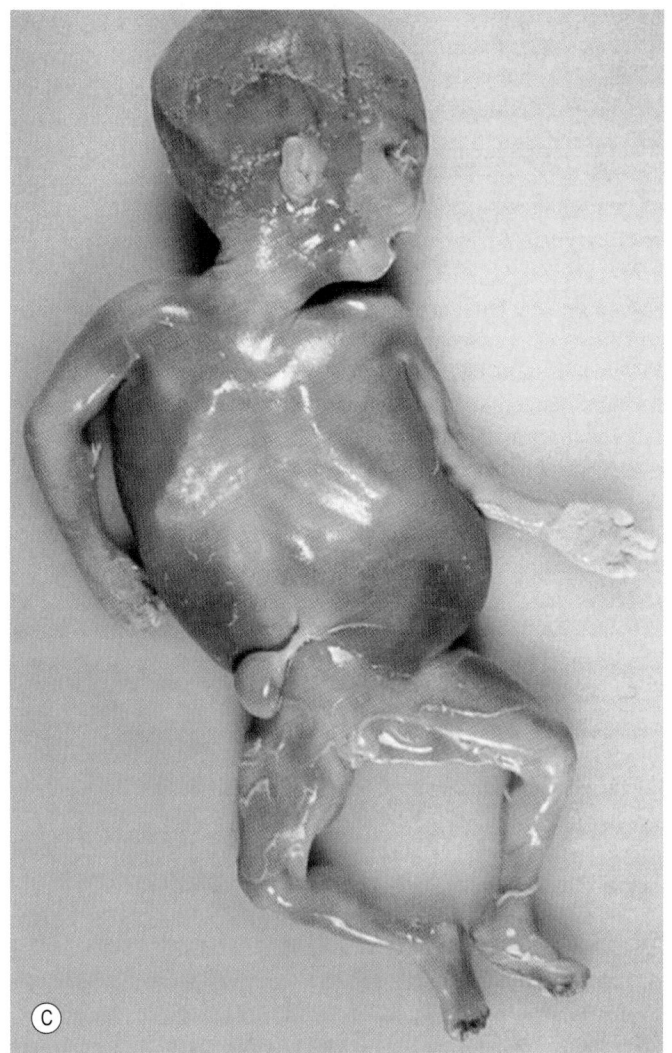

TABLE 7.7 INFANT MORTALITY RATE PER 1000 LIVE BIRTHS IN SELECTED DEVELOPED COUNTRIES

Country	Infant mortality rate (Year of data)
USA	6.9 (2000)
Cuba	6.2 (2000)
Israel	5.8 (1999)
	5.6 (2000)
Canada	5.3 (1999)
Australia	4.9 (2000)
Germany	4.4 (2000)
Italy	4.4 (2000)
France	4.4 (2000)
Sweden	3.2 (2000)
Singapore	2.9 (2000)

From Arias et al 2003,[5] with permission.

FIGURE 7.17 (cont'd) (C) Fetus retained for ≥ 1 week. The skin is olive-brown. (From Potter and Gilbert-Barness 1997,[115] with permission.)

Neonatal deaths

Infant mortality is one of the most widely used general indices of health in the world. The USA has a higher IMR than most developed countries (Table 7.7). This is in part due to ethnic diversity in the USA, but the IMR is also related to the policies of health care which adversely affect those in lower socio-economic circumstances.

Low birth weight, prematurity and complications

Neonatal morbidity and mortality are profoundly affected by LBW and premature birth. The mortality rate is increased more than 10-fold when the birth weight is less than 2500 g, 50-fold for infants of very low birth weight (1500 g or less), and almost 200-fold for infants with birth weights of 500 g or less[5] (Table 7.8). More recent studies show little if any improvement in these data.[117]

Most infants with LBW are premature. Prematurity constitutes 12% of all live births in the USA.[5] Very low birth weight infants weighing 1500 g or less account for about 1–2% of all live births. Moderate to severe functional handicap is noted in 66–80% of survivors at age 4 years if born at 24 weeks or less.[118]

The major risk factors for prematurity are PROM before labor begins, chorioamnionitis, low uteroplacental blood flow, and multiple gestation.[14] The overall outcome depends on the gestational age. Fetal movements that strike the placental membranes and coitus appear to predispose to PROM. Markers for vigorous motor activity by the fetus, a long umbilical cord, and diffuse subchorionic fibrin correlate with PROM.[119] Complications of PROM are prolapse of the umbilical cord, abruptio placentae, and oligohydramnios.[120] The incidence of hypoplastic lungs is more than 80% in neonates when oligo-

gastrointestinal tract (1 week), adrenal (1 week), and kidney (4 weeks). Maternal fever or a delay of more than 24 h in refrigerating the body or fetal hydrops may accelerate these changes. Conversely, extreme prematurity (< 25 weeks gestation) may decelerate some of the expected autolytic findings.[112–114]

Despite several days of postmortem retention in the uterus, the autolyzed bone marrow may retain good hematoxyphilia. The brain, even if semiliquid, will also have reasonable histologic features and should always be processed by putting such soft specimens in a cassette lined with lens paper.

Fresh stillbirths are the result of intrapartum death. The external features often include meconium staining of skin, fingernails, and the fetal surface of the placenta as well as petechial hemorrhages.[116] Internal gross features are mainly congestion and petechial hemorrhages of internal organs (heart, parietal pleura, thymus, and liver). Non-specific histologic findings include acute congestion, hemorrhages, and aspiration of amniotic fluid.

TABLE 7.8 NEONATAL MORTALITY RATES AT VARIOUS BIRTH WEIGHTS

Birth weight (g)	Neonatal mortality rate deaths per 1000 live births
All weights	4.5
< 2500	47.6
< 1500	213.8
< 500	838.3
500–749	411.1
750–999	115.9
1000–1249	50.0
1250–1499	34.0
1500–1999	17.4
2000–2499	6.0
2500–2999	1.7
3000–3499	0.8
4000–4499	0.5
≥ 4500	1.4

From Arias et al 2003,[5] with permission.

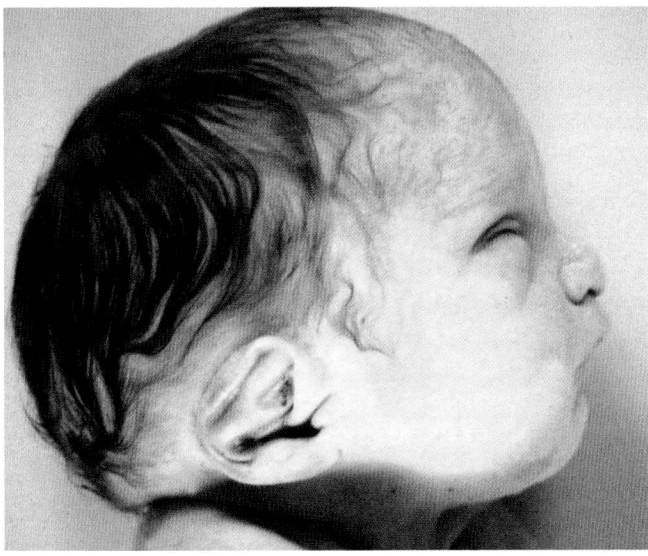

FIGURE 7.18 'Potter's facies' with low-set, posteriorly rotated ears, a beaked nose, and a small, receding chin. The pregnancy was complicated by severe oligohydramnios.

hydramnios develops and is persistent in the first trimester of pregnancy, 10% when oligohydramnios starts at 25 weeks, but nearly zero if it occurs after 28 weeks of gestation.[121, 122] The oligohydramnios tetrad includes Potter facies, IUGR, limb positioning defects, and pulmonary hypoplasia (Fig. 7.18).

Congenital malformations and genetic abnormalities

Once independent of the mother and placenta, severely malformed infants are at risk of early death, especially if they have cardiopulmonary lesions. Malformations of the central nervous system, heart, lungs, diaphragm, abdominal wall, and kidneys cause most of the neonatal deaths in any series. Chromosomal and genetic abnormalities associated with neonatal death are listed in Table 7.9.[123]

Neonatal infections

Most neonatal infections are similar to those described in the sections on maternal, fetal, and placental conditions. The liveborn infant has additional risk factors, namely hospital acquired infections or those acquired in the home. Late onset GBS appears after 96 h with signs of meningitis. The mortality rate is much lower than with early onset GBS. Coagulase negative and coagulase positive staphylococci figure prominently in postnatal infections. *Haemophilus influenzae* and *S. viridans* are other important pathogens as are *E. coli*, and *Enterococcus faecium*. *E. faecium* has the added hazard of resistance to vancomycin.[124] *Pseudomonas aeruginosa* can infect the respiratory tract in infants who receive respirator therapy. Indwelling catheters are another source of infection, often with out-of-the-ordinary organisms. Neonatal bacterial infections manifest as pneumonia, septicemia, meningitis, cerebritis, septic arthritis, and visceral or cutaneous abscesses.[23]

Neonatal respiratory distress syndrome

The neonatal respiratory distress syndrome (RDS) affects premature infants and near-term infants born to diabetic mothers. In past decades, this condition was responsible for about 20% of neonatal deaths. The basis of the disease is failure to maintain expansion of the lung because of inadequate surface active lipids. The treatment of RDS has improved with mechanical ventilation, monitoring of blood gases, and insufflation of the lungs with exogenous surfactant. Refinements include reducing carbon dioxide in the trachea and large bronchi by insufflating this dead space with continuous fresh air or oxygen. Complications with tracheal gas insufflation include pneumothorax, overinflated lungs, poor humidity control, and mechanical irritation with increased mucus production.[125] Insufflated surfactant reduces the incidence of chronic lung disease and allows for quicker extubation.[126] Careful monitoring is necessary since transient but significant surges in cerebral blood flow have been documented along with elevated pCO_2 levels in the minutes and hours following a bolus of intratracheal surfactant.[127] A multicenter study has also shown that babies with birth weights > 1249 g do as well without surfactant therapy as those with it.[128] Corticosteroids can be administered to mothers at risk for premature delivery (vaginal bleeding, excessive intermittent uterine contractions, etc.). This treatment accelerates maturation of surfactant-producing pneumocytes. Betamethasone is preferred since dexamethasone has been associated with an increased incidence of cerebral intraventricular hemorrhage in the offspring.[129] Bronchopulmonary dysplasia or chronic lung

TABLE 7.9 MALFORMATION SYNDROMES ASSOCIATED WITH NEONATAL DEATH EXCLUDING CHROMOSOME AND METABOLIC DISORDERS

McKusick no.		Lethality	Genetics
MULTIPLE SYSTEM ANOMALIES			
100300	Adams-Oliver syndrome	Occasionally	AD
217100	Amnion rupture sequence	Sporadic	
118450	Alagille syndrome	Rarely	AD
130650	Beckwith-Wiedemann syndrome (EMG -exomphalos-macroglossia-gigantism)	Occasionally	Mostly sporadic, rarely AD. Chromosome 11p15.5
211180	Bowen-Conradi syndrome	Often	AR
122470	Cornelia de Lange syndrome	Often	Mostly sporadic, rarely AD. Chromosome 5p13.1
113650	Branchio-otorenal (BOR) dysplasia	Occasionally	AD
188400	DiGeorge syndrome	Rarely	Sporadic or AD with variable expressivity and reduced penetrance; del 22q11.2
213300	Joubert syndrome type 1	Occasionally	AR
256710	Elejalde syndrome	Always	AR
134780	Femoral-facial syndrome	Rarely	AD and sporadic forms; 35% in infants of diabetic mothers
193700	Freeman-Sheldon syndrome	Occasionally	AD
229850	Fryns syndrome	Usually	AR
312870	Golabi-Behmel syndrome	Occasionally	XR
164210	Goldenhar syndrome	Rarely	Mostly sporadic, AD with variable expressivity
142900	Holt-Oram syndrome	Rarely	AD
236680	Hydrolethalus	Always	AR
208530	Asplenia with cardiovascular anomalies syndrome	Often	AR
243800	Johanson-Blizzard syndrome	Occasionally	AR
244400	Kartagener syndrome	Occasionally	AR
236700	McKusick-Kaufman syndrome	Rarely	AR
309800	Lenz microphthalmia	Rarely	XR
151050	Lenz-Majewski syndrome	Often	Sporadic
246200	Leprechaunism (Donahue syndrome)	Usually	AR
169170	Patterson pseudo leprechaunism syndrome	Usually	Uncertain, sporadic
265000	Multiple pterygium syndome, Escobar variant	Occasionally	AR
248700	Marden-Walker syndrome	Rarely	AR
154780	Marshall (Marshall-Smith) syndrome	Rarely	AD
249210	Megacystic microcolon–intestinal hypoperistalsis syndrome	Often	AR
309350	Melnick-Needles syndrome	Rare in females, usually in males	XD
156610	Michelin tire baby syndrome	Rarely	AD
253250	Mulibrey nanism	Frequently	AR
163950	Noonan phenotype	Rarely	AD; sporadic phenotype associated with intra-uterine hydrops
300000	Opitz syndrome	Rarely	XR (and AD phenocopy)
311300	Otopalatodigital (OPD) type I (Taybi)	Rarely	XR
304120	Otopalatodigital (OPD) type II (Fitch)	Occasionally	XR
146510	Pallister-Hall syndrome	Frequent	AD
208150	Pena-Shokeir phenotype (fetal akinesia sequence)	Frequent	AR
263650	Popliteal pterygium (severe lethal) (Bartsocas-Papas type)	Usually	AR
264090	Progeroid syndrome, neonatal form	Usually	AR
268300	Roberts (pseudothalidomide) syndrome	Usually	AR
180849	Rubinstein-Taybi syndrome	Rarely	AD
180860	Silver-Russell syndrome	Occasionally	Usually sporadic; rarely XR
274000	Thrombocytopenia-absent radius (TAR)	Rarely	AR
107480	Townes-Brocks syndrome	Rarely	AD

TABLE 7.9 MALFORMATION SYNDROMES ASSOCIATED WITH NEONATAL DEATH EXCLUDING CHROMOSOME AND METABOLIC DISORDERS (*CONT'D*)

McKusick no.		Lethality	Genetics
ASSOCIATIONS			
214800	CHARGE association (Colobomas-Heart-Atretic choanae- Restricted growth or mental development-Genital –Ear)	Fairly often	AD
601076	MURCS association (müllerian aplasia or hypoplasia – Renal agenesis or ectopy- Cervicothoracic vertebral defects-Short stature)	Rarely	Sporadic
–	Schisis association Midline defects neural tube, oral clefts, omphalocele, diaphragmatic hernia, and congenital heart disease	Occasionally	Sporadic but associated
192350	VATER association (Vertebral anomalies-Anal atresia,-Tracheoesophageal fistula, Radial Renal anomalies), cardiac defects	Occasionally	Sporadic
CRANIOFACIAL DEFECTS			
101200	Apert syndrome (acrocephalosyndactyly)	Occasionally	AD
218600	Baller-Gerold syndrome	Rarely	AR
211750	C-trigonocephaly syndrome	Occasionally	AR
117650	Cerebrocostomandibular syndrome	Fairly often	AR or AD
214150	Cerebrooculofacioskeletal syndrome (COFS)	Usually	AR
304110	Craniofrontonasal syndrome	Rarely	XD
136760	Frontonasal dysplasia	Rarely	Most cases sporadic
154400	Acrofacial dysostosis 1, Nager type	Occasionally	AD
311200	Orofaciodigital (OFD) syndrome type 1	Rarely	XD lethal in males
261800	Pierre Robin syndrome	Occasionally	Sporadic and part of other syndromes
311900	TARP syndrome	Often	X-linked
154500	Treacher Collins–Franceschetti (mandibulofacial dysostosis)	Rarely	AD
CENTRAL NERVOUS SYSTEM DISORDERS			
164180	Delleman syndrome	Often	AD
213300	Joubert syndrome 1	Often	AR
247200	Miller-Dieker lissencephaly syndrome	Occasionally	AD, del (17p13.3)
249000	Meckel syndrome type 1	Always	AR
256520	Neu-Laxova syndrome	Always	AR
209880	Ondine curse (congenital failure of autonomic control)	Frequent	AD vs AR?
305450	Opitz-Kaveggia (FG) syndrome	Occasionally	XR
236670	Walker-Warburg syndrome	Always	AR
307000	X-linked hydrocephalus	Usually	XR
CONNECTIVE TISSUE DISORDERS			
154700	Marfan syndrome (severe)	Rarely	AD
DYSPLASIAS			
257350	Familial nuchal bleb syndrome	Always	AR, often in Turner syndrome
176920	Proteus syndrome	Rarely	AD
191100	Tuberous sclerosis	Rarely	AD, many new mutations
GENITOURINARY DISORDERS			
143400	Bilateral multicystic renal dysplasia syndrome	Always	AD
191830	Hereditary urogenital adysplasia syndrome	Depends on renal malformation	AD
219000	Fraser syndrome	~50%	AR
194080	Denys-Drash syndrome	Rarely	AD; del (11p13)
600057	Exstrophy of bladder syndrome	Often	AD
263200	Autosomal recessive polycystic kidney disease	Always	AR
242700	Nezelof syndrome	Almost always	AR, rarely XR
100100	Prune-belly syndrome	Often	AD?, AR?
258040	OEIS Complex	Often	Mostly sporadic

TABLE 7.9 MALFORMATION SYNDROMES ASSOCIATED WITH NEONATAL DEATH EXCLUDING CHROMOSOME AND METABOLIC DISORDERS (*CONT'D*)

McKusick no.		Lethality	Genetics
SKELETAL DYSPLASIAS			
200600	Achondrogenesis type 1A	Always	AR
200610	Achondrogenesis type II	Always	AD
207410	Antley-Bixler syndrome	Occasionally	AR
208500	Asphyxiating thoracic dystrophy (Jeune)	Often	AR
114290	Campomelic dysplasia	Often	AD
302950	Chondrodysplasia punctata 1 (severe rhizomelic form)	Usually	XR
121050	Congenital contractural arachnodactyly (Beals)	Occasionally	AD
256050	De la Chapelle neonatal osseous dysplasia 1	Always	AR
222600	Diastrophic dwarfism	Rarely	AR
224400	Dyssegmental dysplasia	Often	AR
225500	Ellis-van Creveld syndrome	Rarely	AR
228520	Fibrochondrogenesis	Always	AR
239200	Hyperparathyroidism, neonatal, severe primary	Rarely	AD
146000	Hypochondroplasia	Always	AD
103300	Aglossia-adactylia (Hanhart syndrome)	Occasionally	AD
241500	Hypophosphatasia, infantile	Often	AR
308050	Congenital hemidysplasia with icthyosiform erythroderma and limb defects	Usually	XR
277300	Jarcho-Levin syndrome	Often	AR
245190	Kniest-like dysplasia, lethal	Often	AD
245600	Larsen syndrome (severe)	Rarely	AR
250600	Metatropic dwarfism	Variable	AD and AR non-lethal, and AR lethal forms
160900	Myotonic dystrophy (severe congenital form)	Often	AD, CTG trinucleotide expansion
166210	Osteogenesis imperfecta (OI) congenita type II	Always	AD, most new mutations, occasionally germline mosaicism
259775	Raine syndrome	Always	AR
269250	Schneckenbecken dysplasia	Usually	AR
263530/263510	Short rib polydactyly type 1 (Saldino-Noonan)	Usually	AR
263520	Short rib polydactyly type 2 (Majewski)	Usually	AR
263510	Short rib polydactyly type 3 (Naumoff)	Usually	AR
183900	Spondyloepiphyseal dysplasia congenital (severe lethal forms)	Often	AD
108720	Spondylohumerofemoral dysplasia (atelosteogenesis type 1)	Rarely	Sporadic
187600	Thanatophoric dysplasia (and variants)	Always	AD
SKIN DISORDERS			
219150	Cutis laxa, severe lethal form	Usually	AR
219250	Cutis marmorata (telangiectasia congenital)	Rarely	AR
226700	Epidermolysis bullosa letalis (Herlitz)	Almost always	AR
226730	Epidermolysis bullosa with pyloric atresia	Rarely	AR
305600	Focal dermal hypoplasia (Goltz syndrome)	Rarely lethal in males	XD
242500	Ichthyosis congenita (harlequin baby)	Always	AR
308300	Incontinentia pigmenti	Rarely in females, usually lethal in males	XD
163200	Linear sebaceous nevus (nevus sebaceous of Jadassohn)	Rarely	Sporadic
275210	Restrictive dermopathy	Always	AR
TERATOGENIC DISORDERS			
–	Aminopterin/ methotrexate exposure	Rarely	
–	Fetal alcohol syndrome (FAS)	Rarely	
–	Trimethadione exposure	Rarely	
–	Valproate exposure	Rarely	
	Warfarin embryopathy	Rarely	

AD, Autosomal dominant; AR, autosomal recessive; XR, X-linked recessive; XD, X-linked dominant
Revised from Hall 1992,[123] and Kalousek and Gilbert-Barness 1997,[100] with permission.

disease still develops in some of these babies, especially those with a very low birthweight.[130] In the past corticosteroids have been prescribed for neonates to reduce the incidence of chronic lung disease. This is now considered unwise since long-term effects include short stature, reduced head circumference, poor motor development and coordination, and low IQ scores.[131]

While RDS is a problem with premature infants, idiopathic pulmonary hemorrhage is noted in infants born at term. Most such cases are found in infants beyond the first month of life and some have been attributed to inhaled fungal spores, such as those of *Stachybotrys chartarum*. A more likely cause is a clotting disorder such as von Willebrand factor antigen.[132]

Amniotic fluid and meconium aspiration

Amniotic fluid aspiration before or during birth is most likely to occur in a hypoxic term or near-term infant. Meconium inhibits pulmonary surfactant function and may produce pulmonary hemorrhage. Aspiration of thick meconium has a frequency of 9 per 1000 births; 59% have been attributed to severe acute chorioamnionitis, less frequently to low uteroplacental blood flow and abruptio placentae.[133] Assisted ventilation in these infants may lead to interstitial emphysema or even pneumothorax and pneumomediastinum.

Necrotizing enterocolitis

Necrotizing enterocolitis (NEC) develops in 10% of premature infants whose birth weights are < 1500 g and death results in about 25% of these infants. Full-term infants are rarely affected.[134] Ischemia/hypoxia of the intestinal mucosa is a factor. Early oral feeding may 'overwork' the bowel in susceptible infants.[135] Inflammatory cytokines including platelet activating factor, tumor necrosis factor α, and lipopolysaccharides interact in the development of NEC and reactive oxygen species also play a role in experimental models.[134] Severe thrombocytopenia predicts which infants will require surgery to remove necrotic bowel, which ones will have cholestasis, and which ones will die, but paradoxically, platelet transfusions may aggravate the condition.[136] Hyperglycemia exceeding 12 mM/L is associated with death in almost 30% of patients versus only 2% in infants with normal glucose levels. Late onset of NEC (> 10 days) is another risk factor.[137] Infants with NEC frequently have complicating periventricular leukomalacia and septic shock.[138]

Central nervous system lesions

Cerebral intraventricular hemorrhage (IVH) occurs in stillborn fetal brains and in full-term infants, but is found mostly in premature infants hours or days after birth. Periventricular leukomalacia (PVL) is another serious complication of prematurity. RDS often precedes the development of these lesions, suggesting that hypoxia is involved in the pathogenesis. Bacterial infections also seem to enhance the development of both IVH and PVL.[139, 140] Indomethacin tocolysis for women in premature labor was thought to be a factor but the data have proved unconvincing.[140] Lenticulostriate vasculopathy (LSV) is demonstrated radiographically with mineral-dense streaks along small vessels in the thalamostriate region of the brain. These lesions often accompany IVH and may be related to magnesium sulfate tocolysis.[141] Pathologic studies of LSV are not reported.

Neonatal blood dyscrasias

Neonatal blood dyscrasias include hemolytic diseases of the newborn due to blood group incompatibility, vitamin K deficiency (hemorrhagic disease of the newborn), anemia due to hemorrhage, maternal transfer of antiplatelet antibodies, factor V Leiden, and deficiencies of protein S, protein C, and antithrombin III. Anemia of prematurity and that due to withdrawing blood for laboratory tests are continuing problems. Blood transfusions carry a small risk of transmitting infectious agents or a hemolytic reaction. Widness and colleagues have used exogenous erythropoietin to good effect and have been able to reduce the frequency of transfusions.[142] Their studies indicate that acute hemorrhage or a severe hemolytic episode produce elevations of endogenous erythropoietin within hours, which peak at 3–5 days but the reticulocyte response lags by about 2 days.[142] Fetuses from pregnancies complicated by hypertension are subjected to chronic hypoxia as reflected in elevated erythropoietin concentrations in the amniotic fluid and umbilical cord blood.[13]

Mortality and morbidity in very premature infants

The survival of premature infants whose birth weights are < 1500 g (including infants weighing < 500 g) is now more than 80% but complications are numerous; chronic lung disease in 4%; periventricular leukomalacia in 12%; pneumothorax 15%; intraventricular hemorrhage 15%; retinopathy 2%.[143] Considering those born at or before 24 weeks and weighing 500 g, death occurs in 67% due to intraventricular hemorrhage and respiratory distress. Survivors often have chronic lung disease retinopathy of prematurity, necrotizing enterocolitis, periventricular leukomalacia, and/or intraventricular hemorrhage.[130]

Mortality and morbidity in postmature infants

Postmature infants are those born after 42 weeks' gestation. They have wrinkled, desquamating skin, absence of lanugo, decreased vernix caseosa, decreased subcutaneous fat, long nails, and abundant scalp hair. They appear wizened and aged, like ancient little men or women. The amniotic fluid, nails, and skin are frequently meconium stained. Early death is a special risk when gestation is prolonged beyond 43 weeks, being three times that of control infants.[144]

BOX 7.2 SOME METABOLIC DISORDERS THAT MAY RESULT IN NEONATAL DEATH

Urea cycle defects

    Ornithine transcarbamylase and arginase deficiency

    Citrullinemia and argininosuccinic aciduria

    Tyrosinemia type I

    Hypervalinemia

    Hyper-β-alaninemia

    Phenylketonuria

Disorders of amino acid metabolism

    Maple syrup urine disease, propionic acidemia and methylmalonic academia

    Non-ketotic hyperglycinemia

Disorders of carbohydrate metabolism

    Galactosemia and hereditary fructose intolerance Fructose-1, 6-diphosphatase deficiency

    Glycogen storage disease type I (von Gierke)

    Glycogen storage disease type II (Pompe)

    Glycogen storage disease type III (debrancher enzyme deficiency)

Disorders of pyruvate metabolism

    Pyruvate carboxylase and pyruvate dehydrogenase deficiencies

Mitochondrial disorders

    Medium- and long-chain coenzyme A dehydrogenase deficiencies

    Multiple coenzyme A dehydrogenase deficiency

    Glutaric acidemia type 2

    Respiratory chain defects (complexes I-V)

    Encephalomyopathy with multiorgan defects

    Subacute necrotizing encephalopathy

    Progressive neuronal degeneration of childhood (Alpert syndrome)

    Pure myopathic disease with chronic progressive external ophthalmoplegia (CPEO)

    Multiple carboxylase deficiency

    Short-chain acyl dehydrogenase deficiency

Defects of mitochondrial DNA

    Kearns-Sayre syndrome (KSS)

    Pearson syndrome

    Leber hereditary optic atrophy (LHOA)

    Neuropathy, ataxia, and retinitis pigmentosa (NARP)

    Mitochondrial encephalomyelopathy with lactic acidosis and strokelike episodes (MELAS)

    Myoclonus epilepsy and ragged red fibers (MERRF)

Lipid storage diseases

    GM$_1$, gangliosidosis type 1

    GM$_2$, gangliosidosis type 2

    Niemann-Pick disease type A

    Gaucher disease

    Infantile type Wolman disease (acid lipase deficiency)

    Krabbe disease (globoid leukodystrophy)

    Metachromatic leukodystrophy

Mucopolysaccharide and mucolipid storage diseases

    Mucopolysaccharidosis VII

    Mucolipidosis (I-cell disease)

Sialic acid storage diseases

    Severe infantile form type 2

Farber disease (lipogranulomatosis)

Peroxisome defects

    Zellweger syndrome

    Neonatal adrenoleukodystrophy

    Pipecolic acidemia

    Rhizomelic chondrodysplasia punctata

Defects in cholesterol metabolism

    Smith-Lemli-Opitz syndrome

    Mevalonic academia

α_1 antitrypsin deficiency (neonatal cirrhosis)

Congenital adrenal hyperplasia

Cystic fibrosis (meconium ileus)

Carnitine deficiency primary

Defects of metal metabolism

    Menkes kinky hair syndrome

    Neonatal iron storage disease (neonatal cirrhosis)

Maternal metabolic disorders

    Phenylketonuria

    Diabetes mellitus

    Thyrotoxicosis

After Behrman and Vaughan 1992,[150] and Kalousek and Gilbert-Barness 1997,[100] with permission.

Trauma and fetal/neonatal death

Connolly et al evaluated 476 cases of significant trauma during pregnancy which resulted in 27 perinatal deaths (5.6%). They found that 54.6% of such cases are the result of motor-vehicle accidents. Domestic violence accounted for 22.3% and tended to occur early in gestation, < 18 weeks. Falls occurred in 21.8% and were concentrated in mid gestation, 20–30 weeks. The remaining 1.3% of trauma cases was due to burns, puncture wounds, bites, etc. While concern for the fetal outcome is concentrated on placental injuries with abruption, this occurred in only 1.6% of pregnancies in which the placental condition was recorded.[145] Birth trauma, including skull fractures; extracranial, extradural, and intraparenchymal hemorrhages; and occipital diastasis may result in neonatal death. Face and breech presentations generate a high risk of trauma to the infant.

Sudden infant death

Sudden infant death in neonates includes accidental suffocation in soft mattresses, soft bedding, and pillows; hyperthermia; and rebreathing with carbon dioxide narcosis in infants sleeping in the prone position.[146] A number of infections may result in sudden death: myocarditis, pneumonia, and meningitis, especially those caused by adenovirus.[147] Cardiac defects may result in sudden death in the neonate, in particular hypoplastic left heart syndrome, anomalous origin of the left coronary from the pulmonary artery, hypoplastic right heart complex, and cardiac conduction defects. SIDS is rarely a cause of death in neonates, and other causes should be excluded before attributing sudden death in the neonatal period to SIDS.[148]

Metabolic disorders

A number of inherited disorders have been related to unexpected death in newborns.[149] In these disorders, there is usually a normal period immediately after birth followed by hypoglycemia, respiratory difficulty, vomiting, and acidosis. Those disorders that may be associated with neonatal death are summarized in Box 7.2.[150]

Pathologist's role in determining cause of fetal and neonatal death

Complete and detailed postmortem fetal and placental examinations and clinicopathologic correlation are necessary to understand the causes of stillbirth and neonatal death. Maceration, while it presents a special challenge, does not preclude a thorough autopsy with meaningful diagnoses. Bacteriologic and viral studies, radiographs and photographs are important adjuncts. Chromosome analyses have uncovered chromosomal abnormalities in 5–10% of all stillborn fetuses and

more if fetuses have anomalies. Placental tissues remain viable after fetal death and should be sampled for karyotype in all cases of unexplained stillbirth. Cultured cells may be banked frozen and archived tissue in paraffin blocks or formalin can be analyzed for specific DNA or probed by fluorescence in situ hybridization.

Counseling parents

The emotional well-being of the mother and father when losing a 'silent child' or a newborn infant should concern pathologists. Meetings with parents to review the findings at autopsy are now commonplace.[151] Such meetings are usually arranged by a social worker or a nurse, sometimes by the attending physician, and sometimes by the pathologist. Any or all of these health care professionals attend. A relative or friend may accompany the mother and/or the father. When the mother is a minor, a grandparent of the fetus or baby usually attends. On rare occasions, the parents are accompanied by their lawyer in which case the hospital's risk manager is notified. The meeting may then have to be postponed until the hospital's legal counsel is available. After introductions, the pathologist starts with an expression of sympathy and a statement such as 'let us review the pertinent clinical and autopsy findings'. Parents are allowed to ask as many questions as they wish. Pertinent negative findings should be emphasized as well as the positive findings. Either may allay a parent's suspicions or feelings of guilt. At the conclusion of the meeting, the parents are asked if they have any more questions and are given the pathologist's office telephone number should a question arise later. These meetings usually last 15–30 min. Parents are given a copy of the final autopsy report.

References

Definitions of fetal and neonatal death

1. Chiswick ML. Commentary on current World Health Organization definitions used in perinatal statistics. Br J Obstet Gynaecol 1986; 93:1236–1238.
2. WHO/FRH/MSM/96.7. Perinatal mortality. A listing of available information. Maternal Health and Safe Motherhood Program. Geneva: World Health Organization; 1996.
3. Dayal AK, Manning, FA, Berck DJ, et al. Fetal death after normal biophysical profile score: An eighteen-year experience. Am J Obstet Gynecol 1999; 181:1231–1236.
4. Singer DB, Macpherson T. Fetal death and the macerated stillborn fetus. In: Wigglesworth JS, Singer DB, eds. Textbook of fetal and perinatal pathology. Malden: Blackwell Science; 1998:246.
5. Arias E, MacDorman MF, Strobino DM, et al. Annual summary of vital statistics – 2002. Pediatrics 2003; 112:1215–1230.

Vital statistics: fetal and neonatal death

6. Bell R, Glinianaia SV, Rankin J, et al. Changing patterns of perinatal death 1982–2000: a retrospective cohort study. Arch Dis Child Fetal Neonatal Ed 2004; 89:F531–F536.

Underlying causes of fetal and neonatal death

7. Bendon RW. Review of some causes of stillbirth. Pediatr Dev Pathol 2001; 4:517–531.
8. Driscoll SG. Autopsy following stillbirth: a challenge neglected. In: Ryder OA, Byrd ML, eds. One medicine . Berlin: Springer-Verlag; 1984:19–31.
9. Yudkin PL, Wood L, Redman CWG. Risk of unexplained stillbirth at different gestational ages. Lancet 1987; 1:1192–1194.
10. Shankar M, Navti O, Amu O, et al. Assessment of stillbirth risk and associated risk factors in a tertiary hospital. J Obstet Gynaecol 2002; 22(1):34–38.
11. Fretts RC, Usher RH. Causes of fetal death in women of advanced maternal age. Obstet Gynecol 1997; 89:40–45.
12. Huang DY, Usher RH, Kramer MS, et al. Determinants of unexplained antepartum fetal deaths. Obstet Gynecol 2000; 95(2):215–221.
13. Teramo KA, Schwartz R, Clemons GK, et al. Amniotic fluid erythropoietin concentrations differentiate between acute and chronic causes of fetal death. Acta Obstet Gynecol Scand 2002; 81(3):245–251.
14. Frøen JF, Arnestad M, Vege A, et al. Comparative epidemiology of sudden infant death syndrome and sudden intrauterine unexplained death. Arch Dis Child Fetal Neonatal Ed 2002; 87:F118–F122.
15. Garite TJ, Clark R, Thorp JA. Intrauterine growth restriction increases morbidity and mortality among premature neonates. Am J Obstet Gynecol 2004; 191(2):481–487.
16. Resnik R. Intrauterine growth restriction. Obstet Gynecol 2002; 99:490–496.

Maternal factors in fetal and neonatal death

17. National vital statistics reports 2004; 52(22):12.
18. Ozalp S, Mete TH, Sener T, et al. Health risks for early (≤ 19) and late (≥ 35) childbearing. Arch Gynecol Obstet 2003; 268:172–174.
19. Petersson K, Bremme K, Bottinga R, et al. Diagnostic evaluation of intrauterine fetal deaths in Stockholm, 1998–99. Acta Obstet Gynecol Scand 2002; 82(4):284–292.
20. Astolfi P, DePasquale A, Zonta LA. Late paternity and stillbirth risk. Hum Reprod 2004; 19(11):2497–2501.
21. Allen VM, Joseph KS, Murphy KE, et al. The effect of hypertensive disorders in pregnancy on small for gestational age and stillbirth: a population based study. BMC Pregnancy Childbirth. 2004; 4:17. Online 6 August 2004.
22. Goldenberg RL, Hauth JC, Andrews WW. Intrauterine infection and preterm delivery. N Engl J Med 2000; 342:1500–1507.
23. Singer DB. Infections of fetuses and neonates. In: Wigglesworth JS, Singer DB, eds. Textbook of fetal and perinatal pathology. Malden: Blackwell Science; 1998:454–511.
24. Baker CJ. Inadequacy of rapid immunoassays for intrapartum detection of group B streptococcal carriers. Obstet Gynecol 1996; 88(1): 51–55.
25. Davies HD, Miller MA, Faro S, et al. Multicenter study of a rapid molecular-based assay for the diagnosis of group B Streptococcus colonization in pregnant women. Clin Infect Dis 2004; 39(8):1129–1135.
26. Arisoy AS, Altinisik B, Tunger O, et al. Maternal carriage and antimicrobial resistance profile of group B streptococcus. Infection 2003; 31(4):244–246.
27. Das A, Ray P, Sharma M, et al. Rapid diagnosis of vaginal carriage of group B β haemolytic streptococcus by an enrichment cum antigen detection test [abstract]. Indian J Med Res 2003; 117:247–252.
28. Gilbert GL, Hewitt MC, Turner CM, et al. Epidemiology and predictive values of risk factors for neonatal group B streptococcal sepsis [abstract]. Aust N Z J Obstet Gynaecol 2002; 42(5):497–503.
29. American Academy of Pediatrics Committee on Infectious Diseases and Committee on Fetus and Newborn: Revised guidelines for prevention of early-onset group B streptococcal (GBS) infection. Pediatrics 1997; 99:489–496.
30. American Academy of Obstetrics and Gynecology: Group B streptococcal infections in pregnancy. ACOG Tech Bull 170:1992.
31. Platt JS, O'Brien WF. Group B streptococcus: prevention of early-onset neonatal sepsis. Obstet Gynecol Surv 2003; 58(3):191–196.
32. Gilbert GL, Hewitt MC, Turner CM, et al. Compliance with protocols for prevention of neonatal group B streptococcus sepsis: practicalities and limitations. Infect Dis Obstet Gynecol 2003; 11(1):1–9.
33. Baltimore RS, Huie SM, Meek JI. Early-onset neonatal sepsis in the era of group B streptococcal prevention. Pediatrics 2001; 108:1094–1098.
34. Singer DB , Campognone P. Perinatal group B streptococcus infection in mid gestation. Pediatr Pathol 1986; 5:271–276.
35. Baker CJ, Rench MA, McInnes P. Immunization of pregnant women with group B streptococcal type III capsular polysaccharide-tetanus toxoid conjugate vaccine. Vaccine 2003; 21(24)3468–3472.
36. Gust DA, Levine WC, St Louis ME, et al. Mortality associated with congenital syphilis in the United States, 1992–1998. Pediatrics 2002; 109(5):E79–9.
37. Pillay T, Khan M, Moodley J, et al. Perinatal tuberculosis and HIV-1: considerations for resource-limited settings. Lancet Infect Dis 2004; 4(3):155–165.
38. Fairley CK, Smoleniec JS, Caul OE, et al. Observational study of effect of intrauterine transfusions on outcome of fetal hydrops after parvovirus B19 infection. Lancet 1995; 346(8986):1335–1337.
39. Harger JH, Adler SP, Koch WC, et al. Prospective evaluation of 618 pregnant women exposed to parvovirus B19:risks and symptoms. Obstet Gynecol 1998; 91:413–420.
40. Nunoue T, Kusuhara K, Hara T. Human fetal infection with parvovirus B19: maternal infection time in gestation, viral persistence and fetal prognosis. Pediatr Infect Dis J 2002; 21(12):1133–1136.
41. Reef SE, Frey TK, Theall K, et al. The changing epidemiology of rubella in the 1990s: on the verge of elimination and new challenges for control and prevention. JAMA 2002; 287(4): 464–472.
42. Wen LZ, Xing W, Liu LQ, et al. Cytomegalovirus infection in pregnancy. Int J Gynaecol Obstet 2002; 79(2):111–116.
43. Hartert TV, Neuzil KM, Shintani AK, et al. Maternal morbidity and perinatal outcomes among pregnant women with respiratory hospitalization during influenza season. Am J Obstet Gynecol 2003; 189(6):1705–1712.
44. Rogers BB, Mark Y, Oyer CE. Diagnosis and incidence of fetal parvovirus infection in an autopsy series: I. Histology. Pediatr Pathol 1993; 13:371–379.
45. Joshi VV, Oleske JM, Connor EM . Morphologic findings in children with acquired immune deficiency syndrome: pathogenesis and clinical implications. Pediatr Pathol 1990; 10(1–2):155–165.
46. Connor EM, Sperling RS, Gelber R, et al. Reduction of maternal-infant transmission of human immunodeficiency virus type 1 with zidovudine treatment. N Engl J Med 1994; 331:1173–1180.
47. Tuomala RE, Shapiro DE, Mofenson LM, et al. Antiretroviral therapy during pregnancy and the risk of an adverse outcome. N Engl J Med 2002; 346(24):1863–1870.
48. Benirschke K, Raphael SI. Candida albicans infection of the amniotic sac. Am J Obstet Gynecol 1958; 75:200–202.
49. van Geertruyden J-P, Thomas F, Erhart A, et al. The contribution of malaria in pregnancy to prenatal mortality. Am J Trop Med Hyg 2004; 71:35–40.
50. Greco P, Vimercati A, Angelici MC, et al. Toxoplasmosis in pregnancy is still an open subject. J Perinat Med 2003; 31(1):36–40.
51. Hermann E, Truyens C, Alonso-Vega C, et al. Congenital transmission of Trypanosoma cruzi is associated with maternal enhanced parasitemia and decreased production of interferon-γ in response to parasite antigens. J Infect Dis 2004; 189(7):1274–1281.
52. Torrico F, Alonso-Vega C, Suarez E, et al. Maternal Trypanosoma cruzi infection, pregnancy outcome, morbidity, and mortality of congenitally infected and non-infected newborns in Bolivia. Am J Trop Med Hyg 2004; 70(2): 201–209.
53. Ugwumadu AH. Bacterial vaginosis in pregnancy. Curr Opin Obstet Gynecol 2002; 14(2):115–118.
54. McGrady GA, Daling JR, Peterson DR. Maternal urinary tract infection and adverse outcomes. Am J Epidemiol 1985; 121:377–381.
55. Ueberrueck T, Koch A, Meyer L, et al. Ninety-four appendectomies for suspected acute appendicitis during pregnancy. World J Surg 2004; 28(5):508–511.

56. Petrova A, Demissie K, Rhoads GG, et al. Association of maternal fever during labor with neonatal and infant morbidity and mortality. Obstet Gynecol 2001; 98:20–27.

57. Kujovich JL. Thrombophilia and pregnancy complications. Am J Obstet Gynecol 2004; 191:412–424.

58. Nurk E, Tell GS, Refsum H, et al. Associations between maternal methylenetetrahydrofolate reductase polymorphisms and adverse outcomes of pregnancy: the Hordaland Homocysteine Study. Am J Med 2004; 117(1):26–31.

59. Sebire NJ, Backos M, El Gaddal S, et al. Placental pathology, antiphospholipid antibodies, and pregnancy outcome in recurrent miscarriage patients. Obstet Gynecol 2003; 101(2):258–263.

60. Brenner B. Thrombophilia and fetal loss. Semin Thromb Hemost 2003; 29(2):165–170.

61. Triplett DA, Brandt JT, Musgrave KA, et al. The relationship between lupus anticoagulants and antibodies to phospholipids, JAMA 1988; 259:550–554.

62. Rappaport VJ, Velazquez M, Williams K. Hemoglobinopathies in pregnancy. Obstet Gynecol Clin North Am 2004; 31:287–317.

63. Cohen AR, Galanello R, Pennell DJ, et al. Thalassemia Hematology. Am Soc Hematol Educ Program 2004; 14–34.

64. Oyer CE, Singer DB. The hematopoietic system. In: Wigglesworth JS, Singer DB, eds. Textbook of fetal and perinatal pathology. Malden: Blackwell Science; 1998:1149–1153.

65. Sheiner E, Levy A, Yerushalmi R, et al. β-thalassemia minor during pregnancy. Obstet Gynecol 2004; 103:1273–1277.

66. Cao A, Rosatelli MC, Monni G, et al. Screening for thalassemia: a model of success. Obstet Gynecol Clin North Am 2002; 29:305–328, vi–vii.

67. Serjeant GR, Loy LL, Crowther M, et al. Outcome of pregnancy in homozygous sickle cell disease. Obstet Gynecol 2004; 103(6):1278–1285.

68. Garcia-Patterson A, Erdozain L, Ginovart G, et al. In human gestational diabetes mellitus congenital malformations are related to prepregnancy body mass index and to severity of diabetes. Diabetologia 2004; 47(3):509–514.

69. Kabiru W, Raynor BD. Obstetric outcomes associated with increase in BMI category during pregnancy. Am J Obstet Gynecol 2004; 191(3):928–932.

70. Neave C. Congenital malformation in offspring of diabetics. Perspect Pediatr Pathol 1984; 8:213–222.

71. Versiani BR, Gilbert-Barness E, Giuliani LR, et al. Caudal dysplasia sequence: severe phenotype presenting in offspring of patients with gestational and pregestational diabetes. Clin Dysmorphol 2004; 13(1):1–5.

72. Wren C, Birrell G, Hawthorne G. Cardiovascular malformations in infants of diabetic mothers. Heart 2003; 89(10):1217–1220.

73. Gutgesell HP, Speer ME, Rosenberg HS. Characterization of cardiomyopathy in infants of diabetic mothers. Circulation 1980; 61:441–450.

74. Nold JL, Georgieff MK. Infants of diabetic mothers. Pediatr Clin North Am 2004; 51(3):619–637.

75. Lappas M, Permezel M, Rice GE. Release of proinflammatory cytokines and 8-isoprostane from placenta, adipose tissue, and skeletal muscle from normal pregnant women and women with gestational diabetes mellitus. J Clin Endocrinol Metab 2004; 89(11):5627–5633.

76. Hockett PK, Emery SC, Hansen L, et al. Evidence of oxidative stress in the brains of fetuses with CNS anomalies and islet cell hyperplasia. Pediatr Dev Pathol 2004; 7(4):370–379.

77. Salim R, Hasanein J, Nachum Z, et al. Anthropometric parameters in infants of gestational diabetic women with strict glycemic control. Obstet Gynecol. 2004; 104(5):1021–1024.

78. Leipold H, Kautzky-Willer A, Ozbal A, et al. Fetal hyperinsulinism and maternal one-hour postload plasma glucose level. Obstet Gynecol 2004; 104(6):1301–1306.

79. Kjos SL, Berkowitz KM, Kung B. Prospective delivery of reliably dated term infants of diabetic mothers without determination of fetal lung maturity: comparison to historical control. J Matern Fetal Neonatal Med 2002; 12(6):433–437.

80. Sarkar S, Hagstrom NJ, Ingardia CJ, et al. Prothrombotic risk factors in infants of diabetic mothers. J Perinatol 2004; 25:134–138.

81. Walker MC, Murphy KE, Pan S, et al. Adverse maternal outcomes in multifetal pregnancies. Brit J Obstet Gynaecol 2004; 111(11):1294–1296.

82. Horon H, Cheng D. Enhanced surveillance for pregnancy-associated mortality- Maryland, 1993-1998. JAMA 2001; 285:1455–1459.

83. Lacey M. For Africa's poor, pregnancy is often life threatening. New York Times International Section 12 December 2004:14.

Fetal and placental conditions associated with stillbirth

84. De Paepe ME, Friedman RM, Gundogan F, et al. The histologic fetoplacental inflammatory response in fatal perinatal group B-streptococcus infection. J Perinatol 2004; 24:441–445.

85. Nadra L, Ariel I, Singer DB. Infections, preterm delivery, and perinatal death in midgestation. R I Med J 1991; 74(1):25–29.

86. Ananth CV, Berkowitz GS, Savitz DA, et al. Placental abruption and adverse perinatal outcomes. JAMA 1999; 282(17):1646–1451.

87. Machin GA, Ackerman J, Gilbert-Barness E. Abnormal umbilical cord coiling is associated with adverse perinatal outcomes. Pediatr Dev Pathol 2000; 3(5):462–471.

88. Bowman JM, Lewis M, deSa DJ. Hydrops fetalis caused by massive maternofetal transplacental hemorrhage. J Pediatr 1984; 104:769–772.

89. Chen JC, Davis BH, Wood B, et al. Multicenter clinical experience with flow cytometric method for fetomaternal hemorrhage detection. Cytometry 2002; 50:285–290.

90. Owen J, Stedman CM, Tucker TL. Comparison of predelivery versus postdelivery Kleihauer-Betke stains in cases of fetal death. Am J Obstet Gynecol 1989; 161:663–666.

91. Lackman, F, Capewell, V, Richardson, B, et al. The risks of spontaneous preterm delivery and perinatal mortality in relation to size at birth according to fetal versus neonatal growth standards. Am J Obstet Gynecol 2001; 184: 946–953.

92. Salafia CM. Placental pathology of growth restriction. Clin Obstet Gynecol 1997; 40(4):740–749.

93. Ohyama M, Itani Y, Yamanaka M, et al. Maternal, neonatal, and placental features associated with diffuse chorioamniotic hemosiderosis, with special reference to neonatal morbidity and mortality. Pediatrics 2004; 113:800–805.

94. De Paepe ME, Friedman RM, Poch M, et al. Placental findings after laser ablation of communicating vessels in twin-to-twin transfusion syndrome. Pediatr Dev Pathol 2004; 7:159–165.

95. Redline RW, Ariel I, Baergen RN, et al and the Society for Pediatric Pathology, Perinatal Section, Fetal Vascular Obstruction Nosology Committee. Fetal vascular obstructive lesions: nosology and reproducibility of placental reaction patterns. Pediatr Dev Pathol 2004; 7:443–452.

96. Kraus FT, Acheen VI. Fetal thrombotic vasculopathy in the placenta:cerebral thrombi and infarcts, coagulopathies and cerebral palsy. Hum Pathol 1999; 30:759–769.

97. Nelson K, Holmes LB. Malformation due to presumed spontaneous mutations in newborn infants, N Engl J Med 1989; 320:19–23.

98. Simpson JW, Geppert LJ. The responsibility of the obstetrician to the fetus. 1: an analysis of fetal and neonatal mortality in 10,000 deliveries. Am J Obstet Gynecol 1951; 62:1062–1070.

99. Jacobs PA, Hassold TJ. Chromosome abnormalities: origin and etiology in abortions and livebirths. In: Vogel F, eds. Human genetics. New York: Springer-Verlag; 1987:233.

100. Kalousek DK, Gilbert-Barness E. Causes of stillbirth and neonatal death. In: Potter EL, Gilbert-Barness E, eds. Potter's pathology of the fetus and infant. 1st edn. St Louis: Mosby;1997.

101. McFadden DE, Kalousek DK. Fetal triploid phenotypes: correlation with parental origin of the tetraploid set. Am J Med Genet 1991; 38: 535–538.

102. McKusick VA. Mendelian inheritance in man. 11th edn. Baltimore; The Johns Hopkins University Press; 1994.

103. Kalousek DK. Confined placental mosaicism. Pediatr Pathol 1990; 10:69–77.

104. Kalousek DK, Barrett IJ. Confined placental mosaicism and stillbirth. Pediatr Pathol 1994; 14:151–159.

105. Stetten G, Escallon CS, South ST, et al. Reevaluating confined placental mosaicism. Am J Med Genet 2004; 131(A):232–239.

106. Cattanach BM, Kirk M. Differential activity of maternally and paternally derived chromosome regions in mice. Nature 1985; 315:496–498.

107. Gilbert-Barness EF, Opitz JM. Chromosome abnormalities In: Wigglesworth JS, Singer DB, eds. Textbook of fetal and perinatal pathology. Malden: Blackwell Science; 1998:332–333.

108. Gibson BR, Muir-Padilla J, Champeaux A, et al. Mesenchymal dysplasia of the placenta. Placenta 2004; 25:671–672.

109. Ohto H, Miura S, Ariga H, et al. Collaborative study group. The natural history of maternal immunization against foetal platelet alloantigens. Transfus Med 2004; 14:399–408.

110. Harkness UF, Spinnato JA. Prevention and management of RhD isoimmunization. Clin Perinatol 2004; 31:721–742.

111. Kaaja E, Kaaja R, Hiilesmaa V. Major malformations in offspring of women with epilepsy. Neurology 2003; 60:575–579.

Effects of intrauterine retention after fetal death

112. Genest DR, Williams MA, Green MF. Estimating the time of death in stillborn fetuses: I. Histologic evaluation of fetal organs; an autopsy study of 150 stillborns. Obstet Gynecol 1992; 80(4):575–584.

113. Genest DR. Estimating the time of death in stillborn fetuses: II. Histologic evaluation of the placenta; a study of 71 stillborns. Obstet Gynecol 1992; 80(4):585–592.

114. Genest DR, Singer DB. Estimating the time of death in stillborn fetuses: III. External fetal examination; a study of 86 stillborns. Obstet Gynecol 1992; 80(4):593–600.

115. Potter EL, Gilbert-Barness E, eds. Potter's pathology of the fetus and infant. 1st edn. St Louis: Mosby; 1997.

116. Wigglesworth JS: Pathology of intrapartum and early neonatal death in the normally formed infant. In: Wigglesworth JS, Singer DB, eds. Textbook of fetal and perinatal pathology. Malden: Blackwell Science; 1998:75–86.

Neonatal deaths

117. Serenius F, Ewald U, Farooqi A, et al. Short-term outcome after active perinatal management at 23–25 weeks of gestation. A study from two Swedish perinatal centres. Part 3: neonatal morbidity. Acta Paediatr 2004; 93:1090–1097.

118. Johnson A, Townsend PA, Yudkin P, et al. Functional abilities at 4 years of children born before 24 weeks of gestation. BMJ 1993; 306:1715–1718.

119. Naeye RL. Disorders of the placenta, fetus, and neonate: diagnosis and clinical significance. St Louis: Mosby-Year Book; 1992.

120. Nelson DM, Stempel LE, Zuspan FP. Association of prolonged, preterm premature rupture of the membranes and abruptio placentae. J Reprod Med 1986; 31:249–253.

121. Liggins D, Thurlbeck WM. Conditions altering normal lung growth and development. In: Thibeault DW, Gregory GA, eds. Neonatal pulmonary care. 2nd edn. Norwalk: Appleton-Century-Crofts; 1986:3–9.

122. Rotschild A, Ling EW, Puterman ML, et al. Neonatal outcome after prolonged preterm rupture of the membranes. Am J Obstet Gynecol 1990; 162:46–52.

123. Hall JG. Developmental defects in stillborn and newborn infants. In: Dimmick JE, Kalousek DK, eds. Developmental pathology of the embryo and fetus. Philadelphia; JB Lippincott; 1992.

124. Treitman AN, Yarnold PR, Warren J, et al. Emerging incidence of Enterococcus faecium among hospital isolates (1993–2002). J Clin Microbiol 2005; 43:462–463.

125. Miller TL, Blackson TJ, Shaffer TH, et al. Tracheal gas insufflation-augmented continuous positive airway pressure in a spontaneously breathing model of neonatal respiratory distress. Pediatr Pulmonol 2004; 38:386–395.

126. Hammond M, Al-Kazmi N, Alshemmiri M, et al. Randomized clinical trial comparing two natural surfactant preparations to treat respiratory distress syndrome. J Matern Fetal Neonatal Med 2004; 15:167–175.

127. Kaiser JR, Gauss CH, Willims DK. Surfactant administration acutely affects cerebral and systemic hemodynamics and gas exchange in very-low-birth-weight infants. J Pediatr 2004; 144:809–814.

128. Escobedo MB, Gunkel JH, Kennedy KA, et al. Texas Neonatal Research Group. Early surfactant for neonates with mild to moderate respiratory distress syndrome: a multicenter, randomized trial. J Pediatr 2004; 144:804–808.

129. Spinillo A, Chiara A, Bergante C, et al. Obstetric risk factors and persistent increases in brain parenchymal echogenicity in preterm infants. Brit J Obstet Gynaecol 2004; 111:913–918.

130. McElrath TF, Robinson JN, Ecker JL, et al. Neonatal outcome of infants born at 23 weeks' gestation. Obstet Gynecol 2001; 97:49–52.

131. Yeh TF, Lin YJ, Lin HC, et al. Outcome of school age after postnatal dexamethasone therapy for lung disease of prematurity. N Engl J Med 2004; 350:1304–1313.

132. Center for Disease Control: Morbidity Mortality Weekly Report 10 September 2004; 53:817–820.

133. Naeye RL. Functionally important disorders of the placenta, umbilical cord and fetal membranes, Hum Pathol 1987; 7:680–691.

134. Hsueh W, Caplan MS, Qu XW, et al. Neonatal necrotizing enterocolitis: clinical considerations and pathogenetic concepts. Pediatr Dev Pathol. 2003; 6:6–23.

135. Ostlie DJ, Spilde TL, St Peter SD, et al. Necrotizing enterocolitis in full-term infants. J Pediatr Surg 2003; 38:1039–1042.

136. Kenton AB, Hegemier S, Smith EO, et al. Platelet transfusions in infants with necrotizing enterocolitis do not lower mortality but may increase morbidity. J Perinatol 2005; 3:173–177.

137. Hall NJ, Peters M, Eaton S, et al. Hyperglycemia is associated with increased morbidity and mortality rates in neonates with necrotizing enterocolitis. J Pediat Surg 2004; 39:898–901.

138. Goepfert AR, Andrews WW, Carlo W, et al. Umbilical cord plasma interleukin-6 concentrations in preterm infants and risk of neonatal morbidity. Am J Obstet Gynecol 2004; 191:1375–1381.

139. Graham EM, Holcroft CJ, Rai KK, et al. Neonatal cerebral white matter injury in preterm infants is associated with culture positive infections and only rarely with metabolic acidosis. Am J Obstet Gynecol 2004; 191:1305–1310.

140. Suarez RD, Grobman WA, Parilla BV. Indomethacin tocolysis and intraventricular hemorrhage. Obstet Gynecol 2001; 97:921–925.

141. Mittendorf R, Kuban K, Pryde PG, et al. Antenatal risk factors associated with the development of lenticulostriate vasculopathy (LSV) in neonates. J Perinatol 2004; 25:101–107.

142. Widness JA, Seward VJ, Kromer IJ, et al. Changing patterns of red blood cell transfusion in very low birth weight infants. J Pediatr 1996; 129(5):680–687.

143. Ozkan H, Duman N, Kumral A, et al. Synchronized ventilation of very-low-birth-weight infants; report of 16 years' experience. J Matern Fetal Neonatal Med 2004; 15:261–265.

144. Overall JC Jr. The fetus and the neonatal infant. In: Behrman RE, Vaughan VC, eds. Nelson textbook of pediatrics. 14th edn. Philadelphia: WB Saunders; 1992:358–435.

145. Connolly AM, Katz VL, Bash KL, et al. Trauma and pregnancy. Am J Perinatol 1997; 14:331–336.

146. Gilbert-Barness E, Barness L. Sudden infant death syndrome: is it a cause of death? [editorial]. Arch Pathol Lab Med 1993; 117:1246–1248.

147. Oyer CE, Ongcapin EH, Ni J, et al. Fatal intrauterine adenoviral endomyocarditis with aortic and pulmonary valve stenosis. Diagnosis by polymerase chain reaction. Hum Pathol 2000; 31:1433–1435.

148. Krous HF, Beckwith JB, Byard RW, et al. Sudden infant death syndrome and unclassified sudden infant death: a definitional and diagnostic approach. Pediatrics 2004; 114:234–236.

149. Clarke LA, Dimmick JE, Applegarth DA. Pathology of inherited metabolic diseases. In: Dimmick JE, Kalousek DK, eds. Developmental pathology of the embryo and fetus. Philadelphia: JB Lippincott; 1992:199.

150. Behrman RE, Vaughan VC III, eds. Nelson textbook of pediatrics. 14th edn. Philadelphia: WB Saunders; 1992.

Counseling parents

151. Valdes-Dapena M. The postautopsy conference with families. Arch Pathol Lab Med 1984; 108(6):497–498.

Hydrops, cystic hygroma, hydrothorax, pericardial effusions, and fetal ascites

8

Geoffrey A. Machin

But a water-baby is contrary to nature.   Charles Kingsley The Water-Babies, 1863

Hydrops fetalis

'General dropsy of the foetus was the disease which in 1887 first attracted my attention to the study of antenatal pathology; and since that year I have had the extraordinary opportunity of examining eleven specimens of the malady. . . . The result of these opportunities and of all this writing is, that I now feel far less certain about the pathogenesis of the disease than I did shortly after I examined my first specimen! Of this, however, I have become increasingly persuaded: general dropsy of the foetus is not a pathological entity, but a group of structural alterations due to several different causes, and really representing several different diseases in the ordinary sense of the word. . . . It is the "hydropsie généralisée du foetus" of the French, and the "Haut-und allgemeine Wassersucht" of the German writers.' [1, p. 288]

Hydrops fetalis (HF) is the end stage of many fetal diseases that cause **fetal anemia, hypoproteinemia, and cardiac failure**; in fully developed HF, there is subcutaneous edema with fluid accumulations in peritoneal, pleural, and pericardial cavities (Fig. 8.1). The umbilical cord and placenta are also edematous with marked placental thickening and there is polyhydramnios. Various degrees of 'incipient' HF are also recognized, in which fluid accumulations are not present in all compartments. This can make diagnosis difficult since effusions caused by local events in these cavities may also lead to HF. There is also considerable overlap between HF, nuchal cystic hygroma, and accumulations of lymph fluid in body cavities resulting from malformation and/or obstruction of the major lymphatic vessels. When the causation for hydrops is not obvious, lymphatic obstruction should be considered, and can be confirmed histologically. Such obstruction may be limited to the thorax, without cystic hygroma, but with localized 'atlas-like' lymphedema of the subcutaneous tissues of the torso.

The investigation of HF and related conditions is a diagnostic challenge to clinician and pathologist alike. Many cases are diagnosed prenatally by ultrasound, and urgent prenatal investigation of exact causes is carried out to ascertain potentially treatable cases; therapeutic options consist of fetal transfusions in cases of anemia, medical (and rarely surgical) treatment in cases of arrhythmias and drainage of pulmonary cysts and pleural effusions. Many cases are now treated empirically, and there are reported survivals even with diseases hitherto considered lethal. Until recently the most common cause of HF in the Western world was blood group isoimmunization, usually involving the Rhesus blood group antigens. The success of isoimmunization prevention programs has been such that most cases of HF are now **non-immune.**[2] In recent times **congenital syphilis** has re-emerged as a potent cause of HF.[3] In Southeast Asia the most common cause of HF remains **homozygous α-thalassemia.** Worldwide, this disease is probably the most common cause of HF today, and its diagnosis should always be suspected when parents are of Southeast Asian origin.

HF is caused by three main mechanisms: anemia, hypoproteinemia, and cardiac failure (Fig. 8.2); most cases fit within this classification, although some cases remain unsolved under the name *idiopathic HF*. In some complex cases there may be more than one candidate as the cause of HF. There is frequently underlying genetic disease such as **chromosomal abnormalities, single gene defects** (including genetic metabolic diseases), and other syndromes. Mendelian Inheritance in Man currently lists 90 genetic disorders that may cause hydrops. Protocols have been developed for prenatal diagnosis, and these can be applied equally well at the perinatal autopsy. Of the 10 major categories

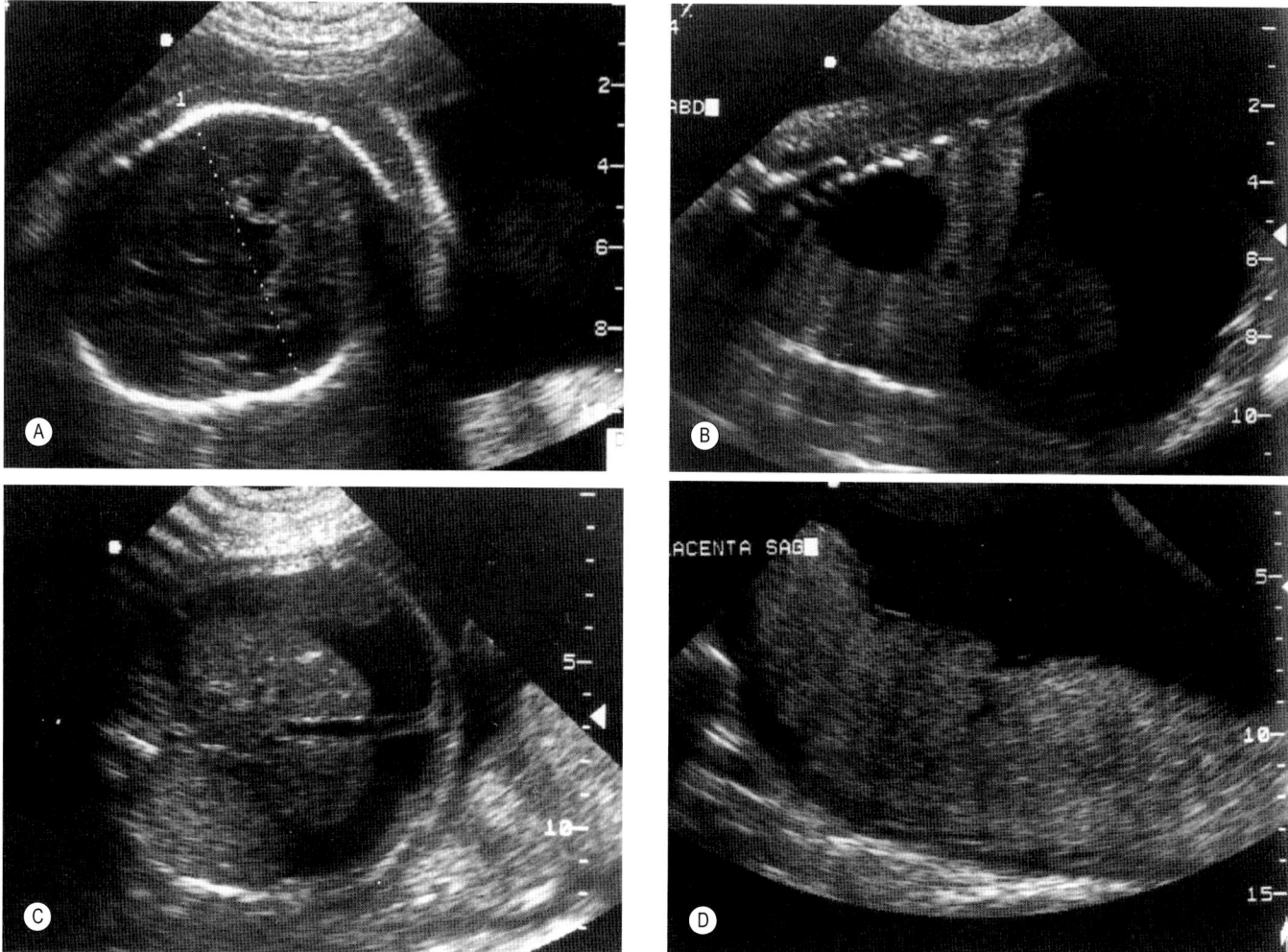

FIGURE 8.1 Fetal ultrasound appearances of hydrops fetalis. (A) Scalp edema. (B) Pericardial effusion in hydropic fetus. (C) Ascites in hydrops. The umbilical vein is dilated as it crosses the peritoneal cavity into the liver. (D) Placentomegaly in hydrops.

of fetal disease amenable to in utero surgery, the following six cause HF:[4]

- congenital cystic adenomatoid malformation of lung;
- hydrothorax/chylothorax;
- laryngeal atresia/stenosis;
- congenital heart block (which is nevertheless more frequently treated medically);
- sacrococcygeal teratoma; and
- twin-to-twin transfusion.

Unfortunately the causal diagnosis is often difficult to determine at autopsy if there has been prolonged fetal death, but attempts should still be made to diagnose malformations, other genetic diseases, and infections. Thorough investigation of HF is necessary for genetic counseling.

Causes

The principal causes and associations of HF are shown in Table 8.1.[5–15] The map in Figure 8.2 is only approximate since actual clinical situations are sometimes complex. For example, as shown in Figure 8.2, one lesion, **generalized lymphatic vascular dysplasia,** can cause HF in at least three ways:

- by sequestration of plasma proteins in subcutaneous lymphedema and lymph effusions in body cavities (and hence hypoproteinemia);
- by direct compression of the developing heart by hydrothorax/chylothorax; and
- by reduced systemic venous return to the heart caused by hydrothorax/chylothorax.

Likewise, **metabolic storage diseases** can cause hypoproteinemia through liver cell dysfunction as well as by impinging on hepatic sinusoids, causing ascites and plasma protein sequestration; in turn, high-pressure ascites could impede placental and systemic venous return to the thorax; hepatomegaly itself might also impede venous return. **Large neoplasms** can cause high-output cardiac failure, obstructed venous return, and acute anemia secondary to microangiopathy or hemorrhage into the tumor. **Parvovirus infection** can involve red cell precursors and cardiac myocytes. **Chromosomal aneuploidy** can cause

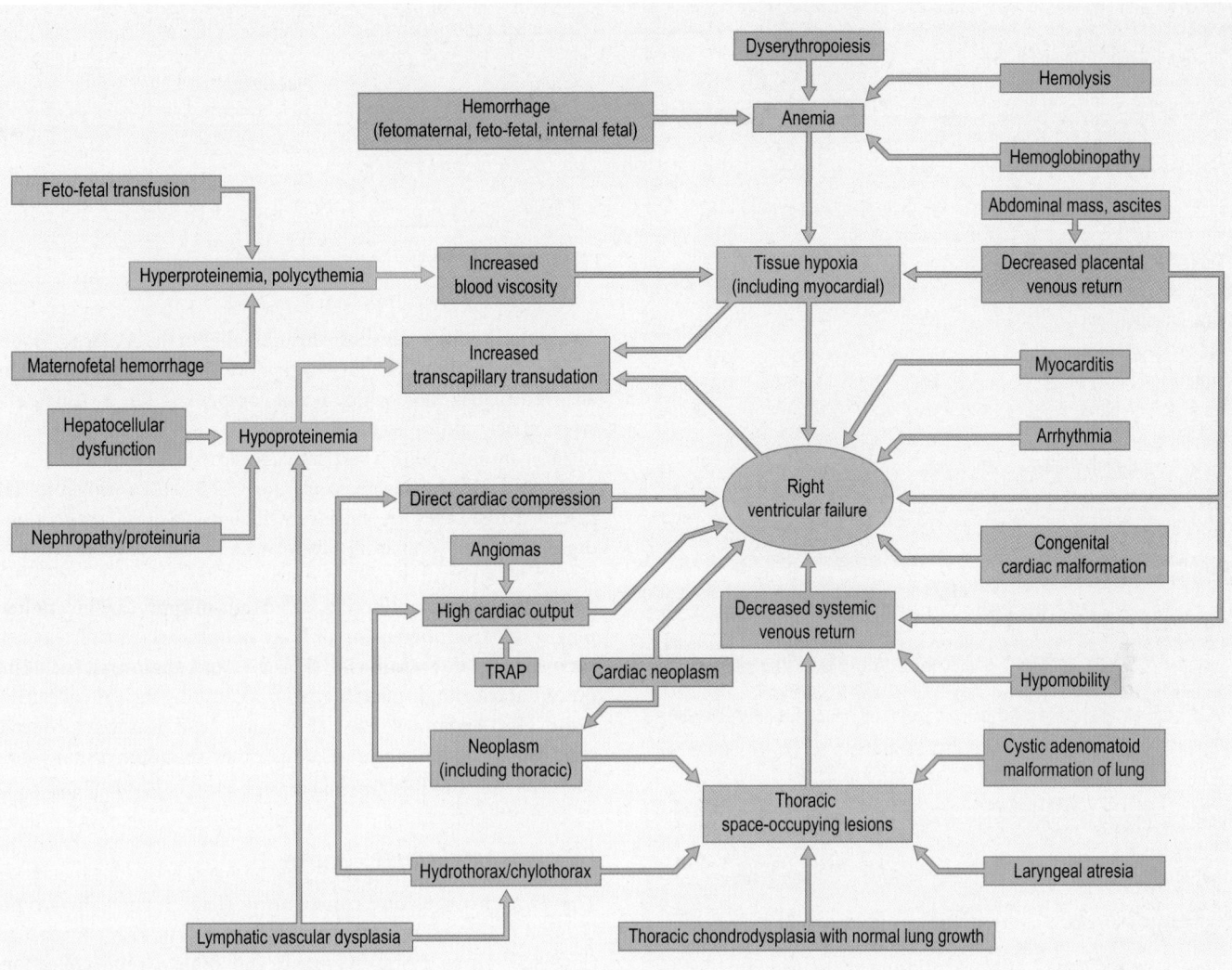

FIGURE 8.2 Mechanisms of hydrops fetalis. A flowchart of important and likely factors causing hydrops. TRAP, twin reversed arterial perfusion.

congenital heart disease, cystic hygroma, and transient abnormal myelopoiesis. There are several single-gene disorders that have similar pleiotropic effects, any one of which may cause hydrops. Hence, it is not uncommon to find in a given case more than one potential cause of HF, such as the presence of chondrodysplasia and cystic hygroma, or fetal hypomobility and congenital cardiac anomaly.

HF is a pathophysiologic process; thus, while convincing structural anomalies may be present, these are often combined with functional abnormalities (e.g. structural congenital heart disease with cardiac arrhythmia). Occasionally, structural congenital heart disease may be found of types that do not usually cause HF; caution should be used before ascribing hydrops to such anomalies, when some other functional cause, such as fetomaternal hemorrhage, might be the real cause of HF.

The first six causes of HF listed in Table 8.1 account for about two-thirds of cases. In 20% no specific causes are found, or miscellaneous rare causes and associations are ascertained. Thus **the most frequent routes leading to HF are cardiovascular, chromosomal, thoracic, anemic, cystic hygroma, and com-plications of monochorionic twinning**. Recognition of these main causes is straightforward, using a simple protocol of investigations of the living fetus or at fetal autopsy. In vivo, obstetric ultrasound, fetal echocardiography, fetal blood sampl-ing, fetal effusion study, or early amniocentesis, together with maternal blood sampling will together yield structural and/or functional lesions in most cases. Some pointers may allow distinc-tion at prenatal diagnosis between anemic and non-anemic causes of HF.[9] **Anemia more commonly causes placentomegaly, while non-anemic cases are often characterized by pleural effusions and more marked subcutaneous edema.** At autopsy only the strictly structural causes will be confirmed or ascertained.

The importance of identifying causes of HF lies at least as much in prognosis for subsequent pregnancies as it does with providing explanations for the current adverse outcome.

Cardiac causes (Table 8.2)

Cardiac malformations are found in about 40% of cases of cardiogenic hydrops and include atrioventricular canal, left and

TABLE 8.1 MAJOR CAUSES AND ASSOCIATIONS OF HYDROPS FETALIS IN 1644 REPORTED CASES

Cause	No.	Percentage
Cardiovascular	362	22
Chromosomal	208	13
Thoracic	160	10
Anemia	132	8
Cystic hygroma	116	7
Monochorionic twinning	97	6
Fetal infection	88	5
Ascites/peritonitis	40	2
Urinary tract malformation	41	2
Fetal hypomobility	18	1
Hepatic pathology	11	0.6
Genetic metabolic disease	7	0.4
Nephrosis	1	0.0
Miscellaneous	34	2
Not determined	329	20
TOTAL	1472	100

After Machin, 1989[5] with permission. Based on this review and 11 subsequently reported series.[6-14] In some series, cardiovascular causes account for 8% of fetal hydrops (3/4 supraventricular tachyarrhythmia, 1/4 complete heart block), and immune causes account for 13% of cases.[14] Aneuploidy accounts for nearly half of cases of fetal hydrops diagnosed prior to 24 weeks.[15] Fetal outcome depends on the primary pathology, but is favorable in 15/55 (27%) of non-immune hydrops.[14]

TABLE 8.2 CARDIAC PATHOLOGY IN HYDROPS FETALIS

Pathology	Percentage
Malformation, 40% of which are due to	
Left ventricular hypoplasia	25
Atrioventricular canal	20
Right ventricular hypoplasia	11
Other	44
Tachyarrhythmia, 25% of which are due to	
Atrial flutter	20
Paroxysmal atrial tachycardia	17
Wolff-Parkinson-White syndrome	15
Other	48
High-output cardiac failure, 15% of which are due to	
Sacrococcygeal teratoma	50
Large fetal angioma	40
Other	10
Bradyarrhythmia, 7% of which are due to	
Complete heart block	54
Maternal connective tissue disease	8
Other	38
Other, 13%	

right ventricular hypoplasia, and primary closure of the foramen ovale. It is generally accepted that in most cases, it is not the structural malformation (e.g. atrial septal defect, ventricular septal defect, tetralogy of Fallot, right or left ventricular hypoplasia, etc.) which causes the hydrops, but rather the associated

TABLE 8.3 CHROMOSOMAL ABNORMALITIES IN HYDROPS FETALIS

Abnormality	Percentage
45,X	42
Trisomy 21	34
Trisomy 18	9
Triploidy	5
Other	10

dysrhythmia which results from anomalies in the AV or SA nodes of the conduction system. Exceptions include stenosis of an atrioventricular valve which is not compensated by a sufficiently large atrial and/or ventricular shunt (e.g. in some cases of Ebstein anomaly with a restrictive foramen ovale).

Tachyarrhythmias account for 75% of cardiogenic HF cases.[14] Most cases are supraventricular and are managed with digoxin and/or verapamil. Bradycardia (7–25% of cases) may be caused by structural cardiac disease or transplacental maternal connective tissue antibodies.[14, 16] **High-output cardiac failure may result from perfusion of large neoplasms** (most frequently **sacrococcygeal teratomas**)[17] (Fig. 8.3) **and angiomas**, including **placental chorangiomas** (Fig. 8.4), accounting for 15% of cardiogenic HF. Angiomas may also cause fetal **Kasabach-Merritt syndrome**.[18] Rarer causes include cardiac **rhabdomyomas** (often indicative of fetal tuberous sclerosis)[19] and **cardiomyopathies**.

Chromosomal causes (Table 8.3)

The *45,X* **chromosome constitution** (fetal Turner phenotype) is lethal in the second trimester in about 90% of 45,X conceptuses (Fig. 8.5). Large cystic hygromas and other lymph collections accumulate, and global cardiac hypoplasia is reported.[20] HF occurs from any or all of these causes. **Trisomies 21 and 18** commonly result in hydrops, some cases having cystic hygromas. **Triploid fetuses** may be hydropic, but trisomy 13 is rare as a cause of HF.

Thoracic causes (Table 8.4)

Thoracic space-occupying lesions may cause raised intrathoracic pressure of such degree as to obstruct systemic venous return ('fetal Valsalva maneuver'). **Congenital cystic adenomatoid malformation of lung** (*CCAM*, also called congenital pulmonary airway malformation, or *CPAM*) (Fig. 8.6) is the most frequent lesion (30% of thoracic HF).[21] A **right-sided diaphragmatic hernia** may impinge on inferior vena caval flow as well as allowing space-occupying organs into the chest. **Pleural effusions** may be primary, usually as part of lymphatic vessel dysplasia. In the **short-rib chondrodysplasias** normal lung growth and pulmonary fluid production within the confines of the dysplastic thoracic skeleton may obstruct systemic venous return causing HF (Fig. 8.7). **Intrathoracic neoplasms** can also cause HF (Fig. 8.8).

Intrathoracic pressure may be so high that effusions do not accumulate in pericardial or pleural cavities. CCAM of the lung

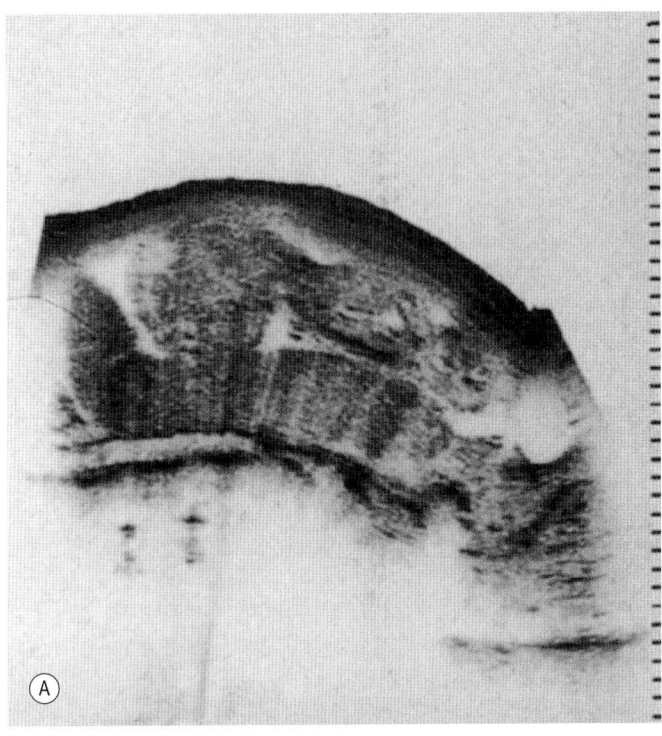

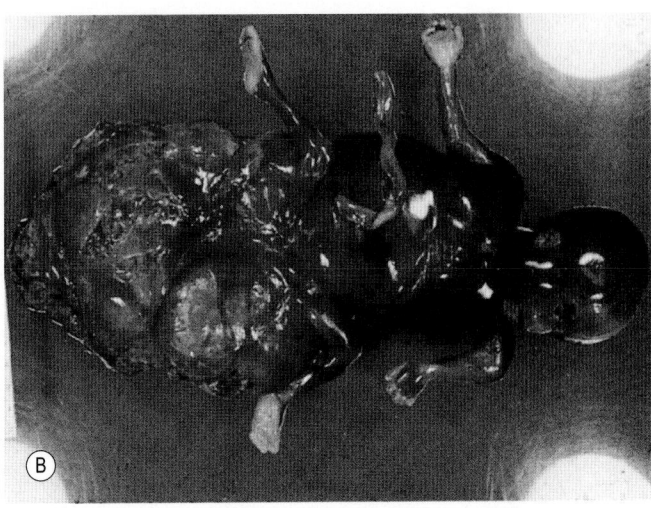

FIGURE 8.3　Sacrococcygeal teratoma. (A) Fetal ultrasound shows sacrococcygeal mass. (B) Termination of pregnancy for maternal hyperplacentosis, with very large sacrococcygeal teratoma and hydropic fetus.

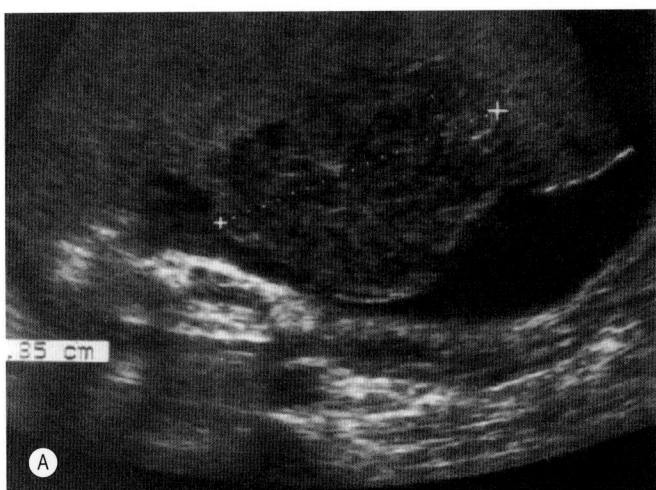

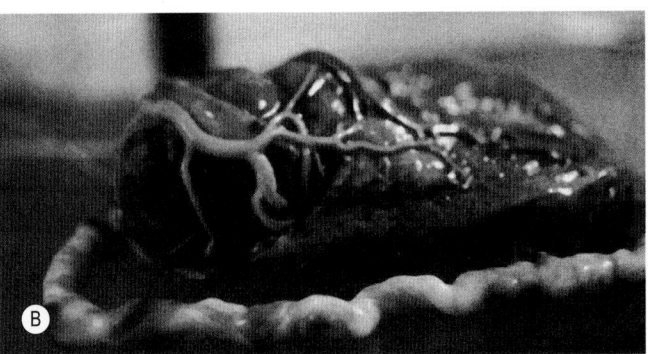

FIGURE 8.4　Placental chorangioma. (A) Placental ultrasound showing multiloculated parenchymal mass. (B) Gross appearance of placenta, with injection of feeder vessels. (C) Gross cut section of chorangioma, corresponding with (A).

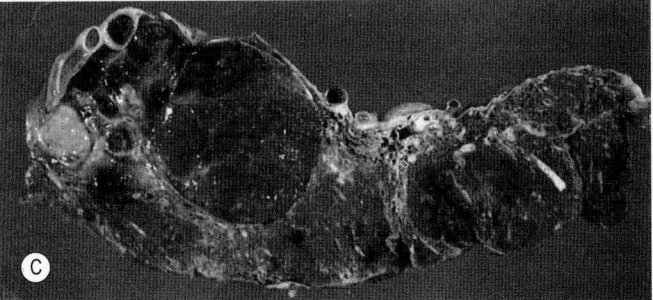

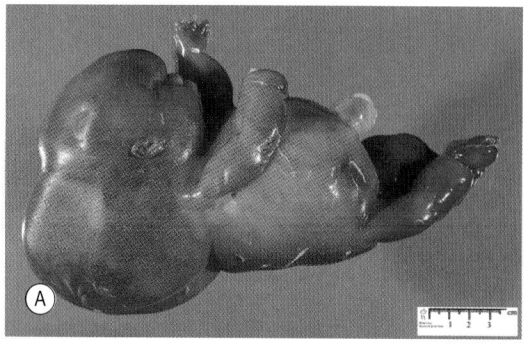

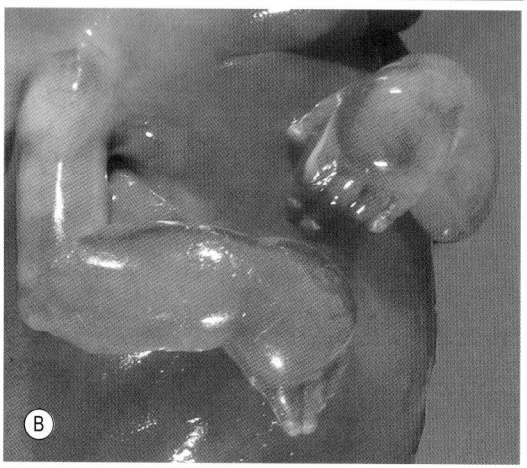

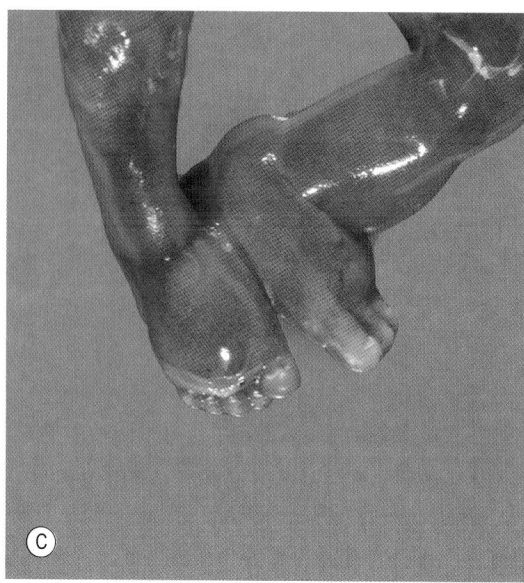

FIGURE 8.5 Hydrops in Turner syndrome. (A) There is generalized subcutaneous edema in addition to the obvious cystic hygromas. (B) and (C) Edema is most marked on dorsum of hands and feet.

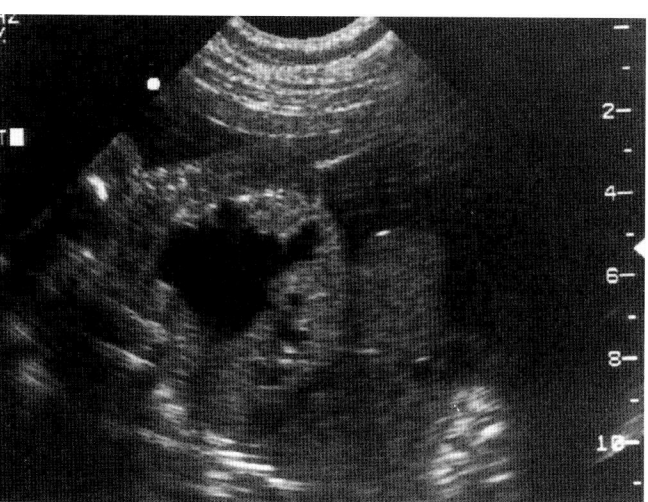

FIGURE 8.6 Ultrasound appearance of congenital cystic adenomatoid malformation of lung, causing hydrops.

TABLE 8.4 THORACIC PATHOLOGY IN HYDROPS FETALIS

Abnormality	Percentage
Congenital cystic adenomatoid malformation of lung	30
Chondrodysplasia	25
Right-sided diaphragmatic hernia	15
Other intrathoracic mass	9
Pulmonary sequestration	8
Other	13

TABLE 8.5 MONOCHORIONIC TWINNING AND HYDROPS FETALIS

Mechanism	Percentage
Donor, TTT	9
Recipient, TTT	9
TTT, not specified	77
Pump twin, TRAP	5

TTT, Twin-to-twin transfusion; TRAP, twin reversed arterial perfusion.

may thus present clinically as fetal ascites with or without generalized hydrops.

Monochorionic twinning (Table 8.5)

In prenatal **twin-to-twin transfusion** (*TTT*), either donor or recipient may develop HF (Fig. 8.9). Although both anemia and polycythemia can cause HF in singleton fetuses, other more subtle and sudden hemodynamic changes may precipitate HF in the context of anastomotic vessels in monochorionic placentas. Transient hydrops may occur in the donor twin after **laser therapy** for TTT and it may also be seen transiently in the survivor following **fetal demise** of one twin.

In **twin reversed arterial perfusion** (*TRAP*), the normal (or 'pump') twin perfuses the whole placenta and the acardiac co-twin in addition to the normal cardiac output. One of the main indications for active management of twin transfusion and TRAP is the onset of cardiac failure in a viable and structurally normal twin.

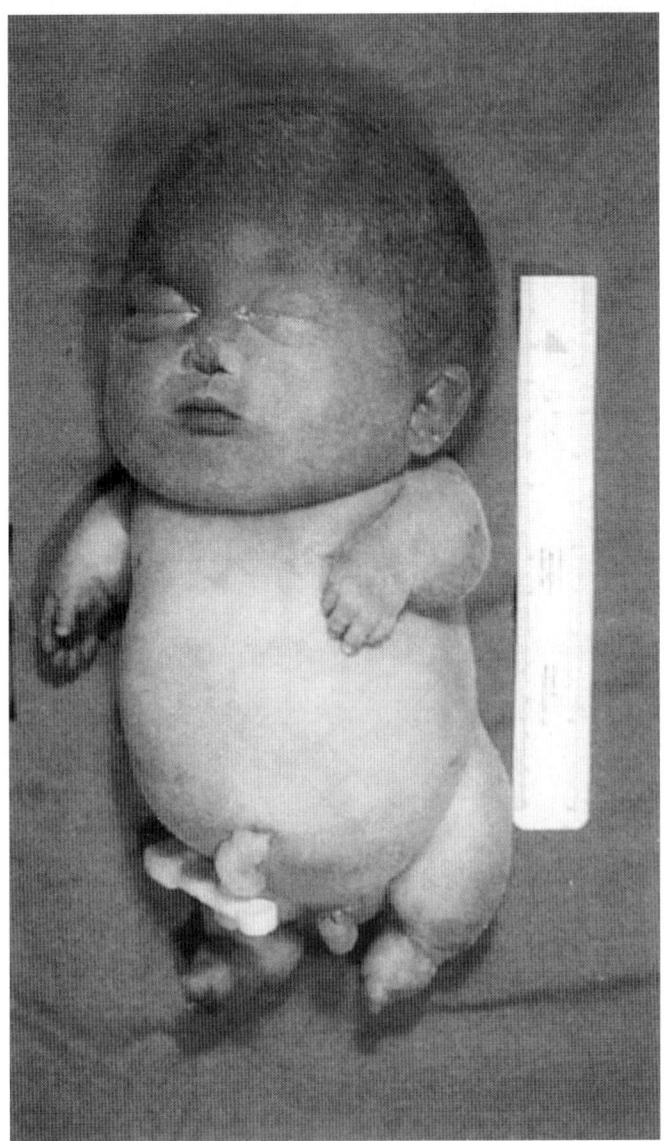

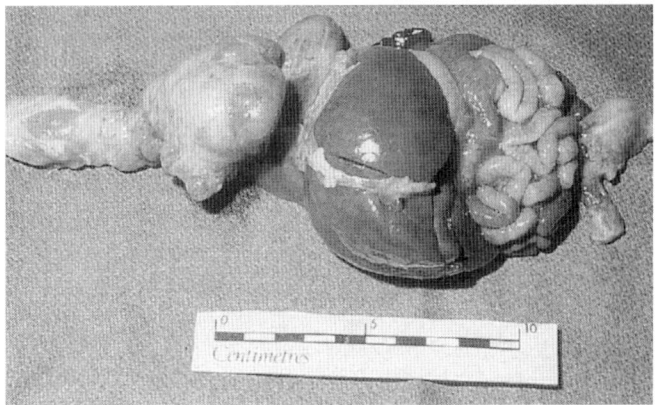

FIGURE 8.8 Mediastinal teratoma, causing hydrops.

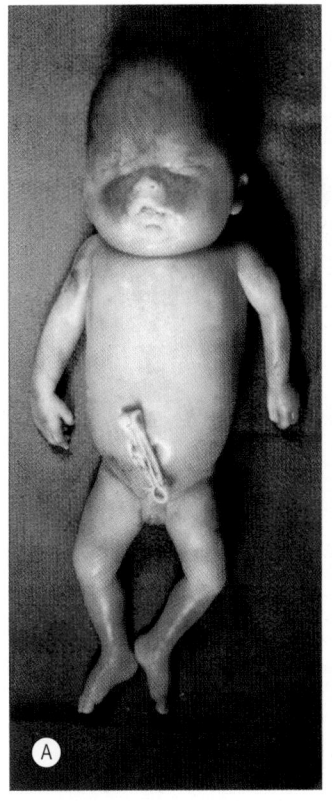 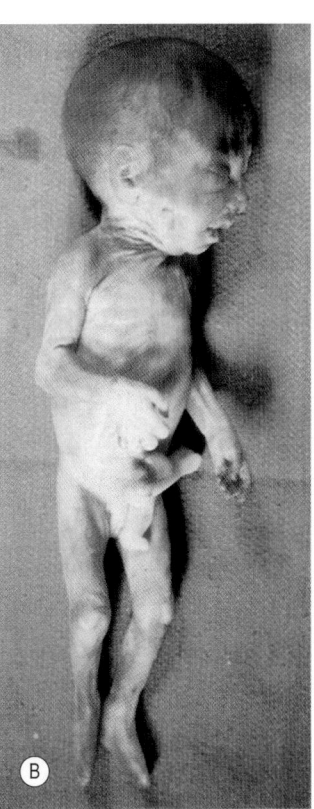

FIGURE 8.7 Chondrodysplasia. Achondrogenesis type II with hydrops.

FIGURE 8.9 Hydrops in twin-to-twin transfusion. (A) The recipient is hydropic. (B) The donor was a 'stuck' twin.

Anemia (Table 8.6)[14, 23, 23]

In some parts of the world, **homozygous α-thalassemia** (Fig. 8.10) is the most common cause of HF as a whole, representing up to 55% of all anemia-related hydrops fetalis.[22] Isoimmunization continues to be an important cause. More recently transplacental infection with **parvovirus B19** has been frequently diagnosed.[14, 23–25] The virus causes erythema infectiosum (**fifth disease**) in adults and children. After respiratory transmission the virus replicates in erythrocyte precursors, with transient arrest in erythrocyte production; there is also a hemolytic component. In immunocompromised patients, pure red cell aplasia may develop after parvovirus infection. The virus enters red blood cell lines via a receptor, the erythrocyte P antigen, which is also expressed in megakaryocytes, endothelial cells, placenta, fetal liver, and fetal heart.[26] Lack of the P antigen prevents infection with parvovirus. Immunoglobulin M (IgM) antibodies

to parvovirus are detected by day 10 after infection, with immunoglobulin G (IgG) antibodies developing at about 2 weeks after infection.

Transplacental transmission of the virus causes aplastic and hemolytic anemia and HF in susceptible fetuses. The virus can be seen in red blood cell precursor nuclei (Fig. 8.11), and the virus can also be demonstrated by in situ hybridization, and by polymerase chain reaction (PCR). Other tissues may be affected, most notably the myocardium.[27] In a review of 1018 cases of acute maternal parvoviral B19 infection in pregnancy, the fetal death

TABLE 8.6 ANEMIA AS A CAUSE OF HYDROPS FETALIS

Cause	No. of cases	Percentage
Immune: Anti-D	5	~ 25
Immune: Anti-Kell	1	~ 5
Immune: Anti-C	1	~ 5
Parvovirus infection	8	~ 45
Twin-twin transfusion	2	~ 10
Transplacental hemorrhage	1	~ 5

From Ismail et al 2001,[14] with permission – review of 63 consecutive cases of fetal hydrops seen in Birmingham Women's Hospital (UK) between 1996 and 1999. Note that results vary between populations (e.g. homozygous α-thalassemia accounts for 55% of all anemia-related fetal hydrops is some parts of Asia),[22] and according to gestational age.[14, 23] Fetomaternal transfusions account for 17% of cases in some series.

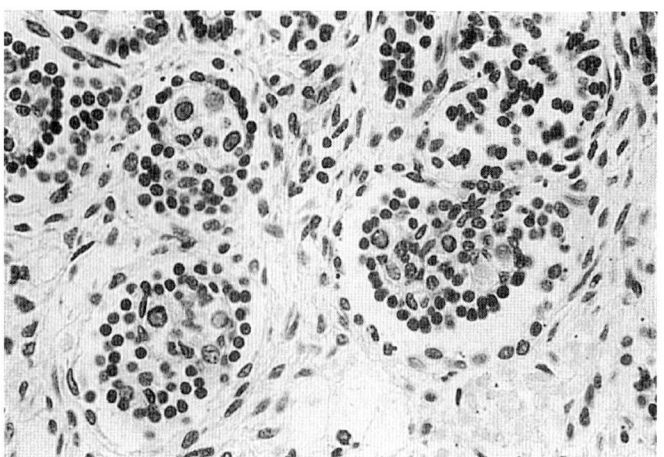

FIGURE 8.11 Parvovirus causing hypoplastic anemia and hydrops. Normoblasts in glomerular capillaries contain intranuclear parvovirus inclusions.

TABLE 8.7 FETAL INFECTION IN HYDROPS FETALIS (EXCLUDING PARVOVIRUS)*

Infection	Percentage
Cytomegalovirus	30
Bacterial, various	9
Toxoplasmosis	6
Rubella	3
Herpes	3
Other presumed, not specified	49

Ismail et al's review of 63 consecutive cases of fetal hydrops seen in Birmingham Women's Hospital (UK) between 1996 and 1999 identified eight cases (12.6%) due to *parvovirus infection*, and no other infectious cause.[14]

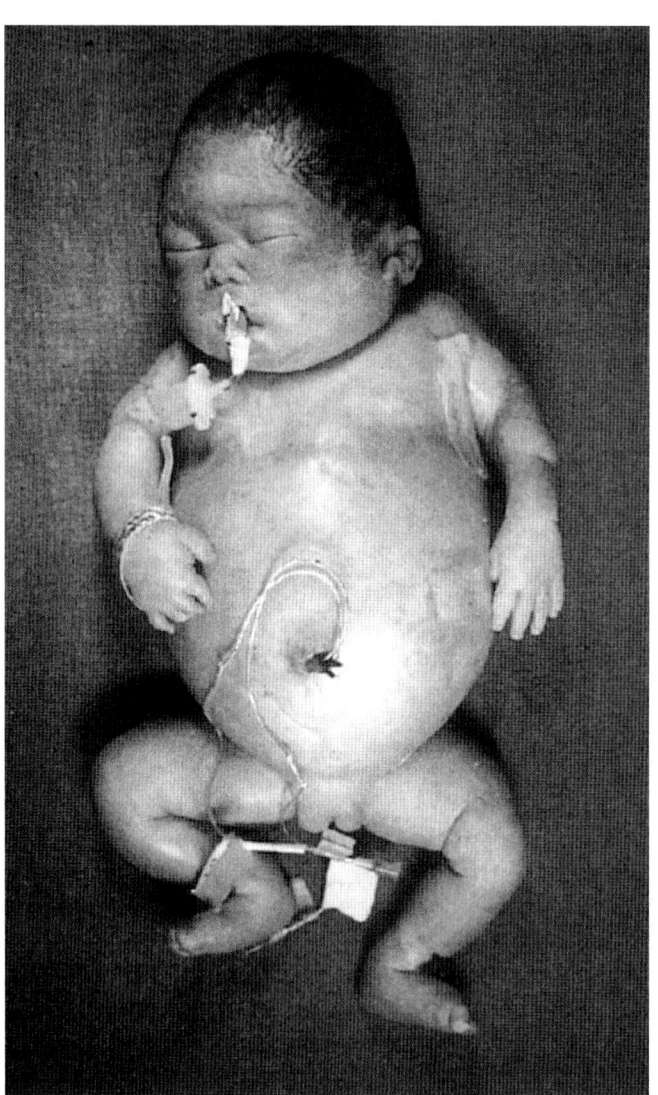

FIGURE 8.10 Hydropic fetus of Southeast Asian origin with homozygous α-thalassemia.

rate was 11% in infections before 20 weeks of gestation. Also, 3.9% of pregnancies developed fetal hydrops. Of fetuses with severe hydrops who received intrauterine transfusions, 85% survived. A small number of fetal deaths did not take place via hydrops.[28]

Fetal infections (Table 8.7)[14]

In most centers, parvovirus (discussed previously) now accounts for the majority of infectious fetal hydrops.[14, 23] Although other infections can be investigated as a cause of HF, results in the literature are meager and difficult to interpret. At autopsy, the characteristic findings of **TORCHS** (toxoplasmosis, 'others', rubella, cytomegalovirus, herpes, and syphilis) include a hydropic fetus and placenta, hepatosplenomegaly, hepatitis, myocarditis in some cases, purpura, and the placenta shows a plasma cell villitis. Characteristic viral inclusions or the **Treponema** of syphilis can often be identified histologically. Results from the **maternal serology** must be sought in cases of hydrops of undetermined etiology.

Parvovirus and syphilis should be diagnosed. The remaining agents can cause myocarditis and hepatitis as well as cerebral pathology.

TABLE 8.8 URINARY TRACT MALFORMATIONS IN HYDROPS FETALIS

Malformation	Percentage
Urethral obstruction	35
Upper urinary tract obstruction	12
Cloacal malformation	12
Other, not specified	41

Urinary tract malformation and neoplasia (Table 8.8)

Megacystis secondary to **urethral stenosis/atresia** can impinge on the umbilical circulation causing hypoxia. Upper urinary tract malformations, such as large **multicystic or polycystic kidneys**, may impede venous return, both inferior caval and umbilical. **Cystic or hydronephrotic kidneys** may rupture, with the formation of urinomas and urinary ascites, in turn leading to HF.

HF is also described in congenital Wilms tumor and congenital mesoblastic nephroma, but the pathway is not well understood. Hydrops does not appear to be caused by high-output cardiac failure in these cases.

Other causes

There are few reports of **fetal akinesia/hypomobility** in HF, so the relative frequency of specific causative diseases cannot be given accurately. Specific diseases are given in Box 8.1.[3, 10, 17, 19, 21, 22, 24–26, 29–131] Peritonitis/ascites can cause HF. Mechanisms include hypoproteinemia, while many cases are caused by intestinal or urinary tract obstruction (Box 8.1).

Similarly, genetic metabolic diseases are rare causes of HF, but their diagnosis is important for reproductive prognosis (Boxes 8.1 and 8.2).[132] There are miscellaneous syndromal diseases that sometimes present as HF. Some of these are listed in Box 8.1 which also gives appropriate reference for further reading on individual causes and associations of HF. The 50 genetic diseases associated with hydrops fetalis in Online Mendelian Inheritance in Man, February 2005 are listed in Box 8.3. HF may be a final common pathway in male fetuses of mothers who have X-linked dominant disorders such as myotonic dystrophy type I (Box 8.1) and incontinentia pigmenti.[133]

Investigation and treatment

Prenatal diagnosis of causes of HF involves the following tests, used in an algorithmic fashion, and depending on any history of HF:

- detailed (level 3) fetal and placental ultrasound, including fetal echocardiography;
- fetal karyotyping by early amniocentesis, fetal blood sampling, or sampling of cystic hygroma or pleural effusion fluid;
- fetal blood sampling and/or amniocentesis for investigation of hemoglobin gene or red blood cell enzyme mutations, parvovirus investigation, suspected genetic metabolic diseases, hemoglobin and serum protein levels, viscosity studies;

- maternal blood sampling for Kleihauer stain for fetomaternal transfusion, blood grouping and antibody screen, serology for infectious agents, connective tissue antibodies, hemoglobinopathies and red blood cell enzymopathies.

Considerations at perinatal autopsy are similar, bearing in mind that functional causes of HF, such as cardiac arrhythmias, are not always caused by identifiable anatomic lesions. Special attention should be focused on the heart, parenchymal organs (genetic metabolic diseases), neuromuscular system (fetal hypomobility), and placenta. Radiology should be used if there are skeletal anomalies. Effusions should be analyzed for lymphocyte count, since this may indicate primary lymphatic dysplasia. Frozen sections can be used during the autopsy, so as to exclude certain diseases and guide the thorough investigation in a problem-oriented manner. Infectious diseases should be studied by culture, Southern blots, in situ hybridization, PCR, and light and electron microscopy. Fetal DNA should be stored for investigation of syndromes (known and unknown), and investigation and confirmation of likely or actual genetic diseases that are diagnosed after the completion of the autopsy and during compilation of other test results.

Autopsy findings may be modified by fetal interventions for diagnosis and treatment. Indications for fetal surgery have been previously discussed.[4] Empirical therapy of fetal anemia and hypoproteinemia has been partially successful;[7, 11, 134–137] albumin and packed red blood cells can be transfused into the fetal peritoneal cavity or bloodstream. Fetal transfusion with packed red blood cells lacking the appropriate red blood cell antigen has long been used for treatment of fetomaternal isoimmunization; the rationales are that there is no primary fetal disease, and that ongoing isoimmunization is cured by delivery. Such methods cannot be used indiscriminately, but there have been some surprisingly good early results from empirical treatment of α-thalassemia[89, 90] and parvovirus infection.[14, 23] Intrapleural infusion of OK-432 has been used successfully to treat fetal chylothorax,[15] but surgical treatment consists of intrauterine drainage of the effusion into the amniotic cavity.

Cystic hygroma: Nuchal edema

'The curious deforming malady known as congenital cystic elephantiasis is probably nearly related to fetal dropsy. It is, however, a disease which chiefly affects the subcutaneous tissue, leading to an increase in its dimensions and the formation in it of cysts of various sizes, with clear serous or curd-like contents. It may implicate the subcutaneous tissue all over the body, but frequently it is very pronounced in a special region, e.g. the back of the head and neck. Fluid in the body cavities is sometimes but not always met with, and in this character the disease differs from general fetal dropsy. . . . details regarding microscopic appearances. . . . The skin was fairly normal, but the lymphatics of it and the subcutaneous and intermuscular structures were greatly dilated and tortuous, and here and there formed real cystic spaces.'[1], p. 297

BOX 8.1 CAUSES OF HYDROPS FETALIS: A SOURCE LIST WITH REFERENCES

1. **Cardiovascular**

   Malformation

   Left ventricular hypoplasia[29, 30]

   Atrioventricular canal[31]

   Right ventricular hypoplasia[32]

   Restricted foramen ovale[33]

   Endocardial fibroelastosis[34, 35]

   Arrhythmia

   Tachyarrhythmias[36–40]

   Bradyarrhythmias[41–43]

   High output

   Sacrococcygeal teratoma[17, 44, 45]

   Fetal angioma[46, 47]

   Chorangioma[48, 49]

   Other neoplasm[50–54]

   Other

   Cardiac rhabdomyoma[19, 55, 56]

   Cardiomyopathy[57, 58]

2. **Chromosomal Abnormalities**

   45,X[59–62]

   Trisomy 21[63–65]

   Trisomy 18[66]

   49,XXXXY[67]

   7q deletion[68]

   Trisomy 13[69, 70]

   Tetraploidy[71]

   17q deletion[72]

   Miscellaneous

3. **Thoracic**

   Congenital cystic adenomatoid malformation[21, 73–75]

   Pulmonary sequestration[76, 77]

   Intrathoracic teratoma[78, 79]

   Other intrathoracic neoplasm[80]

   Enterogenous, bronchogenic cysts[81]

   Dyschondroplasias[82–84]

   Laryngeal atresia with congenital pulmonary hyperinflation[85]

   Hydro/chylothorax[86–88]

   Right-sided diaphragmatic hernia[10]

4. **Anemia**

   α-thalassemia[22, 89, 90]

   Parvovirus infection[24–26]

   Fetomaternal transfusion[91, 92]

   Isoimmunization[93–95]

   Dyserythropoiesis[96, 97]

   Red blood cell enzymopathy[99, 99]

   Intrafetal hemorrhage[100, 101]

   Microangioipathy/hemophagocytosis[102, 103]

   Other[104–107]

5. **Monochorionic Twinning**

   Twin-to-twin transfusion[108–110]

   Twin reversed arterial perfusion[111]

6. **Fetal Infection**

   Syphilis[3, 112, 113]

   Herpes[114]

   Cytomegalovirus[115]

   Listeria[116]

   Toxoplasmosis[117]

7. **Genitourinary Tract Malformation/Neoplasia**

   Urethral obstruction[118]

   Cloacal malformation[119]

   Recessive polycystic kidney disease[120]

   Kaufman-McKusick syndrome[121]

8. **Fetal Hypomobility**

   Myotonic dystrophy type I[122, 123]

   Neu-Laxova syndrome[124]

   Multiple pterygium syndrome[125]

   Congenital muscular dystrophy[126]

9. **Genetic Metabolic Diseases**

   Infantile Gaucher disease[127]

   Niemann-Pick disease[128]

   β-glucuronidase deficiency[129, 130]

   Mucopolysaccharidosis type VII[131]

Development of the lymphatic system is complex and variable, even more so than that of the systemic venous system. In broad outline the major lymphatic trunks develop in close proximity to the large neck veins.[138] The lymphatic vessels continue to develop by processes of centrifugal extension and branching. The lymphatic primordia are regarded as being of venous origin; however, this does not readily explain failure or delay in lymphatico-jugular connection.

Major **lymphatic vessel dysplasia** is a common and serious anomaly and may arise in two major ways: through reduced or absent development of peripheral lymphatics and by delayed or absent lymphatico-venous connection, with dilated peripheral

BOX 8.2 GENETIC METABOLIC DISEASES IN HYDROPS FETALIS

Mucopolysaccharidosis type IVA (Morquio)

Mucopolysaccharidosis type VII (Sly)

Sialic acid storage

Mucolipidosis type I (sialidosis)

Mucolipidosis type II (I-cell disease)

Galactosialidosis

Gaucher

GM_1 gangliosidosis

Niemann-Pick type C

Farber

Congenital disorders of glycosylation

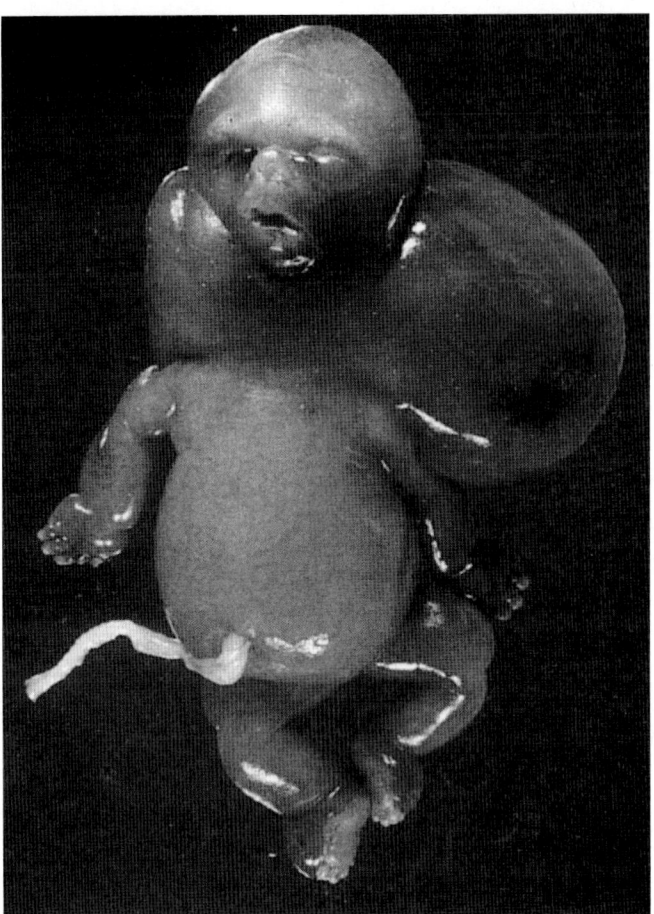

FIGURE 8.12 Cystic hygroma with hydrops. The fetus was euploid.

and central lymphatic vessels. In the case of delayed connection, it is generally assumed that the lymphatic trunks are abnormally developed, but insufficient attention has been paid to the question of primary venous malformation.

Cystic hygroma colli is the most obvious manifestation of lymphatic vessel dysplasia and represents the most extreme form of **nuchal edema** (Fig. 8.12). Many cases have **chromosomal anomalies**; in fact, the prenatal diagnosis of cystic hygroma yields a higher proportion of chromosomally abnormal fetuses than any other fetal anomaly. Apart from chromosomal disorders, cystic hygroma is a component of a variety of pleiotropic maldevelopmental syndromes, often with other potentially lethal anomalies. Therefore the prenatal diagnosis of cystic hygroma demands careful further investigation of precise causes, because the prognosis depends to a large degree on the specific causative disease, as well as on the gestational age at onset. Even so, a policy of expectant management is best for chromosomally normal cases, since the disease course is unpredictable. Some authors feel that unilocular and multilocular, septate cystic hygromas (Fig. 8.13) have different prognoses, but not all agree on this point. Whether chromosomally abnormal or normal, many cases **resolve spontaneously**, leaving the fetuses with residual mechanical deformities such as **neck skin webbing, hypoplastic hearts and aortic arches, and pulmonary hypoplasia**. Surprisingly, some cases show no residual dysmorphology.

Cystic hygroma colli represents large collections of lymph in the major lymphatic trunks (principally the thoracic duct) in the regions of the lymphatico-venous connections at the confluences of the subclavian and jugular veins. As a consequence, fluid also tends to collect in the serous cavities; HF may ensue. As mentioned in the section on hydrops, it is important to recognize that serous cavity lymphatic effusions may actually cause hydrops, and their removal may be curative. The matter is usually resolved by analysis of the fluid for protein and lymphocyte content.

Thus there are several complex issues in the diagnosis and management of lymphatic dysplasia. Even when precise causes are identified, prognosis remains uncertain.

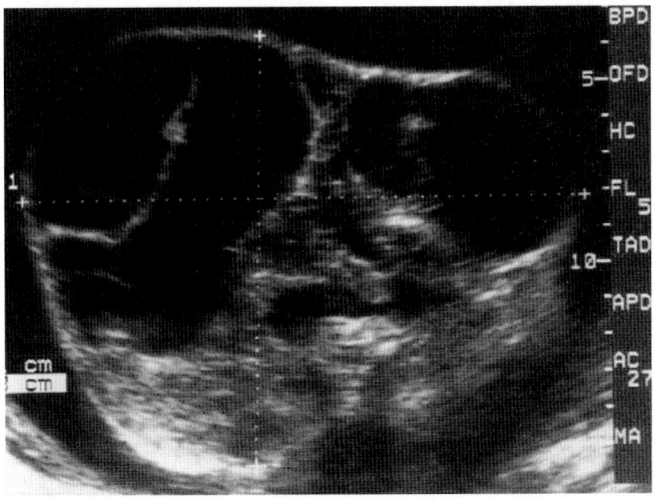

FIGURE 8.13 Ultrasound appearance of a septate cystic hygroma.

Underlying causes

Chromosome analysis of fetuses with severe nuchal edema shows that 60% are aneuploid (Table 8.9).[139–173] Of the aneuploid fetuses, 52% have a 45,X chromosome constitution and variations

BOX 8.3 SINGLE GENE DISEASES LISTED IN 'ONLINE MENDELIAN INHERITANCE IN MAN' AS BEING ASSOCIATED WITH HYDROPS FETALIS

Osteochondrodysplasias

Moth-eaten skeletal dysplasia (Greenburg) 215140

Short rib-polydactyly syndrome type I (Saldino-Noonan) 263530

Short rib-polydactyly syndrome type II (Majewski) 263520

Short rib-polydactyly syndrome type IV (Beemer-Langer) 269860

Chondrodysplasia Blomstrand type 215045

Achondrogenesis type Ia (Houston-Harris) 200600

Achondrogenesis type Ib (Fraccaro) 600972

Achondrogenesis type II (Langer-Saldino) 200610

Fibrochondrogenesis 228520

Chondrodysplasia punctata 2, X-linked dominant (Conradi-Hünermann) 302960

Lethal Kniest-like dysplasia 245190

Osteogenesis imperfecta congenital type II 166210

Metabolic diseases

Mucopolysaccharidosis type VII 253220

Sialidosis type I 256550

Sialic acid storage 269920

Galactosialidosis 256540

Gaucher type II 230900

Perinatal lethal Gaucher disease (subtype of type II) 608013

Neonatal hemochromatosis 231100

Glycogen storage type IIb 300257

Glycogen storage type IV (Andersen) 232500

Analbuminemia (suggested) 103600

Congenital disorder of glycosylation type Ia 212065

Lymphangiectasia

Autosomal recessive congenital pulmonary lymphangiectasia 265300

Hypotrichosis-lymphedema-telangiectasia syndrome 607823

Lymphedema, ASD, facial changes 601927*

* Only one report each, may represent 'private' genetic diseases

Yellow nail syndrome 153300

Hennekam lymphangiectasia-lymphedema syndrome 235510

Campomelia, Cumming type 211890

Acrocephalopolydactylous dysplasia 200995

Familial nuchal bleb syndrome 257350

Akinesia

Lethal multiple pterygium syndrome 253290

Lethal congenital contracture syndrome type I 253310

Simpson-Golabi-Behmel type I 312870

Dystrophia myotonica type I 160900

Multiple pterygium syndrome, X-linked 312150

Cardiac

Ulnar agenesis endocardial fibroelastosis 276822*

Developmental cardiac valve defect 212093*

Left ventricular noncompaction 605906

Supravalvular aortic stenosis (? Williams) 185500

Anemia

α-thalassemia 141800

Glucose 6-phosphate isomerase 172400

Pyruvate kinase 266200

Congenital dyserythropoietic anemia type I 224120

Congenital erythropoietic porphyria 263700

Rhesus antigen D 111680

Spherocytosis type I (spectrin Providence) 182870

Thoracic

Laryngeal atresia, encephalocele and limb defects 607132

Pleiotropic syndromal

Fryns 229850

McKusick-Kaufman 236700

TABLE 8.9 CHROMOSOME CONSTITUTION OF 900 KARYOTYPED FETUSES WITH CYSTIC HYGROMA[139-173]

	45,X	Trisomy 21	Trisomy 18	Trisomy 13	Other abnormality	Normal
All fetuses	282 [52]*	136 [25]	66 [12]	23 [4]	35 [6]	358 (40)
First trimester	41 [22]	72 [30]	46 [25]	10 [5]	16 [9]	151 (45)
Second trimester	241 [67]	64 [18]	20 [6]	13 [4]	19 [5]	207 (37)

[ ], Percentage of chromosomal abnormalities; ( ), percentage total.

(such as mosaicism, structural X-chromosome abnormalities). The so-called fetal Turner phenotype includes large cystic hygromas of the neck and trunk, generalized subcutaneous lymphedema, very marked on the dorsa of the hands and feet, and with characteristic constriction zones at the wrists and ankles

(Fig. 8.14). All the serous cavities contain **effusions of lymph fluid with high lymphocyte counts**. There is usually HF. **Severe forms of congenital heart disease include hypoplastic aortic arch**. Fetal mortality of 45,X conceptuses without mosaicism has been calculated to be nearly 100%; this implies that survivors

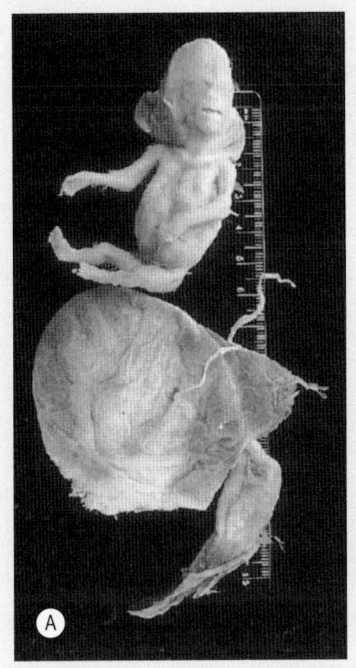

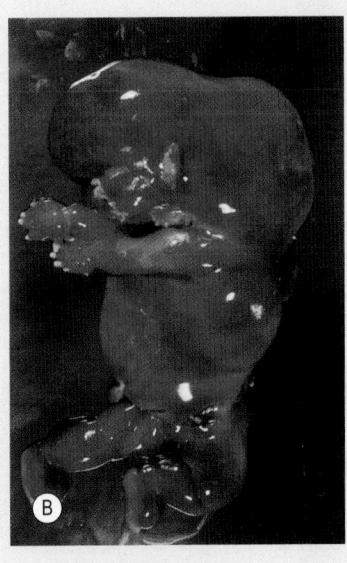

FIGURE 8.14 Phenotype of 45,X conceptuses.
(A) Spontaneous miscarriage at 10 weeks. The fetus has very large cystic hygromas and mild general lymphedema.
(B) Classic appearances of 'fetal Turner syndrome'. There are cystic hygromas, generalized edema, and constrictions at wrists and ankles.

TABLE 8.10 SEPTATION AND CHROMOSOME STATUS IN FETUSES WITH CYSTIC HYGROMA

Septate			Non-septate		
Euploid	Aneuploid	Total	Euploid	Aneuploid	Total
54 (44)	69 (56)	123	182 (69)	80 (31)	262

( ), Percentages of septate and non-septate hygromas.

BOX 8.4 NON-CHROMOSOMAL SYNDROMES WITH CYSTIC HYGROMA AS COMMON OR REPORTED COMPONENT

Noonan syndrome[174–176]

Multiple lethal pterygium syndrome[177, 178]

Fryns syndrome[179]

Achondrogenesis type Ia[180]

Brachmann-de Lange syndrome[181]

Fraser (syndromal cryptophthalmos) syndrome[182]

Roberts syndrome

Lymphedema-distichiasis syndrome

Greenburg chondrodysplasia

If cystic hygromas are analyzed by gestational age at diagnosis, slightly different patterns are found in the first and second trimesters (Table 8.9). Slightly fewer (55%) are chromosomally abnormal, and **autosomal trisomies are more common at this early gestational age**.

In attempts to predict prenatally those fetuses with good outcomes, some authors have found that **unilocular hygromas are less frequently aneuploid** and consequently do well (Table 8.10). However, not all workers agree, and Table 8.10 is somewhat skewed by three series with statistically significant results. All authors agree that poor prognosis is generally associated with very large hygromas, aneuploidy, presence of other malformations, and onset of HF.

Many euploid cases resolve spontaneously at 17 to 18 weeks of gestation and thus represent delayed rather than failed jugulolymphatic connection. A minority of euploid fetuses has persistent, even massive hygromas and some of these represent other developmental diseases with cystic hygromas as components. Such disorders are listed in Box 8.4.[174–182] Among the most frequent are fetuses with various forms of **fetal akinesia** (Fig. 8.16). However, spontaneous fetal resolution of cystic hygroma is also reported in aneuploid fetuses; thus resolution is not an indication of euploidy and good outcome.

The anatomic distribution and severity of lymphatic vascular dysplasia varies with the underlying disorder: **45,X fetuses have very distended cervical and lumbar hygromas and deficient or absent peripheral lymphatics** (Fig. 8.17A). Other fetuses generally have generalized dilatation of peripheral lymphatics in addition to cervical hygromas (Fig. 8.17B). Subcutaneous edema and serous effusions are present in both types. Hence subcutaneous edema of 45,X fetuses is actually a standard

with less severe features of Turner syndrome have lesser degrees of chromosomal abnormalities, including mosaicism for normal cell lines and structural X-chromosome abnormalities.

Cystic hygromas are also regularly found in fetuses with trisomies 21 (Fig. 8.15), 18, and 13 (Table 8.9).

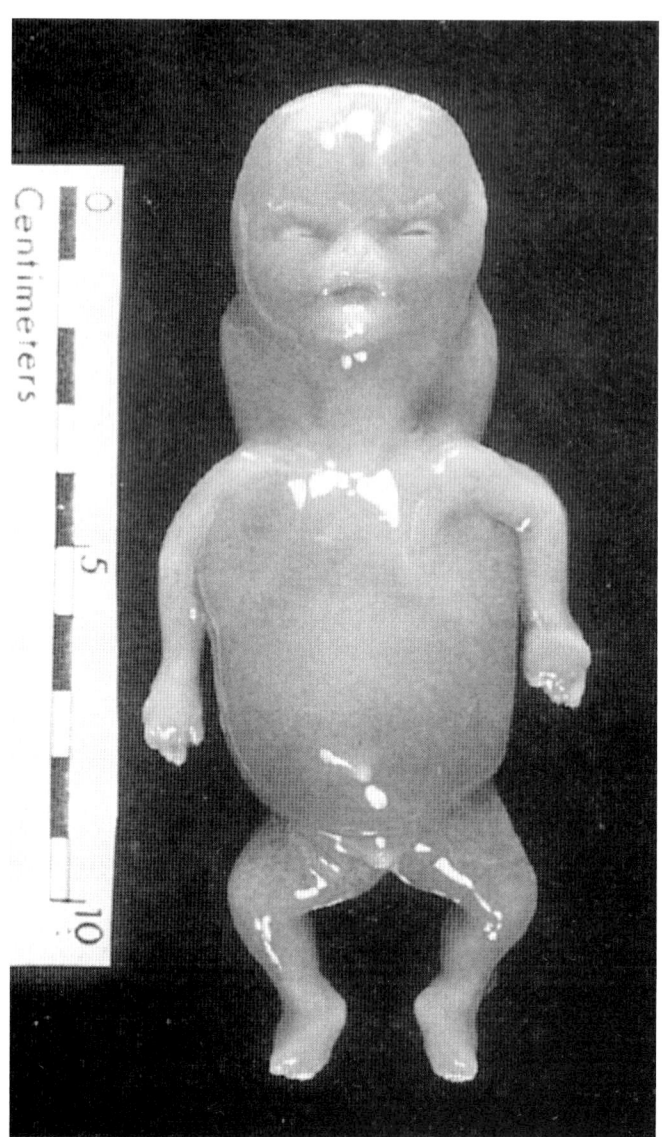

FIGURE 8.15 Termination of pregnancy of a fetus with trisomy 21 with cystic hygromas.

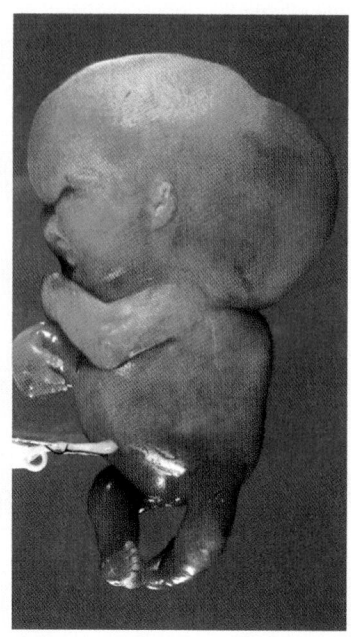

FIGURE 8.16 Multiple lethal pterygium syndrome with cystic hygroma and hydrops.

interstitial soft tissue edema, whereas the other fetuses have distended lymphatics and interstitial edema.

Jugulo-lymphatic misconnection is a specific malformation that may be a component of many developmental disorders. Prenatal and autopsy investigation is aimed at chromosome analysis and detection of other malformations. Rapid chromosome analysis (3 days) can be achieved using lymphocytes derived from aspirated hygroma fluid.[146, 183–185]

Fetal hydrothorax

Pleural effusions may be components of HF of all causes, manifestations of lymphatic dysplasia, or secondary to other

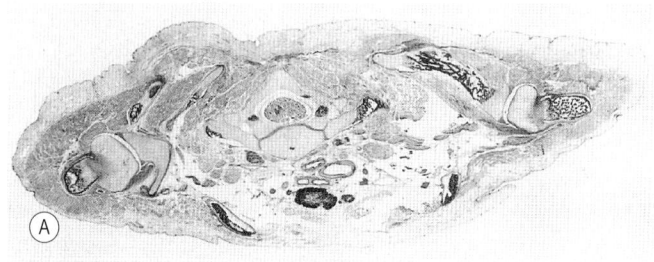

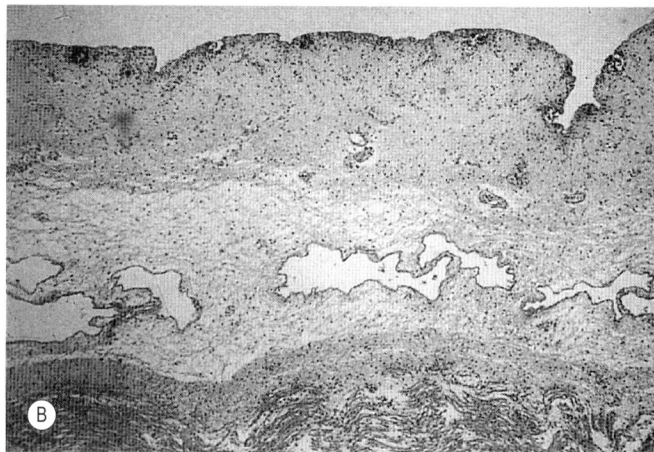

FIGURE 8.17 Histology of lymphatic vascular dysplasia. (A) Histologic transverse section of 45,X fetus at level of humeral heads. Numerous confluent lymph-filled spaces are present outside of the lymphatic vasculature (i.e., interstitial edema is present), and lymphatic vessels are sparse. (B) Dilated subcutaneous lymphatics in a euploid fetus with cystic hygroma.

346

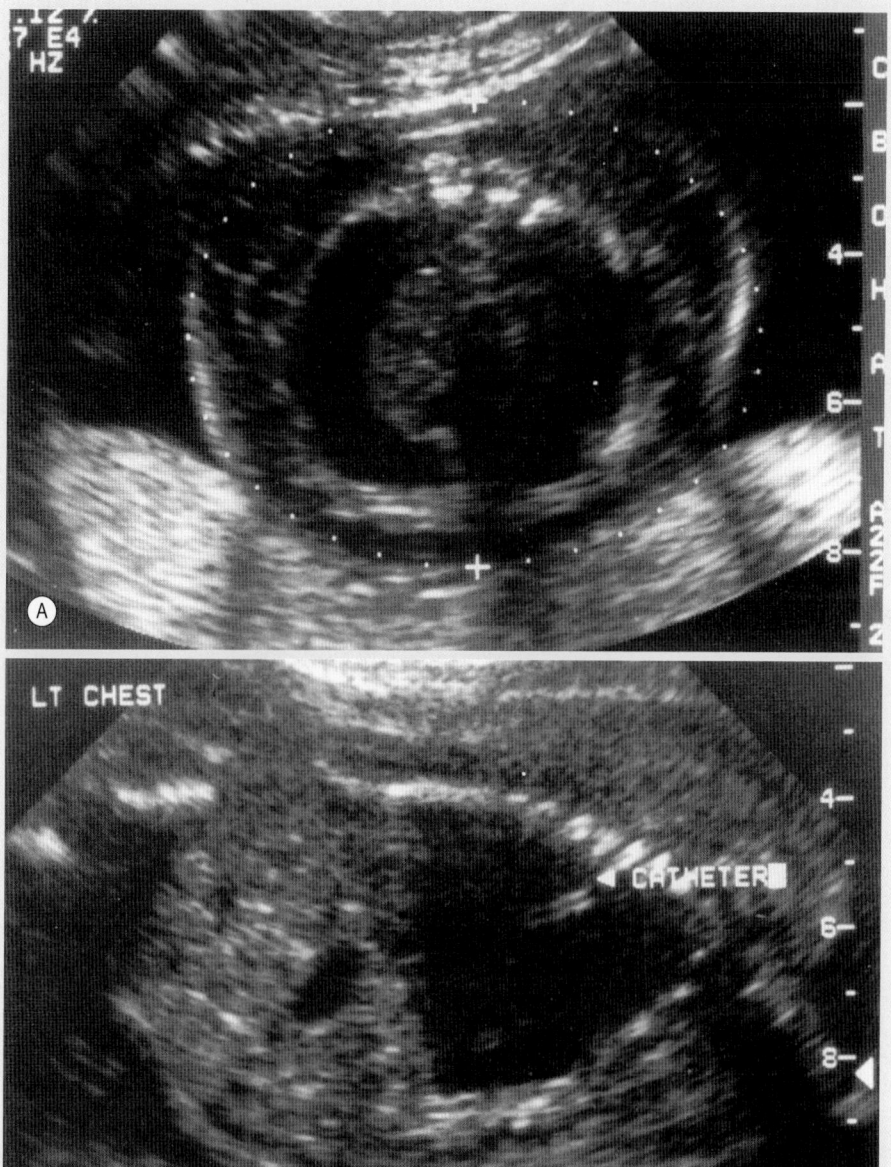

intrathoracic pathology. **Hydrothorax causes pulmonary hypoplasia** and it may be unilateral or bilateral. Prenatal diagnosis of hydrothorax (Fig. 8.18A) permits empirical treatment to prevent pulmonary hypoplasia, and a specific diagnosis may emerge during treatment. Therapy includes multiple sequential thoracocenteses, the insertion of pleuro-amniotic pigtail catheters (Fig. 8.18B), and treatment with OK432. However, some cases resolve spontaneously, and others may be managed without fetal intervention.[186] Thoraco-amniotic shunting of pleural effusions with hydrops has a survival rate of approximately 60%.[187, 188]

Analysis of **protein levels** and cell content of pleural fluid is important in reaching specific diagnoses. In **chylothorax/** **hydrothorax** secondary to localized lymphatic obstruction, the **lymphocyte count is high** (Fig. 8.19).

Causes

It is difficult to give the relative frequency of causes of hydrothorax, but it seems that lymphatic obstruction is the most common. Reported causes and associations of hydrothorax are listed in Box 8.5.[75, 189–194] In a literature review of 124 cases of lymphatic hydrothorax,[195] only 54% survived (Table 8.11): 81 cases were documented as bilateral and 33 as unilateral. Factors

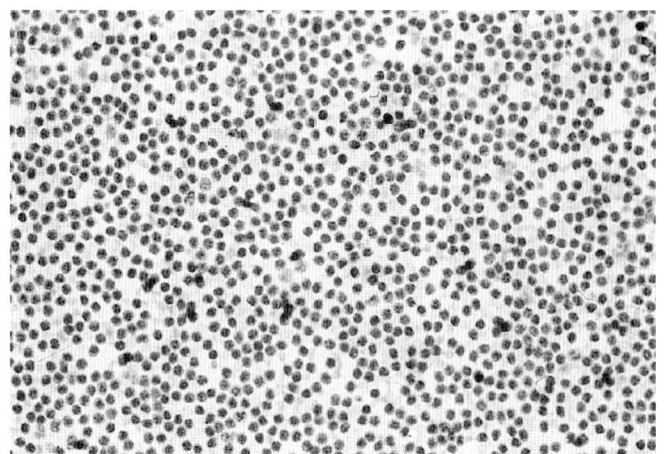

FIGURE 8.19 Lymphocytes in chylothorax.

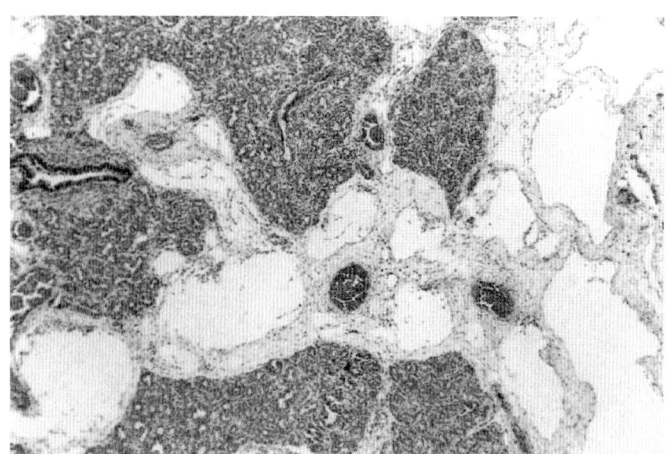

FIGURE 8.20 Pulmonary lymphangiectasia in a case of chylothorax.

BOX 8.5 CAUSES OF FETAL HYDROTHORAX COMPONENT OF HYDROPS FETALIS

Component of hydrops fetalis of other, non-thoracic causes

Localized intrathoracic lymphatic dysplasia[189, 190]

Congenital cystic adenomatoid malformation of lung[75]

Pulmonary sequestration[191–193]

Foregut duplication cysts[194]

Pulmonary lymphangiectasia

TABLE 8.11 OUTCOMES IN LYMPHATIC FETAL HYDROTHORAX

Variable	Good outcome	Poor outcome
Gestation at < 31 weeks	24/59 (41%)	35/59 (59%)
Gestation at > 32 weeks	29/47 (62%)	18/47 (38%)
Diagnosis at < 31 weeks	2/18 (11%)	16/18 (89%)
Diagnosis at > 32 weeks	51/84 (61%)	33/84 (39%)
Hydrops		
Present	13/42 (31%)	29/42 (69%)
Absent	32/40 (80%)	8/40 (20%)
Antenatal therapy		
None	35/70 (50%)	35/70 (50%)
Thoracocentesis	7/12 (58%)	5/12 (42%)
Shunting	18/23 (78%)	5/23 (22%)

After Weber and Philipson 1992,[195] with permission.

associated with good outcome were later gestational age at diagnosis and at delivery, no development of HF, and successful fetal therapy by thoracocentesis or shunting. The main complications were preterm delivery and pulmonary hypoplasia. Careful measurements of cardiac components by fetal echocardiography showed that primary hydrothorax actually compresses cardiac structures, and that the compression is more pronounced when hydrops has developed.[196]

Fetal chylothorax may be associated with pulmonary lymphangiectasia (Fig. 8.20), in which case treatment of the chylothorax alone may not be successful. Unlike cystic hygroma, **isolated fetal chylothorax is not usually associated with chromosomal or non-chromosomal syndromes**. Investigation of hydrothorax is aimed at delineating focal thoracic causes or confirming chylothorax by lymphocyte counts.

Rarely is hydrothorax a complication of monochorionic twin pregnancy; twin transfusion syndrome resulted in fetal death of one of the twins, following which the survivor developed right-sided pleural effusion.[197] The survivor died in the neonatal period, and pulmonary remodeling was noted at autopsy; the likely cause was pulmonary infarction.

It seems likely that many cases of 'idiopathic' hydrops fetalis actually have fetal hydrothorax, but it is not recognized that the hydrothorax is the primary cause of the hydrops, rather than merely being a component of hydrops.

Fetal pericardial effusions

Pericardial effusions are almost invariably components of HF and are reliable early guides to incipient hydrops. **Isolated chylopericardium** is rare.[198] **Intrapericardial teratomas** are usually accompanied by pericardial effusions.[199] **Congenital central eventration of the diaphragm** can result in herniation of abdominal organs into the pericardial sac, accompanied by effusion.[200]

Fetal ascites

'Fetal ascites may be defined as the effusion of fluid into the peritoneal cavity, with consequent abdominal distension due to several different causes, accompanied by various lesions of the viscera, and leading usually to delay in labor and intranatal or early postnatal death of the affected infant. It is, just as in the adult, a symptom or effect of different morbid processes rather than a disease per se; but the morbid processes which produce the

TABLE 8.12 CAUSES OF FETAL AND NEONATAL ASCITES[201]

	Fetal ascites	Neonatal ascites
Urinary tract obstruction	9	66
Chylous ascites	2	36
Hepatic disease	0	10
Intestinal perforation	2	7
Pancreatic disease	0	8
Infection	1	3
Congenital heart disease	2	4
Miscellaneous	13	4
No cause identified	8	8
TOTAL	37	146

TABLE 8.13 CAUSES OF PRENATALLY-DIAGNOSED FETAL ASCITES WITHOUT HYDROPS[202]

Cause	Number	Percentage
Urinary	15	26
Cloacal dysgenesis	7	12
Cardiac	7	12
Thoracic	6	10
Intestinal	5	9
Infection	3	5
Chylous	2	3
Unidentified	8	8

antenatal form are almost certainly different from those which lead to the adult variety.[1, p. 355]

As with other serous effusions, fetal ascites may cause or be a component of HF. Isolated ascites is usually caused by intra-abdominal pathology, but this is not always so.

Causes

In a literature review of 146 cases of fetal and neonatal ascites, the most frequent causes were **urinary tract obstruction (urinary ascites), chylous ascites**, and **hepatogastrointestinal diseases**[201] (Table 8.12). A recent series of 58 cases of fetal ascites without hydrops diagnosed prenatally produced a somewhat different range and frequency of causes (Table 8.13).[202] **Congenital cystic adenomatoid malformation of the lung**[75] and other congenital lung malformations regularly present with ascites and without subsequent development of HF. It is not known whether this represents a local transdiaphragmatic effect, or whether the intra-thoracic pressure is too elevated by the space-occupying lesion to permit pleural effusions to accumulate. The prenatal investigation of fetal ascites usually reveals intra-abdominal primary pathology. Since the early literature review,[201] subsequent case reports have confirmed and amplified the general trends, as well as adding more sophisticated methods to investigate precise pathology.

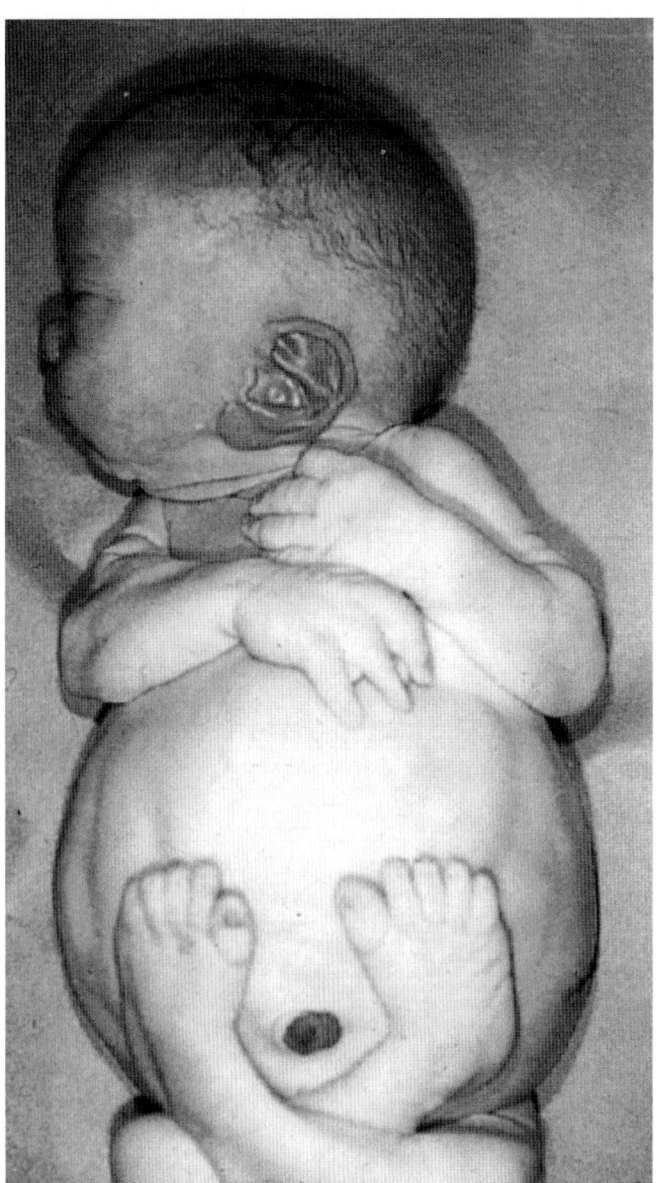

FIGURE 8.21 Fetus with urinary ascites. There was bilateral ureteric obstruction, with cystic dysplastic kidneys, urinomas, and urinary ascites. As renal function failed, the urinary ascites regressed, leaving a prune-belly appearance. Positional deformities, large ears and the Potter facies are manifestations of the oligohydramnios sequence.

Urinary ascites

Urinary tract obstructive malformations include **posterior urethral valves, urethral atresia, ureterocele, and ureteric obstruction/hypoperistalsis** as well as **retroperitoneal neoplasia** (Fig. 8.21). Rupture of the urinary tract may occur at the level of the bladder, but is more common in the kidneys. Urine collects in the perinephric tissues as a **urinoma** and ultimately leads to urinary ascites. The diagnosis may be made by fetal ultrasound, with oligohydramnios and urinary tract dilatation. The outcome is likely to be poor because of pulmonary hypoplasia secondary to oligohydramnios. **Perlman syndrome** (MIM 267000,

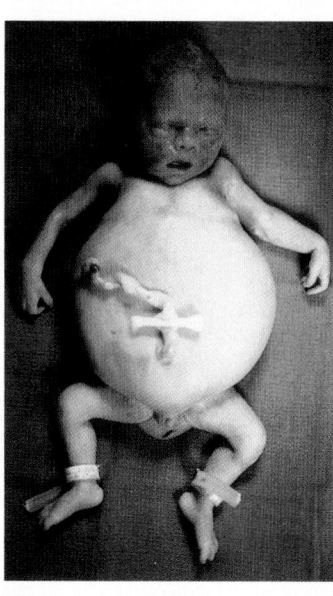

FIGURE 8.22 Fetal ascites secondary to lysosomal storage disease.

characterized by renal hamartomas, nephroblastomatosis, Wilms tumor and fetal gigantism) is also associated with ascites.[203]

Chylous ascites

Chylous or 'isolated' **ascites** implies **intra-abdominal lymphatic obstruction.**[204] The disease may cause severe ascites with potential abdominal dystocia, and **prenatal paracentesis** may be indicated in the presence of diaphragmatic elevation and pulmonary hypoplasia.[205] However, some cases do resolve spontaneously.

Intestinal perforation

Intestinal perforation liberates **meconium** into the peritoneal cavity, leading to a meconium peritonitis (Fig. 21.15). Ascites and peritoneal calcification follow. Progression from meconium extrusion, ascites, and calcification has been documented by serial ultrasound.[206] The causes of bowel perforation include **single or multiple atresias, volvulus,** and **meconium ileus.** In the case of meconium ileus, the newborn can be rapidly investigated for cystic fibrosis. In one reported case[207] the δF508 mutation was found in the CFTR gene, using DNA amplified by PCR from small amounts of peripheral white blood cells and cells from urine sediment.

Spontaneous perforation of the extrahepatic **biliary tree** is a rare cause of fetal ascites.[208]

Congenital infection

Congenital infections causing ascites include **syphilis, toxoplasmosis,** and particularly **cytomegalovirus.** The pathogenesis is not clear but may include hepatitis or fibrosis with portal hypertension.[209]

Genetic metabolic diseases

Fetal ascites is an important presenting feature of several **genetic metabolic diseases** including the following (Fig. 8.22):

- infantile sialidosis,[210]
- GM_1 gangliosidosis,[211]
- α_1-antitrypsin deficiency,[212]
- infantile Gaucher disease,[213]
- generalized *N*-acetylneuraminic acid storage disease,[214]
- Niemann-Pick disease type C[215] and
- Wolman disease.[216]
- Chondrodysplasia punctata[217]
- Fraser syndrome[218]

As already mentioned, cells in fetal ascitic fluid can be used for chromosome analysis or other methods of genetic diagnosis.

The investigation of fetal and neonatal ascites is challenging because causes may be simple, with spontaneous resolution, or may be complex, requiring a sophisticated diagnostic approach.

References

Hydrops fetalis

1. Ballantyne JW. Manual of antenatal pathology and hygiene: the foetus. Edinburgh: William Green; 1902.
2. Potter EL. Universal edema of the fetus unassociated with erythroblastosis. Am J Obstet Gynecol 1943; 46:130.
3. Berkowitz K, Baxi L, Fox HE. False-negative syphilis screening: the prozone phenomenon, non-immune hydrops, and diagnosis of syphilis during pregnancy. Am J Obstet Gynecol 1990; 163:975–977.
4. Adzick NS, Harrison MR. Fetal surgical therapy. Lancet 1994; 343:897–902.
5. Machin GA. Hydrops revisited: literature review of 1414 cases published in the 1980s. Am J Med Genet 1989; 34:366–390.
6. Boyd PA, Keeling JW. Fetal hydrops. J Med Genet 1992; 29:91–97.
7. Hansmann M, Gembruch U, Bald R. New therapeutic aspects of non-immune hydrops based on 402 prenatally diagnosed cases. Fetal Ther 1989; 4:29–36.
8. Santolaya J, Alley D, Jaffe R, et al. Antenatal classification of hydrops fetalis. Obstet Gynecol 1992; 79:256–259.
9. Salzman DH, Frigoletto FD, Harlow BL, et al. Sonographic evaluation of hydrops fetalis. Obstet Gynecol 1989; 74:106–111.
10. Ruiz Villaespesa A, Suarez Mier MP, Lopez Ferrer P, et al. Nonimmunologic hydrops fetalis: an etiopathogenetic approach through the postmortem study of 59 patients. Am J Med Genet 1990; 25:274–279.
10d. Wy CA, Sajous CH, Loberiza F, et al. Outcome of infants with a diagnosis of hydrops fetalis in the 1990s. Am J Perinatol 1999; 16:561–567.
10e. Recep A. Non-immune hydrops fetalis in the first trimester: A review of 30 cases. Clin Exp Obstet Gynecol 2001; 27:187–190.
11. Shimokawa H, Hara K, Maeda H, et al. Intrauterine treatment of idiopathic hydrops. J Perinat Med 1988; 16:133–138.
12. Rodriguez MM, Chavez F, Romaguera RL, et al. Value of autopsy in nonimmune hydrops fetalis: series of 51 stillborn fetuses. Pediatr Dev Pathol 2002; 5:365–374.
13. Sohan K, Carroll SG, De La Fuente S, et al. Analysis of outcome of hydrops fetalis in relation to gestational age at diagnosis, cause and treatment. Acta Obstet Gynecol Scand 2001; 80:726–730.
14. Ismail KM, Martin WL, Ghosh S, et al. Etiology and outcome of hydrops fetalis. J Matern Fetal Med 2001; 10:175–181.
15. Jorgensen C, Brocks V, Bang J, et al. Treatment of severe fetal chylothorax associated with severe hydrops with intrapleural injection of OK-432. Ultrasound Obstet Gynecol 2003; 21:66–69.

16. Litsey SE, Noonan JA, O'Connor WN, et al. Maternal connective tissue disease and congenital heart block. N Engl J Med 1985; 312:98–100.

17. Nakayama DK, Killian A, Hill LM, et al. The newborn with hydrops and sacrococcygeal teratoma. J Pediatr Surg 1991; 26:1435–1438.

18. Anai T, Miyakawa I, Ohki H, et al. Hydrops fetalis caused by fetal Kasabach-Merritt syndrome. Acta Paediatr Jpn 1992; 34:324–327.

19. Scurry J, Watkins A, Acton C, et al. Tachyarrhythmia, cardiac rhabdomyomata and fetal hydrops in a premature infant with tuberous sclerosis. J Paediatr Child Health 1992; 28:260–262.

20. Barr M, Oman-Gaines L. Turner syndrome and small heart: a cause of death in utero. Proceedings, Interim Meeting. Pediatric Pathology Society; 1988.

21. Revillon Y, Jan D, Plattner V, et al. Congenital cystic adenomatoid malformation of the lung: prenatal management and prognosis. J Pediatr Surg 1993; 28:1009–1011.

22. Hsieh FJ, Ko TM, Chen HY. Hydrops fetalis caused by severe α-thalassemia. Early Hum Dev 1992; 29:233–236.

23. Sohan K, Carroll SG, De La Fuente S, et al. Analysis of outcome in hydrops fetalis in relation to gestational age at diagnosis, cause and treatment. Acta Obstet Gynecol Scand 2001; 80:726–730.

24. Rogers BB, Mark Y, Oyer CE. Diagnosis and incidence of fetal parvovirus infection in an autopsy series: I. Histology. Pediatr Pathol 1993; 13:381–386.

25. Mark Y, Rogers BB, Oyer C. Diagnosis and incidence of fetal parvovirus infection in an autopsy series: II. DNA amplification. Pediatr Pathol 1993; 13:381–386.

26. Brown KE, Hibbs JR, Gallinella G, et al. Resistance to parvovirus B19 infection due to lack of virus receptor (erythrocyte P antigen). N Engl J Med 1994; 330:1192–1196.

27. O'Malley A, Berry-Kinsella C, Hughes C, et al. Parvovirus infects cardiac myocytes in hydrops fetalis. Pediatr Dev Pathol 2003; 6:414–420.

28. Enders M, Weidner A, Zoellner I, et al. Fetal morbidity and mortality after acute human parvovirus B19 infection in pregnancy: a prospective evaluation of 1018 cases. Prenat Diagn 2004; 24:513–518.

29. Sahn DJ, Shenker L, Reed KL, et al. Prenatal ultrasound diagnosis of hypoplastic left heart syndrome associated with hydrops fetalis. Am Heart J 1982; 104:1368–1372.

30. Weinberg PM, Peyser K, Hackney JR. Fetal hydrops in newborn with hypoplastic left heart syndrome. J Am Coll Cardiol 1985; 6:1365–1369.

31. Chitayat D, Lao A, Wilson RD, et al. Prenatal diagnosis of asplenia syndrome. Am J Obstet Gynecol 1988; 158:1085–1087.

32. Vintzileos AM, Campbell WA, Deaton JL, et al. Hydrops fetalis associated with immunologic and non-immunologic factors. Am J Perinatol 1987; 4:115–120.

33. Porcelli PJ, Saller DN, Duwaji MS, et al. Nonimmune hydrops with isolated premature restriction of foramen ovale. J Perinatol 1992; 12:37–40.

34. Wolfson DJ, Pepkowitz SH, van de Velde R, et al. Primary endocardial fibroelastosis associated with hydrops fetalis in a premature infant. Am Heart J 1990; 120:708–711.

35. Newbould MJ, Armstrong GR, Barson AJ. Endocardial fibroelastosis in infants with hydrops. J Clin Pathol 1991; 44:576–579.

36. Hijazi ZM, Rosenfeld LE, Copel JA, et al. Amiodarone therapy of intractable atrial flutter in a premature hydropic neonate. Pediatr Cardiol 1992; 13:227–229.

37. Smoleniec JS, Martin R, James DK: Intermittent fetal tachycardia and fetal hydrops. Arch Dis Child 1991; 66:1160–1161.

38. Hallak M, Neerhof MG, Pery R, et al. Fetal supraventricular tachycardia and hydrops fetalis: combined intensive, direct, and transplacental therapy. Obstet Gynecol 1991; 78:523–525.

39. Sherer DM, Sadovsky E, Menashe M, et al. Fetal ventricular tachycardia associated with nonimmunologic hydrops fetalis: a case report. J Reprod Med 1990; 35:292–294.

40. Khositseth A, Ramin KD, O'Leary PW, et al. Role of amiodarone in the treatment of fetal supraventricular tachycardia and hydrops fetalis. Pediatr Cardiol 2003; 24:454–456.

41. Harris JP, Alexson CG, Manning JA, et al. Medical therapy for the hydropic fetus with congenital complete heart block. Am J Perinatol 1993; 10:217–219.

42. Chua S, Ostman-Smith I, Sellers S, et al. Congenital heart block with hydrops fetalis treated with high-dose dexamethasone. Eur J Obstet Gynecol Rep Biol 1991; 42:2155–2158.

43. Watson WJ, Katz VL. Steroid therapy for hydrops associated with antibody-mediated congenital heart block. Am J Obstet Gynecol 1991; 165:553–554.

44. Kapoor R, Saha MM. Antenatal sonographic diagnosis of fetal sacrococcygeal teratoma with hydrops. Australas Radiol 1989; 33:285–287.

45. Langer JC, Harrison MR, Schmidt KG, et al. Fetal hydrops and death from sacrococcygeal teratoma: rationale for fetal surgery. Am J Obstet Gynecol 1989; 160:1145–1150.

46. Gonen R, Fong K, Chiasson DA. Prenatal sonographic diagnosis of hepatic hemangioendothelioma with secondary hydrops fetalis. Obstet Gynecol 1989; 73:485–487.

47. Drut R, Sapia S, Gril D, et al. Nonimmune hydrops fetalis, hydramnios, microcephaly, and intracranial meningeal hemangioendothelioma. Pediatr Pathol 1993; 13:9–13.

48. Hirata GI, Masaki DI, O'Toole M, et al. Color flow mapping and Doppler velocimetry in the diagnosis and management of a placental chorangioma associated with nonimmune fetal hydrops. Obstet Gynecol 1993; 81:850–852.

49. Chazotte C, Girz B, Koenigsberg M, et al. Spontaneous infarction of placental chorangioma and associated regression of hydrops fetalis. Am J Obstet Gynecol 1990; 163:1180–1181.

50. McGinnis M, Jacobs G, el Naggar A, et al. Congenital peribronchial myofibroblastic tumor (so-called 'congenital leiomyosarcoma'). A distinct neonatal lung lesion associated with nonimmune hydrops fetalis. Mod Pathol 1993; 6:487–492.

51. Sherer DM, Abramowicz JS, Eggers PC, et al. Prenatal ultrasonographic diagnosis of intracranial teratoma and massive craniomegaly with associated high-output cardiac failure. Am J Obstet Gynecol 1993; 168:97–99.

52. Kazzi NJ, Chang CH, Roberts EC, et al. Fetal hepatoblastoma presenting as nonimmune hydrops. Am J Perinatol 1989; 6:278–280.

53. Lam PM, Leung TN, Ng PC, et al. Congenital cervical fibrosarcoma with hydrops fetalis. Acta Obstet Gynecol Scand 2004; 83:773–776.

54. Castellino SM, Powers R, Kalwinsky D, et al. Abdominal rhabdoid tumor presenting as hydrops fetalis: a case report. J Pediatr Hematol Oncol 2001; 23:258–259.

55. Calhoun BC, Watson PT, Hegge F. Ultrasound diagnosis of an obstructive cardiac rhabdomyoma with severe hydrops and hypoplastic lungs. A case report. J Reprod Med 1991; 36:317–319.

56. Geva T, Santini F, Pear W, et al. Cardiac rhabdomyoma. Rare cause of fetal death. Chest 1991; 99:139–142.

57. Steenhout P, Elmer C, Clercx A, et al. Carnitine deficiency with cardiomyopathy presenting as neonatal hydrops: successful response to carnitine therapy. J Inherit Metab Dis 1990; 13:69–75.

58. Sardesai MG, Gray AA, McGrath MM, et al. Fatal hypertrophic cardiomyopathy in the fetus of a woman with diabetes. Obstet Gynecol 2001; 98:925–927.

59. Saller DN, Canick JA, Schwartz S, et al. Multiple-marker screening in pregnancies with hydropic and nonhydropic Turner syndrome. Am J Obstet Gynecol 1992; 167:1021–1024.

60. Nicolaides KH, Azar G, Snijders RJ, et al. Fetal nuchal oedema: associated malformations and chromosomal defects. Fetal Diagn Ther 1992; 7:123–131.

61. Mostello DJ, Bofinger MK, Siddiqi TA. Spontaneous resolution of fetal cystic hygroma and hydrops in Turner syndrome. Obstet Gynecol 1989; 73:862–865.

62. Schwanitz G, Zerres K, Gembruch U, et al. Rate of chromosomal aberrations in prenatally detected hydrops fetalis and hygroma colli. Hum Genet 1989; 84:81–82.

63. Hendricks SK, Sorensen TK, Baker ER. Trisomy 21, fetal hydrops, and anemia: prenatal diagnosis of transient myeloproliferative disorder? Obstet Gynecol 1993; 82:703–705.

64. Ilagan NB, Liang KC, Delaney-Black V, et al. Hydrops fetalis, polyhydramnios, pulmonary hypoplasia, and Down syndrome. Am J Perinatol 1992; 9:9–10.

65. Sherer DM, Miller KS, Woods JR. Prenatal sonographic diagnosis of severe nonimmune hydrops in a Down syndrome fetus at 16 weeks of gestation. Am J Med Genet 1991; 39:458–460.

66. Szabo J, Gellen J, Szemere G. Non-immune hydrops in trisomy-18. Diagnosis by vaginosonography and chorionic villus sampling in the first trimester. Case report. Br J Obstet Gynaecol 1990; 97:955–956.

67. Hovav Y, Nadjari M, Dagan J, et al. Nonimmune hydrops fetalis in a 49,XXXXY fetus at 16 menstrual weeks. Am J Med Genet 1993; 47:529–530.

68. Finley BE, Seguin JH, Bennett TL, et al. Terminal deletion of 7q presenting in utero with a truncus arteriosus and nonimmune hydrops. Am J Med Genet 1993; 47:221–222.

69. Greenberg F, Carpenter RJ, Ledbetter DH. Cystic hygroma and hydrops fetalis in a fetus with trisomy 13. Clin Genet 1983; 24:389–391.

70. Milner S, Mayo J, Klein R. Ultrasonic diagnosis of a fetal cardiac malformation. A case report. S Afr Med J 1982; 62:105–106.

71. Fryns JP, Vandenberghe K, Moerman F, et al. Tetraploidy with hydrops fetalis, cystic nuchal hygroma and 90,XX karyotype. Clin Genet 1987; 31:158–160.

72. Williamson RA, Weiner CP, Patil S, et al. Abnormal pregnancy sonogram: selective induction for fetal karyotype. Obstet Gynecol 1987; 69:15–20.

73. Sherer DM, Abramowicz JS, Metlay LA, et al. Nonimmune fetal hydrops caused by bilateral type III congenital cystic adenomatoid malformation of the lung at 17 weeks' gestation. Am J Obstet Gynecol 1992; 167:503–505.

74. Pinson CW, Harrison MW, Thornburg KL, et al. Importance of fetal fluid imbalance in congenital cystic adenomatoid malformation of the lung. Am J Surg 1992; 163:510–514.

75. Morris E, Constantine G, McHugo J. Cystic adenomatoid malformation of the lung: an obstetric and ultrasound perspective. Eur J Obstet Gynecol Rep Biol 1991; 40:11–15.

76. Brus F, Nikkels PG, van Loon AJ, et al. Non-immune hydrops fetalis and bilateral pulmonary hypoplasia in a newborn with extralobar pulmonary sequestration. Acta Paediatr 1993; 82:416–418.

77. Meizner I, Carmi R, Mares AJ, et al. Spontaneous resolution of isolated fetal ascites associated with extralobar lung sequestration. J Clin Ultrasound 1990; 18:57–60.

78. Rheuban KS, McDaniel NL, Feldman PS, et al. Intrapericardial teratoma causing nonimmune hydrops fetalis and pericardial tamponade: a case report. Pediatr Cardiol 1991; 12:54–56.

79. Weinraub Z, Gembruch U, Fodisch HJ, et al. Intrauterine mediastinal teratoma associated with non-immune hydrops fetalis. Prenat Diagn 1989; 9:369–372.

80. Khong TY, Keeling JW. Massive congenital mesenchymal malformation of the lung: another cause of non-immune hydrops. Histopathology 1990; 16:609–611.

81. Franzek DA, Strayer SA, Hull MT, et al. Enteric cyst as a cause of non-immune hydrops fetalis: fetal thoracentesis with a fluid analysis. J Clin Ultrasound 1989; 17:275–279.

82. Chen H, Yang SS, Gonzalez E, et al. Short rib-polydactyly syndrome, Majewski type. Am J Med Genet 1980; 7:215–222.

83. Greenberg CR, Rimoin DL, Gruber HE, et al. A new autosomal recessive lethal chondrodystrophy with congenital hydrops. Am J Med Genet 1988; 29:623–632.

84. Passarge E. Familial occurrence of a short rib syndrome with hydrops fetalis but without polydactyly. Am J Med Genet 1983; 14:403–405.

85. Machin GA, Popkin JS, Zacks D, et al. Case report: fetus with asymmetric parietal encephalocele, and hydrops secondary to laryngeal atresia. Am J Med Genet 1987; 3:311–321.

86. Dubos JP, Bouchez MC, Kacet N, et al. Non-immunologic hydrops fetalis and congenital chylothorax. Arch Fr Pediatr 1985; 42:537–538.

87. Rodeck CH, Fish NM, Fraser DI, et al. Long-term in utero drainage of fetal hydrothorax. N Engl J Med 1988; 319:1135–1138.

88. Sacks LM, Polin JL, Breckenbridge J. Congenital chylothorax presenting as hydrops fetalis. J Reprod Med 1983; 28:341–344.

89. Bianchi DW, Beyer EC, Stark AR, et al. Normal long-term survival with α-thalassemia. J Pediatr 1986; 108:716–718.

90. Liang ST, Wong VCW, So WWK, et al. Homozygous α-thalassemia: clinical presentation, diagnosis and management. A review of 46 cases. Br J Obstet Gynaecol 1985; 92:680–684.

91. Thorp JA, Cohen GR, Yeast JD, et al. Nonimmune hydrops caused by massive fetomaternal hemorrhage and treated by intravascular transfusion. Am J Perinatol 1992; 9:22–24.

92. Gilbert WM, Scioscia AL. Spontaneous fetal-maternal hemorrhage resulting in hydrops and elevated maternal serum α-fetoprotein levels. J Ultrasound Med 1991; 10:645–648.

93. Sherer DM, Abramowicz JS, Ryan RM, et al. Severe fetal hydrops resulting from ABO incompatibility. Obstet Gynecol 1991; 78:897–899.

94. Moise KJ, Carpenter RJ. Increased severity of fetal hemolytic disease with known rhesus alloimmunization after first trimester transcervical chorionic villus biopsy. Fetal Diagn Ther 1990; 5:76–78.

95. Rouse D, Weiner C, Williamson R. Immune hydrops fetalis attributable to anti-HJK. Obstet Gynecol 1990; 76:988–990.

96. Roberts DJ, Nadel A, Lage J, et al. An unusual variant of congenital dyserythropoietic anaemia with mild maternal and lethal fetal disease. Br J Haematol 1993; 84:549–551.

97. Remacha AF, Badell I, Pujol-Moix N, et al. Hydrops fetalis-associated congenital dyserythropoietic anemia treated with intrauterine transfusions and bone marrow transplantation. Blood 2002; 100:356–358.

98. Hennekam RC, Beemer FA, Cats BP, et al. Hydrops fetalis associated with red cell pyruvate kinase deficiency. Genet Genet Couns 1990; 1:75–79.

99. Ravindranath Y, Paglia DE, Warrier I, et al. Glucose phosphate isomerase deficiency as a cause of hydrops fetalis. N Engl J Med 1987; 316:258–261.

100. Bose C. Hydrops fetalis and in utero intracranial hemorrhage. J Pediatr 1978; 93:1023–1024.

101. Gray ES. Mesoblastic nephroma and non-immunologic hydrops. Pediatr Pathol 1989; 9:607–609.

102. Martinez AE, Robinson MJ, Alexis JB, et al. Kaposiform hemangioendothelioma associated with non-immune hydrops fetalis. Arch Pathol Lab Med 2004; 128:678–681.

103. Malloy G, Polinski C, Alkan S, et al. Hemophagocytic lymphohistiocytosis presenting with non-immune hydrops fetalis. J Perinatol 2004; 24:458–460.

104. Vicente-Gutierrez MP, Castello-Almazan I, Salvia-Roiges MD, et al. Non-immune hydrops fetalis due to congenital xerocytosis. J Perinatol 2005; 25:63–65.

105. Arnon S, Tamary H, Dgany O, et al. Hydrops fetalis associated with homozygosity for hemoglobin Taybe (α 38/39 THR deletion) in newborn triplets. Am J Hematol 2004; 76:263–266.

106. Dunbar AE, Moore SL, Hinson RM. Fetal Diamond-Blackfan anemia associated with hydrops fetalis. Am J Perinatol 2003; 20:391–394.

107. Pannier E, Viot G, Aubrey MC, et al. Congenital erythropoietic porphyria (Gunther's disease): two cases with very early manifestation and cystic hygroma. Prenat Diagn 2003; 23:25–30.

108. Mahone PR, Sherer DM, Abramowicz JS, et al. Twin-twin transfusion syndrome: rapid development of severe hydrops of the donor following selective feticide of the hydropic recipient. Am J Obstet Gynecol 1993; 169:166–168.

109. Achiron R, Rabinovitz R, Aboulafia Y, et al. Intrauterine assessment of high-output cardiac failure with spontaneous remission of hydrops fetalis in twin-twin transfusion syndrome: use of two-dimensional echocardiography, Doppler ultrasound, and color flow mapping. J Clin Ultrasound 1992; 20:271–277.

110. Wax JR, Blakemore KJ, Blohm P, et al. Stuck twin with cotwin nonimmune hydrops: successful treatment by amniocentesis. Fetal Diagn Ther 1991; 6:126–131.

111. Gibson JY, D'Cruz CA, Patel RB, et al. Acardiac anomaly: review of the subject with case report and emphasis on practical sonography. J Clin Ultrasound 1986; 14:541–545.

112. Barton JR, Thorpe EM, Shaver DC, et al. Nonimmune hydrops fetalis associated with maternal infection with syphilis. Am J Obstet Gynecol 1992; 167:56–58.

113. Hallak M, Peipert JF, Ludomirski A, et al. Nonimmune hydrops fetalis and fetal congenital syphilis. J Reprod Med 1992; 37:173–176.

114. Greene D, Watson WJ, Wirtz PS. Non-immune hydrops associated with congenital herpes. S D J Med 1993; 46:219–220.

115. Fadel HE, Ruedrich DA. Intrauterine resolution of nonimmune hydrops associated with cytomegalovirus infection. Obstet Gynecol 1988; 71:1003–1005.

116. Gembruch U, Niesen M, Hansmann M, et al. Listeriosis: a cause of non-immune hydrops fetalis. Prenat Diagn 1987; 7:277–282.

117. Zornes SL, Anderson PG, Lott RL. Congenital toxoplasmosis in an infant with hydrops fetalis. South Med J 1988; 81:391–393.

118. Castillo RA, Devoe LD, Hadi HA, et al. Nonimmune hydrops fetalis: clinical experience and factors related to a poor outcome. Am J Obstet Gynecol 1986; 155:812–816.

119. Holzgreve W, Holzgreve B, Curry CJR. Nonimmune hydrops fetalis. Diagnosis and management. Semin Perinatol 1985; 9:52–67.

120. Kim CK, Kim SK, Yang YH, et al. A case of recurrent infantile polycystic kidney associated with hydrops fetalis. Yonsei Med J 1989; 30:95–103.

121. Rosen RS, Bocian ME. Hydrops fetalis in the McKusick-Kaufman syndrome. Am J Obstet Gynecol 1991; 165:102–103.

122. Afifi AM, Bhatia AR, Eyal F. Hydrops fetalis associated with congenital myotonic dystrophy. Am J Obstet Gynecol 1992; 166:929–930.

123. Curry CJ, Chopra D, Finer NN. Hydrops and pleural effusions in congenital myotonic dystrophy. J Pediatr 1988; 113:555–557.

124. Karimi-Nejad M, Khajavi H, Gharavi MJ, et al. Neu-Laxova syndrome: report of a case and comments. Am J Med Genet 1987; 28:17–23.

125. Moerman P, Fryns J-P, Cornelis A, et al. Pathogenesis of the lethal pterygium syndrome. Am J Med Genet 1990; 35:415–421.

126. Sombekke BH, Molenaar WM, van Essen AJ, et al. Lethal congenital muscular dystrophy with arthrogryposis multiplex congenita: three new cases and review of the literature. Pediatric Pathol 1994; 14:277–285.

127. Sun CC. Hydrops fetalis associated with Gaucher disease. Pathol Res Pract 1984; 179:101–104.

128. Meizner I, Levy A, Carmi R, et al. Niemann-Pick disease associated with nonimmune hydrops fetalis. Am J Obstet Gynecol 1990; 163:128–129.

129. Nelson J, Kenny B, O'Hara D, et al. Foamy changes of placental cells in probable β glucuronidase deficiency associated with hydrops fetalis. J Clin Pathol 1993; 46:370–371.

130. Lissens W, Dedobbeleer G, Foulon W, et al. β-glucuronidase deficiency as a cause of prenatally diagnosed non-immune hydrops fetalis. Prenat Diagn 1991; 11:509–512.

131. Stangenberg M, Lingman B, Roberts G, et al. Mucopolysaccharidosis VII as cause of fetal hydrops in early pregnancy. Am J Med Genet 1992; 44:142–144.

132. Burin MG, Scholz AP, Gus R, et al. Investigation of lysosomal storage diseases in nonimmune hydrops fetalis. Prenat Diagn 2004; 24:653–657.

133. Dufke A, Vollmer B, Kendziorra H, et al. Hydrops fetalis in three male fetuses of a female with incontinentia pigmenti. Prenat Diagn 2001; 21:1019–1021.

134. Maeda H, Koyanagi T, Nakano H. Intrauterine treatment of non-immune hydrops fetalis. Early Hum Dev 1992; 29:241–249.

135. Buckshee K, Bhatla N, Paul VK. Successful ultrasound-guided intrauterine blood transfusion in severe non-immune hydrops fetalis. Int J Obstet Gynecol 1990; 32:153–156.

136. Lingman G, Strangenberg M, Legarth J, et al. Albumin transfusion in non-immune hydrops: Doppler ultrasound evaluation of the acute effects on blood circulation in the fetal aorta and the umbilical arteries, Fetal Ther 1989; 4:120–125.

137. Weiner CP, Pelzer GD, Heilskov J, et al. The effect of intravascular trans-fusion on umbilical venous pressure in anemic fetuses with and without hydrops. Am J Obstet Gynecol 1989; 161:1498–1501.

Cystic hygroma: Nuchal edema

138. van der Putte SCJ. The development of the lymphatic system in man. Adv Anat Embryol Cell Biol 1975; 51:3–60.

139. Schulman LP, Emerson DS, Felker RE, et al. High frequency of cytogenetic abnormalities in fetuses with cystic hygroma diagnosed in the first trimester. Obstet Gynecol 1992; 80:80–82.

140. Gembruch U, Hansmann M, Bauld R, et al. Prenatal diagnosis and management in fetuses with cystic hygroma colli. Eur J Obstet Gynecol Rep Biol 1988; 29:241–255.

141. Chervenak FA, Isaacson G, Blakemore KJ, et al. Fetal cystic hygroma. Cause and natural history. N Engl J Med 1983; 309:822–825.

142. Kalousek DK, Seller MJ. Differential diagnosis of posterior cystic hygroma in previable fetuses. Am J Obstet Gynecol 1987; 3(suppl):83–92.

143. Pijpers L, Reuss A, Stewart PA, et al. Fetal cystic hygroma: prenatal diagnosis and management. Obstet Gynecol 1988; 72:223–224.

144. Garden AS, Benzie RJ, Miskin M, et al. Fetal cystic hygroma colli: antenatal diagnosis, significance and management. Am J Obstet Gynecol 1986; 154:221–225.

145. Schwanitz G, Zerres K, Gembruch U, et al. Rate of chromosomal aberrations in prenatally detected hydrops fetalis and hygroma colli. Hum Genet 1989; 84:81–82.

146. Nicolaides KH, Rodeck CH, Gosden CM. Rapid karyotyping in non-lethal fetal malformations. Lancet 1991; i:283.

147. Johnson MP, Johnson A, Holzgreve W, et al. First-trimester simple hygroma: cause and outcome. Am J Obstet Gynecol 1993; 168:156–161.

148. Redford DHA, McNay MR, Fergusson-Smith ME, et al. Aneuploidy and cystic hygroma detectable by ultrasound. Prenat Diagn 1984; 4:377–382.

149. Nicolaides KH, Azar G, Byrne D, et al. Fetal nuchal translucency: ultrasound screening for chromosomal defects in first trimester pregnancies. BMJ 1992; 304:867–869.

150. Marchese C, Savin E, Dragone E, et al. Cystic hygroma: prenatal diagnosis and genetic counseling. Prenat Diagn 1985; 5:221–227.

151. Abramowicz JS, Warsof SL, Doyle DL, et al. Congenital cystic hygroma of the neck diagnosed prenatally: outcome with normal and abnormal karyotype. Prenat Diagn 1989; 9:321–327.

152. Byrne J, Blanc WA, Warburton D, et al. The significance of cystic hygroma in fetuses. Hum Pathol 1984; 15:61–67.

153. Suchet IB, van der Westhuizen NG, Labatte MF. Fetal cystic hygromas: further insights into their natural history. Can Assoc Radiol J 1992; 43:420–424.

154. van Zalen-Sproch RM, van Vugt JM, van Geijn HP. First-trimester diagnosis of cystic hygroma – course and prognosis. Am J Obstet Gynecol 1992; 167:94–98.

155. Ville Y, Borghi E, Pons JC, et al. Fetal karyotype from cystic hygroma fluid. Prenat Diagn 1992; 12:139–143.

156. Droste S, Hendricks SK, Von Alfrey H, et al. Cystic hygroma colli: perinatal outcome after prenatal diagnosis. J Perinat Med 1991; 19:449–454.

157. Bernstein HS, Filly RA, Goldberg JD, et al. Prognosis of fetuses with cystic hygroma. Prenat Diagn 1991; 11:349–355.

158. Macleod AM, McHugo JM. Prenatal diagnosis of nuchal cystic hygroma. Br J Radiol 1991; 64:802–807.

159. Douvier S, Feldman JP, Nivelon-Chevalier A, et al. Retrocervical cystic hygro-ma: a series of 13 cases. J Gynecol Obstet Biol Reprod Paris 1991; 20:183–190.

160. Cullen MT, Gabrielli S, Green JJ, et al. Diagnosis and significance of cystic hygroma in the first trimester. Prenat Diagn 1990; 10:643–651.

161. Langer JC, Fitzgerald PG, Desa D, et al. Cervical cystic hygroma in the fetus: clinical spectrum and outcome. J Pediatr Surg 1990; 25:58–61.

162. Tannirandorn Y, Nicolini U, Nicolaidis PC, et al. Fetal cystic hygromata; insights gained from fetal blood sampling. Prenat Diagn 1990; 10:189–193.

163. Miyabara S, Sugihara H, Maehara N, et al. Significance of cardiovascular malformation in cystic hygroma: a new interpretation of the pathogenesis. Am J Med Genet 1989; 34:489–501.

164. Bronshtein M, Rottem S, Yoffe N, et al. First-trimester and early second-trimester diagnosis of nuchal cystic hygroma by transvaginal sonography: diverse prognosis of the septated from the nonseptated lesion. Am J Obstet Gynecol 1989; 161:78–82.

165. Pons JC, Diallo AA, Eydoux P, et al. Chorionic villus sampling after first trimester diagnosis of fetal cystic hygroma colli. Eur J Obstet Gynecol Reprod Biol 1989; 33:141–146.

166. Friese K, Merz E. Sonographic detection of hygroma colli in the fetus. Ultraschall Med 1989; 10:25–28.

167. Chitayat D, Kalousek DK, Bamforth JS. Lymphatic abnormalities in fetuses with posterior cervical cystic hygroma. Am J Med Genet 1989; 33:352–356.

168. Trauffer PML, Anderson CE, Johnson A, et al. The natural history of euploid pregnancies with first trimester cystic hygromas. Am J Obstet Gynecol 1994; 170:1279–1284.

169. Toftager-Larsen K, Benzie RJ, Donan TA, et al. α fetoprotein and ultrasound scanning in the prenatal diagnosis of Turner's syndrome. Prenat Diag 1983; 3:35–40.

170. Nadel A, Bromley B, Benacerraf BR. Nuchal thickening or cystic hygromas in first- and early second-trimester fetuses: prognosis and outcome. Obstet Gynecol 1993; 82:43–48.

171. Nicolaides KH, Azar G, Snijders RT, et al. Fetal nuchal edema: associated malformations and chromosomal defects. Fetal Diagn Ther 1992; 7:123–131.

172. Pearce JM, Griffin D, Campbell S. The differential prenatal diagnosis of cystic hygromata and encephalocoele by ultrasound examination. J Clin Ultrasound 1985; 13:317–320.

173. Schulte-Vallentin M, Schindler H. Non-echogenic nuchal edema as a marker in trisomy 21. Lancet 1992; 339:1053.

174. Witt DR, Hoyme HE, Zonana J, et al. Lymphedema in Noonan syndrome: clues to pathogenesis and prenatal diagnosis and review of the literature. Am J Med Genet 1987; 27:841–856.

175. Sonesson SE, Fouron JC, Lessard M. Intrauterine diagnosis and evolution of a cardiomyopathy in a fetus with Noonan's syndrome. Acta Paediatr 1992; 81:368–370.

176. Donnenfeld AE, Nazir MA, Sindoni F, et al. Prenatal sonographic documentation of cystic hygroma regression in Noonan syndrome. Am J Med Genet 1991; 139:461–465.

177. Spearritt DJ, Tannenberg AE, Payton DJ. Lethal multiple pterygium syndrome: report of a case with neurological anomalies. Am J Med Genet 1993; 47:45–49.

178. Moerman P, Fryns JP, Cornelis A, et al. Pathogenesis of the lethal multiple pterygium syndrome. Am J Med Genet 1990; 35:415–421.

179. Bulas DI, Saal HM, Allen JF, et al. Cystic hygroma and congenital diaphragmatic hernia: early prenatal sonographic evaluation of Fryns' syndrome. Prenat Diagn 1992; 12:867–875.

180. Wenstrom KD, Williamson RA, Hoover WW, et al. Achondrogenesis type II (Langer-Saldino) in association with jugular lymphatic obstruction sequence. Prenat Diagn 1989; 9:527–532.

181. Bruner JP, Hsia YE. Prenatal findings in Brachmann-de Lange syndrome. Obstet Gynecol 1990; 76:966–968.

182. Ramsing M, Rehder H, Holzgreve W, et al. Fraser syndrome (cryptophthalmos with syndactyly) in the fetus and newborn. Clin Genet 1990; 37:84–96.

183. Patil SR, Weiner C, Williamson R. Rapid chromosome analysis and prenatal diagnosis using fluid from cystic hygromas. N Engl J Med 1987; 317:1159–1160.

184. Golden WL, Schneider BF, Gustashaw KM, et al. Prenatal diagnosis of Turner syndrome using cells cultivated from cystic hygromas in two pregnancies with normal serum α-fetoprotein. Prenat Diag 1989; 9:683–689.

185. Platt LD, De Vore GR, Horenstein J, et al. Performing cytogenetic studies on ascites, amniotic, and hygroma fluid. J Reprod Med 1990; 35:1145–1146.

Fetal hydrothorax

186. Pijpers L, Reuss A, Stewart PA, et al. Noninvasive management of isolated bilateral fetal hydrothorax. Am J Obstet Gynecol 1989; 161:330–332.

187. Picone O, Benachi A, Mandelbrot L, et al. Thoracoamniotic shunting for fetal pleural effusions with hydrops. Am J Obstet Gynecol 2004; 191:2047–2050.

188. Blaicher W, Hausler M, Gembruch U, et al. Feto-amniotic shunting – experience of six centres. Ultraschall Med 2005; 26:134–141.

189. Mandelbrot L, Dommergues M, Aubry MC, et al. Reversal of fetal distress by emergency in utero decompression of hydrothorax. Am J Obstet Gynecol 1992; 167:1278–1283.

190. Longaker MT, Laberge JM, Dansereau J, et al. Primary fetal hydrothorax: natural history and management. J Pediatr Surg 1989; 24:573–576.

191. Brus F, Nikkels PG, van Loon AJ, et al. Non-immune hydrops fetalis and bilateral pulmonary hypoplasia in a newborn with extralobar pulmonary sequestration. Acta Paediatr 1993; 82:416–418.

192. Hernandez-Schulman M, Stein SM, Neblett WW, et al. Pulmonary sequestration: diagnosis with color Doppler sonography and a new theory of associated hydrothorax. Radiology 1991; 180:817–821.

193. Slotnick RN, McGahan J, Milio L, et al. Antenatal diagnosis and treatment of fetal bronchopulmonary sequestration. Fetal Diagn Ther 1990; 5:33–39.

194. Franzek DA, Strayer SA, Hull MT, et al. Enteric cyst as a cause of non-immune hydrops fetalis: fetal thoracocentesis with fluid analysis. J Clin Ultrasound 1989; 17:275–279.

195. Weber AM, Philipson EH. Fetal pleural effusion: a review and meta-analysis for prognostic factors. Obstet Gynecol 1992; 79:281–286.

196. Bigras JL, Ryan G, Suda K, et al. Echocardiographic evaluation of fetal hydrothorax: the effusion ratio as a diagnostic tool. Ultrasound Obstet Gynecol 2003; 21:37–40.

197. Yancey MK, Brady K, Read JA. Sonographic evidence of fetal hydrothorax after in-utero death of monozygotic twin. J Clin Ultrasound 1991; 19:162–166.

Fetal pericardial effusions

198. Chan BB, Murphy MC, Rodgers BM. Management of chylopericardium. J Pediatr Surg 1990; 25:1185–1189.

199. Reynolds JL, Donahue JK, Pearce CW. Intrapericardial teratoma: a cause of acute pericardial effusion in infancy. Pediatrics 1969; 43:71–78.

200. Iliff PJ, Eyre JA, Westaby S, et al. Neonatal pericardial effusion associated with central eventration of the diaphragm. Arch Dis Child 1983; 58:147–149.

Fetal ascites

201. Machin GA. Diseases causing fetal and neonatal ascites. Pediatr Pathol 1985; 4:195–211.

202. Favre R, Dreux S, Dommergues M, et al. Nonimmune fetal ascites: A series of 79 cases. Am J Obstet Gynecol 2004; 190:407–412.

203. Greenberg F, Copeland K, Gresik MV. Expanding the spectrum of Perlman syndrome. Am J Med Genet 1988; 29:773–776.

204. Winn HN, Stiller R, Grannum PA, et al. Isolated fetal ascites: prenatal diagnosis and management. Am J Perinatol 1990; 7:370–373.

205. Sarno AP, Bruner JP, Southgate WM. Congenital chyloperitoneum as a cause of isolated fetal ascites. Obstet Gynecol 1990; 76:955–957.

206. Chalubinski K, Deutinger J, Bernaschek G. Meconium peritonitis: extrusion of meconium and different sonographical appearances in relation to the stage of the disease. Prenat Diagn 1992; 12:631–636.

207. Macek M Jr, Macek M, Stuhrmann M, et al. The direct early diagnosis of cystic fibrosis by the detection of the δ F508 CFTR gene mutation in a prematurely delivered boy. Clin Genet 1991; 39:219–222.

208. Chilukuri S, Bonet V, Cobb M. Antenatal spontaneous perforation of the extrahepatic biliary tree. Am J Obstet Gynecol 1990; 163:1201–1202.

209. Sun CC, Keene CL, Nagey DA. Hepatic fibrosis in congenital cytomegalovirus infection: with fetal ascites and pulmonary hypoplasia. Pediatr Pathol 1990; 10:641–646.

210. Aylsworth AS, Thomas GH, Hood JL, et al. A severe infantile sialidosis: clinical, biochemical and microscopic features. J Pediatr 1980; 96:662–668.

211. Abu-Dalu KI, Tamary H, Livni N, et al. GM1 gangliosidosis presenting as neonatal ascites. J Pediatr 1982; 100:940–943.

212. Ghishan FK, Gray GF, Greene IIL. α 1-antitrypsin deficiency presenting with ascites and cirrhosis in the neonatal period. Gastroenterology 1983; 85:435–438.

213. Gillan JE, Lowden JA, Gaskin K, et al. Congenital ascites as a presenting sign of lysosomal storage disease. J Pediatr 1984; 104:225–231.

214. Hancock LW, Thaler MM, Horowitz AJ, et al. Generalized N-acetylneuraminic acid storage disease: quantitation and identification of the monosaccharide accumulating in brain and other tissues. J Neurochem 1982; 38:803–809.

215. Maconochie IK, Chong S, Mieli-Vergani G, et al. Fetal ascites: an unusual presentation of Niemann-Pick disease type C. Arch Dis Child 1989; 64:1391–1393.

216. Ben-Haroush A, Yogev Y, Levit D, et al. Isolated fetal ascites caused by Wolman disease. Ultrasound Obstet Gynecol 2003; 21:297–298.

217. Straub W, Zarabi M, Mazer J. Fetal ascites associated with Conradi's disease (chondrodysplasia punctata): report of a case. J Clin Ultrasound 1983; 11:234–236.

218. Thomas IT, Frias JL, Felix V, et al. Isolated and syndromal cryptophthalmos. Am J Med Genet 1986; 25:85–98.

Multiple pregnancies and conjoined twins

9

Geoffrey A. Machin

'What is the use of going to bed early to save money on candles, when the result is twins?'

Ancient Chinese Proverb

The perinatal pathologist has at least four roles in the documentation of biology and pathology of multiple birth:

- Twins make up an excessive component of perinatal deaths,[1-3] the mechanisms of which are to be elucidated.
- In many institutions all placentas of twins and higher-multiple pregnancies are examined by pathologists.[1,4] Clinicopathologic analysis yields information about normal and abnormal outcomes of multiple pregnancy.
- In some multiple pregnancies knowledge of the sex of the multiple set and anatomy of the placenta(s) allow statements about zygosity.
- In an ideal setting, and at little expense, the zygosity of all like-sex (LS) multiples can be determined at birth, using DNA from placental tissues.[5]

This gives valuable biological information to parents and the multiples themselves, as well as laying a firm baseline for genetic and other studies in twins and multiples.

The biology of twinning seems complex, and there is a limited correlation between zygosity and placentation (i.e. chorionicity and amnionicity). However, simple rules solve many of these problems, although there are exceptions to all rules.

Obstetric problems are common to all multiple pregnancies. The major problem is preterm delivery; in many cases this simply reflects the increased mass and volume of the pregnancy,[6] which affects maternal physiology both through hyperplacentosis and toxemia, and because of increased myometrial irritability, cervical dilatation, ascending infection, and premature membrane rupture. But multiple pregnancies containing monochorionic (MC) twins have six- to tenfold rates of these complications in comparison with dichorionic (DC) multiple pregnancies.[1,7-11] In clinical practice, research, and publication, multiple pregnancies are often regarded as a homogeneous group of high-risk pregnancies. This is far from the truth, since **MC pregnancies constitute a very high risk subgroup.** Chorionicity can be diagnosed with some accuracy by first trimester obstetric ultrasound and can be recognized by the pathologist examining placentas.

Dizygotic (DZ) twinning is now understood as often being due to an increased tendency (inherited via the female line) for **simultaneous polyovulation.** However, the genesis of monozygotic (MZ) twinning is far from clear. The perinatal pathologist can provide important materials to investigate this matter. There are several known mechanisms whereby MZ twin pairs may be very dissimilar both in genotype and phenotype. Accurate placental examination and retention of tissues for chromosome and DNA analysis offer opportunities to put these rare cases of MZ discordance into the general context of MZ twinning. The perinatal pathologist can contribute to twin studies by comprehensive and careful studies of multiple pregnancies.

Zygosity in twins and higher-order multiples

There are two main types of twins, MZ and DZ. A third type of twin (so-called polar body twin) may exist, but data are fragmentary. Higher-multiple pregnancies, whether spontaneously conceived (SC) or assisted reproduction (AR), comprise combinations of MZ and DZ twins, triplets, and so forth.

The prevalence of multiple pregnancy varies as to time and place. **The prevalence of SC MZ twins is constant worldwide,** and geographic and ethnic differences in overall prevalence of multiple pregnancy are caused by variations in the prevalence of DZ twinning. Thus in areas with high twinning rates, such as Nigeria, there is a high proportion of DZ twins.[12] In Japan, with a low overall prevalence of twins, the proportion of MZ twins is higher. However, the prevalence of MZ twins varies with time, and there has been a recent slight increase.[13] These considerations apply to SC multiples and are confounded by AR cases.

DZ twins and multiples may be monopaternal or heteropaternal. Several cases of heteropaternal twins have been ascertained by multiple antigen testing and/or DNA testing.[14]

Distinction between spontaneous and induced multiple pregnancies

Since the mid-1980s the numbers of AR multiple pregnancies have increased through the use of ovulation induction, in vitro fertilization, and related procedures.[15] Selective reduction of higher-multiple pregnancies can then be used to bring down the number of fetuses to triplets and twins. In the current literature an optimistic prognosis is given for higher-multiple pregnancies; this is largely because most of these pregnancies are the result of AR.[16] There is a low proportion of MZ, including MC, twins in AR higher multiples, with a corresponding low mortality. However, the prevalence of MZ and MC twins is far from negligible in AR multiples; approximately 10% of AR twins are MZ.[17, 18]

In SC higher-order multiple pregnancies (HOMPs), the majority contain an MZ twin pair, and MC twins are frequently present. SC HOMPs therefore carry high risks because of the multiple fetuses, added to which are the risks inherent in MC twinning.

Prevalence of monozygotic and dizygotic twins

In white populations 30–40% of SC twins are MZ.[1, 19] About one-third of MZ twins are DC, fused or separate, whereas two-thirds of MZ twins are MC. All but a few of these are diamniotic (DA). A small proportion of MC twins are also monoamniotic (MA) (Fig. 9.1). They are at high risk for fetal death through intertwining of their cords. Thus about one-eighth of DC twins are MZ, and one-quarter of like-sex (LS), DC twins are MZ.

The Weinberg law allows the calculation of MZ and DZ frequencies in twin populations; it is assumed that DZ twins contain equal proportions of LS and unlike-sex (ULS) twins; therefore the excess of LS twins gives the prevalence of MZ twins in that population. This law is widely used, but its validity has been questioned.[20] There appears to be an excess of LS over

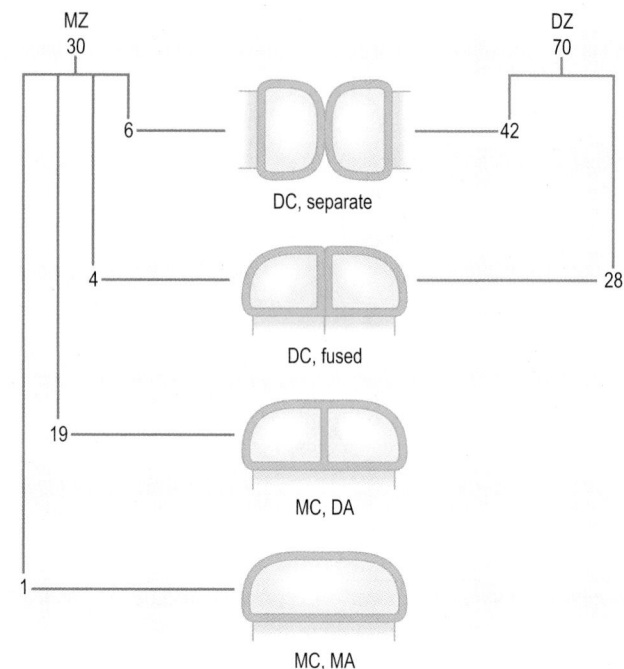

FIGURE 9.1 Diagrammatic representation of approximate distribution of twin zygosity by type of placentation. (After Benirschke and Kim 1973,[27] with permission.)

ULS twins in DZ twin pairs, and this can lead to overestimation of MZ twin frequency. In twin research that depends on precise diagnosis of zygosity and chorionicity, the use of the Weinberg law is inappropriate.

Zygosity testing

Because of variation from the Weinberg law – which, in any case, cannot be applied to individual cases – some researchers advocate that zygosity testing be carried out on all LS twins and multiplets at birth.[5] In the past multiple gene products were used to search for discordance within a pair, thus proving them DZ. The preferred method was a **DNA restriction fragment length polymorphism (RFLP) testing** (Fig. 9.2), which has now been replaced by a PCR-based search for polymorphisms. This method looks for discordance in pairs between variable number tandem repeats (VNTRs) and other polymorphisms at many sites in the genome.[5, 21–26] The method can be applied to **any tissue including blood, placental tissues, tissues obtained at autopsy, and cells swabbed from buccal mucosa.** DNA is well preserved in the event of fetal death[22] and has even been extracted successfully from fetus papyraceus. If necessary, it can also be used in prenatal diagnosis[24] (Fig. 9.3). DNA studies have been important in indicating some of the possible stimuli of MZ twinning. Although it can be assumed that almost **all MC twins are MZ,** there is sufficient interest in the causation of MZ and MC twinning that DNA could be stored from such twin as well as

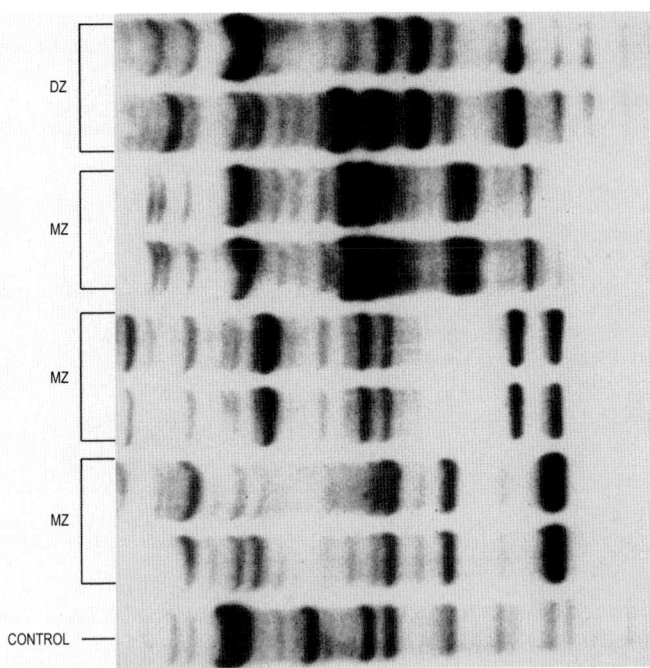

FIGURE 9.2 Diagnosis of zygosity by DNA RFLP testing using probes for VNTRs.

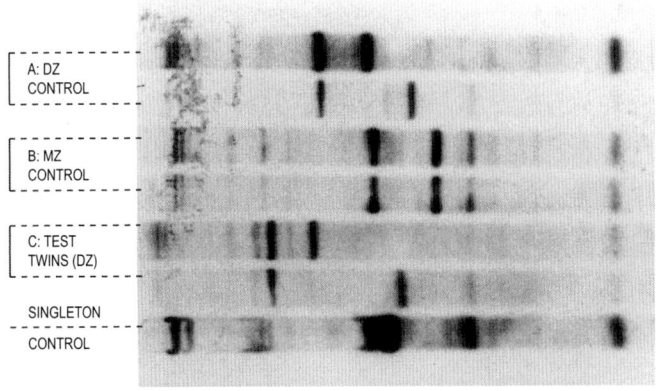

FIGURE 9.3 Prenatal zygosity testing, using amniocytes from each sac, in a twin pregnancy of unknown chorionicity. The twins were like-sexed and one was dying with poor biophysical profiles. The twins were proven to be DZ, hence DC. It was safe to allow one twin to die in utero at 26 weeks of gestation, the pregnancy then continuing to 34 weeks, with intact survival of the second twin.

from LS DC twins. It has recently been found that IVF twins may merge their trophoblast to form an MC placenta, whereas the twins are DZ[25]. It has long been suspected that some DZ twin pairs are more similar than would be expected. It is now clear, from a single case report[25a], that some DZ twins may share their maternal genotype as a result of some type of abnormal splitting of the oocyte and fertilization of the products by 2 sperm. The reported pair were male/female with true hermaphroditism in the girl, and placental anatomy is not known. The frequency of this phenomenon in anatomically normal male/male and female/female pairs remains to be determined.

It is not clear whether zygosity testing will become a routine part of the management of multiple pregnancy and its products, but accurate data are sometimes required for medical and/or research purposes.

Causes of monozygotic twinning

Strictly, MZ twins are the only true twins. They arise from a single zygote at varying intervals between conception (zygosis) and the laying down of the major body axes (e.g. notochord) at about 14 days post conception (pc).[27, 28] To produce twins of roughly appropriate birth weight, the whole conception goes through one extra mitotic cell division and/or less apoptosis. It should not be presumed that equal numbers of blastomeres are allocated to each twin.

It is proposed that the timing of the MZ twinning event, at any time from 0 to 14 days pc, determines the placentation of the twins.[27] Early twinning results in DC placentas that may be separate or fused. It has been reported that there is an excess of fused over separate DC, MZ placentas compared with fused and separate DZ placentas;[4] since the twins are derived from one zygote and travel down the same oviduct, they may therefore be likely to implant close together. Later MZ twinning, after the separation of the inner cell mass from the trophoblast, results in MC, MZ twins. Most MZ twins fall into this category. A later twinning event after the amniotic cavity has separated from the embryo results in MA twins. **Conjoined twinning** represents an incomplete form of twinning in which the limits of a single embryonic zone have been set by one embryonic disk, but an attempt is then made to form two major body axes within that zone. **Conjoined twins (CTs) characteristically have MC, MA placentation.**

Each of these events could have different or overlapping etiologies, but information is scarce. However, there are clear indications that some MZ twin pairs are genotypically and phenotypically discordant; these discordances may be either causes or effects of the twinning event.

Discordance for congenital anomalies and genetic diseases in MZ twins may be classified into three groups.[29]

- **those disorders that are certainly intrinsic to the twinning event itself,** for example, holoacardius acephalus [twin reversed arterial perfusion (TRAP)], conjoined twinning, and mechanical deformation secondary to intrauterine crowding;
- **those epigenetic events that might cause MZ twinning,** for example, postzygotic events leading to discordance for chromosome status, trinucleotide repeat sequence expansion, imprinting and X chromosome inactivation status; and
- **those disorders that might represent cause or effect in MZ twinning,** for example, discordance for major anomalies such as renal agenesis, holoprosencephaly, symmelia, neural tube defect, and amniotic band syndrome.

Although several pathways may lead to the MZ twinning event, intrinsic and extrinsic mechanisms may be considered.

TABLE 9.1 MZ TWIN PAIRS DISCORDANT FOR X-CHROMOSOME ANEUPLOIDY

Author	Twin A fibroblasts	Twin B fibroblasts	Blood chimerism
Edwards et al[31]	UT 45,X	NM 45,X	46,X/46,XY
Karp et al[32]	UT 45,X/46	XY,NM	45,X/46,XY
Schmidt et al[33]	UT 45,X	NM 46,XY	None
Reindollar et al[34]	UT 45,X/46	XY NM 45,X/46,XY	?
Arizawa et al[35]	UT 45,X	NM 46,XY	None
Turpin et al[36]	UT 45,X	NM 46,XY	—
Perlman et al[37]	UT 45,X	NM 46,XY	?
Dallapicolla et al[38]	UT 45,X	NM x 2 (triplets) 46,XY	—
Kurosawa et al[39]	UT 45,X/47,XXY	45,X/47,XXY	—
Deacon et al[40]	TRAP, features UT 45,X	NF pump twin 46,XX	45,X/46,XX
Pedersen et al[41]	UT 45,X	NF	—
Ross et al[42]	UT 45,X/47,XXX	NF 45,X/47,XXX	—
Kaplowitz et al[43]	UT 45,X	NF 46,XX	45,X/46,XX
Neilson et al[44]	UT 45,X	NF 46,XX	—

UT, Ullrich-Turner phenotype; NM, normal male phenotype; NF, normal female phenotype.

Early postzygotic epigenetic events may result in two distinct cell populations in one zygote. These two clones may 'recognize and repel' each other, leading to aggregations of the two cell lines into separate embryonic organization centers and the genesis of MZ twins. Postzygotic events found in discordant MZ twins include chromosomal changes and variations in the patterns of X chromosome inactivation in MZ female twin pairs. Discordance for mutation leading to single gene disease in one MZ twin has recently been described.[30] The range and variety of discordant epigenetic effects within MZ twin pairs offers a valuable window on these events occurring in mitosis.

Discordance for chromosomal abnormality has been reported frequently in MZ twin pairs[31–44] (Table 9.1). The most striking cases involve discordance for external genital development. Thus a 46,XY zygote with a 46,XY and 45,X MZ mosaic twin pair have the result of a genitally normal male and genitally female twin with features of monosomy X (Turner syndrome). It would be theoretically possible for a 47,XXY zygote to result in MZ twins who have 46,XX and 46,XY karyotypes, through two separate non-disjunctional events.

Chromosomal mosaicism in MZ twins probably arises later than the first one to five postzygotic mitotic divisions. In these circumstances at least one of the twins will have two cell lines, implying the incorporation of one or both cell lines into one or both embryos. However, there are two reported cases in which each MZ twin apparently showed no mosaicism, implying that non-disjunction may have occurred at the first postzygotic cell division.

Because most MZ twins are MC, many with interfetal vascular anastomoses, the presence of two cell lines in the blood of a twin may result from the **transfusion of stem cells from the heterokaryotypic co-twin.** Ideally such twins should be investigated also in fixed somatic cell lines such as skin fibroblasts. The banking of placental tissues at birth would aid in these studies.

Heterokaryotypia is frequent in the context of *TRAP*. Although there is no constant pattern, 46,XX or XY/45,X twin mosaicism

has been found more than once. These chromosomally abnormal TRAP cases may represent a subgroup in which the *acardiac fetus* has a primary lethal developmental abnormality, perhaps cardiac; if the fetus were a singleton, fetal death would ensue, but the chromosomally normal pump twin supports the acardiac fetus.

In humans, **X-chromosome inactivation** probably occurs during the **2nd week post conception,** at the 'inner cell mass' (ICM) stage.[45, 46] It is normally nearly random in chromosomally normal females. Very occasionally, females who are heterozygous for X-linked recessive disease (e.g. hemophilia) may actually manifest the disease. In such cases there may be marked skewing of the inactivation of the X chromosome, with the majority of the inactivated X chromosomes carrying the normal allele. Non-random skewing of X-inactivation also occurs in X-autosome translocations. The excessive expression of the mutation-bearing allele on the other X chromosome leads to clinical disease.

Non-random inactivation has been reported several times in female MZ twin pairs (Table 9.2; Fig. 9.4).[47–57] In one type of non-random X-inactivation, there are two cell populations in the zygote, showing reciprocal patterns of X-inactivation. If this process occurs before the twinning event, the two cell populations might form distinct clones and result in two embryonic organizing centers. In the second pattern the cells of one MZ twin show random X-chromosome inactivation, while the co-twin has non-random X-chromosome inactivation, with an excess of activated chromosomes carrying the mutant gene. The cell clones derived from the two cell types are larger in the diseased twin than in normal heterozygous females; the diseased twin may have arisen from a relatively small number of cells and these cells have undergone extra mitoses to reach an almost appropriate body size. This pattern may be due to an extrinsic event leading to unequal allocation of cells from the inner cell mass to the twin pair, after X-inactivation has occurred; such an event could result from the separation of a small segment of cells of the ICM, or the late development of a second organizing primitive streak, accounting

TABLE 9.2 NON-RANDOM X-INACTIVATION IN FEMALE MZ TWIN PAIRS DISCORDANT FOR PHENOTYPIC EXPRESSION OF X-LINKED DISEASES

Author	Disease	Affected twin DNA source		Normal twin DNA source		Possible mechanism
		F	L	F	L	
Tuckerman et al[47]	XLMR	–	Sk to wild	–	Sk to mutant	RSk, pre-T
Burn et al[48]	DMD	Sk to wild	–	Sk to mutant	–	RSk, pre-T
Richards et al[49]	DMD	Sk to wild	Sk to wild	Sk to mutant	Sk to mutant	RSk, pre-T
Lupski et al[50]	DMD	–	Sk to wild	–	R	UBA, post-T
Abbadi et al[51]	DMD	–	Sk to wild	–	Sk to mutant	RSk, pre-T
Jorgensen et al[52]	RGCB	Sk to wild	R	Sk to mutant	R	UBA post-T, blood chimerism
Winchester et al[53]	Hunter	Sk to wild	Sk to wild	–	R	UBA, post-T
Kruyer et al[54]	XLMR	–	Sk to wild	–	Sk to mutant	RSk, pre-T
Levade et al[55]	Fabry	–	Sk to wild	–	Sk to mutant	RSk, pre-T

F, Fibroblasts; L, leukocytes; XLMR, X-linked mental retardation; Sk, skewed; RSk, reciprocal skewed X-inactivation; pre-T, occurs before twinning; DMD, Duchenne muscular dystrophy; R, random X-inactivation; UBA, unequal blastomere allocation; post-T, occurs after twinning; RGCB, red–green color blindness.

TABLE 9.3 PATTERNS OF X-INACTIVATION IN FEMALE TWINS AND TRIPLETS WITHOUT X-LINKED DISEASES

Twin group	X-Inactivation pattern		
	% Random	% Non-random	(%) Total
Dizygotic	21 (95)	1 (5)	22 (100)
Monozygotic, dichorionic	21 (78)	6 (22)	27 (100)
Monozygotic, monochorionic	72 (85)	13 (15)	85 (100)
All monozygotic twins	93 (83)	19 (17)	112 (100)
All twins	114 (85)	20 (15)	134 (100)

for the fact that this segment of cells shows a clonal X-inactivation, resulting in that female having a skewed inactivation pattern.

The striking finding in female MZ twins heterozygous for X-linked diseases is that there have been no reported cases in which both twins are affected by the disease, nor any in which both twins are unaffected. This has led to the hypothesis that **X-inactivation events may be causally linked to twinning in all female MZ twins.** X-inactivation patterns have therefore been analyzed in female MZ twins who are not heterozygous for X-linked diseases; these studies show that random X-inactivation is the most usual pattern, although non-random patterns do occur infrequently (Table 9.3). The mutated genes may themselves somehow cause non-random X-inactivation, but X-inactivation is most commonly random in female MZ twins without X-chromosome gene mutations.

Patterns of X-chromosome inactivation in MZ twins of various chorionic patterns broadly confirm the timing of MZ twinning events in relation to X-inactivation.[58, 59]

The third type of twin

Whereas normal spermatogenesis yields four gametes per primordial germ cell, oogenesis normally results in a single ovum capable of zygosis. The first and second polar bodies represent unequal divisions of oocytic cytoplasm containing the other chromosomal products of first and second meiotic division. Because of recombination (crossing-over) during first meiotic division, the genetic constitutions of the first polar body and secondary oocyte are different; the ovum and second polar body are likewise genetically different, especially for loci remote from the centromeres. Furthermore, fertilization of a first polar body would produce a triploid zygote.

Some DZ twin pairs show closer genetic and phenotypic similarity than others; these might be derived from the same primary oocyte. Such twins have been termed **monovular,** although they may not be truly derived from a single ovum; **mono-oocytic** would be the preferred term. There have been few formal molecular studies of candidates for mono-oocytic twinning, and there are only two fully reported cases.[60, 61] The other examples may represent chance events in which two oocytes have segregated rather similar maternal genomes in their haploid chromosome sets; this happens by chance in successive singleton siblings and is more likely when the mother is homozygous for several of the commonly tested gene products. In the two cases reported[60, 61] the twin pairs were both MC. If the third type of twin does exist, the phenomenon is probably rare. No cases have been documented in the era of DNA-based genetic testing.

Obstetric complications and perinatal mortality in multiple pregnancy

The major complication of twin and multifetal pregnancy is **preterm delivery.** The precipitating factors are **preterm labor, pregnancy-induced hypertension, hydramnios, premature ruptured membranes, and fetal death** (Table 9.4).[62–64] Because of predicted adverse outcomes, many MC twin pregnancies are induced prematurely [e.g. twin-to-twin transfusion (TTT), TRAP, severe growth discordance]. Perinatal mortality in SC twin pregnancies is 6–10 times that for singletons and residual neonatal morbidity is also high, although not significantly higher than for singletons of similar gestational age. As shown in Table 9.4, most of these complications are more frequent in

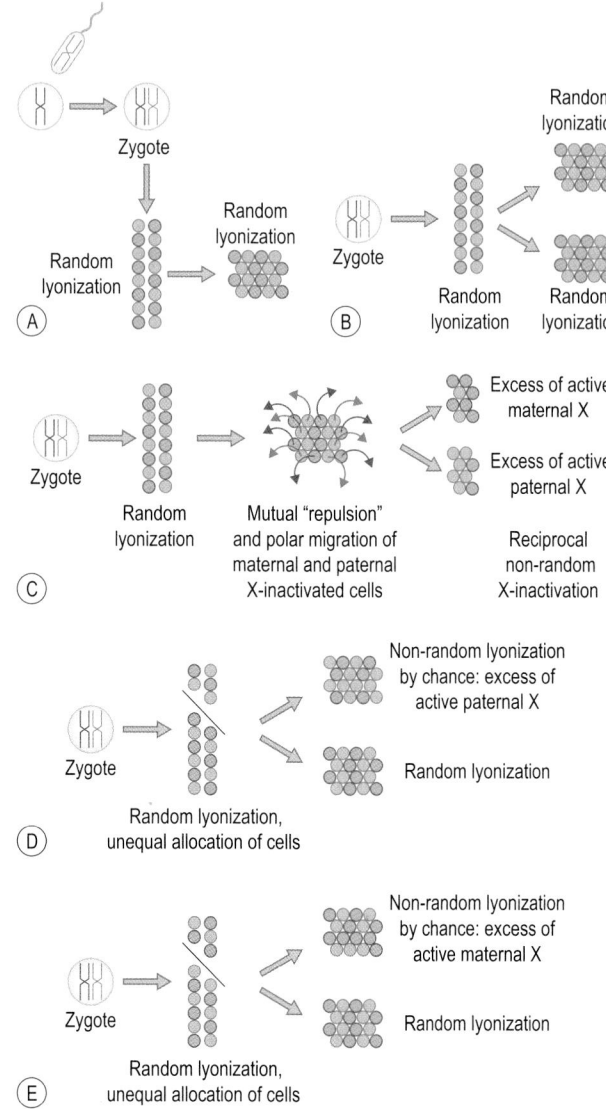

TABLE 9.4 MAJOR COMPLICATIONS (PERCENTAGE) IN TWIN PREGNANCY

Complication	Singleton	Monozygotic twin	Dizygotic twin
Preterm labor	8.4	48	40
Pregnancy-induced hypertension	8.2	18	27
Gestational diabetes	10	8.9	8.7
Pyelonephritis	4.1	4.2	3.0
Spontaneous premature membrane rupture	4.0	3.1	2.4
Anemia	3.5	2.6	2.4
Fetal death	1.0	6.8	2.8
Third trimester hemorrhage	2.8	1.5	2.3
Congenital malformation	2.4	9.4	7.3
Mean birth weight (g)	3297	2358	2430
Neonatal death	5.6	34	33

After Kovacs et al 1989,[62] Spellacy et al 1990,[63] and Fabre et al 1988,[64] with permission.

TABLE 9.5 PLACENTAL ANATOMY IN 2029 TWIN PAIRS

	Number	Percentage
Dichorionic	1515	74.7
Monochorionic, diamniotic	468	23.1
Monochorionic, monoamniotic	46	2.3
Total	2029	100

After Potter 1963,[1] Benirschke 1961,[2] Fujikura and Froehlich 1971,[4] and Cameron et al 1983,[19] with permission.

FIGURE 9.4 (A) X-chromosome inactivation is usually random in singleton female embryos resulting in approximately equal numbers of somatic cells expressing maternal and paternal X-linked genes. (B) Similarly, X-inactivation may be random in each twin in MZ female twin pairs. However, there are female twin pairs with non-random X-inactivation who are discordant for the phenotypic expression of X-linked genetic diseases. (C)This may occur through mutual 'recognition and migration' in the inner cell mass before twinning, resulting in reciprocal patterns of non-random X-inactivation. (D) and (E) Alternatively, one twin of a pair may show random X-inactivation, while the other has non-random X-inactivation. In these cases the twinning process may happen after X-inactivation has occurred, with unequal allocation of blastomeres to each twin, the smaller twin having a larger 'patch' or 'clone' size than the larger twin. See Table 9.2.

Bed rest, tocolytic agents, and cervical cerclage are used in attempts to prevent onset of preterm labor. No definite benefits have been shown. None of these series sought to analyze results by chorionicity and zygosity. Real reductions in twin mortality will follow when MC twins are routinely diagnosed prenatally; when such pregnancies are recognized for their extra high risks, they can be intensively monitored accordingly.

The perinatal risks are increased for HOMPs[65–67] and are probably highest in SC sets containing MZ and MC twins.

Although many deaths in twins are caused by general 'background' materno-utero-placental causes such as toxemia, preterm labor, and premature rupture of membranes, the perinatal pathologist should also seek to identify special problems in twins (particularly MC twins) that may have a basis in the genetic and/or placental constitution of those twins. **Twins constitute 1.2% of births and 10% of perinatal deaths.**

MZ (probably MC) twins than DZ twins.[1, 4, 9] This is largely because of vascular anastomoses in and unequal vascular sharing of the MC placental parenchyma.

Despite advances in prenatal and neonatal care, high-risk multiple pregnancies continue to contribute an excess of perinatal mortality and postnatal morbidity to the newborn population.

Placentation in multiple pregnancy

DZ twins usually have DC placentation and their placentas may be separate or fused (Table 9.5).[1, 2, 4, 7, 8, 10, 11, 19] **The majority of MZ**

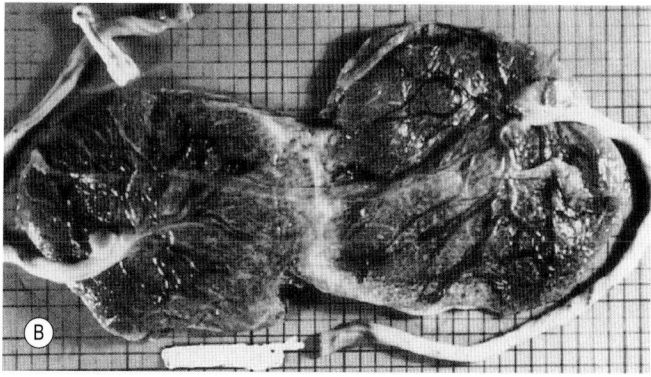

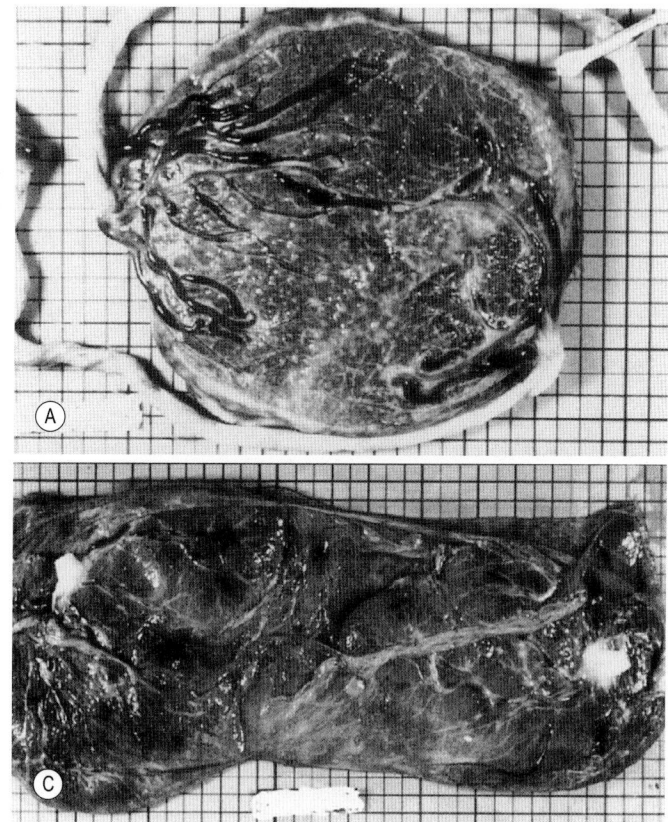

FIGURE 9.5 Monochorionic (MC) placental disks. (A) Typical MC twin placenta with single ovoid disk, resembling a singleton placenta. (B) MC placentas may rarely have nearly separate disks. (C) An MC placenta with completely separate disks.

twins have MC placentas. Hence both MC twins are supported by a truly single (not fused) placenta. Fetal growth rates fall off more significantly in the third trimester in MC twins than in DC twins in comparison with singleton gestations.[68, 69] Separate growth charts have been developed for MC twins.

Growth discordance of equal ranges of severity occurs in both DC and MC twin pairs.[70, 71] Hence growth discordance per se is not a specific diagnostic indicator of TTT. **Growth discordance in DC twins may be caused by unfavorable placental implantation** for the smaller twin (often with velamentous cord insertion) or by **discordant placental disease,** such as extensive infarction and maternal floor infarction.[72, 73] It is often thought that prenatal growth discordance in DC twins simply represents:

- a multifactorial genetic program that will ultimately control adult body weight; or
- a disadvantageous intrauterine environment caused by maternal factors such as implantation site.

However, discordance for placental parenchymal disease such as maternal floor infarction may actually represent fetal genetic disease (thrombophilia) of one DZ twin causing a disadvantageous placental environment, with secondary growth restriction. **Marginal and velamentous cord insertions** are more common in all types of twin placentation than in singleton placentas.[10] The frequencies are highest in MC placentas. The anomalous cord insertions may contribute to growth discordance as well as increasing the risks for vasa previa.[10]

Although the rule generally applies that DZ twins have DC placentation, there is one case of interventional conversion of DC to MC, MA status after perforation of the septum during amnio-

TABLE 9.6 PLACENTATION IN SPONTANEOUSLY CONCEIVED TRIPLET

Author	Cases	Monochorionic	Dichorionic	Trichorionic
Nylander[12]	19	3	8	8
Matayoshi and Yoshida[76]	11	4	6	1
Gonen et al*[77]	5	4		
Gonen et al**[77]	5	0		
Borlum et al[78]	45	12	18	15
Machin and Bamforth[79]	15	2	7	6

*Triplet sets with at least one fetal death.
**Triplet sets without fetal death.

centesis.[74] Cases have recently been reported in which DZ in vitro fertilization (IVF) twins were MC.[25, 75]

In general, MC placentas have single disks, but there are rare exceptions with large succenturiate lobes or true bi-lobation (Fig. 9.5). Thus the presence of two disks is not a reliable sign of DC status and cannot be used as such in prenatal diagnosis. Very rarely, hybrid DC/MC twin placentas are seen.

HOMPs, whether SC or AR, contain any possible combinations of zygosity, chorionicity, and amnionicity. They require careful study, which can be completed only if the cords and/or placentas are identified appropriately. The few detailed studies of placentation in SC triplets show a high proportion of MZ triplets, MZ/DZ twins, and a corresponding high frequency of MC placentas (Table 9.6, Fig. 9.6).[12, 76–79] Data on SC quadruplets are

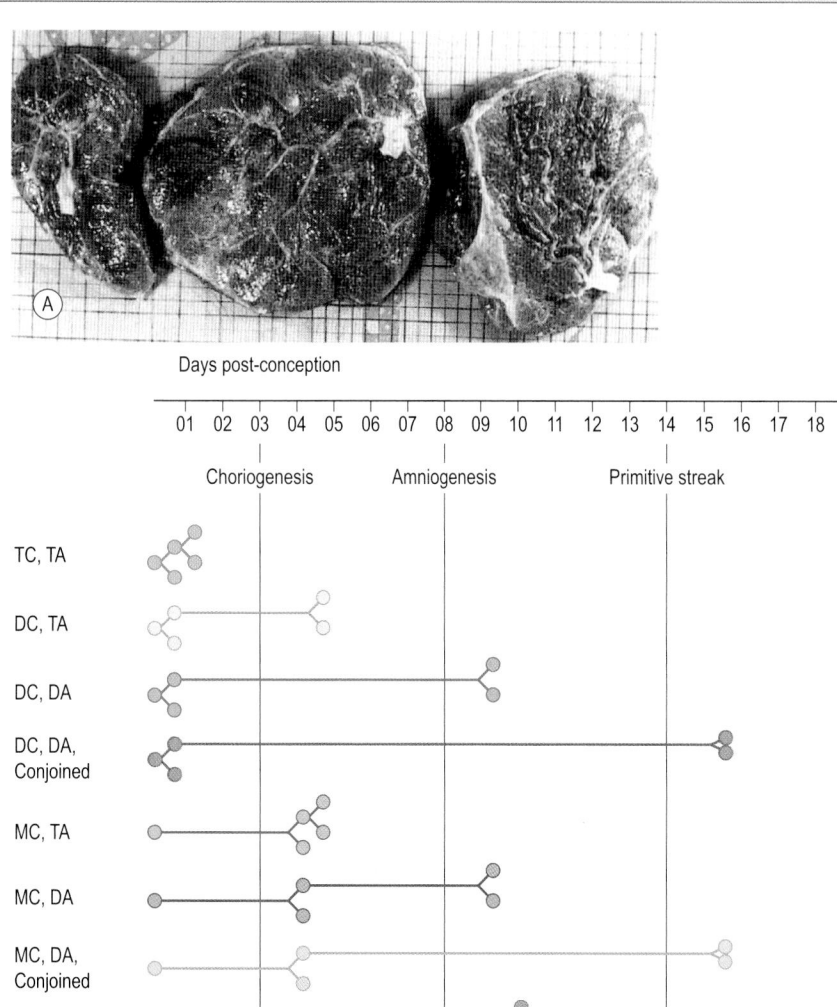

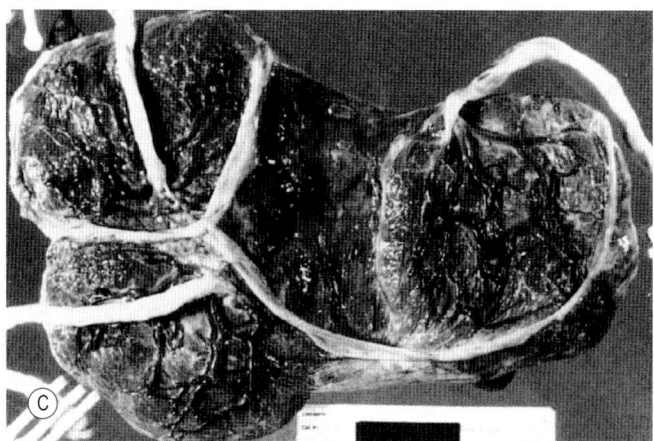

FIGURE 9.6 Placentation in spontaneously conceived triplets and quadruplets. (A) These triplets had three separate placentas. They were found to be trizygotic by DNA RFLP testing. (B) Diagrammatic representation of possible placental arrangements in MZ triplets. When the triplets arise early, before choriogenesis at around 3 days post conception, placentation is trichorionic (TC), either fused or separate. If twinning occurs before choriogenesis and again after choriogenesis, but before amniogenesis, there will be a pair of MC triplets and a DC triplet; the MC triplets will be MA if the second event follows amniogenesis. If twinning events occur after choriogenesis, the triplets are MC, with varying possibilities of amniotic anatomy. MZ triplets may include TTT, TRAP, and conjoined twinning as complications of MC status. (C)This triplet placenta was TC and fused; the triplets were MZ by RFLP testing.

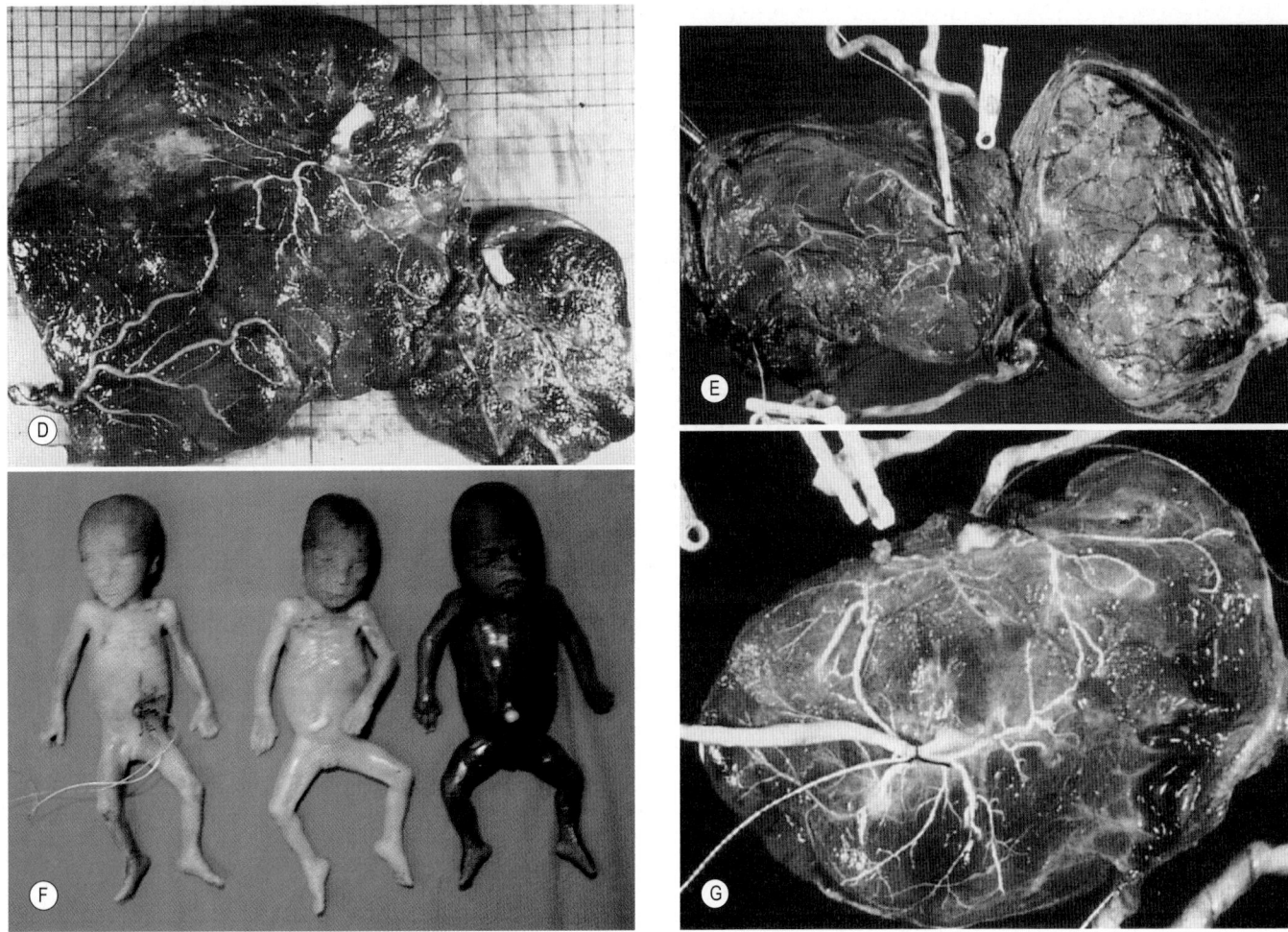

FIGURE 9.6 *(cont'd)* (D) This triplet placenta was MC, TA, with arterio-arterial anastomoses between all three triplets, who survived intact. (E) Triplet placenta with prenatal TTT. Placentation was DC, TA, with MZ status by DNA RFLPs. The triplets sharing the MC, DA placenta died of prenatal TTT at 24 weeks of gestation. The third MZ triplet had a separate placenta (right), and was therefore not affected by TTT but died of complications of prematurity. (F) These MZ, MC, TA triplets died of TTT at 33 weeks of gestation. (G) The MC, TA placenta had arterio-venous anastomosis from A (donor) to C (recipient). Triplet B was not involved in the TTT but died of asphyxia.

scarce, but the same general principles apply (Fig. 9.7). AR higher multiples may contain MZ twins (Fig. 9.8).[17, 18]

Prenatal diagnosis of chorionicity

Most twin and multiple pregnancies are diagnosed prenatally by obstetric ultrasound.[80–88] The zygosity and chorionicity can be determined in a proportion of twins by noting external genital sex and the thickness of the septum. **Septal thickness is best documented in the first trimester** (Fig. 9.9); later in gestation DC septa become quite thin and can be difficult to distinguish from septa of MC twins. Most quote a watershed of 4 mm, with **septa of MC twins measuring less than 4 mm.** Careful inspection of DC septa as they insert into the placental surface often shows tenting of the septum, referred to as the **twin peak, Δ, or Λ.** It results from the collision of the chorionic plates as they turn up into the septum (Fig. 9.10). In some cases the tenting is very marked, and viable chorionic villi and maternal vascular space are present in the base of the septum.

In practice, many septa are reported as '*indeterminate*', mostly because the ultrasound assessment is made after the first trimester. Because the septum of MC twins consists only of two layers of amnion, it may be difficult to find and, if seen, is described as 'hairlike'.[81] Hence MC, DA twin sacs may be misreported as MC, MA. Because of the **high risks of cord intertwining and double fetal death in MC, MA twins,** some advocate further investigation using opaque dye injections. If the dye diffuses throughout the pregnancy sac and is swallowed by both fetuses, MC, MA status is proven.[89–91] The intra-amniotic injection of sterile microbubbles is reported.[92] Cord braids are frequently found in MC, MA twins.

Obstetric ultrasound scan is also used to diagnose the number of placental disks and the degree of growth discordance in the

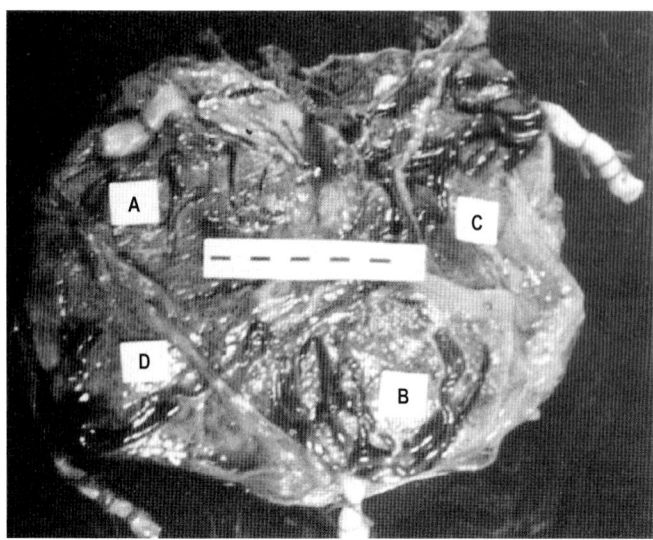

FIGURE 9.7 Spontaneously conceived quadruplets with MC, quadriamniotic placenta (therefore MZ). There was arterio-arterial anastomosis between B and C. The quadruplets survived intact.

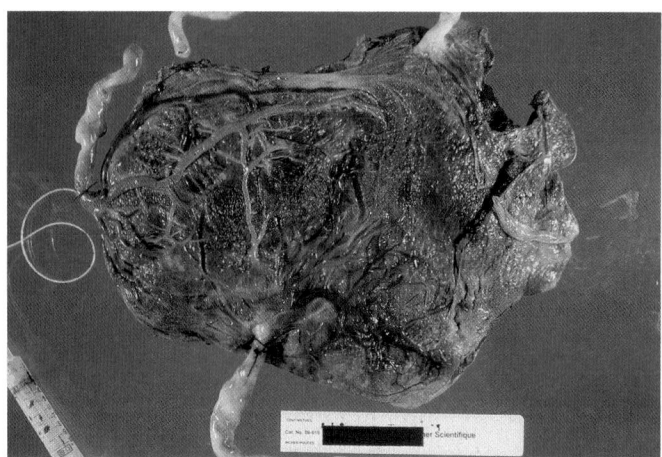

FIGURE 9.8 Multiple pregnancies from assisted reproduction may also contain MZ twins. These triplets were conceived by IVF. The cords on the left and below belong to a pair of MC, DA (MZ) twins. The third triplet was DZ to the twins by DNA RFLP testing; the DC placenta was fused to the MC twin placenta.

twin pairs. **Doppler ultrasound scan is used to document umbilical venous flow patterns.** None of these modalities is reliable for the diagnosis of MC and DC twins; in particular, they cannot be used to diagnose or exclude TTT.

CTs may be diagnosed prenatally by the observation of a constant relationship between the axes of the two bodies.[93]

Practical placental pathology

Clinically relevant test request forms, at a minimum, should include gestational age, major pregnancy complications, mode of delivery, sexes, birth weights and Apgar. Actual and likely mortality and morbidity may be known at the time of birth. The cords should be identified. One standard method is to place the number of cord clamps on the placental end of the cord to reflect the birth order of successively delivered multiplets (one clamp on the cord of the first born, two on the second's, etc).

Placentas should be unfixed. Although it is customary to weigh and measure placentas, little useful information is gained.

DC placentas may have separate disks or may have disk fusion (Fig. 9.11). As received in the laboratory, separate DC placentas may show fusion of membranes or may be completely separate. The septum of DC twins is translucent (not transparent), feels thick between the fingers, and has a fine reticular pattern of sclerosed chorionic vessels. The relevance of separate and fused DC placentas is that there may be greater fetal growth discordance in fused than in separate DC placentas, and the frequency of MZ twinning is higher in fused than in separate DC placentas.

MC placentas are easily diagnosed because the disks usually have the **ovoid shape** of truly single placentas, while the **septa are thin and fully transparent** (Fig. 9.12). Histologic archiving of the DA septum (either as a membrane roll from unfixed placentas or as a T-junction from fixed placentas) leaves an indelible record of

monozygosity, without the necessity for DNA zygosity testing, although exceptional cases of MC, DZ twins are reported.[25] Rare MC placentas have two separate disks (Fig. 9.5). Cases are also reported in which the disc is a hybrid, partially MC in one segment, and DC elsewhere. Because the septa of MC placentas can frequently be stripped from the fetal surface during delivery, care should be taken not to over diagnose MA placentation. Careful examination of the stripped amniotic membranes may show areas where the two amnia are still attached back-to-back, and confirmatory histologic sampling can be made from these areas. MC placentation is not excluded by fetal discordance for genetic disease, for major malformation, or for external genital and/or chromosomal sex. Such cases require careful investigation, and storage of DNA should be considered.

There is an excess of marginal and velamentous cord insertions in twin placentas, especially in MC placentas[94–96] (Table 9.7). This is likely to be particularly dangerous if the velamentous insertion is into a DC septum, constituting a potential vasa previa for the second-born twin (Fig. 9.13). Cord insertion close to the septum of MC twins may be implicated in the genesis and/or progression of prenatal TTT. If hydramnios/ oligohydramnios develops the site of insertion of the septum into the disk may actually move, putting stress on the cord vessels which may also be particularly vulnerable to pressure changes in the two amniotic cavities. However, it should be noted that true septal velamentous insertions do not occur in MC twins because the fetal surface vessels are chorionic and there is no chorionic component in the MC septum.

Most MC placentas have interfetal vascular anastomoses (IFVA). These are of three types: **arterio-arterial (a-aa), veno-venous (v-va), and arterio-venous (a-vc),** whose structure and function is summarized in Table 9.8. A-aa and v-va are superficial, running in the chorionic plate; they may be obvious on initial inspection but are best seen by perfusion studies. A-va anasto-

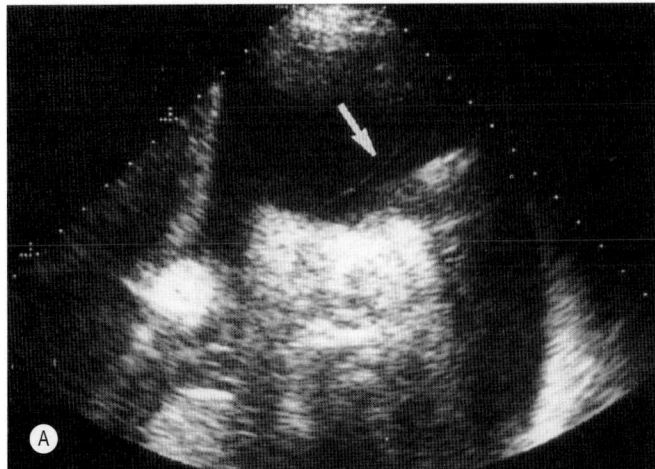

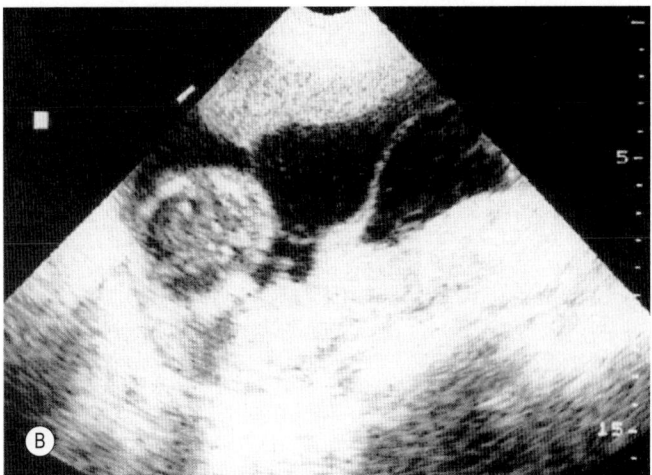

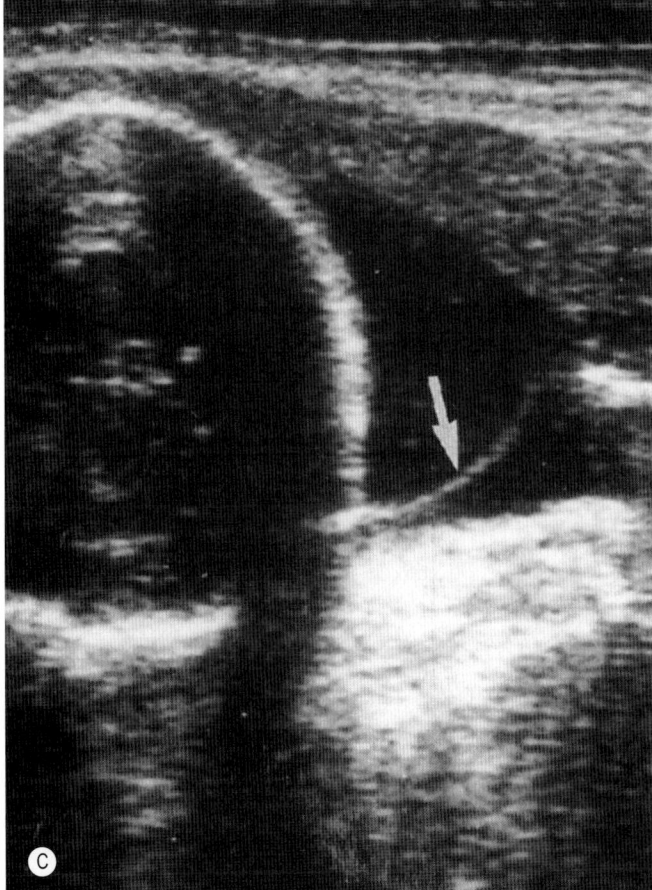

FIGURE 9.9 Prenatal diagnosis of chorionicity by ultrasonography. (A) In MC placentas the septal membranes consist of two layers of amnion only. Septal thickness is at the lower limit of resolution. (B) The DC septum is easily visible by ultrasound scan. (C) Trichorionic triplet septa. All three septa are well seen. [Same case as Fig. 9.6 (C) and (D)].

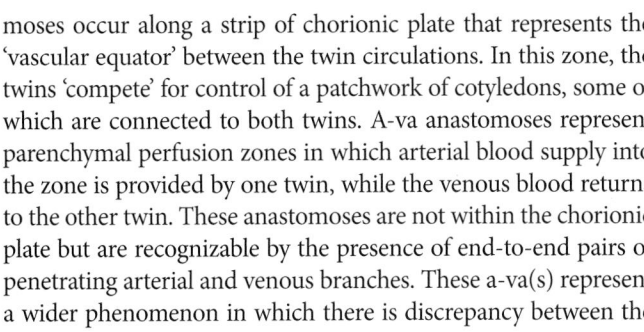

moses occur along a strip of chorionic plate that represents the 'vascular equator' between the twin circulations. In this zone, the twins 'compete' for control of a patchwork of cotyledons, some of which are connected to both twins. A-va anastomoses represent parenchymal perfusion zones in which arterial blood supply into the zone is provided by one twin, while the venous blood returns to the other twin. These anastomoses are not within the chorionic plate but are recognizable by the presence of end-to-end pairs of penetrating arterial and venous branches. These a-va(s) represent a wider phenomenon in which there is discrepancy between the

TABLE 9.7 FREQUENCY OF VELAMENTOUS CORD INSERTION IN TWIN PLACENTAS

Chorionicity	Cords	Velamentous	
		No	Percentage
Dichorionic, separate	482	15	3
Dichorionic, fused	376	58	15
Monochorionic, diamniotic	494	113	23
Monochorionic, monoamniotic	30	7	23
Data from Benirschke and Kaufmann 1995,[94] with permission			
Monochorionic	76	12	16
TTT	22	7	32
No TTT	54	5	9
Data from Fries et al,[95] with permission			
Monochorionic	246	23	9
TTT	52	10	19
No TTT	194	13	7
TTT, Twin-to-twin transfusion.			

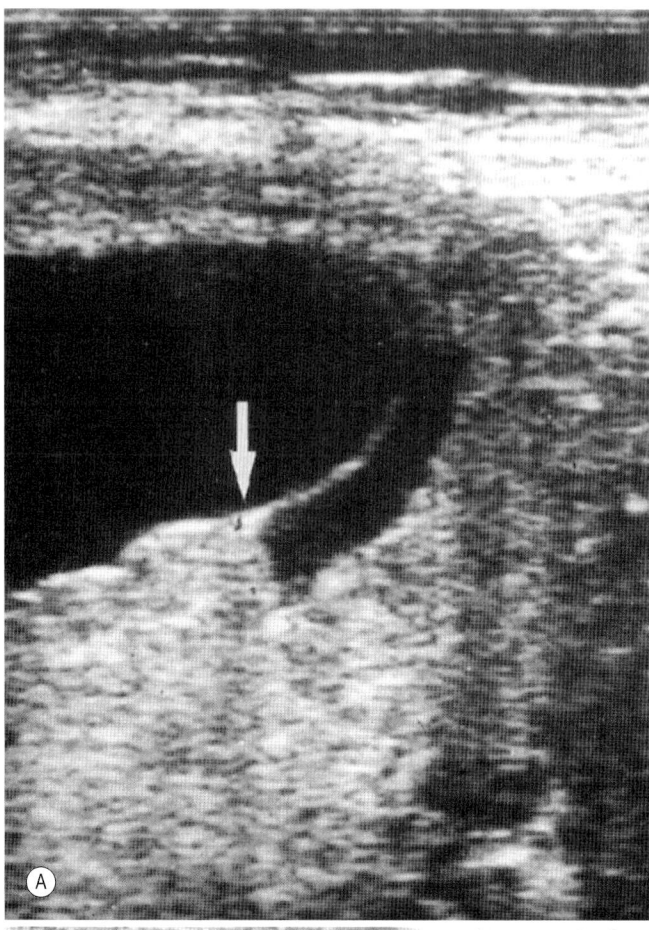

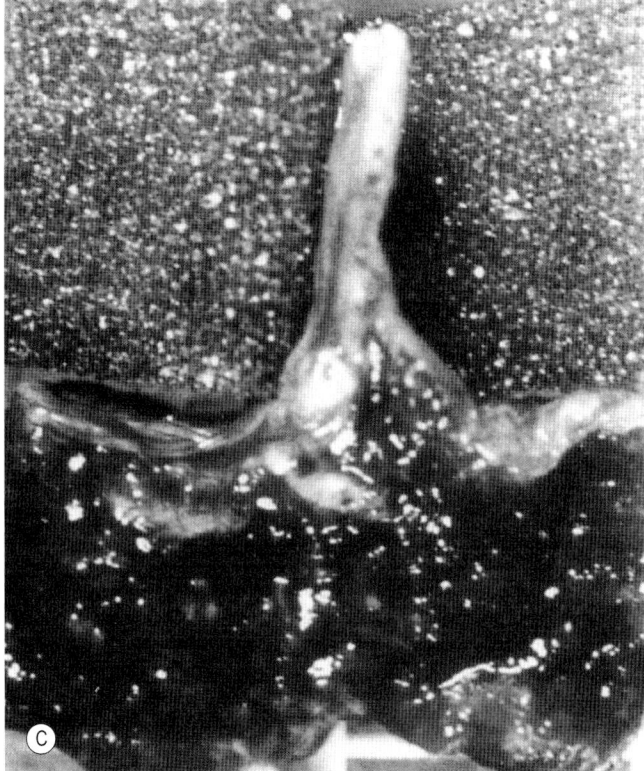

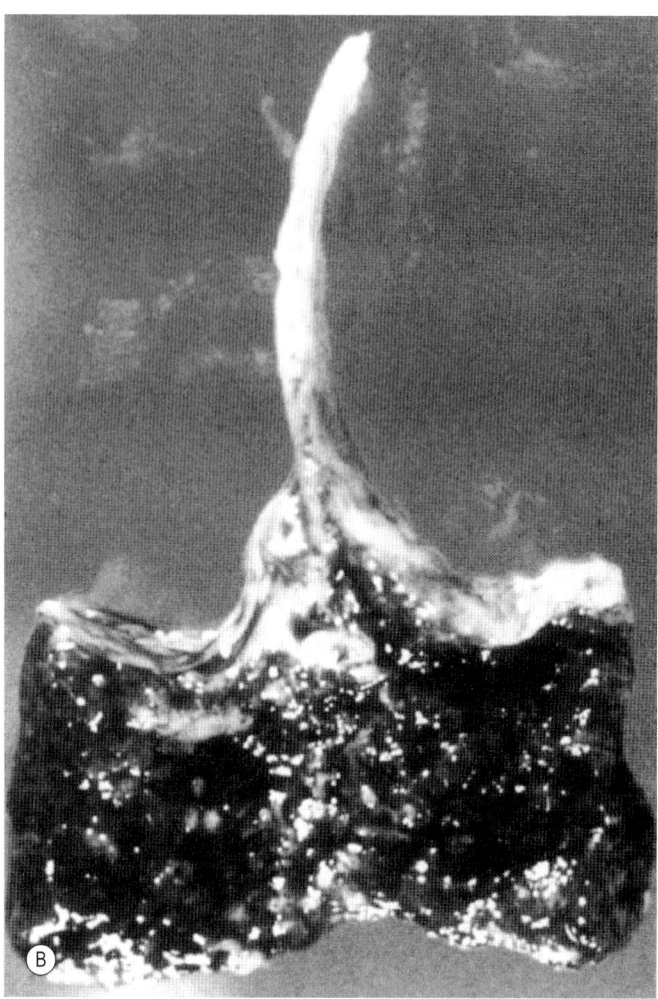

FIGURE 9.10 (A) Appearance of 'Δ sign' on ultrasound scan. (B) Tissue cut section of septal insertion. (C) Orientation of septal base in cassette for histologic confirmation.

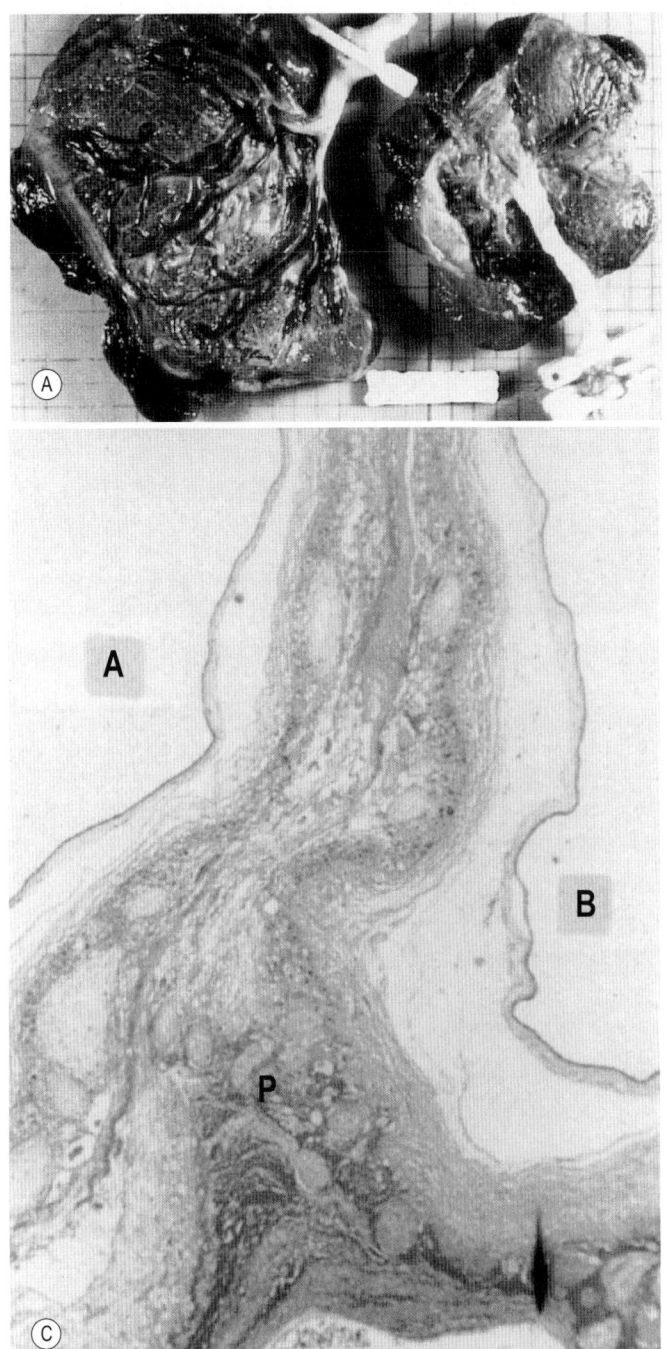

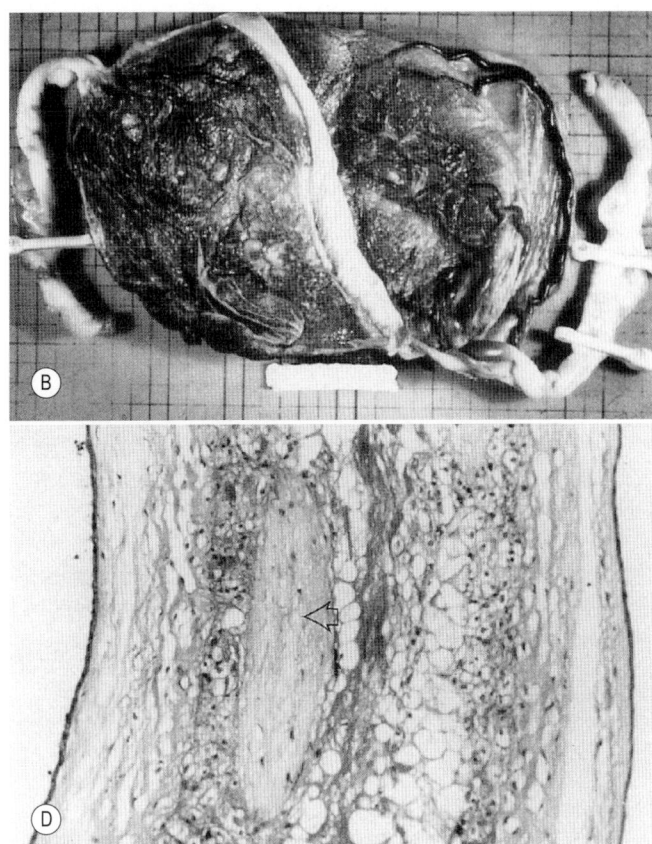

FIGURE 9.11 Dichorionic twin placentation. (A) Separate placental disks. (B) Fused placental disks. The septal membranes are thick, with frequent 'δ' sign (Fig. 9.10). (C) Septal histology, with two chorionic layers and two amniotic layers. The chorionic plates (P) participate in septum formation. [(A) and (B) represent amniotic cavities of the twins.] (D) An atrophic chorionic villus (arrow) in the septum.

size of the zone perfused arterially and that zone drained venously by one twin. If the arterial zone is larger than the venous zone, the twin contributes into the venous zone of the co-twin via the a-va(s) (Fig. 9.14). The superficial a-aa and v-va act as channels for return of transfused blood to the twin with the smaller venous zone. In the absence of superficial anastomoses, the **unopposed flow through a-va perfusion zones results in prenatal TTT.**

The purposes of perfusion studies are to map the sizes of the arterial and venous zones, to document superficial anastomoses, and to find areas of potential a-va. The degree of unequal arterial and venous sharing can be assessed as a percentage of the whole,

and the sizes of anastomoses can be assessed as large (likely of clinical importance) and small (probably of no clinical relevance). Some MC placentas show areas not apparently perfused by any major chorionic vessels; this raises the likelihood that the vascular anatomy seen at birth may not represent the situation that applied during most of the pregnancy. In particular, adverse events such as development of hydramnios and/or prenatal TTT, or fetal death, may cause major changes in the structure and function of placental vessels.

Standard umbilical arterial and venous catheters are inserted by cutting down in the vessels in the cord, near its insertion onto

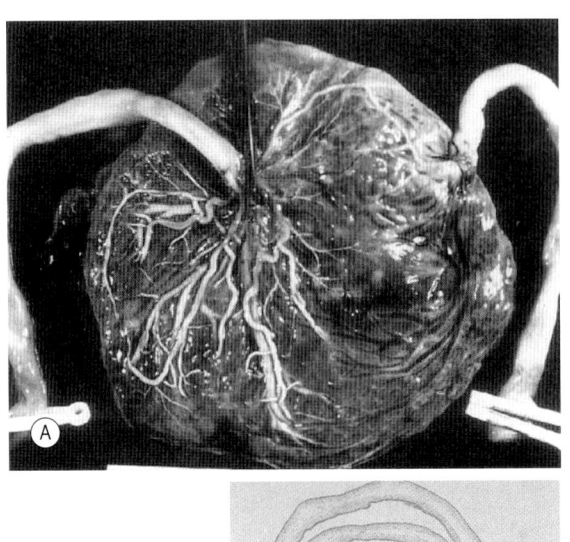

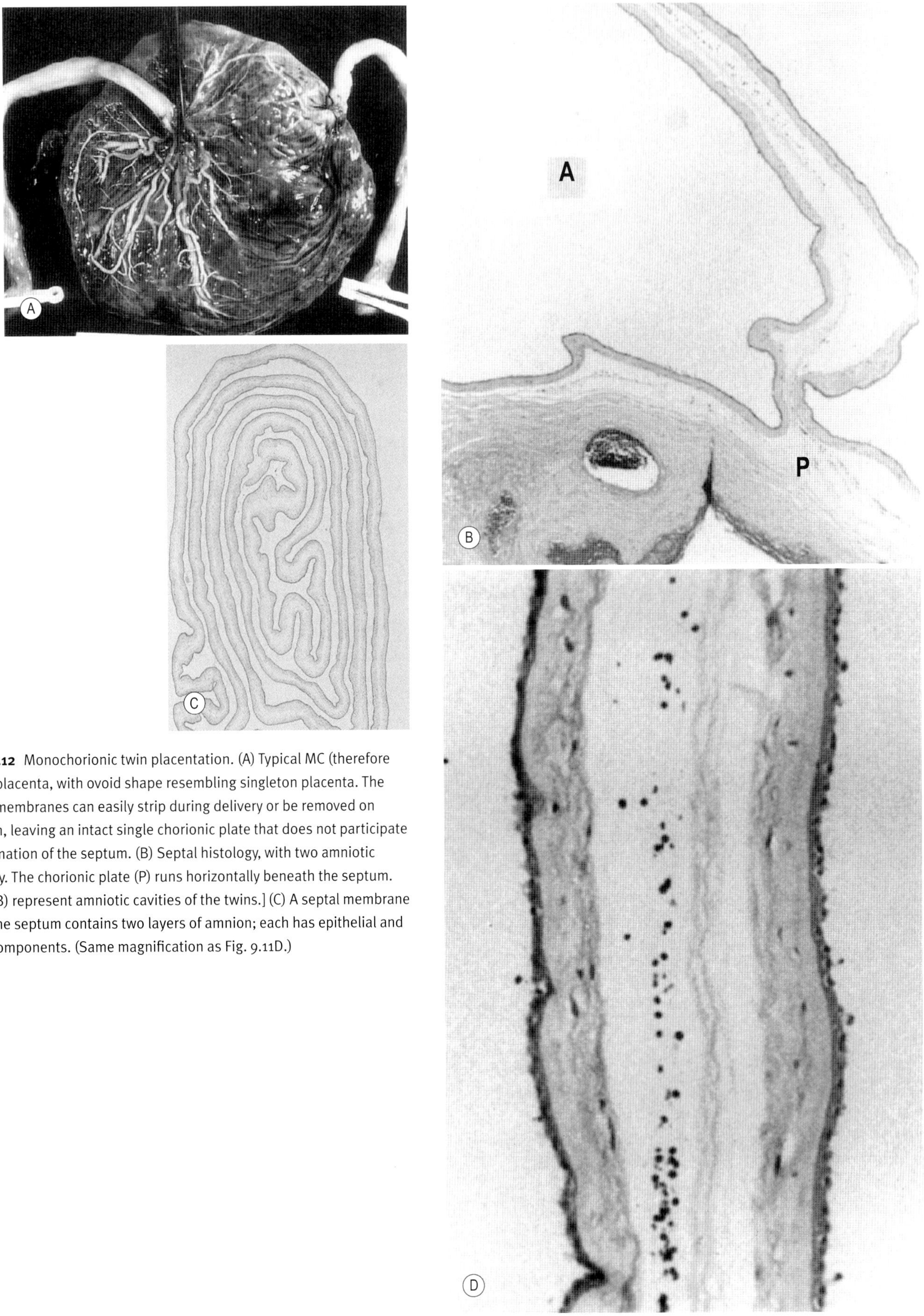

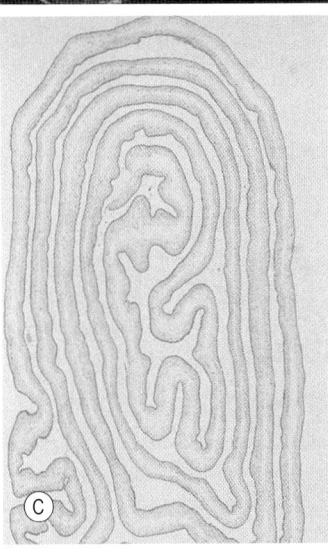

FIGURE 9.12 Monochorionic twin placentation. (A) Typical MC (therefore MZ) twin placenta, with ovoid shape resembling singleton placenta. The amniotic membranes can easily strip during delivery or be removed on inspection, leaving an intact single chorionic plate that does not participate in the formation of the septum. (B) Septal histology, with two amniotic layers only. The chorionic plate (P) runs horizontally beneath the septum. [(A) and (B) represent amniotic cavities of the twins.] (C) A septal membrane roll. (D) The septum contains two layers of amnion; each has epithelial and stromal components. (Same magnification as Fig. 9.11D.)

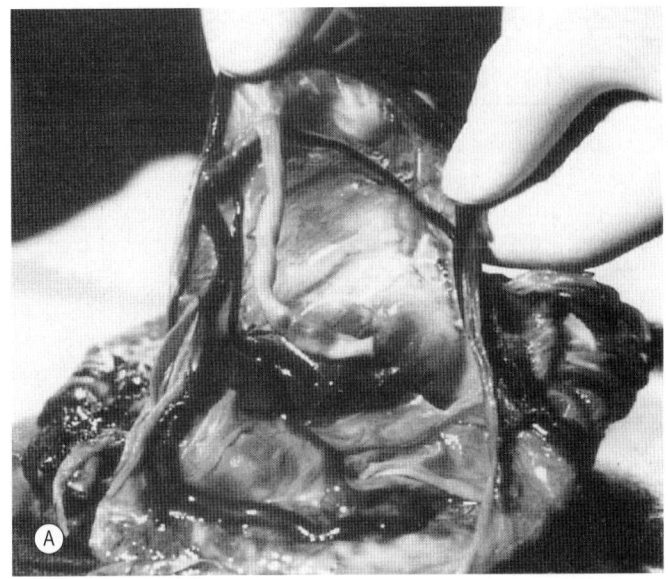

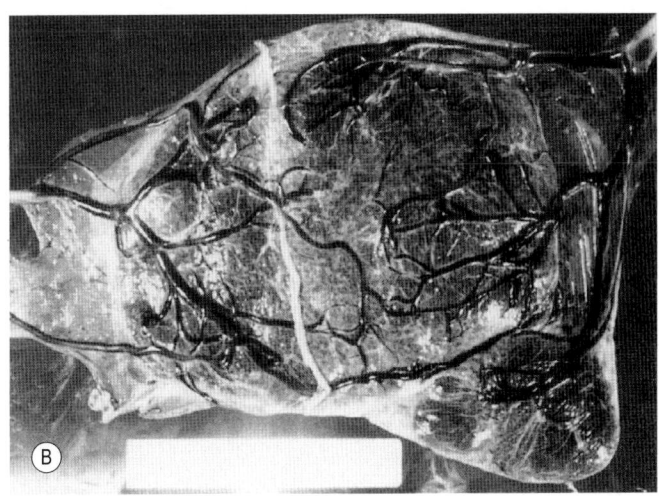

FIGURE 9.13 Velamentous cord insertions in twin placentas. (A) Velamentous insertion of both cords into the septum of DC fused twin placentas. Neither twin survived intact. (B) Velamentous insertions of both cords of MC twins into opposite sides of the disk. Note the markedly unequal vascular sharing of parenchyma.

TABLE 9.8 STRUCTURE AND FUNCTION OF INTER-FETAL VASCULAR ANASTOMOSES IN MC TWIN PLACENTAS

Type of connection	AVC*	AAA*	VVA*
Frequency	Majority of placentas. Up to 2–5 per placenta	Majority of placentas. One per placenta	15-20% of placentas. Up to 2–3 per placenta
Flow/pressure	Always present, low pressure	High pressure. No net flow when twin cardiac outputs are equal, but output eventually becomes unequal due to the law of Laplace (P = QR, Pressure = Flow × Resistance)	Low pressure. No net flow if twin cardiac outputs are equal. Potential for rapid transfusion of large volumes across pressure gradient (e.g. after fetal demise of one twin)
Flow direction	Unidirectional in each AVC, but different AVCs can flow in opposite directions	Bidirectional, minimal, pulsatile	Bidirectional, minimal, non-pulsatile

AVC, Arterio-venous connection; AAA, arterio-arterial anastomosis; VVA, veno-venous anastomosis.

the disk. Different colored dyes can be used (Fig. 9.15). In the case of TTT and/or significant growth discordance, **the venous system of the recipient or larger twin should be perfused first, followed by the arterial tree of the other twin.** Anastomotic patterns can be recorded by photography.

After perfusion studies MC placentas, like DC placentas, can be sampled for histology, principally to:

- confirm the status of the septa;
- look for chorioamnionitis; and
- assess significant differences between villous structure in the two halves of the placenta.

Samples of cord, amnion, and chorion can be stored for later zygosity studies, using VNTRs.

The same principles apply to **triplet and quadruplet placentas.** When these are MC, the anastomotic vascular patterns may be complex. Figure 9.6G shows an MC triplet placenta in which two of the twins died of prenatal TTT. The third twin had an a-aa with the donor but did not show any evidence of having been involved in TTT.

Clinico-pathologic associations should include the diagnosis of MZ status for MC placentas. When there is significant growth discordance in twin pairs, causes may be sought in the placental size and villous pathology of DC twins.[74] In MC twins discordance is more likely to be secondary to unequal sharing of parenchyma; in some cases the arterial and venous tree of one twin is larger than that of the other twin, but there are no anastomoses; growth is simply due to vascular inequality, and TTT is not invoked. TTT may sometimes have rapid clinical onset, without significant growth discordance. However, most twin pairs with prenatal TTT have growth discordance. The

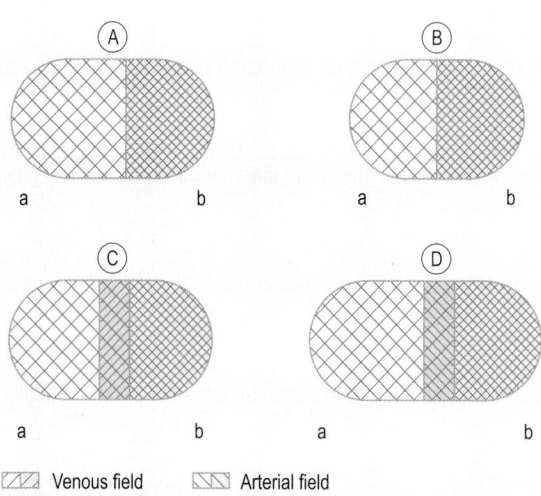

☒ Venous field   ☒ Arterial field

FIGURE 9.14 Theoretical diagram of relative sizes of arterial and venous zones of each twin of MC pair. (A) Arterial and venous zones of twin a are equal in size, and both are larger than the corresponding zones of twin b. There is likely to be growth discordance, but TTT is usually not present. (B) Arterial and venous zones of twin a are equal, and are the same size as those of twin b. Regardless of the presence or absence of vascular anastomoses, the twins will usually be of equal birthweight and of long gestation. (C) In twin a the arterial zone is larger than the venous return zone, while the converse is true of twin b. There is an equatorial band of parenchyma that is perfused arterially by twin a but with venous return to twin b. In this zone arteriovenous transfusion is likely to occur from twin a to twin b. If there are no arterio-arterial or veno-venous anastomotic vessels, unidirectional, uncompensated transfusion will occur. There may not be significant growth discordance. (D) The anatomy is similar, but there is greater discrepancy in the sizes of the venous fields of the twins. Some cases of TTT show little growth discordance [perhaps corresponding with the anatomy of (C)], while others have severe growth discordance, reflecting markedly discrepant venous fields as well as arterio-venous transfusion.

vascular pattern of MC twins may differ, resulting in different phenotypic traits.[97]

The relative frequencies of anastomotic vessels are summarized in Table 9.9.[2, 98–103] The most common is a-aa, which may be found alone or in combination. **The most common pattern is a combination of a-aa and a-va.** V-va is rare, alone or in combination.

Prenatal TTT is only found in cases with a-va, although these may be combined with other anastomoses. One series found that v-va had a poor prognosis;[103] this may be due to rapid transfer of blood volumes in the low-pressure venous system.

With TRAP, **the two cords are inserted close together, and there are large, direct a-aa and v-va.**

Special clinico-pathologic disorders in monochorionic multiples

Several related and overlapping disease processes place MC, MZ multiples at higher risk of perinatal mortality and morbidity. In addition to discordance for chromosome status and expression of X-linked genes, MC multiples can suffer a number of complications of IFVA. The relationship between interfetal vascular connections and various clinical outcomes is summarized in Table 9.10.[104] The frequency of major malformations may also be increased in MC twins. Prenatal TTT and severe GD in MC twin pairs, as well as discordant malformations, can all give rise to discordant amniotic fluid volumes (Table 9.11).

Prenatal twin-to-twin transfusion syndrome

MC, DA twins have a perinatal mortality of 15–25%, mostly as a result of prenatal and perinatal twin-to-twin transfusion syndrome (TTTS). The pathophysiology of TTTS is complex and incompletely understood, but the syndrome primarily results from a net transfusion of whole blood from a chorionic plate artery of the donor to a chorionic plate artery or vein of the recipient in a villous zone of overlapping perfusion at the vascular equator.[105] To some degree the recipient (who is larger because of a larger venous perfusion zone) can compensate for hypervolemia by polyuria;[106] **recipients have high atriopeptin levels.[107] The polyuria produces hydramnios in the amniotic sac of the recipient,** and the discordance in amniotic fluid accumulation between the sacs is thought to play a major role in the development of the syndrome, accounting for amnioreduction and septostomy of the intervening membrane representing therapeutic options.[108] The onset may be rapid and severe, leading to premature ruptured membranes and ascending infection as well as premature labor. Onset of severe prenatal TTTS typically occurs at **18–24 weeks of gestation** and is rare thereafter.

The ultrafiltration of the plasma component of transfused whole blood renders the recipient **polycythemic and hyperviscotic.**[109] This may be severe enough to cause *arterial hypoperfusion*, and many cases evolve into **hydrops fetalis; this may be the result of coronary artery hypoperfusion and myocardial ischemia** (Fig. 9.17F).

The donor is also adversely affected by the whole blood transfusion. There is shutdown in visceral perfusion, and the resulting oliguria causes oligohydramnios. **The donor responds to chronic anemia with raised erythropoietin production.**[110] The fetuses show growth lag and develop mechanical flexion deformities (Fig. 9.17).

Without therapy, almost 100% of cases of TTTS die in the second trimester;[111] death is due either directly to TTTS or is secondary to the complications of preterm delivery. A very few cases may resolve spontaneously; in other rare cases one fetus dies and the other twin reverts to normal, with intact survival.[112, 113] Active intervention may be successful if the membranes are intact and labor can be suppressed. The following methods have been

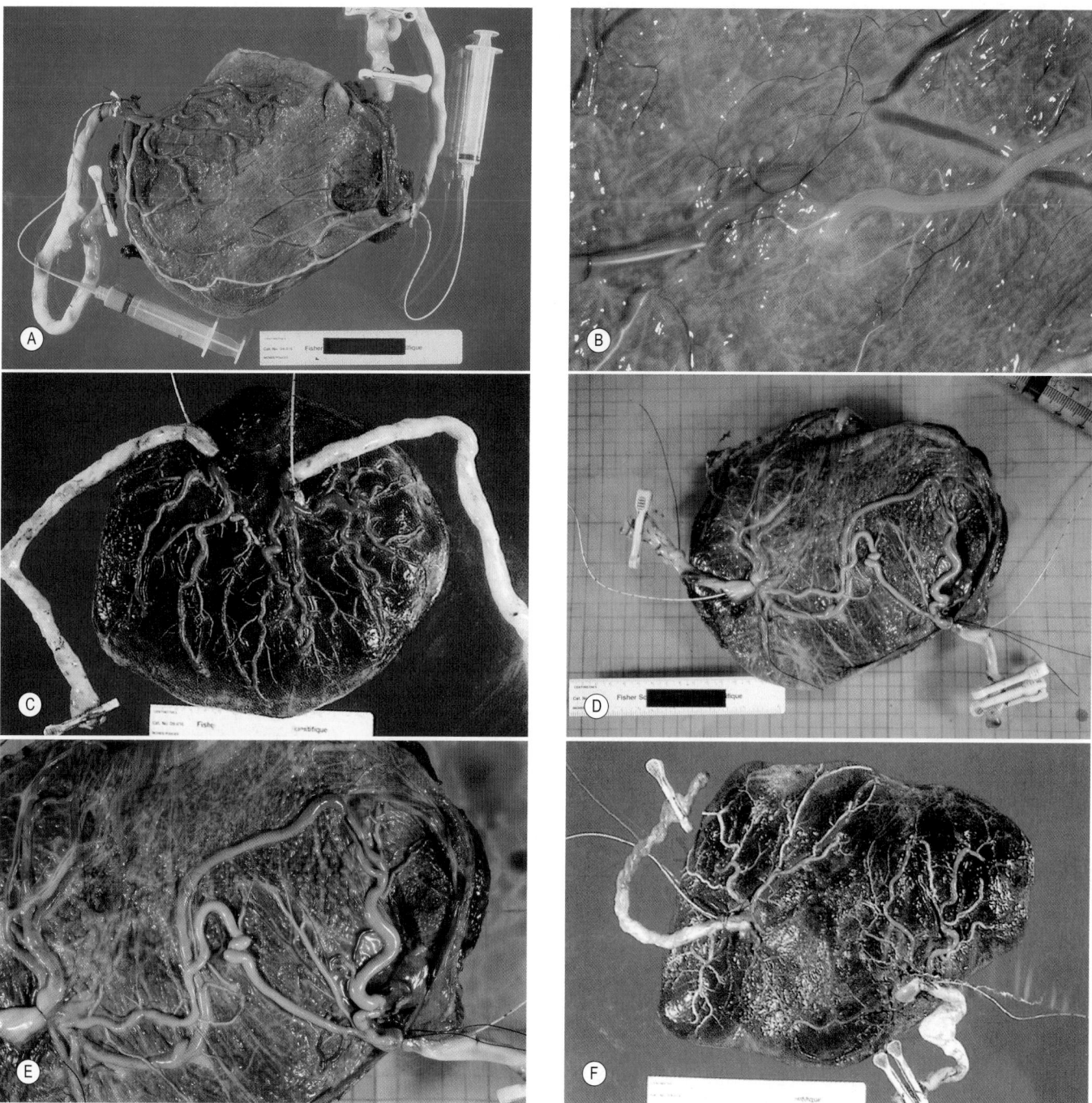

FIGURE 9.15 Perfusion of vascular anatomy in MC twin placentas. (A) Venous perfusion (green) of twin A (left) shows unequal venous sharing, A > B, but without v-v anastomosis. Arterial perfusion (yellow) of twin B shows a single large a-a anastomosis below. (B) Close-up view of (A). In the equatorial zone, there is a parenchymal unit supplied by an artery of twin B (yellow) but drained by a vein of twin A (left). This end-to-end arrangement of artery and vein is typical of major vessel supply to a zone of a-v transfusion. Transfusion occurs through normal capillary loops in the villi, and there is no direct arterio-venous transfusion in the large surface vessels. The a-v anastomosis reflects unequal venous sharing, while the a-a anastomosis acts as a safety valve to return blood to the donor. This combination of a-a and a-v anastomosis is the most common finding in MC placentas. (C) In this case the cords are inserted close together and there is a large proximal a-a anastomosis. The arterial system is virtually syncytial. (D) There is markedly unequal venous sharing, A > B, with a large a-a anastomosis perfused in green. A vein from twin A reaches deep into the territory of twin B, making an a-v anastomosis, with B as donor. (E) Close-up of (D) showing the two anastomoses. There was considerable growth discordance, probably caused by unequal venous sharing. Twin B also had an omphalocele; thus these MZ twins were discordant for a major malformation. (F) This case shows unequal parenchymal sharing, with a single a-a anastomosis (lower). There are no a-v perfusion zones; there was 20% growth discordance, and the twins survived intact.

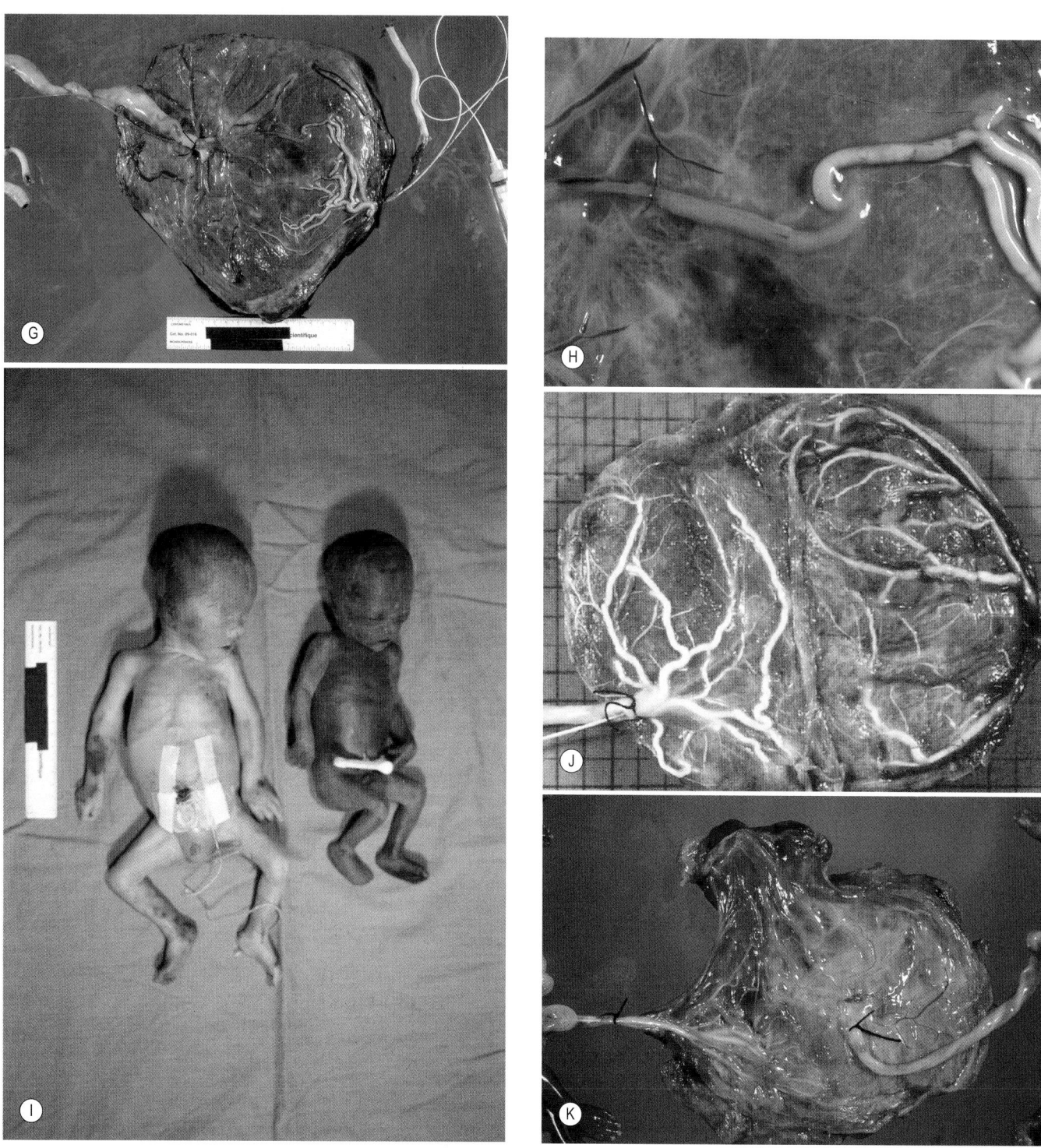

FIGURE 9.15 (*cont'd*) (G) These MC twins died of severe prenatal TTT at 23 weeks of gestation. The cord of twin A (left) is large and edematous compared with the marginally inserted cord of twin B (right). The venous zone (pink) of twin A is large compared with that of twin B (green). There are no a-a or v-v anastomoses. The arterial zone of twin B (yellow) overlaps the venous zone of twin A at the equatorial belt, producing a zone of a-v transfusion. (H) Close-up of the a-v perfusion zone in G. The artery (yellow) of twin B (right) supplies a zone from which the vein of twin A (pink) rather than that of twin B (green) received the venous return. In the absence of a-a or v-v anastomoses, no prenatal TTT occurred. (I) Twin A was delivered first, after which there was acute reversed intrapartum TTT to twin B (Fig. 9.18). (J) This MC placenta has equal arterial and venous sharing. No anastomoses were present. There was no growth discordance, and the twins survived intact. (K) Double fetal death of MC twins from antepartum hemorrhage at 18 weeks of gestation. The circulation of the left twin was perfused with blue (artery) and yellow (venous) dye, while the venous side of the right twin was perfused in orange.

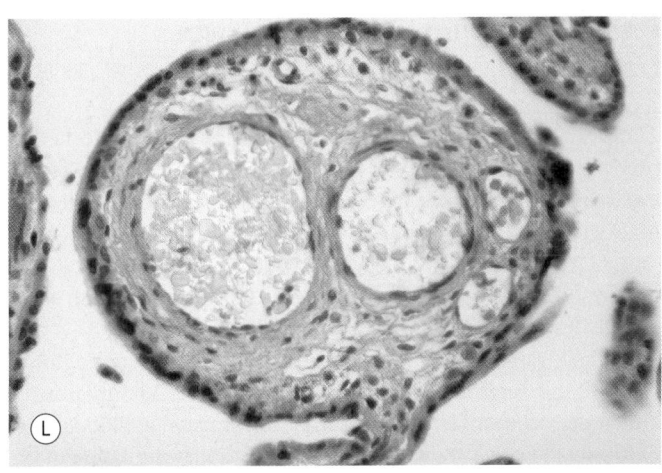
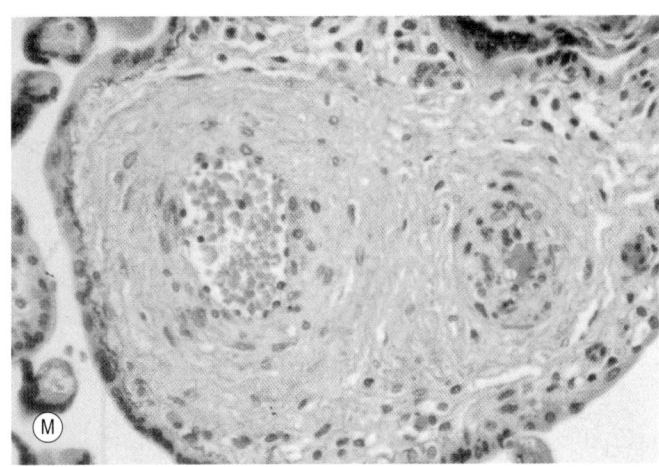

FIGURE 9.15 *(cont'd)* (L) Villus from perfusion zone of left twin, with blue and yellow dye particles in artery and vein. (M) Villous vein of right twin contains orange dye particles. Microscopy can be used to confirm zones of anastomosis.

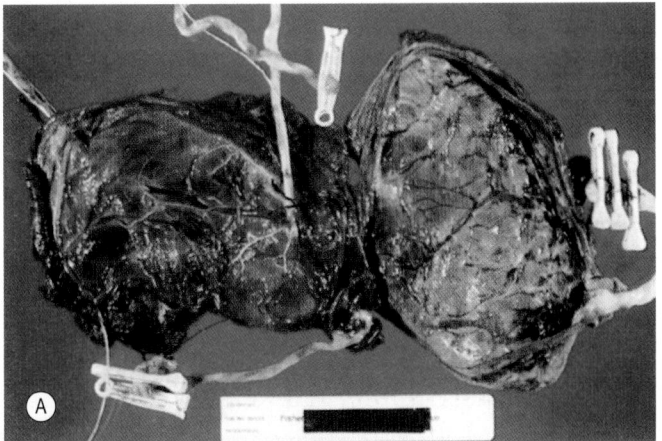
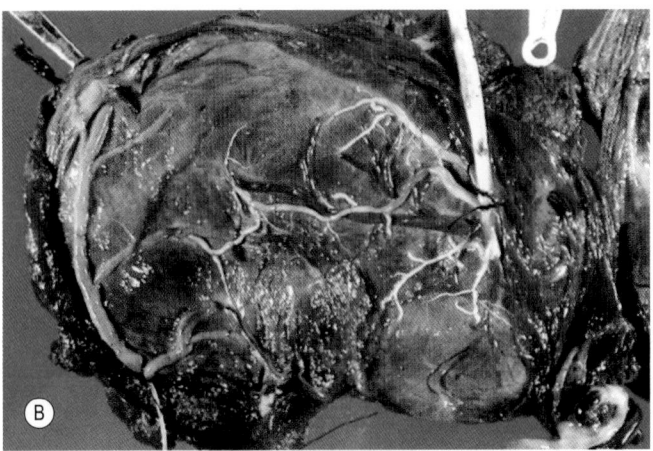

FIGURE 9.16 Death from prenatal TTT in MZ spontaneously conceived triplets. (A) On the left is the MC placenta of triplets A and B. The placenta of triplet C (right) was fused DC to the MC placenta. The triplets were MZ by DNA RFLP testing. (B) Close-up of (A). There is a zone of a-v anastomosis from the yellow arterial tree of triplet A to the green venous zone of triplet B. Triplet C died of complications of prematurity.

TABLE 9.9 PATTERNS AND NUMBERS OF ANASTOMOTIC VESSELS IN MONOCHORIONIC PLACENTAS

Author	Cases	a-a Present	v-v Present	a-v Present	Anastomosis Present	No	%	No	%
Benirschke[2]	60	36	60	8	13	29	48	51	85
Strong and Corney[98]	39	31	79	14	36	29	74	35	90
Galea et al[99]	32	22	71	3	9	2	6	22	69
Arts and Lohman[100]	23	17	74	2	9	15	65	20	87
Sekiya and Hafez[101]	44	33	75	18	41	21	48	–	–
Robertson and Neer[102]	56	–	–	–	–	–	–	55	98
Yoshida and Soma[91]	182	70	86	24	30	19	23	62	31
Total	436	209	55	69	18	115	30	245	62

used, alone or in combination: **maternal digoxin therapy,**[114] **maternal indomethacin therapy to suppress polyuria in the donor,**[115] **selective termination of the least viable fetus,**[116] **serial amniocentesis,**[117] and **selective photocoagulation of vessels on the fetal surface of the placenta** (Fig. 9.18).[118, 119] Of these,

maternal digoxin therapy is not usually effective, while the use of indomethacin is not advised because it causes lasting and sometimes permanent anuria in the donor. Selective termination is not always feasible without inducing labor. Laser photocoagulation of chorionic plate vessels at the intertwin membrane appears

TABLE 9.10 MEAN NUMBERS OF VASCULAR CONNECTIONS IN MC TWIN PAIRS WITH SUBTYPES OF CLINICAL DISEASE

TABLE 9.10 MEAN NUMBERS OF VASCULAR CONNECTIONS IN MC TWIN PAIRS WITH SUBTYPES OF CLINICAL DISEASE

Clinical disease	All connections	AAA	VVA	AVC, both directions
Severe prenatal TTTS	1	0	0	1
Mild prenatal TTTS	2	1	0	1
Severe growth discordance	3	0	0	3
Controls	5	2	1	2

Prenatal diagnosis of twin-to-twin transfusion

There is considerable disagreement about the criteria for prenatal diagnosis of TTT.[70] **Growth discordance per se is not a reliable sign,** because this can occur in DC twins as well as in MC twins with unequal venous sharing but without actual a-va.

Criteria for the diagnosis of MC twinning must be applied first, followed by assessment of growth discordance, hydramnios/oligohydramnios and incipient or actual hydrops. Some advocate **umbilical vessel sampling for measurement of hemoglobin levels, total serum protein levels, viscosity,[109] atriopeptin,[107] and erythropoietin levels.**[110] In addition, infusion of blood group O Rhesus-negative adult red blood cells into the circulation of the presumed donor allows for detection of a-va if such cells are later recovered from the circulation of the presumed recipient.[110, 123]

In general, the presence of hydramnios/oligohydramnios, growth discordance, and hydrops allows the diagnosis of prenatal TTT.[124] Early signs of prenatal TTT to be detected before the onset of the fully established disease would require frequent and detailed ultrasonic assessment of MC pregnancies that had been firmly diagnosed in early gestation.

more effective than serial amnioreduction; selective feticide and intervening membrane septostomy have not been adequately studied.[108, 120, 121]

Amniocentesis leads sometimes to major clinical improvement, with apparent cessation of transfusion and with improved growth and urine production in the donor. In fatal cases placentas almost always show uncompensated a-va. The increased pressure of the hydramniotic sac may be sufficient to close down coexisting v-va, leaving no trace of such IFVA in lethal cases; in successfully treated cases, lowering amniotic fluid pressure may be sufficient to allow some return of function of v-va if these are present. Few v-va have been found in successfully treated cases.

Surviving recipient fetuses may have cardiomyopathy with subendocardial fibroelastosis. This appears to resolve over time, although myocardial infarction may cause neonatal death (Fig. 9.17F). There is no long-term follow-up information on postnatal growth in twin pairs who survive prenatal TTTS.

Twin reversed arterial perfusion

Twin reversed arterial perfusion (TRAP) is a special condition in MC twins **whereby one twin (the pump twin) actively perfuses the co-twin (acardiac twin) via large a-aa and v-va.** A-va is not invoked. Necessary preconditions for the development of TRAP are the appropriate vascular anastomoses, closely apposed umbilical cord insertions, and circulatory failure of the acardiac twin (Fig. 9.20).

At least two mechanisms have been suggested as the etiology of TRAP.[125, 126] One proposes that the anatomically normal pump twin dominates the future acardiac twin by the vascular anastomoses. The acardiac twin is initially anatomically normal, although it may be derived from a smaller inner cell mass by unequal division of the blastomeres. The key finding is that the **arterial supply into the placenta by the pump twin is able to overcome the blood pressure of the co-twin so as to perfuse that twin by reversed flow** (toward the co-twin) in the umbilical arteries of the co-twin. This supplies postductal blood from the pump twin; this blood is normally destined for the placental parenchyma and is relatively hypoxic, hypercarbic, acidotic, poor

Acute perinatal twin-to-twin transfusion

This event may occur with established prenatal TTTS, growth discordance, or no previous vasculogenic pathology.[122] When the umbilical cord of the first-delivered twin is clamped, blood from the whole of the MC placenta is available for venous return to the second-born twin. In the context of established prenatal TTT, this may result in an apparent paradox; the recipient (who is often first-born) appears pale in comparison with the plethoric second-born donor (Fig. 9.19). The combination of prenatal and perinatal transfusions makes the clinical postnatal diagnosis of TTT much less straightforward. In acute perinatal TTT, it is always the second-born twin who is plethoric.

TABLE 9.11 CAUSES OF AMNIOTIC FLUID VOLUME ABNORMALITIES IN MC TWINS

AFV	Twin A	Twin B	Cause
	Polyhydramnios	Oligohydramnios	Prenatal TTTS
	Normal	Oligohydramnios	Severe growth discordance; discordant urinary tract obstruction; membrane rupture
	Normal	Polyhydramnios	Discordant upper gastrointestinal obstruction; hydrops

AFV: amniotic fluid volume

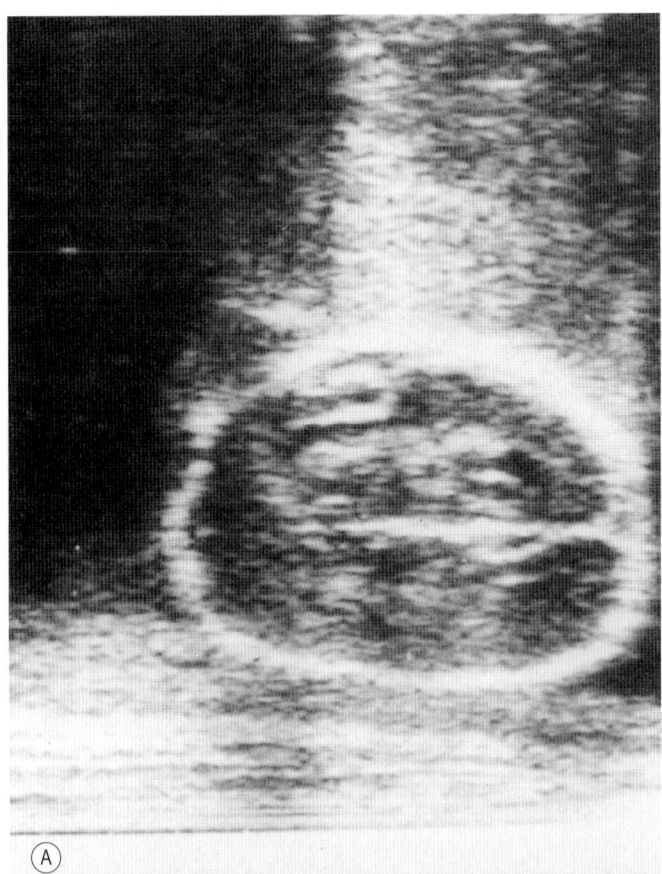

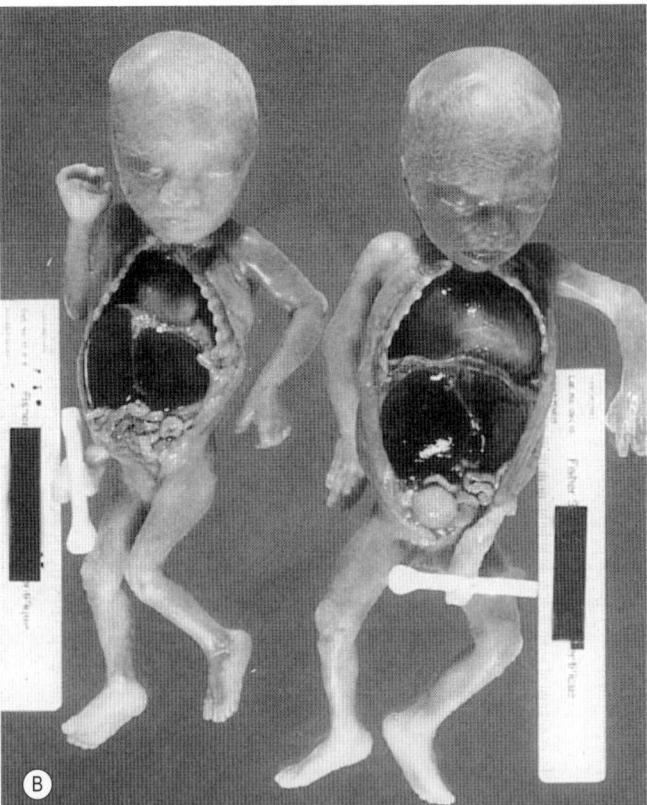

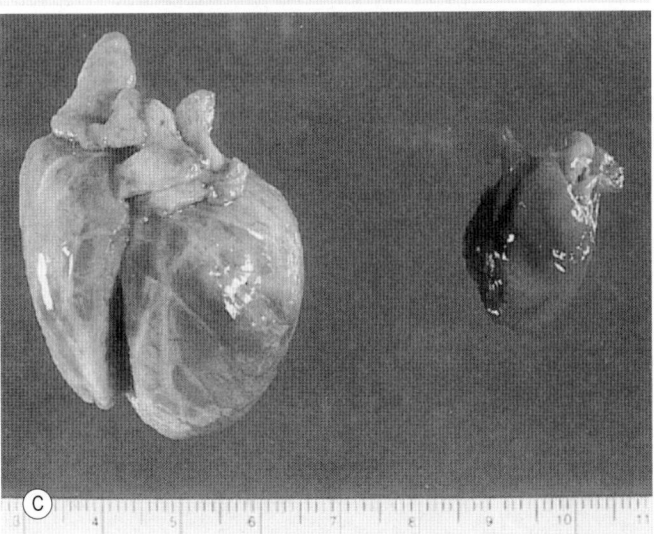

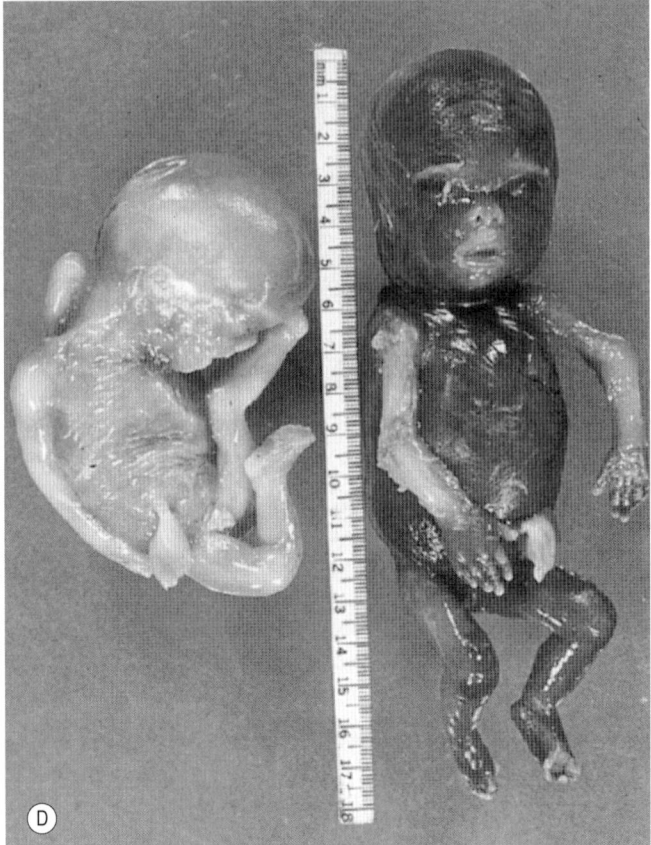

FIGURE 9.17 The fetal pathology of chronic prenatal TTT. (A) Prenatal ultrasound scan of dolichocephalic head of 'stuck' donor twin, compressed against the placenta. (B) The viscera of the donor (left) are smaller than those of the recipient; in particular, the urinary bladder of the recipient is large, indicating polyuria and hydramnios. (C) The heart of the recipient on the left. (D) Typical prenatal TTT. The 'stuck' donor (left) is small, anemic, and flexed because of oligohydramnios. The recipient (right) is large and plethoric.

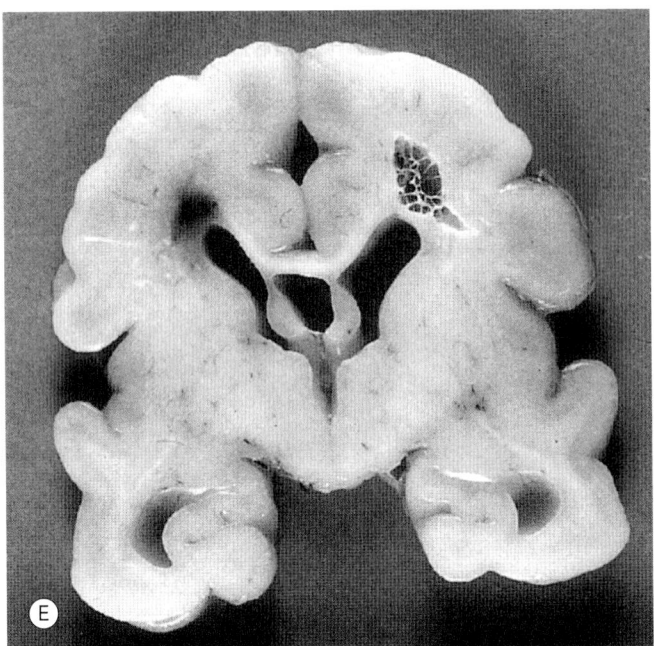

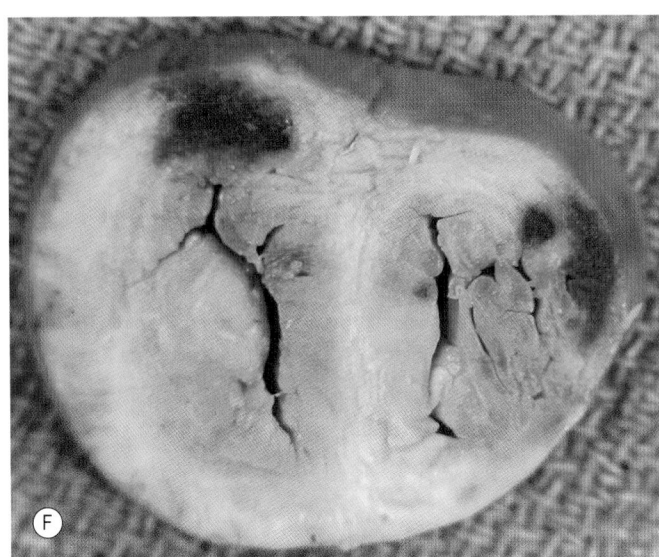

FIGURE 9.17 (*cont'd*) (E) Coronal section of brain of donor, showing multicystic encephalomalacia. (F) Biventricular myocardial infarction in a TTT recipient.

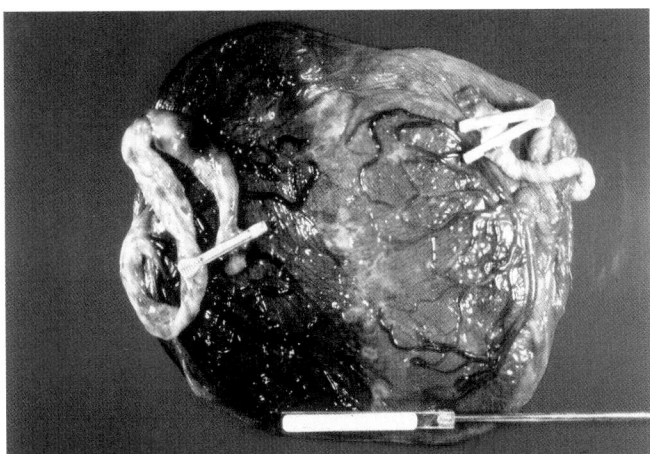

FIGURE 9.18 Management of prenatal TTT by laser coagulation of equatorial chorionic vessels, which are potential sites of a-v anastomosis. (From De Lia et al 1993,[119] with permission.)

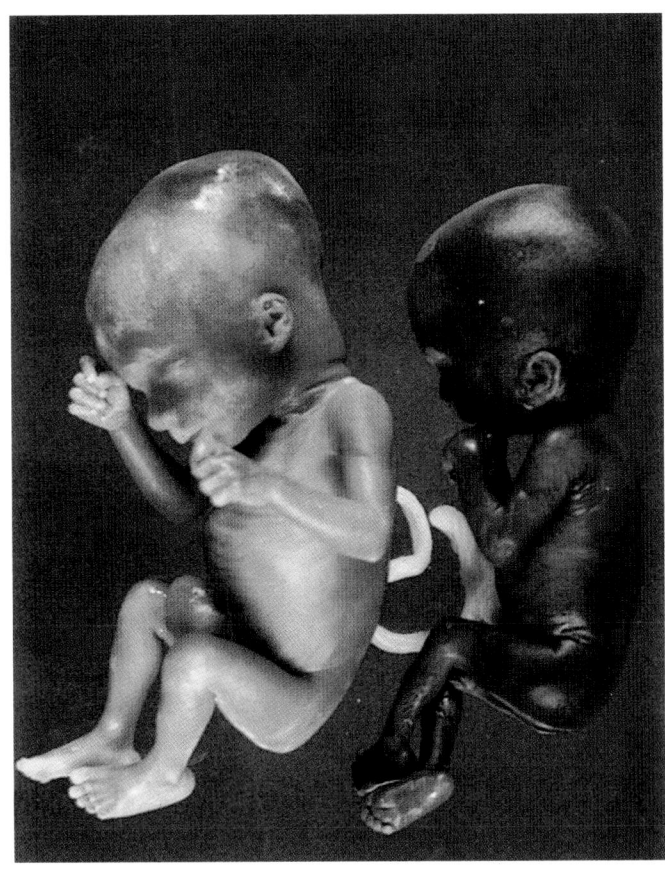

FIGURE 9.19 Acute intrapartum TTT. The larger twin (left) is anemic, while the small donor twin (right) is plethoric.

in nutrients, and rich in waste products. Furthermore, this **blood flows retrogradely** in the arterial tree to the acardiac; **it enters the fetal body via the common iliac arteries and runs retrogradely up the aorta,** the most distal branches of which are the arteries of the head and neck and the coronary arteries. Organ systems with low metabolic requirements and high tolerance of hypoxia/ acidosis will survive to some degree. **The lower limbs usually persist better than the upper limbs** because of the femoral artery takeoff from the common iliacs. The brain, heart, and upper limbs do not tolerate the quality and quantity of blood flow and **undergo ischemic necrosis.** The degree of regression depends on the interval between the onset of reversed flow and the delivery of the fetuses.

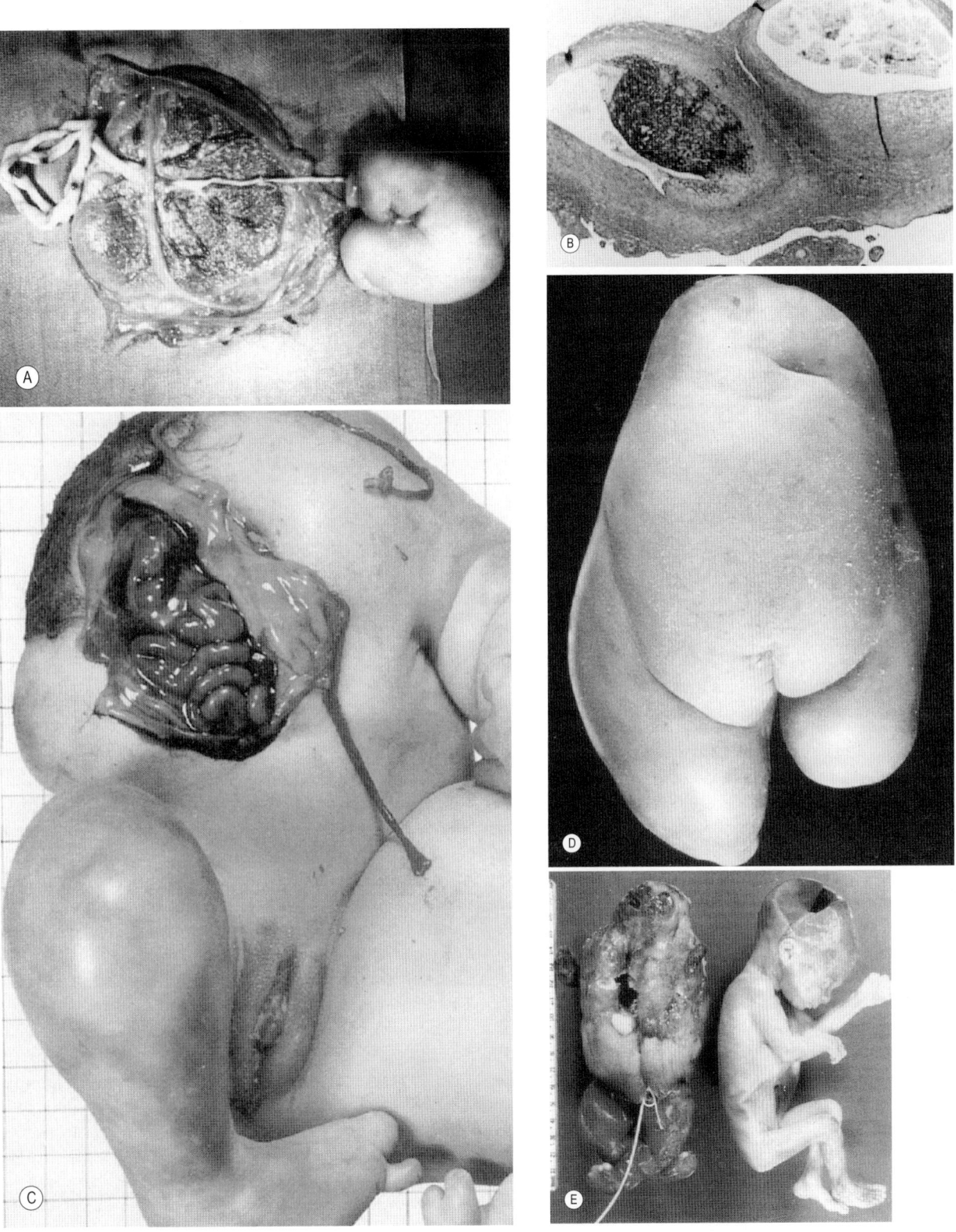

FIGURE 9.20 The pathology of TRAP. (A) The placenta is MC, DA, with cords inserted close together. This facilitates the large, direct a-a and v-v anastomoses, which allow the acardiac fetus to survive. (B) There was a recent mural thrombus in an arterial anastomotic vessel. Such events may endanger the pump twin. (C) Typical acardiac fetus with sternal cleft/omphalocele. The right arm is absent, having been perfused by the subclavian artery most remote for reversed arterial perfusion. This acardiac fetus was one of MZ, MC triplets. The others survived intact. (D) Severely reduced acardiac fetus with lower torso and lower limb remnants only. (E) When the onset of acardius is late, the affected fetus may show quite good preservation of organs.

TABLE 9.12 CHROMOSOMAL ABNORMALITIES IN TWIN REVERSED ARTERIAL PERFUSION

Acardiac fetus	Pump twin
46,XY/47,XY,+C	46,XY
46,XX/47,+min/47,XX,+ring	46,XX/47,XX,+min
46,XY/47,XY,+G	46,XY
45,X	46,XX
70,XXX,+15	46,XY
45,XX,t(4;21),del4p	46,XX
46,XX/47,XX,+11	46,XX
94,XXXXYY	47,XXY
46,XX	45,X/46,XX
45,X,+mar1/47,X,+mar1,+mar2	46,XX

After Wolf et al 1990,[127] with permission.

The second suggested mechanism is that the acardiac twin is constitutionally abnormal, with chromosomal abnormality and/or major malformation, including congenital heart disease or other malformation that compromises cardiac function. Were this embryo a singleton, it would probably undergo early spontaneous miscarriage; the presence of the pump twin allows the continued passive existence of the abnormal embryo, which undergoes ischemic regression because of the reversed arterial perfusion.

Evidence for constitutional abnormality in the acardiac fetus includes a **significant number of cases with major chromosomal abnormality** (Table 9.12).[127] There are several cases in which major malformation can be detected; symmelia is particularly common.[128] To ascertain major malformation, angiography on the acardiac twin and chromosome and DNA studies to look for specific single gene defects may be necessary.

TRAP can be diagnosed prenatally by obstetric ultrasonography.[129] It is sometimes confused with fibroids. Independent leg movements occur because spinal reflexes are intact;[129] the paradox is that an apparently dead fetus (no cardiac activity) moves independently. Retrograde umbilical arterial and aortic flow has been identified by Doppler flow studies.[130–133] The acardiac twin may continue to grow after its first recognition by ultrasonography.[129]

TRAP occurs frequently in triplet pregnancies.[134, 135]

The pump twin is at risk of fetal death because of cardiac failure; the risk is about 50%.[125] Selective removal of the acardiac twin has been attempted by hysterotomy and selective delivery,[136–138] by the use of thrombogenic coils,[139] and by tying off the cord.[140] Any method must ensure that there is no risk of acute hypotension in the pump twin. Pump twins may also have major malformations.[141, 142]

Monoamniotic twins

MA twins occur in about 1–2% of twins and in 1 in 30 MC pairs. Cord origins may be extremely close (Fig. 9.21). All forms of TTT and TRAP occur in MC, MA placentation. The additional cord complications cause a greatly increased risk (30–50%) of fetal and neonatal death.[143, 144]

Because the twins share a single amniotic cavity, **complex knotting and braiding of the cords may occur**[145] (Fig. 9.21). These can be diagnosed by ultrasound and are not necessarily fatal.[146, 147]

A further risk is that a **nuchal cord** of the presenting twin may actually belong to the second twin, who will suffer asphyxia when that nuchal cord is clamped and cut.[148, 149] There are intact survivors from this situation. **The cord of the second-born twin may prolapse** before the birth of the first twin.[150]

Most of the adverse effects in MC, MA twins occur in early pregnancy and few occur after 30 weeks of gestation.[144]

Death of one fetus

Fetal death of one twin occurs in DC and MC pregnancies, but the consequences are far more serious in MC twins because of vascular anastomoses in the MC placentas.

Fetal death may occur in the first trimester, when the dead fetus is usually completely resorbed [vanishing twin (VT)]. **Up to 30% of early twin pregnancies revert to singleton gestations.**[151] There are some reports of questionable remnants of VT, such as hydropic villi.[152, 153] The presence of two chromosomally different populations by placental sampling is not necessarily evidence of VT, since it could also result from placental mosaicism.[154]

In the second trimester the dead fetus is sufficiently large that it usually survives as a **fetus papyraceus** (FP) (Fig. 9.22). FP occurs both in DC and MC twins.[155] The effect of fetal death in the second trimester can be severe on the survivor in MC twins. A particular pattern of tissue damage involves the skin (**widespread aplasia cutis**) and the bowel (**multiple small bowel atresias**).[156–162]

Third trimester fetal death in MC twins can inflict severe hypoxic/hypotensive/ischemic pathology on the survivor (Table 9.13).[163–182] The pattern involves the brain (multicystic encephalomalacia, porencephaly), liver, lungs, and kidneys and results in a high prevalence of cerebral palsy in MC twin survivors.

The fetal death of one MC twin was previously thought to generate thromboplastins that flow or diffuse into the survivor, causing thrombotic organ ischemia and infarction; however, **acute changes in blood pressure and hematocrit** may be more important, such that 'rescue transfusion' of the surviving fetus can be successful, even as the co-twin is dying.[2, 183–186] In the presence of a-aa and v-va, the death of one twin leaves a large proportion of the MC placenta as a low-pressure zone into which the circulation of the survivor may now spread, greatly and acutely increasing the circulation volume of the survivor, leading to severe hypotension.

Organ infarction in the MC survivor has been seen by ultrasound to occur extremely rapidly after the fetal death. Thus decisions about the fate of the surviving twin are best made before the death of the dying twin, from whatever cause.

The impending fetal death of one twin highlights the need to know chorionicity early in pregnancy. In almost all DC pairs, it is safe to allow the dying fetus to die, after which the co-twin can be left in utero until pulmonary maturity is reached.

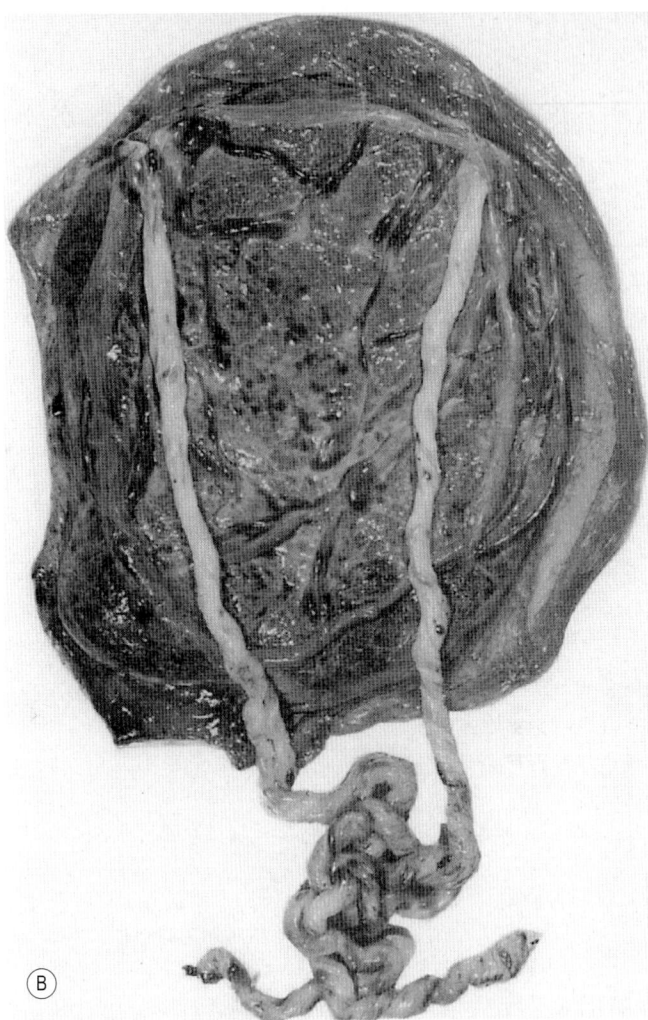

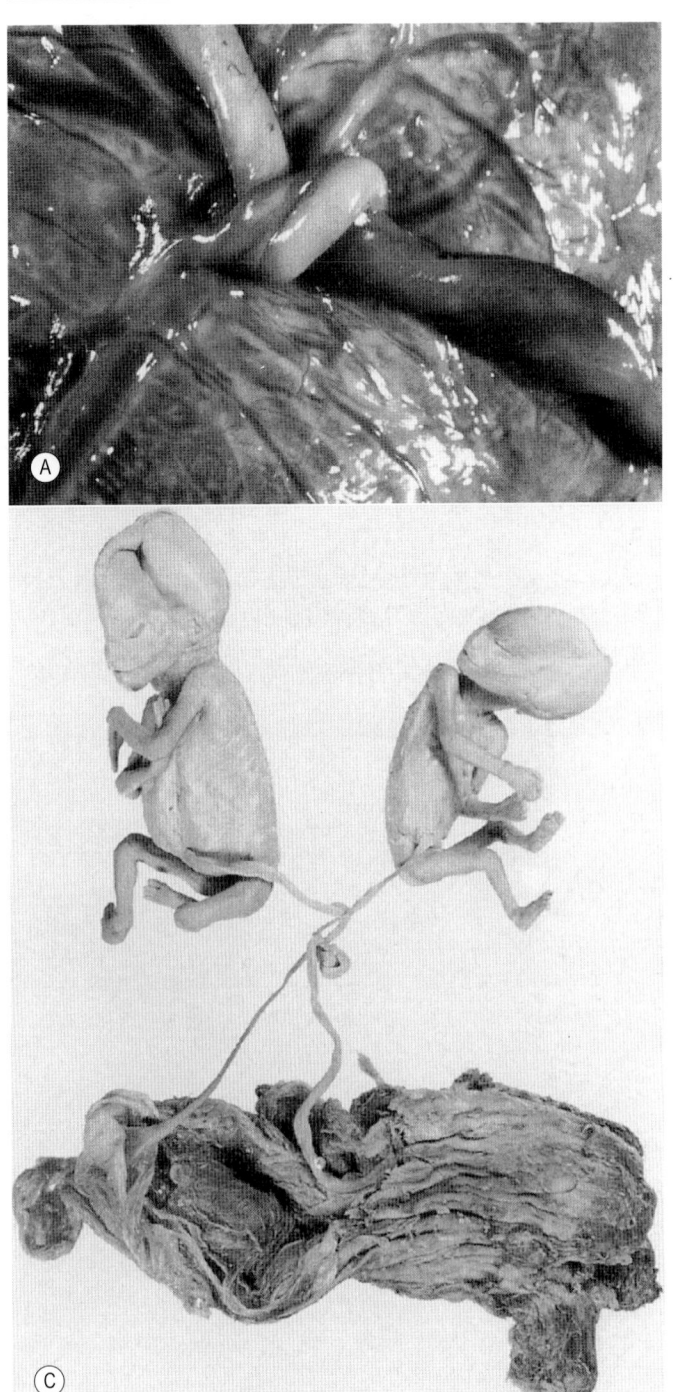

FIGURE 9.21 Complications of monoamniotic twinning. (A) Cords inserted close together, with a single knot. One twin survived with cystic encephalomalacia. (B) Extensive braiding of the cords, which can be seen by ultrasound scan. Both twins survived intact. (C) First trimester asphyxial fetal death of MC, MA twins with cord entanglement.

Discordance for malformation

Major malformation and genetic diseases of types that also occur in singletons may be found in only one of a MZ twin pair (see the earlier section on chromosome mosaicism and non-random X-inactivation). Discordance for other genetic diseases (e.g. Beckwith-Wiedemann syndrome) may reflect differential imprinting of these genes in a twin pair.

Discordances for major malformations such as neural tube defect, holoprosencephaly and symmelia (Fig. 9.23)[187–194] **may be intrinsic to the twinning process itself;** they may result from disturbances of embryogenesis by the twinning event at the time when the major axes are being laid down. Completion of recognition and fusion processes in and around the midline may be arrested or prevented by the twinning event.

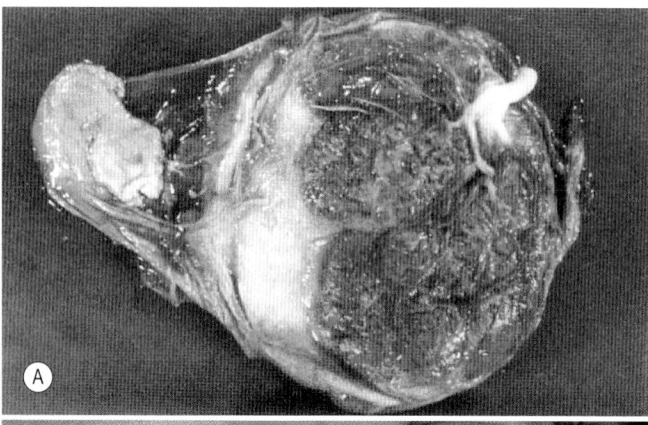

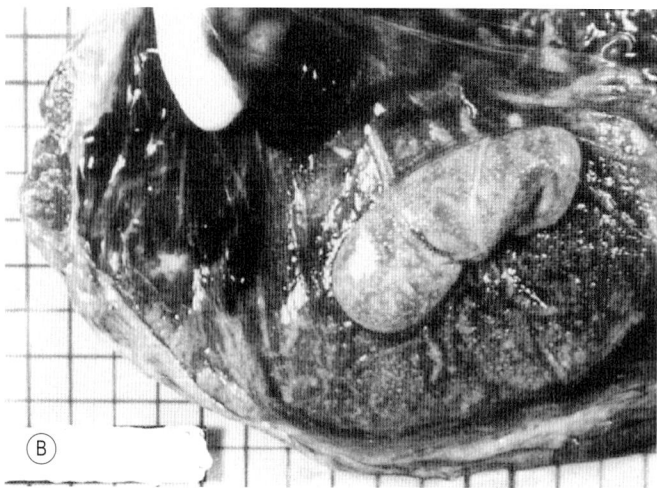

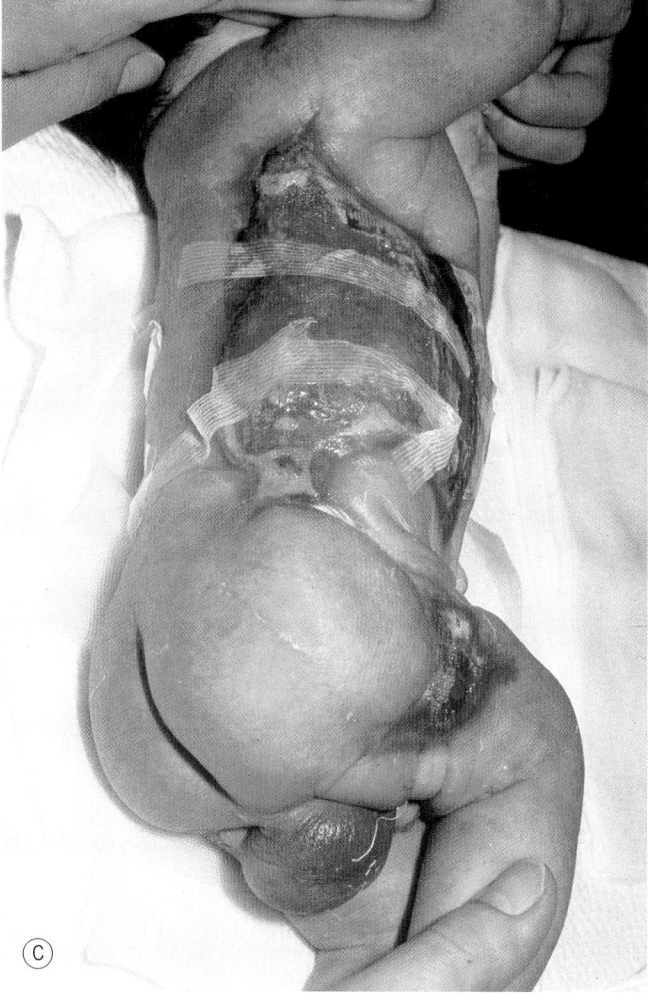

FIGURE 9.22 Fetus papyraceus. (A) Dichorionic fetus papyraceus in peripherally attached sac. Its placenta is shrunken and fibrotic. The co-twin survived intact. (B) Fetus papyraceus on placental surface. Note the amnion nodosum. The twins were MC. (C) The surviving twin had extensive aplasia cutis congenita and multiple small bowel atresias.

Discordance for major malformation in a twin pair does not imply DZ, DC status; attempts can be made to deliver an intact normal MZ co-twin when the other twin is lethally malformed. Little is known about the chorionicity of discordantly malformed MZ twins; such information would help in assessing the timing of the event.

Discordance for congenital heart disease in MC twins may result from unequal distribution of blood flow through placental vascular anastomoses. The heart of recipients of prenatal TTT may remain abnormal for some time postnatally; tricuspid regurgitation, right ventricular hypertrophy, and subendocardial fibroelastosis may occur.

Selective termination of pregnancy

Selective termination of a morbid fetus may be indicated in three circumstances: deteriorating clinical status in severe growth

TABLE 9.13 HYPOXIC/HYPOTENSIVE/ISCHEMIC LESIONS IN SURVIVORS OF THIRD TRIMESTER FETAL DEATH OF CO-TWIN

Author	Multiple pregnancies	Single twin fetal death		Organ infarction in surviving twin	
		No	%	No	%
Benirschke[2]	201			1	
Hagay et al[163]	1192	17	1.4	0	0
Wessel et al[164]	186	8	4.3	1	12.5
Cherouny et al[165]	435	20	4.5	1	5.0
Enbom[166]	40	2	5.0	0	0
Carlson and Towers[167]	642	17	2.6	1	5.9
Hannah and Hill[168]	–	3	2.2		
D'Alton et al[169]	325	15	4.6		
Lumme and Saarikowski[170]			2.2		
Litschgi and Stucki[171]		13	6.8		
Yoshida and Soma[156]	189	5	4.3	1	20

discordance; TTT and TRAP; major malformation causing clinical deterioration or potentially difficult delivery; and multi-fetal reduction in HOMPs resulting from AR. In these situations MC gestations are fraught with risk that both twins will die if one of them is terminated.[195, 196] In MC twins, selective termination of one twin poses high risks to the remaining fetuses due to the presence of vascular anastomoses.[197] The earlier the termination, the less likely that questions of zygosity and chorionicity will be clarified. Empty sacs and fetal remnants may be present, but the arrangements of septal membranes may not be exactly identifiable. Zygosity should be investigated by DNA methods.

Higher-order multiple pregnancies

By Hellin's law, the prevalence of spontaneously conceived triplets and quadruplets is 1 in 80 × 80 and 1 in 80 × 80 × 80 deliveries, respectively. There has been a steady rise in the frequency of HOMPs in the West since the mid-1980s;[12] this is caused by various methods of AR. These gestations contain about 10% MZ twins.

Optimism about the outcome of HOMPs only applies to those cases resulting from AR.[16] SC multiplets contain larger proportions of MZ and MC twins, triplets, and quadruplets, with the attendant risks of TTT, TRAP, and malformation.

Methods of investigation of zygosity and chorionicity resemble those used for twins, but the options are many for various combinations of septal membrane arrangements, vascular anastomoses, and zygosity (Table 9.14).[13, 67, 76–79]

HOMP gestations that are MZ may show various combinations of DC and MC placentations, implying serial twinning events at different times in early embryogenesis. HOMP is associated with lower mean gestational age at delivery and higher mortality than twin pregnancy.

SC quadruplets are rare, and little is known about zygosity and chorionicity. Figure 9.7 shows an MC, tetra-amniotic (TA)

TABLE 9.14 CHORIONICITY AND ZYGOSITY OF 15 SETS OF SPONTANEOUSLY CONCEIVED TRIPLETS

	Monozygotic	Dizygotic	Trizygotic	No.	Total percentage
Monochorionic	2	0	0	2	13
Dichorionic	3	4	0	7	47
Trichorionic	1	3	2	6	40
Total	6	7	2	15	100

The 45 triplets were derived from 26 zygotes. All but two pairs contained at least MZ twins.

quadruplet placenta. There were a-aa between quadruplets B and C. All the female infants survived intact (Fig. 9.7).

Conjoined twins

CTs are particularly important because they may be diagnosed prenatally, may be surgically separable, and can contribute to the understanding of normal and abnormal embryogenesis. There is an unabated and lively debate as to whether CTs arise by incomplete fission of one embryonic axis, or by re-fusion of two axes that were previously completely separate.[198, 199] Classifications address two main issues: how the body axes of the twins are mutually orientated in the embryonic disc, and how the subsequent events of migration, growth, and body folding result in the types of CTs that are actually found in practice.[200–202]

CTs result from relatively late twinning events when the body axes (primitive streak, notochord, neural tube) have been molecularly specified and are beginning to be visible morphologically. It can result from the simultaneous development of two primitive streaks. These events occur **at or about day 14 post fertilization.** Thus two major body plans are laid down within one body, delimited by ectoderm, and with complex relationships

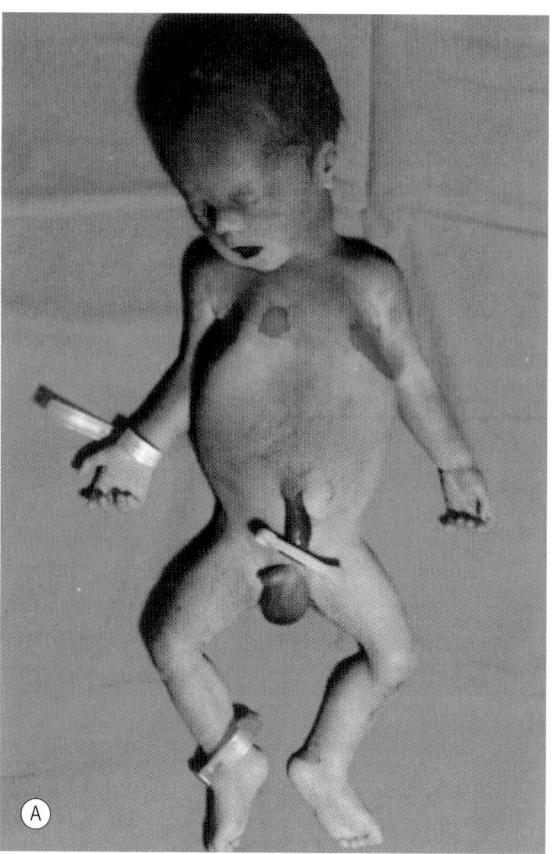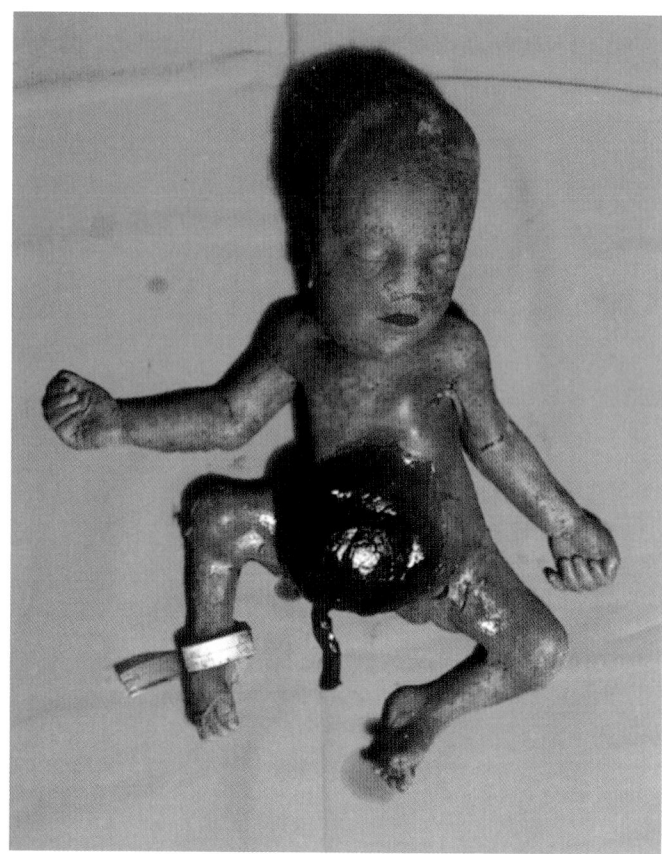

FIGURE 9.23 MZ twins with discordance for major malformations. (A) MC, MZ twins discordant for cloacal exstrophy. There is also acute intrapartum TTT.

to amnion, and intraembryonic and extraembryonic celom. Patterns of coalescence of the body plans seen in clinical practice are limited because other arrangements would probably interfere with development to such a degree that early fetal demise occurs. Although many pairs have severe degrees of overlap with no feasibility of separation, CTs in clinical practice probably represent the least severe examples of all the forms that are possible.

The body axes of most CT pairs are oriented toward each other in ways that suggest that embryogenesis was closely integrated, occurring on a segment-by-segment and field-by-field basis. Specific zones of coalescence or overlap may be identified, and actions of genes (such as Hox and Pax genes) that are implicated in very early embryogenesis may be determined.

There are only two major methods of CT classification: according to the orientation of the two body axes and their degree of complete development (Figs 9.24 and 9.25). Most CTs have **two almost complete notochordal axes,** which are arranged so as to cause minimal mutual interference with development (i.e. cranial-to-cranial, caudal-to-caudal, and ventro-ventral). In the second type the **two notochords are closely side by side with closest apposition caudally;** there is a varying degree of duplication of the bodies, which are more separated cranially than caudally. These types **(dicephalus and diprosopus)** most closely correspond with the older classification of 'catadidymus'. Although

dipygous twins are regarded as the classic form of 'anadidymus', with single representation cranially and duplication caudally, such is not truly the case. The two caudal components are not arranged side-by-side (as in dicephalus/diprosopus), but rather ventro-ventrally. Thus one of the twins represents a parasitic twin.

Classification of CTs as **heteropagus** implies that one body plan is completely laid out, while the other is present as a reduced axis with incomplete formation of fields and zones (so-called heteropagus parasitic twins). It is not clear whether formation of components of the second body axis is incomplete ab initio, or whether there is early normal development, followed by an event (perhaps resembling acardius) that leads to secondary degeneration of the minor body axis. The minor axis may also reflect an unequal allocation of blastomeres. In most examples there is segment-by-segment correspondence between the autosite and parasite. There is no complete line of distinction between CTs of all kinds and zones of more localized organ or zone duplication.

Fetus-in-fetu applies to reduced and parasitic fetuses within the body of the autosite, and are differentiated from teratomas as they contain vertebral segmentation, organogenesis or both.[203–205] Fewer than 100 cases have been reported, most of which are intraabdominal.[205] Such fetuses usually derive their blood supply from the superior mesenteric or renal vessels and are located in the upper retroperitoneum.

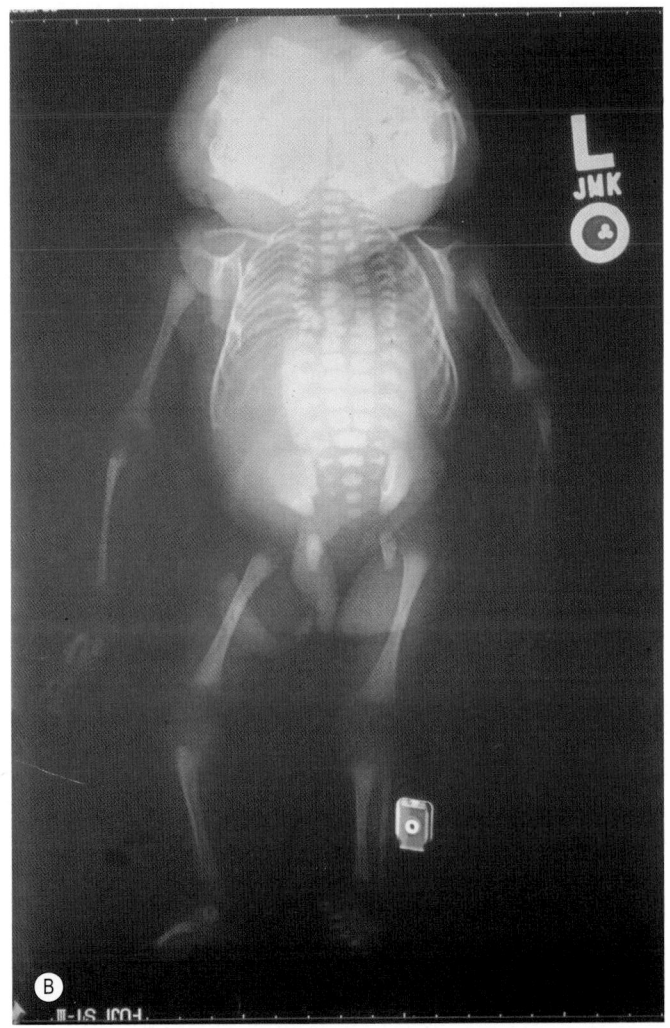

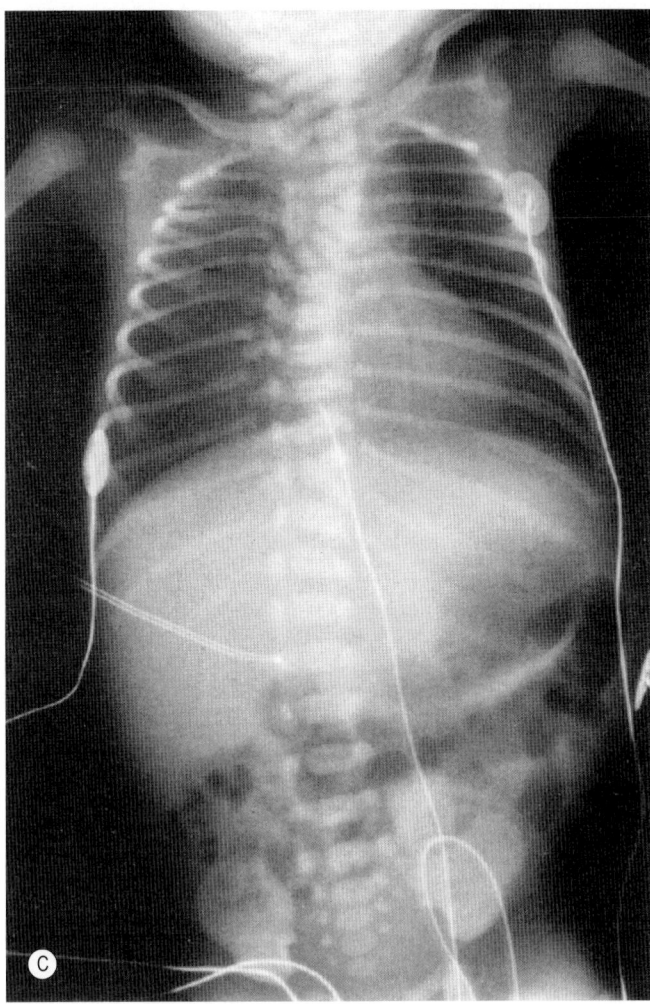

FIGURE 9.23 (*cont'd*) (B) and (C) MC, MZ twins discordant for neural tube defect. One twin has anencephaly, while the other has thoracic hemivertebrae but no other malformations.

There may be considerable overlap between sacrococcygeal teratoma and parasitic conjoined fetus. Some sacrococcygeal teratomas contain very well organized zones and organs, to the extent of formed limbs and suggestions of short segments of body axes.

A working classification of CTs is given in Box 9.1 (Figs 9.26–9.38)[200, 201] These major types represent the stereotypes into which most cases can be classified. Some cases appear to combine features of two or more of the stereotypes, while others seem to defy easy classification. Pathologists will continue to describe cases in detail, accompanied by photography, angiography, and extended dissection. Such investigations should attempt to answer the following kinds of questions:

- **Are both body axes complete or nearly so?**
- **How are the two body axes oriented toward each other,** for example, are they side-by-side (dicephalus/diprosopus) or is there minimal mutual interference, for example, cranio-cranial, caudo-caudal, or ventro-ventral? (Figs 9.24 and 9.25)
- **Are the dorso-ventral midline planes of the two CT axes directly in line (symmetros) or do they meet obliquely (asymmetros)?** (Fig. 9.29)
- **Where are the major zones of organ overlap,** for example, faces, brain segments, branchial arch derivatives, atria, ventricles, great arteries, respiratory tracts, alimentary tracts (especially biliary tracts, midgut), genital and urinary tracts, cloacae, pelvic skeletons? (Figs 9.30 and 9.31)
- **Are new axes formed,** for example, the faces in cephalothoracopagus and the pairs of legs in ischiopagus? (Figs 9.29–9.31)
- **If there are identifiable coalescences or formations of new axes, where do these events occur in terms of embryologic precursors** (e.g. branchial arches, brain segments)?
- **In these zones of interaction and reorientation of viscera, is it possible to postulate abnormal actions of genes that determine major developmental events** (e.g. Hox and Pax genes)?

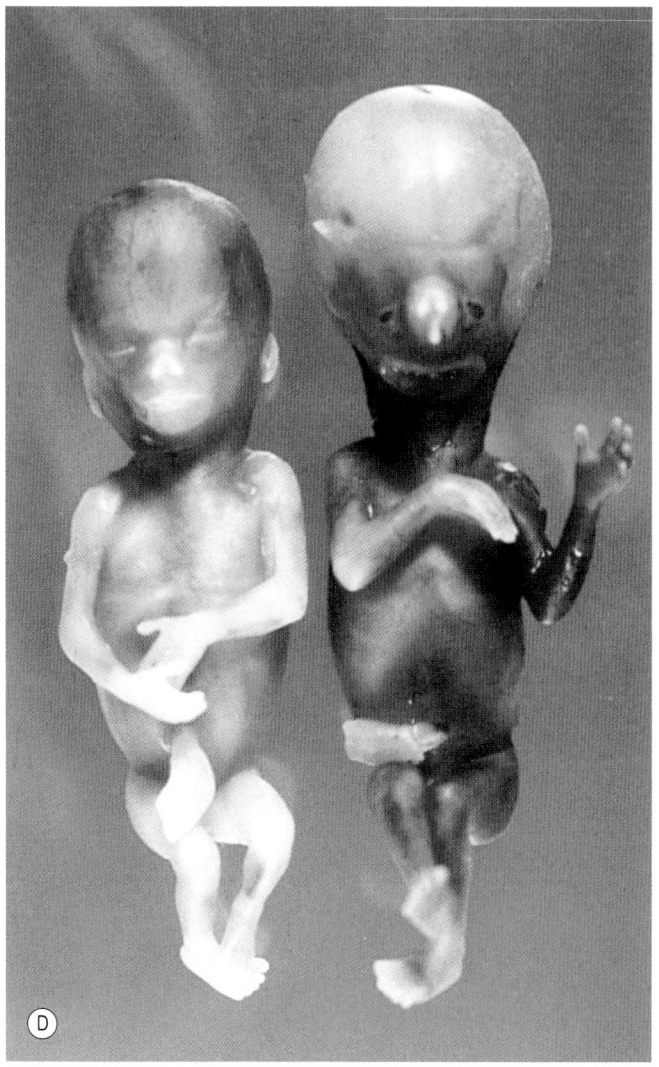

FIGURE 9.23 (*cont'd*) (D) MC, MZ twins discordant for holoprosencephaly. There is also intrapartum TTT.

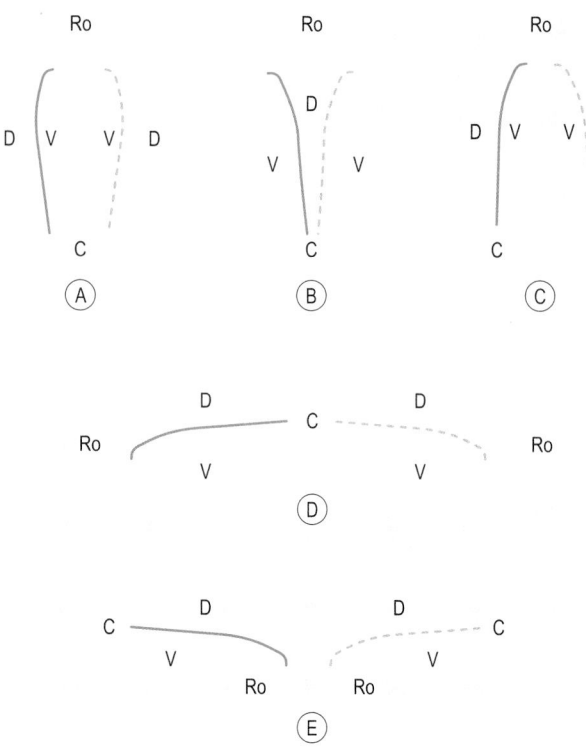

FIGURE 9.24 Tolerated types of notochordal orientations in conjoined twins. (A) Ventro-ventral orientation, as seen in thoracopagus, xiphopagus, etc. (B) Dorso-dorsal with caudal apposition, i.e. pygopagus. (C) Ventro-ventral with cranial apposition, i.e. cephalothoracopagus. (D) Cranio-cranial apposition, i.e. craniopagus. (E) Caudo-caudal apposition, i.e. ischiopagus. D, Dorsal; V, ventral; Ro, rostral/cranial; C, caudal.

Pathology as a basis for genetic studies in twins

Twins are used widely in the investigation of relative effects of genotype and environmental events on the eventual phenotypes of individuals. The general assumptions of such studies are shown in Table 9.15. Recent discoveries in MZ twinning have served to complicate this simple picture in two main ways:

- Many MZ twins are extremely similar in phenotype and genotype.[206] However the existence of postzygotic epigenetic events such as chromosome mosaicism, non-random X chromosome inactivation and discordance for major malformation in MZ twins shows that **many MZ twins are not 'identical'.**

- **The intrauterine environments of MZ and DZ twin pairs may be sufficiently different as to impose major phenotypic differences at birth** that are not caused by genotypic differences.[29] The various

---

BOX 9.1 ANATOMIC CLASSIFICATIONS OF CONJOINED TWINS EACH AXIS FULLY EXPRESSED OR NEARLY SO

Notochordal Axes Face Each Other:

Ventro-ventral:	Thoracopagus (Fig. 9.26), xiphopagus, etc.
Ventro-ventral, cranial:	Cephalothoracopagus (Figs 9.27 –9.30)
Ventro-ventral, caudal:	Ischiopagus (Fig. 9.31)
End-to-end, cranial:	Craniopagus (Fig. 9.32)
End-to-end, caudal:	Pygopagus (Fig. 9.33)

Notochordal Axes Side-by-Side:

Dicephalus (Fig. 9.34): two heads, two complete spines, variable upper limbs up to and including four arms, single pelvic girdle, two legs

Diprosopus (Fig. 9.35): one head, two faces, one spine, two arms

One Axis Incompletely Expressed

Parasitic twins at all sites, including dipygus* and fetus-in-fetu (Figs 9.36–9.38)

*Dipygus has one full axis and one incomplete axis that is ventro-ventral and only expressed caudally. Dipygus does not represent a 'splitting' of the axes caudally.

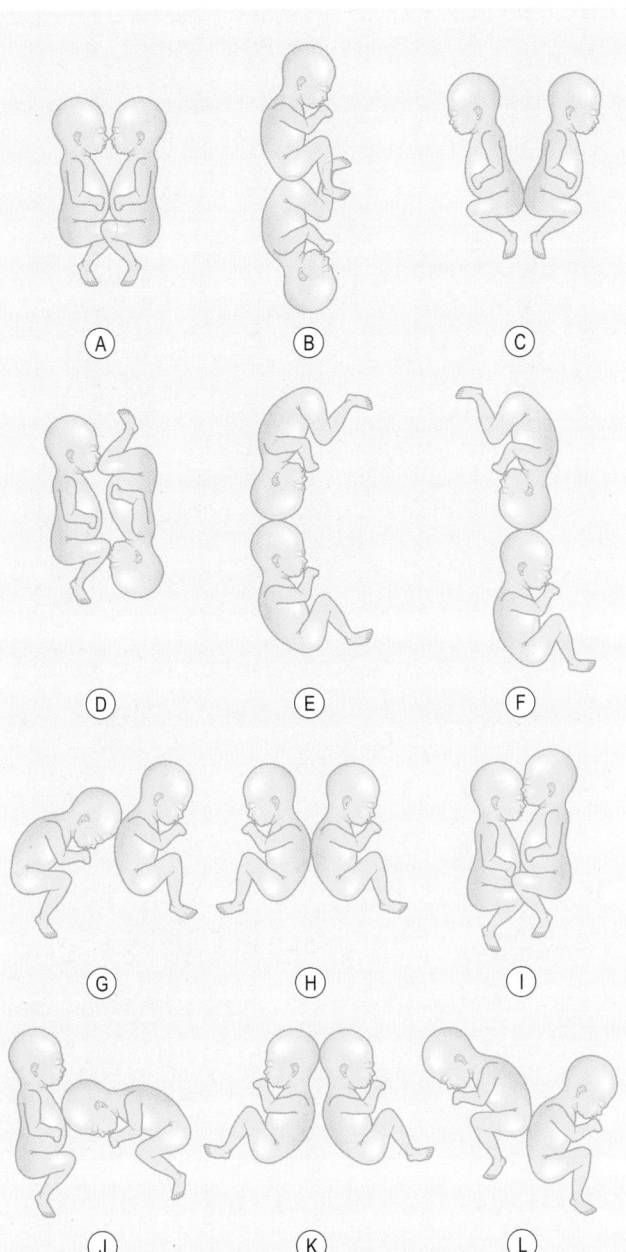

FIGURE 9.25 Tolerated and non-tolerated types of conjoined twins. (A) Ventro-ventral is permitted, e.g. thoracopagus. (B) Caudo-caudal is permitted, i.e. ischiopagus. (C) Dorso-dorsal, caudal apposition is permitted, i.e. pygopagus. (D) Ventro-ventral, with 180-degree rotation on ventro-ventral axis is rare but is an acquired relationship. (E) and (F) Craniopagus is permitted, with and without rotation of one twin on the longitudinal axis, an acquired relationship. (G)–(L) Relationships not seen include cranio-dorsal (G), mid dorso-dorsal (H), ventro-ventral without segmental correspondence (I), cranio-ventral (J), dorsal craniopagus (K), dorso-dorsal without segmental correspondence (L).

TABLE 9.15 IMPACT OF GENOTYPE AND ENVIRONMENT ON PHENOTYPE: ASSUMPTIONS OF TWIN STUDIES

	Similar phenotype	Dissimilar phenotype
MZ twins	Genetic influence	Environmental influence
DZ twins	Environmental influence	Genetic influence

TABLE 9.16 RELATIVE RISKS OF POOR OUTCOMES IN TWIN PREGNANCIES

	Rate per 1000 live births	Relative risk for twins compared with singletons
Very low birth weight, < 1500 g	10.1	9.97
Low birth weight <2500 g, includes very low birthweight	58.2	8.61
Neonatal death	5.86	7.06
Postneonatal death	3.49	2.75
Infant death	9.33	5.43

After Powers and Kiely 1994,[213] with permission.

causes of growth discordance in MC, MZ twins resulting from IFVA ensure that many MZ twin pairs have different body masses at birth. The effects of these discordances on long-term development are unknown.

DC and MC, MZ twinning events occur at different times post conception, and these two types of MZ twins may have significantly different biological characteristics; DC and MC, MZ twins may develop in different ways.

Despite these drawbacks, MZ twins in particular yield impressive evidence of the power of the genotype in determining phenotype. MZ twins separately adopted at birth show striking similarities in physical, intellectual, and psychological constitution.[206] MZ twins are increasingly studied for the natural history of such multifactorial degenerative diseases as atherosclerosis, hypertension, and Alzheimer disease.[207] MZ twins are also studied for their occasional discordance for physiologic constitution such as sexual orientation.[208, 209] Some MZ twin pairs are strikingly discordant for psychiatric disorders.[210, 211] In these situations the discordant aspects of brain function are particularly important.

Summary

The pediatric pathologist has a unique responsibility for recording as much information as possible about the prenatal and perinatal status of the twins and their placenta(s). In particular, aspects of zygosity, chorionicity, parenchymal sharing, and major discordance will be invaluable in clarifying many unsolved questions

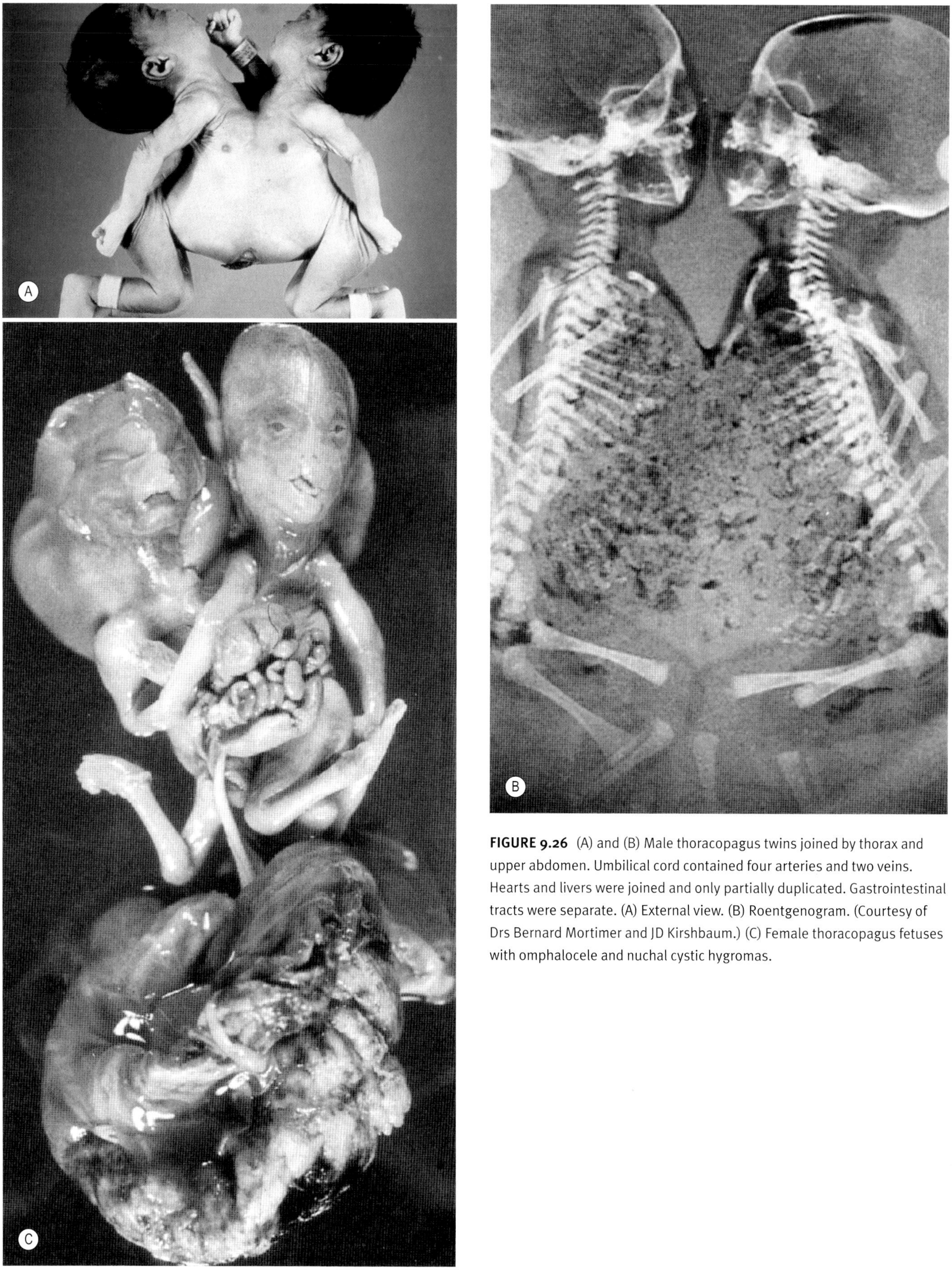

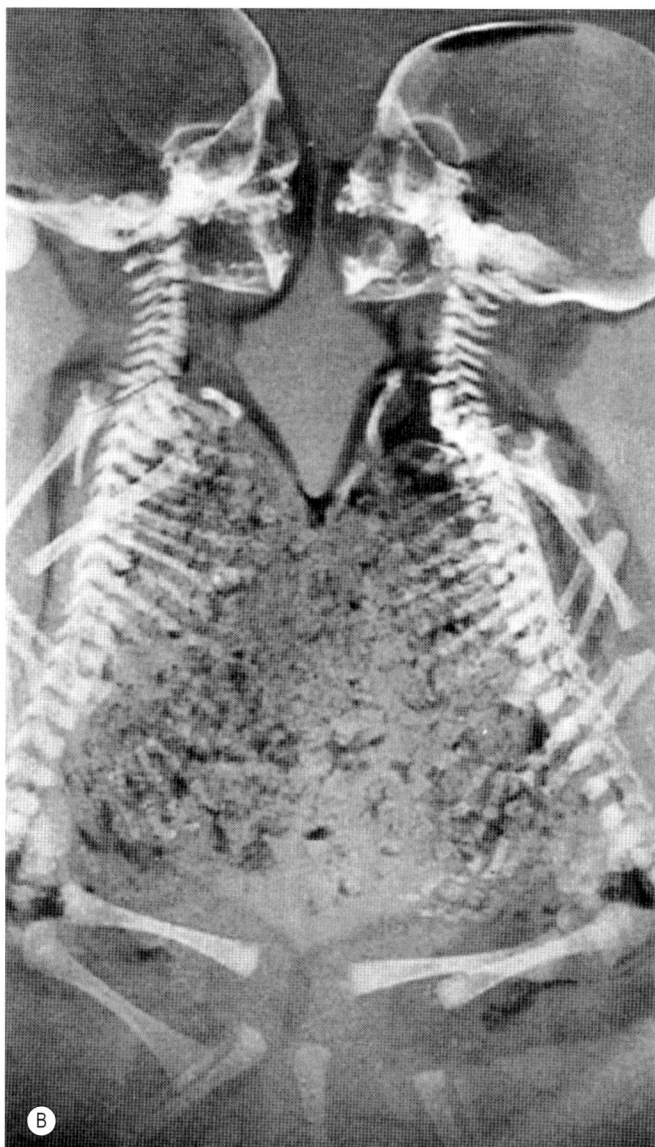

FIGURE 9.26 (A) and (B) Male thoracopagus twins joined by thorax and upper abdomen. Umbilical cord contained four arteries and two veins. Hearts and livers were joined and only partially duplicated. Gastrointestinal tracts were separate. (A) External view. (B) Roentgenogram. (Courtesy of Drs Bernard Mortimer and JD Kirshbaum.) (C) Female thoracopagus fetuses with omphalocele and nuchal cystic hygromas.

TABLE 9.17 COMPARISON OF OBSTETRIC AND NEONATAL OUTCOMES IN MC AND DC TWINS[214–218]

Author	Location	Study type	Outcome measures	MC	DC
214	Nova Scotia, Canada	Population	PND	35/588 (6%)	25/1469 (1.7%)
214			Mean BWD	11.7%	11.0%
214			BWD >25%	8.6%	6.5%
215	Mumbai, India	?Population	PND	18%	9%
215			Mean BWD	35%	14%
216	Tochigi, Japan	Referral	NND to age 1 year	4/88 (4.5%)	6/328 (1.8%)
			Neurologic disability	5.7%	1.8%
217	Birmingham, UK	Referral	PND	3/48 (6.2%)	14/190 (6.2%)
218	Toronto, Canada	Referral	Infants born at 24–30 weeks gestation, surviving 18–24 months; death and neurologic disability	39%	25%

PND, Perinatal death; BWD, birth weight discordance; NND, neonatal death.

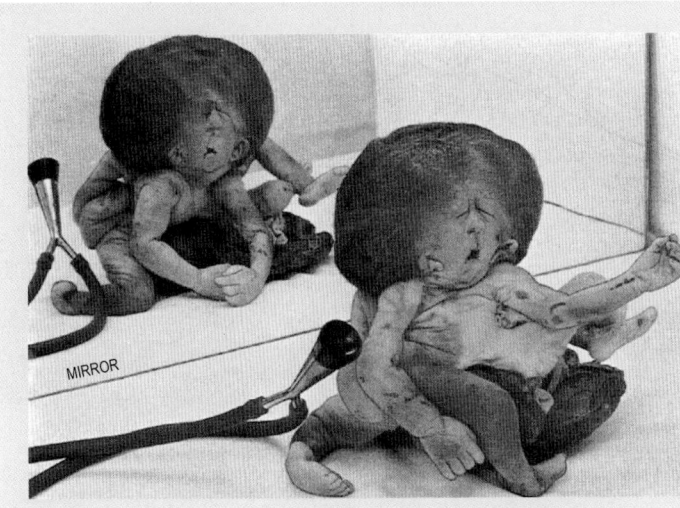

FIGURE 9.27 Cephalothoracopagus janiceps. Fetus has two faces, one of which is visible in the mirror. (Courtesy of Dr Frances Holmes.)

about the process of twinning and its role in adverse perinatal outcomes.[212] Unfortunately, bad outcomes from MC twin pregnancy (unexpected fetal demise, significant neurologic injury in survivors) figure frequently in litigation. Pathologists play a role in explaining these outcomes on the basis of careful placental and fetal examination.

In a study from the Centers for Disease Control and Prevention,[213] relative risks of adverse outcomes were compared for liveborn singletons and twins in a cohort of 7 357 550 singleton and 156 690 twin infants born in 1985 and 1986 (Table 9.16). The relative risks of adverse outcomes for twins were 10.0 for birth weight more than 1500 g, 8.6 for birth weight more than 2500 g, 7.1 for death before 28 days, 2.75 for death between 28 days and 1 year, and 5.4 for death in the first year of life. These outcomes were not stratified for zygosity and chorionicity.

Table 9.17 summarizes the relative frequency of adverse outcomes in MC and DC twin pregnancies.[214–218] MC twins had more frequent bad outcomes than DC twins for all outcome measures. In a reported series of survivors from prenatal TTT, 22% had cerebral palsy.[219] The prime functions of the pediatric pathologist are to distinguish between DC and MC twin placentas and to explain the significantly worse outcomes for MC twins.

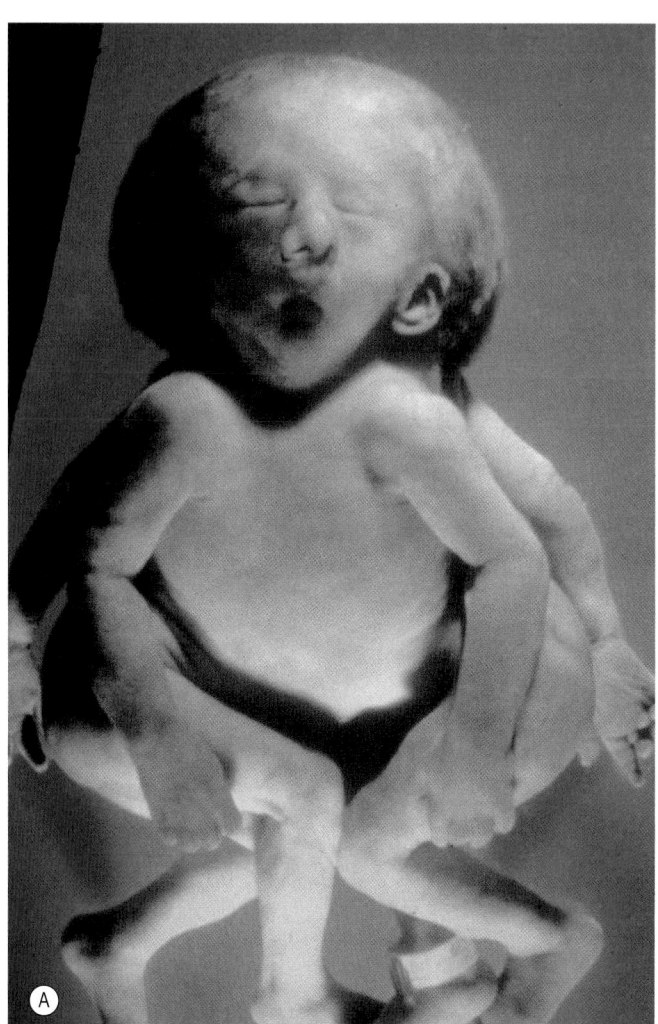 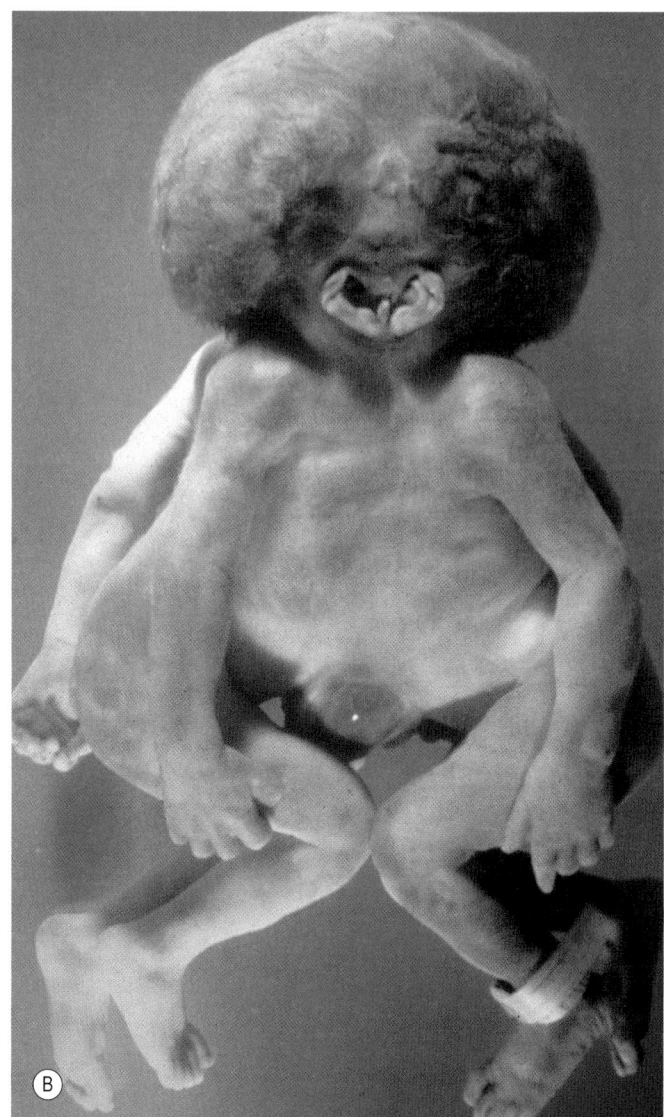

FIGURE 9.28 Cephalothoracopagus syncephalus. (A) Anterior view. (B) Posterior view. These cephalothoracopagus twins are non-symmetric, in the sense that one of the faces consists of ears only. (Courtesy of Drs Harold C Priddle and Charles S Stevenson.)

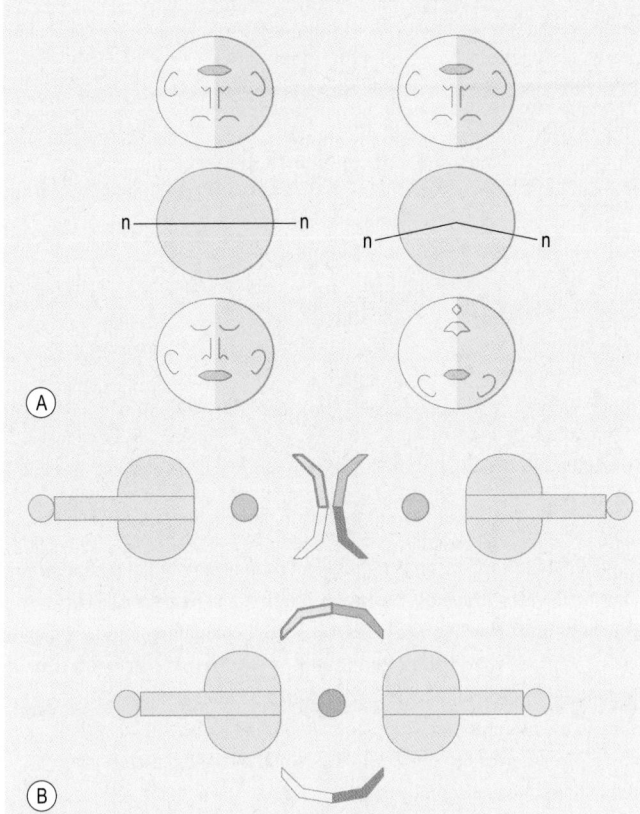

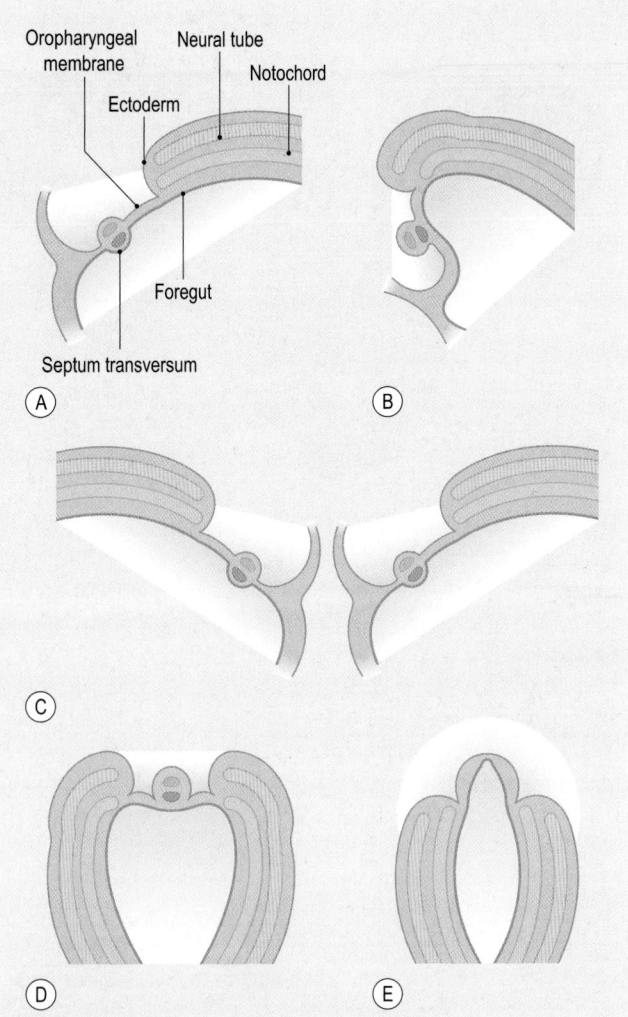

FIGURE 9.29 (A) Plan and side views of non-symmetric cephalothoracopagus twins. If the notochordal axes (n) are facing exactly ventro-ventral (left), both faces are fully represented. If the notochordal axes meet at an angle (right), one face is normal and the other is reduced. (B) Plan view of coalescence zone on embryonic plate of cephalothoracopagus twins. Above, two monoamniotic twin axes are closely apposed caudally but without coalescence. Head folding will occur normally. Below, there is coalescence of the two axes at the oropharyngeal membrane, and the septa transversa are expressed laterally; each new structure (e.g. face, heart, liver) is made up of components from each embryonic axis.

FIGURE 9.30 Lateral view of normal singleton head folding (A) and (B), and head folding in monoamniotic twins closely apposed caudally (C). In thoracopagus twins (D), there is coalescence at the septum transversum, with overlapping fields of development of hearts and livers. In cephalothoracopagus twins (E), coalescence at the oropharyngeal membrane forces derivatives of the septum transversum out of the midline into 'new' lateral zones.

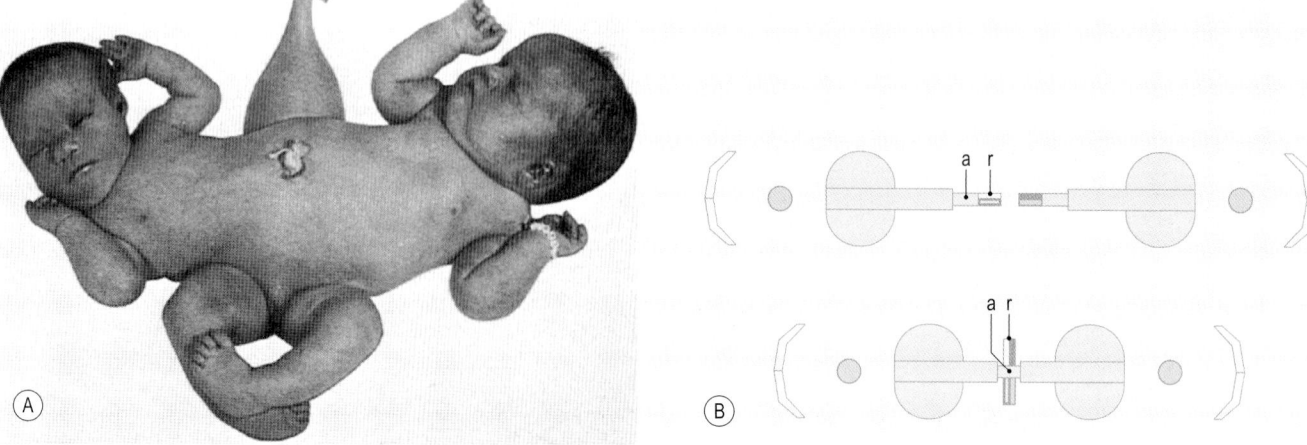

FIGURE 9.31 (A) Ischiopagus twins. Lower abdominal areas are fused and extremities consequently displaced laterally. Only one pelvis is present, associated with single normal external genitalia, the latter located between right leg of left twin and left leg of right twin. The legs are normal except for clubfoot. Opposite legs are fused into a single composite limb. Viscera of one was in situs inversus position. Aortas were fused. The heart of one twin was hypoplastic and circulation through that twin was in reverse direction through arteries and veins. (Courtesy of Dr Hans G. Schlumberger and J. Elmer Gotwals.) (B) Plan view of caudal apposition of embryonic axes. Above are shown monoamniotic twins with caudo-caudal apposition but no coalescence. Below are ischiopagus twins, with coalescence of cloacal membranes as far as anal component. The other cloacal components (genitourinary) are expressed in new, laterally placed axes. Thus genitalia and lower urinary tracts are made up of components from both embryonic axes; considerations are the same as for cephalothoracopagus twins. The sireniform limb seen in Fig. 9.25F corresponds with the reduced side of the coalesced embryonic axes, caused by non-symmetric orientation of the two notochordal axes. a, anus; r, remaining cloacal components.

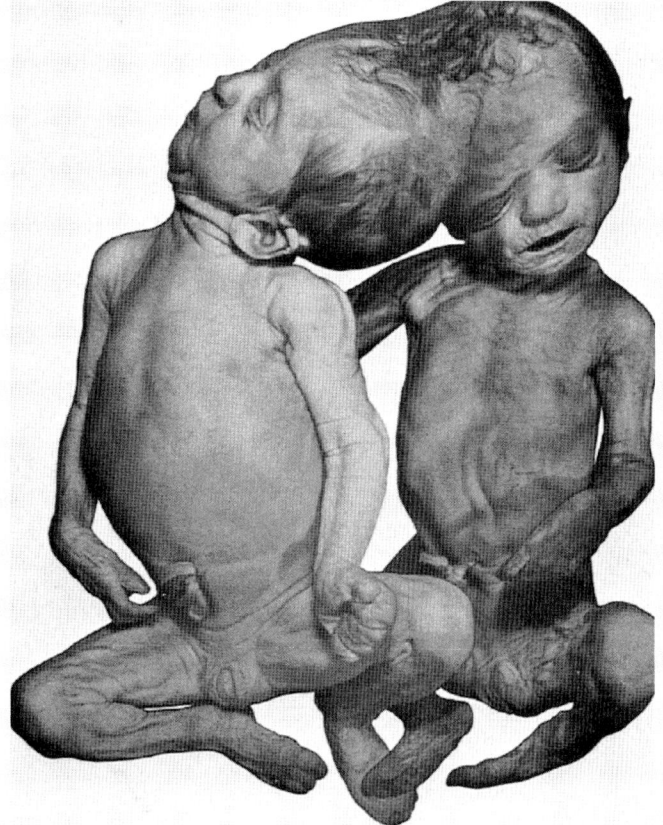

FIGURE 9.32 Craniopagus twins. Median parietal area of right twin is united with right frontoparietal area of left twin. (Courtesy of Dr Charles O McCormick.)

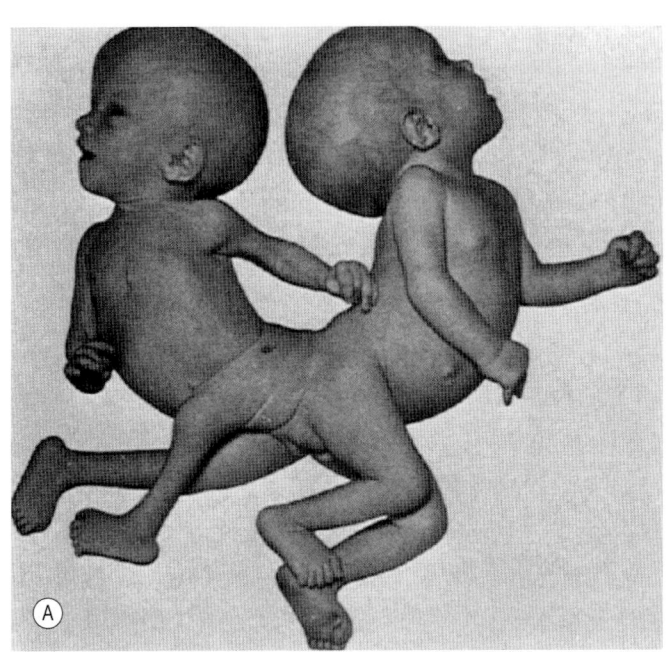

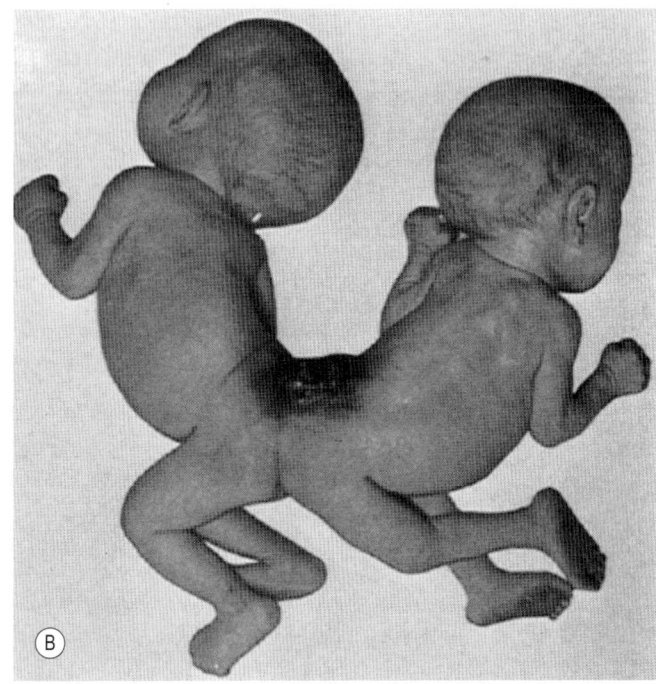

FIGURE 9.33 Pygopagus female twins. Infants joined at sacral areas, each of which was the site of a spina bifida. External genitalia were partially fused, and common vaginal and anal orifices were divided by septa separating the two orifices of the twins. Bladders and all organs were duplicated except the kidneys, of which there were only three. (A) Anterior view. (B) Posterior view. (Courtesy of Dr Helen Dawson.)

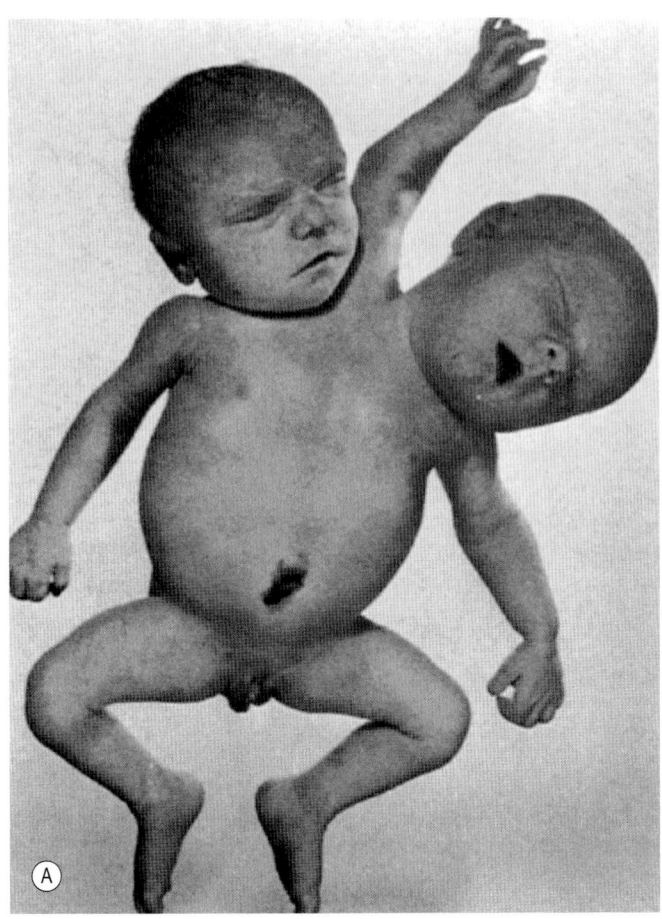

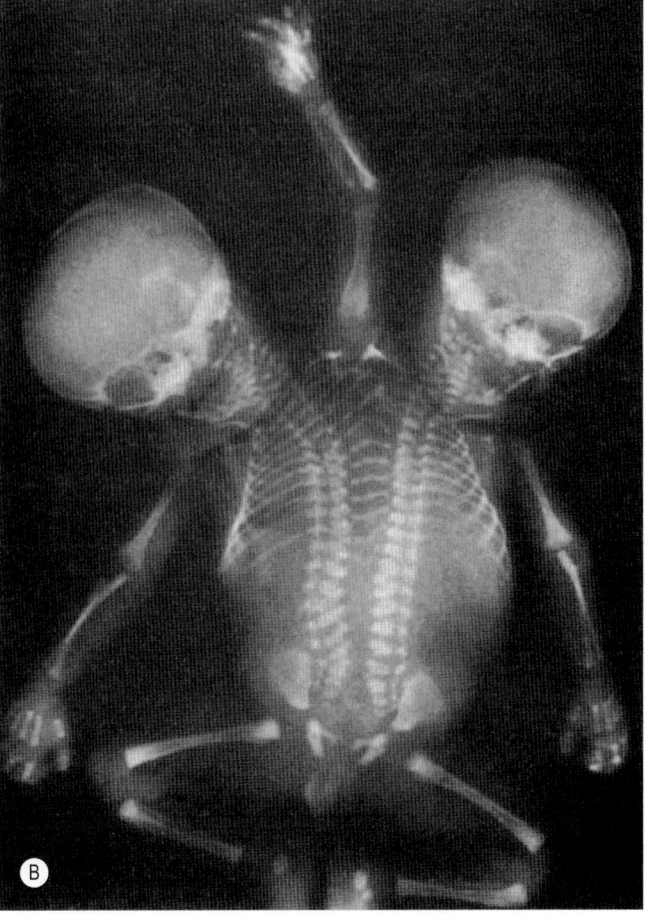

FIGURE 9.34 Dicephalus dipus tribrachius. (A) Anterior body surface. (B) X-ray of skeleton showing common arm with fused humerus and three bones in forearm.

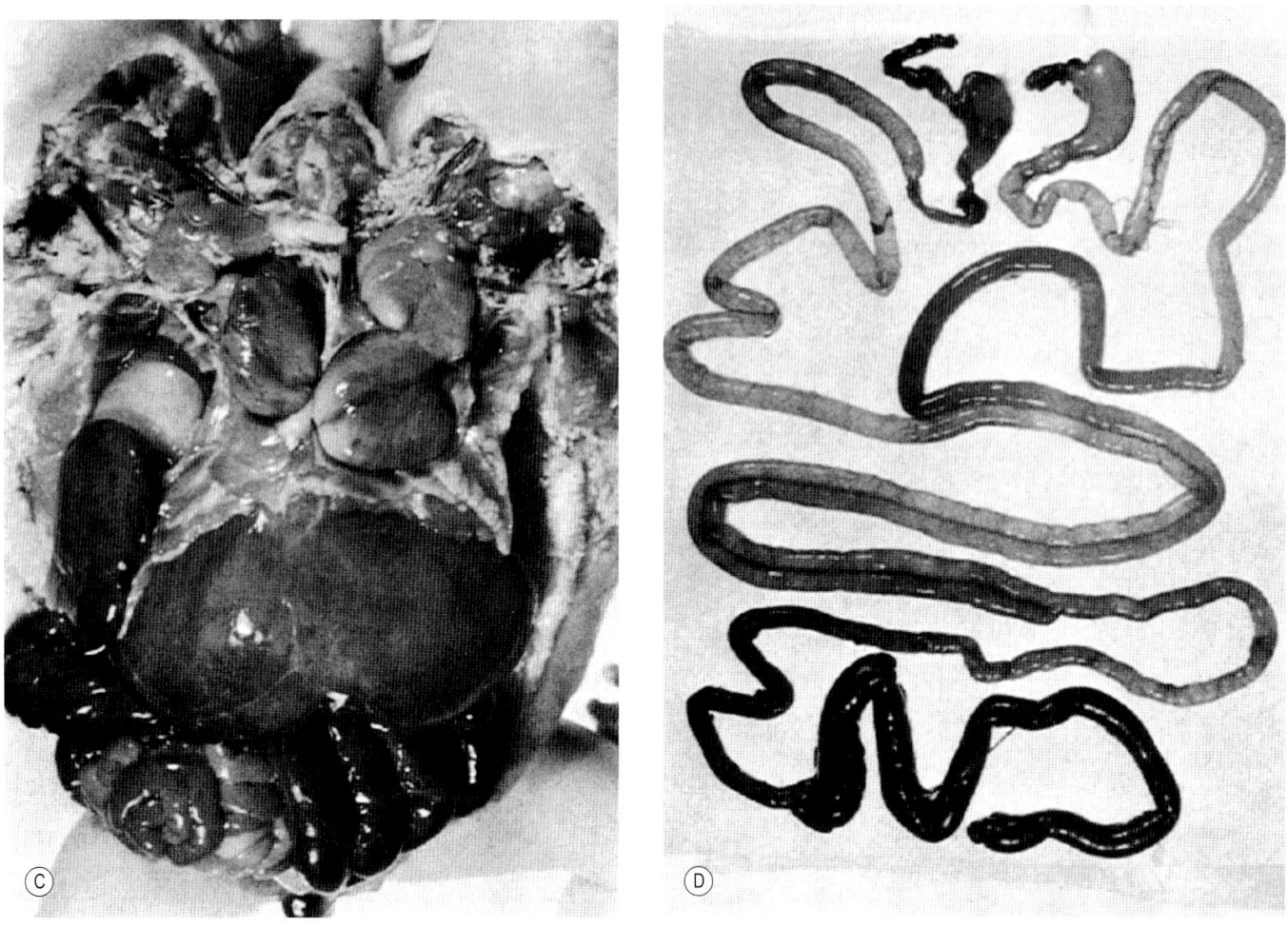

FIGURE 9.34 (*cont'd*) (C) Interior of body cavity, showing two thyroids, two thymuses, two hearts in separate pericardial cavities and one liver with abnormal lobulation caused by right diaphragmatic hernia. (D) Stomachs and intestine with duplication as far as mid ileum. (Specimen courtesy of Dr JB Butler.)

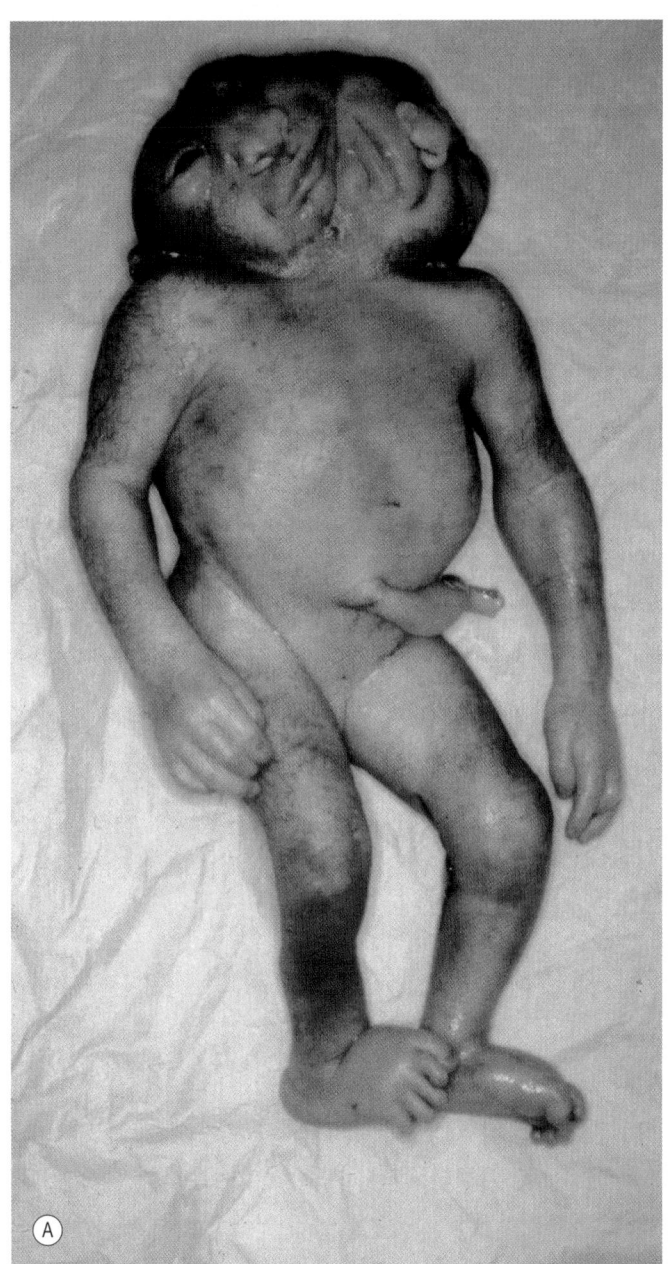

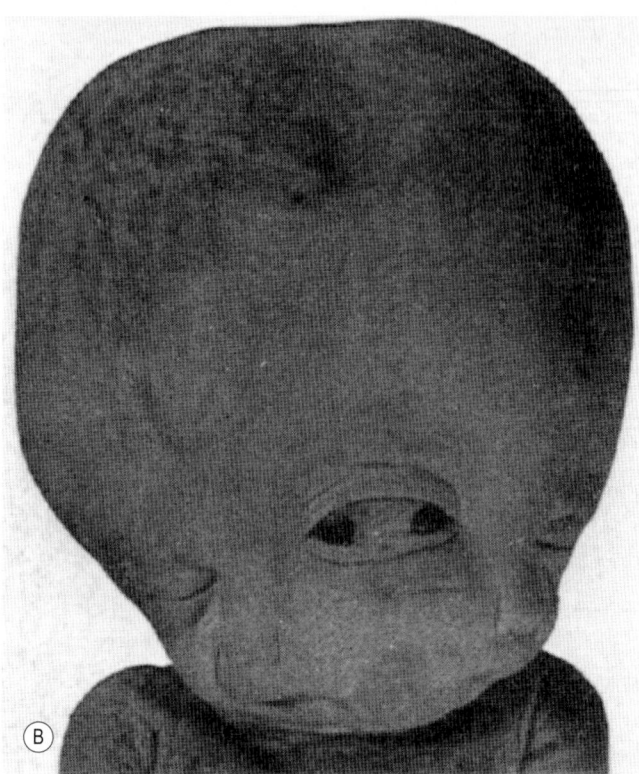

FIGURE 9.35 Monocephalus diprosopus. (A) Anencephalus with two faces and fusion of heads. (Courtesy of Dr Raymond Mitchell.) (B) Duplication of face with a common median orbit. (Courtesy of Dr Henry W Edmonds.)

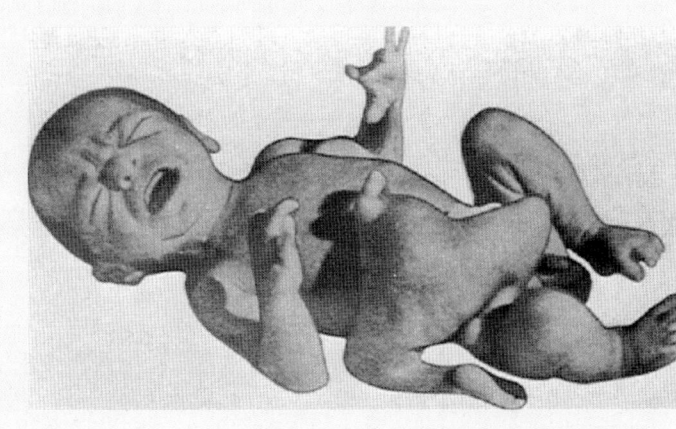

FIGURE 9.36 Parasitic fetus composed of fairly well-developed legs, rudimentary pelvis, and one finger attached to epigastrium of an otherwise normal male infant.

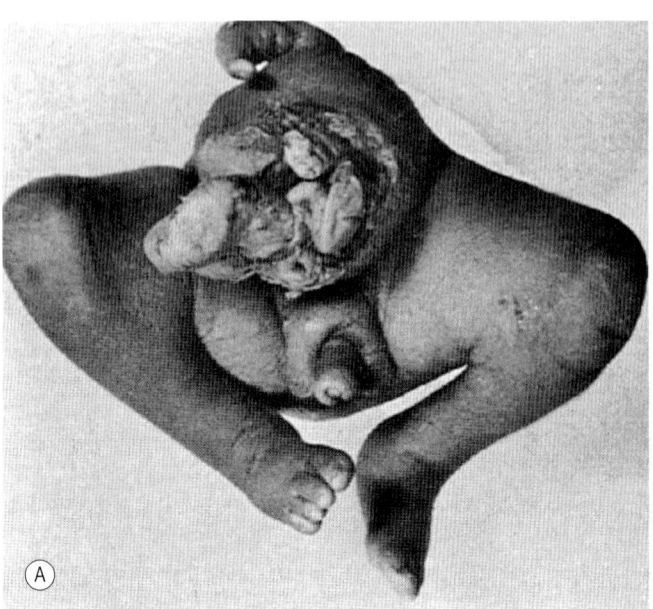

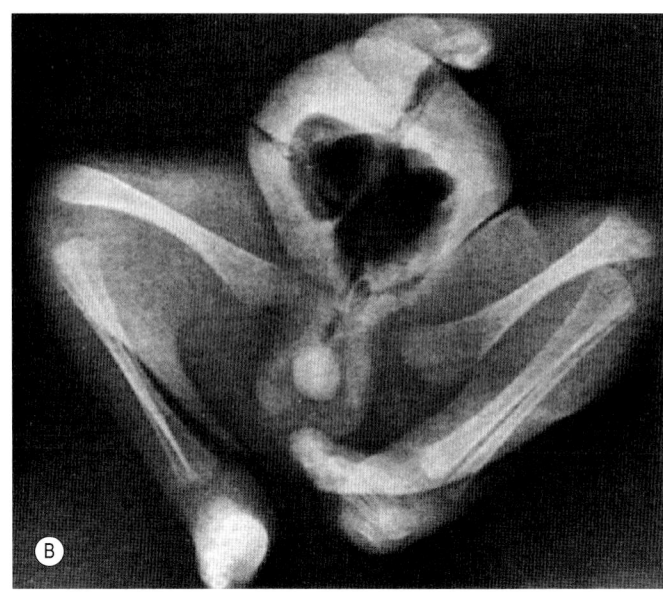

FIGURE 9.37 Parasite shown in Figure 9.36 successfully detached. Abdominal cavity of the parasite contains an isolated portion of intestine, urethra, bladder, one kidney with two ureters, seminal vesicles and prostate. (A) External view. (B) Roentgenogram.

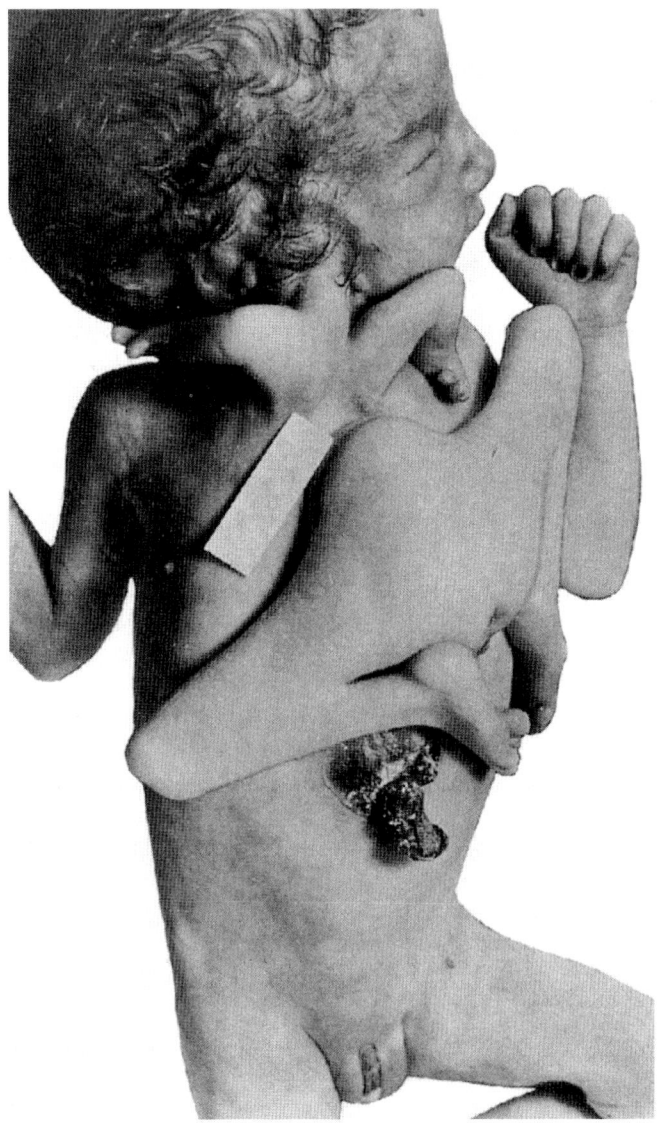

FIGURE 9.38 Parasitic fetus with abnormal arms, pelvis, and legs attached to anterior thorax of autosite. (Courtesy of Dr SA Golberg.)

References

Multiple pregnancies and conjoined twins

1. Potter EL. Twin zygosity and placental form in relation to outcome of pregnancy. Am J Obstet Gynecol 1963; 87:566–577.
2. Benirschke K. Twin placenta in perinatal mortality. N Y State Med J 1961; 61:1499.
3. Fowler MG, Kleinman JC, Keily JL, et al. Double jeopardy: twin infant mortality in the United States, 1983 and 1984. Am J Obstet Gynecol 1991; 165: 15–22.
4. Fujikura T, Froehlich LA. Twin placentation and zygosity. Obstet Gynecol 1971; 37:34–43.
5. Derom R, Vlietinck RF, Derom C, et al. Zygosity testing at birth: a plea to the obstetrician. J Perinat Med 1991; 19(suppl):234.
6. Gardner M, Goldenberg RL, Tucker JM, et al. The origin and outcome of preterm twin pregnancies (abstract). Am J Obstet Gynecol 1994; 170:401.
7. Naeye RL, Tafari N, Judge D, et al. Twins: causes of perinatal death in 12 United States cities and one African city. Am J Obstet Gynecol 1978; 131: 267–272.
8. Gruenwald P. Environmental influences on twins apparent at birth. Biol Neonat 1970; 15:79–93.
9. Myrianthopoulos NC. An epidemiologic survey of twins in a large prospectively studied population. Am J Hum Genet 1970; 22:611–629.
10. Benirschke K, Driscoll SG. The pathology of the placenta. New York: Springer-Verlag; 1967.
11. Bleker OP, Breur W, Huidekoper BL. A study of birth weight, placental weight and mortality of twins as compared to singletons. Br J Obstet Gynaecol 1979; 86:111–118.

Zygosity in twins and higher-order multiples

12. Nylander PPS. Frequency of multiple births. In: McGillivray I, Nylander PPS, Corney G, eds. Human multiple reproduction. London: WB Saunders; 1975: 87.
13. Bressers WMA, Eriksson AW, Kostense PJ, et al. Increasing trend in the monozygotic twinning rate. Acta Genet Med Gemellol (Roma) 1987; 36: 397–408.
14. Wenk RE, Houtz T, Brooks M, et al. How frequent is heteropaternal superfecundation? Acta Genet Med Gemellol 1992; (Roma) 41:43–47.
15. Botting BJ, Davies IM, Macfarlane AJ. Recent trends in the incidence of multiple births and associated mortality. Arch Dis Child 1987; 62:941–950.
16. Lipitz S, Reichman B, Paret G, et al. The improving outcome of triplet pregnancies. Am J Obstet Gynecol 1989; 161:1279–1284.
17. Edwards RG, Mettler L, Walters DE. Identical twins and in vitro fertilization. J In Vitro Fertil Embryo Transfer 1986; 3:114–117.
18. Derom C, Vlietinck R, Derom R, et al. Increased monozygotic twinning rate after ovulation induction. Lancet 1987; 1:1236–1238.
19. Cameron AH, Edwards JH, Derom R, et al. The value of twin surveys in the study of malformations. Eur J Obstet Gynecol Reprod Biol 1983; 14:347–356.
20. James WH. Excess of like-sexed pairs of dizygotic twin pairs. Nature 1971; 232:277–278.
21. Derom C, Bakker E, Vlietinck R, et al. Zygosity determination in newborn twins using DNA variants. J Med Genet 1985; 22:279–282.
22. Derom C, Vlietinck R, Derom R, et al. Genotyping of macerated stillborn fetuses. Am J Obstet Gynecol 1991; 164:797–800.
23. Hill AVS, Jeffreys AJ. Use of minisatellite DNA probes for determination of twin zygosity at birth. Lancet 1985; 2:1394–1395.
24. Kovacs B, Shahbahrami B, Platt LD, et al. Molecular prenatal genetic determination of twin zygosity. Obstet Gynecol 1988; 72:954–956.
25. Souter VL, Kapur RP, Nyholt DR, et al. A report of dizygous monochorionic twins. N Eng J Med 2003; 349:154–158.
25a. Souter VL, Parisi MA, Nyholt DR, et al. A case of the hermaphroditism reveals an unusual mechanism of twinning. Hum Genet 2007; 121:179–185.
26. Akane A, Matsuara K, Shiono H, et al. Diagnosis of twin zygosity by hypervariable RFLP markers. Am J Med Genet 1991; 41:96–98.
27. Benirschke K, Kim CK. Multiple pregnancy. N Engl J Med 1973; 288: 1276–1284.
28. Boklage CE. On the timing of monozygotic twinning events. In: Gedda L, Parisi P, Nance WE, eds. Twin research 3: twin biology and multiple pregnancy. Prog Clin Biol Res 1981; 69A:155–165.
29. Machin GA. Some causes of genotypic and phenotypic discordance in monozygotic twin pairs. Am J Med Genet 1996; 61:216–228.
30. Kondo S, Schutte BC, Richardson RJ, et al. Mutations in IRF6 cause Van der Woude and popliteal pterygium syndrome. Nat Genet 2002; 32:285–289.
31. Edwards JH, Dent T, Kahn J. Monozygotic twins of different sex. J Med Genet 1966; 3:117–123.
32. Karp L, Bryant JI, Tagatz G, et al. The occurrence of gonadal dysgenesis in association with monozygotic twinning. J Med Genet 1975; 12:70–78.
33. Schmidt R, Sobel EH, Nitowsky HM, et al. Monozygotic twins discordant for sex. J Med Genet 1976; 13:64–68.
34. Reindollar RH, Byrd JR, Hahn DH, et al. A cytogenetic and endocrinologic study of a set of monozygotic isokaryotic 45,X/46,XY twins discordant for sex. Mosaicism versus chimerism. Fertil Steril 1987; 47:626–633.
35. Arizawa M, Suehara N, Takemura T, et al. Monozygotic twins discordant for sex. Acta Obstet Gynecol Jpn 1988; 40:1479–1482.
36. Turpin R, Lejeune J, Lafoucade J, et al. Presomption de monozygotisme en depit d'un dimorphisme sexuel: sujet masculin XY et sujet neutre haplo X. CR Acad Sci 1961; [III] 252:2945–2946.
37. Perlman E, Stetten G, Tuck-Muller CM, et al. Sexual discordance in monozygotic twins. Am J Med Genet 1990; 37:551–557.
38. Dallapicolla B, Stomeo C, Ferranti G, et al. Discordant sex in one of three monozygotic triplets. J Med Genet 1985; 22:6–11.
39. Kurosawa K, Kuromaru R, Imaizumi K, et al. Monozygotic twins with discordant sex. Acta Genet Med Gemellol (Roma) 1992; 41:301–310.
40. Deacon JS, Machin GA, Martin JM, et al. Investigation of acephalus. Am J Med Genet 1980; 5:85–99.
41. Pedersen IK, Philip J, Sele V, et al. Monozygotic twins with dissimilar phenotypes and chromosome complement. Acta Obstet Gynecol Scand 1980; 59:459–462.
42. Ross GT, Tjio JH, Lipsett MB. Cytogenetic studies of presumptively monozygotic twin girls discordant for gonadal dysgenesis. J Clin Endocrinol 1969; 29:440–445.
43. Kaplowitz PB, Bodurtha J, Brown J, et al. Monozygotic twins discordant for Ullrich-Turner syndrome. Am J Med Genet 1991; 41:78–82.
44. Neilson JP, Hood VD, Cupples W, et al. Detection by ultrasound of abnormalities in twin pregnancies during the second trimester. Br J Obstet Gynaecol 1982; 89:1035–1040.
45. Ferguson-Smith AC. X inactivation: pre- or post-fertilisation turn-off? Curr Biol 2004; 14:R323–R325.
46. Navarro P, Pichard S, Ciaudo C, et al. Tsix transcription across the Xist gene alters chromatin conformation without affecting Xist transcription: implications for X-chromosome inactivation. Genes Dev 2005; 19:1474–1484.
47. Tuckerman E, Webb T, Bundey SE. Frequency and replication status of the fragile X, fra(X) (q27-28), in a pair of monozygotic twins of markedly differing intelligence. J Med Genet 1985; 22:85–91.
48. Burn J, Povey S, Boyd Y, et al. Duchenne muscular dystrophy in one of monozygotic twin girls. J Med Genet 1986; 23:494–500.
49. Richards CS, Watkins SC, Hoffman EP, et al. Skewed X inactivation in a female MZ twin results in Duchenne muscular dystrophy. Am J Hum Genet 1990; 46:672–681.
50. Lupski JR, Garcia CA, Zoghbi HY, et al. Discordance of muscular dystrophy in monozygotic female twins: evidence supporting asymmetric splitting of the inner cell mass in a manifesting carrier of Duchenne dystrophy. Am J Med Genet 1991; 40:354–364.
51. Abbadi N, Phillipe C, Chery M, et al. Monozygotic twins discordant for Duchenne muscular dystrophy – evidence for mirror X-chromosome inactivation. Proceedings of the Seventh International Congress on Twin Studies, Tokyo, Japan, 1992.
52. Jorgensen AL, Philip J, Rashkind WH, et al. Different patterns of inactivation in MZ twins discordant for red-green color-vision deficiency. Am J Hum Genet 1992; 51:291–298.
53. Winchester B, Young E, Geddes S, et al. Female twin with Hunter disease due

to nonrandom inactivation of the X-chromosome: a consequence of twinning. Am J Med Genet 1992; 44:834–838.

54. Kruyer H, Mila M, Glover G, et al. Fragile X syndrome and the (CGG)n mutation: two families with discordant MZ twins. Am J Hum Genet 1994; 54:437–442.

55. Levade T, Giordano F, Maret A, et al. Different phenotypic expression of Fabry disease in female monozygotic twins. J Inher Metab Dis 1991; 14:105–106.

56. Nance WE. Invited editorial: Do twin Lyons have larger spots? Am J Hum Genet 1990; 46:646–648.

57. Zneimer SM, Schneider NR, Richards CS. In situ hybridization shows direct evidence of skewed inactivation in one of monozygotic twin females manifesting Duchenne muscular dystrophy. Am J Med Genet 1993; 45:601.

58. Monteiro J, Derom C, Vlientinck R, et al. Commitment to X inactivation precedes the twinning event in monochorionic MZ twins. Am J Hum Genet 1998; 63:339–346.

59. Chitnis S, Derom C, Vlietinck R, et al. X chromosome-inactivation patterns confirm the late timing of monoamniotic-MZ twinning. Am J Hum Genet 1999; 65:570–571.

60. Bieber FR, Nance WE, Morton CC, et al. Genetic studies of an acardiac monster: evidence of polar body twinning in man. Science 1981; 213:775–777.

61. Wulfsberg EA, Wassel WC, Polo CA. Monozygotic twin girls with diploid/triploid chromosome mosaicism and cutaneous pigmentary dysplasia. Clin Genet 1991; 39:370–375.

Obstetric complications and perinatal mortality in multiple pregnancy

62. Kovacs BW, Kirschbaum TH, Paul RH. Twin gestations: I. Antenatal care and complications. Obstet Gynecol 1989; 74:313–317.

63. Spellacy WH, Handler A, Ferre CD. A case control study of 1253 pregnancies from a 1982–1987 perinatal data base. Obstet Gynecol 1990; 75:168.

64. Fabre E, de Aquero RG, de Augustin JL, et al. Perinatal mortality in twin pregnancy: an analysis of birth weight-specific mortality rates and adjusted mortality rates for birth weight distributions. J Perinat Med 1988; 16:85–91.

65. Ron-El R, Caspi E, Schreyer P, et al. Triplet and quadruplet pregnancies and management. Obstet Gynecol 1981; 57:458–463.

66. Collins MS, Bleyl JA. Seventy-one quadruplet pregnancies: management and outcome. Am J Obstet Gynecol 1990; 162:1384–1391.

67. Gonen R, Heyman E, Asztalos EV, et al. The outcome of triplet, quadruplet, and quintuplet pregnancies managed in a perinatal unit: obstetric, neonatal and follow-up data. Am J Obstet Gynecol 1990; 162:454–459.

Placentation in multiple pregnancy

68. Naeye RL, Benirschke K, Hagstrom JWC, et al. Intrauterine growth of twins as estimated from live birth-weight data. Pediatrics 1966; 37:409–416.

69. Fliegner JR, Eggers TR. The relationship between gestational age and birth weight in twin pregnancy. Aust N Z J Obstet Gynecol 1984; 24:192–197.

70. Danskin FH, Nielson JP. Twin-to-twin transfusion syndrome: what are appropriate criteria? Am J Obstet Gynecol 1989; 161:365–369.

71. Grennert L, Persson P-H, Gennser G, et al. Zygosity and intrauterine growth of twins. Obstet Gynecol 1980; 55:684–687.

72. Eberle AM, Levesque D, Vintzileos AM, et al. Placental pathology in discordant twins. Am J Obstet Gynecol 1993; 169:931–935.

73. Redline RW, Jiang JG, Shah D. Discordancy for maternal floor infarction in dizygotic twin placentas. Hum Pathol 2003; 34:822–824.

74. Megory E, Weiner E, Shalev E, et al. Pseudomonoamniotic twins with cord entanglement following genetic funipuncture. Obstet Gynecol 1991; 78: 915–917.

75. Ginsberg NA, Ginsberg S, Rechitsky S, Verlinsky Y. Fusion as the etiology of chimerism in monochorionic dizgotic twins. Fetal Diagn Ther 2005; 20: 20–22.

76. Matayoshi K, Yoshida K. Observation of 11 cases of triplets and their outcome. Proceedings of the Sixth International Congress on Twin Studies, Rome, 1989.

77. Gonen R, Heyman E, Asztalos E, et al. The outcome of triplet gestations complicated by fetal death. Obstet Gynecol 1990; 75:175–178.

78. Borlum KG. Third-trimester fetal death in triplet pregnancies. Obstet Gynecol 1991; 77:6–9.

79. Machin GA, Bamforth F. Zygosity and chorionicity of 15 sets of spontaneously conceived triplets. Am J Med Genet 1996; 61:247–252.

80. Mahony BS, Filly RA, Callen PW. Amnionicity and chorionicity in twin pregnancies: prediction using ultrasound. Radiology 1985; 155:205–209.

81. Barss VA, Benacerraf BR, Frigoletto FD. Ultrasonographic determination of chorion type in twin gestation. Obstet Gynecol 1988; 66:779.

82. D'Alton ME, Dudley DK. The ultrasonographic prediction of chorionicity in twin gestation. Am J Obstet Gynecol 1989; 160:557–561.

83. Hertzberg BS, Kurtz AB, Choi HY, et al. Significance of membrane thickness in the sonographic evaluation of twin gestations. AJR Am J Roentgenol 1987; 148:151–153.

84. Winn HN, Gabrielli S, Reeece EA, et al. Ultrasonographic criteria for the prenatal diagnosis of placental chorionicity in twin gestations. Am J Obstet Gynecol 1989; 161:1540–1542.

85. Townsend RR, Simpson GF, Filly RA. Membrane thickness in ultrasound prediction of chorionicity of twin gestations. J Ultrasound Med 1988; 7: 327–332.

86. Monteagudo A, Timor-Tritsch IE, Sharma S. Early and simple determination of chorionic and amniotic type in multifetal gestations in the first fourteen weeks by high-frequency transvaginal ultrasonography. Am J Obstet Gynecol 1994; 170:824–829.

87. Seeds JW. Sonographic evaluation of growth discordance and chorionicity in twin gestation. Am J Perinatol 1991; 8:342–344.

88. Carroll SG, Soothill PW, Abdel-Fattah SA, et al. Prediction of chorionicity in twin pregnancies at 10-14 weeks of gestation. Br J Obstet Gynecol 2002; 109:182–186.

89. Carlan SJ, Angel JL, Sawai SK, et al. Late diagnosis of nonconjoined monoamniotic twins using computed tomographic imaging: a case report. Obstet Gynecol 1990; 76:504–506.

90. Lavery JP, Gadwood KA. Amniography for confirming the diagnosis of monoamniotic twinning. A case report. J Reprod Med 1990; 35: 911–914.

91. Perkins RP, Terry JD. Exclusion of monoamniotic twinning by contrast-enhanced computer tomography. Obstet Gynecol 1992; 79:876–878.

92. Tabsh K. Genetic amniocentesis in multiple gestation: a new technique to diagnose monoamniotic twins. Obstet Gynecol 1990; 75:296–298.

93. Filly RA, Goldstein RB, Callen PW. Monochorionic twinning: sonographic assessment. AJR Am J Roentgenol 1990; 154:459–469.

94. Benirschke K, Kaufmann P. Pathology of the human placenta. 3rd edn. New York: Springer-Verlag; 1995:767.

95. Fries MH, Goldstein RB, Kilpatrick SJ, et al. The role of velamentous cord insertion in the etiology of twin twin transfusion syndrome. Obstet Gynecol 1993; 81:569–574.

96. Boyd T, Blatman T, Greene M, et al. Twin-twin transfusion is related to velamentous cord insertion in monochorionic twins. Proceedings of the Society for Pediatric Pathology, Annual Meeting, San Francisco, March, 1994.

97. Machin GA, Still K, Lalani T. Correlations of placental vascular anatomy and clinical outcomes in 69 monochorionic twin pregnancies. Am J Med Genet 1996; 61:229.

98. Strong SJ, Corney G. The placenta in twin pregnancy. Oxford: Pergamon Press; 1967.

99. Galea P, Scott JM, Goel KM. Feto-fetal transfusion syndrome. Arch Dis Child 1982; 57:781–783.

100. Arts NFT, Lohman AHM. The vascular anatomy of monochorionic diamniotic twin placentas and the transfusion syndrome. Eur J Obstet Gynecol Rep Biol 1971; 1:85.

101. Sekiya S, Hafez ESE. Physiomorphology of twin transfusion syndrome. A study of 86 twin pregnancies. Obstet Gynecol 1977; 50:288–292.

102. Robertson EG, Neer KJ. Placental injection studies in twin gestation. Am J Obstet Gynecol 1983; 147:170–174.

103. Yoshida K, Soma H. A study of twin placentation in Tokyo. Acta Genet Med Gemellol 1984; 33:115–120.

Special Clinico-pathologic disorders in monochorionic multiples

104. Bajoria R. Vascular anatomy of monochorionic twin placenta in relation to discordant growth and amniotic fluid volume. Hum Reprod 1998; 13: 2933–2940.

105. De Paepe ME, DeKoninck P, Friedman RM. Vascular distribution patterns in monochorionic twin placentas. Placenta 2005; 26:471–475.

106. Kirshon B. Fetal urine output in hydramnios. Obstet Gynecol 1989; 73: 240–242.

107. Nageotte MP, Hurvitz SR, Laupke CJ, et al. Atriopeptin in the twin transfusion syndrome. Obstet Gynecol 1989; 73:867–870.

108. Moise KJ Jr, Dorman K, Lamvu G, et al. A randomized trial of amnioreduction versus septostomy in the treatment of twin-twin transfusion syndrome. Am J Obstet Gynecol 2005; 193:701–707.

109. Ludomirski A, Weiner S, Craparo F, et al. Twin to twin transfusion syndrome: role of Doppler flow and fetal hyperviscosity in predicting outcome. Am J Obstet Gynecol 1991; 164:243.

110. Lemery D, Santolaya J, Serre A, et al. Fetal erythropoietin in twin pregnancies with discordant growth, (abstract). Am J Obstet Gynecol 1994; 170: 442.

111. Weir PE, Ratten GJ, Beischer NA. Acute polyhydramnios – a complication of monozygous twin pregnancy. Br J Obstet Gynaecol 1979; 86:849–853.

112. Kirshon B, Moise KJ, Mari G, et al. In utero resolution of hydrops following death of one twin in twin-twin transfusion. Am J Perinatol 1990; 7:107–109.

113. Shapiro I, Sharf M. Spontaneous intrauterine remission of hydrops fetalis in one identical twin: sonographic diagnosis. J Clin Ultrasound 1985; 13: 427–430.

114. De Lia JE, Emery MG, Sheafor SA, et al. Twin transfusion syndrome: successful in utero treatment. Int J Gynaecol Obstet 1985; 23:197–201.

115. Lange IR, Harman CR, Ash KM, et al. Twin with hydramnios: treating premature labor at source. Am J Obstet Gynecol 1989; 160:552–557.

116. Wittman BK, Farquharson DF, Thomas WDS, et al. The role of feticide in the management of severe twin transfusion syndrome. Am J Obstet Gynecol 1986; 155:1023.

117. Saunders NJ, Souidjers RJM, Nicolaides KH. Therapeutic amniocentesis in twin-twin transfusion syndrome appearing in the second trimester of pregnancy. Am J Obstet Gynecol 1992; 166:820–824.

118. De Lia JE, Cruikshank DP. Fetoscopic neodymium YAG laser occlusion of placental vessels in severe twin-twin transfusion syndrome. Obstet Gynecol 1990; 75:1046–1053.

119. De Lia JE, Kuhlman RS, Cruikshank DP, et al. Current topic: placental surgery: a new frontier. Placenta 1993; 14:477–485.

120. Fox C, Kilby MD, Khan KS. Contemporary treatments for twin-twin transfusion syndrome. Obstet Gynecol 2005; 105:1469–1477.

121. Robyr R, Quarello E, Ville Y. Management of fetofetal transfusion syndrome. Prenat Diagn 2005; 25:786–795.

122. Bendon RW, Siddiqi T. Clinical Pathology Conference: Acute twin-to-twin transfusion. Pediatr Pathol 1989; 9:591–598.

123. Bruner JP, Rosemond RL. Twin-to-twin transfusion syndrome. A subset of the twin oligohydramnios-polyhydramnios sequence. Am J Obstet Gynecol 1993; 169:925–930.

124. Reisner DP, Mahoney BS, Petty CN, et al. Stuck twin syndrome: outcome of thirty-seven consecutive cases. Am J Obstet Gynecol 1993; 169:991–995.

125. Van Allen MI, Smith DW, Shepard TH. Twin reversed arterial perfusion (TRAP) sequence: a study of 14 twin pregnancies with acardius. Sem Perinatol 1983; 7:285–293.

126. Gibson JY, D'Cruz CA, Patel RB, et al. Acardiac anomaly: review of the subject with case report and emphasis on practical sonography. J Clin Ultrasound 1986; 14:541–545.

127. Wolf HK, MacDonald J, Bradford WB, et al. Acardius anceps with evidence of intrauterine vascular occlusion: report of a case and discussion of the pathogenesis. Pediatr Pathol 1990; 11:143.

128. Stocker JT, Heifetz SA. Sirenomelia. A morphological study of 33 cases and review of the literature. Perspect Pediatr Pathol 1987; 10:7.

129. Borrell A, Pesarrodona A, Puerto B, et al. Ultrasound diagnostic features of twin reversed arterial perfusion sequence. Prenat Diagn 1990; 10:443–448.

130. Donnenfeld AE, van de Woestijne T, Craparo F, et al. The normal fetus of an acardiac twin pregnancy: Perinatal management based on echocardiographic and sonographic evaluation. Prenat Diagn 1991; 11:235–244.

131. Kirkinen P, Herva R, Rasanen J, et al. Documentation of paradoxical umbilical blood supply of an acardiac twin in the antepartum state. J Perinat Med 1989; 17:63–65.

132. Pretorius DH, Leopold GR, Moore TR, et al. Acardiac twin: Report of Doppler sonography. J Ultrasound Med 1988; 7:413–416.

133. Benson CB, Bieber FR, Genest DR, et al. Doppler demonstration of reversed umbilical blood flow in an acardiac twin. J Clin Ultrasound 1989; 17: 291–295.

134. Al-Malt A, Ashmead G, Judge N, et al. Color-flow and Doppler velocimetry in prenatal diagnosis of acardiac triplet. J Ultrasound Med 1991; 10:341–345.

135. Kirkland JA. An acardiac, acephalic monster in a triplet pregnancy. Aust N Z J Obstet Gynaecol 1982; 22:168–171.

136. Ginsberg NA, Applebaum M, Rabin SA, et al. Term birth after midtrimester hysterotomy and selective delivery of an acardiac twin. Am J Obstet Gynecol 1992; 167:33–37.

137. Goldberg JD. Treatment of acardiac-acephalus twin gestations by hysterotomy and selective delivery (abstract). Am J Obstet Gynecol 1991; 146(suppl):324.

138. Robie GF, Payne GG, Morgan MA. Selective delivery of an acardiac acephalic twin. N Engl J Med 1989; 320:512–513.

139. Porreco RP, Barton SM, Haverkamp AD. Occlusion of umbilical artery in acardiac, acephalic twin. Lancet 1991; 337:326–327.

140. Quintero RA, Reich H, Puder KS, et al. Brief report: umbilical-cord ligation of an acardiac twin by fetoscopy at 19 weeks of gestation. N Engl J Med 1994; 330:469–471.

141. Mulhaus K, Behrens O, Degenhardt F. Antenatal diagnosis of a rare malformation: acardius acephalus and single ventricle of the twin. Am J Perinatol 1991; 8:251–254.

142. Buntinx IM, Bourgeois N, Butaert PM, et al. Acardiac amorphus twin with prune belly sequence in the co-twin. Am J Med Genet 1991; 39:453–457.

143. Tessen JA, Zlatnik FJ. Monoamniotic twinning: a retrospective controlled study. Obstet Gynecol 1991; 77:832–834.

144. Carr SR, Aronson MP, Coustan DR. Survival rates of monoamniotic twins do not decrease after 30 weeks' gestation. Am J Obstet Gynecol 1990; 163:719–722.

145. Annan B, Hutson RC. Double survival despite cord entwinement in monoamniotic twins. Case report. Br J Obstet Gynaecol 1990; 97:950–951.

146. Nyberg DA, Filly RA, Golbus MS, et al. Entangled umbilical cords: a sign of monoamniotic twins. J Ultrasound Med 1984; 3:29–32.

147. Townsend RR, Filly RA. Sonography of nonconjoined monoamniotic twin pregnancies. J Ultrasound Med 1988; 7:665–670.

148. Kassam SH, Tompkins MCT. Monoamniotic twin pregnancy and modern obstetrics. Report of a case with peculiar cord complication. Diagn Gynecol Obstet 1980; 2:213–220.

149. McLeod FN, McCoy DR. Monoamniotic twins with an unusual cord complication. Br J Obstet Gynecol 1981; 88:774–775.

150. Lumme RH, Saarikoski SV. Monoamniotic twin pregnancy. Acta Genet Med Gemellol 1986; 35:99–105.

151. Levi S. Ultrasonic assessment of the high rate of human multiple pregnancy in the first trimester. J Clin Ultrasound 1976; 4:3–5.

152. Sulak LE, Dodson MG. The vanishing twin: pathologic confirmation of ultrasound phenomenon. Obstet Gynecol 1986; 68:811–815.

153. Jauniaux E, Elkazen N, Leroy F, et al. Clinical and morphological aspects of the vanishing twin phenomenon. Obstet Gynecol 1988; 72:577–581.

154. Tharapel AT, Elias S, Shulman LP, et al. Resorbed co-twin as an explanation for discrepant chorionic villus results: non-mosaic 47,XX,+16 in villi (direct and culture) and normal (46,XX) amniotic fluid and neonatal blood. Prenat Diagn 1989; 9:467–472.

155. Kindred JE. Twin pregnancies with one blighted. Am J Obstet Gynecol 1944; 48:642.

156. Yoshida K, Soma H. Outcome of surviving cotwin of a fetus papyraceus or dead twin fetus. Acta Genet Med Gemellol 1986; 35:91–98.

157. Saier F, Burden L, Cavanagh D. Fetus papyraceus: an unusual case with congenital anomaly of the surviving fetus. Obstet Gynecol 1975; 45:217–220.

158. Hoyme HE, Higginbottom MC, Jones KL. Vascular etiology of disruptive structural defects in monozygotic twins. Pediatrics 1981; 67:288–291.

159. Mannino FL, Jones KL, Benirschke K. Congenital skin defects and fetus papyraceus. J Pediatr 1977; 91:559–564.

160. Cruikshank SH, Granados JL. Increased amniotic acetylcholinesterase activity with a fetus papyraceus and aplasia cutis congenita. Obstet Gynecol 1988; 71:997–999.

161. Wagner DS, Klein RL, Robinson HP, et al. Placental emboli from a fetus papyraceus. J Pediatr Surg 1990; 25:538–542.

162. Patten RM, Mack LA, Nyberg DA, et al. Twin embolization syndrome: prenatal sonographic detection and significance. Radiology 1989; 173:685–689.

163. Hagay ZJ, Mazor M, Lieberman JR, et al. Management and outcome of multiple pregnancies complicated by the antenatal death of one fetus. J Reprod Med 1986; 31:717–720.

164. Wessel J, Schmidt-Gollwitzer K. Intrauterine death of a single fetus in twin pregnancies. J Perinat Med 1988; 16:467–476.

165. Cherouny PH, Hoskins IA, Johnson TRB, et al. Multiple pregnancy with late death of one fetus. Obstet Gynecol 1989; 74:318–320.

166. Enbom JA. Twin pregnancy with intrauterine death of one twin. Obstet Gynecol 1985; 152:424–429.

167. Carlson NJ, Towers CV. Multiple gestation complicated by the death of one fetus. Obstet Gynecol 1989; 73:685–689.

168. Hannah JH, Hill JM. Single intrauterine fetal demise in multiple gestation. Obstet Gynecol 1984; 63:126.

169. D'Alton ME, Newton ER, Cetrulo CL. Intrauterine fetal demise in multiple gestation. Acta Genet Med Gemellol (Roma) 1984; 33:43–49.

170. Lumme R, Saarikowski S. Antepartal fetal death of one twin. Int J Gynecol Obstet 1987; 25:331–336.

171. Litschgi M, Stucki D. Course of twin pregnancies after fetal death in utero. Z Geburtshilfe Perinatol 1980; 184:227–230.

172. Melnick M. Brain damage in survivor after in-utero death of monozygous co-twin. Lancet 1977; 2:1287.

173. Szymonowicz W, Preston H, Yu VYH. The surviving monozygotic twin. Arch Dis Child 1986; 61:454–458.

174. Moore CM, McAdams AJ, Sutherland J. Intrauterine disseminated intravascular coagulation: a syndrome of multiple pregnancy with a dead twin fetus. J Pediatr 1969; 74:523–528.

175. Russell LJ, Weaver DD, Bull MJ, et al. In utero brain destruction resulting in collapse of the fetal skull, microcephaly, scalp rugae, and neurological impairment. Am J Med Genet 1984; 17:509–521.

176. Fisher JE, Siongco A. Complications from in utero death of a monozygous co-twin. Pediatr Pathol 1989; 9:765–771.

177. Amiel-Tison C. Multicystic encephalomalacia as a complication in twin pregnancy. Eur J Obstet Gynecol Reprod Med 1983; 15:279.

178. Norman MG. Mechanisms of brain damage in twins. Can J Neurol Sci 1982; 9:339–344.

179. Braat DD, Exalto N, Bernardus RE, et al. Twin pregnancy: case reports illustrating variations in twin transfusion syndrome. Eur J Obstet Gynecol Reprod Med 1985; 19:383–390.

180. Bulla M, von Lilien T, Goecke H, et al. Renal and cerebral necrosis in survivor after in utero death of co-twin. Arch Gynecol 1987; 240:119–124.

181. Clark DA. Hydrops fetalis attributable to intrauterine disseminated intravascular coagulation. Clin Pediatr 1981; 20:61–62.

182. Durkin MV, Kaveggia EG, Pendleton E, et al. Analysis of etiologic factors in cerebral palsy with severe mental retardation. Eur J Pediatr 1976; 123:67–81.

183. Dimmick J, Hardwick D, Ho-Yuen B. A case of renal necrosis and fibrosis in the immediate newborn period. Am J Dis Child 1971; 122:345–347.

184. Feingold M, Cetrulo CL, Newton ER, et al. Serial amniocentesis in the treatment of twin-to-twin transfusion complicated with acute polyhydramnios. Act Genet Med Gemellol (Roma) 1986; 35:107–113.

185. Nicolini U, Pisoni MP, Cela E, et al. Fetal blood sampling immediately before and within 24 hours after death in monochorionic twin pregnancies complicated by single intrauterine death. Am J Obstet Gynecol 1998; 179:800–803.

186. Senat MV, Bernard JP, Loizeau S, et al. Management of single fetal death in twin-to-twin transfusion syndrome: a role for fetal blood sampling. Ultrasound Obstet Gynecol 2002; 20:360–363.

187. Hendry DW, Kohler HG. Sirenomelia ('Mermaid'). Br J Obstet Gynecol Br Emp 1956; 63:865–870.

188. Kohler HG. An unusual case of sirenomelia. Teratology 1972; 6:295–301.

189. Maurer SM, Dobrin RS, Vernier RL. Unilateral and bilateral renal agenesis in monoamniotic twins. J Pediatr 1974; 84:236.

190. Heydanus R, Santema JG, Stewart PA, et al. Preterm delivery rate and fetal outcome in structurally affected twin pregnancies: a retrospective matched control study. Prenat Diagn 1993; 13:155–162.

191. Johnstone HB, Benirschke K. Monozygotic twin discordant for urinary tract anomalies and presenting as hydramnios. Obstet Gynecol 1976; 47:610.

192. Machin GA, Sperber GH, Wootlife J. Monozygotic twin aborted fetuses discordant for holoprosencephaly/synotia. Teratology 1985; 31:203–215.

193. Boles DJ, Bodurtha J, Nance WE. Goldenhar complex in discordant monozygotic twins: a case report and review of the literature. Am J Med Genet 1987; 28:103–109.

194. Fiedler JF, Phelan JP. The amniotic band syndrome in monozygotic twins. Am J Obstet Gynecol 1983; 146:864.

195. Donnenfeld AE, Glazerman LR, Cutillo DM, et al. Fetal exsanguination following intrauterine angiographic assessment and selective termination of a hydrocephalic, monozygotic twin. Prenat Diagn 1989; 9:301–308.

196. Golbus MS, Cunningham N, Goldberg JD, et al. Selective termination of multiple gestations. Am J Med Genet 1988; 31:339–348.

197. Olivennes F, Domerc S, Senat MV, et al. Evidence of early prenatal anastomosis during selective embryo reduction. Fertil Steril 2002; 77: 183–184.

Conjoined twins

198. Spencer R. Conjoined twins. Developmental malformations and clinical implications. Baltimore: The Johns Hopkins University Press; 2003.

199. Beckwith JB. Book review of 198. Pediatr Devel Path 2003; 6:281.

200. Spencer R. Conjoined twins: theoretical embryologic basis. Teratology 1992; 29:181.

201. Machin GA. Conjoined twins: implications for blastogenesis. In: Opitz JM, Paul NW, eds. Blastogenesis: normal and abnormal. March of Dimes Birth Defects Foundation. Birth defects: original article series 1993; 29:141.

202. Weaver DD, Lipson AH, Webster WD, et al. Hypothesis for the pathogenesis of conjoined twins. Proceedings of the Greenwood Genetic Center 1992; 11:79.

203. Knox AJS, Webb AJ. The clinical features and treatment of fetus in fetu: two case reports and a review of the literature. J Pediatr Surg 1975; 10:483–489.

204. Kang YK, Suh Y-L, Kim CW, et al. Fetus in fetu: case with complete umbilical cord and fetal sac. Pediatr Pathol 1994; 14:411–419.

205. Borges E, Lim-Dunham JE, Vade A. Fetus in fetu appearing as a prenatal neck mass. J Ultrasound Med 2005; 24:1313–1316.

Pathology as a basis for genetic studies in twins

206. Bouchard T, Lykken DT, McGue M, et al. Sources of human psychological differences. The Minnesota Study of Twins Reared Apart. Science 1990; 250:223–228.

207. Small GW, Leuchter AF, Mandelkern MA, et al. Clinical, neuroimaging, and environmental risk differences in monozygotic female twins appearing discordant for dementia of Alzheimer type. Arch Neurol 1993; 50:209–219.

208. Garden GM, Rothery DJ. A female monozygotic twin pair discordant for transsexualism. Br J Psychiatry 1992; 161:852–854.

209. King M, McDonald E. Homosexuals who are twins. Br J Psychiatry 1992; 160:407–409.

210. Suddath RL, Christison GW, Torrey EF, et al. Anatomical abnormalities in the brains of monozygotic twins discordant for schizophrenia. N Engl J Med 1990; 322:789–794.

211. Revely AM, Revely MA, Clifford CA, et al. Cerebral ventricular size in twins discordant for schizophrenia. Lancet 1982; 1:540–541.

212. Phillips DIW. Twin studies in medical research: can they tell us whether diseases are genetically determined? Lancet 1993; 341:1008–1009.

213. Powers WF, Kiely JL. The risks confronting twins: a national perspective. Am J Obstet Gynecol 1994; 170:456–461.

214. Dube J, Dodds L, Armson BA. Does chorionicity or zygosity predict adverse perinatal outcomes in twins? Am J Obstet Gynecol 2002; 186:579–583.

215. Hatkar PA, Bhide AG. Perinatal outcome of twins in relation to chorionicity. J Postgrad Med 1999; 45:33–37.

216. Minakami H, Honma Y, Matsubara S, et al. Effects of placental chorionicity on outcome in twin pregnancy. J Reprod Med 1999; 44:595–600.

217. Baghdadi S, Gee H, Whittle MJ, et al. Twin pregnancy outcome and chorionicity. Acta Obstet Gynecol Scand 2003; 82:18–21.

218. Asztalos E, Barrett JF, Lacy M, et al. Evaluating 2 year outcome in twins < or = 30 weeks gestation at birth: a regional perinatal unit's experience. Twin Res 2001; 4:418.

219. Matsuda Y, Kouno S. Fetal and neonatal outcomes in twin oligohydramnios-polyhydramnios sequence including cerebral palsy. Fetal Diagn Ther 2002; 17:268–271.

Infectious diseases

Virginia M. Anderson   R.O.C. Kaschula

How much better it is to get wisdom than gold: to get understanding rather than silver.

Proverbs 15:16

Infection of the fetus and neonate

Acute Chorioamnionitis (See Also Ch. 15)

Intrauterine infection has an adverse effect on the developing fetus and is a major cause of infant mortality.[1-4] Normal amniotic fluid is sterile. Premature onset of labor frequently follows ascending infection from the vagina into the fetal membranes. **Premature rupture of the fetal membranes** for more than 6–24 h is associated with infiltration of the amnion by maternal leukocytes.[5,6] The neutrophil response begins in the subchorionic plate of the placenta with most severe infiltration at the point of rupture of the fetal membranes.

Maternal neutrophil response is best demonstrated by making a membrane roll in which the point of exit of the fetus through the amniotic sac is placed at the center of the roll. A forceps or wooden orange stick is placed parallel to the point of fetal exit. The tissue is then rolled and a perpendicular 2–3 mm slice of the coiled fetal membranes is cut and placed in a tissue cassette. Histologic sections thus cover a broad surface of both the amnion and chorion. Failure to take adequate sections may result in under-reporting of acute chorioamnionitis and underestimation of the intensity of the inflammatory response. Neutrophils in the chorion alone can occur as part of the normal separation of the fetal membranes during labor. Neutrophils must migrate into the amnion proper to merit a diagnosis of chorioamnionitis. Failure to rigorously apply this criterion may result in over diagnosis of chorioamnionitis (Fig. 10.1A, B).

Maternal sepsis accompanied by fever and leukocytosis may have associated villitis, intervillositis, and chorioamnionitis. Villitis may be focal and easily overlooked. Inflammation and necrosis of villi, if extensive, may retard fetal growth.

Organisms responsible for chorioamnionitis include **group B β-hemolytic streptococci and Gram-negative organisms including Escherichia coli and Klebsiella**. Bacteria reside in the vaginal vault. Rupture of the fetal membranes provides a port of entry into the amnion.[7] Less often infectious agents may breach the intact amnion.[8,9]

The incidence of chorioamnionitis, a leading cause of preterm delivery, is directly proportional to gestational age. Inflammation produces cytokines and chemocymes that may induce the fetal systemic inflammatory response syndrome. This can affect brain development and is associated with cerebral palsy. While intrauterine recovery from infectious disease is possible, sequelae such as growth retardation and periventricular leukomalacia may occur. Villitis of unspecified etiology, (VUE), associated with CD3+ T cells in villi can be found in 5% of otherwise normal placentae. VUE is more frequent in cerebral palsy with hypoxic ischemic encephalopathy. Careful identification of this subtle finding can protect the obstetrician from legal action. A putative intrapartum insult may occur much earlier. Clinical diagnosis is impossible and no treatment is available. The identification of VUE is directly proportional to the time spent on histologic evaluation and the experience and interest of the observer.[10] Funisitis (10.1C) and stem vessel vasculitis (Fig. 10.1D) are serious indicators of fetal sepsis which occurs in association with chorioamnionitis, or as a free standing lesion.

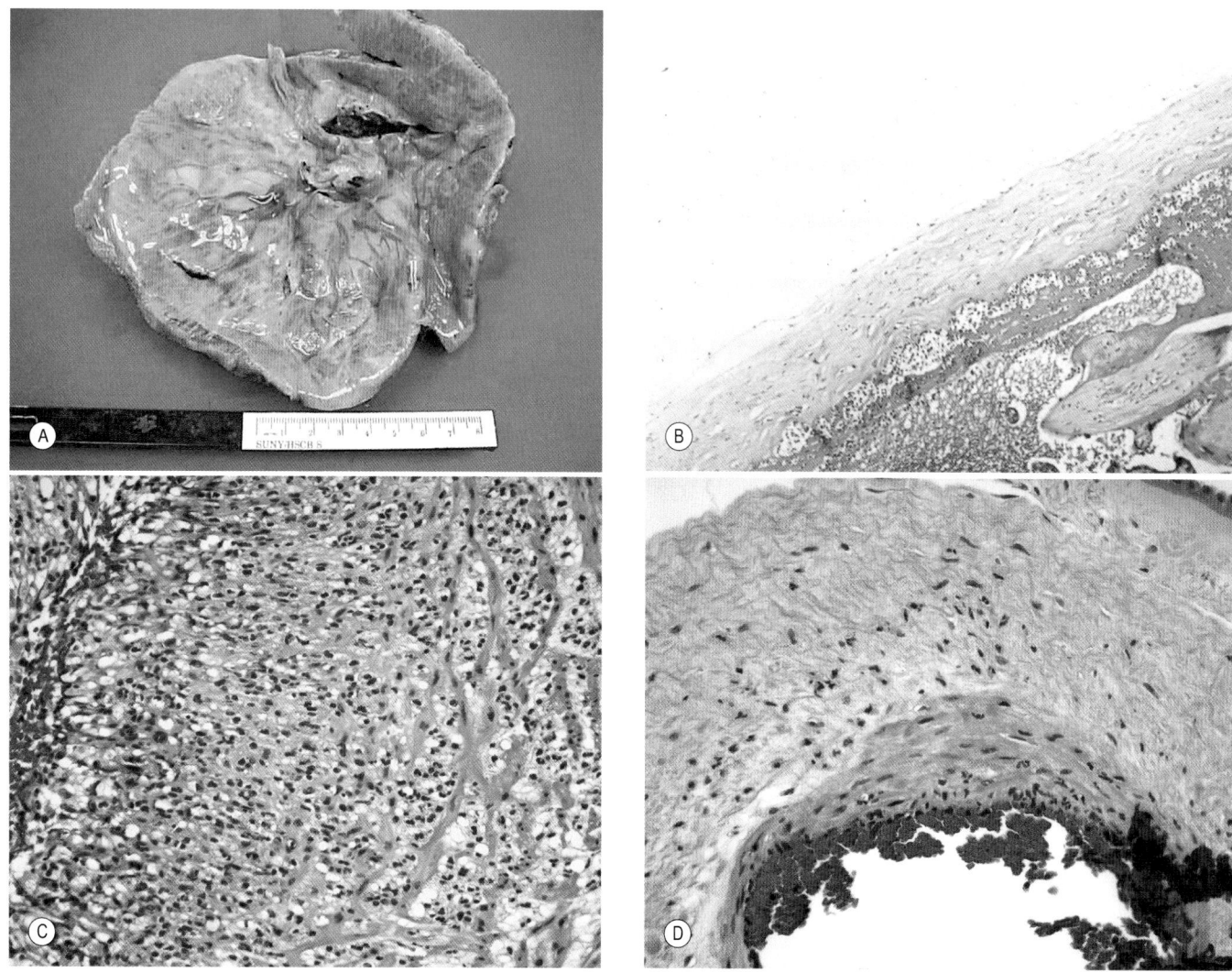

FIGURE 10.1 (A) Yellow–green creamy exudate characteristic of severe chorioamnionitis covers the fetal surface of the placenta. (B) Histologic section shows suppuration of the subchorionic plate with migration of maternal neutrophils into the amnion. (C) Fetal neutrophils migrate into the wall of an umbilical artery indicative of severe fetal sepsis. Usually the umbilical vein alone is involved in funisitis. (D) Stem vessel vasculitis is evidence of a fetal response to bacteria. Inflammatory cytokines may be upregulated in fetal systemic inflammatory response syndrome resulting in in utero injury to the central nervous system.

Aspiration of infected amniotic fluid

The fetus may be encased in a sac of purulent amniotic fluid as maternal neutrophils and bacteria fill the amniotic fluid bath. Fetal distress followed by increased fetal respiration with the **aspiration of maternal neutrophils** into the lung occurs.[11] This can be seen as early as 16 weeks' gestation and is the most frequent cause of perinatal death from immaturity. In the third trimester, pulmonary infection and sepsis follow. Older fetuses may also **aspirate meconium** and excessive amniotic squame cells. At autopsy, sections of lung reveal maternal neutrophils identified by five nuclear lobulations within fetal airspaces (Fig. 10.2A, B). Fetal neutrophils are usually trilobed or bands. Ingestion of maternal white blood cells can sometimes be shown in sections of the stomach or intestines. **Fetal myelopoiesis** may be seen in the interstitium of the lung and the portal areas of the liver and spleen (Fig. 10.2C).[12, 13] Antibiotic treatment of the mother may protect the fetus.[14–16] Steroids used to induce lung maturation may retard the immature fetal inflammatory response. The risk–benefit balance of treating the mother to protect the fetus is fraught with competing concerns. Expectant management of the very low birth fetus has increased survival, morbidity, and health care costs. Practice standards based on clinical trials with careful autopsy studies are essential.

Sepsis neonatorum

Signs of clinical infection are shown in Table 10.1. Clinical signs of sepsis, especially fever, may be absent. Hypothermia is more

TABLE 10.1 CLINICAL SIGNS OF CONGENITAL INFECTION

Stillbirth	Rub; CMV; HSV; Entero; List
Skin	Petechiae/purpura (Rub; CMV; Toxo; HSV; Syph; Entero; List)
	Vesicles (CMV; HSV; Syph)
	Exanthem (Toxo; HSV; Syph; Entero)
Nervous system	Encephalitis (Rub; CMV; Toxo; HSV; Syph; Entero; List)
	Microcephaly (CMV; Toxo; HSV)
	Hydrocephalus (Rub; CMV; Toxo; HSV)
	Intracranial calcification (CMV; Toxo)
	Paralysis (Entero); pseudoparalysis (Syph)
	Hearing loss (Rub; Syph)
Eye	Glaucoma (Rub; Syph)
	Chorioretinitis (Rub; CMV; Toxo; HSV; Syph)
	Cataracts (Rub; Toxo; HSV)
	Optic atrophy (CMV; Toxo)
	Microphthalmia (Rub; Toxo)
	Uveitis (Toxo; Entero)
	Keratoconjunctivitis (HSV; Entero; Chlamydia)
Visceral lesions	Adenopathy (Rub; Toxo; Syph; Entero)
	Myocarditis (Rub; Toxo; HSV; Entero; List)
	Pneumonitis (Rub; CMV; Toxo; HSV; Syph; Entero; List; Chlamydia)
	Hepatosplenomegaly (Rub; CMV; Toxo; HSV; Syph; Entero; List)
	Hepatitis (Rub; CMV; HSV; Syph; Entero; List)
	Jaundice (Rub; CMV; Toxo; HSV; Entero; List)
	Osteochondritis (Rub; Toxo; Syph)
	Congenital heart disease (Rub)

CMV, Cytomegalovirus; Entero, enteroviruses; HSV, herpes simplex virus; List, *Listeria*; Rub, rubella; Syph, syphilis; Toxo, toxoplasmosis.

common. Lethargy, poor feeding, weak cry or suck, cyanosis, and hypotonicity may be present.[17–19] A high index of suspicion with prompt administration of antibiotics is necessary to prevent a fatal outcome. Both humoral and cellular host-defense mechanisms against infection are undeveloped and may be rapidly overwhelmed. Neonates may have a leukemoid reaction or leukopenia with a left shift in the white blood count. Shock and death are often associated with **disseminated intravascular coagulation (DIC) syndrome**. Sepsis is often a sequelae of aspiration of infected amniotic fluid, and severe chorioamnionitis.[20, 21] The neonatal liver and bone marrow are immature. Cholestasis and visceral or cutaneous hemorrhage are not uncommon. Bacterial culture of the blood may identify the organism however the blood sample submitted to the laboratory may be inadequate for culture. The very low neonatal circulating blood volume (80 cc/kg) precludes a larger sample. Antibiotic treatment even without a positive culture prevents pneumonia and meningitis which frequently follow sepsis. Poor peripheral perfusion and splanchnic pooling of blood predisposes the infant to necrotizing enterocolitis, cholestasis and direct reacting hyperbilirubinema.[22] **At autopsy,**

evidence of shock includes intraventricular hemorrhage, periventricular leukomalacia, focal hemorrhages in the skin and viscera, hepatic necrosis, hemorrhage in the renal medulla and adrenal gland, or acute cortical or tubular necrosis of the kidney and granulopoiesis in the liver, bone marrow, and spleen.[23]

Group B streptococcal infection

GBS infection was first identified in the early 1960s.[32] Most often the early-onset form of GBS disease is acquired during vaginal delivery. However, intrauterine infection can also occur.[33] Symptoms of respiratory distress commence soon after birth, and death from septicemia, pneumonia, or meningitis may be rapid.[34–37] At autopsy the gross appearance of GBS pneumonia may be indistinguishable from hyaline membrane disease.[17] Microscopically group B streptococci are found within hyaline membranes (Fig. 10.2A–C and 10.5).

Maternal neutrophils in the infant lung may be numerous or sparse. Necrotizing suppurative intervillositis with trophoblast necrosis may be present. Maternal neutrophils attack and penetrate the chorionic villi. Preterm, low birth weight infants after prolonged labor and preterm rupture of the fetal membranes are particularly at risk. Bacterial cultures of the vagina identify the at-risk fetus and appropriate maternal antibiotic treatment may prevent fetal infection. Concern that maternal penicillin prophylaxis may change the flora of the infant gut and promote overgrowth of Gram-negative pathogens has surfaced. **Late-onset GBS infection** begins 2 weeks to 3 months after birth and is nosocomial or acquired from the mother. Death or serious sequelae may result from suppurative meningitis or septicemia.[38] An extended hospital stay is associated with an increased incidence of late-onset GBS infection. Other bacterial agents, especially *Haemophilus influenzae,* may also produce purple–blue, airless newborn lungs that cannot be distinguished from hyaline membrane disease or GBS infection. **Staphylococcal infections** may incite toxic epidermal necrolysis (**scalded skin syndrome**) (Fig. 10.6).[39] Intrauterine infection with *E. coli* or *Klebsiella* may accompany **maternal urinary tract infection** (Fig. 10.7).[20]

Other neonatal infections

Maternal urinary tract infection may predispose the fetus to hematogenous infection while GBS is acquired during parturition. Stem vessel vasculitis and funisitis in the absence of chorioamnionitis suggests a focus of infection in the mother. Chorioamnionitis may or may not result in fetal infection.[24, 25]In late-onset sepsis additional pathogens include *Staphylococcus aureus, Streptococcus viridans, Enterobacter, Proteus, Pseudomonas, Serratia marcescens, Klebsiella pneumoniae,* and fungal agents – especially *Candida albicans* and *Aspergillus* (Fig. 10.3A, B). Life-saving invasive procedures and broad-spectrum antibiotics are associated with nosocomial infections in the intensive care unit.[26–28] Septic thrombi with candida hyphae can appear in the

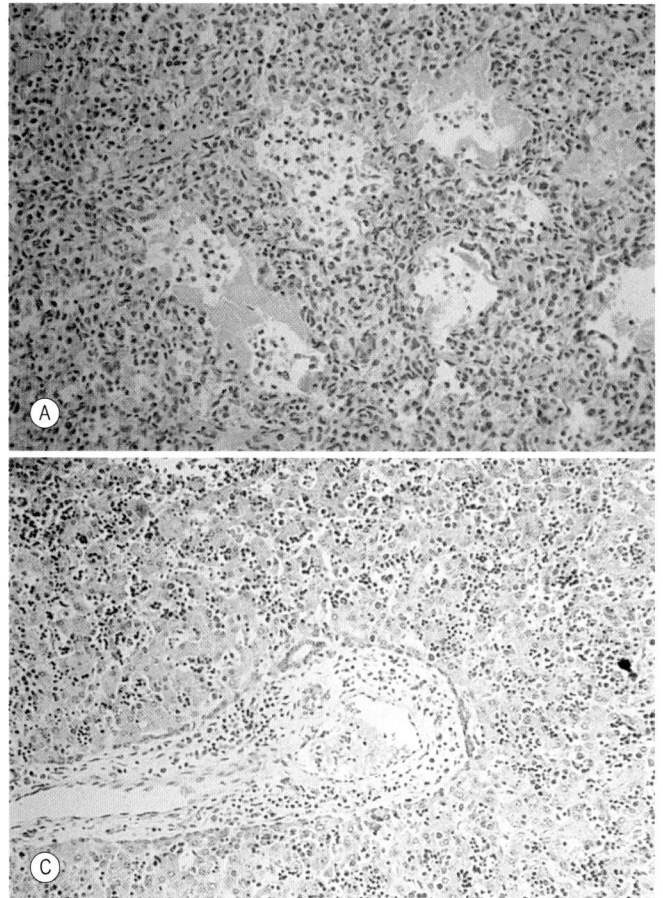

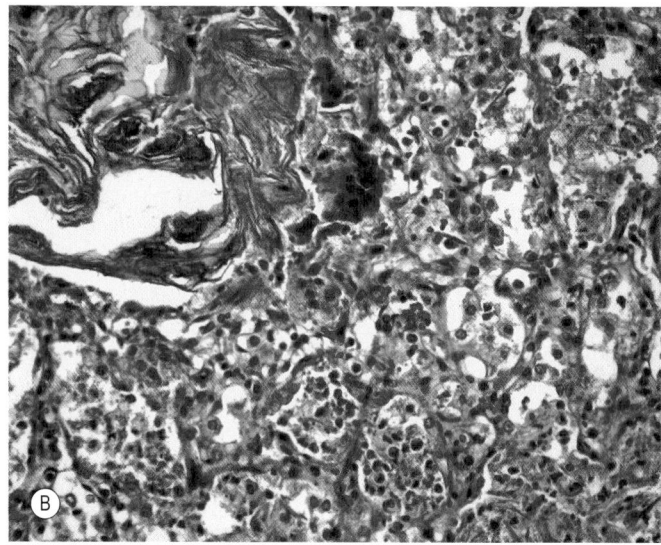

FIGURE 10.2 (A) Chorioamnionitis. Maternal neutrophils and bacteria are aspirated into the fetal lung causing sepsis and congenital pneumonia. Hyaline membranes characteristic of group B streptococcal diseases are seen. (B) Maternal neutrophils fill the immature air spaces of the lung and indicate aspiration of infected amniotic fluid. Squame cell plugs are a sign of fetal distress in the stillborn. (C) Myelopoiesis in the walls of the portal veins of the liver is exuberant in intrauterine infection.

lungs of infants with superior vena cava catheters inserted for total parenteral nutrition. Infants with candida sepsis (Fig. 10.3C, D) often present with thrombocytopenia. *Pseudomonas aeruginosa* (Fig. 10.4) can contaminate the ventilators and cause fatal pneumonia with septicemia, osteomyelitis, empyema, and multiple lung or skin abscesses. *P. aeruginosa*[26–28] invades the blood vessel walls with resultant nodular confluent areas of extensive tissue necrosis.[29–31]

Omphalitis

Omphalitis is acquired after birth. It can progress to peritonitis (Fig. 10.8) and is rapidly fatal if antibiotic treatment is not instituted. In modern hospitals, omphalitis is infrequent, but in the developing world it is a common cause of neonatal death. If asepsis is not practiced, organisms enter the bloodstream directly through the cut end of the umbilical cord vessels and **invade periumbilical tissue**, which becomes red, edematous, and odiferous. Pus may exude around the umbilical stump. In the pre-antibiotic era, septicemia was the usual outcome, even if the umbilicus was only mildly infected. Organisms spread into the blood vessel walls causing pylephlebitis. The thrombosed lumen of the umbilical vein enables organisms to ascend into the liver and sinusoidal channels causing **focal hepatitis**. Localization

of the inflammatory response is sluggish in neonates, and rapid spread of infection is frequent. Intrauterine inflammation of the umbilical cord is called funisitis (Fig. 10.1D).

Listeriosis

Listeria monocytogenes is a worldwide pathogen that affects both humans and wild and domestic animals. Disease in humans is probably transmitted from animals or the soil but the manner of infection is not known. *L. monocytogenes*, a motile, strongly argentophilic, pleomorphic, Gram-positive rod, measures 2–3 μm long and 0.5 μm wide. Animal inoculation or fluorescent antibody technique is required for positive identification. A careful autopsy can strongly support the diagnosis of *Listeria monocytogenes* even if the gold standard of a positive culture is not obtained. Granulomas are seen in the liver, viscera and placenta.[40] A presumptive diagnosis of listeriosis is suggested when a stool smear contains short Gram-positive bacilli. If the Gram stain on control samples distinguishes Gram-positive and Gram-negative organisms, the dearth of Gram-negative and presence of pure Gram-positive rods in stool can only occur in neonatal listeriosis.

The newborn may become infected in utero or during delivery to a mother who harbors the bacteria. *Listeria* organisms can be

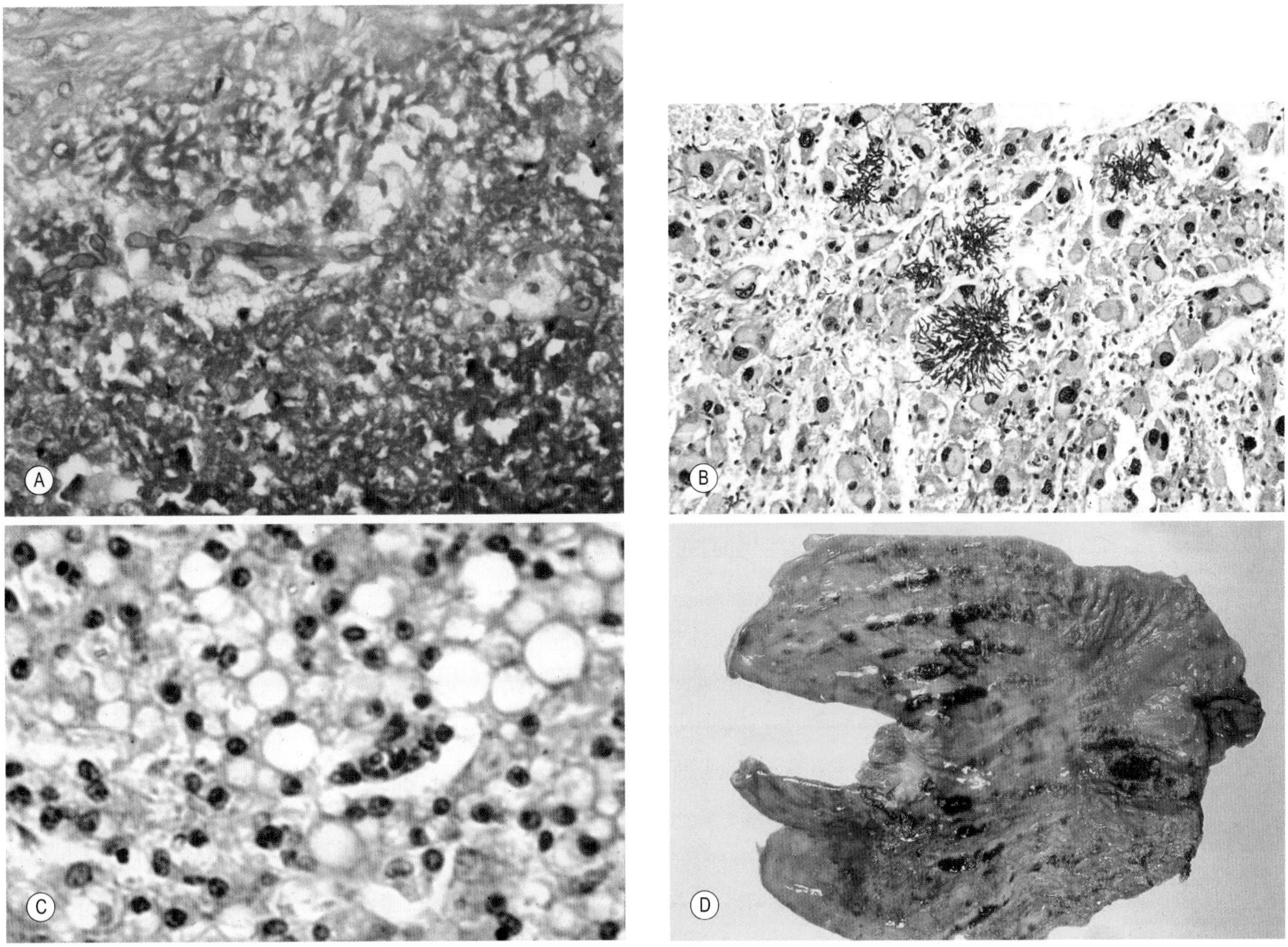

FIGURE 10.3 (A) *Aspergillus* is seen in the kidney in an immunodeficient patient; *Aspergillus* vasculitis as seen with a silver stain. (B) Colonies of candida are present in the liver in an infant with systemic candidiasis. (C) In immunodeficient infants intracellular candida are rarely observed and can mimic leishmaniasis or histoplasmosis. (D) Thrombocytopenia with gastric hemorrhage in systemic candidiasis.

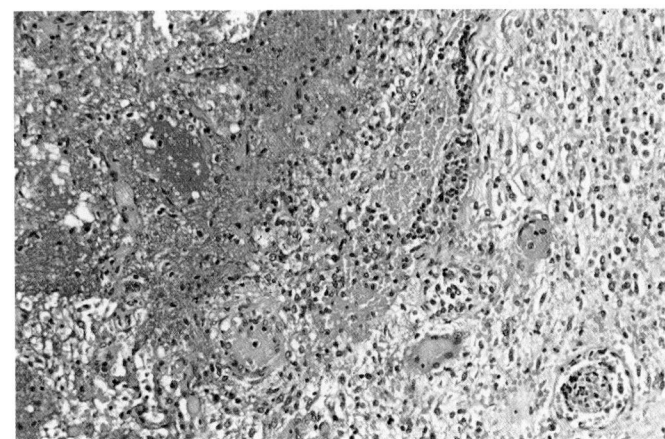

FIGURE 10.4 Necrotizing hemorrhagic pneumonia in an infant with nosocomial pseudomonas infection.

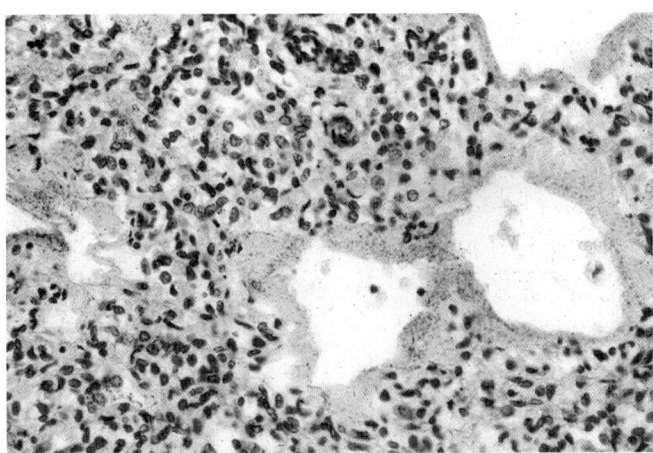

FIGURE 10.5 GBS pneumonia mimics hyaline membrane disease in preterm infants. Note clusters of Gram-positive bacterial colonies in the membranes.

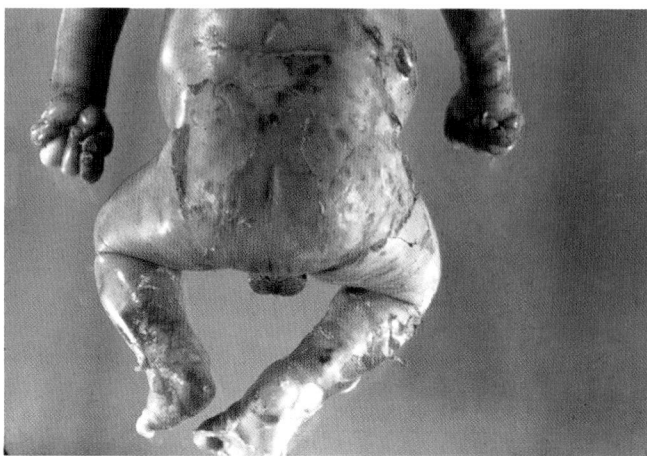

FIGURE 10.6 The staphylococcal scalded skin syndrome mimics severe burns with profound alterations in fluid and electrolyte status.

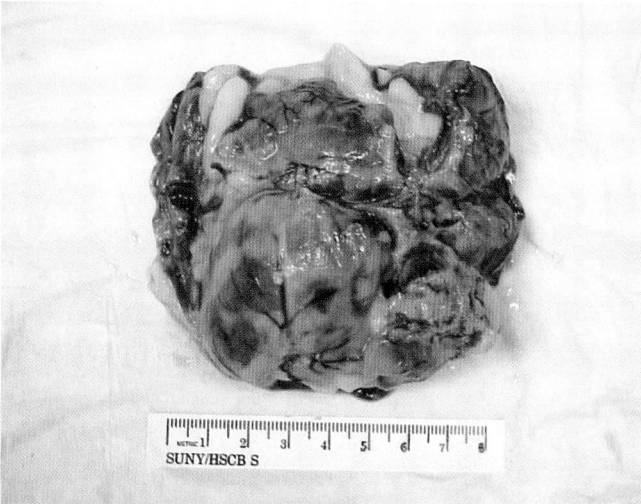

FIGURE 10.7 Intrauterine E coli meningitis in a stillborn. Mother had a urinary tract infection.

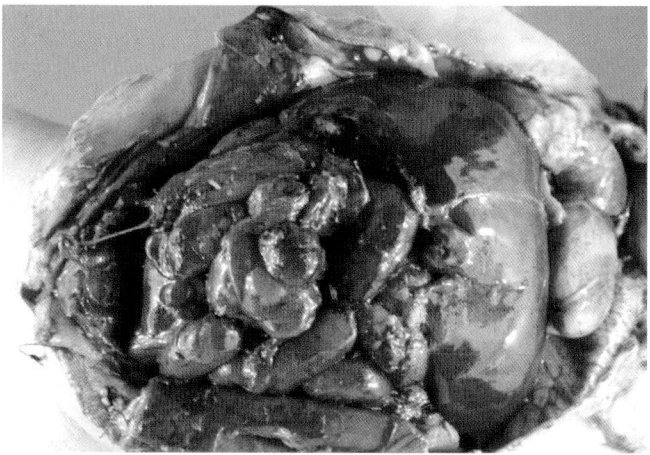

FIGURE 10.8 Plastic peritonitis with bowel necrosis and perforation in severe necrotizing enterocolitis.

found in the mother's vagina. **Stillbirth** or early neonatal death occurs. Non-specific symptoms and **meningoencephalitis** is common and has a 30% mortality rate.

Small yellow foci of necrosis may be found in the liver, spleen, adrenal glands, and lungs.[41] Microscopically **Gram-positive and silver-positive rods** are present in necrotic nodules composed of macrophages and neutrophils (Fig. 10.9) The lesion heals by centripetal scarification. Jaundice and purpuric skin lesions are frequent if liver damage is severe. Early liver lesions may be free of leukocytes and appear as areas of coagulation necrosis. In later stages infiltration with mononuclear and polymorphonuclear cells occurs. Similar **granulomatous lesions** are found occasionally in the placental villi and fetal membranes in disseminated disease. Listeriosis is a disease of developing countries. It is found in the soil and can contaminate vegetation, soft cheese and poorly cooked meats. In the USA 500 deaths occur each year. The mother has a mild illness but the immunologically naive fetus and neonate are susceptible.

Neonatal tetanus

Clostridium tetani spores colonize the umbilical stump of infants born to women who lack prenatal care and were never immunized against tetanus.[42, 43] This is a preventable disease which, like so many infectious diseases, is a measure of the general health of a population.[44, 45] Worldwide over 500 000 infant deaths per year are due to neonatal tetanus. The case fatality rate is 50%.

Exotoxin interferes with neuromuscular transmission, producing **respiratory failure**, abnormalities of the conducting system of the heart, necrosis of skeletal muscle, and bulbar palsy. Death from neonatal tetanus peaks during the second week of life.[31] In some parts of the world, street dust or manure is placed on the newly cut cord and fatal bacterial sepsis or tetanus is frequent. *C. tetani*, like diphtheria, remains localized and secretes a powerful exotoxin that acts on the central nervous system. Hyperirritability and difficulty in swallowing begin to appear 6–14 days after birth. **Nervous system manifestations** start with mild twitching and soon develop into tonic spasms involving the entire body. The jaws become fixed and cannot be pried open. The body maintains a board-like rigidity with back arched, lower limbs extended, arms either extended or tightly flexed, and fists clenched. The facial expression is fixed, with the eyes tightly closed, forehead wrinkled, and contraction of muscles causing a characteristic **sardonic grin**. Treatment was unsuccessful until tracheotomy and hyperbaric oxygen were used. The organisms produce no specific pathologic lesions. Anoxia resulting from cardiac and respiratory depression caused by the severe tonic spasm may produce scattered ecchymoses in the thoracic viscera.

TORCH infections

Torch infections comprise **t**oxoplasmosis, **o**ther (congenital syphilis and viruses), **r**ubella, **c**ytomegalovirus, and **h**erpes

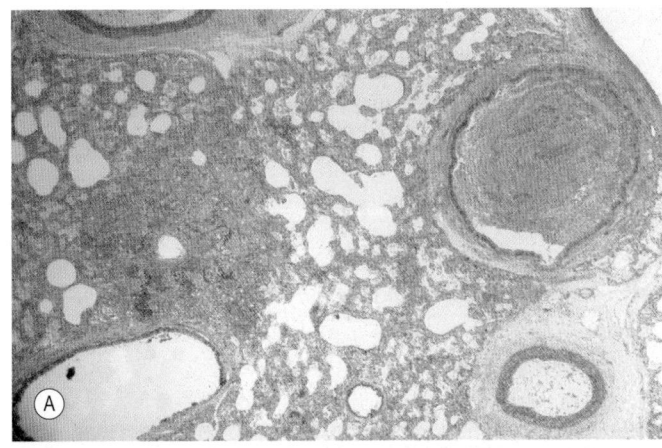

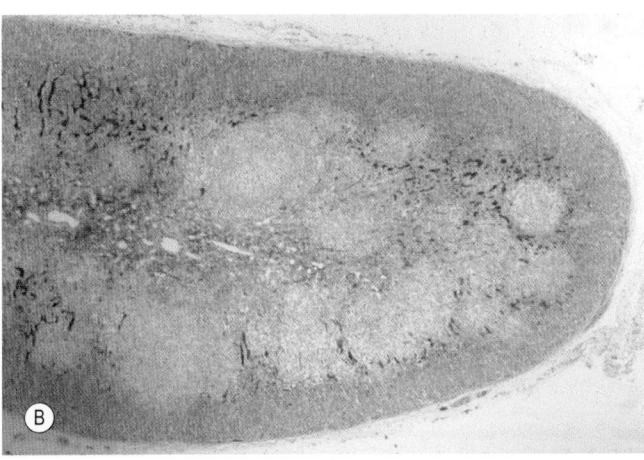

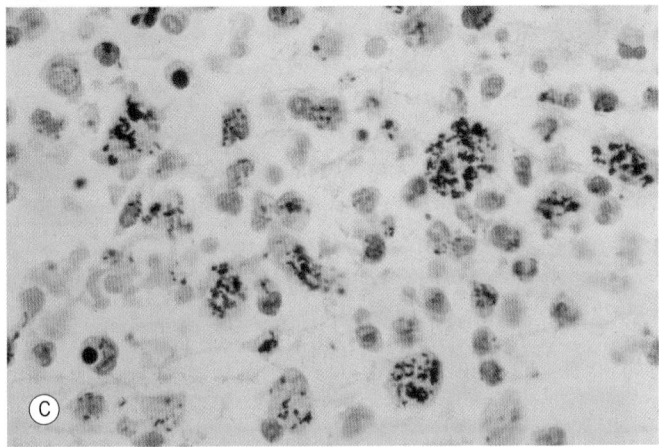

FIGURE 10.9 (A) Listeriosis of the lung with suppuration in a bronchiole. (B) Listeriosis of the adrenal gland. (C) Warthin Starry stain on subarachnoid fluid in *Listeria* meningitis.

simplex virus (HSV). A TORCH screen is often ordered but today this is a limited concept since enteroviruses, especially Coxsackie type B and *Chlamydia* or *Mycoplasma* and other pathogens may be missed. Except for cytomegalovirus (CMV), the other agents in TORCH are extremely rare. Geographic microbiology must direct proper laboratory utilization for endemic pathogens. The cost–benefit relationship where resources are scarce determine which tests are appropriate. A strong argument may be made for the routine identification of CMV in newborn heel blood blots that are mandated for the detection of genetic metabolic diseases. These samples have been used to determine the seroprevalence of human immunodeficiency virus (HIV) in high risk populations.

Congenital toxoplasmosis

Toxoplasmosis,[46–52] an infectious disease caused by protozoa of the genus *Toxoplasma*, affects cats, dogs, sheep, rabbits, guinea pigs, and other animals as well as humans.[53] It was recognized as pathogenic for humans in 1939. Three clinical profiles include:

- a frequently fatal congenital form with the onset of encephalomyelitis in utero, infancy, or childhood;
- an acute febrile adult illness with lymphadenopathy; and
- a latent infection identified by neutralizing antibodies in serum.

Congenital toxoplasmosis is rarely seen in the USA. Organisms have been found in cat feces but maternal or transplacental

human infection is extremely rare. Immigrants from endemic regions of Central America may occasionally present with preterm low birth weight and classical clinical features.

The **tetrad of congenital toxoplasmosis is hydrocephalus** or **microcephalus; chorioretinitis** particularly in the macula; **convulsions**; and **cerebral calcification**. Skin rash, purpura, prolonged jaundice, hepatosplenomegaly, and extramedullary hematopoiesis are also common. The head may appear normal at birth but can increase rapidly in size in the first few days of life. Patients who survive develop progressive hydrocephalus associated with mental retardation.

Chorioretinitis – with small retinal hemorrhages or pathognomonic, flame-like, yellow–white areas studded with black pigment – is seen in 75% of newborns with congenital toxoplasmosis. Impaired vision and searching nystagmus are usually present. In some infants only the eye may be affected. Microphthalmia, autoimmune iridocyclitis, cataracts, glaucoma, and retinal detachment can occur. Organisms may be found within retinal endothelial cells. The disease is often bilateral and associated with optic atrophy and blindness.

Endothelial cells in skeletal muscle and myocardium are frequent targets for tachyzoites of *Toxoplasma*. Dilated cardiomyopathy with focal necrosis and inflammation contain pseudocysts filled with microorganisms. **Immune complex nephrosis or focal glomerulonephritis** may occur. **Giant cell hepatitis, cholestasis**, and involvement of the **endocrine organs** have been

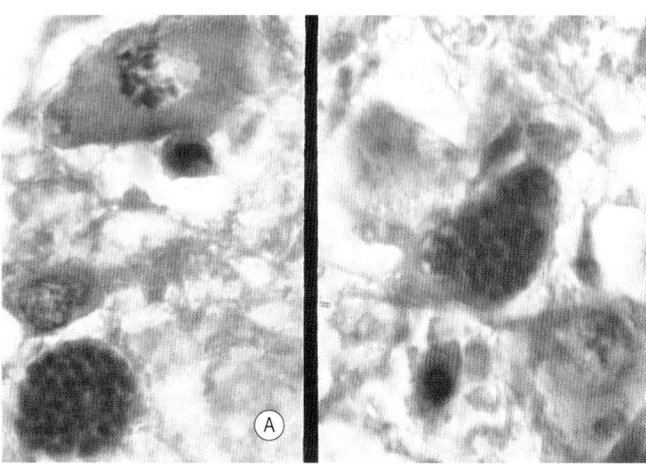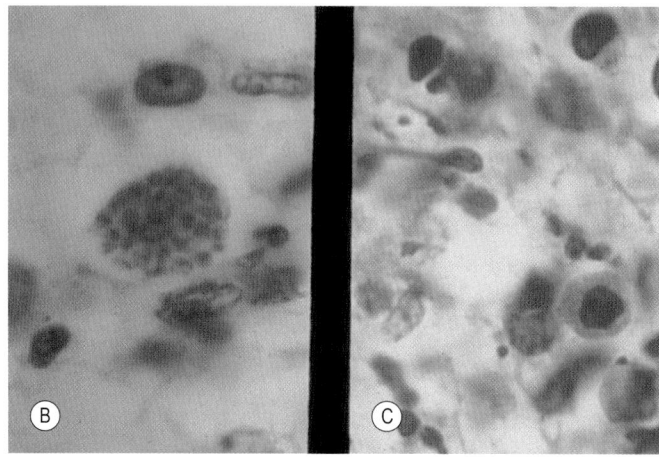

FIGURE 10.10 (A) *Toxoplasma* cysts in congenital cerebral toxoplasmosis. *Toxoplasma gondii* appears in two forms: (B) an encysted form with numerous bradyzoites; (C) tiny trophozoites are free in an area of cerebral necrosis.

reported. **The lung and gastrointestinal tract are rarely involved.** Disseminated disease occurs in 1 per 100 000 deliveries in the USA, but infectious rates may be as high as 6 per 1000 using a type-specific immunoglobulin M (IgM) assay for disease surveillance.[54]

In most cases, *Toxoplasma* organisms are round, piriform, or crescenteric with a distinct nuclear membrane and clear homogeneous cytoplasm. They are 4–7 μm long and 2–4 μm wide in blood smears, but in tissues they are considerably smaller. Obligate intracellular parasites enter a cell, multiply, rupture, and liberate the organisms. When less virulent, multiplication continues and the cell nucleus disappears forming an organism-packed cell known as a pseudocyst (Fig.10.10). Pseudocysts are rarely observed in granulomas.

On postmortem examination the **external surface of the brain** may be covered with **multiple discrete, necrotic yellow nodules** that range in size from a few millimeters to more than 1 cm in diameter.[55] Similar lesions may be present in the **subependymal regions.** Obstruction of cerebrospinal fluid circulation by granulation tissue or necrotic debris leads to **hydranencephaly.** Microscopic examination of the brain reveals **granulomas** with a few epithelioid cells and lymphocytes, or large lesions with central liquefactive necrosis and peripheral cellular infiltration. Free and intracellular parasites are usually numerous, although they may be found with great difficulty. As necrosis continues, calcium is deposited in the brain.

Toxoplasma organisms can be found in many parts of the body without any cellular tissue reaction.[55] **The myocardium, adrenal glands, lungs, subcutaneous tissue, testes, ovaries, pancreas, stomach, kidneys, and liver have been infected.**[56] However, only a few sites are involved in any given case and clinical disease is frequently absent.[57]

In the acute stage of toxoplasmosis, the **brain** is always involved. In chronic, inactive cases specific lesions disappear in the peripheral tissues. Reactivation of latent infection occurs in immunosuppressed individuals. *Toxoplasma* pseudocysts can be found frequently in the umbilical cord and membranes of the placenta. They are less often found in the villi but are associated with plasma cell villitis. The **placenta** may be **large and hydropic.**[58] In the umbilical cord and fetal membranes, there is no cellular reaction. Concurrent congenital human immunodeficiency syndrome (HIV) and toxoplasmosis is rare but reported.[59] The incidence is lower in children than adults since it usually results from reactivation of latent infection.

Congenital syphilis

Transplacental transmission of maternal *Treponema pallidum* infection can harm the fetus.[60–61] Highly motile spirochetes are 10 –15 μm long with 10–15 spirals. Rotary movement made possible by the spirochete shape aids in the passage from the maternal circulation through the walls of the **placental villi** and eventually spirochetes enter the **umbilical vein.** The **liver**, the first organ to contact the spirochetes, can be severely affected.

Primary maternal spirochetemia during the second trimester is most deleterious.[62, 63] The lack of a maternal immune response and the ability of the older fetus to mount an inflammatory response with **plasma cell** infiltration and **fibrosis** of multiple organs maximize tissue destruction in the fetus. Sheets of plasma cells in fetal tissue strongly suggest syphilis even if the maternal serologic tests are negative. In untreated infants spirochetes may be found beneath the endothelium of the umbilical vein on **Warthin Starry stains** (Fig. 10.11) or by immunofluorescence methods.[64] Fetal infection is rare before the fifth month of pregnancy. If anti-syphilitic treatment is begun before the third trimester the infant is usually normal at birth. Mothers who are penicillin allergic and treated with erythromycin may arrest their disease. However, erythromycin does not cross the placenta and the fetus becomes a spirochetal culture with dissemination of organisms in all viscera.

Syphilis may cause stillbirth, or live birth with symptoms, or an asymptomatic infant with positive serology. The clinical manifestations depend on the stage of maternal infection at the time of

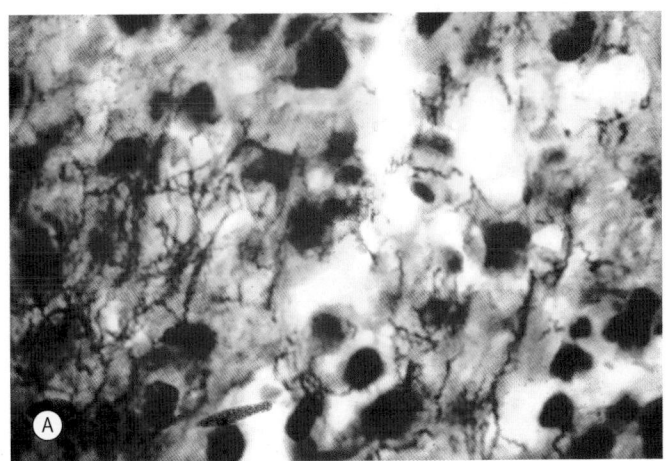
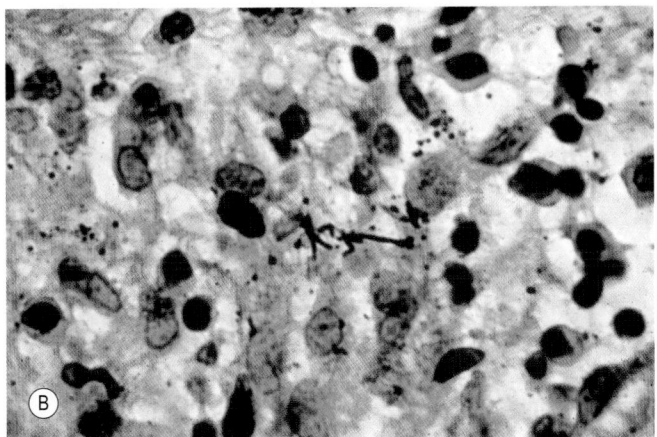

FIGURE 10.11 (A) Warthin Starry stain for spirochetes. (B) Typical *Treponema pallidum* with 6–15 spirals and tapered ends enable corkscrew rotation that facilitates invasion. Similar organisms occur in Lyme disease and leptospirosis.

conception and on treatment during pregnancy. Congenital syphilis is a miliary disease comparable to secondary syphilis in adults (Fig. 10.12). A woman who has been adequately treated before conception and is not reinfected during pregnancy will give birth to a normal infant. A woman who has active syphilis at the time of conception or acquires an infection during pregnancy and is not treated will usually have an affected child.[65, 66]

The spectrum of congenital syphilis ranges from a macerated stillbirth with hydrops fetalis or mild villitis to a normal-appearing infant with subclinical disease. Subtle subperiosteal elevation and **osteochondritis** may be present on radiologic examination, especially of the knee (Fig. 10.13A and B). In some, limb lesions are so painful, pseudoparalysis with decreased spontaneous movements and cries during a diaper change are observed. The syphilitic infant represents a stage of secondary syphilis. Spirochetemia recurs unless antibiotics, usually penicillin, eradicate the infection. Sequelae from **gummatous necrosis** may persist despite treatment. **Late stigmata** of congenital syphilis include saddle nose, Hutchinson teeth, and saber shin. Recognition of the syphilitic infant at birth is essential to minimize these effects.

Prematurity, intrauterine growth retardation, hydrops fetalis, and placental hyperplasia are common.[67] **Hepatosplenomegaly**, conjugated hyperbilirubinemia, and abnormal liver function test results are frequent. **Bleeding disorders** may be attributed to **liver damage** with clotting factor deficiency, autoimmune thrombocytopenia, or disseminated intravascular coagulation (DIC). **Maculopapular skin lesions**, significantly on the palms and soles, may precede a desquamative process. Weeping cutaneous bullae or snuffles, a nasal discharge, may contain large numbers of spirochetes. Rarely, immune complex deposition in the glomeruli is associated with the **nephrotic syndrome**. Hypoalbuminemia with anasarca, ascites, and heart failure may develop in infants over 1 month of age.

Viscera affected by **gummatous necrosis** (Fig. 10.12B–D) in descending order of frequency include the pancreas, liver, bone, lung, gastrointestinal tract, kidneys, and lymphoid tissue. Mesenchymal stroma and extramedullary hematopoiesis are increased and organ maturation is retarded. Mononuclear or plasma cell vasculitis may heal with onionskin fibrosis. Gummas are usually confluent nodular lesions with a central area of amorphous fibrovascular granulation tissue rimmed by inflammatory cells and surrounded by an outer ring of dense fibrous tissue.

In **pneumonia alba** the lung parenchyma is studded with multiple nodules composed of spirochetes; inflammatory cells and connective tissue entrap compressed airspaces. The lungs are pale, voluminous, firm, and airless. White lung refers to endarteritis with impaired circulation and fibrous proliferation in the walls of the airspaces. Similar lesions distort the hepatic parenchyma causing **hepar lobatum**. In the gastrointestinal tract mononuclear cells expand the lamina propria, and vascular compromise follows perivasculitis and fibrosis. Intestinal atresia, stenosis, or perforation with meconium peritonitis is reported. Ulcers may occur in the mouth, tongue, and nose. Gummas may be seen in the heart, pituitary, adrenal glands, testes, meninges, choroid plexus, central nervous system, and eye. In the skin, lymphocytes and plasma cells aggregate around adnexal structures and blood vessels. A similar infiltrate may appear in the interstitium of the kidney.

Osteochondritis with granulation tissue and fibrosis is frequently seen at the growth plate of long bones associated with subperiosteal new bone formation (Fig. 10.13A–B). Congenital syphilis can also present with a miliary rash characteristic of secondary syphilis (Fig. 10.13C). Bone lesions are symmetric and may occur to a lesser extent in other congenital viral infections, especially CMV and rubella. Plasma cells are increased in lymphoid organs, and the thymus may rarely contain a **Dubois abscess**.

The placenta may be large, pale and associated with hydrops fetalis secondary to autoimmune hemolytic anemia. Spirochetes identified with silver stains on placental tissue are uncommon. The villi are immature with evidence of edema, Hofbauer cell proliferation, focal villitis with plasma cells, and obliterative

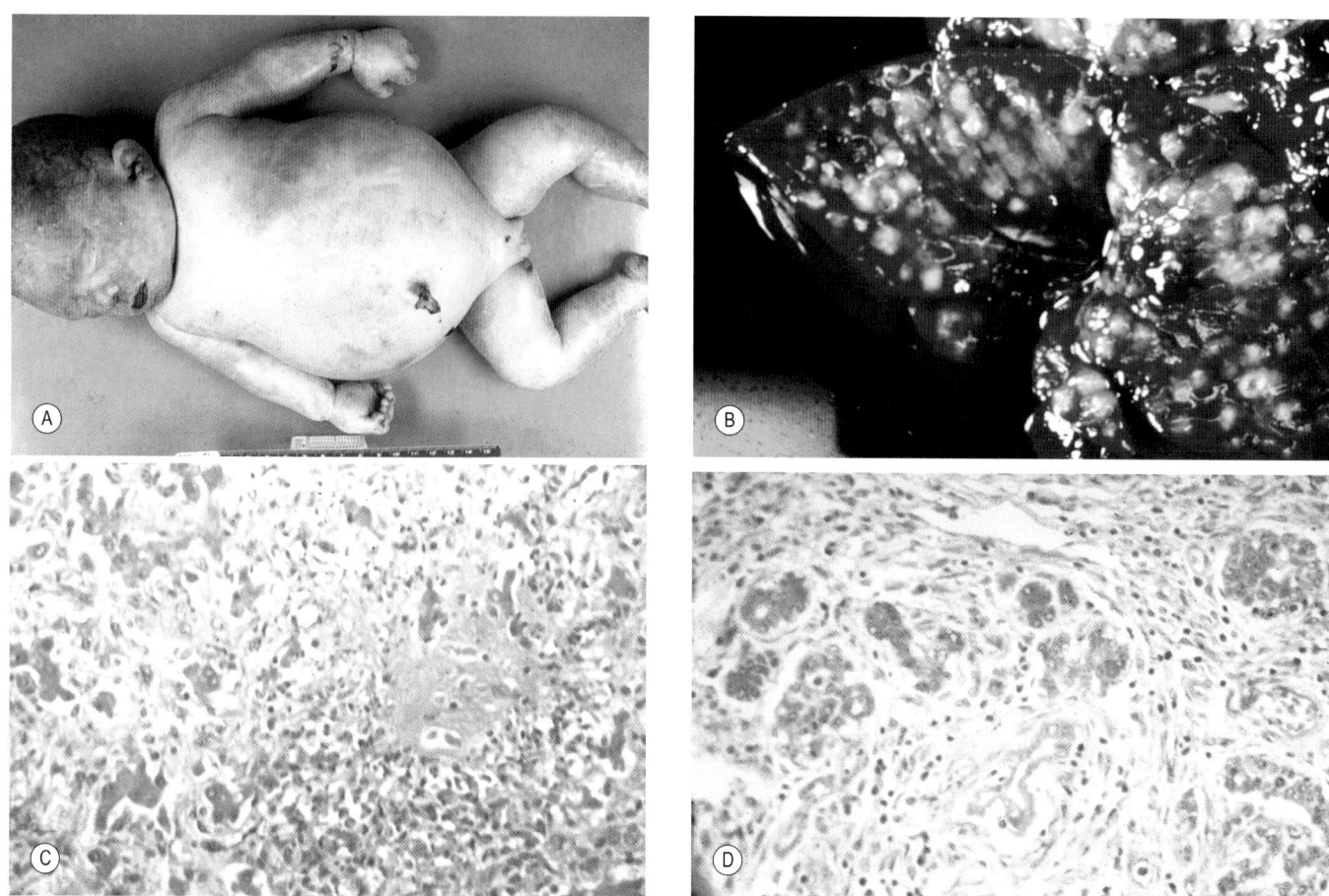

FIGURE 10.12 (A) Hydrops fetalis in congenital syphilis. (B) Pneumonia alba with gummatous necrosis mimics carcinomatosis of the lung. (C) Histologic features of pneumonia alba with obliterative endarteritis, vascularized nodules and fibrosis. Plasma cells are usually present. (D) Gummatous necrosis of the pancreas.

endarteritis.[68, 69] The diagnosis of congenital syphilis is made by a specific IgM antibody with the fluorescent treponema antigen–antibody test. In New York City routine screening serology for syphilis was eliminated due to a low yield of positive tests. The HIV epidemic surged in the early 1990s, and an epidemic of congenital syphilis was superimposed on HIV infected women and their fetuses. The worldwide incidence of congenital syphilis is greater than 500 000 cases per year. The morbidity and mortality rivals HIV infection. A health care delivery system with the economic resources and political will can eliminate this tragedy.[70]

Congenital viral infection

Rubella (German measles) After an epidemic of rubella in Australia in 1942, Gregg[71, 72] found an association between rubella in early pregnancy and **congenital defects of the eyes and heart**.[73–75] Women who contracted rubella during the first 2 months of pregnancy almost invariably gave birth to diseased children (Table 10.2).[76] When the infection occurred later in pregnancy, the infant was less often affected, although eye defects were observed in a few instances following maternal rubella in the third month and ear defects in the fourth month of gestation. The

mother may or may not develop a morbilliform rash and posterior cervical lymphadenopathy. The faint, fleeting macular rash must be distinguished from other viral exanthems including parvovirus B19, human herpesvirus, enteroviruses, and endemic arboviruses.

Infants born following maternal rubella were often small, poorly nourished, and difficult to feed.[77–80] Late eruption of the teeth and abnormalities in enamel production were also reported. Microcephaly and heart disease were rare without accompanying eye or ear defects. Cataracts were found if the mother had rubella in the second month of pregnancy. Ear abnormalities occurred when the disease was contracted late in the second month or early in the third month of gestation.

Viremia during the embryonic period is associated with a 75% incidence of congenital heart disease. Lesions in descending incidence include **patent ductus arteriosus, stenosis of the branch pulmonary arteries** (Fig.10.14A), stenosis of the pulmonary and aortic valves, and cardiac septal defects at the atrial and ventricular level. Microscopic sections of stenotic pulmonary arteries reveal fibromuscular intimal proliferation with elastosis (Fig. 10.14C). Areas of focal fibrosis occur in the heart. **Neonatal hepatitis** with hepatocellular necrosis, giant cell transformation, cholestasis, and biliary atresia can occur in the

TABLE 10.2 FREQUENCY AND DISTRIBUTION OF ABNORMALITIES IN FETUSES WITH RUBELLA

Gestational age at onset of maternal rubella (weeks)	No. of fetuses	Percentage abnormal	Percentage of fetuses with abnormality in specific organs			
			Eye lens	Heart	Ear	Skeletal muscle
0–4	20	80	35	65	12	25
4–8	31	58	48	45	13	16
8–11	6	66	66	50	0	0

From Tondury and Smith 1966,[73] with permission.

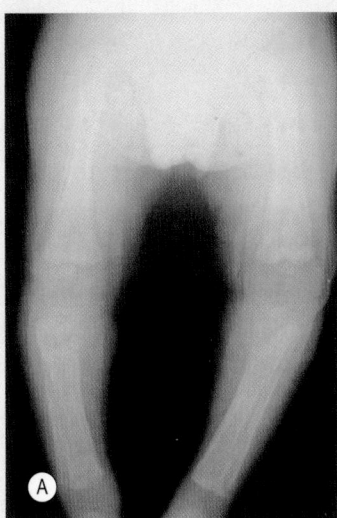

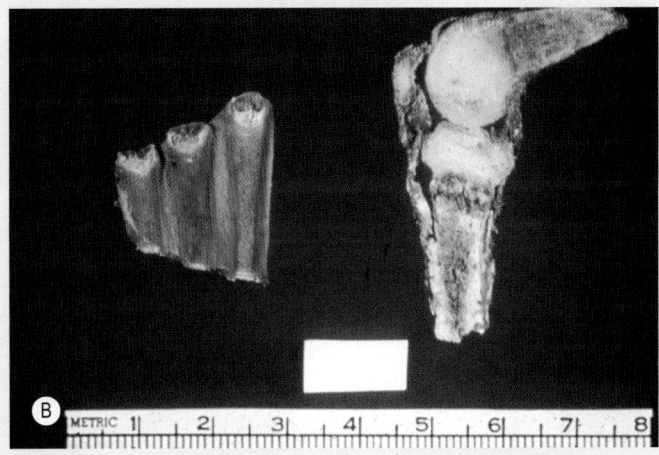

FIGURE 10.13 (A) Radiograph of osteochondritis congenital syphilis. (B) Classical enchondritis of the knee in a syphilitic infant. (C) Morbilliform rash in miliary syphilis in an infant with congenital syphilis.

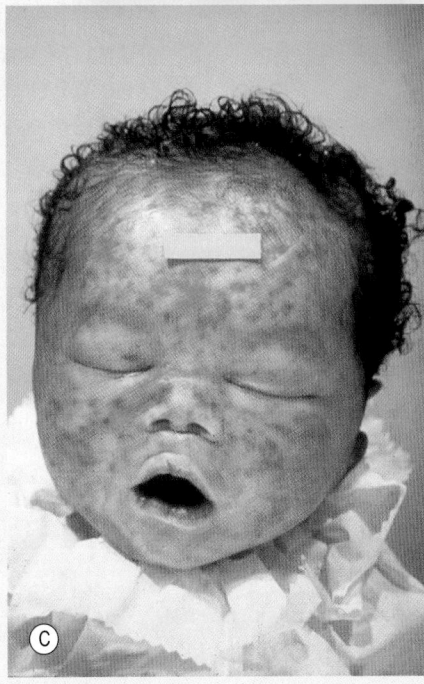

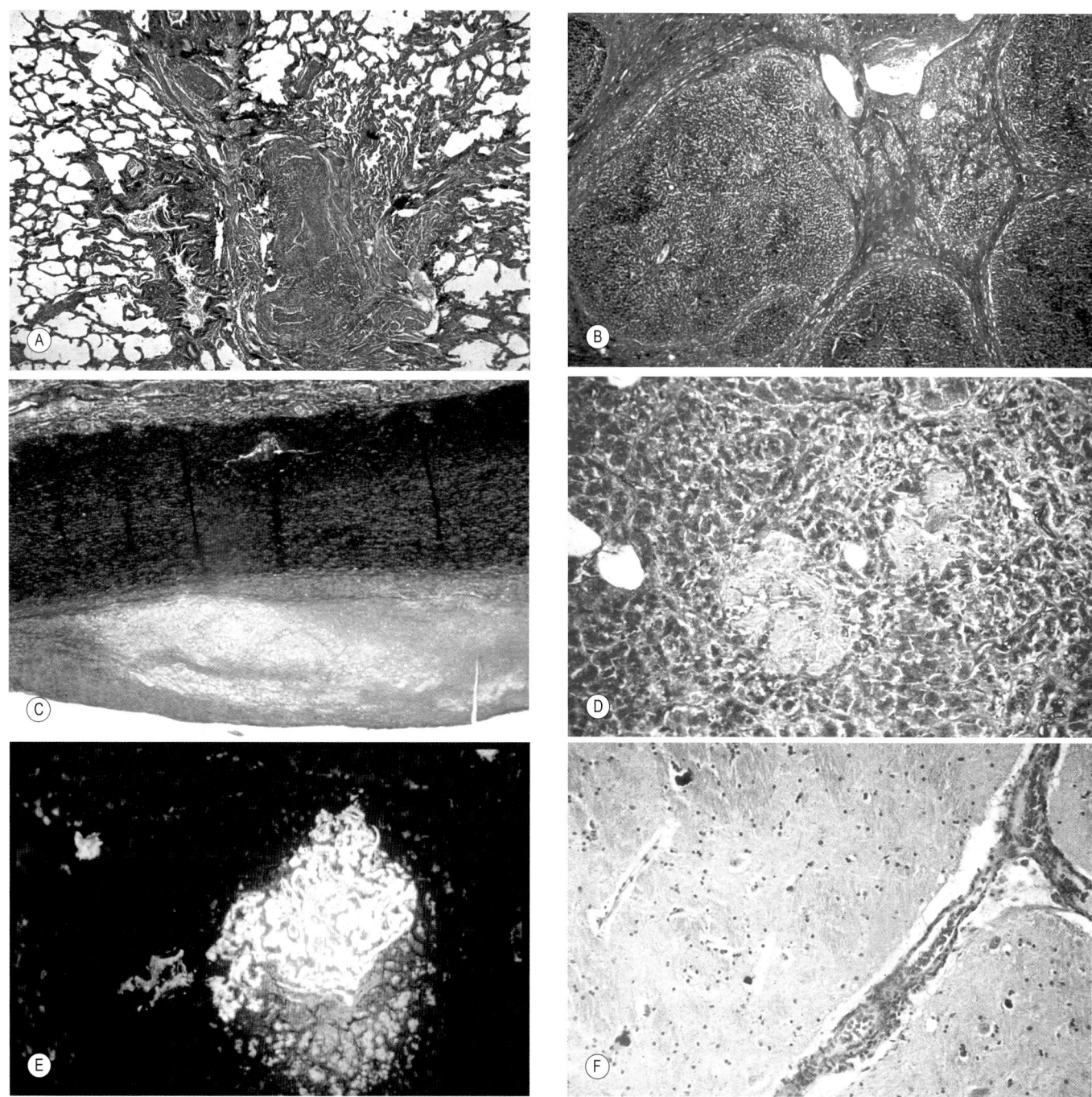

FIGURE 10.14 (A) Pulmonary branch stenosis in a 9-year-old with congenital rubella. (B) Postinfectious hepatic cirrhosis in a child with the congenital rubella syndrome. (C) Elastosis of the thoracic aorta in congenital rubella. (D) Amyloidosis of the pancreatic islets in congenital rubella. (E) Green birefringence confirms presence of amyloid in the pancreatic islets. (F) Chronic encephalitis in congenital rubella.

neonate.[81] Postnecrotic cirrhosis was seen in a 9-year-old who had congenital rubella (Fig. 10.14B). This youngster also had amyloidosis of the pancreatic islets (Fig. 10.14D and E) and subacute sclerotic panencephalitis at autopsy (Fig. 10.14F). Around 20% of congenital rubella survivors develop **diabetes mellitus**.[82, 83] Congenital rubella may be associated with auto-immune hemolytic **anemia** and thrombocytopenia. As in most congenital infections, there is splenomegaly and precocious

development of lymphoid follicles with a decrease in paracortical T cells. The thymus is atrophic, and widespread extramedullary hematopoiesis is present in neonates.[84]

Deafness is attributed to inflammation and degeneration of the cochlear duct with collapse or displacement of the inner ear structures. In the 1970s one-third of adolescents at a college for the deaf had congenital rubella. **Microcephaly** and **micro-calcification**, especially in a perivascular or periventricular region, are frequent. The elastic layer in cerebral arteries may be damaged and associated with ischemic changes such as gliosis and microglial cell proliferation (Fig. 10.14F). **Autoimmune thyroiditis and Addison disease** occur in late survivors.[85] Meningoencephalitis is frequent.

The placenta is hypoplastic with epithelial necrosis and reduction in terminal villi. The stem villi may be enlarged and decidual necrosis is present with cytoplasmic eosinophilic inclusions in the decidua and chorionic villi. The fetus is infected by embolization of necrotic placental endothelium into fetal viscera. Tissue necrosis with a nidus of viral infection without inflammation is seen in multiple viscera. Impaired cellular proliferation leads to growth retardation. Abortus specimens also show **necrotic placental endothelium** with a mild lymphoplasmacytic response in villous stroma.

In the USA, the elimination of congenital rubella syndrome between 1969 and 2004[86, 87] has been remarkable thanks to universal vaccination of teenage girls of childbearing age. The immune status of pregnant women is checked at the onset of prenatal care and prophylaxis provided. Universal vaccination programs in all nations will reduce tragic, needless infant mortality and morbidity.

Cytomegalovirus Congenital CMV infection[88, 89] may be identified in 1 per 100 live births in the USA, but severe brain damage is seen in fewer than 1 per 1000 births. Transmission may be either **intrauterine** or **intrapartum**.[90–93] Youngsters may develop deafness and learning disabilities as sequelae of unrecognized congenital CMV infection. Fewer than 5% of cases of congenital CMV infection are identified at birth, and 80% of CMV infections are subclinical.[94, 95] Laboratory tests must be performed soon after birth to determine if CMV infection is indeed congenital. **Nosocomial infection** is possible, particularly in infants given blood transfusions.

Severely affected infants are growth retarded and have hyperplastic placentas. Microcephaly, hydrocephaly, lissencephaly, and periventricular cerebral calcification occur.[96–98] Giant cell hepatitis[99] with cholestasis is frequent. CMV has a pathognomonic cytopathic effect. A very large cell contains a single dense intranuclear basophilic inclusion surrounded by a clear perinuclear halo called an owl's eye inclusion. Multiple tiny intracytoplasmic inclusions may stain with the periodic acid-Schiff reaction or silver stains.

Cytoplasmic inclusions are easily lost in macerated tissue or degenerating cells. Inclusion-bearing cells may be found in multiple viscera but are common in the kidney, lung, pancreas, liver, and brain (Fig. 10.15; Table 10.3).[100] Epithelial cells and endothelial cells are frequently infected and may be associated with lymphoplasmacytic infiltrate. Molecular techniques and viral culture indicate the incidence of CMV infection to be twice as common as compared with the identification of classic cells on routine histology. Large cells with smudged nuclei may harbor CMV and require **DNA probes** with in situ hybridization or the **polymerase chain reaction (PCR)**[101] to prove infection. The salivary gland is often involved in subclinical infection. In the **brain**, inclusion-bearing cells include neurons,

TABLE 10.3 CLINICAL AND PATHOLOGIC CHARACTERISTICS OF 42 NEWBORN INFANTS WITH CYTOMEGALIC INCLUSION DISEASE

Symptoms	No.	Percentage
Hematologic abnormalities	31	74
Jaundice	30	71
Hepatosplenomegaly	26	62
Prematurity	23	55
Central nervous system abnormalities	16	38
Site of inclusions		
Kidney	37	88
Liver	33	79
Lung	29	69
Pancreas	24	57
Thyroid	18	43
Brain	10	24
Salivary gland	8	19

After Medearis 1957,[100] with permission.

glia, meninges, choroid plexus, or ependyma. Destruction of cerebral gray and white matter with gliosis and dystrophic calcification occurs. In severe infection the subependymal zone of the lateral ventricles of the brain may exhibit diffuse areas of necrosis, cellular infiltration, and calcification.

A wide range of **ophthalmic pathology** occurs in congenital CMV infection (see Ch. 39). Chorioretinitis affects 25% of symptomatic infants. Microphthalmia, cataracts, nystagmus, strabismus, and optic atrophy can develop. Hearing loss is present in asymptomatic children.[102, 103] The kidneys contain inclusion-bearing cells throughout the nephrons. Virus can be cultured from urine, and cytomegalic cells can be identified on microscopic study of cytologic preparations from freshly voided urine specimens. The owl's eye viral inclusion can be identified in sloughed tubular epithelial cells. **Villitis** with classical cells may be occasionally seen in the placenta.[104, 105] **A single inclusion-bearing pathognomonic cell is diagnostic.** Hemolytic anemia, jaundice, hyperbilirubinemia, and purpuric hemorrhages in the skin are common in severe cases. Erythropoiesis is ordinarily marked in liver, spleen, kidneys, and other organs. Immune complex glomerulonephritis, ascites, and pulmonary hypoplasia are rarely seen.[106] Involvement of the biliary tract can cause cholestasis and biliary atresia.[107]

Postneonatal CMV infection is acquired from infected lymphocytes in breast milk or blood transfusion. Transplant recipients are at risk for CMV. Hepatosplenomegaly, pneumonitis, and lymphadenopathy occur, but the manifestations are less severe than the congenital CMV infection. Routine newborn screening could distinguish congenital CMV infection from postnatal infection[108] and antiviral therapy can be prescribed.[108–110] Sensorineural hearing loss in children may be the result of congenital CMV infection (Bradford Detection on the Guthrie card used for routine newborn dried blood heel samples is possible with PCR).[111, 112]

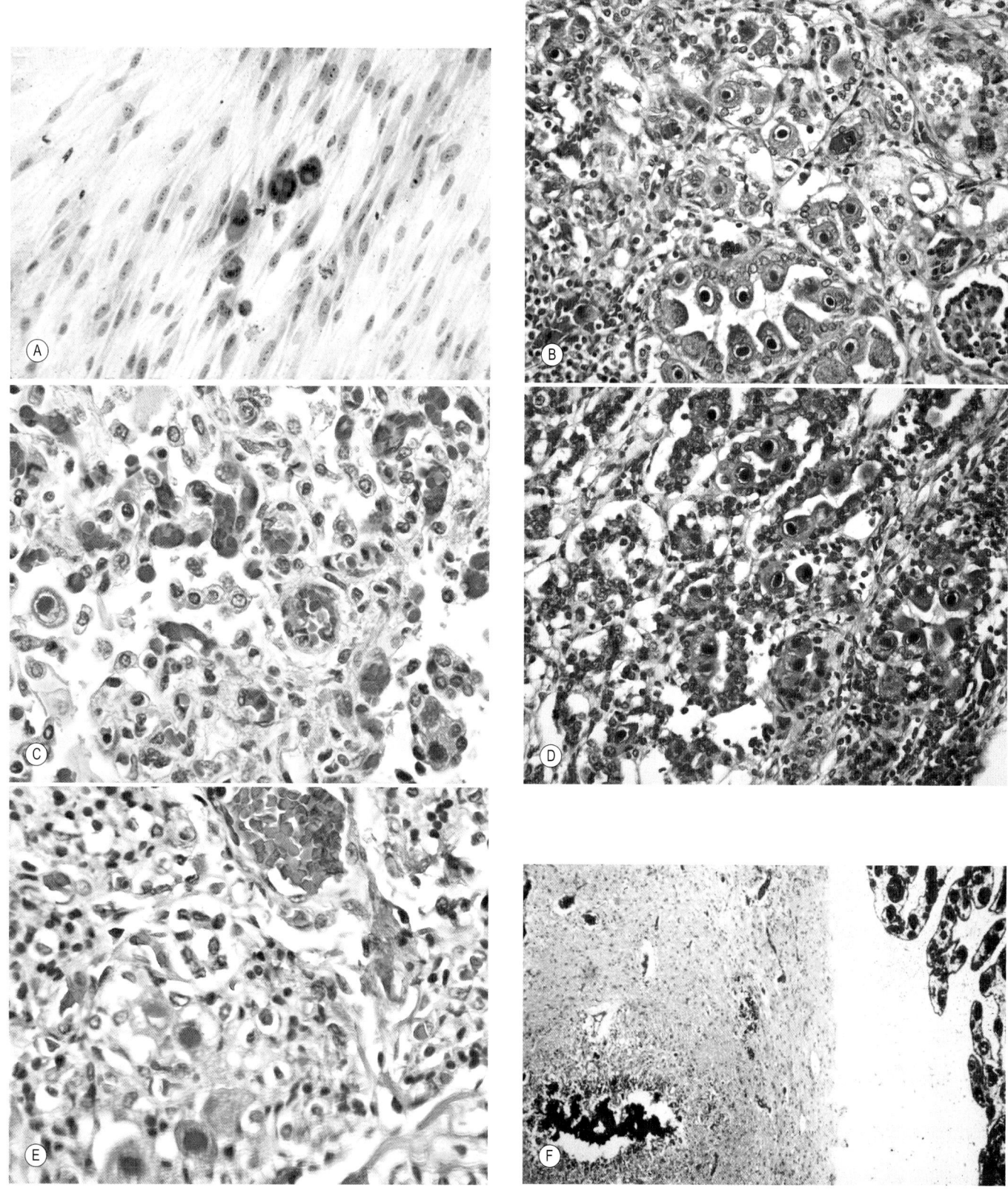

FIGURE 10.15 (A) CMV tissue culture. (B) CMV owl eye inclusions in the kidney. (C) CMV pneumonitis with nuclear and cytoplasmic inclusions. (D) CMV in the pituitary gland. (E) CMV in the thyroid gland. (F) CMV in the brain with characteristic periventricular calcification.

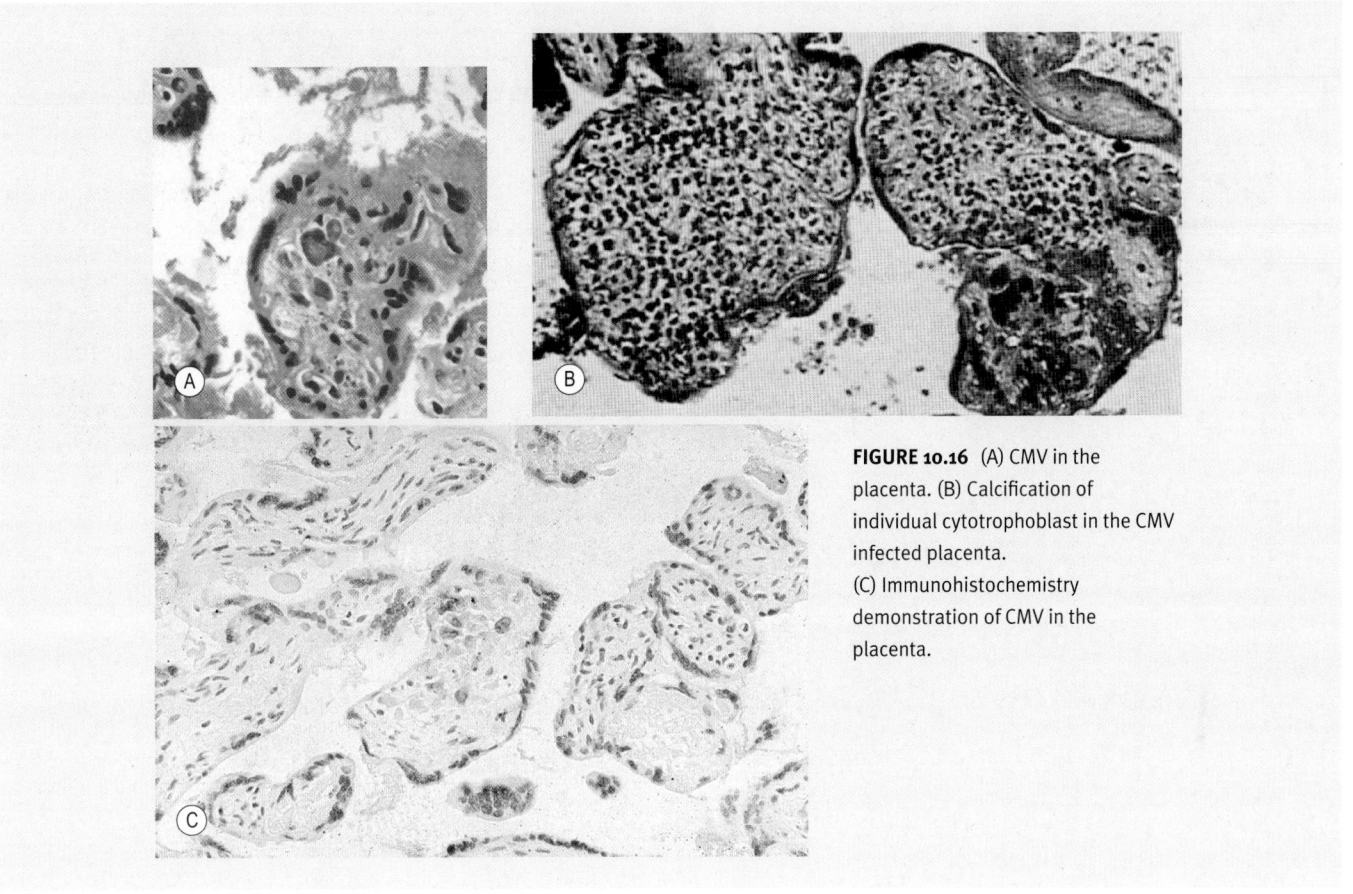

FIGURE 10.16 (A) CMV in the placenta. (B) Calcification of individual cytotrophoblast in the CMV infected placenta. (C) Immunohistochemistry demonstration of CMV in the placenta.

Placental CMV is underdiagnosed. Calcification limited to villous cytotrophoblast with necrotizing lymphocytic vasculitis if strongly suspicious for CMV. Immunostains may be negative if the gene dosage is less than 20 copies and infection is spotty (Fig. 10.16A–C). Acquired maternal immunity reduces the likelihood of CMV in future pregnancies by 69%.[113]

Herpes simplex virus HSV[114–117] causes minor **vesicular epithelial infection** in adults. Fatal viremia or severe disability may result if newborns are exposed to HSV-infected cervical secretions during vaginal delivery. HSV may enter through the conjunctiva, skin, or mucous membranes. In a few cases infection with intact fetal membranes has been established.[118] Herpes genitalis and disseminated disease in the newborn are usually **HSV type 2** (*HSV-2*). The usual perioral strain **HSV type 1** (*HSV-1*) can also cause congenital HSV.[119] Disseminated HSV is more frequent during primary maternal infection.[120, 121] The initial vesicle may not be apparent,[122] and symptoms do not develop until the virus has propagated at 5–7 days of age. Fever or hypothermia, icterus, lethargy, vomiting, dyspnea, cyanosis, and rapidly developing circulatory collapse occur. The spleen and liver are always enlarged. Thick yellow mucus often collects in the throat, and bleeding may be associated with thrombocytopenia, hepatic insufficiency, or DIC, which precedes shock and multiorgan failure.[123]

At autopsy, **the liver and adrenal glands are most often involved**, followed by the lungs,[124] brain,[125, 126] esophagus, tongue, and colon. Less often viral inclusions are present in the spleen, lymph nodes, stomach, bone marrow, conjunctivas, pharynx, and heart. The liver is riddled with pale yellow areas alternating with hemorrhagic, **necrotic nodules** 1–6 mm in diameter. These become confluent and may involve the entire liver. Swollen hepatocytes undergo necrosis with **intranuclear inclusions** at the margin of the necrotic foci (Fig. 10.17). No inflammatory reaction is seen. Early viral inclusions may be large, sharply circumscribed, acidophilic, slightly granular masses surrounded by a clear zone inside the nuclear membrane. Later the entire nucleus may be occupied by the inclusion. Large infected cells may occasionally contain small intracytoplasmic acidophilic granules.

Focal adrenal necrosis with herpetic viral inclusions is frequent. Discrete areas of necrosis may be widespread in the basal ganglia and brainstem. Viral inclusions are found at the margins of the necrotic areas and may involve sympathetic ganglia. Occasionally the brain is the only organ in the body to be affected. HSV-1 has been identified in **paraffin-embedded brain tissue with PCR**.[127] A stat autopsy on a twin who died with congenital herpesvirus infection instigated prompt curative antiviral therapy of the surviving twin.[128] In postnatal HSV the visceral lesions are limited in distribution, and the disease

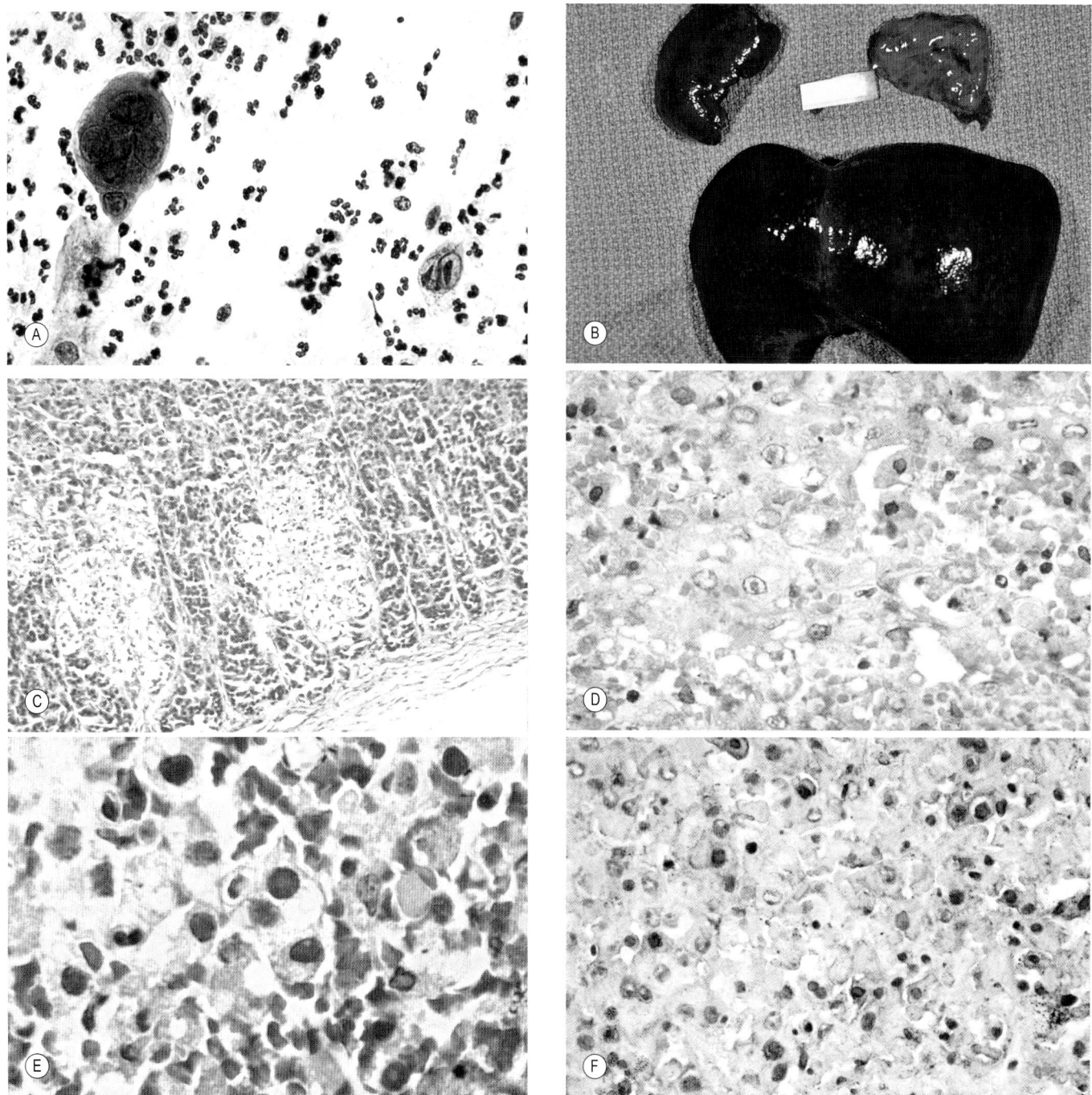

FIGURE 10.17 (A) HSV positive Papanicolaou smear. (B) Classical herpetic necrosis, liver and adrenal gland. (C) HSV with multifocal adrenal necrosis. HSV inclusions in the adrenal gland (D) and liver (E), with demonstration by HSV immunostain in the latter (F) (cont'd over).

is usually less severe than in the newborn.[129] Herpesvirus encephalitis is most often seen in the temporal lobe.[130] The prevention of HSV begins with good prenatal care, expectant management and treatment as needed. Caesarean section delivery can prevent nearly all cases of the disease. Internal fetal monitors during labor has been associated with fetal inoculation if the mother has active herpetic lesions.[131] Disseminated herpesvirus has been acquired by a suckling neonate whose father offered his newborn his finger with a herpetic whitlow.[132] The incidence of

herpesvirus in newborns can be detected by analysis of dried blood blotters obtained for the identification of genetic metabolic disease.[133] Clinical trials for herpes vaccines are under study.[134]

Human herpesvirus 6 (*HHV6*) is associated with **roseola (exanthem subitum)**, which presents with high fever followed by a generalized rash.[135–137] Older infants may develop viremia following herpetic stomatitis. Congenital HHV6 has been identified with PCR. The incidence may be as high as 1% but infants are usually asymptomatic.

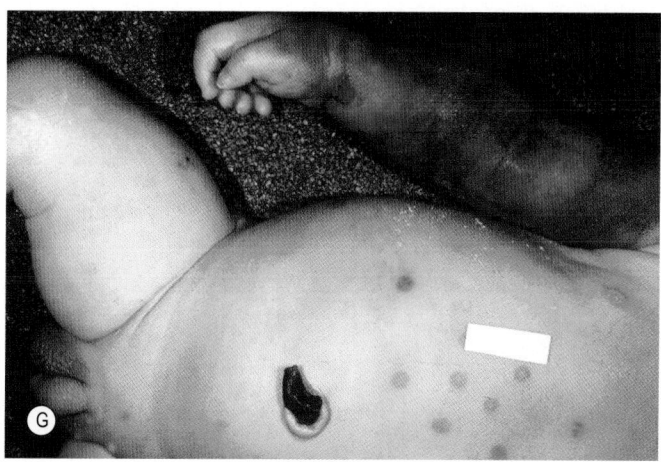
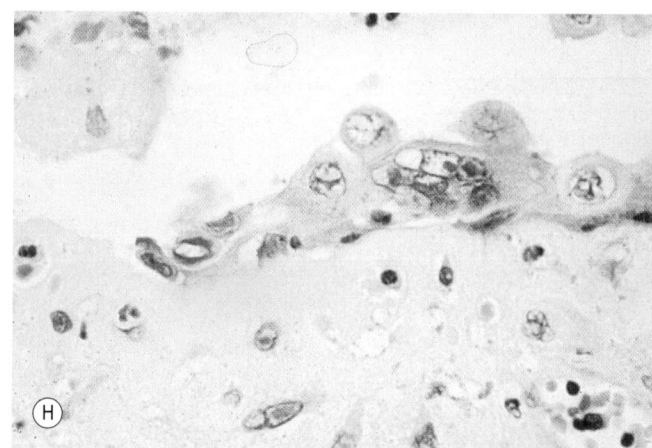

FIGURE 10.17 (*cont'd*) (G) HSV, cutaneous vesicles (H) Herpetic giant cell, skin.

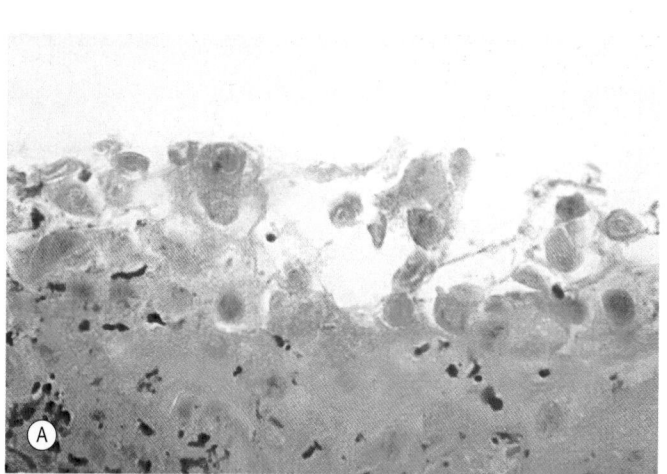
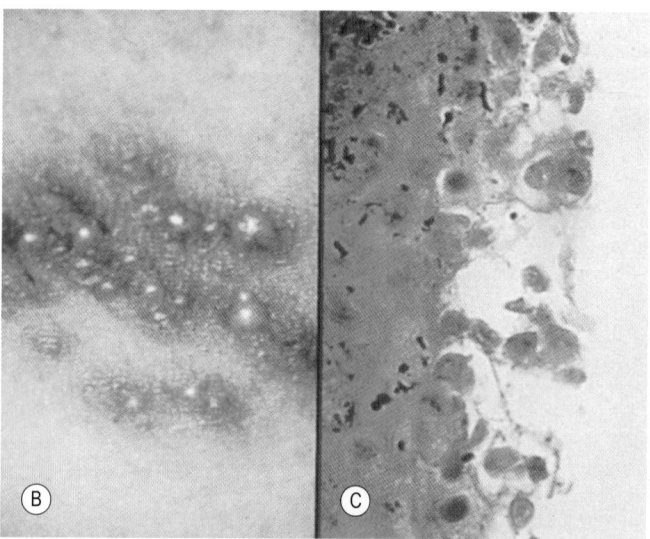

FIGURE 10.18 (A) Chickenpox from a fatal case of Reye syndrome. (B) A crop of early cutaneous vesicles of chickenpox lesions described as 'dew drops on a rose petal'. (C) Necrotic vesicle containing cells with intranuclear inclusions of varicella on the skin from a child with fatal Reye syndrome.

Herpes zoster Neonatal herpes zoster is rare. Pinpoint vesicles have been described in the sciatic and sacral areas. The infection is usually mild and not accompanied by other clinical manifestations. **Dorsal root ganglia** of the affected nerves contain inclusions, and the virus morphology cannot be distinguished from varicella virus.

Varicella (chickenpox) Maternal varicella in early gestation may cause stillbirth or a **fetal syndrome**[138–142] with growth retardation, encephalitis, cataracts, and chorioretinitis.[143, 144] Sharply circumscribed areas of necrosis infiltrated by mononuclear cells have been found in the placenta, lungs, kidneys, liver, pancreas, and skin. In the newborn infant, as in older children, a papulovesicular rash soon follows conjunctivitis. Intraepithelial **vesicles** contain intranuclear inclusions in degenerated cells Necrotic foci in the liver and spleen, and intranuclear inclusions in the skin, esophagus stomach, intestines, lungs, pancreas, adrenal glands, kidneys, and Hassall corpuscles have been reported. Young children who

contract varicella have cutaneous crops of vesicles in various stages of blisters followed by crusts. **Immunodeficient children may have visceral or chronic recurrent skin lesions**. Treatment of acute varicella with aspirin has led to Reye syndrome with hypoglycemia, coma, and microvesicular fatty infiltration of the liver (Fig. 10.18). Prenatal diagnosis by PCR on amniotic fluid has been reported. At autopsy calcified visceral pox were identified. Newborns may have skin lesions in a dermatomal distribution. Passive immunization may reduce the effects of viremia. Subclinical maternal infection may cause neurologic damage in her offspring. Varicella vaccination may prevent this tragedy.[145]

Human papilloma virus Laryngeal or tracheal papillomas[146–150] may develop in infants delivered vaginally to women with **condyloma acuminata**. Lesions unrecognized in the neonatal period may proliferate and develop recurrent papillomas with **airway obstruction** in early infancy and childhood. Warty epithe-

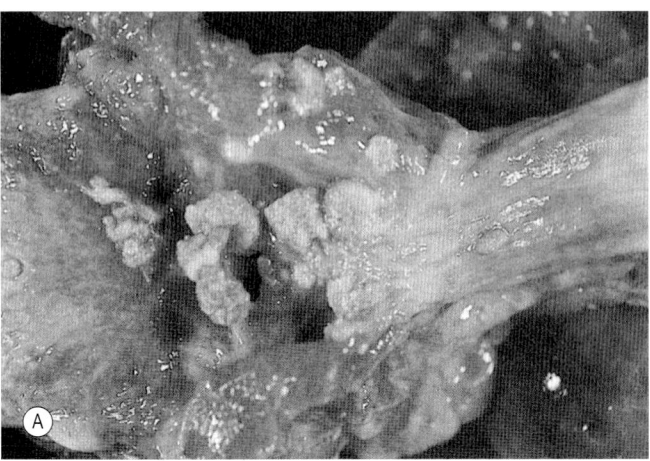
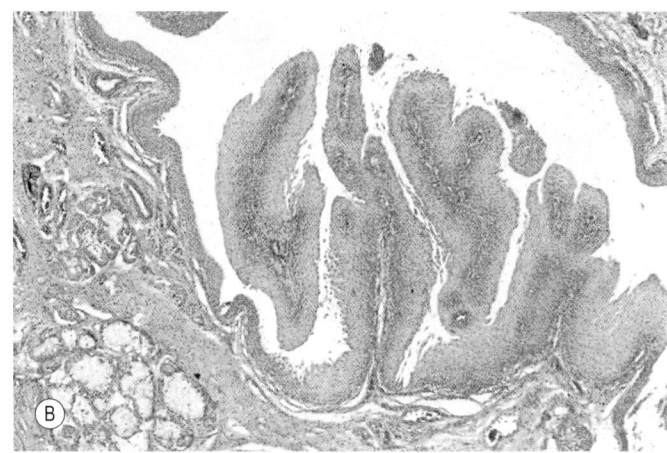

FIGURE 10.19 (A) Fungating growth in upper airway. (B) Laryngeal papilloma in congenital HPV infection. Confirmed by PCR.

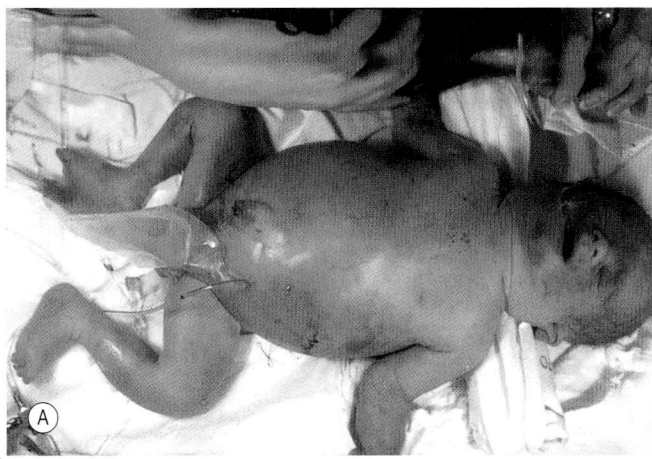

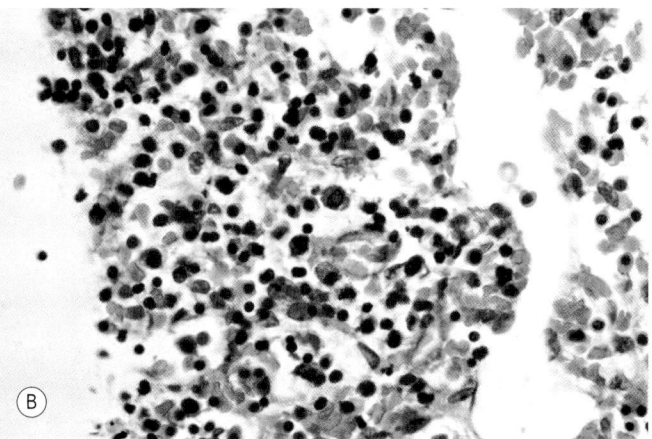

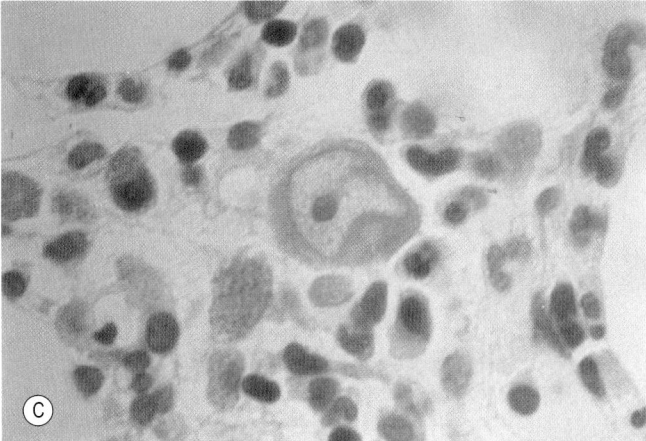

FIGURE 10.20 (A) Hydrops fetalis in parvovirus infection from severe fetal anemia. (B) Parvoviral infection, bone marrow. (C) Parvovirus. Intranuclear inclusions.

lial growths contain characteristic **koilocytic cells** (Fig. 10.19). In 605 of cases the maternal and infant serotype matched. HPV can occur as a result of child sexual abuse but casual non-sexual familial contact may also be responsible. The HPV vaccine may prevent this.

Parvovirus Human parvovirus B19[151–153] is the etiologic agent of *erythema infectiosum*, a benign exanthem of early childhood (*fifth disease*). Children have a slapped-cheek appearance and erythema of the volar surfaces of the forearms. Parvovirus is associated with the aplastic crisis of chronic hemolytic anemia. **Normoblasts with eosinophilic intranuclear viral inclusions** can be seen (Fig. 10.20). In utero, aregenerative anemia leads to heart failure with volume overload. Some fetuses may develop Epstein malformation of the heart. Parvovirus can be identified by immunohistochemistry or PCR on paraffin-embedded tissue.[154–160]

Chlamydia trachomatis

Chlamydia conjunctivitis or **neonatal pneumonia**[161–163] may be acquired during vaginal delivery to a colonized mother. **Inclusions** may be seen in the ocular discharge. **Interstitial and peribronchial infiltrates** with mononuclear cells and eosinophils associated with bronchial necrosis and septal congestion occur in the lung.

Infection in infants
Bacterial infections

Pyogenic bacteria

Gram-positive streptococci are classified by their ability to lyse red blood cells in culture. **α-hemolysis** turns culture media green, with *Streptococcus viridans* found in normal oral bacterial flora. This organism can be pathogenic in children with subacute bacterial endocarditis. **β-hemolytic streptococci** are associated with **impetigo, tonsillitis, and pharyngitis.** Erysipelas or scarlet fever develops if exotoxins are produced. **Rheumatic fever and glomerulonephritis** are disorders of the immune response to streptococcal antigens. **Necrotizing fasciitis** is caused by virulent strains of *Streptococcus,* characterized as flesh-eating bacteria. This explosive reaction may begin with a common puncture wound.

Gram-positive staphylococci also cause **bullous impetigo with furuncles or pneumonia with microabscesses and empyema.** Antimicrobial resistance and nosocomial infection are ominous in hospitalized children.

Streptococcus pneumoniae – previously referred to as *Diplococcus pneumoniae* because of its paired lancet-shaped configuration on Gram stain – is responsible for **lobar pneumonia,** ear infections, meningitis, primary peritonitis, or overwhelming sepsis, especially in children with sickle-cell disease or following splenectomy. Lung infection begins with capillary congestion and edema, called **red hepatization,** and looks like the liver at autopsy. In the later stage of organization (white hepatization) the lung appears firm and pale. **Pneumococcal meningitis** is associated with thick green exudate on the convexities of the cerebrum.

Neisseria

Neisseria organisms are paired Gram-negative cocci. Two main species are pathogenic in humans. *N. gonorrhea* causes venereal disease and **ophthalmia neonatorum** in newborns. Prophylactic instillation of antimicrobials into the eyes at birth has been an effective public health mandate. **Meningococcus** causes septicemia or meningitis in young children or military recruits. Meningococcemia may be complicated by the frequently fatal **Friderichsen-Waterhouse syndrome.** This is associated with clinical shock, obtundation, petechiae, and **ecchymosis. Hemorrhagic infarction of the adrenal gland and fibrin thrombi** in the glomeruli may be seen at autopsy. *Pneumococcus* and Gram-negative infection may also cause Friderichsen-Waterhouse

syndrome (Fig. 10.21B), which is an endotoxic-mediated process that resembles the generalized Schwartzman reaction.[164, 165]

Diphtheria

Diphtheria[166] infection forms a firm white membrane in the airway. In acute disease death may occur through suffocation or pneumonia. **Pseudomembranes** contain fibrin, necrotic epithelial cells, and Gram-positive Löffler bacilli that coat the nasopharynx and larynx. *Corynebacterium diphtheriae* contain bacteriophages that carry genes for **toxins.** Death from abnormalities of the conducting system of the heart and **toxic myocarditis** may occur 2 weeks after the primary infection. Edema, myocytolysis, fatty infiltration, and inflammatory cells may be seen throughout the heart muscle. **Hepatocellular necrosis, interstitial nephritis, and damage to peripheral nerves may occur.**

Pertussis

Bordetella pertussis[167, 168] proliferates in respiratory epithelium and is highly communicable. The entire airway is susceptible, and cuffs of **lymphocytes surround the bronchi and bronchioles.** Sloughed necrotic epithelium is shed into the lumen, and obstructive airway disease with air trapping occurs. Bacterial superinfection is frequent. A protracted course in very young infants is associated with apneic episodes rather than a whooping cough. **Bronchiectasis may develop in survivors. Lymphocytosis** in the peripheral blood and **splenomegaly** are frequent. Pertussis can be prevented by childhood vaccines. A syndrome similar to pertussis can occur with parapertussis and adenovirus infection.

Haemophilus influenzae

H. influenzae[169] is a pleomorphic Gram-negative coccobacillus. Six variants exist as normal flora in the upper respiratory tract in up to 90% of children. **Capsular type b** is responsible for invasive disease, which can be life-threatening in children under 5 years. **Meningitis** peaks at the end of the first year of life and may be fatal or produce serious complications including nerve deafness or mental retardation from obstructive hydrocephalus if prompt antibiotic treatment is not instituted. **Epiglottitis** (Fig. 10.21A) peaks at age 4 with most cases occurring after the second birthday. **Pneumonia** may be mild or similar to staphylococcal infection with empyema, and young infants may develop **septic arthritis** or **orbital cellulitis.** A purple–blue discoloration of the eyelid is characteristic. *H. influenzae* can cause the Friederichsen-Waterhouse syndrome (Fig. 10.20B). In the USA a marked reduction in invasive *H. influenzae* infection is the result of a highly effective vaccine. *H. influenzae* can cause the Waterhouse-Friederichsen syndrome (Fig. 10.21B).

Pseudomonas infections

P. aeruginosa, ubiquitous in soil and water, exists in the normal colonic flora of up to 30% of the population. It can contaminate respiratory equipment used in the intensive care unit. Children

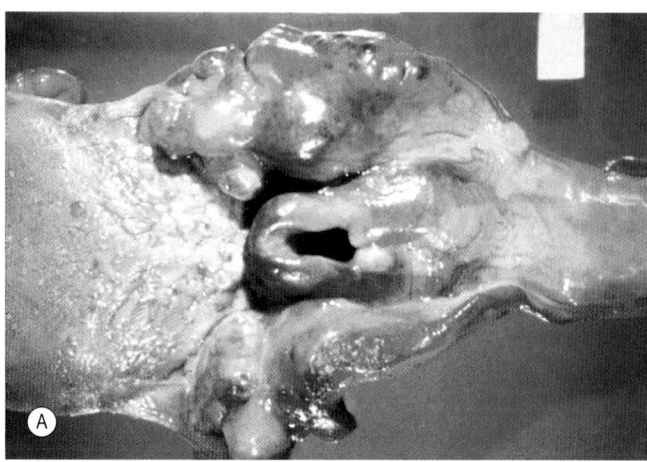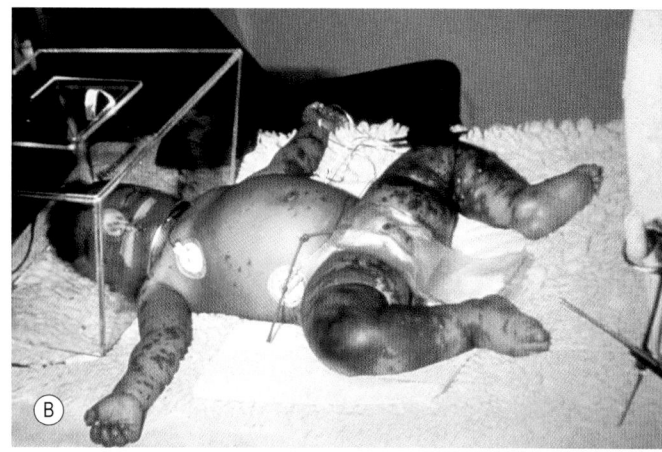

FIGURE 10.21 (A) Epiglottitis secondary to *H. influenza* infection. (B) Friderichsen-Waterhouse syndrome can occur *with H. influenza* and other organisms especially *N. meningitides*.

with **cystic fibrosis** are chronic carriers of this organism, which is resistant to multiple antibiotics. Neonates, burn patients, immunosuppressed patients with **cancer**, and acquired immunodeficiency syndrome **(AIDS)** have a particular risk of nosocomial infection including sepsis and necrotizing hemorrhagic pneumonia.[169–175] *Pseudomonas* may complicate Hirschsprung disease. Pseudomonads are large plump Gram-negative rods that produce a spreading factor that enables the organisms to **invade blood vessel walls,** producing thrombosis and infarction with confluent **abscesses. Ecthyma gangrenosa** can occur.

Mycoplasmal infections

Mycoplasmas are the smallest free-living organisms. A cell wall is absent and the Gram stain is equivocal. *M. pneumoniae* infection of the lung peaks in early childhood and pubescence. Droplet infection paralyses the cilia of **respiratory epithelial cells**. Edema and peribronchial lymphocytes and plasma cells are present. Pharyngitis and otitis media are frequent, and a faint maculopapular rash or conjunctivitis may be seen. *Ureaplasma urealyticum*[176–179] colonizes the urogenital tract and may be sexually transmitted.[180] Involvement of the fetal membranes may be associated with congenital infection.

Respiratory viral infections

Respiratory syncytial virus

Respiratory syncytial virus (RSV)[181–184] is a **recurrent** infection in infants and young children. Symptoms are most severe in the first 6 months of life, especially in hospitalized infants with congenital heart disease. **Necrosis of bronchiolar epithelium** with destruction of the basal cell layer occurs.[185–187] Large cells with intranuclear **inclusions** and vacuolated cytoplasm are rarely seen. Necrotic debris and mucous secretions plug small airways, and **peribronchiolar lymphocytic infiltration** with hypertrophy of smooth muscle may be present (Fig. 10.22). **Bacterial super-**

infection complicates the clinical course. Experimental vaccines[188] and hyperimmune globulin have been proposed for very low birth weight infants.

Influenza

Viral pneumonia secondary to influenza is characterized by **necrosis of bronchiolar epithelium** with peribronchiolar **lymphocytic** infiltrate that extends into the **interstitium** of the lung. **Hyaline membranes** with focal hemorrhage and necrosis are followed by the proliferation of type II pneumocytes during the recovery phase (Fig. 10.23). Mortality is related to **bacterial superinfection**. At autopsy **reactive lymphadenopathy** and focal collections of lymphocytes may be found in several viscera including the heart, liver, meninges, skeletal muscle, and gastrointestinal tract. Cerebral edema, myocarditis, and Reye syndrome with hypoglycemia, coma, and microvesicular fat within hepatocytes may complicate fatal cases. Influenza occurs in epidemics, and protective immunity to new infection is ineffective because of **high mutation rates** and the unique pathogenicity of different strains. Bird flu has been identified in fetal tissue (personal observation).

Parainfluenza

The airway epithelium of infants and young children is susceptible to parainfluenza. **Subglottic edema** and obstruction can produce severe respiratory distress. **Interstitial pneumonia with necrotizing bronchiolitis and hyaline membranes** with multinucleate giant cells are seen. No nuclear or cytoplasmic viral inclusions are present (Fig. 10.24).

Adenovirus

Adenovirus,[189-192] a respiratory DNA virus, attaches to the surface of cells, enters the cytoplasm and integrates into genomic DNA. Transcription of messenger RNA produces virions which include genes that facilitate viral replication, thwart cytotoxic T-cell

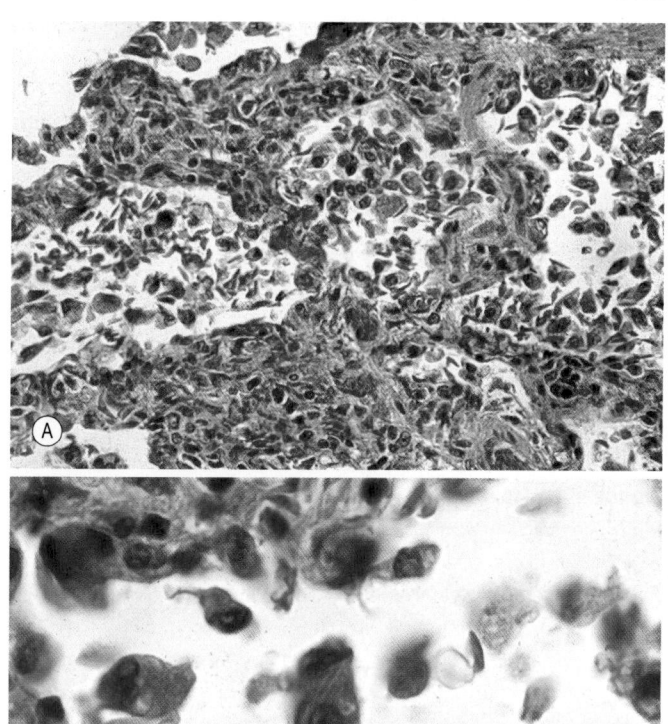

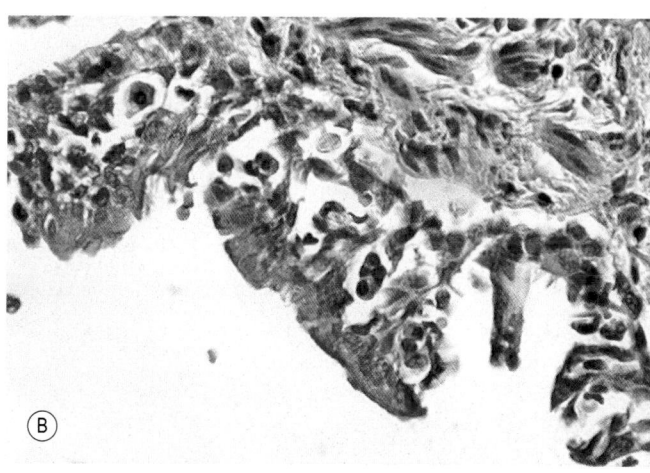

FIGURE 10.22 (A) RSV pneumonia with interstitial infiltrate. (B) Typical bronchiolar necrosis marks the portal of entry of RSV. (C). High power demonstrates the classical RSV inclusion.

defense, and result in cell death. Infective particles spread into contiguous cells in respiratory and lymphoid tissue or during viremia involve the liver or intestinal tract. Different serotypes have particular trophisms, and disseminated disease is most often associated with **either congenital or acquired immuno-deficiency**. Infants, young children, and military recruits are at greatest risk. Adenoviral infection is associated with a high mortality in the post measles interval of impaired cell-mediated immunity.

Intranuclear viral inclusions are most often basophilic but may be amphophilic or eosinophilic with a halo on routine stains (Fig. 10.25). Dark blue smudge cells are suspicious for adenovirus but must be confirmed by culture or immunostaining with in situ hybridization or PCR. Tissue necrosis with **hyaline membranes, interstitial infiltrates** of plasma cells and lymphocytes, and **bronchiolitis obliterans** can produce chronic lung disease in non-fatal cases. **Impaired lung growth** or **bronchiectasis** may result. Serotypes 40 and 41 may be responsible for 5% of infectious infantile diarrhea.

Hepatitis viruses

Neonatal hepatitis B virus (HBV) infection[193–195] is acquired during passage through the birth canal of an infected mother. Most infants are asymptomatic at birth. Lifelong carriage of the virus can spread HBV as an unsuspected sexually transmitted disease. Hyperimmune γ-globulin and the hepatitis vaccine at birth can intercept this outcome. **Immunization of all newborns** would prevent chronic hepatitis B infection and hepatocellular carcinoma[196] in adults. Mothers with active hepatitis and **E antigenemia** may suffer perinatal loss or transmit HBV to the fetus. Mothers who are surface antigen-positive give birth to infants who become asymptomatic carriers with immunologic tolerance to HBV. Blood bank screening for HBV has reduced nosocomial HBV infection.

Hepatitis A is acquired from the **fecal–oral** route. Most cases are subclinical and anicteric; however, severe disease does exist and epidemics occur in institutionalized settings. **Hepatitis C** (previously called 'non-A and non-B' hepatitis) can be acquired during a blood transfusion and occasionally is associated with hepatitis which may progress to chronic liver disease. Hepatitis C with HIV is especially devastating and treatment with interferon is expensive. Vertical transmission of hepatitis C is rare but can occur.

Epstein-Barr virus

Epstein-Barr virus (EBV) is a member of the herpesvirus family. **EBV infectious mononucleosis**[197–199] produces atypical lymphocytes in the peripheral blood with splenomegaly, hepatitis,

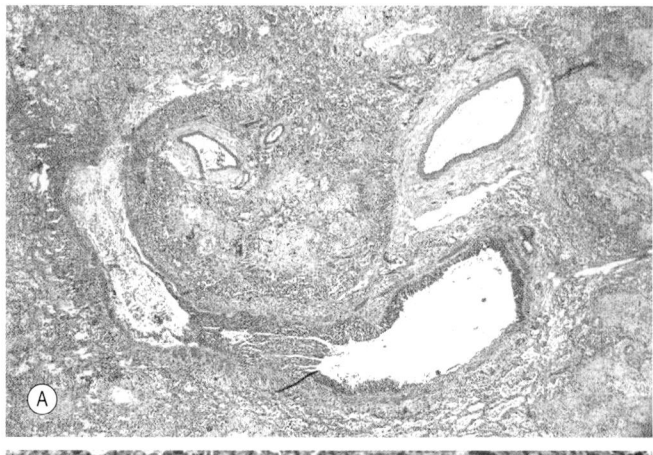

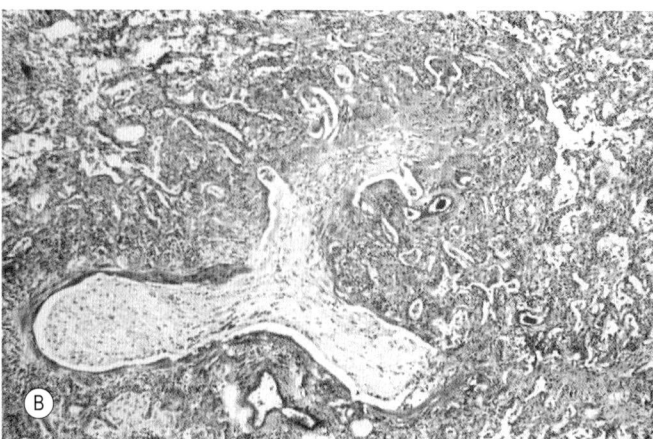

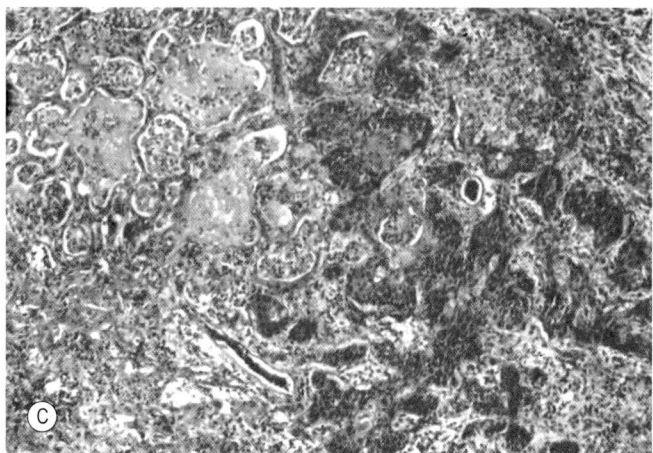

FIGURE 10.23 (A) and (B) Bronchiolitis due to influenza virus infection demonstrating peribronchiolar inflammation with necrosis and regeneration of bronchiolar epithelium. (C) Reparative fibroepithelial nodule in influenza infection of the lung.

enlarged tonsils, and cervical lymphadenopathy. The histology of the lymph node in acute EBV infection may contain **atypical Reed-Sternberg cells** or **immunoblastic proliferation and necrosis**.[200] An EBV reservoir may be present in the parotid gland. Young boys with **X-linked lymphoproliferative syndrome** (Duncan syndrome) cannot put EBV into latency and succumb with a B-cell lymphoproliferative disorder that involves multiple viscera. Progression to lymphoma, especially the Burkitt type, is possible. Acute massive lymphoid infiltration of the spleen may be associated with catastrophic splenic rupture. EBV is frequent in lymphoma, in immunosuppressed patients (e.g. in cases of transplants or from AIDS) developing a lymphoproliferative syndrome, and in the rare fatal cases of hepatitis with acute yellow atrophy.

Diarrheal diseases

Enteroviruses

In the past **polio**[201] epidemics produced severe paralysis in young children. Poliovirus contracted through the fecal–oral route spreads through the bloodstream and localizes in the **anterior horn cells** of the spinal cord. Necrosis, inflammation, and edema occur. Neuronal degeneration results in **spinal muscular atrophy** with loss of entire muscle bundles. In the acute phase involvement of the brainstem, cervical spinal cord, and muscles of respiration can be fatal. During the recovery phase some reinnervation takes place. Despite concern that live polio vaccine may produce disease in an immunosuppressed child, vaccine associated polio has not yet been reported in patients with AIDS. It has been observed in primary immunodeficiency. The post polio syndrome with impaired motor functions develops years after the initial infection.

Coxsackie viruses[202–207] were inadvertently found while the cause of infantile paralysis was being sought. Like polio, the incidence of Coxsackie B peaks in the late summer and fall and involves the anterior horn cells. Necrosis of the liver may be severe. The **heart** is a primary target.[208–210] Necrosis with lymphocytic foci is seen (Fig. 10.26). **Meningoencephalitis** can produce severe sequelae including hydrocephalus. The spectrum of disease includes an erythematous rash, thrombocytopenia, **hemorrhagic pneumonia, enteritis, and hepatitis**. Coxsackie B5 can cause **isletitis** in the pancreas[211–213] and results in juvenile diabetes in children with a genetic predisposition to this disease.

Echovirus[214–219] has a tropism for **brain, liver, kidney, lungs, and adrenal glands**. Hepatic necrosis,[162] disseminated hemorrhage, and intravascular coagulopathy may occur. At autopsy necrotic foci in the heart and skeletal muscle may be extensive. A mononuclear or lymphocytic reaction may be mild or extensive, depending on the duration of illness.

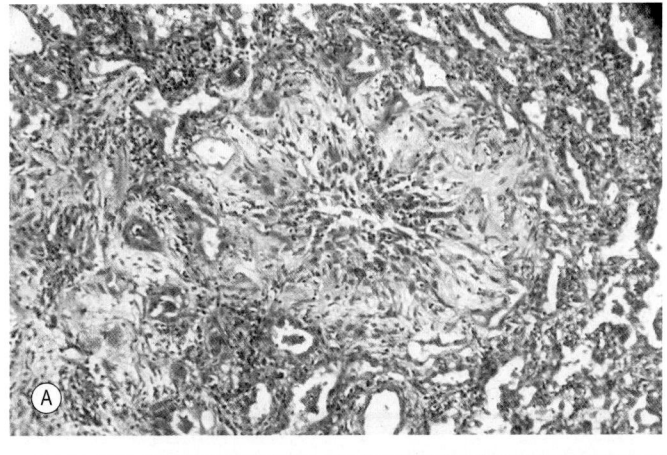

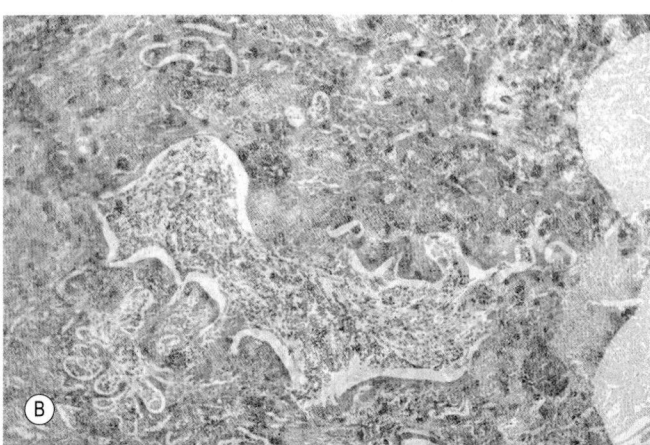

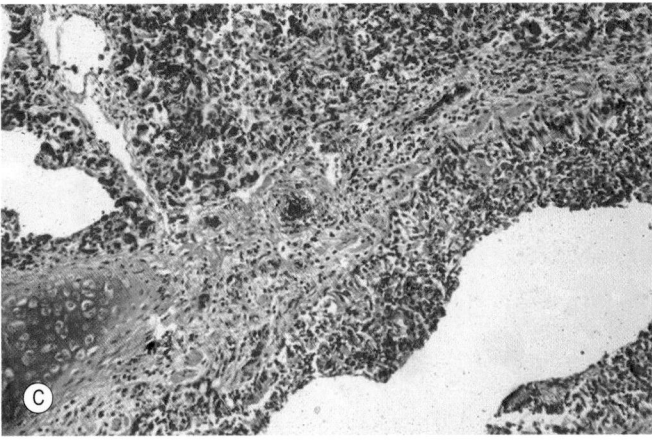

FIGURE 10.24 (A) and (B) Parainfluenza bronchiolitis showing intense edema of bronchiolar walls with giant cell formation and necrosis of epithelium. (C) Rhinovirus associated necrotizing tracheobronchitis.

Infectious diarrhea

Infectious diarrhea of infancy is a leading cause of morbidity and mortality.[220] In industrialized countries **rotavirus** is a frequent pathogen. **Adenovirus, reovirus, astrovirus, picornavirus,** and the **Norwalk agent** have been identified.[221] **Late summer viral syndromes** with bouts of watery diarrhea are common. In developing nations enteropathic bacteria, especially *E. coli* 0157, predominate. *Shigella* and *Salmonella* cause bloody diarrhea with acute inflammation and ulceration. In many cases the etiologic agent of infantile diarrhea is unknown. Survivors of acute infectious diarrhea may develop **chronic diarrhea,** failure to thrive, malabsorption syndrome, and a predilection to infection. Epidemics of cholera can claim many lives in a few days.

Rotavirus causes a self-limited watery diarrhea that is associated with lymphoid infiltrates in the duodenum. Infants are rarely biopsied, and the diagnosis is made by immunoassay or direct electron microscopy of the stool. Rotavirus serotypes are best identified by reverse transcribed PCR.

Tissue effects of enteroviral infection are rarely observed. The histopathologic findings may be non-specific and minimal even during severe clinical disease. **Dehydration and electrolyte imbalance** can prove fatal. Intestinal villi may be edematous with sloughing of the epithelial cells and small numbers of neutrophils in acute infection or show increased lymphocytes and plasma cells during chronic disease. Repair results in **atrophic mucosa** with broad bands of fused villi. This reduces the functional surface area of the small intestine in chronic cases. An increase in mitosis may be present in the crypts. Hyperchromatic cells with reduced numbers of goblet cells cover the flattened mucosa. **Peyer patches may be depleted of lymphocytes.**

Escherichia coli

E. coli is a major component of the normal flora of the colon. **Enteropathic forms**[222, 223] develop adherence factors and secrete toxic substances that cause diarrhea without mucosal destruction on light microscopy. Damage to the brush border may be seen by electron microscopy. **Toxigenic strains** (0157) produce both heat-labile and stable proteins. In some cases verocytoxin similar to *Shigella* toxin, may produce bloody diarrhea associated with mucosal ulceration, headache, myalgia, and abdominal cramps.[224] Rapid onset of septic shock with systemic inflammatory response syndrome is rare but has a high fatality rate. Recovery from diarrhea may be associated with depression of intestinal disaccharidase (especially lactase), mucosal atrophy, and chronic intestinal inflammation.

The **hemolytic-uremic syndrome (HUS)**[225–227] and death during outbreaks of *E. coli* follow the ingestion of contaminated meat. HUS most frequently follows **verocytoxin-producing E. coli** 0157:H7. Thrombotic microangiopathy with hemolytic anemia, bloody diarrhea, and hematuria is common. Fibrin thrombi in

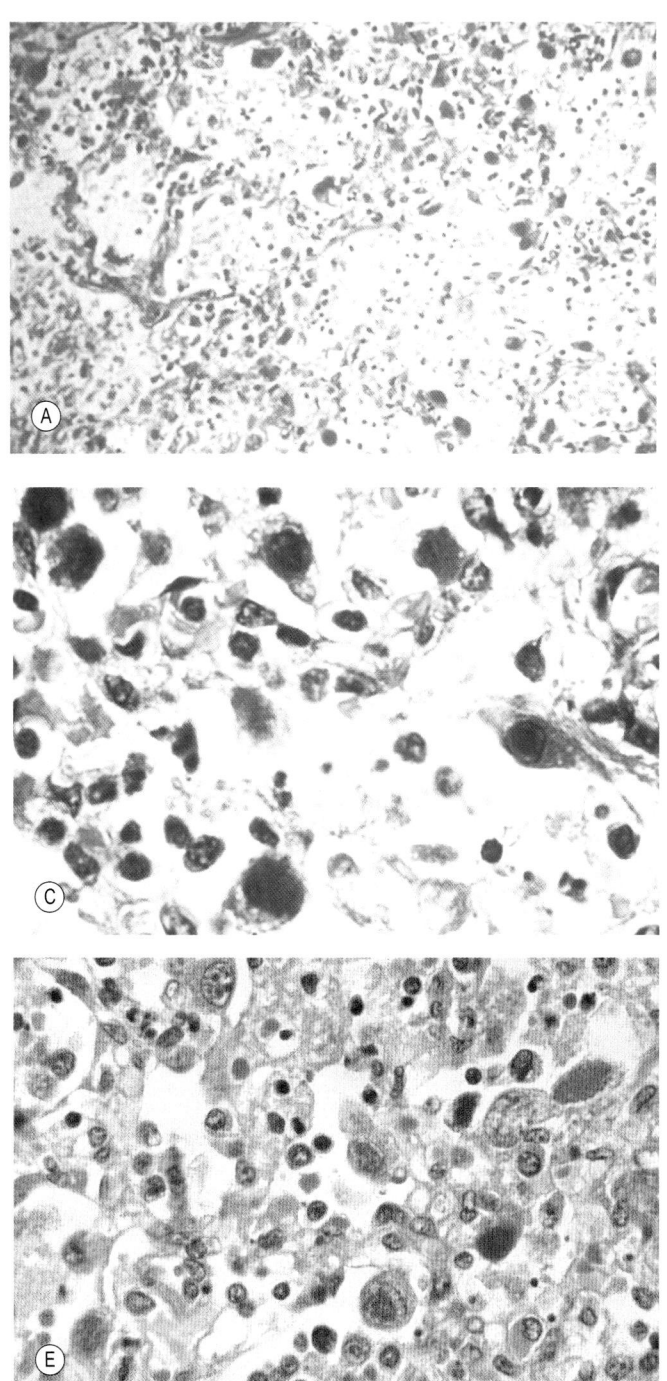

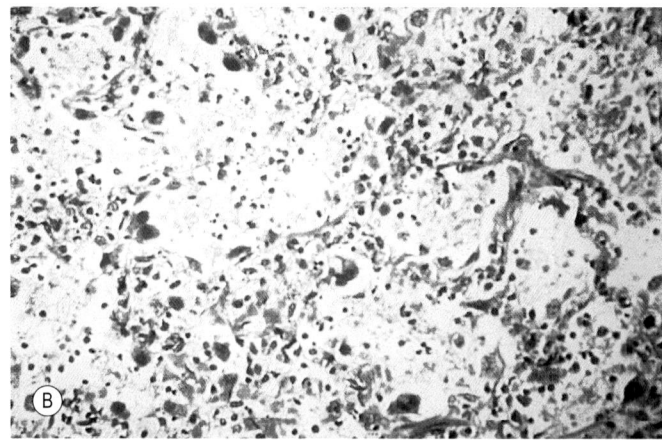

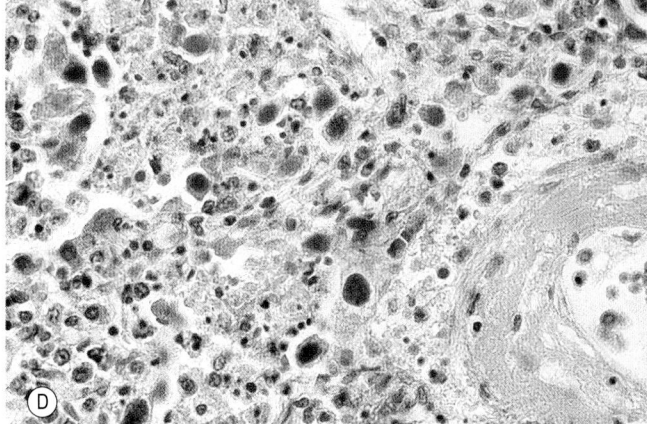

FIGURE 10.25 (A) and (B) Low power photomicrograph of adenoviral pneumonia. (C) High power view of typical smudge cells containing adenoviral inclusions. (D) and (E) Post measles adenovirus infection of the lung showing numerous inclusion with variable staining.

the glomeruli may cause fatal renal failure (Fig. 10.27). Renal transplantation with recurrent HUS in the allograft is reported. HUS has followed other infections and autoimmune diseases (see Ch. 27.1).

Salmonella

Several *Salmonella* species can be responsible for **infantile diarrhea** when sanitary conditions are poor. *Salmonella* **osteomyelitis** occurs in children with **sickle-cell disease**. Recurrent salmonellosis in infants is associated with **HIV infection**. Organisms proliferate within the intestinal lymphoid tissue. Peyer

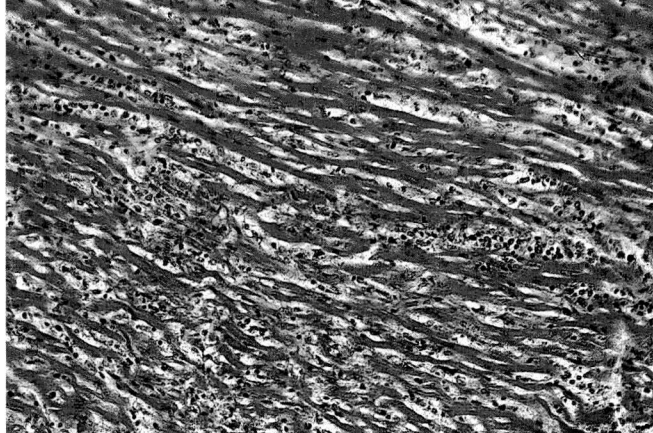

FIGURE 10.26 Congenital Coxsackie virus myocarditis with interstitial lymphocytic infiltration.

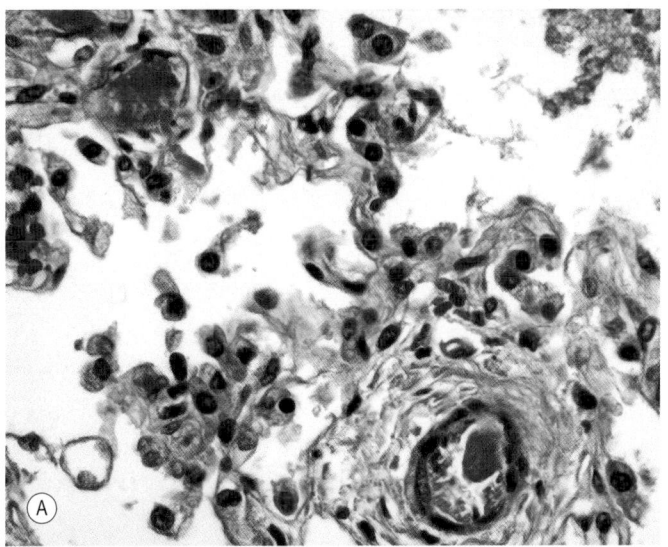
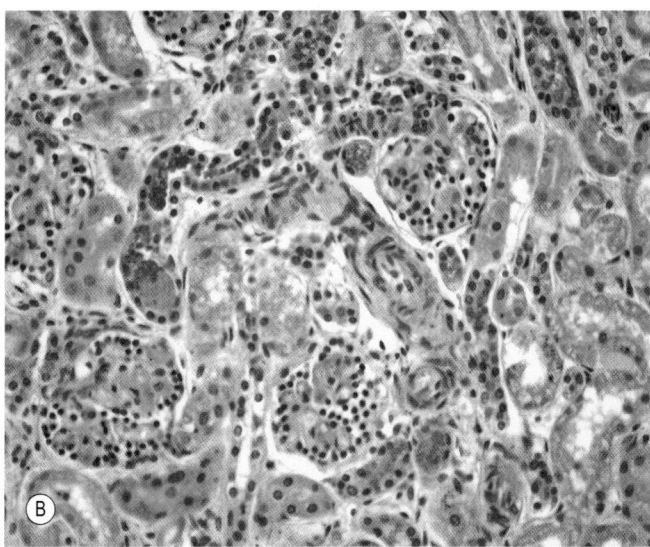

FIGURE 10.27 (A) Fibrin thrombi in the lungs of a teenager with sudden unexpected death secondary to *E. coli* sepsis. (B) Fibrin casts in the kidneys of a teenager with *E. coli* sepsis.

patches may ulcerate and bacteremia occurs in typhoid fever. The mesenteric lymph nodes and spleen enlarge. In advanced disease intestinal perforation and peritonitis may be fatal. **Endotoxin** may cause focal myocardial necrosis. Infection of the meninges and joints occur. Chronic infection of the gallbladder or antibiotic treatment may be responsible for persistent infection and maintenance of the **carrier state**. *Salmonella choleraesuis* produces bacteremia with osteomyelitis and abscess formation. *Salmonella typhi* affects the reticuloendothelial system, but is currently infrequent. *Salmonella paratyphi* A and B is associated with diarrhea, mucosal erosions, and ulceration, especially in the ileum and left side of the colon. Food poisoning with *Salmonella typhimurium* and *Salmonella enteritidis* can result from improper food handling.

Shigella

Shigella dysenteriae group A is associated with severe colitis and hemorrhagic diarrhea. The organism invades superficial epithelial cells, and a pseudomembrane may cover superficial mucosal ulcers (Fig. 10.28). An **exotoxin** produced by the organism may cause mental confusion, convulsions, obtundation, and death. At autopsy mucosal necrosis and crypt abscesses may represent secondary invasion with additional intestinal bacteria. Pronounced tenesmus is associated with **rectal prolapse**. A low white blood cell count with a marked shift to the left is frequent. **Bloody diarrhea** with **leukopenia** and neutrophilic bandemia is presumptive of *Shigella* infection. A Gram stain on the stool may reveal intracellular small Gram-negative rods within sheets of necrotic epithelial cells and polymorphonuclear leukocytes. The organism is spread by the fecal–oral route.

Yersinia enterocolitica

Yersinia enterocolitica[228] can cause enterocolitis with vomiting, watery diarrhea, and fever. **Microabscesses** appear in the Peyer

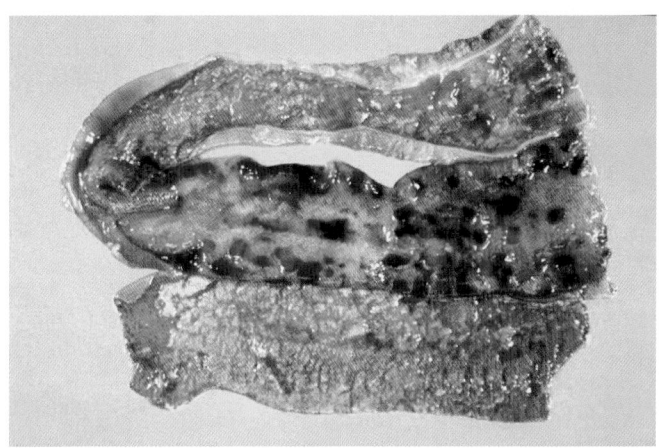

FIGURE 10.28 Superficial mucosal ulcers and pseudomembrane formation in *Shigella* enterocolitis.

patches, and suppurative **mesenteric lymphadenitis** or ileocolitis may be present. Fatal sepsis has been reported, but most cases are self-limited and few develop chronic diarrhea. *Y. pseudotuberculosis* produces **septicemia, erythema nodosum, arthritis, and mesenteric lymphadenitis**. *Y. pestis* causes plague and **presents** with **lymphadenitis, pneumonia, meningitis, and septicemia**.

Helicobacter

Helicobacter jejuni is a frequent cause of **self-limited enteritis** in children under 3 years. In severe cases biopsy reveals hemorrhagic, exudative mucosal lesions with neutrophils, macrophages, and eosinophils. **Crypt abscesses, mucosal ulcers**, and destruction of the mucosa may be present.[229, 230] *Helicobacter* may be responsible for meningitis, arthritis, cholecystitis, endocarditis, pericarditis, peritonitis, and lung abscesses. Intrauterine infection associated

TABLE 10.4 HELMINTHIC DISEASES

Helminths	Disease	Organism	Transmission
Flukes (Trematodes)			
Blood	Schistosomiasis	*Schistosoma mansoni*	Skin to intestines
Intestines	Intestinal fluke	*S. japonicum*	Skin to intestines
Liver	Sheep liver fluke	*S. haematobium*	Larva
		Fasciolopsis buski	Larva
		Fasciola hepatica	
Tapeworms (Cestodes)			
Intestine	Fish tapeworm	*Diphyllobothrium latum*	Raw fish
	Dwarf tapeworm	*Hymenolepis nana*	Egg (fecal–oral)
	Pork tapeworm	*Taenia solium*	Raw pork
	Beef tapeworm	*T. saginatum*	Raw beef
Larvae	Cysticercosis	*T. solium*	Larva
	Hydatid disease	*Echinococcus*	Egg (fecal–oral)
Roundworms (Nematodes)			
Tissue	Ascaris (Fig. 10.35)	*Ascaris lumbricoides*	Egg (fecal–oral)
	Pinworm	*Enterobius vermicularis*	Egg (fecal–oral)
	Whipworm	*Trichuris trichiura*	Egg (fecal–oral)
	Trichinosis	*Trichinella spiralis*	Larvae ingestion
	Visceral	*T. canis*	Egg ingestion
	Larva migrans	*T. cati*	
	Cutaneous	*Ancylostoma braziliense*	Skin
	Larva migrans		
Intestines[241]	Hookworm	*Necator americanus*	Skin
		Ancylostoma duodenale	

with abortion or stillbirth has been reported. *H. pylori* causes chronic antral gastritis and is responsible for peptic ulcer disease which resolves after antibiotic treatment. **Protein-losing enteropathy** occurs in young children.

Cholera

Vibrio cholerae lodges within the brush border of the cell and secretes an enterotoxin within the intact mucosa of the duodenum and jejunum. Rice-water stools appear as flecks of mucus within watery diarrhea. Disturbance of fluid and electrolyte balance may be rapidly fatal and the associated mortality approaches 20% in developing countries. Oral rehydration programs are life-saving.

Other intestinal pathogens

Other bacterial pathogens responsible for infantile diarrhea include *Vibrio parahaemolyticus, Clostridium perfringens, Clostridium difficile,*[231] and staphylococci. Intestinal tuberculosis occurs in developing countries where pasteurization of milk is not performed.

Giardiasis

Giardia lamblia may be acquired from a contaminated water supply. Trophozoites adhere to the surface epithelium of the small intestine, and infestation may cause diarrhea and atrophy of the duodenal and jejunal mucosa with a decrease in the production of immunoglobulin A (IgA).

Amebiasis

Entamoeba histolytica can be devastating in young malnourished children. Invasion of the bowel produces **ulceration** and spread to the liver forms large **abscesses**[232] (Fig. 10.29).

Helminths

Helminths frequently parasitize young infants and children. Examination of the stool is useful when clinical disease is present. It is impossible to completely eradicate parasites, especially those contracted by fecal–oral contamination or insect bites. Table 10.4 lists helminthic diseases and the mode of transmission.[233–241] Infestation with ascaris is shown in Figure 10.36. For morphologic identification of ova and parasites, reference texts should be consulted.

Other infections

Tuberculosis

Pulmonary, intestinal, and disseminated tuberculosis is caused by *Mycobacterium tuberculosis*.[185, 186] Mycobacterial infection in

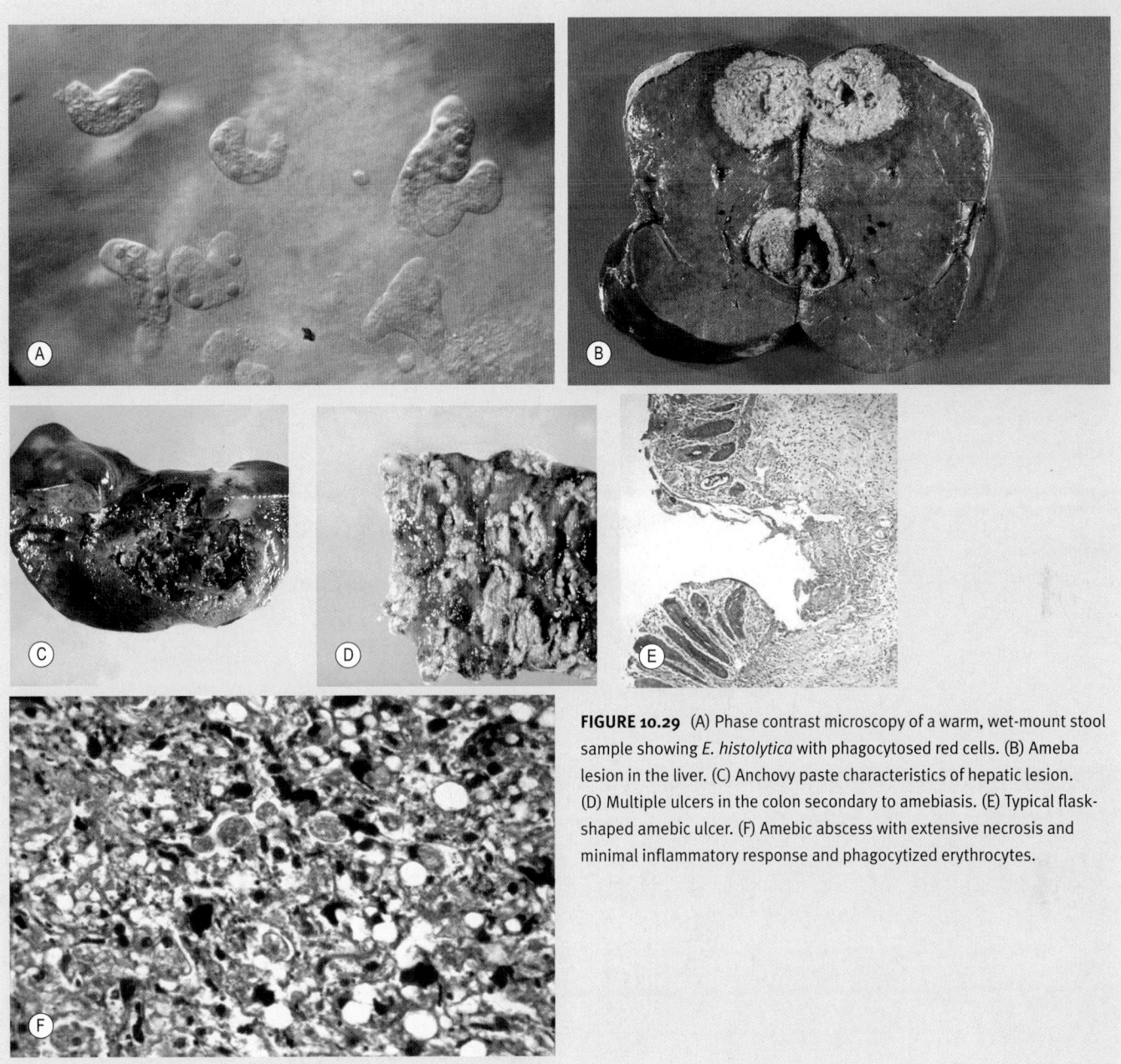

FIGURE 10.29 (A) Phase contrast microscopy of a warm, wet-mount stool sample showing *E. histolytica* with phagocytosed red cells. (B) Ameba lesion in the liver. (C) Anchovy paste characteristics of hepatic lesion. (D) Multiple ulcers in the colon secondary to amebiasis. (E) Typical flask-shaped amebic ulcer. (F) Amebic abscess with extensive necrosis and minimal inflammatory response and phagocytized erythrocytes.

HIV disease is usually caused by *Mycobacterium avium intracellulare.* Lymphadenopathy may be caused by atypical mycobacteria, usually *Mycobacterium fortuitum, Mycobacterium scrofulaceum,* or *M. avium intracellulare.*

Few reported cases of transplacental fetal *M. tuberculosis* exist.[242–245] Fulminant maternal pulmonary or miliary tuberculosis is often fatal soon after delivery. The **rarity of congenital tuberculosis** reflects the infrequency with which tubercle bacilli are present in maternal blood. We have observed an HIV-infected mother who died soon after delivery of a term infant who developed drug-resistant congenital tuberculosis but did not contract HIV infection. An intervillous protein coagulum with neutrophils and acid-fast bacilli is found in **placentas** of infants with congenital tuberculosis. **Thrombosis of fetal vessels** draining the infected area of the placenta may prevent bacilli from entering the fetal circulation. Most infants with congenital tuberculosis survive several months; therefore contact with the infected mother or any other tuberculous person after birth must be excluded before the infection can be assumed to be of prenatal origin.

In the fetus tubercles are usually found in multiple viscera. Tubercle bacilli in the amniotic fluid may be aspirated into the lungs. The umbilical vein is often the site of entry, and the liver can be severely involved. Tubercles may be several millimeters in diameter; **granulomas** appear similar to those found at other age periods, with **giant cells, epithelioid cells, and lymphocytes**.

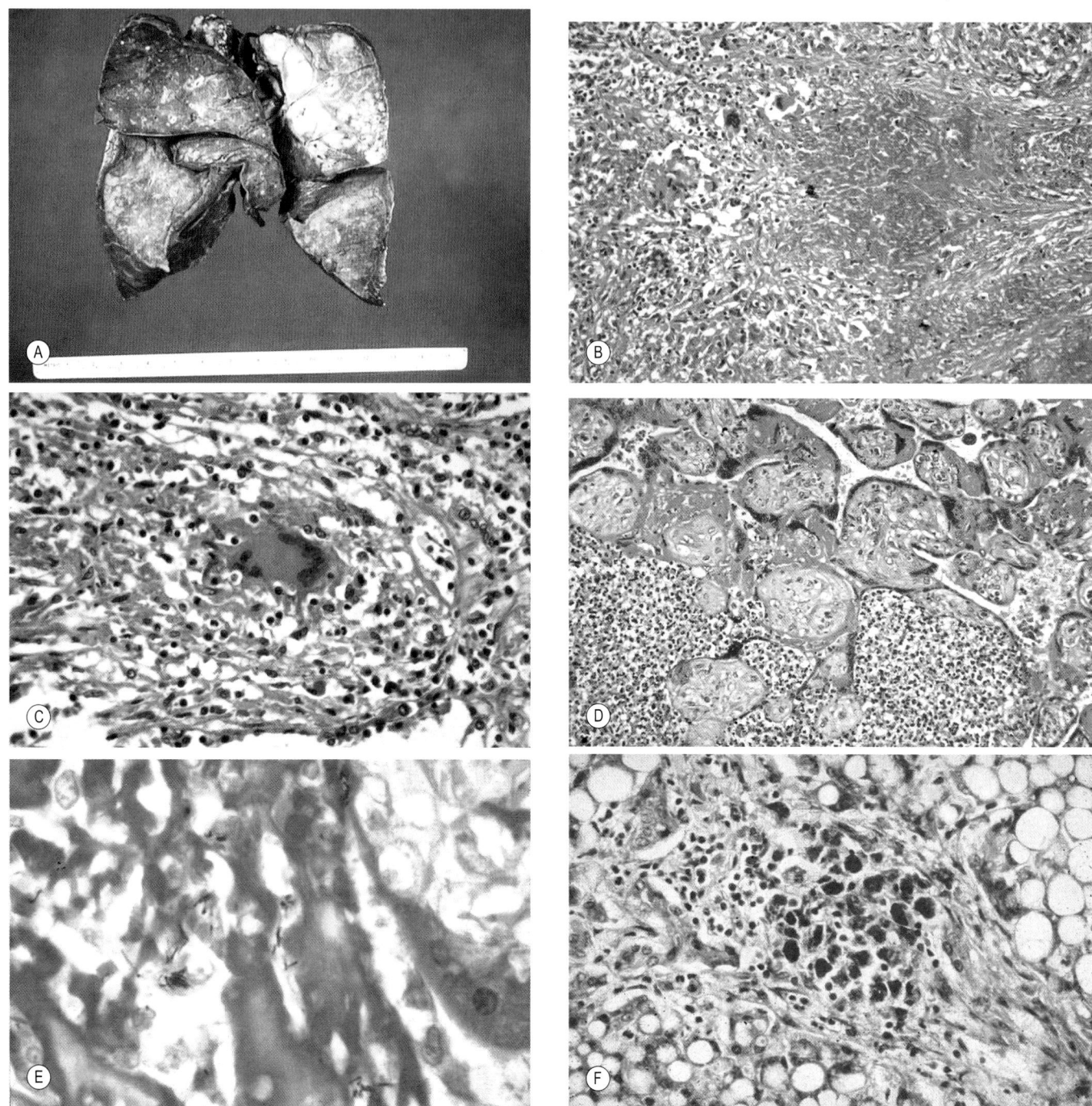

FIGURE 10.30 (A) Confluent caseous nodules in the left upper lobe. (B) Caseating tuberculous granuloma with Langhans giant cells in the lung of fatal miliary tuberculosis. (C) High power photomicrograph of a Langhans giant cell. (D) Suppuration in the intervillous space of the placenta in congenital tuberculosis. (E) Oil power view of beaded mycobacterial organisms in congenital tuberculosis. (F) Intracellular proliferation of atypical *Mycobacterium avium intracellulare* in the portal area of the liver in an HIV infected patient.

Foci of caseous necrosis are less frequent. The relative lack of immunity in young infants increases the likelihood of diffuse tuberculous pneumonia, generalized miliary tuberculosis, or meningitis with a higher mortality as compared with older individuals. In **miliary tuberculosis**, acid-fast bacilli may be difficult to find in granulomas (Fig. 10.30). Granulomas may be widely disseminated in the lungs, liver, spleen, lymph nodes, bone marrow, and the central nervous system.

Tuberculosis in infants has become less common with effective detection and control programs in maternal health clinics.[246] Recently the HIV epidemic and relaxation of public health control measures has led to an increase.[247]

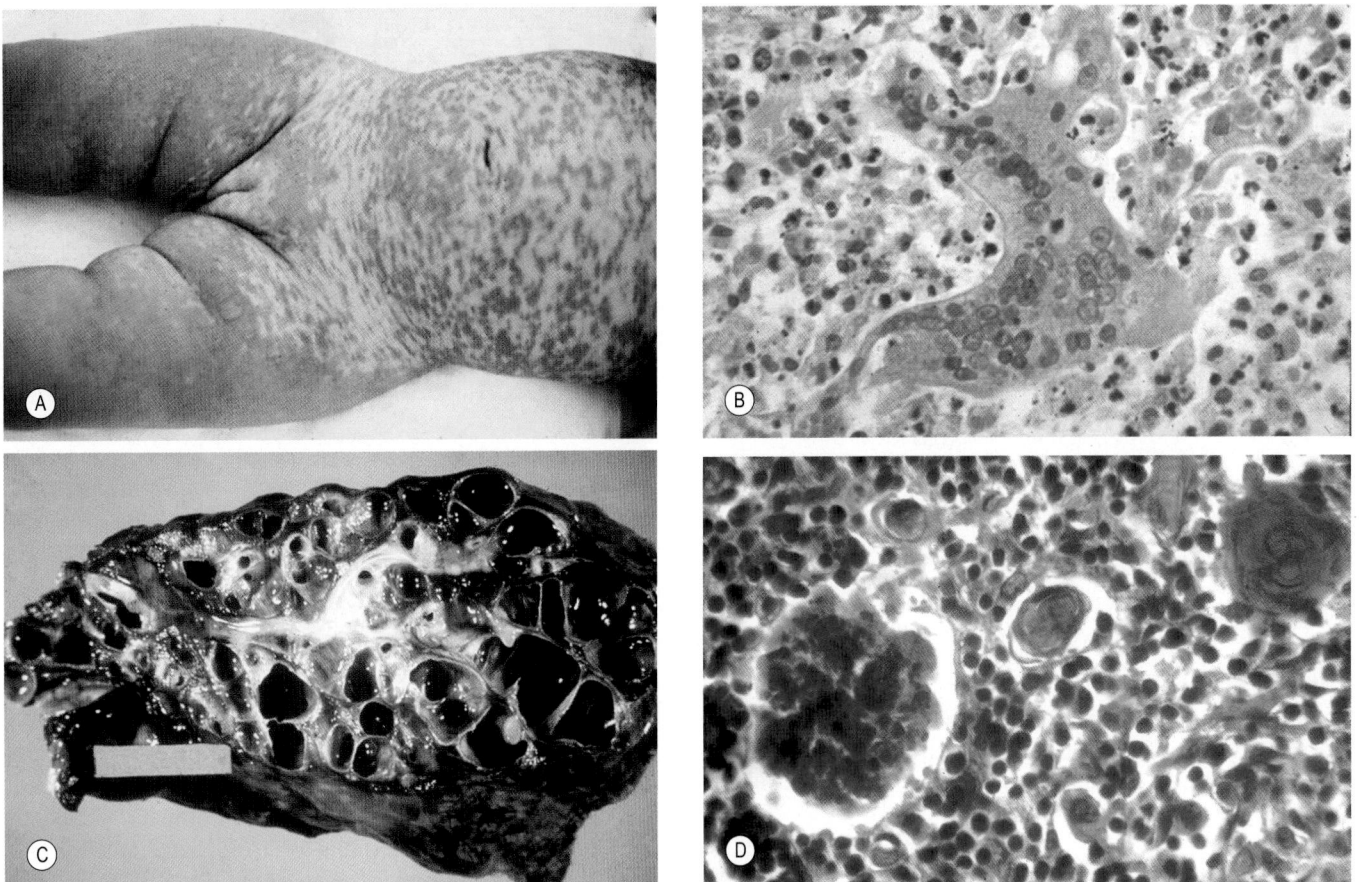

FIGURE 10.31 (A) Morbilliform confluent rash in rubeola infection. (B) Measles giant cell pneumonia with intranuclear inclusions. (C) Post measles bronchiectasis. (D) Fusion giant cells in the thymus in fatal disseminated measles infection frequently seen in vitamin A deficient children.

Rubeola (measles)

Measles is a major cause of infant mortality in developing countries.[248] It is associated with **malnutrition, especially vitamin A deficiency**.[249–252] Measles virus attacks T lymphocytes and **depresses cell-mediated immunity** for 4–6 weeks. This sets the stage for a secondary invader, particularly **(staphylococcus) HSV, or adenovirus infection.** Fatality is reduced with the administration of high doses of vitamin A at the onset of clinical disease. When available, measles vaccine reduces the incidence and complications of measles. Failure to immunize against measles is responsible for outbreaks in inner cities.[253]

Aerosolized droplets infect the conjunctiva or nasopharynx. **Viremia** lasts 2 weeks and secretions are highly infectious. **Multinucleated giant cells** in lymphoid tissue contain intranuclear inclusions called **Warthin-Finkeldey giant cells**. Epithelial measles giant cells appear in the lung as fused type 2 pneumocytes with intranuclear inclusions (Fig. 10.31)[254–256] A morbilliform rash evolves into a brown desquamation. **Koplik spots** composed of epithelial measles giant cells may be present on the buccal mucosa near the orifice of the parotid gland duct and the second molar. This is pathognomonic for rubeola. Before the rash appears, measles giant cells with characteristic **intranuclear inclusions** may be found in lymphoid tissue through-out the body including the **thymus, lymph nodes, tonsils, and appendix**. Anecdotal reports cite the incidental finding of measles giant cells in a routine appendectomy specimen obtained for suspected appendicitis. The pathologist may predict the imminent onset of rubeola before the rash appears. The rash itself may contain epithelial measles giant cells.

Malnourished children under 1 year of age are especially vulnerable to serious rubeola infection. At autopsy pneumonia with squamous metaplasia of the respiratory epithelium is present. This is consistent with vitamin A deficiency in children who have conjunctival keratosis. Gastroenteritis, meningitis, and myocarditis occur. Anergic patients, especially HIV-infected children, may have measles without the exanthem.[257, 258] Autopsy is critical in confirming measles giant cell pneumonia in such patients.

Blindness, hearing loss, mental retardation, or death may follow **acute measles encephalitis**.[259, 260] Perivascular demyelination and inclusion-bearing inflammatory cells are found in the brain. Years after a measles episode, progressive degeneration of the central nervous system with ataxia, seizures, and both mental and motor retardation may result in a persistent vegetative state associated with **subacute sclerosing panencephalitis**. Destruction of the brain is associated with gliosis, perivascular cuffing with lymphocytes and plasma cells, neuronal degeneration, and infil-

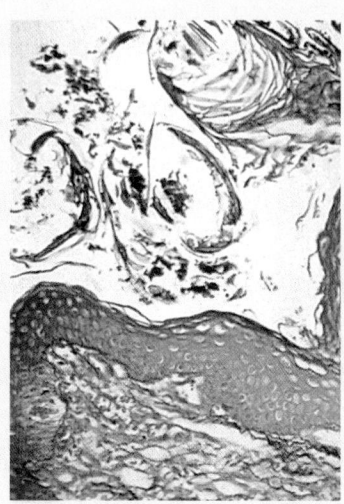

FIGURE 10.32 Mucocutaneous candidiasis of the oropharynx is common in neonates and children with AIDS.

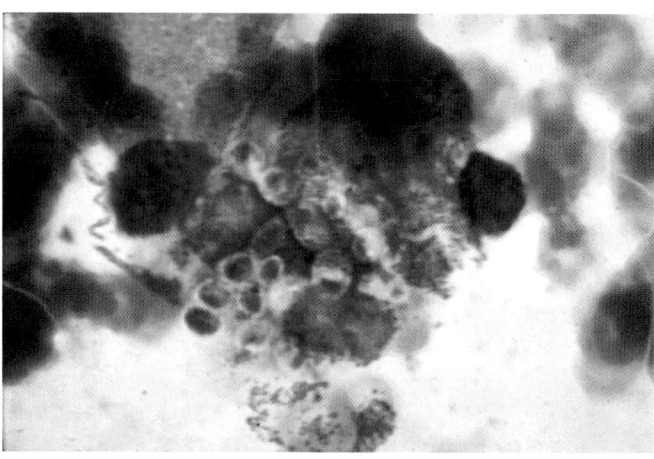

FIGURE 10.33 In inherited immunodeficiency syndromes rare intracellular spores may be found in macrophages. Intracellular histoplasmosis mimics candida.

tration of microglia that may harbor persistent virus. High levels of measles antibodies are frequent in adults with **multiple sclerosis**. Culture of the measles virus from brain tissue is difficult and requires the use of helper viruses.

Candidiasis

Thrush, an infection of the **oral mucosa** with *Candida albicans,* is often secondary to **maternal vaginal infection**.[261–265] Rarely invasion of the amniotic cavity with infection of umbilical cord, placental membranes, and skin occurs.[266] Organisms can be identified by characteristic mycelia and conidiophores (Fig. 10.32), in which oval structures are found separately or attached to mycelial threads.

The tongue, palate, pharynx, and inner surface of the cheeks are covered by a thick white membrane, which when detached leaves a raw bleeding mucosa. The membrane is usually limited to the buccal cavity but may spread into the lung, esophagus, and rarely to the lower gastrointestinal tract. Ulceration with perforation of the intestinal lesions occurs.

In **HIV**, *Candida* of the **gastroesophageal junction** is seen in 30% of cases. A pseudomembranous plaque with spores and pseudohyphae may be seen. In very low birth weight infants with prolonged intensive care, contaminated intravascular catheters may be the source of candidal sepsis.[267] **Invasive systemic disease** produces fungal granulomas in the liver, spleen, kidneys, and brain. Cutaneous candidiasis may occur in epidermolysis bullosa. A mild lymphohistiocytic infiltrate may be present except in the brain, where a neutrophilic infiltrate may predominate.

Histoplasmosis

Infection by *Histoplasma capsulatum*[268, 269] may occur at any age. Death has not been reported in early infancy, but the onset

of symptoms immediately after birth in a few infants suggests possible intrauterine transmission.

The disease attacks the **reticuloendothelial system** and involves multiple viscera. The course is characterized by **irregular fever, enlargement of the spleen and liver, emaciation, anemia, and leukopenia**. Diagnosis often may be confirmed by demonstration of organisms in the sternal marrow or in blood cultures. At autopsy, organisms are found in macrophages in the spleen, liver, lungs, myocardium, adrenal glands, and kidneys. In older individuals small **granulomas** with necrotic centers and peripheral calcification are common, but they are rarely observed in young infants.

In tissues *H. capsulatum* is seen as an oval yeast-like body, 1–5 µm in diameter, with a sharply defined, clear, colorless capsule and a central, dark-staining chromatin mass sometimes possessing a round vacuole (Fig. 10.33). In Sabouraud medium the culture may be a yeast form but is more often seen as white, cottony mycelium with microscopic septate hyphae or filaments bearing small spores.

Coccidioidomycosis

Few cases of coccidioidomycosis have been reported in infants.[270, 271] Congenital infection presents with dyspnea, cyanosis, and non-productive cough. At autopsy the lungs contain multiple yellow granulomas, with irregular **giant cells** and lymphocytes surrounding large endospores, 20–60 µm in diameter. Osteomyelitis and meningitis may also occur.

Aspergillosis

Aspergillosis most often involves the lungs, brain, bone marrow, and liver. Involvement of the nasal passages is associated with a destructive immune mediated sinusitis. A radial array of large septate mycelia branch at a 45-degree angle and surrounds a

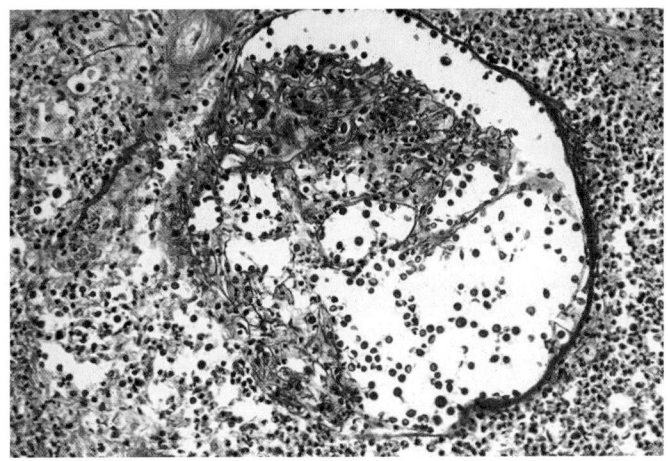

FIGURE 10.34 Cryptococcal infection of the kidney.

central necrotic area or proliferate perpendicular to blood vessels. **Thrombosis, infarction, and hematogenous dissemination** may result. This ubiquitous organism is a threat to immunodeficient patients especially on antileukemic therapy.

Cryptococcus infection

Cryptococcus infection is rare in children (Fig. 10.34) and is associated with **immunodeficiency or severe malnutrition**. The lung, lymph nodes, and brain are most often involved.[272] Meningitis is often fatal. Involvement of the intervillous space can be seen in the placenta. The organism is too large to be transmitted to the fetus.

Pneumocystis carinii pneumonia

Pneumocystis carinii[273] is a unique opportunistic pathogen that has usually been classified as a protozoan parasite, but new molecular analysis suggests it is probably a **fungus**. In the lung it is identified with the Gomori methenamine **silver stain.** Organisms form clusters within foamy proteinaceous material. *Pneumocystis carinii* pneumonia (PCP) accounts for 40% of all deaths in patients with HIV disease. Young malnourished immunodeficient children may acquire PCP, which may be associated with pulmonary plasmacytic infiltrates. Prophylactic antimicrobial therapy can prevent PCP.

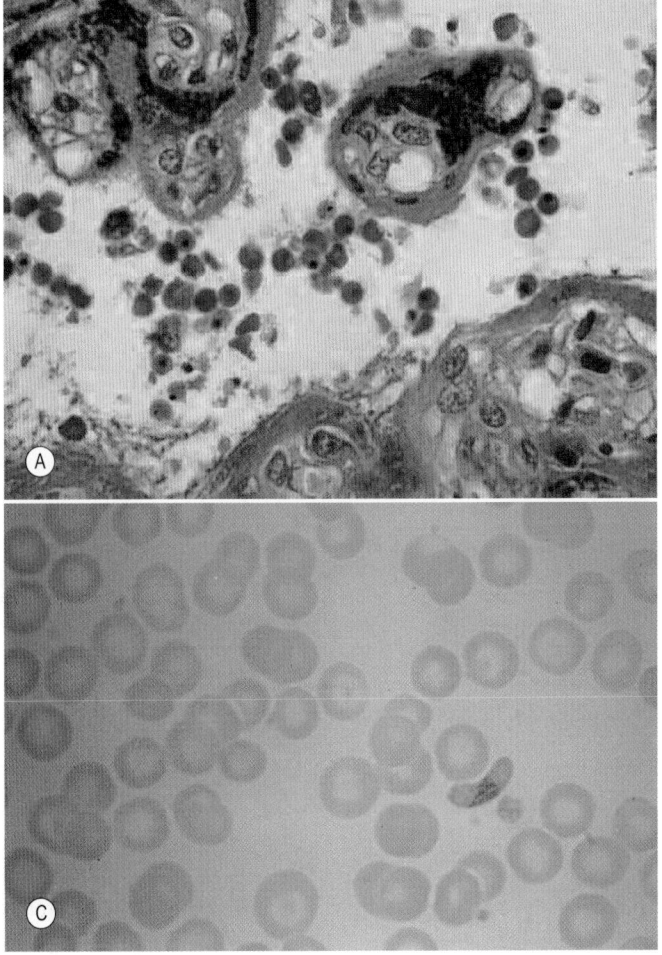

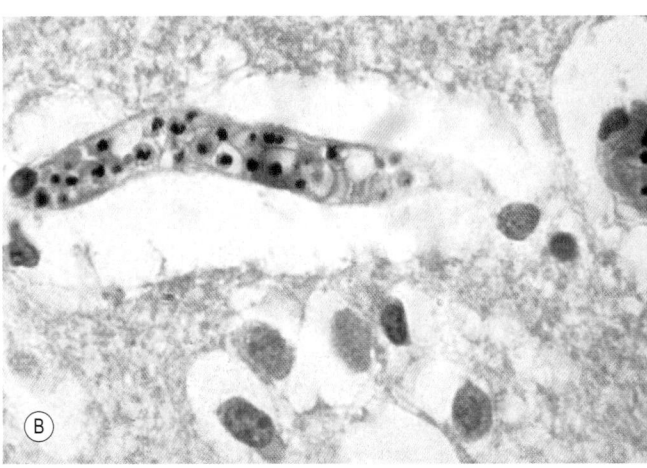

FIGURE 10.35 (A) Placental malaria showing parasitized maternal red blood cells, necrosis of syncytiotrophoblasts and fibrin deposition. (B) Intravascular organisms in the brain. (C) Malaria in peripheral blood showing schizonts.

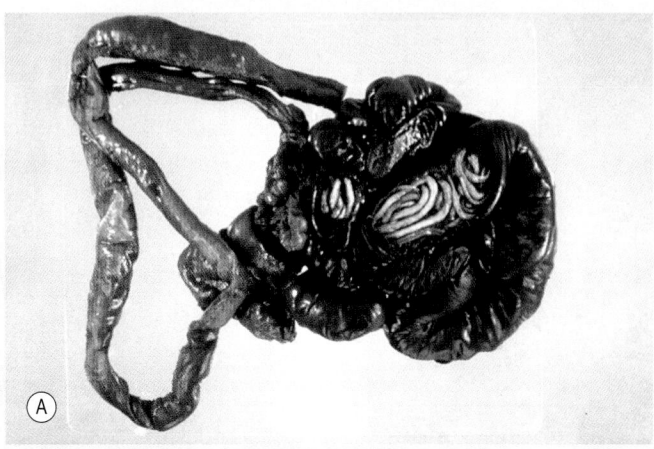

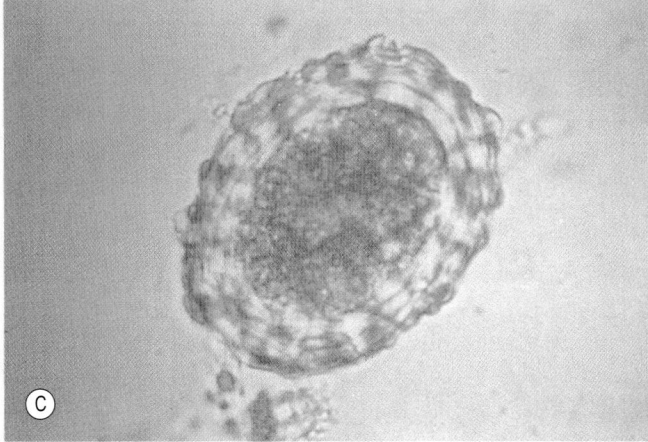

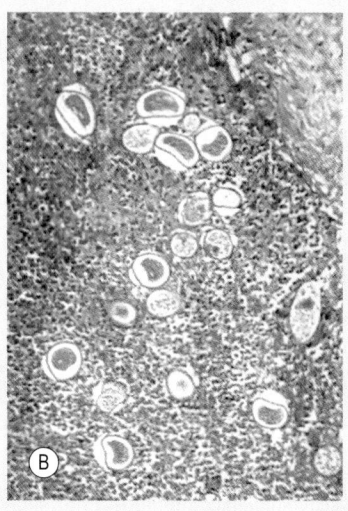

FIGURE 10.36 Infestation with *Ascaris* rarely may cause intestinal obstruction. (B) *Ascaris* ova with a thick cuticle may be found in tissue. (C) *Ascaris* egg.

Malaria

Plasmodium falciparum,[274] the most severe strain responsible for more deaths worldwide than any other form, affects the placenta but **rarely infects the fetus.**[275] *Plasmodium malariae* is less severe and chronic. Anemic children have fewer malarial episodes with fever, shaking chills, and hemolysis than well-nourished children. **Massive hepatosplenomegaly** with **portal triaditis** and accumulation of **malarial pigments** in a perivascular location in an edematous brain may be seen at autopsy (Fig. 10.35). Parasitized red blood cells appear on thick blood smears obtained during febrile episodes. Both *Plasmodium malariae* and *Plasmodium falciparum* may be associated with an **immune complex membranoproliferative glomerulonephritis.**

Intrauterine growth retardation[276] is associated with maternal malaria and pregnancy exacerbates episodes of *P. falciparum* malaria. Acute primary infection late in pregnancy may transmit malarial parasites to the fetus, but most women in endemic areas are infected before pregnancy. Parasites may be found in the umbilical cord blood and viscera in fetal infection. Involvement of the **placenta** is frequent. Maternal histiocytes with erythrophagocytosis of infected red blood cells are seen in the maternal lakes of the placenta. Malarial pigment also accumulates in the intervillous spaces in chronic infection.[277]

Malaria is a formidable infection and is prevalent in tropical countries. Infection is caused by four species of the *Plasmodium* protozoan where infection is transmitted by female Anopheline mosquitos. *P. falciparum*[217] causes the most virulent disease and targets the placenta as a favored site for erythrocyte schizogony. Primigravid maternal infection often leads to premature labor and intrauterine growth retardation that is attributed to maternal anemia. Transplacental spread is rare and is caused by maternal hemorrhage into the fetal circulation.[218] Mothers are usually infected before becoming pregnant and may be asymptomatic but not infrequently develop severe anemia with cerebral involvement. Intrauterine growth retardation and premature birth tend to occur without the fetus being infected. Should transplacental infection occur the fetus becomes anemic and presents with neonatal fever, irritability, jaundice and hepatosplenomegaly some weeks after birth.[218] The placenta may be enlarged and shows chronic intervillositis with parasitized erythrocytes that are confined to the maternal circulation when the fetus is not infected. Fibrinoid necrosis of trophoblast occurs with adherence of parasitized red blood cells to trophoblast in preference to endothelium. Focal necrotizing villitis with or without deposition of malarial pigment is seen when the fetus is infected. Malarial pigment also accumulates in fibrin deposits in the intervillous spaces.[220] Macrophages are a prominent component of the

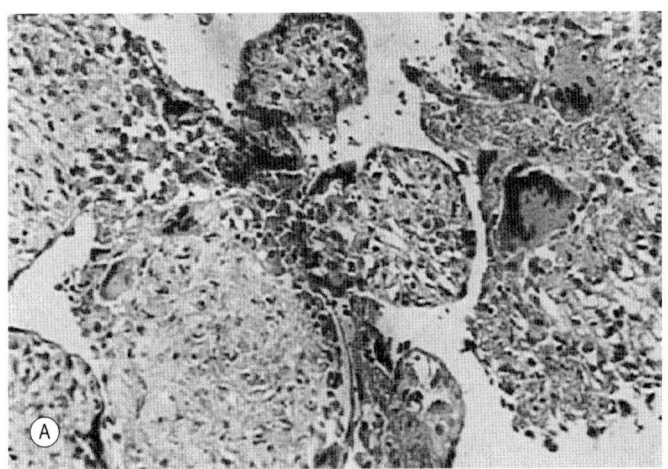
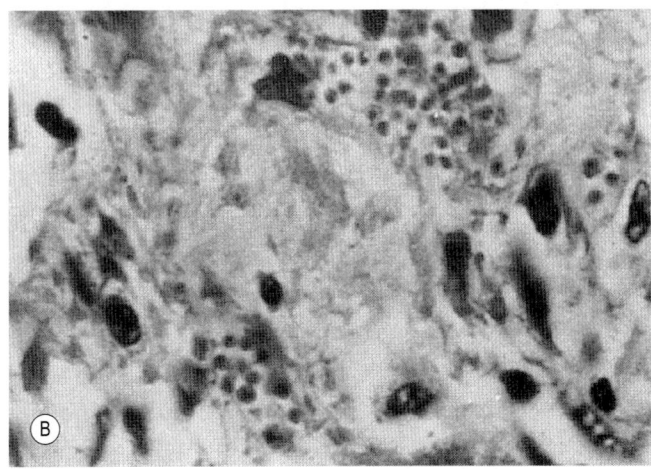

FIGURE 10.37 Placenta of fetus with Chagas disease. (A) Area of necrosis, leukocytic infiltration, and giant cell formation. (B) *Trypanosoma cruzi* in fetal vessels in villi. *(Courtesy Dr. Rita Cardosa.)*

inflammatory reaction as well as in generally associated chronic intervillositis.

Chagas disease

South American trypanosomiasis caused by *Trypanosoma cruzi* is transmitted by the bite of the **reduviid bug**. Congenital infection[279] may be transplacental or follows aspiration of infected amniotic fluid. **Stillbirth or hydrops fetalis** is common. Organisms are seen in the **placenta**, heart, skeletal muscle, nervous system, lung, and gastrointestinal tract. Conjunctivitis and hepatosplenomegaly occur. Trypanosomes may be found in cysts, in free forms called amastigotes, within **granulomas**, or with neutrophils and necrosis. Enlargement of the esophagus, intestines, ureters, and bladder may result from involvement of the **autonomic nervous system** (Fig. 10.37).

Lyme disease

The spirochete *Borrelia burgdorferi* is transmitted by **tick-bite** or rarely by **placental transmission**.[280, 281] **Target skin lesions** herald infection, which may be aborted by prompt antibiotic treatment. Skin rashes, neurologic abnormalities, **arthritis**, or death can follow cryptogenic symptoms and a history of summer exposure in endemic areas. Serologic tests may be helpful. A skin biopsy in the acute phase may reveal a lymphoplasmacytic perivasculitis or lymphocytic dermal infiltrate. Spirochetes may be seen with the **Warthin Starry stain**. Fetal infection occurs.

Botulism

Botulism is not an infectious disease. A rapid onset of vomiting, dysphagia, and respiratory paralysis is a response to a **neurotoxin** produced by the bacterium *C. botulinum*. It is very rare but there is a high case fatality rate. Most human disease follows the ingestion of **infected meat** or **improperly canned food, and honey may harbor the C. botulinum toxin**. The toxin is not degraded by stomach acid, enters the bloodstream, and irreversibly combines with nerve tissue.

References

Infection of the fetus and neonate

1. Christensen KK. Infection as a predominant cause of perinatal mortality. Obstet Gynecol 1982; 59:499–508.
2. Romero R, Mazor M. Infection and preterm labor. Clin Obstet Gynecol 1988; 31:553–584.
3. Minkoff H. Prematurity: infection as an etiologic factor. Obstet Gynecol 1983; 62:137–144.
4. Minkoff H, Grunebaum AN, Schwarz RM, et al. Risk factors for prematurity and premature rupture of membranes: a prospective study of the vaginal flora in pregnancy. Am J Obstet Gynecol 1984; 150:965–972.
5. Perkins RP, Zhou SM, Butler C, et al. Histologic chorioamnionitis in pregnancies of various gestational ages: implications in preterm rupture of membranes. Obstet Gynecol 1987; 70:856–860.
6. Redline RW. Placental inflammation. Sem Neonatol 2004; 9:265–274.
7. St Geme JW Jr, Murray DL, Carter J, et al. Perinatal bacterial infection after prolonged rupture of amniotic membranes: an analysis of risk and management. J Pediatr 1984; 104:608–613.
8. Benirschke K. Routes and types of infections in the newborn. Am J Dis Child 1960; 99:714–721.
9. Naeye RL, Peters EO. Amniotic fluid infections with intact membranes leading to perinatal death: a prospective study. Pediatrics 1978; 61:171–177.
10. Kraus FT, Redline RW, Gersell DJ, et al. Atlas of nontumor pathology. Vol 3. Placental pathology. Armed Forces Institute of Pathology, American Registry of Pathology, 2004.
11. Bernstein J, Wang J. The pathology of neonatal pneumonia. Am J Dis Child 1961; 101:350.
12. Tamiolakis D, Kotini A, Jivannakis T, et al. Induction of hepatic granulopoiesis due to chorioamnionitis during the second trimester of development. Eur J Obstet Gynecol Biol 2003; 110:164–168.
13. Toti P, DeFelice C, Occhini R, et al. Spleen depletion in neonatal sepsis and chorioamnionitis. Am J Clin Pathol 2004; 122:765–771.

14. Edwards RK, Clark P, Sistrom CL, et al. Intrapartum antibiotic prophylaxis 1: relative effects of recommended antibiotics on gram-negative pathogens. Obstet Gynecol 2002; 100:534–539.

15. Sinha A, Yokoe D, Platt R. Intrapartum antibiotics and neonatal invasive infectious caused by organisms other than group B streptococcus. J Pediatr 2003; 142:492–497.

16. Davies PA. Bacterial infection in the fetus and newborn. Arch Dis Child 1971; 46:1–27.

17. Boyle RJ, Chandler BD, Stonestreet BS, et al. Early identification of sepsis in infants with respiratory distress. Pediatrics 1978; 62:744–750.

18. Sinha A, Yokoe D, Platt R. Intrapartum antibiotics and neonatal invasive infections caused by organisms other than group B streptococcus. J Pediatr 2003; 142:492–497.

19. Hauth JC, Gilstrap LC III, Hankins GDV, et al. Term maternal and neonatal complications of acute chorioamnionitis. Obstet Gynecol 1985; 66:59–62.

20. Naeye RL. Causes of the excessive rates of perinatal mortality and prematurity in pregnancies complicated by maternal urinary tract infections. N Engl J Med 1979; 300:819–823.

21. Hillier SL, Martius J, Krohn M, et al. A case-control study of chorioamniotic infection and histologic chorioamnionitis in prematurity. N Engl J Med 1988; 319:972–978.

22. Lamont RF, Rose M, Elder MG. Effect of bacterial products on prostaglandin E production by amnion cells. Lancet 1985; 2:1331–1333.

23. Squire E, Favara B, Todd J. Diagnosis of neonatal bacterial infection: hematologic and pathologic findings in fatal and nonfatal cases. Pediatrics 1979; 64:60–64.

24. Madan E, Meyer MP, Amortequi A. Chorioamnionitis: a study of organisms isolated in perinatal autopsies. Ann Clin Lab Sci 1988; 18:39–45.

25. Saez-Lorens X, McCracken GH. Sepsis syndrome and septic shock in pediatrics: current concepts of terminology, pathophysiology, and management. J Pediatr 1993; 123:497–508.

26. Cordero L, Rau R, Taylor D, et al. Enteric gram-negative bacilli bloodstream infections: 17 years' experience in a neonatal intensive care unit. Am J Infect Control 2004; 32:189–195.

27. Urrea M, Irando M, Thio M, et al. A prospective incidence study of nosocomial infections in a neonatal care unit. Am J Infect Control 2003; 31:505–507.

28. Mehr SS, Sadowsky JL, Doyle LW, et al. Sepsis in neonatal intensive care in the late 1990s. J Paediatr Child Health 2002; 38:246–251.

29. Turkel SB, Pettross CW, Appleman MD, et al. Perinatal mortality associated with intrauterine infection due to pseudomonads. Pediatr Pathol 1986; 6:131–137.

30. Ruvalo C, Bauer CR. Intrauterinely acquired *Pseudomonas* infection in the neonate. Clin Pediatr 1982; 21:664–667.

31. Teplitz C. Pathogenesis of pseudomonas vasculitis and septic lesions. Arch Path 1965; 80:297–307.

32. Larsen CD. Streptococcal puerperal sepsis and obstetrical infections: a historical perspective. Rev Infect Dis 1986; 8:411.

33. Desa DJ, Trevenen CL. Intrauterine infections with group B-haemolytic streptococci. Br J Obstet Gynecol 1984; 91:237–239.

34. Jaureguy F, Carton M, Panel P, et al. Effects of intrapartum penicillin prophylaxis on intestinal bacterial colonization in infants. J Clin Microbiol 2004; 42:5184–5188.

35. Katzenstein A-L, Davis C, Braude A. Pulmonary changes in neonatal sepsis due to group B β-hemolytic streptococcus: relation to hyaline membrane disease. J Infect Dis 1976; 133:430–435.

36. Menke JA, Giacoia GP, Jockin H. Group B β hemolytic streptococcal sepsis and idiopathic respiratory distress syndrome: a comparison. J Pediatr 1979; 94:467–471.

37. Edwards MS, Rench MA, Haffar AAM, et al. Long-term sequelae of group B streptococcal meningitis in infants. J Pediatr 1985; 106:717–722.

38. Baker CJ. Group B streptococcal infections. Adv Int Med 1980; 25:475–501.

39. Melish ME, Glasgow LA. The staphylococcal scalded skin syndrome. N Engl J Med 1970; 282:1114–1119.

40. Ahlfors CE, Goetzman BW, Halsted CC, et al. Neonatal listeriosis. Am J Dis Child 1977; 131:405–408.

41. Evans JR, Allen AC, Stinson DA, et al. Perinatal listeriosis: report of an outbreak. Pediatr Infect Dis J 1985; 4:237–241.

42. Stoll BJ. Tetanus. Pediatr Clin North Am 1979; 26:415–431.

43. Montgomery RD. The cause of death in tetanus. West Indian Med J 1961; 10:84–102.

44. Sheffield JS, Ramin SM. Tetanus in pregnancy. Am J Perinatol 2004; 21:173–182.

45. Chai F, Prevots DR, Wang X, et al. Neonatal tetanus incidence in China, 1996–2001, and risk factors for neonatal tetanus, Guangxi Province, China. Int J Epidemiol 2004; 33:551–557.

46. Dische MR, Gooch WM III. Congenital toxoplasmosis. Perspect Pediatr Pathol 1981; 6:83–113.

47. Frenkel JK. Toxoplasmosis. Pediatr Clin North Am 1985; 32:917–932.

48. McCabe R, Remington JS. Toxoplasmosis: the time has come. N Engl J Med 1988; 318:313–315.

49. Sever JL, Ellenberg JH, Ley AC, et al. Toxoplasmosis: maternal and pediatric findings in 23,000 pregnancies. Pediatrics 1988; 82:181–192.

50. Stagno S. Congenital toxoplasmosis. Am J Dis Child 1980; 134:635–637.

51. Desmonts G, Couvreur J. Congenital toxoplasmosis: a prospective study of 378 pregnancies. N Engl J Med 1974; 290:1110–1116.

52. Desmonts G, Forestier F, Thulliez PH, et al. Prenatal diagnosis of congenital toxoplasmosis. Lancet 1985; 1:500–504.

53. Teutsch SM, Juranek DD, Sulzer A, et al. Epidemic toxoplasmosis associated with infected cats. N Engl J Med 1979; 300:695–699.

54. Daffos F, Forestier F, Capella-Pavlovsky M, et al. Prenatal management of 746 pregnancies at risk for congenital toxoplasmosis. N Engl J Med 1988; 318:271–275.

55. Altshuler G. Toxoplasmosis as a cause of hydranencephaly. Am J Dis Child 1973; 125:251–252.

56. Zuelzer WW. Infantile toxoplasmosis. Arch Pathol 1944; 38:1.

57. Elliott WG. Placental toxoplasmosis: report of a case. Am J Clin Pathol 1970; 53:413–417.

58. Freeman K, Salt A, Prusa A, et al. European Multicentre Study on Congenital Toxoplasmosis. Association between congenital toxoplasmosis and parent-reported developmental outcomes concerns and impairments in 3 year old children. BMC Pediatr 2005; 12:5.

59. O'Donohoe JM, Brueton MJ, Holliman RE. Concurrent congenital human immunodeficiency virus infection and toxoplasmosis. Pediatr Infect Dis J 1991; 10:627–628.

60. Oppenheimer EH, Dahms BB. Congenital syphilis in the fetus and neonate. Perspect Pediatr Pathol 1981; 6:115–138.

61. Mascola L, Pelosi R, Blount JH, et al. Congenital syphilis revisited. Am J Dis Child 1985; 139:575–580.

62. Harter C, Benirschke K. Fetal syphilis in the first trimester. Am J Obstet Gynecol 1976; 124:705–711.

63. Silverstein AM. Congenital syphilis and the timing of immunogenesis in the human fetus. Nature 1962; 194:196–197.

64. Epstein H, King CR. Diagnosis of congenital syphilis by immuno-fluorescence following fetal death in utero. Am J Obstet Gynecol 1985; 152:689–690.

65. McIntosh K. Congenital syphilis: breaking through the safety net. N Engl J Med 1990; 323:1339–1341.

66. Pariser H. Syphilis. Primary Care 1989; 16:603–619.

67. Wendel GD. Gestational and congenital syphilis. Clin Perinatol 1988; 15:287–303.

68. Russell P, Altschuler G. Placental abnormalities of congenital syphilis: a neglected aid to diagnosis. Am J Dis Child 1974; 128:160–163.

69. Qureshi F, Jacques SM, Reyes MP. Placental histopathology in syphilis. Hum Pathol 1993; 24:779–784.

70. Schmid G. Economic and programmatic aspects of congenital syphilis prevention. Bull World Health Organ 2004; 82:402–409.

71. Gregg NM. Congenital cataract following German measles in the mother. Trans Ophthalmol Soc Aus 1941; 3:34.

72. Gregg NM. Occurence of congenital defects in children following maternal rubella during pregnancy. Med J Aust 1945; 2:122.

73. Tondury G, Smith DW. Fetal rubella pathology. J Pediatr 1966; 68:867–879.

74. Dudgeon JA. Maternal rubella and its effect on the fetus. Arch Dis Child 1967; 42:110–125.

75. Driscoll SG. Histopathology of gestational rubella. Am J Dis Child 1969; 118:49–53.

76. South MA, Sever JL. Teratogen update: the congenital rubella syndrome. Teratology 1985; 31:297–307.

77. Singer DB, Rudolph AJ, Rosenberg HS, et al. Pathology of the congenital rubella syndrome. J Pediatr 1967; 71:665–675.

78. Singer DB, South MA, Montgomery JR, et al. Congenital rubella syndrome. Am J Dis Child 1969; 118:54–61.

79. Naeye RL, Blanc W. Pathogenesis of congenital rubella. JAMA 1965; 194: 1277–1283.

80. Menser MA, Reye RDK. The pathology of congenital rubella: a review written by request. Pathology 1974; 6:215–222.

81. Strauss L, Bernstein J. Neonatal hepatitis in congenital rubella: a histo-pathological study. Arch Path 1968; 86:317–327.

82. Rosenberg HS, Oppenheimer EH, Esterly JR. Congenital rubella syndrome; the late effects and their relation to the early lesions. Perspect Pediatr Pathol 1981; 6:183–202.

83. Menser MA, Forrest JM, Bransby RD. Rubella infection and diabetes mellitus. Lancet 1978; 1(8055):57–60.

84. Esterly JR, Oppenheimer EH. Intrauterine rubella infection. Perspect Pediatr Pathol 1973; 1:313–338.

85. Givens KT, Lee DA, Jones T, et al. Congenital rubella syndrome: ophthalmic manifestations and associated systemic disorders. Br J Ophthal 1993; 77: 358–363.

86. Achievements in public health: elimination of rubella and congenital rubella syndrome – United State, 1969–2004. MMWR Weekly 2005; 54:279–282.

87. Banatvala JE, Brown DW. Rubella. Lancet 2004; 363:1127–1137.

88. Becroft DMO. Prenatal cytomegalovirus infection: epidemiology, pathology, and pathogenesis. Perspect Pediatr Pathol 1981; 6:203–241.

89. Hanshaw JB. Congenital cytomegalovirus infection: a fifteen year perspective. J Infect Dis 1971; 123:555–561.

90. Reynolds DW, Stagno S, Hosty TS, et al. Maternal cytomegalovirus excretion and perinatal infection. N Engl J Med 1973; 289:1–5.

91. Stagno S, Pass RF, Dworsky ME, et al. Congenital cytomegalovirus infection. N Engl J Med 1982; 306:945–949.

92. Stagno S, Whitley RJ. Herpes virus infections of pregnancy. Part I. Cyto-megalovirus and Epstein-Barr virus infections. N Engl J Med 1985; 313: 1270–1274.

93. Stagno S, Pass RF, Cloud G, et al. Primary cytomegalovirus infection in preg-nancy: incidence, transmission to fetus, and clinical outcome. JAMA 1986; 256:1904–1908.

94. Stagno S, Pass RF, Dworsky ME, et al. Congenital cytomegalovirus infection. The relative importance of primary and recurrent maternal infection. N Engl J Med 1982; 306:945–949.

95. Stagno S, Pass RF, Dworsky ME, et al. Maternal cytomegalovirus infection and perinatal transmission. Clin Obstet Gynecol 1982; 25:563–576.

96. Alford CA, Stagno S, Pass RF, et al. Congenital and perinatal cytome-galovirus infections. Rev Infect Dis 1990; 12(suppl 7):S745–S753.

97. Bale JF Jr, Murph JR. Congenital infections and the nervous system. Pediatr Clin North Am 1992; 39:669–690.

98. Hayward JC, Titelbaum DS, Clancy RR, et al. Lissencephaly-pachygyria associated with congenital cytomegalovirus infection. J Child Neurol 1991; 6:109–114.

99. Finegold MJ, Carpenter RJ. Obliterative cholangitis due to cytomegalovirus: a possible precursor of paucity of intrahepatic bile ducts. Hum Pathol 1982; 13:662–665.

100. Medearis DN Jr. Cytomegalic inclusion disease. Pediatrics 1957; 19:467–480.

101. Greenfield C, Sinickas V, Harrison LC. Detection of cytomegalovirus by the polymerase chain reaction. A simple, rapid and sensitive non-radioactive method. Med J Aust 1991; 154:383–385.

102. Williamson WD, Demmler GJ, Percy AK, et al. Progressive hearing loss in infants with asymptomatic congenital cytomegalovirus infection. Pediatrics 1992; 90:862–866.

103. Williamson WD, Percy AK, Yow MD, et al. Asymptomatic congenital cytomegalovirus infection. Audiologic, neuroradiologic, and neurodevelop-mental abnormalities during the first year. Am J Dis Child 1990; 144: 1365–1368.

104. Benirschke K, Mendoza GR, Bazeley PL. Placental and fetal manifestations of cytomegalovirus infection. Virchows Arch B 1974; 16:121–139.

105. Hayes K, Gibas H. Placental cytomegalovirus infection without fetal involve-ment following primary infection in pregnancy. J Pediatr 1971; 79: 401–405.

106. Stocker JT. Congenital cytomegalovirus infection presenting as massive ascites with secondary pulmonary hypoplasia, Hum Pathol 1985; 16: 1173–1175.

107. Fjaer RB, Bruu AL, Nordbo SA. Extrahepatic bile duct atresia and viral involvement. Pediatr Transplant 2005; 9:68–73.

108. Balcarek KB, Warren W, Smith RJ, et al. Neonatal screening for congenital cytomegalovirus infection by detection of virus in saliva. J Infect Dis 1993; 167:1433–1436.

109. Reigstad H, Bjerknes R, Markestad T, et al. Ganciclovir therapy of congenital cytomegalovirus disease. Acta Paediatr 1992; 81:707–708.

110. Kimberlin DW, Lin CY, Sanchez PJ, et al. Effect of ganciclovir therapy on hearing in symptomatic congenital cytomegalovirus disease involving the central nervous system: a randomized, controlled trial. J Pediatr 2003; 143:4–6.

111. Binda S, Caroppo S, Dido P, et al. Modification of CMV DNA detection from dried blood spots for diagnosing congenital CMV infection. J Clin Virol 2004; 30:276–279.

112. Bradford RD, Cloud G, Lakeman AD, et al. Detection of cyto-megalovirus (CMV) DNA by polymerase chain reaction is associated with hearing loss in newborns with symptomatic congenital CMV infection involving the central nervous system. J Infect Dis 2005; 191:227–233.

113. Fowler KB, Stagno S, Pass RF. Maternal immunity and prevention of congenital cytomegalovirus infection. JAMA 2003; 290:1709.

114. Corey L, Spear PG. Infections with herpes simplex viruses. Part II. N Engl J Med 1986; 314:749–757.

115. Singer DB. Pathology of neonatal herpes simplex virus infection. In: Rosenberg HS, Bernstein J, eds. Perspectives in pediatric pathology. New York: Masson; 1981:243–278.

116. Nahmias AJ, Alford CA, Korones SB. Infection of the newborn with herpesvirus hominis. Adv Pediatr 1970; 17:185–226.

117. Stagno S, Whitley RJ. Herpes simplex virus and varicella zoster virus infections. Part II. N Engl J Med 1985; 313:1327.

118. Ashley RL, Dalessio J, Burchett S, et al. Herpes simplex virus-2 (HSV-2) type-specific antibody correlates of protection in infants exposed to HSV-2 at birth. J Clin Invest 1992; 90:511–514.

119. Garland SM, Doyle L, Kitchen W. Herpes simplex virus type 1 infections presenting at birth. J Pediatr Child Health 1991; 27:360–362.

120. Arvin AM. Relationships between maternal immunity to herpes simplex virus and the risk of neonatal herpesvirus infection. Rev Infect Dis 1991; 13(suppl 11):S953–S956.

121. Hyde SR, Giacoia GP. Congenital herpes infection: placental and umbilical cord findings. Obstet Gynecol 1993; 81:852–855.

122. Arvin AM, Yeager AS, Bruhn FW, et al. Neonatal herpes simplex infection in the absence of mucocutaneous lesions, J Pediatr 1982; 100:715–721.

123. Whitley RJ, Nahmias AJ, Visintine AM, et al. The natural history of herpes simplex virus infection of mother and newborn. Pediatrics 1980; 66:489–494.

124. Greene GR, King D, Romansky SG, et al. Primary herpes simplex pneu-monia in a neonate. Am J Dis Child 1983; 137:464–465.

125. South MA, Tompkins WAF, Morris RC, et al. Congenital malformation of the central nervous system associated with genital type (type 2) herpesvirus. J Pediatr 1969; 75:13–18.

126. Mirra JM. Aortitis and malacoplakia-like lesions of the brain in association with neonatal herpes simplex. Am J Clin Pathol 1971; 56:104.

127. Nicoll JA, Maitland NJ, Love S. Use of the polymerase chain reaction to detect herpes simplex virus DNA in paraffin sections of human brain at necropsy. J Neurol Neurosur Psychiatry 1991; 54:167–168.

128. Schwartz DA, Bueso-Ramos C, Siegel R. Disseminated herpes simplex infection in a twin: the role of the 'stat' autopsy in immediate therapeutic

intervention for survival of multiple birth neonates. J Perinat Med 1992; 20:281–287.

129. McKenzie D, Hansen JDL, Becker W. Herpes simplex virus infection: dissemination in association with malnutrition. Arch Dis Child 1959; 34:250.

130. Anderson NE, Willoughby EW, Synek BJ, et al. Brain biopsy in the management of focal encephalitis. J Neurol Neurosur Psychiatry 1991; 54: 1001–1003.

131. Brown ZA, Wald A, Morrow RA, et al. Effect of serologic status and cesarean delivery on transmission rates of herpes simplex virus from mother to infant. JAMA 2003; 289:203–209.

132. Schleiss MR. Vertically transmitted herpesvirus infections. Herpes 2003; 10:4–11.

133. Lewensohn-Fuchs I, Osterwall P, Forsgren M, et al. Detection of herpes simplex virus DNA in PCR-based diagnosis and parvovirus B19 in paraffin-embedded heart tissue of children with suspected sudden infant death syndrome. Lab Invest 2003; 83:1451.

134. Hall CB, Caserta MT, Schnabel KC, et al. Congenital infections with human herpesvirus 6 (HHV6) and human herpesvirus 7 (HHV7). J Pediatr 2004; 145:472–477.

135. van Loon NM, Gummuluru S, Sherwood DJ, et al. Direct sequence analysis of human herpesvirus 6 (HHV-6) sequences from infants and comparison of HHV-6 sequences from mother/infant pairs. Clin Infect Dis 1995; 21(4): 1017–1019.

136. Koch WC. Fifth (human parvovirus) and sixth (herpesvirus 6) diseases. Curr Opin Infect Dis 2001; 14:343–356.

137. Dewhurst S, Chandran B, McIntyrne K, et al. Phenotypic and genetic polymorphisms among human herpesvirus-6 isolates from North American infants. Virology 1992; 190:490–493.

138. Alkalay AL, Pomerance JJ, Rimoin DL. Fetal varicella syndrome. J Pediatr 1987; 111:320–323.

139. Greenspoon JS, Masaki DI. Fetal varicella syndrome. J Pediatr 1988; 112: 505–506.

140. Siegel M. Congenital malformations following chickenpox, measles, mumps, and hepatitis: results of a cohort study. JAMA 1973; 226:1521–1524.

141. Sauerbrei A, Wutzler P. The congenital varicella syndrome. J Perinatol 2000; 20:548–554.

142. Hartung J, Enders G, Chaoui R. Prenatal diagnosis of congenital varicella syndrome and detection of varicella-zoster virus in the fetus: a case report. Prenat Diagn 1999; 19:163–166.

143. Magliocco AM, Demetrick DJ, Sarnat HB, et al. Varicella embryopathy. Arch Pathol Lab Med 1992; 116:181–186.

144. Paryani SG, Arvin AM. Intrauterine infection with varicella-zoster virus after maternal varicella. N Engl J Med 1986; 314:1542–1546.

145. Mustonen K, Mustakangas P, Valanne L, et al. Congenital varicella-zoster virus infection after maternal subclinical infection: clinical and neuropathological findings. J Perinatol 2001; 21:141–146.

146. Smith EM, Johnson SR, Cripe TP, et al. Perinatal vertical transmission of human papillomavirus and subsequent development of respiratory tract papillomatosis. Ann Otol Rhinol Laryngol 1991; 100:479–483.

147. Wood CL. Laryngeal papillomas in infants and children. Relationship to maternal venereal warts. J Nurse 1991; 36:297–302.

148. Smith EM, Ritchie JM, Yankowitz J, et al. Human papillomavirus prevalence and types in newborns and parents: concordance and modes of transmission. Sex Transm Dis 2004; 31:57–62.

149. Syrjanen S, Puranen M. Human papillomavirus infections in children: the potential role of maternal transmission. Crit Rev Oral Biol Med 2000; 11: 259–274.

150. Czegledy J. Sexual and non-sexual transmission of human papillomavirus. Acta Microbiol Immunol Hung 2001; 48:511–517.

151. Anand A, Gray ES, Brown T, et al. Human parvovirus infection in pregnancy and hydrops infection. N Engl J Med 1987; 316:183–186.

152. Caul EO, Usher MJ, Burton PA. Intrauterine infection with human parvovirus B19: a light and electron microscopic study. J Med Virol 1988; 24: 55–66.

153. Knisely AS, O'Shea PA, McMillian P, et al. Transmission electron microscopic identification of parvovirus virons within erythroid-line cells in fetal hydrops fetalis. Pediatr Pathol 1988; 8:163.

154. Rogers BB, Mark Y, Oyer CE. Diagnosis and incidence of fetal parvovirus infection in an autopsy series: I. Histology. Pediatr Pathol 1993; 13:371–379.

155. Tolfvenstam T, Papadogiannakis N, Norbeck O, et al. Frequency of human parvovirus B19 infection in intrauterine fetal death. Lancet 2001; 357: 1494–1497.

156. Qian XH, Zhang GC, Jiao XY, et al. Aplastic anaemia associated with parvovirus B19 infection. Arch Dis Child 2002; 87:436–437.

157. Barash J, Dushnitzky D, Sthoeger D, et al. Human parvovirus B19 infection in children: uncommon clinical presentations. Isr Med Assoc J 2002; 4:763–765.

158. Chisaka H, Morita E, Yaegashi N, et al. Parvovirus B19 and the pathogenesis of anaemia, Rev Med Virol 2003; 13:347–359.

159. Lehmann HW, Kuhner L, Beckenlehner K, et al. Chronic human parvovirus B19 infection in rheumatic disease of childhood and adolescence. Clin Virol 2002; 25:135–143.

160. Mark Y, Rogers BB, Oyer CE. Diagnosis and incidence of fetal parvovirus infection in an autopsy series: II. DNA amplification. Pediatr Pathol 1993; 13:381–386.

161. Beem MO, Saxon EM. Respiratory-tract colonization and a distinctive pneumonia syndrome in infants infected with *Chlamydia trachomatis*. N Engl J Med 1977; 296:306–310.

162. Hammerschlag MR, Anderka M, Semine DZ, et al. Prospective study of maternal and infantile infection with *Chlamydia trachomatis*, Pediatrics 1979; 64:142–148.

163. Martin DH, Koutsky L, Eschenbach DA, et al. Prematurity and perinatal mortality in pregnancies complicated by maternal *Chlamydia trachomatis* infections. JAMA 1982; 247:1585–1588.

Infection in infants

164. Powers DR, Rogers ZR, Patch MJ, et al. Purpura fulminans in meningococcemia: association with acquired deficiencies of protein C&S. N Engl J Med 1987; 317:571.

165. Neveling U, Kaschula ROC. Fatal meningococcal disease in childhood: an autopsy study of 86 cases. Ann Trop Paediatr 1993; 13:147–152.

166. Hodes H. Diphtheria. Pediatr Clin North Am 1979; 26:445–459.

167. McGregor J, Ogle JW, Curry-Kane G. Perinatal pertussis. Obstet Gynecol 1986; 68:582–586.

168. Vitek CR, Baughman AL, Murphy TV. Increased deaths from pertussis among young infants in the United States in the 1990s. Pediatr Inf Dis J 2003; 22:628–634.

169. Milne LM, Issacs D, Crook PJ. Neonatal infections with *Haemophilus* species. Arch Dis Child 1988; 63:83–85.

170. Urrea M, Irando M, Thio M, et al. A prospective incidence study of nosocomial infections in a neonatal care unit. Am J Infect Control 2003; 31:505–507.

171. Tan L, Sun X, Zhu X, et al. Epidemiology of nosocomial pneumonia in infants after cardiac surgery. Chest 2004; 125:410–417.

172. Edwards RK, Clark P, Sistrom CL, et al. Intrapartum antibiotic prophylaxis 1: relative effects of recommended antibiotics on gram-negative pathogens. Obstet Gynecol 2002; 100:540–544.

173. Sinha A, Yokoe D, Platt R. Intrapartum antibiotics and neonatal invasive infectious caused by organisms other than group B streptococcus. J Pediatr 2003; 142:492–497.

174. Urrea M, Pons M, Serra M, et al. Prospective incidence study of nosocomial infections in a pediatric intensive care unit. Pediatr Infect Dis J 2003; 22:490.

175. Cordero L, Rau R, Taylor D, et al. Enteric gram-negative bacilli bloodstream infections: 17 years' experience in a neonatal intensive care unit. Am J Infect Control 2004; 32:189.

176. Driscoll S. Genitourinary opportunists: mycoplasmas and chlamydiae. In: Rosenberg HS, Bernstein J, eds. Perspectives in pediatric pathology. Vol 6. New York: Mason:1981; 167.

177. Dische MR, Quinn PA, Czegledy-Nagy E, et al. Genital *Mycoplasma* infection. Intrauterine infection: pathologic study of the fetus and placenta. Am J Clin Pathol 1979; 72:167–174.

178. Kundsin RB, Driscoll SG, Monson RR, et al. Association of *Ureaplasma urealyticum* in the placenta with perinatal morbidity and mortality. N Engl J Med 1984; 310:941–945.

179. Wang EEL, Frayha H, Watts J, et al. Role of *Ureaplasma urealyticum* and other pathogens in the development of chronic lung disease of prematurity. Pediatr Infect Dis J 1988; 7:547–551.

180. McCormack WM, Almeida PC, Bailey PE, et al. Sexual activity and vaginal colonization with genital mycoplasmas. JAMA 1972; 221: 1375–1377.

181. Adams JM, Imagawa DT, Zike K. Epidemic bronchiolitis and pneumonitis related to respiratory syncytial virus. JAMA 1961; 176:1037–1039.

182. MacDonald NE, Hall CB, Suffin SC, et al. Respiratory syncytial virus infection in infants with congenital heart disease. N Engl J Med 1982; 307: 397–400.

183. Hall CB, Powell KR, MacDonald NE, et al. Respiratory syncytial viral infection in children with compromised immune function. N Engl J Med 1986; 315:77–81.

184. McIntosh K. Pathogenesis of severe acute respiratory infections in the developing world: respiratory syncytial virus and parainfluenza viruses. Rev Infect Dis 1991; 13(suppl 6):S492–S500.

185. Toms GL. Respiratory syncytial virus: virology, diagnosis, and vaccination. Lung 1990; 168(suppl):388–395.

186. Caswell SJ, Thomson AH, Ashmore SP, et al. Latent sensitisation to respiratory syncytial virus during acute bronchiolitis and lung function after recovery. Arch Dis Child 1990; 65:946–952.

187. Grimaldi M, Gouyon B, Michaut F, et al. Severe respiratory syncytial virus bronchiolitis: epidemiologic variation associated with the initiation of palivizumab in severely premature infants with bronchopulmonary dysplasia. Pediatr Infect Dis J 2004; 23:1081–1085.

188. Domachowske JB, Rosenberg HF. Advances in the treatment and prevention of severe viral bronchiolitis. Pediatr Ann 2005; 34:35–41.

189. Becroft DMO. Histopathology of fatal adenovirus infection of the respiratory tract in young children, J Clin Pathol 1967; 20:561–569.

190. Nahmias AJ, Griffith D, Snitzer J. Fatal pneumonia associated with adenovirus type 7. Am J Dis Child 1967; 114:36–41.

191. Sun CCJ, Duara S. Fatal adenovirus pneumonia in two newborn infants, one case caused by adenovirus type 30. Pediatr Pathol 1985; 4:247–255.

192. Bowles NE, Ni J, Kearney DL, et al. Detection of viruses in myocardial tissues by polymerase chain reaction: evidence of adenovirus as a common cause of myocarditis in children and adults. J Am Coll Cardiol 2003; 42:466–472.

193. Woo D, Cummins M, Davies PA, et al. Vertical transmission of hepatitis B surface antigen in carrier mothers in two west London hospitals. Arch Dis Child 1979; 54:670–675.

194. Balistreri WF. Viral hepatitism – pediatric gastroenterology II. Pediatr Clin North Am 1988; 35:375–407.

195. Thomas HC. Hepatitis B viral infection. Am J Med 1988; 85(suppl 2A): 135–140.

196. Arevalo JA, Washington E. Cost-effectiveness of prenatal screening and immunization for hepatitis B virus. JAMA 1988; 259:365–369.

197. Seemayer TA, Oligny LL, Gartner JG. The Epstein-Barr virus: historical, biologic, pathologic and oncologic considerations. Perspect Pediatr Pathol 1981; 6:1–33.

198. Morgan DG, Miller G, Niederman JC, et al. Site of Epstein-Barr virus replication in the oropharynx. Lancet 1979; 1:1154–1157.

199. Childs CC, Parham DM, Bernard CW. Infectious mononucleosis: the spectrum of changes simulating lymphoma in lymph nodes and tonsils. Am J Surg Pathol 1987; 11:122–132.

200. Pagano JS. Diseases and mechanisms of persistent DNA virus infection: latency and cellular transformation. J Infect Dis 1975; 132:209–223.

201. Fox JP. Eradication of poliomyelitis in the United States. A commentary on the Salk reviews. Rev Infect Dis 1980; 2:277–281.

202. Fechner RE, Smith MG, Middlekamp JH. Coxsackie B virus infection of the newborn. Am J Pathol 1963; 42:493–505.

203. Kibrick S, Benirschke K. Severe generalized disease (encephalohepatomyocarditis) occurring in the newborn period and due to infection with coxsackie virus, group B: evidence of intrauterine infection with this agent. Pediatrics 1958; 22:857–875.

204. Bates HR Jr. Coxsackie virus B3 calcific pancarditis and hydrops fetalis. Am J Obstet Gynecol 1970; 106:629–630.

205. Euscher E, Davis J, Holzman, et al. Coxsackie virus infection of the placenta associated with neurodevelopmental delays in the newborn. Obstet Gynecol 2001; 98:1019–1026.

206. Dagan R, Jenista JA, Prather SL, et al. Viremia in hospitalized children with enterovirus infections. J Pediatr 1985; 106:397–401.

207. Yoon BH, Park CW, Chaiworapongsa T. Intrauterine infection and the development of cerebral palsy. BJOG 2003; 110 (suppl 20):124–127.

208. Satosar A, Ramirez NC, Bartholomew D, et al. Histologic correlates of viral and bacterial infection of the placenta associated with severe morbidity and mortality in the newborn. Hum Pathol 2004; 35:536–545.

209. Gear JHS, Measroch V. Coxsackievirus infection of the newborn. Prog Med Virol 1973; 15:42–62.

210. Wong SN, Tam AYC, Ng THK, et al. Fatal Coxsackie B1 virus infection in neonates. Pediatr Infect Dis J 1989; 8(9):638–641.

211. Haddad J, Gut JP, Wendling MJ, et al. Enterovirus infections in neonates. A retrospective study of 21 cases. Eur J Med 1993; 2:209–214.

212. Ahmad N, Abraham AA. Pancreatic isletitis with Coxsackie virus B5 infection. Hum Pathol 1982; 13:661–662.

213. Wagenknecht LE, Reosenman JM, Herman WH. Increased incidence of insulin-dependent diabetes mellitus following an epidemic of Coxsackievirus B5. Am J Epidemiol 1991; 133:1024–1031.

214. Krous HF, Dietzman D, Ray CG. Fatal infections with echovirus type 6 and 11 in early infancy. Am J Dis Child 1973; 126:842–846.

215. Modlin JF, Polk BF, Horton P, et al. Perinatal echovirus infection: risk of transmission during a community outbreak. N Engl J Med 1981; 305: 368–371.

216. Modlin JF. Perinatal echovirus infection: insights from a literature review of 61 cases of serious infection and 16 outbreaks in nurseries. Rev Infect Dis 1986; 8:918–926.

217. Philip AG, Larson EJ. Overwhelming neonatal infection with ECHO 19 virus. J Pediatr 1973; 82:391–397.

218. Krous HF, Dietzman D, Ray G. Fatal infections with echovirus types 6 and 11 in early infancy. Am J Dis Child 1973; 126:842–846.

219. Hughes JR, Hanover NH, Wilfert CM, et al. Echovirus 14 infection associated with fatal hepatic necrosis. Am J Dis Child 1972; 123:61–67.

220. Schreiber DS, Blacklow NR, Trier JS. The mucosal lesion of the proximal small intestine in acute infectious nonbacterial gastroenteritis. N Engl J Med 1973; 288:1318–1323.

221. Ford-Jones EL, Mindorff CM, Gold R, et al. The incidence of viral-associated diarrhea after admission to a pediatric hospital. Am J Epidemiol 1990; 131: 711–718.

222. Sack RB, Gorbach SL, Banwell JG, et al. Enterotoxigenic *Escherichia coli* isolated from patients with severe cholera-like disease. J Infect Dis 1971; 123:378–385.

223. Jacobs SI, Holzel A, Wolman B, et al. Outbreak of infantile gastroenteritis caused by *Escherichia coli* 0114. Arch Dis Child 1970; 45:656–663.

224. Cleary TG, Lopez EL. The shiga-like toxin-producing *Escherichia coli* and hemolytic uremic syndrome. Pediatr Infect Dis J 1989; 8:720–724.

225. Drummond KN. Hemolytic uremic syndrome – then and now. N Engl J Med 1985; 312:116–118.

226. Kaplan BS, Proesmans W. The hemolytic uremic syndrome of childhood and its variants. Semin Hematol 1987; 24:148–160.

227. Neild G. The haemolytic uraemic syndrome: a review. J Med 1987; 63: 367–376.

228. Rabson AR, Hallett AF, Koornhof HJ. Generalized *Yersinia enterocolitica* infection. J Infect Dis 1975; 131:447–451.

229. Drumm B. *Helicobacter pylori* in the pediatric patient. Gastroenterol Clin North Am 1993; 22:169–182.

230. George DE, Glassman M. Peptic ulcer disease in children. Gastrointest Endosc Clin N Am 1994; 4:23–37.

231. Han VK, Sayed H, Chance GW, et al. An outbreak of *Clostridium difficile* necrotizing enterocolitis: a case for oral vancomycin therapy. Pediatrics 1983; 71:935–941.

232. Moorthy B, Mehta S, Mitra K, et al. Amoebic liver abscess in a four-month-old infant. Aust Paediatr J 1977; 13:53–55.

233. Warren KS. Schistosomiasis: a multiplicity of immunopathology. J Invest Dermatol 1976; 67:464–469.

234. Smith JH, Christie JD. The pathobiology of *Schistosoma haematobium* infection in humans. Hum Pathol 1986; 12:333–345.

235. Mitchell W, Crawford TO. Intraparenchymal cerebral cysticercosis in children: diagnosis and treatment. Pediatrics 1988; 82:76–82.

236. Brown WJ, Voge M. Cysticercosis: a modern day plague. Pediatr Clin North Am 1985; 32:953–969.

237. Case records of the Massachusetts General Hospital: case 45. N Engl J Med 1987; 317:1209.

238. Gould SE. The story of trichinosis. Am J Clin Pathol 1971; 55:2–11.

239. Dao AH, Virmani R. Visceral larva migrans involving the myocardium: report of two cases and review of the literature. Pediatr Pathol 1986; 6:449–456.

240. Markell EK. Intestinal nematode infections. Pediatr Clin North Am 1985; 32:971–986.

241. Markell EK, Voge M, John DT. Medical parasitology. Philadelphia: WB Saunders; 1986.

Other infections

242. Hudson FP. Clinical aspects of congenital tuberculosis. Arch Dis Child 1956; 31(156):136–139.

243. Reichman LB, O'Day R. Tuberculous infection in a large urban population. Am Rev Respir Dis 1978; 117:705–712.

244. LeRoux FB, Schwersenski J, Greeff MJ. Congenital tuberculosis: a report of a probable case. S Afr Med J 1978; 53:946–948.

245. Hageman J, Shulman S, Schreiber M, et al. Congenital tuberculosis: critical reappraisal of clinical findings and diagnostic procedures. Pediatrics 1980; 66:980–984.

246. Hinman AR, Judd JM, Kolnik JP, et al. Changing risks in tuberculosis. Am J Epidemiol 1976; 103:486–497.

247. Jones DS, Malecki JM, Bigler WJ, et al. Pediatric tuberculosis and human immunodeficiency virus infection in Palm Beach County, Florida. Am J Dis Child 1992; 146:1166–1170.

248. Kaschula ROC, Druker J, Kipps A. Late morphologic consequences of measles: a lethal and debilitating lung disease among the poor. Rev Infect Dis 1983; 5:395–404.

249. Sommer A. Vitamin A status, resistance to infection and childhood mortality. Ann N Y Acad Sci 1990; 587:17–23.

250. Chandra RK. Micronutrients and immune functions: an overview. Ann N Y Acad Sci 1990; 587:9–16.

251. Harris MC, Douglas SD. Nutritional influence on neonatal infections in annual models and man. Ann N Y Acad Sci 1990; 587:246–256.

252. Coutsoudis A, Kiepiela P, Coovadia HM, et al. Vitamin A supplementation enhances specific IgG antibody levels and total lymphocyte numbers while improving morbidity in measles. Pediatr Infect Dis J 1992; 11:203–209.

253. Centers for Disease Control. Measles-United States, first 26 weeks. MMWR 1993; 42:813.

254. Esolen LM, Ward BJ, Moench TR, et al. Infection of monocytes during measles. J Infect Dis 1993; 168:47–52.

255. Radoycich GE, Zuppan CW, Weeks DA, et al. Patterns of measles pneumonitis. Pediatr Pathol 1992; 12:773–786.

256. Kipps A, Kaschula ROC. Virus pneumonia following measles: a virological and histological study of autopsy material. S Afr Med J 1976; 50:1083–1088.

257. Embree JE, Datta P, Stackiw W, et al. Increased risk of early measles in infants of human immunodeficiency virus type 1-seropositive mothers. J Infect Dis 1992; 165:262–267.

258. Palumbo P, Hoyt L, Demasio K, et al. Population-based study of measles and measles immunization in human immunodeficiency virus-infected children. Pediatr Infect Dis J 1992; 11:1008–1014.

259. Pearl PL, Abu-Farsakh H, Starke JR, et al. Neuropathology of two fatal cases of measles in the 1988–1989 Houston epidemic. Pediatr Neurol 1990; 6:126–130.

260. Kipps A, Dick G, Moodie JW. Measles and the central nervous system. Lancet 1983; II:1406–1410.

261. Benirschke K, Raphael SI. *Candida albicans* infection of the amniotic sac. Am J Obstet Gynecol 1958; 75:200–202.

262. Ho CY, Aterman K. Infection of the fetus by *Candida* in a spontaneous abortion. Am J Obstet Gynecol 1970; 106:705–710.

263. Buchanan R, Sworn MJ, Noble AD. Abortion associated with intrauterine infection by *Candida albicans*. Br J Obstet Gynaecol 1979; 86:741–744.

264. Dvorak AM, Gavaller B. Congenital systemic candidiasis: report of a case. N Engl J Med 1966; 274:540–543.

265. Albarracin NS, Patterson WS, Haust MD. *Candida albicans* infection of the placenta and fetus: report of a case. Obstet Gynecol 1967; 30:838–841.

266. Schwartz DA, Reef S. *Candida albicans* placentitis and funisitis: early diagnosis of congenital candidemia by histopathologic examination of umbilical cord vessels. Pediatr Infect Dis J 1990; 9:661–665.

267. Johnson DE, Thompson TR, et al. Systemic candidiasis in very low birth weight infants (<1500 grams). Pediatrics 1984; 73:138–143.

268. Salfelder K, Brass K, Doehnert G, et al. Fatal disseminated histoplasmosis: anatomic study of autopsy cases. Arch Abt A Pathol Anat 1970; 350:303–335.

269. Weinberg GA, Kleiman MD, Grosfeld JL, et al. Unusual manifestations of histoplasmosis in childhood. Pediatrics 1983; 72:99–105.

270. Bernstein DI, Tipton JR, Schott SF, et al. Coccidioidomycosis in a neonate: maternal–infant transmission. J Pediatr 1981; 99:752–754.

271. Richardson HB Jr, Anderson JA, McKay BM. Acute pulmonary coccidioidomycosis in children. J Pediatr 1967; 70:376–382.

272. Siewers CMF, Cramblett HG. Cryptococcosis (torulosis) in children; a report of four cases. Pediatrics 1964; 34:393–400.

273. Bedrossian CWM. *Pneumocystis carinii* infection. Semin Diagn Pathol 1989; 6:191.

274. Galbraith RM, Faulk WP, Galbraith GMP, et al. The human materno-foetal relationship in malaria: I. Identification of pigment and parasites in the placenta. Trans R Soc Trop Med Hyg 1980; 74:61–72.

275. Quinn TC, Jacobs RF, Mertz GJ, et al. Congenital malaria: a report of four cases and a review. J Pediatr 1982; 101:229–232.

276. MacGregor JD, Avery JG. Malaria transmission and fetal growth. Br Med J 1974; 3:433–436.

277. Walter PR, Garin Y, Blot P. Placental pathologic changes in malaria: a histologic and ultrastructural study. Am J Pathol 1982; 109:330–342.

278. Gautam OP, Thawrani YP, Mathur PS. Pattern of malaria in children and its therapeutic evaluation. Indian Pediatr 1980; 17:511–514.

279. Bittencourt AL. Congenital Chagas disease. Am J Dis Child 1976; 130:97–103.

280. Schlesinger PA, Duray PH, Burke BA, et al. Maternal–fetal transmission of the Lyme disease spirochete, *Borrelia burgdorferi*. Ann Intern Med 1985; 103:67–68.

281. MacDonald AB. Gestational Lyme borreliosis: implications for the fetus. Rheum Dis Clin North Am 1989; 15:657–677.

Nutritional diseases

11

Lewis A. Barness

In ancient times, lack of food gave languishing bodies to death. Now, on the contrary, it is abundance that buries them. T. Lucretius Cato *De Rerum Natura*, 55 BC

Modern nutrition in health and disease[1] and pediatric nutrition[2] have been discussed comprehensively.

Utilization of nutrients is important to prevent deficiencies and adapt to environmental stresses. In affluent societies, ingestion in excess of some nutrients results in obesity and, in certain cases, toxicity. In developing societies, protein, carbohydrate, or fat (Table 11.1) may be deficient and starvation, marasmus, or kwashiorkor may occur. In either case, imbalances may mimic deficiency states.

Macronutrients are protein, carbohydrate, fat, and water. The **micronutrients** are vitamins (Table 11.2) and minerals (Table 11.3). **Primary deficiencies** are those due to lack of intake. **Secondary nutrient deficiencies** may be due to malabsorption or to disorders of metabolism.

Nutritional diseases rarely manifest as deficits of single nutrients. Although nutrient deficiencies in humans are usually multiple and complex, each nutrient was discovered in animals, plants, fungi, or humans as a single deficiency. In growing children, deficiency of any or multiple nutrients results in **growth failure**. Even marginal malnutrition causes growth stunting and cognitive and behavioral deficits.[3] Trace elements are essential for gene expression. Genes encode proteins that are involved in transport, storage, and function of the trace elements. Growth and development are dependent on these elements for gene expression at critical stages of embryonal, fetal and postnatal life.[4]

Vitamins

The physical and metabolic properties and food sources of vitamins are listed in Table 11.2.

Vitamin A deficiency

Vitamin A was first believed to be anti-infectious. Vitamin A deficiency was found to cause **squamous cell metaplasia**, resulting in urethritis, vaginitis, or pneumonitis. Alterations in the cells of the cornea with drying (xerosis) and xerophthalmia (Fig. 11.1) result in destruction of the globe of the eye, with clouding of the cornea, keratomalacia; appearance of Bitot spots (dry silver-gray plaques on the bulbar conjunctiva); and finally, leaking of the vitreous and aqueous of the eye.[5]

Vitamin A is found in animal products such as eggs and liver; vitamin A precursors, carotenoids, are found in yellow, orange, and some green vegetables. Vitamin A and carotenoids, like other fats, require bile salts, lipase, and antioxidants for absorption of retinyl esters. Esters are deesterified in the liver to retinol, the alcohol with vitamin A activity. Oxidation yields retinal, an aldehyde, and retinoic acid. Vitamin A is stored as retinyl esters. Retinol released from the liver is bound to retinol-binding protein, transthyretin, which is synthesized in the liver. Membrane surface-specific receptors for retinol-binding protein provide uptake of retinol by cells.[6,7]

Vitamin A-containing pigments are present in rhodopsin in the light-sensitive rods of the eye. *Deficiency* leads to **night blindness**. Iodopsins in the cones respond to different colors. In addition to effects in the eye, vitamin A deficiency produces keratosis in other, mainly mucus-secreting cells, and mucosal surfaces are replaced with keratinizing squamous epithelium. Keratosis of the extensor surfaces of the skin is a late manifestation (Fig. 11.2).

TABLE 11.1 FUNCTIONS OF WATER, PROTEINS, CARBOHYDRATES, AND FATS

Foodstuffs	Functions	Effects of deficiency	Effects of excess	Sources
Water	Solvent for cellular changes; medium for ions; transport of nutrients and waste products; regulation of body temperature	Thirst, dryness of tongue, dehydration, anhydremia, high specific gravity of urine, loss of kidney function (acidosis, oliguria, uremia, death)	Abdominal discomfort, headache, cramps (water without salt), intoxication, convulsions, edema, circulatory failure	Water as such; all foods
Proteins	Supply amino acids for growth and repair of tissue cells; solutes for osmotic equilibrium; buffer. Hemoglobin, albumin, nucleoproteins, glycoprotein, and lipoproteins; enzymes, antibodies; protective structures (nails and hair)	Lassitude, abdominal enlargement, edema, depletion of plasma proteins, kwashiorkor (protein malnutrition); marasmus (protein-calorie malnutrition)	Prolonged high protein intake may aggravate renal insufficiency	Milk, eggs, meat, fish, poultry, cheese, soybeans, peas, beans, cereals, nuts, lentils
Carbohydrates	Readily available source of energy, antiketogenic; structure of cells, antibodies, source of stored calories (glycogen and fat), resynthesis of amino acids, roughage	Ketosis if intake is less than 15% of calories or in starvation; underweight if total calories are low	Overweight if total calories are high. Various syndromes due to inborn errors of sugar metabolism	Milk, cereals, fruits, sucrose, syrups, starches, vegetables
Fats	Concentrated source of energy; physical protection for vessels, nerves, organs; insulation against changes in temperature; cell membranes, and nuclei; vehicle for absorption of vitamins (A, D, E, and K); essential fatty acids; appetite appeal; aids satiety (delays emptying time of stomach)	Lack of satiety (craving for fat); underweight; skin changes with intakes very low in linoleic acid	Overweight; abdominal symptoms in familial hyperlipidemia; high cholesterol intakes may be harmful to selected populations	Milk, butter, egg yolk, lard, bacon, meat, fish, cheese, nuts, vegetable oils. Breast milk usually supplies 4–5% of calories as linoleic acid; vegetable oils vary greatly, safflower, corn, soy, and others being especially rich

Hypervitaminosis A

Acute hypervitaminosis A may occur in infants after ingesting 100 000 μg or more. The symptoms include nausea, vomiting, drowsiness, and, in young infants, bulging of the fontanelle. Diplopia, papilledema, cranial nerve palsies, and other symptoms suggestive of brain tumor (pseudotumor cerebri) may also be present. Toxicity has occurred with supplementation during vitamin administration.

Chronic hypervitaminosis A results from ingestion of excessive doses for several weeks or months. An affected child has anorexia, pruritus, and a lack of weight gain. Irritability, limitation of motion, with tender swelling of the bones, alopecia, seborrheic cutaneous lesions, fissuring of the corners of the mouth, increased intracranial pressure and hepatomegaly may develop. Craniotabes and desquamation of the palms and soles are common. Radiographs show hyperostosis affecting several long bones; it is most notable at the middle of the shafts. A history of

excessive ingestion of vitamin A helps to differentiate vitamin A toxicity from cortical hyperostosis. In addition, the serum vitamin A level is elevated.

Keratosis of the skin occurs and is similar to that of deficiency. Proliferation of bone with **hyperostosis** may occur, clinically presenting with bone pain. Proliferation of cells lining the intracranial ventricles results in **hydrocephalus** and pseudotumor cerebri (Fig. 11.3).

Vitamin A is a teratogen. Deficiency and excess, as well as deficiency or excess of retinoids, result in defects in embryogenesis (see Ch. 4).[8] Severe congenital malformations may occur in infants of mothers who consume large amounts of oral retinoids for treatment of acne.

Retinoids are essential for cell differentiation and participate in the **activation of retinoic acid-responsive genes**. Thus, they are regulators for genes responsive to triiodothyronine, calcitriol, and perhaps other hormones.[7]

TABLE 11.2 PHYSICAL AND METABOLIC PROPERTIES AND FOOD SOURCES OF THE VITAMINS

Names and synonyms	Characteristics	Biochemical action	Effects of deficiency	Effects of excess	Sources
Vitamin A: Retinol (vitamin A) is an alcohol of high molecular weight; 1 μg retinol = 3.3 IU vitamin. Provitamin A: The plant pigments α-, β- and α-carotenes and cryptoxanthin; $1/6$ activity of retinol	Fat soluble; heat stable; destroyed by oxidation, drying; bile necessary for absorption; stored in liver, protected by vitamin E	Component of retinal pigments, rhodopsin and iodopsin, for vision in dim light; bone and tooth development, formation and maturation of epithelia	Nyctalopia, photophobia, xerophthalmia, conjunctivitis, keratomalacia leading to blindness; faulty epiphyseal bone formation; defective tooth enamel; keratinization of mucous membranes and skin-retarded growth; impaired resistance to infection	Anorexia, slow growth, drying and cracking of skin, enlargement of liver and spleen, swelling and pain of long bones, bone fragility, increased intracranial pressure, alopecia, carotenemia	Liver, fish-liver oils, whole milk, milk fat products, egg yolk, fortified margarines. Carotenoids from plants: green vegetables, yellow fruits, vegetables
Carotenoids (primarily β-carotene = $1/6$ activity of retinol)	Converted to retinol in liver and intestinal mucosa; absorptive efficacy decreases with increased doses			Carotenemia	Dark green vegetables, yellow fruits and vegetables, tomato
Vitamin B complex: thiamine vitamin B_1: antiberiberi vitamin; aneurin	Water and alcohol soluble; fat insoluble; stable in slightly acid solution; labile to heat, alkali, sulfites	Component of thiamine pyrophosphate carboxylases, which act in various oxidative decarboxylations, including that of pyruvic acid	Beriberi: fatigue, irritability, anorexia, constipation, headache, insomnia, tachycardia, polyneuritis, cardiac failure, edema, elevated pyruvic acid in blood, aphonia	None from oral intake	Liver, meat (especially pork), milk, whole grain or enriched cereals, wheat germ, legumes, nuts
Riboflavin: Vitamin B_2	Sparingly soluble in water; sensitive to light and alkali; stable to heat, oxidation, acid	Constituent of flavoprotein enzymes important in hydrogen transfer reactions; amino acid, fatty acid, and carbohydrate metabolism and cellular respiration; retinal pigment for light adaptation	Ariboflavinosis; photophobia, blurred vision, burning and itching of eyes, corneal vascularization, poor growth, cheilosis	Excess not harmful	Milk, cheese, liver and other organs, meat, eggs, fish, green leafy vegetables, whole or enriched grains
Niacin: Nicotinamide: nicotinic acid; antipellagra vitamin	Water and alcohol soluble; stable to acid, alkali, light, heat, oxidation	Constituent of coenzymes I and II; NAD/NADP cofactors in a number of dehydrogenase systems	Pellagra, multiple B-vitamin deficiency syndrome, diarrhea, dementia, dermatitis	Nicotinic acid (not the amide) is vasodilator; skin flushing and itching, hepatopathy	Meat, fish, poultry, liver, whole grain and enriched cereals, green vegetables, peanuts
Pantothenic acid	Water soluble, heat stable	Component of CoA, many enzymatic reactions	Observed only with use of antagonists, depression, fatigue, hypotension, muscle weakness, abdominal pain	Unknown	Organ metas, yeast, egg yolk, fresh vegetables, whole grains, legumes
Folacin (folic acid): Group of related compounds containing pteridine ring, para-amino	Slightly soluble in water; labile to heat, light, acid	Concerned with formation and metabolism of one-carbon units;	Megaloblastic anemia (infancy, pregnancy): usually secondary to malabsorption disease;	Toxicity unknown	Liver, green vegetables, nuts, cereals, cheese, fruits, yeast, beans, peas

TABLE 11.2 PHYSICAL AND METABOLIC PROPERTIES AND FOOD SOURCES OF THE VITAMINS (*CONT'D*)

Names and synonyms	Characteristics	Biochemical action	Effects of deficiency	Effects of excess	Sources
benzoic acid, and glutamic acid: pteroylglutamic acid (PGA)		participates in synthesis of purines, pyrimidines, nucleoproteins, and methyl groups	glossitis, pharyngeal ulcers, impaired immunity, irritability, paranoid behavior		
Cobalamin: Vitamin B_{12}	Slightly soluble in water; stable to heat in neutral solution; labile in acid or alkaline destroyed by light	Transfer of one-carbon units in purine and labile-methyl group metabolism; essential for maturation of red blood cells in bone marrow; metabolism of nervous tissue; adenosyl-cobalamin is coenzyme for methylmalonyl CoA mutase	Juvenile pernicious anemia, due to defect in absorption rather than to dietary lack; also secondary to gastrectomy, celiac disease, inflammatory lesions of small bowel, long-term drug therapy (para-aminosalicylic acid, neomycin); methylmalonic aciduria homocystinuria	Unknown	Muscle and organ meats, fish, eggs, milk, cheese
Biotin	Crystallized from yeast; soluble in water	Coenzyme carboxylases; involved in CO_2 transfer	Dermatitis, seborrhea; inactivated by avidin in raw egg white	None known	Yeast, animal products; synthesized in intestine
Vitamin B_6 active forms: pyridoxine, pyridoxal, pyridoxamine	Water soluble; destroyed by UV light and by heat	Constituent of coenzymes for decarboxylation, transamination, transsulfuration; fatty acid metabolism	Irritability, convulsions, hypochromic anemia; peripheral neuritis in patients receiving isoniazid; oxaluria	Sensory neuropathy	Meat, liver, kidney, whole grains, soybeans, nuts, fish, poultry, green vegetables
Vitamin C: Ascorbic acid: antiscorbutic vitamin	Water soluble; easily oxidized, accelerated by heat, light, alkali, oxidative enzymes, traces of copper or iron	Integrity and maintenance of intercellular material; facilitates absorption of iron and conversion of folic acid to folinic acid; metabolism of tyrosine and phenylalanine, activity of succinic dehydrogenase and serum phosphatase in infants, not in adults	Scurvy and poor wound healing	Oxaluria (see also Ch. 17 and discussion of hyperoxaluria), oxalosis	Citrus fruits, tomatoes, berries, cantaloupe, cabbage, green vegetables. Cooking has destructive effect
Vitamin D: Group of sterols having similar physiologic activity; D_2-calciferol is activated ergosterol: D_3 is activated 7-dehydrocholesterol in skin; 1 μg = 40 IU vitamin D	Fat soluble, stable to heat, acid, alkali, and oxidation; bile necessary for absorption. Prohormone for 25-OH cholecalciferol	Regulates absorption and deposition of calcium and phosphorus, by affecting permeability of intestinal membrane; regulates level of serum alkaline phosphatase, which is believed to be concerned with calcium phosphate deposition in bones and teeth	Rickets (high serum phosphatase level appears before bone deformities); infantile tetany, poor growth, osteomalacia	Wide variation in tolerance; over 500 μg/24 hr toxic; when continued for weeks; prolonged administration of 45 μg/24 hr may be toxic; nausea, diarrhea, weight loss, polyuria, nocturia, calcification of soft tissues, including heart, renal tubules, blood vessels, bronchi, stomach	Vitamin D-fortified milk and margarine, fish-liver oils, exposure to sunlight or other UV sources

TABLE 11.2 PHYSICAL AND METABOLIC PROPERTIES AND FOOD SOURCES OF THE VITAMINS (*CONT'D*)

Names and synonyms	Characteristics	Biochemical action	Effects of deficiency	Effects of excess	Sources
Vitamin E: Group of related chemical compounds – tocopherols – with similar biologic activities	Fat soluble; unstable to UV light, alkali, readily oxidized by oxygen, iron, rancid fats	Minimizes oxidation of carotene, vitamin A, and linoleic acid; stabilizes membranes	Requirements related to polyunsaturated fat intake; red blood cell hemolysis in premature infants, loss of neural integrity	Unknown	Germ oils of various seeds, green leafy vegetables, nuts, legumes
Vitamin K: Group of naphthoquinones with similar biologic activities; K_1 is phytoquinone	Natural compounds are fat soluble; stable to heat and reducing agents; labile to oxidizing agents, strong acids, alkali, light; bile salts necessary for intestinal absorption	Prothrombin formation; coagulation factors II, VII, IX, X, and osteocalcin are K dependent, proteins C, S, Z	Hemorrhagic manifestations; bone metabolism	Not established; analogues may produce hyperbilirubinemia in premature infants	Green leafy vegetables, pork liver. Widely distributed

UV, ultraviolet.

TABLE 11.3 PHYSIOLOGY AND SOURCES OF NUTRITIONALLY IMPORTANT MINERALS

Mineral	Function and metabolism	Effects of deficiency	Effects of excess	Sources
Calcium	Structure of bone and teeth, muscle contraction, nerve irritability, coagulation of blood, cardiac action, production of milk	Poor mineralization of bones and teeth; osteomalacia; osteoporosis, tetany; rickets; impairment of growth	Unknown (dietary); heart block and renal stones (parenteral)	Milk, cheese, green leafy vegetables, canned salmon, clams, oysters
Chloride	Osmotic pressure; acid–base balance; HCl in gastric juice. Readily absorbed; about 92% of intake is excreted, mainly in urine, some in feces and sweat; comprises about $2/3$ of blood plasma anions; blood serum level, 99–106 mEq/L; in intracellular and extra cellular fluids; parallels sodium intake and output	Hypochloremic alkalosis may occur with prolonged vomiting or excessive sweating, with parenteral administration of glucose without saline, with excessive ACTH therapy, and with congenital alkalosis	Unknown	Table salt, meat, milk, eggs
Chromium	Glycemia regulation and insulin metabolism	Diabetes in animals	None known	Yeast
Cobalt	Component of vitamin B_{12} (cobalamin) molecule and of erythropoietin	Hypothyroidism	Cardiomyopathy; medicinally it may be goitrogenic or may produce cardiomyopathy	Widely distributed
Copper	Essential for production of red blood cells; transferrin hemoglobin formation; absorption of iron, activities of tyrosinase, catalase, uricase, cytochrome C oxidase, Δ-aminolevulinic acid dehydrase, lysyl oxidase. Absorbed with sulfur-rich proteins; transported bound to "α-2 globulin as ceruloplasmin; present in	May be cause of refractory anemia, osteoporosis, neutropenia, depigmentation and delayed bone age, bone infarctions, pseudoparalysis ataxia; increased serum, cholesterol	Cirrhosis, gastritis, hemolysis	Liver, oysters, meats, fish, whole grains, nuts, legumes

TABLE 11.3 PHYSIOLOGY AND SOURCES OF NUTRITIONALLY IMPORTANT MINERALS (*CONT'D*)

Mineral	Function and metabolism	Effects of deficiency	Effects of excess	Sources
	erythrocytes in a labile form and the more stable hemocuprein; highest concentration in liver and central nervous system (cerebrocuprein); excreted mainly via intestinal wall and bile; deranged metabolism in Wilson disease (hepatolenticular degeneration) and Menkes syndrome			
Fluorine	Tooth and bone structure; retained when intake is above 0.6 mg/day; excreted in urine and sweat; deposited in bones as fluorapatite (dynamic equilibrium)	Tendency to dental caries	Fluorosis: mottling of teeth with intake of more than 4–8 mg/24 hr	Water, seafood, plant and animal foods (dependent on content in soil and water)
Iodine	Constituent of thyroxine (T_4) and triiodothyronine (T_3); readily absorbed from intestine; circulates as inorganic and organic iodide; selectively concentrated about 25:1 in thyroid gland, quickly iodized and incorporated into thyroglobulin; proteolytic enzymes release T_4 and T_3 into blood. Excretion mainly in urine. Antithyroid compounds: goitrins and brassicae; certain drugs interfere with iodine metabolism	Simple goiter, endemic cretinism	Not harmful (less than 1 mg/24 hr); medicinally may cause goiter	Iodized salt, seafood, food grown in non-goitrous areas
Iron	Structure of hemoglobin and myoglobin for O_2 and CO_2 transport; oxidative enzymes; cytochrome C and catalase. Absorbed in ferrous form according to body need, aided by gastric juice and ascorbic acid; hindered by fiber, phytic acid, steatorrhea. Transported in plasma in ferric state bound to transferrin; stored in liver, spleen, bone marrow, and kidney as ferritin and hemosiderin; conserved and reused; minimal losses in urine and sweat; about 90% of intake excreted in stool	Anemia; hypochromic, microcytic, growth failure, hyperactivity (?)	Hemosiderosis in Bantu people of Africa due to low phosphorus and high iron contents of diet. Poisoning by medicinal iron	Liver, meat, egg yolk, green vegetables, whole grains, legumes, nuts
Magnesium	Structure of bones and teeth; activation of enzymes in carbohydrate metabolism;	Occurs in malabsorption and deficiency states; diabetes, may be expressed clinically as	None (dietary); toxicity from intravenous medication	Cereals, legumes, nuts, meat, milk

TABLE 11.3 PHYSIOLOGY AND SOURCES OF NUTRITIONALLY IMPORTANT MINERALS (*CONT'D*)

Mineral	Function and metabolism	Effects of deficiency	Effects of excess	Sources
	muscle and nerve irritability, important intracellular cation, essential to metabolic processes. Principal cation of soft tissue; absorption from small intestine varies with intake; some urinary excretion but excellent renal conservation; antagonist to calcium cation	tetany; associated frequently with hypocalcemia; hypokalemia		
Molybdenum	Component of enzymes; xanthine oxidase for conversion to uric acid and mobilization of ferritin iron in liver, liver aldehyde oxidase. Readily absorbed from intestine; excreted chiefly in urine, some in bile	Not observed in humans	Not established	Legumes, grains, dark-green leafy vegetables, animal organs
Phosphorus	Constituent of bones and teeth; structure of nucleus and cytoplasm of all cells; acid–base balance; energy transformations and transmission of nerve impulses; metabolism of carbohydrate, protein, and fat. About 70% of intake absorbed as free phosphates; vitamin D and parathormone implicated in intestinal absorption and kidney retention; excreted in urine and feces; occurs in blood as phospholipids, organic esters, and inorganic phosphates; inorganic phosphates in blood serum of infants and children, 4–7 mg/dL; ratio of inorganic to organic phosphates in whole blood is about 1:20	Rickets may develop in rapidly growing, very low birth weight babies with low intakes of both P and Ca; muscle weakness	Possibility of tetany during recovery from rickets or in newborn on formula with low Ca:P (1:1) ratio	Milk, milk products, egg yolk, fresh foods, legumes, nuts, whole grains
Potassium	Muscle contraction; nerve impulse conduction; intracellular osmotic pressure and fluid balance; heart rhythm; primarily intracellular; excretion 80% in urine, some in sweat and feces; about 8% retained by growing child; blood serum level 4.0–5.6 mEq/L	In starvation or in such pathologic conditions as diarrhea, diabetic acidosis, ACTH excess; muscle weakness, anorexia, nausea, abdominal distention, nervous irritability, drowsiness, confusion, tachycardia; deficiency exaggerates effects of sodium	Heart block at serum levels of 10 mEq/L; important in Addison disease, renal failure, or administration of vitamin K-containing salts	All foods

TABLE 11.3 PHYSIOLOGY AND SOURCES OF NUTRITIONALLY IMPORTANT MINERALS (*CONT'D*)

Mineral	Function and metabolism	Effects of deficiency	Effects of excess	Sources
Selenium	Cofactor of glutathione peroxidase in tissue respiration	Keshan cardiomyopathy, arthritis (?) Keshan cardiovascular disease, myositis	Alopecia, nail abnormalities, garlic odor to breath	Vegetables, meat
Sodium	Osmotic pressure; acid–base balance; water balance; muscle and nerve irritability. Readily absorbed from intestine; excreted chiefly in urine (98%); parallels chloride intake; renal excretion controlled by adrenocortical hormone; extracellular cation, but small amount in muscle and cartilage; blood serum level 135–145 mEq/L	Nausea, diarrhea, muscle cramps, dehydration, hypotension	Edema if inadequate excretion or excessive parenteral fluids	Table salt, flesh foods, milk, eggs, sodium compounds as baking soda and powder, glutamate, seasonings, and preservatives
Sulfur	Constituent of cellular protein; cocarboxylase; melanin; mucopolysaccharides, vitreous humor, synovial fluid, connective tissues, cartilage, heparin, insulin; metabolism of nerve tissue; detoxification mechanisms; SH (sulfur-hydrogen) group in coenzyme A, cystathionine, and glutathione. Only sources utilized are cystine and methionine; inorganic forms unavailable to body; excreted as inorganic sulfate or ethereal sulfate via urine and bile	Not known; growth failure from protein deficiency may be due in part to deficiency of sulfur-containing amino acids	Not harmful; excreted in urine as sulfates	Protein foods contain about 1%
Zinc	Constituent of several enzymes; carbonic anhydrase (in erythrocytes) essential for CO_2 exchange; carboxypeptidase of intestine for hydrolysis of protein; dehydrogenase of liver. Found in liver and organs, muscles, bones, red and white blood cells; higher tissue concentration in young subjects; excreted chiefly from intestine; competes with copper	Dwarfism, iron deficiency anemia, hepatosplenomegaly, hyperpigmentation and hypogonadism, acrodermatitis enteropathica, depression of immunocompetence, poor wound healing	Gastrointestinal upsets (from galvanized iron cooking utensils); copper deficiency; decreased high-density lipoprotein	Meat, grain, nuts, cheese

ACTH, adrenocorticotropic hormone.

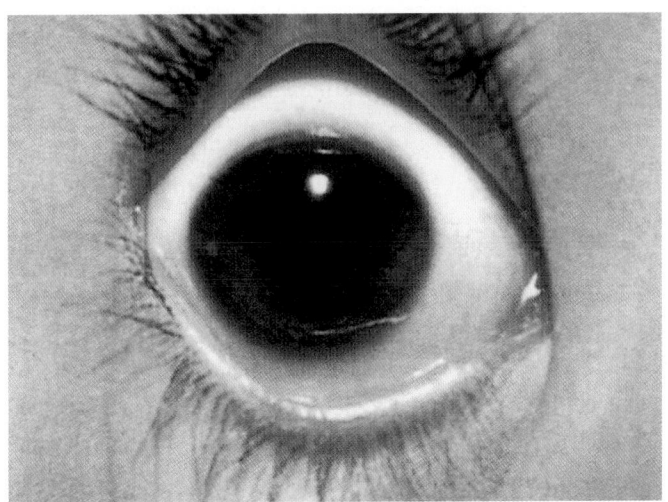

FIGURE 11.1 Early conjunctival xerosis. Dryness and unwettability of the conjunctival surface are characteristic of this early stage of vitamin A deficiency. Wrinkling and increased pigmentation may also be present, as in this case, but are not on their own an indication of vitamin A deficiency. Plasma vitamin A was 9 µg/100 mL (normal 20–50 µg/100 mL). Evidence of night blindness can be elicited by careful history taking and observation of the behavior of the young child at dusk, even at this early stage. (From McLaren DS, ed. A colour atlas and text of diet-related disorders, 2nd edn. London: Wolfe; 1992; with permission.)

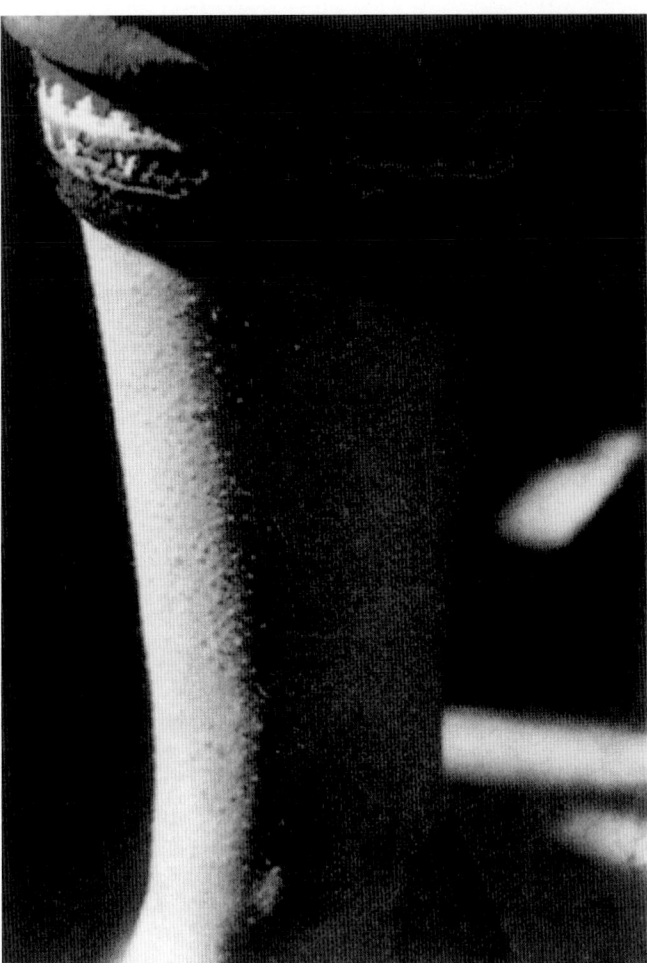

FIGURE 11.2 Perifollicular hyperkeratosis. The shin is a common site. (From McLaren DS, ed. A colour atlas and text of diet-related disorders, 2nd edn. London: Wolfe; 1992; with permission.)

Vitamin A also plays a role in keratinization, cornification, bone metabolism, placental development, growth, spermatogenesis, and mucus formation. Characteristic changes of deficiency in epithelium include proliferation of basal cells, hyperkeratosis, and the formation of stratified, cornified squamous epithelium. Epithelial changes in the respiratory system may result in bronchiolar obstruction. Squamous metaplasia of the renal pelves, ureters, urinary bladder, enamel organs, and pancreatic and salivary ducts may lead to an increase in infections in these areas.

Retinoic acid, one of the metabolic products of vitamin A, is used to treat severe acne. Some evidence suggests that vitamin A or one of its precursors, β carotene, may inhibit the development of certain cancers.[9]

Children not deficient in vitamin A were found to benefit, with lower morbidity and mortality, when given vitamin A during infection with measles.[10] The activity of T lymphocytes is affected by vitamin A;[11] other aspects of immunity may be enhanced.

The B vitamins

Thiamine (vitamin B₁)

Thiamine is water soluble and as thiamine pyrophosphate, is the coenzyme for the decarboxylation of pyruvate and α-ketoglutaric acid. It is essential for carbohydrate metabolism. It also is required for the synthesis of acetylcholine, and deficiency results in impaired nerve conduction. It is the coenzyme in transketolation and in decarboxylation of α-keto acids and participates in the hexose monophosphate shunt that generates nicotinamide adenine dinucleotide phosphate and pentose.

Thiamine deficiency Early manifestations of thiamine deficiency include fatigue, apathy, irritability, depression, drowsiness, poor mental concentration, anorexia, nausea, and abdominal discomfort. Signs of progression include peripheral neuritis with tingling, burning, and paresthesias of the toes and feet, decreased deep tendon reflexes, loss of vibration sense, tenderness and cramping of leg muscles, congestive heart failure, and psychic disturbances. Patients may have ptosis of the eyelids and atrophy of the optic nerve. Hoarseness or aphonia caused by paralysis of the laryngeal nerve is a characteristic sign. Muscle atrophy and tenderness of nerve trunks are followed by ataxia, loss of coordination, and loss of deep sensation. Paralysis occurs in adults but is uncommon in children. Later signs include increased intracranial pressure, meningismus, and coma.

The full-blown deficiency state is beriberi. Two forms exist: wet beriberi and dry beriberi. The child with wet beriberi is

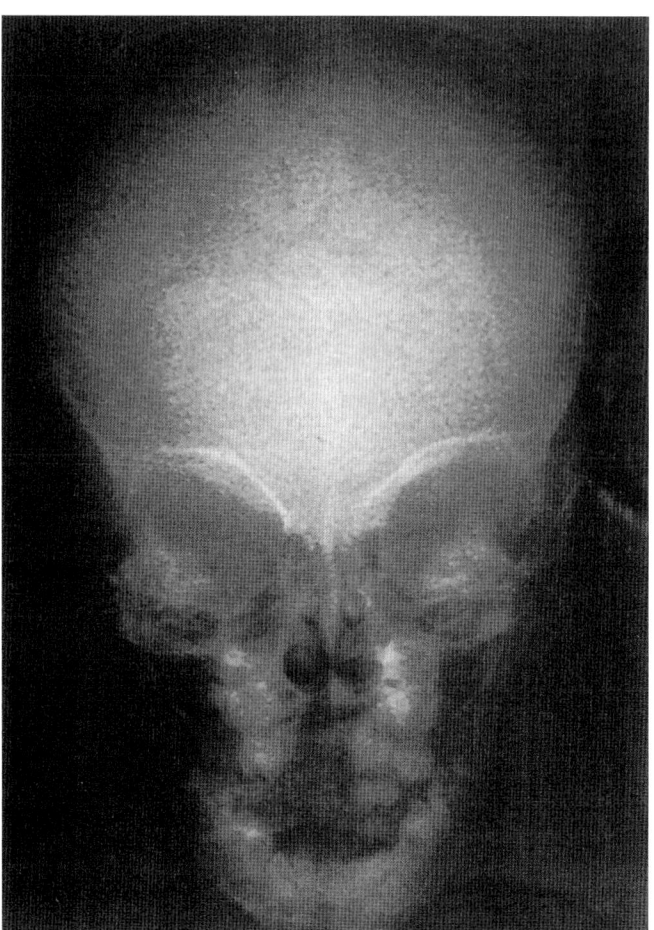

FIGURE 11.3 Skull in hypervitaminosis. Frontal view of a 2-year-old girl showing wide sagittal and coronal sutures. (From McLaren DS, ed. A colour atlas and text of diet-related disorders, 2nd edn. London: Wolfe; 1992; with permission.)

undernourished, pale, edematous with dyspnea, vomiting and tachycardia, and has a waxy skin; the urine often contains albumin and casts. The child with dry beriberi appears plump but is pale, flabby, and listless with dyspnea, tachycardia, and hepatomegaly.

Death from thiamine deficiency usually is secondary to cardiac involvement. The initial signs are cyanosis and dyspnea, but tachycardia, enlargement of the liver, loss of consciousness, and convulsions may develop rapidly. The heart, especially the right side, is enlarged. The electrocardiogram shows an increased QT interval, inverted T waves, and low voltage. These changes as well as the cardiomegaly rapidly revert to normal with treatment, but, without prompt treatment, cardiac failure can develop rapidly and result in death.

Older children develop **meningismus and opisthotonos**. **Seizures** may be present. Wernicke-Korsakoff syndrome is cerebral beriberi and responds to thiamine administration. At autopsy, emaciation, muscle atrophy, edema, and dilation of the heart are found. **Fatty degeneration of myocardial fibers** is noted. Myelin degeneration is found in dry beriberi.

Excess thiamine has no known toxicity.

Diagnosis of thiamine deficiency Low red blood cell transketolase and high blood or urinary glyoxylate levels are useful diagnostic indicators. Measurement of urinary thiamine excretion or urinary excretion of its metabolites, thiaxole or pyrimidine, after an oral loading dose of thiamine may help to identify the deficiency state. Clinical response to administration of thiamine is the best test for thiamine deficiency.

Riboflavin (vitamin B₂)

Riboflavin is a coenzyme for oxidation–reduction reactions as flavin adenine dinucleotide (FAD) and similar flavoproteins. Disease due to riboflavin deficiency is rarely recognized. Deficiency may cause **sore tongue, cheilosis, angular stomatitis**, and occasionally **seborrheic dermatitis**. Superficial keratitis of the conjunctiva may occur, with photophobia, lacrimation, corneal vascularization and seborrheic dermatitis. A normocytic, normochromic anemia with bone marrow hypoplasia is common.

Cheilosis begins with pallor at the angles of the mouth and progresses to thinning and maceration of the epithelium. Superficial fissures, often covered by yellow crusts, develop in the angles of the mouth, and extend radially into the skin for distances of 1–2 cm. With glossitis, the tongue is smooth with loss of papillary structure.

Useful diagnostic tests include urinary excretion of riboflavin below 30 μg/24 hr and low levels of erythrocyte glutathione reductase, a flavoprotein requiring FAD.

Deficiency is usually prevented by a diet that contains adequate amounts of milk, eggs, leafy vegetables, and lean meats.

Niacin

Niacin as nicotine adenine dinucleotide (NAD) and its phosphate (NADP) are essential in biosynthesis and energy generation. At least 200 enzymes require NAD or NADP. Dietary tryptophan can be converted to niacin.

Deficiency results in **pellagra** (pelis, skin; agra, rough), which manifests with diarrhea, dermatitis, dementia, and finally death. The dermatitis appears first as symmetric areas of erythema on exposed surfaces resembling sunburn. Edema and degeneration of the collagen of the dermis occur. The papillary vessels are engorged in the dermis with perivascular infiltration. The **epidermis is hyperkeratotic** and becomes atrophic later. Perivascular changes similar to those in the skin occur in the buccal mucous membranes, tongue, and vagina. **Secondary infections** are common. The wall of the colon is thickened with edema and lymphocytic infiltration, and the mucosa is atrophic. **Demyelinization** occurs in the brain and spinal cord, and degeneration of ganglion cells may be patchy. Sunlight aggravates the skin manifestations.

The cutaneous lesions may be preceded by or accompanied by stomatitis, glossitis, vomiting, and/or diarrhea. Swelling and redness of the tip of the tongue and its lateral margins is often followed by intense redness, even ulceration, of the entire tongue and papillae.

Nervous symptoms include depression, disorientation, insomnia, and delirium.

The classic symptoms of pellagra are usually not well developed in infants but anorexia, irritability, anxiety, and apathy are common. They may also have sore tongues and lips and their skin is usually dry and scaly. Diarrhea and constipation may alternate, and a moderate secondary anemia may occur.

Pellagra occurs chiefly in countries where corn, a poor source of tryptophan, is a basic foodstuff.

Pharmacologic doses of niacin have been used to lower serum cholesterol. Excessive administration results in **flushing of the skin, hyperuricemia**, cholestatic jaundice and **liver failure**.

Pyridoxine (vitamin B₆)

Pyridoxine (vitamin B_6)

The various forms of pyridoxine are constituents of coenzymes for transamination and of several carboxylases and decarboxylases.

Vitamin B_6 is converted to pyridoxal-5-phosphate (or pyridoxamine-5-phosphate).

Pyridoxal phosphate is the coenzyme for both glutamic decarboxylase and aminobutyric acid transaminase, each of which is necessary for normal brain metabolism. Pyridoxine is required for active transport of amino acids across cell membranes, chelation of metals, and synthesis of arachidonic and docosahexaenoic acids from linoleic and linolenic acids, respectively. Prolonged heat processing of milk and cereal destroys it. Diseases with fat malabsorption may contribute to vitamin B_6 deficiency.

Pyridoxine antagonists (e.g., isoniazid used in the treatment of tuberculosis), pregnancy, and drugs such as penicillamine, hydralazine, and the oral progesterone–estrogen contraceptives increase the requirements for pyridoxine.

Deficiency results in a **microcytic hypochromic** and occasionally **sideroblastic anemia**. It may also result in **polyneuritis** or seizures, and in excretion of excess xanthurenic acid. The vitamin is required for the conversion of tryptophan to niacin.

Four clinical disturbances caused by vitamin B_6 deficiency have been described in humans: convulsions in infants, peripheral neuritis, dermatitis, and anemia.

Infants fed a formula deficient in vitamin B_6 for 1–6 months exhibit irritability and generalized seizures. Gastrointestinal distress and an aggravated startle response also are common. Skin lesions include cheilosis, glossitis, and seborrhea around the eyes and nose, and mouth. Microcytic anemia, oxaluria, oxalic acid bladder stones, hyperglycinemia, lymphopenia, decreased antibody formation, and infections also occur.

Convulsions due to vitamin B_6 dependence may occur within several hours to as long as 6 months after birth. In many cases, the mother received large doses of pyridoxine during pregnancy for control of emesis.

In vitamin B_6-dependent anemia, the red blood cells are microcytic and hypochromic. Patients have elevated serum iron concentrations, saturation of iron-binding protein, hemosiderin deposits in bone marrow and liver, and failure of iron utilization for hemoglobin synthesis.

Excessive pyridoxine has resulted in neuropathy.

Folic acid

Folic acid

As tetrahydrofolic acid, folate is essential for DNA synthesis and participates in synthesis of purines, pyrimidines, and methylation reactions.[12] *Deficiency* results in **megaloblastic anemia** and impaired cellular immunity. Symptoms and signs may include a smooth, red tongue and ulceration of the buccal and adjoining mucosa.

Neural tube defects are decreased in infants born of mothers who have received supplemental folate in the preconception and early postconception periods[13] (see Ch. 4).

Vitamin B₁₂ (Cobalamin)

Vitamin B_{12} (Cobalamin)

Vitamin B_{12}, like folic acid, is necessary for DNA synthesis. Deficiency results in **megaloblastic anemia, neurologic deterioration, pernicious anemia, combined system disease, and defective branched-chain amino acid metabolism, with an increase in methylmalonic acid in serum and urine**.[14]

Biotin

Biotin is essential as a coenzyme for many decarboxylases. Biotin deficiency is rare, but when it occurs it manifests predominantly as a **non-specific dermatitis or alopecia**.

Deficiency may occur in those consuming the biotin antagonist avidin, found in raw egg white. Deficiency also has been described in infants and children receiving parenteral nutrition exclusively and in infants whose mothers are biotin deficient.

Brawny dermatitis, oroficial lesions, alopecia, somnolence, hallucinations, hypotonia, and hyperesthesia with accumulation of organic acids are common manifestations of deficiency. Other neurologic signs may occur.

Biotin deficiency is suggested by organic aciduria, particularly propionic and dicarboxylic acids. Response of clinical and biochemical abnormalities to biotin administration is confirmatory.

Vitamin C (Ascorbic acid)

Vitamin C is a water-soluble reducing substance important in collagen metabolism. It facilitates iron absorption and transport and participates in tyrosine metabolism.

Deficiency results in **scurvy**. Scorbutic patients demonstrate capillary fragility with petechial bleeding, especially in skin, gums, and periosteum. Fibroblasts and osteoblasts fail to produce intracellular matrix and osteoid. **Fragility of capillary walls** and decreased strength of periosteal tissue cause subperiosteal hemorrhage (Fig. 11.4). Organization of the hemorrhage leads to deposition of new periosteal bone outside the cortical bone (Fig 11.5). These areas are exquisitely tender and painful.

Changes in the gums are most noticeable after teeth have erupted. These include bluish-purple, spongy swellings of

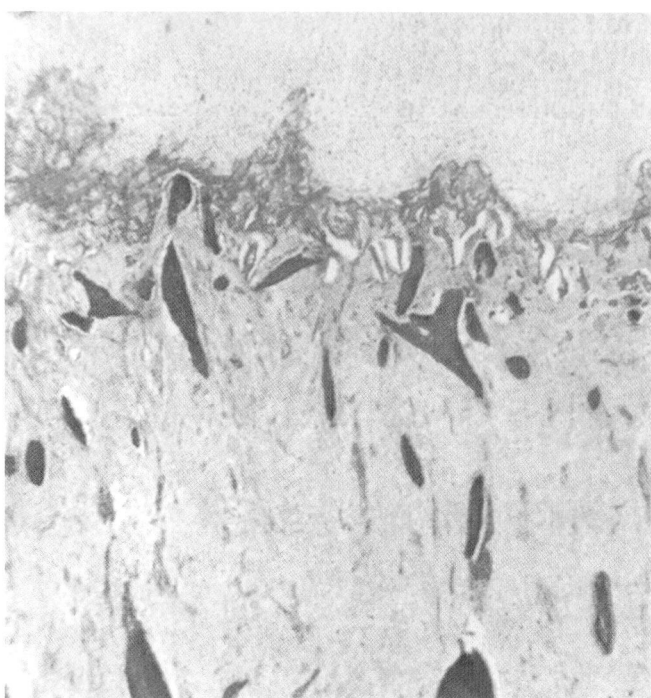

FIGURE 11.4 Bone in scurvy. Defective formation of mesenchymal tissue results from failure of deposition of intercellular ground substance by fibroblasts. In the shafts of long bones, osteoid is not deposited by osteoblasts, the cortex is thin, trabeculae are diminished in size, and hemorrhages occur under the periosteum. (From McLaren DS, ed. A colour atlas and text of diet-related disorders, 2nd edn. London: Wolfe; 1992; with permission.)

the mucous membrane, especially over the upper incisors. A 'rosary' at the costochondral junctions and depression of the sternum are other typical features. The angulation of scorbutic beads is usually sharper than that of a rachitic rosary.

Petechial hemorrhages are often present in the skin and mucous membranes. Hematuria, melena and orbital or subdural hemorrhages may occur. Low-grade fever is usually present. Anemia, if present, may reflect inability to utilize iron or impaired folic acid metabolism. Wound healing is slow, and healed wounds often break down. Swollen joints and follicular hyperkeratosis are features.

In infants with vitamin C deficiency, cartilage and osteoblasts proliferate normally but fail to produce osteoid (Fig. 11.6), in which calcium salts are normally deposited for conversion to bone. Trabeculae of the spongiosa are thin and brittle, and multiple infarctions occur, especially at the lateral borders of the metaphyses.

Excessive vitamin C may result in **oxaluria** in sensitive individuals. Gastritis occurs with excessive vitamin C ingestion.

Vitamin D

Vitamin D_2 and vitamin D_3 are hydroxylated in the kidney to 25-OH-cholecalciferol and, subsequently, in the liver to

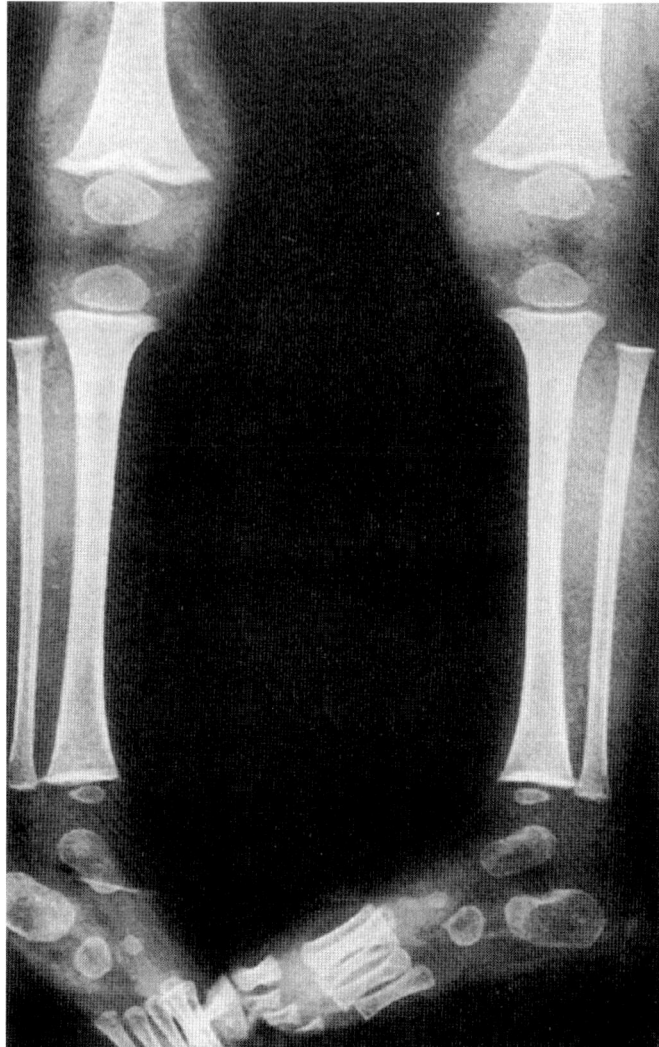

FIGURE 11.5 Bones in active scurvy. The earliest radiographic changes appear at the sites of most active bone growth: sternal ends of the ribs, distal end of the femur, proximal end of the humerus, both ends of the tibia and fibula, and distal ends of the radius and ulna. Several characteristic signs are shown here. A zone of rarefaction immediately shaftward of the zone of provisional calcification gives rise to the 'corner fracture' sign. Atrophy of the trabecular structure and blurring of trabecular markings cause the bone to have a 'ground-glass' appearance. Widening of the zone of provisional calcification causes a dense shadow at the end of the shaft (the white line of Frankel). It also occurs at the periphery of the centers of ossification ('halo' epiphysis or 'penciled effect'). (From McLaren DS, ed. A colour atlas and text of diet-related disorders, 2nd edn. London: Wolfe; 1992; with permission.)

1,25-dihydroxycholecalciferol, which functions as a hormone.[15] Receptors for 1,25-dihydroxycholecalciferol play primary roles in facilitation of intestinal absorption of calcium and phosphorus, renal reabsorption of phosphorus, and have a direct effect on bone deposition. With parathormone and calcitonin, 1,25-dihydroxycholecalciferol plays a major role in calcium and phosphorus homeostasis of both body fluids and tissues.

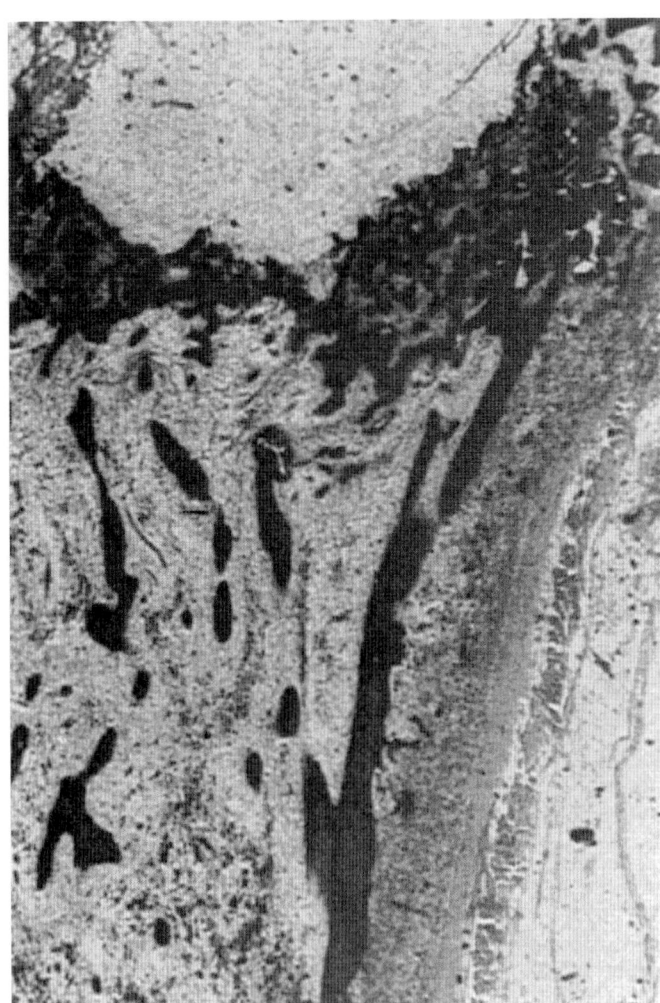

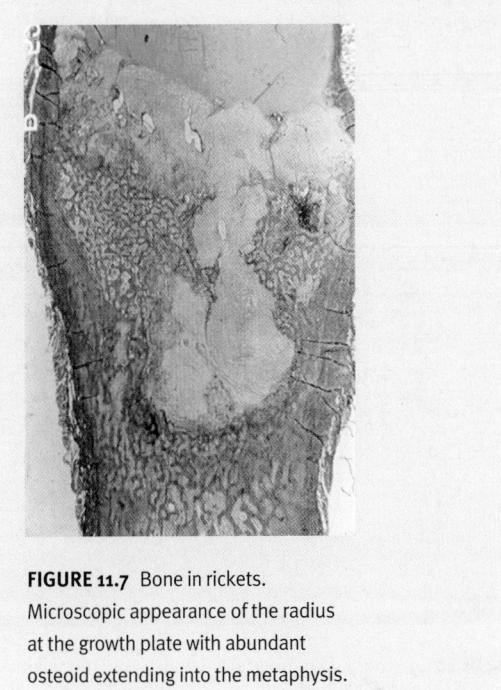

FIGURE 11.7 Bone in rickets. Microscopic appearance of the radius at the growth plate with abundant osteoid extending into the metaphysis.

FIGURE 11.6 Scurvy. Periosteum is elevated from the cortical bone by recent hemorrhage. The marrow spaces are filled with fibrous tissue. There are many fractures of the thin trabeculae next to the epiphyseal plate.

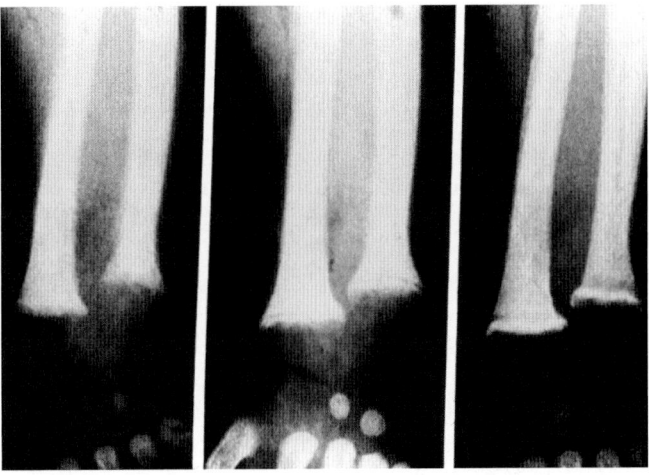

Deficiency results in **rickets** in infants and children, and osteomalacia in non-growing adults with failure to mineralize growing bone or osteoid tissue. Exposure of the skin to sunlight converts cholesterol to active metabolites. Dietary vitamin D is obtained from fish. Low serum calcium levels stimulate parathormone secretion with phosphaturia. Low serum calcium and phosphate levels result in inadequate calcification of cartilage and osteoid in spongiosa and cortical bone (Fig. 11.7). Large masses of uncalcified or irregularly calcified mature cartilage persist in the metaphyseal zone and cause **widening of the metaphyses** (Fig. 11.8). Infarctions are often present. Low ionized extracellular calcium leads to muscle excitation and **hypocalcemic tetany**.

Rickets usually appears towards the end of the first year of life. In infants, gross deformities may be present in the skull (craniotabes) (Fig. 11.9) with **frontal bossing**, and in the ribs with enlargement of the costochondral junctions (rachitic

FIGURE 11.8 There is a failure in deposition of inorganic salts in the matrix of epiphyseal cartilage between rows of hypertrophied cartilage cells, which are not destroyed and pile up irregularly to many times their normal thickness. This gives rise to the bulky mass evident on X-ray examination. This zone is easily compressed, deformed, or displaced. There may be excessive bone destruction as the result of increased parathyroid activity, and the shafts readily bend under pressure. (McLaren DS, ed. A colour atlas and text of diet-related disorders, 2nd edn. London: Wolfe; 1992; with permission.)

rosary). Later, enlargement occurs at the wrist (Fig. 11.10) and ankle. **Bowing of the legs** and pelvic deformity occur after the child begins to walk and bears weight on the skeleton. The sternum with its adjacent cartilage projects forward causing the *pigeon breast* deformity and a horizontal depression, Harrison's groove,

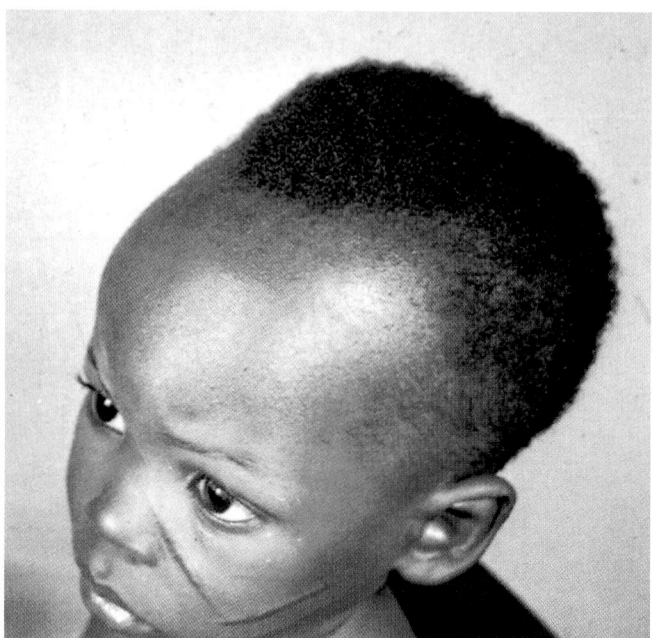

FIGURE 11.9 The skull in rickets. In infancy, the frontal bones are prominent and bossed. The fontanelles are delayed in closing. The skull is soft to the touch and closely resembles pressure on a table tennis (ping-pong) ball; the bone depresses, then comes out again with exactly the same sensation. This is known as craniotabes. It is physiologic at the suture lines and indicative of rickets only when it also occurs away from the suture lines. (From McLaren DS, ed. A colour atlas and text of diet-related disorders, 2nd edn. London: Wolfe; 1992; with permission.)

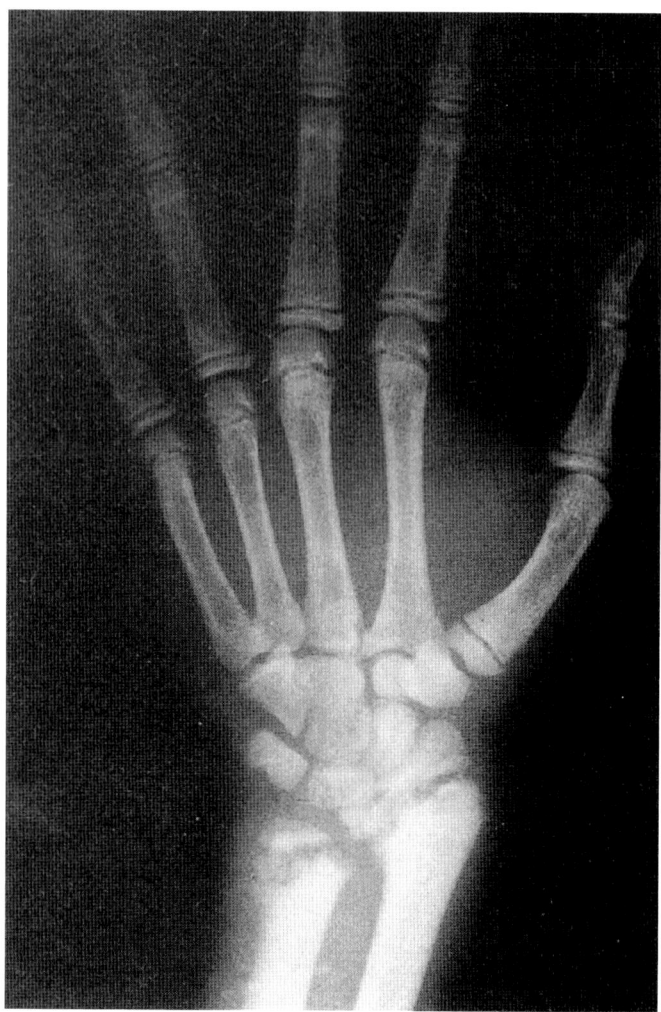

FIGURE 11.10 Rickets. X-ray film showing fragmentation and fraying of the epiphyses of the radius and ulna.

develops along the lower border of the ribs. Eruption of the temporary teeth is delayed and there may be defects of the enamel.

Diagnosis

The serum calcium level of children with rickets may be normal or low, but the serum phosphorus level almost always is less than 4 mg/dL. The serum alkaline phosphatase level and the urinary cyclic AMP level are elevated. Serum 25-hydroxycholecalciferol is low.

Vitamin D is transported bound to an α-globulin, D-binding protein, and is stored mainly in adipose tissue.[15]

These findings of vitamin D deficiency include a generalized aminoaciduria, a low bone citrate level with elevated urinary citrate excretion, impaired renal acidification, phosphaturia, and occasionally, glucosuria. The parathyroid glands hypertrophy. The diagnosis of rickets is based on a history of inadequate intake of vitamin D or inadequate exposure to sunlight and the characteristic clinical signs of the condition. It is confirmed chemically and by radiographic examination.

Early changes of rickets are seen radiographically at the ends of long bones, but evidence of demineralization in the shafts also is present. Non-vitamin-D dependent rickets due to low phosphate may occur.

Ingestion of excessive vitamin D is toxic and results in **hypercalcemia, metastatic calcification, growth failure,** **mental retardation, and renal failure** (Fig. 11.11). Symptoms which develop after 1–3 months of excessive intake include hypotonia, anorexia, irritability, constipation, polydipsia, polyuria, and pallor. Hypercalcemia and hypercalciuria are notable. Aortic valvular stenosis, vomiting, hypertension, retinopathy, and clouding of the cornea and conjunctiva may occur. Proteinuria may be present and, if excessive intake continues, renal damage and metastatic calcification occur. Radiographs of the long bones reveal metastatic calcification and generalized osteopetrosis. Vitamin D excess is **teratogenic**.

Clinical entities that interfere with vitamin D absorption or metabolic conversion include conditions such as steatorrhea, hepatic and renal diseases, or conditions that disrupt calcium and phosphorus homeostasis.

In the absence of vitamin D, less calcium is absorbed from the intestine and with only a slight decrease in serum calcium concentration, parathormone is secreted. This, in turn, leads to mobilization of calcium and phosphorus from the bone. The serum calcium concentration is, thus, maintained, but secondary effects, including the changes of rickets in bone, a low serum

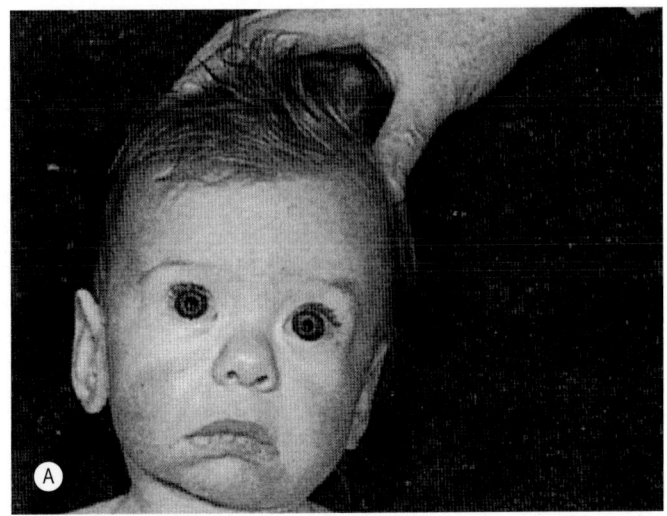

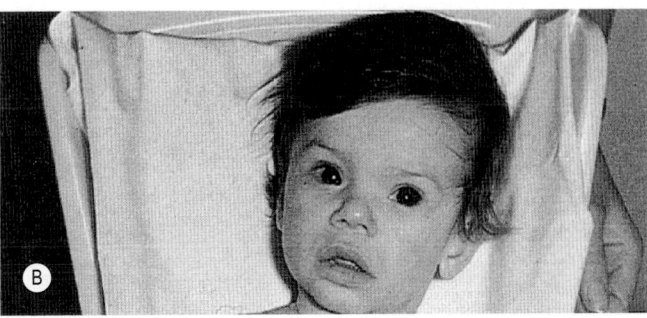

FIGURE 11.11 Elfin facies of idiopathic hypercalcemia. The characteristic facial appearance of the severe form of the disease is shown in these two patients. They are unrelated, but the similarity of features might suggest a family likeness. (From McLaren DS, ed. A colour atlas and text of diet-related disorders, 2nd edn. London: Wolfe; 1992; with permission.)

phosphorus concentration (because parathormone decreases phosphorus reabsorption in the kidneys), and elevated serum phosphatase (due to increased osteoblastic activity), take place.

Craniotabes, one of the early clinical signs of rickets, is caused by thinning of the outer table of the skull. It can be detected as a ping-pong ball sensation when pressing firmly over the occiput or posterior parietal bones.

Vitamin E

Vitamin E, α-tocopherol, is a fat-soluble antioxidant that may be involved in nucleic acid metabolism; deficiency results in **hemolytic anemia in premature infants** between 6 and 12 weeks of age and in nerve degeneration. Platelet adhesiveness increases with deficiency. Except in premature infants fed diets rich in polyunsaturated fatty acids and iron, dietary deficiency is rare. Vitamin E deficiency has been found in those with malabsorption syndromes, particularly infants with biliary atresia, who develop weakness and ataxia. **Neuronal degeneration** consisting of cerebellar ataxia, peripheral neuropathy and posterior column abnormalities are found. Ceroid is deposited in muscles (Fig. 11.12). Excessive iron administration exaggerates signs of vitamin E deficiency. Vitamin E deficiency may be a causative factor in retinitis of prematurity. Vitamin E deficiency is best detected by a serum ratio of α-tocopherol to lipid of less than 0.8 mg/g and/or erythrocyte hemolysis in hydrogen peroxide of more than 10%. Three days should elapse before determination of blood levels in suspected deficiency because orally administered vitamin E may circulate for 1–2 days.

Evidence of toxicity is debatable, but fatigue has occurred.

Vitamin K

Vitamin K is a naphthoquinone that participates in oxidative phosphorylation. Its absence or its failure to be absorbed from

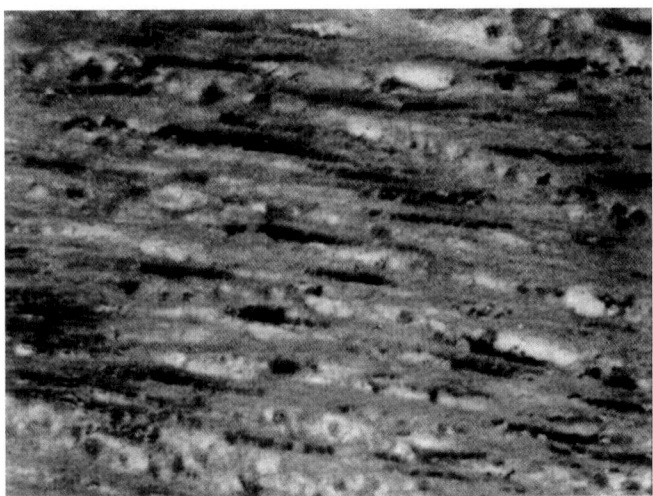

FIGURE 11.12 Brown bowel syndrome: part of the circular layer of the tunica muscularis of the small intestine showing fusiform accumulation of ceroid pigment within muscle cells. Vitamin E deficiency is thought to play a part in this and other disorders in which there is smooth muscle myopathy, probably of mitochondrial origin. (Nile blue stain.) (From McLaren DS, ed. A colour atlas and text of diet-related disorders, 2nd edn. London: Wolfe; 1992; with permission.)

the intestinal tract results in hypoprothrombinemia and decreased hepatic synthesis of proconvertin.

Naturally occurring vitamin K is fat soluble. It is designated vitamin K_1 to distinguish it from vitamin K_2 of bacterial origin and from synthetic naphthoquinones with vitamin K activity. Vitamin K is essential for activating blood clotting factors II, VII, IX, and X and the anticoagulant factors proteins C, S, and Z. Deficiency results in **clotting abnormalities** manifested as hemorrhagic disease.

Breast milk contains little vitamin K. Hydantoins may increase its requirement. Antibiotics inhibit conversion of vita-

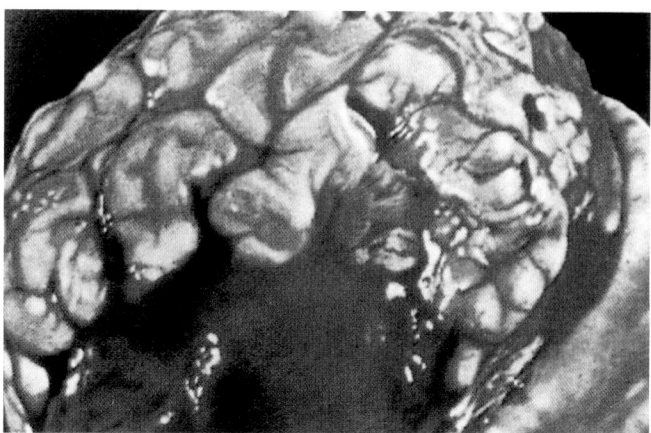

FIGURE 11.13 Hemorrhagic disease of the newborn: fatal subdural hemorrhage. (From McLaren DS, ed. A colour atlas and text of diet-related disorders, 2nd edn. London: Wolfe; 1992; with permission.)

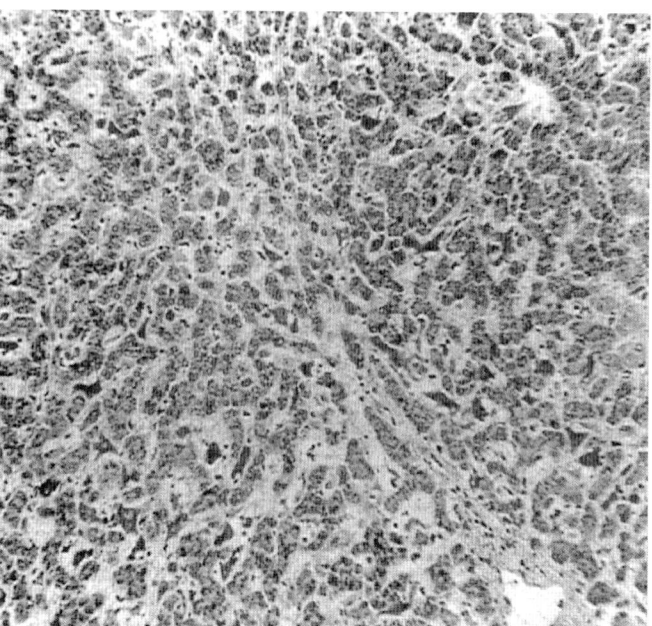

FIGURE 11.14 Hemosiderosis of the liver. Most of the iron staining is confined to the reticuloendothelial (Kupffer) cells in the parasinusoidal spaces. It may also be localized to lungs or kidneys. The term *hemosiderosis* implies absence of tissue damage; when the latter occurs, the term *hemochromatosis* is used. (From McLaren DS, ed. A colour atlas and text of diet-related disorders, 2nd edn. London: Wolfe; 1992; with permission.)

min K in the intestine and may result in vitamin K deficiency, which is also caused by fat malabsorption.

Neonates are prone to vitamin K deficiency, resulting in **hemorrhagic disease of the newborn** with bleeding, especially in the skin, gastrointestinal tract, and central nervous system (Fig. 11.13). The incidence of hemorrhagic disease of the newborn has dropped sharply since prophylactic administration of vitamin K at birth became common. Diarrhea in infants, particularly breast-fed infants, may cause vitamin K deficiency. Diseases of the liver may limit synthesis of prothrombin. Hypoprothrombinemia from this cause usually does not respond to administration of vitamin K.

Hypoprothrombinemia may also result from certain drugs. Dicumarol is thought to prevent the liver from utilizing vitamin K rather than exerting a specific effect on prothrombin.

Salicylic acid, a degradation product of dicumarol, produces hypoprothrombinemia. Large doses of synthetic vitamin K analogues, but not vitamin K_1, may result in hyperbilirubinemia and kernicterus in newborns with glucose-6-phosphate dehydrogenase deficiency and in premature infants.

Dependency states

Vitamin dependencies are described in the Metabolic Diseases section.

Essential fatty acid deficiency

Linoleic acid deficiency in infants causes **dermatitis** and **failure to grow**. Since it is a precursor of arachidonic acid and prostaglandins, blood clotting abnormalities may occur. Linolenic acid is also essential; both essential fatty acid derivatives are present in brain and neural cells and other cellular membranes.[16] These fatty acids can be obtained from cold-water fish and many vegetables.

Minerals

At least 16 minerals are recognized as essential for human nutrition; others are necessary for animal nutrition but have not been proved essential for humans (see Table 11.3). Balance of intake is essential, as excess of one mineral may cause deficiency of others.[17]

Iron

Iron deficiency leads to **microcytic hypochromic anemia**, and children may develop **glossitis, stomatitis, atrophy of gastric mucosa, nail changes** such as white lines in the nailbeds, and **splenomegaly**. Alterations in brain structure are noted in animals and may occur in iron-deficient human infants. Behavioral changes are noted in iron-deficient infants and children.[18,19]

Iron deficiency may occur after ingestion of iron-deficient foods such as cow's milk and strict vegetarian diets. Tea and other chelators may prevent iron absorption. Cow's milk ingestion by infants may result in blood loss via the intestine due to the lack of cytochromes. Cow's milk results in intestinal blood loss in sensitive children.

Excessive dietary iron may be toxic, causing **iron deposits; hemochromatosis; and decreased function in the liver, heart,**

kidney, and other organs (Fig. 11.14). Iron is a corrosive, and acute toxicity results in gastric hemorrhage, liver failure, and brain injury.

Zinc

Zinc is a component of over 200 metalloenzymes. Dietary substances that bind metals, such as phytic acid in cereals, can lead to deficiency. Early parenteral nutrition solutions were deficient in zinc.

Zinc deficiency causes **growth failure, diarrhea, acrodermatitis, anorexia, decreased immunity, and hypogonadism. Congenital malformations** occur in infants born of zinc-deficient women.[20]

Excess dietary zinc causes copper deficiency, a characteristic used to treat children with Wilson disease (hepatolenticular degeneration).

Copper

Copper is an essential cofactor of many enzymes, particularly oxidases. After absorption, copper is transported to the liver, bound to an α-globulin, and forms ceruloplasmin, which catalyzes oxidation of ferrous to ferric iron. Deficiency results in **anemia** and **neutropenia** and defective **elastin, collagen**, and **myelin formation**. Skin and hair depigmentation, osteoporosis, hypotonia, and psychomotor retardation may be present in copper-deficient children.

Copper excess may cause **cirrhosis**. With congenital lack of ceruloplasmin, copper toxicity manifests as Wilson disease, and transport defects as Menkes disease (see Ch. 12).

Iodine

Iodine is essential for formation of thyroxine and triiodothyronine. Iodine deficiency in the young leads to **hypothyroidism** and **cretinism** and is one of the leading causes of mental retardation worldwide. It is also a cause of goiter (Fig. 11.15). Deficiency acts as a teratogen and causes other congenital anomalies and abortion.

Excess iodine ingestion may result in goiter formation or thyrotoxicosis.

Selenium

Selenium is a cofactor of glutathionine peroxidase and, like vitamin E, is an essential antioxidant. Deficiency in young children and pregnant women is associated with **Keshan cardiomyopathy** and **Kashin collagen vascular abnormalities**.

Excess causes **alopecia, garlic odor to breath, and nail abnormalities**.

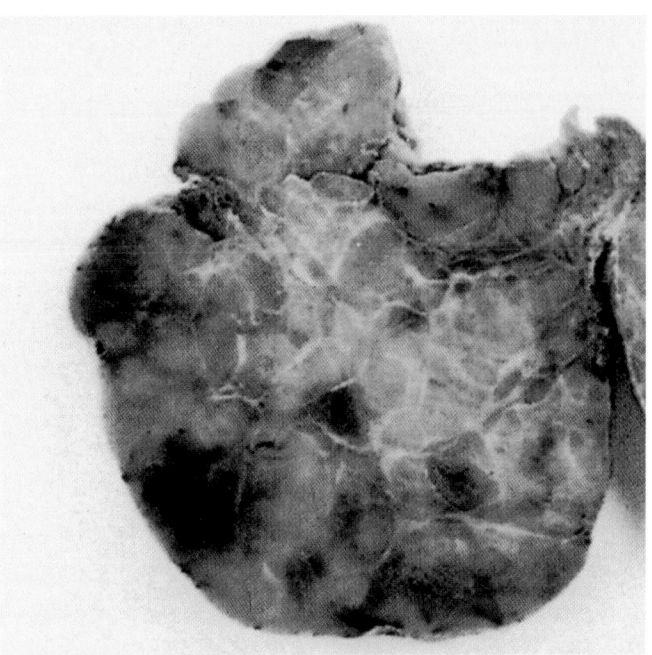

FIGURE 11.15 Colloid goiter. The thyroid gland is considerably enlarged, and follicles of varying size can be seen distended with colloid. (From McLaren DS, ed. A colour atlas and text of diet-related disorders, 2nd edn. London: Wolfe; 1992; with permission.)

Calcium

Dietary calcium deficiency sufficient to cause symptoms is rare. Ionized calcium regulates nerve conduction. Serum calcium is regulated by parathormone, vitamin D metabolites, serum phosphate and magnesium levels, and serum protein levels. Hypocalcemia leads to lack or depression of nerve conduction. This results in **tetany**, which may cause seizures and cardiac failure. With severe, prolonged deficiency, **osteomalacia** occurs. Blood coagulation may become defective. DiGeorge syndrome may also present as tetany with hypocalcemia.

Hypercalcemia occurs with vitamin D excess, malignancies with or without bone metastases, parathormone excess, hyperthyroidism, sarcoid, excess milk ingestion (milk alkali syndrome), and immobilization. Hypercalcemia manifests as **weakness, hyporeflexia, metastatic calcification, constipation**, and **renal failure**. Heart block may occur.

Phosphorus

Together with calcium and magnesium, phosphorus is essential for bone and tooth formation. Phosphorus, as a constituent of adenosine triphosphate (ATP), RNA, and DNA, is in the nucleus and cytoplasm of all cells and is essential for phospholipid and organic ester formation. Intestinal absorption and renal excretion are affected by calcium levels, parathormone, and vitamin D.

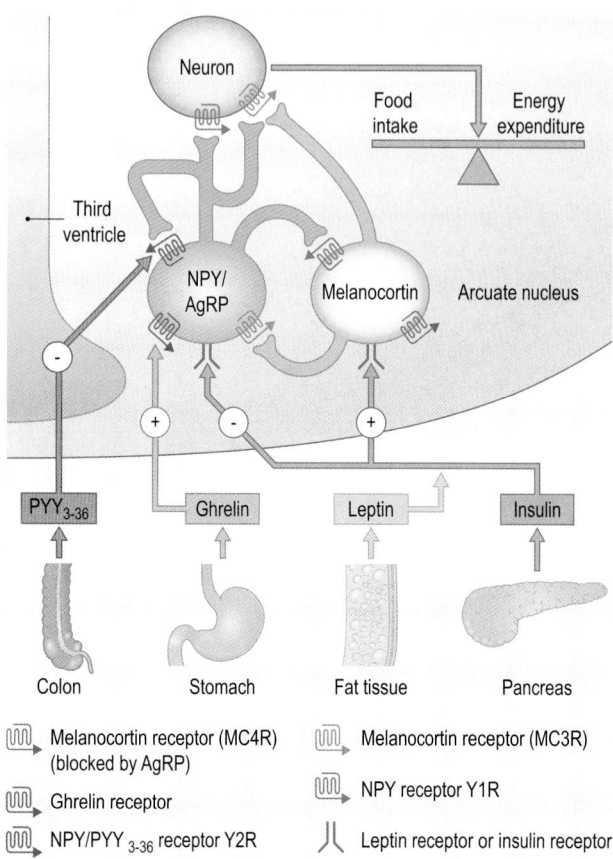

Colon   Stomach   Fat tissue   Pancreas

Melanocortin receptor (MC4R) (blocked by AgRP)

Melanocortin receptor (MC3R)

Ghrelin receptor

NPY receptor Y1R

NPY/PYY₃₋₃₆ receptor Y2R

Leptin receptor or insulin receptor

FIGURE 11.16 Mechanism of obesity. In this schematic diagram the arcuate nuclei in the brain contain neurons that are capable of stimulating or exhibiting food intake through the receptor for melanocortin (MC4R) and NPY/ and AgRP growth hormone secretagogue receptor (agouti-related protein). PYY₃₋₃₆ from the colon, ghrelin from the stomach, leptin from fat tissue, and insulin from the pancreas through receptors regulate the hormonal and control of obesity. (Courtesy of Dr. Frank Diamond.)

Deficiency may result in **rickets**. Excess may produce **tetany** by decreasing ionized calcium.

Magnesium

Magnesium is also essential for bone and tooth formation, and participates in actions with calcium. Dietary toxicity is rare. Deficiency results in **tetany**.

Obesity

Obesity is one of the most common nutrition–genetic disorders of affluent societies. No single definition is adopted; however, it is usually based on body mass index (BMI), and is weight of more than 20% of the 95th percentile for height; BMI, also known as the Quetelet index (weight [kg]/height [m²]), more than 27; and more than 23 for risk of obesity in children after age 1 year. Most authorities accept the appearance of infant or child as a valid definition of obesity. The mechanism of obesity is shown in Figure 11.16 and the genes in Table 11.4.

Nutritional obesity occurs when energy intake exceeds energy expenditure. Sedentary lifestyle together with a diet high in calories explains the occurrence and maintenance of obesity. Approximately 65% of white children in the US are overweight and of those half are obese. Infants, children, and adolescents who are obese are characteristically tall for age, and bone age is consistent with height age. Contrariwise, those overweight infants, children, and adolescents whose obesity is due to metabolic and hormonal diseases or to dysmorphic or genetic syndromes are short for chronologic age.

Marked obesity is a health hazard with a predisposition to many disease states (Table 11.5) including hypertension, non-insulin-dependent diabetes, hyperlipoproteinemia, atherosclerosis, osteoarthritis, and cholelithiasis. In children, hypoventilation, lethargy, and chronic anoxemia are common. Even more destructive are the societal implications: children, and society as a whole, discriminate against obese peers, and obese adults have more difficulty in gaining acceptance to college and obtaining employment than their lean counterparts.

Excess adipose tissue is found in subcutaneous spaces and is usually found in organs such as the liver, heart, and kidney. Weight reduction, particularly recurrent weight reduction followed by weight-regain regimens (the yo-yo effect), produces an increased incidence of biliary stones and other detrimental effects. Obesity in single gene mutations is shown as Table 11.6.

The amount of energy stored in the body as fat exerts potent effects on growth, pubescence, fertility, autonomic nervous system activity, and thyroid function, suggesting that humoral 'signals' reflecting adipose tissue mass interact directly or indirectly with many neuroendocrine systems.[22–26] Weight loss and maintenance of a reduced body weight are accompanied by changes in autonomic nervous system function (increased parasympathetic and decreased sympathetic nervous system tone), circulating concentrations of thyroid hormones (decreased triiodothyronine and thyroxine without a compensatory increase in thyroid stimulating hormone [TSH]), and circulating concentrations of glucocorticoids (increased cortisol)[22,27,28] that are consistent with a homeostatic resistance to altered body weight, acting, in part, through effectors that mediate energy expenditure.[29] Such a neurohumoral system to protect body energy stores would convey clear evolutionary advantages. During periods of undernutrition, the perceived reduction in energy stores would result in hyperphagia, hypometabolism, and decreased fertility (protecting females from the increased metabolic demands of pregnancy and lactation and the delivery of progeny into inhospitable environments).

Traumatic or infectious injury to the human ventromedial hypothalamus results in a syndrome characterized by hyper-

TABLE 11.4 RODENT SINGLE GENE MUTATIONS ASSOCIATED WITH OBESITY

Gene name (rodent); Symbol	Mutation name (rodent) Chromosome	Phenotype	Human chromosome
Agouti (mouse); A	AY (yellow) 2	Adult-onset obesity, yellow coat color, hyperphagia, due to ectopic overexpression of agouti signaling protein (Asp) leading to Mc4 receptor blockade.	20q11.2
Carboxypeptidase E (mouse); Cpe	Cpe/at (fat) 8	Adult obesity, possibly due to impaired processing of prohormones.	4q32
Leptin (mouse); Lep	Lepab (obese) 6	Early-onset obesity, hyperphagia, hypometabolic rate, infertility, diabetes, increased partitioning of stored calories as fat due to leptin deficiency.	7q31.3
Leptin receptor (mouse/rat); Lepr	Leprdb (diabetes) Leppa (fatty rat)	Early-onset obesity, hyperphagia, hypometabolic rate, infertility, diabetes, increased partitioning of stored calories as fat due to deranged leptin signal transduction.	1p31-p22
Tubby (mouse); Tub	Tub (tubby) 7	Impaired Ga-protein coupled receptor (possibly serotonin) signaling in the hypothalamus due to a mutation in this transcription factor may result in earlier cellular apoptosis.	11p15
OLETF (rat); Cckar	Ccka,oLETF	Adult obesity and hyperphagia due to CCK receptor deficiency.	4p15.2-p15.1

Human orthologs are known for all rodent genes that are associated with obesity.
In the case of Lep and Lepr, human mutations associated with obesity have been reported.
From Pediatric nutrition handbook, 5th edn. Am Acad Ped 2002.

phagia, hyperinsulinism,[30] and hyperactivity of the parasympathetic nervous system. The hypothalamus is a part of a complex regulatory system for energy homeostasis through which signals about the nutritional state of the organism, as well as hedonic signals about the palatability of available food, are integrated by a number of neuronal tracts that include the hypothalamus, cerebral cortex, and brain stem.[31]

The hypothalamic proopiomelanocortin (POMC)-melanocortin-4-receptor (MC4R) pathway, by virtue of its constituent arcuate neurons' ability to affect the autonomic nervous system, neuroendocrine axes, pancreatic cell function, and cortical tracts subserving food intake, may provide a central nexus for the integrated effects on energy expenditure and intake that have been detected in weight perturbation experiments.[24,31,32] Human autosomal recessive mutations leading to defects in POMC production result in central hypoadrenalism (due to lack of adrenocorticotropic hormone production), red hair (due to lack of 3-MSH production), hyperphagia due to lack of transduction of leptin-stimulated hypothalamic POMC/3-MSH (melanocyte stimulating hormone) production resulting in lack of MC4R-induced appetite suppression,[31] and obesity.[32] Inactivating mutations of MC4R have been implicated in human obesity. In some studies, up to 5% of individuals with a BMI > 40 kg/m² are heterozygous for such mutations.[32] Arcuate nucleus POMC is processed post-translationally in the hypothalamus to yield multiple neuropeptides including melanocyte-stimulating hormone (3-MSH), 3-MSH, and -endorphin (-EP). -EP inhibits the release of corticotrophin releasing factor (CRF).[33]

Major chemical mediators of ingestive behavior and energy expenditure include peptides, hormones, and neurotransmitters.

LEPTIN: Leptin[34-36] is secreted from adipose tissue and provides a signal linking fat mass to food intake and energy expenditure. Mice homozygous for the Lep[ob] mutation (leptin-deficient) are obese due to increased food intake and reduced energy expenditure. Administration of leptin in the region of the hypothalamus or peripherally to Lep[ob] mice decreases food intake and increases energy expenditure. In contrast to neuropeptide Y (NPY), which is associated with decreased thermogenesis, leptin administration to mice increases thermogenesis. Rare families have been identified with hypoleptinemia (leptin gene mutation, MIM 164160)[37,38] and leptin non-responsiveness (leptin receptor mutation, MIM 601007).[39]

There are rare instances of single gene/locus disorders, which result in human obesity (Table 11.7) (e.g., Prader-Willi syndrome [MIM 176270], Bardet-Biedl syndrome [MIM 209900], Alstrom syndrome [MIM 203800], Cohen syndrome [MIM 216550], in association with other often dysmorphic phenotypes).[32,40]

Obesity is the major risk factor for type 2 diabetes mellitus (DM) in adolescents,[41,42] and adiposity accounts for approxi-

TABLE 11.5 POTENTIAL EFFECTS OF INCREASED ADIPOSITY ON ORGAN SYSTEMS IN CHILDREN

	Nonendocrine
Cardiovascular	Common identifiable cause of pediatric hypertension, ↑ [total cholesterol], ↑ low density lipoproteins, ↓ high density lipoproteins, syndrome X
Respiratory	Abnormal respiratory muscle function and central respiratory regulation, difficulty with ventilation during surgery, lower arterial oxygenation, sleep apnea, pickwickian syndrome, more frequent and severe upper respiratory infections, snoring, daytime somnolence
Orthopedic	Coxa vara, slipped-capital femoral epiphyses, tibia vara, Blount disease, Legg-Calvé- Perthe disease, degenerative arthritis
Dermatologic	Intertrigo, furunculosis, acanthosis nigricans
Immunologic	Impaired cell-mediated immunity, polymorphonuclear leukocyte killing capacity, lymphocyte generation of migration inhibiting factor, and maturation rates of monocytes into macrophages
Gastrointestinal	Gallstones, hepatic steatosis, steatohepatitis
	Endocrine
Somatotroph	↓ basal and stimulated growth hormone release, normal concentration of insulin-like growth factor-I, accelerated linear growth and bone age
Lactotroph	↑ basal serum prolactin but decreased prolactin release in response to provocative stimuli
Gonadotroph	Early entrance into puberty with normal circulating gonadotropin concentrations
Thyroid	Normal serum thyroxine (T4) and increased thyronine levels; normal or elevated serum thyronine levels and decreased release of thyrotropin-stimulated thyroxine
Adrenal	Normal serum cortisol but ↑ cortisol production and excretion, early adrenarche, ↑ adrenal androgens and dehydroepiandrosterone, normal serum catecholamines and 24-hour urinary catecholamine excretion
Gonad	↓ circulating gonadal androgens in males; androgens in females with ↓ sex-hormone binding globulin, dysmenorrhea, dysfunctional uterine bleeding, polycystic ovarian syndrome
Pancreas	increased fasting plasma [insulin], insulin and glucagon release, increased resistance to insulin-mediated glucose transport

Adapted from Pediatric nutrition handbook, 5th edn. Am Acad Ped 2002.

mately 55% of the variance in insulin sensitivity in children.[43] As in adults, 50–90% of children with type 2 DM have a BMI > 85th percentile.[41,42]

Body fat distribution, usually defined on the basis of waist circumference or the ratio of waist-to-hip circumference, is an independent predictor of adiposity-related insulin insensitivity in adolescents and adults.[42,43] There appear to be effects of ethnicity on the relative impact of body fat distribution of hyperinsulinism and insulin secretion during oral glucose tolerance tests (OGTT) and of glucose disposal during glucose clamp studies.[42] In African-American, but not white, prepubertal children, intra-abdominal adipose tissue volume measured by magnetic resonance imaging was significantly correlated with fasting insulin concentrations and with insulin sensitivity as measured by area under the curve (AUC) during oral glucose tolerance testing.[44-46] Other studies of prepubertal children have found that fasting insulin concentrations and insulin sensitivity are significantly correlated with subcutaneous, but not visceral, adipose tissue volume in African-American prepubertal girls.[47] Because of the increasing frequency of type 2 DM among obese adolescents, and the worsening of diabetes-related morbidities that may result from delayed diagnosis, the clinician should be alert to the possibility of type 2 DM in all obese adolescents, and especially those with a family history of early-onset (<40 years of age) type 2 diabetes.[48]

Non-alcoholic steatohepatitis in children can lead to cirrhosis in childhood.[49]

Undernutrition and malnutrition

Undernutrition is due to inadequate dietary intake and results in growth failure. In 2000, 26.7% of preschoolers in the developing world were estimated to be underweight, as reflected by a low weight for age, and 32.5% were estimated to be stunted, based on a low height for age. In the United States and other developed countries, undernutrition as manifested by a low weight for age. It is truism that the prevalence of low height for age (below the 5th percentile) was (by definition) 5% among children from 2 months to 11 year of age.

Severely underweight children (<60% of reference weight for age) have more than an eightfold greater risk for mortality than normally nourished children, and moderately underweight children (60–69% of reference weight for age) have a four- to fivefold greater risk than even mildly underweight children (70–79% of reference weight for age) who have a two- to threefold greater risk.

Undernutrition ranges from a lower than desired intake of one or more nutrients with either no symptoms or only vague symptoms to severe malnutrition.

Severe undernutrition of multiple nutrients produces **marasmus**. Undernutrition of protein compared with calories is **kwashiorkor**. Since both represent deficiency of multiple vitamins, minerals, and calories, symptoms are generalized. Signs and symptoms include growth retardation, diarrhea, mental

TABLE 11.6 HUMAN SINGLE GENE MUTATIONS ASSOCIATED WITH OBESITY

Syndrome	Chromosome	Phenotype
Prader-Willi	Pat (15q11-q12) del	Short stature, small hands and feet, mental retardation, neonatal hypotonia, failure to thrive, cryptorchidism, almond-shaped eyes, and fish-mouth
Alstrom	2p13 (Recessive)	Childhood blindness due to retinal degeneration, nerve deafness, acanthosis nigricans, chronic nephropathy, primary hypogonadism in males only, type 2 diabetes mellitus, infantile obesity, which may diminish in adulthood
Bardet-Biedl	16q21 15q22-q23 (Recessive)	Retinitis pigmentosa, mental retardation, polydactyly, hypothalamic hypogonadism, rarely glucose intolerance, deafness, renal disease
Carpenter	Autosomal recessive	Mental retardation, acrocephaly, poly- or syndactyly, hypogonadism (males only)
Cohen	8q22-q23 (Recessive)	Mental retardation, microcephaly, short stature, dysmorphic facies
Prohormone Convertase	5q15-q21 (Recessive)	Abnormal glucose homeostasis, hypogonadotropic hypogonadism, hypocortisolism, and elevated plasma proinsulin and POMC
Beckwith-Wiedemann	Imprinted 11p15.5 domain	Hyperinsulinemia, hypoglycemia, neonatal hemihypertrophy (Beckwith-Wiedemann syndrome), intolerance to fasting
Nesidioblastosis	11p15.1 (Recessive or Dominant)	Hyperinsulinemia, hypoglycemia, intolerance to fasting
Pseudohypo-parathyroidism (type IA)	20q13.2 (Recessive)	Mental retardation, short stature, short metacarpals and metatarsals, short thick neck, round facies, subcutaneous calcifications, increased frequency of other endocrinopathies (hypothyroidism, hypogonadism)
Leptin	7q31.3 (Recessive)	Hypometabolic rate, hyperphagia, pubertal delay, infertility, impaired glucose tolerance due to leptin deficiency
Leptin receptor	1 p31-p32 (Recessive)	Hypometabolic rate, hyperphagia, pubertal delay due to deranged leptin signal transduction
POMC	2p23.3 (Recessive)	Red hair, hyperphagia, adrenal insufficiency, hyperpigmentation of skin due to impaired α-MSH production
MC4 receptor	18q22 (Dominant)	Obesity, early onset hyperphagia, increased bone density

Adapted from Pediatric nutrition handbook, 5th edn. Am Acad Ped 2002.

TABLE 11.7 OTHER DISEASES AND INJURIES ASSOCIATED WITH OBESITY

Disease	Structural/biochemical lesion	Clinical features
Acquired hypothalamic lesions	Infectious (sarcoid, tuberculosis, arachnoiditis, encephalitis), vascular malformations, neoplasms, trauma	Adipocyte hypotrophy with little hyperplasia, headache and visual disturbance, hyperphagia, hypodipsia, hypersomnolence, convulsions, central hypogonadism-hypothyroidism-hypoadrenalism, diabetes insipidus, hyperprolactinemia, hyperinsulinism, type IV hyperlipidemia
Cushing	Hypercortisolism	Moon facies, central obesity, lean body mass, glucose intolerance, short stature
Growth hormone deficiency	Impaired production of GH (pituitary) or GHRH (hypothalamus)	Short stature, obesity, increased risk of elevated cholesterol (especially in GHRH deficiency), central distribution of body fat
Hypothyroidism	Hypothalamic, pituitary, or thyroidal	Hypometabolic state (constipation, anemia, hypotension, bradycardia, cold intolerance), cretinism (if congenital)

Adapted from Pediatric nutrition handbook, 5th edn. Am Acad Ped 2002.

alterations, pellagra, hair changes, edema, hypoproteinemia, fatty liver, fatigue, lethargy, and increased susceptibility to infection.

Diagnosis of *protein-energy malnutrition* due to inadequate intake of protein and energy (PEM) may be made on the basis of specific measurements, such as determination of serum albumin or serum transferrin levels, creatinine–height ratio, or cell-mediated immunity. Clinical examination, including age, height, and weight measurements, is found to be equally reproducible and diagnostic.[50]

The terms primary and secondary malnutrition refer, respectively, to malnutrition resulting from inadequate food intake and malnutrition resulting from increased nutrient needs, decreased nutrient absorption, and/or increased nutrient losses. Although both primary and secondary malnutrition occur in developing as well as developed countries, primary malnutrition accounts for the major percentage of malnourished children in developing countries, whereas secondary malnutrition accounts for a higher percentage in developed countries.

PEM, whether primary or secondary, is a spectrum ranging from mild undernutrition resulting in some decrease in length and/or weight for age through severe forms of undernutrition resulting in more marked deficits in weight and length for age as well as wasting (i.e., a low weight for length). Historically, the most severe forms of PEM, marasmus and kwashiorkor, were considered distinct disorders. Marasmus was thought to result primarily from inadequate energy intake, whereas kwashiorkor was thought to result primarily from inadequate protein intake. Currently, a third disorder, marasmic kwashiorkor, which has features of both disorders, is recognized. The three conditions have distinct clinical and metabolic disorders, but they also have a number of overlapping features. For example, a low plasma albumin concentration, often thought to be a manifestation of kwashiorkor, is common in children with both clinical marasmus and clinical kwashiorkor. In recognition of the overlapping features of these two clinically distinct conditions, the terms currently preferred are edematous (kwashiorkor), and non-edematous (marasmus) PEM.

In non-edematous PEM (marasmus), initially there is failure to gain weight and irritability, followed by weight loss and listlessness until emaciation results. The skin loses turgor and becomes wrinkled and loose as subcutaneous fat disappears. Loss of fat from the sucking pads of the cheeks may occur late, and the infant's face may retain a relatively normal appearance, compared with the rest of the body, eventually becoming shrunken and wizened. The abdomen may be distended or flat with the intestinal pattern readily visible. There is muscle atrophy and resultant hypotonia. The temperature is usually subnormal and the pulse slow. Infants are usually constipated but may develop a starvation diarrhea with frequent small stools containing mucus.

Edematous PEM (kwashiorkor) may initially present vague manifestations that include lethargy, apathy, or irritability. When well advanced, there is inadequate growth, lack of stamina, loss of muscle tissue, increased susceptibility to infections, vomiting, diarrhea, anorexia, flabby subcutaneous tissues, and edema. The edema is often present in internal organs before it is recognized in the face and limbs. Dermatitis is common, with darkening of the skin in irritated areas but not in areas exposed to sunlight, in contrast to pellagra. The hair is sparse and thin and, in dark-haired children, may become streaky, red or gray. The texture is coarse in chronic disease. Eventually, there is stupor, coma, and death.

It has been proposed that giving excess carbohydrate to a child with clinical marasmus reverses the adaptive responses to low protein intake, resulting in mobilization of body protein stores. Eventually, albumin synthesis decreases, resulting in hypoalbuminemia with edema. Fatty liver also develops secondarily, perhaps to lipogenesis from the excess carbohydrate.

There is a paradox between underweight and obesity in developing countries. Low-cost commercial foods may be nutrient poor and adversely affect the growth of the child but may provide sufficient calories for the adult to gain excess weight. Because intrauterine growth retardation and low birth weight are common in developing countries, this may result in a population of adults who are susceptible to obesity.[51,52]

Dedication

Dedicated with appreciation to Doctors Grant Morrow and the late Frank A. Oski.

References

1. Shils ME, Olson JA, Shike M, et al., eds. Modern nutrition in health and diseases, 9th edn. Baltimore: Williams and Wilkins; 1999:305–483.
2. Kleinman RE, ed. Pediatric nutrition handbook, 5th Edn. Elk Grove, Chicago: Am Acad Ped 2004.
3. Allen LH. The nutrition CRSP: what is marginal malnutrition, and does it affect human function? Nutr Rev 1993; 51:255.
4. Chesters JK. Trace element–gene interaction. Nutr Rev 1992; 50:217.

Vitamins

5. Sommer A. Vitamin A: its effect on childhood sight and life. Nutr Rev 1994; 52:60.
6. Blomhoff R. Transport and metabolism of vitamin A. Nutr Rev 1994; 52:13.
7. Ong DE. Cellular transport and metabolism of vitamin A: roles of the cellular retinoid-binding proteins. Nutr Rev 1994; 52:24.
8. Maden M. Vitamin A in embryonic development. Nutr Rev 1994; 52:3.
9. Kennedy TA, Liebler DC. Peroxyl radical scavenging by β-carotene in lipid layer. J Biol Chem 1992; 267:4658.
10. Hussey GD, Klein M. A randomized control trial of vitamin A in children with severe measles. N Engl J Med 1990; 323:160.
11. Semba RD, Michilal, Ward BJ, et al. Abnormal T-cell subset proportions in vitamin A-deficient children. Lancet 1993; 341:5.
12. Hall JG, Solehdin P. Folate and its various ramifications. Adv Pediatr 1998; 45:1.
13. Horn E. Iron and folate supplements during pregnancy: supplementing everyone treats those at risk and is cost-effective. Br Med J 1988; 297: 1326.
14. Wighton MC, Manson JI, Speed I, et al. Brain damage in infancy and dietary vitamin B_{12} deficiency. Med J Aust 1979; 2:1.
15. DeLuca HF. New concepts of vitamin D functions. Ann NY Acad Sci 1992; 669:59.
16. Hoving EB, van Beusekom CM, Nijeboer HJ, et al. Gestational age dependency of essential fatty acids in cord plasma cholesterol esters and triglycerides. Pediatr Res 1994; 35:461.

Minerals

17. Baumgartner TG. Trace elements in clinical nutrition. Nutr Clin Pract 1993; 8:251.

18. Oski FA. Iron deficiency in infancy and childhood. N Engl J Med 1993; 329:190.

19. Lozoff B. Behavioral alterations in iron deficiencies. Adv Pediatr 1988; 35:331.

20. Nakamura T, Nishiyama S, Futagoishi-Suginohara Y, et al. Mild to moderate zinc deficiency in short children: effect of zinc supplementation on linear growth velocity. J 1993; Pediatr 123:65.

Obesity

21. Rosenbaum M, Leibel RL, Hirsch J. Obesity. N Engl J Med 1997; 337: 396–407.

22. Rosenbaum M, Hirsch J, Murphy E, et al. The effects of changes in body weight on carbohydrate metabolism, catecholamine excretion, and thyroid function. Am J Clin Nutr 2000; 71:1421–1432.

23. Wardlaw SL. Clinical review 127: obesity as a neuroendocrine disease: lessons to be learned from proopiomelanocortin and melanocortin receptor mutations in mice and men. J Clin Endocrinol Metab. 2001; 86:1442–1446.

24. Rosenbaum M, Leibel RL. Leptin: a molecule integrating somatic energy stores, energy expenditure and fertility. Trends Endocrinol Metab 1998; 9:117–124.

25. Ahima RS, Prabakaran D, Mantzoros C, et al. Role of leptin in the neuroendocrine response to fasting. Nature 1996; 382:250–252.

26. Ahima RS, Kelly J, Elmquist JK, et al. Distinct physiologic and neuronal responses to decreased leptin and mild hyperleptinemia. Endocrinol 1999; 140:4923–4931.

27. Aronne LJ, Mackintosh R, Rosenbaum M, et al. Autonomic nervous system activity in weight gain and weight loss. Am J Physiol 1995; 38:R222–R225.

28. Rosenbaum M, Nicolson M, Hirsch J, et al. Effects of weight change on plasma leptin concentrations and energy expenditure. J Clin Endocrinol Metab 1997; 82:3647–3654.

29. Maffeis C, Schutz Y, Pinnelli L. Effects of weight loss on resting energy expenditure in obese prepubertal children. Int J Obes Relat Metab Disord 1992; 16:41–47.

30. Arslanian S, Suprasongsin C. Insulin sensitivity, lipids, and body composition in children: is 'syndrome X' present? J Clin Endocrinol Metab 1996; 81:1058–1062.

31. Schwartz MW, Woods SL, Porte D Jr, et al. Central nervous system control of food intake. Nature 2000; 404:661–671.

32. Leibel RL, Chua SC, Rosenbaum M. Obesity. In: The metabolic and molecular bases of inherited disease. Scriver CR, Beaudet A, Sly WS, et al., eds, vol 1, 8th edn. New York, NY: McGraw-Hill; 2001:3965–4028.

33. Vale W, Rivier C, Brown MR, et al. Chemical and biological characterization of corticotropin releasing factor. Recent Prog Horm Res 1983; 39:245–270.

34. Garrow JS, Webster J. Are pre-obese people energy thrifty? Lancet 1985; 1:670–671.

35. Rosenbaum M, Leibel RL. Pathophysiology of childhood obesity. Adv Pediatr 1998; 35:73–137.

36. Santagata S, Boggon TJ, Baird CL, et al. G-protein signaling through tubby proteins. Science 2001; 292:2041–2050.

37. Farooqi IS, Jebb SA, Langmack G, et al. Effects of recombinant leptin therapy in a child with congenital leptin deficiency. N Engl J Med 1999; 341:879–844.

38. Montague CT, Farooqi IS, Whitehead JP, et al. Congenital leptin deficiency is associated with severe early-onset obesity in humans. Nature 1997; 387:903–908.

39. Clement K, Vaisse C, Lahlou N, et al. A mutation in the human leptin receptor gene causes obesity and pituitary dysfunction. Nature 1998; 392:398–401.

40. Leibel RL, Bahary N, Friedman JM. Genetic variation and nutrition in obesity. In: Simopoulos AP, Childs B, eds. Genetic variation and nutrition. Basel, Switzerland: Karger; 1990:90–101.

41. Young TK, Dean HJ, Flett B, et al. Childhood obesity in a population at high risk for type 2 diabetes. J Pediatr 2000; 136:365–369.

42. Caprio S, Tamborlane WV. Metabolic impact of obesity in childhood. Endocrinol Metab Clin North Am 1999; 28:731–747.

43. Freedman DS, Srinivasan SR, Burke GL, et al. Relationship of body fat distribution to hyperinsulinemia in children and adolescents: the Bogalusa Heart Study. Am J Clin Nutr 1987; 46:403–410.

44. Gower BA, Nagy TR, Trowbridge CA, et al. Fat distribution and insulin response in prepubertal African-American and white children. Am J Clin Nutr 1998; 67:821–827.

45. Gower BA, Nagy TR, Goran MI. Visceral fat, insulin sensitivity, and lipids in prepubertal children. Diabetes 1999; 48:1515–1521.

46. Osei K, Schuster DP. Effects of race and ethnicity on insulin sensitivity, blood pressure, and heart rate in three ethnic populations: comparative studies in African-Americans, African immigrants (Ghanaians), and white Americans using ambulatory blood pressure monitoring. Am J Hypertens 1996; 9:1157–1164.

47. Yanovski JA, Yanovski SZ, Filmer Km, et al. Differences in body composition of black and white girls. Am J Clin Nutr 1996; 64:833–839.

48. Mitchell BD, Kammerer CM, Reinhart LJ, et al. NIDDM in Mexican-American families. Heterogeneity by age of onset. Diabetes Care 1994; 17:567–573.

49. Molleston JP, White F, Teckman J, et al. Obese children with steatohepatitis can develop cirrhosis in childhood. Am J Gastroenterol 2002; 97:2460.

Undernutrition and malnutrition

50. Baker JP, Detsky AS, Wesson DE, et al. Nutritional assessment: a comparison of clinical judgment and objective measurements. N Engl J Med 1989; 306:969.

51. Callabero B. A nutrition paradox – underweight and obesity in developing countries. New Eng J Med 2005; 352:1514.

52. Doak CM, Adair LS, Bentley M, et al. The dual burden household and the nutrition transition paradox. Int J Obes Relat Metab Disord 2005; 29:129.

Further reading

Barness LA, ed. Pediatric nutrition handbook, 3rd edn. Elk Grove Village: American Academy of Pediatrics Committee on Nutrition: 1993.

National Academy of Sciences: Recommended dietary allowances, 10th edn. Washington, DC: National Academy Press; 1989.

Shils ME, Olson JA, Shike M, eds. Modern nutrition in health and disease, 9th edn. Philadelphia: Lippincott, Williams and Wilkins; 1998.

Metabolic diseases

12

Enid Gilbert-Barness   Lewis A. Barness

The mills of God grind slowly but they grind exceedingly small.   Charles Beard

Approach to pathologic diagnosis of metabolic diseases

Garrod coined the term *inborn errors of metabolism* in 1908 and defined them as genetically determined diseases caused by blocks in the metabolic pathways due to deficient activity of an enzyme in each pathway.[1] He described four diseases – alkaptonuria, albinism, cystinuria, and pentosuria – that fit his definition. Beadle and Tatum later developed the concept of one gene, one enzyme.[2] Since 30 000 to 35 000 genes are believed to constitute the human genome, at least the same number of genetic errors are possible and an unestimated but large percentage of these may cause significant disease. Each of these is, or will be, diagnosed by a specific test, whether biochemical, histologic, genetic, or other. Therefore, a strategy is developing for diagnosis of these diseases that is directed to an economically efficient number of tests, equally applicable to metabolic or gene testing.[3]

The strategy consists of meticulous attention to history and physical examinations of relatively low cost, followed by appropriate **screening tests** including **biochemistry, radiology**, or other modalities, and finally **specific enzyme, protein, or gene analysis**.[4]

Most of these disorders are inherited as autosomal recessive traits and some are X-linked. A few are inherited as dominant traits. Mitochondrial disorders form a genetically separate category: mitochondrial enzymes are coded both by the maternal nuclear genome and by the mitochondrial DNA.

Many infants or children with metabolic disease present with neurologic signs and symptoms or fail to thrive either mentally or physically. The newborn presents with signs typical of sepsis or asphyxia, such as irritability, failure to feed or suck, flaccidity, or coma. Previous miscarriages or sudden unexpected death in a sibling may trigger a screening investigation for metabolic disease. Common historical, physical, and laboratory findings are summarized in Box 12.1. Once a presumptive or suggestive diagnosis is made, testing can be pursued. A metabolic disease is diagnosed by demonstrating the underlying biochemical defect. Differential diagnosis in neonates often includes sepsis and asphyxia. Specific genetic probes are available for several diseases.

Even after death, some of the techniques used in the living may be helpful in detecting inborn errors of metabolism. For example, even small amounts of urine may be in the bladder and should be aspirated and saved. Within 6 hours after death, serum, tissues, and body fluids should be obtained and maintained in a state suitable for the tests desired (Box 12.2). Blood samples should be collected in heparin and in fluoride. Plasma should be separated and frozen at −20°C. Red cells should be stored at +4°C. Skin for fibroblast culture should be

BOX 12.1 ABNORMALITIES SUGGESTING INBORN ERRORS OF METABOLISM

Neurologic
Hypo- or hypertonia

Coma

Persistent lethargy

Seizures/movement disorders

Developmental delay

Progressive psychomotor degeneration

Gastrointestinal
Poor feeding

Recurrent vomiting

Jaundice

Failure to thrive

Hepatomegaly

Hydrops, ascites

Eyes
Cataract, corneal clouding

Cherry-red macula

Dislocated lens

Glaucoma/retinitis

Skin
Eczema

Angiokeratoma

Photosensitivity

Xanthoma

Edema

Muscle, joints
Myopathy

Arthritis

Abnormal mobility

Cramps

Other
Dysmorphic features

Neonatal deaths

Consanguinity

Self-mutilation

Abnormal body or urine odor

Abnormal hair

Splenomegaly, cardiomegaly

Recurrent acidosis with or without ketosis

Deafness

Routine laboratory findings abnormal
Blood sugar

Serum pH

Cytopenia, chronic

Liver function tests

Porphyrinuria

Anion gap

Electroencephalography

Radiography of bones

Sweat test

Abnormal odor of urine
Urine odor

Sweaty feet

Mousy or musty

Maple syrup

Tomcat urine

Cabbage

Rotting fish

Rancid fishy or cabbage

Hop-like

Swimming pool

Metabolism disorders
Glutaric (type II), isovaleric acidemia

Phenylketonuria

Maple syrup urine disease

α-methylcrotonylglycinuria

Methionine malabsorption

Trimethylaminuria

Tyrosinemia

Oasthouse disease

Hawkinsinuria

placed in sterile isotonic saline or transport medium at +4°C. Tissue samples for enzyme analysis are stored at −70°C.

An important step between the clinical findings and the biochemical diagnosis is the documentation of anatomic pathology, including histology, histochemistry, immunohisto-chemistry, and electron microscopy. A simple test for screening of **cytoplasmic vacuoles in the lymphocytes of peripheral blood** (Fig. 12.1) may be the first indication of a storage disorder (Table

12.1). A number of metabolic disorders cause liver cirrhosis in infants and children, and some may be suggested or diagnosed by microscopic investigation of the liver sample.[5]

Besides the biochemical tests of **blood and urine, solid tissues and fibroblast cultures** are often needed for biochemical assays. If a biopsy is performed, the specimen should be divided for biochemical analysis and morphologic investigation. This is particularly important in liver, muscle, and intestinal biopsies

BOX 12.2 BIOCHEMICAL TESTS FOR METABOLIC DISORDERS

Urine

Amino acids

Organic acids

Carbohydrates

Indoles

Imidazoles

Mucopolysaccharides (random specimen)

Metachromasia

Methemoglobin, myoglobin

Carnitine and esters

Serum (no anticoagulant)

Enzymes and galactosidase : Fabry: GM1

Arylsulfatase, A: Metachromatic, B: Maroteaux

Biotinidase – Biotin enzymes

Hexosaminidase A & B – Tay-Sachs (GM2 type I gangliosidosis) – Sandhoff (GM2 type 2)

Glucuronidase – MPS VII

Galactocerebrosidase

KrabbeSphingomyelinase – Niemann-Pick

Glucosidase – Gaucher

Iduronidase – Hurler-Scheie

Sialidase – Sialidosis

Glucosaminidase – Sanfilippo B

Oligosaccharidases – Mannosidosis, fucosidosis

Other

Carnitine

Plasma

Amino acids

Cerebrospinal fluid

Amino acids

Lactate

Blood

Chemical

Lactate

Ammonia

Pyruvate

Vacuolated lymphocytes in blood and bone marrow

Other

Chromosomes

DNA technology, RFLP, probes

MPS, mucopolysaccharidosis; RFLP, restriction fragment length polymorphism.

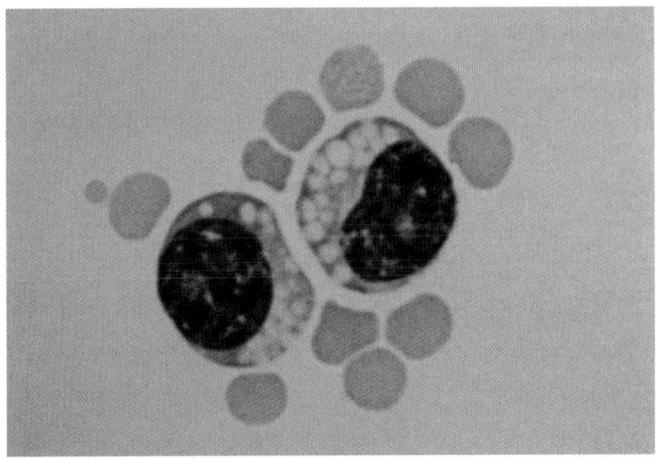

FIGURE 12.1 Vacuolated lymphocytes in peripheral blood in α-mannosidosis

TABLE 12.1 PRESENCE OF VACUOLATED LYMPHOCYTES IN STORAGE DISORDERS

Disease	Vacuolated lymphocytes
GM, gangliosidosis, infantile	Frequent, large
Niemann-Pick A	Occasional, small
Niemann-Pick C	Occasional, small
Sialidosis	Frequent, large
Aspartylglycosaminuria	Frequent, large
Mannosidosis	Frequent, large
Fucosidosis	Occasional, small
Sialic acid storage disorders	Frequent, large
Mucolipidosis types II and III	Frequent, large
Juvenile neuronal ceroid lipofuscinosis	Occasional, variable Occasional, small
Glycogenosis type II	Occasional, small
Wolman disease	Frequent, large
Mucopolysaccharidoses types II and III	Qualify vacuoles

and in skin biopsies made for fibroblast cultures. An electron microscopic (EM) investigation of the skin specimen may reveal changes that direct the biochemical analysis of the fibroblasts (Box 12.3).[6,7] EM investigation of white blood cells (WBCs) and urine sediment may be helpful in diagnosis. Routine placental examination may disclose fetal metabolic storage disease by the presence of vacuolization of syncytiotrophoblast, intermediate trophoblast, and stromal Hofbauer cells.[8]

Some metabolic disorders are rapidly fatal, while some may be asymptomatic but cause episodic crises resulting in death after dehydration, infection, or fasting. The sudden death of an infant may be due to a metabolic disease.

For many hereditary metabolic disorders, no specific therapy is available, but accurate diagnosis is important for prognosis, genetic counseling, and planning of prenatal diagnosis. The lysosomal storage disorders are among those metabolic errors most likely to present with dysmorphic features (Table 12.2).

BOX 12.3 TISSUES USED FOR DIAGNOSIS OF METABOLIC DISORDERS

Skin

Fibroblasts

Lysosomes (EM)

Enzymes

Conjunctiva

Lysosomes (EM)

Intestinal-neurogenic plexus (rectal biopsy)

Gangliosides

Neuronal ceroid lipofuscinosis

Sphyngolipidosis

Niemann-Pick

Peripheral nerve

Fabry

Niemann-Pick

Metachromatic leukodystrophy

Muscle

Carnitine

Glycogen

Enzyme histochemistry

Peripheral lymphocytes (see Table 17.1)

Bone marrow

Cystinosis

Gaucher

Niemann-Pick

Amniocytes

Gaucher

Mucopolysaccharidoses

Gangliosidoses

Brain biopsy

Severe neurologic deterioration when no other method available

Cartilage – bone biopsy

Mucopolysaccharidosis

Skeletal dysplasias (see Chapter 31)

TABLE 12.2 METABOLIC DISEASES ASSOCIATED WITH DYSMORPHOLOGIC FEATURES

Disease	Phenotype
Glutaric aciduria type II	Glomerulopathy
	Renal cystic dysplasia
	Cerebral dysgenesis
	Facial dysmorphism
	Congenital heart disease
	Genital anomalies
Pyruvate dehydrogenase	Microcephaly 'Fetal alcohol' facies
	Agenesis of corpus callosum
Peroxisomal disorders	Renal microcysts
Zellweger syndrome	Epiphyseal calcification
	Facial dysmorphism
	Congenital heart disease
	Cerebral dysgenesis
	Hepatopathy
Infantile Refsum disease	Facial dysmorphism
	Hepatopathy
Rhizomelic chondrodysplasia punctata	Facial dysmorphism
GM$_1$ gangliosidosis	Rhizomelic limb shortening
Congenital adrenal hyperplasia	Frontal bossing, low-set ears
Sialidosis	Ambiguous genitalia
	Coarse facial features, stippled epiphyses
Mucolipidosis type II	Coarse facial features
Mucopolysaccharidoses	Coarse facial features
Infantile sialic acid storage disease	Coarse facial features
Hydroxyisobutyryl-CoA deacylase	Congenital heart defects
	Agenesis of corpus callosum
	Dysmorphic facies
Gaucher-like storage disease	Arthrogryposis
Muscle phosphorylase deficiency	Arthrogryposis

Modified from Dimmick JE, Kalousek DK. Developmental pathology of the embryo and fetus. Philadelphia: JB Lippincott; 1992; with permission.

Storage diseases

Comprehensive references for this group of diseases can be found in the McKusick catalog,[9] *The Metabolic and Molecular Bases of Inherited* Disease,[10] and in *Metabolic Diseases: Foundations of Clinical Management, Genetics and* Pathology.[10a]

The lysosomal storage diseases (LSDs) are individually rare; collectively they affect about 1 in 8000 births.[10b] LSDs occur in all ethnic groups, although some are more prevalent in certain ethnic groups, e.g., Gaucher disease among Ashkenazi Jews and infantile Pompe disease in the African-American population.

There are approximately 400 LSDs. They are characterized by enzyme deficiencies that lead to build-up of large molecules in the lysosome. This accumulation eventually leads to organ dysfunction and life-threatening complications.

The material stored in the various types of affected cells includes **lipid** (neutral lipids such as triglycerides, cholesterol, and cholesterol esters); **sphingolipids** (ceramides, **cerebrosides** and other ceramide hexosides, **sulfatides** and **gangliosides**); **phosphosphingolipids** and the sphingomyelins; **lipofuscins**; **polysaccharides** (glycogen, other **polyglycosans**); **mucopolysaccharides;** and proteins (**glycoproteins** and **lipoproteins**). They can be demonstrated and compared by pathologic methods. For example, histologic and histochemical staining procedures and EM methods are applied to biopsy or autopsy specimens or to cells in specimens such as urine or airway secretions, peripheral blood, spinal fluid, peritoneal or pleural effusions, and cultures

TABLE 12.3 MUCOPOLYSACCHARIDOSES (MPS)

	Inheritance	Defective enzyme	Clinical pathologic features
MPS IH (Hurler)	AR	1-iduronidase	Abnormal facies, visceromegaly, skeletal changes, cardiovascular disease, mental retardation, corneal clouding
MPS IS (Scheie)	AR	1-iduronidase (defect allelic with above)	Cardiac valve disease, corneal clouding, joint stiffness, normal intelligence
MPS IH/Is genetic compound	AR	1-iduronidase	Intermediate between above
MPS IIA (Hunter, clinically severe subset)	XLR	Sulfoiduronate sulfatase	Abnormal facies, growth retardation, hepatosplenomegaly, cardiovascular disease, death by second decade
MPS IIB (Hunter, clinically milder subset)	AR	Sulfoiduronate sulfatase (? defect allelic with IIA)	Features less severe than above with longer survival
MPS IIIA (Sanfilippo A)	AR	Heparan sulfate sulfatase N-Acetyl-D-glucosaminidase	Visceral/skeletal features slight; mental defect severe
MPS IIIB (Sanfilippo B)	AR	Acetyl CoA: glucosaminidase	Similar to above
MPS IIIC (Sanfilippo C)	AR	N-acetyl transferase	Similar to above
MPS IIID (Sanfilippo D)	AR	N-Acetylglucosamine 6-sulfate sulfatase	Similar to above
MPS IVa (Morquio A)	AR	Galactosamine-6-sulfate sulfatase	Thoracic skeletal deformity, aortic valve disease, corneal clouding
MPS IVB (Morquio B)	AR	Galactosidase (presumably allelic with forms of generalized GM1 gangliosidosis)	Skeletal disease, corneal clouding mild, intellect normal
MPS V – now MPS IS MPS VI (Maroteaux-Lamy)	AR	Arylsulfatase B	Skeletal, corneal clouding severe, intellect normal until late in course Short stature, major feature
MPS VII (Sly) MPS VIII	AR	Glucuronidase Glucosamine-6-sulfate sulfatase	Short stature, hepatomegaly, mental retardation, normal corneas

of fibroblasts or other cell types. Determination of the chemical nature of substances in excess in the cells of these specimens, or determination of the levels of activity of enzymes such as lysosomal, mitochondrial, or peroxisomal enzymes or enzymes involved in the pathways of synthesis or breakdown of glycogen is commonly used in the diagnosis of genetic metabolic disease. Pathologic findings often point the direction for such biochemical analysis. DNA analysis is supplementing or supplanting more traditional techniques.

Historically, treatment for LSDs has been symptomatic and supportive. Specific treatments now are available for several LSDs and include enzyme replacement therapy (ERT), stem cell transplantation, and substrate inhibition therapies. The first step in initating therapy is suspecting the diagnosis and pursuing the evaluation.

Mucopolysaccharidoses

Mucopolysaccharidoses (MPSs) are a group of lysosomal storage diseases resulting from a genetic defect of a variety of hydrolases capable of hydrolyzing carbohydrates (Table 12.3). They are distinguished by storage of glycosaminoglycans (mucopolysaccharides) and glycolipids in the lysosomes of different cell types, including fibroblasts; macrophages; WBCs; parenchymal cells of liver, kidneys, brain, and other organs; and neurons, and by excretion of mucopolysaccharide in the urine.[11]

Glycosaminoglycans (GAGs) are long-chain polyanionic carbohydrates with disaccharide repeating units, one component of which consists of D-glucosamine or D-galactosamine and the other of either D-glucuronic or L-iduronic acid. The amino group and the fourth or sixth carbon of hexosamine are often either acetylated or sulfated. Six acidic GAGs are hyaluronic acid, chondroitin 4- and 6-sulfate, keratan sulfate, dermatan sulfate, heparin, and heparan sulfate. These GAGs are present largely as structural constituents of extracellular connective tissue; they are also present in mast cells, granulocytes, and platelets. GAGs attached to proteins are called **proteoglycans**. In pathologic states, intracellular GAGs are free and readily soluble in water or aqueous fixatives.[12]

GAG-synthesizing cells such as fibroblasts, endothelial cells, and leukocytes secrete proteoglycan. Those not secreted enter lysosomes and are degraded by various lysosomal hydrolases, including proteases. With enzyme deficiency, GAGs accumulate within the lysosomes. Proteoglycan or GAG is taken up by endocytic cells, enters lysosomes (heterophagy), and results in lysosomal overloading in the non-GAG-synthesizing cells (e.g., in the liver, spleen, and kidney), causing skeletal deformities, corneal clouding, and hepatosplenomegaly. Free GAGs appear in the urine. In the first year of life, similar compounds may be found in the urine of unaffected infants. The signs and symptoms of mucopolysaccharidoses are shown in Table 12.4.

Diagnosis of mucopolysaccharidoses

The urinary GAG excretion is age-dependent and may be present in normal infants up to 1 year of age. In the MPSs, an increased GAG concentration may be present in amniotic fluid and in urine at birth.

Good screening results have been obtained with a diagnostic test based on dimethylmethylene blue (DMB) as the dye. The test allows direct measurement of GAGs and, in contrast to other methods, keratin sulfate exhibits the same reactivity as dermatan and chondroitin sulfate. Influence of urinary proteins can be prevented by addition of Tris base (DMB-Tris).[13] False-negative screening tests can appear, even in the DMB test.

Positive screening tests for GAGs have been described in mucosulfatidosis and mucolipidosis III, and in a number of acquired diseases and clinical conditions (Table 12.5).

GAG concentrations should be given as GAG–creatinine ratios to avoid the pitfalls in collecting 24-hour urine samples.

Prenatal diagnosis

Prenatal diagnosis is possible for all the MPSs and is common for MPS I and II. All enzyme assays developed for cultured fibroblasts may be used on cells grown from amniotic fluid.

Chorionic villus biopsies are rich in enzymes of MPS II, IIIA, IIIB, IIIC, and IVA. Diagnosis of MPS I presents some difficulty because even normal villi have low activity.[14]

Carrier Testing Using DNA Analysis Is Practical. Homozygous W-402X mutations are indicative of a severe Hurler phenotype. P553R/P553R genotype may be associated with an intermediate, mild, or severe form of Hurler syndrome.

In extraneural tissues fixed in aqueous fixative, affected cells show some **cytoplasmic vacuolization** and cell ballooning (swelling). On EM examination the vacuoles contain fine granular material and, like lysosomes, are limited by a single membrane.[15] When the tissue is fixed in GAG-insoluble fixatives such as alcohol, the accumulated material shows intense **metachromasia** (purple-blue staining) with toluidine blue; it also stains intensely with Alcian blue, stains weakly with periodic acid-Schiff (PAS), and is impregnated with colloidal iron. Lipid is also present and may be abundant. The prototype of MPS is **Hurler syndrome** (Fig. 12.2). The most severe form results from a deficiency of α_1-iduronidase with the accumulation of heparan and dermatan sulfates. The clinical phenotype makes its appearance late in the first year of life with the development of thick, coarse features; prominent supraorbital ridges; thick philtrum; coarse hair; corneal clouding; short, thickened long bones with dwarfism (dysostosis multiplex); a protuberant abdomen due to hepatosplenomegaly; and mental retardation. Most infants die from cardiac complications. The heart is enlarged owing to infiltration of GAGs within the myocardial cells, and the heart valves are thickened and distorted

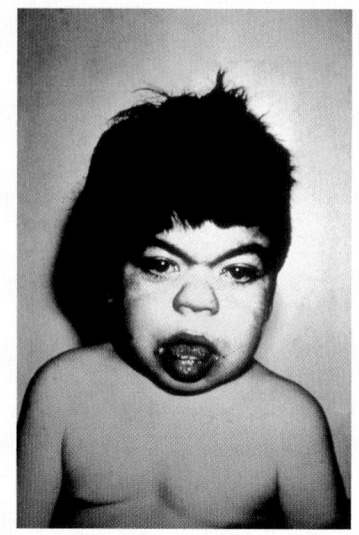

FIGURE 12.2 Hurler syndrome. Phenotypic appearance showing coarse features, prominent supraorbital ridges, and depressed nasal bridge.

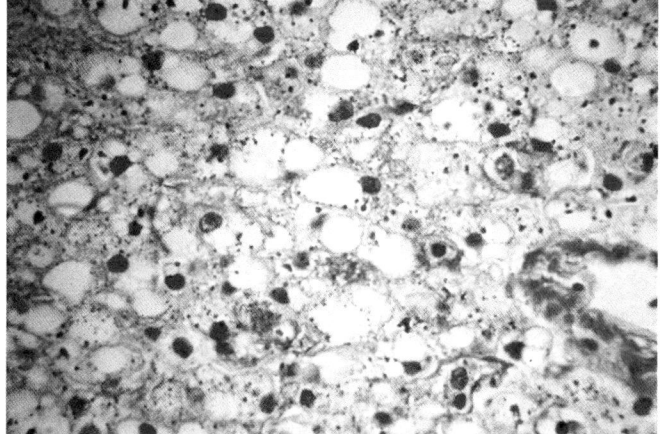

FIGURE 12.3 Microscopic section of liver with granular deposits of mucopolysaccharidosis.

by storage material present within histiocytes. The liver cells and Kupffer cells (Fig. 12.3) and histiocytes of the spleen are distended; storage material is present in histiocytes of the bone marrow and accumulates at the costochondral junctions at the growth plate in the long bones, ribs, and vertebrae, thus impeding linear growth. The brain may be covered by gelatinous exudate resulting from accumulation of GAGs in the leptomeninges. Neurons of the brain and spinal cord accumulate glycolipids (Figs 12.4 and 12.5).[16] The brain is large in infancy but later atrophies. By EM, GAG is characterized by intracytoplasmic membranogranular and reticular electron-dense deposits, while the glycolipids are seen as linear membranous striations.

Since GAG binds strongly with such dyes as Alcian blue, a spot test on filter paper can provide a rough estimation of **mucopolysaccharide excreted in the urine**. Intracellular mucopolysaccharide accumulation can also be found in some other,

TABLE 12.4 GLYCOPROTEIN STORAGE DISEASES*

McKusick no.	Disease	Genetic pattern	Enzyme defect	Clinicopathologic features
230000	Fucosidosis type 1	AR	α-1-fucosidase	Coarse Hurler-like features, skeletal changes, metal retardation, neurologic changes, cutaneous angiokeratomas; lysosomal storage in macrophages, fibroblasts, respiratory tract, bile duct and eccrine gland epithelium, renal tubules, endothelium, neurons; type 1 (onset in first year, death in first decade)
230000	Type 2	AR	α-1-fucosidase	Type 2 (onset in later infancy, survival into second decade)
230000	Type 3	AR	α-1-fucosidase	Type 3 (onset in second decade, survival into third or fourth decades), probably continuous spectrum rather than allelic disorders
248500	α-mannosidosis	AR	α-mannosidase	Coarse Hurler-like features, macroglossia, hypotonia, splenomegaly, deafness, lens cataract; storage in macrophages, lymphocytes, gingiva, retina, myenteric and central neurons (clinical and ? pathologic overlap with mucolipidoses)
248510	β-mannosidosis	AR	β-mannosidase	Coarse facies, mental retardation; hyperactivity, cutaneous angiokeratomas (mannose-N- acetyl glucosamine, heperan sulfate in urine) – cf. MPS 3A (Sanfilippo A)
107400	α₁Antitrypsin	AR	α-1-antitrypsin (protease inhibitor deficiency)	Neonatal cirrhosis, hepatic disease early in life, panacinar emphysema later in life
208400	Aspartylglucosaminuria	AR	N-aspartyl	Coarse Hurler-like features, mental deficiency, mental retardation
269920	Sialic acid storage diseases	AR	β-glucosaminidase	Hypotonia, ocular defects, mental retardation
604369	Salla disease	AR	Sialidase	Hypertonia, ocular defects, mental retardation
269920	Infantile sialic acid storage disease	AR	Sialidase	Hydrops, hepatosplenomegaly, mental retardation
269921	Sialuria		UDP acetylglucosamine epimerase	Sialic acid in urine
271900	Canavan disease	AR	N-acetyl aspartase	Spastic, spongy degeneration
305920	Glutamyl ribose-5-phosphate storage disease	AR	ADP-ribose protein hydrolase	Coarse Hurler-like features, seizures, mental retardation; hypotonia, proteinuria, renal failure, storage in renal epithelium, conjunctiva
232900	Glycoprotein storage disease (Zugibe-Gilbert)	AR	Not known	Splenomegaly, storage in spleen and bone marrow macrophages
231050	Geleophysic dysplasia	AR	Not known	Joint contractures, skeletal changes, short stature, hepatomegaly, cardiomegaly, glycoprotein storage in liver cells, cartilage, macrophages, epidermal and respiratory epithelial cells
212065	Carbohydrate-deficient glycoprotein syndrome	AR	Not known	Dysmorphic features, psychomotor and growth retardation, ataxia, peripheral neuropathy, skeletal and retinal abnormalities, stroke-like episodes, infarcts, liver steatosis, olivopontocerebellar degeneration, microcysts of the kidneys

*A degree of glycoprotein accumulation presumably occurs in some mucopolysaccharidoses and mucolipidoses, in addition to accumulation of polysaccharides and glycolipids.
AR, Autosomal recessive; UDP, uridine diphosphate.

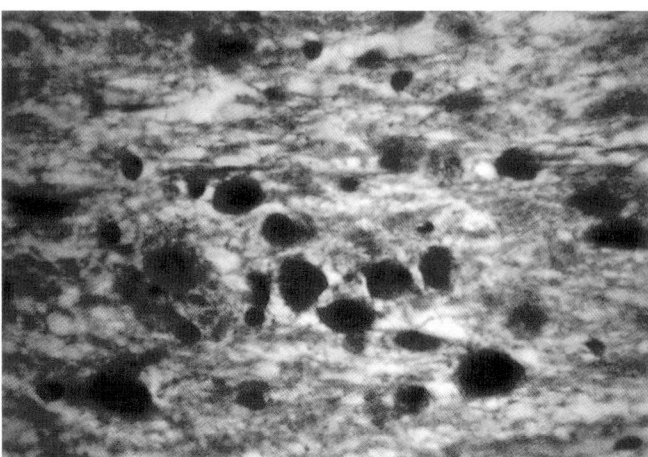

FIGURE 12.4 High magnification of greatly distended neurons of anterior horn cells in the spinal cord.

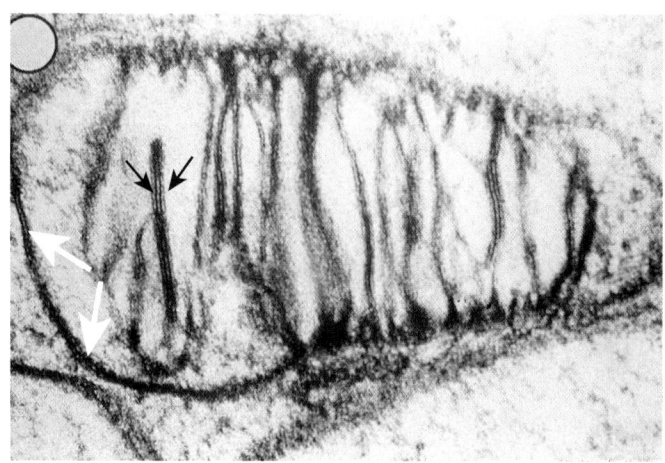

FIGURE 12.6 Electron micrograph of neuron showing stacked lipid lamellae (arrows) (zebra body).

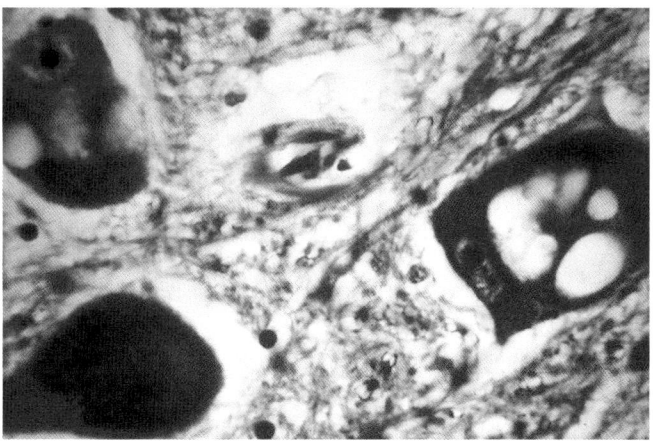

FIGURE 12.5 High magnification of greatly distended (constipated) neurons of anterior horn cells in spinal cord.

clinically quite different diseases such as Fabry disease (a lipid storage disease), Marfan syndrome (a heritable disorder of connective tissue), and cystic fibrosis of the pancreas (a membrane transport disorder).

The storage lysosomes in visceral cells in the MPSs contain GAG and glycolipid seen as membranogranular material and a lamellar pattern of the lipid within lysosomes. Both polysaccharide and glycolipid breakdown are impaired by a single enzyme defect because groups of compounds of carbohydrate chains can have the same terminal sugar, and the inability to be removed prevents further degradation of the molecule. Probably in all these diseases there is also impaired breakdown of glycoprotein. In the neuron the material distending the cytoplasm shows PAS reactivity that is amylase resistant (indicating that the substance is not glycogen), metachromasia with toluidine blue, and staining with Sudan black B, Nile blue, or Alcian blue. The material can be extracted with a chloroform–methanol mixture; these characteristics indicate the glycolipid nature of the accumulated material. Ultrastructurally, the lysosomes are filled with parallel lamellae, usually perpendicular to the limiting membrane, which are appropriately called **zebra bodies** (Fig. 12.6).[17]

A classification of MPSs based on the specific nature of the enzyme deficiency is shown in Table 12.3. Classification of these disorders has been significantly advanced by study of fibroblasts in tissue culture. These cells not only develop GAG accumulation in culture but also show the ability to exchange macromolecules, including the missing enzymes. This unique phenomenon allows in vitro correction of mucopolysaccharide accumulation of affected cells by mixed culture with normal cells or cells of a patient with one disease; e.g., Hurler cells correct the defect of cells from a patient with Hunter disease. Bone marrow transplantation has been performed for some of the MPSs, with variable results.

MPS IS (Scheie-Barness syndrome)

This is a mild form of MPS I characterized by joint stiffness, aortic valve disease, and corneal clouding. The facial features are characteristically coarse, but intelligence and stature are usually normal. MPS IS patients can have stiff fingers and painful feet, pes cavus, and genu valgum. Retinal degeneration with corneal clouding may contribute to significant visual impairment. Aortic valvular disease due to accumulation of mucopolysaccharide deposits on valves and chordae tendineae results in aortic stenosis and regurgitation. The onset of significant symptoms is usually after the age of 5 years, and the diagnosis is usually made between 10 and 20 years of age. Most live a normal life span.

It is caused by a different mutation of the gene for α_1-iduronidase from MPS I (Hurler disease). These allelic diseases are now coded as MPS IH and MPS IS; the genetic compound condition, heterozygosity for both the IH and IS alleles, is also known. Accumulation of dermatan sulfate alone occurs. As a result, the manifestations are considerably milder with a later onset, corneal clouding, and joint involvement, yet with normal

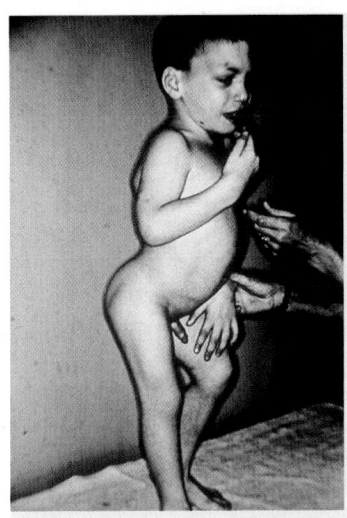

FIGURE 12.7
Mucopolysacchardosis IV (Morquio disease) in a child with severe skeletal deformities.

mentation and stature. Some children have aortic valvular problems, but most live a near-normal life span.

MPS II (Hunter disease) is **X-linked** and less severe than type I. The phenotype and pathologic changes are similar to those of type I.

MPS III (sanfilippo syndrome), MPS IV (Morquio), MPS VI (Maroteaux-Lamy)

The disorders grouped as **MPS III (Sanfilippo syndrome)** have in common severe neurologic damage with few somatic visceral and skeletal features. Of the four different enzyme defects that involve different genes, two are sulfatases (MPS IIIA and IIID), one is a hexosaminidase (MPS IIIB), and one is a hexosamine acetyl transferase (MPS IIIC). In each, the clinical features are similar. Children present around 3 years of age with coarse facial features, developmental delay, and behavioral problems. Mental retardation and progressive central nervous system (CNS) involvement ensue. Although joint stiffness, hepatosplenomegaly, and osseous lesions occur, they are less severe than in Hurler syndrome. Most patients survive about two decades.

MPS IV (Morquio disease) is characterized by severe skeletal deformities (Fig. 12.7) and corneal clouding. Types A and B have been described with different enzyme defects. Type A is due to a deficiency of N-acetylgalactosamine-6-sulfate. The enzyme defect in **MPS IVB (Morquio B syndrome)** involves β-galactosidase, and the abnormal gene is presumably allelic with those causing the three GM_1 gangliosidoses, so that genetic compound disorders may be demonstrated. The cells in Morquio disease store keratan sulfate and chondroitin-6-sulfate; staining is less intense than other forms of MPS, and more lipofuscin is present. This condition predominantly affects the skeleton, resulting in a severe form of dysostosis multiplex. Children present with short stature and joint laxity in the first year of life. Osseous lesions give rise to hearing impairment and restrictive cardiorespiratory problems. Hypoplasia of the odontoid process and atlantoaxial subluxation lead to cervical cord compression, often requiring posterior spinal fusion. Mental development is usually normal. Most patients die in their twenties from cardiorespiratory failure.

The incidence of Morquio syndrome is 1 per 3 000 000.

MPS VI (Maroteaux-Lamy), which is due to arylsulfatase B deficiency, leads to accumulation of dermatan sulfate and is associated with skeletal changes, corneal clouding, and normal intellect until late in the course of the disease. The incidence of Maroteaux-Lamy syndrome is 1 per 216 000 births in British Columbia. An enlarged head and a deformed chest may be present at birth. Umbilical and/or inguinal hernias are common. Claw-hand deformities are not uncommon.[18] Hepatomegaly is always present after the age of 6 years, and an enlarged spleen is found in half of patients.[19] Aortic and mitral valvular dysfunction are due to thickened and calcified stenotic valves.[20,21]

Skeletal changes in severe MPS VI are similar to the Hurler syndrome.

Sly syndrome (MPS VII), MPS VIII

Deficiency of β-glucuronidase results in the accumulation of heparan, keratan, chondroitin 4-sulfate, and chondroitin 6-sulfate. **Sly syndrome (MPS VII)** has a variable phenotype and best resembles a mild form of Hurler syndrome. A newborn with the **severe neonatal form of MPS VII** is often hydropic. This form is one of the very few lysosomal storage diseases that may be recognized in utero or be present at birth.[22] Vacuolization due to storage material occurs in epithelial, neural, and mesenchymal cells; coarse granulocyte inclusions in circulating WBCs are striking. In the placenta, stromal and Hofbauer cells, but not trophoblasts, are vacuolated.

MPS VIII, due to glucosamine 6-sulfatase deficiency with accumulation of keratan and heparan sulfates, is characterized by shortness of stature, hepatomegaly, psychomotor retardation, dysostosis multiplex, and normal corneas.[22–28] It combines the features of Morquio and Sanfilippo syndromes. Lymphocytes show ring-shaped metachromasia when stained with toluidine blue.

For the neurodegenerative forms of MPS, enzyme replacement therapy (ERT), stem cell transplantation are the treatment of choice, if it can be performed before significant neurodegeneration is apparent (usually before age 2). Stem cell transplantation can stabilize brain function.[28a]

For patients with milder disease for whom there is low risk for neurologic involvement, ERT also is available. ERT has effects similar to stem cell replacement except that it does not effectively target the central nervous system and has fewer complications.[28b]

Hyaluronidase deficiency

The clinical, pathologic, and biochemical findings in a child with short stature and multiple periarticular soft tissue masses proved to have a storage disease of hyaluronate (hyaluronic acid) due to a genetic deficiency of hyaluronidase have been reviewed.[29]

The principal abnormalities were periarticular soft tissue masses, unique for the MPSs, composed of nodular aggregates of histiocytes; short stature; and erosions of the acetabula. Hyaluronate concentrations were especially high in synovial fluid. The highest concentrations of hyaluronate in normal solid tissues are in cartilage and skin. Much of the catabolism of hyaluronate in joints occurs locally.

Histologic examination of the patient's ankle and finger masses showed similar pathologic changes. The ankle lesion consisted of synovium with marked villonodular transformation. The villi were bullous and contained many large histiocytes that had abundant cytoplasm filled with clear vacuoles. The vacuoles stained with Alcian blue and colloidal iron, indicating the presence of mucopolysaccharide. The degree of staining was reduced by pretreatment with hyaluronidase.

Ultrastructurally, the histiocytes were nearly filled with numerous large membrane-bound vacuoles consistent with lysosomes. The vacuoles contained a flocculent material. Endothelial cells and vascular smooth-muscle cells appeared normal. Fibroblasts in a separate skin biopsy specimen also showed lysosomes filled with fibrillar material.

The decreased plasma hyaluronidase activity in the patient's parent and in two of her grandparents, together with other data, indicates that the enzyme deficiency is an autosomal genetic disorder.

Glycoprotein storage diseases

Glycoproteins feature a peptide core to which oligosaccharide chains are attached. Deficiency of specific lysosomal acid hydrolases results in failure to remove carbohydrate residues from the oligosaccharide chains. Since similar chains are present in sphingolipids and mucopolysaccharides, several types of material may accumulate in these conditions.

Table 12.4 lists the glycoprotein storage diseases. Possible overlaps with the MPSs and mucolipidoses can be noted, and future studies will undoubtedly lead to refinements in the classification of lysosomal storage diseases. At present, the range of ages of clinical onset in fucosidosis with infantile, late infantile, and adolescent-onset patterns is a reflection of a continuous spectrum of severity of abnormalities in the α_1-fucosidase gene. Patients with the glycoprotein disorders **mannosidosis, fucosidosis, sialidosis, aspartylglycosaminuria,**[30] **glutamylribose-5-phosphate disorder**, and **geleophysic dwarfism** present with a phenotype similar to Hurler disease. **Canavan disease, α_1-antitrypsin deficiency**, and **glycoprotein storage disorder** (Gilbert-Zugibe)[31] phenotypes differ.

Prenatal diagnosis for glycoprotein storage diseases

Identification of affected fetuses by biochemical analysis is reliable and has been demonstrated for α- and β-mannosidosis, fucosidosis, sialidosis, and aspartylglucosaminuria using chorionic villus samples (CVS) or cultured amniotic fluid cells. Although not yet reported, mutation analysis and/or linkage

analysis should be possible for fucosidosis and aspartylglucosaminuria, and for the other disorders as additional molecular information becomes available.

α-mannosidosis

α-mannosidase deficiency[32] is inherited as an autosomal recessive disorder with excretion of abnormal levels of mannose-rich oligosaccharides. The clinical features include a severe infantile phenotype referred to as type I and a milder juvenile–adult phenotype referred to as type II[33,34] with a more slowly progressive course. Virtually all patients have psychomotor retardation, facial coarsening, and some degree of dysostosis multiplex. Frequent findings include recurrent bacterial infections, deafness, hepatomegaly, hernias, and lenticular or corneal opacities. The ocular findings are distinctive and include posterior opacities in a spoke-like pattern in the lens and superficial opacities in the cornea.[35–37] The skeletal dysplasia includes thickening of the calvaria in the majority of patients. The vertebral bodies are prominently involved, with ovoid configurations, flattening, and beak appearance, sometimes in association with gibbous deformity.

The milder juvenile–adult type II phenotype is characterized by more normal early development but appearance of mental retardation during childhood and adolescence. Hearing loss is particulary prominent in type II patients. Hepatocytes contain a foamy cytoplasm. EM demonstrates vacuoles in hepatocytes and Kupffer cells with a reticulogranular pattern. Brain cells appear ballooned. Diagnosis may be made by measuring urinary glycoproteins. A mild form allows for survival into young adulthood.

Laboratory Diagnosis Patients affected with α-mannosidosis excrete increased amounts of several oligosaccharides, the major one being Man(α13) Man(β1i4)G1cNAc. Urinary screening for oligosaccharides[38] should be by high-pressure liquid chromatography (HPLC) for oligosaccharides in urine[39] and in fibroblasts.[40]

Acid α-mannosidase acitivity, determined in WBCs, fibroblasts, or cultured amniotic fluid cells, is severely reduced.[41] Direct measurement of α-mannosidase in plasma has been less reliable than the assay of the cellular enzyme levels because of forms of mannosidase enzymes in plasma that are not decreased in mannosidosis patients.[33,41–43] Activity of α-mannosidase has been demonstrated in trophoblast biopsy.

The gene that codes for both the α and β subunits of this enzyme have been sequenced, and map to 19cen-q12;[43–47] molecular diagnosis is thus possible.

Pathology Vacuolated lymphocytes are present in almost all patients. Most patients have been found not to have mucopolysacchariduria. Decreased serum immunoglobulin G (IgG) can occur, and a decreased PR interval on electrocardiogram (EKG) has been reported.[48] Histiocytes are striking in the bone marrow because their many cytoplasmic, membrane-bound vacuoles, which are variable in size, occupy most of the cytoplasmic space and are frequently intercommunicating. Fibroblasts also contain membrane-bound vacuoles that are similar to those in the histiocytes although they are not as numerous as those in the latter.

The liver demonstrates a granular or foamy cytoplasm in the hepatocytes. PAS staining varies with the histochemical extraction procedure. Ballooned storage cells may be observed in the neurons of the cerebral cortex, brainstem, medulla oblongata, spinal cord, neurohypophysis, retina, and myenteric plexus.[49,50]

Treatment Successful bone marrow transplantation has been reported in a child with a severe form of α-mannosidosis type I. There was complete resolution of the recurrent sinopulmonary disease and organomegaly, improvement in the bony disease, and stabilization of neurocognitive function.[51]

More rarely, **β-mannosidase** may be deficient, with or without an associated reduction of heparan sulfaminidase. A severe form is characterized by status epilepticus, severe quadriplegia, and death by 15 months of age. A milder form features psychomotor retardation with angiokeratomas. The latter phenotype is akin to the Sanfilippo A syndrome. The gene has been sequenced. The enzyme is a lysosomal protein with a molecular mass of 100 kDa. Prenatal diagnosis has been made from cultured amniotic fluid cells and CVS sampling.

Fucosidosis

Fucosidosis is inherited as an autosomal disorder due to deficiency of α-L-fucosidase that leads to the accumulation of fucose-containing sphingolipids, glycoproteins, and oligosaccharides.[52] Affected children are generally of Spanish or Italian descent. Urinary glycoprotein is elevated and the enzyme defect is detected in cultured fibroblasts and leukocytes.

Type 1 fatal infantile fucosidosis presents in infancy with psychomotor retardation, coarse facies, corneal opacities, dysostosis multiplex, neurologic deterioration, growth retardation, and cardiomegaly. Hepatomegaly, splenomegaly, seizures, and increased sweat chloride are found. **Type 2 fucosidosis** is milder; first signs occur at 1–2 years of age and **angiokeratomas** develop. Telangiectasis, pigmentary retinopathy, and tortuous conjunctival vessels may be found. Lymphocytes are vacuolated.

At autopsy, the brain, heart, liver, spleen, and pancreas are large. Hepatocytes and liver cells contain foamy cytoplasm. EM of brain and liver cells reveals heterogeneity, with some cells containing lamellar structures and some storage vacuoles. Sweat glands are vacuolated. Adrenal glands are atrophied.

Urine contains fucose-containing glycopeptides and oligosaccharides.

The fucosidosis gene has been identified at the distal region of 1p34.[53] There are a number of mutations. The enzyme defect results in the accumulation and excretion of a variety of glycoproteins, glycolipids, and oligosaccharides containing fucoside moietes.

Aspartylglycosaminuria

Aspartylglycosaminuria (AGA)[54,55] is an autosomal recessive disease due to deficient activity of aspartylglucosaminidase. AGA results in accumulation of aspartylglycosamine in lysosomes in almost all cells.[56] Aspartylglucosamine is also excreted in large quantities in the urine. The disorder manifests as a dysmorphic syndrome resembling Hurler disease at about 1 year of age. Coarse facies, hypotonia, mental delay, hepatomegaly, and spasticity occur.[57,58] Death occurs in the fourth or fifth decade. This disorder occurs predominantly in Finland.

Enzyme status is measured in skin fibroblasts or leukocytes. Prenatal diagnosis can be made on the basis of amniotic fluid cells, fibroblasts or chorionic villus samples.[59] The gene for AGA resides in the long arm of chromosome 4 (4q32-q33).[60] Because one mutation appears to account for about 98% of the AGA alleles in the Finnish population, a DNA-based test suitable for the detection of the mutation has been developed and is suitable for this population.[61,62]

Carbohydrate-deficient glycoprotein syndrome

Autosomal recessive abnormalities of glycoprotein structure, including increased amounts of carbohydrate-deficient transferrin, are diagnostic of this condition.[54]

Psychomotor retardation, growth failure, dysmorphic features, liver dysfunction, lipocutaneous abnormalities, inverted nipples, ataxia, peripheral neuropathy, skeletal abnormalities, and retinal degeneration are characteristic. Stroke-like episodes and cerebral infarctions may be related to coagulation abnormalities with reduction in factor XI, antithrombin II, and protein C. Hypertrophic cardiomyopathy has been observed in a neonate.[54] Carbohydrate-deficient glycoprotein syndromes (CDGS) may also present as gastrointestinal disorders with hypoglycemia and protein-losing enteropathy.[63]

Pathology Steatosis and fibrosis of the liver that may progress to cirrhosis; lysosomal accumulation of electron-dense and electron-lucent material are seen by EM. Cerebellar atrophy, neuronal loss, in a severe olivopontocerebellar form of the disease have been described. Microcystic changes in the kidneys, and degeneration and loss of photoreceptors of the retina, may occur. Hypertrophic cardiomyopathy may be present. Endocrine abnormalities include, in females, a lack of secondary sex characteristics and hypogonadotrophic hypogonadism. Males exhibit decrease in testicular volume.[64,65]

Four types of CDGS are currently recognized. Two of the four types are associated with known metabolic defects in N-linked oligosaccharide synthesis. Type Ia CDGS is the most common subtype with a frequency of 1 in 80 000; the defect resides in a deficiency of phosphomannomutase (PMM) in the reaction mannose-6-P:mannose -1-P:glycogen conjugates.[66] Type Ib is due to deficiency of phosphomannose isomerase (PMI). Type Ic is due to a deficiency of α-glycotransferase deficiency.

Type II CDGS has affectd only a few families. The index patient had coarse facies, large and low-set ears, widely spaced nipples, a ventricular septal defect, a patent ductus arteriosus, severe developmental delay, generalized hypotonia, and limb weakness.[67]

Type III CDGS has been reported in two unrelated Swedish and German girls. They had perinatal floppiness and a dystrophic appearance. Distinctive features included progression to tetraparesis with brisk reflexes (in contrast to diminished reflexes in type I CDGS), infantile spasms, cerebral and optic atrophy, and pigmentary skin changes reminiscent of incontinentia pigmenti.

Type IV CDGS is due to deficiency of P-mannose synthase.[66] Clinical features include dysmorphic features, seizures, optic atrophy, severe developmental delay with intractable hypsar-rhythmias largely resistant to therapy, and progression from hypotonia to spastic or dystonic tetraparesis. Protein-losing enteropathy may occur with heparan sulfate proteoglycan deficiency.

Other rare variants of CDGS have been reported.[68] All types are characterized by an isoelectric pattern of transferrin abnormalities.[66]

Low serum levels of TBG, haptoglobin, transcortin, apolipoprotein B, cholesterol, coagulation factors, and various peptide and glycopeptide hormones have been noted.

The basic biochemical defect in CDGS has not been identified. Some type I patients manifest a deficiency (to less than 10% of control) of the phosphomannomutase.[69] The known type II patients have exhibited N-acetyglucosamine transferase II deficiency.[70] Types III and IV presumably result from different defects in the N-linked glycan synthetic pathway. It has been suggested[71,72] that CDGS is caused by a defect in some aspect of N-linked oligosaccharide synthesis or transfer.

Diagnosis Serum transferrin by isoelectric focusing shows the presence of abnormally glycosylated serum proteins, typically transferrins. Serum samples as well as blood spots from newborn screens can be used for diagnosis.[73,74]

Plasma amino acids are typically normal, as are urine organic acids and thin-layer chromatography of oligosaccharides.

Prenatal Diagnosis Successful prenatal diagnosis has not been accomplished. In one case, analysis of transferrin fetal blood from an at-risk pregnancy demonstrated primarily the tetrasialo isoform, which suggests that the fetus would be unaffected; however, the fetus was born affected.[75] Mutations in a very large number of different genes can result in CDGS types I and II, making DNA-based diagnosis problematic unless a mutation has been found in a proband.[76a]

Geleophysic Dysplasia

An uncommon form of dwarfism has been described with accumulation of an as yet undefined glycoprotein. The children who inherit this defect were described as having 'happy (geleo) faces (physic).'[77,78] It is characterized by dysostosis multiplex and storage material in the liver, skin, and heart valves. Progressive cardiac valvular disease affects principally the mitral and tricuspid valves. The material accumulates within lysosomes and has the staining properties of a glycoprotein. Radiographic changes are most marked in the hands, feet, spine, tibia, and hips. **Acromicrodysplasia**, geleophysic, and **Moore-Federman syndrome** may be allelic forms of the same disorder that may be due to a defect in glycoprotein metabolism.[79]

Pathology

The liver biopsy showed focal areas of hepatic steatosis containing granular deposits resembling mucopolysaccharide. The most prominent ultrastructural characteristic noted by Lipson et al.[79] is the large number of lysosome-like vesicular bodies in many hepatocytes. These bodies range from 0.3 to 0.9 μm in diameter and are bounded by a single membrane discernible as trilaminar in places, enclosing a generally uniform, granular matrix.

Most cases represent sporadic occurrence, though three sibs described by Spranger et al.[80] and two by Koiffmann et al.[81] suggest autosomal recessive inheritance.

Canavan Disease

Canavan disease (**Canavan Bogaert-Bertrand spongy degeneration**) is an autosomal recessive condition occurring predominantly in Jewish children, owing to deficiency of aspartoacylase with increased amounts of *N*-acetylaspartic acid in urine and plasma.[82] Onset is in the first 6 months of life and is characterized by apathy, loss of motor activity, hypotonia with blindness and optic atrophy, and megacephaly. Spasticity, decerebration, myoclonus, and generalized seizures with impairment of extraocular movements occur by 1 year. Death usually occurs within the first 3 years of life. The brain is heavier than normal with *megacephaly*. The white matter is soft, gelatinous, and gray, with the texture of a wet sponge. The occipital lobe is more involved than the frontal and parietal areas. The globus pallidus is severely involved; the brainstem and spinal cord are less affected.

Microscopically, there is **spongy change, demyelination, proliferation of Alzheimer type II astrocytes**, and **scarce fibrillary gliosis**. Vacuolation involves the arcuate fibers and extends into the deep cortex, vacuoles are round to oval cavities, larger than neurons, and demyelination is moderate with mild gliosis. EM shows abnormality of astrocytic mitochondria. A juvenile form has been described with a later age of onset and sometimes prolonged survival.[83–88]

Prenatal Diagnosis Prenatal diagnosis utilizes quantitation of *N*-acetylaspartate in amniotic fluid and aspartoacylase activity in cells cultured from amniotic fluid or chorionic villous sampling (CVS).[89,90] Isotope dilution methods are more reliable for quantitation of *N*-acetylaspartate.

Levels of aspartoacylase activity in cultured CVS and cultured amniocytes are very low by comparison to cultured skin fibroblasts. Molecular diagnosis is possible, as the gene responsible (*ASPA*) has been sequenced.

TABLE 12.5 COMPARISON OF CLINICAL FINDINGS IN SALLA DISEASE AND INFANTILE SIALIC ACID STORAGE DISEASE (ISSD)

	Salla disease	ISSD
Intrauterine	No findings	Hydrops fetalis 10%
Neonatal	Normal	Hepatosplenomegaly and ascites 50%
Infancy	Hypotonia, ocular nystagmus, ataxia, failure to thrive	Failure to thrive, dysmorphic features
Childhood	Developmental delay, impaired speech, growth retardation	
Adulthood	Severe mental retardation, ataxia, abnormal tendon reflexes, exotropia of eyes	
Age of death	35–72 yr	3 mo–4.5 yr (mean 20 mo)

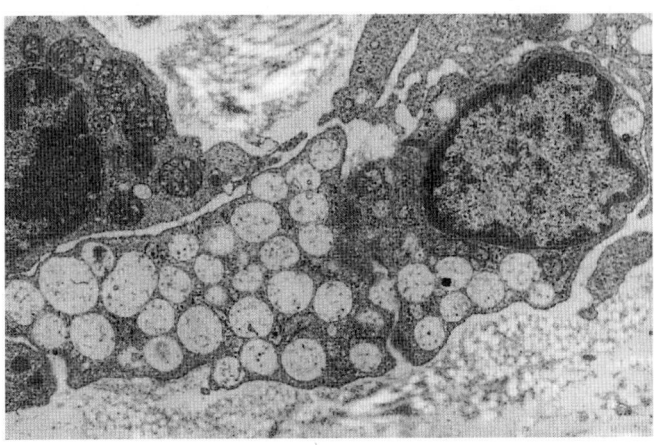

FIGURE 12.8 Salla disease. Peripheral nerve fiber showing abundant storage in lysosomes in the cytoplasm of a Schwann cell (× 4800). (Courtesy of Dr Juhani Rapola.)

Sialic Acid Disorders

Sialic acid storage diseases are characterized by lysosomal storage of sialic acid and excretion of excessive amounts of free N-acetylneuraminic acid (sialic acid) in the urine.

The efflux of free sialic acid through the lysosomal membrane is impaired.[91,92] Cystinosis is based on analogous pathogenesis.[93] The primary gene product mediating the passage of sialic acid through the membrane is called *SLC17A5*.

Sialic acid storage disorders are divided into two main clinical forms, both of which are inherited as autosomal recessive traits. The chronic form with prolonged life span, known also as **Salla disease** (SD) after the area of origin of the first patients, is common in Finland.[94] The more severe **infantile sialic acid storage disease** (ISSD) is less common and does not show ethnic prevalence.[92] Table 12.5 compares SD and ISSD. The diagnosis of both types is made by demonstration of free sialic acid in urine and tissue specimens or cultured fibroblasts in ISSD and sialated oligosaccharide in Salla disease.

Prenatal diagnosis of both SD and ISSD is made by demonstration of increased free sialic acid or sialated oligosaccharides, either in the cultured amniotic fluid cells or in chorionic villus specimens.[95,96]

Decrease of the cerebral white matter, slight ventricular dilation, and a thin corpus callosum were found in two SD patients at autopsy.[97] Microscopic investigation of several tissues, including **liver, skin, kidney, and peripheral blood lymphocytes, conjunctival biopsy, CNS, and myenteric plexus of the gastrointestinal tract** shows enlarged storage lysosomes. **Lymphocytes** show **cytoplasmic vacuoles**. Semithin resin-embedded tissue sections show cytoplasmic vacuoles in several organs (Fig. 12.8). Electron microscopy of skin biopsy specimens shows storage lysosomes. The most affected are dermal fibrocytes, perineural connective tissue cells, and Schwann cells. Sialic acid-binding lectin LPA (*Limulus* polyphenic) accumulates in the cultured fibroblasts of SD.[98]

Clinically, SD shows relatively mild but progressive neurologic signs and retardation, beginning in infancy and leading to a retarded adult with a long life span. No radiologic skeletal changes are evident except a thick calvarium. ISSD shows neonatal and infantile organomegaly and severe retardation, ending in death in infancy or childhood (Table 12.5).

Diagnosis The routine diagnostic test for both SD and ISSD is demonstration of elevated levels of free sialic acid in the urine, generally done by thin-layer chromatography.[99]

The definitive diagnosis of sialidosis is based on the direct measurement of sialidase activity in fresh tissue samples. Tissue samples should not be frozen or exposed to prolonged sonication.[100] The substrate of choice appears to be 4-methylumbelliferyl-β-N-acetylneuraminic acid.[101] Measurement of carboxypeptidase activity should also distinguish galactosialidosis patients who lack this activity from sialidosis patients who have normal levels of this enzyme.[102]

Prenatal Diagnosis Prenatal diagnosis of SD and ISSD can be made definitively by chorionic villus biopsy and/or amniocentesis as early as 9–10 weeks. The cells must be handled with special care because an enzyme activity is quickly destroyed by freezing, sonication, and/or exposure to temperatures of 37°C.[103]

Another rare condition called **French-type sialuria** (McKusick 269921) is caused by defective feedback inhibition of the cytosolic enzyme UDP-N-acetylglucosamine-2-epimerase, with resultant excessive production of sialic acid. This condition is not related to lysosomal storage.

Nephrosialidosis produces cytoplasmic storage with vacuolation in a very wide range of cell types; the pattern of glomerular crescent formation seen in the disease is distinctive.

Sialidosis

Sialidosis1 and 2 are due to neuraminidase deficiency and present with decreasing vision, macular cherry-red spots, normal intelligence, and myoclonus.

There are intermediate neuraminidase levels in parents of affected patients.[104] The neuraminidase deficiency found in a galactosialidosis patient has been shown to be caused by a mutation in a gene located on chromosome 20q13.[105] These findings indicate that sialidosis and the combined deficiencies of galactosialidosis are two distinct and separate genetic disorders.

The majority of type 1 patients have been Italian and those of the more serious type 2 have been Japanese. The age of onset is variable, but is usually in the second decade. Impaired color vision or night blindness[106,107] are found. Ocular cherry-red spot, while consistent, may be atypical; punctuate lenticular opacities occur.[108–110]

Type 2 ISSD is distinguished from the milder type I form by the early onset of a progressive, severe mucopolysaccharidosis-like phenotype with visceromegaly, dysostosis multiplex, and mental retardation.

Nephrosialidosis occurs in type 2 sialidosis with proteinuria progressing to nephritic syndrome in the first few years of life with the storage of sialyloligosaccharides.

Both forms of the disease result from deficiency of a neuraminidase that normally cleaves terminal a(2:3) and a(2:6) sialyl linkages of several oligosaccharides and glycopeptides that are found in increased amounts in tissues and fluids of affected patients. The defect in sialidosis has not been well characterized, but the gene coding for part of this protein maps to chromosome 10pter-q23 and part to chromosome 20.[110a]

Diagnosis Oligosaccharides are excreted in excessive amounts in the urine, as compounds with NANA or *N*-acetlglucosamine, in contrast to SD, in which sialic acid is free. Vacuolated lymphocytes are detected. Mucopolysacchariduria does not occur.

Pathology Vacuolated lymphocytes and bone marrow foam cells are found in type 2 sialidosis. Vacuolation is prominent in Kupffer cells, less so in hepatocytes. Vacuolation is also found in nerve biopsies, tissue fibroblast, and brain cells. Membrane-bound vacuoles may contain reticulogranular material, lipofuscin, and other inclusions. Cytoplasmic inclusions are stored in lysosomes. Sialidase, a lysosomal glycoprotein enzyme, is decreased or absent. EM demonstrates vacuoles of varied sizes bounded by a single membrane. Included material may be electron lucent or granular.

Prenatal Diagnosis and Screening Neuramidase can be measured as in ISSD in amniotic fluid or CVS.

α_1-Antitrypsin (α_1-Antiprotease) Deficiency

α_1-antitrypsin (α_1AT), a glycoprotein of molecular weight 52 kDa, is a major **plasma protease inhibitor** and accounts for 80% of serum α_1-globulin. The physiologic substrate is elastase, particularly important for the integrity of the lower respiratory tract. The **Pi locus** (protease inhibitor) for α_1AT is on **chromosome 14 q31-32.1**, close to the locus for the Pi α_1-chymotrypsin. α_1AT shows considerable genetic variability, with more than 60 genetic variants.[111] For the most common variants, letters are used according to their electrophoretic mobility: F (fast), S (slow), Z (very slow). The normal phenotype is PiMM and has 100% activity.

The phenotype of the most severe form of α_1AT deficiency is **PiZZ** with 10–20% activity. Homozygous PiZZ has an incidence of 1 in 1600 to 2000 live births in North America and Northern Europe. α_1AT is retained in the cytoplasm of the cell.[112] In children, liver involvement is most frequent[113] where the hepatocytes contain **eosinophilic, hyalin-like globules**, usually in periportal hepatocytes (Fig. 12.9A and12.9B). With PAS staining followed by diastase (PASD), the inclusions are easily visualized as brilliant pink globules in the cytoplasm, most prominent in the periportal hepatocytes.[114] In newborn infants the intracytoplasmic inclusions may be fine, granular, and indistinguishable from other granules such as bile. Immunohistochemical stains are useful to confirm the identity of the material, using an antibody to α_1AT. By EM, the storage material is present within the cisternae of the endoplasmic reticulum (Fig. 12.9C).[115] The most common type of liver involvement is characterized by conjugated hyperbilirubinemia, raised serum aminotransferase levels, and often hepatosplenomegaly. In addition to giant cell transformation, hepatocellular injury and fibrosis, cholestasis, and bile duct proliferation can be seen in liver biopsies. There is an increase in the HLA-DR3-Dw25 haplotype in α_1AT-deficient persons with liver disease. Liver injury in α_1AT deficiency is a direct consequence of the intracellular accumulation of mutant α_1AT molecules and does not result from a deficiency in antielastase activity.[116,117] With severe liver disease the treatment has been orthoptic liver transplantation.[118] **Liver cell carcinoma** may occur.[119]

Prenatal Diagnosis Restriction fragment length polymorphisms detected with synthetic oligonucleotide probes[120,121] and family studies[122] allow prenatal diagnosis. There is a 78% chance that a second PiZZ child will have serious liver disease if the older sib had serious liver disease.[124]

Clinical Manifestation of Liver Disease Liver involvement is usually noticed in the first 2 months of life because of persistent jaundice. Serum transaminases are slightly elevated. The liver may be enlarged. These infants are generally admitted with a diagnosis of neonatal hepatitis syndrome. Many of these infants have minimal clinical liver disease but persistent serum transaminase abnormalities for the first few years of life. Approximately 10% of this population has moderate to severe clinical liver disease with complications of liver synthetic dysfunction (bleeding diathesis, ascites, feeding difficulties, poor growth). Bleeding, including intracranial hemorrhage has been a presenting manifestation in the newborn related to the association with vitamin K deficiency.[124] A few infants are recognized initially because of a cholestatic clinical syndrome characterized by pruritus,

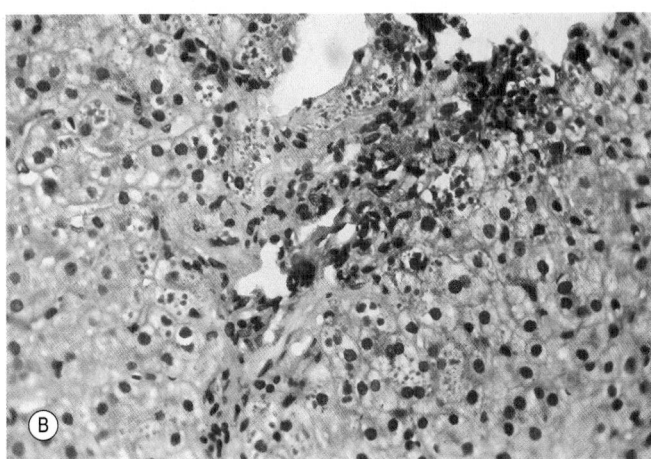

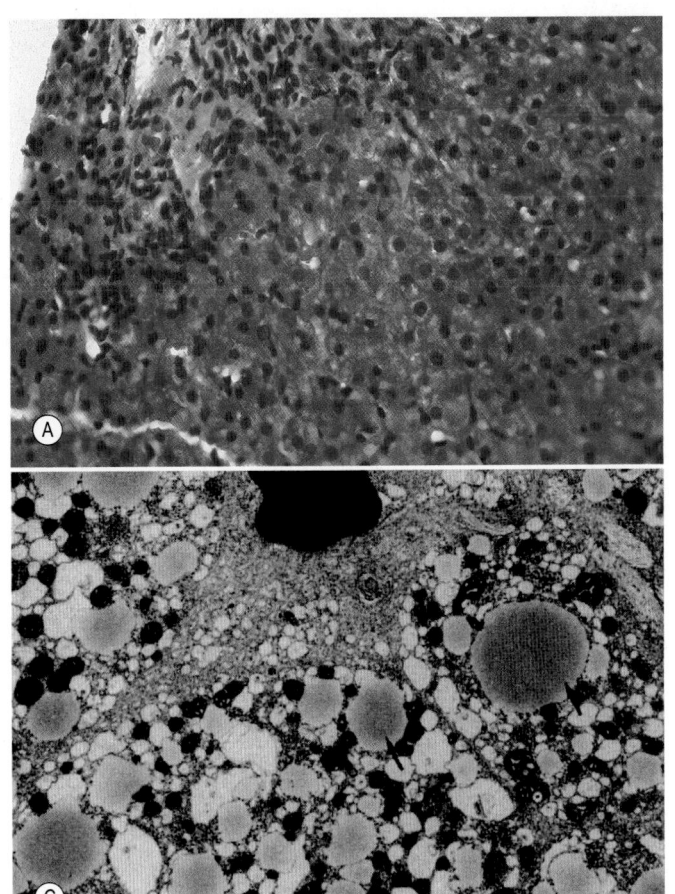

FIGURE 12.9 α-1-antitrypsin deficiency. (A) A liver biopsy in a 4-month-old infant shows globules in periportal hepatocytes there was a mild portal fibrosis. (B) The globules are periodic acid-schiff (PAS)-positive and resist diastase digestion. (C) Electron micrograph shows flocculent pale material within dilated cisternae of rough endoplasmic reticulum (arrows).

hypercholesterolemia, conjugated hyperbilirubinemia, and paucity of intrahepatic bile ducts on histopathologic examination.[125] Congenital cirrhosis may be the first manifestation of α_1AT. Liver disease may also be first manifested in late childhood or early adolescence when there is a history of unexplained prolonged obstructive jaundice in the neonatal period.

Diagnosis of α_1AT Deficiency Diagnosis is established by a serum α_1AT phenotype determination in isoelectric focusing on agarose gel electrophoresis at acid pH. The phenotype should be determined in all cases of neonatal hepatitis or unexplained chronic liver disease in older children.

It is now also possible to detect specific α_1AT variants by amplification of genomic DNA using PCR.[126-128] It should prove useful for confirmation of diagnoses, population screening, and prenatal diagnosis.

In adults, α_1AT is most often associated with **panlobular emphysema** in the lower lobes of the lung. In PiZZ patients, the incidence of cirrhosis or emphysema is approximately 40%.

Galactosialidosis

A similar disease to sialidosis is due to a combined deficiency of neuraminidase and β-galactosidase and referred to as galactosialidosis or Goldberg syndrome.

Galactosialidosis is a lysosomal storage disease associated with a combined deficiency of β-galactosidase and neuraminidase, secondary to a defect of another lysosomal protein, the protective protein.[129]

Galactosialidosis is transmitted as an autosomal recessive trait. The gene encoding the protective protein has been localized on chromosome 10q31.1.

All patients have clinical manifestations typical of a lysosomal disorder, such as coarse facies, cherry-red spots, vertebral changes, foam cells in the bone marrow, and vacuolated lymphocytes and dysostosis multiplex. Two phenotypic subtypes are recognized. The early infantile form is associated with fetal hydrops, edema, ascites, visceromegaly, skeletal dysplasia, and early death. The late infantile type is characterized by hepatosplenomegaly, growth retardation, cardiac involvement, and absence of relevant neurologic signs.

Sialyl-oligosaccharides accumulate in lysosomes and are excreted in body fluids.

The demonstration of a combined deficiency of β-galactosidase and neuraminidase in lymphocytes and/or cultured skin fibroblasts is the preferred method of biochemical diagnosis. The assay of the cathepsin A-like activity of the protective protein might give a false-negative result, because in principle a mutation could affect the protective function but not the catalytic activity. Carrier detection should be based on assays involving the primary defect.[129]

Prenatal diagnosis has been established by demonstrating a combined β-galactosidase–neuraminidase deficiency in cultured amniotic fluid cells.

Glucose transport defects

Glucose transporters move glucose across the plasma membrane of human cells. Defects in glucose transporters cause renal glycosuria and glucose-galactose malabsorption. Alterations in facilitative glucose transporters explain the syndrome of low CNS glucose in the presence of normal blood glucose, causing seizures and developmental delay.[130]

Two main classes of glucose transporters have been identified: active Na+/glucose cotransporters (SGLT) and facilitative glucose transporters (GLUT). Facilitative glucose transporters are regulated by insulin, and variations in their levels are associated with diabetes.

Lysosomal lipid storage diseases

The large number of diseases of lysosomal lipid storage (Table 12.6) reflects a wide variety of molecules – triglycerides, sterols, sphingolipids, sulfatides, sphingomyelins, gangliosides, and lipofuscins – that must be degraded by the lysosomal acid hydrolase system.

Tissues useful in the diagnosis of lysosomal storage diseases are shown in Table 12.7.

Wolman disease and cholesteryl ester storage disease

Both of these diseases are autosomal recessive. Cholesteryl esters are hydrolyzed by lysosomal acid lipase. Deficiency of two allelic forms of the enzymes results in Wolman disease and cholesteryl ester storage disease, in which deficiency of lysosomal acid lipase leads to accumulation of cholesteryl esters. The definitive diagnosis of both disorders is made by assay for lysosomal acid lipase activity in cultured fibroblasts, lymphocytes, or other tissues.[131] The gene encoding lysosomal acid lipase has been linked to chromosome 10q23.3-q23.3.

Wolman disease[132] presents in early infancy and is rapidly progressive with hepatosplenomegaly, jaundice, anemia, failure to thrive, lipid-laden histiocytes in the bone marrow and peripheral blood, and acanthocytosis. Plasma lipids are at the low end of the normal range. Hepatosplenomegaly may be massive. Death occurs by 1 year of age. The liver is enlarged, yellow with foam cells in the periportal areas in both hepatocytes and Kupffer cells. Portal and periportal fibrosis may be marked and cirrhosis may develop. **Cholesteryl and triglycerides** can be identified histochemically.[133] The **adrenal glands** contain necrotic cells and foam cells and become calcified. The **lamina propria of the gastrointestinal (GI) tract** (Fig. 12.10), lung, lymph nodes, spleen, vessel walls,

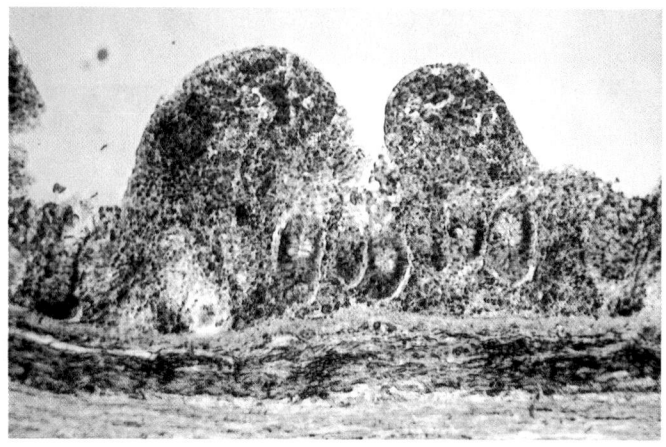

FIGURE 12.10 Wolman disease. Gastrointestinal muscosa contains an abundance of lipid-laden histocytes (oil red O stain). (Courtesy of Dr. Ben Landing.)

oligodendroglia in the brain, Schwann cells, ganglion cells of the GI myenteric plexus, peripheral blood lymphocytes, and histiocytes in the marrow show lipid vacuolization. Lysosomal lipid and cholesteryl ester crystals are demonstrated with birefringent light using unfixed frozen tissue sections and with electron microscopy.[134]

Cholesteryl ester storage disease (CESD) is mild and usually does not present until childhood or later, although it has been diagnosed in a fetus aborted at 17 weeks.[135,136] Syncytiotrophoblasts may show vacuolization in the placenta. Similar changes to Wolman disease occur, but adrenal calcification and foam histocytes in the marrow have not been observed.

Prenatal Diagnosis Prenatal diagnosis of Wolman disease and CESD is established by assays by electrophoresis, and lysosomal and lipase in cultured amniotic fluid cells or chorionic villus cells.

Sphingolipid storage diseases

Sphingolipids that are involved in lipid storage diseases are all based on a long-chain amino alcohol (**sphingosine**) that is combined with a fatty acid to produce complex lipids (**ceramides**). When a sugar is added to a ceramide, a **cerebroside** results. If the sugar is glucose, the lipid is a glucocerebroside. When a polysaccharide is added to the ceramide along with one molecule or more of N-acetyl neuraminic acid, the result is a ganglioside (Fig. 12.11). The structure of sphingolipids is shown in Figure 12.12.

Niemann-Pick disease

Sphingomyelin lipidosis is associated with deficiency of isoelectric forms of sphingomyelinase. Six types of this disorder have been characterized.[137–139] **Type A** is the **infantile form** in which hepatosplenomegaly and CNS degeneration begin within the first year of life. **Type B** is the **non-neuronopathic form** and

TABLE 12.6 LYSOSOMAL LIPID STORAGE DISEASES

McKusick no.	Disease	Inheritance	Deficient enzyme	Clinicopathologic features
Cholesteryl ester storage disease				
278000	Wolman, infantile	AR	Acid lipase (cholesterol ester hydrolase)	Failure to thrive, hepatomegaly, malabsorption, adrenal insufficiency, rapid course, storage of triglyceride, cholesterol ester in liver, spleen, lymphoid tissues, adrenal, marrow, lungs, intestinal lamina propria, renal epithelium, enteric and central neurons, placental trophoblast; adrenal necrosis with calcification
278000	Wolman, late infantile, juvenile	AR	Acid lipase	Later onset, slower course (presumably allelic)
278000	Cholesteryl ester storage disease	AR	Acid lipase	Splenomegaly, atheromas, esophageal varices, pulmonary hypertension, hepatic failure (allelic)
Sphingomyelin storage diseases				
257200	Niemann-Pick A (infantile cerebral type)	AR	Sphingomyelinase	Visceromegaly, cerebral deterioration, rapid course, lysosomal storage in reticuloendothelial cells (foam cells) hepatocytes, bone marrow, lungs, peripheral and central neurons; epicenter in Eastern Europe, with disease most frequent in Ashkenazi Jews; congenital Niemann-Pick disease is variant
607616	Niemann-Pick B (juvenile non-cerebral type)	AR	Sphingomyelinase	Visceromegaly, lung infiltration; storage cells and sea-blue histiocytes, but neurons not involved; survival to at least late first decade
	Niemann-Pick (neonatal malignant cholestatic jaundice)	AR	Presumably sphingomyelinase subset of NP-A	Cholestatic jaundice with giant cell transformation of liver (neonatal hepatitis) early; findings as in NP-A and NP-C or NP-D if survival adequate; possible epicenter in Hispanics in western United States
257220	Niemann-Pick C (subacute juvenile neuronopathic type)	AR	Deficient esterification of exogenous cholesterol	Visceromegaly, cerebellar ataxia, seizures, psychotic features; Western European epicenter; positive OTAN stain of storage cells useful
257220	Niemann-Pick D (subacute juvenile/adult neuronopathic type	AR	Deficient esterification of exogenous cholesterol	Visceromegaly, cerebellar ataxia, seizures, psychotic features; Eastern European epicenter; positive OTAN stain of storage cells useful
257220	Niemann-Pick D (subacute juvenile/adult neuronopathic type)	AR	Same as above	Survival into second decade; epicenter in Nova Scotia
257220	Niemann-Pick E (adult non-cerebral type)	AR	Same as above	Storage cells as in NP-B; possible Mediterranean region epicenter
Other neural lipidoses				
213700	Cerebral dystonic lipidosis	AR	CYP27A1	Onset 4-9 yr, dementia, seizures, dystonic movements, normal fundi; foam cells in marrow

TABLE 12.6 LYSOSOMAL LIPID STORAGE DISEASES (*CONT'D*)

McKusick no.	Disease	Inheritance	Deficient enzyme	Clinicopathologic features
213700	Cerebrotendinous xanthomatosis (cerebral cholesterolosis, normolipemic xanthomatosis)	AR	Mitrochondrial sterol 27-hydroxylase	Onset in second decade; cerebral deterioration, cerebellar ataxia, cataract, atherosclerosis; cholesterol, cholestanol deposits in tendons (especially Achilles tendons) lungs, cerebellar white matter, cerebral peduncles
269600	Neurovisceral disease with supranuclear opthalmoplegia, xanthomatosis	AR	Sphingomyelinase	Supranuclear ophthalmoplegia, hepatic cirrhosis; foam cells, sea-blue histiocytes, in marrow*, neuronal lipid storage
Cerebroside storage diseases				
230800	Gaucher 1 (adult Gaucher disease)	AR	Glucocerebrosidase β-D-glucosyl-*N*-acyl sphingosine hydrolase	Hepatosplenomegaly, osteoporosis with liability to fracture; onset in first decade with survival to sixth decade or later; Gaucher cells are macrophages of spleen, liver, nodes, thymus, marrow; storage lysosomes have elongated tubular shape; Eastern European epicenter, with greater frequency in Ashkenazi Jews (possible West African epicenter)
Note similar disease can be due to saposin C (sphingolipid activator protein 2) deficiency				
230900	Gaucher 2A (infantile cerebral type)	AR	Glucocerebrosidase	Visceral disease similar to type 1, rapidly progressive cerebral damage without neuronal cerebroside storage; short survival; no apparent epicenter
	Gaucher 2B (rapidly progressive with ichthyosis)	AR	Glucocerebrosidase	Neonatal rapidly progressive ichthyosis, non-immune hydrops, death by 5 mo; Gaucher cells in reticuloendothelial system and central nervous system
231000	Gaucher 3 (chronic neuropathic or Norrbottnian type)	AR	Glucocerebrosidase	Both visceral and progressive neurologic dysfunction; survival into second or third decades; storage cells as to Gaucher 1 and adventitia of vessels of cortex and cerebral white matter
230800	Pseudo-Gaucher disease	AR	Glucocerebrosidase	Corneal opacities, hydrocephalus, valvular heart disease, deafness, supranuclear ophthalmoplegia, visceral infiltration mild; caused by a mutation of GBA, which is allelic with Gaucher type 1
245200	Krabbe, infantile type	AR	Galactocerebroside β-Galactosidase	Onset 4-6 mo with rapid severe neurologic damage; storage "globoid body" cells in central white matter
245200	Krabbe, late infantile/juvenile type	AR	Galactocerebroside β-Galactosidase	Onset by 5 yr, course more rapid if onset by 3 yr; visual failure, cerebellar ataxia, spastic hemi/paraparesis, peripheral neuropathy with reduced nerve conduction velocity; storage cells in central and peripheral neural tissue; epicenter in Sicily reported

TABLE 12.6 LYSOSOMAL LIPID STORAGE DISEASES (*CONT'D*)

McKusick no.	Disease	Inheritance	Deficient enzyme	Clinicopathologic features
301500	Farber Lipogranulomatosis			
	a. Early onset	AR	Ceramidase	Subcutaneous nodules, arthritis, laryngeal
	b. Infantile type	AR	Ceramidase	Periarticular, no lung involvement, normal intelligence
	c. Late onset	AR	Ceramidase	Survival into second decade macroglossia, laryngeal, joint but not lung involvement and less cerebral dysfunction
	d. Neonatal type	AR	Ceramidase	Psychomotor retardation, hepatomegaly, debility
	e. Malignant histocytosis type	AR	Ceramidase	Psychomotor retardation at 1–2 yr; hoarseness, arthritis, macular cherry-red spot
301500	Fabry (angiokeratoma corporis diffusum)	XLR	α-galactosidase A (ceramide trihexosidase)	Onset in males in first decade, later with slower course in female heterozygotes; nephrotic syndrome, progressive to renal failure, cardiomegaly with cardiomyopathy (especially in young adult females), episodic abdominal pain, angiokeratomas of skin[†]; storage in renal glomerular and tubular epithelium, cardiac myocytes, enteric and brainstem/spinal cord neurons, blood vessel walls
Gangliosidoses				
230500	GM_1 type 1, gangliosidosis, infantile	AR	β-Galactosidase	Onset birth/early infancy; survival ±1–2 yr; abnormal facies, skeletal changes (especially vertebrae), visceromegaly, cerebral deterioration; storage of ganglioside and/or mucopolysaccharide in reticuloendothelial cells, liver cells, renal glomerular and tubular epithelium, pancreatic and mucoserous gland epithelium, central and peripheral neurons
230600	GM_1 gangliosidosis, type 2 infantile (Derry)	AR	As above, presumably allelic	Onset later, course slower than above; visceromegaly, skeletal changes less marked, neuronal storage as above
230650	GM_1, gangliosidosis type 3, adult	AR	As above, presumably allelic	Mental deterioration, visual loss, myoclonic seizures; angiokeratomas may be early feature
Note above three conditions presumably allelic with mucopolysaccharidosis IVB (Morquio B, q.v.)				
272800	GM_2 type 1 gangliosidosis, infantile (Tay-Sachs disease, B form)	AR	Hexosaminidase A (α-unit mutation)	Rapidly progressive dementia, blindness, macular cherry-red spot; epicenter in eastern Europe with high frequency in Ashkenazi Jews; most frequent gene abnormality is 4 base-pair insertion in Hex A gene, second is G-C substitution
272750	Tay-Sachs disease, AB form	AR	Hexosaminidase activator (saposin)	

TABLE 12.6 LYSOSOMAL LIPID STORAGE DISEASES (*CONT'D*)

McKusick no.	Disease	Inheritance	Deficient enzyme	Clinicopathologic features
272800	Tay-Sachs disease, B1 form, GM2 type 3 (juvenile type)	AR	Hexosaminidase A, α-unit (mutation gives gly 269 ser change in Hex A gene) (allelic with Tay-Sachs α-unit mutations)	Later onset than Tay-Sachs (B form); epicenter in Portugal; Affected persons from other regions genetic compounds for a TS mutation and B1 mutation
268800	GM2 type 2 gangliosidosis, infantile generalized form (Sandhoff)	AR	Hexosaminidases A and B (β-unit mutation)	Neuronal storage like that of Tay-Sachs disease with modest degree of visceral storage
230700	GM₂ gangliosidosis, juvenile, β-unit mutation	AR	As above	Progressive dementia, ataxia; picture can resemble X-linked bulbospinal muscular atrophy
230710	GM₂, gangliosidosis, juvenile, α-unit mutation	AR	Hexosaminidase A α-unit	Similar to above
	GM₂ gangliosidosis, chronic	AR	As above	Can be spinocerebellar degeneration resembling Friedreich ataxia, juvenile spinal muscular atrophy resembling Kugelberg-Welander disease, or like amyotrophic lateral sclerosis
	GM₂ gangliosidosis chronic, α-unit mutation	AR	Hexosaminidases A and B	Dementia, ataxia, pyramidal tract signs, amyotrophy; psychotic features regular; rectal biopsy for neurons useful
256540	Galactosialidosis (Goldberg)	AR	β-Galactosidase, neuraminidase (note early and late infantile forms due to deficiency of 'protector protein' for above lysosomal hydrolases, adult type due to abnormality of processor protein)	Abnormal facies, mental retardation, seizures, corneal clouding, deafness; lysosomal storage, especially in macrophages
Sulfatide storage diseases				
250100	Metachromatic leukodystrophy, infantile	AR	Arylsulfase A (cerebroside sulphate sulfatase) (allele 1 mutation)	Onset at ±2 yr, survival to ±5 yr; hypotonia, muscle weakness, mental deterioration, peripheral nerve involvement (prolonged nerve conduction time); storage cells in liver, kidney, epithelium, rectal lamina propria, central white matter, nerves; sulfatide shows brown metachromasia with cresyl violet, toluidine blue stains
250100	Metachromatic leukodystrophy, juvenile	AR	As above; presumably allelic with above (allele A mutation); genetic compound of allele 1 and allele A mutations presumably occur	As above, clinical onset 4–10 yr, with slower course; reduced nerve conduction velocity
250100	Metachromatic leukodystrophy, adult onset	AR	Same as above (? in spectrum of severity with other forms); pseudodeficiency gene occurs; some patients presumably genetic compound of MLD mutation and pseudodeficiency gene	Onset in second decade with schizophrenia-like behavior; visceral and central nervous system involvement
249900	Metachromatic leukodystrophy	AR	Saposin B (sulfatase activator protein I)	Variably as other forms

TABLE 12.6 LYSOSOMAL LIPID STORAGE DISEASES (*CONT'D*)

McKusick no.	Disease	Inheritance	Deficient enzyme	Clinicopathologic features
272200	Multiple sulfatase deficiency (Austin mucosulfatidosis)	AR	Arylsulfatases A, B and C; clinical type 1: onset in first yr, survival to 6–10 yr; 2: onset in later infancy, survival to second decade; 3: onset in second decade, survival to third–fourth decades; probably due to continuous spectrum of severity rather than allelic differences	Like those of metachromatic leukodystrophy with ichthyosis and somatic features suggesting mucopolysaccharidosis

*Sea blue histiocytes also occur in Hermansky-Pudlak albinism, hemorrhagic tendency, pigmented lipid histiocyte syndrome (q.v.), and Norum lecithin: cholesterol acyltransferase (LCAT) deficiency.

† Cutaneous angiokeratomas also occur in fucosidosis, adult gangliosidosis, GMI, aspartylglycosaminuria, galactosialidosis (Goldberg syndrome), later-onset multiple sulfate deficiency, α-galactosidase β deficiency (Schindler syndrome and Kanzaki glycominoacid storage disease), and β-mannosidosis, fucosidosis.

AR, autosomal recessive; XLR, X-linked recessive.

TABLE 12.7 TISSUES USEFUL IN DIAGNOSIS OF STORAGE DISEASES

Organ or tissue	Manifestation	Disease to be considered	Presumptive test	Diagnostic test
Liver	Increased size; disordered liver function tests may be seen in some, but not all, patients with the disease	α₁-Antitrypsin deficiency	Plasma α₁-antitrypsin	Electrophoresis and Pi typing; liver biopsy, immunopathology, electron microscopy
		Cholesteryl ester storage disease	Liver biopsy	Fibroblast acid lipase
		Mucropolysaccharidoses	Urine mucopolysaccharide quantitation; electron microscopy of conjunctival biopsy	Specific enzyme analysis
		Glycoproteinoses	Urine oligosaccharides; electron microscopy of conjunctival biopsy	Specific enzyme analysis
		Mucolipidoses II, III	Urine oligosaccharides; electron microscopy of conjunctival biopsy	Fibroblast lysosomal enzymes
		Glycogen storage diseases	Conjunctival biopsy (type II); liver biopsy, electron microscopy	Electron microscopy (type II)
		Gaucher disease	Gaucher cells in liver, bone marrow; increased serum total hexosaminidase or acid phosphatase	Leukocyte or fibroblast β-glucosidase; electron microscopy
		Niemann-Pick disease	Conjunctival, liver biopsy, electron microscopy	Leukocyte or fibroblast sphingomyelinase
		Wolman disease	Liver biopsy	Fibroblast acid lipase
Spleen	Increased size	Mucopolysaccharidoses	Urine mucopolysaccharide quantitation; electron microscopy of conjunctival biopsy	Specific enzyme analysis

TABLE 12.7 TISSUES USEFUL IN DIAGNOSIS OF STORAGE DISEASES (*CONT'D*)

Organ or tissue	Manifestation	Disease to be considered	Presumptive test	Diagnostic test
		Gaucher disease	Gaucher cells in bone marrow	Leukocyte or fibroblast β-glucosidase; electron microscopy
		Niemann-Pick disease	Conjunctiva, bone marrow or liver biopsy, electron microscopy	Leukocyte or fibroblast sphingomyelinase
Bone and joint	Dysostosis multiplex, other radiographic changes	Mucopolysaccharidoses	Urine mucopolysaccharide quantitation; electron microscopy of conjunctival biopsy	Specific enzyme analysis
		Glycoproteinoses	Urine oligosaccharide determination; electron microscopy of conjunctival biopsy	Specific enzyme analysis
	Swollen joints, soft tissue nodules	Farber disease	Tissue biopsy for electron microscopy	Fibroblast culture; lysosomal acid ceramidase
Eye	Macular cherry-red spot	Tay-Sachs disease	Serum hexosaminidase A	Leukocyte or fibroblast hexosaminidase A
		Sandhoff disease	Serum total hexosaminidase	Leukocyte or fibroblast total hexosaminidase
		Niemann-Pick disease	Conjunctival, bone marrow, or liver biopsy, electron microscopy	Leukocyte or fibroblast sphingomyelinase
		Generalized gangliosidosis	White cell β-galactosidase; Occasionally urine oligosaccharide increases can be seen by thin layer chromatography; conjunctival, bone marrow biopsy; electron microscopy	Leukocyte or fibroblast, galactosidase
		Sialidoses	Urinary oligosaccharide excretion, conjunctival biopsy for electron microscopy	Fibroblast sialidase
	Corneal clouding	Mucopolysaccharidoses (Hurler, Scheie, Morquio, Maroteaux-Lamy, β-glucuronidase deficiency)	Urine mucopolysaccharides; conjunctival biopsy for electron microscopy	Specific enzyme analysis
		Mucolipidoses II, III	Urinary oligosaccharide excretion; conjunctival biopsy for electron microscopy	Fibroblast lysosomal enzymes
	Crystals in lens	Cystinosis	Cystine crystals in tissues	Cystine in leukocytes/fibroblasts
Adrenal gland	Bilateral adrenal calcification	Wolman disease	Liver biopsy	Fibroblast acid lipase
Muscle-cardiac/skeletal	Cardiomegaly; heart failure; myopathy involving skeletal muscle	Pompe disease	Electron microscopy, conjunctiva, lymphocytes or skin	Lumphocyte or fibroblast α-glucosidase; electron microscopy
		Glycogen storage diseases types III, IV	Liver biopsy for electron microscopy	Specific enzyme analysis
Brain	Progressive mental and motor dysfunction; retardation	Krabbe disease	Conjunctival biopsy for electron microscopy; CSF protein (increased)	Galactocerebroside β-galactosidase, leukocytes, or fibroblast culture

TABLE 12.7 TISSUES USEFUL IN DIAGNOSIS OF STORAGE DISEASES (*CONT'D*)

Organ or tissue	Manifestation	Disease to be considered	Presumptive test	Diagnostic test
		Metachromatic leukodystrophy	Conjunctival biopsy for electron microscopy	Arylsulfatase A, fibroblast culture
		Neuronal ceroid lipofusinoses	CSF protein (increased); sural nerve biopsy; nerve conduction studies	Peripheral blood lymphocytes, skin, conjunctival biopsy for electron microscopy
		Niemann-Pick disease	Conjunctival, bone marrow, or liver biopsy	Leukocyte or fibroblast sphingomyelinase
		Gaucher disease	Gaucher cells in bone marrow, liver	Leukocyte or fibroblast, β-glucosidase; electron microscopy
		Mucopolysaccharidoses	Urine mucopolysaccharide quantitations; electron microscopy of conjunctival biopsy	Specific enzyme analysis
		Glycoproteinoses	Urine oligosaccharide determination; electron microscopy of conjunctival biopsy	Specific enzyme analysis
		Tay-Sachs disease	Serum hexosaminidase A	Leukocyte or fibroblast hexosaminidase A
		Sandhoff disease	Serum total hexosaminidase	Leukocyte or fibroblast total hexosaminidase
		Generalized gangliosidosis	White cell β-galactosidase;	Leukocyte or fibroblast β-galactosidase
			GM_1	Urine oligosaccharide thin layer chromatography; conjunctival, bone marrow biopsy for electron microscopy

is less severe than type A. **Type C,**[139] the **juvenile form**, is characterized by CNS degeneration beginning after the first year of life, with less severe hepatosplenomegaly than is found in type A, and is often accompanied by predominance of cerebellar symptoms. Macular cherry-red spots are seen in types A and C. In type C, defects in the esterification of cholesterol have been identified.[140,141]

The most common and severe variant is type A, the acute neuronopathic form. These patients, often of Eastern European Jewish ancestry, present early in life with hepatosplenomegaly and a rapidly progressive deterioration of the CNS. Often the skin has a yellow-brown pigmentation, lymph nodes are enlarged, and ocular manifestations (cherry-red macula and corneal opacifications) are evident. Few children survive beyond 4 years of age.

The type B variant (an allelic variant of type A) features a pattern of visceral involvement similar to type A yet spares the CNS. These children present at a later age with isolated splenomegaly. In time, a more generalized visceral pattern of involvement is manifest, yet many patients survive several decades. Neonates may present with ascites and meconium ileus, and some have developed biliary atresia or, more commonly, neonatal hepatitis.[142] Storage cells are more prominent in type A. Storage material is found in **reticuloendothelial cells, hepatocytes,**[143] **syncytiotrophoblasts,** and **villus stromal cells.**[144]

Twelve mutations have been identified in the sphingomyelin gene that cause types A and B. Three mutations – R496L, L302P, and fsP330 – account for about 92% of the mutant alleles in Ashkenazi Jewish type A. A single mutation, Δ-R608, accounts for 50% of the Ashkenazi Jewish type B patients. The diagnosis of types A and B Niemann-Pick Disease (NPD) can readily be made by enzymatic determination of sphingomyelinase activity in cell and/or tissue extracts. Prenatal diagnosis can be accomplished by enzymatic and/or molecular analysis of cultured amniocytes or chorionic villus samples.

The chronic neuronopathic form (type C) presents with diverse neurologic symptoms (ataxia, seizures, loss of previously learned speech) at about 5 years of age. Although hepatosplenomegaly is present, it is less pronounced than that in types A and B. Studies of cell lines from these patients have revealed a block in cholesterol esterification. The diagnosis may also be established by cytochemical staining with filipin, which demonstrates an intravesicular cholesterol storage material. Foam cells or **sea-blue histiocytes** are found in many tissues. Although the condition is not rapidly fatal, few patients survive beyond 15 years. An adult-onset form of type C has been reported.[145]

Niemann-Pick type C can result from mutations of the genes *NPC1* and *NPC2*. Unesterified cholesterol, sphingomyelin,

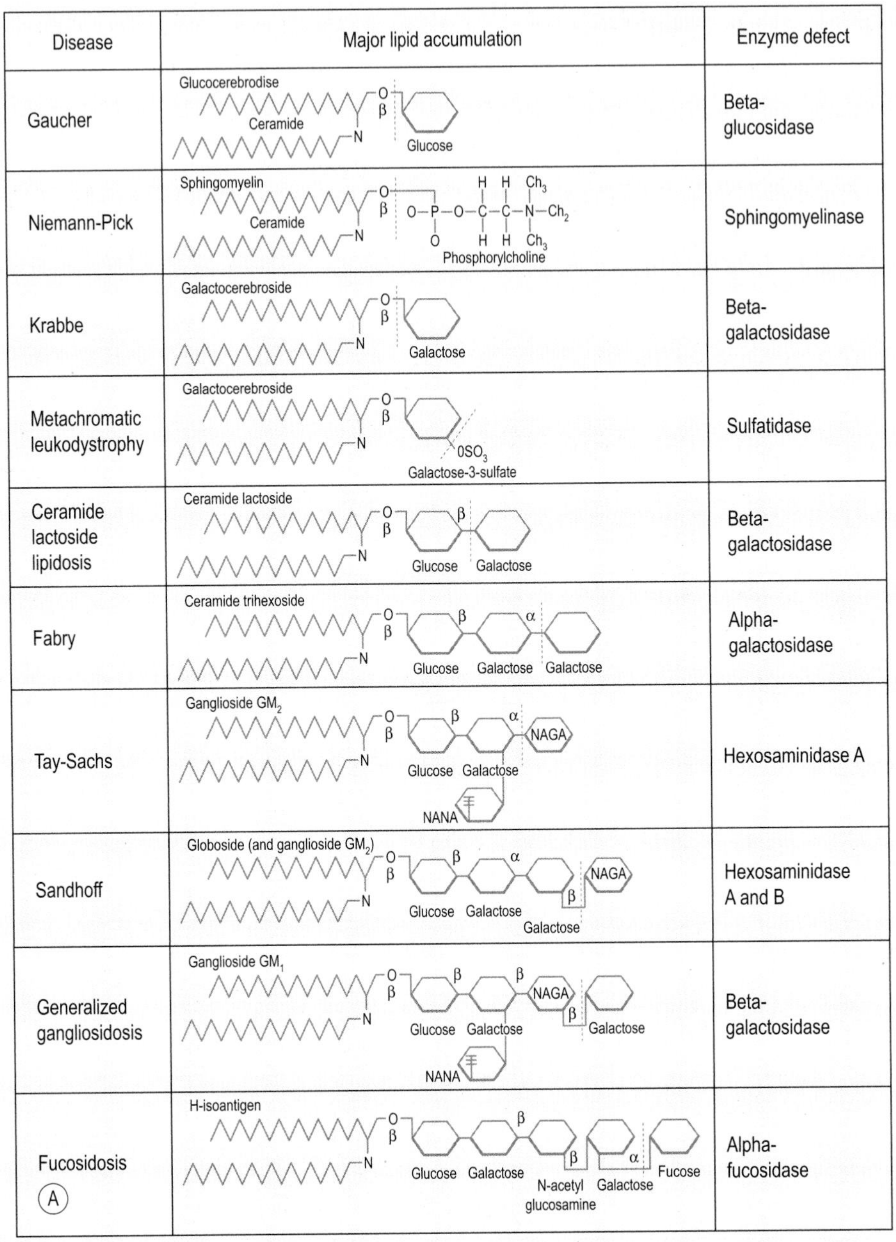

Disease	Major lipid accumulation	Enzyme defect
Gaucher	Glucocerebrodise / Ceramide / Glucose	Beta-glucosidase
Niemann-Pick	Sphingomyelin / Ceramide / Phosphorylcholine	Sphingomyelinase
Krabbe	Galactocerebroside / Galactose	Beta-galactosidase
Metachromatic leukodystrophy	Galactocerebroside / Galactose-3-sulfate	Sulfatidase
Ceramide lactoside lipidosis	Ceramide lactoside / Glucose Galactose	Beta-galactosidase
Fabry	Ceramide trihexoside / Glucose Galactose Galactose	Alpha-galactosidase
Tay-Sachs	Ganglioside GM$_2$ / Glucose Galactose NAGA / NANA	Hexosaminidase A
Sandhoff	Globoside (and ganglioside GM$_2$) / Glucose Galactose NAGA / Galactose	Hexosaminidase A and B
Generalized gangliosidosis	Ganglioside GM$_1$ / Glucose Galactose NAGA Galactose / NANA	Beta-galactosidase
Fucosidosis (A)	H-isoantigen / Glucose Galactose N-acetyl glucosamine Galactose Fucose	Alpha-fucosidase

FIGURE 12.11 (A) Lipid storage diseases with major lipid accumulation.

phospholipids, and glycolipids are stored in excess in the liver and spleen. Only glycolipids are elevated in the brain. Partial sphingomyelinase deficiency, observed only in cultured cells, represents a variable, secondary consequence of lysosomal cholesterol esterification. Cultured fibroblasts show a unique disorder of cellular cholesterol processing, in which delayed homeostatic responses to exogenous cholesterol loading are associated with cholesterol accumulation in lysosomes.[146]

Diagnosis The diagnosis of NPD-C requires both measurement of cellular cholesterol esterification and documentation of a characteristic pattern of filipin–cholesterol staining in cultured fibroblasts during LDL uptake. Candidates for such testing are identified by clinical presentation and findings from neurophysiologic tests and tissue biopsies. There is considerable variability in the degree of impairment of cholesterol esterification in NPD-C. Consequently, antenatal diagnosis is currently restricted to families in which the index case has very low esterification levels.

Type D occurs in patients of **Nova Scotian ancestry**[147] who otherwise have a course similar to patients with type C. **Type E** has been included as an **indeterminate form in adults**[148–150]

Disease	Signs and symptoms	Enzyme defect
Gaucher disease	Spleen and liver enlargement Erosion of long bones and pelvis Mental retardation only in infantile form	Beta-glucosidase
Niemann-Pick disease	Liver and spleen enlargement Mental retardation About 30% with red spot in retina	Sphingomyelinase
Krabbe disease Globoid leukodystrophy	Mental retardation Almost total absence of myelin Globoid bodies in white matter of brain	Beta-galactosidase
Metachromatic leukodystrophy	Mental retardation Psychological disturbances in adult form Nerves stain yellow brown with cresyl violet dye	Arylsulfatase A
Ceramide lactoside lipidosis	Slowly progressing brain damage Liver and spleen enlargement	Beta-galactosidase
Fabry disease	Reddish purple skin rash Kidney failure Pain in lower extremities	Alpha-galactosidase
Tay-Sachs disease	Mental retardation Red spot in retina Blindness Muscular weakness	Hexosaminidase A
Tay-Sachs variant (Sandhoff disease)	Same as Tay-Sachs disease but progressing more rapidly	Hexosaminidase A and B
Generalized gangliosidosis	Mental retardation Liver enlargement Skeletal deformities About 50% with red spot in retina	Beta-galactosidase
Fucosidosis	Cerebral degeneration Muscle spasticity Thick skin	Alpha-fucosidase

FIGURE 12.11 (cont'd) (B) Lipid storage diseases with signs, symptoms and enzyme defects.

and biochemically appears to be closely related to type C. Types D and E have normal levels of sphingomyelinase; the two differ since neurologic involvement is present in type D but not in type E. The deficient enzyme has not been characterized for types D and E. **Type F** is characterized by childhood onset of splenomegaly, lack of neurologic involvement, diminished activity of a heat-labile sphingomyelinase, and **'sea-blue' histiocytes**.[151]

Many variant types have been reported.[152–155] A form of lipid storage disease was described[152] in which four sibs with a slowly progressive lipidosis had marked hepatosplenomegaly. Three of these patients began to show mental and motor deterioration in the second and fourth years of life, with hepatosplenomegaly present at birth in one infant. One child died at age 9 years, and a 14-year-old girl with splenomegaly and foam cells in the marrow had entirely normal mental and physical development. A glycerophospholipid was identified in liver and spleen in a child who died with a visceral sphingomyelinosis and decreased activity of sphingomyelinase. Wiedemann and colleagues[152] considered these cases to be variant forms of NPD.

Another variant of sphingomyelin lipidosis has been reported with unexplained cirrhosis, CNS involvement, and vertical supranuclear ophthalmoplegia.[154,155] One case was associated with hepatocellular carcinoma.[155] The association of hepatic storage and cirrhosis in infants or children should prompt bone marrow examination.

Further biochemical studies with more specific characterization of isoelectric forms of sphingomyelinase continue to define other variant forms of sphingomyelin storage disease.

Pathologically, light microscopic and EM changes are similar in all forms of NPD. The storage cell ranges in diameter from 20

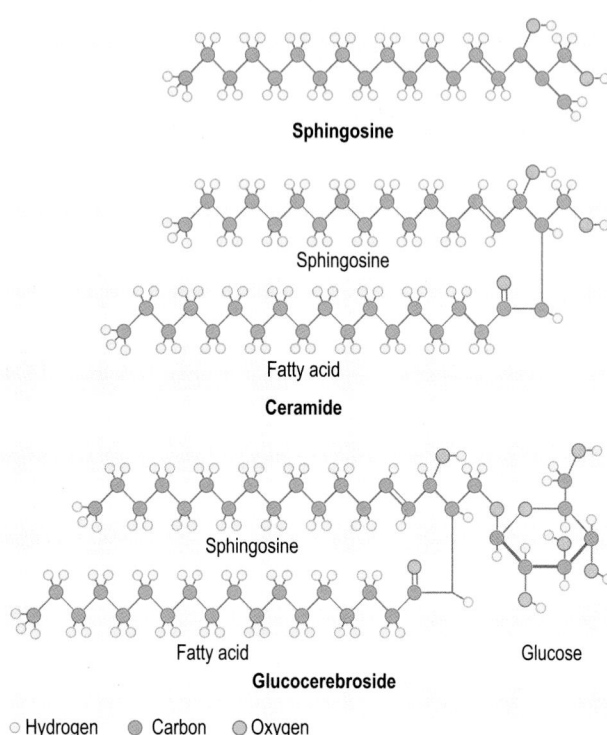

FIGURE 12.12 Structure of sphingolipids. Sphingosine (top) attached to a fatty acid forms ceramide (middle); ceramide attached to a single sugar forms a glucocerebroside (bottom); if ceramide is combined with a polysaccharide (complex sugar) with one or more molecules of N-acetyl-neuraminic acid, the result is a ganglioside. (From Brady RO, Hereditary fat metabolism diseases. Sci Am 1973; 229;88; with permission.)

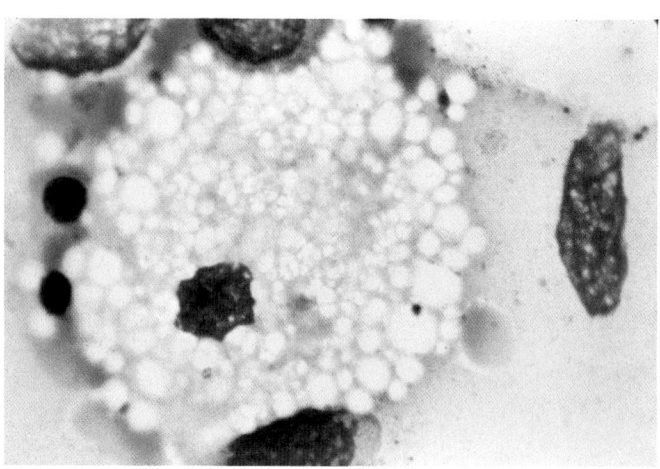

FIGURE 12.13 Niemann-Pick disease. Histocyte in bone marrow has a 'soap bubble' appearance.

myelin, and lesser quantities of cholesterol and gangliosides.[140] The histochemical staining reactions confirm the presence of a complex phospholipid (Table 12.8). Differential staining characteristics of Gaucher disease, NPD, and the gangliosidoses are shown in Table 12.8. The NP cells stain positively with oil red O, Nile blue sulfate, Luxol-fast blue and the OTAN (osmium tetroxide α naphthylamine) reaction after pretreatment with NaOH. The ultrastructural appearance of the lipid inclusions consists of concentrically laminated, myelin-like figures with a periodicity of approximately 50 nm, resembling membranous cytosomes and other pleomorphic lipid profiles in the nervous system (Fig. 12.15A). In the viscera, lipid inclusions are frequently membrane bound and contain stacked membranes, concentrically laminated membranes, and pleomorphic profiles with both electron-dense and electron-lucent cores.[140,150–158] **Cultured fibroblasts** have similar inclusions, and cultured amniotic cells contain storage material (Fig. 12.15B). Histochemical staining of NPD, Gaucher disease, and gangliosidosis is shown in Table 12.9.

Unlike other lipid storage disorders in which the predominant storage substance is the substrate of the deficient enzyme

to 90 μm, and the cytoplasm is filled with lipid droplets that impart a '**soap bubble**' appearance with the nucleus displaced to the periphery (Fig. 12.13). Cells in the viscera, predominantly liver, spleen, lungs, and **ganglion cells of the myenteric plexus** (Fig. 12.14), may contain lipofuscin pigment, sphingo-

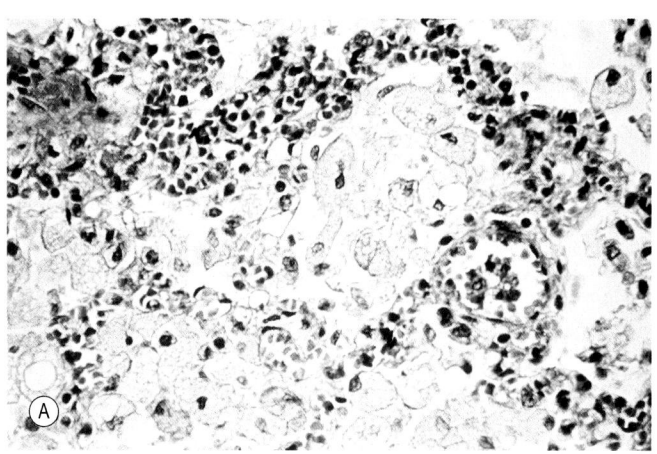

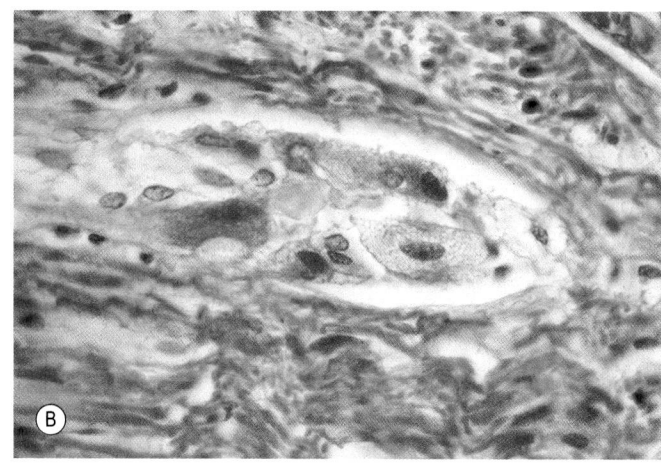

FIGURE 12.14 Nieman-Pick disease. Characteristic histiocytes are filled with lipid material. (A) Lung. (B) Spinal.

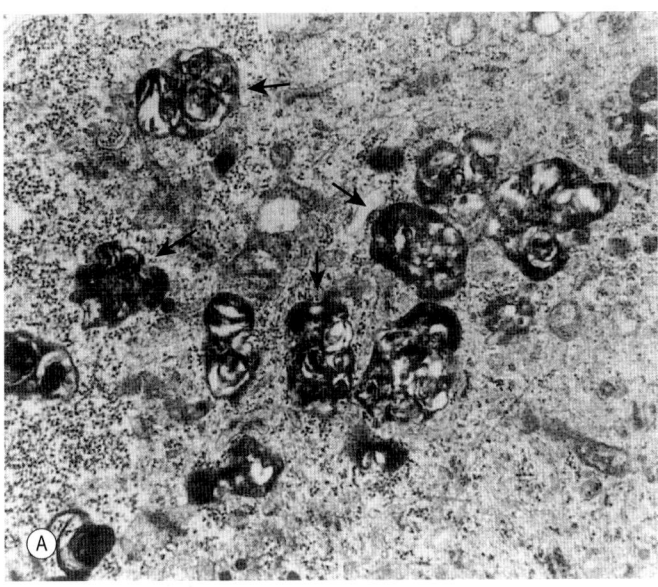
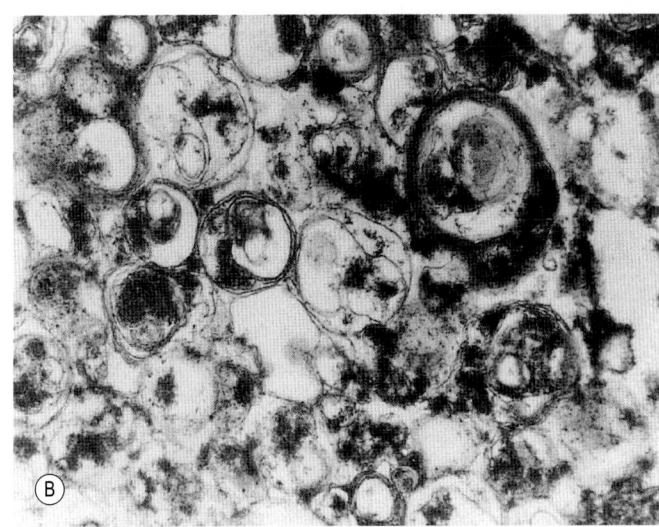

FIGURE 12.15 Niemann-Pick disease electron micrographs. (A) Pleomorphic lipid profiles in the liver. (B) Cultured fibroblast with pleomorphic lipid profiles.

TABLE 12.8 HISTOCHEMICAL PROFILE IN NIEMANN-PICK DISEASE

	Neural tissue	Visceral organs	Bone marrow
Luxol fast blue	+++	++	++
PAS	++	+++	+++
After NaOH	++	+++	+++
After KBr	++	+++	+++
Sudan black B	++	++	++
Oil red O	+	+	+
After hot acetone	+	+	+
After cold acetone	+	+	+
OTAN (osmium tetroxide α napthylamine)	+	+	+
NaOH-OTAN	+	+	+
Ferric hematoxylin	++	++++	++++
After NaOH	++	++++	++++
Schultze reaction for cholesterol	+	++	++
AZO dye reaction for acid phosphatase	++	++	++
Autofluorescence	+++	++	+

TABLE 12.9 HISTOCHEMICAL STAINING OF THREE TYPES OF LYSOSOMAL LIPIDOSES

	Gaucher disease	Niemann-Pick disease	gangliosidoses GM$_1$ and GM$_2$ (types 1 and 2)
PAS	**+++**	o to +	+ to +++
PAS-amylase	**+++**	o to +	+++
Schultz cholesterol technique	o	++	–
Oil red O	+ to ++	+++	++
Oil red O after cold acetone extraction	+ to ++	+++	++
Oil red O after hot acetone extraction	o	+++	+ to ++
Oil red O after pyramidine extraction	o	o	o
Luxol-fast blue	o	+++	++
OTAN	o	+++	++
NaOH-OTAN	o	+++	o to +
Alcian blue	Adult o to +/ infantile ++	+	o
Acid phosphatase	++	o to +	++
Cells involved	RE cells (neuron in infantile)	RE cells (neuron in infantile)	Neurons
Biopsy tissues of choice	Spleen, marrow	Marrow or spleen	Nerve cells

PAS, periodic acid-Schiff; OTAN, Osmium tetroxide α-napthylamine; RE, reticuloendothelial.

responsible for the disease, many of the lipids that accumulate in NPD are not substrates for sphingomyelinase. In addition to sphingomyelin, cholesterol, *bis*-(monoacyl-glycerol) phosphate, and glycosphingolipid are also significantly elevated in types A and C NPD. The predominant lipid in NPD is phospholipid.

In 1966, Brady and colleagues[159] first demonstrated that sphingomyelinase activity was low in tissues from patients with the infantile form of NPD. Callahan and co-workers[160,161] and Besley[162] separated, by isoelectric focusing, multiple components of sphingomyelinase.

Some workers, utilizing [16]C-sphingomyelin or a chromogenic analogue of sphingomyelin, demonstrated sphingomyelinase activities between 51% and 63% of normal in cultured skin fibroblasts from patients with type C NPD.[163] The chromogenic analogue of sphingomyelin has been used successfully in the diagnosis of type A NPD[164] and is hydrolyzed by the enzyme purified from placenta.[165]

Greenbaum and associates[166] documented that total extracts of brain glycolipids in NPD type A contain increased levels of glucosylceramide, di- and trihexoside, and GM_2, changes identical with findings in some cases of NPD type C. Kamoshita and colleagues[150] found a glucocerebroside together with GM_2 and GM_3. In type A, there is mostly neuronal, less so vascular, sphingomyelin storage, while neutral glycolipid dominates in the vascular wall.[167] In type C, glycolipid is stored in the neurons.

Schoenfeld and colleagues[144] reported placental ultrasonographic, biochemical, and histochemical studies in human fetuses affected with NPD type A. Differences in the echo pattern of the placental tissue have been described,[168] but these usually appear in late pregnancy, near term. Focal, opaque, strong echoes in placental tissue with thick and irregular chorionic plates have been observed as early as 18.5 weeks in placentas of NPD fetuses.[145]

Non-neuronopathic forms of NPD involve cholesterol processing and are not due to defective sphingomyelinase activity. This accounts for the relatively long survival of these patients.

Gaucher disease

Gaucher disease, the most common of the lysosomal storage disorders, is autosomal recessive. The gene frequency in the Jewish population is between 0.035 and 0.040. Three types represent different allelic disorders with different mutations in the structural gene of the deficient enzyme β-glucocerebrosidase.[169,170] In the absence of this enzyme, glucocerebroside cannot be catalytically converted into ceramide and glucose, and thus accumulates in organs and tissues, particularly those of the reticuloendothelial system (RES).

The pathophysiology of Gaucher disease with accumulation of storage material in macrophages is shown in Figure 12.16A. The enzymatic defect is shown in Figure 12.16B.

The gene coding acid β-glucosidase has been cloned to chromosome 1q21-q31. A pseudogene that has maintained a high degree of homology is 16 kb downstream from the active gene. The most common mutation in the Ashkenazi Jewish population is at the cDNA nucleotide 1226, where an A to G transition results in an N370S amino acid substitution in acid β-glucosidase. The clinical features of the three forms of Gaucher disease are shown in Table 12.10.

Type I (non-neuronopathic) is the chronic form of Gaucher disease. Clinical manifestations are highly variable. It has been diagnosed in infancy, but more commonly in later childhood and adolescence and sometimes not until adulthood. Painless **splenomegaly, thrombocytopenia, anemia, and leukopenia** are the usual initial presenting symptoms of type I. Platelet counts may be less than 50×10^9/L without an accompanying

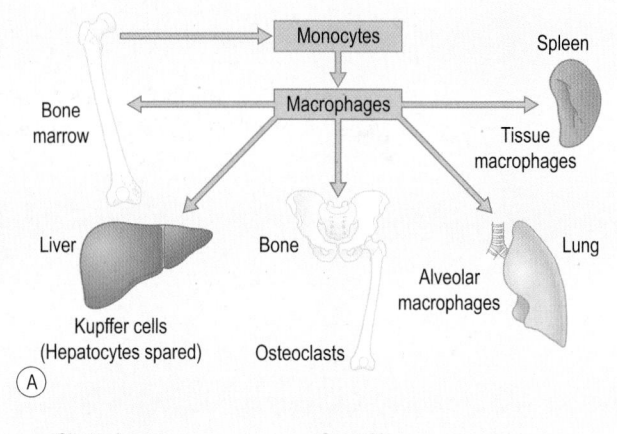

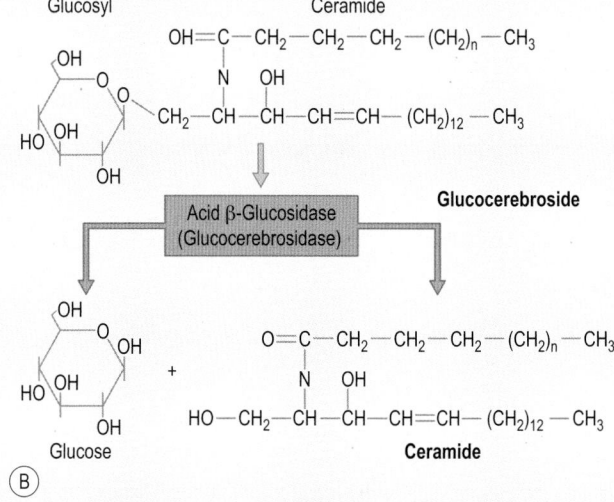

FIGURE 12.16 (A) the pathophysiology of Gaucher disease. (B) the enzymatic defect in Gaucher disease. (From Gaucher Disease Diagnosis Evaluation and Treatment, Genzyme Therapeutics, Parsipanny, NJ with permission.)

bleeding diathesis. The liver frequently does not become significantly enlarged until later in the course of the disease. **Erlenmeyer flask deformity** of the distal ends of the femur (Fig. 12.17) is considered diagnostic of Gaucher disease.[169] Diffuse, yellow-brown skin pigmentation may involve the face and legs. Renal involvement, pulmonary hypertension, and cardiac abnormalities are less common. Patients with type I disease have normal life expectancy. A complex allele of the glucocerebrosidase gene has a milder clinical course.[173]

Enzyme assay for heterozygote detection is being superseded by molecular techniques that can efficiently detect heterozygotes once the mutation of an affected homozygote is known. Testing of family members using enzyme assay remains useful to identify asymptomatic homozygous individuals, particularly where the gene defect remains unknown. In utero diagnosis of Gaucher disease can be made by applying enzyme assay techniques or mutation analysis to cultured amniocytes.[174]

The diagnosis of Gaucher disease should be considered in any patient with unexplained splenomegaly and is strongly

TABLE 12.10 GAUCHER DISEASE: CLINICAL TYPES

Clinical features	Type I	Type II	Type III
Age at onset	Childhood/adulthood	Infancy	Childhood
Splenomegaly	+ → +++	++	+ → +++
Hepatomegaly	+ →+++	++	+ → +++
Skeletal disease	– →+++	–	++ → +++
Primary CNS disease	Absent	+++	+ → +++
Life span	6–80+ years	Approx 2 years	2–60 years
Ethnicity	Ashkenazi Jewish/Panethnic	Panethnic	Norrbottnian/Panethnic
Frequency	Ashkenazi Jewish population 1/450–1/1000 General population1 60 000–1/200 0000	<1/100 000	<1/50 000

From Gaucher Disease Diagnosis Evaluation and Treatment, Genzyme Therapeutics, with permission, (Genzyme Therapeutics. 100 Lackawanna Ave., Parsipanny, NJ 07054; Ph; 800/745-4447, ext. 7664; Fax: 617/374-7357; www.genzyme.com/prodserv/welcome.htm)

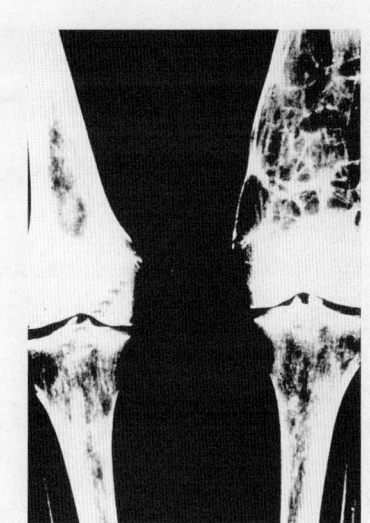

FIGURE 12.17 Gaucher disease. Radiograph of a femur showing Erlenmeyer deformity and radioluceny due to replacement of bone by storage cells containing glucocerebroside.

TABLE 12.11 DIAGNOSIS OF GAUCHER DISEASE

Gold standard for making the diagnosis
- β-glucocerebrosidase activity is measured in peripheral blood leukocytes
- Leukocytes are disrupted, incubated with a commercially available fluorescent substrate, and the resulting fluorescence is measured with a fluorometer
- A reduction of 30% or less in measured activity is diagnostic of the disease
- A lesser degree of reduction is characteristic of the carriers, who average about 50% of normal β-glucocerebrosidase activity
  - This assay has a substantial rate of false-negative readings among carriers
  - Some 20% of carriers demonstrate enzyme activity in the normal range
- Cultured skin fibroblasts, amniotic fluid cells, and chorionic villi can also be used for diagnosis

indicated by levels of serum non-tartrate inhibitable acid phosphatase and the presence of typical Gaucher cells in bone marrow. It is confirmed with results of an assay of white blood cells, fibroblast culture,[175] or urine.[176] Carrier detection fails in 5–20% of known heterozygotes who have no clinical symptoms.[177] Results of amniocentesis or chorionic villus sampling accurately detect the condition prenatally.

Diagnosis of Gaucher Disease See Tables 12.11 and 12.12.

Type II (acute neuronopathic, infantile) Gaucher disease is rare and has no ethnic predilection. It is rapidly progressive, with severe neurologic complications and signs of cranial nerve nuclei and extrapyramidal tract involvement beginning 3–6 months after birth. Although neuronal cerebroside storage is not a feature, the brain is the site of extensive neuronal cell death, reactive gliosis, and the perivascular accumulation of Gaucher cells. CNS deterioration is manifested by strabismus, trismus, and retroflexion of the head. Death occurs by 2 years of age.[169] The condition is believed to stem from an unstable enzyme precursor.

Type III Gaucher disease (subacute juvenile neuronopathic, Swedish, or Norrbottnian [a county in northern Sweden])[178] has a variable age of onset but usually begins in later childhood. Characteristics include ataxia, spasticity, akinetic and myoclonic seizures, and variable degrees of dementia. Patients with types II and III disease share the same mutation (444 leu to pro) in the gene. The phenotypic differences are ascribed to a nonfunctional allele in type II patients.

The diagnosis of Gaucher disease should be considered in any patient with unexplained splenomegaly, and is strongly indicated by **elevated levels of serum non-tartrate inhibitable acid phosphatase** and the presence of typical **Gaucher cells** in bone marrow. It is confirmed with results of an assay of WBCs, fibroblast culture,[179] or urine.[180] Carrier detection fails in 5–20% of known heterozygotes who have no clinical symptoms.[181] Amniocentesis and chorionic villus sampling (CVS) accurately detect the condition prenatally. The gene for glucocerebrosides has been mapped to chromosome 1q21-q31.[182] Hypersplenism may necessitate splenectomy.

TABLE 12.12 DIAGNOSIS OF GAUCHER DISEASE – DNA ANALYSIS

Has some advantages over enzymatic diagnosis
   Results are qualitative rather than quantitative
   Provides greater accuracy in detection of heterozygotes
Polymerase chain reaction (PCR) is the most widely used molecular
diagnostic approach used to detect Gaucher mutations
Allele-specific oligonucleotide (ASO) hybridization
   Regions containing mutations are amplified via PCR
   ASO probes are added and will hybridize only to complementary
   alleles
     Mutant ASO will only hybridize to a mutated allele
     Normal ASOs only hybridize to normal alleles
Serum levels of some enzymes may be elevated
   Acid phosphatase
     Lysosomal enzyme that may reflect overall macrophage activity
     Elevation is suggestive of Gaucher disease when possibility of
     metastatic prostate carcinoma has been eliminated
   Angiotensin-converting enzyme
Elevated plasma ferritin levels are commonly seen
Decreased plasma cholesterol levels may be seen in unsplenectomized
patients

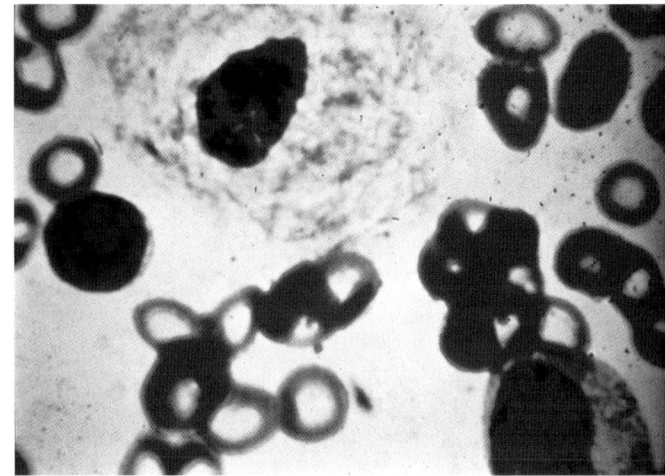

FIGURE 12.19 Gaucher cells. Histiocyte from the bone marrow showing cytoplasmic striations, a 'crinkled tissue' appearance.

Pathologically, the glucocerebroside accumulates in histiocytes of the RES, including *spleen* (Fig. 12.18), **lymph nodes, and bone marrow and in Kupffer cells of the liver**. Late in the disease, portal fibrosis may progress to **cirrhosis**. The pathognomonic feature is the Gaucher cell – 60–80 μm in size – a large, vacuolated histiocyte seen in the bone marrow, liver, spleen, and lymph nodes with striated cytoplasm (wrinkled tissue paper) (Fig. 12.19), best demonstrated with trichrome or aldehyde fuchsin staining.[183] **Erythrophagocytosis** by Gaucher cells is common, and hemosiderin is frequently found in the cell. Marked acid phosphatase activity accompanies the lysosomal accumulation of the storage material. Ultrastructurally, the Gaucher cell measures 60–80 μm in diameter. The cytoplasm is packed with rod-shaped inclusions bound by a single membrane. The inclusions contain tubules that run parallel to their long axes and are branched. The tubules have an anticlockwise spiral (Fig. 12.20). The iron is dispersed in individual micelles of ferritin.[184]

Placenta and Fetal Pathology The placenta may be edematous in Gaucher disease, and storage cells may be found within intravillus and Hofbauer (placental histiocyte) cell vessels.[185] Fetuses at 17 weeks gestation may have storage cells, particularly in liver and spleen.

Intravenous administration of macrophage-targeted placental glucocerebrosidase has been effective in producing clinical improvement in patients with type I Gaucher disease.[186] Alglycerase has been approved by the US Food and Drug Administration as an 'orphan drug' for the treatment of type I disease and allows patients to lead an essentially normal adult life.[186a]

Bone marrow transplantation may also result in improvement.[187]

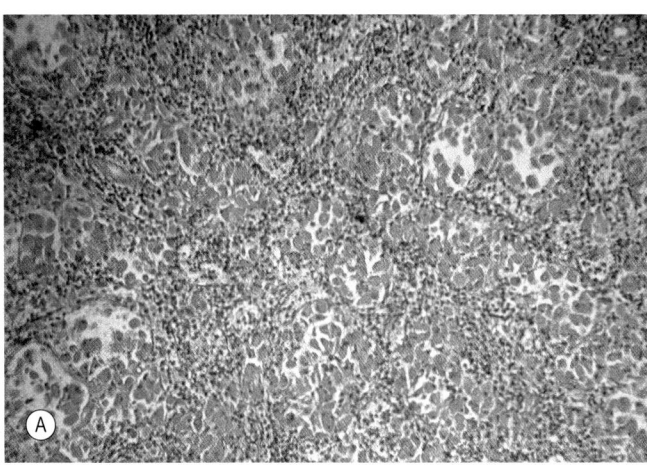

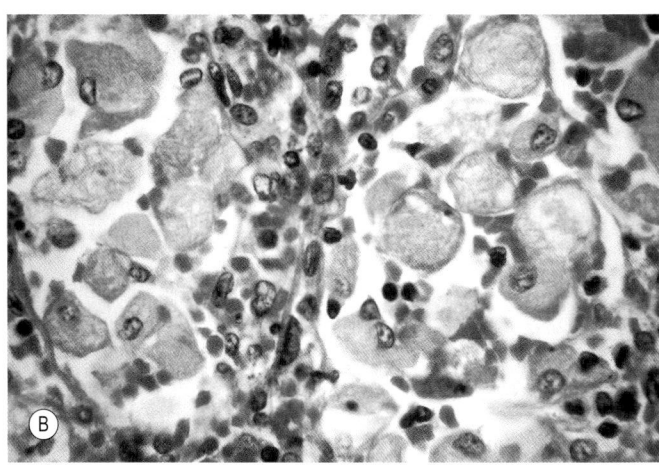

FIGURE 12.18 (A) Microscopic section of spleen showing distended histiocytes in the splenic pulp. (B) High-power view of Gaucher cells.

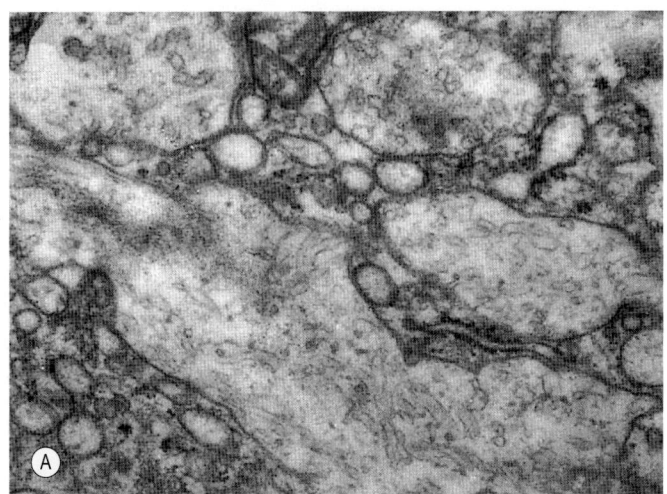

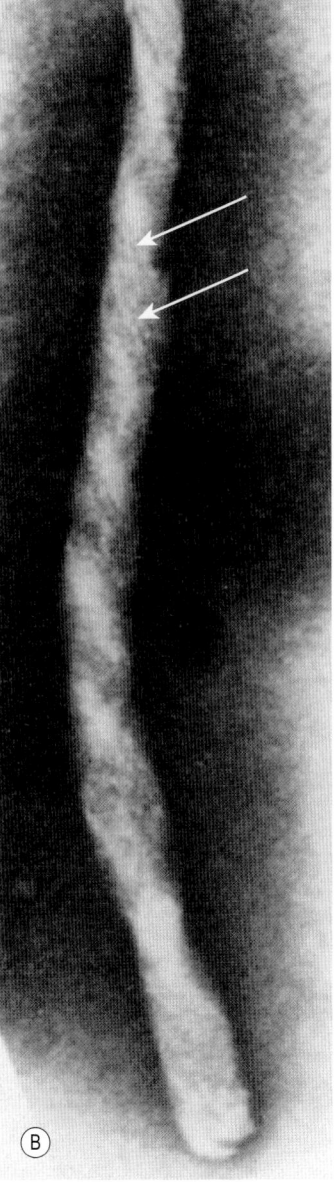

FIGURE 12.20 Gaucher cell electron micrographs. (A) Branching tubular profiles in lysosomes (× 60 000). (B) High magnification of a tubule with spirals in a clockwise direction (× 60 000).

Krabbe disease (globoid cell leukodystrophy)

This autosomal recessive disorder usually presents between 3 and 6 months of life after a normal neonatal period with a rapidly progressive course. It is due to a **deficiency of galacto-cerebrosidase** activity and the accumulation of galactosylceramide in the peripheral and central nervous systems. Diagnosis is made by enzyme assay of leukocytes, cultured fibroblasts; prenatal diagnosis is from amniotic fluid cells, or CVS.

The infantile form is rapidly progressive, with spasticity and irritability progressing to hypotonia, blindness, deafness, seizures, and peripheral neuropathy. The brain is the site of severe atrophy, gliosis, demyelination, and accumulation of the diagnostic cell. The onset is usually between 3 and 6 months and death occurs by 2 years of age. The late-onset variants present in childhood and subsequently undergo diverse, progressive neurologic complications. The gene has been mapped to chromosome 14q24.3-32.1 and cloned.[188]

The lesions are confined to the CNS and are characterized by **cerebral atrophy, loss of myelin, gliosis, and globoid cells** (Fig. 12.21).[189] The globoid cells are multinucleated, microglial macrophages distended with storage material. There is diffuse demyelination of the white matter and numerous calcifications. An intense gliosis is present in the cortex and basal ganglia, and especially around the perivascular spaces of the white matter. The perivascular spaces contain an accumulation of rounded mononuclear or binuclear PAS-positive globoid cells 15–20 μm in diameter. The cells are Sudan positive and glial fibrillary acidic protein (GFAP) negative; they stain strongly for *Ricinus communis* agglutinin and less strongly for peanut agglutinin and wheat germ agglutinin. EM shows tubular structures similar to those observed in Gaucher disease.

Transplantation of umbilical cord blood from unrelated donors in newborns with infantile Krabbe disease has favorably altered the natural history of the disease. Transplantation in babies after symptoms had developed have not resulted in substantive neurologic improvement.[189a]

Farber disease (lipogranulomatosis)

This rare autosomal recessive disorder is due to deficiency of lysosomal ceramidase, resulting in accumulation of ceramide. During infancy, hoarseness, respiratory difficulty, vomiting, skin nodules (Fig. 12.22), swollen painful joints failure to thrive, and death due to respiratory infections occur. Five types have been described (see Table 12.6). Pathologically, **foam cells** with granulomatous reaction occur in the **respiratory system, soft tissues**, and **joints** (Fig. 12.23).[190] **Ganglion cells are vacuolated** and foam cells are present in lymph nodes (Fig. 12.24), bone marrow, spleen, and liver as well as renal proximal tubular epithelial and glomerular cells. The liver is enlarged and pale. The hepatocytes are distended with lipids and the sinusoids are filled with lipid-laden histiocytes. Ceramide, mucopolysaccharides, and gangliosides accumulate. EM demonstrates foam cells containing curvilinear tubular structures and membrane-bound reticulogranular material; mucopolysaccharides and zebra bodies have

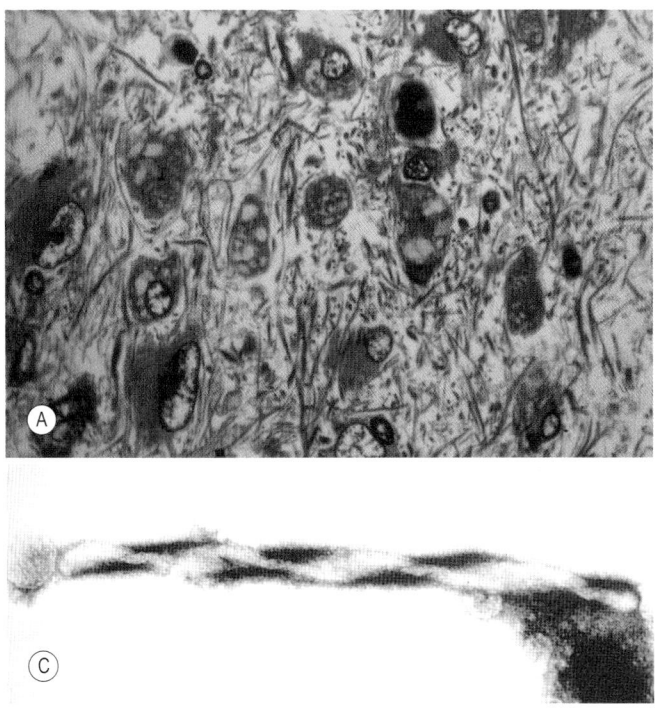

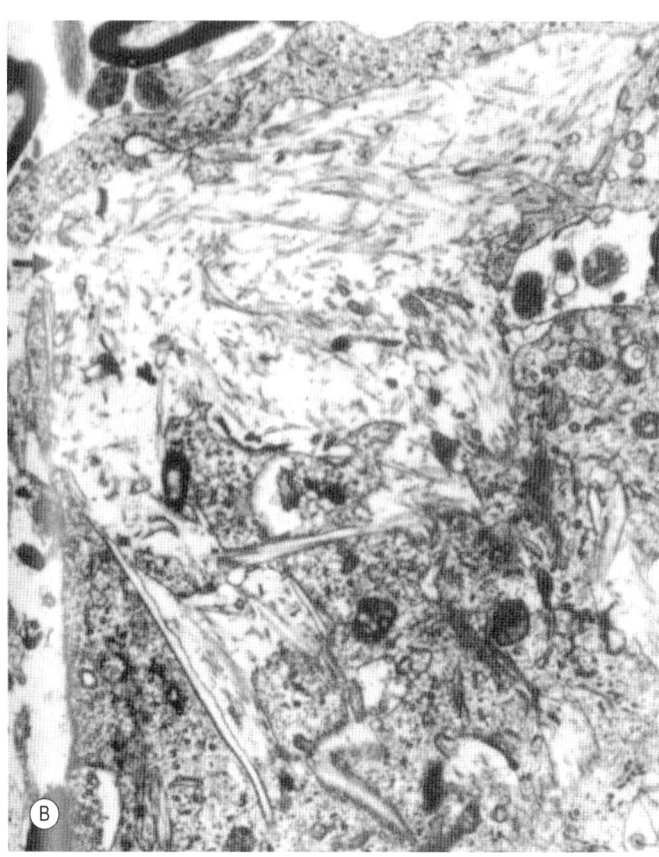

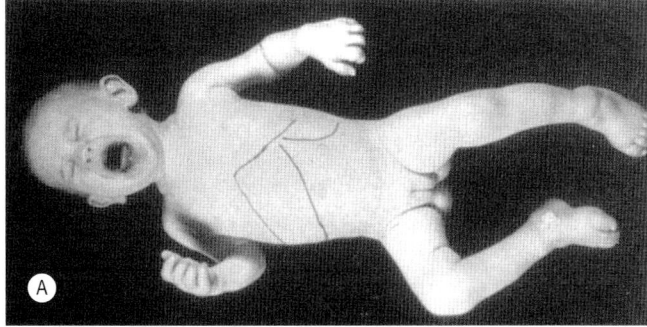

FIGURE 12.21 (A) Krabbe disease. Globoid cells in white matter. (B) Electron micrograph of brain. A globoid cell containing tubules with electron-dense deposits. (C) High magnification of the twisted tubule with a counterclockwise spiral.

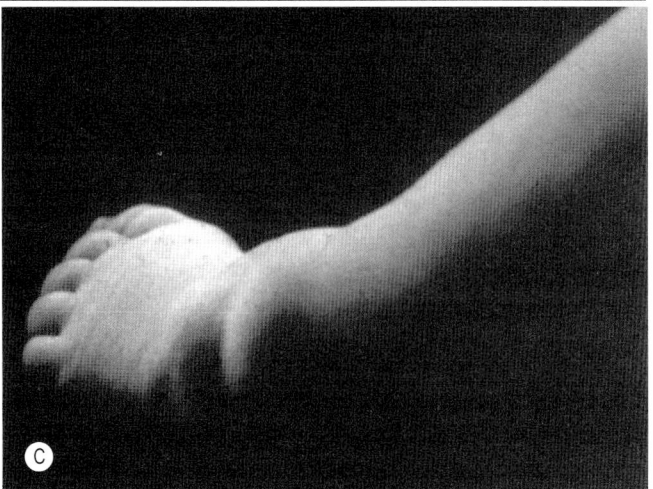

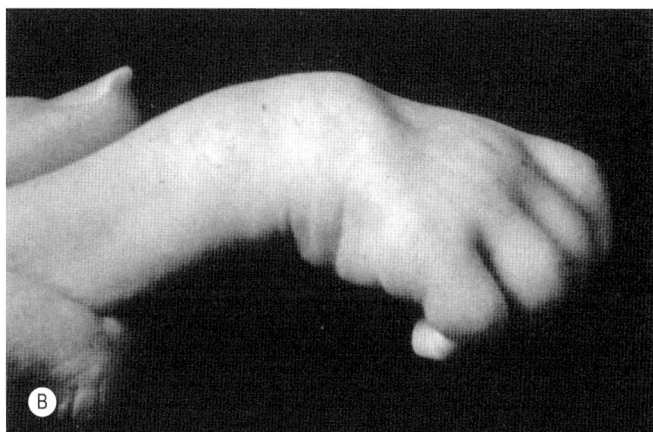

FIGURE 12.22 Farber disease. (A) Child with multiple skin nodules. (B) Large nodules on the wrist and on the ankle (C). (Courtesy of Dr. Stephen Qualman.)

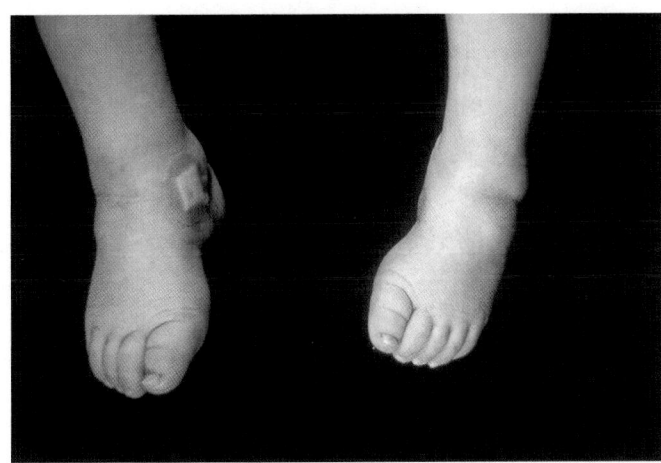

FIGURE 12.23 Farber disease. Nodules on feet and ankles.

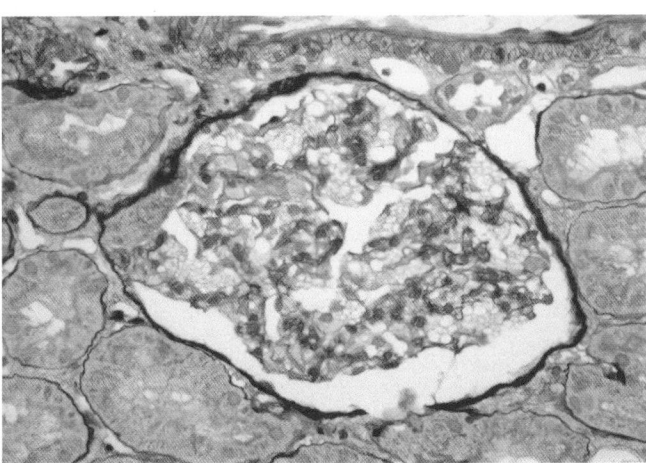

FIGURE 12.25 Fabry disease. Foamy glomerular cells in kidney.

been described.[191] 'Banana bodies' have been reported in Schwann cells.[192]

In the female, the vocal cords may be narrow due to the lipid infiltration and the heart may have epicardial nodules and the lungs, histiocytes infiltration.

Definitive diagnosis is by lysosomal ceramidase activity and ceramide content in cultured fibroblasts or in white blood cells. Biopsy of periarticular tissues may be diagnostic. Acid ceramidase activity in heterozygotes is usually reduced. Prenatal diagnosis is by reduced ceramidase activity in cultured amniotic fluid cells.

Fabry disease

The primary biochemical defect of Fabry disease is **deficiency of lysosomal α-galactosidase A**, an enzyme that hydrolyzes ceramide to sphingosine and a free fatty acid.[193] It is an X-linked disorder mapped to Xq22. Heterozygous female carriers have an intermediate level of enzyme activity. Glycosphingolipid, principally the trihexosyl ceramide-globotriasyl-ceramide, occurs in all organs and tissues[194] and may be up to 300-fold higher than normal levels.[195] The greatest accumulation is observed in **the kidney** (Fig. 12.25), **lymph nodes, blood vessels, prostate, and autonomic ganglia**.[194] The storage has a predilection for vascular endothelium and smooth muscle cells, which is different from that seen in other forms of glycosphingolipidoses.[194] The major abnormalities of **vessels** are narrowness, dilation, and motor unresponsiveness. In addition to endothelial proliferation, the swollen endothelial cells may be the precursor of thromboses, ischemia, and infarction and there may be progressive aneurysmal dilation of the weakened vessel walls. **Microaneurysm formation of retinal and conjunctival vessels** may occur, and in the skin a transition from telangiectasia to a frank **angiokeratoma** is one of the hallmarks of the disease.[194] The involvement of peripheral and central autonomic nerve cells may be responsible for paresthesias, severe pain, GI symptoms such as nausea and diarrhea, and other vague neurologic symptoms.[96] Similar pathologic changes in the kidney with accumulation of glycosphingolipid in the glomerular visceral and tubular

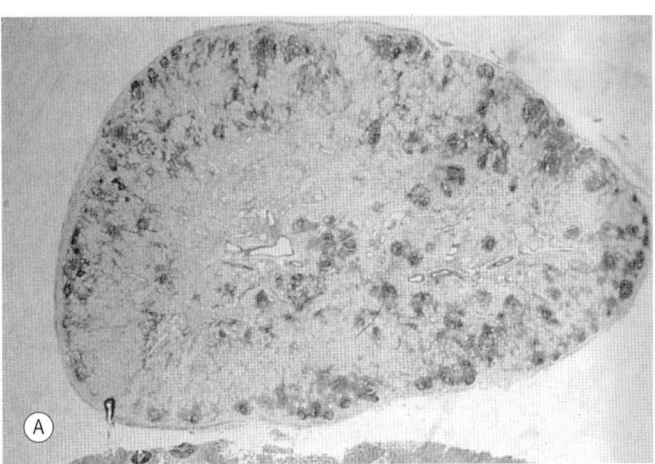

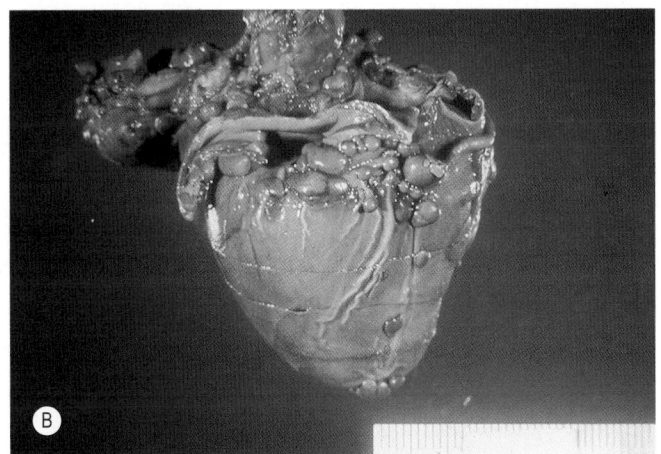

FIGURE 12.24 Farber disease. (A) Microscopic section of a lymph node showing PAS-positive storage histiocytes. (B) Heart showing nodules on epicardial surface. (Courtesy of Dr. Stephen Qualman.)

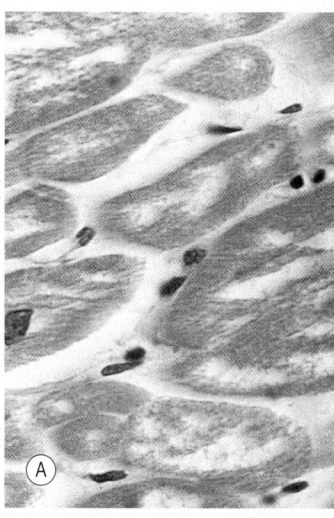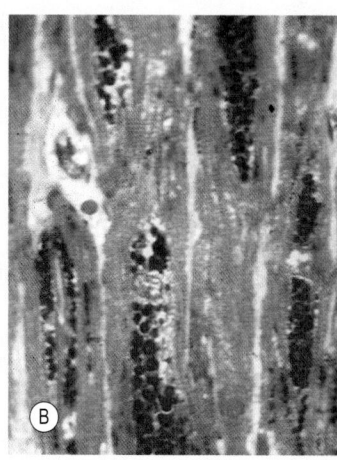

FIGURE 12.26 Fabry disease. Microscopic appearance of heart (A) with vacuolated fibers (B), osmiun staining of myocardial fibers by glycolipid.

epithelial cells, have also been observed in mucolipidosis II and in generalized GM$_1$ gangliosidosis.

The histopathologic changes frequently involve the heart (Fig. 12.26), especially the myocardial cells, specialized tissues of the **atrioventricular conduction system**, and the valves[195] and coronary arteries, due to deposition of glycosphingolipid. **Hypertrophic obstructive cardiomyopathy** has been noted.[196] The aorta may show changes suggestive of **cystic medionecrosis**.

In histologic sections[197] the deposits of ceramide trihexoside appear as vacuoles, and in frozen sections they are sudanophilic, PAS positive, and strongly birefringent. In cardiac muscle the deposits occupy the central perinuclear areas of the cytoplasm, displacing the contractile elements to the periphery. This results in the histologic appearance of a lacework pattern similar to that seen in type II glycogenosis. Ultrastructurally, the storage material is deposited in lysosomes with concentric or parallel lamellae with a periodicity of 4–55 nm (Fig. 12.27).[194] The lamellae react positively with periodate-thiosemicarbazide silver proteinate and periodate-thiosemicarbazide-osmium tetroxide.[194] These structures can also be demonstrated on freeze-fractured preparations.[194]

The severity of this disorder appears to be related to the total amount of glycosphingolipid stored in the tissues, which in turn depends on time, the presence or absence of residual α-galactosidase A activity, and the individual's ABO blood type. Hemizygotes and heterozygotes who are type B and AB are more severely affected owing to the additional accumulation of B-specific glycosphingolipid.

The cutaneous lesion angiokeratoma is not distinctive for Fabry disease. Angiokeratomas also occur in fucosidosis, adult β-galactosidase deficiency, gangliosidosis type I, aspartyl-glycosaminuria, α-N-galactosidase deficiency (Schindler neuro-axonal dystrophy syndrome), Goldberg galactosialidosis syndrome, and Kawasaki disease.

Diagnosis Confirmation of the clinical diagnosis in hemizgotes and heterozygotes requires the demonstration of deficient α-galactosidase A activity in plasma, leukocytes, or tears, or increased levels of galactosylceramide in plasma or urinary sediment. Heterozygous females may have intermediate levels of enzyme activity and accumulated substrate. More accurate diagnosis of heterozygous females can be accomplished by detection of the molecular lesion in the α-galactosidase A gene or by linkage analysis in families with an affected male.[198]

The disease progresses slowly, eventually leading to death from renal or heart complications.[198a] ERT has been approved for Fabry disease. It appears that early treatment is essential to maximize the therapeutic effects.

Prenatal Diagnosis Prenatal diagnosis can be accomplished by demonstration of deficient α-galactosidase A activity and XY karyotype, by linkage analysis, and/or by demonstration of the specific α-galactosidase A mutation in chorionic villi or cultured amniotic cells.[198]

Gangliosidoses

Structural mutations in the gene for acid β-glucosidase are central to diverse phenotypes within this group.

These disorders are autosomal recessive conditions and are divided into two groups, GM$_1$ and GM$_2$.[199] The diverse clinical phenotypes stem from mutations in the genes coding for β-hexosaminidases or a sphingomyelin activator protein. As a consequence, the accumulation of lysosomal GM$_2$ gangliosides and glycosphingolipids leads to progressive cerebral degeneration. The number of phenotypes relates to the structure of β-hexosaminidase, which has an α subunit and a β subunit, each encoded by separate genes. Combinations of these subunits leads to isoenzyme diversity. To stabilize the enzyme–substrate complex, a GM$_2$ activator protein is essential.

GM$_1$ type I gangliosidosis (generalized) is an autosomal recessive disorder that presents in early infancy with coarse facies, macroglossia, depressed nasal bridge, large ears, frontal bossing, hepatosplenomegaly, dysostosis multiplex, and rapidly

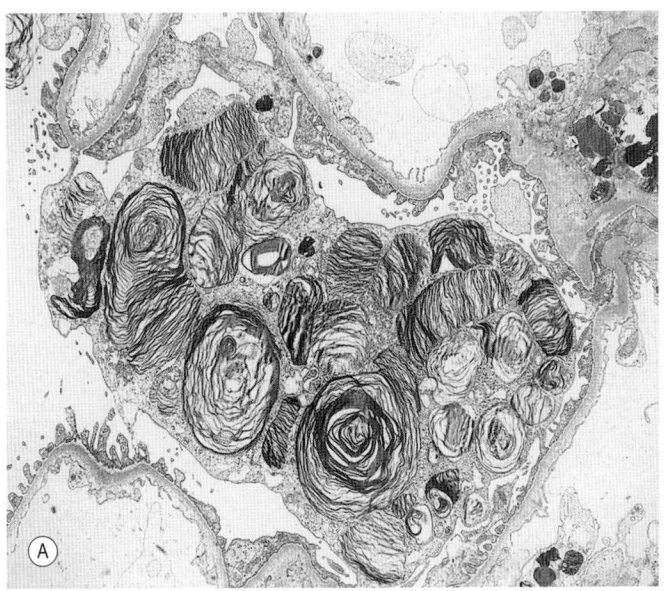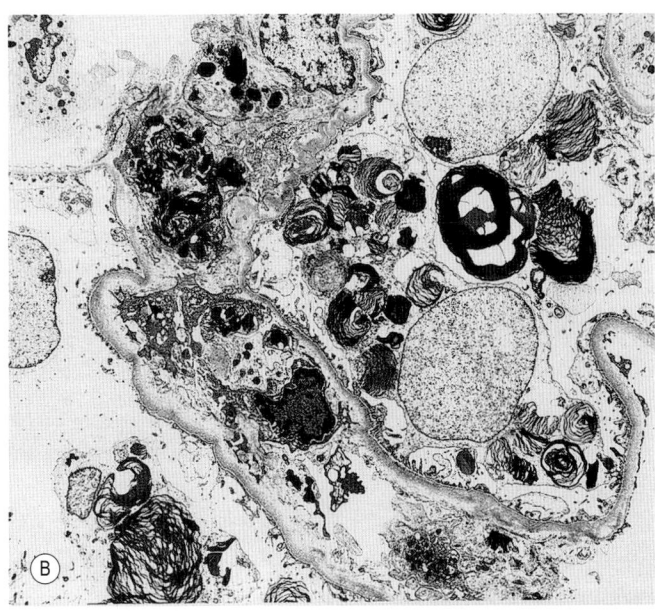

FIGURE 12.27 Fabry disease. (A) Glomerular visceral epithelial cells containing myelin-like figures (× 8250). (B) Glomerular parietal epithelial cells showing pleomorphic lipid inclusions (× 8250).

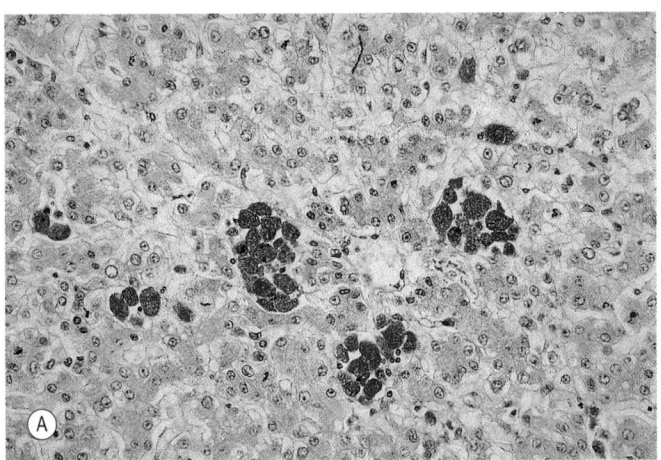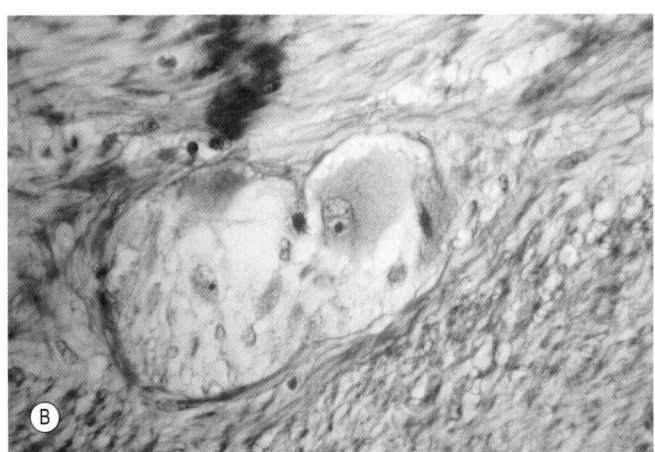

FIGURE 12.28 GM1 gangliosidosis. (A) Liver; some hepatocytes are swollen and contain storage material. (B) Myenteric plexus showing distended neuron.

progressive psychomotor deterioration, with seizures and death by 2 years of age. A macular cherry-red spot occurs in 50% of cases. The human galactosidase has been mapped to chromosome 3 and the cDNA for this enzyme has been cloned.

Deficient activity of β-galactosidase results in accumulation of ganglioside in neurons, and in other sites the defect causes accumulation of mucopolysaccharides.[200] In the **brain** there is **progressive atrophy** with **neuronal swelling** and loss of neurons and gliosis. Neurons contain sudanophilic material (ganglioside) and some PAS-positive material (Fig. 12.28), whereas other viscera accumulate strongly PAS-positive material owing to the presence of mucopolysaccharides. By EM[201] **membranous concentric bodies** (MCBs) are seen in skin or conjunctival biopsy, and reticulogranular material is seen in cultured skin fibroblasts and/or endothelial cells of skin biopsies. Peripheral

blood and bone marrow lymphocytes, and syncytiotrophoblasts of the placenta are vacuolated. The diagnosis can be made in the fetus.[202] Definitive diagnosis by enzyme assay is established using leukocytes, fibroblasts, or amniocytes. In the placenta, trophoblastic cells are vacuolated. The same enzyme deficiency is found in type IV MPS (Morquio); and a variant of sialidosis has both sialidase and β-galactosidase deficiencies.

GM$_1$ type II gangliosidosis (juvenile) usually becomes apparent at about 1 year of age and is clinically and pathologically similar to type I gangliosidosis.[203]

GM$_2$ type I gangliosidosis (Tay-Sachs disease) was first described by the British ophthalmologist Warren Tay and the American neurologist Bernard Sachs at the end of the nineteenth century. There are three forms: **Tay-Sachs disease and variants**, resulting from mutations of the *HEXA* gene, associated with

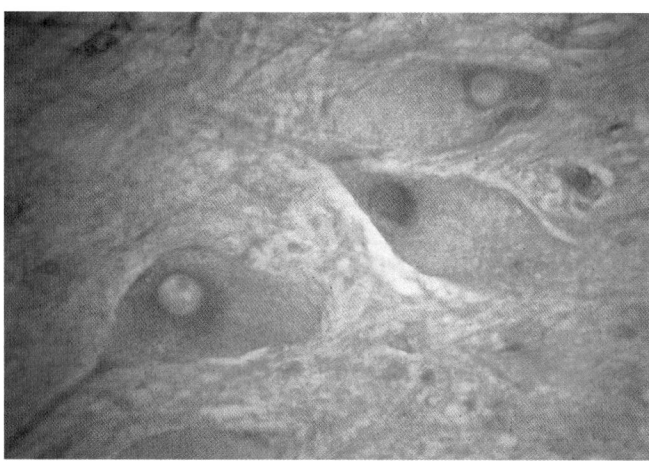

FIGURE 12.29 Tay-Sachs disease (GM$_2$ gangliosidosis) in a brain with swollen neurons.

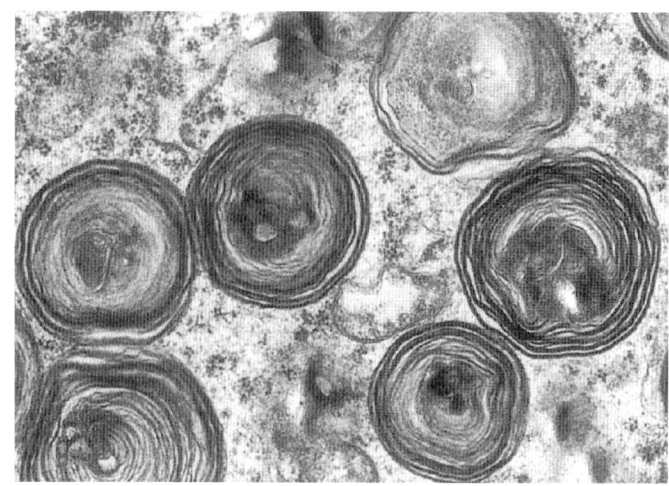

FIGURE 12.30 Tay-Sachs disease. EM of characteristic membraneous concentric bodies.

deficient activity of *HEXA* but normal HEXB; **Sandhoff disease and variants**, resulting from mutations of the *HEXB* gene and is associated with deficient activity of both *HEXA* and *HEXB*; and **GM$_2$ activator deficiency**, due to mutation of the GM2A gene and characterized by normal *HEXA* and *HEXB* but the inability to form a functional ganglioside GM$_2$–GM$_2$ activator complex. Two forms feature mutations of the α subunit of β-hexosaminidase (types B and B1) and another stems from mutation of the gene for saposin, the hexosaminidase activator protein (AB form). The prototype, type B, manifests a striking incidence in children of Eastern European Jewish origin. Since the α but not β subunit is mutated, the total amount of β-hexosaminidase is normal. Although normal at birth, affected infants develop rapidly progressive psychomotor deterioration in the first year of life, seizures, hypotonia, and blindness with **cherry-red spot in the macula**, and dementia and death by age 3–5 years.[204] It is noteworthy that the red macula represents a normal segment of the retina rendered vivid by contiguous white areas, which contain the stored material. In this uniformly fatal autosomal recessive disorder, gangliosides accumulate in the brain and result in the characteristic neuropathologic finding of 'ballooning' of neurons with massive intralysosomal accumulation of lipophilic membranous bodies (Fig. 12.29) and MCBs visible by EM (Fig. 12.30). The brain is first enlarged due to the accumulation of storage material in the neurons. Carrier screening and prenatal diagnosis have been established.[205] The carrier rate in the Ashkenazi Jewish population is 1 in 30 to 40 for Hex A mutations, with an incidence of disease of 1 in 4000. *HEXA* maps to 15q23-q24. Genetic counseling and monitoring of at-risk pregnancies have reduced the incidence of Tay-Sachs disease in the Ashkenazi Jewish population by 90%.

GM$_2$ type II gangliosidosis (Sandhoff disease) includes five phenotypes and features a total deficiency of β-hexosaminidase, leading to extensive neuronal and visceral storage of GM$_2$ gangliosides, glycolipids, glycoproteins, and oligosaccharides.[206] Both α and β subunit mutations are described for the β-hexosaminidase gene. To date, the number of known patients

is approximately 100. The pattern of inheritance is autosomal recessive. The reported heterozygote frequency (0.0020) for Sandhoff disease indicates a birth incidence of about 1 in 1 million among Jewish infants in North America and about 1 in 700 000 among non-Jewish infants (heterozygote frequency, 0.00360). One would expect a Jewish infant to be born with Sandhoff disease in North America about once every 10–15 years.[207] Most patients are non-Jewish. *HEXB* map to 5q13.[208]

The ganglioside content of visceral organs is not significantly increased, but the pattern is abnormal in that GM$_2$ contains a higher proportion of the total gangliosides than normal.[207] The clinical course is similar to that of Tay-Sachs[209] in addition to the CNS involvement as in type I. The cerebral hemispheres appear symmetrical and there are atrophic gyri. On serial coronal sections through the cerebrum, the cortex and white matter are atrophic. The pons, medulla, cerebellum, and spinal cord are atrophic and rubbery in consistency. The aortic and mitral valve leaflets are thickened and distorted. There is also **extraneural visceral storage in histiocytes of the spleen, lymph nodes, bone marrow, lung, gastrointestinal tract, and pancreatic acinar cells**.[207] A derivative of the ganglioside GM$_2$ and GA$_2$ accumulates to levels about 20 times normal. Much higher amounts of GA$_2$ accumulate in the brain and viscera in Sandhoff disease than in Tay-Sachs disease. Globoside accumulates in large quantities in the viscera, especially in the kidney and spleen in Sandhoff disease, and oligosaccharides accumulate in the tissues and are excreted. Oligosaccharides appear to be derived from degradation of glycoproteins and they accumulate because of absence of *HEXA* and *HEXB*.[210–214] All the gangliosidoses and their variants can be diagnosed prenatally from amniotic fluid or chorionic villus biopsies.[215]

Four of the GM$_2$ gangliosidoses may have the clinical picture of brainstem or spinal cord disease, and one may have psychosis and other neurological manifestations with onset in adult life. Similarly, adult-onset metachromatic leukodystrophy may clinically suggest schizophrenia.

TABLE 12.13 INHERITED CONDITIONS WITH ABNORMAL SERUM LIPIDS

Hypercholesterolemia, familial (LDL receptor disorder)	Increased LDL and cholesterol from deficient binding of LDL to receptor; xanthomas
Hyperlipidemia, combined	Increased VLDL, triglycerides; apparently heterogeneous; xanthomas rare
Hyperlipidemia type 5	Increased prebetalipoproteins, triglycerides (carbohyrdate-inducible hyperlipidemia) with APO C2 deficiency
Hyperlipidemia type 6	Increased chylomicrons (Bürger-Grutz disease); xanthomas
Hyperlipoproteinemia 1a-chylomicronemia	Low α and β-lipoproteins, due to deficient lipoprotein lipase, 1b-anapolipoproteinemia C, deficient apolipoprotein C2, activator of lipoprotein lipase; 1c-chylomicronemia from circulating inhibitor of lipoprotein lipase; xanthomas
Hyperlipoproteinemia 2	Increased β-lipoprotein and cholesterol with (type B) or without (type A) increased triglyceride; can have decreased 3 HO-3-methylglutaryl-CoA reductase (HMGC reductase); xanthomas (increased β-lipoprotein [LDL] is phenotype of familial hypercholesterolemia)
Hyperlipoproteinemia 3	Increased β- and pre β-lipoproteins with deficiency of APO E
Hyperlipoproteinemia 4 (carbohydrate inducible hyperlipidemia)	Increased VDL and triglyceride, usually with normal cholesterol and phospholipids; atherosclerosis; xanthomas can occur
Hyperlipoproteinemia 5	Increased VDL, chylomicrons (seen especially with diabetes mellitus); xanthomas
Analphalipoproteinemia (Tangier disease)	Low HDL – involvement of recticuloendothelial cells and vessels; xanthomas
Hypoalphalipoproteinemia	Seen with lecithin:cholesterol acyl transferase (LCAT)deficiency (fish-eye disease) and familial LCAT deficiency; lipid deposits, especially corneal
Abetalipoproteinemia (Bassen Kornzweig disease)	Celiac syndrome, retinal damage, ataxia, acanthocytosis
Hypobetalipoproteinemia with lipid transport defect (Andersen)	Lipid in intestinal epithelium (white villous disease)
Hepatic lipase deficiency	Increased triglyceride in LDL and HDL lipoproteins, xanthomas.

Therapeutic interventions are being investigated for several additional LSDs, including Tay-Sachs disease, Niemann-Pick types B and C, and Pompe disease, MPS II, MPS VI and Wolman disease/cholesterol ester storage disease.[215a]

Serum lipid or lipoprotein abnormalities

These include the neutral lipid triglycerides and cholesterol diseases (Table 12.13) and are characterized by **non-lysosomal lipids in macrophages, walls of blood vessels, cornea, and other cell types.**[216]

In the conditions variously called **hypercholesterolemia, hyperlipidemia,** and **hyperlipoproteinemia,** the lipids commonly accumulate in macrophages, presumably primarily by pinocytosis. The lipid vacuoles, which are dissolved by the usual methods of processing of tissue specimens for microscopic sections, give the cytoplasm of affected cells a bubbly or 'foam cell' appearance. In such disorders the foam cells are usually widely distributed in the RES in the spleen, lymph nodes, thymus, tonsils, lamina propria of the large and small intestines, bone marrow, portal tracts, and Kupffer cells of the liver. A clinically important site of accumulation of such cells is the dermis. The clusters of lipid-laden macrophages are visible on physical examination of patients as yellowish nodules called xanthomas.[217]

Another important site of accumulation of such lipids, both within and external to macrophages, is the walls of arteries and arterioles and, in some patients, in heart valves and endocardium. Coronary artery atheromatosis leading to episodes of myocardial ischemia is a major cause of death in some of these conditions, such as **familial hypercholesterolemia** (FH), in which the cholesterol of **low-density serum lipoprotein** (LDL) is raised because of deficient binding of LDL to receptors in hepatocytes and other cell membranes that normally bind these lipids for intracellular transport into the cells. This was the first genetic condition linked to myocardial infarction. Moreover, the description of a receptor molecule defect in FH served as a prototype for a group of diseases attributed to receptor abnormalities; this discovery was honored by the Nobel Prize in medicine and physiology.

Another mechanism by which the neutral lipids are diverted to cells that do not normally contain them in large amounts is deficiency of the apoprotein precursor of a lipoprotein. Hyperlipoproteinemia similar to lipoprotein lipase deficiency is due to deficiency of apolipoprotein (APO) C-II, the activator of lipoprotein lipase, and of APO E. The former deficiency leads to a chylomicronemic type of syndrome and features recurrent episodes of abdominal pain stemming from pancreatitis. The latter deficiency leads to the accumulation of very-low-density lipoproteins (VLDLs), which are taken up by macrophages, resulting in massive accumulation of cholesterol and premature atherosclerosis.

Analphalipoproteinemia (Tangier disease)[218] and abetalipoproteinemia (Bassen-Kornzweig disease)[219] are disorders of APO A-I and APO A-II, respectively; hypercholesterolemia also occurs with lecithin-cholesterol acyltransferase (LCAT) deficiency (**Norum disease**) and high-density lipoprotein (HDL)-LCAT deficiency (**fish-eye disease**).

Conditions with increased lipid in hepatocytes, with or without involvement of skeletal muscle cells and cardiac myocytes, are listed in Table 12.13. Particularly important in causing hepatic steatosis are the short-chain (SCAD), medium-chain (MCAD), and long-chain (LCAD) fatty acid acyl-CoA dehydrogenase deficiency diseases. MCAD may cause severe hypoglycemia and result in sudden death.

A high proportion of conditions with increased lipid in skeletal muscle fibers, with or without involvement of cardiac myocytes, are mitochondrial disorders, a group of diseases causing lactic and pyruvic acidemia. Several of these cause the fatal CNS disease Leigh, subacute infantile necrotizing encephalopathy (ISNE).[220,221] Pathologic features resemble those of Wernicke encephalopathy of thiamine deficiency with involvement of the mamillary bodies.

Smith-Lemli-Opitz Syndrome

Smith-Lemli-Opitz Syndrome (SLOS) (see Ch. 2) is an autosomal recessive disorder of multiple congenital anomalies due to defective cholesterol biosynthesis. SLOS is a true metabolic malformation syndrome.[222] The syndrome is considered an autosomal recessive, single-gene defect. The incidence of this disease has been estimated at 1:20 000 to 1:40 000; however, Lowery et al. have suggest a minimal birth incidence of 1:20 000. Others estimate a rate as high as 1:9000.[222] It is the second most frequent genetic disorder after cystic fibrosis.[223a] Plasma cholesterol levels are markedly low and 7-dehydrocholesterol reductase (7-DHR) activity is defective.[223b] The gene is mapped to chromosome 11q12-q13.

Patients typically present with microcephaly, a narrow forehead, strabismus, ptosis, apparently low-set, posteriorly angulated ears, broad anteverted nares, micrognathia, cleft and highly arched and rugose palate, broad alveolar ridges, cleft uvula, and cataracts. Ambiguous genitalia and syndactyly are usually present with hypospadius, cryptorchidism, and frequently inguinal herniae in the male; in females, external genitalia are normal.[223c]

Metachromatic leukodystrophy

This autosomal recessive disorder, metachromatic leukodystrophy (MLD), is due to **deficiency of arylsulfatase A**, which hydrolyzes galactocerebroside sulfatide (GCS) to galactocerebroside. The incidence is estimate to be 1 in 40 000. Three phenotypes are defined; all stem from allelic mutations in the gene encoding arylsulfatase A. Genetic heterogeneity is manifested in some patients with later-onset disease which features normal activity of arylsulfatase A but decreased levels of the corresponding activator protein, saposin B. The cortex, brainstem, cerebellum, and spinal cord are affected. A profound deficiency of arylsulfatase A occurs in all tissues from patients with the late infantile, juvenile, and adult forms of MLD. The gene maps to chromosome

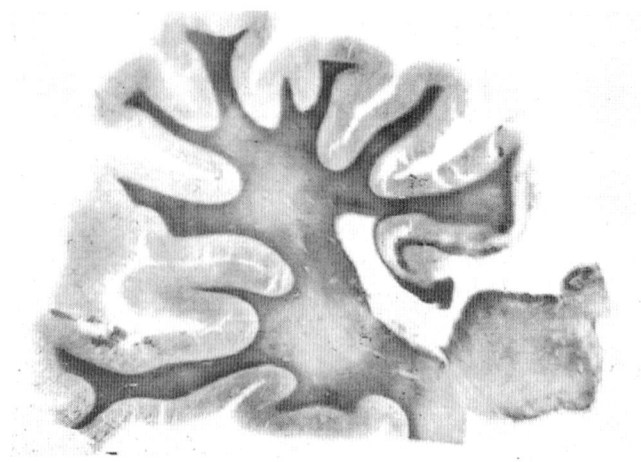

FIGURE 12.31 Metachromatic leukodystrophy. The cerebral cortex is atrophic and the white matter stains brown with cresyl violet.

22q12. Cortical atrophy of the white matter is severe and there is **accumulation of sulfatide** in the neurons and other sites, notably in the lamina propria of the gallbladder that may become polypoid,[224] bile ducts, Kupffer cells, and renal tubular epithelial cells. Sulfatide is found in the urinary sediment. Rarely, this disorder presents in the neonatal period. In the brain, there is loss of myelin and accumulation of **metachromatic material**[224a] that stains brown with the cresyl-violet (Hirsch-Pfeiffer) stain (Figs 12.31 and 12.32). Ultrastructurally, cytoplasmic inclusions are seen in oligodendrocytes and astrocytes that may have a herringbone pattern (Fig. 12.33), amorphous material, and lamellar structures. Pathologic findings are summarized in Table 12.14. Diagnosis is by enzyme assay, although some patients may have normal activity attributed to deficiency of the enzyme activator protein or a Km mutant. In addition, some normal individuals may have low enzyme activity (pseudo-arylsulfatase A deficiency). A cerebroside sulfate loading test, a nerve biopsy, or the presence of urinary sulfatide excretion detected by brown metachromasia on a urine spot on filter paper stained with cresyl violet, may be used for diagnosis.

The human arylsulfatase A gene structure has been determined, several polymorphisms defined, and a number of disease-related mutations identified. The gene, located near the end of the long arm of chromosome 22, is relatively small (3.2 kb) and consists of 8 exons specifying the 507 amino acid enzyme subunit.

The prevention of MLD relies mainly on identifying carriers in known MLD families and providing genetic counseling with the possibility of prenatal diagnosis. Prenatal diagnosis based on arylsulfatase A activity in cultured amniotic fluid or chorionic villus cells appears to be reliable.

Multiple sulfatase deficiency (Austin disease)

This[225] disorder is caused by a deficiency of anylsulfatase A, B and C. The phenotype resembles that of late infantile MLD. Increased

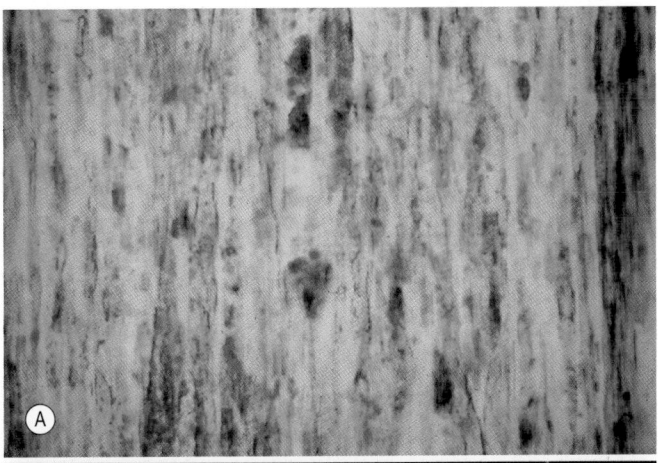

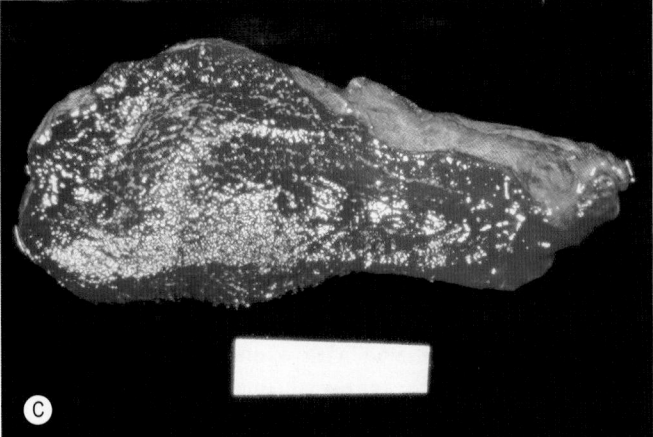

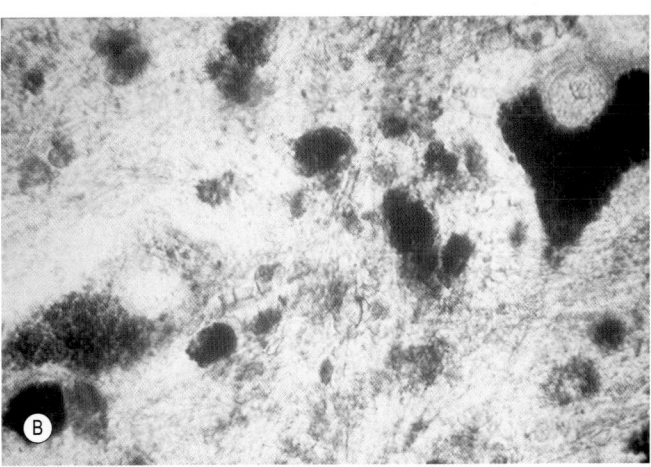

FIGURE 12.32 Metachromatic leukodystrophy. (A) Peripheral nerve showing brown metachromasia (cresyl violet stain). (B) Spinal cord showing neurons with brown metachromasia (cresyl violet stain). (C) Gall bladder showing brown metachromasia (cresyl violet stain).

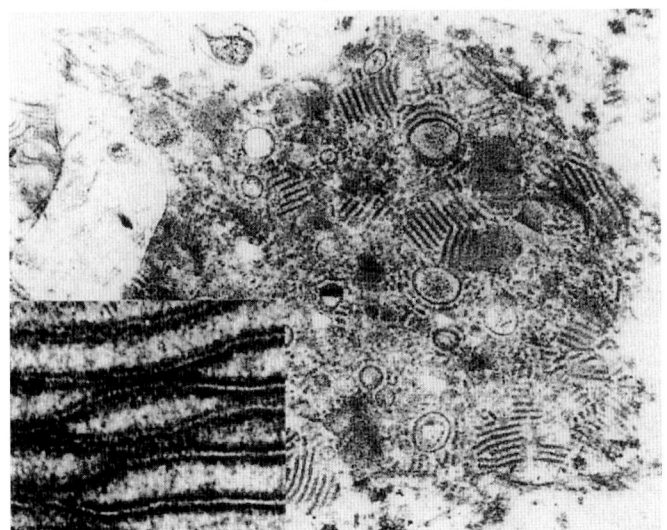

FIGURE 12.33 Metachromatic leukodystrophy. EM of a neuron of the white matter of the brain showing pleomorphic and parallel lipid profiles (× 21 000) inset parallel arrays (× 221 000).

TABLE 12.14 METACHROMATIC LEUKODYSTROPHY: PATHOGENIC FINDINGS

- Destruction of myelin in the cerebral and cerebellar white matter
- Gliosis
- Ballooned macrophages (vacuolated)
- Metachromatic staining of accumulated sulfatides in macrophages and in the white matter
  - Basic dyes (e.g. acidified cresyl violet and toluidine blue) stain different color when they react with the tissue
  - Frozen section tissue must be used
- Subcortical arcuate fibers may be spared
- EM: Prismatic inclusions can be seen in all cell types, representing accumulated sulfatides

amounts of MPS and sulfatide are found in the affected tissues and in the urine. Hurler-type features are mild and there is rapid psychomotor deterioration. Peripheral nerve biopsies show **brown metachromasia**. The manifestations may have onset in the neonatal period. **Hydrocephalus** present at birth, mild **chondrodysplasia calcificans**, and **heart abnormalities** have been described; patients may later develop ichthyosis and features of MPS. Most patients die in their first decade.

TABLE 12.15 MUCOLIPIDOSES (ML)

McKusick no.	Disease	Enzyme defect or deficiency	Storage
256550	ML I (sialidosis III)	GlcNAc	Sialyloligo-saccharides
252500	ML II (I-cell)	N-acetyl-glucosamine-1 phosphotransferase (GlcNAc-phosphotransferase)	Oligosaccharides
252600	ML III (pseudo-Hurler)	N-acetyl-glucosamine-1 phosphotransferase (GlcNAc-phosphotransferase)	Oligosaccharides
252650	ML IV (sialolipidosis)	Ganglioside sialidase	Gangliosides GM_3 and GD_3

Neuroaxonal dystrophy and leukodystrophy (Seitelberger syndrome)

Infantile neuroaxonal dystrophy is an autosomal recessive condition characterized by symptoms appearing around the second year of life with weakness, hypotonia, and areflexia. As the disease progresses, rigidity, spasticity, cerebellar signs, deafness, blindness, and mental deterioration occur. Death typically occurs before the age of 6 years.

Diagnosis is made by pathologic examination of brain, peripheral nerve, conjunctiva, skin, or rectal biopsy. The characteristic axonal swellings are sought by histochemical and ultrastructural techniques. Macroscopically, the brain of affected infants shows atrophy of the cerebral hemispheres with ventricular dilation and cerebellar atrophy. Histologically, axonal spheroids are seen in the gray matter of the nervous system with degeneration of corticospinal and spinobulbar tracts associated with reactive astrocytosis. An infant with cerebellar localization has been described. Neuroaxonal leukodystrophy is characterized by pronounced demyelination associated with the presence of spheroids in the axons of the white matter of the cerebral hemispheres. Ultrastructure shows amorphous electron-dense material in unmyelinated axons. Autosomal recessive neuroaxonal dystrophy due to lysosomal α-N-acetylgalactosaminidase deficiency has been described.

Late infantile, juvenile, and adult neuroaxonal dystrophy typically present with rigidity, ataxia, dysarthria, motor weakness, psychiatric disorders, and later dementia. Case descriptions have been collated by Seitelberger.[226] Macroscopically and histologically, appearances overlap with those described for Hallervorden-Spatz disease.

Hallervorden-Spatz Disease

Hallervorden-Spatz disease (HSD) is a progressive neurodegenerative condition in which prominent *neuroaxonal dystrophy* is associated with movement disorders. This autosomal recessive disease is caused by a mutation of the *PANK2* gene.

HSD has been considered a part of the spectrum of neuroaxonal dystrophy. Alternatively, it has been proposed as an iron storage disease with a central role for iron in causing free radical-mediated damage.[227] Neurochemical abnormalities have been found, with markedly **elevated levels of cystine** and **glutathione–cysteine mixed disulfide** in the **globus pallidus** associated with **reduced activity of cysteine dioxygenase**, the enzyme that converts cysteine to cysteine sulfinic acid. It has been suggested that accumulated cysteine may act as a chelating agent and may be responsible for the **accumulation of iron**.

The disease usually manifests before the age of 15 years and presents as a gait disorder with **rigidity of legs, dystonia, motor slowing, dysarthria, mental deterioration, and a high incidence of choreoathetosis**. Most patients with this pattern of disease die by the age of 35 years. In older patients, the disease usually presents as an extrapyramidal movement disorder with development of dementia.[228]

There is accumulation of iron-containing pigment and destruction of the globus pallidus and pars reticularis of the substantia nigra associated with **axonal spheroids.** Macroscopically, these areas appear shrunken and have a rust-brown discoloration. Spheroids may also be seen outside these main areas of pathology; in the cerebral cortex and in the brainstem nuclei the pigment is present within neurons, including some in spheroids, astrocytes, and microglial cells, while some appears free, often around blood vessels. The **pigment contains lipofuscin, neuromelanin, and iron. Sea-blue histiocytosis** has been seen in bone marrow in some cases. Brown pigment may also be present in the renal tubular epithelium.[229] In some cases there have been associated **neurofibrillary tangles**. Lymphocytes from bone marrow contain dense osmiophilic deposits.

Mucolipidoses

The mucolipidoses (MLs) are a group of recessively inherited lysosomal storage diseases characterized by intracellular accumulation of both mucopolysaccharides and lipids in the lysosomes. They have been divided by McKusick[9] into four main groups: I, II, III, and IV (Table 12.15).

ML is suspected clinically because of the phenotypic appearance of the child, including **coarse facial features, mental retardation, dysostosis multiplex**, and the **lack of mucopolysacchariduria**. It is confirmed histopathologically and biochemically by identification of the substrates.[230] Deficiency of N-acetyl neuraminidase has been identified in ML I, also called sialidosis III.[231-233] Hepatocytes, macrophages, hepatic and splenic sinusoidal lining cells, neurons, renal glomerular, and collecting tubular epithelial cells are most severely affected in ML I. ML II more severely affects mesenchymal tissues (e.g., cartilage), whereas neurons show the most striking changes at the ultrastructural level. Both placental trophoblast and stromal cells are involved in ML I, II,[234,235] and IV.[236] Multiple cellular lysosomal enzyme deficiencies in conjunction with elevated serum levels of specific enzymes are features of ML II and III. In ML II and III the defect is the targeting of the lysosomal enzymes to the lysosome. For some of the hydrolases to act completely, once in the lysosome, activator proteins (APs) must be present. Mutations affecting APs lead to multiple hydrolase deficiencies. Few tissues have been studied from cases of ML III and IV.

The accumulated cytoplasmic acid mucopolysaccharide exhibits histochemical characteristics of a weakly sulfated compound, producing a positive reaction with Hale's colloidal iron, Alcian blue at pH 2.5, and toluidine blue at pH 2.0, but a negative reaction with Alcian blue at pH 1.0.[230]

EM studies show that **lysosomes** contain **finely granular to flocculent**, moderately electron-dense material as the ponderant component of stored mucopolysaccharides. **Osmiophilic multilamellar** bodies and fragments of membrane-like profiles are typical of lipid compounds. The membranous structures are typically within lysosomes of visceral tissues in the classic forms of MPS, but are more common in the MLs that contain both MPS and lipid. The storage vacuoles in brain cells in the mucolipidoses, as in the lipidoses and MPSs, are filled dominantly with osmiophilic membranous bodies and lamellar arrays.[230]

Mucolipidosis I (galactosialidosis; sialidosis III)

A congenital form manifests as hydrops and is lethal within the first 2 years of life.[231a,232a,233a] Clinical features incude facial dysmorphism, psychomotor retardation, dysostosis multiplex, renal failure, corneal clouding, macular cherry-red spots, and cardiomegaly. Pathologic findings are most prominent in placental trophoblast, hepatocytes, neurons, glomerular epithelium, and mononuclear phagocytes.[234a]

A **late infantile** form includes patients who are normal or minimally abnormal at birth[235a,236a,238–246] except for an occasional patient with a hernia. Motor retardation with axial hypotonia and peripheral hypertonicity, hepatosplenomegaly, and coarse facial appearance develop at 6–12 months and are followed by progressive neurologic deterioration, skeletal abnormalities, recurrent infections, and death in early childhood. Occasional renal involvement with glomerular storage and renal failure has prompted the name 'nephrosialidosis.'

A **juvenile form** presents in late infancy or early childhood with progressive neurologic degeneration and progresses in early adulthood to a mild Hurler phenotype. Patients develop ataxia, myoclonus, macular cherry-red spots, hepatosplenomegaly, and dysostosis multiplex, resembling mucopolysaccharidosis. Storage material is present in fibroblasts, hepatocytes, glomerular epithelium, neurons, and histiocytes. A neuraminidase deficiency was first identified in the juvenile form.

An **adult form** presents in adolescence with progressive myoclonus, bilateral macular cherry-red spots, insidious visual loss, hepatosplenomegaly, and normal or only slightly impaired intelligence. Most patients survive into at least their fourth decade. Before its clinical delineation, this disorder was called the 'cherry-red-spot-myoclonus syndrome.'

The enzyme defect is a **deficiency of a neuraminidase**, coded by a locus on chromosome 22[248] that normally cleaves terminal 2:3 and 2:6 sialyl linkages of several oligosaccharides and glycoproteins.[249–251] Combined deficiency of neuraminidase and β-galactosidase results from the primary loss of a protein required to protect the galactosidase and neuraminidase complex from proteolytic degradation.[252]

Diagnosis

Urine samples yield abnormal levels of MPS in all forms of ML I, including those of newborns with the congenital or hydropic form of the disorder.[246,253] Definitive diagnosis of ML I is based on the measurement of neuraminidase and β-galactosidase activity in skin fibroblasts, cultured amniotic fluid cells, or white blood cells, and on the ultrastructural morphology.

Prenatal diagnosis

Neuraminidase and galactosidase activity are detectable in **cultured normal amniotic fluid cells**. The amniotic fluid cells require special handling since freezing, sonication, or exposure to temperatures above 37°C quickly destroy enzyme activity.[254]

Mucolipidosis II (I-Cell disease)

I-cell disease was first differentiated from the Hurler syndrome by the **absence of mucopolysacchariduria**.[255] It was designated I-(inclusion) cell disease because of numerous phase-dense inclusions in the cytoplasm of cultured fibroblasts from affected individuals (Fig. 12.34).[255] Similar inclusions have since been seen in cells from patients with ML I and pseudo-Hurler polydystrophy (ML III).[256]

Multiple lysosomal enzymes in ML II are deficient in cultured fibroblasts,[257,258] with an increased concentration in culture medium,[259,260] serum, and other body fluids. **Mannose-6-phosphate is the recognition marker** for internalization of lysosomal acid hydrolase receptors that is absent in ML II.[261,262]

The diagnosis of both ML II and ML III can be confirmed by measuring the activities of lysosomal enzymes in serum or in cultured fibroblasts.[263] Ten- to twentyfold increases in β-hexosaminidase, iduronate sulfatase, and arylsulfatase A are characteristic of both ML II and ML III.[264]

ML II, like Hurler syndrome, is characterized by severe psychomotor retardation with coarse facial features (Fig. 12.35). Gingival hypertrophy is a more striking feature than in Hurler syndrome. Hepatomegaly is prominent, but splenomegaly is

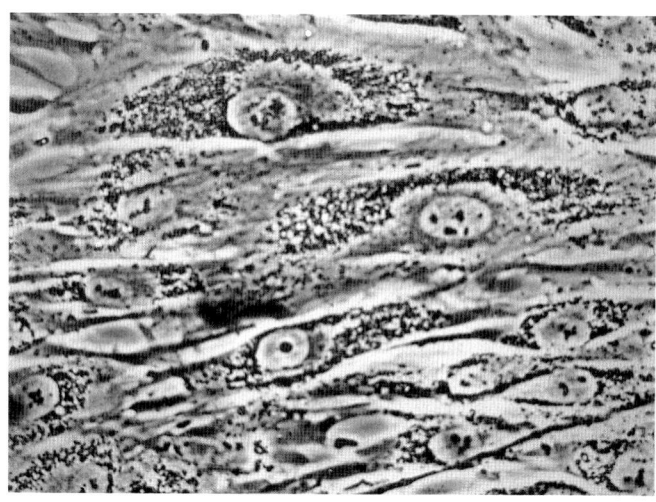

FIGURE 12.34 Mucolipidosis II (ML II I-cell disease). Cultured fibroblasts under polarized light showing coarse granules.

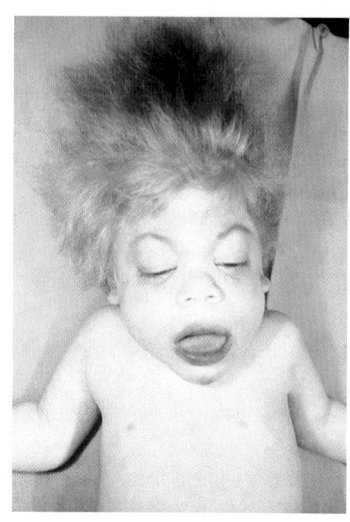

FIGURE 12.35 ML II in a 5-year-old child with Hurler features and brushed out appearance of the hair.

BOX 12.4 PATHOLOGIC FEATURES OF ML II, I-CELL DISEASE

Gross features

Hurler-like facial appearance

Hypertrophy of gingiva

Thick tongue

Dermal nodules

Short neck and thoracic cage

Broad and flat ribs

Knob-like costochondral junctions

Cardiovascular

Pericardium thick and opaque

Cardiomegaly

Valves thick, rigid, and retracted

Subendocardial lipid streaks

Lipid plaques in aorta and major vessels

Storage histiocytes in pericardium, endocardium, and heart valves

Vacuolization of myocardial fibers

Aortic subintimal nodular accumulation of lipid

Lungs

Lipid granulomas throughout parenchyma

Liver

Lipid in Kupffer cells

Lipid in hepatocytes

Histiocytic granulomas in portal tracts

Kidneys

Vacuolization of visceral epithelial cells of glomeruli

Thickening of glomerular basement membrane

Vacuolization of proximal tubular epithelial cells

Focal, interstitial aggregates of storage histiocytes

Brain

Weight below normal

Meninges thick, opaque, gelatinous

Slight atrophy of cerebral cortex

Slight atrophy of cerebellar vermis

Pia–arachnoid thickly infiltrated by storage histiocytes, particularly around blood vessels

Numerical decrease in neurons of cerebral cortex

Some loss of Purkinje cells and granular neurons

PAS-positive material in anterior horn and cerebrocortical neurons

Spleen and lymph nodes

Scattered storage histiocytes

Musculoskeletal system

Tongue: subepithelial nodular accumulations of storage histiocytes

Focal nodular aggregates of storage histiocytes in skeletal muscle

Bones

Growth arrest at epiphyseal growth plate and many storage histiocytes

Skin

Focal nodular aggregates of storage histiocytes and dense collagen in dermis

Peripheral blood

Vacuolated lymphocytes

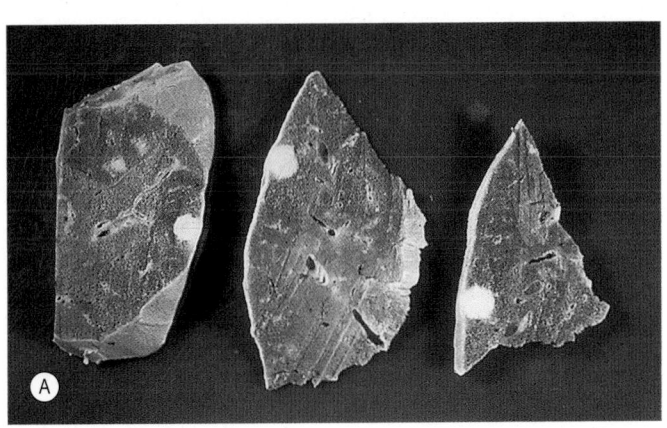
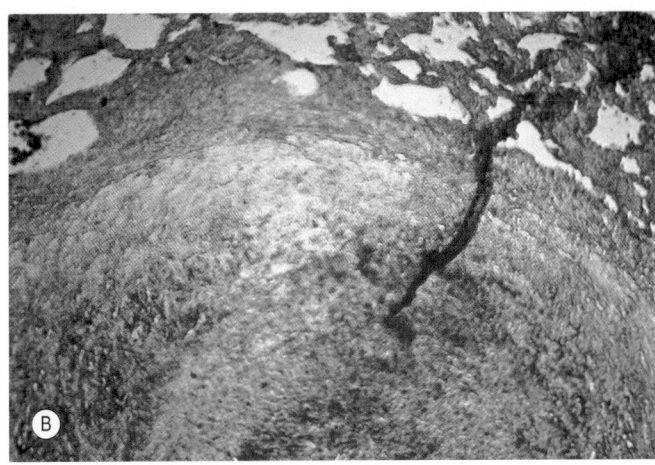

FIGURE 12.36 ML II. (A) The lung contains lipid granulomas. (B) Microscopic appearance of lipid granuloma (× 100).

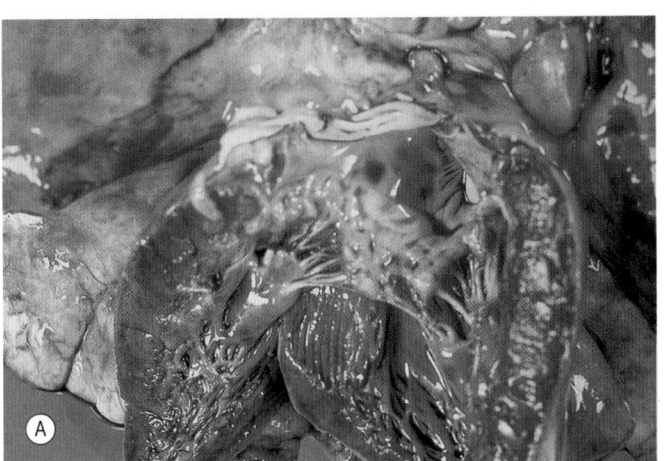
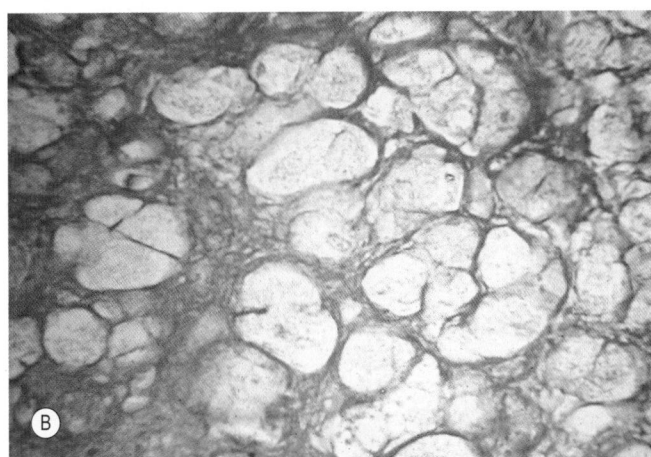

FIGURE 12.37 ML II. (A) The heart valves are thickened and distorted. (B) Myocardial cells are distended with storage material.

minimal. Cardiomegaly, cardiac murmurs, and aortic insufficiency are common.[265]

The pathologic features of I-cell disease[266] are summarized in Box 12.4.

Lipid granulomas may be found in the lungs (Fig. 12.36). The heart (Fig. 12.37) is uniformly hypertrophied. The **mitral and aortic valve leaflets** are extremely thick, rigid, retracted, and distorted. The aorta, the major aortic branches, and the coronary vessels are thickened by yellow subintimal plaques.

The individual myocardial cells appear vacuolated owing to the accumulation of lipid and mucosubstances. The ultrastructure of the myocardial cells is distorted by sarcolemmal inclusions of osmiophilic dense bodies and membranous lamellar bodies, ring-like structures, and reticulogranular deposits (Fig. 12.38). The pulmonary arteries may show similar changes.

Hepatocytes, Kupffer cells, glomerular and tubular epithelial cells, and bone marrow lymphocytes show inclusions.[266] EM demonstrates lysosomal accumulation of reticulogranular material and laminated membranous bodies arranged in parallel or concentric lamellae, some in myelin-like configurations with a periodicity of 50–60 nm.

If death occurs after 5 years of age, the brain (Fig. 12.39A) is small. The leptomeninges over the cerebral convexity are usually thickened, opaque, and gelatinous. There may be **atrophy of the cerebral cortex** with widening of sulci and slight atrophy of the vermis of the cerebellum. Cortical neurons are diminished in number. Most anterior horn motor neurons of the spinal cord contain PAS-positive granules.

The intensity of the staining reactions in formalin-fixed histologic section is consistently greater in collagen and fibroblasts than elsewhere. The histiocytes apparently responsible for the accumulation of the stored material frequently stain faintly or not at all, suggesting that they have disgorged their content, which appears to stimulate the deposition of collagen.

The tinctorial characteristics of the storage material indicate a complex glycolipid since it remains insoluble after treatment with hot or cold acetone and with xylene, suggesting the presence of a ceramide moiety. The strong aniline blue reaction

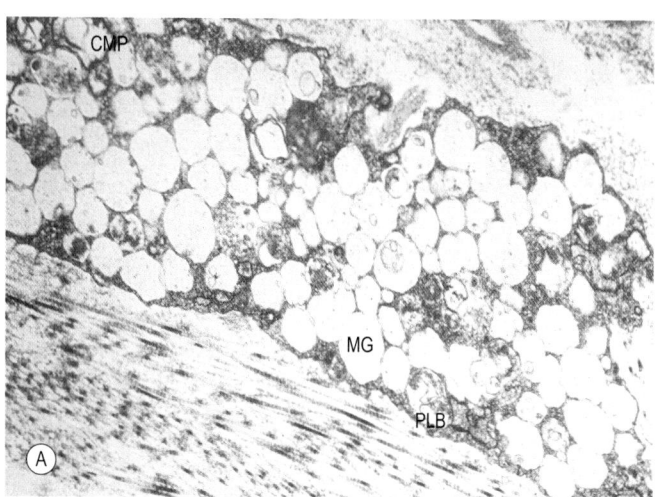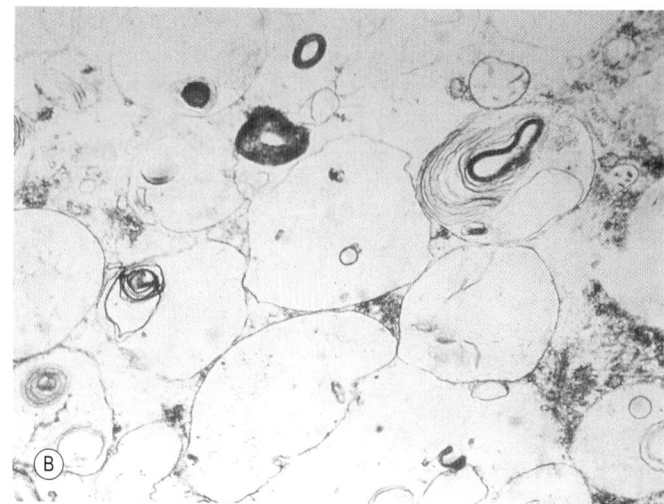

FIGURE 12.38 I-cell disease. (A) Electron micrograph of heart valve showing vacuoles and membranogranular deposits (MG) and pleomorphic lipid bodies (PLB). (B) EM of renal tubular epithelial cell with large membrane-bound vacuoles containing an array of profiles with concentrically laminated bodies and stacked membranes.

indicates the presence of acid phosphatase. The staining reaction with Luxol fast blue may represent phospholipids.

By EM, nerve cells and Purkinje cells contain scattered pleomorphic inclusions of 0.6–2.0 μm in greatest dimension. Some inclusions contain stacked linear membranes, circular and hemicircular profiles, and crystalline structures (Fig. 12.39B).

The eyes may have corneal opacities due to the accumulation of storage substrate.

Diagnosis

The diagnosis of ML II and ML III can be confirmed[267] by measuring the activities of lysosomal enzymes in serum or in cultured fibroblasts. Tenfold to twentyfold increases in β-hexosaminidase, iduronate sulfatase, and arylsulfatase A are characteristic of both ML II and ML III.[268–270] The pattern of lysosomal enzyme deficiencies in cultured fibroblasts and the ratio of extracellular to intracellular enzyme activities are characteristic,[268,271–273] but lysosomal enzyme activities in white blood cells are not as reliable for diagnosis.[274,275] The level of N-acetyl-glucosamine 1 (GlcNAc) phosphotransferase activity in white blood cells or cultured fibroblasts can be measured directly with commercially available substrates.[276–278]

Prenatal diagnosis by amniocentesis or CVS has been accomplished in ML I, II, and IV and is possible in ML III.

ML II is characterized by a mild Hurler phenotype. **The deficiency of GlcNAc phosphotransferase** results in a defective phosphorylation of mannoses of oligosaccharide side chains of multiple lysosomal enzymes.

Mucolipidosis III (Pseudo-Hurler Polydystrophy)

ML III has been corrected in vitro by **gene transfer**.[279] Two siblings have been reported with a very mild form of ML III

with no clinical signs but isolated involvement of the hip and very mild abnormalities of the spine. This indicates that a storage disease, in particular ML III, should be considered in any case of isolated bilateral hip dysplasia.[280] Three patients with ML III (two girls and one boy) were referred to a pediatric rheumatology clinic because of progressive stiffness of their hands and flexion contractures of fingers, accompanied by additional musculoskeletal changes.[281]

Pathology

The pathology of ML III is not as well documented as that of ML II. Fibroblasts cultured from ML III patients contain inclusion bodies similar to, but not as prominent as, those of ML II cells.

Mucolipidosis IV (Sialolipidosis; Ganglioside–Sialidase deficiency)

ML IV, also known as sialolipidosis, is transmitted as an autosomal recessive trait most often in Askenazi Jews. ML IV is characterized by severe visual impairment with corneal clouding. Retinal degeneration often produces visual impairment within the first year of life before corneal opacities are sufficient to impair vision. Although patients may live beyond 10 years of age,[282] maximum developmental level achieved is 12–15 months.

The clinical diagnosis is made by demonstration of the lysosomal storage by EM of skin or conjunctiva. No radiologic changes have been identified in the skeleton. There is no cellular metachromasia in cultured fibroblasts and no mucopolysacchariduria. Assays for a considerable number of lysosomal enzymes have been normal in cultured fibroblasts and in leukocytes.

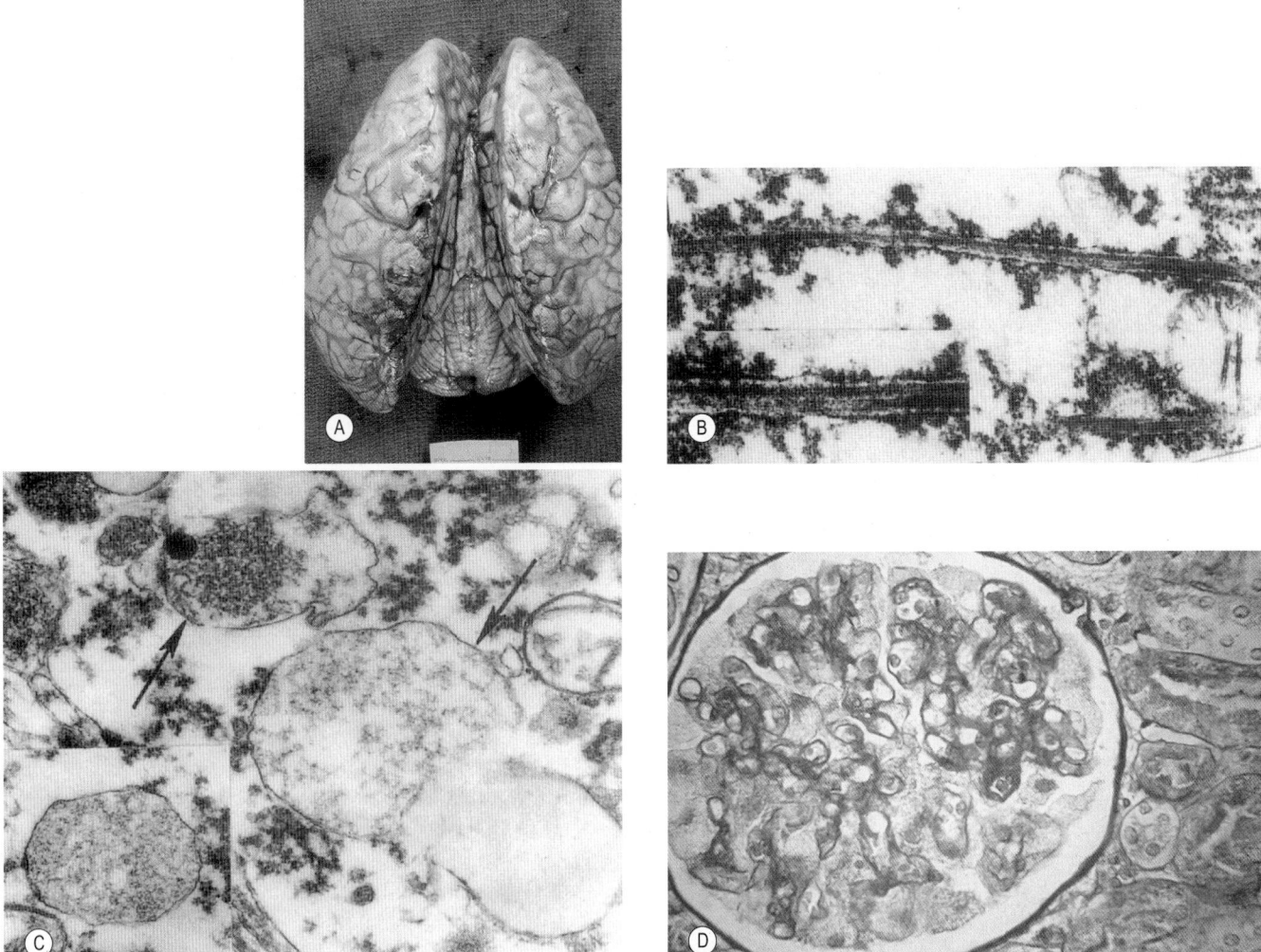

FIGURE 12.39 I-cell disease. (A) Gross appearance with cortical atrophy and gelatinous exudate over the meningeal surface. (B) EM of a neuron with crystaline inclusions (inset at high magnification). (C) EM of a cortical neuron: there are two lysomes, one ruptured, with fine fibrillar inclusions (arrows) (× 35 000). (D) Glomerulus of kidney showing vacuolated epithelial cells (H & E stain).

Pathologic findings in ML IV

Inclusions in epithelial cells, e.g., in conjunctival biopsies, are particularly striking. Ganglioside is the main lipid that accumulates but mucopolysaccharide, particularly hyaluronic acid, also accumulates, probably due to a secondary catabolic shock. Mutation of the gene *MUCOLIPIN 1* results in lysosomal accumulation of storage material which can be visualized in leukocytes and tissue biopsies. In the central nervous system, neuronal loss in the cerebral cortex, basal ganglia, deep cerebellar nuclei, and brainstem nuclei was marked by astrocytosis; the cytoplasm or residual neurons have brown granules positive with PAS, Concanavalia ensiformis, and Sudan black, but not with Luxol fast blue. Ultrastructurally, neurons contain lysosomes laden with osmiophilic, amorphous, and granular material, and few lamellated membranous structures. Hepatocytes, epithelia, endothelia, chondrocytes, and tissue macrophages also stain positively with Datura stramonium and Ricinus communis-I agglutinins.

Ceroid storage diseases

Neuronal ceroid lipofuscinosis (Batten disease)

Neuronal ceroid lipofuscinoses (NCLs) were so named because of the **autofluorescent lipopigment** that showed tinctorial characteristics of **ceroid** and **lipofuscin** in histologic specimens.[283] This group of neurologic disorders share features of progressive psychomotor retardation and accumulation of large amounts of lipopigments in neural and extraneural cells. The disorder was originally called familial neurovisceral lipidosis, characterized by progressive neurologic disease, impaired psychomotor development, blindness, and early death.[284] Several forms of this disorder have been described, depending

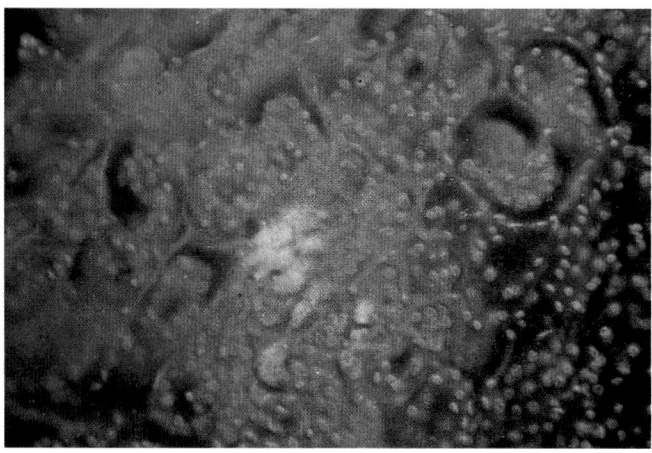

FIGURE 12.40 Neuronal ceroid lipofuscinosis. Autofluorescence of storage material.

TABLE 12.16 ELECTRON-MICROSCOPIC TYPES OF CYTOSOMES IN NEURONAL CEROID LIPOFUSCINOSIS (NCL)

Cytosome disease	Abbreviation	Predominant association
Granular osmiophilic deposits	GROD	INCL
Cytosomes with curvilinear bodies	CCP	LINCL
Cytosomes with fingerprint profiles	CFP	JNCL
Combination of CCB and CFP	Adult	NCL, variant types
Non-specific electron-dense inclusions		All types

INCL, infantile; LINCL, late infantile; JNCL, juvenile NCL.

on the age of onset: infantile (INCL), late infantile (LINCL), juvenile (JNCL), and adult.[285,286] Only the first two forms are within the scope of this text. For a comprehensive review see *Proceedings* of the Fifth International Conference on NCL[287] and *Metabolic Diseases, Foundations of Clinical Management, Genetics and Pathology.*

NCL occurs worldwide and appears to be the most common hereditary neurodegenerative disorder in children, with an estimated incidence of 1 in 12 500 in the United States.[288] The lipopigments in NCL accumulate in the lysosomes, and results from a mutation of the gene *CLN3*, located on 16p12.1;[290] INCL is caused by mutations of *CLN1*, which maps to 1p32.[291] Mutations in the palmitoyl-protein thioesterase gene have been identified.[292] The gene for LINCL is on chromosome 11p15. The gene for LINCL (*CLN2*), maps to 11p15.5; the gene for the Finnish variant (*CLN5*) has been mapped to 13q21.1-q32.

The accumulating lipopigment is autofluorescent (Fig. 12.40) and stains positively with PAS, Sudan black B, oil red O, and acid fuchsin. Only slight differences are noted in the staining characteristic of the lipopigment in different syndromes.[293] The lipopigment granules show intense acid phosphatase activity and are encased by a trilaminar unit membrane seen by EM, indicating lysosomal residual body structure. Lipopigments are very resistant to polar and non-polar solvents, rendering them visible in ordinary paraffin sections.

The lipopigment containing residual bodies or cytosomes shows considerable variability on EM. According to the fine structural characteristics, the cytosomes can be divided into three principal types (Table 12.16). The first type consists of homogeneous, electron-dense, finely granular material without any, or with only occasional, membranous structures. Some of the cytosomes seem to be formed by spherical globules about 0.2–0.5 μm in diameter, called **granular osmiophilic deposits** (GRODs) (Fig. 12.41A). The deposits of the second type are more elaborate and show crescentic or horseshoe-shaped dark profiles. The curved profiles consist of stacks of lamellae with alternating dark and light lines about 4 μm in thickness. Each

stack contains two to six pale, dark lines, and these lamellae are called cytosomes with **curvilinear bodies** (Fig. 12.41B) (CCBs). The third type forms structures superficially resembling fingerprints, named **cytosomes with fingerprint profiles** (CFPs) (Fig. 12.41C). They are composed of groups of curved, parallel, paired dark lines separated by a thin clear space. The fine structure of the NCL cytosomes may occasionally be modified or distorted, and in some cases different so-called membranous bodies may be seen,[294] but one of the basic patterns usually prevails.

Diagnosis of a clinical syndrome based solely on the ultrastructural findings is not warranted.[295]

Clinical and neurophysiologic features of the different forms of NCL are shown in Table 12.17.

Infantile NCL (Santavuori-Haltia)

The clinical onset is between 8 and 14 months of age and runs a relentless rapid course of psychomotor deterioration. Patients become unresponsive at about 3 years of age and bedridden until death ensues between 6 and 15 years of age.[296] Muscular hypotonia, delayed psychomotor development and progressive microcephaly are followed by severe neural retardation, visual failure, myoclonic jerks, hyperexcitability, and ataxia. Magnetic resonance imaging (MRI) shows generalized brain atrophy by 1 year of age with basal ganglia that are hypointense in relation to the hyperintense white matter that is highly suggestive if not pathognomonic of INCL.

The neuropathologic appearance[297,298] is that of an extremely atrophic brain weighing about 250–400 g at autopsy. Extreme degrees of gyral atrophy are present, and the atrophic cortex can hardly be distinguished from the shrunken and tough white matter encircling the dilated ventricles. The cerebellum is likewise very atrophic.

Early, the **neurons accumulate lipopigments** showing signs of neuronal destruction with **astrocytosis and macrophagocytosis**. Both astrocytes and macrophages harbor lipo-

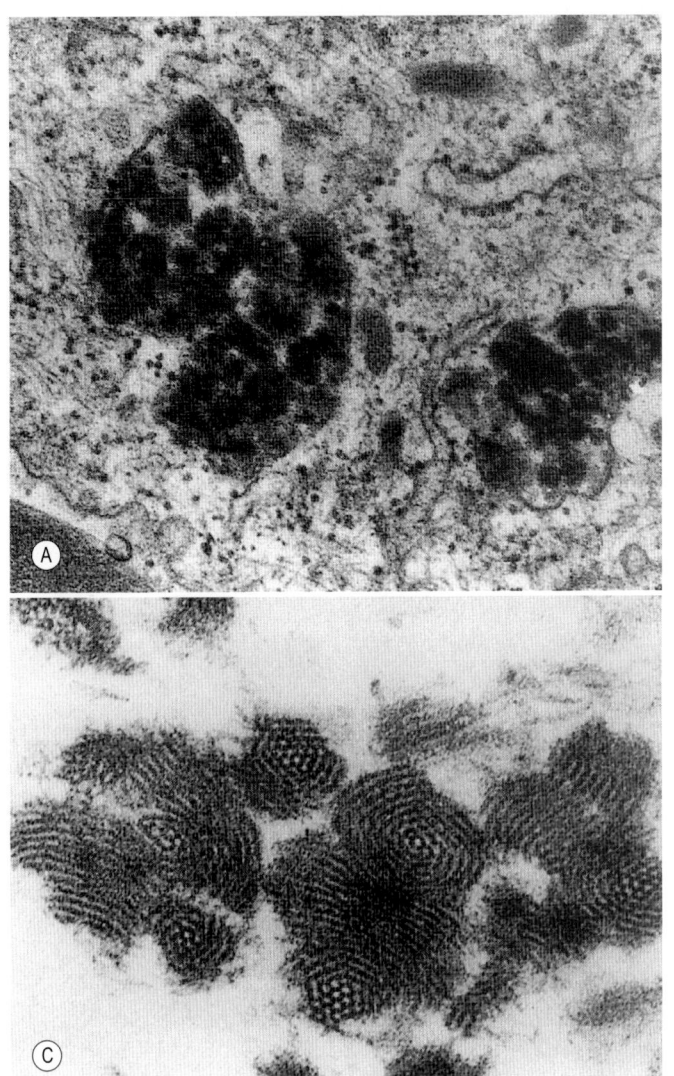

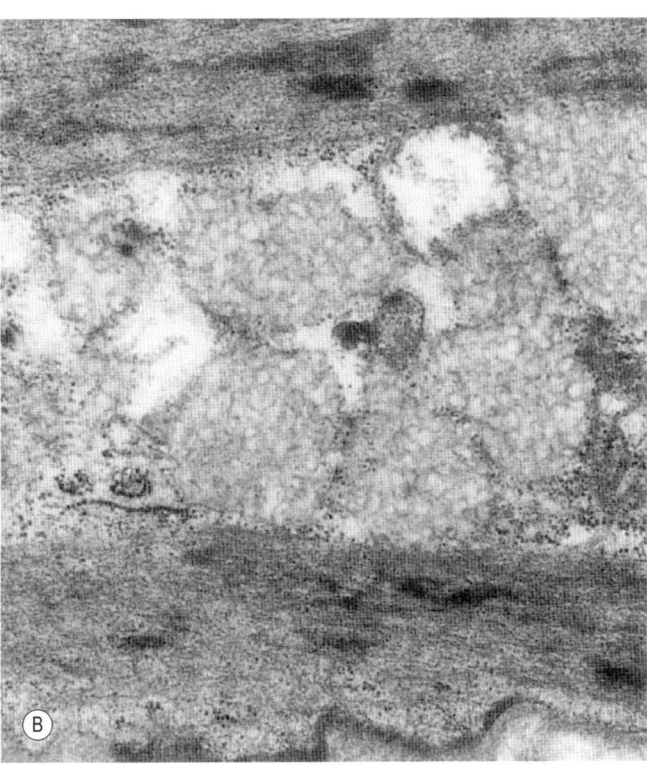

FIGURE 12.41 Neuronal ceroid lipofuscinosis. EMs of (A) granular osmiophilic deposits, (B) curvilinear bodies, and C) fingerprint profiles. (Courtesy of Dr. Juhani Rapola.)

pigments. Up to 4 years of age, subtotal loss of cortical neurons is evident and the cortex is occupied by astrocytes and numerous macrophages. The white matter undergoes demyelinization. After 4 years of age, the cerebral cortex is totally devoid of neurons, axons, and myelin sheaths. The retina degenerates to the same extent as the cerebral cortex. In the spinal cord and autonomic ganglion cells, the cytoplasm is filled with the storage material, but neuronal destruction is not seen.

The storage cytosomes can be detected by EM of ocular conjunctiva,[299] skeletal muscle,[300] rectal mucosa,[301] and lympho-cytes.[295] EM investigation of the skin biopsy specimen is the most useful diagnostic method.[302,303] Diagnostic cytosomes of INCL are most easily found in the cytoplasm of the endothelial cells in different organs, including the autonomic ganglion cells of rectal mucosal biopsies.[301]

The storage cytosomes from brain tissue of patients with INCL contains a high amount of Safosia A and D proteins.

Late infantile NCL (Jansky-Bielschowsky)

Classic LINCL has its clinical onset between 2 and 4 years with seizures, followed by rapid deterioration of vision and psychomotor functions. The patient enters a vegetative stage 2–4 years after the onset and dies soon thereafter.[304]

The macroscopic neuropathologic findings are similar to those of INCL but considerably milder. The neuroepithelium and ganglionic nerve cells of the retina are destroyed and accompanied by **optic atrophy**.[305] The skull bones are abnormally thick. The cerebellum is severely atrophic with atrophy of the pons and spinal cord and optic nerve. The cortical gray matter is narrow and discolored brown. The white matter is demyelinated and gelatinous; reactive gliosis is prominent.

Diagnosis is made by EM investigation[306] of skin, conjunctiva, rectal mucosa, or lymphocytes. The prevailing inclusion is that of CCB. The inclusions are most common in the epithelium of the secretory coils of sweat glands and in various cells of skin specimens. Immunochemical studies suggest that a subunit C of

TABLE 12.17 CLINICAL AND NEUROPHYSIOLOGIC FEATURES OF NEURONAL CEROID LIPOFUSCINOSIS (NCL)

	INCL	LINCL	JNCL	Adult NCL
Age of onset	8–18 mo	2–4 yr	4–8 yr	30 yr
Mental retardation	Early	Late	Late	Late
Visual failure	Relatively early	Late	Early, leading symptom	Not present
Ataxia	Moderate to marked	Marked	Marked	Variable
Myoclonus	Constant	Constant	Mild to marked	Severe, symptom in some patients
Nonambulant	8–30 mo	3–5 yr	13–28 yr	Over 35 yr
Retinal pigment aggregations	Not present	Rare	Constant	Not present
Electoencephalograph	Isoelectric by 3 yr	Spikes inducible by low photic stimulation	Not specific	Sensitivity to low photic stimulation
VEP*	Abolished by 2-4 yr	Early high	Early abnormal	High
SEP†	Low	High	Variable	Variable, high
Vacuolated lymphocytes	Negative	Negative	Positive	Negative
Age at death	8–14 yr	6–15 yr	13–40 yr	Over 40 yr

* Visual evoked potential.

† Somatosensory evoked potential in cases from the past have been designated SEP.

mitochondrial ATP synthase is stored.[306] It results from a mutation of *CLN2*.

Prenatal Diagnosis of NCL Typical cytosomes have been demonstrated by EM in free-floating amniotic cells of a pregnancy at risk for LINCL[308] and another at risk for JNCL; fingerprint inclusions were found in the trophoblastic cells of a CVS sample.[309] CVS biopsy specimens in many pregnancies at risk for INCL were studied by EM and DNA studies. The affected fetuses showed typical GROD in the endothelial cell cytoplasm of the chorionic villi. GRODs are found in the CNS and visceral organs of the fetuses after termination of the pregnancy.[310,311] Prenatal diagnosis of INCL has been made simultaneously with EM and DNA studies in increasing numbers of high-risk pregnancies with fully concordant results.[311]

Juvenile NCL (Spielmeyer-Sjögren-Vogt) (See also Ch. 39)

The gene for juvenile NCL (*CLN3*) is localized to chromosome 16p21.1, a 438 amino acid protein with linkage to the haptoglobin locus.[312]

JNCL is slowly progressive with impaired vision becoming evident between 4 and 7 years. Mental retardation develops slowly and is often first noticed at school. Compulsive speaking and mumbling become evident in the first half of the second decade and severe dysarthria develops a few years later. Dementia often becomes profound later in the course of the disease. Ocular manifestations include macular degeneration of the optic fundi, optic atrophy, and retinal degeneration. Blindness usually occurs.

Pathology The gross appearance of the brain may be near normal but with moderately or even severely decreased weight. Loss of neurons affects all parts of the brain and is associated with reactive astrogliosis. The neurons are distended by perikaryonal granular lipopigment. Microglia harbor lipopigments, best appreciated with appropriate stains, such as PAS.

Vacuolated lymphocytes that stain for lipids in peripheral blood are of diagnostic importance and are seen only in the classic form of JNCL. Sea-blue histiocytes in the bone marrow may be seen.

Adult NCL (KUFS)

This is the least common form of NCL. It is clinically and genetically heterogenous. Its onset is over 30 years with myoclonic epilepsy or dementia.

Distribution of NCL

All types of NCL are found worldwide, but some are clustered in certain populations.[313–315] JNCL has an unusually high prevalence in Sweden.[316] A cluster of LINCL and a variant of JNCL are found in a small population of Newfoundland.[317] INCL is common in the population of Finland with an incidence of 1 in 20 000.[318] Worldwide, JNCL and LINCL are the most common types.

Carbohydrate disorders

Galactosemia

Galactosemia is an autosomal recessive disorder with a frequency of 1 in 60 000 live births. The classic form of galactosemia is a

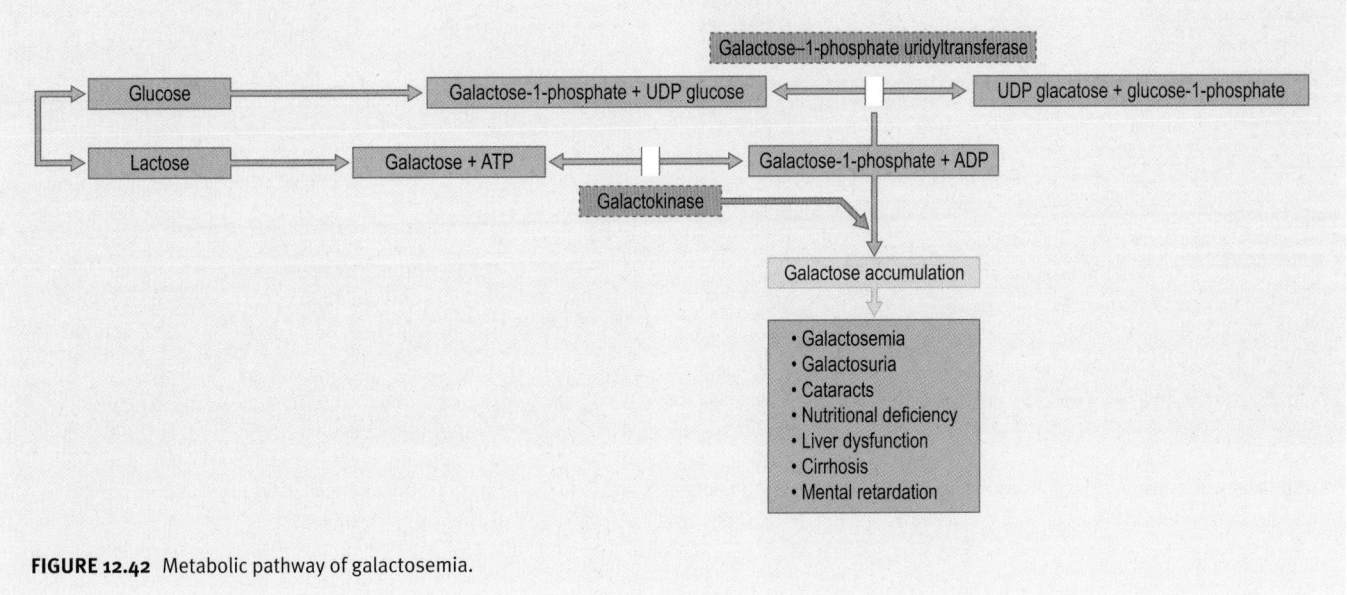

FIGURE 12.42 Metabolic pathway of galactosemia.

deficiency of galactose-1-phosphate uridyltransferase (G1PUT) that results in the accumulation of galactose, galactose-1-phosphate, and galactitol in tissues (Fig. 12.42).[319] Besides red blood cells, the deficiency of the enzyme has been demonstrated in white blood cells, fibroblasts of mucosa, and liver. If the newborn infant diet includes galactose or lactose, vomiting, diarrhea, hyperbilirubinemia, hepatosplenomegaly, renal tubular dysfunction, liver failure, and cataracts develop. **Newborn screening** includes the test for the presence of galactose in the infant's blood. Confirmatory diagnosis is by the **assay of red cell galactose-1-phosphate-uridyltransferase**. The latter is not reliable if the infant has received red blood cell transfusions. Sepsis is common, particularly with *Escherichia coli*. Neutrophil function is depressed by galactose.[320] Hemolysis, coagulopathy, acidosis, aminoaciduria, and proteinuria occur. Only if the infant is receiving galactose will there be galactosuria. Reducing substances in the urine are not reactive to a glucose-specific test. Galactical accumulation accounts for cataract formation, hepatomegaly, ascites and mental retardation.

The pathologic changes are a marked steatosis of the hepatocytes and a progressive **pseudoacinar change of hepatic architecture** (Fig. 12.43) **with ductular proliferation, cholestasis, focal necrosis, and finally cirrhosis.**[321] Pancreatic islet cell hyperplasia and vacuolization of renal tubular epithelial cells occur. The pathologic changes in galactosemia simulate those seen in hereditary fructose intolerance and tyrosinemia (Fig. 12.44). In the brain at autopsy, edema, gliosis, and neuronal necrosis have been attributed to hypoxic–ischemic damage. Pathologic changes in the fetus have been limited to incipient cataracts.

Prenatal diagnosis relies on measuring the enzyme in a cultured chorionic villus sample or amniotic fluid. More than 130 mutations of the *GALT* gene have been found in galactosemia, but 2 account for 70% of mutations in American white people; in African Americans, one mutation accounts for 62% of abnormal alleles.

Restriction of lactose in the diet prevents most of the pathologic changes and the progression of the disease. However, even with good management, children develop difficulty with mathematics, and girls have or develop ovarian failure.

Less common forms of galactosemia with similar clinical and pathological findings are due to galactokinase and galactose epimerase deficiencies. The incidence of heterozygotes for deficiency of galactokinase is 1 in 100; for homozygous births it is 1 in 40 000. The gene is located on chromosome 17q21-q22. In galactose epimerase deficiency the enzyme activity is absent in both erythrocytes and leukocytes but normal in cultured fibroblasts and liver biopsy. The gene has been mapped to chromosome 1p36-p35.

Disorders of fructose metabolism

Hereditary fructose intolerance (**fructose-1-phosphate aldolase deficiency**) and **fructose-1,6-phosphatase deficiency** are autosomal recessive disorders that present in the newborn or in infants when fructose is introduced into the diet.[322] Aldolase B is located on chromosome 9q22.3 has been cloned and sequenced. Ominous signs of severe disease include hemorrhage with coagulopathy, metabolic acidosis, hyperinsulinemia, renal Fanconi syndrome, shock, and seizures. Manifestations that may be fulminant in newborns include vomiting, hepatomegaly and liver failure, hypoglycemia, and lactic acidosis. Steatosis, cholestasis, portal fibrosis, and ductular proliferation progress to cirrhosis and

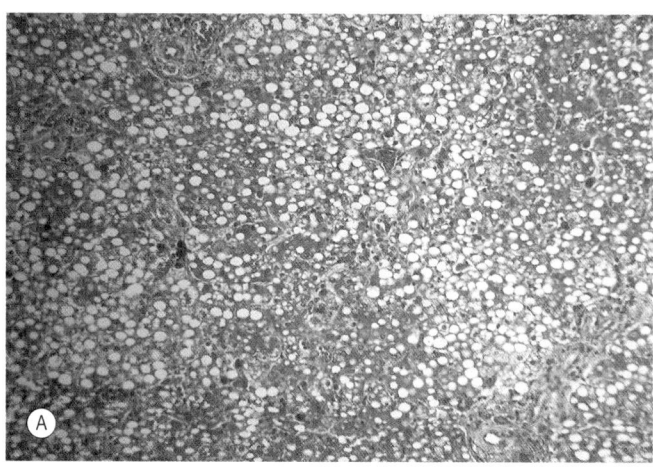
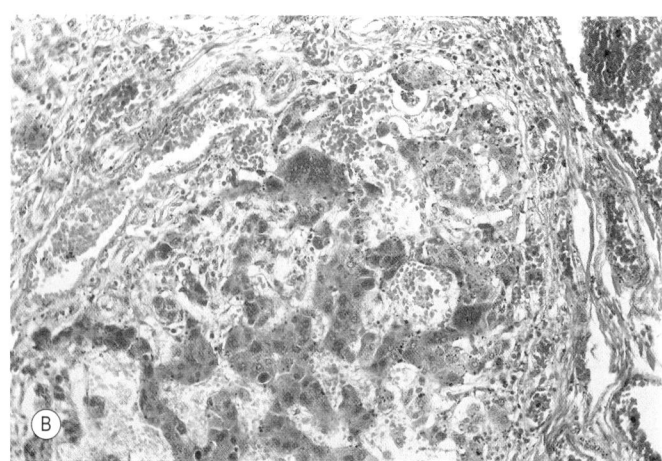

FIGURE 12.43 Galactosemia. (A) Liver with a mild diffuse increase in interlobular connective tissue, a mild diffuse deposit of fat pseudoacinar structures and a circumscribed nodule of liver cells with greatly increased fat. (B) Liver with pseudoacinar structures and periportal fibrosis.

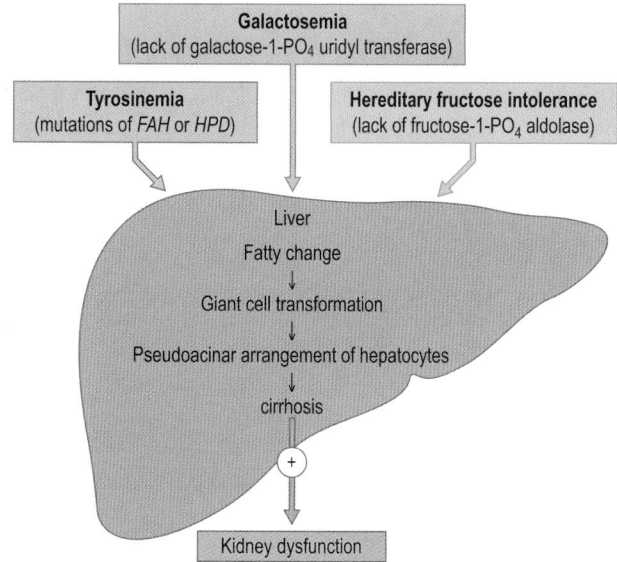

FIGURE 12.44 Similar pathogenic changes in galactosemia, hereditary fructose intolerance, and tryosinemia.

pathologic changes similar to galactosemia and tyrosinemia. Ultrastructural studies reveal hepatocytes and Kupfer cells with polymorphous cytoplasmic inclusions containing electron-dense masses surrounded by an electron-lucent halo ('fructose holes').

Glycogen storage diseases

The many enzymatic steps in the synthesis and breakdown of glycogen (Fig. 12.45) explain the large number of glycogenoses (Table 12.18).[323] The comparative pathology of the glycogen storage diseases (GSDs) has been delineated by McAdams and colleagues.[324]

Type I GSD

Type I glycogen storage disease, the classic **type I glycogenosis (von Gierke disease)** due to **deficiency of glucose-6-phosphatase** (G6P; Fig. 12.46), is characterized by massive hepatomegaly, failure to thrive, severe hypoglycemia, ketosis, increased plasma lactic acid, and marked lipidemia leading to eruptive xanthomas.[325] Administration of epinephrine or glucagon causes a smaller than normal rise in the blood glucose level and a greater elevation in the lactic acid level. Hyperuricemia results from reduced tubular urate secretion and leads to tophi, arthritis, and nephropathy. Microscopic examination shows **massive accumulation of glycogen in hepatocytes and in the renal tubular epithelial cells** (Fig. 12.47).

In the second decade, **hepatic adenomas** may occur. With newer methods of controlling the hypoglycemia, progression to carcinoma and renal insufficiency is rare. Successful liver transplantation has been performed.[326] The Chiquoine stain for G6P is useful.

Several variants of type IA glycogenosis have been described. One, type IB, features a defect in the G6P transport system that shuttles G6P across the microsomal membrane. Another, type IC, stems from defects in translocases. While both variants share clinical features of the classic type IA, those with transporter defects may also manifest neutropenia, recurrent infections, and Crohn disease.

Pathology There is uniform distension of liver cells by glycogen. Normally, glycogen concentration should not exceed 6% of the wet tissue weight in liver and 1.5% in skeletal muscle. Glycogen within the liver cell is uniformly distributed. Lipid vacuoles are frequent and often large. The liver cells are pale

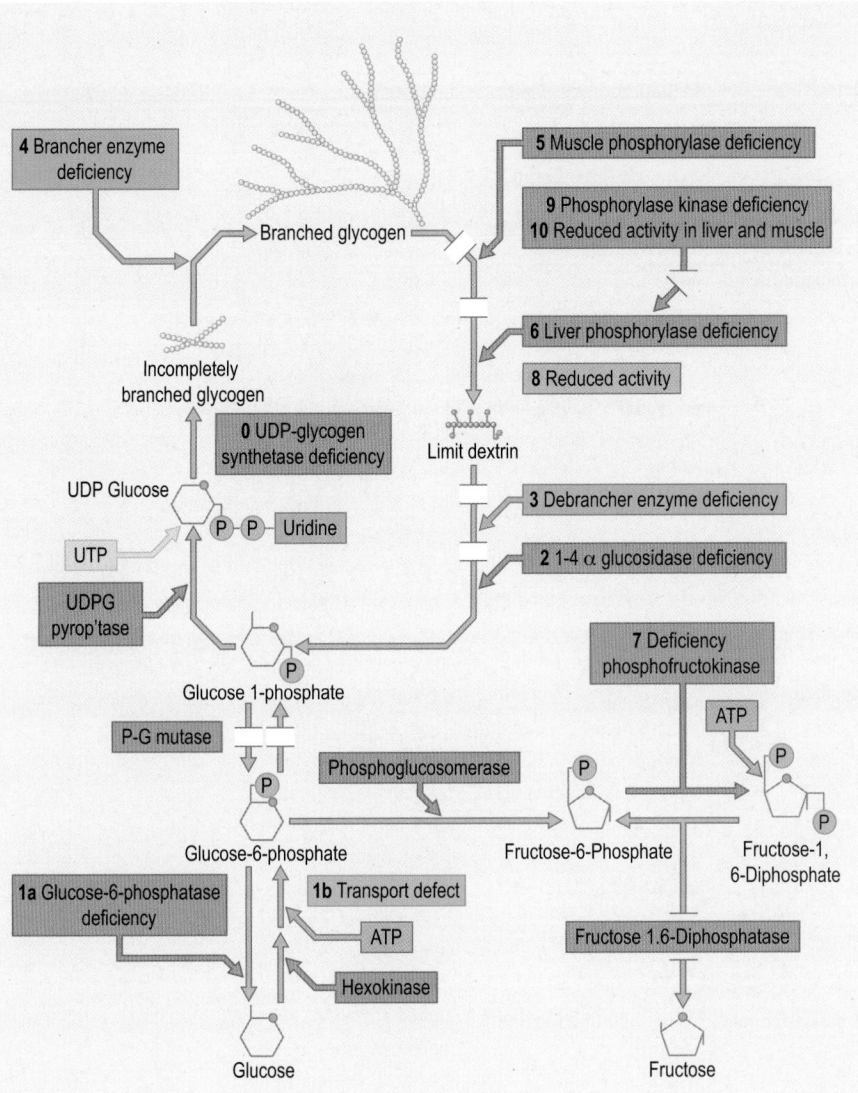

FIGURE 12.45 Metabolic pathway of glycogen storage diseases. Disease types in bold; pyrop'tase: pyrophosphatase.

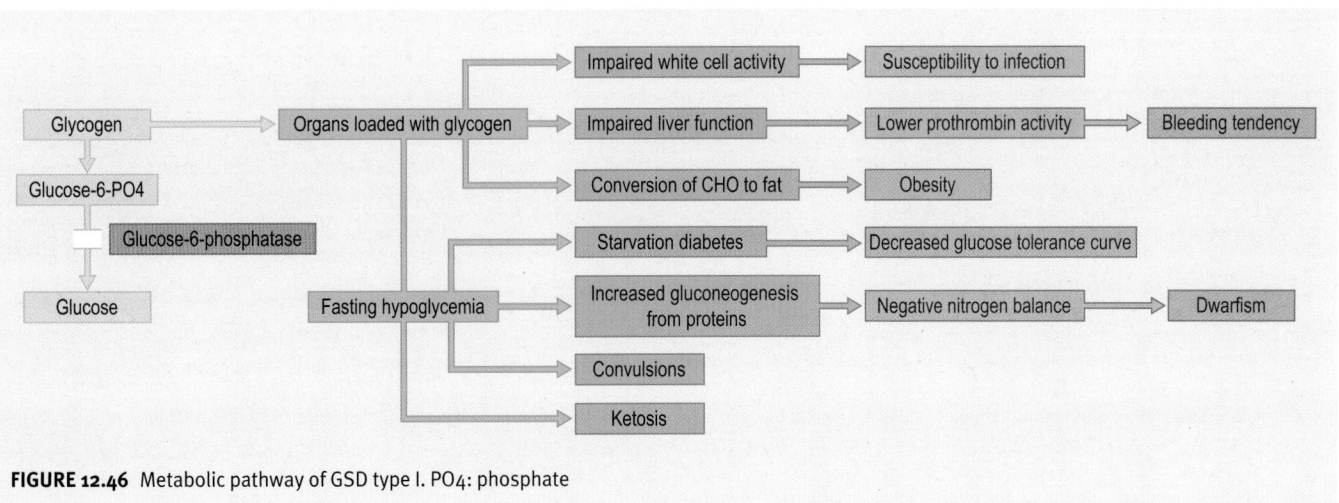

FIGURE 12.46 Metabolic pathway of GSD type I. PO4: phosphate

TABLE 12.18 GLYCOGEN STORAGE DISEASES

McKusick no.	Type	Inheritance	Enzyme defect	Clincopathologic features	Pathology	Tissue for diagnosis
Glycogen storage diseases						
240600	0	AR	Glycogen synthetase	Hypoglycemia, failure to thrive, liver fibrosis	Glycogen is present	Liver, muscle; WBC
23220	IA (von Gierke)	AR	Glucose-6-phosphatase Stabilizing protein for glucose-6-phosphatase	Hepatosplenomegaly, hypoglycemia, hyperlipidemia, acidosis, eruptive xanthomas, hepatic adenomas, hepatocellular carcinoma; no response to glucagon epinephrine, kidney and GI mucosa involved	Uniform distribution of glycogen with distension of liver cells, mosaic pattern, small and large fat vacuoles, nuclear glycogenation; electron microscopy – uniform increase in normal-appearing glycogen, lipid droplets with glycogen particles within them; muscle – normal	Liver
	IS GSD (1aSp)	AR	Stabilizing protein for glucose b-phosphatase	Very early clinical onset		Liver
232220	IB	AR	Glucose-phosphate transporter protein	Like IA plus neutropenia, recurrent infections, Crohn disease	Similar to GSD IA	Liver
232230	II (Pompe)	AR	α-1, 4-glucosidase (acid maltase)	Cardiomegaly, hepatomegaly, hypotonia, hypoglycemia, macroglossia, generalized glycogenosis, CNS involvement, death usually by 1–2 yr	Uniform slight distension of liver cells, microvacuolation due to glycogen accumulation, non-mosaic pattern, fat absent; electron microscopy – glycogen vesicles surrounded by membranes (so-called lysosomes). Muscle – marked glycogen deposition; muscle EM – excessive glycogen (free and in vesicles), loss of myofibrils	Liver, muscle, WBC, amniocytes, fibroblasts
	IIB	XLR	LAMP2 (lysosome-associated membrane protein 2)	Cardiac glycogenosis with survival to second decade	Similar to GSD II	Liver, muscle, WBC, amniocytes,
232230	II (skeletal muscle type)	AR	Acid maltase	Childhood/adult onset, muscle weakness, cerebral aneurysms in adults	Changes in muscle similar to GSD II	Muscle, WBC, amniocytes, fibroblasts
232400	III (GSD) (Forbes/Cori/ limit dextrinosis)	AR	Amylo 1,6-glucosidase (debrancher enzyme)	Liver, skeletal muscle, heart involvement, hypoglycemic response to glucagon	Uniform distension of liver cells due to glycogen, mosaic pattern, nuclear glycogenation, fibrous septa formation, small droplets of fat; electron microscopy – same as type I (lipid vacuoles less frequent), muscle – normal or subsarcolemmal glycogen	Liver and muscle, WBC

TABLE 12.18 GLYCOGEN STORAGE DISEASES (*CONT'D*)

McKusick no.	Type	Inheritance	Enzyme defect	Clincopathologic features	Pathology	Tissue for diagnosis
232500	IV (Anderson – amylopectinosis)	AR	Amylo-1, 4- to 1, 6-transglucosidase (brancher enzyme)	Cirrhosis, jaundice, hepatosplenomegaly, CNS involvement, portal hypertension, sudden death in infancy; adult females with cardiomyopathy are heterozygotes; allelic form with clinical picture like muscular dystrophy in adults	Liver pale; amphophilic hyaline, or vacuolated PAS-positive, diastase-resistant material (amylopectin), particularly in periportal hepatocytes with large lipid vacuoles; prominent septa formation progressing to cirrhosis; EM – fibrillar appearance of amylopectin; muscle – amylopectin deposits	Muscle, WBC, amniocytes, fibroblasts
232600	V (McArdle)	AR	Myophosphorylase (1, 4α-D-glucan-orthophosphatate-α-D-glycosyl transferase) D gluconortho-phosphatase – α-D-glucosyl transferase	Muscle pain, weakness after exercise, myoglobinuria, good prognosis	Muscle subsarcolemmal glycogen; EM – same as light microscopy; liver normal	Muscle enzyme histochemistry
232700	VI (Hers)	AR	Hepatophosphorylase	Hepatomegaly, mild to moderate hypoglycemia, good prognosis	Liver – non-uniform distension of hepatocytes due to glycogen, mosaic pattern, septa formation, small fat droplets; EM – burse appearance of glycogen, rosettes, lipid vacuoles with glycogen; muscle – normal	Liver, WBC, RBC
232800	VII (Tarui)	AR	Muscle phosphofructokinase	Muscle cramps, myoglobinuria, good prognosis	Muscle – subsarcolemmal glycogen, EM – same as light microscopy	Muscle enzyme histochemistry, WBC, fibroblasts
261750	Phosphorylase deficiency of liver and muscle	AR	Hepatic phosphorylase b kinase	Hepatomegaly, growth retardation, lipidemia, progressive neurologic deterioration	Nonuniform distension of hepatocytes due to glycogen, mosaic pattern, electron microscopy – same as type VI, less frequently lipid vacuoles containing glycogen muscle subsarcolemmal glycogen, EM same as light microscopy	Liver, CNS, glycogen in axons and synapses
306000	VIII	XLR	Hepatic phosphorylase kinase, alpha-2 subunit	Marked hepatomegaly, mild hypoglycemia, good prognosis, mild motor development delay	Non-uniform distension of hepatocytes due to glycogen, mosaic pattern, septa formation, small lipid droplets; EM – same as in type VI, frequent lipid vacuoles containing glycogen; muscle – normal	Liver

TABLE 12.18 GLYCOGEN STORAGE DISEASES (*CONT'D*)

McKusick no.	Type	Inheritance	Enzyme defect	Clincopathologic features	Pathology	Tissue for diagnosis
	X	AR	Cyclic 3', 5'-AMP-dependent kinase	Hepatomegaly, liver and muscle involvement, good prognosis	Non-uniform distension of hepatocytes due to glycogen, mosaic pattern, septa formation, small lipid droplets, EM –same as in type VI; muscle – subsarcolemmal glycogen	Liver, muscle
Other forms of glycogen storage diseases						
	Cardiac glycogenosis	AR	Cardiac phosphorylase kinase	Causes early death	Cardiac glycogenosis	Cardiac muscle
	Glycogenosis of liver/ skeletal muscle	AR AR	Phosphorylase kinase Phosphoglucomutase	Hepatomegaly, muscle weakness	Glycogenosis of liver and skeletal muscle	Liver, skeletal muscle
	Glycogen myopathy with hemolytic anemia	AR	Hexokinase	Muscle weakness	Glycogenosis of muscle	Muscle
	Hepatic glycogenosis, hemolytic anemia, mental retardation	AR	Aldolase 1 (aldolase A)	Hepatomegaly, hemolytic anemia	Hepatic glycogenosis	Liver
	Cerebral glycogenosis	AR	Brain glycogen phosphorylase	CNS symptoms	Involvement of cerebral cortex, deep nuclei, cerebellar cortex; glycogen in neurons and astrocytic processes, PAS positive, diastase sensitive	Brain

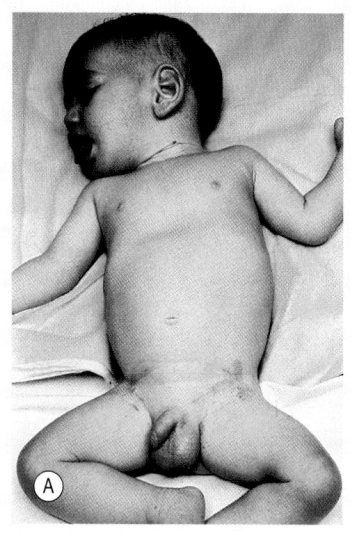

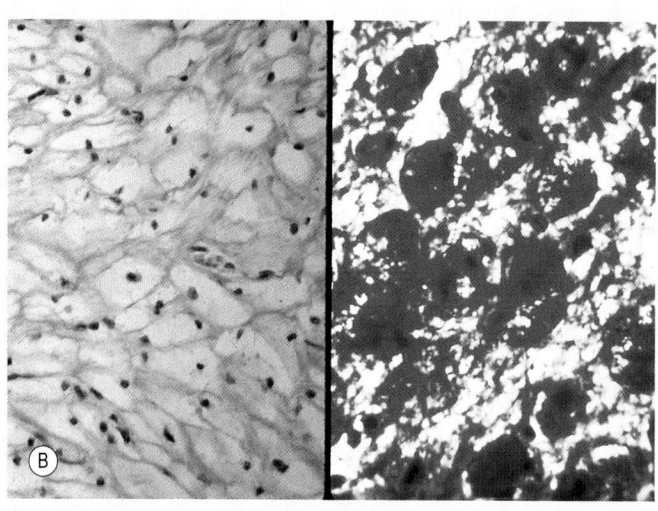

FIGURE 12.47 Glycogen storage disease type II. (A) Infant with extreme hypotonia. (B) Liver. Vacuolated hepatocytes (left), glycogen with PAS stain (right).

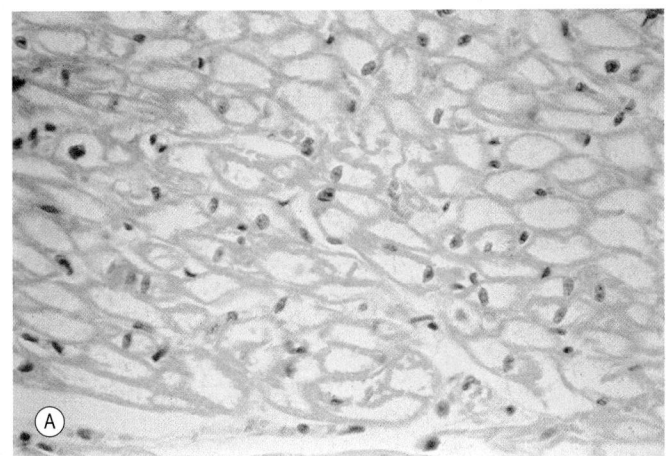
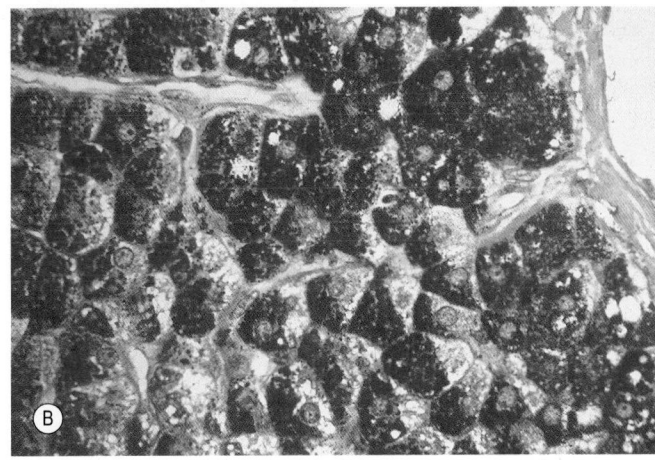

FIGURE 12.48 Glycogen storage disease type II. (A) Vacuolated myocardial cells in heart. (B) Skeletal muscle showing glycogen accumulation in muscle fibers (PAS stain).

staining and have a mosaic appearance that obscures the normal architecture. Nuclear glycogen is commonly seen in hepatocytes of normal children, but in type I glycogenosis (and also in type III), the nuclei are greatly enlarged, a phenomenon referred to as hyperglycogenation. Periodic acid-Schiff stain is strongly positive for glycogen and is digested with diastase. Glycogen is increased in kidney and intestine.

The EM appearance is a uniform increase in normal glycogen particles with displacement of intracellular organelles, glycogenated nuclei, and numerous large lipid droplets.

Type II GSD

Type II (Pompe disease) is the only type in which the stored glycogen is within lysosomes. It is due to **deficiency of α-1,4-glucosidase (acid maltase)**; it affects all tissues and is referred to as generalized glycogenosis. Functional disturbances, however, are focused on the **heart and skeletal muscles** (Fig. 12.48) with massive cardiomegaly, hypotonia and muscle wasting. The *CNS* may be severely affected. Death usually results from cardiac failure before 2 years of age. Microscopic examination shows accumulation of glycogen in the liver, myocardium, skeletal muscle, smooth muscle of vessels, in the neurons of the CNS and anterior horn cells of the spinal cord, and in the stromal cells of the chorionic villi of the placenta.[327] It is important to fix the tissues in alcohol to preserve glycogen that is demonstrated by PAS stains and digested by diastase. With formalin fixation, the hepatocytes appear empty and vacuolated and have a plant-like pattern. EM shows the glycogen in packets within the lysosomes (Fig. 12.49).

In addition to the infantile form, there is a childhood/adult variant in which skeletal muscle is preferentially involved; biopsy reveals excessive muscle lysosomal glycogen and acid maltase deficiency. Since the heart is unaffected, these patients have variable degrees of solely skeletal muscle weakness. Definitive diagnosis rests on finding deficient activity of lysosomal acid α-glucosidase.

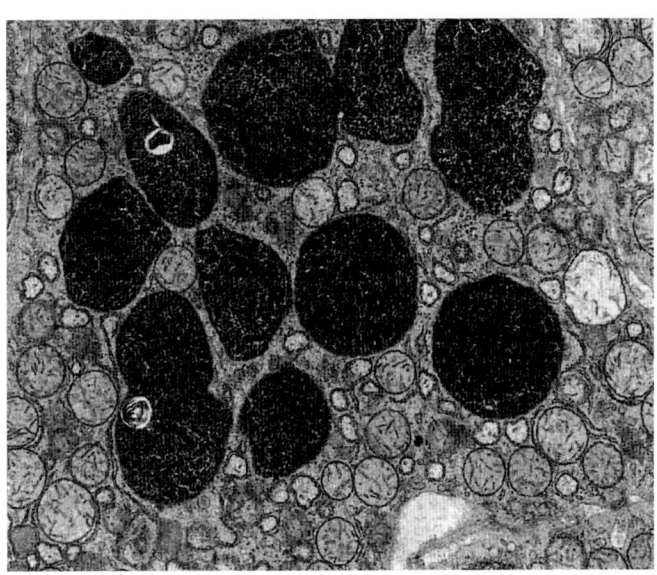

FIGURE 12.49 GSD type II. EM shows dense lysosomes filled with glycogen.

Type III GSD

Type III GSD (Forbes disease, Cori disease, debrancher enzyme amylo-1,6-glucosidase deficiency) is characterized clinically by massive hepatomegaly[328] with both liver and skeletal muscle involvement; in rare instances, only the heart is involved. Six subtypes have been described. At affected sites, the glycogen molecule contains an excessive number of branching points. The clinical features are mild, and most patients survive into adulthood; in a few, hepatic fibrosis and even cirrhosis may develop. Hepatocellular carcinoma has been associated with end-stage cirrhosis.[329] Hypoglycemia and responses to epinephrine and glucagon are variable. With the intravenous glucagon test in the immediate postprandial period there is usually a rise in blood glucose in type III but not in type I GSD.

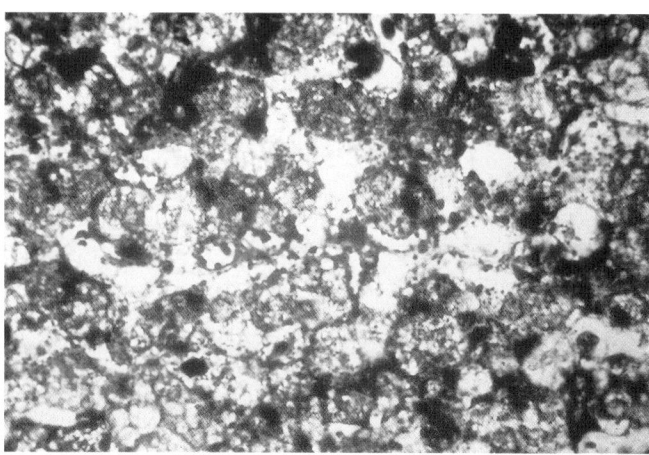

FIGURE 12.50 Glycogen storage disease type IV. Dense masses of diastase-resistant material in cells (PAS-D stain).

Pathology The liver is similar in appearance to that seen in type I glycogenosis with uniform distension of hepatocytes producing a mosaic architecture and periportal nuclear hyperglycogenation. The distinctions from type I glycogenosis are the formation of fibrous septa and the paucity of fat.

Type IV GSD

Type IV GSD (**Andersen disease, brancher enzyme deficiency, amylo-1,4- to 1,6-transglucosidase disease**) produces storage of a starch-like linear glucose polymer with distinctive histologic and histochemical features: strong PAS stain resistant to diastase, positive Langhans iodine stain giving a bluish color to the deposits, and positive colloidal iron stain (Fig. 12.50).[330,331] It is characterized by progressive cirrhosis, hepatosplenomegaly, and ascites. Death is caused by hepatic failure and usually occurs before 2 years of age. Liver transplantation has been successful in some cases.

Type V GSD

Type V GSD due to **muscle phosphorylase deficiency** is characterized by painful cramps on strenuous exercise. The symptoms do not usually appear until about 20 years of age.[332]

Pathology In alcohol-fixed biopsies of skeletal muscle, PAS preparations show glycogen accumulation, which is maximal in subsarcolemmal locations seen in a pattern in both LM and EM similar to the muscle of patients with type III glycogenosis. The abnormality in type V glycogenosis is limited to skeletal muscle.

The diagnosis is established histochemically by demonstrating the absence of phosphorylase activity in cryostat sections using the Takeuchi reaction or one of its modifications. The biochemical diagnosis is made by demonstrating the absence of muscle phosphorylase activity. DNA-based molecular diagnosis is possible.

Type VI GSD

Type VI GSD (**Hers disease with hepatophosphorylase deficiency**) is considered by some to be the most common of the hepatic glycogenoses in Europe. A histochemical procedure for this enzyme is available. Patients have increased liver glycogen and do not clearly fit into any of the other defined types. The clinical syndrome is that of mild hypoglycemia, hepatomegaly, and growth retardation. The prognosis is good.

Pathology Histologically, the parenchyma shows a mosaic of glycogen-distended liver cells. Cell membranes are coarse and may have an undulated appearance. Scattered cytoplasmic vacuoles are present. There is slight septa formation in portal areas, as seen in type III glycogenosis, but nuclear hyperglycogenosis, prominent in type V, is absent in type VI glycogenosis.

Type VII GSD

Type VII GSD (**Tarui disease**) is clinically identical to type V in that exercise causes cramping pain in peripheral skeletal muscles, accompanied by myoglobinuria. It is due to deficiency of phosphofructokinase. Some patients experience hemolysis, a fact explained by the presence of a closely related mutated enzyme in erythrocytes. A histochemical method using fructose-6-phosphate as a substrate demonstrates deficiency of phosphofructokinase.[333]

Type VIII GSD

Hepatomegaly from very early childhood with progressive degeneration of the CNS characterizes type VIII glycogenosis. Initial truncal ataxia, nystagmus, hypotonia, and catecholaminuria are typically followed by spasticity and progress to decerebration. The disease is fatal in childhood. There is no hypoglycemia, and the blood glucose response to epinephrine or glucagon is normal.[334]

Pathology Irregularity in the size of the glycogen-distended cells is particularly prominent. Zones of spectacularly large liver cells produce localized mosaics (Fig. 12.51), which have a tendency to be at the lobular periphery. There is no fibrosis or nuclear hyperglycogenation.

By EM, there are excessive stores of cytoplasmac glycogen and a frayed appearance of particles. Lipid bodies are inconspicuous (Fig. 12.52). In the CNS, there is excessive accumulation of glycogen of the α form, often giant-sized, in axon cylinders and synaptic vesicles.

GSD VIII is the only X-linked glycogenosis. The defect, a deficiency of hepatic phosphorylase kinase, results in one of the mildest of the glycogenoses. In addition to hepatomegaly and growth retardation, there is mild elevation of serum cholesterol and triglycerides. By adulthood, these biochemical abnorma-

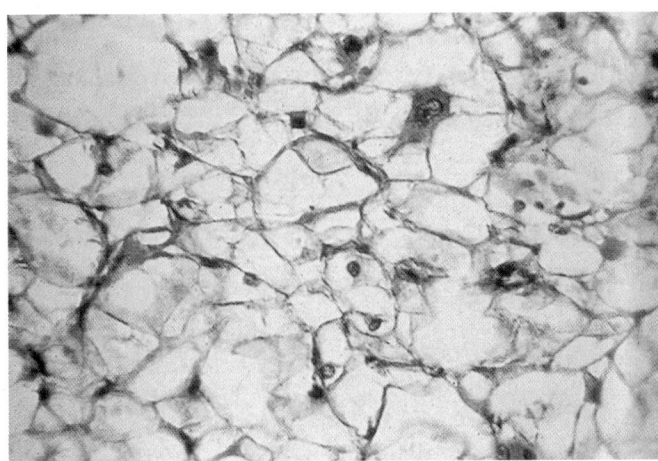

FIGURE 12.51 Liver in type VIII glycogenosis; high-power view. The non-uniform glycogen distention of hepatocytes with cell membranes that are exceptionally coarse. Nuclear glycogenation is not a feature and fibrous sepation is not present.

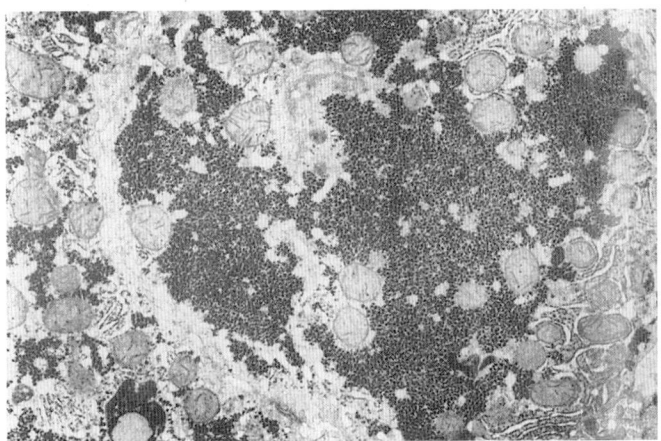

FIGURE 12.52 Electron micrograph of liver in type VIII GSD. This hepatocyte contains excessive glycogen having a frayed appearance but otherwise it is normal. Lipid bodies are absent. Note the glycogen-free zone beneath the cell membrane, a feature that may contribute to the coarse appearance of cell membranes in paraffin sections.

lities disappear. A rare variant is also described with a cerebral palsy-like phenotype.

Type IX glycogenosis (liver phsophorylase kinase deficiency)

Type IX glycogenosis is now known to be part of the GSD VIII spectrum. It is no longer a separate entity.

Type X glycogenosis

Asymptomatic hepatomegaly with no hypoglycemia and no blood glucose rise following glucogen administration characterizes this type of glycogenosis.

Pathology Irregularity in the size of glycogen-distended hepatocytes is the most prominent alteration, with the largest cells appearing adjacent to portal areas similar to types VI, VIII, and IX.

Definitive diagnosis is by the demonstration in liver and muscle of normal total activity of phosphorylase in the inactive form.

Type O GSD

A rare condition, features fasting hypoglycemia and hyperketonemia because of a deficiency of hepatic glycogen synthase. The liver shows a sharp reduction of glycogen stores.

Hypoglycemia does not respond to glucogon. Glycogen content and enzymes are low in liver and normal in muscle. Forms of glycogen storage diseases are summarized in Table 12.18.[337]

Other polysaccharide storage diseases

This group of disorders is characterized by the presence of cytoplasmic bodies called **Lafora bodies**, considered to be composed of polyglycosans. Three types of Lafora body disease are described.[338] All are neurologic diseases: one causes myoclonic epilepsy, one causes a motor neuron defect progressing to tetraparesis as well as peripheral neuropathy, and the third is characterized by bulbar signs. At least three genes underlie Lafora disease, of which two have been isolated and mutations characterised: *EPM2A* and *NHLRC1*. The *EPM2A* gene product laforin is a protein phsophatase while the *NHLRC1* gene product MALIN is an E3 ubiquitin ligase that ubiquitinates and promotes the degradation of laforin. Analyses of the structure and function of these gene products suggest defects in post-translational modification of proteins as the common mechanism that leads to the formation of Lafora inclusion bodies, neurodegeneration and the epileptic phenotype of Lafora disease.[338a] Skin biopsy contains inclusion bodies in acini sweat glands and duct cells. Distinct intraneuronal inclusions (Lafora bodies) are found in the substantia nigra, globus pallidus, dentate nuclei, parts of the reticular system and cerebral cortex as well as the liver, myocardium, skeletal, and smooth muscle that stain with PAS, carmine red, Lugol's iodine, methenamine, and silver nitrate.

Amino acid disorders

Morphologic signs in infants and children with amino acid disorders are rarely apparent.

Phenylketonuria

Inherited as an autosomal recessive trait, phenylketonuria (PKU) has an incidence of 1 in 10 000 live births.[339] The classic

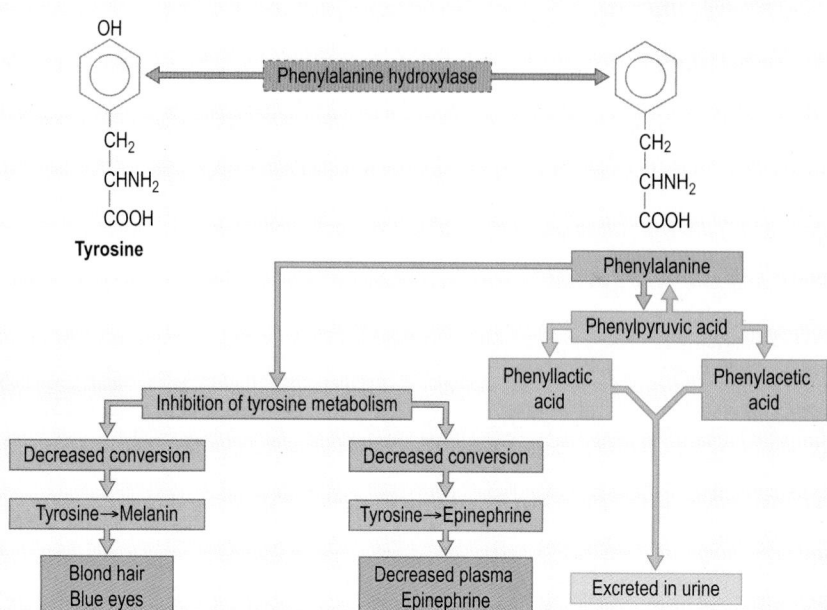

FIGURE 12.53 Metabolic pathway of phenylketonuria (PKU).

form is due to deficiency of **phenylalanine hydroxylase (type 1)** (Fig. 12.53). The chromosomal region involved is 12q22q24.1. Variants include a deficiency of phenylalanine hydroxylase cofactor, **tetrahydrobiopterin (type 2) and dihydropteridine reductase (type 3)**. In the classic form, untreated infants become mentally retarded and develop seizures, a mousy odor to the urine, eczema, and impaired hair pigmentation.

Pathologically, both gray and white matter changes are noted,[340] including lobar disproportion and gyral abnormalities; demyelination and gliosis occur in the white matter (Fig. 12.54) with lipid-laden macrophages. Ulegyria, presumably secondary to ischemia, may occur. Extensive neuronal loss occurs with a reduction in the number of dendritic processes on the Purkinje cells. Vacuolation involves the central white matter of the cerebrum and cerebellum, optic tracts, and fornix. The Guthrie test, based on the requirement of phenylalanine for the growth of *Bacillus subtilis*, is a screening test in the newborn infant. Ferric chloride added to the urine in the presence of phenylalanine metabolites results in a dark green color. Plasma levels of phenylalanine are increased. A biopterin defect is diagnosed by determination of the amount of biopterins present in urine and a blood sample for the assay of dihydropteridine reductase.

Girls treated for PKU who reach reproductive age may give birth to infants with severe abnormalities, including microcephaly, low birth weight, mental and growth retardation, and congenital cardiac defects. Phenylalanine is concentrated by the placenta and may inhibit protein synthesis in fetal liver, brain, and heart.[341]

Prenatal diagnosis is feasible by various combinations of DNA analysis, enzyme assay and measurement of metabolites in amniotic fluid in all forms of hyperphenylalaninemia.

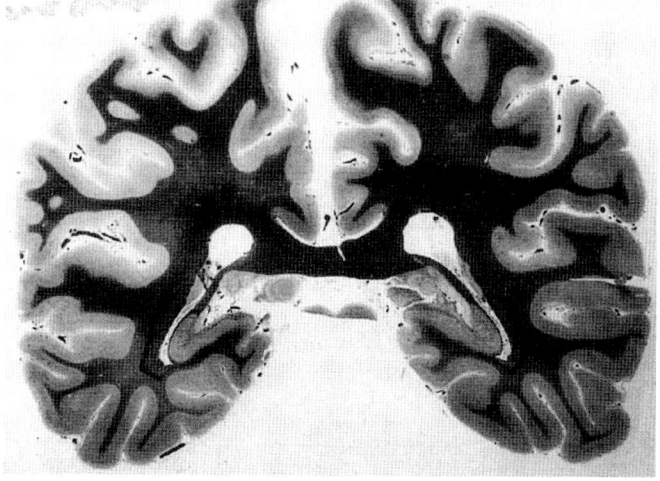

FIGURE 12.54 PKU. Myelin stain of an adolescent brain with focal areas of palor (demyelination).

Hereditary tyrosinemia

Type I hereditary tyrosinemia

Type I hereditary tyrosinemia has an incidence of 1 per 100 000 to 200 000, except in Quebec where the incidence is 8 per 100 000 live births. It is an autosomal recessive disorder due to deficiency of fumarylacetoacetate hydrolase,[342] leading to accumulation of maleylacetoacetate and fumarylacetoacetate, intermediates in tyrosine catabolism. These intermediates are natural alkylating agents with characteristics to make them

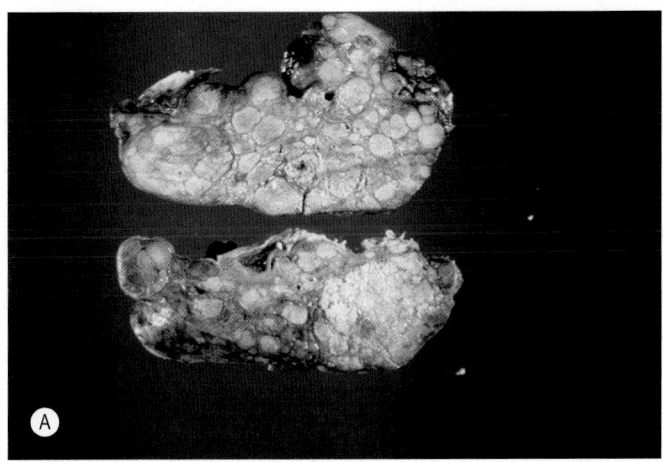
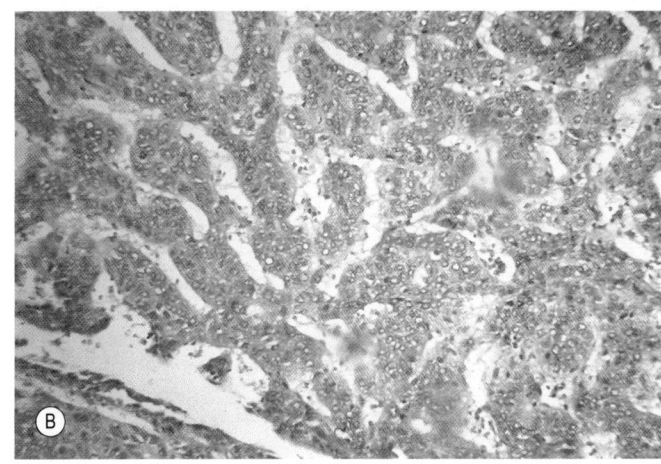

FIGURE 12.55 Tyrosinemia. (A) Micronodular cirrhosis (above). Nodules of hepatocellular carcinoma (below) B: Microscopic appearance of liver showing trabecular pattern of hepatocellular carcinoma.

candidates for carcinogenesis. They are also presumed to directly cause other cellular damage. They cannot be measured directly, but their levels are reflected in the accretion of succinylacetone. In the acute form of tyrosinemia, infants present within the first weeks of life with failure to thrive, vomiting, fever, diarrhea, hepatomegaly, and decreasing liver function. A **fishy odor** may be detected. Patients with the chronic form of tyrosinemia carry the risk of developing **hepatocellular carcinoma**.[343] Infants with this disorder have increased levels of plasma methionine, prolonged prothrombin time, increased α-fetoprotein (AFP), and urinary excretion of succinylacetone and succinylacetoacetate. Elevated levels of methionine and tyrosine in serum, generalized aminoaciduria, and large increases in tyrosine metabolites (4-hydroxyphenyllactic and 4-hydroxyphenylpyruvic acids) in urine may develop in many hepatocellular diseases, such as hereditary tyrosinemia, galactosemia, hereditary fructose intolerance, fructose-1,6-diphosphatase deficiency, glycogenosis type IV (amylopectinosis), and α_1-AT deficiency. **Prenatal detection** is possible by definitive enzyme analysis of cultured amniotic fluid cells or from CVS. The presence of succinylacetone in amniotic fluid and high concentrations of AFP in cord blood of an affected newborn infant suggests that liver changes occured.[344]

The major pathologic changes in tyrosinemia occur in the **liver and kidney**. The liver is typically enlarged, yellow, firm, and nodular (Fig. 12.55A). Microscopic changes (Fig. 12.55B) include formation of areas of fibrosis alternating with nodules of regeneration or preserved parenchyma that shows striking **fatty metamorphosis, cholestasis**, and **pseudogland transformation**. Iron pigment may accumulate in Kupffer cells and hepatocytes with giant cell transformation. These changes are similar to those in galactosemia and hereditary fructose intolerance. **Hepatocellular carcinoma** (Fig. 12.55B) is common in patients with tyrosinemia who survive beyond age 2 years. Regenerative nodules that are frequently dysplastic occur, from which hepatocellular carcinoma may arise. A diffuse fibrosis or cirrhosis

may develop.[345] The kidneys may be enlarged with cortical tubular ectasia and focal tubular calcification with generalized aminoaciduria and glycosuria. Islet cell hyperplasia of the pancreas, hypophosphatemic rickets, and mineralization of blood vessels may occur. Hepatic encephalopathy, meningitis, or liver failure is the usual fatal outcome. In the kidneys, irregular dilatation of the proximal tubular epithelial cells and glycogen accumulation in the collecting tubules are present. **Chromosomal instability**, with increased chromosome breakage in hereditary tyrosinemia type I, was demonstrated in cultured skin fibroblasts.[346] This suggests that the development of **hepatoma** is related to genetic instability caused by accumulation of intermediates of tyrosine catabolism. Liver or liver/kidney transplantation is possible.[347]

Laboratory Findings Demonstration of the presence of succinylacetone on dried filter paper of samples of plasma or urine is pathognomonic.[348] AFP can be assayed in lymphocytes[349] and erythrocytes[350] as well as on liver tissue.

High concentrations of α-fetoprotein in umbilical cord blood of affected neonates suggests that liver disease may be present in late gestation.

AFP activity is also measurable to some extent in kidney, lymphocytes, erythrocytes, fibroblasts, and chorionic tissue.[349] The final diagnosis is made by enzyme determinations in liver, lymphocytes, or cultured skin fibroblasts.[352]

Genetics Heterozygotes for hereditary tyrosinemia are asymptomatic and have normal levels of tyrosine-related metabolites.

Neonatal screening for tyrosinemia can be performed using blood samples dried on filter paper. A blood tyrosine level greater than 248 µmol/L (4.5 mg/dL) is detected.

Prenatal Diagnosis Prenatal diagnosis of tyrosinemia is possible by measuring succinylacetone in the amniotic fluid and by FAH assay using cultured amniocytes or chorionic villus

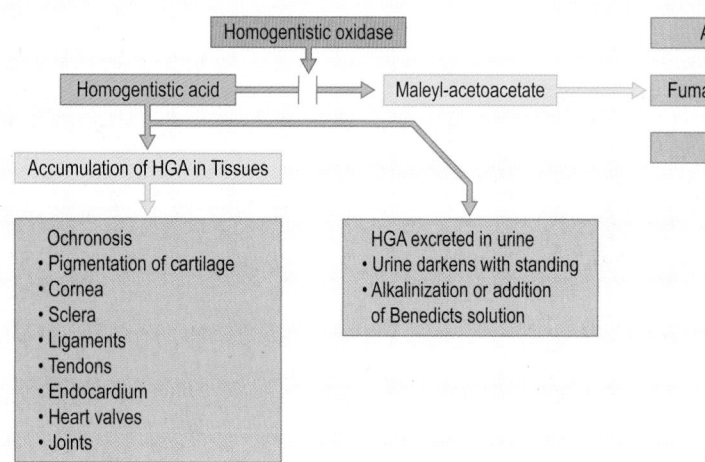

FIGURE 12.56 Metabolic pathway of homocystine in alkaptonuria.

cells.[352] In most cases, both succinylacetone determination and enzyme assay are performed.

Tyrosinemia type II (oculocutaneous tyrosinemia, Richner-Hanhart)

Tyrosinemia type II is also inherited as an autosomal recessive trait due to a **deficiency of hepatic tyrosine aminotransferase**.[342] Children demonstrate mental retardation, corneal ulcers, and palmar and plantar hyperkeratosis. Skin biopsy may show acanthosis or hyper- and parakeratosis. On EM 2–3 µm lipid-like granules with 10 nm filaments intermixed with myelin-like figures may be seen. Mitochondria may appear edematous. Conjunctival biopsy reveals increased keratofibrils and Alcian blue-positive inclusions. Fibroblasts show fine needle crystals. Tyrosinemia and tyrosinuria are present. Treatment consists of a low-phenylalanine, low-tyrosine diet.

Tyrosinemia type III

Only a few patients suffering from tyrosinemia type III have been documented. Episodes of ataxia, severe convulsions, and cerebral atrophy have been reported.

The disease is caused by a deficiency of 4-OH-phenylpyruvate dioxygenase in the liver. Blood tyrosine levels are markedly elevated. In urine, pyruvate and 4-OH-phenylacetate is increased. Treatment consists of tyrosine restriction.

Transient tyrosinemia of the newborn

During the first 2 weeks of life, the tyrosine plasma level may rise to 3000 µmol/L or higher, particularly in low birth weight infants fed a high-protein diet. Symptoms are similar to those of tyrosinemia I. Plasma phenylalanine is also increased, and the infant may be suspected of having PKU. The condition is believed to be due to immaturity of 4-hydroxyphenylpruvate dioxygenase. Infants respond to a low-protein diet (1–1.5 g/kg body weight) and ascorbic acid (200–500 mg/day).

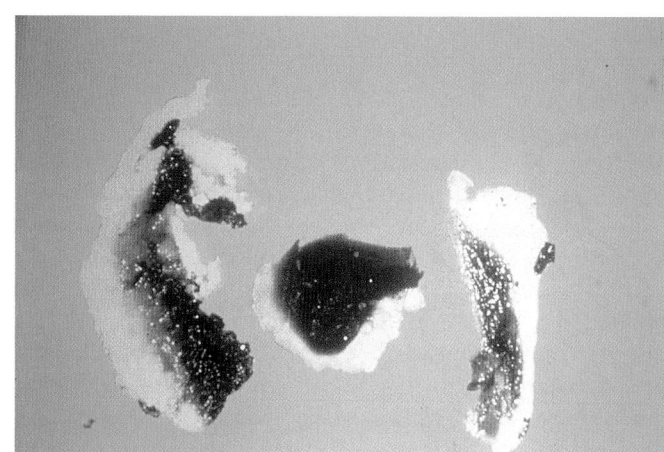

FIGURE 12.57 Pigmented cartilage in alkaptonuria.

Alkaptonuria

Alkaptonuria is inherited as an autosomal recessive trait and is due to the **accumulation of homogentisic acid**, a product in the metabolism of phenylalanine and tyrosine, which in turn is due to a defect or **absence of the enzyme homogentisic acid oxidase** (Fig. 12.56).[353] The connective tissues have generalized pigmentation, usually gray to bluish-black. Usually the deposition of pigment does not occur until the end of the first decade of life. Pigmentation is visible in the **sclera, ear, cartilage**, and **joints** (Fig. 12.57); deposition of homogentisic acid results in arthritis and atherosclerosis of the aorta and coronary vessels, and frequently leads to myocardial infarction.[354] Homogentisic acid itself is not colored, but when exposed to light it is polymerized and results in the formation of a melanin-like pigment. Addition of Benedict solution yields a yellow-orange spot that darkens on exposure to light. Paper chromatography of the urine is a simple technique to identify homogentisic acid in urine, blood, and other tissues.

Non-ketotic hyperglycinemia (NKH)

Non-ketotic hyperglycinemia is an autosomal recessive disorder with an incidence of 1 in 55 000 births and 1 in 12 000 in Finland. Defective glycine cleavage activity in the brain and diminished enzyme activity in the liver cause the accumulation of glycine in blood, cerebrospinal fluid (CSF), and brain.[355,356] Diagnosis is made by the determination of plasma glycine, which may be only slightly elevated, and elevated CSF glycine. Infants with this disorder develop severe mental retardation, seizures, hypotonia, myoclonic jerks, apnea, coma, and death usually in the first 6 months of life. Some forms of the disease have a later onset with varying degrees of retardation. CNS pathologic changes include **hypomyelination and spongiosis**. The liver may appear normal or show **non-specific steatosis**.

Mutations in several genes in the mitochondrial glycine cleavage system (GCS) have been found to cause NKH. These include the genes encoding P protein (GLDC), T protein (GCST), and, in one case, the H protein (GCSH). Most patients with NKH have a defect in the GLDC gene.

Diagnosis

Diagnosis is made by calculating the CSF–plasma glycine concentration ratio. A value of 0.08 or more is diagnostic. Plasma glycine may be only slightly elevated. Confirming the diagnosis necessitates measuring the activity of the GCS in liver tissue.

Prenatal

Prenatal diagnosis is possible by measuring glycine cleavage activity using chorionic villus samples. DNA-based diagnosis is possible.

Pathology

Infants with NKH have spongiform degeneration of the white matter and dysgenesis of the corpus callosum ranging from excessive thinness (1 mm, rather than the usual 5–9 mm) to complete agenesis.[357]

EM of areas of spongy myelinopathy reveal vacuoles formed by splitting of the myelin lamellae. The liver may appear normal or show non-specific steatosis.

Diseases of sulfur-containing amino acids

These include cystinosis (a lysosomal storage disease), cystinuria, homocystinuria, and sulfite oxidase deficiency.

Cystinosis

There are three forms of cystinosis, which share a **defect in carrier-mediated transport of cystine**.[202] Children with the nephropathic form of cystinosis are usually normal at birth and develop renal tubular damage similar to Fanconi urinary syndrome within the first year. Polyuria, growth failure, rickets, photophobia, and decreased pigmentation occur. Renal failure is a common cause of death.

In North America, the incidence of infantile nephropathic cystinosis is approximately 1 per 100 000 to 1 per 1 000 000 births, with a carrier frequency of roughly 1 in 200 in the general population.

Cystinosis is the most identifiable cause of renal tubular Fanconi syndrome in children.

The Fanconi urinary syndrome results in polyuria and excessive urinary losses of glucose, amino acids, phosphate, calcium, magnesium, sodium, potassium, bicarbonate, carnitine, water, and other small molecules. Although blood glucose levels are normal, glucosuria and polyuria can lead to the mistaken diagnosis of juvenile-onset diabetes mellitus. Acidosis can be profound. Hyponatremia and hypokalemia, with risk of arrhythmias, also occur. Hypocalcemia, and occasionally hypomagnesemia, can result in tetany. Phosphaturia leads to hypophosphatemic rickets with typical metaphyseal widening, rachitic rosary, frontal bossing, genu valgum, and failure to walk.

The pancreas may be affected by longstanding cystine accumulation, and insulin-dependent diabetes mellitus has developed in patients after the age of 10.[358]

Patients with the juvenile form develop similar signs and symptoms later in life. Benign cystinosis has minimal cystine accumulation and carries a normal life expectancy.

Untreated patients with nephropathic cystinosis usually die at about 10–12 years of age. Cystine accumulates and forms crystals within the lysosomes of most organs, but particularly in tissues of the reticuloendothelial system (RES) and kidneys (Fig. 12.58).[203] Cystinosis is diagnosed by elevated cystine content of leukocytes or cultured fibroblasts. **Cystine crystals** are most readily seen in the **cornea and bone marrow** (Fig. 12.59). The retina may demonstrate retinopathy with depigmentation; hypothyroidism occurs in some. Cysteamine administration helps decrease cystine. Renal transplantation is effective in treating the renal disease. Prenatal diagnosis can be performed on either cultured amniocytes following amniocentesis at 14–18 weeks of gestation[360] or on chorionic villus samples obtained at 6–8 weeks of gestation.[361,362]

Diagnosis can be made at birth by measuring the cystine content of cord blood leukocytes or of the placenta.[363]

Dello Strologo et al proposed a classification system based on the molecular genetics of the disorder: type A, due to mutation in the SLC3A1 gene; type B, due to mutation in the SLC7A9 gene; and type AB, due to a mutation in both the SLC3A1 and SLC7A9 genes.[364]

Cystinuria

Cystinuria is an **inborn error of transport of the amino acids cystine, ornithine, lysine, and arginine**.[366] Excess urinary excretion of these products results in the formation of **cystine calculi**. No other pathology has been detected. Untreated patients may

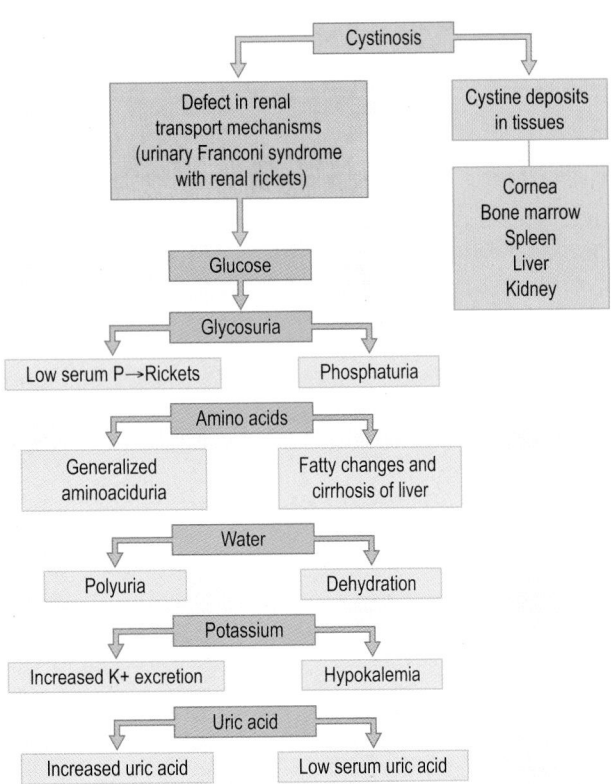

FIGURE 12.58 Pathogenesis of cystinosis.

develop renal failure. The expression of rBAT protein in the proximal renal tubules has been identified. This is the first gene determined to be involved in an inherited amino acid transport disorder.[366] Treatment is symptomatic and includes ingestion of large quantities of water.

Homocystinuria

Three distinct pathophysiologic mechanisms may underlie homocystinuria (HCU), an autosomal recessive disorder. Classic homocystinuria (type I) is due to a deficiency of **cystathionine β-synthetase**. Homocystinuria is also due to defects in **methylcobalamin (type II)** reactions and may respond to vitamin B_{12} administration, or may be due to deficiency of **methylene tetrahydrofolate reductase (type III)**.[367] In each type, homocysteine and other metabolites of methionine accumulate in the body (Fig. 12.60 and 12.61). Patients are usually tall and marfanoid and develop anterior dislocation of the optic lenses, arachnodactyly, osteoporosis, mental retardation, and **thromboemboli** in small and large vessels. Inheritance is autosomal recessive. Treatment includes dietary restriction of sulfur-containing amino acids, supplemental vitamin B_6, folate, and betaine. Pathologically, infarcts are found in the brain and elsewhere. Changes in the eyes and skeleton correspond to the clinical findings.[206] Arterial walls demonstrate marked fibrous thickening of the intima, splitting of the muscle fibers of the media, and elastic fragmentation, resulting in a basket-weave pattern (see Fig. 12.60).[354] The vascular changes may progress to advanced arteriosclerosis. The mutated gene is cystathionine beta-synthase, located on 21q22.3.

Diagnosis Methionine and homocystine are both elevated in body fluids. Cystine is low or absent in plasma. Increased urinary homocystine excretion can be measured by the cyanide–nitroprusside test, paper chromatography, and column chromatography.[368] Cystathionine synthase can be assayed in cultured fibroblasts, lymphocytes, or liver biopsy tissue. Prenatal diagnosis can be determined by enzyme measurement in amniotic cells or chorionic villi.

Pathology The coronary arteries show intimal fibrosis and narrowing of the lumen and frequent thrombosis. Pulmonary vessels show similar changes.

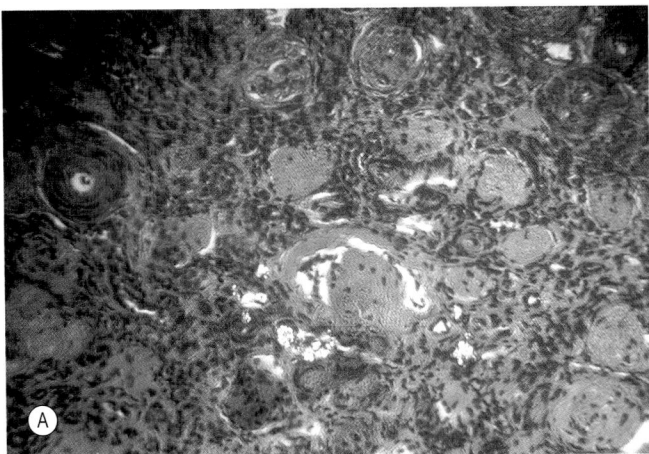
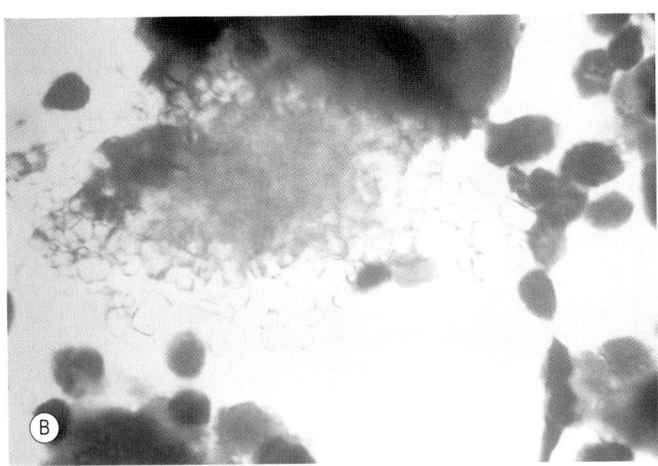

FIGURE 12.59 Cystinosis. (A) Kidney showing glomerular sclerosis, hyalinization and fibrosis. (B) Cystine crystals in bone marrow.

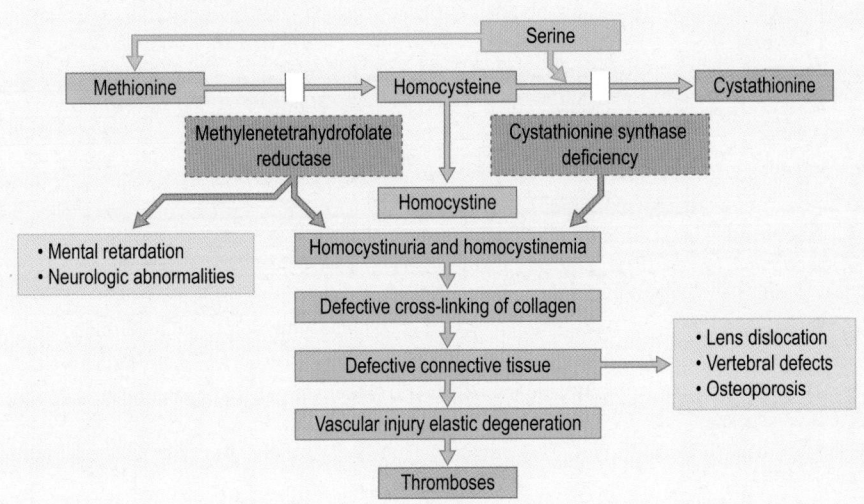

FIGURE 12.60 Homocystinuria. Clinical effects.

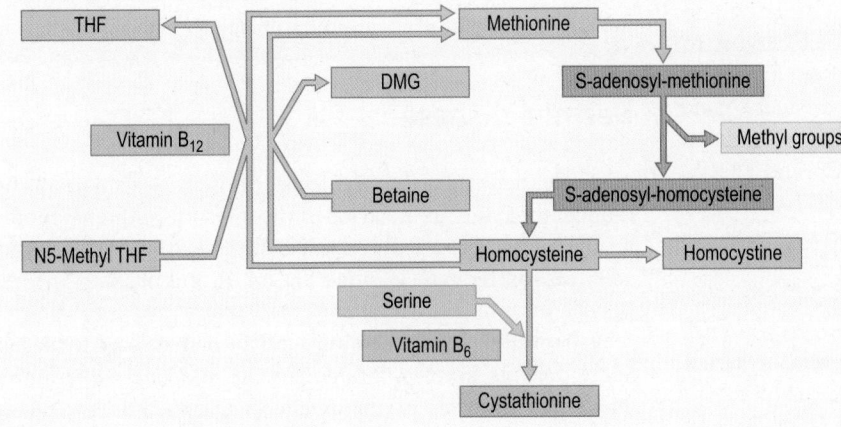

FIGURE 12.61 Homocystinuria. Metabolic pathway.

Fatty change of the liver may be seen. Gluten enteropathy has been reported in a few cases.

Mild fibrosis of the left atrial endocardium, dilatation of the ascending aorta and pulmonary artery, and aortic insufficiency are less frequent in HCU than in Marfan syndrome. Thinness of the aortic media with abnormal elastic tissue has a 'basket-weave' pattern.

Homocystinemia due to Methylenetetrahydrofolate Reductase Deficiency This enzyme reduces 5, 10-methylenetetrahydrofolate to 5-methyltetrahydrofolate, which provides the methyl group for the remethylation of homocysteine to methionine. The gene for this enzyme is located on 1p36.3.[369]

The neonate may present with apneic episodes, myoclonic seizures, coma, and death. Older children may present with developmental retardation, seizures, microcephaly, and spasticity. Vascular thromboses and peripheral neuropathy occur. Demyelination is prominent.[370,371]

Homocystinemia and HCU are moderate, and plasma methionine is decreased. Diagnosis is confirmed by enzyme assay in fibroblasts and leukocytes.

Treatment consists of administration of folic acid, vitamin B_6, vitamin B_{12}, betaine, and methionine. In some patients, intramuscular hydroxocobalamin may be beneficial.

Albinism (see also Ch. 39)

Albinism is due to defects and distribution of melanin. The incidence varies in different populations and is estimated at 1 in 16 000 to 1 in 20 000 in the United States. The gene carrier rate is 1–2%. Melanin is synthesized in melanocytes from tyrosine by tyrosinase, a copper-dependent enzyme, and is responsible for pigmentation of skin, hair, and eyes. Dopa and dihydroxyindole are substrates for tyrosinase. Oculocutaneous albinism (OCA) is the most common form of albinism.[372]

TABLE 12.19 OCULOCUTANEOUS ALBINISM TYPES

Type	Gene locus	Hair color	Retinal pigment	Iris color	Vision
I	TYR 11q14-21	White	None	Blue/gray	Poor
II	TYR 11q14-21	Minimal	Minimal	Blue/tan	Poor
Hermansky-Pudlak[a]	at least 9 different genes	Variant	Decreased	Blue/brown	Poor
Chediak-Higashi[b]	MSH-R	Blonde	Vary	Blue/brown	Vary
Prader-Willi	SNRPN and NECDIN 15q12	Silver		Blue/brown	
Angelman	UBE3A 15q11-q13	Normal-light	Vary	Blue/brown	Normal
Piebald	C-KIT 4q11-q13	Normal	Vary	Blue/gray	Normal
Waardenburg	PAX3 2q35	White	Vary	Normal	Poor

Other albinism genes have been identified in mice.

[a] Generalized albinism with platelet abnormalities and ceroid in tissues.

[b] Partial albinism with granules in leukocytes and susceptibility to infection.

Oculocutaneous (generalized) albinism

Two major forms are identified, type I, tyrosinase-negative and type II, tyrosinase-positive, based on the hair bulb's ability to form melanin when incubated with tyrosine. Both types are inherited as autosomal recessive traits. The tyrosinase gene TYR is mapped to chromosome 11q14-q21; it has two related variants, TYRP1 which maps to chromosome 9p23, and TYRP2 (dopachrome tautomerase) which maps to 13q311-q32.[373–380] Dopa tautomerase converts dopachrome to dihydroxyindole-2-carboxylic acid.

Type I is the most severe form with no visible pigment, caused by the absence of tyrosinase.

Type II is the most common form with several different mutations. In OCA II, the basic metabolic defect in which tyrosinase activity is present (tyrosinase-positive OCA) has not been identified. It is attributed to the lack of a melanosomal polypeptide, the P protein, which is a transmembranal transporter of small molecules such as tyrosine. The P protein is coded by the P gene, which is mapped to chromosome 15q11.2-q12. All present with decreased pigmentation of skin, hair, and eyes; with type II, visible pigment may be variable. Forms of oculocutaneous albinism are presented in Table 12.19. Prenatal diagnosis can be made by histologic or electron microscopic examination of fetal skin biopsies; however, a molecular genetic approach has become possible by the identification of two mutated alleles of the TYR gene coding for tyrosinase; over 60 mutations have been identified.[380]

Treatment is limited to protection of eyes from light exposure.

Ocular albinism

Ocular albinism (OA) is limited to the irises and retina. Photophobia and nystagmus are common. One form of ocular albinism and ocular albinism with deafness are inherited as X-linked traits. The gene causing Nettleship-Falls OA has mapped to Xp22.2-p22.3, and the Forsius-Errikson form to Xp21.1-p21.3. A mild variant is inherited as an autosomal recessive trait, and a form with multiple lentigines and deafness is inherited as an autosomal dominant trait.

Hartnup disease

A single defect in the transport of neutral (mono-amino-monocarboxylic) amino acids in the intestine and renal tubules results in this autosomal recessive inherited disease. The amino acid transporter gene is called *SLC6A19*, and maps to 5p15. Its prevalence is of approximately 1 to 25 000.[381]

Patients develop a pellagra-like rash when exposed to the sun. Some patients develop chronic eczema and rarely intermittent ataxia, but most are asymptomatic.[382] Diarrhea or low protein intake may exacerbate symptoms.[381] Some patients may be mildly mentally retarded. Psychiatric symptoms may occur.[383]

The diagnosis is suggested by finding excretion of neutral amino acids, particularly alanine, glutamine, serine, and histidine but also leucine, isoleucine, phenylanine, tyrosine, and tryptophan.

Glutaric acidemia type I

Glutaric academia type I (GAI) is due to a deficiency of glutaryl-CoA dehydrogenase (GCDH). This deficiency usually presents in infancy and is characterized by acidosis and dystonia. It may simulate Huntington disease in infancy.

The disease usually presents after a period of normal development with the sudden onset of hypotonia, loss of head control, seizures, opisthotonos, grimacing, fisting, tongue thrusting, rigidity and dystonia, with slow and incomplete recovery.[384] Neurologic manifestations may then progress slowly, punctuated by episodes of ketosis, vomiting, hepatomegaly, and encephalopathy brought on by infection, or may remain static, with the condition taking the form of extrapyramidal cerebral palsy.

Macrocephaly at birth is common. Whatever the type of onset, there is relative preservation of intellect. Death can occur during the first decade from intercurrent illnesses or Reye-like episodes.

Laboratory studies

Most routine laboratory studies, including serum electrolyte and pH measurements, are normal except during acute episodes, when acidosis, hypoglycemia, ketonemia and ketonuria, hyperammonemia, and mild parenchymal liver disease may become apparent.[385–387]

Urine organic acids are usually abnormal at diagnosis, showing large quantities of glutaric acid and smaller amounts of 3-hydroxyglutaric acid and occasionally glutaconic acid. Excretion of glutaconic acid may become prominent during episodes of ketosis.[385–387] Glutaric acid concentrations are increased in blood and CSF.

Diagnosis

The diagnosis is made on the basis of increased glutaric and 3-hydroxyglutaric acids in urine, and is confirmed by deficiency of GCDH in cultured fibroblasts. The gene is cloned, and molecular diagnosis is possible.

Genetics

Heterozygous carriers are clinically normal; two carriers did not excrete detectable glutaric acid even after oral loads of L-lysine.[388]

The gene has been mapped to human chromosome 19p13.2.[392]

Prenatal Diagnosis

Prenatal diagnosis is made by increased glutaric acid concentration in amniotic fluid and decreased GCDH activity in cultured amniotic cells[282] or by chorionic villus sampling.[393,394]

Pathology

Striatal degeneration, in particular of the caudate nucleus and putamen, moderate fatty changes in the neurons of the caudate, and increased numbers of astrocytes in the putamen have been observed.[395] Degeneration of globus pallidus and spongy degeneration of cortical white matter is present.

Microvesicular fatty infiltration of liver parenchymal cells, cells of the proximal renal tubules, and myocardium have been observed.[386,396]

Oculocerebrorenal syndrome of Lowe

The oculocerebrorenal syndrome of Lowe (OCRL) is an X-linked disorder characterized by congenital cataract, hypotonia, metabolic acidosis, hyperaminoaciduria, proteinuria, growth

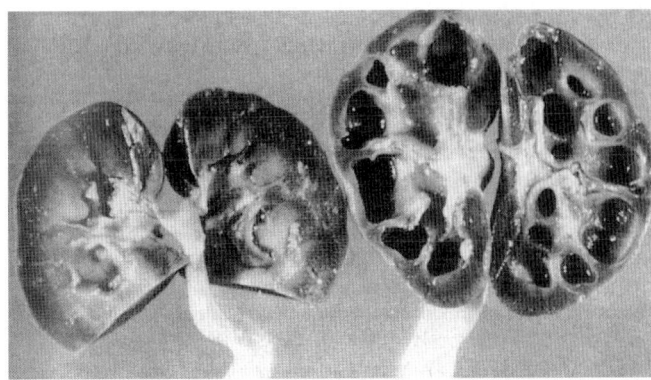

FIGURE 12.62 Lowe syndrome. Kidneys shows bilateral hydroureters and hydronephorosis (left (lower part of kidney was cut). (Courtesy of Dr. Y. Hayashi and Taylor and Francis Publishing.)

retardation, rickets, and mental retardation.[397–402] A chromosome map has assigned OCRL to Xq26.1.

The metabolic disturbances characteristic of Lowe syndrome are not present at birth but the eye changes are already evident.[397,403]

Pathology

In the eye, maldevelopment of the angle (responsible for the glaucoma), the ciliary body, and the peripheral retina may be secondary to a microphakia.[404] The kidneys show hydronephrosis and hydroureters (Fig. 12.62). In the first months of life, the kidney appears normal; later, tubule changes develop without glomerular involvement and then, by mid-childhood, glomerular scarring occurs. Metabolic manifestations of the disease represented by acidosis and aminoaciduria are attributed to the malfunction of renal tubules.[405] Some cases of OCRL show various pathologic findings of the brain – widespread demyelination with spongy degeneration,[406] cerebral edema, and neuronal degeneration of variable severity – whereas some other cases demonstrate no pathologic changes of the brain.[407–409]

Prenatal diagnosis

Prenatal diagnosis for Lowe syndrome[410] has been made by measuring phosphatidylinositol 4,5-biphosphate 5-phosphatase activity in cultured aminocytes. The causative gene is *OCRL1*, and molecular diagnosis is possible.

Sulfite oxidase deficiency

Sulfite oxidase deficiency is due to **deficiency of molybdenum cofactor**[411] and is inherited as an autosomal recessive trait. Patients have severe **neurologic abnormalities**, including mental retardation, and develop dislocated ocular lenses. Sulfite, thiosulfate, sulfocystine, taurine, xanthine, and hypoxanthine are

TABLE 12.20 LEUCINE, ISOLEUCINE, VALINE METABOLITES

MIM#	Disorder	Chromosomal location	Tissue distribution
248600	Maple syrup disease (branched chain α-keto acid dehydrogenase complex deficiency)		WBC, FB
	decarboxylase (E1)		
	E1 α subunit (gene: *BCKDHA*)	19q13.1-q13.2	
	E1 β subunit (gene: *BCKDHB*)	6q14	
	dihydrolipoyl acyltransferase (E2) (gene: *DBT*)	1p31	
	lipoamide dehydrogenase (E3) (gene: *MSUD3*)	7q31	
243500	Isovaleric acidemia (isovaleryl-CoA dehydrogenase deficiency)	15q12-15	WBC, FB
210200	3-methylcrotonyl-CoA carboxylase deficiency		WBC, FB
250950	3-methylglutaconic aciduria type 1 (3-methylglutaconyl-CoA hydratase deficiency)		WBC, FB
250950	(type I) 3-methylglutaconic aciduria,	Chromosome 9 (gene: *AUH*)	WBC, FB, muscle
302060	(type II – Barth syndrome)	Xq28 (gene: *TAFAZZIN*)	
258501	(type III – Costeff syndrome)	19q13.2-q13 (gene: *OPA3*)	
250951	(type IV – unclassified)	Gene unknown	
246450	3-OH-3-methylglutaric aciduria (3-OH-3-methylglutaryl-CoA lyase deficiency)	1p35-36	WBC, PLT, FB
251170	Mevalonic aciduria (mevalonate kinase deficiency)	12q24.1	WBC, FB

Defects not conclusively identified.

WBC, white blood cells; FB, cultured fibroblasts; PLT, platelets.

From Gibson KM, Elpeleg ON, Wappner RS. Disorders of leucine metabolism. In: Blau NM, Blaskovics ME, eds. Physician's guide to the laboratory diagnosis of metabolic diseases. London: Chapman and Hall; 1996.

excreted in the urine. Marked **neuronal loss, demyelination of the white matter, gliosis, and diffuse spongiosis** are manifested as a severe encephalopathy. Prenatal diagnosis is made by a sulfite oxidase assay in a culture of amniotic cells or from CVS. Effective treatment is unknown.

Disorders of branched-chain amino acid metabolism/organic acidemias

The **branched-chain** amino acids **leucine, isoleucine, and valine** are detected in excess in serum and urine in infants and children with certain organic acidemias (Table 12.20).[412]

Organic acidemias and organic acidurias are due to **defects of amino acid or fatty acid metabolism**. If symptoms begin in the neonatal period, the course may be fulminant with severe CNS dysfunction, coma, seizures, and death (Table 12.21). In older infants and children the course may be episodic, with exacerbations following infections that may be reminiscent of Reye syndrome. Acidosis with hyperammonemia and hypoglycemia may be present.

Maple syrup urine disease

Maple syrup urine disease (MSUD) is an autosomal recessive disorder of the mitochondrial multienzyme complex branched-chain α-ketoacid dehydrogenase with an estimated incidence of 1 in 120 000 to 1 in 400 000 live births.[413] A classical form, an intermediate form, an intermittent form, and a thiamin-responsive form have been described. In untreated infants the disease is manifested during the first week of life with vomiting, seizures, and coma. Intermittent and late forms of the disease may be precipitated by a high-protein diet or by infection. The odor of maple syrup is detected in urine, sweat, and saliva, and the diagnosis is made by plasma amino acid analysis and urinary organic acid determinations. Analysis of the branched-chain decarboxylase may be performed on leukocytes, fibroblasts, or amniotic fluid cells. Pathologically, the **liver, kidney, and brain** may be enlarged and the **liver contains increased amounts of glycogen. Renocortical cysts** may be present and the brain shows **hypomyelinization**, particularly in the **pons and medulla**. On frozen sections, crystals within vacuoles may be seen in the liver and other organs.[414] Two women with organic acidemias, one with classic MSUD and another with mild propionic acidemia, on protein-restricted diets and carnitine supplementation, delivered healthy infants without maternal metabolic decompensation.[415]

Pathologically, the liver, kidney, and brain may be enlarged, and the liver contains increased amounts of glycogen. Renal cortical cysts may be present.[416]

Spongy changes in the white matter and delayed myelination occur involving principally the pyramidal tracts of the spinal cord. Loss of myelin around the dentate nucleus,

TABLE 12.21 BRANCH-CHAIN AMINOACIDEMIA

General symptoms common to all disorders
Decreased resistance to infections
Intermittent coma, Reye-like syndrome
Vomiting and failure to thrive
Hypotonia and lethargy
Hypoglycemia
Athetosis or ataxia
Peculiar odor
Myopathy
Neutropenia and thrombocytopenia
Isovaleric acidemia
Propionic acidemia
Methylmalonic acidemia
2-methylacetoacetyl-CoA thiolase deficiency
Hypoglycemia
Maple syrup urine disease
3-hydroxy-3-methylglutaconyl-CoA lyase deficiency
Methylmalonic acidemia
Glutaric acidemia types I and II
Carnitine deficiency
Pyruvate carboxylase deficiency
Pyruvate dehydrogenase deficiency
Myopathy
Glycerol kinase deficiency
Carnitine deficiency
Glutaric acidemia type II

the corpus callosum, and the cerebral hemispheres is present.[417,418]

Prenatal diagnosis relies on measurement of branched-chain amino acids (BCAAs) or keto acids of leucine decarboxylation in cultured amniotic cells.

Isovaleric acidemia

Isovaleric acidemia (IVA) is autosomal recessive and is characterized by intermittent acidosis, vomiting, ketosis, coma, and **sweaty foot odor**.[419] Urinary isovaleryl glycine and hydroxy isovaleric acid are elevated. Enzyme analysis of fibroblasts, leukocytes, or amniocytes reveals deficiency of isovaleryl-CoA dehydrogenase. Hematologic abnormalities include pancytopenia, arrested maturation of hematopoietic precursors, and thrombocytopenia.[420] A chronic intermittent form of IVA is manifested during the first year of life. Pathologic changes are non-specific, although **hepatic steatosis and hemorrhages may occur in the viscera, cerebellum and cerebral ventricles**. Treatment includes a low-protein diet with added glycine and carnitine.

IVA results from mutations of the gene ISOVALERYL COA DEHYDROGENASE, which maps to 15q14-q15.[421]

Pathology

Spongiform changes in the white matter and cerebellar edema with hematuria may occur. The liver frequently shows fatty change.

Diagnosis

Diagnosis of isovaleric acidemia from assay of the metabolites can be confirmed by assay of fibroblasts, leukocytes, or amniocytes for a deficiency of isovaleryl-CoA dehydrogenase by either the tritium release[422] or fluorometric[423,424] assays. Molecular diagnosis is possisble.

Propionic acidemia

This defect is a rare autosomal recessive disorder due to an **enzyme deficiency or cofactor deficiencies of biotin propionyl-CoA carboxylase**.[425] In the newborn, vomiting, respiratory distress, seizures, coma, and death may occur. Less severe forms have a later onset and may be associated with lactic acidosis, ketosis, hyperammonemia, and hypoglycemia. Blood and urine contains excessive glycines and propionate, hence the alternate name **ketotic hyperglycinemia**. Bone marrow depression and pancytopenia occur. Organic acids are present in plasma and urine. Definitive enzyme analysis may be performed on leukocytes, fibroblasts, or amniocytes. Prenatal diagnosis is possible. The **liver shows steatosis**, and ultrastructurally the **mitochondria** may be **enlarged with decreased cristae**, with **amorphic substance within the matrix**.[425]

Genetics

Propionyl-CoA carboxylase is composed of subunits α and β;[426,427] biotin is a coenzyme that binds to subunit α, and the gene is on chromosome 13.[428] The β subunit is on a gene on chromosome 3; genetically distinct deficiencies occur at 4 loci.

Diagnosis

Urinalysis reveals excess propionate, 3-hydroxypropionate, methylcitrate, and triglycine. Serum glycine and carnitine esters are elevated. Propionyl-CoA carboxylase is assayed in leukocytes, fibroblasts, cord blood leucocytes, or amniotic fluid cells.[429]

Pathology

Hepatomegaly and steatosis are reported. Cerebral atrophy is noted after repeated episodes of acidosis.

The mitochondria may be enlarged with decreased cristae and amorphous material within the matrix.

Methylmalonic acidemias

Methylmalonic acidemia (MMA)[430] results from methylmalonyl-CoA mutase deficiency that may be due to many mutations required for the biosynthesis of adenosylcobalamin (AdoCbl). Cobalamin, vitamin B_{12}, is a cofactor for the mutase and for methionine synthase (MeCbl), 5-methyltetrahydrofolate homocysteine methyl transferase.[431]

Deficiency of mutase results in signs and symptoms similar to those of propionic acidemia with infantile or neonatal ketoacidosis, whereas those with methionine synthase deficiency present with no ketoacidosis but with megaloblastosis and homocystinuria. Characteristic features include a high forehead; a broad nasal bridge; epicanthal folds; a long, smooth philtrum; and a triangular mouth. Most deficient patients present with failure to thrive, hypotonia, vomiting, and respiratory distress. Later, developmental retardation, liver failure, hyperammonemia, and coma may occur. A variety of skin lesions may occur, principally mucocutaneous moniliasis with cracking and erythema at the angles of the mouth and eyes. Leukopenia, thrombocytopenia, anemia, and frequent infections occur with periods of acidosis. Some patients are reported with no symptoms. Chronic renal failure is a common long-term complication in non-B_{12}-responsive MMA.

Diagnosis

MMA is elevated in serum and urine. Propionate and hydroxypropionate may also be increased. High protein intake increases their levels. Serum cobalamin is normal or slightly elevated. Prenatal diagnosis has been made by detecting MMA in amniotic fluid and maternal urine at mid-trimester.[432]

Pathology

Diffuse gliosis in the white matter, Alzheimer type II cells, and cerebellar hemorrhage have been observed.

Glutaric acidemia

Type I glutaric acidemia (GA) is due to a **deficiency of glutaryl-CoA dehydrogenase** usually presenting in infancy with acidosis and dystonia. It may simulate Huntington disease in infants. GA type II is due to a defect in the electron transfer from acyl-CoA dehydrogenases to coenzyme Q of the electron transport (ET) chain[433] involved in fatty acid oxidation. **Congenital anomalies** are associated with ET factor dehydrogenase deficiency and include prominent forehead, flat nasal bridge, malformed ears, intrauterine growth retardation, macrocephaly, hypospadias, cryptorchidism, simian creases, and abnormal whorl dermatoglyphic patterns. Kidneys may be enlarged and cystic.[434] Glomerular basement membrane is irregular with areas of thinning or thickening, and the **brain** may have a 'warty' **dysplasia**.[435] **Portobiliary dysplasia and paucity of intrahepatic**

TABLE 12.22 BRANCHED-CHAIN ORGANIC ACIDURIAS

Types	Features
Maple syrup urine disease	Seizures, coma, odor
Propionic acidemia	Vomiting, acidosis, ketosis, coma
Methylmalonic acidemia	Vomiting, acidosis, ketosis
Isovaleric acidemia	Vomiting, acidosis, ketosis
3-Methylcrotonyl-Co-A	Vomiting, acidosis, ketosis, hypoglycemia, coma
3-Methylglutaconic aciduria	Vomiting, hypoglycemia, coma, acidosis
3-Hydroglutaconic aciduria	Vomiting, hypoglycemia, coma, acidosis
Mevalonic aciduria	Ataxia, diarrhea, anemia, hepatosplenomegaly
3-Hydroxyisobutyryl-CoA deacylase deficiency	?
3-hydroxy-3 methylglutaric aciduria	Reye Syndrome
2-methylacyl-CoA thiolase	Vomiting, sweet odor, ketosis
Acetyl-CoA thiolase	Neurologic signs

bile ducts have been noted in a few cases. **Steatosis occurs in liver, myocardium, and renal tubular epithelium; retinal hemorrhages have been described.**[436] It is important to recognize and distinguish this disorder from shaken baby syndrome. GA type II caused by a defect in riboflavin metabolism has been reported in pregnancy.

The defect involves either electron transfer flavin (ETF) or ETF dehydrogenase. The gene for α-ETF is on chromosome 15q23-25 for β-ETF on chromosome 19q13.3,[437] and the gene of ETF:QO is on 4q33.[437] and for ETF on chromosome 4.[437]

Other organic acidurias due to branched-chain disorders are listed in Table 12.22.

Urea cycle defects

The urea cycle consists of five enyzmes responsible for the elimination of ammonia as urea: carbamoyl phosphate synthetase I (CPS I), ornithine transcarbamylase (OTC), argininosuccinate synthetase (AS), argininiosuccinate lyase (argininosuccinase; AL) and arginase (Fig. 12.63). CPS I and OTC are localized in the mitochondrial matrix, whereas the other three enzymes are in the cytosol. The complete urea cycle is found only in the liver where all five enzymes are induced in the perinatal period in a coordinated manner. Induction of the urea cycle enzymes is stimulated by dietary protein and hormones such as glucagons and glucocorticoids. In extrahepatic tissues, CPS I and OTC are expressed strongly in the kidney and weakly in many other tissues.[439] These disorders may present in the neonatal period as a catastrophic illness or later with intermittent **hyperammonemia** episodes and neuropsychiatric

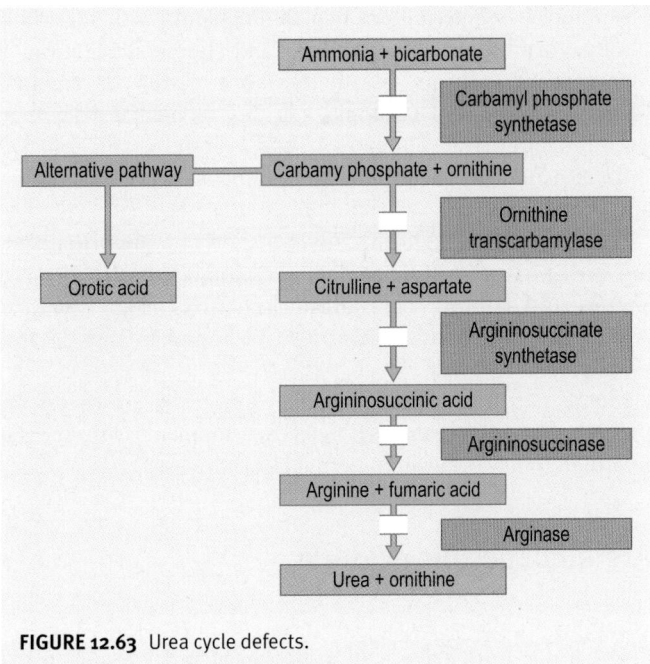

FIGURE 12.63 Urea cycle defects.

signs, including ataxia, hyperactivity, headache, and behavior disorders.[440–442] Argininosuccinate synthetase and argininosuccinate lyase deficiencies maintain the ability to excrete nitrogen in the form of citrulline, arginine, and argininosuccinic acid; therefore, these patients usually present later in infancy. Protein-restricted diets may be beneficial. Analysis of urine and plasma is helpful in diagnosing urea cycle enzyme deficiencies. Liver biopsy may provide the definitive diagnosis in demonstrating decreased levels of the enzyme activity.

Ornithine transcarbamylase deficiency

Ornithine transcarbamylase (OTC) deficiency is an **X-linked recessive disorder**. The gene locus has been mapped to Xp.21.1.[443] The incidence is 1 in 100 000. Two forms exist – a severe neonatal form (40%) and a late-onset form (60%). Hemizygous males pursue a fulminant neonatal course with hypotonia, lethargy, coma, and seizures; heterozygous females have a variable expression and may have a less severe form of the disease. In infants, hyperammonemia and orotic aciduria are noted with reduction in plasma citrulline. The diagnosis may be made by enzyme assay of liver tissue. Prenatal diagnosis is possible by analysis of amniocytes.[444] Heterozygotes can be detected by administration of allopurinol, which leads to marked increase in urinary excretion of orotic acid, and/or restriction fragment length polymorphism (RFLP) and linkage analyses in informative families or DNA studies in non-informative families.[445] The pathology in neonates is non-specific. In males, the **liver** is enlarged with **focal cellular necrosis and steatosis**. In older heterozygous females, there may be focal piecemeal necrosis, inflammation, steatosis, and fibrosis.

Peroxisomal swelling and matrix rarefaction are the usual ultrastructural changes observed; mitochondria are usually normal. CNS changes[446] include **Alzheimer type II astrocytes**, particularly in the segmental area of the pons and midbrain, with **spongiosis, hypomyelination, and cerebellar heterotopias**. Changes of hypoxic–ischemic injury are frequent, with cystic lesions presumed to be infarcts acquired before birth.

Carbamoyl phosphate synthetase deficiency

Carbamoyl phosphate synthetase I (CPS I) is an enzyme found in the liver in the inner mitochondrial matrix; it catalyzes the formation of carbamyl phosphate from ammonia and bicarbonate. It is the first, committed step of urea synthesis.

CPS I deficiency is a rare, **autosomal recessive disease**. The human CPS I gene has been mapped to 2q35.[447] The disease is characterized by **markedly elevated ammonia levels and reduced plasma citrulline and arginine**. Liver function test results are normal.[448] Symptoms usually appear within 24 hours after birth and include vomiting, lethargy, hypothermia, hypotonia, irritability, and opisthotonos. Pulmonary and GI hemorrhage are common terminal complications.[448]

There are two forms of CPS deficiency. In the neonatal-onset form, CPS I activity has varied from 0% to 50% of controls, and ammonia levels are markedly elevated. Symptoms in patients with the late-onset form (CPS II) are similar but milder than in the neonatal-onset form.[448] The diagnosis of CPS I deficiency is made by exclusion. The definitive diagnosis is made by determination of enzyme activity in liver parenchyma obtained by biopsy.

Pathologic changes in the liver are variable: it may show mild steatosis and focal cellular necrosis and progress to mild portal fibrosis, although in light microscopy this is not always observed. Ultrastructurally, mitochondria may be normal, swollen, or pleomorphic with dense deposits in the matrix, and have abnormal cristae. Concentric endoplasmic reticulum with loss of microvilli may be present. **Alzheimer type II astrocytic** changes and **spongiosis** are the usual CNS findings (Fig. 12.64).[446] OTC and CPS are present in significant amounts only in liver and intestine; therefore, prenatal diagnosis made by measuring enzyme activity by enzyme histochemistry can be performed only via fetal liver biopsy. DNA probes are now available for OTC and CPS genes.

Therapy consists of hemodialysis, restriction of dietary protein intake, and activation of other pathways of waste nitrogen synthesis and excretion. Despite therapy, the mortality rate is high, and morbidity, primarily brain damage, is significant.[449] Liver transplant has been attempted in two patients with CPS I deficiency. It was successful in correcting the ammonia levels of both patients, but one patient died of pneumonia 18 months after transplant. The second patient was still alive 40 months after the transplant, but mental and physical development were slightly retarded.[450]

Prenatal diagnosis is possible by DNA analysis of amniocytes and enzyme assay of liver tissue.[451] Enzyme histochemistry can be performed by fetal liver biopsy.

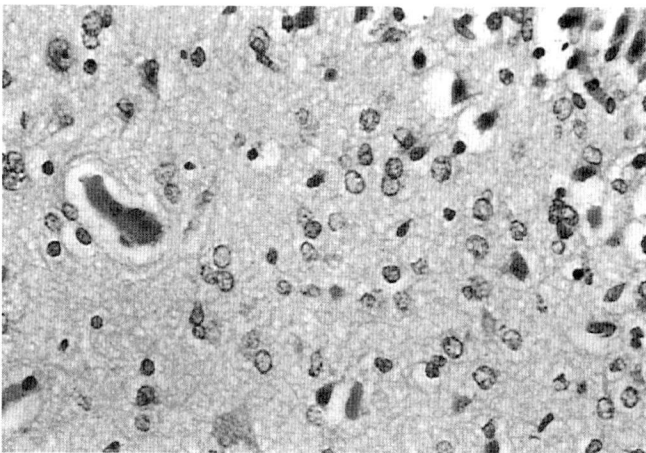

FIGURE 12.64 Carbamoyl phosphate synthetase (CPS) deficiency. Alzheimer type II cells in the white matter of an infant who died at 3 days of age. The nuclei are swollen with few chromatin granules at nuclear margins (naked nuclei gliosis).

Citrullinemia

This disorder is autosomal recessive and characterized by marked **hyperammonemia** with low arginine and **high plasma citrulline** levels due to **deficiency of argininosuccinate synthetase**.[451] Enzyme assays may be performed on fibroblast or amniotic cell cultures. Neuropathologic changes are similar to those of the other urea cycle disorders. **Steatosis and cellular necrosis** may be found in the **liver**, although cholestasis is more common.

Hyperornithinemia, hyperammonemia, homocitrullinuria disease

Hyperornithinemia, hyperammonemia, homocitrullinuria (HHH) disease is an autosomal recessive syndrome characterized by postprandial or intermittent hyperammonemia with increased plasma ornithine concentration and homocitrullinuria.[452] Symptoms may begin in the newborn period or anytime through adulthood. Hypotonia, seizures, or mental delay may occur. Ornithine acculumates in the cytoplasm and reduced intramitochondrial ornithine causes impaired urea formation and orotic aciduria.

Liver biopsy on light microscopy shows no abnormalities, but on EM **liver mitochondria are elongated with bizarre shapes and contain crystalloid structures** (Fig. 12.65).[453] Abnormal mitochondria may also be found in muscle and leukocytes.

Some patients develop normally on a diet restricted in protein, but disturbance in fetal development with mental retardation may occur in maternal HHH disease.[454]

Argininosuccinic aciduria

Argininosuccinic aciduria (ASA) is an autosomal recessive disorder due to **deficiency of argininosuccinic lyase**.[455] In the newborn, **hyperammonemia** develops with **increased argininosuccinic acid in plasma and urine and elevation of plasma citrulline levels**. Hepatomegaly and increased levels of transaminases are present. **Microvesicular steatosis** may be confused with Reye syndrome. Severe septal fibrosis may occur. However, the mitochondrial changes seen in Reye syndrome are not present. Trichorrhexis nodosa is found in a late-onset form, usually without hepatomegaly. In the brain, **hypomyelination and Alzheimer type II cells** are present.

Argininemia

This is an inherited autosomal recessive disorder[456] due to **deficiency of arginase** and characterized by progressive spastic

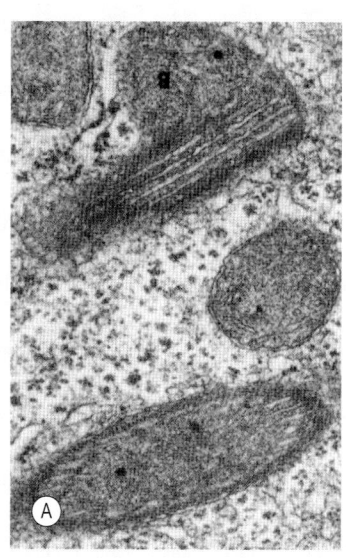
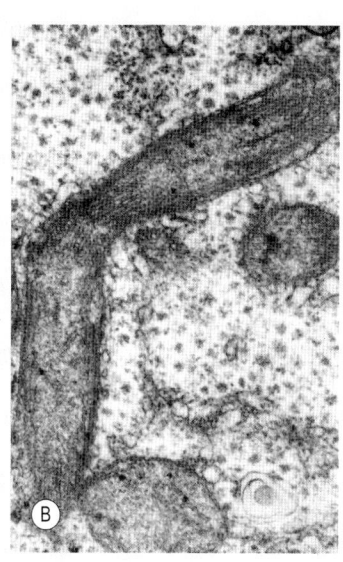

FIGURE 12.65 Hyperornithinemia, hyperammonia, homocitrullinuria (HHH disease). (A) Increased number of mitochondria in the perinuclear region of a hepatocyte display altered form and length. The long forms show tubules running parallel to the longitudinal axis, a thick structure applied to the inner mitochondrial membrane with sieve-like appearance on a slightly tangential cut and several small bulges protruding from the surface (× 15 000). (B) The internal structure of three large electron-opaque mitochondria from a cultured fibroblast of skin. Although difficult to resolve, it shows unusual arrays in addition to probable degenerative changes.

diplegia, mental retardation, hyperammonemia that is usually mild with hepatomegaly, and elevation of transaminase levels. Onset is usually between 2 and 3 years of age. The hepatocytes may be swollen and steatosis and periportal fibrosis may occur. **Mitochondria are normal.** Symptoms usually do not occur until after infancy in this disorder.

Lysinuric protein intolerance

Lysinuric protein intolerance is due to a **defect in transport of dibasic amino acids** with decreased serum lysine, arginine, ornithine, and urea and increased urine excretion of the same amino acids and orotic acid.[457] It results from mutations in the amino acid transporter gene *SLC7A7*, which maps to 14q11.2. Patients present with hypotonia, mental delay, hyperelastic skin, osteoporosis, lens opacities, and intermittent elevation of serum ammonia. Improvement occurs with diets low in protein and most infants do well on breast milk. Besides effects on the CNS, the pathological effects are predominantly in the bones and kidneys. Fractures due to osteoporosis and renal rickets have occurred.

High-protein formula or other high-protein foods can cause severe hyperammonemia. At about 1 year of age, failure to thrive and mild growth retardation occur. The child may present with alopecia, diminished subcutaneous fat and loose skin folds, anemia and leukopenia. Skin lesions may be reminiscent of acrodermatitis enteropathica. Serum lactate dehydrogenase and ferritin concentrations are almost always markedly elevated. Most patients develop pulmonary changes that first resemble mild interstitial pneumonia but may suddenly progress to fatal or life-threatening pulmonary failure, charactertized histoligically by alveolar proteinosis.

Plasma cationic amino acids are decreased and glutamine, alanine, glycine, and citrulline are increased. There is an increase in postprandial serum ammonia and orotic aciduria, and an increase in serum lactic dehydrogenase and ferritin.

Prenatal diagnosis can be accomplished by examination of cultured fibroblasts or from chorionic villus sampling.

Transient hyperammonemia of the newborn

Elevated serum ammonia with concomitant characteristics of hyperammonemia, lethargy, and coma may occur in otherwise normal newborns. There is a striking response to measures to lower serum ammonia. With vigorous correction, there are no permanent ill effects. The condition probably represents an immaturity of urea cycle enzymes.

Biotinidase deficiency

Patients with this disorder are **acidotic and ketotic** and develop **hyperammonemia, hypoglycemia, and hyperglycinemia.** They may develop seizures and become comatose.[458,459] A **tomcat odor** and an erythematous rash characterize the disorder. **Carboxylase enzyme activities are diminished** and are determined by culture of fibroblasts or amniocytes. Assay of this enzyme may be included in neonatal screening.

Vitamin therapy of some metabolic diseases

Several of the metabolic diseases respond to pharmacologic doses of vitamins (Table 12.23).

Purine disorders

Purines are the essence of DNA and RNA, but recognized deficiencies, although severe, are somewhat less all-encompassing.

Adenosine deaminase deficiency (ADA) is an autosomal recessive disorder that results in **reduced DNA synthesis in T- and B-cell precursors**[460] (see Ch. 30). Severe combined immunodeficiency results with multiple life-threatening infections in the first 2 years of life. Enzyme activity is depressed in erythrocytes, lymphocytes, plasma, and fibroblasts. Bone marrow transplantation is beneficial, and modified ADA given by injection results in improvement. Prenatal diagnosis is available.

Lesch-Nyhan syndrome is an **X-linked inherited** disease due to **hypoxanthine guanine phosphoribosyl transferase deficiency**, which results in **hyperuricemia** (Fig. 12.66).[461] The gene is located on Xq26-q27. Four HPRT pseudogenes are present. Two are located on chromosome 11, one located on chromosome 3, and another on 5p13-q11. Infants present in the first few weeks with yellow-orange crystalluria. **Choreoathetosis, spasticity,** and *self-mutilation* (Fig. 12.67) are common. After several months, hyperuricemia is prominent and gouty tophi may occur. There are forms with varying severity. Hematologic abnormalities may include megaloblastic anemia, abnormal platelet morphology, and increased peripheral blood T cells.

Phosphoribosylpyrophosphate synthetase overactivity is inherited as a rare X-linked recessive disorder coded by a gene on chromosome Xq22-24, that results in overproduction of purines and uric acid.[462] It is one cause of **gout**, and in some cases causes developmental delay, deafness, and hypotonia. Heterozygous females may have gout and/or hearing loss.

Purine-nucleotide phosphorylase (PNP) deficiency is inherited as an autosomal recessive disease and manifests in infancy with repeated infections **due to T-cell deficiency.** Death due to generalized vaccinia has followed vaccination.[463] Failure to thrive, developmental delay, neurologic abnormalities including spastic diplegia, ataxia and tremor, psychomotor retardation, and hypotonia may occur. Plasma and urine uric acid are decreased. The absolute lymphocyte count is frequently less than 500/µL with a profoundly decreased T-cell count.

TABLE 12.23 VITAMIN THERAPY OF SOME METABOLIC DISORDERS

Vitamin	Disease	Untreated state	Daily dosage
A	Darier	Hyperkeratosis follicularis	7500 μg
B_1	Leigh-pyruvic-lactic acidosis	Ataxia, mental retardation	600 μg
	Thiamine-responsive anemia	Megaloblastic anemia	20 mg
	Maple syrup urine disease	Hypotonia, seizures	10 mg
Riboflavin	Pyruvate kinase deficiency	Hemolysis	10 mg
	Glutaric acidemia (II)	Hypoglycemia	100–300 mg
Niacin	Hartnup	Ataxia, eczema	200 mg
B_6	Cystathioninuria	No symptoms	200 mg
	Homocystinuria	Mental retardation	200 mg
	B_6 anemia	Hypochromic microcytic anemia	10 mg
	B_6 seizures	Seizures	25 mg
	Xanthurenic aciduria	Mental retardation	10 mg
	Gyrate atrophy of choroid	Blindness	100 mg
	Oxaluria	Oxalate crystals	100 mg
Folic acid	Formiminotransferase deficiency	Retardation	5 mg
	Folate reductase deficiency	Megaloblastic anemia	5 mg
	Homocystinuria	Mental retardation	10 mg
B_{12}	Methylmalonic acidemia	Mental retardation	1 mg
Biotin	Propionic acidemia	Mental retardation	10 mg
	β-methylcrotonyl glycinuria	Coma	10 mg
	Biotinase deficiency	Seizures	5–20 mg
	Holocarboxylase deficiency	Hypotonia	10 mg
C	Chédiak-Higashi	Infections	50 mg
	Alkaptonuria	Increased pigment	300 mg
D	Vitamin D dependency	Rickets	100 μg
	Familial hypophosphatemia	Rickets	2500 μg

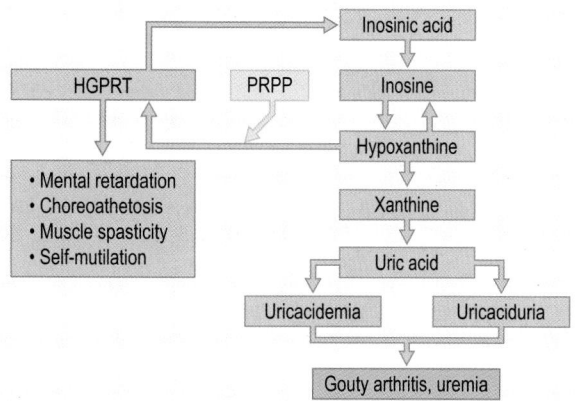

FIGURE 12.66 Lesch-Nyhan syndrome.

Prenatal diagnosis is available. The gene has been assigned to chromosome 14[464] with a number of point mutations. The diagnosis is made by a specific assay (radiochemical or spectrophotometric) of PNP enzymatic activity in red blood cells.[465]

Adenine phosphoribosyl transferase (APRT) deficiency is an autosomal recessively inherited disease that results in **renal stone formation** in the second or third decade.[239] The gene is located on chromosome 16q24. Plasma and urine uric acid are normal. The enzyme is measurable in red cells, leukocytes, and fibroblasts. APRT deficiency may become clinically manifest in childhood or even from birth.[466] Acute renal failure may be the presenting symptom.

Adenylosuccinase deficiency is an autosomal recessively inherited disease that may be associated with autism and psychomotor delay in young children.[467] The majority of children have epilepsy and some have autism and muscular wasting.[468] **Self-mutilation, hypotonia**, and **cerebellar hypoplasia** occur. **Plasma and urine succinyladenosine** are elevated. The gene, *ADSL*, maps to chromosome 22q13.1. Diagnosis is made by assaying succinyl purines in CSF and urine or adenylsuccinase in fresh biopsy specimens of liver or kidney; molecular diagnosis is possible.

Myoadenylate deaminase deficiency is inherited as an autosomal recessive disorder and is associated **with muscle cramps after exercise**.[469] Creatine kinase may be elevated. Muscle ATP is decreased. **Malignant hyperthermia** may occur. The gene is located on chromosome 1p21-p13. Diagnosis is made by histochemical or biochemical assay in a muscle biopsy. DNA diagnosis is also possible.

Xanthine oxidase deficiency is an autosomal recessively inherited disease that may cause **xanthine renal stones**.[470]

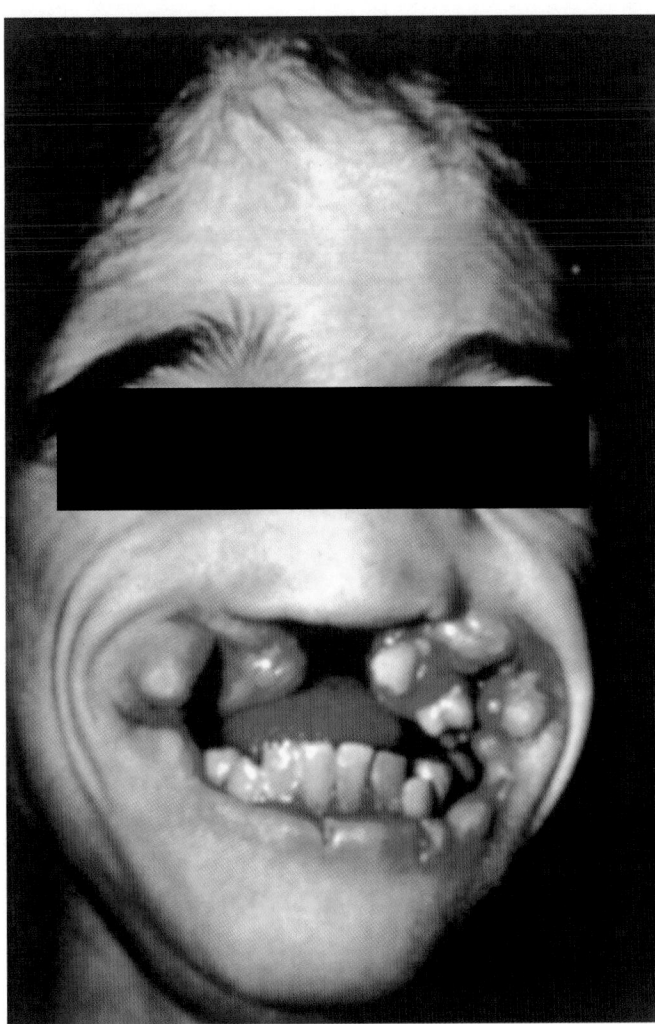

FIGURE 12.67 Self-mutilation in Lesch-Nyhan syndrome.

Urinary uric acid is reduced. The enzyme can be assayed in liver and intestinal mucosal biopsy specimens.

Adenylate kinase deficiency is an autosomal recessively inherited disorder that causes red blood cell hemolysis[471] resulting in hemolytic anemia. There are no other significant symptoms except for the development of splenomegaly.

Pyrimidine disorders

Orotic aciduria is inherited as an autosomal recessive disorder and is distinct from the orotic aciduria that accompanies disorders of the urea cycle.[472] Hereditary orotic aciduria manifests in the first year of life with **hypochromic anemia, megaloblastosis, varying degrees of neutropenia and lympho-penia, immunodeficiency and crystalluria**. Defects in orotate phosphoribosyltransferase and orotidine 5-monophosphate decarboxylase are detectable in liver biopsy specimens and in leukocytes, erythrocytes, and fibroblasts. Enzymatic diagnosis can be performed on red blood cells.

In **pyrimidine 5-nucleotidase deficiency** elevated pyrimidine nucleotides in blood are associated with a **non-spherocytic-hemolytic anemia**, and **basophilic stippling of the erythrocytes**; it is inherited as an autosomal recessive disorder.[473] The gene, *UMPH1*, is located on 7p15-p14, and molecular diagnosis is possible.[474] Diagnosis can also be achieved through assays of enzyme activity in erythrocytes. Diagnosis is confirmed by measurement of erythrocyte enzyme activity.

Fatty acid β-oxidation defects

The major metabolic flux of long-chain fatty acids is through the β-oxidation system of the mitochondria present in all cells except the mature erythrocyte. Access of the fatty acid to the β-oxidation enzymes requires a carnitine-dependent transport system to cross the mitochondrial membrane.

Fatty acids are activated to acyl-CoAs at the outer mito-chondrial membrane, converted to acylcarnitines by carnitine palmitoyl transferase (CPT) I, and transported across the inner mitochondrial membrane by a translocase, and the fatty acid acyl-CoA is regenerated by CPT II (see later discussion of carnitine deficiency). The fatty acid acyl-CoA then undergoes β oxidation to generate acetyl-CoA. β oxidation proceeds through a series of steps resulting in the release of acetyl-CoA and a fatty acid acyl-CoA derivative that is shorter by two carbon groups than the original fatty acid.

Defects of nine proteins have been identified in mitochondrial β-oxidation. These include defects of plasma membrane carnitine transport, CPT I, CPT II, carnitine/acylcarnitine translocase, LCAD, MCAD, SCAD, 2,4-dienoyl-CoA reductase, long-chain-3-hydroxy-acyl-CoA dehydrogenase (LCHAD), and very-long-chain acyl-CoA dehydrogenase (VLCAD).

The disorders of the β-oxidation pathway are characterized by skeletal and/or cardiac muscle weakness and are all inherited as autosomal recessive traits. In some of these disorders, unique metabolites can be identified in blood or urine; exceptions are CPT deficiencies and the carnitine transport defect, in which no abnormal metabolites are excreted. Hypoketotic hypoglycemia characterizes all these disorders.

Enzyme defects can be demonstrated in fibroblasts and leukocytes. Characteristics of fatty acid oxidation defects are shown in Table 12.24.

Clinical findings in intramitchondrial fatty acid oxidation defects are shown in Table 12.25 and laboratory findings common to disorders of fatty acid oxidation in Table 12.26.

Carnitine esters are increased and free carnitine levels are low in plasma, skeletal muscle, and liver. Coma may be a presenting sign. Pathologically, there is fatty infiltration of the liver cells (Fig. 12.68), muscle cells, and cardiac myocytes. Enzyme defects can be demonstrated in fibroblasts and leukocytes. MCAD occurs in 1 in 5000 to 10 000 live births, primarily in white children of Northern European descent. Carrier frequency for the most common genetic mutation, A985G, is 1 in 68 in the United States and Great Britain. Infants,

TABLE 12.24 CHARACTERISTIC FEATURES OF FATTY ACID OXIDATION DEFECTS

MIM no.	Disorder	Tissue distribution	Chromosome location	Symptoms and signs	Laboratory findings
212140	Carnitine deficiency	Kidney, heart, muscle, FB, liver	5q31.1	Cardiomyopathy, coma, muscle weakness, Reye-like syndrome, sudden infant death	Glucose (P)↓, ammonia (B)↑, acidosis+, carnitine (P)↑, long – chain acylcarnitine (P) n, cellular carnitine uptake ↓
255120	Carnitine palmitoyl transferase I	Liver, FB	11q13	Coma, liver insufficiency, hepatomegaly	Glucose (P)↓. Ammonia (B) n-↑. Acidosis +, carnitine (P), long-chain acylcarnitine (P) ↑
212138	Acylcarnitine translocase	FB, liver, heart muscle	3p21.31	Coma, cardiac abnormalities, liver insufficiency, vomiting	Glucose (P)↓, ammonia (B)↑, acidosis ±, free carnitine (P)↓, acylcarnitine (P)↑, long-chain acylcarnitine (P)↑. Seizures ±
255110	Carnitine palmitoyl transferase II Very-long-chain acyl-CoA dehydrogenase	Muscle, heart, liver FB	1p32	Coma, Reye-like syndrome, hepatomegaly, exercise intolerance, myalgia, cardiomyopathy, developmental delay ±, sudden death, respiratory arrest, muscle weakness	Glucose (B)↓, ketosis, liver enzymes (P)↑. Creatine kinase (P)↑, myoglobin (P,U), dicarboxylic acids (U) ±. carnitine (P)↓. Acidosis +, CK (P)↑. $C_{14:1}$ acylcarnitine (P)↑, long chain acylcarnitine (P)↑
201475	Very-long-chain acyl-CoA-dehydrogenase	Muscle, heart, liver, CNS	17p13	Hypertrophic cardiomyopathy, sudden cardiac death, hepatomegaly, hepatic steatosis, hepatocellular necrosis, hypotonia, muscle weakness, rhabdomyolysis, lethargy	Glucose (B) ↓, acidosis +, CK (P) ↑, $C14:1$ acylcarnitine (P) ↑, carnitine (P) ↓, long chain acylcarnitine (P) ↑
201450	Medium-chain acyl-CoA dehydrogenase	Liver muscle, FB, WBC decreased	1p31	Coma/lethargy, hepatopathy, hypotonia, apnea/respiratory arrest, sudden death, seizures ±, mental retardation, attention deficit disorder	Glucose (B)↓, ketosis ±, Acidosis +, transaminases (P)↑, ammonia (B)↑, uric acid (P)↑, dicarboxylic acids (U)↑, glycine conjugates (U,P)↑ decanoate (P)↑, acylcarnitines (U)↑, carnitine (P) n-↓, long-chain acylcarnitine
201470	Short-chain acyl-CoA dehydrogenase	Muscle, liver, FB, WBC decreased	12q22-qter	Muscle weakness, lethargy, failure to thrive, mental retardation	Ketosis+, Acidosis +, ethylmalonic acid (U) n-↑, carnitine (P)↓-n
143450	Long-chain 3-hydroxyacyl-CoA dehydrogenase	Liver, muscle, heart, FB, WBC decreased	2p23	Coma/lethargy, hepatopathy, cardiomyopathy, neuropathy, retinopathy, muscle weakness, sudden death	Glucose (B)↓, acidosis, lactate (P)↑, myoglobin ↑ (P,U), CK (P)↑, hydroxy-dicarboxylic acids (U)↑, long-chain 3-hydroxy-fatty acids (P)↑, carnitine (P)↓, long-chain acylcarnitine (P)↑

TABLE 12.24 CHARACTERISTIC FEATURES OF FATTY ACID OXIDATION DEFECTS

MIM no.	Disorder	Tissue distribution	Chromosome location	Symptoms and signs	Laboratory findings
609016	Long-chain 3-hydroxyacyl-Co-A dehydrogenase deficiency	Muscle, FB	2p23	Cardiomyopathy, muscle weakness, lethargy	Glucose (B)↓, myoglobinuria +, CK (P)↑, AST/ALT (P)↑, ketosis +, ketones (U)↑, dicarboxylic acids (U) n-↑

B, blood; U, Urine; P, Plasma; FB, Fibroblasts; WBC, white blood cells; AST, aspartate transferase; ALT, alanine transferase; n, normal; CK, creatine phosphokinase.

TABLE 12.25 CLINICAL FINDINGS IN INTRAMITOCHONDRIAL FATTY ACID OXIDATION DEFECTS

Medium-chain-acyl-CoA dehydrogenase deficiency

1. Reye-like or sudden infant death syndrome (SIDS)-like syndrome with hypoketotic hypoglycemia secondary to lack of oral intake, usually within the first 2 years of life
2. Ammonia and liver enzymes (may or may not be elevated)
3. Possible mild hepatomegaly because of fat accumulation in hepatocytes
4. Increased levels of urinary N-hexanoglycine, 3-phenylpropionyl glycine, and suberylglycine during episode
5. Elevated C_6-C_{12} – dicarboxylic acids in urine during episode
6. Acylcarnitine profiles also reflect increased medium-chain fatty acid CoA thioesters during episode
7. Increased octanoyl carnitine after 100 mg/kg of oral carnitine intake during asymptomatic period

Short-chain acyl-CoA dehydrogenase deficiency

1. Reye-like symptoms (acute)
2. Failure to thrive and muscle weakness chronically
3. Lipid in muscle and liver tissue (triglyceride)
4. Low muscle carnitine with low-normal plasma carnitine levels

Long-chain acyl-CoA dehydrogenase deficiency

1. Reye-like or SIDS-like symptoms
2. Hypoketotic hypoglycemia, hepatomegaly, cardiomegaly, and hypotonia usually presenting between 2 and 4 months of age
3. Possible muscle cramps and myoglobinuria in chronic disease
4. Possible failure to thrive
5. Hepatomegaly with or without elevated hepatocellular enzyme or ammonia level
6. Fatty liver with low carnitine levels
7. Low plasma carnitine with high esterification

Carnitine palmitoyl transferase deficiency

1. Seizures and coma from fasting hypoglycemia and hypoketonemia
2. Normal liver tests and ammonia level
3. Normal carnitine levels
4. Fatty liver but no accumulation of triglycerides in muscle tissue

Systemic carnitine deficiency

1. Recurrent episodes of Reye-like or SIDS-like syndrome during infancy or early childhood
2. Muscle weakness progressing to atrophy
3. Eventual development of cardiomyopathy with abnormal echocardiogram
4. Fatty liver
5. Low serum carnitine levels with disproportionately high urine levels

usually in the neonatal period, develop episodes of hypoketotic hypoglycemia, vomiting, lethargy, seizures, and coma and some succumb to **sudden infant death**. If survival is beyond 2 years, developmental and behavioral disability, chronic muscle weakness, failure to thrive, and cerebral palsy may become manifest.

LCAD deficiency

The human LCAD gene has been localized to chromosome 2q34-q35.

Elevated long-chain acylcarnitines, mainly $C_{14:1}$ acylcarnitine, are present in plasma.[475]

TABLE 12.26 LABORATORY FINDINGS COMMON TO DISORDERS OF FATTY ACID OXIDATION

Hypoglycemia
    Hypoketosis (negative or 1+ urine ketones)
    Elevated plasma FFA
    Plasma FFA > β-hydroxybutyrate
Acidosis
    Mild to moderate
    Increased lactate (especially in LCHAD deficiency)
Mild to moderate increase in AST and ALT usually without hyperbilirubinemia
PT, PTT normal or mildly elevated
Elevated CPK
    Cardiac and skeletal muscle
    Marked with episodic muscle weakness
    Rhabdomyolysis, myoglobinuria
Mild elevation of ammonia
Marked hyperuricemia
Low plasma carnitine (except in CPT I deficiency)
    Elevated acylcarnitine (except in CPT I deficiency)
    Specific accumulating acylcarnitines

FFA, free fatty acids; LCHAD, long-chain 3-hydroxyacyl-CoA dehydrogenase; AST, aspartate aminotransferase; ALT, alanine aminotransferase; PT, prothrombin time; PTT, partial thromboplastin time; CPK, creatine phosphokinase; CPT, carnitine palmitoyl transferase.

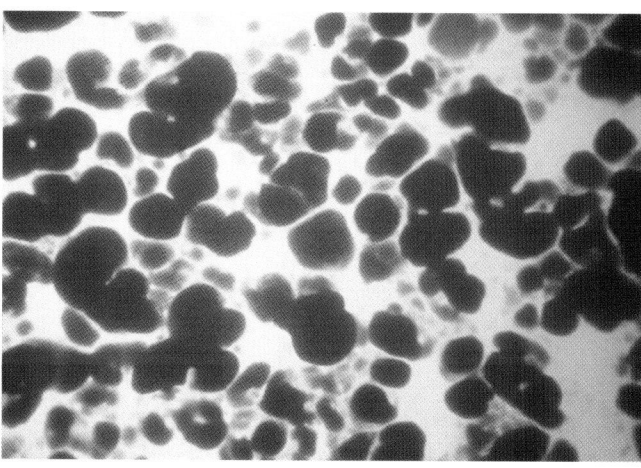

FIGURE 12.68 Medium-chain acyl-dehydrogenase deficiency (MCAD) liver showing marked fatty change (oil red O stain).

There is considerable clinical similarity to patients with MCAD deficiency. LCAD-deficient patients are hypoglycemic, hypoketotic, and acidotic, and they have abnormal liver function tests and hyperuricemia.

VLCAD deficiency

The enzyme deficiency has been found in fibroblasts, platelets, and skeletal muscle. Low levels of palmitoyl-CoA dehydro-genase activity are found by immunoblot analysis.[476] The clinical presentation of VLCAD deficiency[477] is characterized by onset of symptoms soon after birth with ventricular fibrillation, respiratory arrest, and metabolic acidosis. Sudden death may occur with massive hepatic steatosis.

SCAD deficiency

SCAD deficiency has been identified in only a few patients[478–484] with highly variable clinical and laboratory findings. Persistent hypotonia is a common symptom.[485,486] Lactic acidosis may occur.

Pathologic findings may be limited to muscle and include lipid vacuolation, especially in type I fibers.[487] The liver may show ultrastructural evidence of both microvesicular and macro-vesicular steatosis; mitochondrial changes reminiscent of those seen in MCAD deficiency, with increased matrix density, and crystalloids are found.[475]

Diagnosis of SCAD deficiency is made by measuring acyl-CoA dehydrogenase activities in available tissues, including fibroblasts. Activity of palmitoyl-CoA and octanoyl-CoA are normal. Heterozygotes have intermediate SCAD activity.

SCHAD deficiency

In SCHAD deficiency the enzyme defect can be demonstrated in fibroblasts.

Patients may have recurrent hypoglycemic encephalopathy, recurrent myoglobinuria, and cardiomyopathy. It has been associated with HELLP syndrome (hemolysis, elevated liver enzymes, low platelets) during pregnancy.[479]

Lactic acidosis

Lactic acid is produced in the anaerobic metabolism of glucose through pyruvate and is converted in the liver to glucose. Insufficient oxygen in this latter reaction is the most common cause of lactic acidemia. The hepatic glucose is used by all tissues and generates ATP.

Of the metabolic errors causing lactic acidosis, deficiency of pyruvate dehydrogenase complex is the most common.

Pyruvate dehydrogenase deficiency

Pyruvate dehydrogenase (PDH) is required for complete oxidation of glucose and fatty acids and provides acetyl-CoA for the citric acid cycle. **Pyruvate dehydrogenase is a protein complex with three main catalytic domains: E_1, E_2, and E_3.**[488] Defects of the E_1 α subunit are inherited in an X-linked fashion. Males with E_1 α deficiency have a partial deficiency; females may carry a more severe mutation. A defect of pyruvate dehydrogenase results in a variable phenotype, including lactic acidosis in the early neonatal period, ataxia, and developmental delay in infancy.[488,489] Subtle dysmorphic features are similar to those of the fetal alcohol syndrome, including a narrow head with frontal bossing, a wide nasal bridge, an upturned nose, a long philtrum, and flared nostrils. An abnormal gyral pattern with polymicrogyria, poor myelination, agenesis of the corpus callosum, and cardiac defects has occurred. Pyruvate dehydrogenase deficiency has been found in Leigh encephalopathy. PDH can be assayed in a number of tissues including cultured fibroblasts as well as in muscle biopsy. The $E_1 \alpha$ subunit is located at Xp22.1-p22.2.

Pyruvate carboxylase deficiency

Pyruvate carboxylase deficiency may present in the neonate or in the first few months as mild lactic acidemia with developmental delay, or in a severe form with **hyperammonemia, hypoglycemia, hyperlysinemia**, and **citrullinemia**.[490] In either type, **decreased neurons** are noted in the **cerebral cortex with gliosis, thin corpus callosum, increased astrocytes, and ventricular enlargement. Lipid droplets accumulate in hepatocytes. Leigh encephalopathy** may be the clinical presentation.[491,492] The biochemical and clinical lesions are similar to those of pyruvate decarboxylase deficiency.

Defects in the mitochondrial respiratory chain are also associated with chronic lactic acidemia (see below). Defects in other enzymes in the Krebs and Cori cycles also cause lactic acidosis.

Lactic acidemia with normal or decreased pyruvate values leading to an increased lactate–pyruvate ratio indicates defects in oxidative phosphorylation or severe pyruvate carboxylase defect. Lactic acidemia with increased pyruvate value and normal or decreased lactate–pyruvate ratio suggests defective pyruvate dehydrogenase complex function or certain glycogenoses if associated with hypoglycemia. **Lactic acidosis** with abnormal urinary organic acids should direct further investigations toward defects in fatty acid oxidation and organic acidurias.

Lactic acidemia is a common laboratory finding in mitochondrial dysfunction. Lactate must be measured under well-controlled conditions, and simultaneous measurements of pyruvate, organic acids, amino acids, ketone bodies, and carnitine in blood and urine are of value.[493–495] Pyruvate carboxylase is intramitochondrial and has its highest activity in liver and kidney. The gene is located at chromosome 11q13. Prenatal diagnosis is by enzyme analysis of amniotic fluid.

Pathology

Hepatomegaly with vesiculation of hepatocytes, cholestasis, hepatocyte swelling, mild ductular proliferation as well as edema, hemorrhage and infarcts in the brain,[496] poor myelination and paucity of neurons in the cerebral cortex and gliosis, ventricular enlargement, and thinning of the corpus callosum are present.

Mitochondrial disorders

A disease caused by abnormal mitochondrial energy production was first described in 1962.[497] Mitochondria are present in all eukaryotic cells dependent on aerobic metabolism and generate most of the cellular ATP. They also regulate cytoplasmic calcium levels. By EM, mitochondria show a smooth, spherical outer membrane and an inner membrane with numerous infoldings, known as cristae. The cristae are usually perpendicular to the long axis of a mitochondrion. The membranes divide the contents of mitochondria into separated compartments, each harboring specific biochemical structures for transportation and processing of chemical compounds. The outer membrane is permeable to many small molecules and contains receptors for transporting macromolecules from the cytosol to the inner parts of the mitochondrion. The inner membrane is impermeable and contains special transporters for small molecules, controlled by several specific translocase systems. The four complexes of the ET chain are embedded in the inner membrane. The **mitochondrial matrix** contains many **enzymes, including the citric acid (Krebs) cycle, fatty acid oxidation pathways**, and many others. The mitochondrial genome and its protein synthetic machinery for mitochondrially coded polypeptides is also confined to the matrix.

Mitochondrial genome

Mitochondria are unique cytoplasmic organelles by virtue of having their own genome, the mitochondrial DNA (mtDNA). The mtDNA of all cells has its origin in the unfertilized ovum. Although spermatozoa contain mitochondria, no paternal mtDNA has been demonstrated in the human zygote. Consequently, mtDNA is inherited exclusively from the mother.[498] **Maternal or cytoplasmic inheritance** has several unique features differing from mendelian traits.[499] When mutant mtDNA is present in the ovum, it is transmitted to all offspring, resulting in larger numbers of affected individuals than in autosomal dominant traits.

The pathways of the oxidation of substrates connected with the synthesis of ATP may be divided into two major classes of chemical reactions:

1. **Oxidation of pyruvate and fatty acids to CO_2** with generation of reduced forms of nicotinamide adenine dinucleotide (NADH) and flavine adenine dinucleotide ($FADH_2$). The processes in this set of reactions include pyruvate dehydrogenase complex and β oxidation of fatty acids succeeded by reactions of the citric acid cycle.

2. **Oxidative phosphorylation**, which includes transfer of electrons from NADH and $FADH_2$ to oxygen linked to creation of an electrochemical gradient across the inner membrane of the mitochondrion. The electrons are transported through macromolecular complexes (I, II, III, IV) ET or respiratory chain, resulting in reduction of molecular oxygen to water in complex IV. (Table 12.27) The electrochemical gradient is utilized by the proton translocating ATP synthase in complex V to synthesize ATP from ADP and inorganic phosphorus (Pi). The ATP is then exchanged for the cytosolic ADP by adenine nucleotide translocase (ANT).

TABLE 12.27 STRUCTURAL GENE PRODUCTS OF MTDNA IN RESPIRATORY CHAIN COMPLEXES

Complex	Structural protein
I	NADH: ubiquinone oxidoreductase
II	Succinate: ubiquinone oxidoreductase
III	Cytochrome $b_1 c_1$ complex
IV	Cytochrome c oxidase
V	ATP synthase

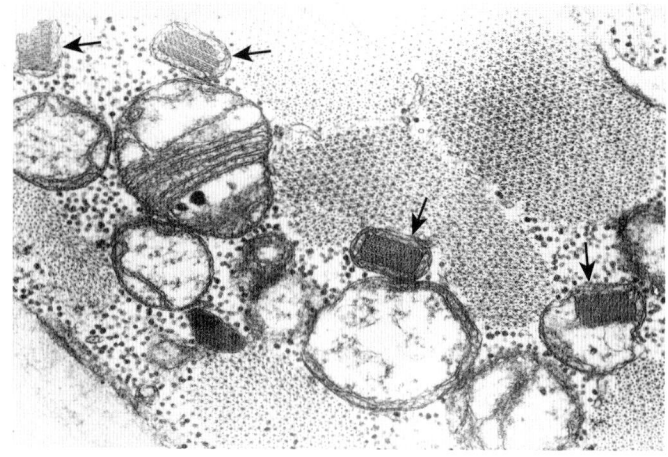

FIGURE 12.69 Crystalline inclusions (arrows) in mitochondria seen in mitochondrial disorders (courtesy of Dr Juliani Rapola).

Mitochondrial diseases

Inherited defects are known for each of the main biochemical sets of reactions in mitochondria, most of which are inherited as autosomal recessives.

The contemporary classification[500] is based on the biochemical defects linked with the molecular genetic findings of the patients (Table 12.27). All disorders caused by mtDNA defects and intergenomic signaling defects that **impair respiratory chain and/or oxidative phosphorylation**.

Pathologic changes of mitochondrial diseases

The morphologic changes associated with mitochondrial dysfunction are divided into two groups: (1) abnormalities associated directly with altered number and structure of the mitochondria; and (2) secondary degenerative and destructive changes due to impaired function of the mitochondria.

EM reveals a number of mitochondrial alterations in mitochondriopathies. The number and size of the mitochondria are often increased. **Giant mitochondria with concentric tubular, reticular, lamellar, or otherwise dissociated cristae** are characteristic.[501] The mitochondrial matrix may be swollen and contain large, spherical dense bodies, vacuoles, or crystals. The rectangular crystals are often arranged in blocks of parallel crystals, with a 'parking lot' configuration (Fig. 12.69).[501] They contain proteins, and at least two different types of crystals are known.

Light microscopic and EM investigation of suspected mitochondrial disorders shows changes confined to defects of the respiratory chain or of oxidation–phosphorylation coupling, but not in disorders of substrate utilization.[502] Several examples of disorders of oxidative phosphorylation have no morphologic mitochondrial changes. On the other hand, **ragged red fibers** (RRFs) and accompanying EM findings are occasionally seen in a small proportion of muscle fibers in neuromuscular disorders other than mitochondriopathies. Zidovudine, a drug used to treat AIDS, causes myopathy with RRFs.[503] Absent or weak histochemical cytochrome oxidase (COX) activity is seen in some, but not all, mitochondrial disorders due to complex IV defects. Moderately increased fat droplets and glycogen are often seen in association with RRFs, but extensive fatty infiltration of the muscle and liver is more characteristic of carnitine transport defects and impaired fatty acid oxidation.[504]

Leigh syndrome

Leigh syndrome (subacute necrotizing encephalomyelopathy [SNE]) is an encephalopathy of infancy. Four major causes have been well established: (1) **pyruvate dehydrogenase deficiency** transmitted as an autosomal recessive or an X-linked recessive trait, depending on the subunit affected; (2) **COX deficiency** inherited as an autosomal recessive trait; (3) **pyruvate carboxylase deficiency**; and (4) **maternally inherited point mutation at nt 8993 in the ATPase 6 gene of mtDNA**. Beside the CNS, heart involvement has been described in all four forms and consists of hypertrophic cardiomyopathy with electrocardiographic evidence of concentric left ventricular hypertrophy.[505,506]

Leigh syndrome is characterized by symmetric basal lesions extending from the thalamus to the pons, inferior olives of the medulla, substantia nigra and posterior columns of the spinal cord.[507] Histologically, SNE shows necrosis, astrocytosis, and vascular proliferation, particularly involving the mamillary bodies. The lesions are gray-brown in color and may become cystic or cavitated. Proliferation of capillaries resembles Wernicke's encephalopathy.[508]

A distinctive pattern of destructive brain lesions is seen in mitochondriopathies caused by deletions and point mutations of the mtDNA, and includes **Kearns-Sayre syndrome**; myopathy, encephalopathy, lactic acidosis, neurologic weakness, ataxia, retinitis pigmentosa (NARP), Leber hereditary optic neuropathy (LHON), stroke (MELAS); and myoclonic epilepsy, ragged red fibers (MERRF) syndromes.[509–511] Status spongiosus, neuronal degeneration, gliosis, demyelinization, necrosis, and mineral deposits are seen in these disorders. Malignant hyperthermia is seen in those with primary myopathies rather than in mitochondrial defects.

A distinct late-onset mitochondrial disorder with mitochondrial myopathy, anemia, cardiomyopathy, lactic acidosis, and stroke-like episodes is characterized by deficiencies of complexes IV and II.[512]

Barth syndrome (MIM 302060) is a congenital dilated cardiomyopathy and mitochondrial myopathy with growth retardation.

BOX 12.5 CLINICAL AND LABORATORY FINDINGS OF MITOCHONDRIAL DISORDERS

General
Congenital anomalies and dysmorphic features

Coma

Hypotonia

Respiratory difficulties

Failure to thrive

Symptoms are episodic, related to fasting, strenuous exercise, and infection

Nervous system
Migraine-like headache

Epilepsy

Ataxia

Myoclonus

Stroke-like episodes

Mental retardation

Hearing impairment

Polyneuropathy

Eyes
Ptosis

Progressive external ophthalmoplegia

Pigmentary retinopathy

Optic atrophy

Skeletal muscle
Myalgia

Weakness

Muscle cramps

Hypotonia

Wasting

Heart
Conduction defect

Cardiomyopathy

Hematopoietic
Anemia

Thrombocytopenia

Granulocytopenia

Kidney
Fanconi nephropathy

Liver
Fatty liver

Hepatomegaly

Jaundice

Endocrine function
Short stature

Delayed puberty

Hypoparathyroidism

Infertility

Diabetes mellitus

Laboratory findings
Lactic acidemia

Non-ketotic hypoglycemia

Dicarboxylic aciduria

Organic aciduria

Aminoaciduria

Myoglobinuria

Mitochondria are abnormal and there is neutropenia. This genetic defect has been mapped to chromosome Xq28[513] and involves mutation in the TAZ (G4.5) gene that encodes the tafassin protein. Seventy-three different disease-causing mutations have been identified.[513a] Diagnostically important laboratory findings include 3-methylglutaconic aciduria and acidemia, increased urinary excretion of citric acid cycle intermediates and 2-ethylhydracrylic acid, hypocholesterolemia, low levels of tetralinoleoyl cardiolipin in muscle, platelets and cultured fibroblasts, and mutation of Xq28-linked G4.5 (TAZ1) gene (see also Ch. 23).

Clinical and laboratory findings in mitochondrial disorders are shown in Box 12.5.

Diagnosis of mitochondrial disorders is multidisciplinary.[514–516] The key diagnostic procedures include detailed enzyme determinations and molecular analysis of mtDNA. The enzyme defects are usually assayed in fresh muscle samples, but cultured fibroblasts provide fresh cells for repeated enzyme measurements. PCR clarifies changes in the mtDNA from very small samples. Old paraffin-embedded tissue specimens can be used to study mtDNA.

Carnitine deficiency

Carnitine deficiency is transmitted as an autosomal recessive trait and results in a **defect in fatty acid transport across the inner mitochondrial membrane** (Fig. 12.70).[517] Carnitine is synthesized from peptide-bound lysine to trimethyllysine and further to α-butyrobetaine (Fig. 12.71). Carnitine also regulates the intra-mitochondrial CoA/acetyl-CoA ratio. Fatty acids are transported to liver and other tissues and form acyl-CoA esters (see earlier discussion of fatty acid oxidation defects). Primary carnitine deficiency is classified as **myopathic, systemic, and mixed forms.**[518] The myopathic form is manifested as progressive skeletal muscle weakness. Serum carnitine is normal but muscle carnitine

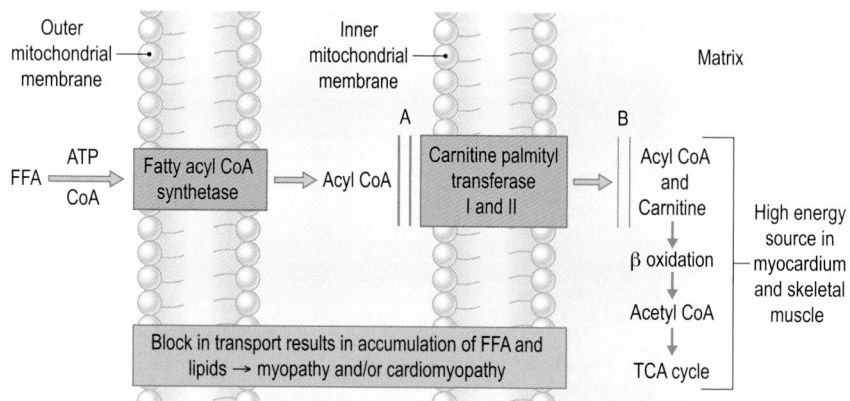

FIGURE 12.70 Transport of free fatty acids (FFA) across the inner mitochondrial membrane in carnitine metabolism. (A) Results in myopathy. (B) Results in cardiopathy (TCA, tricarboxylic acids).

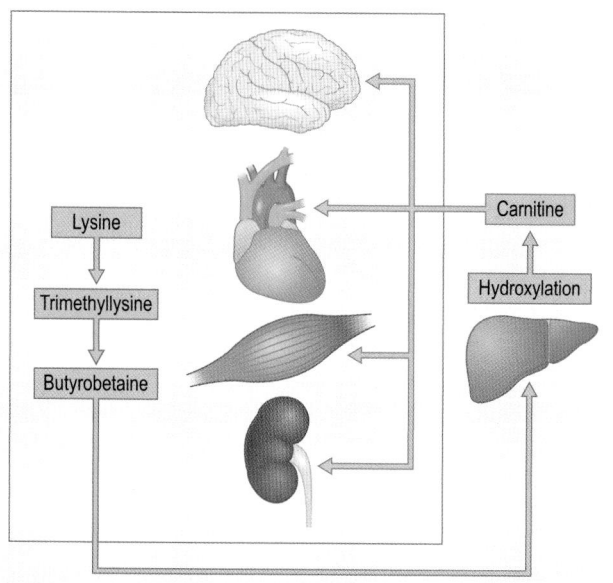

FIGURE 12.71 Transport of carnitine.

TABLE 12.28 CLINICAL FEATURES OF CARNITINE DEFICIENCY

	MCD	SCD	MxCD
Average age at onset (years)	15	3.5	4.5
Familial occurrence	+	+	+
Progressive weakness	Common	Frequent	Frequent
Encephalopathy	–	+	+
Cardiomyopathy	Rare	+	+
Respiratory symptoms	+	Rare	Rare
Myoglobinuria	+	–	+
Peripheral neuropathy	+	–	+
Serum carnitine	Normal	Decreased	Decreased
Increased serum CK	Usual	Usual	Usual
Lipid storage in muscle	+	+	+
Abnormal EMG	+	+	+
Response to carnitine	Usually good	Variable	Variable

MCD, myopathic carnitine deficiency; SCD, systemic carnitine deficiency; MxCD, mixed carnitine deficiency; CK, creatine kinase; EMG, electromyogram.

is low. Systemic carnitine deficiency is characterized by low serum and tissue carnitine concentrations. Abnormality of the CoA/acetyl-CoA ratio results in accumulation of acetyl-CoA compounds. The gene maps to chromosome 5q31.2-32.

Clinical features of carnitine deficiency are shown in Table 12.28.

Symptoms of cardiomyopathy, muscle weakness, hypotonia, hypoglycemia, hypoketonemia, and coma implicate a deficiency in many tissues, including heart, skeletal muscle, and liver. **Lipid accumulates in skeletal muscle in type I myocytes**, in liver, and frequently in the **cardiac muscle cells**.[519] EM demonstrates **abnormal mitochondria**. The pathologic features of carnitine deficiency are summarized in Box 12.6. Diagnosis is readily made by plasma carnitine levels or muscle biopsy. Treatment is administration of carnitine. **Secondary carnitine deficiency** may be associated with varied **defects of intermediary metabolism** (Box 12.7).[520]

Carnitine palmitoyl transferase deficiency

Carnitine palmitoyl transferase (CPT) deficiency results in two different clinical variants, one with hepatic (CPT I) and one with muscular symptoms (CPT II).

CPT I is important in the transfer of long-chain fatty acids into mitochondria where all the enzymes for β-oxidation are located. This enzyme is present in the outer mitochondrial membrane. CPT II is present on the inner mitochondrial membrane and catalyzes the regeneration of carnitine and the long-chain-fatty-acyl-CoA when they undergo β-oxidation.

CPT I deficiency

The clinical presentation is characterized by coma, seizures, hepatomegaly, and hypoketotic hypoglycemia following fasting, a viral infection or diarrhea. There is no evidence of chronic muscle weakness, and cardiomyopathy has not been noted. The onset is between 8 and 18 months.

BOX 12.6 PATHOLOGIC FEATURES OF SYSTEMIC CARNITINE DEFICIENCY

Heart

Gross – usually cardiomegaly, biventricular hypertrophy, mild endocardial fibrosis

Microscopic – myocardial fibers containing vacuoles of lipid (stains positively for neutral lipid)

EM – disruption of myofibrils by accumulation of frequently bizarrely shaped mitochondria; disrupted and twisted mitochondrial cristae with electron-dense inclusions

Liver

Microscopic – extensive fatty metamorphosis (microsteatosis)

EM – proliferation of endoplasmic reticulum and increased numbers of peroxisomes, lipid vacuoles

Skeletal muscles

Microscopic – accumulation of lipid droplets (type I fibers); positive neutral lipid (oil red O, Sudan black B, Nile blue sulphate); type I fibers, granular appearance with subsarcolemmal basophilic staining (ragged red fibers with Gomori trichrome stain)

EM – lipid vacuoles without limiting membrane adjacent to mitochondria; alteration of mitochondria – indistinct or concentric cristae, dense or paracentric inclusions

BOX 12.7 SECONDARY CARNITINE DEFICIENCY

Defects of intermediary metabolism

Methylenetetrahydrofolate reductase deficiency

Propionyl-coenzyme A carboxylase deficiency

Cytochrome C oxidase deficiency

Methylmalonyl-coenzyme A apomutase deficiency

Nicotinamide adenine dinucleotide-ubiquinone reductase deficiency

Fatty acyl-coenzyme A dehydrogenase deficiencies

  Long-chain deficiency

  Medium-chain deficiency

  Multiple deficiencies associated with ornithine transcarbamylase deficiency

  Isovaleric acidemia

  Glutaric acidemia

Carnitine octanoyltransferase deficiency

Mitochondrial adenosine triphosphatase deficiency

Kearns-Sayre syndrome

Secondary to other conditions

Chronic renal failure treated with hemodialysis

Myxedema, hypopituitarism, and adrenal insufficiency

Valproate-induced Reye syndrome

Hyperammonemia associated with valproic acid therapy

Kwashiorkor

Total parenteral nutrition in premature infants

Renal Fanconi syndrome

Chronic severe myopathies

Cirrhosis with cachexia

Pregnancy

High plasma carnitine levels (both total and free) distinguish CPT I deficiency from the other known carnitine defects.

The definitive diagnosis of CPT I deficiency is made by measuring enzyme activity in fibroblasts, leukocytes, or solid tissues. Long-term treatment with medium-chain triglyceride oil appears to prevent the recurrence of metabolic crises. The prognosis of CPT I deficiency with treatment is good.[521]

CPT II deficiency

Lethal deficiency of CPT II in newborns has been described. Neonatal onset of lethal multiorgan deficiency with dysmorphic features, cardiomyopathy, and cystic dysplasia of the kidney occurs. A late-onset form is more benign with myopathy. The enzyme defect is expressed in skeletal muscle, liver fibroblasts, and leukocytes. The gene is on chromosome 1p32.

Peroxisomal disorders

The peroxisomal diseases are a group of genetically determined disorders in which the major cause of pathology is either the **failure to form or maintain the peroxisome, or a defect in the function of a single enzyme** that is normally located in the peroxisome.

Peroxisomal enzymes oxidize d-amino acids, uric acid, 2-hydroxy acids, and very-long-chain fatty acids (VLCFAs)[522–524] and synthesize glycerolipids, glycerol ether lipids, and plasmalogens. Catalase in the peroxisome catalyzes the conversion of hydrogen peroxide to oxygen and water. Peroxisomal fatty acid oxidation is not dependent on carnitine.[522] **Abnormally high levels of VLCFAs in tissues and body fluids occur** in patients with many peroxisomal disorders.

Peroxisomal disorders can be subdivided into two major groups. In the first group the organelle fails to be formed or maintained and results in defective function of multiple peroxisomal enzymes. In the second group there is a genetically determined deficiency of a single peroxisomal enzyme, and peroxisome structure is intact. **Rhizomelic chondrodysplasia punctata** (RCDP) is placed in a separate third group, since there is at present no general agreement concerning the peroxisomal defect in this disorder. Abnormalities found in peroxisomal disorders are shown in Table 12.29.[525]

By complementation studies, these disorders are determined to be genetically heterogeneous, and the relationships between phenotype and genotype are complex. For instance, Zellweger syndrome with its characteristic and consistent phenotype can be associated with at least four distinct genotypes.

TABLE 12.29 GENERAL CHARACTERISTICS AND SPECIFIC BIOCHEMICAL FINDINGS IN PEROXISOMAL DISORDERS

Characteristics	X-linked ALD (adult form)	Refsum disease	Acatalasemia	Zellweger syndrome	Neonatal aid	Infantile Refsum disease	Chrondrodysplasia punctata	Hyperpipecolic acidemia
Inheritance	X-linked	AR	AR	AR	AR	AR	AR	AR
Sex	Male	M & F	M & F	M & F	M & F	Male	M & F	Male
Survival	Variable – usually adolescent	Adult	Adult	Usually <1 yr	1 to 6–8 yr	–	Usually <2 yr	Mostly <2 yr
Minor facial anomalies	Absent	Absent	Absent	Present	Absent	Present	Typical facial appearance	Present
Renal cysts	Absent	Absent	Absent	Present	Absent	–	+	–
Patellar calcification	–	–	–	Present	–	–	+	Calcific stippling
Eye abnormalities								
Cataracts	–	–	–	+	–	–	+	+
Retinal degeneration	–	+	–	+	–	+	+	+
Oral involvement	–	–	+	–	–	–	–	–
Pathologic changes								
Adrenals	Atrophy	Not involved	Not involved	Not involved	Atrophy	Not involved	Not involved	Not involved
Liver								
Fibrosis and micronodular cirrhosis	Absent	–	–	+++	Periportal fibrosis (mild)	Absent	–	Not involved
Hepatic siderosis	Absent	Absent	Absent	+	Absent	Absent	Absent	Absent
Brain demyelination	+	–	–	+	+	–	–	–
Neuronal heterotopia	–	–	–	+	–	–	–	+
Ultrastructural lamellar inclusions	In brain/adrenals	–	–	–	++	–	–	–
Peroxisomes Liver	Normal	Normal	Normal	Absent	Decreased	Absent	Decreased or absent, sometimes enlarged	Decreased
Biochemical abnormalities (body fluids)								
Very-Long-chain fatty acids (C26/C22)	Elevated	Normal	–	Elevated	Elevated	Elevated	–	Elevated
Pipecolic acid	Normal	Elevated	–	Elevated	Elevated	Elevated		Elevated
Phytanic acid	Normal	Elevated	–	Elevated	Elevated	Elevated		Elevated
Intermediates of bile acid synthesis	Normal	Normal	–	Elevated	Elevated	Elevated		–
Plasmalogen contents in tissues	Normal	–	–	Decreased	–	Decreased	Decreased	Decreased
De novo synthesis	Normal	–	–	Decreased	–	Decreased	–	–
Enzyme activity								
Dihydroxyacetone acyl transferase	Normal	–	–	Deficient	Deficient	Deficient	Deficient	Deficient
Alkyl dihydroxyacetone synthetase	–	–	–	Deficient	–	Deficient	–	–

ALD, adrenoleukodystrophy; AR, autosomal recessive; M & F, male and female; –, not reported.

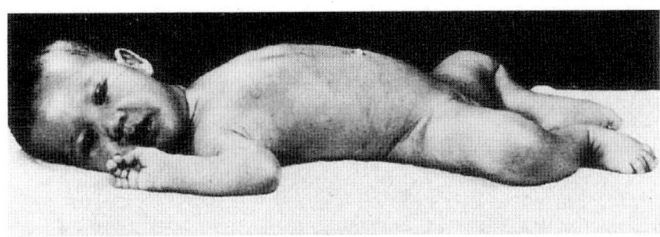

FIGURE 12.72 Zellweger syndrome.

Heterozygote identification is only available for X-linked ALD using VLCFA analysis or restriction fragment length polymorphism.[526]

The morphologic identification of a peroxisomal disorder requires histochemical, immunochemical, and EM techniques. Transmission EM allows identification of peroxisomes in the liver where the organelle normally is large and plentiful. The alkaline–diaminobenzidine reaction, applicable to light microscopy or EM, has been used to localize catalase and identify the peroxisomes.[527]

Except for type I hyperoxaluria, all peroxisomal disorders can be identified prenatally in the first or second trimester of pregnancy by measurement of VLCFAs, bile acid intermediates, and assays of plasmalogen synthesis[528] in cultured amniocytes or cultured chorionic villus cells.[529]

The prenatal diagnosis of type I hyperoxaluria requires measurement of alanine-glyoxylate aminotransferase (AGT) activity in biopsies of fetal liver.

Zellweger syndrome

Zellweger (cerebrohepatorenal) syndrome is inherited as an autosomal recessive trait. Newborn infants have a typical phenotype with high forehead, up-slanting palpebral fissures, hypoplastic supraorbital ridges, epicanthal folds, micrognathia, severe weakness and hypotonia (Fig. 12.72), seizures, and eye abnormalities including cataracts, glaucoma, corneal clouding, Brushfield spots, pigmentary retinopathy, and optic nerve dysplasia. They rarely live more than a few months with liver and renal involvement.

A microdeletion involving 7q11.12-q11.13 has been identified.[530] The incidence is 1 in 25 000 to 1 in 50 000.[531]

Some atypical patients with Zellweger syndrome (Versmold variant) have hypertonia and may live longer.[532,533] **Increased serum iron content** and evidence of **tissue siderosis** can be established in most cases before death and are diagnostically helpful.[534] Biochemical abnormalities include hypoglycemia, elevated serum iron, siderosis, hyperpipecolic acidemia, hepatic and cerebral glycogen storage, elevated VLCFAs, abnormal bile acids, dicarboxylic aciduria, and hypocarnitinemia. EM examination reveals **absence of demonstrable peroxisomes in the liver and kidney.**[535] The defect is also present in cultured skin fibroblasts[536] and amniocytes.[537] The brain shows a striking and characteristic disorder of neuronal migration involving the cerebral hemispheres, cerebellum, and inferior olivary nucleus.[538,539] **Brain** abnormalities include focal **lissencephaly and other cerebral gyral abnormalities, heterotopic cerebral cortex, olivary nuclear dysplasia,** defects of the corpus callosum, **numerous lipid-laden macrophages and histiocytes in cortical and periventricular areas, and dysmyelination.**[538]

Pathologically, the **liver** is enlarged and **fibrotic** in 76% of cases, and 37% show **micronodular cirrhosis** (Fig. 12.73A)[540] and hepatic **lobular disarray, biliary dysgenesis, and siderosis.** Excessive iron deposits are present in the youngest patients but diminish with time.[541] The kidneys show persistent fetal lobulations, and **corticorenal cysts** are frequent (Fig. 12.73B).[540] The cysts vary from glomerular microcysts to large cortical cysts of glomerular and tubular origin.[541] The **adrenal glands** show **cytoplasmic lamellar inclusions** that consist of cholesterol esterified with VLCFAs.[542] Eye pathology includes corneal clouding, congenital cataracts, and glaucoma. The posterior segment shows ganglion cell loss, gliosis of the optic nerve fiber layer, optic atrophy, and changes resembling retinitis pigmentosa.[543] The interstitial cells of the testis contain trilaminar lamellae. Malformations of the heart include ventricular septal defect, atrial septal defect, tetralogy of Fallot, and patent ductus arteriosus. Pancreatic islet cell hyperplasia, pancreatic fibrosis, thymic aplasia or hypoplasia, and mitochondrial myopathy have been described. The brain may show **pachygyria** or **lissencephaly** (Fig. 12.73C). Calcific stippling of the epiphyses occurs in 50% of Zellweger patients.[544, 545] The **DiGeorge syndrome** has been seen in several infants with Zellweger syndrome.[546]

Neonatal adrenoleukodystrophy

Neonatal adrenoleukodystrophy (NALD) is a slightly less severe illness than Zellweger syndrome, and the dysmorphic features are less striking. Peroxisomes in liver[543] or cultured skin fibroblasts[547] are diminished in number and VLCFA accumulation is less than in Zellweger syndrome. NALD may show **micropolygyria**[548] or only mild neuronal migrational defects and heterotopias.[549, 549a] Renal cysts are not observed.

Most NALD patients have an impaired adrenal cortisol response to ACTH stimulation, but overt adrenal insufficiency is infrequent.

NALD shows the same biochemical abnormalities as Zellweger syndrome.

Infantile Refsum disease

The mode of inheritance of infantile Refsum disease is **autosomal recessive**. It results from mutations of the *PEX1*, the *PEX2*, or the *PEX26* genes. Patients have moderately dysmorphic features, including epicanthal folds, deafness, retinal pigment abnormalities, developmental delay, flat bridge of the nose, and low-set ears. Early hypotonia and enlarged liver with impaired function are frequent. The level of **plasma phytanic acid is elevated** and cholesterol and lipoproteins are often moderately

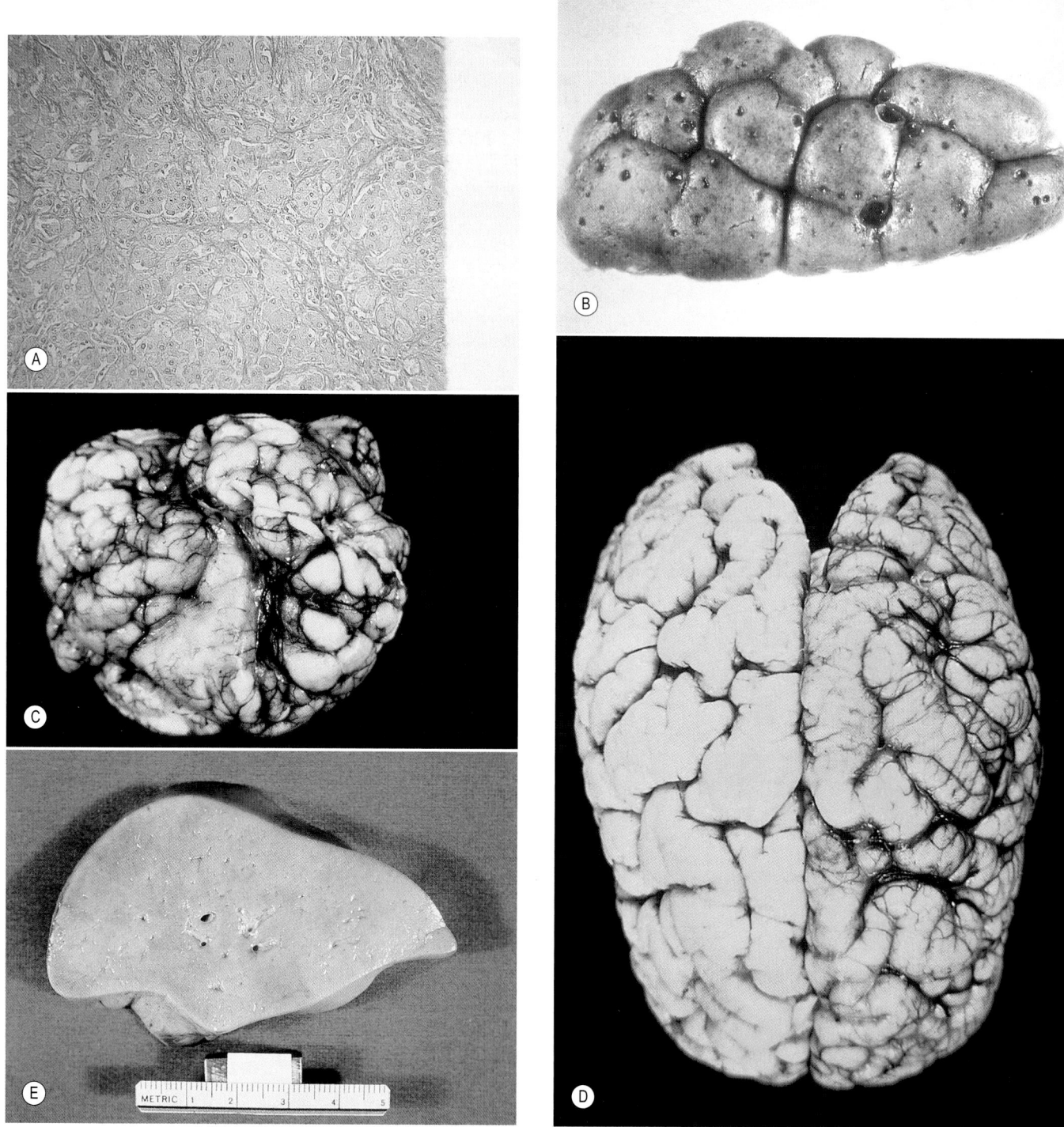

FIGURE 12.73 Zellweger syndrome. (A) Section of liver showing cirrhosis. (B) Kidney with multiple cortical cysts. (C) Brain with abnormal gyral pattern and lissencephaly. (D) Brain with pachygyria. (E) Liver with brown discoloration due to iron deposition.

reduced. Chondrodysplasia punctata and renocortical cysts are not present. The autopsy of a 12-year-old child[550] showed micronodular liver cirrhosis and small hypoplastic adrenals. The brain showed no malformations except for severe hypoplasia of the cerebellar granular layer and ectopic location of the Purkinje cells in the molecular layer.

X-linked adrenoleukodystrophy

X-linked adrenoleukodystrophy (ALD) was the first and most common peroxisomal disorder to be described. Depending on age of onset of symptoms, a number of types have been identified, including childhood, adolescent, and adult cerebral

ALD; adrenomyeloneuropathy (AMN); and asymptomatic ALD. The differential features of neonatal and X-linked ALD are shown in Table 12.30. The basic defect in X-linked ALD is a specific **impairment in the capacity to degrade VLCFAs**.[551] The defect involves impaired capacity to activate VLCFAs, i.e., defective function of the enzyme lignoceroyl-CoA synthetase.[552]

In childhood ALD, development is usually normal until age 4–8 years. Males exhibit a behavioral deficit that is progressive with emotional outbursts. Later, dementia, seizures, visual deficits due to cortical or optic nerve involvement, loss of coordination, and paralysis develop with progressive deterioration until death, usually by 10 years.[553,554] Adrenal insufficiency is the presenting manifestation in 15–30% of boys.[554] Pathologic changes[555] of X-linked and neonatal ALD are shown in Table 12.31.

The **adrenal glands are small**. The cells in the adrenal cortex, particularly the zona fasciculata, contain **cytoplasmic lipid inclusions** (Fig. 12.74A) with a characteristic **lamellar structure** seen in the ultrastructure (Fig. 12.74B).[555] These inclusions consist of cholesterol esterified with saturated VLCFAs, such as hexacosanoic (C26:0) and tetracosanoic (C24:0) acids. The same types of lipids accumulate in the CNS associated with a **severe demyelinative process** that in 85% of cases initially affects the posterior parietal or occipital regions. Perivascular infiltration by lymphocytes is similar to that observed in multiple sclerosis. White matter involvement causes characteristic abnormalities in computed tomographic (CT) or MRI studies owing to demyelination in the posterior portion of the brain, with a garland of accumulated contrast material.[556]

The X-linked ALD gene has been mapped to the terminal segment of the long arm of the X chromosome (Xq28).[557] It is caused by a mutation of the *ABCD1* gene, and molecular diagnosis is possible.[558]

Hyperpipecolic acidemia

The clinical features of hyperpipecolic acidemia closely resemble those of Zellweger syndrome, with hepatomegaly, hypotonia, eye changes, and excretion of pipecolic acid. However, EM shows peroxisomes in the liver, suggesting a functional disorder of the peroxisome.[559] Complementation studies suggest that hyperpipecolic acidemia is allelic with one form of Zellweger syndrome and with infantile Refsum syndrome.

Hyperoxaluria, primary oxalosis

There are two types of genetically determined hyperoxaluria. In the somewhat more common **type 1**, hyperoxaluria is accompanied by increased excretion of glycolic and glyoxylic

TABLE 12.30 ADRENOLEUKODYSTROPHY (ALD): DIFFERENCES BETWEEN X-LINKED ALD AND NEONATAL ALD

Characteristics	X-linked	Neonatal
Age of onset	Prepubertal boys	Neonatal
Clinical course	Slowly progressive, death in adolescence	Death by 6 yr
Storage material	VLCFA (C26–C24) in tissues	Same
Pathology		
Organs involved	Brain, adrenals	Brain, adrenals, liver, macrophages
Biochemical abnormalities		
1. Plasma concentration of VLCFA	Increased	Increased
2. Ratio of C26:0: C22:0	Abnormal	Abnormal
3. Hepatic catalase activity	Normal; 50% is sedimented (10.3 nmol/mL)	Abnormal, increased, 12% is sedimented (8 nmol/mL)
4. Total serum bile acids	Normal	Normal
5. Trihydroxycoprostanic acid (THEA) (normally absent)	Absent	Serum bile acids

VLCFA, very-long-chain fatty acids.

TABLE 12.31 ADRENOLEUKODYSTROPHY (ALD): PATHOLOGIC CHANGES

Characteristics	X-linked	Neonatal
Brain	Demyelination (centripetally spreading)	Diffuse demyelination
	Perivascular inflammatory infiltrates follow margin of demyelination	Perivascular inflammation, not intense
	Diffuse gliosis	Mild primary maldevelopment of cerebral cortex
	Relative neuronal and axonal preservation	
	Normal cytoarchitecture of cortex	
Adrenal glands	Atrophy of zona fasciculata and reticularis	Same
	Ballooning adrenocortical cells with or without striations	Usually not present
Ultrastructure	Bilamellar and laminar lipid inclusions	Same
Liver	Normal	Periportal fibrosis, macrophages, PAS-positive material
Ultrastructure peroxisomes	Peroxisomes identified	Reduced

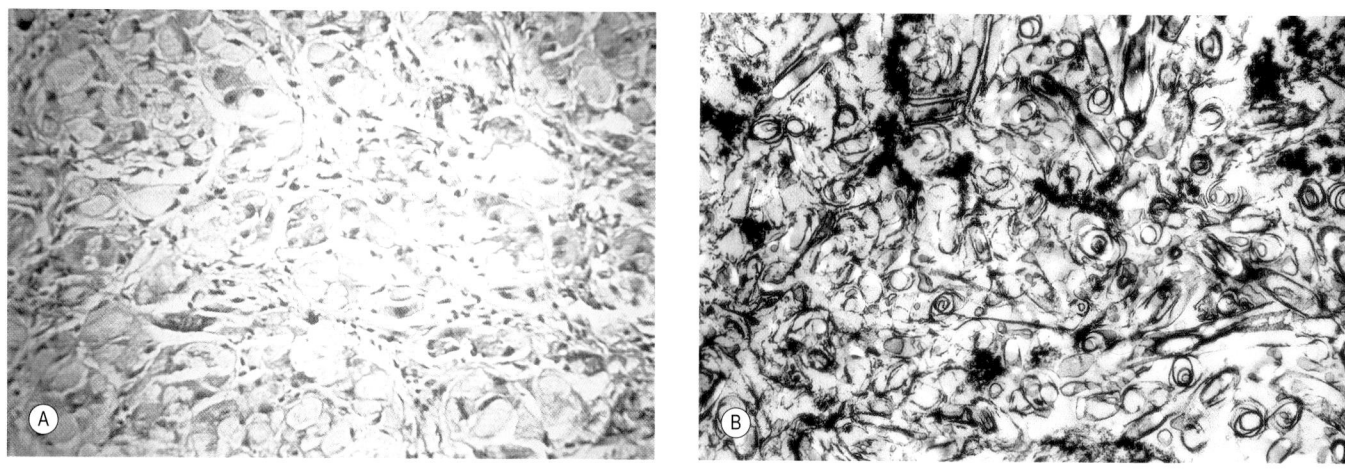

FIGURE 12.74 X-linked adrenleukodystrophy. (A) Microscopic section of adrenal gland. The cells are large with pink granular cytoplasm and striations. (B) EM of adrenocortical cells showing linear bilaminar intracytoplasmic inclusions (× 800).

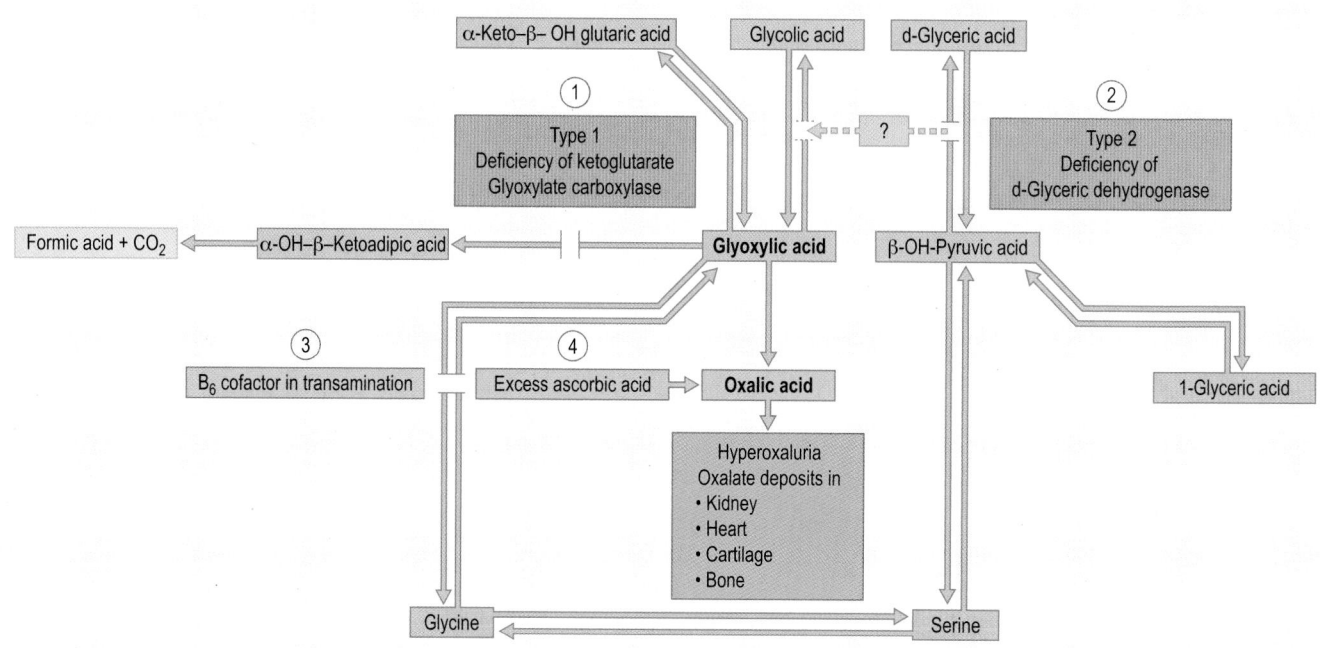

FIGURE 12.75 Metabolic pathway of oxalosis.

acid, while in **type 2** it is accompanied by increased excretion of L-glyceric acid (Fig. 12.75).[560] The mode of inheritance is autosomal recessive.

Patients have a **deficiency of the enzyme alanine-glyoxylate aminotransferase** that catalyzes the conversion of glyoxylate to glycine. This reaction results in the accumulation of glyoxylate, which is converted to oxalic acid. The enzyme is in the peroxisome.[561]

Nephrolithiasis, renal tubular acidosis, growth failure, progressive renal failure, recurrent fractures, and frequently cardiac arrhythmia with death before age 20 years characterize the course of the disease. The calcium salt of oxalate is deposited in the kidneys, bones, conduction system of the heart, soft tissues, CNS, and rete testis. The crystals have a rosette pattern with radial striations, giving a starburst appearance, and are best seen with polarized light (Fig. 12.76).

Diagnosis depends on demonstration of excessive quantities of glyoxylate, oxalate, and glycolic acid in the urine. The specific enzyme defect can be demonstrated by percutaneous liver biopsy. A combined hepatic and renal transplantation represents a sub-optimal option; as for most other metabolic diseases, gene replacement therapy is not yet feasible.[562,563]

Causes of **secondary oxalosis** include **ethylene glycol and dioxane poisoning, pyridoxine deficiency, inflammatory bowel**

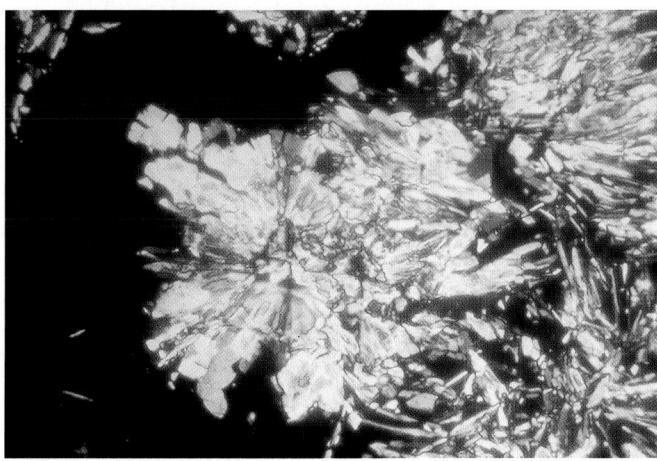

FIGURE 12.76 Oxalate crystals in bone showing a starburst appearance under polarized light.

disease, methoxyflurane anesthesia, diabetes mellitus, sarcoidosis, **excessive vitamin C ingestion, and jejunoileal bypass surgery.**[564]

Acatalasemia

Most people with acatalasemia are free of symptoms,[565] although gum ulceration may occur. The disorder appears to be heterogeneous. The human catalase gene has been cloned[566] and mapped to chromosome 11p13. Deletions in this region may be associated with Wilms tumor, aniridia, and hypocatalasemia.[567]

Classic Refsum disease

Classic Refsum disease is autosomal recessive, with an isolated **defect of phytanic acid oxidation**. This leads to accumulation of phytanic acid in tissues and body fluids.[568] Peroxisome structure and function are intact.[569] Manifestations include **retinitis pigmentosa, hearing loss, peripheral neuropathy, and cerebellar ataxia. Cardiac arrhythmias or conduction defects** may occur when phytanic acid levels are very high. A diet low in phytanic acid and plasmapheresis result in improvement.

Rhizomelic chondrodysplasia punctata

Rhizomelic chondrodysplasia punctata (RCDP) (see Ch. 34) is autosomal recessive and differs from the single-enzyme disorders since at least two and possibly three separate peroxisomal functions are deficient. In RCDP there is a profound **defect in plasmalogen synthesis**, more severe than that in Zellweger syndrome, defective phytanic acid oxidation, and failure to process the thiolase enzyme.[571–573] Levels of VLCFAs, bile acids, and pipecolic acid are normal. Peroxisome structure is abnormal. Peroxisomes may be absent, or hepatocytes may contain huge and irregularly shaped peroxisomes.

RCDP is characterized by **stippled foci of calcification** within the hyaline cartilage and is associated with dwarfing and multiple malformations due to contractures of vertebral bodies. **Coronal clefts** are occupied by cartilage and are due to an embryonic arrest. Short stature affects the proximal parts of the extremities (rhizomelia). Metaphyseal cupping, disturbed ossification, cataracts, microcephaly, severe mental retardation, and ichthyosiform erythroderma are present. It is due to a *PEX7* deficiency.[570]

Diagnostic tests for peroxisomal disorders

Diagnostic findings of greatest value include the following:

1. There are **increased levels of very-long-chain saturated fatty acids** in plasma, red blood cells,[574] or cultured skin fibroblasts.[575] Saturated VLCFAs are elevated in peroxisomal disorders,[314] except in RCDP.[568]
2. **Diminished levels of plasmalogen** in red cells and defective plasmalogen synthesis are a feature in all the disorders of peroxisome biogenesis[577–580] and represent the most striking single abnormality in RCDP.[568]
3. **Elevated pipecolic acid levels** in plasma are present in nearly all patients with disorders of peroxisomes.
4. **Elevated levels of plasma phytanic acid** are the prime and characteristic abnormality in **Refsum disease.**[568]
5. EM shows **absent or abnormal peroxisomes in liver biopsy specimens.**[581] An elegant procedure is described in which peroxisomal enzyme activities and immunoblot studies of peroxisomal fatty acid oxidation enzymes are performed in a rectal mucosal biopsy specimen.[320]

Prenatal diagnosis

Except for hyperoxaluria type 1, all peroxisomal disorders can be identified prenatally in the first or second trimester of pregnancy by measurement of VLCFA[583] and assays of plasmalogen synthesis[584] in cultured amniocytes or cultured chorionic villus cells (see also Ch. 14).

Disorders of metal metabolism

Neonatal iron storage disease (neonatal hemochromatosis)

Neonatal iron storage disease or neonatal hemochromatosis is clinically and pathologically defined by severe liver disease of **intrauterine onset** associated with **extrahepatic siderosis that spares the RES.**[585–589] Attempts to identify a primary disorder of iron handling have not been successful. Hemochromatotic siderosis in the perinate may be a sequel of intrauterine liver disease. Infants with neonatal hemochromatosis may be stillborn or born prematurely. Oligohydramnios may be present, and **placental edema or polyhydramnios** may occur. Infants with neonatal hemochromatosis exhibit hypoglycemia, hypoalbuminemia, edema, and frequently a hemorrhagic diathesis with or without evidence of fibrinogen consumption or thrombocytopenia, anemia, and acanthocytosis. Hyperbilirubinemia develops during

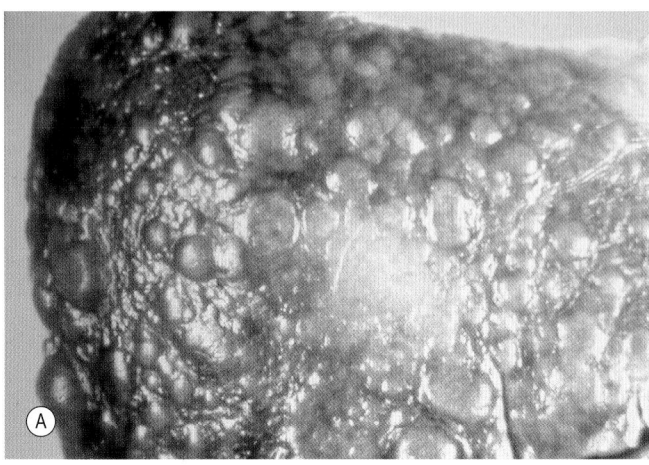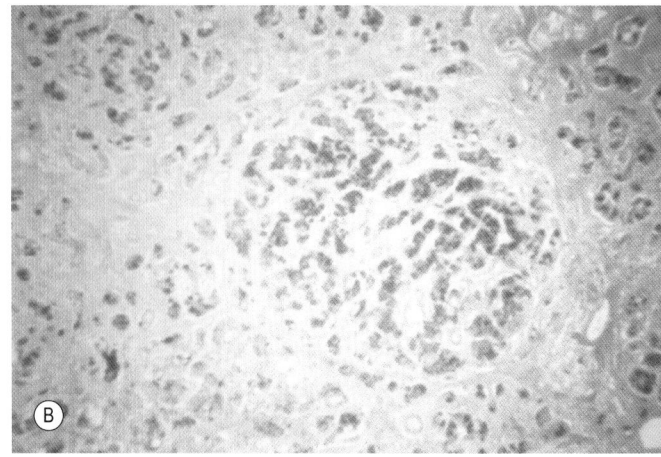

FIGURE 12.77 Neonatal hemochromatosis. (A) Liver of a neonate showing advanced congenital cirrhosis. (B) Iron overload in hepatocytes (Prussian blue stain).

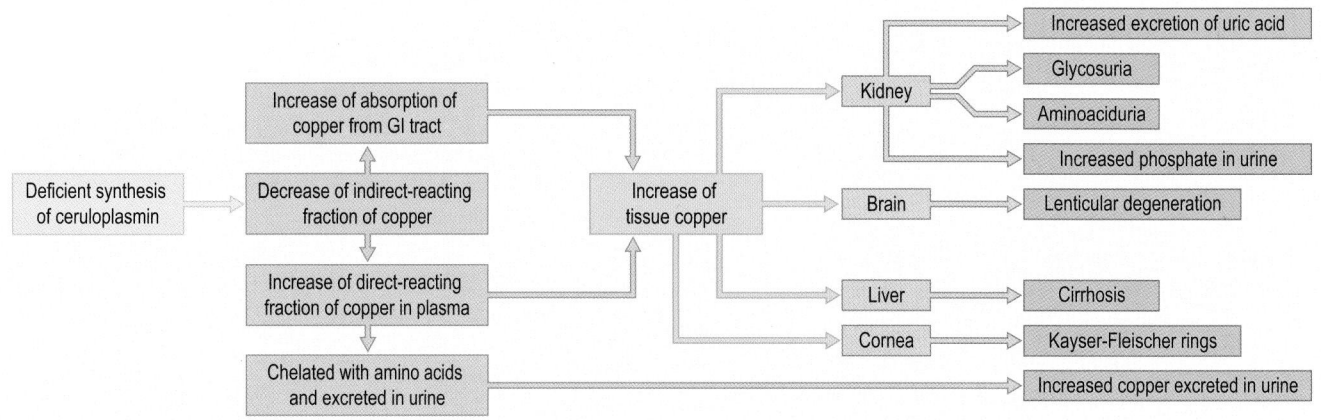

FIGURE 12.78 Wilson disease.

the first few days after birth. Transaminase activities are usually low and serum concentrations of AFP are high. Concentrations of α_1AT and ceruloplasmin may be low. **Hepatocellular injury** results in low levels of clotting factors, hypotransferrinemia, or hypoerythropoietinemia.[590]

The presence of hyperferritinemia supports the diagnosis of neonatal hemachromatosis. Transmission is autosomal recessive. However, this disorder may be related to a latent **maternal viral infection** affecting the fetal liver.[585] Grossly, the **liver** weighs less than normal, is fibrotic and **cirrhotic**, and may be bile stained (Fig. 12.77A). Congestive splenomegaly and esophageal varices occur. **Cholestasis and giant cell transformation** are found in all cases.[586–590] **Iron accumulation is massive in liver cells** (Fig. 12.77B)[591] with lesser quantities in biliary epithelium and Kupffer cells. Diffuse interacinar fibrosis, cholangiolar proliferation, and cirrhosis may be present at birth.[592,593] **Hyperplasia and hypertrophy of the islets of Langerhans** are constant findings. **Extrahepatic sites for iron accumulation** include **pancreatic acinar and islet cells, renal tubules, the adrenal cortex, and the thyroid follicular epithelium.**[593] The RES is spared. Ultrastructurally, hemosiderin accumulates in lysosomes

within hepatocytes and to a lesser extent in Kupffer cells and liver cytoplasm. Electron-dense masses and membranous arrays are observed in the lysosomes.[594]

Neonatal hemochromatosis has been associated with maternal autoantibodies against RO/SS-A and LA/SS-B ribonucleoproteins.[595]

Wilson disease

Wilson disease is an **inborn error of copper metabolism** (Fig. 12.78) with an autosomal recessive pattern of inheritance. **Levels of hepatic copper are elevated and liver and serum ceruloplasmin are decreased**, although in some cases the serum ceruloplasmin values may be normal. Serum copper levels are usually low and copper excretion in the urine is increased. Incorporation of radioactive copper into ceruloplasmin is considered a reliable test for Wilson disease. The gene, *ATP7B*, maps to chromosome 13q14.3.[596]

The Wilson disease gene product is a copper-binding P-type ATPase protein homologous to the Menkes disease

TABLE 12.32 COMPARISON OF MENKES AND WILSON DISEASES

	Menkes	Wilson
Location	Xq13.3/recessive	13q14.3/recessive
Clinical	Onset at birth, cerebral degeneration/MR, abnormal hair and facies, hypopigmentation, bone changes/cutis laxa, arterial rupture/thrombosis, hypothermia, death < 3 yr	Onset late childhood, liver disease, loss of coordination, involuntary movements, dysarthria, Kayser-Fleischer rings (cornea)
Laboratory findings	Decreased serum Cu, decreased serum ceruloplasmin, increased intestinal/kidney Cu, decreased liver Cu	Decreased serum Cu, decreased serum ceruloplasmin, increased urinary Cu, increased liver Cu
Cultured cells	Increased Cu accumulation, decreased Cu release	Normal in most patients
Defect	Intestinal Cu absorption, deficiency of Cu-dependent enzymes	Biliary Cu excretion, Cu incorporation into ceruloplasmin
Treatment	No effective treatment	Chelating agents: penicillamine, zinc salts
Potential animal models	Mottled mouse (Mo)	Toxic milk mouse (tx), Bedlington terriers
Gene product	Cu-binding P-type ATPase	Cu-binding P-type ATPase (60% identity with Menkes [kinky-hair] syndrome)
Expression	All tissues except liver	Liver, kidney, placenta
Mutation	16% deletions	Point mutations, small deletion

From Chelly J, Monaco AP. Cloning the Wilson disease gene. Nat Genet 1993; 5:317, with permission.
Cu, copper.

gene.[333] A comparison of Menkes and Wilson diseases is shown in Table 12.32. In Wilson disease there is a reduction in the rate of incorporation of copper into ceruloplasmin and a reduction in biliary excretion of copper.

Acute hepatitis and hepatic failure may be presenting features in the very young patient. **Hemolytic anemia, CNS signs, and Kayser-Fleischer rings** develop during the course of the disease.

The pathologic effects on the liver, kidneys, and brain are directly related to the accumulation of copper ions.

In the precirrhotic stage of Wilson disease, the changes resemble a chronic, active hepatitis with **focal necrosis, scattered acidophilic bodies**, and **moderate to marked steatosis**.[597] **Glycogenated nuclei** in periportal hepatocytes are a typical finding. Kupffer cells are hypertrophied and may contain **hemosiderin**. In later stages, **periportal fibrosis**, portal inflammation, and finally **cirrhosis** occur.

Submassive or massive hepatocellular necrosis may occur; the clinical and biochemical findings in such cases may resemble those of chronic active hepatitis.[597–599] The cirrhosis of Wilson disease is macronodular or macronodular and micronodular (Fig. 12.79) with periportal fibrosis, cholangiolar proliferation, and lymphocytic infiltration.[600]

The presence of **copper may not be cytochemically demonstrable in the precirrhotic stage**. In young, asymptomatic patients the copper is diffusely distributed in the cytoplasm but later accumulates in lysosomes.[601] Rhodanine and rubeanic acid stains specifically detect the presence of copper.[602] Copper-associated protein can be stained with orcein or aldehyde fuchsin.[603,604]

The ultrastructural changes are pathognomonic.[594] The mitochondria show marked pleomorphism; intracristal spaces widen, and microcysts form at the tips of the cristae. Copper deposits are extremely electron dense.

A major copper-binding protein in Wilson disease is metallothionein.[605] It has been suggested that the liver damage in Wilson disease may be due to the toxic ionic form of copper, which saturates the binding sites of metallothionein.[606]

Penicillamine or succimer chelating agents may be effective treatment. In cases of advanced liver disease, transplantation has been effective and curative.[606]

Menkes syndrome

Inherited as an **X-linked recessive trait of copper metabolism**, Menkes kinky hair syndrome is characterized by a **defect in intestinal copper absorption** resulting in a low serum level of copper and ceruloplasmin in affected male infants.[607,608] Copper is bound intracellularly in excess to metallothionein. All copper-containing enzymes (e.g., cytochrome oxidase, superoxide dismutase, dopamine hydroxylase, and lysyl oxidase) are defective. The gene, *ATP7A*, maps to Xq12-q13. The phenotype is characterized by a sparse, **steel wool appearance of the hair**, which is coarse and brittle (**pili torti**) (Fig. 12.80);[609] pudgy cheeks; skeletal changes including wormian bones and metaphyseal widening (particularly of the ribs and femora and lateral spurs); progressive cerebral deterioration with seizures; and widespread **arterial elongation and tortuosity** due to deficiency of copper-dependent cross-linking in the internal elastic membrane of the arterial wall.[610] By histofluorescence for the identification of catecholamines, peculiar, torpedo-like swellings of catecholamine-containing axons are seen in the peripheral nerve tracts, and reduced numbers of adrenogenic fibers in the middle forebrain.[610] Progressive neurologic deterioration leads to death in infancy.

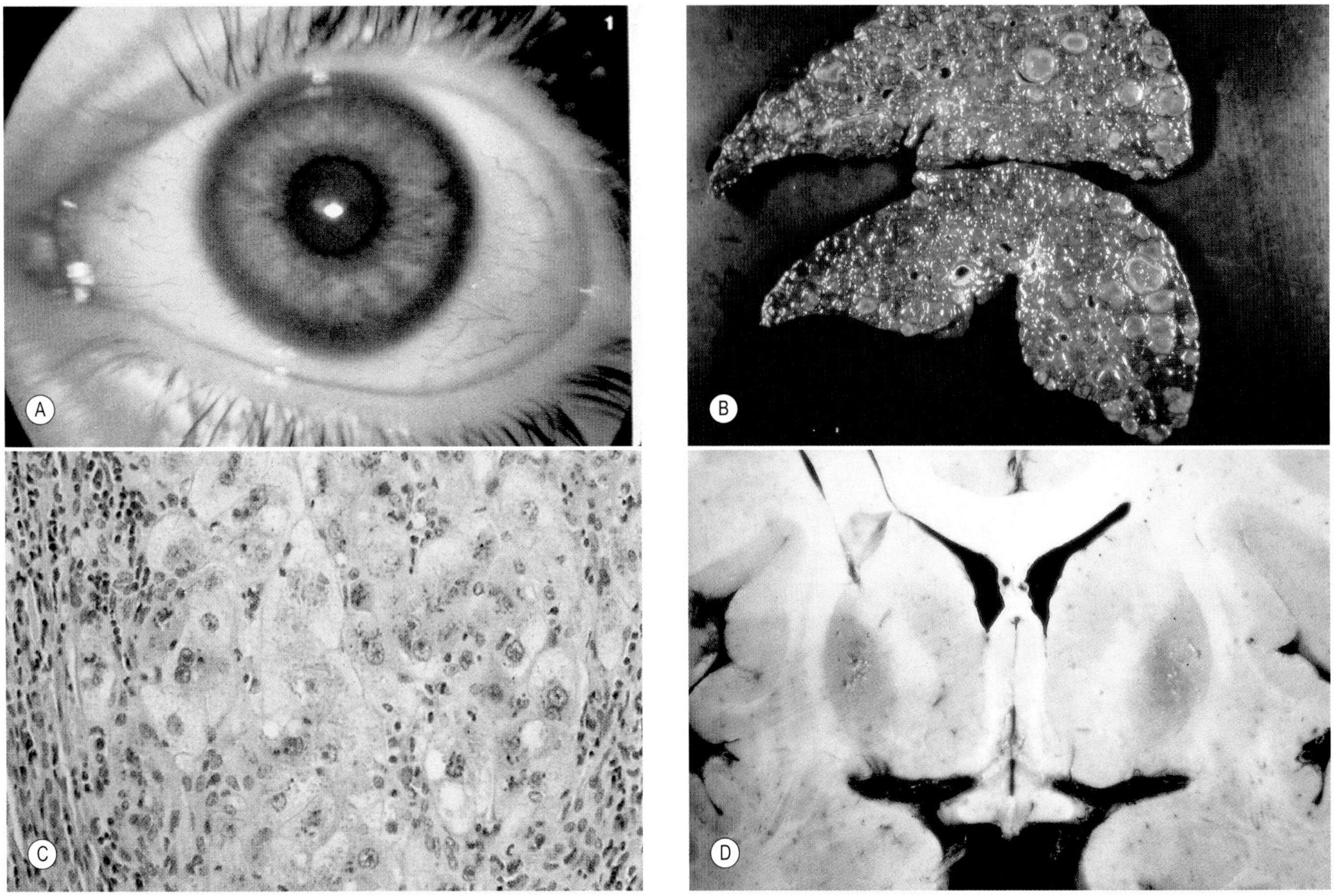

FIGURE 12.79 Wilson disease. (A) Kayser-Fleischer ring. (B) Liver cirrhosis. (C) Copper stain in section of liver. (D) Coronal section of brain through basal ganglia showing lesions in putamen.

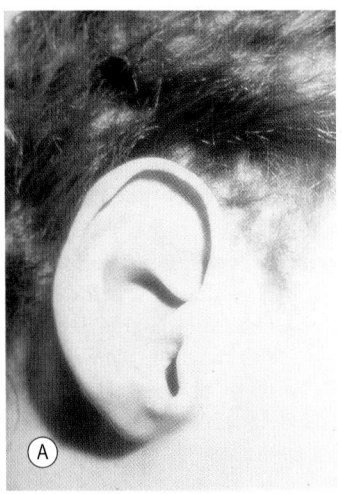

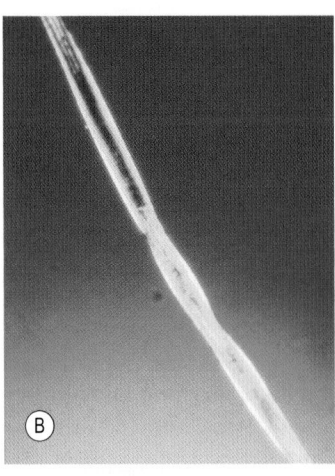

FIGURE 12.80 Menkes kinky hair syndrome. (A) Child with typical coarse kinky hair. (B) Hair under polarized light shows pili torti.

Occipital horn syndrome

A **variant of Menkes disease** is **type IX Ehlers-Danlos syndrome**, known as X-linked cutis laxa or **occipital horn syndrome**, in reference to the pathognomic **wedge-shaped calcification that forms within the trapezium and sternocleidomastoid muscles** at their attachment to the occipital bone in affected individuals.[611] Clinical findings include lax skin and joints, bladder diverticula, inguinal hernia, vascular tortuosity, and normal or slightly subnormal intelligence. Biochemically, plasma copper and ceruloplasmin levels are in the low to normal range, copper egress in cultured fibroblasts is impaired to the same degree as in classic Menkes disease, and the activity of fibroblast lysyl oxidase is markedly reduced.

Cystic fibrosis

Cystic fibrosis is a common metabolic disorder inherited as an **autosomal recessive trait** and characterized by steatorrhea and malnutrition resulting from pancreatic exocrine insufficiency, severe pulmonary disease, and disturbances in sweat- and mucus-secreting glands. In whites, it is estimated to occur in 1 in 2000 to 1 in 3000 liveborn infants with equal sex occurrence.

The defect is identified as a mutation of the **cystic fibrosis transmembrane regulator (CFTR) gene on chromosome 7**.[612] The most common mutation results in a protein defective in phenylalanine at position 508, referred to as ΔF508; more than 400 other mutations have been identified.

The pathology has been extensively reviewed.[613] It may present in the perinatal period as a **meconium ileus**, in which meconium is so viscid that it results in intestinal obstruction and even rupture in the fetus or newborn, leading to meconium peritonitis (see Ch. 25). The pancreas in severe cases contains **dilated and cystic ducts** filled with inspissated secretion. The acini may be completely destroyed by fibrosis; the islets are usually intact. **Nasal polyps, salivary glands, duodenum, small bowel, and appendix** are the sites of **accumulation of eosinophilic secretions**. The lung presents a wide spectrum of changes (see Ch. 24). Grossly, **zones of emphysema alternate with areas of atelectasis**, depending on whether the obstruction by viscid secretions has been partial or complete. Secondary infection is usually due to *Staphylococcus aureus* or *Pseudomonas aeruginosa* and leads to **bronchiectasis**. In long-standing cases in which **vitamin A deficiency** and infection co-exist, there is often **squamous metaplasia of the tracheobronchial mucosa**. At the time of death, the entire tracheobronchial tree is usually filled with dense purulent material. In 90% of cases, this yields a pure culture. In the liver, **focal biliary cirrhosis** occurs in 10% of infants up to 3 months of age and 25% over 1 year of age.[614] Myocardial lesions have been related to mitochondrial deficiency secondary to malabsorption. The gallbladder and the cystic duct may be filled with mucus. Severe anemia, hepatic dysfunction, and respiratory failure may occur in early infancy.[614] Young children are predisposed to salt depletion, especially with salt loss due to vomiting

and diarrhea. Mild mutations are found in males with congenital bilateral absence of the vas deferens. Almost all newborn males have vasoepidermal abnormalities. This is a disruption, not a developmental anomaly.

Methods of presumptive diagnosis rely on detection of either abnormal chloride secretion in sweat or, in newborns, elevated immunoreactive trypsinogen;[614,615] and for prenatal diagnosis, measurement of microvillar enzymes in amniotic fluid.[352] **DNA probes** are valuable for diagnosis. DNA can be isolated via PCR and used to detect the ΔF508 (the most common mutation in the white population), Δ1507, G551D, R553X, and S549N mutations. With these DNA analyses, up to 95% of cystic fibrosis mutations can be detected.

Porphyrias

Porphyrias are due to **errors in heme synthesis**.[616] They have variable forms of inheritance and are classified according to the site of their main effect as either erythroid or hepatic types (Table 12.33).

Congenital erythropoietic porphyria

Patients with congenital erythropoietic porphyria (CEP) have marked skin **photosensitivity**. Bullae may form and the fluid may fluoresce. The genetic defect, inherited as an autosomal recessive characteristic, is a **deficiency of uroporphyrinogen III cosynthetase**. Hemolysis is common and improves after splenectomy, sunscreens, or β-carotene administration. Skin infections are common. Teeth and urine may be reddish-brown. Urinary porphyrins are increased.

Bone marrow reveals erythroid hyperplasia. Normoblasts and reticulocytes fluoresce.

Erythropoietic protoporphyria

Patients with erythropoietic protoporphyria (EPP) may have no symptoms or may have mild photosensitivity. **Reduced ferrochetalase** is inherited as an **autosomal dominant** feature. Some patients develop liver disease that may progress to cirrhosis and protoporphyrin-containing gallstones. Stool protoporphyrins are increased.

A severe hepatic form is inherited as an **autosomal recessive** condition with signs and symptoms similar to CEP. Scarring and scleroderma-like skin changes occur early in life; hypertrichosis and red teeth are common. The **red blood cells** in peripheral smears **fluoresce under polarized light**. Urinary uroporphyrin is increased. Severe liver disease may progress to **cirrhosis** (Fig. 12.81).[617]

Skin biopsy shows subepidermal bullae and other signs similar to those of porphyria cutanea tarda (PCT).

TABLE 12.33 CLASSIFICATION AND CHARACTERISTICS OF CONGENITAL PORPHYRIAS

McKusick no.	Disease	Inheritance	Enzymatic defect	Metabolites present in excess		
				Urine	Feces	Erythroid cells
263700	Congenital erythropoietic porphyria	AR	Uroporphyrinogen 1 synthetase and uroporphyrinogen III cosynthetase	Uroporphyrin I ++++ Coproporphyrin I +++	Coproporphyrin I ++++ Uroporphyrin I ++	Uroporphyrin I ++++ Coproporphyrin ++
177000	Congenital erythropoietic Protoporphyria	AD	Ferrochetalase	Normal	Protoporphyrin ++++ Coproporphyrin ++	Protoporphyrin ++++ Coproporphyrin + Coproporphyrin III ++++
176000	Intermittent acute porphyria	AD	Uroporphyrinogen I synthetase	δ-aminolevulinic acid ++++ Porphobilinogen ++++	Normal	Normal
121300	Hereditary coproporphyria	AD	Coproporphyrinogen synthetase	Coproporphyrin III +++	Coproporphyrin III +++ Protoporphyria +	Normal
176200	Variegate porphyria	AD	Protoporphyrinogen oxidase	δ-aminolevulinic acid ++ Porphobilinogen ++	X-porphyrin ++++ Protoporphyrin ++++ Coproporphyrin ++++	Normal
176100	Porphyria cutanea tarda	AD	Uroporphyrinogen decarboxylase	Uroporphyrin I and III ++++	Protoporphyrin N to ++ Coproporphyrin N to ++	Normal

Acute intermittent porphyria

Acute intermittent porphyria (AIP) is the most common porphyria but is rarely symptomatic before puberty. It is inherited as an **autosomal dominant** trait due to **porphobilinogen deaminase deficiency**. Severe intermittent abdominal pain, particularly after ingestion of drugs, is the striking clinical feature. Vomiting, constipation, diarrhea, muscle pains, weakness, and seizures may occur. Signs and symptoms may be confused with those of psychiatric illness. King George III of Britain had this disorder.

Edema and irregularity of the myelin sheaths of autonomic and peripheral nerves and axonal vacuolization are found on histologic examination. In the CNS, reddish fluorescence is found in the white matter. Neuronal loss and gliosis are present in other parts of the brain.

Hereditary coproporphyria

Hereditary coproporphyria (HCP) is an **autosomal dominantly inherited** disease with neurologic symptoms similar to, but milder than, those in AIP, and is due to **deficiency of coproporphyrinogen oxidase**. Photosensitivity is also present. Urinary aminolevulinic acid and porphobilinogen are increased. Coproporphyrins may be found in the urine.

Variegate porphyria (VP)

Variegate porphyria (VP) is an **autosomal dominantly inherited** disease due to **protoporphyrinogen oxidase deficiency** with signs and symptoms similar to HCP. Aminolevulinic acid and porphobilinogen are found in the urine and stools.

Porphyria cutanea tarda

Porphyria cutanea tarda (PCT) may be inherited but is more commonly acquired, and is due to decreased activity of uroporphyrinogen decarboxylase. **Cutaneous photosensitivity is marked, with large bullae formation. Uroporphyrins are found in the urine.** Vessels in the dermis are PAS positive. Immunofluorescence reveals immunoglobulins G and M. **Liver biopsy reveals siderosis and fatty changes. Cytoplasmic inclusion bodies due to crystallized porphyrins emit red fluoresence.**

Bone metabolic inborn errors
Hypophosphatasia

Alkaline phosphatase functions to release phosphate ions. Deficiency results in defects of bone mineralization (see also

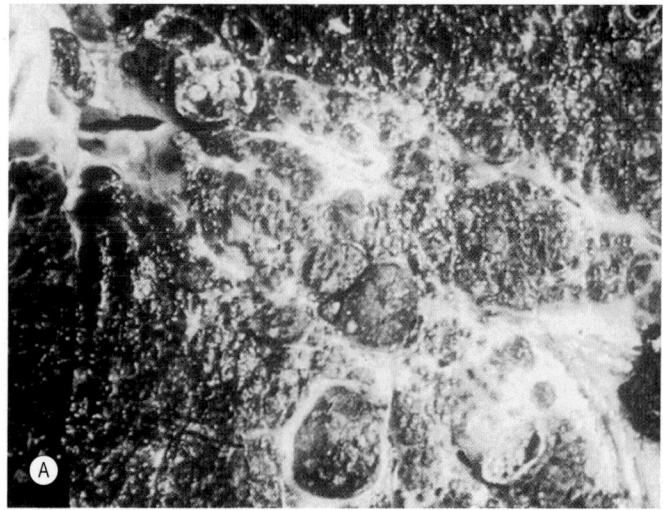
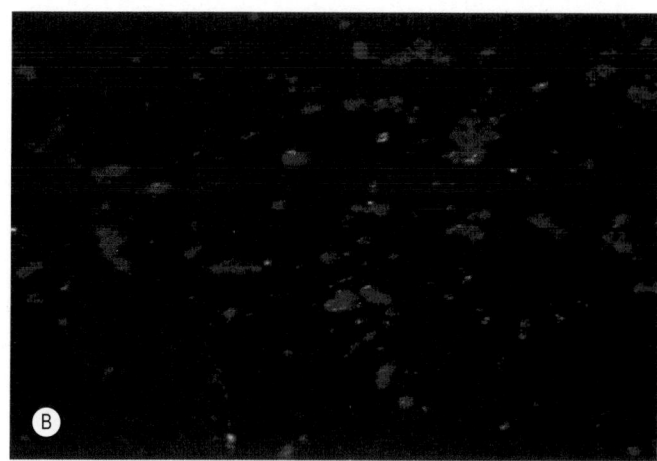

FIGURE 12.81 Erythropoietic protoporphyria. (A) Gross appearance of reddish brown cirrhotic liver in a 9-year-old child who died from liver failure. (B) Red fluorescence of porphyrin pigment in hepatocytes.

Ch. 31). **Serum alkaline phosphatase levels are low and urinary phosphoethanolamine, pyridoxal phosphate, and inorganic pyrophosphate are increased.**[618]

In the infantile autosomal recessively inherited form, short extremities, fractures, hypercalcemia, hypercalciuria, nephrocalcinosis, and cranial synostosis are found. Skeletal demineralization is marked on X-ray examination. Treatment to decrease serum calcium is helpful.

Other forms of hypophosphatasia are either autosomal recessive or autosomal dominant and are milder, becoming symptomatic with **fractures, loss of teeth, and rachitic bone changes** after 3–4 years of age. Some individuals have similar bone and urinary findings with normal serum levels of alkaline phosphatase (pseudohypophosphatasia).

Vitamin D-resistant rickets

Rickets may develop in infants with adequate intake of vitamin D or adequate exposure to sunlight.[619] Clinical and pathologic findings are similar to those found in children with vitamin D deficiency. Hereditary **deficiency of renal 1-α-hydroxylase** results in **deficiency of 1,25-dihydroxy-D** with normal serum levels of 25-hydroxy-D. These patients respond to physiologic doses of 1,25-dihydroxy-D. Deficiency of receptor sites of 1,25-dihydroxy-D results in a more severe form of rickets, which responds poorly or not at all to pharmacologic doses of 1,25-dihydroxy-D. This disorder has been mapped to the short arm of X chromosome at Xp22.1 and the gene PHE[x] has been cloned.

A related disorder, hereditary hypophosphatemic rickets with hypercalciuria has high serum 1,25-dihydroxy-D and intestinal absorption of calcium and hypercalciuria. This disorder is autosomal recessive, and is linked to chromosome 5. Vitamin D-resistant rickets shows genetic heterogeneity.

Dedication

Dedicated to the Immortal Memory of JAMES CHRISTIAN GILBERT (born 3 January 1960, died 11 July 1983) …who realized early that "The earth is full of things that permit man a partnership with God …" and that "Man's inner liberation is God's justification."

References

1. Garrod AE. Inborn errors of metabolism. London: Oxford Press; 1909.
2. Beaudet AL, Scriver CR, Sly WS, et al. Genetics biochemist and molecular basis of variant human phenotypes. In: Scriver CR, Beaudet AL, Sly WS, eds. The metabolic and molecular bases of inherited disease, 8th edn. New York: McGraw-Hill; 2001.
3. Fernandez J, Saudubray J-M, Tada K, eds. Inborn metabolic diseases. Diagnosis and treatment. Berlin: Springer-Verlag; 1990.
4. Applegarth DA, Dimmick JE, Toone JR. Laboratory detection of metabolic disease. Pediatr Clin North Am 1989; 36:49–65.
5. Ishak KG, Sharp HL. Metabolic errors and liver disease. In: MacSween RNM, Anthony PP, Scheuer PJ, eds. Pathology of the liver. Edinburgh: Churchill Livingstone; 1987.
6. Vogler C, Rosenberg HS, Williams JC, et al. Electron microscopy in the diagnosis of lysosomal storage diseases. Am J Med Genet Suppl 1987; 3:243–255.
7. O'Brien JS, Bernett J, Veath ML, et al. Lysosomal storage disorders. Diagnosis by ultrastructural examination of skin biopsy specimens. Arch Neurol 1975; 32:592–599.
8. Roberts DJ, Ampola MG, Lage JM. Diagnosis of unsuspected fetal metabolic storage disease by routine placental examination. Pediatr Pathol 1991; 11:647–656.

Storage diseases

9. McKusick VA, et al. Mendelian inheritance in man. A Catalogue of human genetics and genetic disorders autosomal dominant recessive and X-linked phenotypes, 12th edn. Baltimore: Johns Hopkins University Press; 1998.

10. Scriver CR, Beaudet AL, Sly WS, et al., eds. The metabolic and molecular bases of inherited disease, 18th edn. New York: McGraw-Hill; 2001.

10a. Gilbert-Barness E, Barness LA. Metabolic diseases: foundations of clinical management, genetics and pathology. South Natick, MA: Eaton Publishing Co.; 2000.

10b. Meikle PJ, Hopwood JJ, Clague AR, et al. Prevalence of lysosomal storage disorders. JAMA 1999; 281(3):249–254.

Mucopolysaccharidoses

11. Neufeld EF, Muenzes J. The mucopolysaccharidoses. In: Scriver CR, Beaudet AL, Sly WS, et al., eds. The metabolic and molecular bases of inherited disease, 8th edn. New York: McGraw-Hill; 2001.

12. Sly WS. The mucopolysaccharidoses. In: Bondy PD, Rosenberg LE, eds. Metabolic control and disease, 8th edn. Philadelphia: WB Saunders; 1980.

13. Clements PR, Brooks DA, Saccone GPT, et al. Human a-$_L$-iduronidase 1. Purification, monoclonal antibody production and subunit molecular mass. Eur J Biochem 1985; 152:21–28.

14. Young EP. Prenatal diagnosis of Hurler disease by analysis of a-$_L$-iduronidase in chorionic villi. J Inherit Metab Dis 1992; 15:224–230.

15. Dimmick JE, Applegarth DA. Inherited metabolic diseases. In: Stocker JT, Dehner LP, eds. Pediatric pathology. Philadelphia: JB Lippincot; 1992.

16. Gilbert EF. The effects of metabolic diseases on the ctardiovascular system. Am J Cardiovasc Pathol 1987; 1:189–213.

17. Van de Kamp JJP, Niermeyer MF, Von Figura K, et al. Genetic heterogeneity and clinical variability in the Sanfilippo syndrome. Clin Genet 1981; 20:152.

18. Taylor HR, Hollows FC, Hopwood JJ, et al. Report of a mucopolysaccharidosis occurring in Australian aborigines. J Med Genet 1978; 15:455–461.

19. Guffon N, Souillet G, Maire I, et al. Follow-up of nine patients with Hurler syndrome after bone marrow transplantation. J Pediatr 1998. 133:119–125.

20. Marwick TH, Bastian B, Hughes CF, et al. Mitral stenosis in the Maroteaux-Lamy syndrome: a treatable cause of dyspnoea. Postgrad Med J 1992; 68:287–288.

21. Tan CT, Schaff HV, Miller FA Jr, et al. Valvular heart disease in four patients with Maroteaux-Lamy syndrome. Circulation 1992; 85:188–195.

22. Machin GA. Hydrops revisited: literature review of 1414 cases published in the 1980s. Am J Med Genet 1989; 34:366–390.

23. Irani D, Kim HS, El-Hibri H, et al. Postmortem observations on β-glucuronidase deficiency as a cause of fetal hydrops. Ann Neurol 1983; 14:486–490.

24. Kagie MJ, Kleijer WJ, Huijmans JGM, et al. β-glucuronidase deficiency as a cause of fetal hydrops. Am J Med Genet 1992; 42:693–695.

25. Strangenberg M, Lingman G, Roberts G, et al. Mucopolycassharidosis VII as cause of fetal hydrops in early pregnancy. Am J Med Genet 1992; 15:142–144.

26. Clarke LA, Dimmick JE, Applegarth DA. Pathology of inherited metabolic diseases. In: Dimmick JE, Kalousek DK, eds. Developmental pathology of the embryo and fetus. Philadelphia: Lippincott; 1992: 199.

27. Ginsburg LC, DiFerrnati DR, Caskey CT, et al. Glucosaurine-6-SO4 sulfatase deficiency: a new mucopolysaccharidosis (abstract). Clin Res 1977; 25:471A.

28. DiFerrante N. N-acetylglucosamine-6-sulfate sulfatase deficiency reconsidered (letter). Science 1980; 210:448.

28a. Staba SL, Escolar ML, Poe M, et al. Cord-blood transplants from unrelated donors in patients with Hurler's syndrome. N Engl J Med 2004; 350(19):1960–1969.

28b. Wraith JE. The clinical presentation of lysosomal storage disorders. Acta Neurol Taiwan 2004; 13(3):101–106.

29. Natowicz MR. Clinical and biochemical manifestations of hyaluronidase deficiency. N Engl J Med 1996; 335:1029–1033.

Glycoprotein storage diseases

30. Spranger J, Gilbert EL, Aria S, et al. Geleophysic dysplasia. Am J Med Genet 1984; 19:487–499.

31. Zugibe FT, Gilbert EL, Gaziano D. Glycoprotein storage disease: a new entity. Am J Med 1969; 47:135–140.

32. Dickerson GR, Lott IT, Kolodny EH, et al. A light and electromicroscope study of mannosidosis. Hum Pathol 1980; 11:245–256.

33. Hug G. Nonbilirubin genetic disorders of the liver. In: Gall ED, Mostofi FK, eds. The liver. International Academy of Pathology Monograph No 13. Baltimore: Williams and Wilkins; 1972:21.

34. Hug G, Schubert WK, Schwachman H. Imbalance of liver phosphorylase and accumulation of hepatic glycogen in a girl with progressive disease of the brain. J Pediatr 1965; 67:741–751.

35. Murphree AL, Beaudet AL, Palmer EA, et al. Cataract in mannosidosis. Birth Defects Orig Artic Ser 1976; 12:319–334.

36. Arbisser AI, Murphree AL, Garcia CA, et al. Ocular findings in mannosidosis. Am J Ophthalmol 1976; 82:465–471

37. Letson RD, Desnick RJ. Punctate lenticular opacities in type II mannosidosis. Am J Ophthalmol 1978; 82:218–224.

38. Warner TG, Mock AK, Nyhan WL, et al. α-Mannosidosis: analysis of urinary oligosaccharides with high performance liquid chromatography and diagnosis of a case with unusually mild presentation. Clin Genet 1984; 25:248–255.

39. Hommes FA, Varghese M. High performance liquid chromatography of urinary oligosaccharides in the diagnosis of glycoprotein degradation disorders. Clin Chim Acta 1991; 203:211–224.

40. Blom HJ, Anderson HC, Krasnewich DM, et al. Pulsed amperometric detection of carbohydrates in lysosomal storage disease fibroblasts: a new screening technique for carbohydrate storage diseases. J Chromatogr 1990; 533:11–21.

41. Thomas GH. Disorders of glycoprotein degradation and structure: α-mannosidosis, β-mannosidosis, fucosidosis, sialidosis, aspartyglucosaminuria, and carbohydrate-deficient glycoprotein syndrome. In: Scriver CR, Beaudeet AL, Sly WS, et al., eds. The metabolic and molecular bases of inherited disease, 8th edn. New York: McGraw-Hill; 2001:2529,

42. Prence EM, Natowicz MR. Diagnosis of α-mannosidase in plasma. Clin Chem 1992; 38:501–503.

43. Champion MJ, Shows TB. Mannosidosis: assignment of the lysosomal α-mannosidase B gene to chromosome 19 in man. Proc Natl Acad Sci USA 1977; 74:2968–2972.

44. Ingram PH, Bruns GAP, Regina VM, et al. Expression of α-D-mannosidase in man–hamster somatic cell hybrids. Biiochem Genet 1977; 15:455–476.

45. Brooks JD, Shaw DJ, Meredith L, et al. Localization of genetic markers and orientation of the linkage group of chromosome 19. Hum Genet 1994; 68:282.

46. Martiniuk F, Ellenbogen A, Hirschhorn K, et al. Further regional localization of the genes of human acid α glucosidase (GAA), peptidase D (PEPD), and α-mannosidase B (MANB) by somatic cell hybridization. Hum Genet 1985; 69:109–111.

47. Kaneda Y, Hayes H, Uchida T, et al. Regional assignment of five genes on human chromosome 19. Chromosoma 1987; 95:8–12.

48. Mehta J, Desnick RJ. Abbreviated PR interval in mannosidosis. J Pediatr 1978; 92:599–601.

49. Kjellman B, Gamstorp I, Brun A, et al. Mannosidosis: a clinical and histopathologic study. J Pediatr 1969; 75:366–373.

50. Ormos J, Monus Z, Szabo L, et al. Die beduetung der elektronenmikrosckepischen. Untersuchung der Leberbiopsie bei der Beurteilung der verschiedenen mucopolysaccharidosen. Verh Dtsch Ges Pathol 1971; 55: 399–405.

51. Wall DA, Grange DK, Goulding P, et al. Bone marrow transplantation for the treatment of α-mannosidosis. J Pediatr 1998; 133:282–285.

52. Labrisseau A, Brouchu P, Jasmin G. Fucosidose de type 1: étude anatomique. Arch Fr Pediatr 1979; 36:1013–1023.

53. Fowler ML, Nakai H, Byers MG, et al. Chromosome 1 localization of the human α-L-fucosidase structural gene with a homologous site on chromosome 2. Cytogenet Cell Genet 1986; 43:103–108.

Aspartylglycosaminuria

54. Thomas GH. Disorders of glycoprotein degradation and structure: α-mannosidosis, β-mannosidosis, fucosidosis, sialidosis, and aspartylglucosaminuria, and carbohydrate-deficient clycoprotein syndrome. In: Scriver CR, Beaudet AL, Sly WS, et al,. eds. The metabolic and molecular bases of inherited disease, 8th edn. New York: McGraw-Hill; 2001.

55. Ikonen E, Aula P, Gron K, et al. Spectrum of mutations in aspartylglucosaminuria. Prod Natl Acad Sci USA 1991; 88:11222–11226.

56. Haltia M, Palo J, Autio S. Aspartylglucosaminuria: a generalized storage disease. Morphological and histochemical studies. Acta Neuropathol (Berl) 1975; 31:243–255.

57. Autio S, Visakorpi JK, Järvinen H: Aspartylglucosaminuria. Further aspects on its clinical picture, mode of inheritance and epidemiology based on a series of 57 patients. Ann Clin Res 1973; 5:149–155.

58. Hreidarsson S, Thomas GH, Valle DL, et al. Aspartylglucosaminuria in the United States. Clin Genet 1983; 23:427–435.

59. Aula P, Mattila K, Piiroinen O, et al: First-trimester prenatal diagnosis of aspartylglucosaminuria. Prenat Diagn 1989; 9:617–620.

60. Aula P, Astrin KH, Francke U, et al. Assignment of the structural gene encoding human aspartylglucosaminidase to the long arm of chromosome 4 (4q21-4qter). Am J Hum Genet 1984; 36:1215–1224.

61. Ikonen E, Syvanen A-C, Peltonen L. Dissection of the molecular pathology of aspartylglucosaminuria provides the basis for DNA diagnostics and future therapeutic interventions. Scand J Clin Lab Invest 1993; 53:19–27.

62. Enoma N, Heiskanen T, Halila R, et al. Human aspartylglucosaminidase. A biochemical and immunocytochemical characterization of the enzyme in normal and aspartylglucosaminuria. Biochem J 1992; 286:613.

Carbohydrate-deficient glycoprotein syndrome

63. Freeze HH. Disorders in protein glycosylation and potential therapy: tip of an iceberg? J Pediatr 1998; 133:593–600.

64. Stromland K, Hagberg B, Kristiansson B. Ocular pathology in disialotransferrin developmental deficiency syndrome. Ophthalmic Paediatr Genet 1990; 11:30090.

65. Kristiansson B, Stibler H, Wide L. Gonadal function and glycoprotein hormones in the carbohydrate-deficient glycoprotein (CDG) syndrome. Acta Paediatr 1995; 84:655–659.

66. Freeze H. Carbohydrate deficient glycoprotein deficiency and their enzymatic defects. In: Society for Inherited Metabolic Disorders Annual Meeting, Lake Lanier Islands, GA, March 12–15, 1999.

67. Ramaekers VT, Stibler H, Kint J, et al. A new variant of the carbohydrate deficient glycoproteins syndrome. J Inherit Metab Dis 1991; 25:385–388.

68. Krasnewich D, Gahl W. Carbohydrate-deficient glycoprotein syndrome. In: Barness LA, ed. Advances in pediatrics. St. Louis: Mosby-Yearbook; 1997:109.

69. Van Schaftingen E, Jaeken J. Phsophomannmutase deficiency is a cause of carbohydrate deficient glycoprotein syndrome type I. FEBS Lett 1995; 377:318–320.

70. Jaeken J, Schachter H, Carchon H, et al. Carbohydrate deficient glycoprotein syndrome type II: a deficiency in Golgi localized N-acetyl-glucosaminyl transferase II. Arch Dis Child 1984; 71:123.

71. Jaeken J, Stibler. A newly recognized herited neurological disease with carbohydrate deficient secretory glycoproteins. In: Wetterberg L, ed. Genetics of neuropsychiatric diseases, vol. 51. Wenner-Green International Symposium Series. London: MacMillan Press; 1989:69.

72. Wada Y, Niskikawa A, Okamoto N, et al. Structure of serum transferrin in carbohydrate-deficient glycoprotein syndrome. Biochem Biophys Res Commun 1992; 1889:832–836.

73. Aula P, Autio S, Raivio K, et al. Detection of heterozygotes for aspartylglucosaminuria (AGU) in cultured fibroblasts. Humangenetik 1974; 25:307–314.

74. Van Pelt J, Bakker JA, Velmans MH, et al. Carbohydrate-deficient transferrin values in neonatal and umbilical cord blood. J Inherit Metab Dis 1996; 19:253–256.

75. Clayton P, Winchester B, Di Tomaso E, et al. Carbohydrate-deficient glycoprotein syndrome: normal glycosylation in the fetus. Lancet 1993; 341:956.

76. Martinsson T, Bjursell C, Stibler H, et al. Linkage of a locus for carbohydrate-deficient glycoprotein syndrome type I (CDG1) to chromosome 16p, and linkage disequilibrium to microsatellite marker D16S406. Hum Mol Genet 1994; 3:2037–3042.

Geleophysic dysplasia

77. Spranger JW, Gilbert EF, Tuffli GA, et al. Geleophysic dwarfism – a 'focal' mucopolysaccharidosis? (letter). Lancet 1971; 1:97–98.

78. Spranger J, Gilbert EF, Flatz S, et al. Acrofacial dysplasia resembling geleophysic dysplasia. Am J Med Genet 1984; 19:501–506.

79. Lipson AH, Kan AE, Kozlowski K.Geleophysic dysplasia–acromicric dysplasia with evidence of glycoprotein storage. Am J Med Genet Suppl 1987; 3:181–189.

80. Spranger J, Gilbert EF, Flatz S, et al. Acrofacial dysplasia resembling geleophysic dysplasia, Am J Med Genet 1984; 19:501–506.

81. Koiffmann CP, Wajntal A, Ursich MS, et al. Familial recurrence of geleophysic dysplasia. Am J Med Genet 1984; 19:483–486.

Canavan disease

82. Metalon R, Kaul R, Casanova J, et al. Aspartoacylase deficiency: the enzyme defect in Canavan disease. J Inherit Metab Dis 1989; 12(suppl 2):329.

83. Von Moers A, Sperner J, Michael T, et al. Variable course of Canavan disease in two boys with infantile aspartoacylase deficiency. Dev Med Child Neurol 1991; 33:824.

84. Zelnik N, Luder AS, Elpeleg ON, et al. Protracted clinical cures for patients with Canavan disease. Dev Meded Child Neurol 1993; 35:355–358.

85. Adachi M, Volk BW. Protracted form of spongy degeneration of the central nervous system (van Bogaert and Bertrand type). Neurology 1968; 18:1084–1092.

86. Brucher M, Dom R, Robin A. Degerescence spongieuse juvenile du systeme nerve central. Ses rapports avec la maladie d'Hallervorden-Spatz et let dystrophies neuroaxnales. Rev Neurol 1968; 119:425.

87. Jellinger K, Seitelberger F. Juvenile form of spongy degeneration of the CNS. Acta Neuropathol 1969; 13:276–281.

88. Goodhue WW, Couch RD, Nakimi H. Spongy degeneration of the CNS. An instance of the rare juvenile form. Arch Neurol 1979; 36:481–484.

89. Kelly RI. Prenatal detection of Canavan disease by measurement of N-acetyl-L-asparate in amniotic fluid. J Inherit Metab Dis 1983; 16:918.

90. Matalon R, Michals K, Gashkoff P, et al. Prenatal diagnosis of Canavan disease. J Inherit Metab Dis 1992; 15:392–394.

Sialic acid disorders

91. Renlund M, Tietze F, Gahl WA. Defective sialic acid egress from isolated fibroblast lysosomes of patients with Salla disease. Science 1986; 232: 759–762.

92. Mancini GMS, Verheijen FW, Beerens CEMT, et al. Sialic acid storage disorders: observations on clinical and biochemical variation. Dev Neurosci 1991; 13:327.

93. Gahl WA. Disorders of lysosomal membrane transport – cystinosis and Salla disease. Enzyme 1987; 38:154–160.

94. Aula P, Autio S, Raivio KO, et al. 'Salla disease:' a new lysosomal storage disorder. Arch Neurol 1979; 36:88–94.

95. Renlund M, Aula P. Prenatal detection of Salla disease based upon increased free sialic acid in amniocytes. Am J Med Genet 1987; 28:377–384.

96. Vamos E, Libert J, Elkhazen N, et al. Prenatal diagnosis and confirmation of infantile sialic acid storage disease. Prenat Diagn 1986; 6:437–446.

97. Autio-Harmainen H, Oldfors A, Sourander P, et al. Neuropathology of Salla disease. Acta Neuropathol (Berl) 1988. 75:481–490.

98. Virtanen I, Ekblom P, Laurila P, et al. Characterization of storage material in cultured fibroblasts by specific lectin binding in lysosomal storage diseases. Pediatr Res 1980; 14:1199–1203.

99. Wenger DA, Williams C. Screening for lysosomal disorders. In: Hommes FA, ed. Techniques in diagnostic human biochemical genetics. A laboratory manual. New York: Wiley-Liss; 1991:587.

100. Thomas GH, Reynolds LW, Miller CW. Characterization of neuraminidase activity of cultured human fibroblasts. Biochem Biophys Acta 1979; 568:39–48.

101. Myers RW, Lee RT, Lee YC, et al. The synthesis of 4-methylumbel-liferyl α-ketoside of N-acetyl neuraminic acid and its use in a fluorometric assay for neurominidase. Anal Biochem 1980; 101:166–174.

102. Tranchemontagne J, Michaud L, Poitier M. Deficient lysosomal carboxypeptidase activity in galactosialidosis. Biochem Biophys Res Commun 1990; 168:22–29.

103. Thomas GH, Renolds LW, Miller CW. Characterization of neuraminidase activity of cultured human fibroblasts. Biochim Biophys Acta 1979; 568:39–48.

Sialidosis

104. Lowden JA, O'Brien JS. Sialidosis: a review of human neuraminidase deficiency. Am J Hum Genet 1979; 31:1–18.

105. Mueller OTA, Henry WM, Hale LL, et al. Sialidosis and galactosialidosis: chromosomal assignment of two genes and associated with neuraminidase deficiency disorders. Proc Natl Acad Sci USA 1985; 83:1817.

106. Thomas GH, Tipton RE, Ch'ien LT, et al. Sialidase (a-N-acetyl neuraminidase) deficiency: the enzyme defect in an adult with macular cherry-red spots and myoclonus without dementia. Clin Genet 1978; 13:369–379.

107. Steinman L, Tharp BR, Dorfman LJ, et al. Peripheral neuropathy in the cherry-red spot myoclonus syndrome (sialidosis type I). Ann Neurol 1980; 7:450–456.

108. Durand P, Gatti R, Cavalieri S, et al. Sialidosis (mucolipidosis I). Helv Pediatr Acta 1977; 32:391–400.

109. Rapin I, Goldfisher S, Katzman R, et al. The cherry red spot myoclonus syndrome. Ann Neurol 1978; 3:234–242.

110. Thomas PK, Abrams JD, Swallow D, et al. Sialidosis type I: cherry red spots myoclonus syndrome with sialidosis deficiency and altered eletrophoretic mobilities of some enzymes known to be glycoproteins. J Neurol Neurosurg Psychiatry 1979; 42:873–880.

110a. Loren DJ, Campos Y, d'Azzo A, Wyble L, Grange DK, Gilbert-Barness E, White FV, Hamvas A. Sialidosis Presenting as Severe Nonimmune Fetal Hydrops is Associated with Two Novel Mutations in Lysosomal α-Neuraminidase. J of Perinatology 2005; 25:491.

α_1-Antitrypsin (α-antiprotease) deficiency

111. Cox DW. α-1-antitrypsin deficiency. In: Scriver CR, Beaudet AL, Sly WS, et al., eds. The metabolic and molecular bases of inherited disease, 8th edn. New York: McGraw-Hill; 2001.

112. Perlmutter DH. The cellular basis for liver injury in α-1-antitrypsin deficiency. Hepatology 1991; 13:172–185.

113. Cario WB. Liver disease in α-1-antitrypsin deficiency in children. J Gastroenterol 1990; 49:141.

114. Quizilbash A, Young-Pong O. α-1-antitrypsin liver disease differential diagnosis of PAS-positive, diastase-resistant globules in liver cells. Am J Clin Pathol 1983; 79:697.

115. Cutz E, Cox DW. α-1-antitrypsin deficiency. Perspect Pediatr Pathol 1979; 5:1–39.

116. Carlson JA, Rogers BB, Sifers N, et al. Accumulation of PiZ antitrypsin causes liver damage in transgenic mice. J Clin Invest 1988; 82:1183.

117. Dycaico JM, Grant SGN, Felts K, et al. Neonatal hepatitis induced by α-1-antitrypsin: a transgenic mouse model. Science 1988; 242:1409.

118. Esquivel CO, Iwatsuki S, Gordon RD, et al. Indications for pediatric liver transplantation. J Pediatr 1987; 111:1039–1045.

119. Lieberman J. Emphysema, cirrhosis, and hepatoma with α-1-antitrypsin deficiency. Ann Intern Med 1974; 81:850–852.

120. Kidd VJ, Golbus MS, Wallace RB, et al. Prenatal diagnosis of α-1-antitrypsin deficiency by direct analysis of the mutation site in the gene. N Engl J Med 1984; 310:639–642.

121. Cox DW, Mansfield T. Prenatal diagnosois of α-1-antitrypsin deficiency and estimates of fetal risk for disease. J Med Genet 1987; 24:52–59.

122. Nukiwa T, Brantly M, Graver R, et al. Evaluation of 'at risk' α-1-antitrypsin genotype SZ with synthetic oligonucleotide gene probes. J Clin Invest 1986; 77:528–537.

123. Psacharopoulos HT, Mowat AP, Cook PJL, et al. Outcome of liver disease associated with α-1-antitrypsin deficiency (PiZ). Arch Dis Child 1983; 58:882–887.

124. Israels SJ, GilFix BM. α-l-antitrypsin deficiency with fatal intracranial hemorrhage in a newborn. J Pediatr Hematol Oncol 1999; 21:447–450.

125. Hadchouel M, Gautier M. Histopathologic study of the liver in the early cholestatic phase of α-1-antitrypsin deficiency. J Pediatr 1976; 89:211–215.

126. Dermer SJ, Johnson EM. Methods in laboratory investigation: rapid DNA analysis of α-1-antitrypsin deficiency. Lab Invest 1988; 59:403–408.

127. Petersen KB, Kolvroa S, Bolund L, et al. Detection of α-1-antitrypsin genotypes by analysis of amplified DNA sequences. Nucleic Acids Res 1988; 16:352.

128. Saiki RK, Scharf S, Foloona F, et al. Enzymatic amplification of γ-globulin genomic sequences and restriction site analysis for diagnosis of sickle cell anemia. Science 1985; 280:1350–1354.

Galactosialidosis

129. d'Azzo A, van der Spoel A, Bonten E. Molecular characterization of the enzyme deficient in both sialidosis and galactosialidosis: lysosomal neuraminidase [abstr W47]. Vienna, Austria: Society for Inborn Errors of Metabolism; 1997.

Glucose transport defects

130. Longo N, Elsas LJ. Human glucose transporters. Adv Pediatr 1998; 45:293–313.

Wolman disease and cholesteryl ester storage disease

131. Kyriakides EC, Paul B, Balin JA. Lipid accumulation and acid lipase deficiency in fibroblasts from a family with Wolman's disease, and their apparent correction in vitro. J Lab Clin Med 1972; 80:810–816.

132. Assmann G, Seedorf U. Acid lipase deficiency: Wolman disease and cholesteryl ester storage disease. In: Scriver CR, Beaudet AL, Sly WS, et al., eds. The metabolic and molecular bases of inherited disease, 8th edn. New York: McGraw-Hill; 2001.

133. Schaub J, Janka GE, Choestomanou H, et al. Wolman's disease: clinical, biochemical and ultrastructural studies in an unusual case without adrenal calcification. Eur J Pediatr 1980; 135:45–53.

134. Miller R, Bialer MG, Rogers JF, et al. Wolman's disease. Arch Pathol Lab Med 1982; 106:41.

135. Desai PK, Astrin KH, Thung SN, et al. Cholesteryl ester storage disease. Pathologic changes in an affected fetus. Am J Med Genet 1987; 26:689–698.

136. Kelly DR, Hoeg JM, Demosky S, et al. Characterization of plasma lipids and lipoproteins in cholesteryl ester storage disease. Biochem Med 1985; 33:29–37.

Niemann-pick disease

137. Crocker AC. The cerebral defect in Tay-Sachs disease and Niemann-Pick disease. J Neurochem 1961; 7:69–80.

138. Schuchman EH, Desnick RJ. Niemann-Pick disease types A and B: acid sphingomyelinase deficiencies. In: Scriver CR, Beaudet AL, Sly WS, et al., eds. The metabolic and molecular bases of inherited disease, 8th edn. New York: McGraw-Hill; 2001.

139. Patterson MC, Vanier MT, Suzuki K, et al. Niemann-Pick disease type C: a cellular cholesterol lipidosis. In: Scriver CR, Beaudet AL, Sly WS, et al., eds. The metabolic and molecular bases of inherited disease, 8th edn. New York: McGraw-Hill; 2001.

140. Gal AE, Brady RO, Hibbert SR, et al. A practical chromogenic procedure for the detection of homozygotes and heterozygous carriers of Niemann-Pick disease. N Engl J Med 1975; 293:632–636.

141. Gilbert EF, Callahan J, Viseskul C, et al. Niemann-Pick disease type C: pathological, histochemical, ultrastructural and biochemical studies. Eur J Pediatr 1981; 136:263–274.

142. Maconochie IK, Chong S, Mieli-Vergani G, et al. Fetal ascites: an unusual presentation of Niemann-Pick disease type C. Arch Dis Child 1989; 64:1391–1393.

143. Barness LA, Wiederhold S, Chandra S, et al. Clinicopathological conference: one-year-old infant with hepatosplenomegaly and developmental delay. Am J Med Gen 1987; 28:411.

144. Schoenfeld A, Abramovici A, Klibanski C, et al. Placental ultrasonographic biochemical and histochemical studies in human fetuses affected with Niemann-Pick disease type A. Placenta 1985; 6:33–43.

145. Hulette CM, Earl NL, Anthony DC, et al. Adult-onset Niemann-Pick disease type C presenting with dementia and absent organomegaly. Clin Neuropathol 1992; 6:293–297.

Gaucher disease

146. Pentchev PG, Vanier MT, Suzuki K, et al. Niemann-Pick disease type C: a cellular cholesterol lipidosis. In: Scriver CR, Beaudet AL, Sly SW, et al., eds. The Metabolic bases of inherited disease, 7th edn. New York: McGraw-Hill; 1995.

147. Vethamany VG, Welch JP, Vethamany S. Ultrastructure of blood, skin fibroblasts and bone marrow. Arch Pathol 1972; 93:537.

148. Pilz H. Niemann-Picksche Krankheit im Erwachsenenalter. Dtsch Med Wochenschr 1970; 38:1905–1910.

149. Attal HC, Grover S, Jiwane AD. Familial lipidosis – report of a rare form of Niemann-Pick disease (type E) with a review of literature. J Assoc Physicians India 1977; 25:829–831.

150. Kamoshita S, Aron AM, Suzuki K. Infantile Niemann-Pick disease. A chemical study with isolation and characterization of membranous cytoplasmic bodies and myelin. Am J Dis Child 1969; 117:379–394.

151. Schneider EL, Pentchev PG, Hibbert SR, et al. A new form of Niemann-Pick disease characterized by temperature-labile sphingomyelinase. J Med Genet 1978; 15:370–374.

152. Wiedemann HR, Debuch H, Lennert K, et al. Über eine infantil-juvenile, subchronische verlaufende, den Sphingomyelinosen (Niemann-Pick) anzureihende Form der Lipidosen – ein neuer Typ. Z Kinderheilk 1972; 112:187–225.

153. Hagberg B, Haltia M, Sourander P. Neurovisceral storage disorder simulating Niemann-Pick disease. Neuropädiatrie 1978; 9:59–73.

154. Wenger DA, Barth G, Githens JH. Nine cases of sphingomyelin lipidosis, a new variant in Spanish-American children. Juvenile variant of Niemann-Pick disease with foamy and sea-blue histiocytes. Am J Dis Child 1977; 131:955–961.

155. Witzleben CL, Palmieri MJ, Watkins JB, et al. Sphingomyelin lipidosis variant with cirrhosis in the pediatric age group. Arch Pathol Lab Med 1986; 110:508–512.

156. Luse S. The fine structure of the brain and other organs in Niemann-Pick disease. In: Aronson SM, Volk BW, eds. Inborn disorders of sphingolipid metabolism. Oxford: Pergamon Press; 1967.

157. Lynn R, Terry RD. Lipid histochemistry and electron microscopy in adult Niemann-Pick disease. Am J Med 1964; 37:987–994.

158. Gumbinas M, Larsen M, Lui H. Peripheral neuropathy in classic Niemann-Pick disease: ultrastructure of nerves and skeletal muscles. Neurology 1975; 25:107–113.

159. Brady RO, Kanfer JN, Mock MB, et al. The metabolism of sphingomyelin. II. Evidence of an enzymatic deficiency in Niemann-Pick disease. Proc Natl Acad Sci USA 1966; 55:366–369.

160. Callahan JW, Khalil M, Gerrie J. Isoenzymes of sphingomyelinase and the genetic defect in Niemann-Pick disease, type C. Biochem Biophys Res Commun 1974; 58:385–390.

161. Callahan JW, Khalil M, Philippart M: Sphingomyelinases in human tissues. II. Absence of a specific enzyme from liver and brain of Niemann-Pick disease, type C. Pediatr Res 1975; 9:908–913.

162. Besley GTN. Sphingomyelinase defect in Niemann-Pick disease, type C, fibroblasts. FEBS Lett 1977; 80:71–74.

163. Gal AE, Brady RO, Hibbert SR, et al. A practical chromogenic procedure for the detection of homozygotes and heterozygous carriers of Niemann-Pick disease. N Engl J Med 1975; 293:632–636.

164. Gal AW, Fash FJ. Synthesis of 2-hexadecanoylamino-4-nitrophenyl phosphorylcholine-hydroxide, a chromogenic substrate for assaying sphingomyelinase activity. Chem Phys Lipids 1976; 16:71,

165. Pentchev PG, Brady RO, Hibbert SR, et al. Purification and properties of sphingomyelinase from human placental tissue. Biochim Biophys Acta 1977; 488:312.

166. Greenbaum M, Hoffman LM, Schneck L, et al. Ceramide hexosides in Niemann-Pick diseased brain. J Neurol 1976; 213:251–255.

167. Elleder M, Jirásek A. Neuropathology of various types of Niemann-Pick disease. Acta Neuropathol 1981; 7:201–203.

168. Winsberg F. Echographic changes with placental aging. J Clin Ultrasonog 1973; 1:182–189.

169. Beutler E, Grabowski GE: Glucosylceramide lipidoses: Gaucher disease. In: Scriver CR, Beaudet AL, Sly WS, et al., eds. The metabolic and molecular bases of inherited disease, 8th edn. New York: McGraw-Hill; 2001.

170. Ginns EL, Brady RO, Perruccello S, et al: Mutations of glucocerebrosidase. Proc Natl Sci USA 1982; 79:5607.

171. Smith RRI, Hutchins GM, Sack GH, et al. Unusual cardiac, renal and pulmonary hypertension and fatal bone marrow embolization. Am J Med 1978; 65:352–360.

172. Roberts WC, Fredrickson DS; Gaucher's disease of the lung causing severe pulmonary hypertension with associated acute recurrent pericarditis. Circulation 1967; 35:783–789.

173. Zimran A, Horowitz M. RecTL: a complex allele of the glucocerebrosidase gene associated with a mild clinical course of Gaucher disease. Am J Med Genet 1994; 50:74–78.

174. Beutler E, Kay A, Sven A, et al. Enzyme replacement therapy for Gaucher disease. Blood 1991; 78:1183–1189.

175. Daniels LB, Glew RH. β-glucosidase assays in the diagnosis of Gaucher's disease. Clin Chem 1982; 28:569–577.

176. Aerts JMFG, Donker-Koopman WE, Koot M, et al. Deficiency activity of glycocerebrosidase in urine from patients with type I Gaucher disease. Clin Chem Acta 1986; 158:155–163.

177. Daniels LB, Glew RH. β-glucosidase assays in the diagnosis of Gaucher" disease. Clin Chem 1982; 28:569–577.

178. Dreborg S, Erikson A, Hagberg B. Gaucher disease – Norrbottnian type I: general clinical description. Eur J Pediatr 1980; 133:107–118.

179. Daniels LB, Glew RH. β-glucosidase assays in the diagnosis of Gaucher's disease. Clin Chem 1982; 28:569–577.

180. Aerts JMFG, Donker-Koopman WE, Koot M, et al. Deficiency activity of glycocerebrosidase in urine from patients with type I Gaucher disease. Clin Chem Acta 1986; 158:155–163.

181. Martin BM, Sidransky E, Ginns EL. Gaucher's disease: advances and challenges. In: Barness LA, ed. Advances in pediatrics. St. Louis, MO: Mosby-Year Book; 1989.

182. Barneveld RA, Keijzer W, Tegelaers FPW, et al. Assignment of the gene coding for human β-glucocerebroidase to the region q21-q31 of chromosome 1 using monoclonal antibodies. Hum Genet 1983; 64:227–231.

183. Ishak KG. Pathology of inherited metabolic disorders. In: Balistreri WF, Stocker JT, eds. Pediatric hepatology, New York, Hemisphere Publishing; 1990.

184. Lorber M, Nemes JL. Identification of ferritin within Gaucher cells. Acta Haematol 1967; 37:189–197.

185. Spranger J, Gilbert EF, Flatz S, et al. Acrofacial dysplasia resembling geleophysic dysplasia, Am J Med Genet 1984; 19:501–506.

186. Barton NW, Brady RO, Dambrosia JM, et al. Replacement therapy for inherited enzyme deficiency macrophage-targeted glucocerebrosidase for Gaucher's disease. N Engl J Med 1991; 324:1464–1470.

186a. Grabowski GA. Gaucher disease: gene frequencies and genotype/phenotype correlations. Genet Test 1997; 1(1):5–12.

187. Beutler E. Gaucher's disease. N Engl J Med 1991; 325:1354–1360.

Krabbe disease

188. Inui K, Fu L, Nishigaki T, et al. Molecular defects in Krabbe disease. Hum Mol Genet 1995; 4:1865–1868.

189. Wenger DA, Suzuki K, Suzuki Y, et al. Galactosylceramide lipidosis: globoid cell leukodystrophy (Krabbe disease). In: Scriver CR, Beaudet AL, Sly WS, et al., eds. The metabolic and molecular bases of inherited disease, 8th edn. New York: McGraw-Hill; 2001.

189a. Escolar ML, Poe MD, Provenzale JM, et al. Transplanation of umbilical-cord blood in babies with infantile Krabbe's Disease. N Engl J Med 2005; 382:2069–2081.

Farbe disease

190. Tanaka T, Takahashi K, Hakozakih H, et al. Farber's disease (disseminated granulomatosis). Acta Pathol Jpn 1979; 29:135.

191. Qualman SJ, Moser HW, Valle D, et al. Farber disease: pathologic diagnosis in sibs with phenotypic variability, Am J Med Genet 1987; 3(Suppl):233–241.

192. Rauch HJ, Aubock L: Banana bodies and disseminated lipogranulomatosis (Farber's disease), Am J Dermatopathol 1983; 5:263–266.

Fabry disease

193. Brady RO, Gal AE, Bradley RM, et al. Enzymatic defect in Fabry's disease: ceramide trihexosidase. N Engl J Med 1967; 276:1163–1167.

194. Abreo K, Oberley T, Gilbert E, et al. Clinicopathological conference: a 29-year-old man with recurrent episodes of fever, abdominal pain, and vomiting. Am J Med Genet 1984; 18:249–264.

195. Schibanoff JM, Kamoshita S, O'Brien JS: Tissue distribution of glycosphingolipids in a case of Fabry's disease. J Lipid Res 1969; 10:515–520.

196. Gilbert-Barness E. Metabolic cardiomyopathy in childhood. In: Pomerance HH, Bercu BB, eds. Topics in pediatrics. Lewis A. Barness Festschrift. New York: Springer-Verlag; 1990.

197. Ferrans VJ, Hibbs RG, Burda CD. The heart in Fabry's disease. A histochemical and electron microscopic study. Am J Cardiol 1969; 24:95–110.

198. Brady RO, Gal AE, Bradley RM, et al. Enzymatic defect in Fabry's disease: ceramide trihexosidase deficiency. N Engl J Med 1967; 276:1163–1167.

198a. Reis M, Grupta S, Moore DF, et al. Pediatric Fabry disease. Pediatrics 2005; 115(3):344.

Gangliosidoses

199. Gravel RA, Kaback MM, Proia RL, et al. The GM_2 gangliosidoses. In: Scriver CR, Beaudet AL, Sly WS, et al., eds. The metabolic and molecular bases of inherited disease, 8th edn. New York: McGraw-Hill; 2001.

200. Landing BH, Silverman FN: Familial neurovisceral lipidosis. Am J Dis Child 1964; 108:503–522.

201. Severi F, Magrini U, et al. Infantile GM_1 gangliosidosis. Histochemical, ultrastructural and biochemical studies. Helv Paediatr Acta 1971; 26:192–209.

202. Yamano T, Shimada M, et al. Ultrastructural study on nervous system of fetus with GM_1 gangliosidosis type I. Acta Neuropathol (Berl) 1983; 61:15–20.

203. Gilbert E, Varakis J, Opitz JM, et al. Generalized gangliosidosis II type II (juvenile GM_1 gangliosidosis). A pathological, histochemical and ultrastructural study. Z Kinderheilk 1975; 120:151–180.

204. Sandhoff K, Andreae U, Jatzkewita H. Deficient hexosaminidase activity in an exceptional case of Tay-Sachs disease with additional storage of kidney globoside in visceral organs. Pathol Eur 1968; 3:278–285.

205. Kaback M, Lim-Steele J, Dabholkar D, et al. Tay-Sachs disease-carrier screening, prenatal diagnosis, and the molecular era. JAMA 1993; 270:2307–2315.

206. Krivit W, Desnick RW, Lee J, et al. Generalized accumulation of neutral glycosphingolipids with GM_2 ganglioside accumulation in the brain; Sandhoff's disease (variant of Tay-Sachs disease). Am J Med 1972; 52:763–770.

207. Barness LA, Henry K, Kling P, et al. Clinico-pathological report: A 7-year-old white male boy with progressive neurological deterioration. Am J Med Genet 1991; 40:271.

208. Warner TG, De Kremar RD, Applegarth D, et al. Diagnosis and characterization of GM_2 gagliosidosis type II (Sandhoff disease) by analysis of the accumulating N-acetyl-glucosaminyl oligosaccharides with high performanace liquid chromatography. Clin Chem Acta 1986; 154:151–164.

209. Schulte FJ. Clinical course of GM_2 gangliosiodses. A correlative attempt. Neuropediatrics 1984; 15:66–70.

210. Warner TG, De Kremar RD, Applegarth D, et al. Diagnosis and characterization of GM_2 gagliosidosis type II (Sandhoff disease) by analysis of the accumulating N-acetyl-glucosaminyl oligosaccharides with high performanace liquid chromatography. Clin Chem Acta 1986; 154:151–164.

211. Sonderfeld S, Conzelmann E, Schwarzmann G, et al. Incorporation and metabolism of ganglioside GM_2 gangliosidosis subjects. Eur J Biochem 1985; 149:247–255.

212. Barness LA, Henry K, Kling P, et al. Clinco-pathological report: a 7-year-old white male boy with progressive neurological deterioration. Am J Med Genet 1991; 40:271.

213. Gustavson KH, Hagberg B. The incidence and genetics of metachromatic leukodystrophy in Northern Sweden. Acta Pediatr Scand 1971; 60:585–590.

214. Von Specht B, Geiger B, Arnon B, et al. Enzyme replacement in Tay-Sachs disease. Neurology 1979; 29:848–854.

215. Gravel RA, Clarke JTR, Kabach MM, et al. The GM_2 gangliosidoses. In: Scriver CR, Beaudet AL, Sly WS, et al., eds. The Metabolic bases of inherited disease, 7th edn. New York: McGraw-Hill; 1995:2339.

Serum lipid or lipoprotein abnormalities

216. Havel RJ, Kane JP. Introduction: structure and metabolism of plasma lipoprotein. In: Scriver CR, Beaudet AL, Sly WS, et al., eds. The Metabolic bases of inherited disease, 7th edn. New York: McGraw-Hill; 1995:2339.

217. Tall AR, Breslow JL, Rubin EM. Familial disorders of high density lipoprotein metabolism. In: Scriver CR, Beaudet AL, Sly WS, et al., eds. The metabolic and molecular bases of inherited disease, 8th edn. New York: McGraw-Hill; 2001.

218. Assmann G, von Eckardstein A, Brewer HB Jr. Familial high density lipoprotein deficiency: Tangier disease. In: Scriver CR, Beaudet AL, Sly WS, et al., eds. The Metabolic bases of inherited disease, 7th edn. New York: McGraw-Hill; 1995:2339.

219. Kane JP, Havel RJ. Disorders of biogenesis and secretion of lipoproteins containing the B apolipoproteins. In: Scriver CR, Beaudet AL, Sly WS, et al., eds. The metabolic and molecular bases of inherited disease, 8th edn. New York: McGraw-Hill; 2001.

220. Robinson BH. Lactic acidosis. In: Scriver CR, Beaudet AL, Sly WS, et al., eds. The metabolic and molecular bases of inherited disease, 8th edn. New York: McGraw-Hill; 2001.

221. Gilbert EL, Arya S, Chun R. Leigh's necrotizing encephalopathy with pyruvate carboxylase deficiency. Arch Pathol Lab Med 1983; 107:162–166.

Smith-Lemli-Opitz syndrome

222. Lowry R, Yong SL. Borderline normal intelligence in the Smith-Lemli-Opitz syndrome. Am J Med Genet 1980; 5:137–143.

223. Opitz JM, De La Cruz F. Cholesterol metabolism in RSH/Smith-Lemli-Opitz syndrome: summary of an NICHD conference. Am J Med Genet 1994; 50:326–338.

223a. Putman AR, Szakacs JG, Opitz JM, Byrne JLB. Prenatal death in Smith-Lemli-Opitz syndrome. Am J Med Genet 2005; A; 138:61–65.

223b. Opitz JM, Gilbert-Barness E, Ackerman J, et al. Cholesterol and development: the RSH ('Smith-Lemli-Opitz') syndrome and related conditions. Pediatri Pathol Mol Med 2002; 21:153–181.

223c. Opitz JM. RSH (so-called Smith-Lemli-Opitz) syndrome. Curr Opin Pediatr 1999; 11(4):353–362.

Metachromatic leukodystrophy

224. Burgess J, Kalfayan B, Gilbert EL. Papillomatosis of gallbladder in metachromatic leukodystrophy. Arch Pathol Lab Med 1985; 109:79–81.

224a. von Figura K, Gieselmann V, Jaenken J. Metachromatic leukodystrophy. In: Scriver CR, Beaudet AL, Sly WS, et al., eds. The metabolic and molecular bases of inherited disease, 8th edn. New York: McGraw-Hill; 2001.

Multiple sulfatase deficiency

225. Burch M, Fensom AH, Jackson M, et al. Multiple sulfatase deficiency presenting at birth. Clin Genet 1986; 30:409–415.

Neuroaxonal dystrophy and leukodystrophy

226. Seitelberger F. Neuroaxonal dystrophy: its relations to aging and neurological disease. In: Vinken P, Bruyn G, Klawans H, eds. Handbook of clinical neuropathology, extrapyramidal disorders, vol. 5. Amsterdam: Elsevier; 1986:391.

Hallervorden-Spatz disease

227. Olanow C. Hallervorden Spatz syndrome: an iron storage disease. In: Calne D, ed. Neurodegenerative diseases. Philadelphia: WB Saunders; 1994:807.

228. Jankovic J, Kirkpatrick JB, Blomquist KA, et al. Late-onset Hallervorden-Spatz disease presenting as familial parkinsonism. Neurology 1985; 35:227–234.

229. Antoine JC, Tommasi M, Chalumeau A. Hallervorden-Spatz disease with Lewy bodies. Rev Neurol 1985; 141:806–809.

Mucolipidoses

230. Gilbert-Barness E, Barness LA: The mucolipidoses. In: Landing B, Haust M, Bernstein J, et al., eds. Genetic metabolic diseases. Basel: Karger; 1993.

231. Aylsworth A, Thomas G, Hood J, et al. A severe infantile sialidosis: clinical, biochemical, and microscopic features. J Pediatr 1980; 96:662–668.

231a. Aylsworth AS, Thomas GH, Hood JL, et al. A severe infantile sialidosis: clinical, biochemical, and microscopic features. J Pediatr 1980; 96:662–668.

232. Spranger J, Gehler J, Cantz M. Mucolipidosis I – a sialidosis. Am J Med Genet 1977; 1:21.

232a. Johnson WG, Thomas GH, Miranda AF, et al. Congenital sialidosis: biochemical studies: clinical spectrum in four sibs; two successful prenatal diagnoses. Am J Hum Genet 1980; 32:43A.

233. Spranger J. Mini review: inborn errors of complex carbohydrate metabolism. Am J Med Genet 1987; 28:489–499.

233a. Beck M, Bender SW, Reiter H-L, et al. Neuraminidase deficiency presenting as nonimmune hydrops fetalis. Eur J Pediatr 1984; 143:135–139.

234. Powell H, Benirschke K, Favara B, et al. Foamy changes of placental cells in fetal storage disorders. Virchows Arch Pathol 1976; 396:191–196.

234a. Hug G, Schubert WK, Schwachman H. Imbalance of liver phosphorylase and accumulation of hepatic glycogen in a girl with progressive disease of the brain. J Pediatr 1965; 67:741–751.

235. Rapola J, Aula P. Morphology of the placenta in fetal I-cell disease. Clin Genet 1977; 11:107–113.

235a. Maroteaux P, Poissonnier M, Tondeur M, et al. Sialidose par deficint en α-(2,6)-neuraminidase sans atteinte neurologique. Arch Fr Pediatr 1978; 35:280.

236. Sekeles E, Ornoy A, Cohen R, et al. Mucolipidosis IV: fetal and placental pathology. Monogr Hum Genet 1978; 10:47–50.

236a. Sec G, Stanescu R, Lyon G. Un nouveau type de silidose avec atteinte renale. II. Etude anatomique. Arch Fr Pediatr 1978; 35:830–844.

237. Kelly T, Graetz G. Isolated acid neuraminidase deficiency: a distinct lysosomal storage disease. Am J Med Genet 1977; 1:31–46.

238. Maroteaux P. A new type of sialidosis with kidney disease: nephrosialidosis. I. Clinical, radiological and nosological study. Arch Fr Pediatr 1978; 35:819–829.

239. Cantz M, Gehler J, Spranger J. Mucolipidosis I: increased sialic acid content and deficiency of an α-N-acetylneuraminidase. Biochem Biophys Res Commun 1977; 74:732–738.

240. Spranger J, Cantz M. Mucolipidosis I, the cherry-red-spot-myoclonus syndrome and neuraminidase deficiency. Birth Defects 1978; 14:105–112.

241. Winter RM, Swallow DM, Baraitser M, et l. Sialidosis type 2 (acid neuraminidase deficiency): clinical and biochemical features of a further case. Clin Genet 1980; 18:203–210.

242. Oohira T, Nagata N, Akaboshi I, et al. The infantile form of sialidosis type II associated with congenital adrenal hyperplasia: possible linkage between HLA and the neuraminidase deficiency gene. Hum Genet 1985; 70:341–343.

243. Laver J, Fried DK, Beer SI, et al. Infantile lethal neuraminidase deficiency (sialidosis). Clin Genet 1983; 23:97.

244. Young ID, Young EP, Mossman J, et al. Neuraminidase deficiency: case report and review of the phenotype. J Med Genet 1987; 24:283–290.

245. Kelly TE, Bartoshesky L, Harris DJ, et al. Mucolipidosis I (acid neuraminidase deficiency). Am J Dis Child 1981; 135:703–708.

246. Louis JJ, Marie I, Hermier M, et al. Une observation de mucolipidose de type I par deficit primaire en α D neuraminidase. J Genet Hum 1983; 31:79.

247. Spranger J. Mini review: inborn errors of complex carbohydrate metabolism. Am J Med Genet 1987; 28:489–499.

248. Mueller OT, Henry WM, Haley LL, et al. Sialidosis and galactosialidosis: chromosomal assignment to two genes associated with neuraminidase deficiency disorders. Proc Natl Acad Sci USA 1985; 83:1817.

249. Frisch A, Neufeld EF. A rapid and sensitive assay for neuraminidase: application to cultured fibroblasts. Anal Biochem 1979; 95:222–227.

250. Cantz MH. Sialidoses. In: Schauer R, ed. Sialic acids, chemistry, metabolism and functions. Cell Biology Monography 10. Vienna: Springer; 1982.:307.

251. Cantz MH. Oligosaccharide and ganglioside neuraminidase activities of mucolipidosis I (sialidosis) and mucolipidosis II (I-cell disease) fibroblasts. Eur J Biochem 1979; 97:113.

252. D'Azzo A, Hoogeveen A, Reuser AJJ, et al. Molecular defect in combined β-galactosidase and neuraminidase deficiency in man. Proc Natl Acad Sci USA 1982; 29:4535–4539.

253. Lowden JA, O'Brien JS. Sialidosis: a review of human neuraminidase deficiency. Am J Hum Genet 1979; 31:1–18.

254. Thomas GH, Reynolds LW, Miller CS. Characterization of neuraminidase activity of cultured human fibroblasts. Biocem Biophys Acta 1979; 568:39–48.

Mucolipidosis II

255. DeMars RI, LeRoy JG. The remarkable cells cultured from a human with Hurler's syndrome: an approach to visual selection for in vitro genetic studies. In Vitro 1967; 2:107.

256. Taylor HA, Thomas GH, Miller CS, et al. Mucolipidosis III (pseudo-Hurler polydystrophy): cytological and ultrastructural observations of cultured fibroblast cells. Clin Genet 1973; 4:388–397.

257. Leroy JG, Jo M, McBrinn MC, et al. I-cell disease: biochemical studies, Pediatr Res 1972; 6:752.

258. Hickman S, Neufeld EF. A hypothesis for I-cell disease: defective hydrolases that do not enter lysosomes. Biochem Biophys Res Commun 1972; 49:999–999.

259. Wiesmann UN, Lightbody J, Vasella F, et al. Multiple lysosomal deficiency due to enzyme leakage. N Engl J Med 1971; 284:109–110.

260. Kaplan A, Achord DT, Sly WS. Phosphohexosyl components of a lysosomal enzyme are recognized by pinocytosis receptors on human fibroblasts. Proc Natl Acad Sci USA 1977; 74:2026–2030.

261. I-cell disease

262. Distler J, Hieber V, Sahagian G, et al. Identification of mannose 6-phosphate in glycoproteins that inhibit the assimilation of β-galactosidase by fibroblasts. Proc Natl Acad Sci USA 1979; 76:4325–4239.

263. Gabel CA, Costello CE, Reinhold VN, et al. Identification of methyl-phosphomannosyl residues as components of the high mannose oligo-saccharides of Dictyostelium discoideum glycoproteins. J Biol Chem 1984; 259:13762–13769.

264. Herd JK, Dvorak AD, Wiltse HE, et al. Mucolipidosis type III – multiple elevated serum and urine enzyme activities. Am J Dis Child 1978; 132:1181–1186.

265. Satoh Y, Sakamoto K, Fujibayashi Y, et al. Cardiac involvement in mucolipidosis: importance of non-invasive studies for detection of cardiac abnormalities. Jpn Heart J 1983; 24:149–159.

266. Gilbert EF, Dawson G, ZuRhein GM, et al. I-cell disease, mucolipidosis II, pathological, histochemical, ultrastructural and biochemical observations in four cases. Z. Kinderheilk 1973; 114:259–292.

267. Gabel CA, Costello CE, Reinhold VN, et al. Identification of methyl-phosphomannosyl residues as components of the high mannose oligo-saccharides of Dictyostelium discoideum glycoproteins. J Biol Chem 1984; 259:13762–13769.

268. Kelly TE, Thomas GH, Taylor HA. Mucolipidosis III (pseudo-Hurler polydystrophy): clinical and laboratory studies in a series of 12 patients. Johns Hopkins Med J 1975; 137:156–175.

269. Herd JK, Dvorak AD, Wiltse HE, et al. Mucolipidosis type III – multiple elevated serum and urine enzyme activities. Am J Dis Child 1978; 132:1181–1186.

270. Liebaers I, Neufeld EF. Iduronate sulfatase activity in serum, lymphocytes and fibroblasts – simplified diagnosis of the Hurler syndrome. Pediatr Res 1976; 10:733.

271. Leroy JG, Jo M, McBrinn MC, et al. I-cell disease: biochemical studies, Pediatr Res 1972; 6:752.

272. Hall CW, Liebaers I, Dinatale P, et al. Enzymatic diagnosis of the genetic mucopolysaccharide storage disorders. Methos Enzymol 1978; 50:439–456.

273. Like KK, Thomas GH, Taylor HA, et al. Analysis of N-acetyl-β-D-glucosaminidase in mucolipidosis II (I-cell disease). Clin Chem Acta 1978; 45:243.

274. Kato E, Yokoi T, Taniguchi N. Lysosomal acid hydrolases in lymphocytes of I-cell disease. Clin Chem Acta 1979; 95:285–290.

275. Tanaka T, Kobayashi M, Fukuda T, et al. Nine lysosomal enzyme levels in lymphocytes and granulocytes. Hiroshima J Med Sci 1979; 28:190.

276. Ben-Yoseph Y, Potice M, Mitchell DA, et al. Altered molecular size of N-acetylglycosaminyl phosphotransferase in I-cell disease and pseudo-Hurler polydystrophy. In: Berlin: 7th International Congress on Human Genetics; 1986.

277. Ben-Yoseph Y, Baylerian MS, Nadler HL. Radiometric assays of N-acetylglucosaminyl-phosphodiesterase with substrates labeled in the glucosamine moiety. Anal Biochem 1984; 142:297–304.

278. Griffiths GM, Isaaz S. Granzymes A and B are targeted to the lytic granules of lymphocytes by the mannose-6-phosphate receptor. J Cell Biol 1993; 120:885–896.

Mucolipidosis III

279. Fowler ML, Fan YS, Mueller OT, et al. Correction of mucolipidosis III in vitro by gene transfer. Genome 1993; 18:236–243.

280. Freisinger P, Padovani JC, Maroteaux P. An atypical form of muco-lipidosis III. J Med Genet 1992; 29:834–836.

281. Brik R, Mandel IH, Aizin A, et al. Mucolipidosis III presenting as a rheumatological disorder. J Rheum 1993; 20:133–136.

Mucolipidosis IV

282. Amir N, Zlotogora J, Bach G. Mucolipidosis type IV: clinical spectrum and natural history. Pediatrics 1987; 79:953–959.

Ceroid storage diseases

283. Zeman W, Dyken P. Neuronal ceroid-lipofuscinosis (Batten's disease): relationship to amaurotic family idiocy? Pediatrics 1969; 44:570–583.

284. Zeman W. Historical development of the nosological concept of amau-rotic familial idiocy. In: Vinken PJ, Bruyn GW, eds. Handbook of neurology. Amsterdam: North-Holland; 1970:212.

285. Dyken PR. The neuronal ceroid lipofuscinoses. J Child Neurol 1989; 4:165–174.

286. Rapola J. Neuronal ceroid-lipofuscinoses in childhood. In: Landing BH, Haust MD, Bernstein J, et al., eds. Perspectives in pediatric pathology, Basel: Karger; 1993:7.

287. Proceedings of the Fifth International Conference on Neuronal Ceroid Lipofuscinoses. Am J Med Genet 1995; 57:12J.

288. Rider JA, Rider DL. Batten disease: past, present and future. Am J Med Genet Suppl 1988; 5:21–26.

289. Hall NA, Lake BD, Patrick AD. Recent biochemical and genetic advances in our understanding of Batten's disease (ceroid-lipofuscinosis). Dev Neurosci 1991; 13:339–344.

290. Callen DF, Baker E, Lane S, et al. Regional mapping of the Batten disease locus (CLN3) to human chromosome 16p12. Am J Hum Genet 1991; 49:1372–1377.

291. Järvelä I, Schleutker J, Haataja L, et al. Infantile neuronal ceroid lipofuscinosis (CLN1) maps to the short arm of chromosome 1. Genomics 1991; 9:170–173.

292. Peltonen L, Vesa J, Hellsten LA, et al. Mutations in the palmitoyl-protein thioesterase gene lead to a severe brain disorder, infantile neuronal ceroid lipofuscinoses (INCL). Minneapolis, Minn: American Society of Human Geneticists meeting; Oct. 1995.

293. Lake BD. Lysosomal enzyme deficiencies. In: Adams JH, Corsellis JAN, Duchen LW, eds. Greenfield's neuropathology. London: Edward Arnold; 1984:491.

294. Goebel HH, Zeman W, Patel VK, et al. On the ultrastructural diversity and essence of residual bodies in neuronal ceroid-lipofuscinosis. Mech Ageing Dev 1979; 10:53–70.

295. Haynes ME, Manson JI, Carter RF, et al. Electron microscopy of skin and peripheral blood lymphocytes in infantile (Santavuori) neuronal ceroid lipofuscinosis. Neuropädiatrie 1979; 10:245–263.

Infantile NCL

296. Santavuori P. Clinical findings in 69 patients with infantile type of neuronal ceroid lipofuscinosis. In: Armstrong D, Koppang N, Rider JA, eds. Ceroid-lipofuscinosis (Batten's disease). Amsterdam: Elsevier Biomedical Press; 1982:230.

297. Haltia M, Rapola J, Santavuori P. Infantile type of so-called neuronal ceroid-lipofuscinosis. Histological and electron microscopical studies. Acta Neuropathol (Berl) 1973; 26:157–170.

298. Haltia M. Infantile neuronal ceroid-lipofuscinosis: neuropathological aspects. In: Armstrong D, Koppang N, Rider JA, eds. Ceroid-lipofuscinosis (Batten's disease). Amsterdam: Elsevier Biomedical Press; 1982:105.

299. Libert J. Diagnosis of lysosomal storage disorders by the ultrastructural study of conjunctival biopsies. Pathol Annu 1980; 15(Part 1):37–66.

300. Carpenter S, Karpati G, Andermann F. Specific involvement of muscle, nerve, and skin in late infantile and juvenile amaurotic idiocy. Neurology 1972; 22:170–186.

301. Rapola J, Santavuori P, Savilahti E. Suction biopsy of rectal mucosa in the diagnosis of infantile and juvenile types of neuronal ceroid lipofuscinoses, Hum Pathol 1984; 15:352–360.

302. Martin JJ, Jacobs K. Skin biopsy as a contribution to diagnosis in late infantile amaurotic idiocy with curvilinear bodies. Eur Neurol 1973; 10:281–291.

303. Ceuterick CH, Martin JJ, Casaer P, et al. The diagnosis of infantile generalized ceroid-lipofuscinosis (type Hagberg-Santavuori) using skin biopsy. Neuropädiatrie 1976; 7:250–260.

Late infantile NCL

304. Boustany R-MN, Alroy J, Kolodny EH. Clinical classification of neuronal ceroid-lipofuscinosis subtypes, Am J Med Genet Suppl 1988; 5:47–58.

305. Goebel H, Zeman W, Damaske E. An ultrastructural study of the retina in the Jansky-Bielschowsky type of neuronal ceroid lipofuscinosis. Am J Ophthalmol 1977; 83:70–79.

306. Buhl L, Muirhead D, Litthander J, et al. Late infantile neuronal ceroid lipofuscinosis: an ultrastructural investigation. Pediatr Pathol 1994; 14:397–404.

307. Sleat DE, Donnelly RJ, Lackland H, et al. Association of mutations in a lysosomal protein with classical late-infantile neuronal ceroid lipofuscinosis. Science 1997; 277:1802–1805.

308. MacLeod P, Dolman C, Nickel R, et al. Prenatal diagnosis of neuronal ceroid lipofuscinosis. N Engl J Med 1984; 310:595.

309. Conradi NG, Uvebrant P, Hökegård K-H, et al. First-trimester diagnosis of juvenile neuronal ceroid lipofuscinosis by demonstration of fingerprint inclusions in chorionic villi. Prenat Diagn 1989; 9:283–287.

310. Rapola J, Salonen R, et al. Prenatal diagnosis of the infantile type of neuronal ceroid lipofuscinosis by electron microscopic investigation of human chorionic villi. Prenat Diagn 1990; 10:553–559.

311. Järvelä I, Rapola J, Peltonen L, et al. DNA-based prenatal diagnosis of the infantile form of neuronal ceroid lipofuscinosis (INCL, CLN1). Prenat Diagn 1991; 11:323–328.

Juvenile NCL

312. Järvelä I, Autti T, Lamminranta S, et al. Relationship between genotype and phenotype in juvenile-onset neuronal ceroid lipofuscinosis (JNCL, Batten disease) – analysis of the major mutation (1.02 kb deletion) [abstr W34]. In: 7th International Congress of Inborn Errors of Metabolism. Vienna, Austria: May21–25, 1997.

Adult NCL

313. Santavuori P, Rapola J, Nuutila A, et al. The spectrum of Jansky-Bielschowsky disease. Neuropediatrics 1991; 22:135.

314. Goebel HH, Schulz F. The ultrastructural variability of non-specific lipopigments. Acta Neuropathol (Berl) 1979; 48:227–230.

315. Carpenter S. Morphological diagnosis and misdiagnosis in Batten-Kufs disease. Am J Med Genet Suppl 1988; 5:85–91.

316. Sjögren T. Die juvenile amaurotische Idiotie. Klinische unter blichkeit-smedizinische Untersuchungen. Hereditas 1931; 14:197.

317. Andermann E, Jacob JC, Andermann F, et al: The Newfoundland aggregate of neuronal ceroid-lipofuscinosis. Am J Med Genet Suppl 1988; 5:111–116.

318. Santavuori P. Neuronal ceroid-lipofuscinoses in childhood. Brain Dev 1988; 10:80–83.

Galactosemia

319. Holton JB, Walter JH, Tyfield LA. Galactose metabolism. In: Scriver CR, Beaudet AL, Sly WS, et al., eds. The metabolic and molecular bases of inherited disease, 8th edn. New York: McGraw-Hill; 2001.

320. Kobayashi RH, Kettelbut BV, Kobayashi AL. Galactose inhibition of neonatal neutrophil function. Pediatr Infect Dis 1983; 2:442–445.

321. Smetana HL, Olen E. Hereditary galactose disease. Am J Clin Pathol 1962; 38:3.

Disorders of fructose metabolism

322. Steinmana B, Gitzelmann R, Van den Berghe G. Disorders of fructose metabolism. In: Scriver CR, Beaudet AL, Sly WS, et al., eds. The metabolic and molecular bases of inherited disease, 8th edn. New York: McGraw-Hill; 2001.

Glycogen storage diseases

323. Chen Y-T. Glycogen storage diseases. In: Scriver CR, Beaudet AL, Sly WS, et al., eds. The metabolic and molecular bases of inherited disease, 8th edn. New York: McGraw-Hill; 2001.

324. McAdams AJ, Hug G, Bove KE. Glycogen storage disease types I–X. Hum Pathol 1974; 5:463–487.

325. Hufton BR, Wharton BA. Glycogen storage disease (type I) presenting in the neonatal period. Arch Dis Child 1982; 57:309–311.

326. Malatack JJ, Finegold DN, Iwatsuki S, et al. Liver transplantation for type I glycogen storage disease. Lancet 1983; I:1073–1075.

327. Bendon RW, Hug G. Morphologic characteristics of the placenta in glycogen storage disease type II. Am J Obstet Gynecol 1985; 152: 1021–1026.

328. Reifen RM, Nadjari M, Hurvitz H, et al. Hepatomegaly in utero in type III glycogenosis. Acta Paediatr Scand 1989; 78:954–955.

329. Fellows IW, Lowe JS, Ogilvie AL, et al. Type III glycogensosis presenting as liver disease in adults with atypical histological features. J Clin Pathol 1983; 36:431–434.

330. Ferguson IT, Mahon M, Bieminery WJK.An adult case of Andersen's disease-type IV glycogenesis: a clinical, histochemical ultrastructural and biochemical study. J Neurol Sci 1983; 60:337–351.

331. van Noort G, Straks W, Van Diggelen OP, et al. A congenital variant of glycogenosis type IV. Pediatr Pathol 1993; 13:685–698.

332. Milstein JM, Herron TM, Haas JE. Fatal infantile muscle phosphorylase deficiency. J Child Neurol 1989; 4:186–188.

333. Bonilla E, Schotland DL. The histochemical diagnosis of muscle phosphofructokinase deficiency. Arch Neurol 1970; 22:8–12.

334. Hug G, Schubert WK, Chuck G, et al. Liver phosphorylase. Deactivation in a child with progressive brain disease, increased hepatic glycogen and increased urinary catecholamines. Am J Med 1967; 42:139–145.

335. Minassian BA. Progressive myoclonus epilepsy with polyglucason bodies: Lafora disease. Adv Neurol 2002; 89:199–210.

336. Ganesh S, Puri R, Singh S, et al. Recent advances in the molecular basis of Lafora's progressive myoclonus epilepsy. J Hum Genet 2006; 51:1–8.

337. Eishi Y, Takemura T, Sone R, et al. Glycogen storage disease confined to the heart with deficient activity of cardiac phosphorylase kinase: a new type of glycogen storage disease. Hum Pathol 1985; 16:193–197.

338. Greene CM, Weldon DE. Juvenile polysaccharidosis with cardioskeletal myopathy. Arch Pathol Lab Med 1987; 111:977.

Phenylketonuria

339. Scriver CR, Kaufman S. The hyperphenylalaninemias. In: Scriver CR, Beaudet AL, Sly WS, et al., eds. The metabolic and molecular bases of inherited disease, 8th edn. New York: McGraw-Hill; 2001.

340. Malamud N. Neuropathology of phenylketonuria. J Neuropathol Exp Neurol 1966; 25:254–268.

341. Levy HL. Maternal phenylketonuria. In: Scarpelli DG, Migaki G, eds. Transplacental effects in fetal health. Bethesda, MD: Proceedings of a Symposium; 1988.

Hereditary tyrosinemia

342. Mitchell GA, Grampe M, Lambert M, et al. Hypertyrosinemia. In: Scriver CR, Beaudet AL, Sly WS, et al., eds. The metabolic and molecular bases of inherited disease, 8th edn. New York: McGraw-Hill; 2001.

343. Weinberg AG, Mize CE, Worthen HG. The occurrence of hepatoma in the chronic form of hereditary tyrosinemia. J Pediatr 1976; 88:434–438.

344. Hostetter MK, Levy HL, Winter HS, et al. Evidence for liver disease preceding amino acid abnormalities in hereditary tyrosinemia. N Engl J Med 1983; 308:1265–1267.

345. Hardwick DF, Dimmick JE. Metabolic cirrhoses of infancy and early childhood. Perspect Pediatr Pathol 1976. 3:103–144.

346. Gilbert-Barness E, Barness LA, Meisner LF. Chromosomal instability in hereditary tyrosinemia type I. Pediatr Pathol 1990; 10:243–252.

347. Tuchman M, Freese DK, Sharp HL, et al. Contribution of extrahepatic tissues to biochemical abnormalities in hereditary tyrosinemia type I: study of three patients after liver transplantation. J Pediatr 1987; 110:399–403.

348. Grenier A, Lescault A, Laberge C, et al. Detection of succinylacetone and use of measurement in mass screening for hererditary tyrosinemia. Clin Chem Acta 1982; 123:93–99.

349. Kvittingen EA, Brodtkorb E. The pre- and postnatal diagnosis of tyroseinemia type I and the detection of the carrier state by assay of fumarylacetoacetase. Scand J Clin Lab Invest Suppl 1986; 184:35–40.

350. Laberge C, Grenier A, Valet JP, et al. Fumarylacetoactase measurement as a mass-screening procedure for hereditary tyrosinemia type I. Am J Hum Genet 1990; 47:325–328.

351. Phaneuf D, Labelle Y, Bérubé D, et al. Cloning and expression of the cDNA encoding human fumarylacetoacetate hydrolase, the enzyme in hereditary tyrosinemia: assignment of the gene to chromosome 15. Am J Hum Genet 1991; 48:525–535.

352. Jakobs C, Stellard F, Kvittingen EA, et al. First trimester prenatal diagnosis of tyrosinemia type 1 by amniotic fluid succinylacetone determination. Prenat Diagn 1990; 10:133–134.

Alkaptonuria

353. La Du BN. Alkaptonuria. In: Scriver CR, Beaudet AL, Sly WS, et al., eds. The metabolic and molecular bases of inherited disease, 8th edn. New York: McGraw-Hill; 2001.

354. Gilbert-Barness E: Metabolic cardiomyopathy in childhood. In: Barness LA, Festschrift-Pomerance HH, Bercu BB, eds. Topics in pediatrics. New York: Springer-Verlag; 1990.

Non-ketotic hyperglycinemia

355. Perry TL, Urquhart N, MacLean J, et al. Nonketotic hyperglycinemia. Glycine accumulation due to absence of glycine cleavage in brain. N Engl J Med 1975; 292:1269–1273.

356. Tada K, Hayasaka K. Non-ketotic hyperglycinaemia: clinical and biochemical aspects. Eur J Pediatr 1987; 146:221–227.

357. Dobyns WB. Agenesis of the corpus callosum and gyral malforations are frequent manifestations of nonketotoic hyperglycinemia. Neurology 1989; 39:817–820.

Cystinosis and cystinuria

358. Chantler C, Carter JE, Bewick M, et al. 10 years' experience with regular haemodialysis and renal transplantation. Arch Dis Child 1980; 55:435–445.

359. Koizumi F, Koeda T. Cystinosis with marked atrophy of the kidneys and thyroid. Acta Pathol Jpn 1985; 35:145–155.

360. Schneider JA, Verroust FM, Kroll WA, et al. Prenatal diagnosis of cystinosis. N Engl J Med 1974; 290:878–882.

361. Smith ML, Pellett OL, Cass MMJ, et al. Prenatal diagnosis utilizing chorionic villus sampling. Prenat Diagn 1986; 6:195.

362. Patrick AD, Young EP, Mossman J, et al. First trimester diagnosis of cystinosis using intact chorionic villi. Prenat Diagn 1987; 7:71–74.

363. Smith ML, Clark KF, Davis SE, et al. Diagnosis of cystinosis with use of the placenta. N Engl J Med 1989; 321:397–398.

364. Dello Strologo L, Pras E, Ponteselli C, et al. Comparison between SLC3A1 and SLC7A9 cystinuria patients and carriers: a need for a new classification. J Am Soc Nephrol 2002; 13:2547–2553.

365. Town M, Jean G, Cherqui S, et al. A novel gene encoding an integral membrane protein is mutated in nephropathic cystinosis. Nat Genet 1998; 18:319–324.

366. Palacin M, Goodyer P, Nunese V, et al. Cystinuria. In: Scriver CR, Beaudet AL, Sly WS, et al., eds. The metabolic and molecular bases of inherited disease, 8th edn. New York: McGraw-Hill; 2001.

Homocystinuria

367. Beckman DR, Hoganson G, Gilbert EF. Pathological findings in 5,10-methylene tetrahydrofolate reductase deficiency. Birth Defects 1987; 23: 47–64.

368. Emery AH, Rimoin DL. Principles and practice of medical genetics. Edinburgh: Churchill Livingston; 1985.

369. Tonstad S, Refsum H, Ose L, et al. The C677T mutation in the methylenetetrahydrofolate reductase gene predisposes to hyperhomocystinemia in children with familial hypercholesterolemia treated with cholestyramine. J Pediatr 1998; 132:365–368.

370. Kang SS, Passen EL, Ruggie N, et al. Thermolabile defect of methylenetrahydrofolate reductase in coronary artery disease. Circulation 1993; 88:1463–1469.

371. Kanwar YS, Manaligod JR, Wong PWK. Morphologic studies in a patient with homocystinuria due to 5,10-methylenetetrahydrofolate reductase deficiency. Pediatr Res 1976; 10:598–609.

Albinism

372. King RA, Hearing VJ, Creel DJ, et al. Albinism. In: Scriver CR, Beaudet AL, Sly WS, et al., eds. The metabolic and molecular bases of inherited disease, 8th edn. New York: McGraw-Hill; 2001.

373. Tripathi RK, Strunk RM, Giebel LB, et al. Tyrosinase gene mutations in type I (tyrosinase deficient) oculocutaneous albinism define two clusters of missense substitutions. Am J Med Genet 1992; 43:865.

374. Lee ST, Nicholls RD, Bundley S, et al. Mutations of the P gene in oculocutaneous albinism, ocular albinism, and Prader-Willi syndrome plus albinism. N Engl J Med 1994; 330:529–534

375. Spritz AR, Hearing VJ. Genetic disorders of pigmentation. Adv Hum Genet 1994; 22:1.

376. Oetting WS, King RA. Molecular basis of oculocutaneous albinism. J Invest Dermatol 1994; 103:131S–136S.

377. Oetting WS, Brilliant MH, King RA. The clinical spectrum of albinism in humans. Mole Med Today 1996; 2:330–335.

378. Spritz RA. Molecular genetics of oculocutaneous albinism. Semin Dermatol 1993; 12:167–172.

379. Spritz RA. Molecular genetics of oculocutaneous albinism. Hum Mol Genet 1994; 3:1469–1475.

380. Rosenmann E, Rosemann A, Ne'eman Z, et al. Prenatal diagnosis of oculocutaneous albimism type I: review and personal experience. Perspect Pediatr Pathol 1999; 2:404.

Hartnup disease

381. Levy HL. Hartnup disorder. In: Scriver CR, Beaudet AL, Sly WS, et al., eds. The metabolic and molecular bases of inherited disease, 8th edn. New York: McGraw-Hill; 2001.

382. Haim S, Gilhar A, Cohen A. Cutaneous manifestations associated with aminoaciduria. Report of two cases. Dermatologica 1978; 156:244–250.

383. Mori E, Yamadori A, Tsutsumi A, et al. Adult-onset Hartnup disease presenting with neuropsychiatirc symptoms but without skin lesions. Clin Neurol 1989; 29:687–692.

Glutaric acidemia

384. Kimura S, Hara M, Nezu A, et al. Two cases of glutaric aciduria type 1: clinical and neuropathological findings. J Neurol Sci 1994; 123:38–43.

385. Floret D, Divry P, Dingeon N, et al. Acidurie glutarique: une nouvelle observation. Arch Fr Pediatr 1979; 36:462–470.

386. Goodman SI, Norenberg MD, Shikes RH, et al. Glutaric aciduria: biochemical and morphologic consideration. J Pediatr 1977; 90:746–750.

387. Gregersen N, Brandt NJ. Ketotic episodes in glutaryl-CoA dehydrogenase deficiency (glutaric aciduria). Pediatr Res 1979; 13:977–981.

388. Goodman SI, Markey SP, Moe PG, et al. Glutaric aciduria: a 'new' disorder of amino acid metabolism. Biochem Med 1975; 12:12–21.

389. Gregersen N, Brandt NJ, Christensen E, et al. Glutaric aciduria: clinical and laboratory findings in two brothers. J Pediatr 1977; 90:740–745.

390. Whelan DR, Hill R, Ryan ED, et al. L-Glutaric academia: investigation of a patient and his family. Pediatrics 1979; 63:88.

391. Leibel RL, Shih VE, Goodman SI, et al. Glutaric academia: a metabolic disorder causing progressive choreoathetosis. Neurology 1989; 30:1163.

392. Goodman SI, Kratz LE, Frerman FE. Pork and human cDNAs encoding glutaryl-CoA dehydrogenase. In: Coates PM, Tanaka K, eds. New developments in fatty acid oxidation. New York: Wiley-Liss; 1992:169.

393. Christensen E. First trimester prenatal exclusion of glutaryl-CoA dehydrogenase deficiency (glutaric aciduria type I). J Inherit Metab Dis 1989; 12:277–279.

394. Holme E, Kyllerman M, Lindstedt S. Early prenatal diagnosis in two pregnancies at risk for glutaryl-CoA dehydrogenase deficiency. J Inherit Metab Dis 1989; 12:280–282.

395. Iafolla AK, Kahler SG. Megalencephaly in the neonatal period as the initial manifestation of glutaric aciduria type I. J Pediatr 1989; 114:1004–1006.

396. Benett MJ, Marlow N, Pollitt RJ, t al. Glutaric aciduria type I: biochemical investigations and postmortem findings. Eur J Pediatr 1986; 145:403–405.

Oculocerebrorenal syndrome of lowe

397. Abbassi V, Lowe CU, Calcagno PL. Oculo-cerebro-renal syndrome: A review. Am J Dis Child 1968; 115:145–168.

398. Lowe CU, Terry M, MacLachan EA. Organic aciduria, decreased renal ammonia production, hydropthalmos, and mental retardation: a clinical entity. Am J Dis Child 1952; 85:164–184.

399. Bickel H, Thursby-Pelham DC. Hyperaminoaciduria in Lignac-Fanconi disease, in galactosaemia and in an obscure syndrome. Arch Dis Child 1954; 29:224–231.

400. Lamy M, Frezal J, Rey J, et al. Etude metabolique du syndrome de Lowe. Rev Fr Etude Clin Biol 1962; 7:271–283.

401. Le Febvre G, Biserte G, Woillez M, et al. Etude clinique, genetique and biologique du syndrome de Lowe-Bickel. Pediatr 1957; 12:527–534.

402. Richards W, Donnel GN, Wilson WA, et al. The oculocerebrorenal syndrome of Lowe. Am J Dis Child 1965; 109:185–203.

403. Hooft C, Valcke R, Herpol J. Etude clinique du syndrome de Lowe. Acta Pediat Belag 1964; 18:197–270.

404. Curtin VT, Joyce EE, Ballin N. Ocular pathology in the oculo-cerebro-renal syndrome of Lowe. Am J Ophthamol 1967; 64:533–543.

405. Witzleben CL, Schoen EJ, Tu WH, et al. Progressive morphologic renal changes in the oculo-cerebro-renal syndrome of Lowe. Am J Med 1968; 44:319–324.

406. Habib R, Bargeton E, Brissaud H-E, et al. Constatations anatomiques chex un enfant attaint d'un syndrome de Lowe. Arch Fr Pediatr 1962; 19:945–960.

407. Matin MA, Sylvester PE. Clinicopathological studies of oculo cerebrorenal syndrome of Lowe, Terrey and MacLachlan. J Ment Defic Res 1980; 24:1–16.

408. Chutorian A, Rowland LP. Lowe's syndrome. Neurology 1966; 16:115–122.

409. Banerjee AK, Allen IV, McKee P. Oculo-cerebro-renal syndrome: failure to demonstrate specific neuropathological abnormalities in four cases. Ir J Med Sci 1982; 15:42–45.

410. Suchy SF, Lin T, Horwitz JA, et al. First report of prenatal biochemical diagnosis of Lowe syndrome. Prenat Diagn 1998; 18:1117–1121.

411. Johnson JL, Duran M. Molybdenum cofactor deficiency and isolated sulfite oxidase deficiency. In: Scriver CR, Beaudet AL, Sly WS, et al., eds. The metabolic and molecular bases of inherited disease, 8th edn. New York: McGraw-Hill; 2001.

Disorders of branched-chain amino acid metabolism/organic acidemias

412. Sweetman L, Williams JC. Branched chain organic acidurias. In: Scriver CR, Beaudet AL, Sly WS, et al., eds. The metabolic and molecular bases of inherited disease, 8th edn. New York: McGraw-Hill; 2001.

Maple syrup urine disease

413. Chaung DT, Shih VE. Maple syrup urine disease or branched chain ketoaciduria. In: Scriver CR, Beaudet AL, Sly WS, et al., eds. The metabolic and molecular bases of inherited disease, 8th edn. New York: McGraw-Hill; 2001.

414. Scriver CR, Clow CL, George H. So-called thiamine responsive maple syrup urine disease: 15-year follow-up of the original patient. J Pediatr 1985; 107:763–765.

415. Van Calcar SC, Harding CO, Davidson SR, et al. Case reports of successful pregnancy in women with maple syrup urine disease and propionic acidemia. Am J Med Genet 1992; 44:641–646.

416. Diezel PB, Martin K. Die Ahornsirupkrankheit mit familiaren Befall. Virchows Arch 1964; 337:425.

417. Feign I, Budzilovich G, Pena C. The infantile spongy degeneration. J Neuropathhol Exp Neurol 1968; 27:158–159.

418. Riviello JJ Jr, Rezvani I, DiGeorge AM, et al. Cerebral edema causing death in children with maple syrup urine disease. J Pediatr 1991; 119:42–45.

Isovaleric acidemia

419. Duran M, Bruinvis L, Ketting D, et al. Isovaleric acidemia presenting with dwarfism, cataracts and congenital abnormalities. J Inherit Metab Dis 1982; 5:125–127.

420. Kelleher JF, Yudkoff M, Hutchinson RJ, et al. The pancytopenia of isovaleric acidemia. Pediatrics 1980; 65:1023–1027.

421. Kraus JP, Matsubara Y, Barton D, et al. Isolation of cDNA clones coding for rat isovarleryl-CoA dehydrogenase and assignment of the gene to human chromosome 15. Genomics 1987; 1:264–269.

422. Hyman DB, Tanaka K. Isovaleryl-CoA deydrogenase activity in isovaleric academia fibroblasts using an improved tritium release assay. Pediatr Res 1986; 20:59–61.

423. Frerman FE, Goodman SI. Fluorometric assay of acyl-CoA dehydrogenase in normal and mutant human fibroblasts. Biochem Med 1985; 33:38–44.

424. Hine DG, Hack AM, Goodman SI, et al. Stable isotope dilution analysis of isovaleryglycine in amniotic fluid and isovaleric academia. Pediatr Res 1986; 20:222–226.

Propionic acidemia

425. Fenton WA, Gravel RA, Rosenberg LE, et al. Disorders of propionate and methylmalonate metabolism. In: Scriver CR, Beaudet AL, Sly WS, et al., eds. The metabolic and molecular bases of inherited disease, 8th edn. New York: McGraw-Hill; 2001.

426. Kalousek F, Darigo MD, Rosenberg LE. Isolation and characterization of propionyl-CoA carboxylase from normal human liver: evidence for a protomeric tetramer of nonidentical subunits. J Biol Cem 1980; 255:60–65.

427. Gravel RA, Lam KF, Mahuran D, et al. Purification of human liver propionyl-CoA carboxylase by carbon tetrachloride extratction and monometric avidin affinity chromatography. Arch Biochem Biophys 1980; 201:669–673.

428. Lamhonwah AM, Barankiewics TJ, Willard HF, et al. Isolation of cDNA clones coding for the α and β chains of human propionyl-CoA carboxylase: chromosomal assignments and DNA polymorphisms associated with PCCA and PCCB genes. Proc Natl Acad Sci USA 1986; 83:4864–4868.

429. Rosenberg LE. The inherited methylmalonic acidemias: a model system for the study of vitamin metabolism and apoenzyme–coenzyme interactions (MilnerLecture). In: Belton NR, Toothill C, eds. Transport and inherited disease. Lancester: MTP; 1981.

Methylmalonic acidemias

430. Barness LA, Morrow F. Methylmalonic aciduria – a newly discovered inborn error. Ann Int Med 1968; 69:633–635.

431. Fenton WA, Gravel RA, Rosenberg LE. Disorders of propionate and methylmalonate metabolism. In: Scriver CR, Beaudet AL, Sly WS, et al., eds. The metabolic and molecular bases of inherited disease, 8th edn. New York: McGraw-Hill; 2001.

432. Morrow G, Schwartz RH, Hallock JA, et al. Prenatal detection of methylmalonic academia. J Pediatr 1970; 77:120.

Glutaric acidemia

433. Goodman SI, Frerman FE. Organic acidemias due to defects in lysine oxidation: 2-ketoadipic acidemia and glutaric acidemia. In: Scriver CR, Beaudet AL, Sly WS, et al., eds. The metabolic and molecular bases of inherited disease, 8th edn. New York: McGraw-Hill; 2001.

434. Mitchell G, Sauduleray JM, Gubler MC, et al: Congenital anomalies in glutaric acidemia type 2. J Pediatr 1984; 104:961–962.

435. Bohm N, Kiessling M, Lehner JW. Multiple acyl-CoA dehydrogenation deficiency (glutaric aciduria type II), congenital polycystic kidneys, symmetric warty dysplasia of the cerebral cortex in two newborn brothers. Eur J Pediatr 1982; 139:60–65.

436. Goodman SI, Stene DO, McCabe ER, et al. Glutaric academia type II: clinical, biochemical and morphologic considerations. J Pediatr 1982; 100(6):946–950.

437. Goodman SI, Binard RJ, Woontner MR, et al. Glutaric academia type II: gene structure and mutations of the electron transfer flavoprotein: ubiquinone oxidoreductase (ETF:QO) gene. Mol Genet Metab 2002; 77(1–2):86–90.

438. Goodman SI, Bemelen KF, Frerman FE. Human cDNA encoding ETF dehydrogenase (ETF:ubiquinone oxidoreductase), and mutations in glutaric academia type II. Prog Clin Biol Res 1992; 375:567–572.

Urea cycle defects

439. Masataka M. Regulation of the urea cycle genes in urea and nitric oxide synthesis (abstract). In: Advances in Inherited Urea Cycle Disorders; Vienna, Austria: May 20–21, 1997.

440. Batshaw ML. Inborn errors of urea synthesis. Ann Neurol 1994; 35:133–141.

441. Ozand PT, Gascon GG. Organic acidurias: a review. Part 1. J Child Neurol 1991; 6:196–219.

442. Ozand PT, Gascon GG. Organic acidurias: a review. Part 2. J Child Neurol 1991; 6:288–303.

Ornithine transcarbamylase deficiency

443. Fox JE, Rosenberg LE. Toward a molecular understanding of ornithine transcarbamylase deficiency. Adv Neurol 1988; 48:71–81.

444. Old JM, Briand PL, et al. Prenatal exclusions of ornithine transcarbamylase deficiency by direct gene analysis. Lancet 1985; 1:73–75.

445. Spence JE. Prenatal diagnosis and heterozygote detection by DNA analysis in ornithine transcarbamylase deficiency. J Pediatr 1989; 114:582–588.

446. Zimmerman A, Bachmann C, Colombo JP. Ultrastructural pathology in congenital defects of the urea cycle: ornithine transcarbamylase and carbamoylphosphate synthetase deficiency. Virchows Arch 1981; 393:321.

Carbamyl phosphate synthetase deficiency

447. Adcock MW, O'Brien WE. Molecular cloning of cDNA for rat and human carbamyl phosphate synthetase I. J Biol Chem 1984; 259:13471–13476.

448. Brusilow SW, Horwich AL. Urea cycle enzymes. In: Scriver CR, Beaudet AL, Sly WS, et al., eds. The metabolic and molecular bases of inherited disease, 8th edn. New York: McGraw-Hill; 2001.

449. Su TS, Bock HGO, O'Brien W, et al. Cloning of a DNA for arginosuccinate synthase in RNA and study of enzyme overproduction in a human cell line. J Biol Chem 1981; 256:11826–11831.

450. Todo S, Starzl TF, Tzakis A, et al. Orthotopic liver transplantation for urea cycle enzyme deficiency. Hepatology 1992; 15:419–422.

Citrullinemia

451. Spence JE. Prenatal diagnosis and heterozgote detection by DNA analysis in ornithine transcarbamylase deficiency. J Pediatr 1989; 114:582–588.

Hyperornithinemia, hyperammonemia, homocitrullinuria disease

452. Haust DM, Gordon BA. Possible pathogenetic mechanism in hyperornithinemia, hyperammonemia and homocitrullinuria syndrome. Birth Defects 1987; 23:17–45.

453. Wong P, Lessick M, Kang S, et al. Maternal hyperornithinemia-homocitrullinemia-hyperammonemia (HHH syndrome). Am J Hum Genet 1989; 45:A14.

454. Clarke LA, Dimmick JE, Applegarth DA. Pathology of inherited metabolic disease. In: Dimmick JE, Kalousek DK, eds. Developmental pathology of the embryo and fetus. Philadelphia: JB Lippincott; 1993.

Argininosuccinic aciduria

455. Simard L, O'Brien WE, McInnes RR. Argininosuccinate lyase deficiency. Proc Natl Acad Sci USA 1984; 81:44.

Argininemia

456. Fuehshuber A, Marescau LB, Roth B, et al. Hemodialysis and continuous veno-venous hemofiltration in a patient with hyperargininemia and acute renal failure. J Inherit Metab Dis 1993; 16:909–910.

Lysinuric protein intolerance

457. Cox RP. Errors of lysine metabolism. In: Scriver CR, Beaudet AL, Sly WS, et al., eds. The metabolic and molecular bases of inherited disease, 8th edn. New York: McGraw-Hill; 2001.

Biotinidase deficiency

458. Wolf B. Disorders of biotin metabolism. In: Scriver CR, Beaudet AL, Sly WS, et al., eds. The metabolic and molecular bases of inherited disease, 8th edn. New York: McGraw-Hill; 2001.
459. Wolf B, Grier RE, Allen RJ, et al. Phenotypic variation in biotinidase deficiency. J Pediatr 1983; 103:233–237.

Purine disorders

460. Bluese RM. Genetic immunodeficiency syndromes with defects in both T- and B-lymphocyte function. In: Scriver CR, Beaudet AL, Sly WS, et al., eds. The metabolic and molecular bases of inherited disease, 8th edn. New York: McGraw-Hill; 2001.
461. Jinnah HA, Friedmann T. Lesch-Nyhan disease and its variants. In: Scriver CR, Beaudet AL, Sly WS, et al., eds. The metabolic and molecular bases of inherited disease, 8th edn. New York: McGraw-Hill; 2001.
462. Becker MA, Roessler BJ. Hyperuricemia and gout. In: Scriver CR, Beaudet AL, Sly WS, et al., eds. The metabolic and molecular bases of inherited disease, 8th edn. New York: McGraw-Hill; 2001.
463. Virelizier JL, Hamet M, Ballet JJ, et al. Impaired defense against vaccine in a child with T-lymphocyte deficiency associated with isosine phosphorylase defect. J Pediatr 1978; 92:358–362.
464. Cregan RP, Tan YH, Chen S, et al. Mouse/human somatic cell hybrids utilizing human parental cells containing a (14:22) translocation. Assignment of a gene for nucleoside phosphorylase to chromosome 14. In: Bergsma D, ed. Human gene mapping. New York: National Foundation, March of Dimes; 1973.
465. Hershfield MS, Mitchell BS. Immunodeficiency diseases caused by adenosine deaminase deficiency and purine nucleoside phosphorylase deficiency. In: Scriver CR, Beaudet AL, Sly WS, et al., eds. The metabolic and molecular bases of inherited disease, 8th edn. New York: McGraw-Hill; 2001.
466. Kamatani N, Terai C, Kuroshima S, et al. Genetic and clinical studies on 19 families with adenine phosphoribosyltransferase deficiencies. Hum Genet 1987; 75:163–168.
467. Meyer RA, Teryung RL. Differences in ammonia and adenylate metabolism in contracting fast and slow muscle. Am J Physiol 1979; 237:C111–C118.
468. Jaeken J, Wadman SK, Duran M, et al. Adenylosuccinase deficiency: an inborn error of purine nucleotide synthesis. Eur J Pediatr 1988; 148:126–131.
469. Fishbein WN, Armbrustmacher VW, Griffin JL. Myoadenylate deaminase deficiency: a new disease of muscle, Science 1978; 200:545–548.
470. Roesel RA, Bowyer F, Blankenship PR, et al. Combined xanthine and sulfate oxidase defect due to deficiency of molybdenum cofactor. J Inherit Metab Dis 1986; 9:343–347.
471. Hirono A, Kanno H, Miwa S, et al. Pyruvate kinase and other enzymopathies of the erythrocyte. In: Scriver CR, Beaudet AL, Sly WS, et al., eds. The metabolic and molecular bases of inherited disease, 8th edn. New York: McGraw-Hill; 2001.

Purine disorders

472. Becroft DMO, Webster DR, Simmonds HA, et al. Hereditary orotic acidemia, further biochemistry. Adv Exp Med Biol 1986; 195A:67–70.
473. Valentine DM, Fink K, Paglia DE, et al. Hereditary hemolytic anemia with human erythrocyte pyrimidine 5-nucleotidase deficiency. J Clin Invest 1974; 54:866–879.

474. Marinaki AM, Escuredo E, Duley JA, et al. Genetic basis of hemolytic anemia caused by pyrimidine 5-prime-nucleotidase deficiency. Blood 2001; 97:3327–3332.

Fatty acid b-oxidation defects

475. Roe CR, Ding J. Mitochondrial fatty acid oxidation disorders. In: Scriver CR, Beaudet AL, Sly WS, et al., eds. The metabolic and molecular bases of inherited disease, 8th edn. New York: McGraw-Hill; 2001.
476. Yamaguchi S, Indo Y, Coates PM, et al. Identification of very long chain acyl-CoA dehydrogenase deficiency in three patients previously diagnosed with long chain acyl-CoA dehydrogenase deficiency. Pediatr Res 1993; 34:111–113.
477. Bertrand C, Largilliere C, Zabot MT, et al. Very long chain acyl-CoA dehydrogenas deficiency: identification of a new inborn error of mitochondrial fatty acit oxidation in fibroblasts. Biochem Biophys Acta 1993; 1180:327–329.
478. Turnbull DM, Shepherd IM, Barlett K, et al. Short-chain acyl-CoA dehydrogenase deficiency. In: Tanaka K, Coates PM, eds. Fatty acid oxidation: clinical, biochemical, and molecular aspects. New York: Alan R. Liss; 1990:313.
479. Treem W. Inborn errors in mitochondrial and fatty acid oxidation. In: Suchy FJ, ed. Liver disease in childhood. St. Louis: Mosby; 1994.
480. Clarke L, Dimmick JE, Applegarth DA. Pathology of inherited metabolic disease. In: Dimmick JE, Kalousek DK, eds. Developmental pathology of the embryo and fetus. Philadelphia, JB Lippincott; 1992:199.
481. Suchy FJ, ed. Short chain acyl dehydrogenase deficiency. In: Liver disease in children. St. Louis: Mosby; 1994.
482. Coates PM, Hale DE, Finochiarro, et al. Genetic deficiency of short chain acyl-CoA dehydrogenase in cultured fibroblasts from a patient with muscle carnitine deficiency and severe skeletal muscle weakness. J Clin Invest 1987; 81:171.
483. Bhala A, Willi SM, Rinaldo P, et al. Clinical and biochemical characterization of short-chain acyl-coenzyme A dehydrogenase deficiency. J Pediatr 1995; 126:910–915.
484. Dawson DB, Waber L, Hale DE, et al. Transient organic aciduria and persistent lacticacidemia in a patient with short-chain acyl-coenzyme A dehydrogenase deficiency. J Pediatr 1995; 126:69–71.
485. Boles RG, Buck EA, Blitzer MG, et al. Retrospective biochemical screening of fatty acid oxidation disorders in postmortem livers of 418 cases of sudden death in the first year of life. J Peediatr 1998; 132:924–933.
486. Rebouche CJ, Ppaulson DJ. Carnitine metabolism and function in humans. Annu Rev Nutr 1986; 6:41–66.
487. Turnbull DM, Bartlett K, Stevens DL, et al. Short chain acyl-CoA dehydrogenaase deficiency associated with a lipid-storage myopathy and secondary carnitine deficiency. N Engl J Med 1984; 311:1232–1236.

Pyruvate dehydrogenase deficiency

488. Robinson BH, Macmillan H, Petrova-Benedict R, et al. Variable clinical presentation in patients with deficiency of pyruvate dehydrogenase complex. J Pediatr 1987; 111:525–533.
489. Stansbie D, Wallace SJ, Marac C. Disorders of the pyruvate dehydrogenase complex. J Inherit Metab Dis 1986; 9:105–119.

Pyruvate carboxylase deficiency

490. Farrel DF, Clark AF, Scott CR, et al. Absence of pyruvate decarboxylate activity in man: A cause of congenital lactic acidosis. Science 1975; 187:1082–1084.
491. Farmer TW, Veath L, Miller AL, et al. Pyruvate decarboxylase deficiency in a child with subacute necrotizing encephalopathy. Neurology 1973; 23:429.

492. Gilbert EF, Arya S, Chin R. Leigh's necrotizing encephalopathy pyruvate decarboxylase deficiency. Arch Pathol Lab Med 1983; 107:162–166.

493. Trijbels JM, Sengers RC, Ruitenbeek W, et al. Disorders of the mitochondrial respiratory chain: clinical manifestations and diagnostic approach. Eur J Pediatr 1988; 148:92–97.

494. Robinson BH. Lactic acidemia (disorders of pyruvate carboxylate pyruvate dehydrogenase). 481. Suchy FJ, ed. Liver disease in children. St. Louis: Mosby; 1994

495. Sergers RCA, Stadhouders AM, Trijbels JMF. Mitochondrial myopathies: clinical, morphological and biochemical aspects. Am J Pediatr 1984; 141: 192–207.

496. Murphy JV, Isohasi F, Weinberg MG. Pyruvate carboxylase deficiency –an alleged biochemical cause of Leigh's disease. Pediatrics 1981; 88:401–404.

Mitochondrial disorders

497. Luft R, Ikkos D, Palmieri G, et al. A case of severe hypermetabolism of nonthyroid origin with a defect in the maintenance of mitochondrial respiratory control: a correlated clinical, biochemical, and morphological study. J Clin Invest 1962; 41:1776–1804.

498. Giles RE, Blanc H, Cann HM, et al. Maternal inheritance of human mitochondrial DNA. Proc Natl Acad Sci USA 1980; 77:6715–6719.

499. Wallace DC. Diseases of the mitochondrial DNA. Annu Rev Biochem 1992; 61:1175–1212.

Mitochondrial diseases

500. De Vivo DC. The expanding clinical spectrum of mitochondrial diseases. Brain Dev 1993; 15:1–22.

501. Stadhouders AM, Sengers RC. Morphological observations in skeletal muscle from patients with a mitochondrial myopathy. J Inherit Metab Dis 1987; 1:62–80.

502. DiMauro S, Bonilla E, Lombes A, et al. Mitochondrial encephalomyopathies. Neurol Clin 1990; 8:483–506.

503. Arnaudo E, Dalakas M, Shanske S, et al. Depletion of muscle mitochondrial DNA in AIDS patients with zidovudine-induced myopathy. Lancet 1991; 337:508–510.

504. Hale DE, Bennett MJ. Fatty acid oxidation disorders: a new form of metabolic diseases. J Pediatr 1992; 121:1–11.

Leigh syndrome

505. Rutledge JC, Haas JE, Monnat R, et al. Hypertrophic cardiomyopathy in a component of subacute necrotizing encephalomyelopathy. J Pediatr 1982; 101:706–710.

506. Servidei S, Bertini E, DiMauro S. Hereditary metabolic cardiomyopathies. In: Barness LA, ed. Advances in pediatrics, vol. 41. St. Louis: Mosby-Year Book; 1994.

507. van Erven PMM, Cillessen JP, Eekhoff EM, et al. Leigh syndrome, a mitochondrial encephalo(myo)pathy: A review of the literature. Clin Neurol Neurosurg 1987; 89:217–230.

508. Lombes A, Nakase H, Tritschler HJ, et al. Biochemical and molecular analysis of cytochrome C oxidase deficiency in Leigh's syndrome. Neurology 1991; 41:491–498.

509. Müller-Höcker J, Hübner G, Bise K, et al. Generalized mitochondrial microangiopathy and vascular cytochrome C oxidase deficiency. Arch Pathol Lab Med 1993; 117:202–210.

510. Van Hove JLK, Shanske S, Ciacci F, et al. Mitochondrial myopathy with anemia, cardiomyopathy, and lactic acidosis: a distinct late-onset mitochondrial disorder. Am J Med Genet 1994; 51:114–120.

511. Tritschler HJ, Bonilla E, Lombes A, et al. Differential diagnosis of fatal and benign cytochrome C oxidase-deficient myopathies of infancy: an immunohistochemical approach. Neurology 1991; 41:300–305.

512. Sparaco M, Bonilla E, DiMauro S, et al. Neuropathology of mitochondrial encephalomyopathies due to mitochondrial DNA defects. J Neuropathol Exp Neurol 1993; 52:1–10.

513. Ades LC, Gedeon AK, Wilson MJ. Barth syndrome: clinical features and confirmation of gene localization to distal Xq28. Am J Med Genet 1993; 45:327–334.

513a. Gonzalez IL. Barth Syndrome: TAZ gene mutations, mRNAs, and evolution. Am J Med Genet 2005; 134A:409–414.

514. Munnich A, Rustin P, Rotig A, et al. Clinical aspects of mitochondrial disorders. J Inherit Metab Dis 1992; 15:448–455.

515. De Vivo DC, DiMauro S. Mitochondrial defects of brain and muscle. Biol Neonate 1990; 1:54–69.

516. Salo MK, Rapola J, Somer H, et al: Reversible mitochondrial myopathy with cytochrome C oxidase deficiency. Arch Dis Child 1992; 67: 1033–1035.

Carnitine deficiency

517. Roe CR, Ding J. Mitochondrial fatty acid oxidation disorders. In: Scriver CR, Beaudet AL, Sly WS, et al., eds. The metabolic and molecular bases of inherited disease, 8th edn. New York: McGraw-Hill; 2001.

518. Rebouche CJ, Paulson DJ. Carnitine metabolism and function in humans. Annu Rev Nutr 1986; 6:41–66.

519. Gilbert EF. Carnitine deficiency. Pathology 1985; 17:161–171.

520. Roe CR, Millington DS, Maltley DA. Diagnostic and therapeutic implications of acylcarnitine profiling in organic acidurias with carnitine deficiency. In: Borum PR, ed. Clinical aspects of human carnitine deficiency. New York: Pergamon; 1986.

Carnitine palmotyl transferase deficiency

521. Salazar D, Wilcox WR. Carnitine palmitoyl transferase type I deficiency – a recognizable phenotype with a favorable prognosis. In: Society for Inherited Metabolic Disorders Annual Meeting, March 12–15, 1999.

Peroxisomal disorders

522. Moser HW. Peroxisomal diseases. In Barness LA, ed. Advances in pediatrics, vol. 36. St. Louis: Mosby-Year Book; 1989.

523. Brown FR, Voigt R, Singh A, et al. Peroxisomal disorders: neurodevelopmental and biochemical aspects. Am J Dis Child 1993; 147:617–626.

524. Lazarow PB. Rat liver peroxisomes catalyze the β oxidation of fatty acids. J Biol Chem 1978; 253:1522–1528.

525. Fournier B, Smeitink L, Dorland R, et al. Peroxisomal disorders: a review. J Inherit Metab Dis 1994; 17:481.

526. Aubourg PR, Sack GH, Meyers DA, et al. Linkage of adrenoleukodystrophy to a polymorphic DNA probe. Ann Neurol 1987; 21:349–352.

527. Roels F, Pauwels M, Poll-The BT, et al. Hepatic peroxisomes in adrenoleukodystrophy and related syndromes: cytochemical and morphometric data. Virchows Atch 1988; 413:275–285.

528. Beard ME, Moser AB, Sapirstein V, et al. Peroxisomes in infantile phytanic acid storage disease: a cytochemical study of skin fibroblasts. J Inherit Metab Dis 1986; 9:321–334.

529. Poll-The BT, SAudubray JM. Peroxisomal disorders. In: Fernades J, Saudubray JM, Van den Berghe G, eds. Inborn metabolic diseases, 2nd edn. Berlin: Springer; 1996.

Zellweger syndrome

530. Naritomi K, Hyakuna N, Suzuki Y, et al. Zellweger syndrome and a microdeletion of the proximal long arm of chromosome 7. Hum Genet 1988; 80:201–202.

531. Zellweger H. The cerebro-hepato-renal (Zellweger) syndrome and other perixosomal disorders. Dev Med Child Neurol 1987; 29:821–829.

532. Singh I, Moser AE, Goldfischer S, et al. Lignoceric acid is oxidized in the peroxisome: implications for the Zellweger cerebro-hepato-renal syndrome and adrenoleukodystrophy. Proc Natl Acad Sci USA 1984; 81:4203–4207.

533. Friedman A, Betzhold J, Hong R, et al. Clinico-pathologic conference: a three-month-old infant with failure to thrive, hepatomegaly and neurological impairment. Am J Med Genet 1980; 7:171–186.

534. Versmold HT, Bremer HJ, et al. A metabolic disorder similar to Zellweger syndrome with hepatic acatalasemia and absence of peroxisomes, altered content and redox state of cytochromes, and infantile cirrhosis with hemosiderosis. Eur J Pediatr 1977; 124:261–275.

535. Goldfischer S, Moore CL, Johnson AB, et al. Peroxisomal and mitochondrial defects in the cerebro-hepato-renal syndrome. Science 1973; 182:62–64.

536. Arias JA, Moser AB, Goldfischer SL. Ultrastructural and cytochemical demonstration of peroxisomes in cultured fibroblasts from patients with peroxisomal deficiency disorders. J Cell Biol 1985; 100:1789–1792.

537. Lazarow PB, Small GM, Santos M, et al. Zellweger syndrome amniocytes: morphological appearance and a simple sedimentation for prenatal diagnosis. Pediatr Res 1988; 24:63–67.

538. Volpe JJ, Adams RD. Cerebro-hepato-renal syndrome of Zellweger: an inherited disorder of neuronal migration. Acta Neuropathol 1972; 20:175–198.

539. Evrard P, Caviness VS Jr, Prats-Vinas J, et al. The mechanism of arrest of neuronal migration in the Zellweger malformation, an hypothesis based upon cytoarchitectonic analysis. Acta Neuropathol (Berl) 1978; 41:109–117.

540. Heymans HS. Cerebro-hepato-renal (Zellweger) syndrome: clinical and biochemical consequences of peroxisomal dysfunction. University of Amsterdam: Thesis; 1984.

541. Bernstein J, Brough AJ, McAdams AJ. The renal lesions of syndromes of multiple congenital malformations: cerebro-hepato-renal syndrome, Jeune asphyxiating thoracic dystrophy, tuberous sclerosis, Meckel syndrome. Birth Defects 1974; 10:35–43.

542. Goldfischer S, Powers JM, Johnson AB, et al. Striated adreno-cortical cells in cerebro-hepato-renal (Zellweger) syndrome. Virchows Arch (Pathol Anat) 1983; 401:355–361.

Neonatal adrenoleukodystrophy

543. Cohen SMZ, Brown FR III, Martyn L, et al. Ocular histopathological and biochemical studies of the cerebro-hepato-renal (Zellweger) syndrome and its relation to neonatal adrenoleukodystrophy. Am J Ophthalmol 1984; 96:488.

544. Poznanski AK, Nosanchuk JS, Baublis J, et al. The cerebro-hepato-renal syndrome (CHRS) Zellweger's syndrome. Am J Roentgen 1970; 109:313–322.

545. Williams JP, Secrest L, Fowler GW, et al. Roentgenographic features of the cerebro-hepato-renal syndrome of Zellweger. Am J Roentgen 1972; 115:607–610.

546. Hong R, Horowitz SD, Borzy MF, et al. The cerebro-hepato-renal syndrome of Zellweger: similarity to and differentiation from the DiGeorge syndrome. Thymus 1981; 3:97–104.

547. Vamecq J, Draye JP, van Hoof F, et al. Multiple peroxisomal enzymatic deficiency disorders: a comparative biochemical and morphological study of Zellweger cerebro-hepato-renal syndrome and neonatal adrenoleukodystrophy. Am J Pathol 1986; 125:524–535.

548. Ulrich J, Herschkowitz N, Heitz P, et al. Adrenoleukodystrophy: preliminary report of a connatal case. Acta Neuropathol 1978; 43:77.

549. Aubourg P, Scotto J, Rocchiccioli F, et al. Neonatal adrenoleukodystrophy. J Neurol Neurosurg Psychiatry 1986; 49:77–83.

549a. Powers JM. Adreno-leukodystrophy: a personal historical note. Acta Neuropathol 2005; 109:124–127.

Infantile refsum disease

550. Torvik A, Torp S, Kase BF, et al. Infantile Refsum's disease: a generalized peroxisomal disorder: report of a case with postmortem examination. J Neurol Sci 1988; 85:39–53.

X-linked adrenoleukodystrophy

551. Singh I, Moser AB, Moser HW, et al. Adrenoleukodystrophy: impaired oxidation of very long chain fatty acids in white blood cells, cultured skin fibroblasts and amniocytes. Pediatr Res 1984; 18:286–290.

552. Lazo O, Contreras M, Hashmi M, et al. Peroxisomal lignoceroyl-CoA ligase deficiency in childhood adrenoleukodystrophy and adrenomyeloneuropathy. Proc Natl Acad Sci USA 1988; 85:7647–7651.

553. Moser HW, Moiser AB, Singh I, et al. Adrenoleukodystrophy: survey of 303 cases: biochemistry, diagnosis and therapy. Ann Neurol 1984; 16:628–641.

554. Moser HW, Naidu S, Kumar AJ, et al. Adrenoleukodystrophy: toward a biochemical definition of a disease with varied presentations. CRC Crit Rev Neurobiol 1987; 3:29.

555. Barness LA, Chandra S, Gilbert-Barness E. Progressive neurologic deterioration in a nine-year-old male. Am J Med Genet 1990; 37:489–503.

556. Kumar AJ, Rosenbaum AE, Naidu S, et al. Adrenoleukodystrophy: correlating MR imaging with CT. Radiology 1987; 165:497–504.

557. Migeon BA, Moser HW, Moser AB, et al. Adrenoleukodystrophy: evidence for X-linkage, inactivation, and selection favoring the mutant allele in heterozygous cells. Proc Natl Acad Sci USA 1981; 78:5066–5070.

558. Kemp S, Pujol A, Waterham HR, et al. ABCD1 mutations and the X-linked adrenoleukodystrophy mutation data base: role in diagnosis and clinical correlations. Hum Mutat 2001; 18:499–515.

Hyperpipecolic acidemia

559. Brul S, Westerweld A, Strijland A, et al. Genetic heterogeneity in the cerebrohepatorenal (Zellweger) syndrome of other inherited disorders with a generalized impairment and peroxisomal functions: a study using complementation analysis. J Clin Invest 1988; 81:1710–1715.

Hyperoxaluria, primary oxalosis

560. Danpure CJ, Purdue PE. Primary hyperoxaluria. In: Scriver CR, Beaudet AL, Sly WS, et al., eds. The metabolic and molecular bases of inherited disease, 8th edn. New York: McGraw-Hill; 2001.

561. Danpure CJ, Jennings PR. Peroxisomal alanine: glyoxylate aminotransferase deficiency in primary hyperoxaluria type I. FEBS Lett 1986; 201:20.

562. Browski AE, Longman CB. Hyperoxaluria and systemic oxalosis: current therapy and future directions. Expert Opin Pharmacother 2006; 7:1887–1896.

563. Rosenblatt GS, Jenkins RD, Barry JM. Treatment of primary hyperoxaluria type 1 with sequential liver and kidney transplants from the same living donor. Urology 2006; 68:427–428.

564. Gelhart DR, Brewer LL, Fajardo LF, et al. Oxalosis and chronic renal failure after intestinal bypass. Arch Intern Med 1977; 137:239–243.

Acatalasemia

565. Wanders RJA, Jacobs C, Skjeldal OH. Single peroxisomal enzyme deficiencies. In: Scriver CR, Beaudet AL, Sly WS, et al., eds. The metabolic and molecular bases of inherited disease, 8th edn. New York: McGraw-Hill; 2001.

566. Quan F, Komeluk RG, Tropak MB, et al. Isolation and characterization of the human catalase gene. Nucleic Acids Res 1986; 14:5321–5335.

567. Junien C, Turleau C, de Grouchy J, et al. Regional assignment of catalase (CAT) gene to band 11p13: association with the aniridia-Wilms' tumor-gonadoblastoma (WAGR) complex. Ann Genet 1980; 23:165.

Classic refsum disease

568. Wanders RJA, Jacobs C, Skyeldal OH. Refsum's disease. In: Scriver CR, Beaudet AL, Sly WS, et al., eds. The metabolic and molecular bases of inherited disease, 8th edn. New York: McGraw-Hill; 2001.

569. Wanders RJA, Heymans HSA, Schutgens RBH, et al. Peroxisomal functions in classical Refsum's disease: comparison with infantile form of Refsum's disease. J Neurol Sci 1988; 84:147–155.

Rhizomelic chondrodysplasia punctata

570. Purdue PE, Zang IW, Skoneczny M, et al. Rhizomelic chondrodysplasia punctata is caused by deficiency of PEX7, a homologue of the yeast PTS2 receptor. Nat Genet 1997; 15:381–384.

571. Heymans HSA, Oorthuys JWE, Nelck G, et al. Rhizomelic chondro-dysplasia punctata: another peroxisomal disorder. N Engl J Med 1985; 313:187–188.

572. Heymans HSA, Oorthuys JWE, Nelck G, et al. Peroxisomal abnor-malities in rhizomelic chondrodysplasia punctata. J Inherit Metab Dis 1986; 9(Suppl 2):329.

573. Hoefler G, Hoefler S, Watkins PA, et al. Biochemical abnormalities in rhizomelic chondrodysplasia punctata. J Pediatr 1988; 112:726–733.

574. Tsuji S, Suzuki M, Ariga T. Abnormality of long chain fatty acids in erythrocyte membrane sphingomyelin from patients with adreno-leukodystrophy. J Neurochem 1981; 36:1046–1049.

575. Moser HW, Moser AB, Kawamura N, et al. Adrenoleukodystrophy: elevated C26 fatty acid in cultured skin fibroblasts. Ann Neurol 1980; 7:542–549.

576. Moser AE, Singh I, Brown FR III, et al. The cerebro-hepato-renal (Zellweger) syndrome: increased levels and impaired degradation of very long fatty acid and prenatal diagnosis. N Engl J Med 1984; 310:1141–1146.

577. Datta NS, Wilson GN, Hajra AK. Deficiency of enzymes catalyzing the biosynthesis of glycerol-ether lipids in Zellweger syndrome: a new category of metabolic disease involving the absence of peroxisomes. N Engl J Med 1984; 311:1080–1083.

578. Schrakamp G, Roosenboom CFP, Schutgens RBH. Alkyl dihydroxy-acetone phosphate synthase in human fibroblasts and its deficiency in Zellweger syndrome. J Lipid Res 1985; 26:867–873.

579. Wanders RJA, van Weringth G, Schrakamp G, et al. Deficiency of acyl-CoA dihydroxyacetone phosphate acyltransferase in thrombocytes of Zellweger patients: a simple postnatal test. Clin Chim Acta 1985; 151:217.

580. Roscher A, Molzer B, Bernheimer H, et al. The cerebro-hepato-renal (Zellweger) syndrome: an improved method for the biochemical diagnosis and its potential for prenatal diagnosis. Pediatr Res 1985; 19:930–933.

581. Roels F, Goldfischer S. Cytochemistry of human catalase: the demon-stration of hepatic and renal peroxisomes by a high temperature procedure. J Histochem Cytochem 1979; 27:1471–1477.

582. Shimozawa N, Suzuki Y, Orii T, et al. Diagnosis of Zellweger syndrome by rectal biopsy: Immunoblot of peroxisomal β oxidation enzyme and activity of dihydroxyacetone phosphate acyltransferase in rectal mucosa. Clin Chim Acta 1988; 175:345–347.

583. Bjorkhem I, Folk O. Assay of the major bile acids in serum by isotope dilution-mass spectrometry. Scand J Clin Invest 1983; 43:163.

584. Hajra AK, Datta NS, Jackson LG, et al. Prenatal diagnosis of Zellweger cerebro-hepato-renal syndrome. N Engl J Med 1985; 312:445–446.

Neonatal iron storage disease

585. Knisely AS, Magid MS, Dische MR, et al. Neonatal hemochromatosis. In: Gilbert EF, Opitz JM, eds. Genetic aspects of development pathology. New York: Alan R. Liss; 1987.

586. Silver MM, Beverley DW, Valberg LS, et al. Perinatal hemochromatosis: clinical, morphologic, and quantitative iron studies. Am J Pathol 1987; 128:538–554.

587. Witzleben CL, Uri A. Perinatal hemochromatosis: entity or end result? Hum Pathol 1989; 20:335–340.

588. Knisely AS. Neonatal hemosiderosis. In: Barness LA, ed. Advances in pediatrics, vol. 37. St. Louis: Mosby-Year Book; 1990.

589. Moerman P, Pauwels P, Vandenberghe K, et al. Neonatal hemochromatosis. Histopathology 1990; 17:345–351.

590. Hamill RL, Woods JC, Cook BA. Congenital atransferrinemia. A case report and review of the literature. Am J Clin Pathol 1991; 96: 215–218.

591. Bassett ML, Halliday JW, Powell LW. Value of hepatic iron measurements in early hemochromatosis and determination of the critical iron level associated with fibrosis. Hepatology 1986; 8:24–29.

592. Silver E, Cutz LS, Valberg M, et al. Hepatic morphology in perinatal hemochromatosis compared with liver disease in the newborn caused by proven and presumptive inborn metabolic errors. Pediatr Pathol Abs 1992; 12:248.

593. Hoogstraten J, DeSa DG, Knisely AS. Fetal liver disease may precede extrahepatic siderosis in neonatal hemochromatosis. Gastroenterology 1990; 98:1699.

594. Phillips MJ, Poucell S, Patterson J, et al. The liver. An atlas and text of ultrastructural pathology. New York: Raven Press; 1987.

595. Schoenlebe J, Buyon JP, Zitelli BJ, et al. Neonatal hemochromatosis associated with maternal autoantibodies against Ro/SS-A and La/SS-B ribonucleoproteins. Am J Dis Child 1993; 147:1072–1075.

Wilson disease

596. Chelly J, Monaco AP. Cloning the Wilson disease gene. Nat Genet 1993; 5:317–318.

597. Scheinberg IH, Sternlieb I. Wilson's disease. Philadelphia: WB Saunders; 1984.

598. Archer GJ, Monie RDH. Wilson's disease and chronic active hepatitis. Lancet 1977; 1:486–487.

599. Scott J, Gollan JL, Samourian S, et al. Wilson's disease presenting as chronic active hepatitis. Gastroenterology 1978; 74:645.

600. Ishak KG. Pathology of inherited metabolic disorders. In: Balisteri WF, Stocker JT, eds. Pediatric hepatology, Washington, DC: Hemisphere Publishing: 1990.

601. Goldfischer S, Sternlieb I. Changes in the distribution of hepatic copper in relation to the progression of Wilson's disease (hepatolenticular degeneration). Am J Pathol 1968; 53:883–901.

602. Irons RD, Schenk EA, Lee JCK. Cytochemical methods for copper. Arch Pathol Lab Med 1977; 101:298–301.

603. Jain S, Scheuer PJ, Archer BB, et al. Histological demonstration of copper and copper-associated protein in chronic liver diseases. J Clin Pathol 1978; 31:784–790.

604. Salaspuro M, Sipponen P. Demonstration of an intracellular copper-binding protein by orcein staining in long-standing cholestatic liver disease. Gut 1976; 17:787–790.

605. Nartey NO, Frei JV, Cherian MG. Hepatic copper and metallothionein distribution in Wilson's disease (hepatolenticular degeneration). Lab Invest 1987; 57:397–401.

606. Schilsky ML, Scheinberg H, Sternlieb I, et al. Liver transplantation for Wilson's disease: indications and outcome. Hepatology 1994; 19:583–587.

Menkes syndrome

607. Danks DM, Campbell PE, Stevens BJ, et al. Menkes kinky hair syndrome. An inherited defect in copper absorption with widespread effects. Pediatrics 1972; 50:188–201.

608. Kaler SG. Menkes disease. In: Barness LA, ed. Advances in pediatrics, vol. 41. St. Louis: Mosby-Year Book; 1994.

609. Menkes JH, Alter M, Steigleder GK, et al. A sex-linked recessive disorder with retardation of growth, peculiar hair, and focal cerebral and cerebellar degeneration. Pediatrics 1962; 29:764–779.

610. Uno H, Arya S. Neuronal and vascular disorders of the brain and spinal cord in Menkes kinky hair disease. In: Opitz JM, Bernstein J, eds. Topics in pediatric genetic pathology. The Enid Gilbert-Barness Festschrift. New York: Alan R. Liss; 1987.

Occipital horn syndrome

611. Kaler SG. Menkes disease. In: Barness LA, ed. Advances in pediatrics, vol. 41. St. Louis: Mosby-Year Book; 1994.

Cystic fibrosis

612. Riordan JR, Rommens JM, et al. Identification of the cystic fibrosis gene: cloning and characterization of complementary DNA. Science 1989; 245:1066–1073.
613. Oppenheimer EH, Esterly JR. Pathology of cystic fibrosis: review of the literature and comparison with 146 autopsied cases. Perspect Pediatr Pathol 1975; 2:241–278.
614. Farrell P, Gilbert-Barness E, Bell J, et al. Progressive malnutrition, severe anemia, hepatic dysfunction and respiratory failure in a three-month-old white female. Am J Med Genet 1993; 45:725–738.
615. Davidson AGF, Wong LTK, Kirby LT, et al. Immunoreactive trypsin in cystic fibrosis. J Pediatr Gastroenterol 1984; 3(Suppl 1):S79–S88.

Porphyrias

616. Anderson KE, Sassa S, Beshop DF, et al. Disorders of hemebiosynthesis: X-linked sideroblastic anemia and the porphyrias. In: Scriver CR, Beaudet AL, Sly WS, et al., eds. The metabolic and molecular bases of inherited disease, 8th edn. New York: McGraw-Hill; 2001.

Erythropoietic proto porphyria

617. Cripps DJ, Gilbert LA, Goldfarb SS. Erythropoietic protoporphyria. Juvenile protoporphyrin hepatopathy, cirrhosis and death. J Pediatr 1977; 91:744–748.

Bone metabolic inborn errors

618. Whyte MP. Hypophosphatasia. In: Scriver CR, Beaudet AL, Sly WS, et al., eds. The metabolic and molecular bases of inherited disease, 8th edn. New York: McGraw-Hill; 2001.

Vitamin D-resistant rickets

619. Marx SJ: Vitamin D and other calciferols. In: Scriver CR, Beaudet AL, Sly WS, et al., eds. The metabolic and molecular bases of inherited disease, 8th edn. New York: McGraw-Hill; 2001.

Appendix 1

EXAMPLES OF REFERENCE LABORATORIES FOR STUDIES OF METABOLIC DISEASES

DISEASE OR METABOLITE	LABORATORY DIRECTOR	PHONE NUMBER
Galactose Metabolism:	Chunli Yu, MD Emory University Emory Biochemical Genetics Laboratory Decatur, GA	(404) 778-8552 Fax: (404) 778-8557
Porphyrias	Piero Rinaldo, MD, PhD Mayo Clinic Biochemical Genetics Laboratory Rochester, MN	(507) 266-8158 Fax: (507) 266-2888
Urea cycle defects	V Reid Sutton, MD Baylor College of Medicine Biochemical Genetics Laboratory Houston, TX	(800) 411-GENE Fax: (713) 798-6584
Glycogen storage disease	Yuan-Tsong Chen, MD, PhD Duke University Medical Center Glycogen Storage Disease Laboratory Research Triangle Park, NC	(919) 684-2036 Fax: (919) 684-0414
Crigler-Najjar	[Not Found]	
Mitochondropathies	Georgirene D. Vladutiu, PhD The Women's and Children's Hospital of Buffalo Robert Guthrie Biochemical Genetics Laboratory Buffalo, NY	(716) 878-7513 Fax: (716) 878-7980
HMG-CoA lyase	Milan Elleder, MD, PhD Charles University 1st Faculty of Medicine Institute of Inherited Metabolic Disorders Praha 2, Czech Republic	(+420) 2-24967691 Fax: (+420) 2-24919392
Glutaric Aciduria	Stephen I. Goodman, MD UCHSC Biochemical Genetics Laboratory Department of Pediatrics University of Colorado Health Sciences Center at Fitzsimons Aurora, CO 80010	(303)724-3826 Fax: (303)724-3827
Acyl CoA dehydrogenase	Donald Chace, PhD, MFS Pediatrix Screening Bridgeville, PA	(866) 463-6436 Fax: (412) 220-0785
Peroxisomal disorders	Dr. Paul Lazarow Mt. Sinai School of Medicine New York, NY	(212) 241-1505 Fax: (212) 860-1174
Niemann-Pick C	Edwin H Kolodny, MD New York University School of Medicine NYU at Rivergate New York, NY	(212) 263-8344 (212) 263-1018
Fatty Acid Oxidation Disorders	Sihoun Hahn, MD, PhD Mayo Clinic Biochemical Genetics Laboratory Rochester, MN	(507) 266-8158 Fax: (507) 266-2888
MCAD Deficiency [Medium Chain Acyl-Coenzyme A Dehydrogenase Deficiency]	William J Rhead, MD, PhD Medical College of Wisconsin Fatty Acid Oxidation Laboratory Milwaukee, WI	(414) 266-2906 (414) 266-1616
Carnitine/ Acylcarnitine Profile	David S Millington, PhD Duke University Medical Center Pediatric Biochemical Genetics Lab Research Triangle Park, NC	(919) 684-2036 (919) 684-8944
Canavan Disease	Edwin H Kolodny, MD New York University School of Medicine NYU at Rivergate New York, NY	(212) 263-8344 Fax: (212) 263-1018

Mitochondrial Disorders	Georgirene D Vladutiu, PhD The Women's and Children's Hospital of Buffalo Robert Guthrie Biochemical Genetics Laboratory Buffalo, NY	(716) 878-7513 Fax: (716) 878-7980
Biotinidase Deficiency	Donald Chace, PhD, MFS Pediatrix Screening Bridgeville, PA	(866) 463-6436 Fax: (412) 220-0785
Menkes Kinky Hair Syndrome	Nina Horn, PhD, DMSc John F Kennedy Institute Medical Genetics Laboratory Center Glostrup, Denmark	(+45) 4326-0100 (+45) 4343-1130
Lysosomal Storage Disease	Jerry N Thompson, PhD, FACMG University of Alabama at Birmingham Metabolic Disease Center Birmingham, AL	(205) 934-6370 (205) 975-2742
Ketothiolase Deficiency	Milan Elleder, MD, PhD Charles University 1st Faculty of Medicine Institute of Inherited Metabolic Disorders Praha 2, Czech Republic	(+420) 2-24967691 (+420) 2-24919392
Neuronal ceroid lipofuscinosis	Katherine B Sims, MD Massachusetts General Hospital Neurogenetics DNA Diagnostic Laboratory Charlestown, MA	(617) 726-5721 (617) 724-9620
	John J Hopwood, PhD Adelaide Women's and Children's Hospital National Referral Laboratory North Adelaide, Australia	(+61) 8-8161-8062 (+61) 8-8161-7100

LABORATORIES PERFORMING SPECIALIZED STUDIES

A list of a number of laboratories performing metabolic studies can be accessed at:

http://biochemgen.ucsd.edu/

A web list of biochemical genetics laboratory services

LABORATORIES OFFERING MOLECULAR AND BIOCHEMICAL TESTING FOR SPECIFIC GENETIC DISORDERS.

http://www.genetests.org/

A directory of medical genetics laboratories.

Phone: 206 616-4033

Fax: 206 221-4679

E-mail: genetests@genetests.org

INFORMATION SITES FOR INHERITED DISORDERS

http://www.ncbi.nlm.nih.gov/

Directories of gene information from the National Center for Biotechnology Information

http://archive.uwcm.ac.uk/uwcm/mg/hgmd0.html

Human Gene Mutation Database at the Institute of Medical Genetics in Cardiff.

http://www3.ncbi.nlm.nih.gov/entrez/query.fcgi?db=OMIM

OMIM™ - Online Mendelian Inheritance in Man™

Complications of perinatal care

Glenn Taylor   Enid Gilbert-Barness

'To know truly is to know by causes.'   Francis Bacon: De Augmentis Scientiarum

Introduction

The survival of ever younger neonates in the developed countries resulting from the remarkable improvements in obstetric and perinatal care of the past four decades has been accompanied by a dramatic reduction in morbidity and mortality from birth associated complications. Whereas in the 1930s and 1940s birth trauma accounted for nearly 19% of neonatal mortality, in the 1980s it dropped to under 3% and at the end of the last millennium less than 1%.[1, 2] However, the fragile, physiologically immature fetus or infant remains at risk for iatrogenic injury related to these increasingly more sophisticated and more invasive interventions. The adverse consequences of perinatal care can relate to antepartum, intrapartum, or postpartum procedures or events, which may occur during therapeutic or diagnostic activities or, fortunately much less often, through the consequences of accidental or intentional trauma. Major forms of traumatic injury related to birth are listed in Box 13.1. The injury arising can be a recognized complication, a previously unrecognized event, an accident, or a potentially litigious misadventure. The injury may be the sole, a contributory, or an incidental factor in the mortality or morbidity. The best opportunity for evaluation, documentation, and correlation of the morphologic sequelae of injurious perinatal care lies with the pathologist autopsying the infant with a thorough, systematic technique that acknowledges not just the distinct anatomic features of the neonate but also anticipates the potential consequences of the therapeutic and diagnostic interventions.[3–5]

Complications of antenatal care

In the first and second trimesters diagnostic procedures comprise the most frequent iatrogenic risks for the fetus, while in the third trimester therapeutic and monitoring interventions become more important.

Diagnostic procedures

Fetal diagnostic procedures are generally performed to determine chromosomal abnormalities and to confirm or exclude inherited metabolic conditions. In most North American jurisdictions they are done in the second trimester before or around 18 weeks of gestational age, in order to allow for decisions on maintenance of pregnancy. In experienced hands, the procedures are safe for mother and fetus, with only a small incidence of serious complications.[6]

Amniocentesis

Sampling of the amniotic fluid usually is done transabdominally using a long needle, 18–22 gauge. Amniocentesis carries an estimated risk of fetal loss of 0.2–1.0%.[7] Cell culture failure occurs in less than 1% of cases where the specimen is taken at 16 weeks.[8] Invasive procedures such as amniocentesis may **elevate the maternal α-fetoprotein concentration**; therefore blood samples for screening should be obtained before amniocentesis is performed.

A small risk is present in amniocentesis even in experienced hands. The fetus may be damaged directly or the placenta may be punctured, resulting in hemorrhage. Stimulation of uterine contractions with the induction of premature labor, chorioamnionitis, or maternal sensitization to fetal blood may occur.[9,10] **Massive fetomaternal transfusion** is a potential complication. **Perforation of an umbilical vein**[11] has been reported with exsanguination and stillbirth. **Placental abruption** with fetal death has been related to this procedure.[12]

Tears of the amnion may result in amniotic band syndrome.[13] Distal limb **constrictions and amputations secondary to amniotic bands** have been attributed to amniocentesis.[14] Foot deformities have been associated with first trimester amniocentesis.[15,16]

Amniocentesis-related leakage of amniotic fluid during the canalicular stage of lung development (16–24 weeks of gestation) has been linked to lung hypoplasia.[17]

Collaborative studies in Canada,[18] Europe,[19] and the USA [National Institutes of Child Health and Human Development (NICHD)] found no increase in fetal wastage over the natural level expected at that stage of gestation. In the UK, the Medical Research Council Collaborative Study in 1978 found an **increase in fetal loss of 1–1.5%** over controls and a similar increase in infant morbidity.

A NICHD study found that post amniocentesis abortion was significantly associated with use of a needle larger than 18 gauge without relationship to the volume of fluid removed.[20] The needle may cause **fetal skin puncture** with healing to form small scars or dimples.[21] Needle punctures have resulted in fetal hemothorax, ileal atresia and peritoneal adhesions, intestinal–cutaneous fistulae, and ileal atresia.[22,23] Other **puncture injuries** include temporal and occipital skin lesions and porencephalic cysts, and severe brain injury.[24,25]

In the third trimester the most frequent complication of amniocentesis is premature rupture of membranes with risk for development of **chorioamnionitis**. However, perinatal death rarely complicates such amnionitis.[9,26] Factors in fetal injury during a third trimester amniocentesis is the large size and relative immobility of the fetus. Fatal intracranial hemorrhage, ocular trauma necessitating enucleation, hemothorax and hemopericardium, and pneumothorax are rare complications.[27–30]

To obviate the risks of amniocentesis non-invasive techniques for obtaining fetal cells such as isolating fetal cells from maternal blood or cervical mucous plugs have been tried and continue to be evaluated.[31,32]

Chorionic villus sampling

Depending on the location of the placenta, chorionic villi may be obtained by aspiration through a transcervical catheter or ultrasound guided transabdominal needle. Chorionic villus sampling (CVS) provides earlier availability of results than amniocentesis. The procedure is generally **performed between 9 and 12 weeks of gestation**. Results based on a direct preparation of spontaneously dividing cells are usually available in 24–48 h and final results from cultured cells in 10–14 days. Another advantage of CVS is that more tissue is obtained than by amniocentesis. This is useful when **DNA analysis** or **enzymatic diagnosis** is necessary. Amniocentesis must be used, however, for assays for which amniotic fluid is essential, such as measurement of α-fetoprotein concentration. Rate of **fetal loss with CVS is reported as 2.3–2.5%.**[33]

Firth and colleagues[34] reported **transverse limb-reduction defects** (TLDs) in five infants born to a group of 289 women who underwent CVS 56–66 days after the beginning of the last menstrual period (Fig. 13.1). **Oromandibular hypogenesis** was present in four of the five infants. The proposed mechanism is a form of vascular insult leading to hypoperfusion of the fetus.

The Italian Multicentric Birth Defect Registry and other studies found that CVS is a risk factor for fetal TLDs and

Therapeutic procedures

Fetal blood transfusion

Fetal peritoneal transfusion was first described for use in fetuses with erythroblastosis.[44] Although not now done for erythroblastosis fetalis, intrauterine fetal transfusions are still occasionally used when direct cord transfusion is not practical.[39] Preliminary precise localization of the placenta is essential. Blind traversal of an anteriorly placed placenta may result in laceration of a major fetoplacental vascular channel with subsequent fetal exsanguination.[45] Direct trauma to the fetus has resulted in **laceration of the heart, liver, and spleen, hemothoraces**, and **needle injuries to the brain, heart, and lung**. Instances of the accidental injection of contrast medium into the body or extremities of a fetus are reported.[46] Tension pneumothorax, subcutaneous emphysema, and hemothorax are rare complications.[46]

Currently, the treatment of **fetal anemia by intrauterine intravascular transfusion (cordocentesis)** permits a term delivery in the majority of cases and is associated with high perinatal survival and low perinatal morbidity.[47] Bleeding from uterine and umbilical cord puncture sites has not been of clinical significance; however, fetal bradycardia may occur.[48]

Perinatal transfusion

Hazards in administering blood products include transmission of hepatitis virus, cytomegalovirus (CMV), Epstein-Barr virus, and human immunodeficiency virus (HIV).[49–51]

The majority of transfusion-induced hepatitis cases have been due to hepatitis C. This is not usually as severe as hepatitis B, but it may lead to persistent elevation of liver enzymes and chronic liver disease.

Persons with serologic evidence of past infection can transmit CMV in their donated blood. **Antibody-screened, seronegative blood should be used in any perinatal transfusion.**[52]

Acquired immunodeficiency syndrome (AIDS) in infants and children has been acquired via perinatal blood transfusion.[49, 50] **HIV antibody screening is 98–99% sensitive**, but it may not detect antigen-positive, antibody-negative blood.

Graft-versus-host disease (GVHD) may be a complication of blood transfusion to the fetus that is immunodeficient. Acute GVHD usually occurs in babies who receive blood that differs at the HLA-D locus. **Blood or leukocytes should be irradiated before transfusion to inactivate the T cells.**[50] This is clinically essential for any infant considered a candidate for organ transplantation. In an intrauterine transfusion the exchange transfusion donor cells may cause GVHD.[53]

Fetal surgery

Fetal surgical procedures have been successfully performed for a number of defects.[54] Fetal surgical treatment for **diaphragmatic hernia** performed at the end of the second trimester, before pulmonary hypoplasia progresses too far, has been successful.[55] A major complication has been acute obstruction to the ductus venosus when the left lobe of the liver is reduced back into the

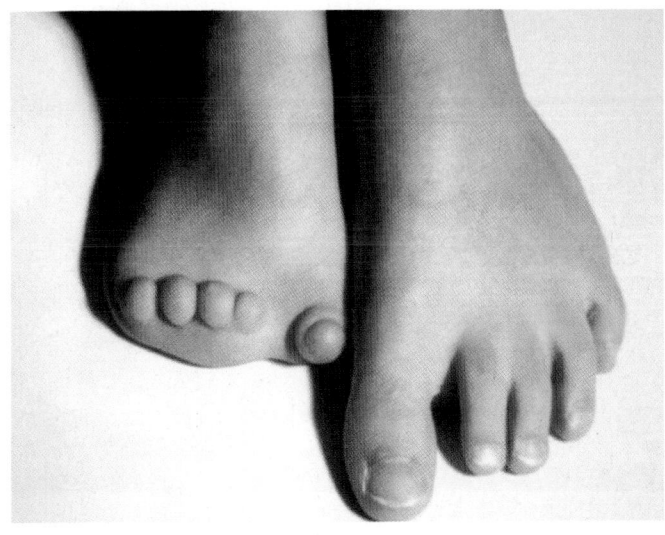

FIGURE 13.1 Transverse digital defects associated with chorionic villus sampling.

oromandibular-limb hypogenesis complex, particularly if performed before 70 gestational days.[35, 36] However, other studies have not confirmed this.[16, 37]

Percutaneous umbilical blood sampling

Beginning at approximately **18 weeks of gestation**, fetal blood can be obtained by a 20- or 22-gauge spinal needle inserted under ultrasound guidance into the umbilical cord. This technique was developed for the diagnosis of toxoplasmosis, but it permits the assessment of other **viral, bacterial, and parasitic infections by serologic testing, polymerase chain reaction, and culture**.[38] Access to the fetal circulation allows the prenatal evaluation of many **fetal hematologic abnormalities including isoimmunization, hemoglobinopathy, thrombocytopenia, and coagulation factor abnormalities**.[39] Fetal blood can be used for the prenatal diagnosis of some inborn errors of metabolism. Cytogenetic results from short-term fetal lymphocyte cultures are usually available within 48–72 h.

The rate of fetal loss with experienced operators is about 1%.[40, 41] Because percutaneous umbilical blood sampling entails a greater risk of pregnancy loss than amniocentesis, it should be reserved for situations requiring rapid diagnosis or diagnostic information that cannot be obtained by safer means.

Fetal biopsy

Certain **genetic skin disorders**, such as **epidermolysis bullosa**, that cannot now be diagnosed by DNA analysis require fetal skin sampling. **Fetal liver biopsy** was used in the past to diagnose ornithine transcarbamylase deficiency.[42] **Fetal muscle biopsy** has been used to diagnose Duchenne muscular dystrophy in a family in which DNA studies were uninformative.[43] However, the procedure carries risk of injury and hemorrhage to the fetus.

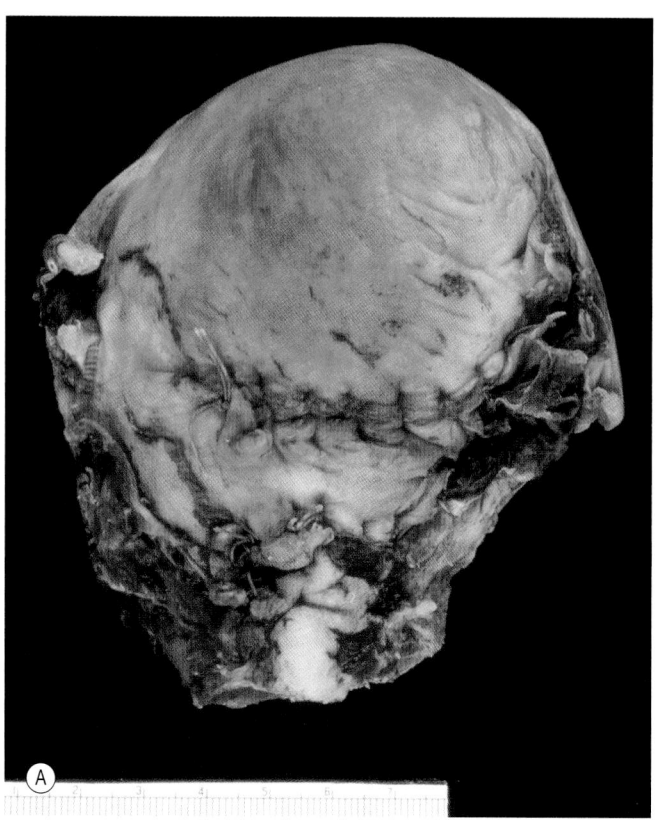

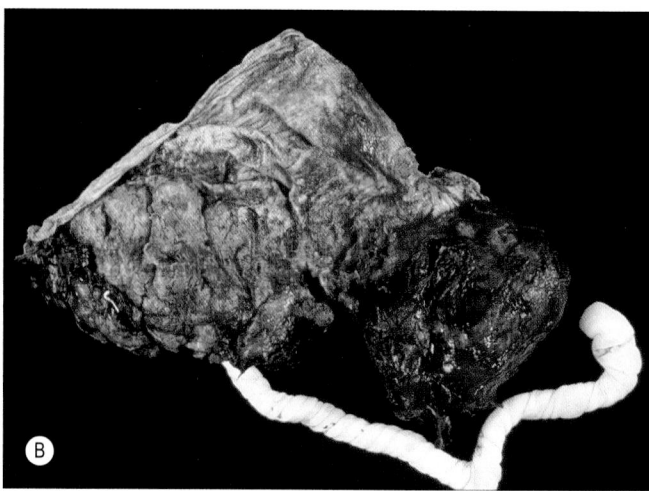

FIGURE 13.2 Maternal motor vehicle accident. (A) Sutured, surgically removed ruptured uterus. The fetus was expelled into mother's abdominal cavity. (B) Maternal surface of disrupted placenta with retroplacental hematoma (abruption).

abdomen. Gradual restoration of the liver to its intra-abdominal position has yielded better results.[56]

A technique using a plug placed in the trachea to prevent the egress of fetal lung fluid and consequently expand the compressed lung has been experimentally validated.[57] The pressure in the internally produced fluid displaces the herniated bowel. Clinical trials have had mixed results.[58]

For certain congenital heart defects surgical therapy in utero with cardiopulmonary bypass has resulted in increased placental vascular resistance, causing decreased placental blood flow with hypoxia to the infant. This may be related to the production of vasoactive prostaglandins after fetal cardiac bypass.[59]

Intrauterine fetal lobectomy and aspiration of cystic lesions and cystoamniotic shunts have been performed for congenital cystic lesions of the lung. One series reported death in four of six fetuses.[60] Because of this mortality risk and acknowledgement of the natural history of antenatally diagnosed congenital cystic adenomatoid malformation, fetal surgery for cystic lung lesions becomes a stronger option when there are associated complications like non-immune hydrops fetalis.[61]

In utero stem cell transplantation from human fetal liver or from cord blood has been used for the treatment of immunodeficiencies and thalassemia major. Fetal cells are infused into the umbilical vein or intraperitoneally (R Good, personal communication, 1995). This technique provides increased probability of graft take, ideal isolation of the fetus (in utero), and optimal environment for fetal cell development. Potential injuries include bleeding into the umbilical cord, abdominal injury, and premature labor.

Maternal factors in fetal injury

Maternal abdominal trauma

Fetal death and injury in utero due to maternal trauma sustained as an automobile passenger is a significant cause of perinatal death. The most common direct injuries occurring in the fetus have been **intracranial hemorrhage** and **skull fractures**.[62] Such injuries to the fetus implicate the conventional automobile lap belt as the causative agent in many cases. Therefore it has been recommended that the gravid patient should wear seat belt restraints under the uterus rather than over the fundus.[63]

Blunt abdominal trauma to the gravid uterus has resulted in fetal injury and death due to a variety of etiologies including: uterine rupture (Fig. 13.2A); intracranial hemorrhage – subarachnoid and intraventricular; abruptio placentae (Fig. 13.2B); **cord rupture; skull fracture; and other skeletal fractures including those of extremities**.[64]

Maternal drug administration

Medications that may adversely affect the fetus are discussed in Chapter 4. Medications administered late in gestation may affect the newborn (Table 13.1). Non-prescription drugs can also be hazardous to the fetus.[65] No drugs should be prescribed during pregnancy without weighing maternal need against the risk of fetal damage.

TABLE 13.1 MATERNAL MEDICATIONS THAT MAY AFFECT THE FETUS AND NEWBORN ADVERSELY – EXCLUDING TERATOGENIC EFFECTS*

Maternal medication	Fetal effects
Antacids	
Sodium bicarbonate	Metabolic alkalosis
	Circulatory overload
	Edema, congestive heart failure
Magnesium trisilicate	Damage to fetal kidneys
Antihistamines	Hypotension
Dimenhydrinate (Dramamine)	Liver toxicity
Diphenhydramine	Respiratory depression
Chlorpheniramine	
Belladonna derivatives	Tachycardia
Atropine	Respiratory depression
Scopolamine	
Camphor	Convulsions
Chloramphenicol	Gray-baby syndrome
Dapsone	Hemolysis in G6PD deficiency
Dextromethorphan	Respiratory depression
	Withdrawal symptoms
Dicumarol	Fetal bleeding, death, hypoplasia of nasal structures
Furazolidone	Hemolysis in G6PD deficiency
Iodides	Goiter
Laxatives	Increased intestinal peristalsis resulting
Aloe	in release of meconium in utero
	Kidney damage
Mepivacaine	Bradycardia, death
Methimazole	Goiter
Methyltestosterone	Masculinization of female fetus
Nitrofurantoin	Hemolysis in G6PD deficiency

Maternal medication	Fetal effects
Norlutin	Masculinization of female fetus
Para-aminophenol	Anemia
Acetaminophen	Methemoglobinemia
Phenacetin	Liver toxicity
	Hypotension
	Respiratory depression
Phenols	Liver toxicity
Thymol	Bone marrow depression
Hexylresorcinol	Convulsions
Phenytoin (Dilantin)	Malformations, IUGR, tumors
Primaquine	Hemolysis in G6PD deficiency
Propylthiouracil	Goiter
Quinine	Eighth cranial nerve dysfunction; limb malformations
Radioactive iodine	Destruction of fetal thyroid
Diethylstilbestrol	Vaginal adenosis and very rarely adenocarcinoma in adolescents
Sulfonamide	Hemolysis in G6PD deficiency; hyperbilirubinemia
Sympathomimetics	Palpitations
Ephedrine	Central nervous system irritability
Pseudoephedrine	Alkalosis; gastroschisis malformations
Phenylpropanolamine	
Xanthines	Tachycardia
Caffeine	Liver damage
Theophylline	Clotting deficiencies
Theobromine	

*Data from multiple sources. G6PD, glucose 6-phosphate dehydrogenase; IUGR, intrauterine growth retardation.

Complications of intrapartum care

Birth injuries

Birth injury represents neonatal trauma sustained during labor and delivery. The incidence of **birth injuries is estimated at 2–7 per 1000 live births**.[66, 67] Predisposing to birth trauma are large size of the infant, cephalopelvic disproportion, dystocia, prolonged labor, and breech presentation.[68, 69] Of all methods of delivery, **breech extraction** is the most hazardous to the infant (see below).

Extracranial edema and hemorrhages

Subcutaneous edema and hemorrhage

The presenting part of the fetus is surrounded and compressed by the uterus and late in labor by the cervix, except in the region of the cervical os; this usually results in edema of the presenting part. The part underlying the cervical os is subject to exudation of fluid and extravasation of blood into the subcutaneous tissues.

If the head is the presenting part, the area of maximal edema is usually over the vertex, a **caput succedaneum**. Microscopic examination of tissue from a caput succedaneum reveals an excessive amount of fluid and mild extravasation of blood cells around the smaller blood vessels. Generally the tissues return to normal in a few days. However, more extensive caput succedaneum can result from prolonged and traumatic vertex deliveries, often with associated **subgaleal hemorrhage** (Fig. 13.3).

In face presentation the subcutaneous tissues of the eyelids, cheeks, nose, and lips are edematous and hemorrhagic. Similar areas of edema and hemorrhage are present over the buttocks when the infant has been in a breech position. The scrotum or labia are usually also extremely congested, and in severe cases the testes and epididymis may show extensive interstitial extravasations.

An arm or a leg that is prolapsed through the cervix becomes edematous and discolored. Gangrene has been reported as a rare sequela to prolonged circulatory obstruction caused by constriction of the cervix around the proximal portion of a prolapsed extremity.

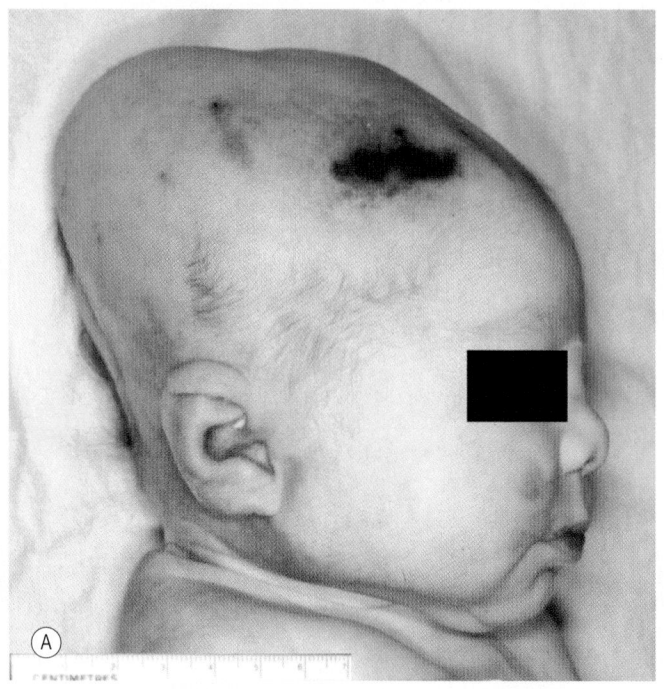

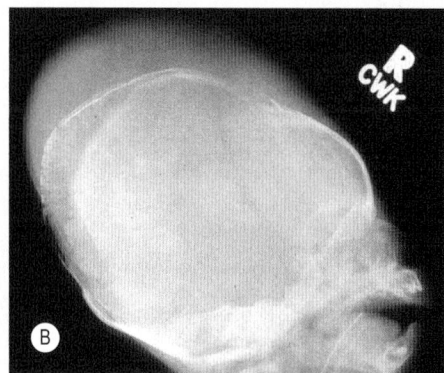

FIGURE 13.3 Traumatic vertex delivery. (A) Large caput succedaneum and subgaleal hemorrhage deforming head. (B) X-ray reveals associated skull fracture.

The use of a vacuum extractor (see below), especially when rigid vacuum cups are used, may result in a circumscribed area of soft tissue edema with localized hemorrhage called chinon (chignon) (Fig. 13.4). Excoriation of the overlying skin may occur. Healing without scarring usually ensues but occasionally permanent baldness results.

Subgaleal hemorrhage and cephalhematoma

Subgaleal hemorrhage forms in the tissue plane between the scalp aponeurosis and the periosteum of the skull (Fig. 13.5), whereas **cephalhematoma is an accumulation of blood between the surface of a calvarial bone and the periosteum** (Fig. 13.6). Both are most often associated with vacuum assist delivery (see below), but occasionally cephalhematoma is recognized antenatally.[70] Blood loss with subgaleal hemorrhage can lead to hypovolemic shock.[71] The collection of blood may be sufficient to deform the calvaria and compress the underlying brain.[72] However, as each bone of the calvaria is completely enveloped by an individual sheath of periosteum, blood loss with cephalhematoma is limited in surface area to the bone involved. Blood may be present over one or both parietal bones or over the squamous portion of the occipital bone, and one, two, or three individual elevations may be produced. These are easily differentiated from a caput succedaneum in a living child because they never extend over a suture line. The overlying scalp is not discolored, and the swelling may not be visible for hours after birth.

During the first few days the blood of a cephalhematoma is fluid and the mass is soft and fluctuant. The blood eventually clots and may be absorbed slowly or become organized and

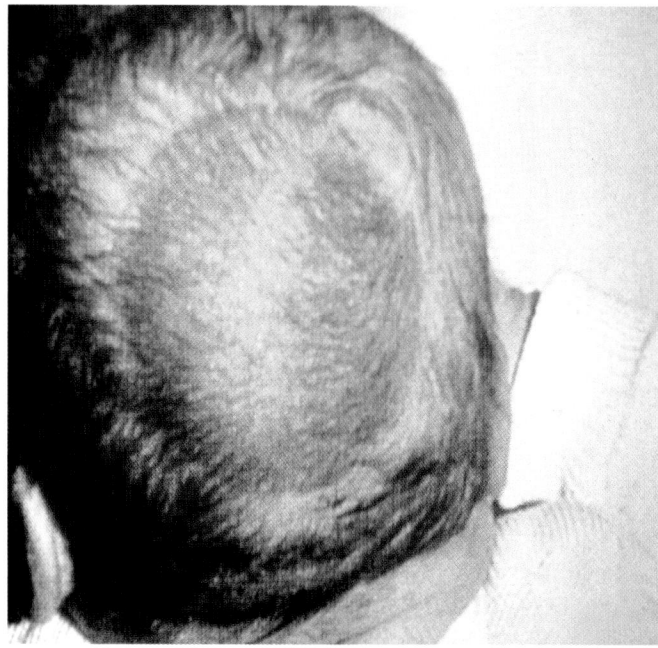

FIGURE 13.4 Chinon. Suction applied to vertex of head to facilitate delivery has resulted in a circumscribed area of edema and scalp hemorrhage.

eventually calcified. Bony elevations disappear only as the skull increases in size and thickness. Calcium is often deposited around the outer margin of the hemorrhage and forms a thin, hard rim that may make the bone beneath the cephalhematoma seem thinner than that of the rest of the skull. Most such

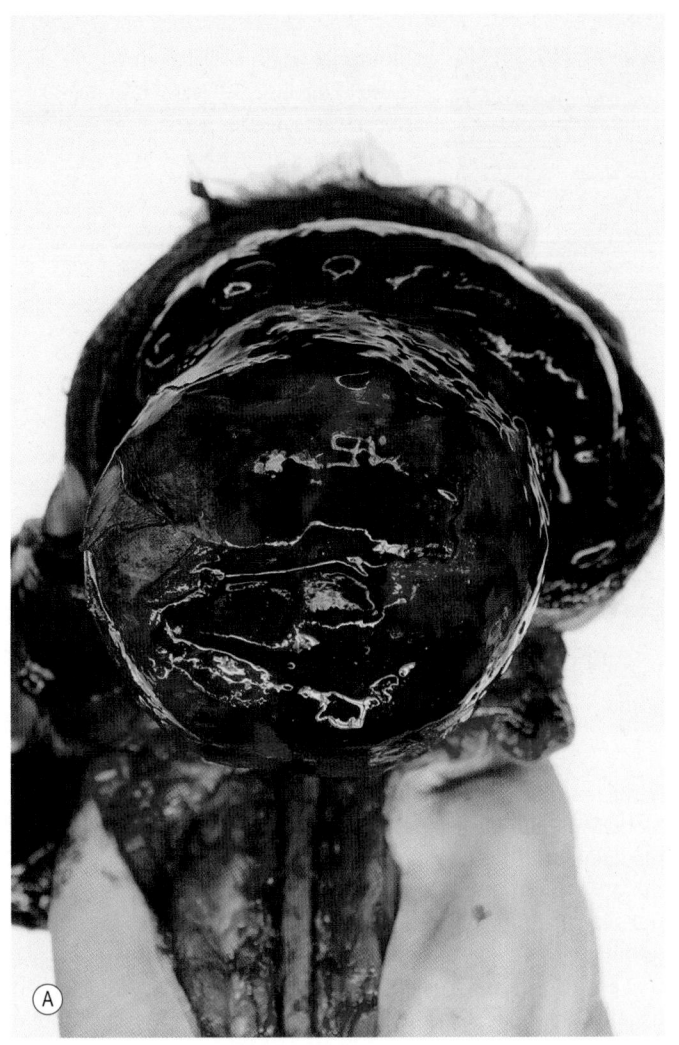
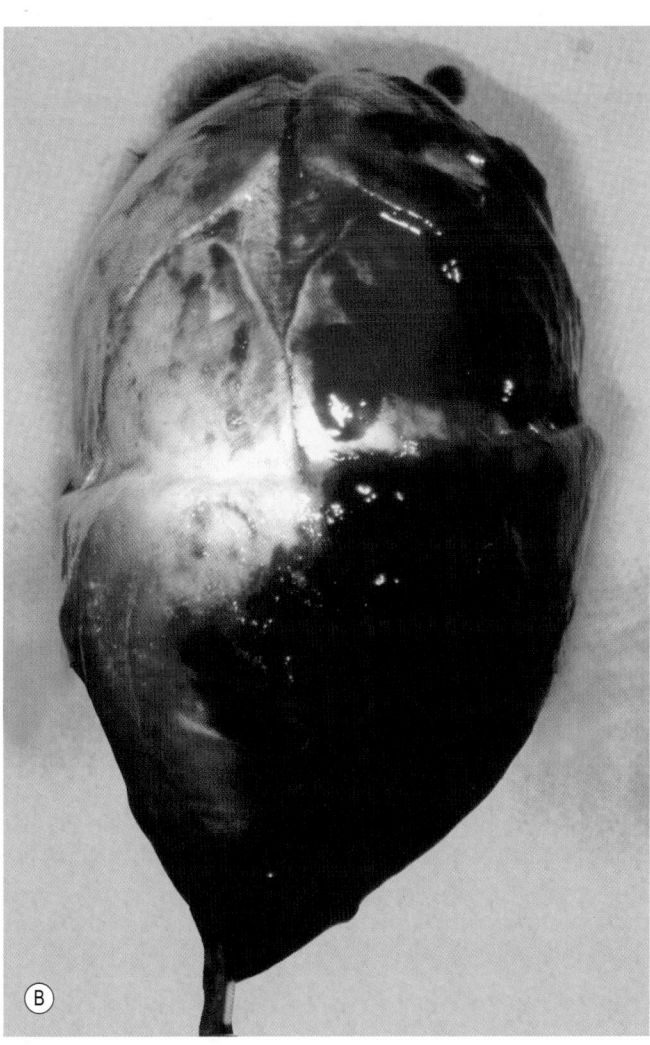

FIGURE 13.5 Subgaleal hemorrhages. (A) Extensive hemorrhage accumulates between the skull periosteum and the fibrous aponeurosis of the scalp. In this case there was associated occipital skull fracture. (B) The hemorrhage extends over sutures, often overlying multiple skull bones, here demonstrated by reflecting the scalp posteriorly.

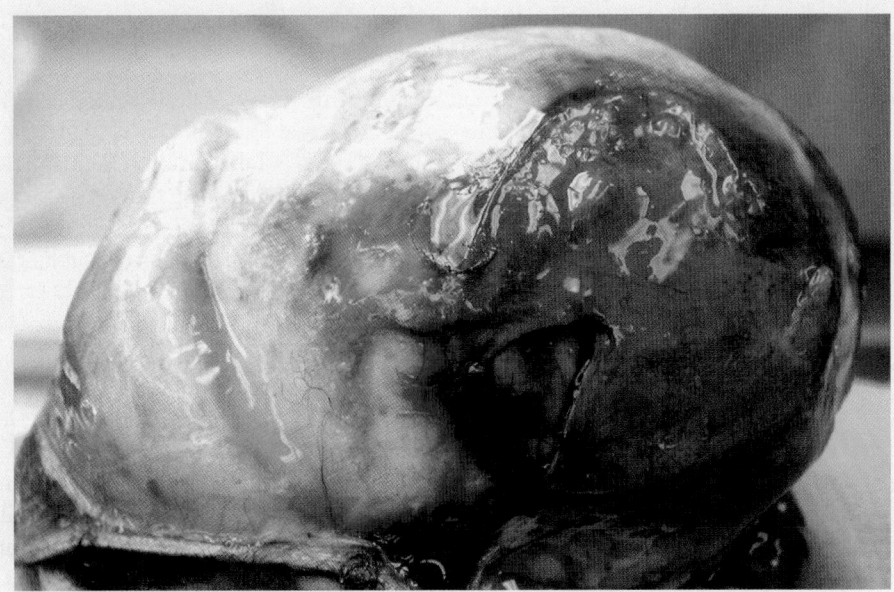

FIGURE 13.6 Cephalhematoma over left parietal bone. The hemorrhage demonstrated with the scalp reflected is confined by the sutures of the bone. The hematoma has been cut into, showing the accumulation of blood between the skull and the external periosteum.

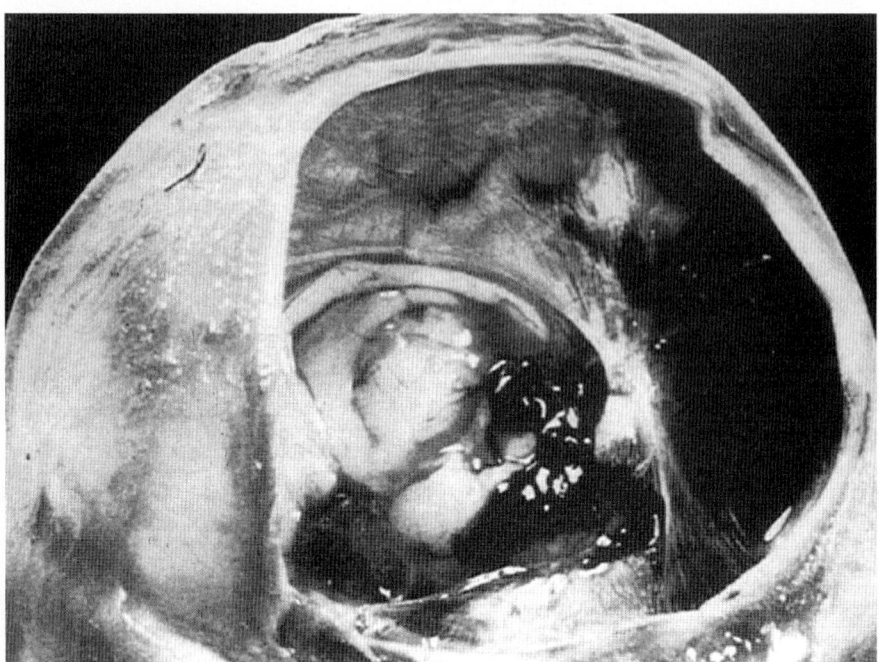

FIGURE 13.7 Intracranial hemorrhage caused by rupture of left leaf of tentorium cerebelli with extension into straight sinus.

collections of blood are resorbed within 2 weeks to 3 months. Occasionally, especially in a small, premature infant, a large cephalhematoma may result in excessive resorption of blood products, hyperbilirubinemia, and anemia. An underlying skull fracture, usually linear and not depressed, is frequently associated and easily overlooked.

Intracranial hemorrhages

Laceration of tentorium cerebelli

The brain is encased in a tough membrane – the dura mater. A midline extension of the dura grows downward from the superior sagittal suture to form a somewhat crescentic sheet separating the cerebral hemispheres, helping to hold them in place; this is the falx cerebri. In the posterior portion of the skull, the falx cerebri divides into the two leaves of the tentorium cerebelli, which form a roof over the cerebellum. The margins of the falx cerebri and tentorium cerebelli are reinforced with fibers designated 'bands of stress' because, like the selvedge on a piece of cloth, they can withstand more strain than the rest of the membrane. The falx is usually thinner than the tentorium and often has penetrations anteriorly, which should not be confused with traumatic lacerations.

As long as the force increases gradually and is directed toward the midline or is equally distributed on both sides of the head, there is little danger that the margin of either the falx or the tentorium will give way. If force is applied asymmetrically, one leaf of the tentorium is relaxed while the other is placed under excessive tension, and if the force is sufficient, especially if suddenly applied, the leaf of the tentorium that is under tension will rupture (Fig. 13.7). A simple laceration of the anterior margin of the tentorium does no harm in itself for this region contains no blood vessels. However, as the tentorium tears, the rent extends medially into the straight sinus that runs anteroposteriorly along the apex of the tentorium or laterally into the portion of the transverse sinus that lies just below the attachment of the tentorium to the dura mater. If one of these sinuses ruptures, the ensuing hemorrhage increases intracranial pressure and usually causes death. The major bleeding is subtentorial, but a thin layer is often present over the surface of the brain in the subdural space. The lower edge of the falx cerebri carries the inferior sagittal sinus, and rupture of the margin leads to immediate bleeding. Fortunately the tensions within the head are such that the margin of the falx seldom tears.

Rupture of the vein of Galen

The other structure subject to injury is the internal cerebral vein, commonly called the great vein of Galen, which is a **confluence of the internal veins of both cerebral hemispheres** and is somewhat **less than 1 cm long**. Arising near the posterior margin of the area in which the two cerebral hemispheres unite, it **empties into the straight sinus**. It is unsupported and literally hangs in space during its brief course (Fig. 13.8A). If the anteroposterior diameter of the head is abnormally increased, excessive tension may cause rupture of the wall of the vein of Galen with blood loss into the space around the base of the brain and between the cerebral hemispheres (Fig. 13.8B), with extension over the surface of the brain under the dura mater.[73]

Hemorrhage from the vein of Galen or from the transverse or straight sinus is **usually fatal** owing to the compression of vital centers of the brainstem with bleeding into the subtentorial space. **The location makes surgical treatment impossible**.

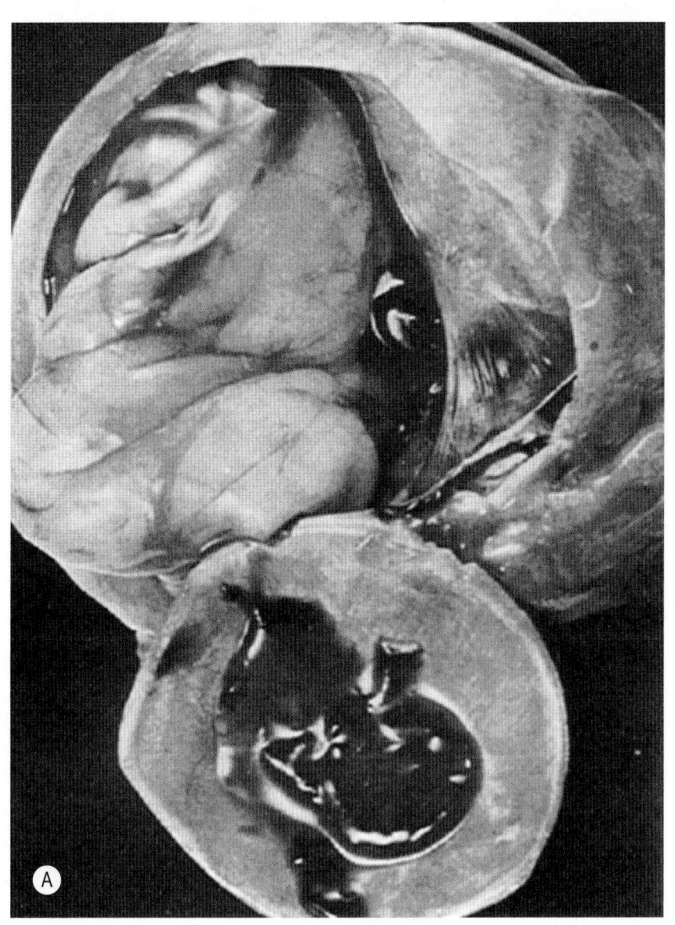

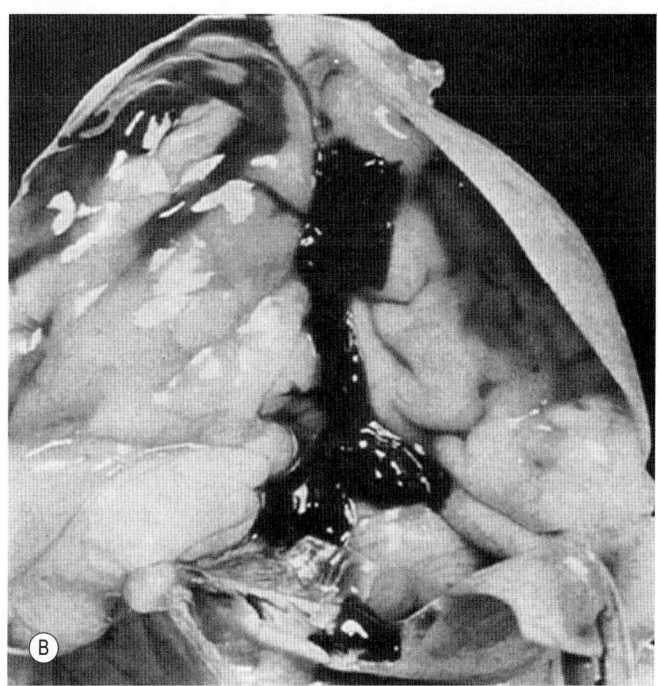

FIGURE 13.8 Rupture of vein of Galen. (A) Blood in region of vein of Galen and under dura. (B) Blood extending forward between cerebral hemispheres.

Massive subdural hemorrhage

Massive subdural hemorrhage (Fig. 13.9) is encountered particularly with high **forceps delivery** in babies born at term rather than in premature infants.[74] It is the most common form of intracranial birth injury occurring in the term neonate.[75] However, small subdural hemorrhages are identified in normal, vaginally born infants, without apparent neurologic sequelae.[76] A subdural hematoma may result from a **tear in the tentorium cerebelli** at its junction with the falx cerebri or from rupture of connecting veins over the vertex. If allowed to accumulate, it may destroy underlying brain tissue and extend into the ventricular system. If less severe the blood may remain in the meninges and only as a result of pressure may the brain be injured. The surface of the blood clot is often converted into a layer of granulation tissue that acts as a dialyzing membrane. Fluid is drawn into the clot, increasing its size and intensifying the symptoms resulting in a subdural hygroma. By means of a needle inserted through one of the cranial sutures, several milliliters of blood may be obtained on successive days. After a short time the material removed usually changes from pure blood to blood-tinged fluid. A subdural hematoma may be evacuated; if undisturbed it becomes organized and gradually converts into fibrous tissue that may calcify. Small subdural hygromas may spontaneously resorb. The destruction of blood

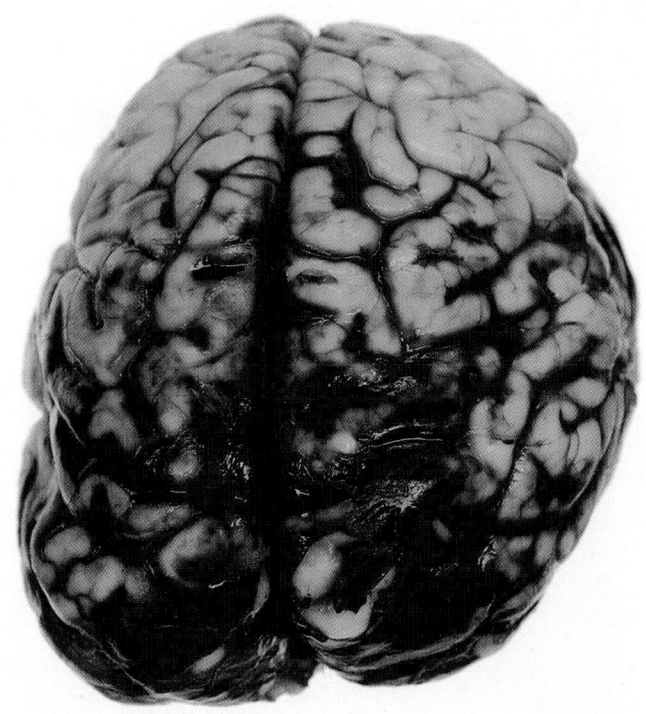

FIGURE 13.9 Posterior subdural hematoma associated with forceps assisted delivery. There was accompanying subgaleal hemorrhage and skull fracture.

cells in a hematoma may increase the serum bilirubin sufficiently to cause jaundice.

Subarachnoid hemorrhage

Hemorrhage into the subarachnoid space is usually mild, consisting principally of slight extravasation of cells in the areas around the major blood vessels, and is not uncommon. **Large subarachnoid hemorrhages are invariably a result of hypoxia, not caused by mechanical injury.** If small, it is usually not clinically recognized or seen on ultrasound scan.

Intraventricular and parenchymal hemorrhage

Intraventricular bleeding may accompany traumatic hemorrhage in other parts of the head (Fig. 13.10). Intraventricular hemorrhage is rare in term infants, but is relatively common in very low birth weight prematurely born infants (Fig. 13.11). When found alone it is **usually a result of hypoxia with hemorrhage beginning in the germinal matrix** (see Ch. 36). In rare cases the fourth ventricle may be the only site of hemorrhage and a massive hematoma may excavate the interior of the cerebellum.

Intracranial hemorrhage before onset of labor

In addition to small subdural hemorrhages seen by imaging studies in infants born by non-traumatic vaginal delivery, occasionally infants who are stillborn or die soon after birth have hemorrhagic areas in the brain that antedate birth. These areas are usually small, but may be 1–2 cm in diameter. Although some fresh blood may still be present in the central

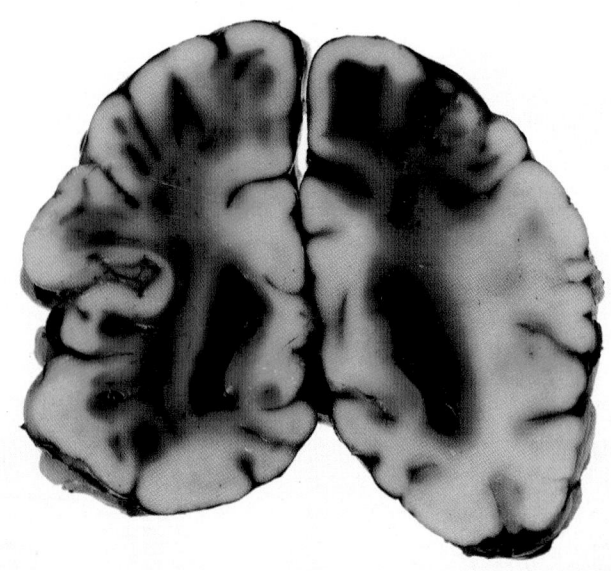

FIGURE 13.10 Intraventricular hemorrhage occurring with traumatic delivery of a term infant. There is associated subdural and intraparenchymal hemorrhage.

portions, the periphery of the lesion usually consists predominantly of large macrophages. Some areas contain blood pigment and others have lipid material derived from destroyed brain tissue. The cause of such bleeding is almost impossible to prove but is usually attributed to rupture of an aneurysm or hypoplastic blood vessel. It may be associated with stroke-like events in **offspring of cocaine-abusing mothers**.[77]

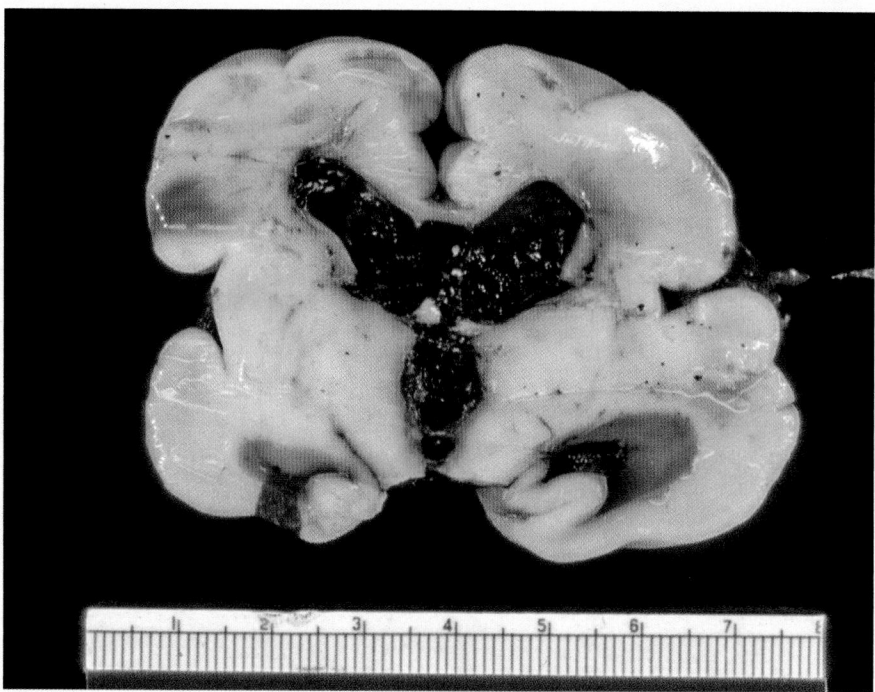

FIGURE 13.11 Extensive intraventricular hemorrhage in a premature infant.

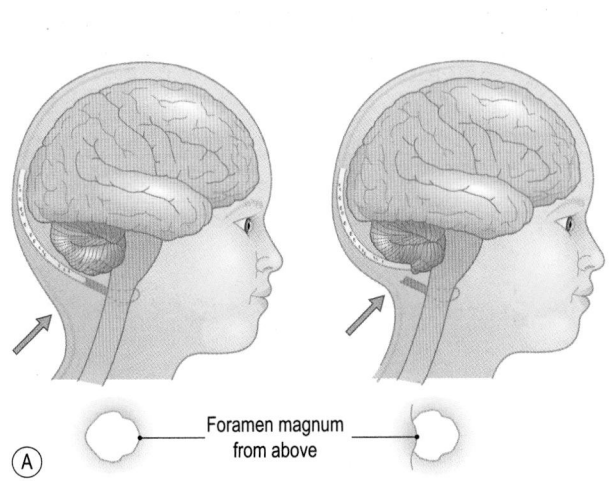

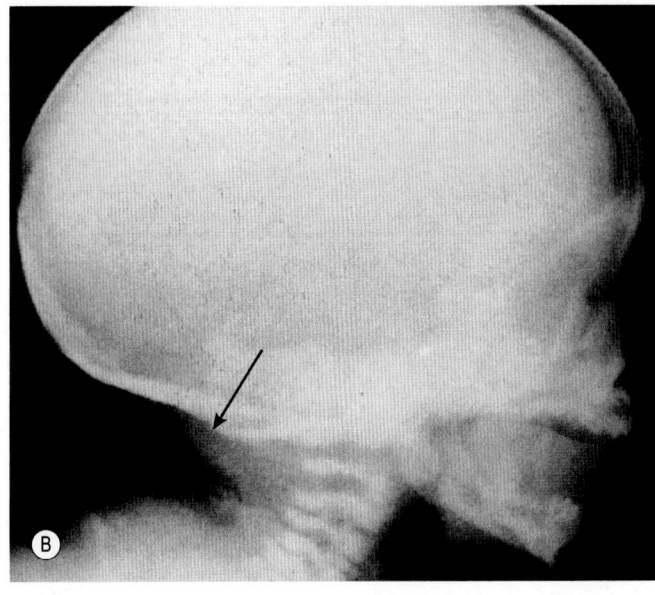

FIGURE 13.12 Occipital osteodiastasis. (A) Mechanism of injury. (From Pape 1979,[79] with permission.) (B) Lateral skull radiograph showing occipital osteodiastasis (arrow). (From Wigglesworth and Husemeyer 1977,[78] with permission.)

Epidural hemorrhage

Epidural hemorrhages are collections of **blood between the dura and overlying bone** usually due to **rupture of the middle cerebral artery**. They are rare in the newborn and are of **traumatic origin**.

Occipital osteodiastasis

Occipital diastasis (**separation of the squamous and lateral parts of the occipital bone**) is the most important form of disruption of the cranial bones but is missed at autopsy unless specifically sought.[78] At autopsy, reflection of the scalp downward as far as the foramen magnum is necessary to explore fully the occipital bone. A posterior approach to the intracranial autopsy facilitates recognition of this injury and of soft tissue disruptions in the posterior neck and upper back.[3] The squamous and lateral parts of the occipital bone are widely separated by cartilage until about 36 weeks' gestation and do not fuse until the second year of life. The lower margin of the squamous occipital bone forms the posterior boundary of the foramen magnum centrally and is closely related to the occipital sinuses on each side. Excessive pressure on the suboccipital region during birth causes **traumatic separation of the cartilaginous joint between the squamous and lateral parts of the bone on one or both sides**. The lower edge of the squamous occipital bone is then displaced and rotated forward. The dura and occipital sinuses are torn, resulting in **subdural hemorrhage in the posterior fossa and laceration of the cerebellum** (Fig. 13.12).[79]

The infant is most at risk during vaginal breech delivery but injury may occur in a persistent occipitoposterior presentation. A minor separation of the occipital bone with little displacement may be without consequence; however, a few millimeters' difference in the severity of displacement may result in distortion and obstruction of the venous sinuses in the posterior fossa or direct pressure on the cerebellum and brainstem, with rapid fatal outcome.

Fractures

Skull fracture

Skull fracture is usually attributed to **application of forceps** or pressure against the maternal symphysis pubis, sacral promontory, or ischial spines. Rarely, linear skull fracture has been reported with spontaneous vaginal delivery, attributed to an intrauterine event.[80] A portion of one parietal bone may become depressed. This is not a true fracture, for an actual break in continuity almost never occurs; it consists rather of a snapping inward of a thin resilient external table of bone. Symptoms are seldom produced, but the depressed area is usually elevated surgically because of fear that long-continued pressure might injure the underlying cortex. Linear fractures occurring over the prominence of the calvaria are usually in the parietal bone, at right angles to and adjoining the sagittal suture. However, they usually cause no symptoms and require no treatment.[73]

Linear fractures of the parietal bone have been described with **overlying cephalhematoma in an association as great as 25%**.[81] Leptomeningeal cysts may form along the fracture line. Such cysts appear as a 'growing fracture of the skull' and are associated with dural tears and significant neurologic morbidity as the cranial defect forms and enlarges.[82]

A serious complication following the application of forceps is a **bilateral multiradiate fracture of the parietal bones** (Fig. 13.13A), which may lead to exsanguination under the scalp within a few hours of birth even though the underlying dura remains intact.[83]

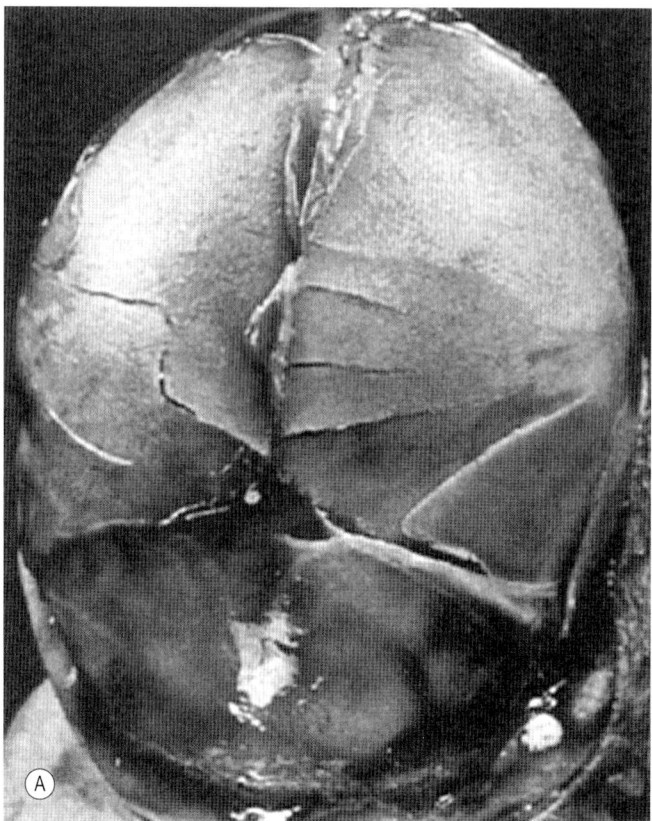
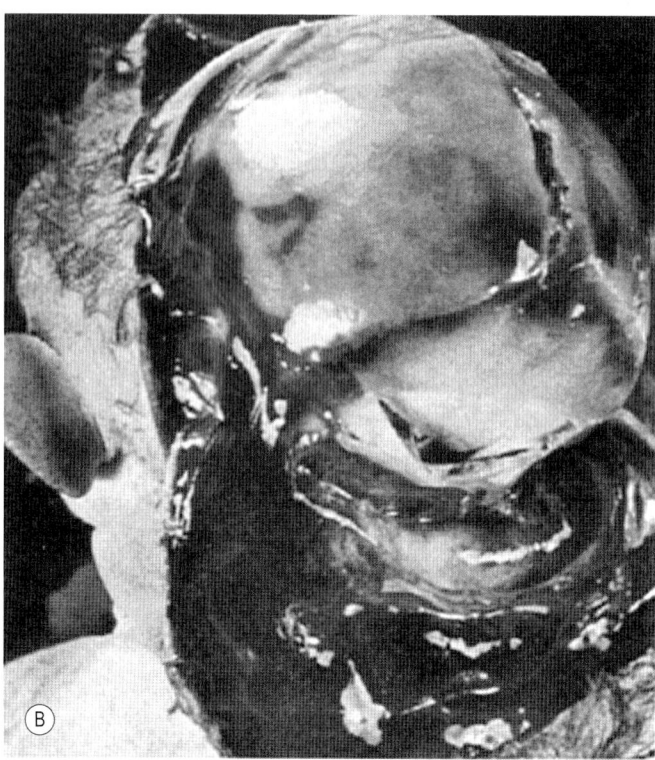

FIGURE 13.13 Severe birth trauma in infant stillborn at term. (A) Multiple skull fractures along normal planes of cleavage. The one fracture at right angles required more force for its production than did the others. (B) Fracture separating squamous and basal portions of occipital bone, responsible for hemorrhage under scalp and for laceration of cerebral sinuses with resultant massive intracranial hemorrhage. This type of hemorrhage may be seen in child abuse. Professor John Emery has seen this in a newborn baby who was swung by the heels, hitting the head on a mantelpiece and also on a bedrail.

Fracture of the occipital bone with separation of the basal and squamous portions is a form of injury frequently mentioned in the older literature but rarely observed with modern obstetric techniques. It is invariably fatal because the underlying vascular sinuses are disrupted by the separation of the two parts of the bone (Fig. 13.13B). It almost never occurs except in **breech deliveries** and ordinarily results when traction is applied to the hyperextended spine of the infant while the head remains fixed in the maternal pelvis. The squamous portion of the occipital bone is held beneath the symphysis pubis, and if the infant's body is pulled upward, the basal portion of the occipital bone moves with the spine and separates from the squamous portion, which is fixed in the pelvis. The line of separation is a suture formed earlier in fetal life and for this reason is weaker than any other part of the bone. If the infant's spine is not hyperextended during breech delivery at the same time as traction is exerted, such a fracture will not occur.

Depressed skull fractures may or may not be birth-associated injuries.[84] Depressions of the frontal or parietal bones may occur: in association with circumstances producing pressure of the fetal head against the maternal symphysis pubis, promontory of the sacrum, or ischial spines;[85] in association with difficult forceps delivery and possible misapplication of forceps; as deformities of the skull caused by intrauterine

position of fetal limbs, particularly if oligohydramnios is present;[86] or even as residua of prenatal fractures caused by abdominal trauma to the mother during the pregnancy.[87]

Fractures of the clavicle

Fractures of the clavicle are perhaps the most common orthopedic injury in the perinatal period and occur primarily in association with the delivery of **large infants, with breech presentation, or with shoulder dystocia**.[88, 89] A 3-year retrospective study of all deliveries in a residency program revealed that the incidence of clavicular fractures was 7.2 per 1000 term deliveries.[90]

The clavicle is fractured more frequently than any other bone (Fig. 13.14) during labor and delivery, particularly when difficulty is encountered in delivering the shoulders in a vertex presentation or arms are extended in breech deliveries. The arm portion of the Moro reflex is absent on the affected side. Of all deliveries, 4.3% may produce secondary injuries to the brachial plexus.

Fractures of the extremities

The femur and humerus are the only other bones fractured during a normal delivery. Approximately three-quarters of

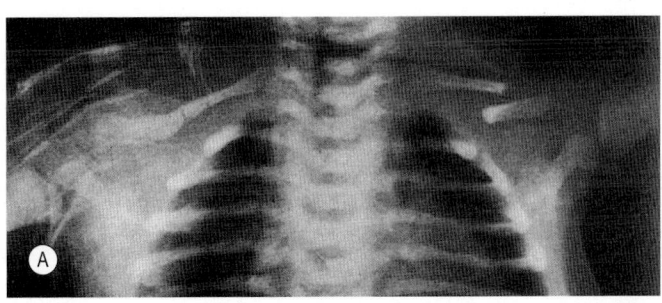 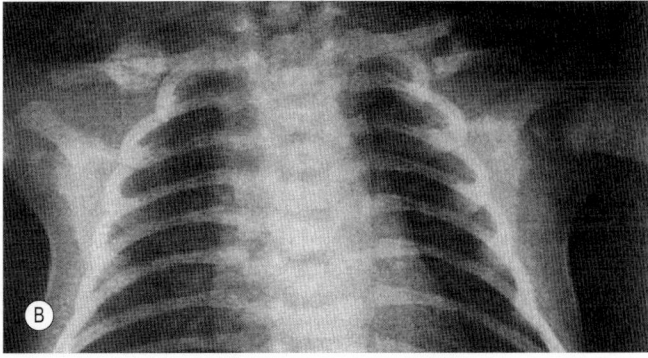

FIGURE 13.14 Bilateral fracture of the clavicles. (A) At age 2 days right clavicle well aligned; left, severely displaced. (B) At age 10 days callus deposited around both fractures.

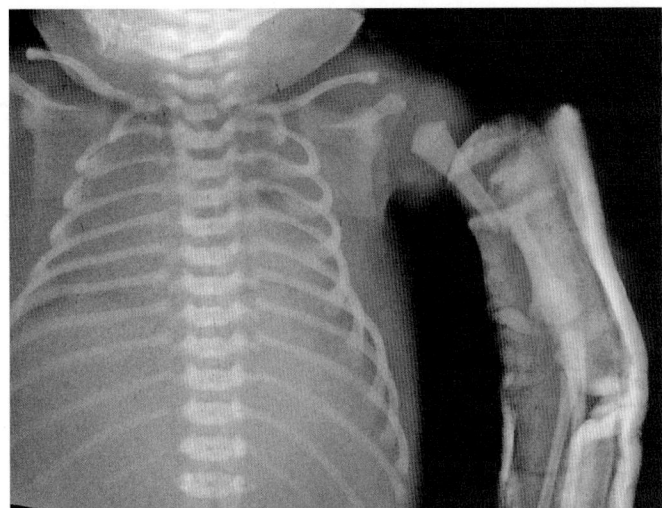

FIGURE 13.15 Mid shaft fracture of the left humerus in a neonate delivered from breech presentation.

birth-associated fractures occur with **breech presentation**. Fractures are rare with cephalic deliveries but may occur during an internal version. The fractures are usually located in the middle third of the bone and are ordinarily diagonal or spiral (Fig. 13.15).[91] There is usually marked overriding but often little or no lateral displacement. Callus forms rapidly. With appropriate therapy the prognosis for complete recovery is excellent, except for those with an associated neurologic injury such as a plexus injury.

Shoulder dislocations may occur in association with traction application without an associated fracture.[92] Traumatic epiphyseal separation of the distal humerus and dislocation of the radial head may occur at birth.[93] The latter is usually associated with delivery from the breech presentation.[94]

Neonatal traumatic proximal femoral epiphysiolysis is a complication of difficult and traumatic breech delivery of large infants.[95] This fracture of the upper epiphysis of the femur is believed to be caused by torsion injury to the femur during a footling breech delivery.

Fractures of the vertebrae

Vertebral fractures are most commonly associated with **breech delivery** or, at high cervical levels, with difficult obstetric forceps rotations. Fractures of spinous processes, the odontoid, or even fracture dislocation of vertebral bodies may occur. Almost uniformly such fractures occur when excessive force has been applied. **Lesions above C3 paralyze the diaphragm and lead to immediate fatality** unless ventilatory support is initiated. Those fractures and fracture dislocations that occur at a **lower cervical or upper thoracic level** usually result in **flaccidity of the legs and portions of the arms** with classic neurologic findings of paraparesis or quadriparesis.

Other fractures

Differentiation of birth trauma from **child abuse** may be necessary when fractures are diagnosed in the late neonatal period. Cumming pointed out that **calcification of most birth-associated fractures are apparent on radiographs by 9 or 10 days of life**.[96] If no calcification is present later than 11 days after birth, there is a high likelihood that the fracture represents trauma after birth. Skull fractures that appear to have been sustained during birth can simulate those of child abuse.

Rib fractures seen in the neonatal period result from either the problems of metabolic bone disease in association with prematurity, resuscitation, or some genetically determined bone dystrophies such as osteogenesis imperfecta.

Subluxation or fracture of the nasal septum in the newborn consists of dislocations or fractures of nasal bones and/or septum and usually occurs following persistent occiput posterior presentation and delivery.[97] When an alternate unilateral compression test of the nose is carried out as part of the normal newborn examination, 3.2% of deliveries are associated with dislocation of the nasal septal cartilage.[98]

Spine and spinal cord injuries

Injuries to the spine and spinal cord may occur when difficulty is encountered in delivering the shoulders in cephalic pre-

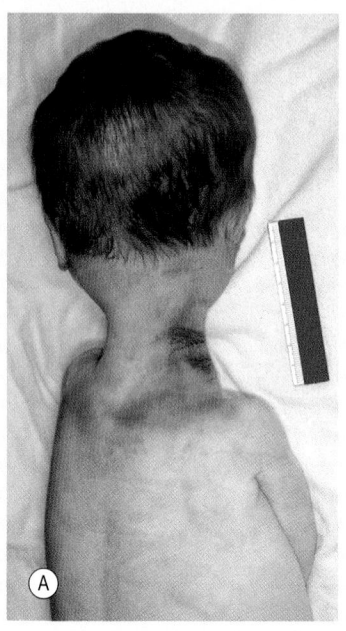

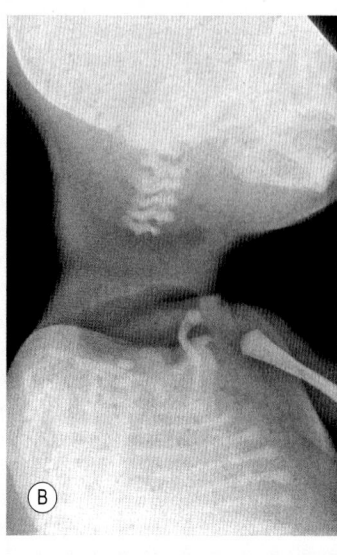

FIGURE 13.16 Cervical spinal column separation and cord transection. (A) High forceps were used to extract the infant from a delivery impeded by massive fetal ascites, resulting in excessive stretching of the neck. (B) The postmortem X-ray demonstrates separation of the vertebral column at the lower cervical level.

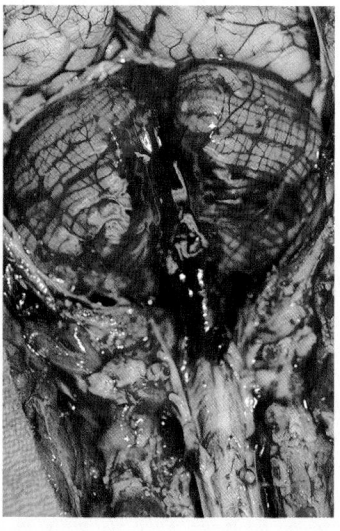

FIGURE 13.17 Traumatic breech delivery. Subdural and subarachnoid bleeding at the base of the brain, exposed by a posterior dissection approach.

are the maneuvers that most often produce fracture and separation of the vertebrae.[67]

Injuries include vertebral fracture with spinal cord transection, avulsion of the cord, subdural hemorrhage of the cord, and edema (Fig. 13.16). Most infants with severe spinal cord injuries die soon after birth. Postmortem examination may reveal a fracture and separation of the vertebrae; less often, blood in the spinal canal is the only evidence of injury (Fig. 13.17). If vertebrae have been dislocated, blood is usually present in the spinal subdural space or external to the spine in the connective tissue immediately surrounding the site of fracture.

Injury to the cervical region of the spinal cord may occur if the neck is overextended during delivery or with forceps rotations of 90 degrees or more.[100] **During an autopsy, it is necessary to excise the cervical portion of the vertebral column with the spinal cord in situ to examine the whole area for evidence of injury by slicing the specimen transversely after fixation and decalcification.**

sentations or the head in **breech presentations**. The latter is **especially dangerous when the head is hyperextended.**[99] These injuries may result in complete motor and sensory loss in the lower half of the body. The spinal cord can withstand considerable tension, and it has been stated that elongation of 2 cm or more produces no injury as long as the direction of traction is in the straight axis of the spine. Injury most frequently occurs at the **level of the seventh cervical and first thoracic vertebrae.** Strong traction exerted when the spine is hyperextended or when the direction of the pull is lateral, or longitudinal traction on the trunk while the head is still firmly engaged in the pelvis

Peripheral and cranial nerve injuries

Brachial plexus paralysis

Brachial plexus injury occurs when lateral traction is exerted on the head and neck during delivery of the shoulders in a vertex presentation, or when the arms are extended over the head in a **breech presentation**, sometimes with excessive traction on the shoulders. The reported incidence varies from approximately 1 to 5 per 1000 births.[101, 102] Babies with birth weights in excess of 4000 g are more susceptible to brachial plexus injury.[103]

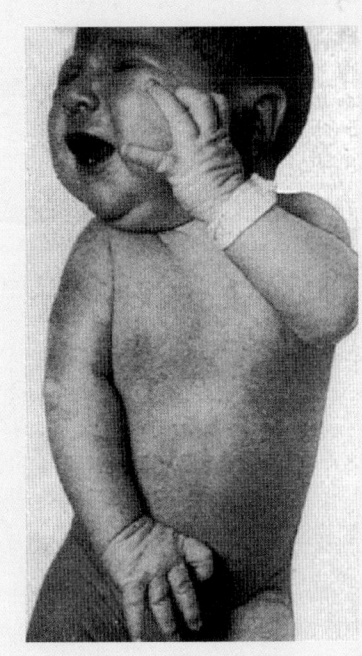

FIGURE 13.18 Erb's palsy. Paralysis of right arm showing characteristic position assumed after injury to 5th and 6th cervical roots of brachial plexus. Infant aged 7 days.

When the fifth and sixth cervical nerves are damaged (**Erb's palsy**) (Fig. 13.18), the **Moro reflex is absent** on the arm of that side. When the seventh and eighth cervical and first thoracic nerves are injured (**Klumpke paralysis**), the hand is paralyzed and produces ipsilateral ptosis, and meiosis (**Horner syndrome**) if the sympathetic fibers of the first thoracic root are injured. Fetal distress is a common concomitant and is present in 44% of instances.[104] The diaphragm may be paralyzed on the same side, and some infants also have facial paralysis.[104]

Phrenic nerve palsy

Phrenic nerve palsy is usually unilateral and associated with **upper brachial palsy on the same side**. The infant may become cyanotic and have irregular, labored respiration. Breathing is intercostal in type with no protrusion of the abdomen during inspiration.

Facial nerve palsy

Most facial nerve injuries result either from compression of the facial nerve against the rigid cervical spine during rotation or from direct pressure effects in the application of either mid or outlet forceps. **Facial nerve palsy often occurs with multiple birth injuries.**[97] The overall incidence is approximately 0.25% of live births and occurs not only with vaginal deliveries but with cesarean section. This suggests that the lesion may be produced by in utero positioning of the fetus as, for example, by pressure against the maternal sacral promontory or ischial spines.[105]

In virtually all affected infants there is rapid resolution of transient facial nerve palsy. **Nuclear agenesis (Moebius syn-**drome), **facial muscle agenesis**, as well as **pseudoparalysis secondary to in utero positioning of the fetus may be confused with facial nerve palsy**.

Visceral injuries

Types of visceral injuries are listed in Table 13.2.

Pericardial hemorrhage

Pericardial hemorrhage is rare. In a case from the Chicago Lying-In Hospital, a stillborn fetus – observed 2 days after the mother had fallen down a flight of stair – had an extensive pericardial hemorrhage.

Liver damage and subcapsular hematomas

The mildest type of hepatic damage, subcapsular hematoma, usually results from pressure exerted on the liver during delivery of the head in a **breech delivery**. If it follows cephalic presentations, it is usually caused by trauma sustained during **attempts at resuscitation**. No symptoms are produced as long as the capsule remains intact, but later manipulation of the infant during bathing, feeding, or examination may cause the hematoma to rupture; blood escapes into the abdomen and release of pressure permits fresh hemorrhage (Fig. 13.19). The infant can exsanguinate from loss of blood into the abdominal cavity and die before medical aid can be obtained or a diagnosis established. Small hematomas probably disappear without rupturing, although organized clots or areas in the liver suggesting earlier injuries are almost unknown. The small, unruptured hematomas occasionally found at autopsy cannot be considered a cause of death.

Gross laceration or rupture of the liver is uncommon[106]; it may also be associated with splenic rupture.[107]

Adrenal hemorrhages

The central part of the fetal zone of the adrenal gland is composed of anastomosing cords of cells separated by sinusoidal spaces somewhat like those in the liver. When these are dilated, as is common with anoxia or early maceration, the central portion of the gland appears hemorrhagic on gross inspection.[108] Even on microscopic examination this dilatation may be mistaken for hemorrhage.

Adrenal hemorrhages occur especially during **breech deliveries**.[109] An accumulation of as much as 30–40 mL of blood may remain in the capsule, but with greater bleeding the capsule generally ruptures and blood escapes into the surrounding tissues, producing perirenal hemorrhage (Fig. 13.20A). Such hemorrhage is usually unilateral, although occasionally both glands are involved. **They may calcify** within a few days. In older individuals calcified areas that have resulted from earlier hematomas may distend the central portion of the gland (Fig. 13.20B).[110] Adrenal

TABLE 13.2 TYPES OF VISCERAL INJURIES

Organ	Injury	Clinical features
Liver	Laceration; rupture; subcapsular hematoma	Pallor; tachycardia
		Tachypnea
		Low or falling hematocrit
		Hypovolemic shock
		Distention
		Cullen sign
		Hemoscrotum
		Diagnosis, radiology
Spleen	Rupture of capsule; avulsion of splenic vein	Ileus diagnosis; abdominal X-ray + liver or spleen scan + body CT scan
		Quadrant paracentesis
Kidney	Laceration; rupture	Hematuria; flank mass, abdominal distention
		Diagnosis, umbilical arteriogram/intravenous pyelogram
Subserosal hematoma of bowel	Obstruction of ileum	Obstruction; vomiting; diagnosis by plain/contrast radiograph
Adrenal	Obliterative hemorrhage, unilateral or bilateral	Flank mass; adrenal insufficiency; low hematocrit; ?body scan; later adrenal calcification
Retroperitoneal hemorrhage	Diffuse spreading hemorrhage	Abdominal distention; low hematocrit; DIC; decreased renal output/hematoma; body scan

CT, Computed tomography; DIC, disseminated intravascular coagulation.
From Curran 1985,[105] with permission.

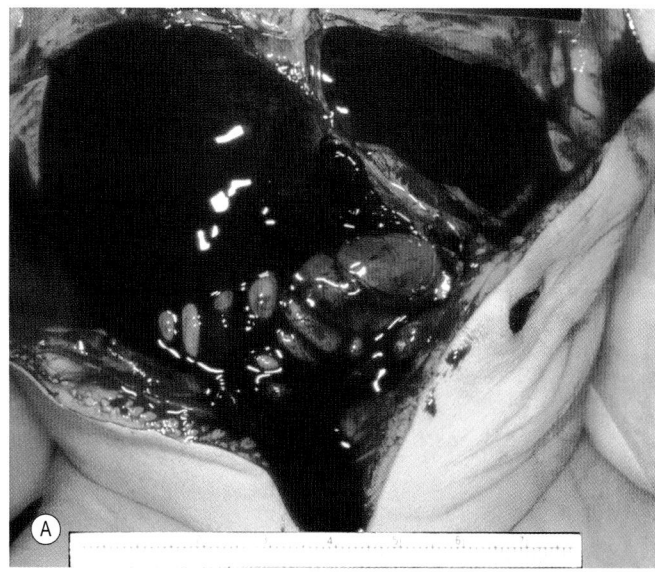

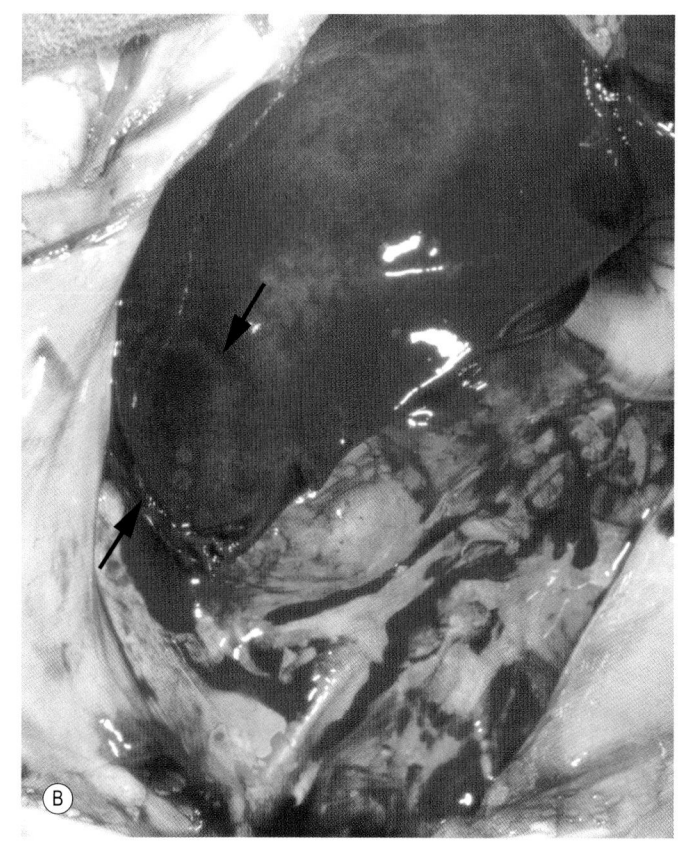

FIGURE 13.19 Ruptured subcapsular hematoma of the liver. (A) Significant fresh hemoperitoneum. (B) Site of the ruptured right hepatic lobe subcapsular hematoma (arrows) revealed after blood removed from the peritoneal cavity.

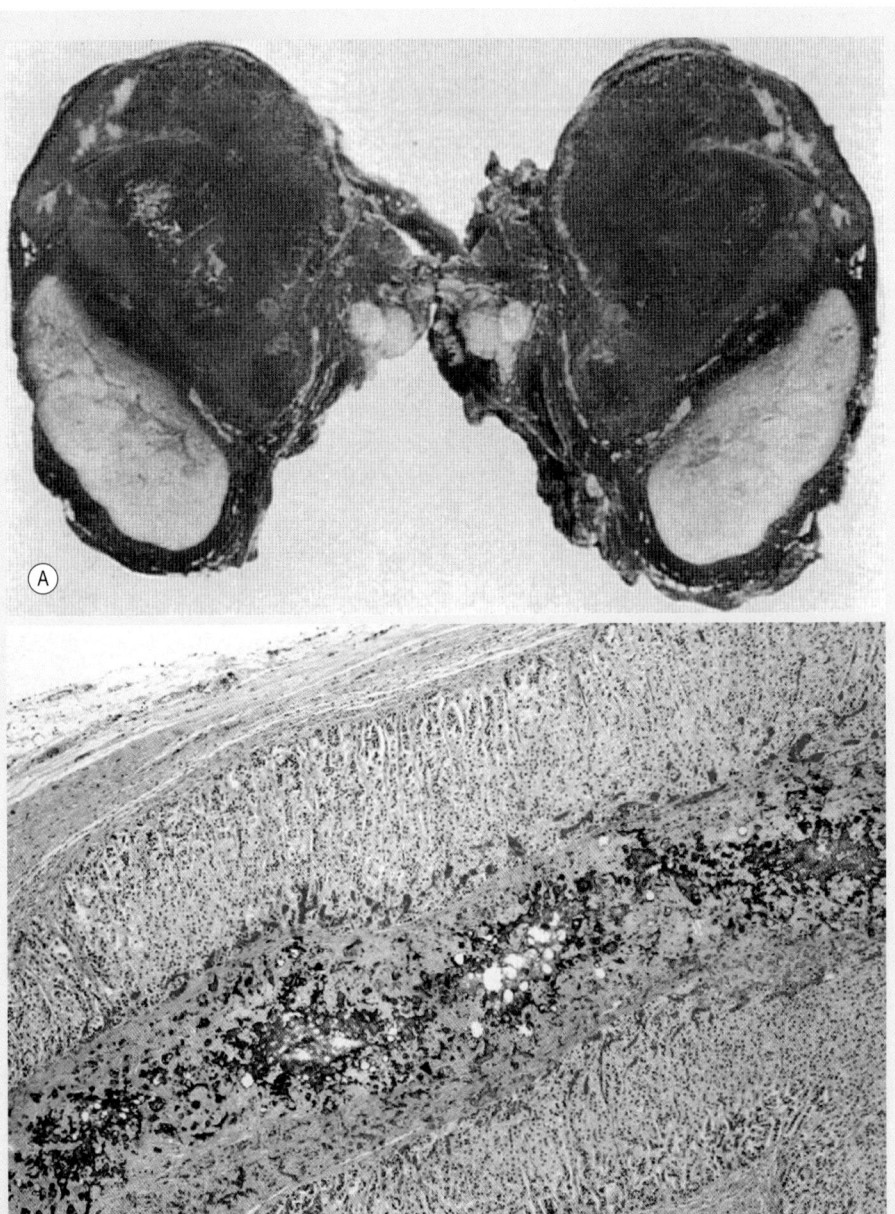

FIGURE 13.20 Adrenal hemorrhages acute and old. (A) Extension of acute adrenal hemorrhage into perirenal tissues. The white masses are halves of the kidney. (B) Remote adrenal hematoma represented by fibrosis and calcification in center of adrenal gland, from an infant aged 6 months.

hemorrhages, unless massive, are usually not fatal and because they are usually unilateral may be asymptomatic. **Adrenal insufficiency may result if the lesion is bilateral**.

Muscle injuries

Muscles are rarely injured during birth, but damage to the sternocleidomastoid muscle may occur with **breech or forceps delivery** (Fig. 13.21).[111] Clinically, this may present as a **small mass, 1–2 cm, in the sternocleidomastoid muscle** soon after birth or when the child is several days old. It may regress and leave the muscle with normal function, persist without producing symptoms, or cause permanent inclination of the head toward the affected side. **Torticollis** in older individuals rarely dates from birth, and injury sustained at birth seldom is responsible for permanent torticollis.

Microscopic examination of such a mass in the sternocleidomastoid muscle reveals atrophy and partial absence of muscle cells with proliferation and hyalinization of intervening fibrous tissue (Fig. 13.21C). The lesion is also referred to as fibromatosis colli.

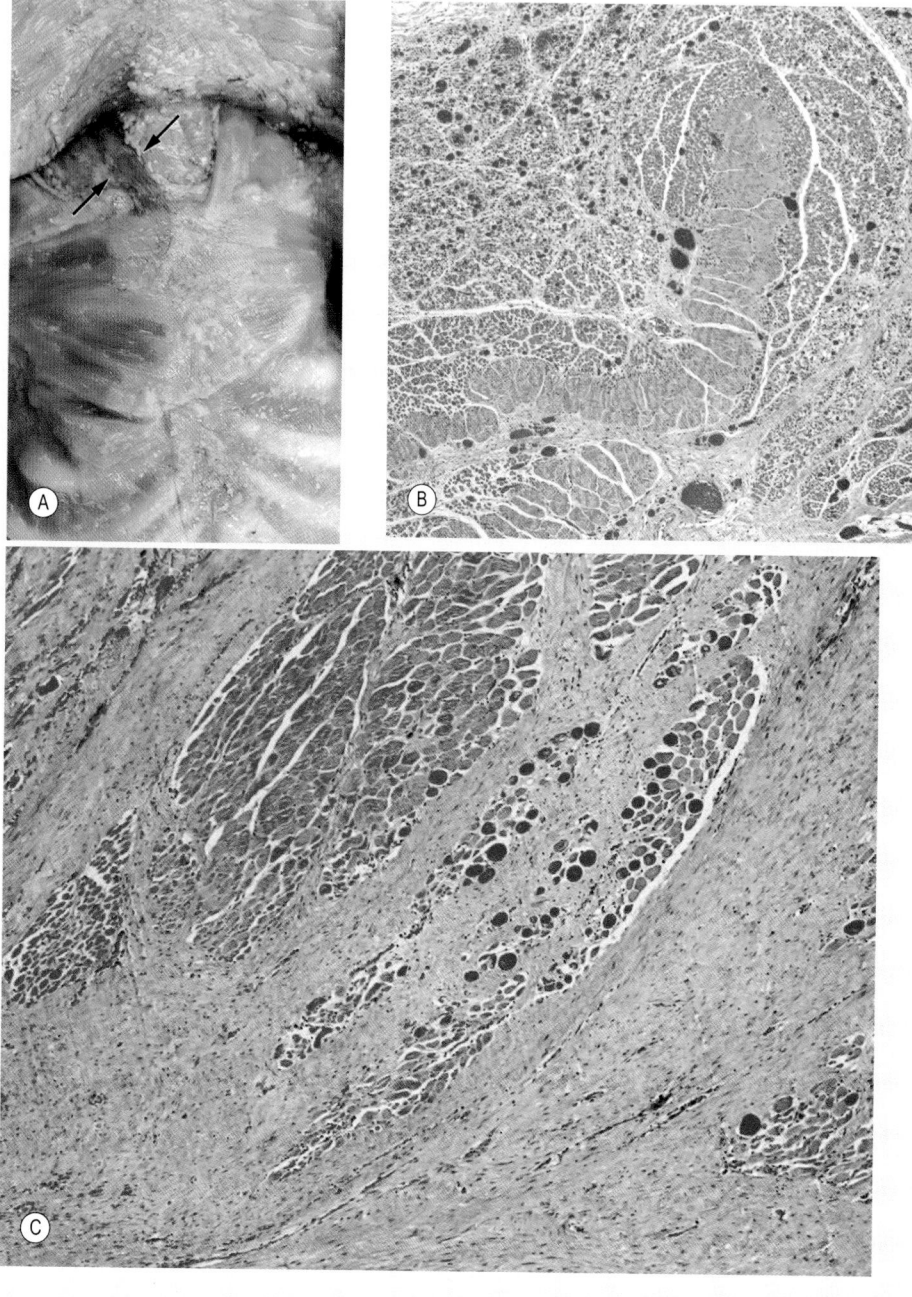

FIGURE 13.21 Birth-related sternocleidomastoid (SCM) muscle injury. (A) Hemorrhage in the right SCM muscle (arrows) in a neonate dying 2 weeks after difficult delivery. (B) Histology of the SCM muscle reveals muscle disruption and atrophy, granulation tissue, and early fibrosis. (C) Fibromatosis colli from a 1-year-old with a slowly growing SCM muscle mass. Proliferative fibrosis invades and replaces atrophic muscle. The child had breech delivery.

Interventional and complicated deliveries

Breech delivery

The hazards of vaginal delivery from breech presentation relate to compression of structures in the birth canal and/or traction, manual or assisted, applied to deliver the baby. The potential injuries are listed in Box 13.2 and many have been mentioned above. Other injuries include testicular interstitial hemorrhage with potential testicular loss if the testes have descended at the time of breech delivery.[112] Intrapartum hypoxic damage to the pituitary has resulted in growth hormone deficiency

following breech deliveries. The safety of vaginal delivery compared with cesarean section delivery for breech presentation remains debated, although current trends favor the latter.[113, 114]

Cesarean section delivery

The infant morbidity and mortality associated with emergency cesarean section delivery generally relate to the disorder affecting the fetus that precipitated the procedure. Direct trauma to the fetus, such as skin laceration, extremity fracture or direct penetrating injury, is rare.[115] A high percentage of infants delivered by cesarean section have an **increase in intracranial fluid and an increase in frequency of neonatal respiratory distress syndrome** (RDS). RDS is an important complication of preterm birth before fetal lung maturation (Ch. 24). Awaiting the onset of spontaneous labor to determine the timing of repeat cesarean section for women at term is an effective means of preventing neonatal RDS.[116]

Forceps assisted delivery

Midpelvic forceps assisted delivery and deliveries where more than 45 degrees rotation must be applied have significant risk for fetal injuries.[117] These include extracranial and intracerebral hemorrhages, skull and extremity fractures, facial lacerations, and brachial plexus and spinal cord injuries, as detailed above. Forceps delivery with rotation 45 degrees or less and from low in the pelvis or the birth outlet is much safer, but still retains some risk for injury to the baby.[118]

Vacuum assisted delivery

Subgaleal hemorrhage now most often occurs with application of the vacuum extractor (ventouse) rather than with other types of delivery. With use of soft vacuum cups, the incidence is about 0.5%.[71] It is slightly higher when rigid cups are applied. The bleeding may be sufficient to cause hemorrhagic shock. Lesser hemorrhages may be responsible for development of jaundice. **Chinon, cephalhematoma**, and **epidural, subdural and intracranial hemorrhage** have occurred with vacuum extraction.[119–121] Other complications include **retinal hemorrhage, skull fracture** including growing fracture and Erb's palsy.[122]

Monitoring of labor and delivery

Intrapartum monitoring

Use of scalp electrodes for continuous intrapartum fetal heart rate monitoring may result in **abrasions or puncture of the scalp, scalp or eyelid laceration, abscess, or osteomyelitis**.[123] D'Souza and colleagues recognized an increase in neonatal jaundice following scalp bruising.[124] Fatal herpes simplex infection has followed intrapartum monitoring at 34 weeks of gestation.[125]

Complications of postnatal care

The current expectation is that 84% of infants with a birth weight between 500 and 1500 g, including just over half of those with a birth weight between 500 and 750 g, will survive to be discharged from the neonatal nursery.[126] Much of the pathology affecting infants in the newborn period relates to **consequences of prematurity or perinatal hypoxia–ischemia** that is expressed with the facilitated survival of the infant beyond the initial postnatal period. These conditions are discussed fully in other chapters and include bronchopulmonary dysplasia (Ch. 24), necrotizing enterocolitis (Ch. 25) and hypoxic ischemic encephalopathy (Ch. 36). This section focuses more specifically on the injuries complicating the provision of neonatal care, acknowledging that the immature physiologic state of the newborn infant often factors in the development of such injuries.

Neonatal cardiopulmonary resuscitation

Complications of cardiopulmonary resuscitation occur with airway intubation and ventilation, endovascular catheterization (both discussed below), overzealous drug administration and trauma from the external application of force for cardiac compressions.[127] Significant examples of the latter are rare even in premature babies and **include rib and sternal fractures, lacerations of the viscera with subsequent hemorrhage and retinal hemorrhage**.[128, 129]

Respiratory therapy

Injuries caused by endotracheal intubation

For a comprehensive review of injuries due to intubation in the newborn see Joshi.[130] The most important and life-threatening complication of **endotracheal (ET) intubation is obstruction of the tube by mucus or secretions** (Fig. 13.22).[131] Suctioning of the tube can precipitate cardiorespiratory arrest. The **ET tube may perforate the nasopharynx** and dissect into the chest or the esophagus; both accidents may be difficult to diagnose.[132] A **vertical row of shallow ulcers** may be found in the midline anteriorly **over tracheal rings** following endotracheal intubation. Squamous metaplasia of the anterior half of the tracheal

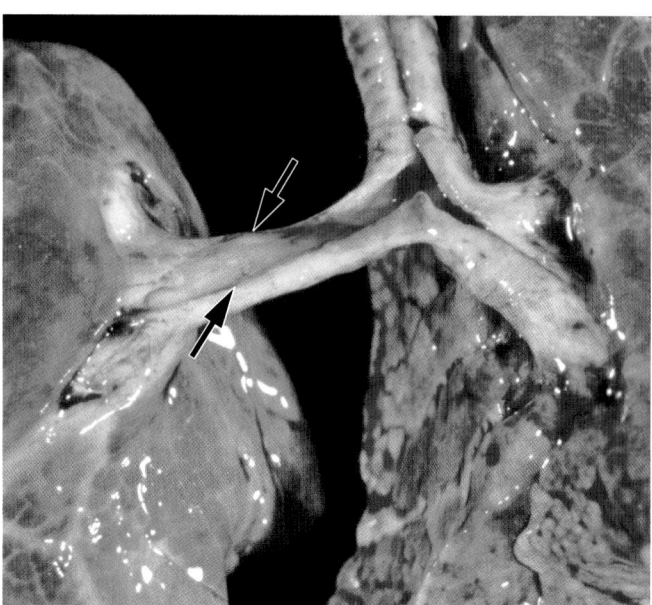

FIGURE 13.22 Excessive mucus production in an intubated and ventilated infant. Frequent suctioning of the endotracheal tube was required. At autopsy a mucous plug (arrows) obstructed the right main stem bronchus, causing atelectasis of the right lung.

epithelium may develop in that part of the trachea in contact with the tube.

Pharyngeal, tracheal or esophageal perforation is an infrequent complication of endotracheal intubation.[133, 134]

Ulceration of the vocal cords or subglottic region may heal without sequelae.[135] However, deep ulceration stimulates fibrosis, and scarring can narrow the airway necessitating tracheostomy or operative repair.[136] **Intubation-acquired subglottic mucous cysts** in the neonate may mimic features of chronic lung disease.[137] Early identification of the cysts with flexible bronchoscopy is important since airway compromise may progress and surgical intervention may be life-saving. These cysts have occurred in extreme preterm and very low birth weight infants with a mean duration of intubation of 28 days. **Perichondritis and chondromalacia may affect the arytenoid and cricoid cartilages** after prolonged intubation.[135, 136] It has been estimated that **laryngeal or tracheal stenosis** occurs in 1.5% of infants intubated for longer than 4 weeks. Studies have demonstrated potential prevention by use of tubes properly sized for gestation.

Excessive heating and condensation of water from humidification have been linked to tracheobronchial burns, water aspiration, and infection.[138]

Necrotizing tracheobronchitis

Morphologically, necrotizing tracheobronchitis is distinctive. It is most striking in the lowermost portion of the trachea, and it extends down into the major bronchi (Fig. 13.23A). It arises

below the distal end of the ET tube and hence cannot be attributed to mechanical trauma. The affected area appears cobblestoned and either total denudation of the mucosa or a 'pseudomembrane' replaces the mucosa.[139] The exact etiology is unknown.[140] **Hypotheses include thermal burn, toxic insult** (from some chemical component of the tube), **and drying**. It is more severe with **high-frequency jet ventilation** than it is with conventional mechanical ventilation. Muscle trauma is not a factor. It does, however, depend on the presence of an ET tube and the use of mechanical ventilation plus high mean pressure of ventilation.[141] A **pseudomembrane** (Fig. 13.23B) **can become occlusive**, resulting in respiratory compromise.

The lesions may extend to the true vocal cords and subglottic region of the trachea proximally, and into the bronchi distally. Contamination particularly with *Pseudomonas* and *Candida* may occur with prolonged endotracheal intubation.

Long-term sequelae include the formation of granulation tissue, polypoid lesions of fibrous tissue covered by metaplastic squamous epithelium, submucosal fibrosis, and stenosis.[142] **Obstructive lesions may result in acquired lobar emphysema.**[143]

Pulmonary interstitial emphysema (see also Ch. 24)

The pressure of mechanical ventilation imposed on immature or hypoplastic lungs may result in rupture of alveoli and passage of gas into the interstitial tissue. The **gas dissects along interlobular septa, bronchovascular connective tissue sheaths and beneath the pleura and accumulates in lymphatics and interlobular fissures** (Fig. 13.24). It tracks into the mediastinum and may continue into the retroperitoneal tissues. Crepitation identifies extension of air into subcutaneous tissues over the head and neck. The common predisposing factors to pulmonary interstitial emphysema (PIE) are listed in Box 13.3.

PIE may occur spontaneously or as a complication of ET tube displacement but more frequently it develops in neonates receiving mechanical ventilation. Large air collections in the extra-alveolar spaces result in decreased perfusion and ventilation of the affected lung, compression of adjacent pulmonary parenchyma and mediastinum and possible air embolism. Usually PIE is less severe and spontaneously regresses, but in some instances the process is self-perpetuating, leading to an air block syndrome. Lobectomy or segmental resection may be necessary.[144] PIE, if bilateral and complicated by tension pneumothorax (Fig. 13.25), has a high mortality.[145] **Pneumothorax** is a common and life-threatening complication of PIE and may occur in up to 20% of infants receiving intermittent positive pressure ventilation.

Air may extend along the lymphatics and rupture into the mediastinum (**pneumomediastinum**) or pericardial sac (**pneumopericardium**). It can track into the retroperitoneum and lead to pneumoperitoneum (Fig. 13.26). These complications are life-threatening in the newborn. At autopsy the **chest should be opened under water or be assessed by needle aspiration to detect intrapleural air**.[4] Lung perforation may occur in patients treated by aspiration of air for pneumothorax (Fig. 13.27).[146]

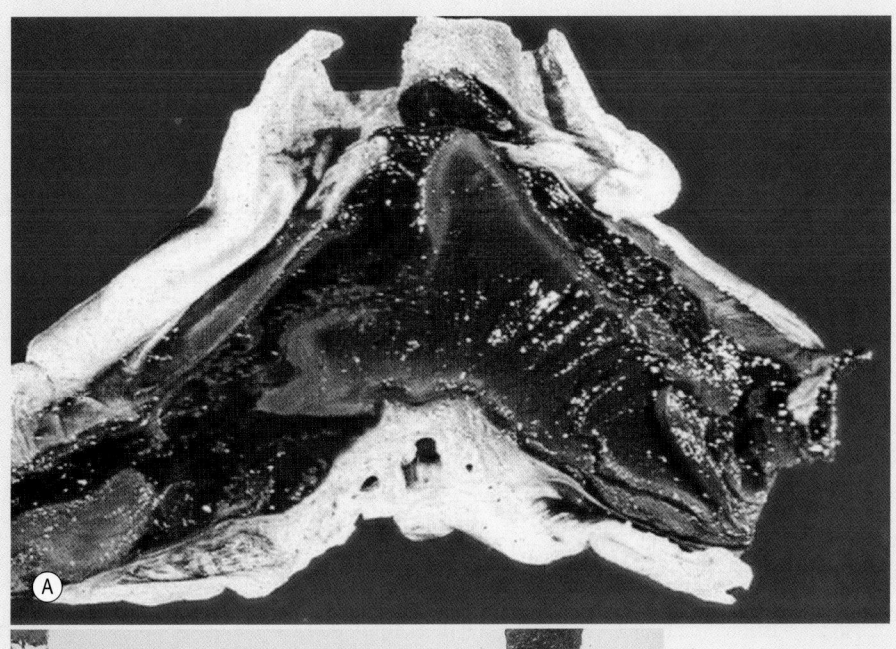

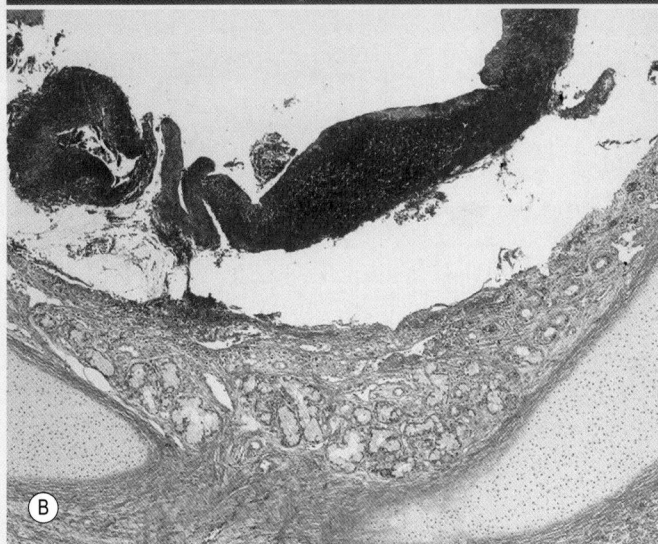

FIGURE 13.23 Necrotizing tracheobronchitis. (A) The hemorrhagic pseudomembrane extends from the trachea into the major bronchi. (B) Microscopically, the pseudomembrane is formed by necrotic mucosa, which can slough, leaving an ulcerated surface, and potentially obstructs the airway.

Pulmonary air leaks in preterm infants requiring extreme mechanical ventilation may lead to systemic gas embolism with gas within the heart resulting in shock and death. In addition to arising from mechanical ventilation, **air embolism may occur by introduction of air into a vessel via a three-way stopcock during exchange transfusion.**[147] Large quantities of air are ordinarily required to cause death; relatively small amounts introduced during routine intravenous (IV) therapy are not of major significance if they dissolve rapidly in the plasma, but may produce embolic events in very low birth weight infants. Air has been recognized not only in the heart but also in the aorta, in hepatic and other veins, in the lateral ventricles of the brain, and in cerebral arteries.[147]

If air embolism is suspected, a postmortem roentgenogram before commencing the autopsy provides accurate docu-

mentation of that complication. The pathologist should **open the heart under water (right side of the heart first) or look carefully** for **froth in the chambers of the heart as it is opened.**

Persistent loculated pulmonary interstitial emphysema

Persistent loculated pulmonary interstitial emphysema occurs when pseudocysts develop within interstitial tissue.[148] These are related to either continuous positive airway pressure or mechanical ventilation. Premature and very low birth weight infants are predisposed to this lesion.[149] Stocker and colleagues divide these cases into two types: those with **localized** disease and those with **diffuse** disease.[150] In the former, lesions in one or more

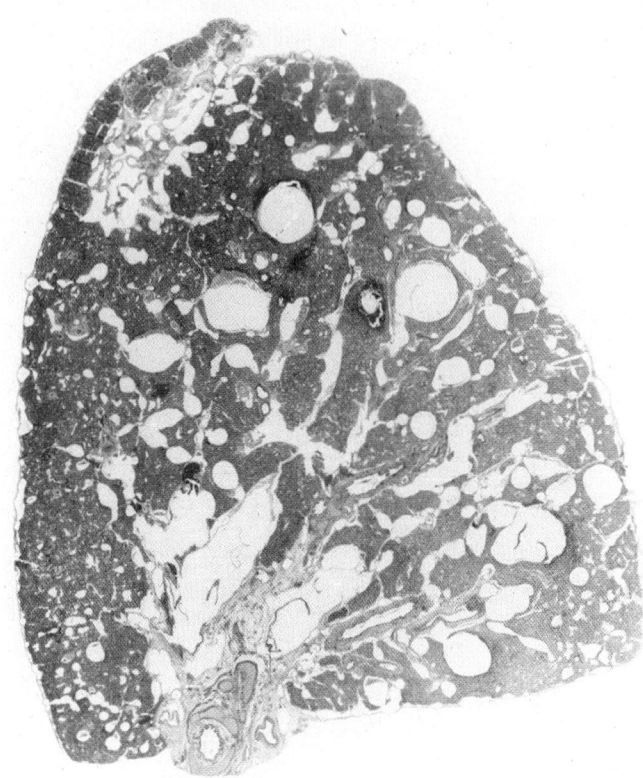

FIGURE 13.24 Pulmonary interstitial emphysema demonstrated by a whole mount slide of lung. Airspaces are overdistended and gas has dissected along lobular septa.

Immaturity of the lung
  Increased connective tissues and interstitial fluid
  Atelectasis

Respiratory distress syndrome

Aspiration syndromes (fetal hypoxia with excessive aspiration of amniotic fluid)

Pulmonary infection

Anomalies of the lung
  Hypoplasia of the lung, with or without diaphragmatic hernia
Overzealous resuscitation at birth

Intubation of a mainstem bronchus followed by positive pressure ventilation

Needle puncture of lung in attempting to relieve pneumothorax

Assisted ventilation
  Excessive peak inspiratory pressure and tidal volume
  Excessive artificial respiration
  Non-homogeneity of surfactant development
  Asynchronous breathing
  Continuous positive airway pressure (CPAP) >10 cm H_2O
  Positive end expiratory pressure (PEEP) >10 cm H_2O
  Invasive inadvertent PEEP
    Fast frequency of breathing
    Small diameter of intubation tubes
    Increased airway resistance
    Peribronchial edema
    Prolonged time constant pressure
    Absent pores of Kohn

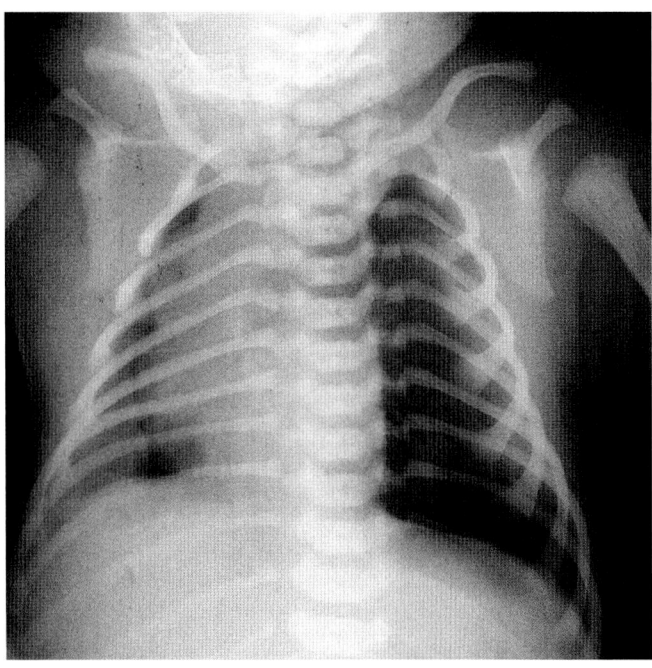

FIGURE 13.25 Left side tension pneumothorax displacing mediastinal organs into the right chest. A small right side pneumothorax is also present.

lobes cause expansion of the lung, which tends to push the mediastinum toward the opposite side of the chest. The localized form of the disease may require surgical resection of the affected portion of the lung. In the diffuse form, all lobes of both lungs are involved. The diagnosis was made only at autopsy in all of 12 cases reported by Stocker and colleagues.[149] In addition, 11 of these 12 infants had bronchopulmonary dysplasia.

The **pseudocysts** range in size from 0.1 cm to 3.0 cm in diameter (Fig. 13.28A). They are often arranged radially in the interlobular septa, extending from the hilus to the pleura. Subpleural regions are rarely involved. A smooth and glistening membrane lines the cysts. Lung parenchyma surrounding the lesions is atelectatic. The walls of the pseudocysts are composed of a layer of septal fibrous tissue surrounded by pulmonary parenchyma. Characteristically many **foreign-body giant cells are present along the inner surface of the cysts** (Fig. 13.28B). These clustered giant cells cover 10–35% of the inner aspect of the pseudocyst and are more prominent in the localized than in the diffuse form of the disease.[150]

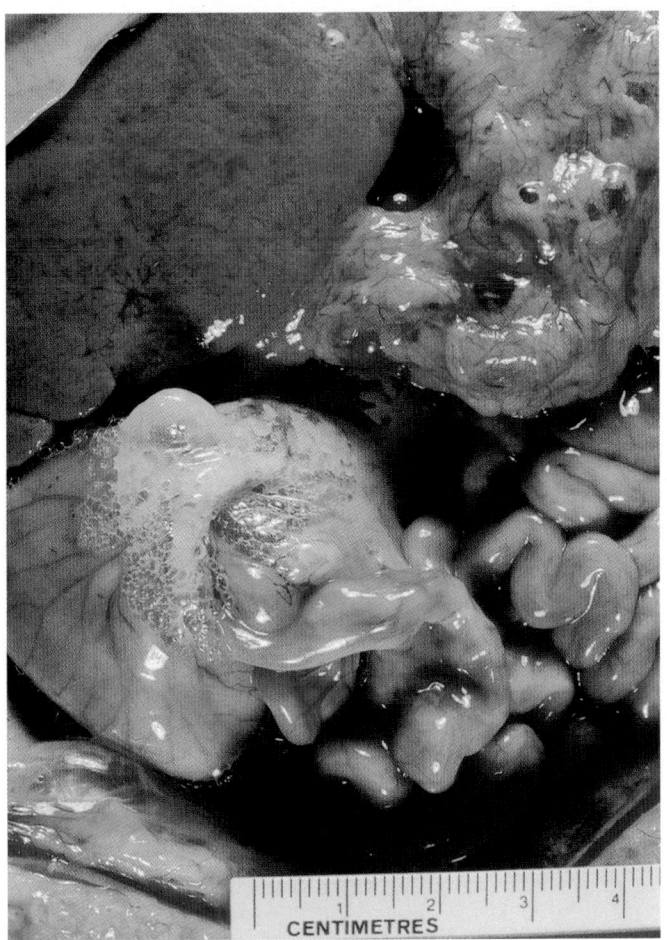

FIGURE 13.26 Multiple gas bubbles of abdominal tissues resulting from extension of pulmonary interstitial emphysema. Pneumoperitoneum was radiologically identified.

Atrophy of the diaphragm (see also Ch. 24)

Mechanical ventilation prolonged for 12 days or more may result in reduced diaphragmatic muscle mass with small size of muscle fibers probably due to disuse atrophy.[151] Recent animal studies have shown the onset of diaphragm myofiber degenerative changes within 3 days of mechanical ventilation.[152] This acquired diaphragm dysfunction may impede weaning from ventilatory support.

Oxygen toxicity (see also Ch. 24)

The two most recognized complications of oxygen toxicity are its effects on the eye and the lung. **Retinopathy of prematurity** (see Ch. 39) occurs in the preterm infant of early gestation with incomplete retinal vascular development when PO_2 is elevated for a period that stimulates neovascularization of the retina.[153] Retinal detachment and fibroblast proliferation in the vitreous may occur.

High oxygen concentration in the premature lung may damage the lining cells of alveoli with thickening of the alveolar walls by **fibroblastic proliferation resulting in bronchopulmonary dysplasia** (BPD) (see Ch. 24). Oxygen damage alone may result in BPD; however, it is **accelerated by high peak airways pressure**, intubation, and increased ventilatory rates. All the histologic features of human BPD can be produced in animals that are exposed to high levels of oxygen, without the need for mechanical ventilation.[154] If the oxygen concentration is kept below 80%, these complications rarely occur. The classic histopathology of bronchopulmonary dysplasia includes severe airway damage with smooth muscle hyperplasia and epithelial metaplasia, alveolar

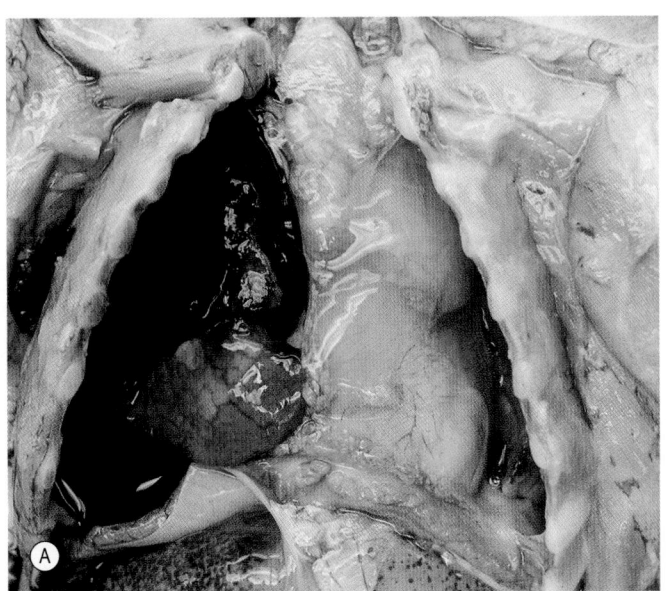
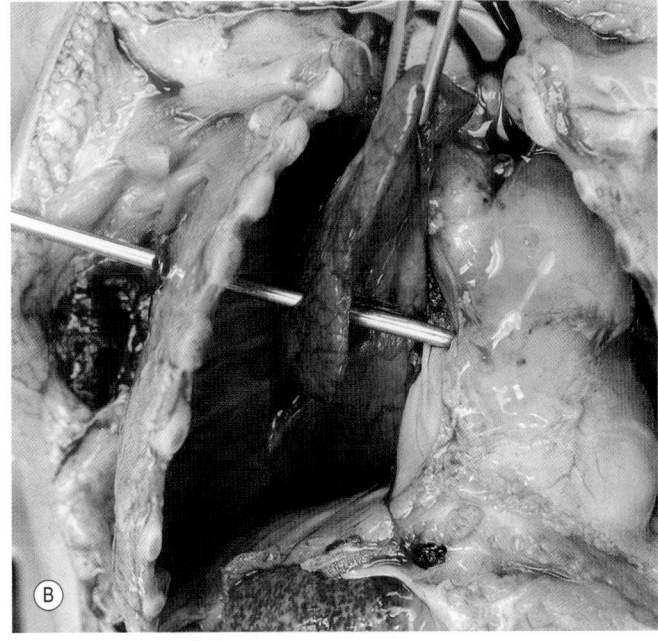

FIGURE 13.27 Traumatic chest tube injury. (A) Large right hemothorax. (B) The chest tube track, demonstrated by a probe after the hemothorax has been removed, perforates the right lung.

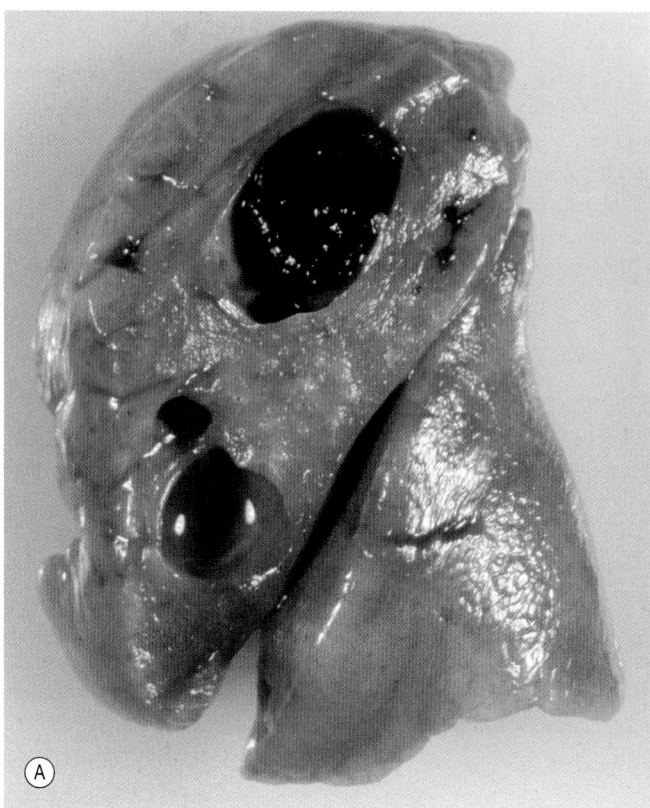

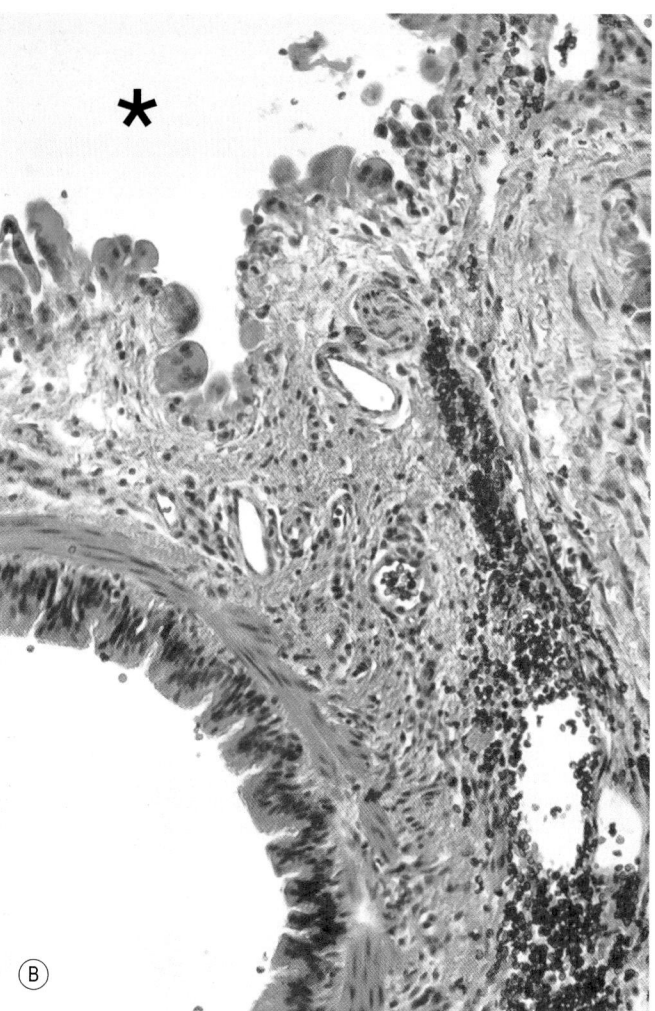

FIGURE 13.28 Persistent loculated pulmonary interstitial emphysema in the lung of a premature infant. (A) Hemorrhage into one of the cysts has occurred. (B) The pseudocyst (asterisk) is lined by foreign-body-type giant cells.

interstitial fibrosis, and alternating areas of airspace collapse and overdistension.[155] Contemporary management of neonatal respiratory distress syndrome has altered this pathology of chronic lung disease, which is now more characterized by enlargement and simplification of alveoli, reduction of the alveolar vascular bed, and variable, generally minimal interstitial fibrosis.[156]

Other airways

Positive-pressure ventilation delivered by nasal prongs or face mask can result in significant interference with gastrointestinal (GI) tract function from overdistention, and damage from rupture of viscera.[157]

Cameron and Lupton reported that during routine nasal intubation of a premature infant, the nasotracheal tube penetrated the brain. Blood-stained cerebrospinal fluid and neural tissue emerged. The infant later developed extensive intracranial hemorrhage.[158]

Surfactant and nitric oxide therapy

Nitric oxide (NO), a targeted pulmonary vasodilator, and exogenous surfactant have contributed to improved outcomes in the management of newborn infants with respiratory distress syndrome and persistent pulmonary hypertension. A 40% reduction in mortality is attributed to the use of surfactant for treatment or prophylaxis of neonatal respiratory distress syndrome.[159] Initial experience with exogenous surfactant raised concerns for the development of pulmonary hemorrhage in treated infants. Subsequent studies have demonstrated a slight or no increased risk for this potential complication.[160] The pulmonary toxicity of NO remains unresolved, however potential adverse affects include formation of cytotoxic oxidants and other chemical irritants of the lung, interference with surfactant function and extrapulmonary vascular dilatation.[161]

Suction catheters

Secretions in the newborn are suctioned from the pharynx, upper respiratory tract, esophagus, and stomach. Suction catheters may cause **mucosal and submucosal erosions** and **transient but severe esophagitis** with ulceration more severe in the upper esophagus.[162] **Secondary pneumothorax** after **bronchial perforation** due to deep endotracheal suction is reported.[163] This should be suspected in an infant who suddenly deteriorates during or after such a suction procedure.

Extracorporeal membrane oxygenation

Extracorporeal membrane oxygenation (ECMO) makes use of prolonged extracorporeal cardiopulmonary bypass via extra-thoracic cannulation and provides partial or complete heart–lung function using a membrane oxygenator while the underlying disease resolves. Catheters are placed in the jugular vein and in the common carotid artery (venoarterial bypass) or a single cannula with double lumen is placed in the right atrium from the jugular vein (venovenous bypass), and the blood is then diverted through a bypass circuit.[164]

ECMO is used for those infants in whom there is an 80% or greater expected mortality risk and the indications include severe **air leak syndrome (pneumothorax, pneumomediastinum, pneumopericardium, persistent interstitial pulmonary emphysema, or a persistent air leak), meconium aspiration pneumonia, respiratory distress syndrome with persistent fetal circulation, pulmonary hypertension syndrome, sepsis, diaphragmatic hernia, B-surfactant protein deficiency before lung transplantation and certain congenital heart malformations before heart transplantation.**[165]

Pathologic findings include **interstitial and intra-alveolar hemorrhage** with **hyaline membrane** formation during the first few days of therapy, **hyperplasia of type II alveolar cells and bronchial epithelial cells after 2 days of ECMO** therapy and by **7 days with interstitial fibrosis in all patients.** Squamous metaplasia of bronchial epithelium is also seen in most cases. **Clusters of calcified material may be present in the alveoli.**[166]

Complications[167, 168] include the following:

- **Hemorrhage.** Because active heparinization is used to maintain the circuit and platelets are destroyed in the circuit, patients are at risk for intracranial, retroperitoneal, incisional, GI, endobronchial, and intrapleural hemorrhages.[169, 170]
- **Non-hemorrhagic neurologic damage.** Edema, generalized atrophy, and porencephalic cysts, infarcts, sagittal sinus thrombosis, and multifocal ischemic neuronal necrosis are documented, in part associated with ligation of the carotid artery used for arterial cannulation. Long-term effects include microcephaly, seizures, and neurologic impairment.[171]
- **Hypertension.** Systolic hypertension is a serious side effect of ECMO related to elevations in plasma renin activity, aldosterone, epinephrine, norepinephrine, prostaglandin E_2, thromboxane, and antidiuretic hormone.[172]
- **Infection.** Local and systemic infections are rare. However, strict aseptic techniques, daily cultures of blood, urine, and tracheal aspirates, daily white blood cell counts, and routine antibiotic coverage are employed to minimize risk.
- **Renal failure.** Volume overload and electrolyte imbalance complicate ECMO.[173]
- **Pulmonary changes.** Intra-alveolar hemorrhage, hyaline membrane disease, bronchopulmonary dysplasia (BPD), interstitial fibrosis, bronchiolar calcification and mucinous metaplasia of bronchiolar and alveolar epithelium and cystic lesions are described.[174, 175] However, these lesions may be related

or enhanced by the underlying condition for which ECMO is given.[176]

- **Thromboemboli.** Multiple fibrin- or aluminum-containing thromboemboli may lodge in arteries, arterioles, and capillaries in infants who are receiving ECMO for more than 1 week;[177] these occur principally in extrapulmonary sites and are characteristically basophilic (in contrast to eosinophilic fibrin emboli) when they contain aluminum salts.[178]
- **Hypercalcemia.** Hypercalcemia frequently develops in neonates undergoing ECMO; in one series more than a third of patients became hypercalcemic.[179] The frequency of calcium metabolic problems rises with the duration of EMCO. Among other problems the hypercalcemia can predispose to dystrophic calcification of damaged tissues or result in metastatic calcification of otherwise viable structures such as pulmonary alveoli (Fig. 13.29).

Nutritional support

Nasogastric intubation

Nasogastric intubation of an infant with respiratory compromise may cause **overdistention of the stomach** leading to elevation of the diaphragm and a **fall in functional residual capacity** that can result in **hypoxemia and apnea.** Patients maintained on full GI rest with gastric suction are at risk for development of **mucosal lesions, hemorrhage, and stress ulcerations. Perforations of the pharynx, esophagus, stomach, and even the urinary bladder** have been reported.[180, 181]

Intravenous alimentation

Intravenous alimentation (**total parental nutrition, TPN**) is frequently instituted in very low birth weight infants, infants requiring bowel rest, for example in the management of necrotizing enterocolitis, and in babies with intractable diarrhea. Complications relate to metabolic alterations consequent to the constituents of the fluid and the physiology of the neonate and to the apparatus delivering the infusate. **Liver dysfunction** is the most common metabolic complication of intravenous alimentation, occurring in up to half of very low birth weight infants.[182] The incidence and severity correlate inversely with the weight of the infant and directly with the duration of treatment. The liver injury is characterized by **canalicular and ductular cholestasis, ductular proliferation and portal fibrosis that may progress to cirrhosis** (see Ch. 26).[183]

Intravenous alimentation solutions containing fat emulsions may lead to **pulmonary lipid embolism** in both preterm and mature infants.[184] In addition, **lipid accumulation in the intima of pulmonary arteries** with involvement of the media and adventitia may occur with narrowing of the lumina and may potentiate pulmonary hypertension.[185] The administration of fat emulsions to neonates may overload the reticuloendothelial system and lipid droplets can be demonstrated in macrophages; this may compromise control of bacteria.[186]

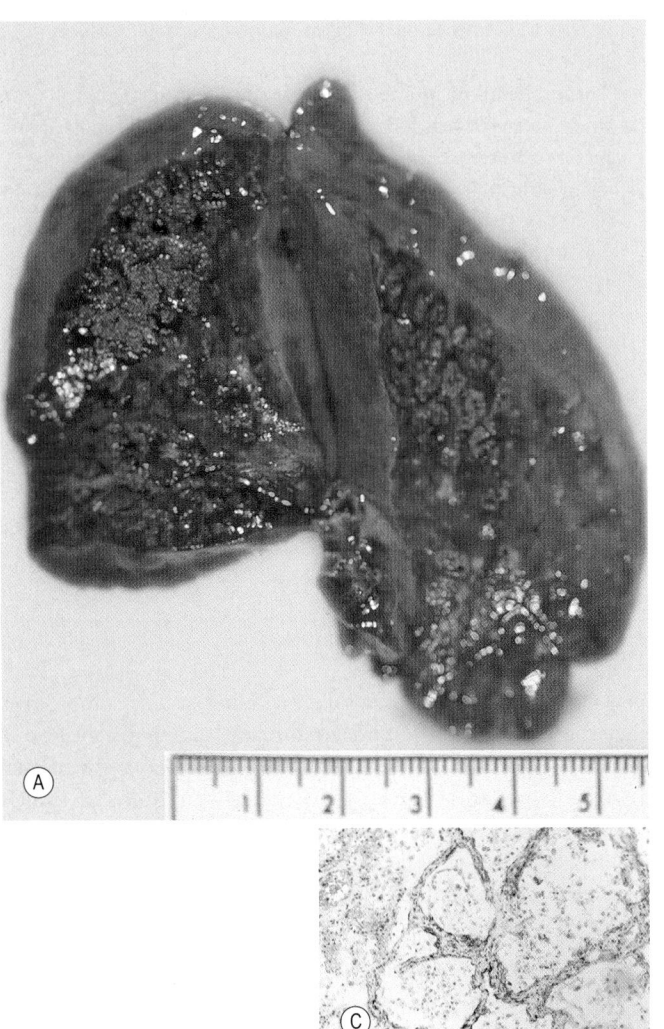

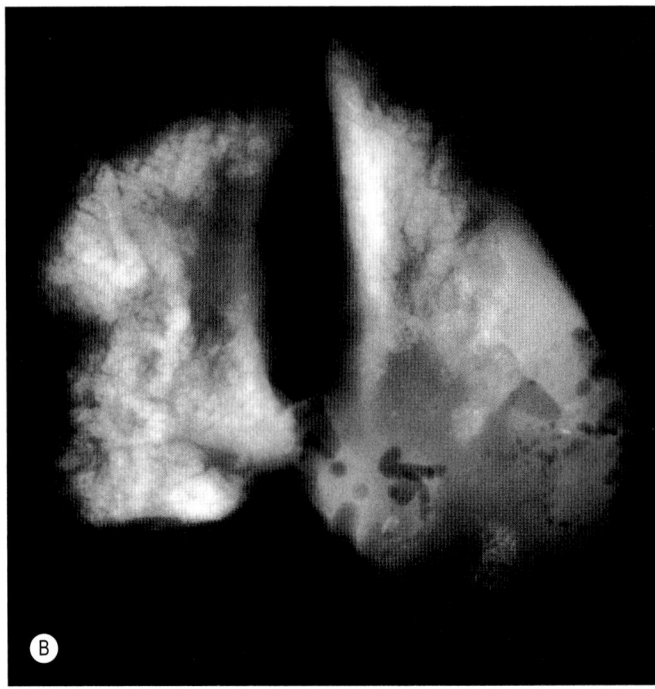

FIGURE 13.29 Lung calcification in a neonate on prolonged extracorporeal membrane oxygenation. (A) Cut section of the lung reveals multiple areas of consolidation and necrosis. (B) Specimen X-ray demonstrates extensive calcification corresponding to the damaged areas. (C) Lung away from the necrotic foci shows patchy alveolar septal calcification. (von Kossa stain)

Malassezia furfur infection may develop in TPN.[187] This fungus requires high concentrations of fatty acids for its growth. These organisms in the lung cause vasculitis, and fat stains demonstrate deposition of fat in the affected vessel wall. Other complications of TPN relate more directly to the central venous catheter (see Central catheters, below).

Nutritional rickets

Low intake of both calcium and vitamin D compounded by the administration of sodium bicarbonate and furosemide[188, 189] have been related to the development of nutritional rickets in preterm infants with respiratory problems. **Expansion of epiphyses and costochondral junctions, rib fractures, and bizarre angulation** of the ribs occur.

Necrotizing enterocolitis (see Ch. 25)

A variety of iatrogenic factors has been tentatively implicated in the development of necrotizing enterocolitis (NEC), including infant feeding practices, drugs, exchange transfusion via umbilical vessels with rapid changes in pressure in the splanchnic circulation resulting in ischemia, and others.[190] NEC in term neonates following aortic catheterization and angiography in the investigation of congenital heart disease may be caused by vascular spasm with reduced splanchnic blood flow. Hyperviscosity of blood may result from the use of hyperosmolar contrast medium that also has a diuretic effect, with resultant sluggish or obstructed blood flow in newborns of low birth weight.[191]

Intravascular catheters

Catheterization for the purposes of sampling blood, monitoring hemodynamic status or delivering fluids, drugs, and nutrients into the circulation can be made into either the venous side or arterial side, depending on the purpose. Umbilical, central, or peripheral vessels may be cannulated. Each route of access bears specific risks and complications in addition to those generally related to presence of an intravascular catheter.

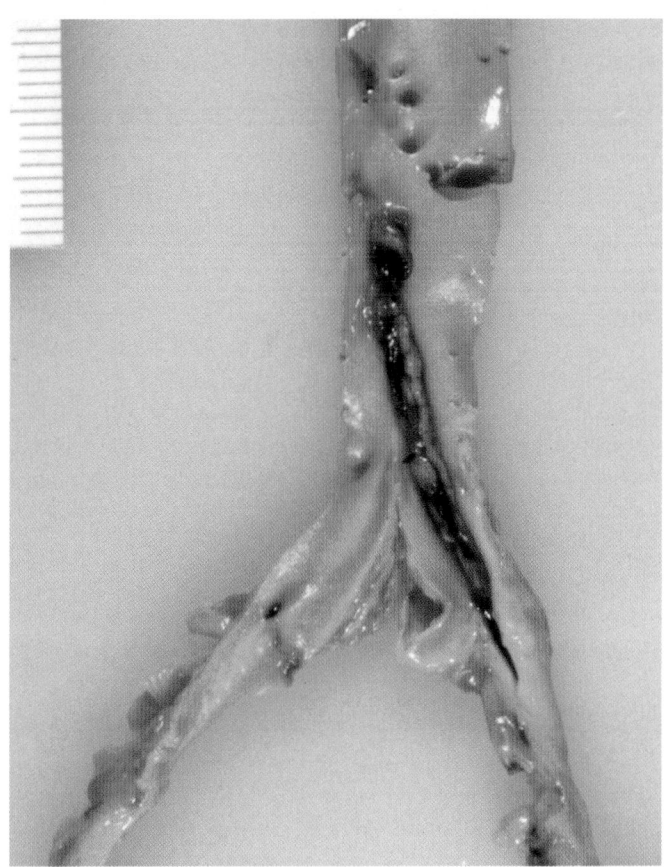

FIGURE 13.30 Large but non-occlusive thrombus of the right iliac artery and lower abdominal aorta resulting from an umbilical artery catheter.

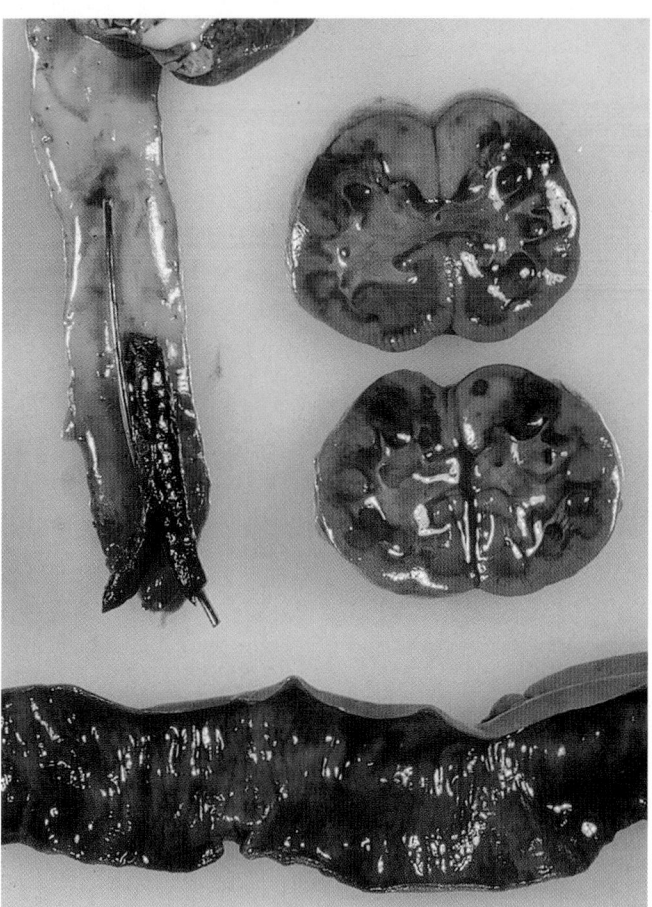

FIGURE 13.31 Umbilical artery-associated occlusive thrombus of the abdominal aorta and both iliac arteries resulting in infarcts of the kidneys and bowel.

Umbilical vein catheterization

Venous catheterization is now rarely performed because of the high frequency of complications and is generally only used in emergencies to obtain a blood sample or for urgent infusion of fluid or drugs. **Umbilical vein thrombosis** is common and particularly likely to follow the infusion of **hypertonic solutions**,[192] presence of the catheter for **longer than 2 days**, and failure to ensure that the tip of the catheter is in the inferior vena cava.[193] If the catheter extends into the portal vein or into the right atrium, **portal vein thrombosis, patchy hepatic necrosis, ventricular dysrhythmias, and pulmonary thromboembolism** are possible complications.[194] An infrequent late complication of umbilical venous catheterization is **portal hypertension**; the patient presents with **splenomegaly or hematemesis**.[195] NEC is reported following umbilical venous catheterization.[196]

Umbilical artery catheterization

Thrombosis of the aorta may rarely result from umbilical catheterization (Fig. 13.30). Technically difficult insertion of a catheter may perforate an umbilical artery near the umbilicus and lead to hemorrhage into the tissues of the abdominal wall, **perforation of the aorta, or occlusion of a mesenteric vessel with** the **development of NEC**.[197] Localized intestinal perfora-

tion is more likely to be associated with an umbilical artery catheter in place within 48 h and in infants who have received doses of indomethacin.[198]

Duration of catheterization does not appear to be related to the development of thrombosis, although most thromboses develop within 36 h after insertion of the catheter. Not all aortic thrombosis or thromboembolism in the neonate is iatrogenic. Massive aortic thrombosis as a result of propagation of a thrombus in the ductus arteriosus has been observed. **Aortic aneurysm** is an infrequent complication of aortic catheterization. **False aneurysms of the aorta** have been described[199] and are related to infection, particularly *Pseudomonas*, from the catheter. **Mycotic aneurysms** following umbilical arterial catheterization in preterm infants have been due to *Staphylococcus aureus*, *Klebsiella pneumoniae*, or *Candida albicans*.[200] A late, infrequent complication of umbilical arterial catheterization is hypertension.[201] Inadvertent **urachal catheterization may result in urinary ascites**.[202]

Mural thrombi may occlude the ostia of major branches of the abdominal aorta. Occlusion of the renal artery results in infarction of the kidney and renal hypertension (Fig. 13.31). Occlusion of the ostium of the superior or inferior mesenteric

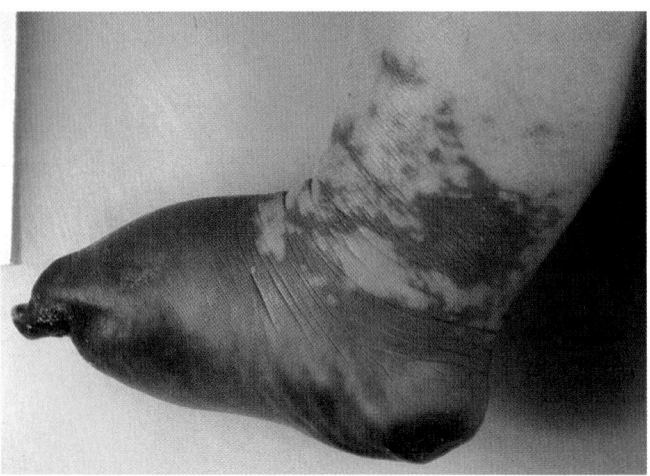

FIGURE 13.32 Gangrene of the foot resulting from embolism of an iliac artery thrombus that developed around an umbilical catheter.

arteries leads to infarction of the small or large intestine that may be mistaken for NEC.[203] Peritoneal perforation and rupture of the urinary bladder have been reported.[204, 205] **Minute thrombi on the catheter tips of umbilical artery catheters may become dislodged, and blanching or small infarcts of the toes may occur.** Occasionally larger thrombi develop and may propagate or dislodge, occluding major arterial branches of the leg (Fig. 13.32).

Gangrene of the perineum or buttocks may follow a single injection of hyperosmotic solutions into the umbilical artery at birth if the catheter is in the iliac artery extending into the gluteal artery.[206]

Central catheters

Catheterization of the thoracic aorta or pulmonary artery trunk, the central parts of the arterial circulation, is usually performed for the purpose of monitoring hemodynamic status. Catheterization of the central venous system, with the tip in either the superior or inferior vena cava close to the heart, provides long-term access for delivering fluids and nutrients and for repeated venous blood sampling. The catheters can be placed percutaneously via a peripheral vessel (peripherally inserted central catheter, PICC), or through a surgical cutdown procedure.

Complications occur in up to one-third of infants receiving central catheters.[207] A frequent serious complication is catheter-related **bloodstream infection**. The usual organism is of the skin flora. However, infection from less common nosocomial organisms, such as **candidemia**, also occurs.[208] Some of these bloodstream infections are associated with **right-sided endocarditis**.[185] Others occur with infected pericatheter thrombi (Fig. 13.33). Another common complication is catheter thrombotic occlusion. To prevent this obstruction to the delivery of therapeutic solutions critically required by the sick infant heparin is often added to the infusate. The anticoagulation can potentially augment any bleeding tendency that the infant may have.

Thrombosis can complicate placement of arterial catheters, with the risk for visceral or extremity ischemia. Pulmonary artery catheters, like central venous catheters where tips are malpositioned within the heart, may stimulate ventricular dysrhythmias. Pulmonary microembolic events or ischemia from continuous wedging of a pulmonary artery catheter may occur.

Inadvertent arterial insertion of a PICC line can cause arterial spasm, laceration with bleeding and thrombosis, jeopardizing the limb. Other serious, though less common, complications of PICC lines include **migration of the catheter with the risk for cardiac perforation and tamponade** (Fig. 13.34), vascular perforation with resultant extravasation of infusate into the pleura, mediastinum, peritoneum or retroperitoneum, dislodgement or inadvertent removal of the catheter, breakage of the catheter with potential embolism and insertion site phlebitis. **Caval thrombosis** is rare, but whether bland or infected has risk for significant pulmonary thromboembolism (Fig. 13.35).

Peripheral catheters

The most important complications of peripheral intravenous catheters are infection and **phlebitis with thrombosis**. The infection begins in the skin and soft tissues at the site of insertion of the catheter. It may remain localized, forming an abscess, or lead to bacteremia or septicemia. Catheterized peripheral veins frequently thrombose, although embolism is rare. Because of the occurrence of repeated thromboses of peripheral veins and eventual loss of vascular access, central lines are placed when possible in the infant requiring prolonged intravascular cannulation. Local hematoma and extravasation of infusate complicate perforation of the vessel either during insertion of the catheter or with partial dislodgment.

Skin puncture for blood sampling

Skin puncture for blood sampling ('**heel sticks**') can leave residua in the **form of abscesses and calcaneal chondritis**.[209] Calcified nodules may develop in scars from heel skin punctures that are eventually extruded through the epidermis. These lesions most often occur in **preterm infants below 1500 g** who have needed ventilatory support and who have had multiple heel sticks. Microscopically, these lesions are **calcified cysts in the superficial dermis**. Careful selection of the site and depth of newborn heel skin puncture have been recommended.[209]

Other causes of perinatal complications
Infections

Infections can occur in almost every organ system and are almost exclusively associated with some type of invasive monitoring or life-support system. Infants and children are particularly susceptible to **nosocomial infections**. Their cellular and humoral immunity may not be fully mature when they are under 2 years of age.[210] **Vascular access, urethral catheterization,**

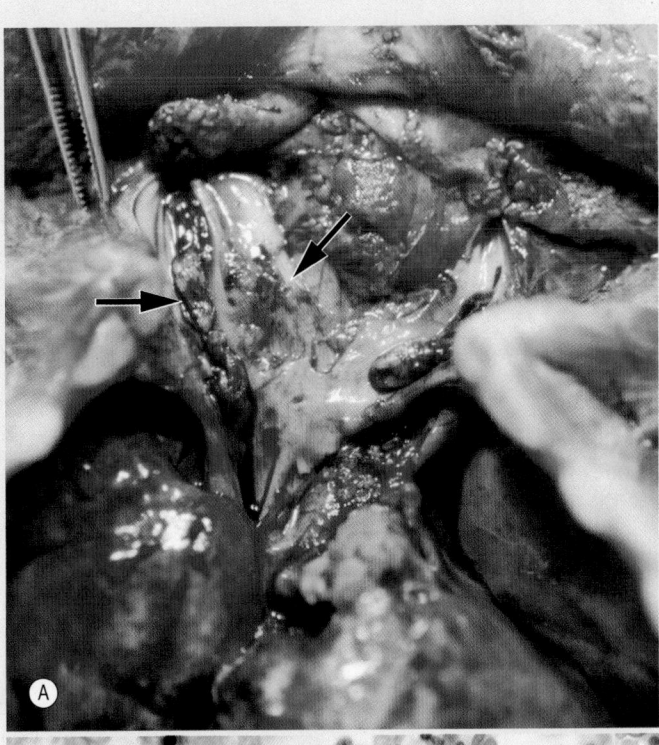

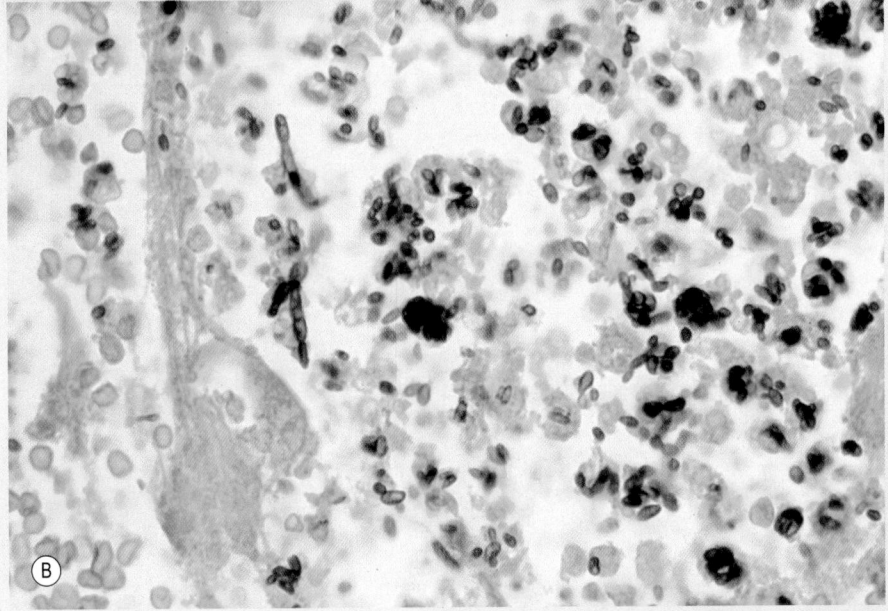

FIGURE 13.33 Infected central catheter thrombus. (A) Near occlusive superior vena caval thrombus (arrows). (B) Proliferation of *Candida* within the thrombus. (Grocott methenamine silver stain)

and **intubation of the trachea** are common procedures that disrupt the natural barriers of host defense. Coupled with the liberal use of antibiotics, which can select for resistant organisms, infectious complications are common.

Hazards of instrumentation

Modern pediatric critical care cannot function without **electrical monitoring devices. Improper grounding of equipment** can result in electrical injury. There are case reports of injury and

death from electric shock resulting from faulty ground wires or the use of a two-wire extension cord to connect a three-wire instrument power cord to the voltage source.[211]

Burns have been reported from the use of **transilluminators, radiant warmers, incubators, cardiogram leads, and transcutaneous oxygen monitors**. The patient who may be most susceptible to thermal injury is the infant with reduced skin integrity or poor perfusion. We have observed extensive burns to the skin and subcutaneous tissue by the use of heated infusion bags used to warm the infant (Fig. 13.36A).

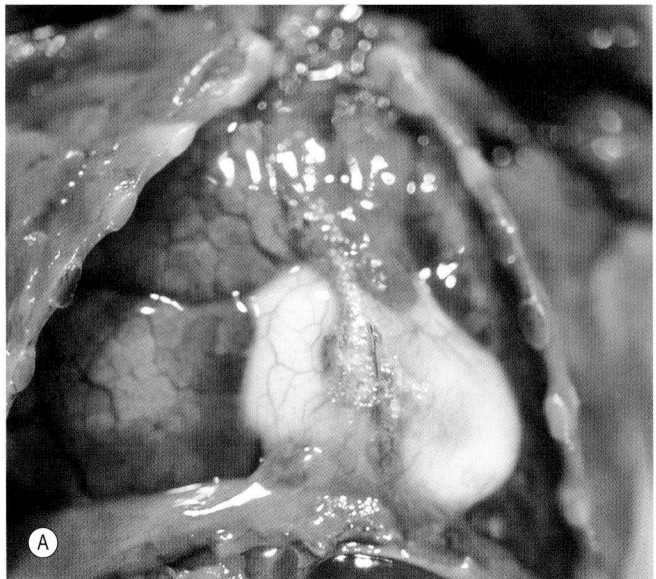

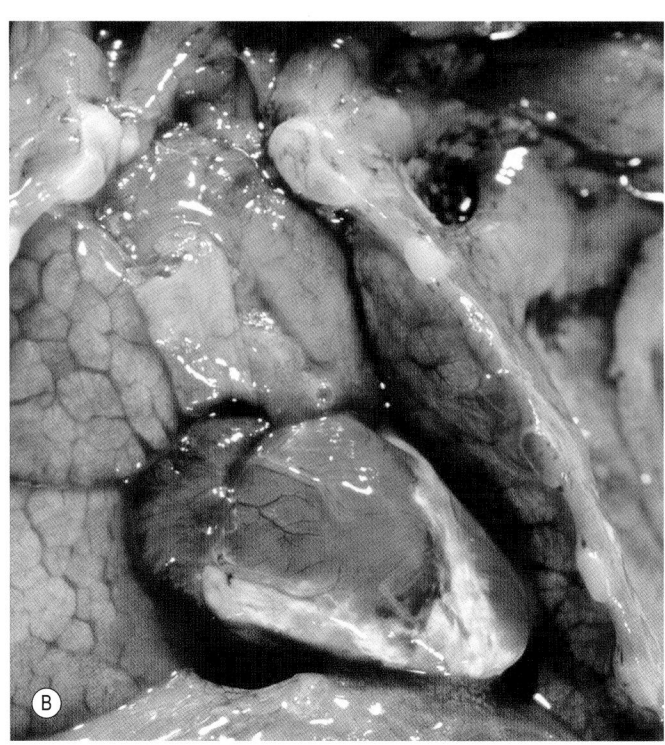

FIGURE 13.34 Perforation of the heart by peripherally inserted central catheter. (A) The pericardial sac is filled with milky parenteral alimentation fluid, causing cardiac tamponade. (B) Perforation site near the apex of the right ventricle, with alimentation fluid staining the epicardium.

FIGURE 13.35 Massive pulmonary 'saddle' thromboembolus originating from a central catheter.

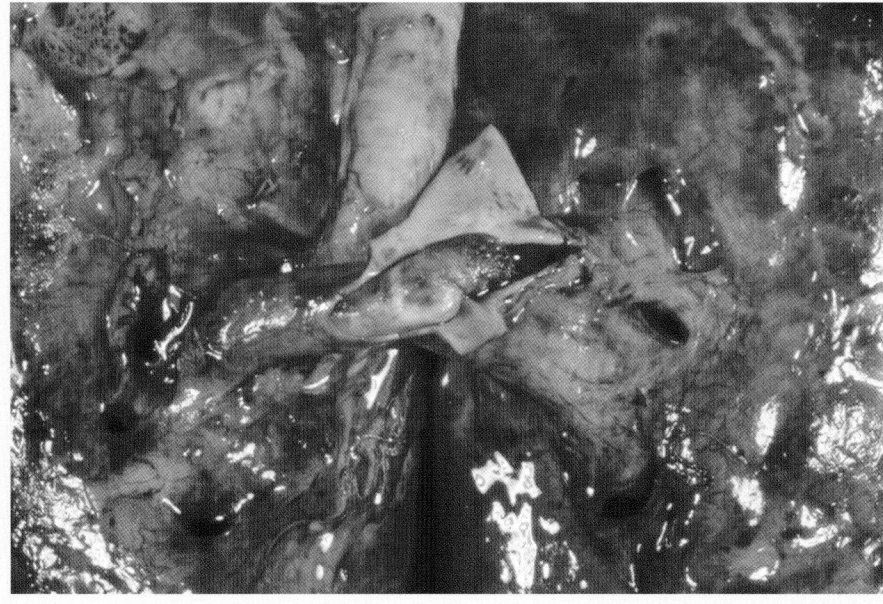

Medications used in the newborn

It is estimated that one-third of babies admitted to the intensive care nursery will have an adverse drug reaction.[212] These occur with agents given intravenously, orally and topically. Drugs easily tolerated by adults and older children may pose significant hazard to the newborn, especially those born prematurely, because of immaturity of hepatic and renal physiology.[213]

Neuropathologic abnormalities with spongy degeneration of both brain and spinal cord followed topical applications of hexachlorophene.[214] Excessive absorption of hexachlorophene has been related to prematurity and the presence of pathologic abnormalities of the skin. Hexachlorophene is no longer in clinical use in neonatal units.

Furosemide, a diuretic used frequently in BPD therapy, is a well-recognized cause of **renal calcification**, which can also occur with **prolonged dexamethasone therapy**.[215] **Dexamethasone therapy may result in hypertrophic cardiomyopathy**. This appears to be transient and resolves after discontinuation of the drug.

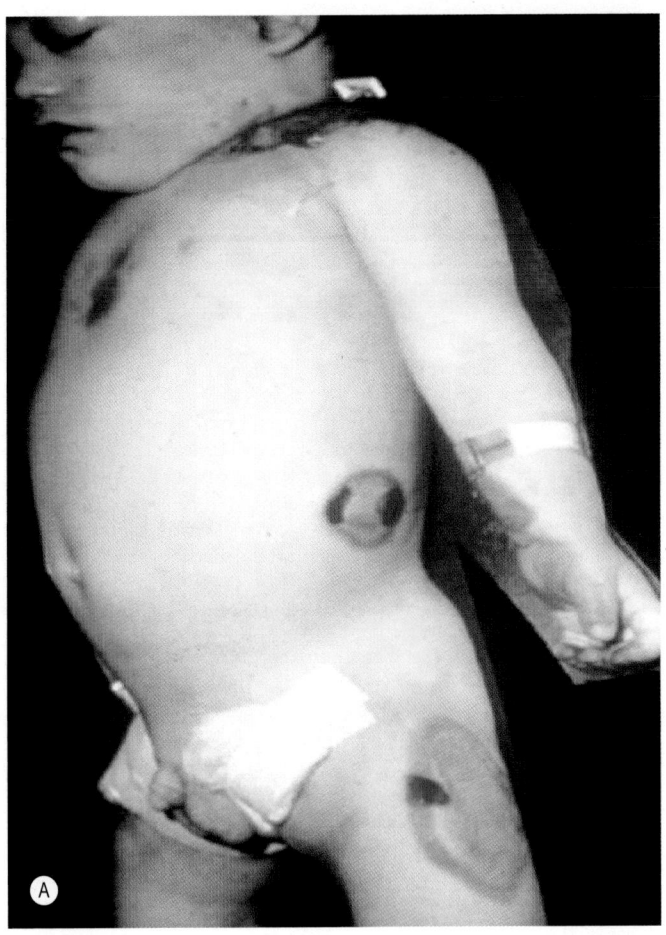
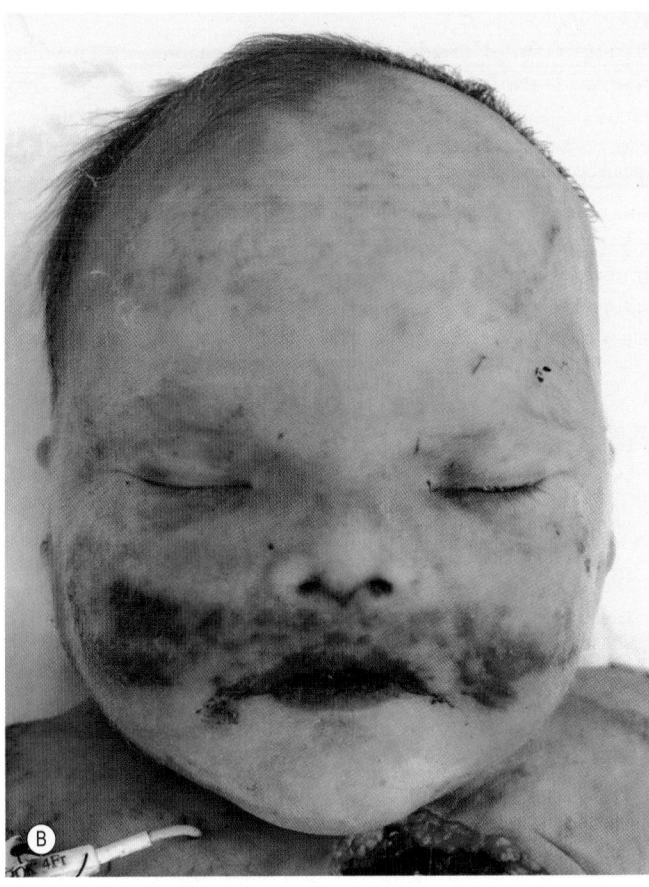

FIGURE 13.36 Iatrogenic skin injuries. (A) Extensive burns to skin and subcutaneous tissues in a hypothermic infant after application of heated infusion bag to increase body temperature. (B) Facial abrasions from adhesive tape used to hold endotracheal and nasogastric tubes in place.

Prostaglandin synthetase inhibitors used to inhibit labor and prolong pregnancy may result in **oligohydramnios and fetal and neonatal oliguria/anuria as well as pulmonary hypertension.**[216]

Indomethacin is used to promote closure of the patent ductus arteriosus in small preterm infants.[216] Complications include **intracranial hemorrhage, NEC, and perforations of the gut.** Decreased mesenteric blood flow occurs with indomethacin therapy.[217]

Prostaglandin E₁ used for perinatal patency of the ductus arteriosus in some types of congenital heart disease, in particular tetralogy of Fallot and pulmonary stenosis and hypertension, may cause **hyperplasia of the gastric antrum and result in gastric outlet obstruction and bone changes identical to infantile cortical hyperostosis.**[218]

Skin injuries

The poor cutaneous keratinization and relatively large surface area of infants may more readily permit transcutaneous absorption of drugs than might occur in the mature infant. Superficial **skin necrosis** may occur in infants who have had **prolonged application of alcoholic solutions** to the skin. Phenothiazines,

sulfonamides, and tetracyclines may cause an allergic or toxic reaction in the skin, and toxic epidermal necrolysis (Ritter disease) may be elicited by drugs such as **aspirin, barbiturates, penicillin, phenytoin, and sulfonamides**. These drugs, as well as **codeine, phenobarbital, and tetracycline cause erythema multiforme**. Exfoliative dermatitis may be associated.[197]

Skin lesions that occur as a result of IV infiltration or extravascular infusion of a sclerosing substance are not uncommon in infants. **Hypertonic fluids**, parenteral alimentation solutions, calcium (especially the chloride salt), potassium, bicarbonate, sodium pentothal, paraldehyde, and α-adrenergic agonists are all potentially damaging when they **extravasate into the tissues**.

The fragility of the immature infant's skin renders it susceptible to abrasion, laceration, and bruising from rubbing by the various tubes and catheters inserted into the sick child and from the removal of the adhesive tapes or bandages used to hold them in place (Fig. 13.36B). In the premature infant with poorly keratinized skin, ulceration around the nose or mouth can easily occur if the ET tube or face mask is not securely fixed. **Fastening of face masks by means of a Velcro band may result in deformity of the skull and cerebellar hemorrhage due to venous infarcts.**[219]

Conclusion

As illustrated repeatedly throughout this chapter, the very care that saves and nourishes these vulnerable lives, sophisticated, technologically advanced, and given with only the best intention, can come with its own cost to the wellbeing of the child. As always, it is the health care provider's responsibility to balance this cost with the benefit to be derived. The pediatric pathologist's charge is to carefully and thoroughly document these iatrogenic injuries, strive to understand their cause, and hopefully return information to those caring for the living patients that leads to ways to prevent or minimize their recurrence.

Acknowledgements

The authors gratefully acknowledge Dr William Halliday for contributing Figures 13.5, 13.6, 13.9, 13.10, 13.11 and 13.17, and Michael Starr for his assistance with the illustrations.

References

Introduction

1. Golding J. Epidemiology of fetal and neonatal death. In: Keeling J, ed. Fetal and neonatal pathology. 3rd edn. London: Springer-Verlag; 2001: 175–190.
2. de Galan-Roosen AE, Kuijpers JC, van der Straaten PJ, et al. Evaluation of 239 cases of perinatal death using a fundamental classification system. Eur J Obstet Gynecol Reprod Biol 2002; 103(1):37–42.
3. Giannini C, Okazaki H. Nervous system. In: Ludwig J, ed. Handbook of autopsy practice. 3rd edn. Totowa: Humana Press; 2002:65–84.
4. Gilbert-Barness E, Debich-Spicer DE. Handbook of pediatric autopsy pathology. Totowa: Humana Press; 2005.
5. Squier W, Cowan FM. The value of autopsy in determining the cause of failure to respond to resuscitation at birth. Semin Neonatol 2004; 9(4):331–345.

Complications of antenatal care

6. Ball RH. Invasive fetal testing. Curr Opin Obstet Gynecol 2004; 16(2): 159–162.
7. Nassar AH, Martin D, Gonzalez-Quintero VH, et al. Genetic amniocentesis complications: is the incidence overrated? Gynecol Obstet Invest 2004; 58(2):100–104.
8. D'Alton ME, DeCherney AH. Prenatal diagnosis. N Engl J Med 1993; 328(2):114–120.
9. Brinsmead MW. Complications of amniocentesis. Med J Aust 1976; 1:379–385.
10. Roper EC, Konje JC, De Chazal RC, et al. Genetic amniocentesis: gestation-specific pregnancy outcome and comparison of outcome following early and traditional amniocentesis. Prenat Diagn 1999; 19(9):803–807.
11. Behrman RE. The fetus and the neonatal infant. In: Vaughan VC, McKay RH, Behrman RE, eds. Nelson textbook of pediatrics. 11th edn. Philadelphia: WB Saunders; 1979.
12. Cook LN, Shott RJ, Andrews BF. Fetal complication of diagnostic amniocentesis: a review and report of a case with pneumothorax. Pediatrics 1974; 53(3):421–424.
13. Strauss A, Hasbargen U, Paek B, et al. Intra-uterine fetal demise caused by amniotic band syndrome after standard amniocentesis. Fetal Diagn Ther 2000; 15(1):4–7.
14. Rehder H. Fetal limb deformities due to amniotic constrictions (a possible consequence of preceding amniocentesis). Pathol Res Pract 1978; 162: 316–326.
15. Tredwell SJ, Wilson D, Wilmink MA, et al. Review of the effect of early amniocentesis on foot deformity in the neonate. J Pediatr Orthop 2001; 21(5):636–641.
16. Cederholm M, Haglund B, Axelsson O. Infant morbidity following amniocentesis and chorionic villus sampling for prenatal karyotyping. Br J Obstet Gynaecol 2005; 112(4):394–402.
17. Moessinger AC, Collins MH, Blanc WA, et al. Oligohydramnios-induced lung hypoplasia: the influence of timing and duration in gestation. Pediatr Res 1986; 20(10):951–954.
18. Simpson NE, Dallaire L, Miller JR, et al. Prenatal diagnosis of genetic disease in Canada: report of a collaborative study. Can Med Assoc J 1976; 115:739–748.
19. Galjaard H. European experience with prenatal diagnosis of congenital disease: a survey of 6121 cases. Cytogenet Cell Genet 1976; 16:453–467.
20. Karp LE, Hayden PW. Fetal puncture during midtrimester amniocentesis. Obstet Gynecol 1977; 49:115–117.
21. Morrison WA, Hurley JV, Ahmad TS, et al. Scar formation after skin injury to the human foetus in utero or the premature neonate. Br J Plast Surg 1999; 52(1):6–11.
22. Rickwood AMK. A case of ileal atresia and ileocutaneous fistula caused by amniocentesis. J Pediatr 1977; 91(2):312.
23. Therkelsen AJ, Rehder H. Intestinal atresia caused by second trimester amniocentesis. Br J Obstet Gynaecol 1981; 88:559–562.
24. Squier M, Chamberlain P, Zaiwalla Z, et al. Five cases of brain injury following amniocentesis in mid-term pregnancy. Dev Med Child Neurol 2000; 42(8):554–560.
25. Youroukos S, Papadelis F, Mastaniotis N. Porencephalic cysts after amniocentesis. Arch Dis Child 1980; 55:814–815.
26. Liley AW. The technique and complications of amniocentesis. Northwest Med 1960; 59:581–586.
27. Creasman WT, Lawrence RA, Thiede HA. Fetal complications of amniocentesis. JAMA 1968; 204(11):949–957.
28. Grove CS, Trombetta GC, Amstey MS. Fetal complications of amniocentesis. Am J Obstet Gynecol 1973; 115(8):1154.
29. Hyman CJ, Depp R, Pakravan P, et al. Pneumothorax complicating amniocentesis. Obstet Gynecol 1973; 41:43–46.
30. Portman MA, Brouillette RT. Fatal intracranial hemorrhage complicating amniocentesis. Am J Obstet Gynecol 1982; 144:731–733.
31. Adinolfi M. Non- or minimally invasive prenatal diagnostic tests on maternal blood samples or transcervical cells. Prenat Diagn 1995; 15(10):889–896.
32. Steele CD, Wapner RJ, Smith JB, et al. Prenatal diagnosis using fetal cells isolated from maternal peripheral blood: a review. Clin Obstet Gynecol 1996; 39(4):801–813.
33. Rhoads GG, Jackson LG, Schlesselman SE, et al. The safety and efficacy of chorionic villus sampling for early prenatal diagnosis of cytogenetic abnormalities. N Engl J Med 1989; 320:609–617.
34. Firth HV, Boyd PA, Chamberlain P, et al. Severe limb abnormalities after chorion villus sampling at 56–66 days' gestation. Lancet 1991; 337(8744): 762–763.
35. Burton BK, Schulz CJ, Burd LI. Limb anomalies associated with chorionic villus sampling. Obstet Gynecol 1992; 79(5 Pt 1):726–730.
36. Froster-Iskenius UG, Baird PA. Limb reduction defects in over one million consecutive livebirths. Teratology 1989; 39(2):127–135.
37. Schloo R, Miny P, Holzgreve W, et al. Distal limb deficiency following chorionic villus sampling? Am J Med Genet 1992; 42:404–413.
38. Daffos F, Capella-Pavlovsky M, Forestier F. Fetal blood sampling during pregnancy with use of a needle guided by ultrasound: a study of 606 consecutive cases. Am J Obstet Gynecol 1985; 153(6):655–660.
39. Ralston SJ, Craigo SD. Ultrasound-guided procedures for prenatal diagnosis and therapy. Obstet Gynecol Clin North Am 2004; 31(1):101–123.
40. Ghidini A, Sepulveda W, Lockwood CJ, et al. Complications of fetal blood sampling. Am J Obstet Gynecol 1993; 168(5):1339–1344.
41. Weiner CP, Okamura K. Diagnostic fetal blood sampling-technique related losses. Fetal Diagn Ther 1996; 11(3):169–175.

42. Shulman LP, Elias S. Percutaneous umbilical blood sampling, fetal skin sampling, and fetal liver biopsy. Semin Perinatol 1990; 14:456–464.

43. Evans MI, Greb A, Kunkel LM, et al. In utero fetal muscle biopsy for the diagnosis of Duchenne muscular dystrophy. Am J Obstet Gynecol 1991; 165:728–732.

44. Liley AW. Intrauterine transfusion of foetus in hemolytic disease. Br Med J 1963; 5365:1107–1109.

45. Cassady G, Barnett R, Ceballos R. Dangers of fetal transfusion: importance of placental location. Am J Obstet Gynecol 1971; 110:672–673.

46. Spackman TJ. Pediatric trauma: medical abuse of infants. Radiol Clin North Am 1973; 11:633–656.

47. Van Kamp IL, Klumper FJ, Oepkes D, et al. Complications of intrauterine intravascular transfusion for fetal anemia due to maternal red-cell alloimmunization. Am J Obstet Gynecol 2005; 192(1):171–177.

48. Weiner CP, Williamson RA, Wenstrom KD, et al. Management of fetal hemolytic disease by cordocentesis. II. Outcome of treatment. Am J Obstet Gynecol 1991; 165:1302–1307.

49. Curran JW, Lawrence DN, Jaffe H, et al. Acquired immunodeficiency syndrome (AIDS) associated with transfusion. N Engl J Med 1984; 310(2):69–75.

50. Macpherson TA, Shen-Schwarz S, Valdes-Dapena M. Prevention and reduction of iatrogenic disorders in the newborn. In: Guthrie RD, ed. Neonatal intensive care. New York: Churchill Livingstone; 1988.

51. Oleske J, Minnefor A, Cooper R, Jr, et al. Immune deficiency syndrome in children. JAMA 1983; 249:2345–2349.

52. Sloan SR, Benjamin RJ, Friedman DF, et al. Transfusion medicine. In: Nathan DG, Orkin SH, Ginsburg D, et al, eds. Nathan and Oski's hematology of infancy and childhood. 6th edn. Philadelphia: WB Saunders; 2003:1709–1756.

53. Parkman R, Mosier D, Umansky I, et al. Graft versus host disease after intrauterine and exchange transfusions for hemolytic disease of the newborn. N Engl J Med 1974; 290:359–363.

54. Cortes RA, Farmer DL. Recent advances in fetal surgery. Semin Perinatol 2004; 28(3):199–211.

55. Harrison MR, Adzick NS, Longaker MT, et al. Successful repair in utero of a fetal diaphragmatic hernia after removal of herniated viscera from the left thorax. N Engl J Med 1990 31; 322(22):1582–1584.

56. Ford WD, Cool J, Derham R. Intrathoracic silo for the potential antenatal repair of diaphragmatic herniae with liver in the chest. Fetal Diagn Ther 1992; 7:75–81.

57. Hedrick MH, Estes JM, Sullivan KM, et al. Plug the lung until it grows (PLUG): a new method to treat congenital diaphragmatic hernia in utero. J Pediatr Surg 1994; 29(5):612–617.

58. Davis CF, Sabharwal AJ. Management of congenital diaphragmatic hernia. Arch Dis Child Fetal Neonatal Ed 1998; 79(1):F1–3.

59. Sabik JF, Assad RS, Hanley FL. Prostaglandin synthesis inhibition prevents placental dysfunction after fetal cardiac bypass. J Thorac Cardiovasc Surg 1992; 103:733–741.

60. Kuller JA, Yankowitz J, Goldberg JD, et al. Outcome of antenatally diagnosed cystic adenomatoid malformations. Am J Obstet Gynecol 1992; 167(4 Pt 1):1038–1041.

61. Adzick NS, Harrison MR, Crombleholme TM, et al. Fetal lung lesions: management and outcome. Am J Obstet Gynecol 1998; 179(4):884–889.

62. Breysem L, Cossey V, Mussen E, et al. Fetal trauma: brain imaging in four neonates. Eur Radiol 2004; 14(9):1609–1614.

63. Connor E, Curran J. In utero traumatic intra-abdominal deceleration injury to the fetus – a case report. Am J Obstet Gynecol 1976; 125(4):567–569.

64. Raney EH. Fetal death secondary to nonpenetrating trauma to the gravid uterus. Am J Obstet Gynecol 1970; 106(2):313–314.

65. Schenkel B, Vorherr H. Non-prescription drugs during pregnancy: potential teratogenic and toxic effects upon embryo and fetus. J Reprod Med 1974; (12):27–45.

Complications of intrapartum care

66. Salonen IS, Uusitalo R. Birth injuries: incidence and predisposing factors. Z Kinderchir 1990; 45(3):133–135.

67. Valdes-Dapena M. Iatrogenic disease in the perinatal period as seen by the pathologist. In: Naeye RL, Kissane JM, Kaufman N, eds. Perinatal disease. Baltimore: Williams & Wilkins; 1981:382–418.

68. Oral E, Cagdas A, Gezer A, et al. Perinatal and maternal outcomes of fetal macrosomia. Eur J Obstet Gynecol Reprod Biol 2001; 99(2):167–171.

69. Perlow JH, Wigton T, Hart J, et al. Birth trauma. A five-year review of incidence and associated perinatal factors. J Reprod Med 1996; 41(10):754–760.

70. Petrikovsky BM, Schneider E, Smith-Levitin M, et al. Cephalhematoma and caput succedaneum: do they always occur in labor? Am J Obstet Gynecol 1998; 179(4):906–908.

71. Benaron DA. Subgaleal hematoma causing hypovolemic shock during delivery after failed vacuum extraction: a case report. J Perinatol 1993; 13(3):228–231.

72. Amar AP, Aryan HE, Meltzer HS, et al. Neonatal subgaleal hematoma causing brain compression: report of two cases and review of the literature. Neurosurgery 2003; 52(6):1470–1474.

73. Zelson C, Lee SJ, Pearl M. The incidence of skull fractures underlying cephalhematomas in newborn infants. J Pediatr 1974; 85:371–373.

74. Hayashi T, Hashimoto T, Fukuda S, et al. Neonatal subdural hematoma secondary to birth injury. Clinical analysis of 48 survivors. Childs Nerv Syst 1987; 3(1):23–29.

75. Pollina J, Dias MS, Li V, et al. Cranial birth injuries in term newborn infants. Pediatr Neurosurg 2001; 35(3):113–119.

76. Holden KR, Titus MO, Van Tassel P. Cranial magnetic resonance imaging examination of normal term neonates: a pilot study. J Child Neurol 1999; 14(11):708–710.

77. Dusick AM, Covert RF, Schreiber MD, et al. Risk of intracranial hemorrhage and other adverse outcomes after cocaine exposure in a cohort of 323 very low birth weight infants. J Pediatr 1993; 122(3):438–445.

78. Wigglesworth JS, Husemeyer RP. Intracranial birth trauma in vaginal breech delivery: the continued importance of injury to the occipital bone. Br J Obstet Gynaecol 1977; 84:684–691

79. Pape KE, Wigglesworth JS, eds. Hemorrhage, ischemia and the perinatal brain. Philadelphia: Lippincott, 1979.

80. Heise RH, Srivatsa PJ, Karsell PR. Spontaneous intrauterine linear skull fracture: a rare complication of spontaneous vaginal delivery. Obstet Gynecol 1996; 87(5 Pt 2):851–854.

81. Kendall N, Woloshin H. Cephalhematoma associated with fracture of the skull. J Pediatr 1952; 41:125.

82. Huisman TA, Fischer J, Willi UV, et al. 'Growing fontanelle': a serious complication of difficult vacuum extraction. Neuroradiology 1999; 41(5):381–383.

83. Norman MG. Perinatal brain damage. In: Rosenberg HS, Bolande RP, eds. Perspectives in pediatric pathology. Chicago: Year Book Medical Publishers; 1978:41–92.

84. Dupuis O, Silveira R, Dupont C, et al. Comparison of 'instrument-associated' and 'spontaneous' obstetric depressed skull fractures in a cohort of 68 neonates. Am J Obstet Gynecol 2005; 192(1):165–170.

85. Garza-Mercado R. Intrauterine depressed skull fractures of the newborn. Neurosurgery 1982; 10:694–697.

86. Theander G, Thunander J. Congenital deformities of skull caused by fetal limbs. Acta Radiol Diagn (Stockh) 1980; 21:309–313.

87. Alexander E, Jr, Davis CH, Jr. Intra-uterine fracture of the infant's skull. J Neurosurg 1969; 30(4):446–454.

88. Beall MH, Ross MG. Clavicle fracture in labor: risk factors and associated morbidities. J Perinatol 2001; 21(8):513–515.

89. Lam MH, Wong GY, Lao TT. Reappraisal of neonatal clavicular fracture: relationship between infant size and neonatal morbidity. Obstet Gynecol 2002; 100(1):115–119.

90. Cohen AW, Otto SR. Obstetric clavicular fractures. A three-year analysis. J Reprod Med 1980; 25(3):119–122.

91. Morris S, Cassidy N, Stephens M, et al. Birth-associated femoral fractures: incidence and outcome. J Pediatr Orthop 2002; 22(1):27–30.

92. Babbitt DP, Cassidy RH. Obstetrical paralysis and dislocation of the shoulder in infancy. J Bone Joint Surg 1968; 50(7):1447–1452.

93. Raupp P, Haas D, Lovasz G. Epiphyseal separation of the distal humerus. J Perinat Med 2002; 30(6):528–530.

94. Danielsson LG, Theander G. Traumatic dislocation of the radial head at birth. Acta Radiol Diagn (Stockh) 1981; 22:379–382.

95. Theodorou SD, Ierodiaconou MN, Mitsou A. Obstetrical fracture-separation of the upper femoral epiphysis. Acta Orthop Scand 1982; 53:239–243.

96. Cumming WA. Neonatal skeletal fractures: birth trauma or child abuse? J Can Assoc Radiol 1979; 30(1):30–33.

97. Hughes CA, Harley EH, Milmoe G, et al. Birth trauma in the head and neck. Arch Otolaryngol Head Neck Surg 1999; 125(2):193–199.

98. Jazbi B. Subluxation of the nasal septum in the newborn: etiology, diagnosis, and treatment. Otolaryngol Clin North Am 1977; 10(1):125–138.

99. Svenningsen NW, Westgren M, Ingemarsson I. Modern strategy for the term breech delivery – a study with a 4-year follow-up of the infants. J Perinat Med 1985; 13(3):117–126.

100. Menticoglou SM, Perlman M, Manning FA. High cervical spinal cord injury in neonates delivered with forceps: report of 15 cases. Obstet Gynecol 1995; 86(4 Pt 1):589–594.

101. Christoffersson M, Rydhstroem H. Shoulder dystocia and brachial plexus injury: a population-based study. Gynecol Obstet Invest 2002; 53(1):42–47.

102. Hoeksma AF, Wolf H, Oei SL. Obstetrical brachial plexus injuries: incidence, natural course and shoulder contracture. Clin Rehabil 2000; 14(5):523–526.

103. Chauhan SP, Rose CH, Gherman RB, et al. Brachial plexus injury: a 23-year experience from a tertiary center. Am J Obstet Gynecol 2005; 192(6):1795–1800.

104. Gordon M, Rich H, Deutschberger J, et al. The immediate and long-term outcome of obstetric birth trauma. Am J Obstet Gynecol 1973; 117:51–56.

105. Curran JS. Factors predisposing to birth associated injuries. In: Milunsky A, Friedman EA, Gluck L, eds. Advances in perinatal medicine. New York: Plenum Medical Book Company; 1985.

106. Goodman JM. Liver trauma in the newborn: a case report. J Trauma 1974; 14:427–428.

107. Sokol DM, Tompkins D, Izant RJ Jr. Rupture of the spleen and liver in the newborn: a report of the first survivor and a review of the literature. J Pediatr Surg 1974; 9:227–229.

108. Koplewitz BZ, Daneman A, Cutz E, et al. Neonatal adrenal congestion: a sonographic–pathologic correlation. Pediatr Radiol 1998; 28(12):958–962.

109. Tank ES, Davis R, Holt JF, et al. Mechanisms of trauma during breech delivery. Obstet Gynecol 1971; 38(5):761–767.

110. Bergman SM, Scouras GP. Incidental bilateral adrenal calcification. Urology 1983; 22(6):665–666.

111. Ho BC, Lee EH, Singh K. Epidemiology, presentation and management of congenital muscular torticollis. Singapore Med J 1999; 40(11):675–679.

112. Mathews R, Sheridan ME, Patil U. Neonatal testicular loss secondary to perinatal trauma in breech presentation. BJU Int 1999; 83(9):1069–1070.

113. Rietberg CC, Elferink-Stinkens PM, Brand R, et al. Term breech presentation in The Netherlands from 1995 to 1999: mortality and morbidity in relation to the mode of delivery of 33824 infants. Br J Obstet Gynaecol 2003; 110(6):604–609.

114. Kayem G, Goffinet F, Clement D, et al. Breech presentation at term: morbidity and mortality according to the type of delivery at Port Royal Maternity Hospital from 1993 through 1999. Eur J Obstet Gynecol Reprod Biol 2002; 102(2):137–142.

115. Durham JH, Sekula-Perlman A, Callery RT. Iatrogenic brain injury during emergency cesarean section. Acta Obstet Gynecol Scand 1998; 77(2):238–239.

116. Bowers SK, MacDonald HM, Shapiro ED. Prevention of iatrogenic neonatal respiratory distress syndrome: elective repeat cesarean section and spontaneous labor. Am J Obstet Gynecol 1982; 143(2):186–189.

117. Robertson PA, Laros RK, Jr, Zhao RL. Neonatal and maternal outcome in low-pelvic and midpelvic operative deliveries. Am J Obstet Gynecol 1990; 162(6):1436–1442.

118. Hagadorn-Freathy AS, Yeomans ER, Hankins GD. Validation of the 1988 ACOG forceps classification system. Obstet Gynecol 1991; 77(3):356–360.

119. Hall SL. Simultaneous occurrence of intracranial and subgaleal hemorrhages complicating vacuum extraction delivery. J Perinatol 1992; 12:185–187.

120. Okuno T, Miyamoto M, Itakura T, et al. A case of epidural hematoma caused by a vacuum extraction without any skull fractures and accompanied by cephalohematoma. No Shinkei Geka (Neurol Surg) 1993; 21:1137–1141.

121. Uchil D, Arulkumaran S. Neonatal subgaleal hemorrhage and its relationship to delivery by vacuum extraction. Obstet Gynecol Surv 2003; 58(10):687–693.

122. Miksovsky P, Watson WJ. Obstetric vacuum extraction: state of the art in the new millennium. Obstet Gynecol Surv 2001; 56(11):736–751.

123. Lauer AK, Rimmer SO. Eyelid laceration in a neonate by fetal monitoring spiral electrode. Am J Ophthalmol 1998; 125(5):715–717.

124. D'Souza SW, Black P, MacFarlane T. Fetal scalp damage and neonatal jaundice: a risk of routine fetal scalp electrode monitoring. J Obstet Gynaecol 1982; 2:161.

125. Goldkrand JW. Intrapartum inoculation of herpes simplex virus by fetal scalp electrode. Obstet Gynecol. 1982; 59:263–265.

Complications of postnatal care

126. Lemons JA, Bauer CR, Oh W, et al. Very low birth weight outcomes of the National Institute of Child health and human development neonatal research network, January 1995 through December 1996. NICHD Neonatal Research Network. Pediatrics 2001; 107(1):E1.

127. Powner DJ, Holcombe PA, Mello LA. Cardiopulmonary resuscitation-related injuries. Crit Care Med 1984; 12(1):54–55.

128. Bush CM, Jones JS, Cohle SD, et al. Pediatric injuries from cardiopulmonary resuscitation. Ann Emerg Med 1996; 28(1):40–44.

129. Polito A, Au Eong KG, Repka MX, et al. Bilateral retinal hemorrhages in a preterm infant with retinopathy of prematurity immediately following cardiopulmonary resuscitation. Arch Ophthalmol 2001; 119(6):913–914.

130. Joshi VV. Endotracheal injuries, perinatal iatrogenic diseases. Common problems in pediatric pathology. New York: Igaku-Shoin; 1994.

131. Stoll BJ, Kliegman RM. Respiratory tract disorders. In: Behrman RE, Kliegman RM, Jenson HB, eds. Nelson textbook of pediatrics. 17th edn. Philadelphia: Saunders; 2004:573–588.

132. De Espinosa H, Garcia de Paredes C. Traumatic perforation of the pharynx in a newborn baby. J Pediatr Surg 1974; 9(2):247–248.

133. Clarke TA, Coen RW, Feldman B, et al. Esophageal perforations in premature infants and comments on the diagnosis. Am J Dis Child 1980; 134(4):367–368.

134. Mahieu HF, de Bree R, Ekkelkamp S, et al. Tracheal and laryngeal rupture in neonates: complication of delivery or of intubation? Ann Otol Rhinol Laryngol 2004; 113(10):786–792.

135. Gould SJ, Howard S. The histopathology of the larynx in the neonate following endotracheal intubation. J Pathol 1985; 146(4):301–311.

136. O'Neill JA, Jr. Experience with iatrogenic laryngeal and tracheal stenoses. J Pediatr Surg 1984; 19(3):235–238.

137. Downing GJ, Hayen LK, Kilbride HW. Acquired subglottic cysts in the low-birth-weight infant. Characteristics, treatment, and outcome. Am J Dis Child 1993; 147(9):971–974.

138. Graff TD, Benson DW. Systemic and pulmonary changes with inhaled humid atmospheres: clinical application. Anesthesiology 1969; 30(2):199–207.

139. Mimouni F, Ballard JL, Ballard ET, et al. Necrotizing tracheobronchitis: case report. Pediatrics 1986; 77(3):366–368.

140. Boros SJ, Mammel MC, Lewallen PK, et al. Necrotizing tracheobronchitis: a complication of high-frequency ventilation. J Pediatr 1986; 109(1):95–100.

141. Kirpalani H, Higa T, Perlman M, et al. Diagnosis and therapy of necrotizing tracheobronchitis in ventilated neonates. Crit Care Med 1985; 13(10):792–797.

142. Ratner I, Whitfield J. Acquired subglottic stenosis in the very-low-birth-weight infant. Am J Dis Child 1983; 137(1):40–43.

143. Azizkhan RG, Grimmer DL, Askin FB, et al. Acquired lobar emphysema (overinflation): clinical and pathological evaluation of infants requiring lobectomy. J Pediatr Surg 1992; 27(8):1145–1151.

144. Drew JH, Landau LI, Acton CM, et al. Pulmonary interstitial emphysema requiring lobectomy. Complications of assisted ventilation. Arch Dis Child 1978; 53(5):424–426.

145. Boglino C, Inserra A, Ciprandi G, et al. Interstitial pulmonary emphysema. Combined therapeutic approach in a retrospective multidisciplinary study. Minerva Pediatr 1991; 43(11):675–683.

146. Richter A, Tegtmeyer FK, Moller J. Air embolism and pulmonary interstitial emphysema in a preterm infant with hyaline membrane disease. Pediatr Radiol 1991; 21(7):521–522.

147. Rudd PT, Wigglesworth JS. Oxygen embolus during mechanical ventilation with disappearance of signs after death. Arch Dis Child 1982; 57(3):237–239.

148. Magilner AD, Capitanio MA, Werthemier I, et al. Persistent localized intrapulmonary interstitial emphysema: an observation in three infants. Radiology 1974; 111(2):379–384.

149. Stocker JT, Madewell JE. Persistent interstitial pulmonary emphysema: another complication of the respiratory distress syndrome. Pediatrics 1977; 59(6):847–857.

150. Stocker JT, Drake RM, Madwell JE. Cystic and congenital lung disease in the newborn. In: Rosenberg HS, Bolande RP, eds. Perspectives in pediatric pathology. Chicago: Year Book Medical Publisher; 1978:93–154.

151. Knisely AS, Leal SM, Singer DB. Abnormalities of diaphragmatic muscle in neonates with ventilated lungs. J Pediatr 1988; 113(6):1074–1077.

152. Gayan-Ramirez G, Decramer M. Effects of mechanical ventilation on diaphragm function and biology. Eur Respir J 2002; 20(6):1579–1586.

153. Weinberger B, Laskin DL, Heck DE, et al. Oxygen toxicity in premature infants. Toxicol Appl Pharmacol 2002; 181(1):60–67.

154. DeLemos R, Wolfsdorf J, Nachman R, et al. Lung injury from oxygen in lambs: the role of artificial ventilation. Anesthesiology 1969; 30(6):609–618.

155. Northway WH, Jr, Rosan RC, Porter DY. Pulmonary disease following respirator therapy of hyaline-membrane disease. Bronchopulmonary dysplasia. N Engl J Med 1967; 276(7):357–368.

156. Coalson JJ. Pathology of new bronchopulmonary dysplasia. Semin Neonatol 2003; 8(1):73–81.

157. Garland JS, Nelson DB, Rice T, et al. Increased risk of gastrointestinal perforations in neonates mechanically ventilated with either face mask or nasal prongs. Pediatrics 1985; 76(3):406–410.

158. Cameron D, Lupton BA. Inadvertent brain penetration during neonatal nasotracheal intubation. Arch Dis Child 1993; 69(1 Spec No):79–80.

159. Suresh GK, Soll RF. Exogenous surfactant therapy in newborn infants. [Review] [134 refs]. Ann Acad Med Singapore 2003; 32(3):335–345.

160. Pinar H, Makarova N, Rubin LP, et al. Pathology of the lung in surfactant-treated neonates. Pediatr Pathol 1994; 14(4):627–636.

161. Weinberger B, Laskin DL, Heck DE, et al. The toxicology of inhaled nitric oxide. Toxicol Sci 2001; 59(1):5–16.

162. Deneyer M, Goossens A, Pipeleers-Marichal M, et al. Esophagitis of likely traumatic origin in newborns. J Pediatr Gastroenterol Nutr 1992; 15(1): 81–84.

163. Jaw MC, Soong WJ, Chen SJ, et al. Pneumothorax: a complication of deep endotracheal tube suction: report of 3 cases. Zhonghua Yi Xue Za Zhi (Taipei) 1991; 48:313–317.

164. Cook LN. Update on extracorporeal membrane oxygenation. Paediatr Respir Rev 2004; 5 (suppl A):S329–337.

165. Kim ES, Stolar CJ. ECMO in the newborn. Am J Perinatol 2000; 17(7): 345–356.

166. Chou P, Shen-Schwartz S, et al. Pulmonary epithelial changes with extracorporeal membrane oxygenation (ECMO) therapy. Analysis of 17 autopsy cases. Mod Pathol 1991; 4:2.

167. Vogler C, Sotela C, Fulling K. Extracorporeal membrane oxygenation (ECMO) therapy: an analysis of 23 autopsies (abstract). Pediatr Pathol 1987; 7:498.

168. Zwischenberger JB, Nguyen TT, Upp JR, Jr, et al. Complications of neonatal extracorporeal membrane oxygenation. Collective experience from the Extracorporeal Life Support Organization. J Thorac Cardiovasc Surg 1994; 107(3):838–848.

169. Sell LL, Cullen ML, Whittlesey GC, et al. Hemorrhagic complications during extracorporeal membrane oxygenation: prevention and treatment. J Pediatr Surg. 1986; 21(12):1087–1091.

170. McManus ML, Kevy SV, Bower LK, et al. Coagulation factor deficiencies during initiation of extracorporeal membrane oxygenation. J Pediatr 1995; 126(6):900–904.

171. Taylor GA, Fitz CR, Miller MK, et al. Intracranial abnormalities in infants treated with extracorporeal membrane oxygenation: imaging with US and CT. Radiology 1987; 165(3):675–678.

172. Sell LL, Cullen ML, Lerner GR, et al. Hypertension during extracorporeal membrane oxygenation: cause, effect, and management. Surgery 1987; 102(4):724–730.

173. Sell LL, Cullen ML, Whittlesey GC, et al. Experience with renal failure during extracorporeal membrane oxygenation: treatment with continuous hemofiltration. J Pediatr Surg 1987; 22(7):600–602.

174. Goretsky MJ, Martinasek D, Warner BW. Pulmonary hemorrhage: a novel complication after extracorporeal life support. J Pediatr Surg 1996; 31(9):1276–1281.

175. Taylor GA, Lotze A, Kapur S, et al. Diffuse pulmonary opacification in infants undergoing extracorporeal membrane oxygenation: clinical and pathologic correlation. Radiology 1986; 161(2):347–350.

176. Ehren H, Palmer K, Eriksson M, et al. Pediatric ECMO for pulmonary support: experience from 12 cases. Acta Paediatr 1995; 84(4):442–446.

177. Vogler C, Sotelo-Avila C, Lagunoff D, et al. Aluminum-containing emboli in infants treated with extracorporeal membrane oxygenation. N Engl J Med 1988; 14; 319(2):75–79.

178. Maloney NA, Ott SM, Alfrey AC, et al. Histological quantitation of aluminum in iliac bone from patients with renal failure. J Lab Clin Med 1982; 99(2):206–216.

179. Fridriksson JH, Helmrath MA, Wessel JJ, et al. Hypercalcemia associated with extracorporeal life support in neonates. J Pediatr Surg 2001; 36(3):493–497.

180. Mattar MS, al-Alfy AA, Dahniya MH, et al. Urinary bladder perforation: an unusual complication of neonatal nasogastric tube feeding. Pediatr Radiol 1997; 27(11):858–859.

181. Pulzer F, Bennek J, Robel-Tillig E, et al. Gastric perforation in a newborn. Lancet 2004; 363(9410):703.

182. Schwimmer J, Balistreri WF. Liver disease associated with systemic disorders. In: Behrman RE, Kliegman RM, Jenson HB, eds. Nelson textbook of pediatrics. 17th edn. Philadelphia: Saunders; 2004:1333–1335.

183. Mullick FG, Moran CA, Ishak KG. Total parenteral nutrition: a histopathologic analysis of the liver changes in 20 children. Mod Pathol 1994; 7(2):190–194.

184. Levene MI, Wigglesworth JS, Desai R. Pulmonary fat accumulation after intralipid infusion in the preterm infant. Lancet 1980; 2(8199):815–818.

185. Dahms BB, Halpin TC, Jr. Pulmonary arterial lipid deposit in newborn infants receiving intravenous lipid infusion. J Pediatr 1980; 97(5): 800–805.

186. Joshi VV, Wang NS. Repeated pulmonary embolism in an infant with subacute Candida endocarditis of the right side of the heart. Am J Dis Child 1973; 125(2):257–259.

187. Redline RW, Redline SS, Boxerbaum B, et al. Systemic Malassezia furfur infections in patients receiving intralipid therapy. Hum Pathol 1985; 16(8):815–822.

188. Chudley AE, Brown DR, Holzman IR, et al. Nutritional rickets in 2 very low birthweight infants with chronic lung disease. Arch Dis Child 1980; 55(9):687–690.

189. Oppenheimer SJ, Snodgrass GJ. Neonatal rickets. Histopathology and quantitative bone changes. Arch Dis Child 1980; 55(12):945–949.

190. Hsueh W, Caplan MS, Qu XW, et al. Neonatal necrotizing enterocolitis: clinical considerations and pathogenetic concepts. Pediatr Dev Pathol 2003; 6(1):6–23.

191. Hakanson DO, Oh W. Necrotizing enterocolitis and hyperviscosity in the newborn infant. J Pediatr 1977; 90(3):458–461.

192. Kitterman JA, Phibbs RH, Tooley WH. Catheterization of umbilical vessels in newborn infants. Pediatr Clin North Am 1970; 17(4):895–912.

193. Larroche JC. Umbilical catheterization: its complications. Anatomical study. Biol Neonate 1970; 16(1):101–116.

194. Scott JM. Iatrogenic lesions in babies following umbilical vein catheterization. Arch Dis Child 1965; 40:426–429.

195. Junker P, Egeblad M, Nielsen O, et al. Umbilical vein catheterization and portal hypertension. Acta Paediatr Scand 1976; 65(4):499–504.

196. Orme RL, Eades SM. Perforation of the bowel in the newborn as a complication of exchange transfusion. Br Med J 1968; 4(627):349–351.

197. Wigger HJ. Influence of perinatal management. In: Wigglesworth JS, Singer DB, eds. Textbook of fetal and perinatal pathology. London: Blackwell Scientific Publishing; 1991.

198. Buchheit JQ, Stewart DL. Clinical comparison of localized intestinal perforation and necrotizing enterocolitis in neonates. Pediatrics 1994; 93(1):32–36.

199. Spangler JG, Kleinberg F, Fulton RE, et al. False aneurysm of the descending aorta: a complication of umbilical artery catheterization. Am J Dis Child 1977; 131(11):1258–1259.

200. Lobe TE, Richardson CJ, Boulden TF, et al. Mycotic thromboaneurysmal disease of the abdominal aorta in preterm infants: its natural history and its management. J Pediatr Surg 1992; 27(8):1054–1059.

201. Plumer LB, Kaplan GW, Mendoza SA. Hypertension in infants – a complication of umbilical arterial catheterization. J Pediatr 1976; 89(5):802–805.

202. Vordermark JS, 2nd, Buck AS, Dresner ML. Urinary ascites resulting from umbilical artery catheterization. J Urol 1980; 124(5):751.

203. Joshi VV, Draper DA, Bates RD, 3rd. Neonatal necrotizing enterocolitis. Occurrence secondary to thrombosis of abdominal aorta following umbilical arterial catheterization. Arch Pathol 1975; 99(10):540–543.

204. Diamond DA, Ford C. Neonatal bladder rupture: a complication of umbilical artery catheterization. J Urol 1989; 142(6):1543–1544.

205. Van Leeuwen G, Patney M. Complications of umbilical vessel catheterization: peritoneal perforation. Pediatrics 1969; 44(6):1028–1030.

206. Mann NP. Gluteal skin necrosis after umbilical artery catheterisation. Arch Dis Child 1980; 55(10):815–817.

207. Pettit J. Assessment of infants with peripherally inserted central catheters: Part 1. Detecting the most frequently occurring complications. Adv Neonatal Care 2002; 2(6):304–315.

208. Weese-Mayer DE, Fondriest DW, Brouillette RT, et al. Risk factors associated with candidemia in the neonatal intensive care unit: a case-control study. Pediatr Infect Dis J 1987; 6(2):190–196.

209. Blumenfeld TA, Turi GK, Blanc WA. Recommended site and depth of newborn heel skin punctures based on anatomical measurements and histopathology. Lancet 1979; 1(8110):230–233.

210. Holzman BH, Scott GB. Control of infection and techniques of isolation in the pediatric intensive care unit. Pediatr Clin North Am 1981; 28(3): 703–721.

211. Stanley PE. Instrumentation, instrument safety. In: Zschoche DA, ed. Mosby's comprehensive review of critical care. St Louis: Mosby Year Book; 1981.

212. Kumar SP. Adverse drug reactions in the newborn. Ann Clin Lab Sci 1985; 15(3):195–203.

213. Stoll BJ, Kliegman RM. The high-risk infant. In: Behrman RE, Kliegman RM, Jenson HB, eds. Nelson textbook of pediatrics. 17th edn. Philadelphia: Saunders; 2004:547–559.

214. Powell H, Swarner O, Gluck L, et al. Hexachlorophene myelinopathy in premature infants. J Pediatr 1973; 82(6):976–981.

215. Kamitsuka MD, Peloquin D. Renal calcification after dexamethasone in infants with bronchopulmonary dysplasia. Lancet 1991; 337(8741):626.

216. Cantor B, Tyler T, Nelson RM, et al. Oligohydramnios and transient neonatal anuria: a possible association with the maternal use of prostaglandin synthetase inhibitors. J Reprod Med 1980; 24(5):220–223.

217. Nagaraj HS, Sandhu AS, Cook LN, et al. Gastrointestinal perforation following indomethacin therapy in very low birth weight infants. J Pediatr Surg 1981; 16(6):1003–1007.

218. Ueda K, Saito A, Nakano H, et al. Cortical hyperostosis following long-term administration of prostaglandin E_1 in infants with cyanotic congenital heart disease. J Pediatr 1980; 97(5):834–836.

219. Pape KE, Armstrong DL, Fitzhardinge PM. Central nervous system pathology associated with mask ventilation in the very low birthweight infant: a new etiology for intracerebellar hemorrhages. Pediatrics 1976; 58(4):473–483.

Further reading

deSa DJ. Pathology of neonatal intensive care. An illustrated reference. London: Chapman and Hall Medical; 1995.

Howatson AG. Iatrogenic disease. In: Keeling J, ed. Fetal and neonatal pathology. 3rd edn. London: Springer-Verlag; 2001:349–380.

Nikkels PGJ. Iatrogenic damage in the neonatal period. Semin Neonatol 2004; 9:303–310.

Pinar H. Pathology of perinatal and neonatal care. In: Wigglesworth JL, Singer DB, eds. Textbook of fetal and perinatal pathology. 2nd edn. Oxford: Blackwell Science; 1998:41–74.

Examination of the fetus and infant

PART

Prenatal diagnosis and neonatal screening

14

Philip M. Farrell   Sherman Elias

Every physician's first duty is to diagnose – accurately and promptly.
Diagnosis is the first step of treatment.[1]

The purpose of this chapter is to review selected genetic disorders and the diagnostic methods used to identify them prenatally or in the early neonatal period. Prenatal and neonatal diagnostic technologies have evolved gradually over four decades, but they are expanding dramatically in the twenty-first century, as is their application in population-based screening and/or targeted assessment of at-risk couples. Clearly, the demand for prenatal genetic screening tests will continue to increase as a result of individual and organizational advocacy efforts. Therefore, the authors are providing an overview with emphasis on prenatal diagnosis and suggest more comprehensive references in the bibliography.[2–5] We also recommend that the reader consults practice guideline publications of The American College of Obstetricians and Gynecologists (ACOG)[6,7] and the American Academy of Pediatrics (AAP).[8] For a variety of reasons, this review has focused almost exclusively on the situation in the United States, where the complexity is generally greater than in other countries such as Canada which has relatively limited newborn screening programs in all the provinces.

Evolution of prenatal and neonatal genetic screening

Prenatal and perinatal medicine advanced dramatically, though incrementally, during the second half of the twentieth century because of the combination of research discoveries and technological developments applicable to the fetus and newborn. The important discoveries and their translation into patient care depended on interdisciplinary science and teamwork among health care providers. Perhaps no other area of medical practice has been so immediately and profoundly influenced by the genetics revolution, as cellular and molecular biology techniques developed in research laboratories have become widely available in clinical practice. Thus, recent years have witnessed an extraordinary improvement in our ability to diagnose genetic conditions either prenatally or in the early neonatal period; almost all of these depend upon collaboration with clinical laboratories.

Prenatal genetics emerged in the 1960s and 1970s with amniocentesis used to assess fetal conditions. During the 1980s, chorionic villus sampling technology with cell culture emerged as an important step forward. This was followed during the next decade by ultrasound-based assessment of fetal morphology, originally applied by radiologists and subsequently by maternal–fetal specialists and reproductive geneticists. As cytogenetics, genomics, and proteomics are applied, the precision of diagnostic technologies has improved dramatically and non-invasive screening methods now predominate in prenatal genetics practice. The interval from laboratory discovery to bedside application is no longer measured in years, as previously has been the case in medicine, but in months or even weeks. In recent years, the most significant advances have come about by combining high-resolution ultrasonography with maternal serum markers for first-trimester screening for Down syndrome and other aneuploidies. In addition, in relevant ethnic and racial populations, offering carrier screening for sickle cell anemia, the thalassemias, Tay-Sachs disease, Canavan disease, familial dysautonomia, and cystic fibrosis has become standard practice. The burgeoning field of prenatal diagnosis has fostered a host of specialty journals, most notably *Prenatal Diagnosis*, books, and internet sites. Thus, driven by a combination of excellent diagnostic technologies and patient demand, and also augmented by growing proportion of first pregnancies in women beyond 30 years of age, a new era in prenatal diagnosis of genetic disease has been well established worldwide.[9]

In parallel, the diagnosis of genetic disorders in newborn infants has improved for both conditions associated with dysmorphology and a wide variety of inborn errors of metabolism due to single gene defects. Cytogenetics technology played a key role in the former, while biochemical tests applied to neonatal blood specimens catalyzed the latter advances. The advent of newborn screening is historically interesting because it depended primarily on development of a neonatal blood sampling technique rather than analytical biochemistry advances.[10] Specifically, to promote early diagnosis of phenylketonuria (PKU) in newborn populations, Robert Guthrie devised a technique for routine procurement of blood using a 'heel stick' to obtain about 0.4 mL of blood on filter paper. During the early 1960s, the potential opportunity to prevent mental retardation through early diagnosis aroused great interest, and Guthrie was motivated to focus his attention on PKU using blood phenylalanine levels determined microbiologically to ensure early diagnosis through population-based screening of all newborns. Driven by parent advocacy groups, mandatory statewide screening for PKU was first instituted in Massachusetts and Oregon during 1963, and two years later 28 more states had statutory requirements for PKU screening of all newborns. Next, galactosemia screening was implemented on the same dried blood specimens using microbiologic determinations, and in the early 1970s congenital hypothyroidism followed. Many other genetic disorders classified as inborn errors of metabolism were added in the 1980s and 1990s. With the recent advent of tandem mass spectrometry, more than 50 inborn errors of metabolism can be readily diagnosed using dried blood specimens. The analytical methods extended in the 1990s to DNA analyses for carrier screening and diagnosis of cystic fibrosis (CF). Because these congenital metabolic and endocrine disorders have a latent period from onset to irreversible pathology, the opportunity exists for intervention with preventive therapies.

Diagnostic strategies

Diagnosis of disease typically depends on history, physical examination, and laboratory studies confirming pre-existing suspicion. In the case of the fetus and asymptomatic neonate, laboratory tests become predominant. Screening for early detection of disease is especially valuable in prenatal and neonatal practice. According to Hennekens and Buring,[11] 'screening refers to the application of a test to people who are as yet asymptomatic for the purpose of classifying them with the respect to their likelihood of having a particular disease ... the screening procedure itself does not diagnose illness ... those who test positive are sent on for further evaluation by a subsequent diagnostic test or procedure to determine whether they do, in fact, have the disease.' As modern laboratory methods improve, however, some screening tests can actually become diagnostic tests as in the case of CF when DNA analyses on neonatal blood specimens reveal two ΔF508 mutations of the cystic fibrosis transmembrane conductance regulatory (CFTR) gene.[12]

There are important differences between prenatal diagnostic strategies practiced by obstetricians and the early diagnosis of genetic disorders in newborns through population-based screening. In general, the former has relied on the traditional medical model of intervention in individuals (pregnant women), although the interventions are usually triggered by risk factors rather than illnesses. Population-based screening has also being applied increasingly to pregnant women ever since the era of maternal serum α-fetoprotein (MSAFP) screening for neural tube defects was introduced in the mid 1970s, followed by Merkatz et al.[13] expanding the use of MSAFP screening for fetal Down syndrome, and later augmented by other tests.[14]

Important screening test characteristics include two measures of validity, namely sensitivity and specificity, and also measures of probability. Sensitivity and specificity are inherent characteristics of screening tests with a defined cut-off value and are not affected by disease prevalence, whereas the predictive values (probability measures) of the tests are influenced by prevalence. The most important consideration in prenatal and neonatal genetics practice is that screening tests achieve close to 100% sensitivity, i.e., avoidance of false-negative results. Unfortunately, it is impossible to achieve 100% sensitivity over a long duration because even when there are no biologic false negatives, the possibility always exists for laboratory or human error. Therefore, health care providers should always assume that no screening test is perfect, just as no laboratory test is infallible. Test specificity, or the true negative rate, indicates the probability that a person without the disease will have a negative test result. As with sensitivity, specificity should ideally approach 100%. Finally, the positive predictive value of (PPV) should be regarded as extremely important because it provides a measure of the post-test probability or likelihood of disease following a positive screening test. PPV indicates a proportion of persons with positive test results who have the disease.

Methods of prenatal diagnosis

A brief overview of the well-known conventional techniques is provided below and is followed by comments about newer preimplantation techniques.

Sampling techniques

Chorionic villus sampling

Since amniocentesis (discussed below) is most commonly performed in the mid-second trimester (15–16 weeks), fetal diagnosis cannot usually be established prior to 17–18 weeks' gestation. A technique that could be performed during the first trimester is most desirable to reduce the psychological stress of awaiting results until mid-pregnancy and to allow a safer method of pregnancy termination. Chorionic villus sampling (CVS) is such a technique. Following fertilization, the zygote differentiates first into the blastocyst, which contains an inner cell mass that develops into the fetus, and an outer trophoblastic layer that develops into non-fetal structures such as amnion, chorion, and placenta. The genetic complement of the outer cell mass nearly always reflects the genetic constitution of the inner cell mass (i.e., the fetus) because both are derived from the same zygote. It follows that cytogenetic, DNA, or biochemical analysis on trophoblastic cells should provide information comparable with that obtained from cultured amniotic fluid cells. The one major exception is that assays requiring amniotic fluid, specifically AFP, require amniocentesis. CVS is usually performed between 10 and 14 weeks' gestation. Under ultrasound guidance, chorionic villi are aspirated either by passing a catheter transcervically into the placenta or passing a needle through the maternal abdomen and uterus into the placenta.[15,16] There is a risk of approximately 1% for loss of pregnancy truly associated with CVS. The risk for fetal limb defects following CVS has not been determined unequivocally.[17]

Mosaicism in CVS is a recently recognized but extremely important phenomenon, since prenatal interpretation of a fetal karyotype may result in irreversible decisions to continue or terminate a pregnancy. If the interpretation is inaccurate, the decision can have permanently devastating effects upon the family's life. Chromosomal mosaicism is found in vivo most frequently in sex chromosomal abnormalities, occasionally in autosomal abnormalities, and is usually a postconceptional, postmitotic event. It occurs in about 1 in 1000 newborn infants. Several mechanisms can result in mosaicism observed prenatally, including the true phenomenon. For example, so called pseudomosaicism can occur in amniotic cells. It is artifactual and can usually be excluded by finding different karyotypes in several different culture flasks. The contamination of fetal by maternal cells can also result in confusion but should be eliminated by discarding the first amniotic fluid withdrawn at amniocentesis. If a fetus is suspected of having a karyotype of 46,XY/46,XX, other techniques such as DNA analysis, or polymorphisms can be used for clarification. In CVS, three mechanisms can result in mosaicism. It is possible that twinning is more common at conception than observed at birth, and some of the early discrepancies might reflect this. Maternal cell contamination has also been observed, as in amniocentesis. By far the most important is the phenomenon of confined placental mosaicism (CPM), described by Kalousek in 1983.[18] CPM generally results from an aneuploid germ cell generating a trisomic zygote, followed by loss of the extra chromosome by one of the cells of the blastula, which thus consists of two distinct cell lines. The reason for the discrepancy between chromosomes in extraembryonic tissues and those in the fetus proper is, briefly and superficially, caused by the difference between cells from the cytotrophoblast (usually used for direct or 12-hour, short-term CVS cultures) and cells from the inner cell mass that gives rise to the mesenchymal core from which cells are grown in long-term (72-hour) cultures, after enzymatic digestion of the outer layers. The long-term culture reflects the fetal karyotype, whereas the short-term or direct culture more frequently reflects the syncitiocytotrophoblast. Unfortunately, there are several forms of CPM, depending on the timing and location of the event causing the karyotypic change. Practically, mosaicism in CVS cells occurs about 10 times more frequently than in newborn karyotypes. Because of the possibility of CPM occurring, the potential need for confirmatory or clarifying amniocentesis or other tests should be discussed during the pre-CVS counseling session. The reader is referred to a detailed review of the subject by Schreck and colleagues.[19] The possibility of single gene mosaicism, which could occur through the same mechanism and result in similar confusion during prenatal detection of single gene disorders, raises an interesting, hitherto unaddressed question.

Amniocentesis

Biological specimens obtainable include amniotic fluid and cells. The procedure is performed from 14 weeks' gestation onward. The technique involves passing a needle transabdominally into the amniotic cavity under continuous ultrasound monitoring. Analyses are the same as for CVS. AFP can also be evaluated in amniotic fluid, as can additional metabolites (e.g., proteins, hormones). The procedure has a risk of 0.5% or less for pregnancy loss, depending on the expertise of the physician performing the procedure.[3,20]

Percutaneous umbilical blood sampling

Access to the fetal circulation was initially accomplished by fetoscopy, a method of directly visualizing the fetus, umbilical cord, and chorionic surface of the placenta, using endoscopic instruments.[21] Fetoscopy for this purpose has now been replaced by ultrasound-directed percutaneous umbilical blood sampling (PUBS), also termed cordocentesis or funipuncture. Fetal blood chromosome analysis has been used to help clarify purported chromosome mosaicism detected in cultured amniotic fluid cells[22] or chorionic villi. Rapid assessment of fetal chromosome complement has been accomplished by 'direct' cytogenetic analysis of uncultured nucleated blood cells.[23] Short-term fetal lymphocyte cultures can provide a cytogenetic result within 72 hours; direct analysis of spontaneously dividing fetal cells (probably nucleated red blood cells) can provide a karyotype result within 24 hours. This proves particularly useful for patients presenting late in the second trimester, when results from amniocentesis would be available before 24 weeks' gestation. In most centers, 24 weeks' gestation is usually the most advanced stage of pregnancy when termination remains an option if a fetal abnormality is diagnosed. Also, in cases of fetal structural abnormalities or intrauterine growth retardation (IUGR) presenting in the third trimester, rapid results may prove useful for decision-making concerning the mode of delivery.[24,25] More recently, fluorescent in situ hybridization (FISH) with chromosome-specific DNA probes has also been used for rapid prenatal diagnosis of aneuploidy using nucleated fetal blood cells from umbilical cord blood, as well as chorionic villus and amniotic fluid cells.[26] Fetal blood sampling appears to be a relatively safe procedure when performed by experienced physicians, albeit carrying more risk than CVS or amniocentesis. Collaborative data from 14 North American centers, sampling 1600 patients at varying gestational ages and for a variety of indications, revealed an uncorrected fetal loss rate of 1.6%.[27]

Maternal serum screening

Second trimester maternal serum screening is a non-invasive way to identify women whose risk of having children with neural tube defects (usually open spina bifida or anencephaly) or Down syndrome or trisomy 18 is high enough to warrant amniocentesis.[28] Screening should be offered to all pregnant women. When amniocentesis is recommended, some women older than 35 years request serum screening before they agree to the procedure, so that risk of fetal abnormalities can be more precisely defined. Results are most accurate when the initial sample is obtained between 16 and 18 weeks of pregnancy, although screening can be done from about 15 to 20 weeks. Normal values vary with gestational age. Corrections for maternal weight, diabetes mellitus, race, and other factors are necessary.

Maternal α-fetoprotein levels are measured first; elevated levels suggest open spina bifida, anencephaly, increased risk of pregnancy complications (e.g., intrauterine growth restriction, abruptio placentae), or, occasionally, twins or other multifetal pregnancy. Closed spina bifida is usually not detected. Designating a cut-off value to determine whether further testing is warranted involves weighing the risk of missed abnormalities against the risk of complications from unnecessary testing. Usually, a cut-off value in the 95th to 98th percentile or 2.0–2.5 times the normal pregnancy median (multiples of the median, or MOM) is used. This value is about 80% sensitive for open spina bifida and 90% sensitive for anencephaly. When this value is used, amniocentesis is eventually required in 1–2% of women originally screened. Lower cut-off values increase sensitivity but decrease specificity, resulting in more amniocenteses.

If further testing is warranted, ultrasonography is the next step. It can confirm gestational age (which may be underestimated) or detect multiple gestation, fetal death, or congenital malformations. In some women, ultrasonography cannot identify a cause for elevated α-fetoprotein levels. Some experts believe that if high-resolution ultrasonography done by an experienced sonographer is normal, further testing is unnecessary. However, because this test occasionally misses neural tube defects, many experts recommend further testing regardless of ultrasonography results.

Subsequent testing includes amniocentesis and measurement of α-fetoprotein and acetylcholinesterase levels in amniotic fluid. Elevated α-fetoprotein in amniotic fluid suggests a neural tube defect, another malformation (e.g., omphalocele, congenital nephrosis, cystic hygroma, gastroschisis, upper GI atresia), or contamination of the sample with fetal blood. Presence of acetylcholinesterase in amniotic fluid suggests a neural tube defect or another malformation. Elevated α-fetoprotein plus presence of acetylcholinesterase in amniotic fluid is virtually 100% sensitive for anencephaly and 90–95% sensitive for open spina bifida. High-resolution ultrasonography can detect most of these malformations. However, even if a malformation cannot be detected, abnormal amniotic fluid markers indicate that a malformation is likely, and parents should be informed.

Second trimester maternal serum levels of α-fetoprotein, human chorionic gonadotropin (hCG), and unconjugated estriol (triple screening), adjusted for gestational age, are measured to refine estimates of Down syndrome risk. With triple screening, sensitivity for Down syndrome is about 65%, with a false-positive rate of about 5%. Some laboratories also measure inhibin A, increasing sensitivity to 75%. If screening suggests Down syndrome, ultrasonography is done to confirm gestational age, and risk is recalculated. If the original blood sample was drawn too early, another one must be obtained later at the appropriate time. Amniocentesis is offered if risk exceeds the usual threshold for doing amniocentesis (1 fetal loss in 270), which is about the same as when maternal age is greater than 35 years.

Triple screening can also detect risk of trisomy 18, indicated by low levels of all three serum markers. The sensitivity for trisomy 18 is 60–70%; the false-positive rate is about 0.5%. Combining ultrasonography and serum screening increases sensitivity to about 80%.

Ultrasound screening combined with serum analytes in the first trimester

The use of ultrasound for first-trimester screening for fetal Down syndrome and trisomy 18 has begun to gain wide acceptance in Europe and North America. The association of prominent nuchal translucency (NT) and increased risk for fetal chromosome abnormalities has been well documented;[29,30] however, it was Nicolaides and colleagues[31] who proposed the use of first-trimester nuchal measurement and first trimester maternal serum analytes in a screening paradigm for fetal Down syndrome. Among 1273 women carrying singleton pregnancies who were undergoing first-trimester CVS, a nuchal measurement of >3 mm could identify more than 85% of trisomy fetuses with a false-positive rate of approximately 5%.

Further studies have shown that the incorporation of two serum analytes, pregnancy-associated plasma protein A (PAPP-A) and free β-hCG, can improve the screening of pregnancies for Down syndrome and trisomy 18. A large multicenter trial[32] incorporating biochemical and ultrasound measurements showed a detection rate for Down syndrome of 79% at a positive screening rate of 5% and for trisomy 18 a detection rate of 91% at a positive screening rate of 2%. A recent study from the UK demonstrated a 93% detection rate for fetal Down syndrome at a positive screening rate of 5.9% and a 96% detection rate for all chromosome abnormalities at a 6.3% positive screening rate.[33]

The optimal protocol for fetal Down syndrome screening must take into account the obstetrical circumstances and preferences of the patient along with the available ultrasound and laboratory services. Ferguson-Smith[34] has summarized the possible options:

1. A combination of maternal serum markers and NT measurement at 11–13 weeks' gestation for women who want an early risk assessment (FPR of 2–6% for a DR of 85%).
2. A four-marker screening test at 15–19 weeks for women who first attend for prenatal care after 13 weeks (FPR of 6–10% for a DR of 85%).
3. An 'integrated' test in which (1) and (2) are combined and the result reported after (2), as a single risk incorporating all markers (FPR of 1–2% for a DR of 85%).

However, there continues to be considerable discussion concerning the optimal approach to integrating and reporting first- and second-trimester screening data. Women who choose prenatal screening must balance the advantages of an early risk assessment with a higher amniocentesis/CVS rate against a later result with a lower amniocentesis. The key is individualizing the needs of each patient. Regardless of the screening approach chosen, first-trimester screening provides improved detection rates compared to second-trimester screening; however, important clinical issues require further study and clarification before first-trimester screening becomes standard obstetrical care. According to the American College of Obstetricians and Gynecologists,[35] the following criteria are required to offer first-trimester screening as an option:

Special ultrasound training and an ongoing quality monitoring program (e.g., Fetal Maternal Foundation) are required to properly implement this screening program.

Sufficient information and resources are available to provide comprehensive counseling regarding the different screening options and limitations of these tests as well as to provide appropriate follow-up.

Access to an appropriate diagnostic test (e.g., CVS) is available when screening tests are positive and an invasive prenatal test is elected.

New first-trimester maternal serum markers continue to be investigated. One marker that holds promise is ADAM12-S, a pregnancy-associated metalloprotease, which has been shown to be markedly reduced in maternal serum during the first trimester in women carrying fetuses with Down syndrome and trisomy 18.[36, 37] In addition, first-trimester nuchal translucency measurements and maternal serum PAPP-A and free β-hCG have been used to identify pregnancies at increase risk for adverse obstetrical outcomes, including fetal loss, low birth weight, preeclampsia, gestational hypertension, preterm birth, and stillbirth.[38]

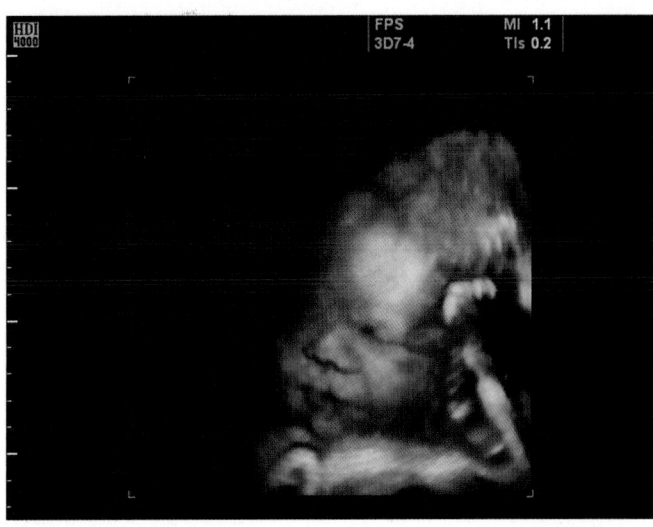

FIGURE 14.1 Ultrasound figure: 3-D ultrasound of a normal fetus at 30 weeks' gestation. (Courtesy of Leeber Cohen, M.D.)

Visualization techniques: advances through ultrasonography

Indications for ultrasonography during pregnancy are many and diverse and include estimation of gestational age by biometric measurements, estimation of fetal growth, bleeding from the vagina, determination of fetal growth, suspected multiple gestation, adjunct to an invasive procedure (e.g., CVS or amniocentesis), suspected uterine or adnexal abnormality, suspected fetal demise, and many others. In the context of prenatal diagnosis, many major, and even some minor, fetal structural anomalies can now be reliably detected. It is unrealistic, however, to expect 100% accuracy in detecting fetal anomalies, even with the most expert and thorough scanning. Some anomalies are more readily diagnosed than others. For example, anencephaly and marked hydrocephaly are rarely misdiagnosed, whereas others are more difficult to diagnose and may be overlooked, such as heart defects, facial clefts, diaphragmatic hernias, skeletal abnormalities, and neural tube detects.[39]

Although there is no question that high-resolution ultrasonography is invaluable in detecting fetal anomalies, accuracy of diagnosis will vary depending on the experience of the sonographer, as well as on equipment, gestational age at time of scanning, and the a priori risk of the abnormality in question. As such, the limitations of diagnostic ultrasonography must be recognized. It is inappropriate for a given clinical program to make any claims about diagnostic accuracy unless their own experience has been analyzed critically. However, the excellent imaging capability of high-resolution ultrasonography, as illustrated by Figure 14.1, will continue to improve diagnostic accuracy.

Controversy persists as to whether ultrasound monitoring of all obstetric patients should be routine to screen for fetal structural anomalies. These issues have been addressed in a report from the NICHD-sponsored Routine Antenatal Diagnostic Imaging with Ultrasound (RADIUS) study.[40] Low-risk pregnant women with no indication for ultrasonography were randomly assigned to have either two screening sonograms (15–22 weeks and 31–35 weeks) or conventional obstetric care with ultrasonography used only on a selective basis as determined by the clinical judgment of the patient's physician. Major congenital anomalies occurred in 2.3% of the 15 281 fetuses and infants. Antenatal ultrasonography detected 35% of the anomalous fetuses in the screened group versus only 11% of the control population (relative detection rate 3.1; 95% CI 2.0–5.1). Surprisingly, ultrasonography did not significantly influence the management or outcome of pregnancies complicated by fetuses with congenital malformations. Moreover, ultrasonography screening had no significant impact on survival rates among infants with potentially treatable, life-threatening anomalies despite the opportunity to take precautionary measures such as delivery at a tertiary center. The RADIUS study also provided some insight into the content and limitations of obstetric ultrasound examinations. For example, a four-chamber view of the heart permitted detection of only 43% of fetuses with complex heart disease, and only 30% of fetuses with cleft lip and palate were detected. Finally, it was estimated that a public health policy of routine ultrasonographic screening would increase US health care costs by at least US$500 million. This study concluded that 'given this extraordinary cost and the lack of measurable benefit, ultrasonographic screening for fetal anomaly detection cannot be justified.'

Many groups and centers have reevaluated the RADIUS findings as well as their own experience and have come to the opposite conclusion. DeVore[41] reported that the RADIUS study demonstrated that second-trimester ultrasonography could be provided in a cost-effective fashion to low-risk women. The Eurofetus Study[42] combined the ultrasound and clinical outcomes of 61 European centers over a 3-year period and found that systematic ultrasound during pregnancy detected a large proportion of fetal malformations.

Providing ultrasonographic services to all women regardless of risk will continue to be a contentious issue. More research is needed on the potential added value and cost effectiveness.

Preimplantation genetic diagnosis

Preimplantation genetic diagnosis (PGD) is an attractive newer addition to the prenatal diagnostic armamentarium.[43, 44] Many couples choose PGD rather than traditional prenatal genetic diagnostic approaches for assessing mendelian disorders, aneuploidy, or chromosomal imbalance. Unlike early amniocentesis, chorionic villus sampling, and other invasive techniques, PGD is not just an earlier option for prenatal diagnosis. It allows genetic diagnosis prior to the establishment of a pregnancy, a preconceptional approach that has unique advantages. Moreover, potential application of PGD extends beyond traditional prenatal genetic diagnosis and improved pregnancy rates in assisted reproductive technology (ART).

A successful preimplantation genetics diagnostic program requires: (1) high-quality ART, (2) micromanipulation skills sufficient to obtain a specimen (polar body or blastomere) for analysis, and (3) molecular technology more sophisticated than that required for traditional prenatal diagnosis. Preimplantation genetic diagnosis requires access to gametes (oocyte) or embryos before 6 days post conception, the time when implantation occurs. There are three potential approaches: (1) polar body biopsy, (2) blastomere biopsy or aspiration of 1 or 2 blastomeres from the 6–8 cell embryos (2–3 days), and (3) trophectoderm biopsy from the 5- to 6-day blastocyst.

Blastomere (6–8 cells) biopsy

Biopsy at this stage was the first technique developed. The approach is to aspirate 1 or 2 of the 6–8 cells contained within the zona pellucida. This can be accomplished by mechanical (razor) or chemical (pronase, EDTA) dissociation of the zona pellucida, followed by aspiration with a second pipette.

Polar body biopsy

A second general approach is to remove either the first or second polar biopsy, or both. Polar body biopsy (PBB) is technically similar to blastomere biopsy, but the embryo is not entered per se. Literally, this constitutes preconceptional diagnosis, as opposed to preimplantation diagnosis per se. Suppose a woman and her mate were both heterozygous for the same autosomal recessive disorder. A first polar body having the mutant allele should be complemented by a primary oocyte presumed to have the normal allele. The normal oocyte could thus be allowed to fertilize in vitro and then be transferred for potential implantation. Conversely, if the first polar body were normal, fertilization would not be allowed to proceed because the oocyte would contain the mutant allele. The same reasoning would apply for detecting of aneuploidy. A polar body containing only one chromosome 21 (as determined by fluorescent in situ hybridization with a chromosome-specific probe) should be complemented by a primary oocyte also containing a single number 21 chromosome. If the first polar body failed to show a 21, the oocyte can be presumed to have two number 21 chromosomes, which would lead to a trisomic zygote.

Disadvantages include inability to assess the paternal genotype, precluding application if a father has an autosomal dominant disorder. Lacking information about paternal transmission also results in reproductive inefficiencies. Presence of a mutant autosomal recessive allele in the second polar body precludes allowing that oocyte to be fertilized, whereas in reality the embryo resulting from fertilization of that oocyte would be affected only if the sperm also contained the father's mutant allele. If it were known that the father's normal allele were transmitted, the embryo would be heterozygous and phenotypically normal.

Another disadvantage is recombination, the meiotic phenomenon that occurs routinely between homologous chromosomes. Diagnostic hazards resulting from recombination are a greater problem for genes located nearer the telomeres because these genes display recombination frequencies approximating 50%.

Blastocyst (trophectoderm) biopsy

An underlying difficulty when aspirating either the polar body or a blastomere from the 6–8 cell embryo is that diagnosis must depend upon only a single cell, or occasionally two. Many more cells would be available if one biopsied the 5- to 6-day blastocyst, which contains hundreds of cells. The strategy is to biopsy the trophectoderm overlying the anembryonic pole. One major problem is that blastocysts are less readily obtainable as 6–8 cell embryos. Blastocysts can be obtained by culture in vitro, but this process has traditionally proved very inefficient. After 3–4 days in vitro, embryonic development is not sustained efficiently to the blastocyst stage.

Cytogenetic analysis in preimplantation genetic diagnosis would clearly be useful for a variety of reasons. Sex determination (XX or XY) may be desirable for couples at risk for X-linked recessive disorders in which an exact diagnosis is not possible. Aneuploidy, translocations, or other chromosomal rearrangement could be excluded. Cytogenetic methodologies are well established in traditional prenatal genetic diagnosis (CVS, amniocentesis); however, accuracy is more an issue in PGD because of the inherent limitation of analyzing only one or two cells.

In PGD, diagnosis may depend upon information from a single cell. There is little margin for error. Metaphase analysis is possible for only a single cell, but this is not optimal. Other approaches to determine chromosomal status include comparative genome hybridization (CGH).[45] The preferable approach for chromosomal analysis in PGD involves fluorescence in situ hybridization (FISH) with chromosome-specific probes. FISH is a molecular genetic technique based on analysis of DNA sequences that are chromosome specific. Chromosome-specific probes can hybridize to denatured DNA, in either metaphase or interphase. In interphase cells the number of FISH signals should equal the number of a given chromosome. Using a chromosome 21-specific probe would detect trisomy 21 if three signals were visualized in the nucleus. Simultaneous use of probes for more than one chromosome is possible using different colored fluorochromes, as illustrated in Figure 14.2. This approach is also well suited for sex determination, X and Y probes being utilized concurrently. A diagnostic dilemma unique to PGD is the very high frequency of mosaicism in the early embryos.

Molecular analysis of a single cell requires techniques more sensitive than those necessary for analyzing chorionic villi or amniotic fluid cells. The small amount of DNA in one cell (6 pg), is insufficient for conventional multi-cell molecular diagnostic approaches. In traditional polymerase chain reaction (PCR) methods, a targeted DNA sequence flanked by specific primers is amplified to increase numbers of copies, usually 10^5 to 10^6 fold. Amplification from a single cell using a single set of primers is successful if a repetitive DNA sequence is being evaluated (e.g., Y-chromosome). However, technical modifications are necessary

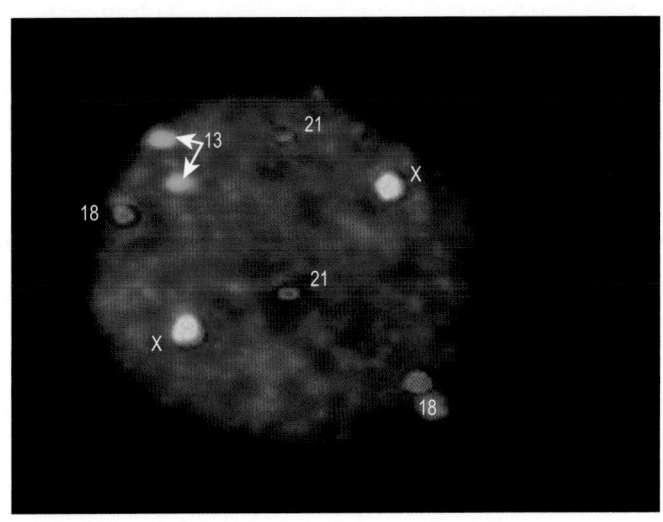

FIGURE 14.2 FISH: multicolor fluorescent in situ hybridization on human blastomeres for preimplantation genetic diagnosis. (Courtesy of Ferideh Bischoff, Ph.D.)

when analyzing unique sequence mutations because sensitivity for detecting unique sequence DNA cannot be readily achieved below approximately 100 pg DNA. Rather than a single round of PCR (20–30 cycles), nested primers are required. The second set of primers is constructed internal to the first. Following approximately 20 cycles of PCR with the outer primers, the product is subjected to PCR with a second (internal) set of primers. Using nested PCR, as little as 1 pg of DNA suffices for diagnosis.

The list of mendelian disorders for which PGD has been clinically used has grown rapidly in recent years. These include cystic fibrosis (ΔF508 homozygosity), Tay-Sachs disease, Rh (D), sickle cell anemia, certain β-thalassemias, phenylketonuria, spinal muscular atrophy and myotonic dystrophy, and adenosis polyposis coli and Li-Fraumeni syndrome. Of special note is that PGD has been accomplished for a variety of adult-onset autosomal dominant disorders, including Huntington disease and Marfan syndrome. Any mendelian disorder whose gene is localized or whose molecular basis is known is potentially detectable by linkage analysis if not otherwise.

Genetic conditions of special concern and prenatal identification

Within the context of this chapter, **prenatal diagnosis** is defined as a process that rules out or detects and manages embryonic and fetal abnormalities or disease and that provides information to parents and physicians to optimize both pregnancy outcome and family well-being. Although prenatally diagnosable disorders may be categorized in many ways, it is simplest to consider only two groups of couples or families who may benefit from prenatal testing. Theoretically, the two groups encompass all types of embryonic or fetal disorders that may be amenable to prenatal testing or management.

The first are those patients who themselves, or whose physicians, are (or theoretically can be) aware **before conception** of a known risk for fetal abnormality or unfavorable pregnancy outcome. This is the group of families in whose medical, family, or personal history there are known factors that might result in prenatally detectable or even preventable fetal disorders. They might include families of increased parental age, those with previous infants with chromosomal abnormalities or other genetically determined disorders, or families of specific ethnic origin that might increase their risk for abnormal pregnancy outcome.

The second are those who **during pregnancy**, without previously recognizable known risk factors, have an unexpected risk of fetal abnormality or potential for unfavorable outcome identified. Examples include those in whom a routine blood test or prenatal ultrasound reveals an unexpected abnormal finding.

Couples at recognizable risk before conception

Indications for prenatal testing can be divided into several categories. The most common is the need for fetal or, more recently, embryonic karyotyping. Consequently, basic cytogenetic principles are summarized below prior to reviewing the genetic conditions and how they can be diagnosed.

Basic cytogenetic principles and chromosomal abnormalities

Chromosomal abnormalities are not uncommon. They occur in about two-thirds of early spontaneously aborted pregnancies[46–48] (trisomy 16, monosomy X, and triploidy are the most common) and in 5.6–6% of stillborn infants (20 weeks or older). This has been confirmed by findings among the more than 1000 infants evaluated to date by the Wisconsin Stillbirth Service Program (WiSSP).[49] Even among the 0.6% liveborn infants with chromosomal abnormalities,[50] those with trisomies 13 and 18 rarely survive beyond the first weeks or months of life.

Chromosomal abnormalities can be divided into those that affect the number and those that affect the structure of chromosomes. Ultrasound markers for fetal chromosome abnormalities have been published.[46]

Numerical Abnormalities Numerical abnormalities result in a change in the total number of chromosomes per cell. They account for a little more than half of the 0.6% of chromosomal abnormalities in live births.

TRISOMY. The most frequent numerical abnormality is trisomy, in which three copies of a given chromosome exist instead of two, resulting in a total of 47 chromosomes per cell.

The most frequent cause of trisomy is a phenomenon known as non-disjunction; instead of the separation of a pair of

chromatids to opposite poles of the cell during anaphase, they migrate to the same pole. This occurs in maternal meiosis I and II and paternal meiosis I and II, in decreasing order of frequency. Approximately 10–15% of supernumerary chromosomes resulting from non-disjunctional events are of paternal origin.[52] They are usually present in offspring of younger parents, as opposed to maternal non-disjunction, which tends to occur more frequently (but not always) during gametogenesis of women older than 35 years (the maternal age effect). The most frequent complete (i.e., involving a whole additional chromosome) autosomal trisomies in liveborn infants are trisomies 21, 18, and 13. Trisomy 16 and other rarer autosomal trisomies are infrequently seen in spontaneous abortions but never in liveborns. The most frequent sex chromosomal trisomies are 47,XXY, 47,XXX, and 47,XYY, all occurring in less than 1 in 1000 live births.

MONOSOMY. Monosomy means that only one of a given chromosome pair is present instead of two. The only monosomy known in humans that is compatible with life is monosomy X, the most common chromosomal complement associated with Turner syndrome. It is written as 45,X and occurs, not as a result of nodisjunction like trisomies, but during a meiotic process known as anaphase lag. Even in this unique situation, most conceptions with a missing X chromosome are aborted spontaneously, under rather specific circumstances, while 4–6% are liveborn with the characteristic clinical picture of girls and women with Turner syndrome.[53]

PARTIAL MONOSOMY OR TRISOMY. Partial monosomy and partial trisomy are more common. They usually involve loss or gain of part of a short, p, or long arm of a chromosome. For example, a male patient with additional material from the short arms of chromosome 9 may have a characteristic phenotype, and his chromosome complement would be written 46,XY,9p+. If an entire additional chromosome is present or missing the plus or minus sign is written *before* the number of the chromosome in question – e.g., 47,XX,+13. If a partial abnormality is present, the sign is written *after* the chromosome number and arm designation – e.g., 46,XY,5p– (missing portion of the short arm of 5). The nomenclature that describes a specific abnormality of a portion of the chromosome uses the banding patterns. Prominent bands, acquired technically through trypsin digestion and various types of staining, are called regions; they are numbered consecutively starting from the centromere up on the short arm (p), down on the long arm (q). Smaller bands within the larger ones are numbered similarly. Thus, if the terminal band of the long arm of chromosome 14 is missing, the designation would be 46,XX or XY, 14q32.3– or 46,XX or XY, del(14)(q32.3).

TRIPLOIDY (TETRAPLOIDY). Triploidy and tetraploidy (69 or 92 chromosomes per cell) rarely exist in viable humans. Triploidy, however, is one of the three most common findings in spontaneous abortions (along with trisomy 16 and monosomy X). Triploidy is usually associated with a partial hydatidiform mole. It may arise as the result of one of four phenomena, which include a tetraploid spermatogonium or oogonium, an error in first or second meiotic division, or a result of dispermy (fertilization with two spermatozoa).

MOSAICISM. Non-disjunction also can occur postmitotically and result in mosaicism. This means that at least two cell lines are present, the original one, derived from the zygote, and the second, derived after the non-disjunctional event. The degree of mosaicism depends on the percentage of cells and the number of tissues in which it is present. It may be written as follows: 46,XY (50%)/47,XY,+21. Whenever mosaicism is suspected, it is essential to evaluate as many tissues as possible, because it is the predominant cell line, and probably the tissues in which it occurs (e.g., the brain), that are clinically and phenotypically significant. Chromosome mosaicism for autosomal trisomies is relatively rare; it is much more frequent in sex chromosomal abnormalities. The phenomenon of confined placental mosaicism, discovered relatively recently with the advent of chorionic villus sampling (CVS), is mentioned in the section on techniques used in prenatal diagnosis, and is discussed in Chapter 5.

Structural Abnormalities Structural chromosomal rearrangements, which occur in about 1 in 500 live births, are among the most challenging situations. Except for the short arms of the acrocentric chromosome, no matter what the arrangement or rearrangement of chromosomal material, none must be missing or additionally present for an individual to be *un*affected. There must be a complete set of the material of 46 chromosomes within the cells; that is, the chromosomal complement must be balanced. If material is missing or additionally present, the chromosomal complement is unbalanced and results in phenotypic effects. However, the opposite does not apply. While an individual with abnormal amounts of chromosomal material almost always is affected, someone with completely normal chromosomes is not necessarily genetically perfectly healthy and normal. Most genetic disorders do not result from an imbalance in chromosomal material; hence, not all (in fact very few) pathologic processes are detectable through a structural abnormality of the chromosomes. There are two basic types of structural rearrangements or translocations: robertsonian and reciprocal. Each can be either inherited (familial) or occur de novo for the first time in an individual.

ROBERTSONIAN TRANSLOCATIONS. Robertsonian translocations result in the centric fusion (with usually one centromere or two, with one inactivated) of two arms of chromosomes, involving most frequently the acrocentric (number 13, 14, 15, 21 and 22) chromosomes. The most common are 13;14 and 14;21. A robertsonian translocation may be balanced, with no phenotypic or clinical effects except reproductive risks associated with the birth of an infant with an unbalanced karyotype. It also may be unbalanced, in which case trisomy or monosomy of one of the fused chromosomes usually results. Figure 14.3 shows that if a parent is a healthy (e.g., 14;21) translocation carrier, theoretically six possible types of gametes and zygotes can be formed. They are normal (Fig. 14.3, A1), balanced 14;21 translocation carriers (like parent) (Fig. 14.3, A2), trisomy 21 (Fig. 14.3, B3), monosomy 21 (Fig. 14.3, B4), trisomy 14 (Fig. 14.3, C5), and monosomy 14

(Fig. 14.3, C6). Of these, the first three instances can result in a viable infant, of which two will be normal, and one will have Down syndrome (DS) from an unbalanced 14;21 translocation. Phenotypically, patients with this type of DS, while microscopically different, are like every other patient with DS caused by the effects of an additional chromosome 21. The remaining three gametes resulting in monosomy 21, trisomy, and monosomy 14 are not compatible with life and may be spontaneously aborted. Hence, the risk for a parent who is a balanced 14;21 translocation carrier is theoretically 50% for a viable infant, one-third of which (about 15%) could result in DS and 50% spontaneous miscarriage. The couple's risk for having a child with DS (since that is the only viable possibility for an affected child) is theoretically 33% if the fetus goes to term. Note that a balanced translocation carrier father's karyotype is written as 45,XY,−14,−21, +t(14q;21q), where 45 is the total number of chromosomes (including XY), a normal 14 and 21 is missing and replaced by the translocated chromosomes. His DS son's karyotype is written as 46,XY,−14, t(14q;21q).

The practical situation is, fortunately, very different from what would be expected from segregation analysis. Statistical studies have shown more favorable empirical risks. If the parental carrier is the mother, her risk for translocation DS in her offspring is about 11%; if the carrier is the father, his risk is around 2.4%.

Similar situations apply to other robertsonian translocations (e.g., 13;14), in which the chance of normal (or balanced carrier) offspring is usually greater than would be expected theoretically. However, if a balanced translocation carrier is identified within a family, usually through the birth of a malformed infant with an unbalanced karyotype, it is imperative that other family members be evaluated, their chromosomes analyzed, information and supportive genetic counseling provided, and prenatal diagnosis offered as applicable. One of the few situations in medical genetics in which there is a 100% risk for an abnormal outcome is in the presence of a homologous robertsonian translocation, such as that in a balanced 21;21 translocation carrier. Unless such a carrier is mosaic for the translocation and has some cells (gonadal or other) with the normal chromosomal complement, the resulting zygotes will be either trisomic or monosomic for chromosome 21 and result in an abnormal pregnancy outcome. This type of translocation (if balanced) cannot be inherited from a normal parent, unless that parent is mosaic for the translocation; if it were (inherited), the carrier would be trisomic for chromosome 21. Therefore, no one else in the family is at risk for carrying or transmitting such a translocation. If balanced, it is always a de novo event. Prenatal diagnosis in this situation will reveal either a monosomic or trisomic fetus. On the other hand, recurrence risks for a couple that has had an infant with aneuploidy resulting from a spontaneous, noninherited, or de novo robertsonian translocation are empirically comparable to the recurrence risks for a non-disjunctional event, about 1–2% or less. Prenatal diagnosis is indicated in all such situations during a subsequent pregnancy.

RECIPROCAL TRANSLOCATIONS. If chromosomes from two different pairs exchange segments without loss or addition of

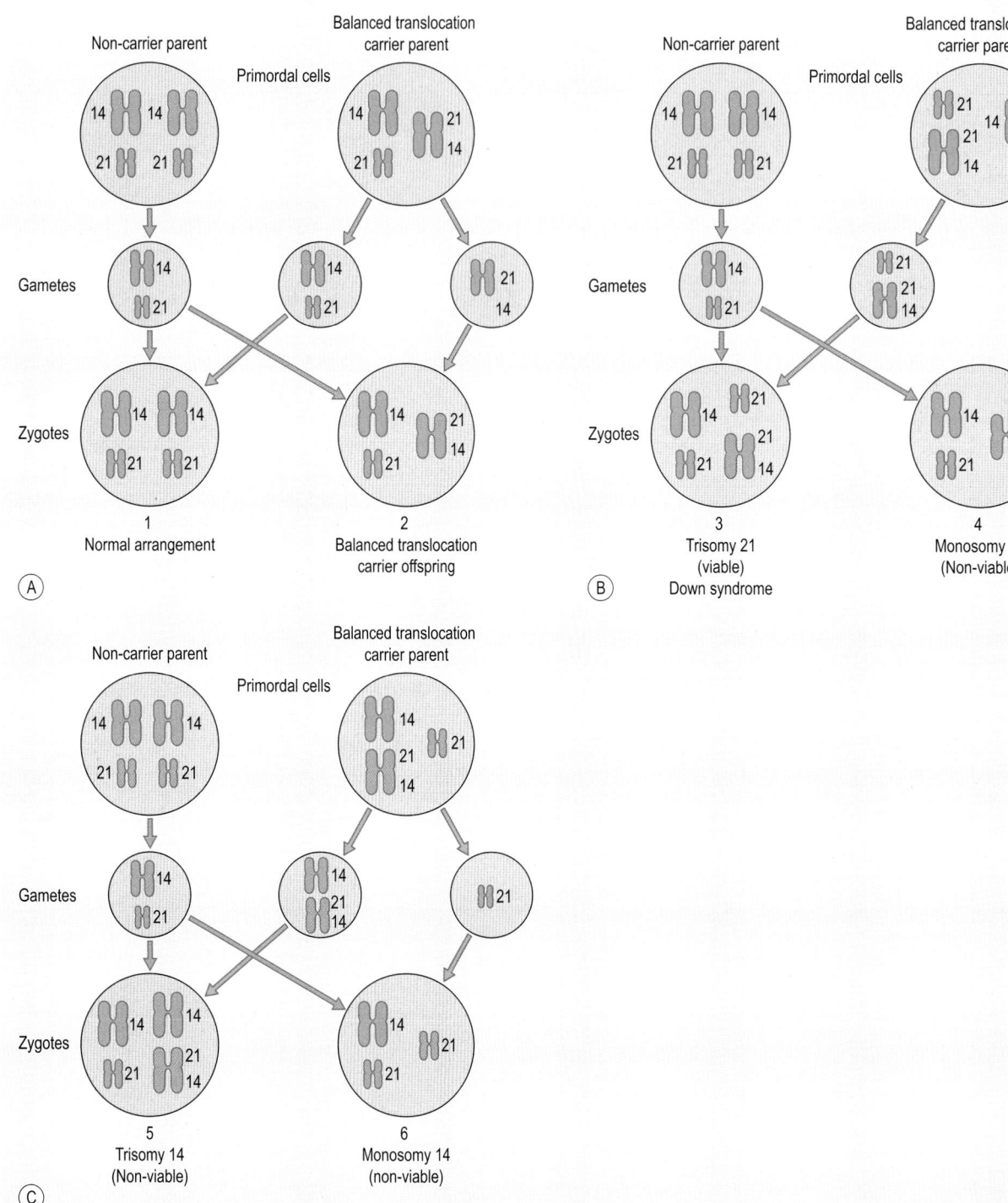

FIGURE 14.3 Diagrammatic transmission of a 14; 21 translocation.

chromosomal material, the phenomenon is known as a balanced reciprocal translocation. During gametogenesis, there are four possibilities (Fig. 14.4): a normal chromosomal complement (Fig. 14.4, 1); a balanced rearrangement, as in the parent carrier (Fig. 14.4, 2); too much of one chromosome (partial trisomy) and too little of the other (partial monosomy) (Fig. 14.4, 3); or too little of one and too much of the other (Fig. 14.4, 4). Once a couple has had an infant with an unbalanced karyotype resulting from a parental reciprocal translocation, theoretically they have a 50% risk for another pregnancy resulting in an unbalanced (one or

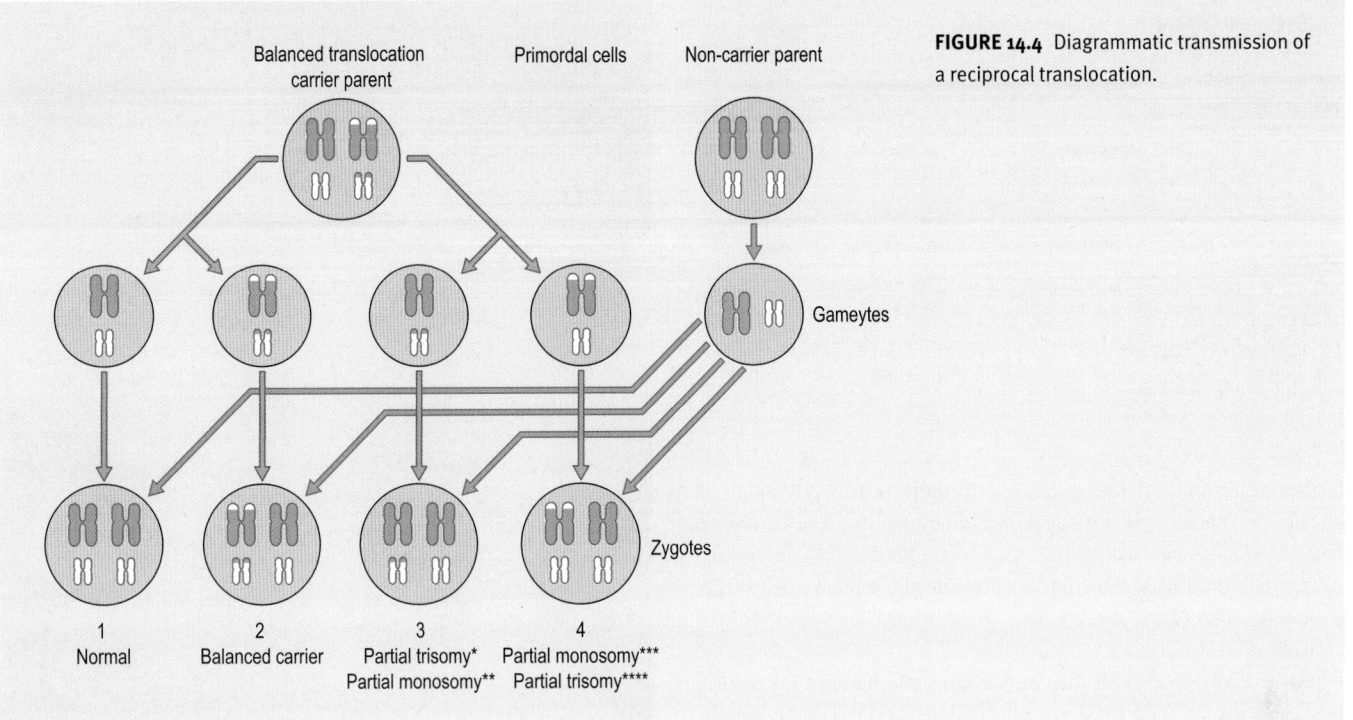

Balanced translocation carrier parent | Primordal cells | Non-carrier parent

FIGURE 14.4 Diagrammatic transmission of a reciprocal translocation.

Gameytes

Zygotes

1 Normal

2 Balanced carrier

3 Partial trisomy* Partial monosomy**

4 Partial monosomy*** Partial trisomy****

the other) karyotype. Practically, little is known about the actual risks for specific translocations because they are individually rare and involve so many different segments of different chromosomes. It is recommended in counseling a couple in which one partner is a known carrier of a reciprocal translocation that general principles be explained but that current information be sought on the specific translocation in question. Prenatal diagnosis is strongly indicated in all instances of translocation, and family studies are recommended.

CHROMOSOME BREAKS. Chromosome breaks, resulting in deletions, and therefore in the loss of genetic material, are usually associated with phenotypic manifestations. Deletions, the phenotypic effects of which are known and recognizable, include 46,XX or XY 5p−, or cri-du-chat syndrome; 46,XX or XY 4p−, or Wolf-Hirschhorn syndrome; 46,XX or XY 18p−, 18q−; 17p− (Miller-Dieker syndrome if the deletion is terminal, namely, 17p13.3, or Smith-Magenis syndrome if it is 17p11.2).[54,55] Unless caused by a parental reciprocal translocation, deletions in a previous infant usually are not associated with an increased risk for recurrence, although prenatal diagnosis usually is offered for reassurance. Balanced inversions and duplications of chromosomal material also may be encountered. The former are usually without phenotypic effect. Duplications, on the other hand, are often associated with deleterious phenotypic effects, although they depend on the specific segment in question (e.g., euchromatin vs heterochromatin).

Any type of chromosomal rearrangement, however balanced it appears cytogenetically, can result in deletion or disruption of (a) gene(s), and have deleterious effects. For example, constitutional loss of a tumor suppressor gene (e.g. translocations involving chromosomal segment 13q14 which disrupts the Rb gene of retinoblastoma) can result in cancer.[56]

Cytogenetic indications for prenatal diagnosis

Families at risk of having an infant with a chromosomal abnormality can be divided into the following groups: (1) those associated with increased parental age; (2) those who have had a previous child with a de novo or inherited chromosomal abnormality; and (3) those in which one of the parents is a carrier of a balanced translocation.

Parental Age Mothers aged 35 years or older are at increased risk for having an infant with an additional chromosome as a result of a non-disjunctional event. The risks for such an event are given in Table 14.1 and are compared with the proportion of DS births. Despite the validity of the maternal age effect, most infants with additional chromosomes are born to women younger than 35 years. The reason is that only about 6% of all pregnancies are in women aged 35 or older; approximately 5% are between ages 35 and 39, and 1% are 40 or older. This proportion of pregnancies (6%) results in about 28%, 30%, and 32% of all infants with DS, trisomy 18, and Klinefelter's syndrome, respectively. The remaining 94% of women younger than age 35 give birth, respectively, to 72%, 70%, and 68% of infants with the above syndromes. Half the specific age-related risk is for trisomy 21; the remaining half is for any other non-disjunctional event.

The effect of increased paternal age is more controversial. The risk for dominant mutations in offspring of older fathers is

TABLE 14.1 CHROMOSOMAL ABNORMALITIES DETECTED DURING SECOND TRIMESTER AMNIOCENTESIS IN 17 859 WOMEN AGED 35 OR OVER

Age	All chromosome abnormalities detected		Trisomy 21 only	
	No.	Percent	No.	Percent
35–39	148	1.54	76	0.79
40	305	3.99	185	2.42
Total	453	≈2.5	261	≈1.5

Adapted from Milunsky A, ed. Genetics disorders and the fetus. Plenum; 1979:97; with permission.

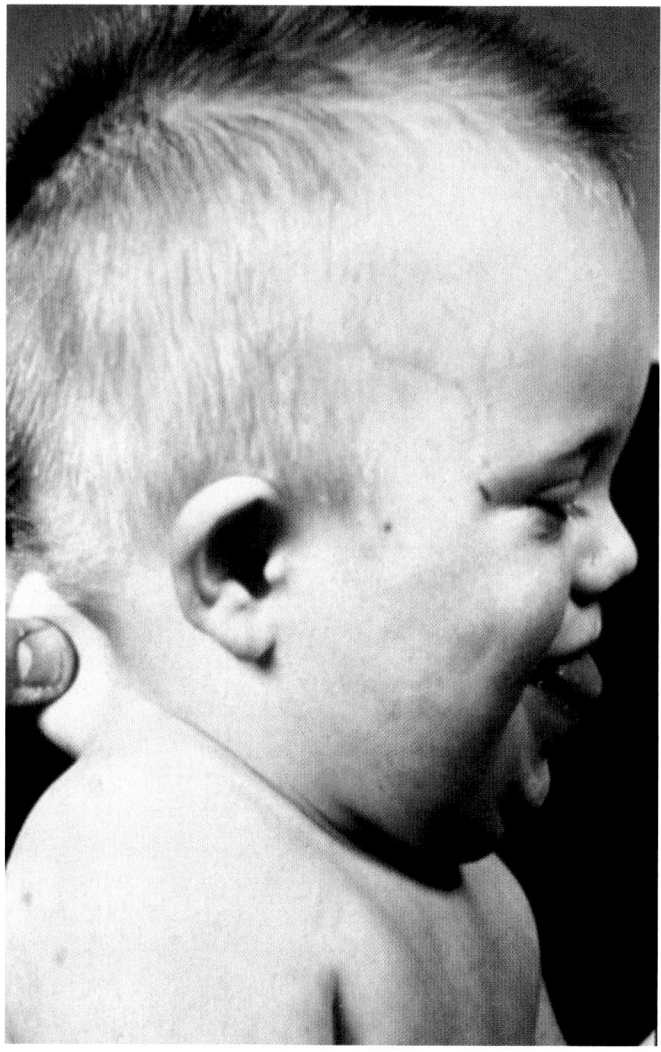

FIGURE 14.5 Phenotypic appearance of a child with Down syndrome caused by trisomy 21.

higher than that in the general population, and, although it should be mentioned during prenatal counseling to a couple at risk, there is no technique that can prenatally detect an otherwise undefined dominant mutation in the fetus, unless it is a severe structural abnormality that might be detected on routine ultrasound.

At the other end of the spectrum, pregnancies in young teenagers are at higher risk for prematurity and low birth weight infants. There is weak evidence that age alone predisposes teenaged mothers to a higher risk than the general population for infants with non-disjunctional events.

DOWN SYNDROME. Trisomy 21 is the most common of all age-related chromosomal abnormalities, constituting about half the overall maternal age-related risk; at ages 35, 40, and 45 it is about 1 in 270, 1 in 135, and 1 in 50, respectively. The other half of the maternal age-related risk is, as previously mentioned, cumulatively for other autosomal (18, 13) and sex chromosomal (XXY, XXX) trisomies.

The cytogenetic prenatal diagnosis of these abnormalities, through CVS, usually performed between 10 and 12 weeks, or amniocentesis between 14 and 16 weeks of gestation, is relatively straightforward, accurate, and unequivocal.

Numerical chromosomal abnormalities by definition are often associated with multiple congenital malformations. They are mentioned briefly in the following material. DS, or trisomy 21, is among the most common and best-known forms of developmental delay in children, occurring in 1 in 700 to 1000 live births. It is always associated with an additional number 21 chromosome (i.e., with complete [or partial] trisomy 21), irrespective of whether it arises through non-disjunction or a familial or de novo translocation rearrangement.

The postnatal phenotypic appearance of mature infants and children with DS is well known (Fig. 14.5). Prenatally, however, the phenotype is much more subtle; several clues may suggest the diagnosis, even if the conclusive cytogenetic finding of 47,XX or XY 21 is unavailable. Clues may be detected from several ultrasonographic signs (in utero), externally (after early pregnancy termination or delivery), or internally (on autopsy). On ultrasound, the fetus is usually proportionately mildly growth retarded.[57] Although this is neither a specific nor an unequivocal sign, proportionate or disproportionate intrauterine growth

retardation (IUGR), if accurately measured and coordinated with accurate estimates of gestational age, is always a somewhat alarming sign that should be factored into the differential diagnosis before completion of chromosome analysis or if the latter is unavailable. A cystic hygroma of the neck or at least thickening of the neck in the nuchal area (Fig. 14.6) may also be suggestive of trisomy 21 (or another chromosomal abnormality) and is in itself an indication for chromosome analysis. A flat facial profile is less easily detectable, unless the ultrasonographer is highly experienced. The presence of a double bubble, indicating duodenal obstruction or atresia, may be highly suggestive of trisomy 21; 20% of infants with trisomy 21 are born with gastrointestinal obstructions. The most common group of congenital malformations, known to be present in 40–50% of fetuses and infants with DS, are congenital heart defects, the more severe of which (e.g., endocardial cushion defect) are reliably detectable on ultrasound by fetal echocardiography. Apart from possibly small palpebral fissures (by objective

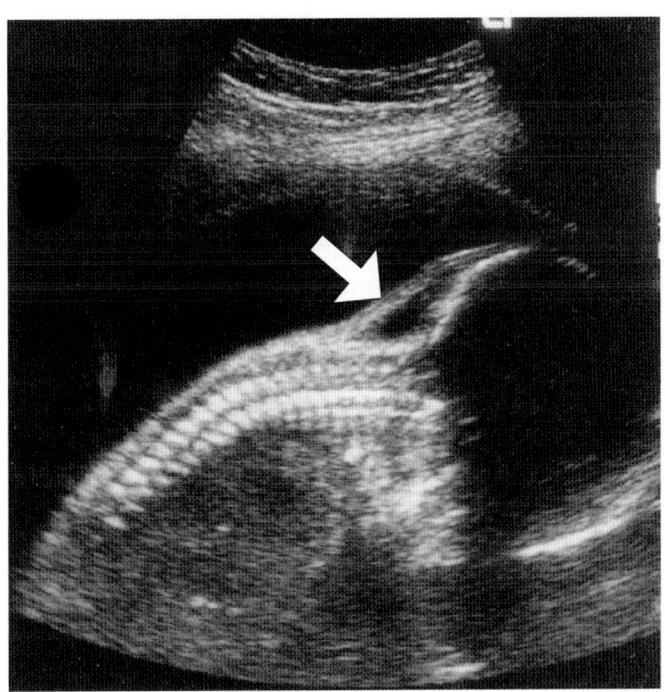

FIGURE 14.6 Nuchal thickening in a fetus at 18 weeks' gestation subsequently found to have trisomy 21.

measurement and comparison with norms for gestational age) a somewhat 'beaky'-appearing nasal apex, possibly fifth clinodactyly and, occasionally, a four-finger palmar crease, there are few external physical features suggestive of fetal DS.

These comments and description apply equally to fetuses with non-disjunctional and those with translocational trisomy 21. No clinical or physical differences have been observed between the two groups, as long as the fetus has a whole additional long arm of chromosome 21.

Of all conceptions with trisomy 21, about 60% are lost spontaneously before birth. Thus, a proportion of those diagnosed prenatally may not result in a live birth, and theoretically this should be factored into parental decision-making. In addition, of all conceptions with trisomy 21, 94% have standard, non-inherited non-disjunctional trisomy 21, 4% have a robertsonian translocation (e.g., 14/21, 21/22), half of which (2% of the total) are inherited, and 2% occur de novo. The remaining 2% of infants with DS have mosaicism. In total, then, 98% of all infants with DS have a non-inherited type. Approximately one-third of these are born to mothers who are 35 years old or older and are therefore prenatally detectable. The remaining (about two-thirds) are born to younger mothers. Theoretically, a proportion of these is also detectable through screening tests.

TRISOMY 18. Trisomy 18 is the second most common maternal age-related non-disjunctional event (about 1 in 2000 to 3000 liveborn infants). It, too, is characterized by multiple malformations. Severe IUGR upon ultrasound is probably the most obvious sign. If observed together with an unusually configured hand with digits 2, 4, and 5 overlapping digit 3, and possibly a horseshoe or otherwise structurally abnormal kidney,

it may be almost pathognomonic for trisomy 18. A fetal echocardiogram may reveal severe congenital heart disease. After pregnancy termination or stillbirth, the infant, like that with trisomy 21, may not have an immediately recognizable characteristic appearance to the untrained observer. However, the hands, feet, and subsequently the autopsy usually leave little doubt about the diagnosis, even before or in the absence of the completion of chromosome analysis.

TRISOMY 13 (PATAU SYNDROME). With an incidence of about 1 in 5000 to 6000 liveborns, this is perhaps the most easily prenatally recognizable of the trisomies. No organ system has been spared in the complex picture, beginning with the central nervous system (CNS), in which holoprosencephaly or alobar holoprosencephaly is most typical, through proboscis, ocular and midline facial clefting malformations, severe congenital heart disease, kidney and limb malformations, postaxial polydactyly, neural tube and abdominal wall defects (AWDs), and others. All of these are easily recognizable on ultrasound scans, and with cytogenetic confirmation there is no doubt as to the diagnosis. A careful autopsy can also be almost unequivocally diagnostic.

Trisomy 18 or 13 has a grave prognosis. Approximately 92 and 94%, respectively, of children with trisomies 18 and 13 die within the first 6 months of life, most of them within days or weeks of birth, most of complex congenital heart disease and brain malformations. The few who survive are invariably severely mentally retarded, dysmorphic, and have complicated medical needs. It is essential, however, that even this apparently dismal prognosis be conveyed to the parents because those who decide to continue the pregnancy must be prepared for the chance, albeit slim, of their infant's postnatal survival.

It is difficult to predict, even postnatally, which of the children might survive. The severity of congenital heart disease and of the CNS malformations probably play a role, as may the sex of the infant, girls possibly surviving more frequently than boys.

SEX CHROMOSOMAL ABNORMALITIES. Sex chromosomal abnormalities resulting from non-disjunctional events are much less easily detected prenatally by techniques other than cytogenetic analysis. There are no phenotypic signs to provide clues on ultrasound or at delivery, nor is the autopsy particularly suggestive apart from possible indications on gonadal histology. The two more common maternal age-related sex chromosomal abnormalities are 47,XXY (Klinefelter syndrome) and 47,XXX (triple X syndrome).

KLINEFELTER SYNDROME. Some boys and men with Klinefelter syndrome have a recognizable, though subtle, physical phenotype. They may have mildly upslanting palpebral fissures, flared nostrils, and a somewhat square-shaped face. Klinefelter's syndrome patients may also show chronic pulmonary disease. Germ cell tumors of both gonadal and extragonadal origin occur with increased frequency. Gonadal tumors include Leydig cell neoplasia. Gynecomastia predisposes to breast carcinoma, which is 20–50 times more frequent than among normal males. In 47,XXY Klinefelter syndrome IQ is definitely lowered. Overt mental retardation is uncommon. The consensus is that IQ is decreased about 15 points. Treatment in Klinefelter syndrome is directed toward the androgen deficiency. Replacement can take the form of intramuscular testosterone injections or topical application of testosterone.

NON-INHERITED CHROMOSOMAL REARRANGEMENTS. A spontaneous non-disjunctional event resulting in trisomies 21, 18, and 13, sex chromosomal aneuploidy, and trisomies associated with a de novo robertsonian translocation all have an empirical recurrence risk of approximately 1%. It is possible that this overall, statistically derived number encompasses some situations in which the risk for recurrence is higher, as it must be, for example, if one member of a couple has gonadal mosaicism, or if there is a tendency toward non-disjunction within a family. Half the 1–2% risk for recurrence of a non-disjunctional event, such as that associated with increased maternal age, is for trisomy 21, and the remaining half for other trisomies. Cytogenetic prenatal diagnosis should be offered to all such families.

Non-inherited reciprocal translocations are not known to be associated with an increased recurrence risk; they result from breaks rather than from non-disjunctional events and are not likely to recur. Similarly, de novo interstitial deletions would not be expected to recur in subsequent pregnancies. Thus, fetal karyotyping, although usually offered, is not as strongly indicated during subsequent pregnancies, because the outlook is no less favorable than that in the general population.

Occasionally, the detection of an unexpected cytogenetic finding that is completely different from and unrelated to the basic indication for fetal or embryonic chromosome analysis raises difficult technical and ethical issues. Examples of such chance findings might include a de novo rearrangement, deletion, or duplication; counseling in these instances is extremely difficult and filled with anguish and ambiguity. The question of whether a seemingly balanced de novo reciprocal translocation is truly balanced and without phenotypic effect can never be answered with certainty. Even more difficult is the question of the nature of the phenotypic effects, if any, because the rearrangements seen in most reciprocal translocations are individually rare, sometimes unique, and have little precedent in the literature. Information as to an identical occurrence and its outcome is rarely available, and empirical risks that are non-specific and unsatisfactory have to be used. A detailed anomaly scan with ultrasound can rule out severe abnormalities of anatomy or growth but is by no means completely reassuring as to the absence of mental retardation or other future problems. Empirically, the risk of abnormality in a de novo reciprocal, seemingly balanced translocation is 6–10%.

Furthermore, the finding of an unexpected deletion or duplication in the chromosomes of a fetus whose karyotype was evaluated for different reasons can also be painful and difficult for the parents and the geneticist. The parents' question of the significance of the finding can rarely be answered with accuracy. If the deletion (duplication) is on a chromosome site that is not associated with a known clinical picture, it is probably rare (even unique) and unlikely to have been clearly and unequivocally delineated in the literature in association with specific clinical manifestations. Also, if it has been reported,

the chromosomal segments involved, while similar, usually differ in size. Even a series of reported patients with a duplication of part of 4q, for example, will have different clinical manifestations, sometimes correlated to the size of the segment.[58]

MOLECULAR CYTOGENETICS. In recent years exciting advances have resulted from merging molecular techniques with traditional cytogenetics leading to the new field of molecular cytogenetics. The basic principle is first identifying a DNA sequence specific for a given chromosome and then rendering the sequence fluorescent for cytologic identification. With in situ hybridization (ISH) or fluorescent in situ hybridization (FISH), a single-stranded DNA probe will hybridize to its complementary DNA sequence (if the latter is present). The DNA probe may be labeled directly with a fluorochrome or labeled indirectly. If labeled indirectly, another compound (e.g., biotin) is attached to the probe, and it is this compound that is capable of conjugating with a fluorochrome. If the probe is directly labeled, the fluore intercalates into the DNA. Irrespective, FISH can be used to derive information from interphase cells (e.g., uncultured amniotic fluid cells).

Chromosome-specific probes can be used to determine chromosomal status of interphase nuclei. Using different fluorochromes allows simultaneous analysis of more than one chromosome in a given interphase cell. At least three is routine and five is readily possible. In addition, more than 3 or 5 different chromosomes can be assessed at once. Rehybridization is especially applicable for preimplantation genetic diagnosis to exclude aneuploidy.

Mixing varying proportions of the limited number of primary fluorescent colors (fluores) can produce enough distinct colors to allow identification of all 22 autosomes and the sex chromosomes (X,Y). This is termed spectral karyotyping (SKY) The fluorochromes used can be non-isotopic. This technique is especially useful for identifying rearrangements not easily recognizable on high-resolution karyotypes. The principle is that an unexpected color on a given chromosome would indicate a previously unsuspected excess of DNA. Cancer cytogeneticists find spectral karyotyping especially useful.

The availability of sequence-specific DNA probes which can be amplified by PCR and tagged with fluorochrome reporter molecules has bridged the gap between microscope and molecule. Probes can be constructed enabling hybridization of specific chromosomal regions, or even of a single gene.

In chromosomal painting, composite probes can be coupled with suppressive hybridization to allow selected whole chromosomes or chromosomal segments to be 'painted' and uniquely visualized. This technique can be used if more easily subtle rearrangements or deletions exist.

A variant of this technique is comparative genome hybridization (CGH). A metaphase or interphase nucleus from a normal individual is labeled with a fluorochrome of one color (e.g., red). DNA from the patient is labeled with a different fluore (e.g., green) and mixed with the control DNA; the mixture is then hybridized to normal metaphases onto a slide. If the DNA content is equal in the reference and the patient; the result is uniformly yellow (red plus green). If the patient has more DNA than the reference (e.g., trisomic) an area of green highlight will exist; if deletion exists the highlight will conversely be red.

INHERITED CHROMOSOMAL REARRANGEMENTS. If an infant is born with an unanticipated chromosomal rearrangement, parental chromosomal analysis is imperative, so that inherited abnormalities and risks for other relatives can be identified. If one parent is a balanced translocation carrier, evaluation of the relevant grandparents and (if positive) other relatives is indicated. If grandparents are not available, all siblings of the translocation carrier must be evaluated. Recurrence risks for subsequent pregnancies would be the same as for those in the following group.

For families at risk because one parent is a balanced translocation carrier (see Fig. 14.3), theoretical and practical recurrence risks are given above. The literature should be consulted for each individual rearrangement encountered, because, apart from the situation associated with the most common translocations (e.g., 14; 21, 13; 14), many are unique for the family in question and recurrence risks differ within each family.

In families with a known incidence of a chromosomal abnormality, the only parents to whom prenatal diagnosis must be offered are those who are known to be at increased risk. They include those who have had a previous infant with a non-disjunctional event and those in which one member of a couple has been found to be carrying a familial chromosomal rearrangement.

Family History of Suspected Chromosomal Abnormality A family history of infants with multiple congenital malformations who have died or are not available for chromosome analysis, or of several miscarriages in one or more relatives, might be suggestive of an inherited chromosomal rearrangement and prenatal diagnosis should be offered to such parents. If an abnormality is detected by lymphocyte culture (from peripheral blood), prenatal testing is indicated in all who are carriers.

Occasionally, miscarriages, if evaluated cytogenetically, are found to be aneuploid. Although evidence for increased risk of recurrence after a chromosomal abnormality in a nonviable conception is controversial, and in the opinion of some authors the risk for a viable abnormal outcome is no higher than that for the general population, it is still appropriate to offer the option of prenatal cytogenetic testing.

Family History of Disorder Necessitating Fetal Sex Determination Fetal sex determination by chromosome analysis is a crucial first step in some disorders affecting preferentially only one sex. Further testing is frequently possible in the fetus if the high-risk sex is determined. Examples of such disorders include Duchenne muscular dystrophy (DMD) and fragile X and other X-linked mental retardation syndromes.

Summary of ACOG recommendations on prenatal diagnosis of fetal chromosomal abnormalities[6]

The following recommendation is based on good and consistent scientific evidence (Level A):

Early amniocentesis (<13 weeks) is not recommended because of the higher risk of pregnancy loss and complications compared with traditional amniocentesis (15–17 weeks).

The following recommendations are based primarily on consensus and expert opinion (Level C):

Women with singleton pregnancies who will be age 35 years or older at delivery should be offered prenatal diagnosis for fetal aneuploidy.

Patients with a risk of fetal aneuploidy high enough to justify an invasive diagnostic procedure include women with a previous pregnancy complicated by an autosomal trisomy or sex chromosome aneuploidy, a major fetal structural defect identified by ultrasonography, or either parent with a chromosome inversion or parental aneuploidy.

A combination of one major or two or more minor ultrasound markers of Down syndrome substantially increases risk and warrants further counseling regarding invasive testing.

The use of ultrasonographic screening for Down syndrome in high-risk women (e.g., women age 35 years and older) to avoid invasive testing should be limited to specialized centers.

With an isolated choroid plexus cyst, testing is indicated only if serum screening results are abnormal or the patient will be older than 32 years at delivery.

Cervical infections with *Chlamydia* or herpes are contraindications to transcervical CVS.

Counseling for amniocentesis in a twin pregnancy in women age 33 years is indicated because the mid-trimester risk of fetal Down syndrome is approximately the same as for that of a singleton pregnancy at age 35 years.

Non-directive counseling before genetic amniocentesis does not require a patient to commit to pregnancy termination if the result is abnormal.

Metabolic single gene disorders detectable by biochemical analysis

In considering pregnancy in association with biochemical disorders, most of which are inherited in autosomal recessive fashion, it is important to take into account the type of disorder, whether it is a parent who is affected or a fetus who is at risk, and whether and by what method the disorder is prenatally detectable. Clinical consideration of biochemical disorders can be divided into two categories: (1) carrier (heterozygote) screening to identify couples at risk for having an affected fetus and thereby candidates for prenatal diagnosis, and (2) diagnosis and management, of a first affected child.

Tay-Sachs disease, a lysosomal sphingolipid storage disorder, is a typical example of a **disorder that is detectable in the first pregnancy of a couple at risk**. Its clinical manifestations, occurring more frequently in the Ashkenazi Jewish, Cajun, and some French-Canadian populations, are caused by the absence of the α subunit of the enzyme hexosaminidase A (Hex A), which is a normal gene product. The clinical course of the infantile form is relentlessly fatal, usually within 4–6 years after birth. It is characterized by loss of developmental skills and milestones in an initially healthy-appearing infant; a typical cherry-red spot on the ocular macula; gradual deterioration (associated with intracellular accumulation of the abnormal metabolite, GM_2 ganglioside) of visual, auditory, and motor function; and frequent seizures. Hex A levels in the serum of heterozygotes are decreased by approximately 50% in comparison to those in unaffected homozygotes and are easily detectable in populations at risk. In women who are pregnant or on oral contraceptives, measurement of serum Hex A levels may lead to false-positive results. Therefore, a leukocyte Hex A assay is used for these women.

The International Tay-Sachs Disease Network, through the participation of many centers around the world with well-organized, targeted, and accurate screening surveys, has been indirectly responsible for the dramatic reduction of this fatal disorder from about 60 newly diagnosed patients per year in the United States around 1970 to 3 per year in 1992.[59] Most cases were prevented through prenatal diagnosis and pregnancy termination of affected fetuses of couples found through screening to be at 25% risk. The fetal diagnosis was initially established by quantitative Hex A determination in amniocytes or chorionic villus tissue. More recently it has become molecularly based and several mutations, as well as multiple forms of disease in addition to the infantile one, are known to exist. Thus, Tay-Sachs disease has become not only a preventable, but in its severe, infantile form, now almost extinct disorder. In addition to Tay-Sachs disease, it is recommended that Ashkenazi Jewish individuals be offered screening for Canavan disease, familial dysautonomia, and cystic fibrosis. Additional tests that may be added to a screening panel include Fanconi anemia group C, mucolipidosis IV, Bloom syndrome, and Gaucher disease.[60]

For most inborn errors of metabolism, carrier screening is not available. After the birth of an affected child the parents are identified as heterozygotes for a particular disease and prenatal diagnosis may be an option in subsequent pregnancies. Examples of metabolic single gene disorders detectable by biochemical analysis are given in Table 14.2, together with the specific enzyme deficiency, the tissue in which it is prenatally detectable, their mechanism of inheritance, and the feasibility of heterozygote detection. Table 14.2 is not all-inclusive.

Single gene disorders detectable by direct molecular analysis

There is an ever increasing list of disorders detectable by molecular analysis, which permits identification of the mutation directly in fetal (or embryonic) tissue. However, this should not be offered to any couple unless the couple is known to be at risk for the disorder in question, and unless testing is preceded by extensive, supportive, and informative counseling of all aspects and implications of potential results, as well as complications and ambiguities. Table 14.3 provides a selective list of disorders prenatally diagnosable by direct identification of the mutation, as well as the chromosomal location and mechanism of inheritance. Prototypes of more commonly occurring disorders within this group include cystic fibrosis (CF), sickle cell disease, Duchenne muscular dystrophy (DMD), fragile X syndrome, and Huntington disease (HD).

Cystic Fibrosis Cystic fibrosis is a multisystem disease inherited in autosomal recessive fashion. In the white population approximately 1 in 4000 individuals in North American and northern Europe are affected. The frequency of heterozygous carriers is about 1 in 30 individuals in Caucasians (Northern European origin) and Ashkenazi Jews. The heterozygote is lower in Hispanic, Asians, and African-Americans. CF is a disease of exocrine glands that results in viscid secretions which most commonly and most severely affect the respiratory and gastrointestinal system. In 1989, the CF gene was mapped to chromosome 7.[61] Its gene product, a transport protein called cystic fibrosis transmembrane conductance regulator (CFTR), functions as a chloride channel activated by cAMP-dependent protein kinase A phosphorylation.[61] More than 1400 different mutations have been discovered that result in an abnormal CFTR, the most common being ΔF508, which is a deletion of 3 base pairs that code for phenylalanine. The only other mutation present in high frequency in any ethnic group is W1282X, the most common mutant allele in Ashkenazi Jews.

The pathogenesis in cystic fibrosis involves a blocked or closed chloride channel in the epithelial cell membrane. As a result, chloride ions are trapped inside the cell. This draws sodium ions and water into the cell resulting in dehydration of mucus secretions. In the lungs, this can lead to airway obstruction and predisposition to infection, dyspnea, bronchiectasis, and pulmonary fibrosis. The major cause of morbidity and mortality in these individuals is progressive, chronic bronchopulmonary disease. In the pancreas, the dehydrated secretions are also insufficiently alkalinized, hence causing not only duct obstruction but also a reduction in digestive enzymes and fibrosis. The fibrosis can involve the endocrine cells and may lead to not only pancreatic insufficiency but also diabetes mellitus. In the intestinal tract, the lack of digestive enzymes leads to malabsorption of fats and protein and the altered mucus can lead to bowel obstruction. Infants born with meconium ileus have a significantly higher risk of subsequent malnutrition. Sweat electrolytes are also abnormal, with elevated concentrations of sodium and chloride. This in turn can lead to heat intolerance, hyponatremia, and a hypochloremic metabolic alkalosis.

The clinical presentation and course of individuals affected with CF is highly variable. The median age at diagnosis by traditional methods is 6–8 months. Some individuals have severe pulmonary and/or gastrointestinal disease, whereas others have mild expression with presentation in adolescence and young adulthood. There is a close correlation of genotype with phenotype in relation to pancreatic function; however, identification of the specific CFTR mutation has not proved highly predictive of the severity of pulmonary disease. Modifier genes and environmental factors undoubtedly play roles in this varied expressivity.

With advances in medical treatment, the prognosis for individuals affected with CF has improved. In the United States, median survival has reached 37.8 years for men and 34.2 years for women. Data from the Cystic Fibrosis Foundation indicate that about a third of affected individuals are 18 years or older, and survival into the fourth or fifth decades is not uncommon.[62]

TABLE 14.2 PRENATAL DIAGNOSIS OF SOME METABOLIC DISORDERS

Metabolism	Disorder	Enzyme deficiency	Mechanism of inheritance	Technique	Cvs	Amnio	Heterozygote detection	Approx. Locus	Comment
Amino acid	PKU	Phenylalanine hydroxylase	AR	Cells, molecular	+	+	Mutation	12q24.1	Beware maternal PKU
	Maple syrup urine disease	Branched-chain 2-ketoacid dehydrogenase	AR	Fluid, cells, enzyme linkage	+	+	RFLP	19q13.1	Odor of maple syrup in urine of affected patients; several types
	Homocystinuria	Cystathionine-α-synthetase	AR	Linkage	+	+	+	21q22	Several types; responsive to vitamin B$_6$
Organic acid	Propionic acidemia	Propionyl-CoA carboxylase	AR	Fluid, methylcitrate mutations	+	+	+ Mutations	13q32	Different mutations, types A and B —more?
	Glutaric acidemia Type I	Glutaryl-CoA dehydrogenase	AR	Fluid, glutaric acid	−	+			
	Type II	Fatty acid oxidation	AR	Fluid, cells, glutaric acid	−	+		15q14	Dysmorphism in affected infants; more than 1 type
	Methylmalonic acidemia	Methylmalonyl-CoA mutase	AR	Fluid, cells, methylcitrate, methylmalonate	+	+		6p21	
	B$_{12}$ defect		AR	Fluid, cells, methylcitrate, methylmalonate	+	+			Effective prenatal maternal treatment with vitamin B$_{12}$
Mucopoly-saccharide	MPS I-HHurler	α$_1$-Iduronidase	AR	Cells, enzyme			a.b.	4p16.3	MPS I-H and S are allelic
	MPS I-SScheie	α$_1$-Iduronidase	AR	Same linkage?					Milder course than I-H
	MPS II Hunter	Iduronate	XLR	Cells			a.b.	Xq28	
	MPS III A Sanfilippo	Heparin sulfatase	AR	Cells, enzyme			b.b.		
	MPS III B	Acetyl-CoA-glucosaminidase	AR	Cells, fluid					
	MPS III C	N-acetyl-transferase glucosaminidase N-acetyl transferase	AR	Cells					
	MPS III D	Acetylglucosamine-6-sulfatase	AR	Cells				12q14	
	MPS IV Morquio A	N-acetylgalactosamine-6-sulfate sulfatase	AR	Cells, enzyme					Type A placental enzyme cloned and sequenced; variable expression; more forms possible
	B	β-galactosidase							
	MPS VI Maroteaux-Lamy	Arylsulfatase B	AR	Cells, linkage	+	+	a.b.	5q11-q13	

TABLE 14.2 PRENATAL DIAGNOSIS OF SOME METABOLIC DISORDERS (*CONT'D*)

Metabolism	Disorder	Enzyme deficiency	Mechanism of inheritance	Technique	Cvs	Amnio	Heterozygote detection	Approx. Locus	Comment
	MPS VII Sly	β-glucuronidase, incorporation of S	AR	Cells	+	+		7q21.11	
	Multiple sulfatase deficiency	Iduronate sulfate sulfatase, arylsulfatase A, B, C	AR	Cells	+	+	a.b.	Xpter-p22.32	
Carbohydrate	Glycogen storage								
	Type I von Gierke	Glucose-6-phosphatase	AR	AFP?	?	?			
	Type II Pompe	α-glucosidase	AR	Enzyme in cells, EM on uncultured cells enzymes	+	Cells + fluid		17q23	Liver dysfunction
	Type III, IV		AR		+	+	b.b.		Rare forms
	Galactosemia Classic	Galactose-1-uridylphospho-transferase	AR	Enzymes in cells	+	+		9p13	
Glycoprotein	Mannosidosis	α-mannosidase	AR	Enzyme in cells	+	+	a.b.	19p13.2-q12	Not a single entity
	Mucolipidosis I-Sialidosis	Neuraminidase + oligosaccharides	AR	Enzyme	+	+	a.b.		
	Mucolipidosis II-I cell disease	Multiple lysosomal enzymes	AR	Multiple enzyme deficiencies in cells, EM inclusions	+	+		4q21-q23	Total elevation of Hex A and B in maternal serum during pregnancy
Sphingolipid	Niemann-Pick A, B	Sphingomyelinase	AR	Enzyme in cells	+	+		11p15	
	Gaucher (several forms)	β-glucosidase	AR	Enzyme in cells, molecular	+	+	b.b. in some forms	1q21	Many mutations; population screening possibly feasible
	Fabry	α-galactosidase	XLR	Enzyme, molecular	+	+		Xq22	
	GM, gangliosidosis	β-galactosidase	AR	Enzyme in cells	+	+		3p21-p14	
	Tay-Sachs (several forms)	Hexosaminidase	AR	Enzyme in cells, molecular	+ +	+ +	b.b.	15q23	Population screening feasible
	Sandhoff	Total hexosaminidase	AR	Enzyme in cells, molecular			a.b.	5q11	
Peroxisome	Adrenoleuko-dystrophy	Lignoceroyl-CoA ligase deficient in peroxisomes	XLR	VLCFAs in amniotic cells	+	+	a.b.	Xq28	Variable expression
	Zellweger		AR	As above	+	+	a.b.	7q11	
Other	Congenital adrenal hyperplasia	Steroid 21-hydroxylase	AR	VLCFAs	+	+		6p21.3	

VLCFAs, very long chain fatty acids; a.b., detectable after birth of affected child; b.b., detectable before birth of first affected child; MPS, mucopolysaccharidosis; EM, electron microscope; AR, autosomal recessive; XLR, X-linked recessive.

Both women and men have compromised fertility. Women show delayed onset of menarche; those with malnutrition and advanced lung disease often have anovulatory cycles with secondary amenorrhea. Dehydrated and thickened cervical secretions also may pose a physical barrier to sperm penetration of the cervical os. Nonetheless, as more women with CF enter reproductive age, they should be appropriately counseled about contraception, pregnancy, and the potential increased risks

TABLE 14.3 CURRENT LIST OF DISORDERS ASSOCIATED WITH UNSTABLE TRINUCLEOTIDE REPEATS

Disorder	Mechanism of inheritance	Chromosome location	Trinucleotide	Gen. pop	Number of repeats* Premutation/carrier	Mutation
Dystrophia myotonica	AD	19q13.3	CTG	5–35	50–80	>80
Fragile X syndrome FRA-X-A	XLD	Xq27.3	CGG	6–50	51–200	>200
FRA-X-E syndrome	XL	Xq27-28	GCC	<30	≈200	≈700
Huntington disease	AD	4p16.3	CAG	9–34	?	30–140
Kennedy disease (spinobulbar muscular atrophy	XL		CAG	11–31	?	40 to >60
Dentatorubral-pallidoluysian atrophy	AD	12	CAG	25–36	?	43 to ≈80
Spinocerebellar ataxia I	AD	6p	CAG	7–23	?	49 to ≈750
Others to follow? e.g., hereditary nonpolyposis colon cancer (HNPCC)	AD					

* The number of repeats is approximate and differs among studies. It should *not* be used as an unequivocal cutoff for prenatal diagnosis. It is important that individual laboratories and geneticists provide physicians with careful interpretation of results.
AD, autosomal dominant; XL, X-linked; XLD, X-linked dominant.

associated with CF. Pregnancy rates among CF women have increased. During pregnancy these women are at risk for respiratory and cardiac compromise because their underlying lung disease has the potential to be further exacerbated by gestationally related hypoxemia and pulmonary hypertension. The changes in ventilatory drive, cardiac function, blood volume, and increased nutritional requirements all pose potential problems for the woman with CF.[63] Most women with CF can complete a successful pregnancy. Careful monitoring of lung function and ensuring adequate energy intake is recommended. Affected women should be counseled about the symptoms and signs of preterm labor and routine cervical exams should be considered.

As mentioned above, over 1400 mutations have been identified in the CFTR gene. The ΔF508 mutation is represented in almost all populations, although its relative frequency varies among different geographic locations. The highest frequency for ΔF508 is observed in white populations, especially of Northern European origin, where it accounts for 70–75% of the CF alleles. ΔF508 is present in 48% of CF alleles in African-Americans, 46% in Hispanics, and 30% in Asian-Americans, and 30% in Ashkenazi Jews. About 15–20 other mutations account for 2–15% of the other CF alleles, depending on the ethnic group studied. Most remaining mutations are rare. A panel of 25 mutations will detect 87% in Caucasians and differing frequencies in other ethnic groups. In several populations, the combination of ΔF508 with other ethnic-specific mutations allows for a 90–95% detection rate: Ashkenazi Jews, Celtic Britons, French Canadians from Quebec, and some Native Americans.[64] In Ashkenazi Jews, ΔF508 and W1282X alone account for 85% of CF alleles.

An important implication of the various mutation detection rates among different populations is the number of couples in whom both partners can actually be identified as CF carriers, thereby enabling unequivocal prenatal diagnosis. For example, if the mutation detection rate is 75% and one partner is determined to be a carrier and the other not, the risk of having an affected

offspring is 1 in 400. By contrast, if the mutation detection rate is 90% and one partner is determined to be a carrier and the other not, the risk for an affected offspring is 1 in 1000. If both partners are screen negative, the risk is 1 in 240 000.[65]

If amniotic fluid analysis were possible for the cystic fibrosis gene product (i.e., mutant protein), the inability to detect all mutations would not matter so much in situations where one parent carries an identified CF mutation and the other is screen negative, but still has a residual risk of carrying an unidentified CF mutation. Unfortunately, no such assay exists, meaning prenatal diagnosis is not possible except to exclude the fetus who inherited the mutation from the known heterozygous parent. Measuring microvillus intestinal enzymes in amniotic fluid is specifically not helpful, for a low value is more likely to connote a false-positive than a true-positive value.

Another issue with carrier screening is genotype–phenotype correlations. Predictions of the severity and course of pulmonary disease is variable for specific mutations, especially for fetuses detected to be compound heterozygotes; however, prediction for pancreatic function is generally reliable.[66] The issue of phenotype being different from CF with pancreatic and pulmonary insufficiency becomes most relevant when one is confronted with a male having two CF alleles that results in congenital bilateral absence of the vas deferens (CBAVD).

Males with classic CF are virtually always sterile due to CBAVD. There is an increased frequency of CF mutations in otherwise healthy men with CBAVD. About 25% of these men with CBAVD are compound heterozygotes for two mutant alleles (one being a 'mild' mutation); half have one identifiable mutation, and the remainder have no identifiable mutation.[67] Eighty-four percent with no identifiable mutation carry this splice site variant for a CF mutation called the 5T allele and 25% with no identifiable mutation carry this splice site variant. The 5T refers to the number of thymines present at the end of intron 8, which alters the likelihood of proper splicing of exon 9. The

7T allele is associated with normal splicing. The 5T allele is present in men with CBAVD at a fourfold higher frequency than the general population.[68–70]

Recommendations for Cystic Fibrosis Carrier Screening
Population-based programs offering CF carrier screening were introduced as standard of care in the US in 2001.[71] The following guidelines and recommendations have been provided:[72]

- CF carrier screening should be offered to all couples with a positive family history of CF. All partners of individuals with CF and all Caucasian couples of European or Ashkenazi Jewish descent planning a pregnancy or seeking prenatal care. Ideally screening is performed prior to conception or during the first or early second trimester. Information about CF screening should also be provided to patients in other ethnic and racial groups. Counseling and screening should be provided and made available to individuals in the lower risk groups upon their request.

- The clinician should identify couples to whom screening should be offered based on family history and ascertainment of the ethnicity and race of the partners during the initial history. Counseling and standardized written educational material or other formats such as videos, and/or interactive computer programs should be used to inform the woman and, whenever possible, her partner. In the event that her partner does not accompany the woman to a prenatal or preconception visit, written educational material should be provided for her to give to her partner. Women and their providers may elect to use either a simultaneous or sequential carrier screening strategy for CF. Simultaneous testing may be particularly important when there are time constraints for making a decision regarding prenatal diagnosis or on the availability of termination of affected pregnancies.

- The obstetrical care provider should offer CF screening when appropriate and may choose to provide or refer for pre-test counseling. Post-test counseling for couples with positive/negative, positive/untested, or positive/positive screening results requires special knowledge of CF with regard to range of severity, prognosis, treatment options, etc., and calculation of genetic risk. Referral to a geneticist or a provider with special expertise with CF testing may be considered in these situations. Referral to a geneticist or individual with special expertise with CF testing should also be considered when there is a family history of CF, when carriers are identified with CF mutations that may be associated with congenital absence of the vas deferens in the male offspring, or when an affected adult or an affected fetus is identified.

To implement these guidelines a minimum panel of 25 mutations was recommended to be included in CF screening. Provider educational materials, patient pamphlets, and model informed consent forms are available.

Sickle Cell Disease Sickle cell disease, is an autosomal recessive disorder occurring commonly (1 in 400 to 500) in the African-American population, with heterozygote frequency of about 1 in 10. Heterozygotes are detected by hemoglobin electrophoresis. Sickle cell disease is attributable to the SS hemoglobin molecule's instability, which leads to anemia, blood flow reduction, and increased susceptibility to pneumococcal infections that can be prevented with penicillin prophylaxis.[73] Historically, the discovery of the prenatal diagnosis of sickle cell disease with restriction endonucleases[74] was one of the more dramatic breakthroughs in prenatal diagnosis. Direct detection of the mutation at the specific site within the β-globin gene on chromosome 11, resulting in exchange from glutamine to valine, is one of the simplest and most accurate tests available. It utilizes polymerase chain reaction, and needs no adjuvant family studies, apart from the identification of (a) parent(s) at risk.

Fragile X Syndrome Fragile X syndrome is thought to be one of the most common causes of an inherited form of mental retardation, rivaled only by the incidence of Down syndrome, and possibly by the effects of intrauterine exposure to maternal alcohol ingestion. It is inherited in X-linked dominant fashion, affecting about 1/4,500 and 1/9,000 males and females, respectively, with no male-to-male transmission. The syndrome is defined by a combination of a characteristic phenotype and behaviors, cognitive impairment, the presence of a fragile site (gap) detectable cytogenetically in folate-free culture medium on Xq27.3, called FRA-X-A. Molecularly, it is caused by transcriptional inhibition, through overmethylation, of a messenger ribonucleic acid (mRNA) protein binding gene called *FMR-1* (fragile X mental retardation-1; see Ch. 5).

The characteristic but subtle phenotype includes elongated face and mandible, large ears, macrocephaly with bizygomatic pinching, soft skin, inconsistent mitral valve prolapse, macro-orchidism, mildly shortened stature in adulthood, and occasional seizures. Characteristic behaviors may resemble autism and attention deficit disorders. Intellectual impairment in affected individuals varies from mild to severe with most affected males within the moderate range of cognitive disability. However, 20% of males who have the fragile X mutation are phenotypically and intellectually unaffected. They are called transmitting males. Female heterozygotes may be indistinguishable from the general population or may have subtle signs of both physical and intellectual impairment.

The mutation is characterized by varying lengths of DNA fragments, consisting of varying numbers of repeats of the trinucleotide CGG, located 5' to the gene (FMR-1) itself. The trinucleotide is repeated approximately 6–45 times in the normal population, approximately 55–200 times in unaffected individuals with a so-called premutation, who are at risk for expansion and transmission to offspring in expanded form, and over 200 times in individuals who are (usually) affected and said to have a full mutation. These CGG repeats are called unstable (their numbers change) tandem (they are next to one another) repeats, and there are several disorders the molecular basis of which includes such unstable tandem repeats.[75]

Prenatal diagnosis of fragile X syndrome should be contemplated only in families with (a) member(s) in whom the diagnosis has been unequivocally confirmed by DNA analysis. The next step is the determination, first from the family history, then by DNA analysis, whether one of the parents of the pregnancy is at risk. If the mother is a heterozygote with a premutation (≈50–200 repeats), she could be at risk for transmitting it in similar (i.e., premutational) or expanded (i.e., mutational) form, or not at all, by transmitting her normal X.

Expansion occurs only during oogenesis, not spermatogenesis; therefore if the father is a transmitting male (i.e., unaffected, symptomless, with a premutation), it is unlikely that his daughters would be affected. They would all have premutations also, and it would be their offspring (more frequently sons, less frequently daughters) who would be at risk for having a full mutation and therefore clinical manifestations of the syndrome.

Direct DNA analysis of fetal tissue either by CVS or amniocentesis can differentiate between a normal, a premutational, and a mutational number of CGG repeats. Although males are affected more frequently than females, carrier mothers can have affected offspring of both sexes, and awareness of fetal sex can sometimes be helpful in attempts to provide the parents with prognostic information about the severity of the disorder, if present in their future child.

Muscular Dystrophies **Duchenne muscular dystrophy** (DMD) and Becker muscular dystrophy (BMD) are allelic X-linked recessive (XLR) disorders, caused by a gene on Xp21, the malfunction of which results in a deficiency of the muscle protein DYSTROPHIN. The two disorders can occur within members of the same family and differ in severity. While boys with DMD are usually wheelchair bound by age 8–10 years, those with BMD are sometimes ambulatory into their twenties and thirties. Their life expectancy also differs significantly, and may not exceed 20 years in patients with DMD, whereas patients with BMD frequently live into middle age or longer. In contrast to fragile X syndrome, the genetic transmission of DMD and BMD is straightforward XLR. Thus, with very few exceptions, only males are affected within the family and in most cases they are sons of carrier females. The exceptions may include females with X autosomal chromosomal translocations involving the crucial segment of Xp21, females with a 45,X (Turner syndrome) karyotype, or, rarely, those in whom the active X is the abnormal one, enhancing the expression of the gene.

The prenatal diagnosis of DMD and BMD begins, as in all other instances, with an accurately confirmed diagnosis, usually including a muscle biopsy in an affected family member. Wherever possible, the identification of carrier status in the mother should also be established. Localization of the DYSTROPHIN gene to Xp21 now allows prenatal diagnosis for DMD and BMD. Many affected boys with the disorder have a deletion, at the molecular level, of the DYSTROPHIN gene,[76] as do their carrier mothers and other female relatives. In the simplest instance, then, prenatal diagnosis in such families is based on the detection, by direct DNA analysis, of a deletion in a male fetus of a known carrier mother. Such a result is accurate and reliable. Occasionally, an affected infant with a deletion is born to an apparent non-carrier mother (she does not have a detectable gene deletion). If the birth of her affected son were the result of a new mutation (the remainder of the family history is negative), there should be no increased risk for recurrence, and prenatal diagnosis would ordinarily not be indicated for a subsequent pregnancy. However, the possibility of maternal gonadal mosaicism cannot be ruled out, and has indeed been confirmed in several instances[77] in which two affected boys have been born to mothers whose carrier status had been undetectable by currently available techniques. Since it is not possible to rule out gonadal mosaicism, it is advisable to offer prenatal diagnosis to all couples who have had an affected child with DMD, even if the family history is negative and the mother appears not to be a carrier.

A third scenario is even more confusing. Not all affected boys have a molecularly detectable deletion, even though they are unequivocally affected. The technique of choice in such families is then by linkage – that is, the tracking of the crucial chromosomal segment with molecular markers and comparison among known affected and unaffected individuals. If a mother and her male fetus have inherited the same X chromosome as her affected brothers, sons, or maternal uncles, the probability that the fetus is affected is high, but never certain. It is inversely proportionate to the probability of recombination (crossing over) between homologous chromosomal segments. The closer the compared markers are, the lower the probability of crossing over, and the higher the probability of the presence of the gene in question.

Myotonic dystrophy, or **dystrophia myotonica** (DM), is thought to be the most common form of muscular dystrophy that affects adults. It is a systemic disease inherited in an autosomal dominant manner, but the well-known congenital form that is most severe occurs only in children of affected mothers.

Like all pleiotropic dominant disorders, adult-onset DM varies in phenotype, age of onset, and degree of involvement of different organ systems. It can be so mild that its presence in an elderly grandfather may not be recognized until the birth of a grandchild with the severe congenital form. The disorder is characterized by progressive muscle weakness, myotonia (inability of the muscles to relax after contraction), cataracts, frontal alopecia, cardiac conduction defects, endocrine failure with subsequent infertility in males, dilatation of the gastrointestinal tract with absence of peristalsis, progressive dementia, and respiratory failure. The congenital form may be suspected prenatally by reports – and ultrasonic evidence – of lack of fetal movement and polyhydramnios. At birth the infant is frequently immobile, with a characteristic myopathic open-mouthed face and inability to suck or swallow. Gradually these signs tend to improve and the child begins to move and develop gross motor skills, though very slowly. Such children are almost always not only physically but also psychometrically delayed. Historically, **anticipation** (namely, increasing severity of the disease in successive generations) was recognized as early as 1946[78] but was attributed mostly to ascertainment bias.[79] The discovery of heritable unstable trinucleotide repeats (CTG) finally provided a molecular explanation not only for the phenomenon of anticipation but also for some of the variable expression of the disease.[80] The gene is now known to be located on chromosome 19q; before that it was found to be linked to the Lutheran blood group and secretor status genes, and this was used in the early 1970s for prenatal diagnosis, but the recombination rate was high and many families were uninformative. As more markers became available, linkage was the prenatal diagnostic method of choice, using family parental and fetal (amniotic) material. The breakthrough in 1992 by Aslanidis and colleagues[81] resulted in the possibility of direct molecular prenatal diagnosis without the need for extensive family studies. It consists of the detection of a CTG triplet located in the 3' untranslated region of a mRNA-encoded polypeptide of the protein kinase family. The triplet is repeated between about 5 to 27 times in the general (unaffected) population; mildly affected patients with DM may have 50 or more, while severely affected ones have over 1000 repeats.

It seems, therefore, that the size of the expansion is correlated with the severity of the disease and age of onset, but contraction (or mosaicism) has been observed in male somatic cells as well as in sperm.[82] Thus, patients with DM may have gonosomal mosaicism and contraction in sperm; and this may account for the presence of congenital DM only in infants of affected mothers. This explanation, however, is probably incomplete.

Hecht and colleagues[80] investigated directly several fetal tissues and chorionic villi (after CVS and pregnancy termination). They found no heterogeneity or mosaicism in lengths of repeats among tissues or villi thus evaluated. However, expansion did occur during culture of CVS cells. The authors therefore recommend that prenatal diagnosis for DM be performed on direct rather than cultured cells. More experience is needed before these findings enable the provision of unequivocal and unambiguous information to parents who request not only prenatal diagnosis for DM but who, in the case of maternal transmission, may wish to know early during the pregnancy whether or not their fetus has the congenital or adult-onset form. The clinical severity and progression of the disease in the affected parent might also be considered by the couple, as they plan their future and that of their family.

Huntington Disease Huntington disease (HD) is an autosomal dominantly inherited, mostly adult-onset, progressive neurodegenerative disorder characterized by initial involuntary movements, gradual psychological changes, and cognitive and emotional decline. Before the onset of recognizable signs of HD, some young adults may occasionally receive a diagnosis of schizophrenia. The disorder leads relentlessly to death, within, variably, 10–20 years after onset of symptoms. Until recently, the diagnosis of HD has been based on the family history, careful clinical and finally pathologic evaluation at autopsy of the CNS, which grossly is characterized by atrophy of the caudate, putamen, and internal capsule. Microscopically, severe diffuse neuronal loss and gliosis are observed in the caudate, putamen, and globus pallidus.

The HD gene has been located to 4p16.3.[83] Prior to the discovery of the molecular basis of HD, prenatal diagnosis of this devastating disease did not exist, and genetic counseling had little to offer apart from the explanation of autosomal dominant inheritance with its concomitant 50% and 25% risk of development of symptoms in children and grandchildren, respectively, of affected patients. The first breakthrough in molecular genetics research came in 1983 when Gusella and colleagues,[84] through the extensive study of large Venezuelan kindreds, found that the gene for HD was linked to the short arm of chromosome 4p. HD belongs to the group of disorders charac-

terized by trinucleotide repeats (see Table 14.3). The triplet in question is CAG; superficially, unaffected individuals have a range of about 9 to 34, while affected patients have a range from 34 to about 140 repeats.[85] There is a significant negative correlation between the number of repeats on the HD chromosome and the age of onset of the disease, regardless of the sex of the transmitting parent. However, it also appears that this negative correlation (i.e., the higher the number of repeats, the lower the age of onset) applies to the number of repeats on the paternal (normal) allele and age of onset of offspring of affected mothers. The abnormal repeat is unstable – it can expand and decrease in size during meiosis of either sex, with the largest expansions occurring in abnormal paternal alleles. In summary, the larger the abnormal parental allele, the earlier the age of onset (and death) in offspring. Paternal expansions seem to be more extensive than maternal ones, hence the prognosis is probably worse if the abnormal allele is inherited from the father with the number of repeats nearer to the upper end of the abnormal range.

Presymptomatic predictive testing and prenatal diagnosis for HD have been available since 1993 by direct mutation analysis. A large European collaborative study has shown that presymptomatic predictive tests for HD far exceeds that for prenatal testing.[86] Another option is preimplantation genetic diagnosis for couples who do not wish investigation of an established pregnancy.[87] Recent studies of Europeans at reproductive ages have shown that predictive DNA testing has a significant impact on subsequent reproduction; specifically, 14% of HD carriers had one or more subsequent pregnancies compared to 28% of the non-carriers.[88]

Single gene disorders detectable by indirect molecular analysis or linkage studies

Linkage analysis is the technique usually used for the diagnosis of disorders that have been assigned to a specific chromosomal segment, but the gene itself has not been isolated. For example, linkage studies were used for presymptomatic prenatal testing for HD for 9 years, because, although the gene was known to be somewhere on distal 4p, its exact location had not been determined.

Linkage is the step that precedes direct analysis, but it has several disadvantages, the most significant of which are probably: (1) recombination – the more distant the markers from the gene, the greater the probability of recombination between the locus of the marker and that of the mutated gene, and the lower the accuracy of the test; (2) not all markers are highly polymorphic and if they are not, they may not be helpful in the identification of parental origins of chromosomal segments; (3) linkage studies necessitate the collaboration of several family members and sometimes their unrelated spouses; (4) not all families are cooperative; (5) not all families are large enough; and (6) not all families are molecularly informative.

Despite its disadvantages, linkage analysis represented a breakthrough in the prenatal diagnosis of single gene disorders for which none was previously available. Parents at risk were dependent only on statistical risks based on classical mendelian

TABLE 14.4 EXAMPLES OF DISORDERS UTILIZING DNA ANALYSIS FOR PRENATAL DIAGNOSIS

Disorder	Locus	DNA analysis	Direct	Linkage
			Other technique or comment	
Achondroplasia	4p16.3	+	+	Ultrasound
Batten disease	16P12		+	
Breast cancer – early	17q21		+	
Cystic fibrosis	7q31.3	+		
DiGeorge syndrome	22q11	+	+	Ultrasound
Duchenne/Becker muscular dystrophy	Xp21.2	+	+	
Fragile X syndrome	Xp27.3	+		
Huntington disease	4p16.3	+		
Miller-Dieker syndrome	17p13.3	+	+	Cytogenetic
Myotonic dystrophy	19q13.3	+		Ultrasound rule out congenital
Neurofibromatosis I	17q11.2		+	
Neurofibromatosis II	22q		+	
Sickle-cell disease	11p15.5	+		
Tay-Sachs disease	15q23.3		+	Enzyme assay
Tuberous sclerosis	12q23.3		+	Other types, other loci
Waardenburg syndrome	2q37.3	+		
X-linked mental retardation	X		+	Many types

inheritance. It is still useful, for example for families with a known incidence of X-linked mental retardation without a specific diagnosis. The predominance of males among the mentally retarded population is not accounted for by those with fragile X syndrome only (they comprise about half). There are many genes on the X chromosome that cause mental retardation, with or without other symptoms, the exact location of which are not yet known. Linkage studies enable the tracking of the X chromosome in some of these families and may distinguish between affected and unaffected fetuses. DMD itself is not always caused by a definable molecular deletion of the gene; consequently, this disorder must, in some families, be prenatally diagnosed by linkage.

Table 14.4 lists several disorders for which linkage analysis might be an appropriate prenatal diagnostic technique. Of these, it may be helpful to mention the neurocutaneous disorders in more detail. This group of mostly autosomal dominantly inherited disorders has always been among the clinical geneticist's greatest challenges. Clinical heterogeneity, lack of strict diagnostic criteria, difficult differentiation within families between instances of inherited forms of the disorders and those occurring as a result of new mutations or gonadal mosaicism in a parent resulted in confusing information for families about recurrence risks (which ranged from 0% to 50%), and no availability of prenatal diagnosis. Even today, after localization and partial molecular characterization of at least some of the genes causing, for example, neurofibromatosis (NF) and tuberous sclerosis (TS), much confusion and uncertainty persists.

Neurofibromatosis Neurofibromatosis (NF), or von Recklinghausen's disease, is characterized by at least seven or more different but related forms, possibly caused by as many genes. Only the best known form, or NF1, is associated with von Recklinghausen's name. An excellent analysis of NF is the monograph on the subject by Riccardi.[89] Like all forms of NF, NF1 and NF2 are associated with pathology of cells that are neural crest derivatives. NF1, localized to chromosome 17q11.2, occurs in about 1 in 3000 individuals. It is characterized by diagnostic criteria established by consensus in 1988.[90] They include two or more of the following seven features: (1) six or more café au lait macules; (2) two or more neurofibromata or one plexiform neurofibroma; (3) axillary or inguinal freckling; (4) optic glioma; (5) two or more iris Lisch nodules; (6) distinctive osseous lesion; and (7) a first-degree relative with NF1. On the other hand, NF2, the gene for which has been localized to chromosome 22q, has different manifestations from NF1. They include: (1) bilateral eighth (acoustic) nerve masses seen on computed tomographic (CT) scans or magnetic resonance imaging (MRI); and (2) a first-degree relative with NF2 and either a unilateral acoustic neuroma or two of the following: neurofibroma, meningioma, glioma, schwannoma, or juvenile posterior subcapsular lenticular opacity.[90]

Despite these criteria, the diagnosis is frequently very difficult to establish. Thus, molecular geneticists have invested efforts to identify mutations that cause NF1 and NF2. Both have been isolated, and the NF1 product is called NEUROFIBROMIN. Collins and colleagues[91] estimated that the *NF1* gene was very long (290–390 kb), and the finding of homology with a gene, coding for a guanosine triphosphatase-activating protein (GAP) led to recognition of at least one function of the NF1 gene. It is thought that this part of the gene, called NF1-GAP-related domain,[92] is in some way associated with the activation of a *ras* oncogene, and although intragenic probes for this part of the NF1 gene exist,[93] they have not been used routinely for prenatal or postnatal diagnostic or clinical purposes. At present, the molecular prenatal and postnatal diagnosis of NF1 and NF2 utilizes linkage strategies with DNA probes, which hybridize to relevant segments of chromosome 17q and 22q, respectively. As more genes (as well as the whole NF1 gene) are characterized, it will become possible to determine, by using several probes, which form of NF is present in a family, which individual or fetus is affected, and who is at risk for tumorigenesis. It is theoretically possible to consider prenatal ultrasound to rule out the presence of large facial plexiform neurofibromas or bony deformations. However, these are so rare congenitally that their absence and the finding of a healthy-appearing fetus on ultrasound does not preclude the presence of NF.

Tuberous Sclerosis Tuberous sclerosis (TS), an autosomal dominant mutation, is associated with neurocutaneous hamartomas. It occurs in about 1 in 10 000 individuals and is characterized by: (1) mental retardation, typical infantile spasms, and hypsarrhythmia on electroencephalogram (EEG), sometimes followed by variable seizures later in life; (2) skin changes in the form of angiofibroadenomata, shagreen patches, hyperpigmented and hypopigmented macules, ungual fibromata; and (3) hamartomatous lesions in potentially any organ, particularly the kidneys (angiomyolipomata), heart, retina, or CNS. Congenital cardiac rhabdomyoma has been observed in stillborn infants or those who have died shortly after birth, as well as in young infants in whom – unrecognized – it has resulted in what initially appeared to be sudden infant death syndrome.

As with NF, variable expression, questions of accurate diagnosis, progression, and new mutations versus gonadal mosaicism – all resulting in vague information about recurrence risks and prognosis – are difficult issues to address with affected families. Even less is known about the nature of the genes, localized to chromosome 9q and 16p13.3. It is estimated that about 60% of patients with TS (now called TS2) have the form caused by an abnormal gene at the latter locus, on chromosome 16, which is linked to and possibly allelic to the gene for adult-onset polycystic kidney disease.[94] Prenatal diagnosis can be attempted either through ultrasound in a fetus of an affected parent to rule out hamartomatous lesions, particularly of the heart, kidneys, or CNS, or by linkage analysis tracing the relevant chromosomal segment. The latter also necessitates two generations of affected and unaffected individuals. Neither is particularly reliable in ruling out the disorder.

Exposure to potentially hazardous agents

It is estimated that 10–15% of birth defects are the result of maternal exposure to exogenous agents known as teratogens.[95] It is important to consider environmental factors in a chapter dealing with causes and detection of fetal malformations. Literally, a teratogen is a 'producer of monsters' (Greek). The definition, however, is any exogenous agent, chemical or physical, that can produce a permanent abnormality of structure or function in an organism exposed during embryonic or fetal life. Teratogenic effects therefore may include structural malformations, and functional and behavioral deficits which may or may not be associated with visible malformations of the brain. For example, alcohol is a potent teratogen. A mutagen, on the other hand, is an agent that can alter the genetic material in somatic or germ cells (e.g., radiation is a mutagen).

Most pregnancies at risk because of maternal exposure to potentially hazardous agents come to attention unexpectedly during gestation. The exposure is either inadvertent or most frequently occurs before the mother knows she has conceived. Many teratogenic effects are preventable. There are relatively few definitive teratogens (in total probably fewer than 50), the effects and risks of which have been clearly documented and defined. As far as possible, all drugs should be avoided during pregnancy, since the potential teratogenicity is frequently unknown. The great majority of exposures, however, is associated with little or no risk for teratogenicity, and most mothers can be reassured that the exposure in question is not known to be associated with risks to the fetus. Many unnecessary elective abortions can be avoided if pregnant women and their physicians obtain accurate, applicable, and carefully analyzed information about the specific exposure within the context of the individual concerned. Such information is available from Teratogen Information Services (TIS).

Not every pregnant woman who is exposed even to a known teratogen faces an increased risk. Many factors must be considered to determine the magnitude of the risk. They include the type, timing, route of administration, dosage, and duration of the exposure – all within the context of a family, the individual, and knowledge and interpretation of the literature.

Exposures that potentially occur before conception, and the hazards of which are therefore known, include medications, addictive agents, maternal diseases, and infections. In considering chronic medications, it is important to weigh the risk to the health of the mother of discontinuation or modification against the usually minimal risks to the fetus. For example, lithium, with a predilection for the right side of the heart, is teratogenic only at the specific time of embryonic vulnerability (i.e., at the time of cardiac development), and in the second and third trimester is not teratogenic. Fetal echocardiography is indicated prenatally to rule out lithium effects. Other antidepressants are usually not teratogenic or are minimally teratogenic. Anticonvulsants (e.g., hydantoin, less probably valproate) can result in the so-called fetal hydantoin or valproate syndrome, which may include ocular hypertelorism, cleft palate, and digital anomalies. If a change in maternal treatment is desired, it is indicated before, *not* during pregnancy; complications of changes in treatment can have more severe effects on a pregnancy than the anticonvulsant itself. Only a few medications are absolutely contraindicated during pregnancy. They include isotretinoin (Accutane), warfarin, thalidomide, and chemotherapeutic drugs.

Treatment of addiction before conception can prevent adverse effects of exposure to alcohol, cocaine, nicotine, or caffeine; decrease in or cessation of ingestion at any time during the pregnancy is always beneficial. Of these agents, alcohol has by far the most devastating effects on the exposed fetus. Intrauterine exposure to alcohol is estimated to be the most frequent cause of learning, behavior, and developmental disability. Most information available on alcohol use during pregnancy is based on data gathered from chronic and heavy alcohol use (i.e., 10–12 drinks per day) throughout pregnancy. Children born to women drinking this amount have approximately a 30–40% risk of being born with fetal alcohol syndrome (FAS, see Fig. 2.18). Heavy alcohol use throughout the first trimester has also been known to result in FAS, but accurate percentage risks are not available.

The following components must be present for a diagnosis of FAS to be made:[77]

- Growth retardation – decreased rate of growth both before and after birth. Even under optimal conditions, babies with FAS do not appear to 'catch up.' They remain smaller than average (both in height and weight) throughout their lives. This delayed growth includes a smaller head size.
- CNS abnormalities – abnormalities of the brain and spinal cord. Individuals diagnosed with FAS usually have some degree of mental retardation. The degree of mental retardation varies.
- Characteristic facial features – although subtle, characteristic facial features associated with FAS are recognizable to a trained clinician. They create no medical concerns in themselves.

Children with FAS are at increased risk for having limb defects, heart problems, spina bifida, and other structural abnormalities.

Not all individuals who are adversely affected by prenatal exposure to alcohol have all the characteristics of FAS. Women who consume large amounts of alcohol or who 'binge' drink during pregnancy are also at increased risk for having a child who is growth retarded, or who has structural defects or CNS abnormalities, but not the full-blown syndrome. These adverse effects are termed fetal alcohol effects (FAE). A child may be born with mental retardation alone as a result of alcohol exposure. There is also a risk for second trimester pregnancy loss even after alcohol use has stopped. When the amounts of alcohol consumed are less than chronic use, estimates become more difficult to make. Given the uncertainty in the literature, our best estimate is that the risks for FAE are slightly increased.

Prenatally in pregnancies at risk, fetal growth can be followed as can head measurements, and the presence of gross structural anomalies excluded. It is rarely possible to diagnose FAS, and impossible to determine prenatally which infant will have FAE.

Fetal cells and fetal DNA in maternal blood

The concept of identifying and isolating fetal cells or fetal DNA in maternal blood is one that has been evaluated by numerous groups around the world for the past three decades. Such technology would ostensibly permit more effective screening for a wide variety of chromosome and mendelian disorders and allow for the non-invasive diagnosis of certain detectable fetal abnormalities. The presence of fetal cells in maternal blood was first documented by Walknowska et al.[96] when they found XY metaphases in maternal blood of pregnant women carrying male fetuses. During the late 1970s, Herzenberg et al.[97] and Iverson et al.[98] applied flow sorting technology to enrich for fetal cells. Their experimental design used HLA-A2-negative women who had an HLA-A2-positive spouse (heterozygote or homozygote). Any A2-positive cells recovered by flow sorting presumably must be fetal in origin, that antigen having been inherited from the father. Subsequently, a number of centers around the world have investigated isolation and analysis of intact fetal cells from mother's blood for prenatal diagnosis. The Elias group was successful in detecting fetal aneuploidies, including trisomies 18 and 21, by sorting for CD 71, glycophorin-A positivity, cell size, and cell granularity followed by interphase fluorescent in situ hybridization with chromosome-specific probes.[99, 100] However, more recent work failed to develop techniques or processes that would provide a consistent number of fetal cells amenable to successful diagnostic protocols. Indeed, a National Institute of Child Health and Human Development conference recently reviewed the current status of work in the field of fetal cells in maternal blood and provided a clear consensus of the inadequacy of the methods used to date.[101] The rarity of fetal cells in maternal blood is likely an important factor in the inability to develop an effective screening program. However, this could be overcome by fetal cell culture, which if successful could obviously increase the absolute number of fetal cells present.

In contrast to diagnosis of fetal aneuploidy using intact fetal cells isolated from maternal blood, detection of fetal mendelian disorders by analysis of fetal cells does not necessarily require enrichment procedures.[102] PCR-based technology alone may suffice since DNA from any fetal cell should be reflective of fetal status. A circumstance permitting detection of a mendelian disorder through analysis of fetal cells or fetal DNA in maternal blood arises when the father is heterozygous (Aa) and the mother homozygously abnormal (aa) for an autosomal recessive trait. The normal allele, which may or may not be transmitted by the heterozygous father, should be readily detectable. If blood from the homozygous mother reveals DNA of the normal paternal allele (A), the fetus could be deduced to be heterozygous. An example of PCR in maternal blood to detect autosomal recessive disorder is identifying pregnancies at risk for fetal Rh(D) disease. The molecular basis for an individual being Rh(D)-negative (dd) is usually a gene deletion, d representing lack of the DNA sequence that if present encodes D. If the mother is Rh-negative and the father is homozygous for Rh(D) (Rh-positive), all fetuses must be heterozygous (Dd); every pregnancy would then be a risk for RhD-isoimmunization. If the father is heterozygous, however, the likelihood is 50% that the fetus would inherit his RhD gene and, hence, be affected; the other 50% of pregnancies would not be at risk for Rh-isoimmunization. Nested primers can be constructed so that the CE sequence is concurrently amplified, allowing an 'internal control' that assures lack of D is not the result of primers failing to anneal or absence of cellular DNA in the sample tested. Using such a strategy, Lo and coworkers[103, 104] studied 57 RhD-negative women throughout pregnancy. All RhD-positive fetuses in the second and third trimesters were correctly identified; 10 of 12 in the first trimester were also detected.

Initially, the discussion regarding RhD and other mendelian conditions implied that the fetal DNA to be analyzed is present in the nucleus. Actually, cell-free DNA is also present in maternal plasma and serum.[105, 106] The Elias group,[107] as well as others[108] have shown Rh(D) DNA in maternal serum of Rh negative women (dd) carrying heterozygous (Dd) fetuses. Indeed, the detection of free fetal DNA in maternal serum for prenatal RhD genotyping in cases of maternal alloimmunization is now beginning to be used clinically in Europe[109, 110] and is actively being studied in the United States.[111]

In the future, uses of fetal DNA and fetal cells in maternal blood for prenatal diagnosis will undoubtedly continue to expand. For example, preliminary reports have already shown applications for the prenatal diagnosis of such genetic disorders as cystic fibrosis, Huntington disease, Hb Bart disease, and β-thalassemia.[112–114] In addition, elevated levels of fetal DNA in maternal plasma may be predictive in the early development of preeclampsia.[115]

Newborn screening: principles and practices

Newborn screening may be defined as 'a population-based public health service applying preventive medicine systematically in defined regions to reduce newborn morbidity and mortality from certain biomedical and genetic disorders by using presymptomatic detection/diagnosis with dried blood specimens analyzed in central laboratories and employing automated procedures and linked to clinical follow-up programs. It should be emphasized that each aspect of the system from blood collection to follow-up care is essential for assurance of quality.

The fundamental principle for achieving benefits through newborn screening is illustrated in Figure 14.7. In essence, early diagnosis through newborn screening provides children with an opportunity for better outcomes when there is a detectable preclinical stage of a congenital disorder, ideally soon after birth, and effective, accessible therapy exists that prevents irreversible abnormalities such as severe morbidity (e.g., mental retardation) or death. Often, the biologic onset and symptomatic onset are chronologically close, and only limited time (days to weeks) exists from that stage to a 'point of no return' where irreversible pathology has supervened. The goals of newborn screening are summarized in Table 14.5. For most genetic diseases included in newborn screening programs, prevention of mental retardation and developmental disabilities has been the primary objective and indeed was the driving force for the advent of this

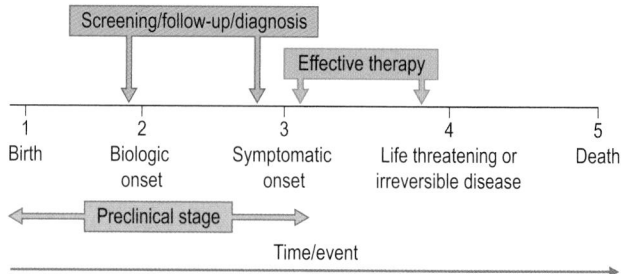

FIGURE 14.7 Principle of achieving benefits for infants through early diagnosis and therapy.

TABLE 14.5 GOALS OF NEONATAL SCREENING

PKU* and hypothyroidism – prevent MR/DD

Biotinidase – prevent DD and possibly deaths

Congenital adrenal hyperplasia – prevent neonatal deaths in males at risk for salt-wasting crisis and prevent incorrect gender assignment

Galactosemia – prevent MR/DD and infant deaths

Sickle cell disease – prevent deaths

Cystic fibrosis[†] – prevent malnutrition, hyponatremia, deaths and early progressive respiratory disease

Maple syrup urine disease[†] – prevent infant deaths and DD

Homocystinuria[†] – prevent MR/DD, thromboembolic episodes, and death

* PKU, phenylketonuria; MR, mental retardation; DD, developmental disabilities.
[†] Goals may not be fully achievable.

---

model public health initiative. Also, most of these disorders are autosomal recessive and very difficult to diagnose using the traditional history/physical exam strategy; even the very best pediatricians will fail to diagnose 'accurately and promptly' enough to prevent long-term adverse consequences.[1]

As described previously, the first newborn screening programs were implemented in the early 1960s for PKU,[10] a disorder associated with phenylalanine hydroxylase deficiency. Initially voluntary, the PKU test became mandatory by legislative actions throughout the US, such that by 1973 a total of 43 states had formal statutes. In general, state health departments, particularly their maternal and child health programs funded by Title V of the Social Security Act, assumed responsibility for implementing the new laws and ensuring neonatal blood collection and analysis. Thus, PKU became the prototype[116, 117] genetic disorder for newborn screening because it is very difficult to diagnose early in primary care practice, has a relatively short latent (preclinical) stage, a high risk for serious, irreversible pathology (mental retardation), and can be effectively treated using dietary phenylalanine restriction.[118] Although early implementation efforts were fraught with problems, attention to the entire newborn screening system led to quality improvement as centralized laboratories became responsible for the lab tests and a network of centers assumed the essential follow-up

TABLE 14.6 INCIDENCE OF GENETIC DISEASES INCLUDED MOST COMMONLY IN US NEWBORN SCREENING PROGRAMS

Condition[a]	Prevalence in US (approximate)
Congenital hypothyroidism	1:3000
Sickle cell disease	1:3000
Cystic fibrosis	1:4000
MCAD deficiency[b]	1:10 000
Congenital adrenal hyperplasia	1:15 000
Phenylketonuria	1:20 000
Galactosemia	1:70 000
Biotinidase deficiency	1:70 000
Homocytinuria	1:225 000 (?)
Maple syrup urine disease (branched-chain ketoaciduria)	1:250 000 (?)

[a] All autosomal recessive, except for some varieties of congenital hypothyroidism.
[b] MCAD, Medium-chain acyl-CoA dehydrogenase.

role. All states screen every newborn for PKU, but the analytical tests vary considerably from the original bacterial inhibition assay of Guthrie[5] to automated methods using sophisticated tandem mass spectrometry (MS/MS).[4] As described below under 'The Future of Newborn Screening' it is likely that the antiquated methods from the 1960s will be replaced by MS/MS.

All states also screen their newborn populations for congenital hypothyroidism using the same dried blood specimen and a variety of radioimmunoassay methods.[4] The testing protocols have varied and included simple measurement of blood thyroxin, a combination of thyrotropin and thyroid stimulating hormone (TSH), or TSH alone. There has been a trend to use primary TSH screening in recent years because it can be both effective and cost-effective.[5] As shown in Table 14.6, congenital hypothyroidism is almost seven times more common than PKU, and thus was very attractive in the 1970s to add to newborn screening panels, especially in view of the curative therapy available (thyroxine).[119] In the US, about 1200 confirmed cases per year are identified with an assumed sensitivity of 100%, specificity of 98.5%, and PPV of about 2%, i.e., 50 false positives for every diagnosis.[120] A variety of problems were encountered quite rapidly as implementation occurred nationwide[5,121,122] (e.g., imperfect sensitivity of laboratory protocols and follow-up problems), but congenital hypothyroidism screening has been a great success. In retrospect, the lessons learned from flawed implementation of PKU screening promoted an expeditious, constructive response of leaders that was very effective. AAP guidelines include the recommendations provided below.[123]

- Every infant should be tested before discharge from the nursery.
- In instances such as home births, or in the case of a critically ill or premature neonate, blood should be obtained within 7 days after birth.
- The responsibilities for transmission of screening test results back to the physician or hospital identified on the screening filter paper card should rest with the authority or agency that performed the test.

- Infants with low T_4 and elevated TSH concentrations have congenital hypothyroidism until proved otherwise.
- Administration of *l*-thyroxine is the treatment of choice.
- Routine clinical examination, including assessment of growth and development, should be performed at regular intervals, approximately every few months during the first 3 years.

Another hereditary endocrinopathy, congenital adrenal hyperplasia (CAH), is now tested for in about half the states as part of newborn screening programs. The goal of early diagnosis through neonatal screening is to prevent deaths associated with the salt-wasting form of the disease. This disorder is identified by radioimmunoassay of 17-hydropyprogesterone and is readily treated with cortisol replacement.[5,124] The major problem with CAH screening is the relatively low PPV of 0.5%, which leads to a large proportion of false-positive tests, especially in premature infants,[5] i.e., 200 for each diagnosis.[120]

Most states also screen newborns for galactosemia in an effort to prevent mental retardation (see Table 14.5). A variety of methods are used.[4] Classical galactosemia is caused by a deficiency of galactose-1-phosphate uridyl-transferase. A growing number are now screening for biotinidase deficiency, which develops because of an ability to recycle biotin. Both of these disorders occur with an incidence of 1:70 000 and thus are somewhat infrequently diagnosed, i.e., about 50 cases of each disorder per year among the approximate four million newborns in the USA. Delays in diagnosis, however, can be catastrophic for those 50 infants.

Other hereditary metabolic disorders are being included in newborn screening panels, although the value of early diagnosis is debatable for some conditions. For instance, both homocystinuria, which is caused by defective metabolism of sulfur-containing amino acids, and maple syrup urine disease (branched-chain ketoaciduria) screening were discontinued in Wisconsin because of their very low incidence (about 1:225 000) and uncertain benefits. Indeed, these two disorders do not meet the criteria used in Wisconsin[125,126] (listed below) or the World Health Organization (WHO) criteria.[127] With their low incidence, only about 18 cases of each disorder are likely to be diagnosed per year in the United States. Unfortunately, preventing mental retardation may not be feasible in the 20 states currently screening newborns. On the other hand, these disorders will progress and be life threatening or fatal with long delays in diagnosis, and their detection may be more feasible with new analytical, automated technology.

The implementation of tandem mass spectrometry has promoted screening for numerous disorders of amino acid and organic acid metabolism as well as disturbances in fatty acid oxidation (Table 14.7). Tandem mass spectrometry is arguably the most significant procedural advance in newborn screening since the 'Guthrie card' method of obtaining dried blood specimens was introduced in the 1960s. Consequently, the authors have included a detailed review of this technological advance. Prior to MS/MS, the laboratory strategy was to use a separate biochemical test or even two tests (e.g., congenital hypothyroidism and CF) for each disorder. Automated, computer-assisted MS/MS transformed that paradigm into a modern strategy of using that method to screen for multiple

TABLE 14.7 EXPANDED ACMG CORE PANEL OF NEWBORN SCREENING

1. Amino Acid Disorders
Arginosuccinic aciduria (ASA lyase deficiency)
Carbamoylphosphate synthetase deficiency
Citrulinemia
Galactosemia (classical)
Homocystinuria
Maple syrup urine disease (MSUD)
Phenylketonuria (PKU)
Tyrosinemia (type I)

2. Biotinidase Deficiency

3. Congenital Endocrinopathies
Congenital adrenal hyperplasia
Congenital hypothyroidism

4. Cystic Fibrosis

5. Fatty acid oxidation disorders
Carnitine uptake defect
Multiple acyl-CoA dehydrogenase deficiency (MADD or glutaric acidemia II)
Medium-chain acyl-CoA dehydrogenase deficiency (MCAD)
Trifunctional protein deficiency (TFP)
Very-long-chain acyl-CoA dehydrogenase deficiency (VLCAD)

6. Hemoglobinopathies: sickle cell disease
Sickle cell anemia
HB S/β Thalassemia
HB S/C disease

7. Organic acid disorders
Hydroxymethylglutaric aciduria (HMG-CoA lyase deficiency)
Glutaric acidemia type I (GA-I)
Isovoleric acidemia (IVA)
3-Methylcrotonyl-CoA carboxylase deficiency (3MCC)
Methylmalonic acidemia: methylmalonyl-CoA mutase deficiency (MUT)
Methylmalonic acidemia cBlA and cblB forms
Mitochondrial acetocetyl-CoA thiolase deficiency (Beta-ketothiolase deficiency)
Propionic acidemia (PA)
Multiple CoA carboxylase deficiency

8. Hearing impairment
*http://mchb.hrsa.gov/screening/

hereditary metabolic disorders. Nearly a quarter-century of evolutionary advances, however, was needed to reach the current status of routine MS/MS in newborn screening laboratories. The early phase depended on a combination of liquid chromatography and mass spectrometry detection of metabolite derivatives (analytes). By the 1990s, instrumentation advances with techniques such as fast atom bombardment and fast ion bombardment coupled to a series of units controlling separation, fragmentation, and detection set the stage for creating a high-throughput system employing electrospray ionization as the optimal sample delivery interface. With the addition of computed-assisted data monitoring, it became possible for a newborn screening laboratory to analyze up to 500 samples per day and screen for 30 or more disorders (see Table 14.7).

MS/MS-detectable hereditary metabolic disorders include aminoacidopathies, fatty acid oxidation deficiencies, organic acidemia disturbances, and urea cycle defects. The detection of aminoacidopathies and urea cycle disorders relies on determination of elevated amino acids such as phenylalanine for PKU and leucine/isoleucine/valine for MSUD. The abnormalities in fatty acid oxidation and organic acid metabolism are identified by measuring acylcarnitines, an intermediate metabolite consisting of a fatty acid or organic acid and carnitine, which is required for transfer across the mitochrondrial membrane for oxidation. Each disorder shown in Table 14.7 has a distinct profile of abnormal levels of specific acylcarnitines. Although these disorders are individually uncommon, when MS/MS as a single test is used to facilitate their early diagnosis, the cumulative incidence among newborns is approximately 1:4000 and thus is similar to congenital hypothyroidism and CF (see Table 14.6).

Decisions to add MS/MS and screen newborns with an expanded panel are being made in different regions based on a variety of criteria, including technical capability and financial capacity. When Wisconsin decided to proceed in 2000, it was clear that the predetermined criteria[125] summarized below were met.[128]

- In general, screening should not take place unless the disorder is recognized as an important public health problem for which there will be a commitment of financial support. Benefits to identified infants should outweigh the costs of the screening program.
- Incidence: The identification of 1 case per 100 000 births should be the minimum number of any specific disorder. With an annual birth rate of 70 000–75 000, Wisconsin should expect to identify approximately 1 case per year.
- Morbidity and mortality: Assessment of scientific evidence should support the expectation that benefits of identification in the neonatal period (treatment effective only when started before the age at which clinical diagnosis is usually made) will outweigh adverse consequences such as psychological effects on false-positive populations and the costs of screening.
- Potential for successful treatment: There should be evidence that effective management can be implemented to benefit infants and their families; diagnosis without effective treatment is inappropriate.
- Cost: Laboratory costs of any test to be added should be comparable to the costs of well-established tests such as PKU.
- Laboratory feasibility: Tests must be adaptable to a mass screening program. The health care system and laboratory technology limits tests to those that use blood specimens at this time.

Medium-chain acyl-CoA dehydrogenase deficiency (MACD) is the prototype disorder in this category and causes potentially fatal vomiting, lethargy, encephalopathy, hepatomegaly, seizures, and coma.[129] The approximate incidence is 1:10 000. Effective treatment to prevent crisis depends on a low fat, high carbohydrate diet. Early results of screening are promising.

When it became clear that penicillin prophylaxis could be life-saving for children with sickle cell disease (SCD),[73] hemoglobinopathy screening was incorporated into many programs

TABLE 14.8 NEWBORN SCREENING METHODS FOR CYSTIC FIBROSIS

Testing method	Description	Follow-up sweat testing
1. IRT	IRT analysis of the initial specimen obtained at 24–72 hours of life	Required
2. IRT/IRT	IRT analysis of the initial specimen obtained at 24–72 hours of life *plus* repeat analysis (to reduce false positive results) on a routine recall specimen	Required
3. IRT/DNA (ΔF508)[†]	IRT analysis of the initial specimen, with positive specimens subsequently tested for the ΔF508 mutation	May not be required if ΔF508/ΔF508 is detected but generally is required
4. IRT/DNA (CFTR)[†]	IRT analysis of the initial specimen, with positive specimens subsequently tested for a panel of the most common mutations in the region	Required

IRT, immunoreactive trypsinogen.

[†] Some programs have recently added a third tier with a follow-up IRT determination if the DNA analysis is negative (i.e., IRT/DNA/IRT).

and now is offered in 44 states. Originally depending on protein electrophoresis, after using cellular acetate, programs now use other molecular diagnostic methods such as isoelectric focusing and high pressure liquid chromatography.[4] Prevention of deaths associated with pneumococcal infections can be readily achieved in children with SCD,[73] and thus it seems surprising that some states don't include hemoglobinopathy screening in their panels. Although a lower incidence (e.g., 1:40 000) of SCD associated with regional demographic differences (i.e., a lower proportion of African-Americans) is offered as an explanation, some of these states screen for hereditary metabolic disorders that are even less prevalent.[8] This situation is typical of the regional disparities currently evident in the newborn screening programs of North America and suggests the need for national policy development.[8,126,127]

In the case of CF, approximately a quarter-century of extensive, well-organized research in North America, Western Europe, and Australia[11] led to national recommendations in 2004 by the Centers for Disease Control and Prevention (CDC). The recommendations summarized below are leading in turn to a nationwide expansion, beyond the 2 states with mandatory screening during 2004, as well as more clinical research on aspects ranging from screening protocols, described in Table 14.8, to assessment of follow-up quality and cost-effectiveness studies. The emphasis on prospective research on CF newborn screening is unique because in general only limited systematic outcomes research has occurred regarding other genetic conditions included in newborn screening panels. Other features are also unique, such as the screening test used most commonly which involves DNA analysis. Specifically, a two tiered method employing immunoreactive trysinogen (IRT) is used first and this is followed by DNA analysis for CFTR mutations when the IRT level exceeds a cutoff selected to maximize sensitivity. The IRT/DNA test was the first molecular genetics method applied to complete populations in community-based screening.[125] Because there are more than 1400 CFTR mutations, the DNA component has been challenging but fortunately about 70% of CF chromosomes have the principal and first mutation discovered,[61] namely ΔF508 (deletion of 3 bases at codon 508 and loss of phenylalanine in the mutant chloride channel protein). Furthermore, over 90% of CF patients in the USA have at least one ΔF508 mutation, so that simple IRT/DNA (ΔF508)

testing detects most of them and actually diagnoses half the CF population who are homozygous for ΔF508.[130] The IRT/DNA (ΔF508) screening test has the highest PPV (17%) among disorders on routine newborn screening panels.[125] In addition, there are advantages to using IRT/DNA (CFTR) multimutation analysis, and development of such tests is proceeding rapidly.[131] New analytical technologies such as multiplex, liquid chip methods[132] provide an opportunity to detect more than 50 CFTR mutations simultaneously within a few hours. As shown in Table 14.6, CF is relatively common among disorders included in newborn screening programs. In fact, CF is the most common, life-threatening autosomal recessive disorder among Caucasians, and over 1000 patients per year are diagnosed in the US.

Early diagnosis through IRT/DNA screening provides an opportunity to prevent the potentially fatal salt depletion with sweating, and the severe malnutrition that can cause long-term problems such as growth retardation and cognitive dysfunction.[12, 133] In addition, early diagnosis facilitates therapy of CF lung disease, although currently it can't be prevented.[12, 134] Nevertheless, CF illustrates the challenges that need to be addressed to enhance the quality of newborn screening programs, including: (1) improved testing protocols to optimize both sensitivity and PPV; (2) enhanced quality assurance with consistent policies; (3) better education of families and providers, especially in the prescreening, prenatal period; (4) improved risk communication for both true- and false-positive families, i.e., consistently informative genetic counseling; and (5) determination of cost-effectiveness to confirm the value of screening newborns at public expense. It is likely that CF newborn screening with IRT/DNA methods combined with tandem mass spectrometry will usher in a new era of expansion and accountability. The CDC has recognized the dynamic state of newborn screening with the recommendations summarized below.[135]

- The magnitude of the health benefits from screening for CF is sufficient that states should consider including routine newborn screening for CF in conjunction with systems to ensure access to high-quality care.

- In reaching a decision as to whether to add newborn screening for CF, states should consider available state resources and priorities as well as available national guidelines regarding CF screening, diagnosis, and treatment.

- States that implement newborn screening for CF should collect follow-up data in collaboration with CF care centers and analyze this information to monitor and improve the quality of CF newborn screening. In particular, states should collect, share, and analyze data by using standard protocols to evaluate and optimize laboratory algorithms used to screen for CF. States seeking guidance on optimal laboratory protocols might wish to consult with states having more experience in conducting CF screening of newborns.

- Newborn screening for CF should be accompanied by rigorous infection control practices to minimize the risk to children with CF detected at an early age of acquiring infectious organisms associated with lung disease from older patients. Further research is needed to evaluate and optimize these practices.

- Newborn screening systems should ensure parental and provider education and communication of screening results to primary care providers in a manner that will ensure prompt referral to diagnostic centers. For CF, these should be centers skilled in providing both sweat tests to young, presymptomatic children with CF and accurate and effective counseling to families, including those with infants identified as carriers. States are recommended to work with each other and with professional organizations and federal agencies to develop approaches to provide newborn screening information to parents during the prenatal and perinatal periods on all conditions, including CF, to facilitate informed choices and appropriate responses to positive screen results.

The future of newborn screening

Although the time frame for future evolution of newborn screening programs is difficult to predict, it is clear that more and better tests will be applied to newborn populations to ensure early diagnosis and hopefully reduce health disparities further. More precise and technologically advanced, though not necessarily more expensive, methods are readily available, such as tandem mass spectrometry and DNA analysis; these procedures are likely to be implemented during the next decade.

Clearly, tandem mass spectrometry is an evolution that is already causing a revolution. Not only are more regions implementing MS/MS, but it is causing an expansion of testing panels to literally quadruple overnight the number of congenital disorders being screened for routinely. Completion of the Human Genome Project has provided molecular genetics analytical biotechnology capability far beyond what is currently being used in newborn screening programs, but more DNA-based tests will emerge over time. Indeed, the CDC[136] referred to newborn screening for CF using IRT/DNA analysis as 'a paradigm for public health genetics policy development.' It is safe to predict that as DNA-based assessment of newborns for CF proliferates, other DNA tests will be implemented. For instance, CAH screening programs, because of their low PPV (about 200 false positives for every diagnosis),[120] could be improved quite significantly with a two-tier strategy using 17-

hydroxyprogesterone coupled to detection of 21-hydroxylase mutations.[5]

In addition to more and better tests, the glaring lack of consistencies among regions needs to be addressed effectively and eliminated. The variations relate to policies, financing, testing panels and protocols, follow-up efforts, and education. Consequently, the American Academy of Pediatrics Newborn Screening Task Force[8] has issued 'a call for a national agenda on state newborn screening programs.' Some of their most important recommendations follow.

- Federal agencies must take action to strengthen the public health infrastructure for newborn screening.
- State public health agencies should direct their newborn screening program to be consistent with professional guidelines and recommendations.
- States and state public health agencies should implement mechanisms to inform and involve health professionals and the public.
- States and state public health agencies should provide support for coordination and integration of program activities, including information and services.
- A federally-funded newborn screening research agenda should be outlined that aims to: develop better tests (more sensitive, more specific, and less costly); assess the validity and utility of new technologies (e.g., tandem mass spectrometry, DNA-based testing, and other evolving technologies); and define appropriate uses of residual biologic samples for a population-based research and surveillance.
- Pilot studies should be undertaken to demonstrate the safety, effectiveness, validity, and clinical utility of tests for additional conditions and new testing modalities.
- States should assure adequate financing of all parts of the newborn screening system: screening, short-term follow-up, diagnostic testing, comprehensive medical care/treatment, and evaluation of the system.

The AAP 'call for a national agenda' was followed by a landmark effort under the leadership of the American College of Medical Genetics (ACMG) to address some of the critical issues. Commissioned by the Maternal and Child Health Bureau of the Health Resources and Services Administration (US Department of Health and Human Services), a consensus-developing group of multidisciplinary experts published their analyses, conclusions, and recommendations recently in a document entitled "Newborn Screening: Toward a Uniform screening Panel and System" (*http://mchb.hrsa.gov/screening/*). This group recommended a core panel of 29 genetic conditions based on predetermined criteria "as primary targets for screening that warrant the full breadth of the newborn congenital adrenal hyperplasia, congenital hypothyroidism, cystic fibrosis, three hemoglobinopathies associated with the hemoglobin S allele, five disorders of fatty acid oxidation, six amino acidurias, and nine organic acidurias (see Table 14.7). Mutiplex technologies such as MS/MS will detect blood analyte abnormalities found in 23 of the 29 condtions of the core panel. The group also emphasized that newborn screening "programs are obligated to establish a diagnosis **and** communicate the result to the health care provider and family" and furthermore to make available the information "when newborn screening laboratory resutls definitely establish carrier status."

The AAP list of recommendations describes a wide range of issues that need to be addressed in quality improvement efforts. Enhancing quality assurance is difficult because although newborn screening is a system, its application varies markedly in different regions. In addition, as advances in biotechnology occur, the rate and effectiveness of implementation also vary. Furthermore, the ability of providers and parents to understand the laboratory results, whether they be diagnoses or false positives, is variable at best. Currently, about 5% of newborn screening tests are associated with a reportable result that needs to be explained to the parents. This amounts to 200 000 families per year in the United States or about 4000 per week (ironically, the same number as the total diagnosed through newborn screening on an annual basis). The communication challenges faced by providers are daunting. The content of the message, how and when to deliver the stress-promoting news to parents, and the kind of follow-up required are all difficult issues.[111] It is ironic that the biotechnology has advanced far beyond the capability of the system to meet the most fundamental of human interactions – communication. Clearly, more research is needed to improve risk communication methods and to evaluate their impact.

Despite the need for multidimensional improvement, it should be emphasized that newborn screening programs have been one of the great public health success stories. Thousands of children have benefited with reductions in mortality and morbidity. Even greater success will undoubtedly be achieved in the future.

Acknowledgements

This chapter was written as an expansion and modification of Dr. Renata Laxova's excellent contribution entitled 'Prenatal Diagnosis' (Chapter 7) in the previous edition. We thank Dr. Laxova, Emeritus Professor, University of Wisconsin for her contribution. In addition, we thank Dr. Elaine Zackai, Children's Hospital of Philadelphia (CHOP) for reviewing and approving components reproduced with minor revision herein. We are grateful to Gary Hoffman of the Wisconsin State Laboratory of Hygiene for providing information on advanced methods of newborn screening and to Drs Leeber Cohen and Ferideh Bischoff for providing Figures 14.1 and 14.2, respectively. We are also most grateful to Kathy Holland for expert typing and editorial assistance.

References

Prenatal diagnosis and neonatal screening

1. Farrell PM. Neonatal Screening: Toward earlier diagnosis and improved outcome. In: Doershuk C. Cystic fibrosis in the 20th century. Cleveland: AM Publishing; 2001:120–137.

2. Simpson JL, Elias S. Genetics in obstetrics and gynecology, 2nd edn. Philadelphia: WB Saunders; 2003.

3. Elias S, Simpson JL. Amniocentesis and fetal blood sampling. In: Milunsky A, ed. Genetic disorders and the fetus: diagnosis, prevention, and treatment. Baltimore: The Johns Hopkins University Press; 2004:66–99.

4. Therrell BL Jr. Laboratory methods for neonatal screening. Washington, DC: American Public Health Association; 1993.

5. Allen DB, Farrell PM. Newborn screening. Adv Pediatr 1996; 43:231–270.

6. American College of Gynecology. Prenatal diagnosis of fetal chromosomal abnormalities. Washington, DC: AGOC Practice Bulletin No. 27; May 2001.

7. American College of Gynecology . Neural tube defects. Washington, DC: ACOG Practice Bulletin No. 44; July 2003.

8. Newborn Screening Task Force. Newborn screening: a blueprint for the future. J Pediatr 2000; 106:389.

Evolution of prenatal and neonatal genetic screening

9. Resta RG. Changing demographics of advanced maternal age (AMA) and the impact on the predicted incidence of Down syndrome in the United States. Implications for prenatal screening and genetic counseling. Am J Med Genet 2005; 133A:31–36.

10. Guthrie R. The origin of newborn screening. Screening 1992; 1:5–15.

Diagnostic strategies

11. Hennekens C, Buring J. Epidemiology in medicine. Boston/Toronto: Little, Brown; 1987.

12. Farrell MH, Farrell PM. Newborn screening for cystic fibrosis: Ensuring more good than harm. J Pediatr 2003; 707–711.

13. Merkatz IR, Nitowsky, HM, Marci JN, et al. An association between low maternal serum α-fetoproteina and fetal chromosome abnormalities. Am J Obstet Gynecol 1984; 148:886–894.

14. Mennut MT, Driscoll DA. Screening for Down's syndrome – Too many choices? N Engl J Med 2003; 349;1471–1473.

Methods of prenatal diagnosis

15. Elias S, Simpson JL, Martin AO, et al. Chorionic villus sampling for first trimester prenatal diagnosis: Northwestern University Program. Am J Obstet Gynecol 1985; 152:204–210.

16. Elias S, Simpson JL, Shulman LP, et al. Transabdominal chorionic villus sampling for first-trimester prenatal diagnosis. Am. J. Obstet. Gynecol 1989; 320:609–617.

17. D'Alton ME, DeCherney AH. Prenatal diagnosis. N Engl J Med 1993; 328:114.

18. Kalousek DK, Dill FJ, Pantzar T, et al. Confined chorionic mosaicism in prenatal diagnosis/ Hum Genet 1987; 77:163.

19. Schreck RR, Falik-Borenstein Z, Hirata G. Chromosomal mosaicism in chorionic villus sampling. Clin Perinatol 1990; 17:867.

20. Seeds JW. Diagnostic mid trimester amniocentesis: how safe? Am J Obstet Gynecol 2004; 191:608–616.

21. Elias S.The role of fetoscopy in antenatal diagnosis. Clin Obstet Gynaecol 1980; 7:73.

22. Gosden C, Nicolaides KH, Rodeck CH. Fetal blood sampling in investigation of chromosome mosaicism in amniotic fluid culture. Lancet 1988; 2:613.

23. Tipton RE, Tharapel AT, Change HT, et al. Rapid chromosome analysis using spontaneously dividing cells from umbilical cord blood (fetal and neonatal). Am J Obstet Gynecol 1990; 161:1546.

24. Porreco RP, Harshbarger B, McGavran L. Rapid cytogenetic assessment of fetal blood samples. Obstet Gynecol 1992; 82:242.

25. Liou JD, Chen CP, Breg WR, et al. Fetal blood sampling and cytogenetic abnormalities. Prenat Diagn 1993; 13:1.

26. Bryndorf T, Lundsteen C, Lamb A, et al. Rapid prenatal diagnosis of chromosome aneuploidies by interphase in situ hybridization: a one-year clinical experience with high-risk and urgent fetal and postnatal samples. Acta Obstet Gynecol Scand 2000; 79:8.

27. Nicolaides KH, Thorpe-Beeston JG, Noble P. Cordocentesis in assessment and care of the fetus. In: Eden RD, Boehm FH, eds. Assessment and care of the fetus. Norwalk, CT: Appleton & Lange; 1990:291.

28. American College of Obstetricians and Gynecologists. Neural tube defects. Washington, DC: ACOG Practice Bulletin No. 44; 2003.

29. van Zalen-Sprock, van Vugt JMG, et al. Ultrasound diagnosis of fetal abnormalities and cytogenetic evaluation. Prenat Diagn 1991; 11:655.

30. Nicolaides KH, Azar G, Byrne D, et al. Fetal nuchal translucency: Ultrasound screening for chromosomal defects in first trimester of pregnancy. Br Med J 1992; 304:867.

31. Nicolaides KH, Brizot ML, Snijders RJ. Fetal nuchal translucency: Ultrasound screening for fetal trisomy in the first trimester of pregnancy. Br J Obstet Gynaecol 1994; 101:782.

32. Wapner R, Thom E, Simpson JL, et al. First-trimester screening for trisomies 21 and 18. N Engl J Med 2003; 349:1405.

33. Stenhouse EJ, Crossley JA, Aitken DA, et al. First-trimester combined ultrasound and biochemical screening for Down syndrome in routine clinical practice. Prenat Diagn 2004; 24:774.

34. Ferguson-Smith MA. Which prenatal screening protocol? Prenat Diagn 2004; 24:761.

35. American College of Obstetricians and Gynecologists ACOG Committee Opinion No.296: Committee on Genetics. First-trimester screening for fetal aneuploidy. Washington, DC: ACOG, July 2004.

36. Laigaard J, Sørenson T, Fröchlich C, et al. ADAM-12: A novel first trimester maternal serum marker for Down's syndrome. Prenat Diagn 2003; 23:1086–1091.

37. Laigaard J, Chrisitansen M, Fröchlich C, et al. The level of ADAM-12 in maternal serum is an early first-trimester marker of fetal trisomy 18. Prenat Diagn 2005; 25:45.

38. Dugoff L, Hobbins JC, Malone FD, et al. First-trimester maternal serum PAPP-A and free-β subunit human chorionic gonadotropin concentrations and nuchal translucency are associated with obstetric complications: a population-based screening study (The FASTER trial). Am J Obstet Gynecol 2004; 191:1446.

39. American College of Obstetricians and Gynecologists. Ultrasonography in pregnancy. Washington, DC: ACOG Practice Bulletin. No. 58; 2004.

40. Crane JP, LeFevre ML, Winborn RC. A randomized trial of prenatal ultrasonographic screening: Impact on the detection, management, and outcome of anomalous fetuses. Am J Obstet Gynecol 1994; 171:392–399.

41. DeVore GR The routine antenatal diagnostic imaging with ultrasound study: Another perspective. Obstet Gynecol 1994; 84:622.

42. Grandjean H, Larroque D, Levi S. The performance of routine ultrasonography screening of pregnancies in the Eurofetus Study. Am J Obstet Gynecol 1999; 181:446.

43. Verlinsky Y, Cohen J, Munne S, et al. Over a decade of experience with preimplantation genetic diagnosis. Fertil Steril 2004; 82:295,

44. Grace J, Toukhy T, Braude P. Pre-implantation genetic testing. Br J Obstetr Gynecol 2004; 111:1165.

45. Elias S. Preimplantation genetic diagnosis by comparative genomic hybridization. N Engl J Med 2001; 345:1569–1571.

Genetic conditions of special concern and prenatal identification

46. Boué A, Boué J, Gropp A. Cytogenetics of pregnancy wastage. In: Harris H, Hirschhorn K, eds. Advances in human genetics, Vol 14. New York: Plenum; 1985:1–57.

47. Sanchez JM, Franzi L, Collia F, et al. Cytogenetic study of spontaneous abortions by transabdominal villus sampling and direct analysis of villi. Prenat Diagn 1999; 19:601.

48. Fritz B, Hallermann C, Olert J, et al. Cytogenetic analysis of culture failures by comparative genomic hybridization (CGH): Re-evaluation of chromosome aberration rates in early spontaneous abortions. Eur J Hum Genet 2001; 9:539.

49. Pauli RM, Reiser CA, Lebovitz RM, et al. Wisconsin Stillbirth Service Program: I. Establishment and assessment of a community-based program for etiologic investigation of intrauterine deaths. Am J Med Genet 1994; 50:116.

50. Hook EB, Hamerton JL. The frequency of chromosome abnormalities detected in consecutive newborn studies – differences between studies – results by sex and by severity of phenotypic involvement. In: Hook EB, Porter IH, eds. Population cytogenetics. New York: Academic Press; 1977:63–79.

51. Snidjers RJM, Nicolaides KH, eds. Ultrasound markers for fetal chromosomal abnormalities. New York: Parthenon Pub Group; 1995.

52. Mattei JF, Mattei MG, Aymé S, et al. Origin of the extra chromosome in trisomy 21. Hum Genet 1979; 46:107.

53. Hook E, Warburton D. The distribution of chromosomal genotypes associated with Turner's syndrome: livebirth prevalence rates and evidence for diminished fetal mortality and severity in genotypes associated with structural X abnormalities or mosaicism. Hum Genet 1983; 64:24.

54. van Tuinen P, Dobyns WB, Rich DC, et al. Molecular detection of microscopic and submicroscopic deletions associated with Miller-Dieker syndrome. Am J Med Genet 1988. 43:587.

55. Smith AC, McGavran L, Robinson J, et al. Interstitial deletion of (17)(p11.2p11.2) in nine patients. Am J Med Genet 1986; 24:393.

56. Ehlen T, Dubeau L. Loss of heterozygosity on chromosomal segments 3p, 6q and 11p in human ovarian carcinomas. Oncogene 1990; 5:219.

57. Fitzsimmons J, Droste S, Shepard TH, et al. Growth failure in second trimester fetuses with trisomy 21. Teratology 1990; 42:337.

58. Legare J, Sekhon GS, Laxova R. De novo translocation involving chromosomes 1 and 4 resulting in partial duplication of 4q and partial deletion of 1p. Am J Med Genet 1994; 53:216.

59. Kaback M, Lim-Steele J, Dabholkar D, et al. Tay-Sachs disease – carrier screening, prenatal diagnosis, and the molecular era: an international perspective, 1970–1993. JAMA 1993; 270:2307.

60. ACOG Committee Opinion No. 298, Prenatal and preconceptional carrier screening for genetic diseases in individuals of Eastern European Jewish descent. Washington, DC: ACOG.

61. Kerem B-S, Rommens JM, Buchanan JA, et al. Identification of the cystic fibrosis gene: genetic analysis. Science 1989; 245:1073.

62. Cystic Fibrosis Foundation. Patient Registry 1999 Annual Report. Bethesda, Maryland, September 2000.

63. Frangolias DD, Nakielna EM, Wilcox PG. Pregnancy and cystic fibrosis: A case-controlled study. Chest 1997; 111:963.

64. Genetic Testing for Cystic Fibrosis. NIH Consensus Statement, 1997.

65. Lemna WK, Feldman GL, Kerem B, et al. Mutation analysis for heterozygote detection and the prenatal diagnosis of cystic fibrosis. N Engl J Med 1990; 322:291.

66. Genetic Testing for Cystic Fibrosis. NIH Consensus Statement, 1997.

67. Mercier B, Verlingue C, Lissens W, et al. Is congenital bilateral absence of the vas deferens a primary form of cystic fibrosis? Analyses of CFTR in 67 patients. Am J Hum Genet 1995; 56:272.

68. Costes B, Girodon E, Ghanem N, et al. Frequent occurrence of CFTR intron 8 (TG)n 5T allele in men with congenital bilateral absence of the vas deferens. Eur J Hum Genet 1995; 3:285.

69. Kiesewetter S, Macek M, Davis C, et al. A mutation in CFTR produces different phenotypes depending on chromosomal background. Nat Genet 1993; 5:274.

70. Chillon M, Casals T, Mercier B, et al. Mutations in cystic fibrosis gene in patients with congenital absence of the vas deferens. N Engl J Med 1995; 332:1475.

71. Grody WW, Cutting GR, Klinger KW, et al. Laboratory standards and guidelines for population-based cystic fibrosis carrier screening. Genet Med 2001; 3:149.

72. The American College of Obstetricians and Gynecologist and The American College of Medicine Genetics. Preconception and Prenatal Carrier Screening for Cystic Fibrosis. Washington DC: ACOG; October 2001.

73. Gaston MH, Verter JI, Woods G, et al. Prophylaxis with oral penicillin in children with sickle cell anemia, N Engl J Med 1986; 314:1593.

74. Kan YW, Trecartin RF, Golbus MS, et al. Prenatal diagnosis of β-thalassemia and sickle cell anemia: experience with 24 cases. Lancet 1971; 1:269–271.

75. Hagerman RJ, Silverman AC, eds. Fragile X syndrome: diagnosis, treatment, and research. Baltimore: The Johns Hopkins University Press; 1991.

76. Hoffman EP, Brown RH, Kunkel LM. Dystrophin: the protein product of the Duchenne muscular dystrophy locus. Cell 1987; 51:919.

77. Bakker E, Veenema H, den Dunnen JT, et al. Germinal mosaicism increases the recurrence risk for 'new' Duchenne muscular dystrophy mutations. J Med Genet 1989; 26:553.

78. Bell J. Dystrophia myotonica and allied diseases. Treas Hum Inherit 1947; 4:343.

79. Penrose LS. The problem of anticipation in pedigrees of dystrophia myotonica. Ann Eugen Lond 1948; 14:125.

80. Hecht BK, Donnelly A, Gedeon AK, et al. Direct molecular diagnosis of myotonic dystrophy. Clin Genet 1993; 43:276.

81. Aslanidis C, Jansen G, Amemiya C, et al. Cloning of the essential myotonic dystrophy region and mapping of the putative defect. Nature 1992; 355:548.

82. Jansen G, Willems P, Coerwinkel M, et al. Gonosomal mosaicism in myotonic dystrophy patients: involvement of mitotic events in $(CTG)_n$ repeat variation and selection against extreme expansion in sperm. Am J Hum Genet 1994; 54:575.

83. The Huntington's Disease Collaborative Research Group. A novel gene containing a trinucleotide repeat that is expanded and unstable on Huntington's disease chromosomes. Cell 1993; 72:971.

84. Gusella JF, Wexler NS, Conneally PM, et al. A polymorphic DNA marker linked to Huntington's disease. Nature 1983; 306:234.

85. Andrew SE, Goldberg YP, Kremer B, et al. The relationship between trinucleotide (CAG) repeat length and clinical features of Huntington's disease. Nature Genet 1993; 4:398.

86. Simpson S, Soeteweij MW, Nys K, et al. Prenatal testing for Huntington's disease: a European collaborative study. Eur J Hum Genet 2002; 10:689.

87. Sermon K, Goosens B, Seneca S. Preimplantation diagnosis for Huntington's disease (HD): clinical application and analysis of the HD expansion in affected embryos. Prenat Diagn 1998; 18:1427.

88. Evers-Kiebooms G, Nys K, Harper P, et al. Predictive DNA-testing for Huntington's disease and reproductive decision making: a European collaborative study. European J Hum Genet 2002; 10:167.

89. Riccardi VM. Neurofibromatosis, phenotype, natural history and pathogenesis, 2nd eds. Baltimore: Johns Hopkins University Press; 1992.

90. National Institutes of Health Consensus Development Conference. Neurofibromatosis. Arch Neurol 1988; 45:575.

91. Collins FS, Ponder BAJ, Seizinger BR, et al. The von Recklinghausen's neurofibromatosis region on chromosome 17 – genetic and physical maps come into focus. Am J Hum Genet 1989; 44:1.

92. Martin GA, Viskochil D, Bollag G, et al. The GAP-related domain of the neurofibromatosis type I gene product interacts with ras p21. Cell 1990; 63:843.

93. Xu G, Nelson L, O'Connell P, et al. An Alu polymorphism intragenic to the neurofibromatosis type I gene (NF1). Nucleic Acids Res 1991; 19:3764.

94. Kandt RS, Haines JL, Smith M, et al. Linkage of a major gene locus for tuberous sclerosis to chromosome 16 marker for polycystic kidney disease (Abstract supplement). Am J Hum Genet 1992; 51:A4.

95. Barlow SM, Sullivan FS. Reproductive hazards of industrial chemicals. London: Academic Press; 1982.

Fetal cells and fetal DNA in maternal blood

96. Walknowska J, Conte FA, Grumback MM. Practical and theoretical implications of fetal/maternal lymphocyte transfer. Lancet 1969; 1:119–1122.

97. Herzenberg LA, Bianchi DW, Schroder J. Fetal cells in the blood of pregnant women: detection and enrichment by fluorescence-activated cell sorting. Proc Nat Acad Sci USA 1979; 76:1453–1455.

98. Iverson GM, Bianchi DW, Cann HM, et al. Detection and isolation of fetal cells from maternal blood using the fluorescence-activated cell sorter (FACS). Prenat Diagn 1981; 1:61–73.

99. Price J, Elias S, Wachtel SS, et al. Prenatal diagnosis using fetal cells isolated from maternal blood by multiparameter flow cytometry. Am J Obstet Gynecol 1991; 165:1731–1737.

100. Wachtel SS, Elias S, Price J, et al. Fetal cells in the maternal circulation: isolation by multiparameter flow cytometry and confirmation by PCR. Hum Reprod 1991; 6:1466–1469.

101. Jackson LG. Fetal cells and DNA in maternal blood. Prenat Diagn 2003; 23:837.

102. Lo YMD, Pate P, Sampietro M, et al. Detection of single-copy fetal DNA sequence from maternal blood. Lancet 1990; 335:1463–1464.

103. Lo YMD, Bowell PJ, Selinger M, et al. Prenatal determination of fetal RhD status by analysis of peripheral blood of rhesus negative mothers. Lancet 1993; 341:1147–1148.

104. Lo YM, Hjelm NM, Fidler C, et al. Prenatal diagnosis of fetal RhD status by molecular analysis of maternal plasma. N Engl J Med 1998; 339:1734.

105. Lo YM, Corbatta N, Chamberlain PF, et al. Presence of fetal DNA in maternal plasma and serum. Lancet 1997; 350:458.

106. Lo YM, Tein MS, Lau TK et al. Quantitative analysis of fetal DNA in maternal plasma and serum: implications for noninvasive prenatal diagnosis. Am J Hum Genet 1998; 62:768.

107. Bischoff FZ, Nguyen DD, Marquez D-O, et al. Noninvasive determination of fetal RhD status using fetal DNA in maternal serum. J Soc Gynecol Invest 1999; 6:64.

108. Lo YM, Hjelm NM, Fidler C, et al. Prenatal diagnosis of fetal RhD status by molecular analysis of maternal plasma. N Engl J Med 1998; 339: 1734.

109. Randen I, Hauge R, Kjeldsen-Kragh J, et al. Prenatal genotyping of RhD and SRY using maternal blood. Vox Sang 2003; 85:300.

110. Finning K, Martin P, Daniels G. A clinical service in the UK to predict fetal Rh (Rhesus) D blood group using free fetal DNA in maternal plasma. Ann NY Acad Sci 2004; 1022:119.

111. Harper TC, Finning KM, Martin P, et al. Use of maternal plasma for noninvasive determination of fetal RhD status. Am J Obstet Gynecol 2004; 191:1730.

112. Gonzalez-Gonzalez C, Garcia-Hoyos M, Trujillo-Tiebas MJ, et al. Application of fetal DNA in maternal plasma: a prenatal diagnosis unit experience. Hisochem Cytochem 2005; 53:307.

113. Lau ET, Kwok YK, Luo HY, et al. Simple non-invasive prenatal detection of Hb Bart's disease by analysis of fetal erythrocytes in maternal blood. Prenat Diagn 2005; 25:123.

114. Li Y, Di Naro E, Zimmermann B, et al. Detection of paternally inherited fetal point mutations for β-thalassemia using size-fractioned cell-free DNA in maternal plasma. JAMA 2005; 293:843.

115. Farina A, Sekizawa A, Sugito Y, et al. Fetal DNA in maternal plasma as a screening variable for preeclampsia: A preliminary nonparametric analysis of detection rate in low-risk nonsymptomatic patients. Prenat Diagn 2005; 24:83.

Newborn screening: principles and practices

116. Scriver CR, Clow CL. Phenylketonuria: epitome of human biochemical genetics I. N Engl J Med 1980; 303:1336–1342.

117. Scriver CR, Clow CL. Phenylketonuria: Epitome of human biochemical genetics II. N Engl J Med 1980; 303:1394–1400.

118. Bickel H, Gerrard J, Hickmans EM. Influence of phenylalanine intake on phenylketonuria. Lancet 1953; 2:812–813.

119. Dussault JH, Coulombe P, Laberge C, et al. Preliminary report on a mass screening program for neonatal hypothyroidism. J Pediatr 1975; 86: 670–674.

120. Kwon C, Farrell PM. The magnitude and challenge of false-positive newborn screening test results. Arch Pediatr Adoles Med 2000; 154:714–718.

121. Fisher DA, Dussault JH, Foley TP. Screening for congenital hypothyroidism: Results of screening one million North American infants. J Pediatr 1979; 94:700–705.

122. Allen DB, Hendricks SA, Sieger JE. Screening programs for congenital hypothyroidism: How can they be improved? Am J Dis Child 1989; 142:232–236.

123. AAP Section on Endocrinology and Committee on Genetics, American Thyroid Association Committee on Public Health: Newborn screening for congenital hypothyroidism: Recommended guidelines. Pediatrics 1993; 91:1203–1209.

124. Pang S, Wallace MA, Hofman L, et al. Worldwide experience in newborn screening for classical congenital adrenal hyperplasia due to 21-hydroxylase deficiency. Pediatrics 1988; 81:866–874.

125. Farrell PM, Aronson RA, Hoffman G, et al. Newborn screening for cystic fibrosis in Wisconsin: First application of population-based molecular genetics testing. Wisc Med J 1994; 93:415–421.

126. Stoddard JJ, Farrell PM. State-to-state variations in newborn screening policies. Arch Pediatr Adolesc Med 1997; 151:561–564.

127. Wilson JMG, Junger G, Principles and practice of screening for disease. In: World Health Organization. Public Health Papers, No 34. Geneva: WHO; 1968.

128. Ciske JB, Hoffman G, Hanson K, et al. Newborn screening in Wisconsin: Program overview and test addition. Wisc Med J 2000; 99:38–42.

129. Roe CR, Coates PM. Mitochondrial fatty acid disorders. In: The metabolic basis of inherited disease, 7th edn. Scriver et al., eds. New York: McGraw Hill; 1995:1501–1634.

130. Gregg RG, Simantel A, Farrell PM, et al. Newborn screening for cystic fibrosis in Wisconsin: comparison of biochemical and molecular methods. Pediatrics 1997; 99:819–824.

131. Bobadilla JL, Farrell MH, Farrell PM. Applying CFTR molecular genetics to facilitate the diagnosis of cystic fibrosis through neonatal screening. Adv Pediatr 2002; 49:131–190.

132. Johnson SC, Marshall DJ, Harms G, et al. Multiplexed genetic analysis using an expanded genetic alphabet. Clin Chemistr 2004; 50: 2019–2027.

133. Koscik RL, Farrell PM, Kosorok MR, et al. Cognitive function of children with cystic fibrosis: deleterious effect of malnutrition. Pediatr 2004; 113:1549–1558.

134. Farrell PM, Li Z, Kosorok MR, et al. Bronchopulmonary disease in children with cystic fibrosis after early or delayed diagnosis. Am J Resp Crit Care Med 2003; 168:1100–1108.

135. Centers for Disease Control and Prevention. Newborn screening for cystic fibrosis: Evaluation of benefits and risks and recommendations for state newborn screening programs. MMWR 2004; 53(No. RR-13).

The future of newborn screening

136. Centers for Disease Control and Prevention. Newborn screening for cystic fibrosis: A paradigm for public health genetics policy development-proceedings of a 1997 workshop. MMWR 1997; 456(No. RR-16):11–12.

Pathology of the placenta

15

Theonia K. Boyd   Raymond W. Redline

As flies the wind, as flies the mind, as fly the winged birds, so do thou, O embryo.
Ten months old, fall along with the placenta! May the placenta fall down!

Atharva Veda (final of the four Vedas, ancient Hindu scripture)

Introduction

Why examine the placenta? The placenta provides a tissue record of the intrauterine environment in the evaluation of pregnancy gone awry. In some instances, the placenta is the only tissue present for pathologic evaluation (e.g., anembryonic early miscarriage, complete hydatidiform mole), in some instances both embryofetal and placental tissue are received for evaluation, and in some instances embryofetal tissue is present but not available for examination (e.g., live birth, intrauterine demise without postmortem consent). Except in the circumstance of an anomalous fetus, where the mechanism of aberrant pregnancy may be genetic and thus intrinsic to the conceptus, placental evaluation should no longer be considered an elective component of embryofetal examination. On the contrary, in phenotypically normal fetuses, particularly those lost in the latter half of pregnancy, the mechanism of demise will most likely be revealed not from fetal postmortem examination but from placental evaluation, in the context of maternal history. Fetal pathology in this setting is more useful for determining both the chronicity of stress prior to demise and the interval between demise and delivery.

This chapter addresses topics in placental pathology chronologically, as they arise during gestation. First there is a brief review of early embryogenesis, primarily to delineate the origins and significance of embryonic versus extraembryonic tissue derivatives. Second, there are considerations of placental pathology within the first trimester. Third, there is outlined a systematic approach to placental examination, applicable to second and third trimester singleton placentas (multifetal placentation is covered in Ch. 9). Last covered are placental pathology findings in the context of their clinical significance. Emphasized within this final section are constellations of pathologic features which, when present in combination, indicate specific clinicopathologic conditions; examples include amniotic fluid infection and maternal vascular underperfusion.

Placental origins[1-5]

The earliest cells destined to contribute to placental development are those of the blastocyst outer shell, the trophoblast, which are distinguished from the inner cell mass, the embryoblast, by 4 days postconception. Ultimately, extraembryonic derivatives within the placenta will include the chorionic epithelium and stroma, chorionic villous stroma and endothelium, and all trophoblast subtypes. In contrast, the amniotic epithelium and stroma, and umbilical cord are of embryonic derivation; hence the recognition of any one of these elements in the histologic evaluation of early miscarriage without a recognizable embryo reflects early embryogenesis with subsequent demise.

Blastocyst implantation occurs at about 6 days postconception, as trophoblast cells interdigitate between surface endometrial epithelia. Trophoblasts at the embryonic pole proliferate into two cell layers. By day 8 postconception, the invading front of trophoblast differentiates into a syncytium, thus establishing the syncytiotrophoblast phenotype. In contrast, the inner trophoblast cell layer retains its histologic discrete cell borders and physiologic generative capacity. As the trophoblast syncytium expands, spaces or lacunae form within the syncytium, and the resulting syncytial columns become referred to as trabeculae. By day 12 postconception, the blastocyst is fully embedded within the uterine wall, and although syncytial and trophoblast expansion occur circumferentially, proliferation is more robust at the embryonic pole. It is this region which will form the definitive placental disc.

The cytotrophoblast layer in contact with the blastocyst cavity forms the primary chorionic plate. Trophoblast cell columns derived from the primary chorionic plate invade the syncytial trabeculae, extending eventually to cover the exterior perimeter of the syncytial cells. This outermost layer subsumes the invasive function of the syncytium to establish the definitive implantation site. By this time, syncytial cells have already disrupted superficial endometrial capillaries, resulting in maternal blood cell trafficking into the syncytial lacunae. By day 13, lacunae fuse to form an interconnected reticular network – the primary maternal blood space. Next, outer shell trophoblasts initiate the first wave of invasion into the uterus, eroding spiral arterial walls and plugging the arterial lumens until about 10–12 weeks' gestation, when lumen recanalization establishes the definitive maternal-to-placental circulation (Fig. 15.1).

Primary villi, comprised of cyto- and syncytiotrophoblast, transform into secondary villi when at about 2 weeks postconception extraembryonic mesenchyme, located between the blastocyst cavity and the inner layer of the primary chorionic plate, extend into the primary villi to form the secondary villi. These mesenchymal cells are progenitor cells for the villous stroma, including villous capillaries. Once capillary formation is established, tertiary villi, also called mesenchymal villi, constitute ultimate villous structure. Further villous proliferation and expansion occurs by generational branching. Mature villous phenotypes can be divided into the following: stem villi, mature intermediate, and mature terminal villi. Stem villi are primarily transport villi, which contain muscularized villous vessels designed solely to carry blood. Intermediate villi contain both muscular arterioles and non-muscularized villous vessels surrounded by abundant villous stroma. Thus, the function of intermediate villi appears to be a hybrid of fetal blood transport and maternal–fetal blood constituent transfer. Transfer occurs with greatest efficiency within tertiary villi, where the villous capillaries abut the villous trophoblast membrane, permitting maximal opportunity for oxygen and nutrient transfer between the maternal and fetal circulations. Immature intermediate villi, histologically recognizable as intermediate villi invested by a double layer of cyto- and syncytiotrophoblast, can be seen late in gestation, reflecting the continual proliferative capacity of chorionic villi.

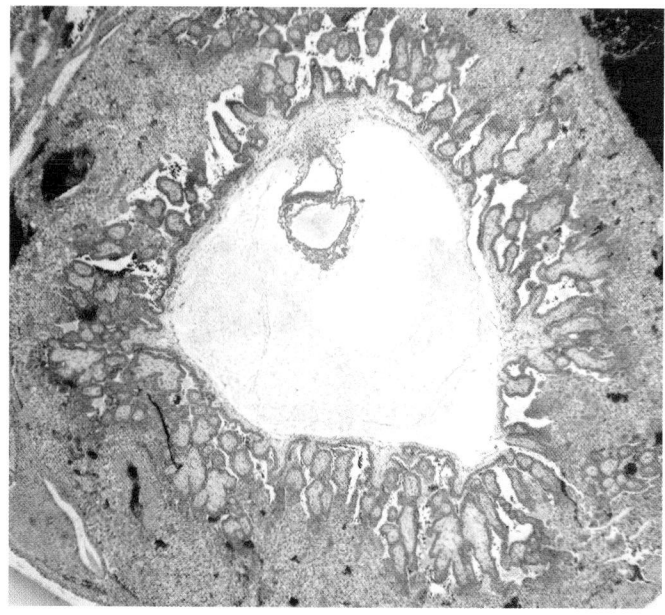

FIGURE 15.1 Blastocyst at about 13 days postconception. Note circumferential trophoblast columns extending centrifugally from secondary villi.

It is well to note that villous capillary formation and nucleated erythrocytes do not necessarily imply embryogenesis. Recent evidence suggests that the placenta, like the yolk sac and the floor of the aorta, constitutes an independent hematopoietic microenvironment.[6,7] The first nucleated erythrocytes appear within villous capillaries at 24 days of gestation. Under normal circumstances placental hematopoiesis ceases during the sixth week postconception, coincident with the onset of a continuous embryonic-to-placental circulation. These observations make it easier to explain why early complete hydatidiform moles may exhibit villous capillary nucleated red cells in the absence of an embryo proper.[8]

With polarized trophoblast proliferation, the definitive placenta localizes to the implantation area within the uterine wall, forming the chorion frondosum, and the remainder of the once-circumferential placenta regresses as the chorion laeve. In this location, within the extraplacental membranes, occasional remnant avascular chorionic villi can be seen throughout the remainder of gestation. Decidua present at the base of the definitive placental disc forms the decidua basalis, while decidua overlying the implanted embryo at the endometrial surface, apposed to the chorion laeve, becomes the decidua capsularis. As embryonic growth proceeds and the decidua capsularis moves into the uterine cavity toward the opposing uterine surface, the decidua capsularis contacts the opposing decidua parietalis. Extraplacental membranes are thus comprised of both these decidual layers, though physiologic degeneration of the decidua capsularis probably renders its contribution as minor.

In general, as placental development proceeds, placental growth occurs by increasing the number of villous generations of the fetal vascular tree, which expands both disc thickness and disc width. As villi mature, the phenotype of each villous type changes, but the maturational changes are most evident in the terminal villi. Circumferentially distributed syncytiotrophoblast nuclei redistribute to form clusters ('knots') which are polarized to one area of the terminal villus perimeter. As the cross-sectional size of terminal villi decreases, terminal villus capillaries become apposed to the cytotrophoblast membrane to form so-called vasculosyncytial membranes. This physiologic change permits maximal capacity of diffusible substances to cross the maternal–fetal blood barrier, comprised solely of cytotrophoblast and capillary endothelial cytoplasmic membranes. Maternal oxygen, nutrients, and protective molecules such as antibodies can thus be transferred efficiently to the fetal circulation. As a bidirectional process, fetal waste products, principally carbon dioxide, are transferred from the fetal to the maternal circulation. Mature villous stroma loses the 'watery' appearance of the immature, e.g., first and second trimester, phenotype, as stromal collagen deposition increases.

The functional compartments of the definitive placental disc are better conceived than seen as histologically discrete areas. Placental cotyledons, observed on the intact maternal surface, can be discriminated microscopically by the presence of placental septae, which represent decidual invaginations of the basal plate. A single cotyledon contains several lobules, which are the functional units of maternal intervillous blood flow as it relates to villous branching. A lobule is comprised of all villi surrounding a single spiral arteriole. Maternal intervillous blood drains into decidual veins, located between lobules. Although the maternal-to-fetal flow relationships are not directly visible microscopically, surrogate findings reflect flow structure. Stem villous trees positioned over oxygen-rich spiral arterial blood inflow tend to show more widely spaced villi, which are histologically less 'mature' than adjacent villi overlying draining maternal veins. Spacing results from spiral arterial inflow pressure, whereas variability in villous 'maturation' reflects the relative degree of intervillous oxygen available for maternal-to-fetal exchange (Fig. 15.2).

The first half of gestation: the first trimester and early second trimester

Early pregnancy rarely has specific placental correlates, since most early pregnancy loss is chromosomal, and thus intrinsic to the entire conceptus, without specific extraembryonic tissue correlates. The exception to this paradigm exists in molar gestations, which are covered in detail below. However, since early pregnancy loss often leads to examination of all products of conception, which are predominantly extraembryonic (villous) due to early embryonic demise, the following paragraphs cover general concepts in early pregnancy failure in addition to some specific pathologic conditions which manifest as early pregnancy loss, namely ectopic pregnancy and recurrent spontaneous abortion. Where relevant, extraembryonic (villous) correlates are discussed.

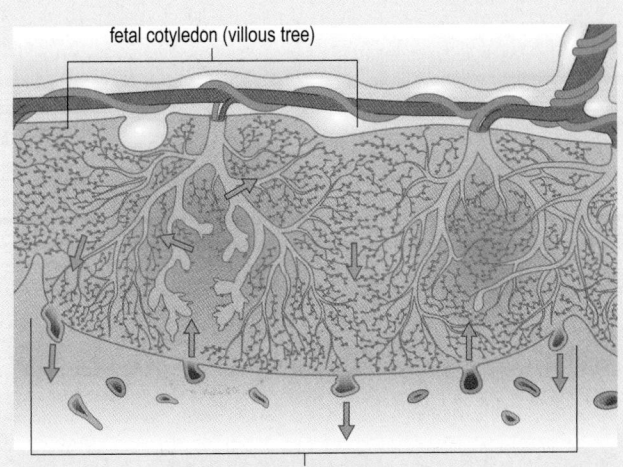

fetal cotyledon (villous tree)

Maternal cotyledon (placental lobule)

FIGURE 15.2 Functional relationship between villous trees emanating from the chorionic plate and maternal intervillous blood flow. All villous parenchyma surrounding a spiral arteriole constitutes a *placental lobule*. In this diagram there are two lobules within the depicted cotyledon. Note also the relative immaturity of villous architecture in contact with arterial inflow, compared to the villous architecture overlying venous drainage.

About half of all conceptions are lost within the first trimester of pregnancy, 50–75% of which are chromosomally abnormal.[9] Pregnancy loss in the first trimester is referred to as early miscarriage, or early spontaneous abortion. Tissues passed or extracted from non-viable early gestations are termed products of conception (POCs), and include both embryonic (embryofetal) and extraembyonic (placental) derivatives. Most of the time, tissue clinically designated as products of conception which have been removed iatrogenically by dilatation and curettage (D&C; dilatation and extraction, D&E) will be comprised, on gross examination, of fragmented chorionic villi, maternal decidua, and clotted blood. Sometimes, placental membranes or an umbilical cord segment will be visible. Less commonly, embryo-fetal fragments are present. In contrast, spontaneously passed products of conception sent to pathology are more likely to be received intact, in one of several forms. A decidual cast represents a gestational sac surfaced by maternal decidua. Internally, the sac may be empty, or it may contain an embryonic remnant ranging in gross appearance from an amorphous nubbin (nodular or cylindrical embryo) to a completely formed embryo (Fig. 15.3). At this gestational age, grossly visible malformations are difficult to identify (see Ch. 6). Rarely, a late first trimester spontaneous abortus will consist of an intact fetus, which may be attached to a grossly recognizable placenta, and which may be contained within an intact amniotic sac. Fetal malformations, if present, are easier to identify once fetal size and organogenesis have reached the limits of unaided visual resolution, or visual resolution using the aid of a dissecting microscope. In contrast, gross placental phenotype in any first trimester loss is, with rare exception, both non-specific and uninformative, except in the case of a partial or complete hydatidiform mole (discussed in

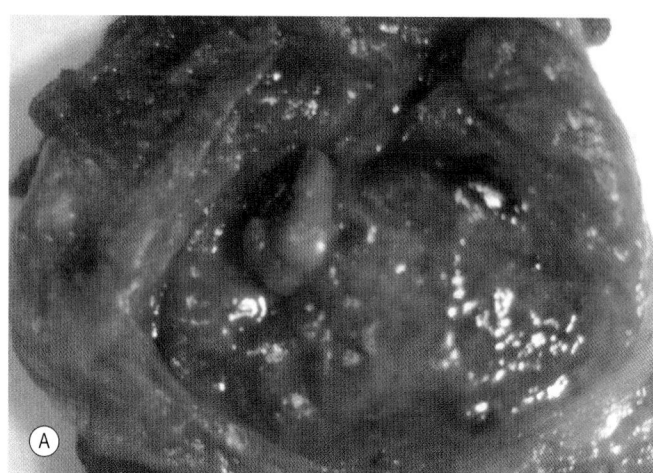

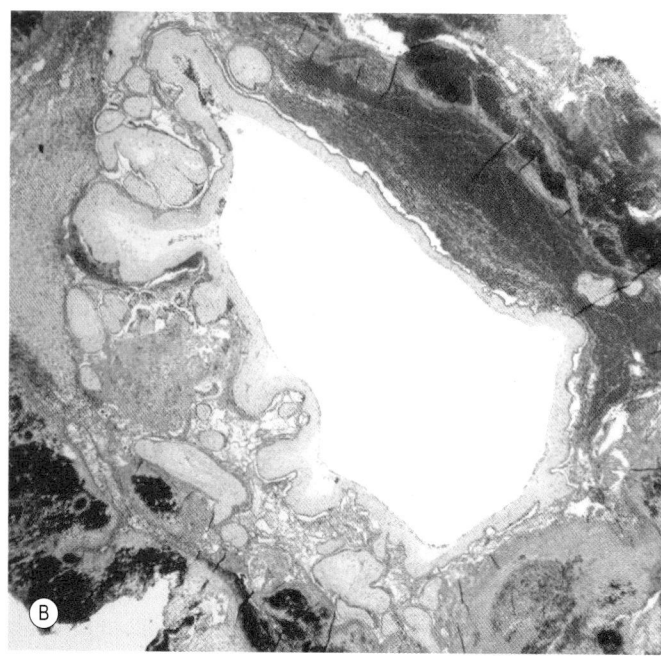

FIGURE 15.3 (A) Gross photograph of a nodular embryo within a decidual cast. (B) Histology of an anembryonic pregnancy ('empty sac') encased within a decidual cast.

detail below). Microscopically, the earliest villous change in a nonviable gestation is villous vascular karyorrhexis, reflecting karyorrhectic nucleated erythrocytes and/or karyorrhectic vascular endothelium. Histologic changes are usually more advanced by the time nonviable gestations are sampled in pathology, and more typically chorionic villi from early pregnancy losses exhibit one of two non-specific patterns, referred to as either hydropic or hyalinized changes. Hydropic villi contain a myxoid, watery stroma, which is paucicellular and usually avascular. Attenuated villous trophoblast surrounds the ballooned and simplified villous contour. Uniformly hydropic villi indicate early anembryonic pregnancy, clinically referred to as a blighted ovum (Fig. 15.4A). Hyalinized villi (also termed fibrotic or sclerotic villi) demonstrate a more collagen-rich, eosinophilic avascular stroma, containing stromal fibroblasts. Villous trophoblast is attenuated, as with hydropic villi, and surround a simplified oval villous contour. Hyalinized villi reflect gestational nonviability occurring after embryogenesis has been initiated (Fig. 15.4B). The two villous patterns of hydropic and fibrotic change can be intermixed. Other than reflecting whether pregnancy loss has preceded or followed embryogenesis, the appearance of chorionic villi in early miscarriage is non-specific; importantly, villous phenotype is an unreliable predictor of karyotype, except in molar gestations.[10–13]

Hydatidiform mole

Molar pregnancy occurs when the number of haploid chromosome sets of paternal origin exceeds that of maternal origin. In complete hydatidiform moles, the karyotype is diploid, reflect-ing the contribution of two haploid chromosome sets. The resulting karyotype contains 46 chromosomes, with 44 autosomes and 2 sex chromosomes. However, in contrast to normal diploid gestations, complete moles are entirely of paternal (androgenic) origin. Partial moles are comprised of three haploid chromosome complements, one of maternal and two of paternal origin. Karyotype contains 69 chromosomes; 66 autosomes and 3 sex chromosomes. In the genesis of a complete or partial mole, an excess of paternal chromosomes occurs in one of two ways: by fertilization of an oocyte with two haploid sperm, or by fertilization of an oocyte with a single sperm having a diploid chromosome complement. The fertilized oocyte is devoid of maternal chromosomes (an anucleate oocyte or 'empty egg') in the case of a complete molar pregnancy, whereas the oocyte contains a normal maternal haploid set of chromosomes at the time of fertilization in a partial mole.

Complete and partial moles have different but overlapping clinical and pathologic phenotypes. In general, patients with complete moles will present with higher maternal serum hCG levels, and by clinical examination will measure larger for dates than patients with partial moles. Ultrasonographically, more abundant molar tissue is present with complete moles, and evidence of embryonic development is absent except in the rare circumstance of a complete mole and coexistent non-molar twin, where evidence of embryogenesis is seen in tissues from the non-molar twin. In contrast, partial molar pregnancies frequently present with ultrasonographic and/or pathologic evidence of embryogenesis. Because excess trophoblast volume is pathogenetically linked to the risk of preeclampsia, patients with complete moles are more likely to manifest early-onset preeclampsia than are patients with partial molar pregnancies.

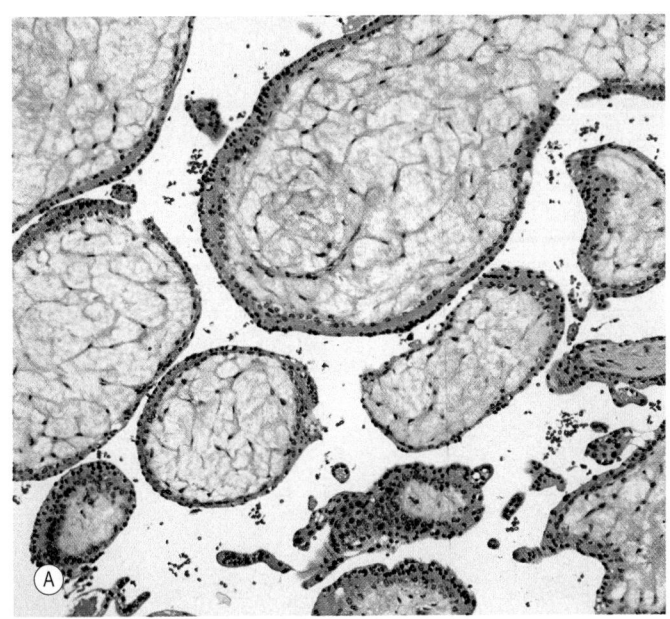

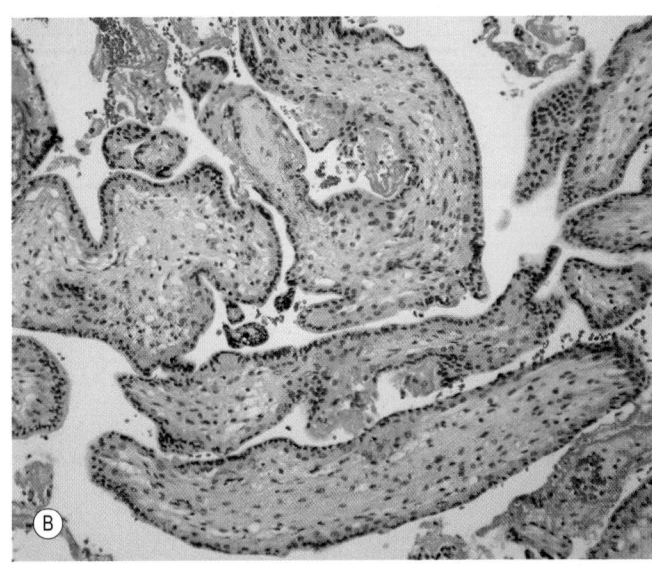

FIGURE 15.4 Characteristic but non-specific villous histology in first trimester losses. (A) Hydropic villi. (B) Fibrotic villi.

The significance of trophoblast proliferation in histologic differentiation of complete from partial moles is discussed in the next paragraph. Finally, patients with complete hydatidiform moles are at greater risk for persistent or recurrent gestational trophoblast diseases, namely persistent mole, invasive or deported mole, and choriocarcinoma, than are patients with partial moles. Recurrence risks for the former are reported in the range of 10–20%, while recurrence risks for the latter are about 3–5%. Post-evacuation monitoring of maternal serum hCG levels is standard practice in all molar pregnancies. Therapeutic intervention of persistent or recurrent disease involves local control, such as repeat dilatation and curettage, and/or systemic chemotherapy with methotrexate. Fortunately, gestational trophoblastic diseases resulting from molar pregnancies are exceedingly sensitive to chemotherapy. Long-term survival using chemotherapy in patients who present with metastatic disease is greater than 90%.[14]

Pathologic evaluation of molar pregnancies usually discriminates between the two phenotypes, complete and partial, without the need for excessive deliberation. Grossly, complete moles have diffusely hydropic and massively enlarged villi (from the Greek *hydatis*, meaning watery cyst), readily visible to the unaided eye (Fig. 15.5). Embryofetal tissues are not present. Partial moles, by contrast, may or may not have patchily distributed hydropic villi sufficiently enlarged to be grossly visible. While evidence of embryogenesis is almost always present microscopically, visible embryonic tissues (embryo proper, umbilical cord, amnionic membranes) may be absent. Microscopically, both complete and partial moles exhibit a constellation of features which characterize their histologic phenotypes. The hallmark feature of the **complete hydatidiform mole** is trophoblast proliferation involving all trophoblast compartments. In fully developed form, villi demonstrate circumferential proliferation of both cyto- and syncytiotrophoblasts. Extravillous trophoblasts are

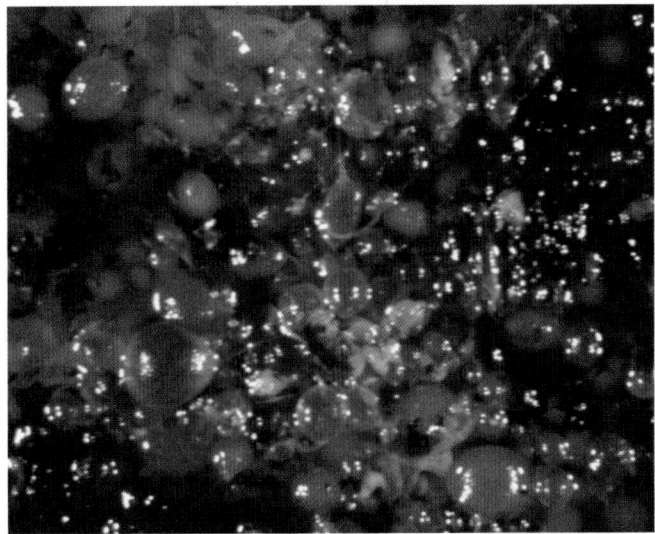

FIGURE 15.5 Gross photograph of a complete hydatidiform mole. Immersion in water has enhanced global villous hydrops. (Courtesy of Daniel Grimmer, MD, former resident, Dept. of Pathology, University of North Carolina Hospitals, Chapel Hill, NC.)

also expanded to produce clusters of cytologically atypical intervillous trophoblasts and proliferation of cytologically atypical implantation site trophoblasts (Fig. 15.6). As an aside, pathologic molar trophoblast proliferation should not be confused with physiologic early villous trophoblast expansion. In the latter, villous cytotrophoblasts demonstrate polarized expansion, in continuity with extravillous trophoblast columns. Cytologic atypia is absent (Fig. 15.7). In the former, villous cytotrophoblast proliferation is circumferential, and independent of excess intervillous cytotrophoblasts; both compartments show cytologic atypia. **Partial hydatidifrom moles** demonstrate

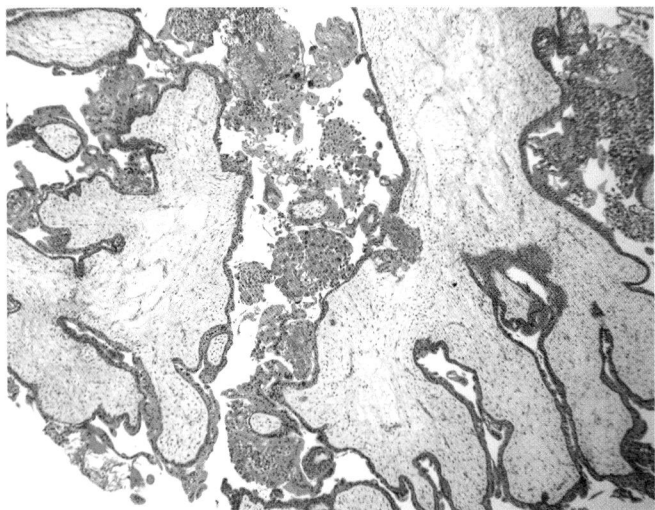

FIGURE 15.6 Complete hydatidiform molar histology. Note markedly enlarged chorionic villi with complex villous contours, circumferential villous cyto- and syncytiotrophoblast hyperplasia, and proliferation of cytologically atypical extravillous trophoblast.

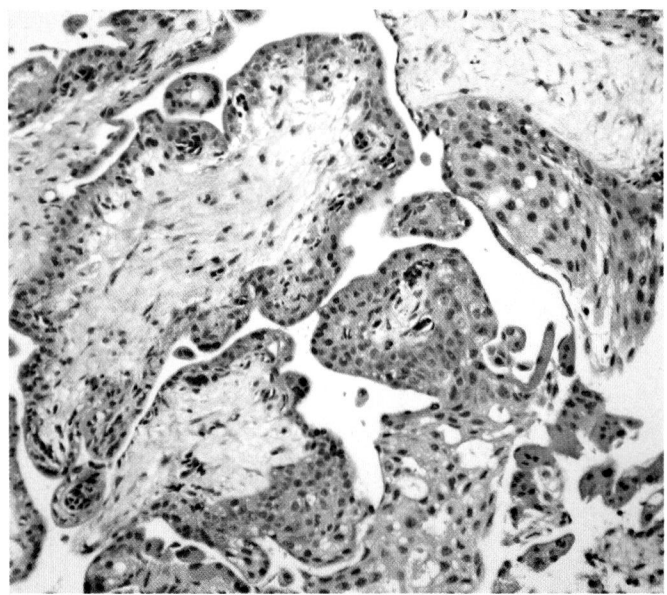

FIGURE 15.7 Normal first trimester villous histology. Note polarized cytotrophoblast columns with uniform trophoblast cytomorphology, in contrast to circumferentially proliferating and cytologically atypical villous trophoblast in complete moles.

variable proliferation of villous syncytiotrophoblasts; villous cytotrophoblast volume appears relatively normal. Intervillous and implantation cytotrophoblast expansion is modest at best, as is any degree of trophoblast cytologic atypia (Fig. 15.8). Villous contours are altered in both complete and partial moles. The complexity of villous infoldings and outpouching produces so-called villous scalloping; the infoldings, when cut perpendicular to their long axis, produce villous trophoblast clusters seemingly invested by villous stroma, resulting in so-called trophoblast pseudo-inclusions. While complete and partial molar villi are enlarged, complete moles show essential diffuse villous enlargement, whereas partial moles are characterized by variably enlarged to normal-sized and normal-appearing villi. Both complete and partial moles can exhibit a peculiar pattern of central villous stromal clearing, with margination of villous stromal cells around the periphery of so-called central cisterns. While villous capillary outlines may persist in both complete and partial moles, only partial moles will routinely exhibit

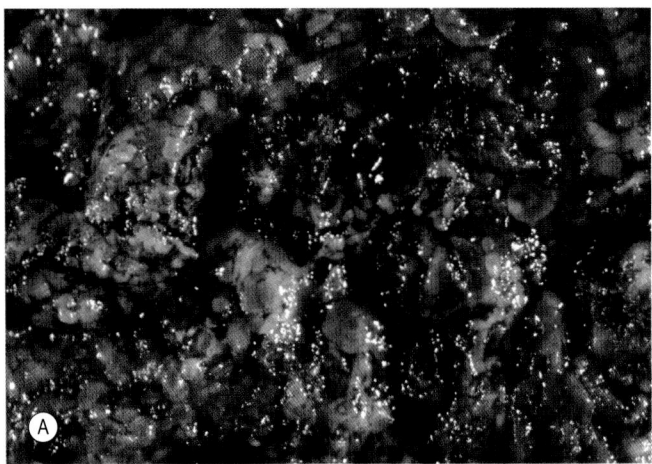

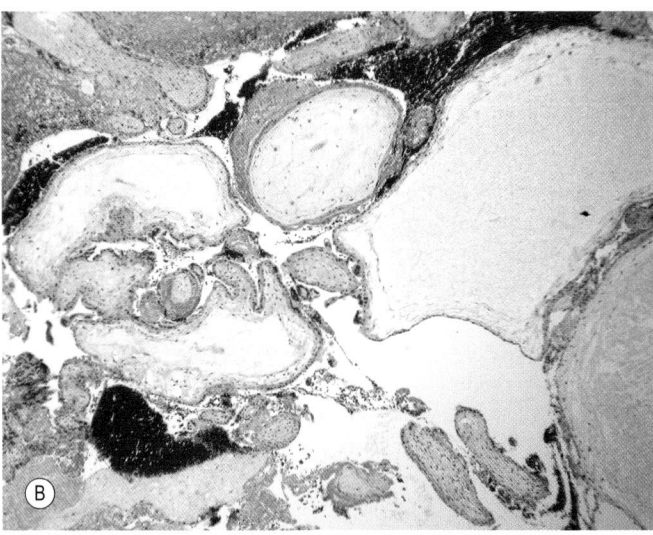

FIGURE 15.8 Partial hydatidiform mole. (A) Grossly, scattered hydropic villi can be identified. (B) Microscopically, a subpopulation of markedly enlarged villi is present; other villi are normal in size. This case demonstrates central villous cisterns and circumferential but modest villous syncytiotrophoblast proliferation.

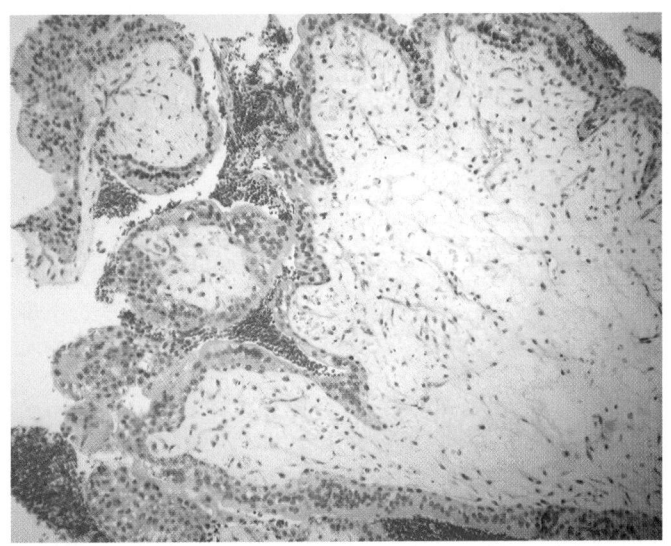

FIGURE 15.9 Very early complete hydatidiform mole. Note bulbous villous contours and the hallmark of complete moles: circumferential proliferation of villous trophoblast.

intravascular nucleated erythrocytes, reflecting embryogenesis. Other microscopic evidence of embryo formation, including somatic tissues, umbilical cord and amnionic membranes, is usually present with partial moles but should be absent in complete moles with two exceptions. First is the simultaneous presence of a complete mole and a non-molar twin, as has been discussed previously. The second exception to the complete mole/absent embryo paradigm occurs in the circumstance of very early complete hydatidiform moles, when on rare occasion inner cell mass derivatives (e.g., nucleated red cells, amnion, yolk sac) may be seen.[8] In these cases, the classic complete molar phenotype may be incompletely developed. Recognition of the following five histologic features is helpful in challenging cases: (1) bulbous terminal villi, (2) hypercellular villous stroma, (3) labyrinthine stromal canaliculi, (4) focal cyto- and syncytiotrophoblast hyperplasia on both villi and the subchorionic plate, and (5) atypical implantation site trophoblasts (Fig. 15.9).[15] In molar gestations, p57(KIP2), a cell cycle inhibitor and tumor suppressor, and the product of *CDKN1C*, an imprinted maternally expressed gene, is absent in complete molar trophoblast and diminished in partial moles, relative to strong expression in non-molar tissues. This differential p57(KIP2) expression can be utilized by immunohistochemistry in difficult cases.[16] Immunohistochemistry for PHLDA2 (also known as IPL and TSSC3), the product of a paternally imprinted, maternally expressed gene can be similarly employed.[17]

Ectopic pregnancy

Ectopic implantation usually occurs in circumstances of anatomic abnormality along the path of oocyte movement, between extrusion from the ovary and the intended destination within the uterine cavity. While on occasion the oocyte fails to enter the fallopian tube following fertilization, implanting somewhere within the pelvis or lower abdomen to produce an abdominal pregnancy, it is much more common for ectopic pregnancies to be identified clinically within the fallopian tube, resulting in so-called tubal ectopics.[18] Many more abdominal pregnancies are probably initiated than come to clinical attention, likely due to limited abdominal surfaces capable of sustaining implantation site maternal-to-placental flow, resulting in undetected early demise. Nevertheless, while sufficient intra-abdominal space exists to theoretically permit fetal growth throughout gestation, the limited capacity of extrauterine vessels to support fetal nutrition and oxygenation has rarely permitted extension of pregnancy until live birth.[19]

Tubal ectopic pregnancies are associated with factors that alter normal tubal anatomy, particularly with respect to the ability to promote movement of the oocyte along the tubal lumen. In current times, active salpingitis due to infectious sexually transmitted diseases (pelvic inflammatory disease, PID) is the most common reason luminal anatomy is distorted. Severe chronic active inflammation gives rise to tubo-ovarian abscesses. Ectopic implantation can occur anywhere along the length of the fallopian tube, including the fimbria. Removal of tubal contents with the intent of preserving integrity of the fallopian tube may make pathologic confirmation of an ectopic gestation problematic, as luminal contents are usually hemorrhagic and may contain only a small amount of gestational tissue relative to the volume of material extracted. Even with partial salpingectomy, it may be difficult to confirm ectopic products of conception, as early embryonic demise without a recognizable embryo often occurs in ectopic gestations. If the embryo or chorionic villi are not identified pathologically, a search for the implantation site by serial sectioning and sampling of the fallopian tube wall may yield diagnostic implantation site trophoblasts (Fig. 15.10). In cases of ruptured tubal ectopic pregnancy, the practice of sampling the area of mural disruption may be essential to identification of the implantation site, as the remaining products of conception may have been extruded into the peritoneal cavity. Finally, since some tubal ectopic implantations occur on the fallopian tube fimbria, thorough sampling of the fimbrial end of the tube may be necessary to identify the implantation area, particularly if the fimbria appear grossly hemorrhagic or disrupted. Microscopically, tubal products of conception appear identical to their intrauterine counterparts, save for implantation site trophoblasts percolating through the tubal rather than the uterine wall. Not surprisingly, gestational karyotype is not related to the likelihood of tubal pregnancy, since the risk factors are host (i.e., maternal) anatomic, not embryonic. Because tubal ectopic gestations are directly related to unmodifiable maternal factors, i.e., permanent tubal tissue damage, patients who have experienced one ectopic tubal pregnancy are at risk for recurrent pregnancy loss by the same anatomic mechanism. This phenomenon is probably heightened by the effects of necessary

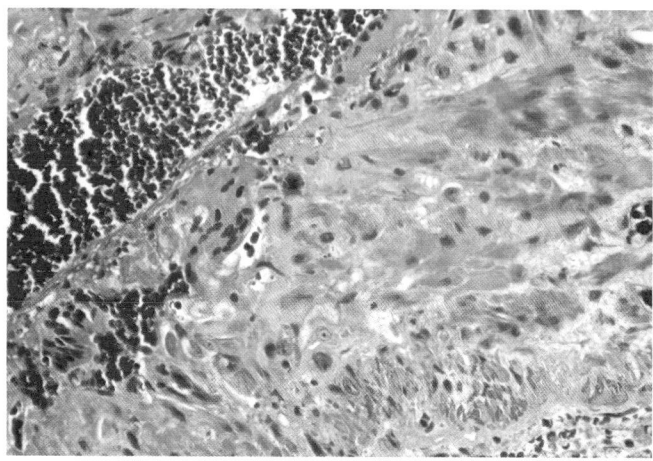

FIGURE 15.10 Fallopian tube implantation site. Note the presence of (1) implantation site trophoblasts interdigitated between smooth muscle fibers, and (2) a few mural surface syncytiotrophoblasts. These cells may be the only pathologic confirmation of ectopic implantation suspected clinically.

iatrogenic surgical intervention in ectopic tubal pregnancies, which further disrupts fallopian tube anatomic integrity.

Recurrent spontaneous abortion

Recurrent pregnancy loss is directly and solely related to parental factors which may recur in subsequent pregnancies. These factors may be chromosomal, anatomic or immune-mediated. In the first trimester, recurrent pregnancy loss may result from any one of these mechanisms. Karyotyped products of conception from patients with recurrent spontaneous abortions are more likely to be chromosomally normal than are karyotypes from sporadic spontaneous abortuses. This is due to the contribution of anatomic and immune-mediated mechanisms in recurrent loss, which operate independent of factors intrinsic to the conceptus, including embryofetal karyotype.

Chromosomal mechanisms which lead to recurrent pregnancy loss can be maternal or paternal in origin, and usually result from a **germ line balanced translocation**, whereby the parental diploid chromosome complement contains all portions of all chromosomes, but where two chromosomes have switched fragments with one another, leading to a portion of one chromosome attached to a portion of another. When chromosomes undergo meiosis, two unbalanced haploid chromosome sets will result if the translocated chromosomes segregate independently, thus producing a partial trisomic region in one germ cell and a partial monosomic segment in the other. Because balanced translocations involve germ line chromosomes, there is an unmodifiable risk for each fertilized embryo to contain unbalanced translocated chromosomes, leading to an embryonic-lethal karyotype. Because demise usually occurs before recog-

nizable embryogenesis, there are no specific embryonic or extraembryonic (villous) features. Approximately 5% of all recurrent pregnancy loss is attributable to parental germ line balanced chromosomal translocations.[20]

A few other rare mechanisms of genetically induced recurrent pregnancy loss have been described. Mothers who repeatedly conceive aneuploid gestations, usually trisomies, represent women with an inherent, presumed genetic, predisposition for **chromosomal non-disjunction**, independent of maternal age.[21] Pedigrees have been described where related women repeatedly conceive molar pregnancies. Apparent genetic heterogeneity exists in **familial hydatidiform moles**, though most consanguineous kindreds appear to bear a recessive locus at 19q13.4. Mutations in what has been postulated as a 'control gene' result in dysregulation of imprinting in the maternal germ line, resulting in unopposed expression of the paternal allelic gene(s) believed to be responsible for trophoblast proliferation.[22, 23]

Anatomic reasons for recurrent pregnancy loss are of course maternal in origin, and are related to the inability of sperm to reach the uterus and fallopian tube for fertilization to occur, or due to defective implantation of the fertilized embryo. The quintessential example of anatomic abnormality, tubal ectopic pregnancy, has already been covered. Rare other anatomic defects include Müllerian anomalies whereby normal fallopian tubes and ovaries are present in conjunction with an anatomically abnormal uterus, resulting in failure of effective embryo implantation and survival. Examples of such **uterine anomalies** include a unicornuate or globally hypoplastic uterus, the latter of which may result from embryofetal DES exposure in utero.[24] Defective implantation results in clinical infertility, whereas implantation with limited survival leads to recurrent early pregnancy loss. Embryofetal or placental tissues, if available for examination in these circumstances, will not manifest specific pathologic changes.

Immune-mediated mechanisms of early pregnancy loss are not well understood, either clinically or pathologically. Some couples experience recurrent early pregnancy losses without definable cause, even after genetic, anatomic, and hormonal causes have been excluded. Clinical treatment in these circumstances is largely empirical, and may include anti-inflammatory agents, steroids, other immune suppressive drugs, or anticoagulants in cases of suspected thrombophilia. However, a few clinical subsets of recurrent pregnancy loss patients have been partially characterized. Rarely, patients with autoimmune disease such as lupus erythematosus will present with early loss which is pathogenetically related to their autoimmunity. In one such case examined pathologically following dilatation and curettage, maternal decidual vessels exhibited severe decidual arteriopathy with fibrinoid necrosis and atherosis.[25] Products of conception did not exhibit specific pathologic features. Another presumed immune-mediated disorder of possible alloimmune etiology associated with recurrent pregnancy loss is **chronic histiocytic intervillositis**.[26–32] The histologic phenotype has also been described in the pathology literature as massive chronic intervillositis. The microscopic hallmark is of intervillous space plugging with an

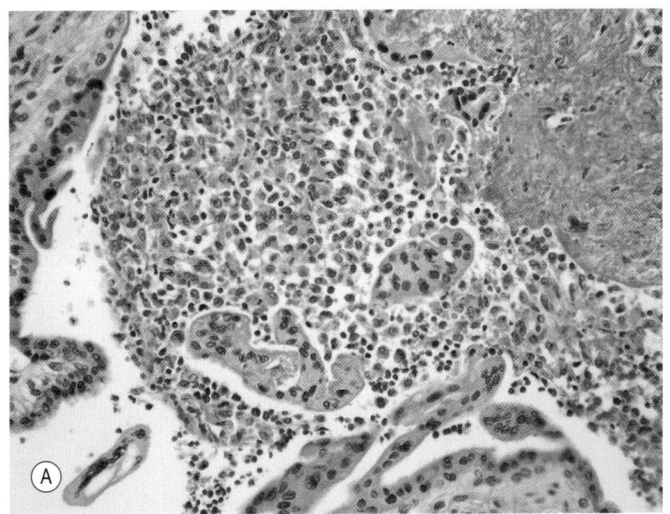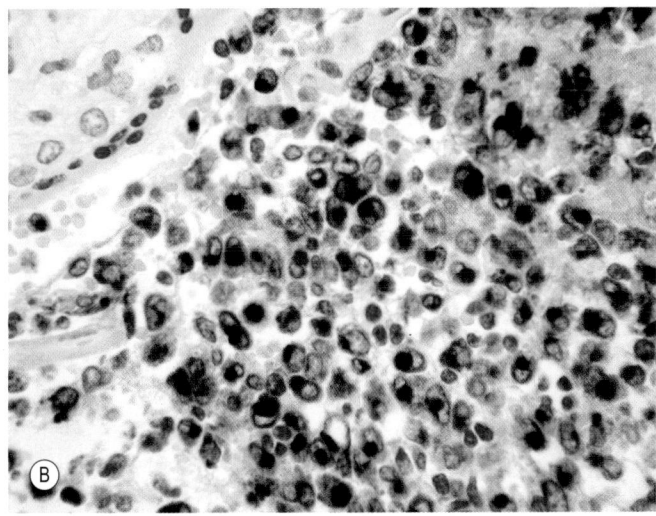

FIGURE 15.11 Chronic histiocytic intervillositis. (A) Intervillous histiocytes of maternal derivation, accompanied by intervillous fibrin. (B) Phenotypically mature histiocytes, demonstrated by CD68 positive cytoplasmic staining.

admixture of histiocytes and fibrinoid. Histiocytes, which are cytologically and antigenically mature (CD68 positive), are of maternal derivation. Intervillous fibrinoid, which accompanies the histiocytes, may lead to ischemic embryonic demise by space-occupying restriction of maternal intervillous blood flow. Chorionic villi encased in histiocyte–fibrinoid material are phenotypically normal, as histiocytes remain restricted to the intervillous space (Fig. 15.11). In other words, chronic villitis is not a feature of the lesion. Chronic histiocytic intervillositis is not confined to the first trimester, although the recurrence rate appears highest in this subset of patients. Chronic histiocytic intervillositis identified in later pregnancy may be associated with fetal growth restriction and stillbirth.

Infection

Infection leading to early pregnancy loss occurs, but much less commonly than in late miscarriages. In early losses, infection is more likely to be hematogenous than ascending, which is the reverse pattern of infection leading to untoward pregnancy outcome later in gestation. Currently in more affluent societies, the most likely hematogenously spread organisms to result in early pregnancy loss are **Parvovirus** and **Cytomegalovirus**. Herpes simplex virus, toxoplasma and other even rarer non-bacterial pathogens may also lead to early miscarriage. Histology in these cases is characteristic for the responsible pathogens, and is covered below, in Constellation Disorders.

Early pregnancy loss due to ascending bacterial infection, resulting in histologic chorioamnionitis, occurs rarely in the first trimester and uncommonly before the window of pregnancy where cervical incompetence manifests, namely the mid-second trimester. Histology is as with routine amniotic fluid infection.

The last half of gestation: systematic placental evaluation

Gross placental examination

Gross examination of the placenta should follow a routine methodology, as has been outlined previously.[33] Ideally, gross placental examination is performed fresh, following brief drainage and removal of non-adherent blood. While untidier than examination of formalin-fixed specimens, the benefits of fresh examination are many. First, lesions best appreciated by recognizing discoloration or abnormal texture can be altered or lost with formalin fixation. Second, special procedures requiring fresh tissue (culture, cytogenetics) cannot be performed on formalin-fixed material. Third, photography of placental lesions is most dramatic in the unfixed state. Fourth, formalin fixation increases placental weight on average about 6–10%; the range is wide, however (2–20%),[34] and therefore fresh weight cannot be reliably calculated from the fixed state.

Tissue procurement, if relevant, should occur prior to gross examination. Culture for infectious organisms is best accomplished by incising the chorionic plate and obtaining culture by swab or tissue removal beneath the amnion, in order to avoid surface contamination. Tissue for genetic studies is obtained sterilely, by incising the fetal or maternal surface of the disc, in order to expose and procure chorionic villi.

Gross examination can be subdivided into portions of the placenta which receive individual consideration and comment: the umbilical cord, the extraplacental membranes, the disc proper and its components: the fetal surface, the maternal surface, and the cut surface of the placental disc. Considering the qualities outlined below, begin by assessing the umbilical cord, then the extraplacental membranes, and the fetal and maternal surfaces. Following removal of the umbilical cord and extraplacental membranes, weigh the trimmed placental disc.

Serially section the disc at approximately 1–2 cm intervals, examining the cut surface of each section. Photograph important or demonstrative lesions. Remember that the most thorough gross examination of any tissue utilizes not only the visual sense but also tactile and, very occasionally, olfactory senses.

Standard sampling of the placenta for microscopy should follow a systematic approach. Two cross-sections of umbilical cord should be submitted, one each from the fetal and placental poles. A membrane roll should be taken, comprised of a narrow strip of a few millimeters in diameter to include the disc margin, which also samples peripheral chorionic villi and the so-called marginal sinus area (peripheral draining maternal veins). Alternatively, and in the authors' experience of lesser utility, some laboratories take a second membrane section which extends from the free membrane edge (point of rupture) inward toward the disc margin. At least two sections of placental disc should be taken centrally. Ideally, each section would include both the fetal and maternal surfaces, but if height prohibits full-thickness sections, then one section should include the fetal surface and the second should include the maternal surface. In addition to standard sections, grossly visible lesions should be sampled, particularly if the lesion is of indeterminate origin (and therefore of indeterminate significance) on gross examination. If multiple identical lesions are present, then representative sections will suffice. Some lesions that are of clear clinical significance but are patchy in distribution and not evident grossly may require multiple sections to examine microscopically. For example, in circumstances where decidual arteriopathy is suspected, generous sampling of the extraplacental membranes may be necessary.

Summarized below for easy reference are the aspects of gross placental examination requiring evaluation. More in-depth discussion of gross findings, in conjunction with microscopic findings and clinical considerations, follows in Pathologic Placental Findings of Clinical Significance in Mid- to Late Gestation and Their Mimics.

Umbilical cord observations:

- Insertion onto the placental disc (central, eccentric, marginal, velamentous, furcate – with distance from margin in centimeters);
- Length in centimeters;
- Number of vessels;
- Coiling; extent (maximum number of coils per 10 cm);
- True knot(s) versus varices (false knot[s]);
- Hue: overall color, discrete discolored lesions;
- Vessel caliber (e.g., ectasia, thrombosis, avolemia);
- Wharton's jelly abnormalities: compression, torsion, edema, deficient stroma; and
- Unusual contents: vitelline and urachal remnants, omphalocele.

Extraplacental membrane observations:

- Complete versus incomplete, intact versus fragmented;
- Insertion onto the placental disc: marginal, circummarginate, circumvallate;
- Hue: overall color, discrete discolored areas;
- Opacity versus transparency;
- Texture: edematous, diffluent (slimy);

- Abnormal structures: aberrant fetal vessels (e.g., vasa previa), fetus papyraceus; and
- Adherent material: surface meconium, retromembranous blood.

General disc observations:

- Weight;
- Dimensions (width × 2 by maximal thickness); and
- Shape (e.g., discoid, multilobate, accessory lobes).

Fetal surface (chorionic plate) observations:

- Arborization pattern of chorionic plate vessels;
- Chorionic plate vessel caliber and texture (e.g., ectasia, thrombosis, avolemia);
- Hue: overall color, discrete discolored areas;
- Opacity versus transparency;
- Texture: edematous, diffluent (slimy);
- Surface lesions: amnion nodosum, squamous metaplasia, yolk sac remnant; and
- Subsurface lesions: membrane cyst or hematoma; subchorionic fibrin, hematoma, chorangioma.

Maternal surface (decidua basalis) observations:

- Contour: normally convex versus regionally concave;
- Completeness: intact versus fragmented/missing cotyledons; and
- Adherent blood: recent versus remote hematoma.

Cut surface observations:

- Hue: color(s) (pale tan to burgundy);
- Texture: by palpation (spongy versus consolidated); and
- Lesions: consistency, location, size or percentage involvement.

Note: the range of visible parenchymal lesions on cut surface is wide, and may vary from clinically inconsequential, such as perivillous fibrin plaques, septal cysts or small chorangiomas, to clinically relevant such as multiple temporally heterogeneous placental infarcts, so-called maternal floor infarction, or a fresh intervillous hematoma in the setting of fetal–maternal hemorrhage. As an additional consideration, not all parenchymal lesions are recognizable on gross examination; microscopic exam is required to correctly identify many lesions which have non-specific gross appearances, such as the firm off-white nodule which may be an old infarct, an area of intervillous fibrin, or a region of avascular villi.

Pathologic placental findings of clinical significance in mid- to late gestation and their mimics

This section follows the order of gross placental observations enumerated in the section above.

The umbilical cord

Insertion onto the placental disc

The normal umbilical cord insertion is central or, more commonly, eccentric (paracentral). Normal cord insertion protects

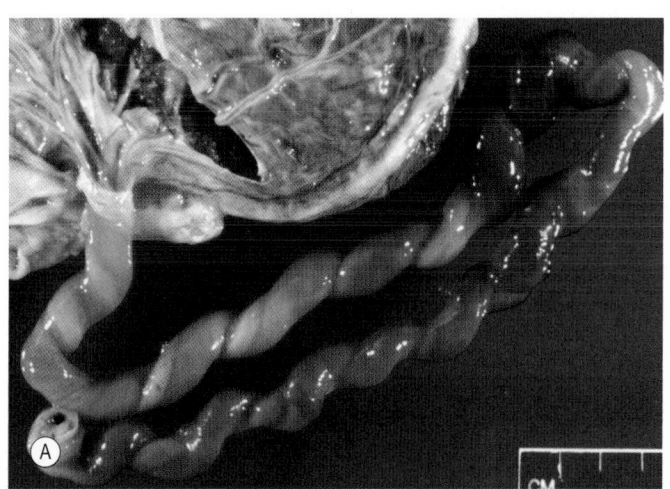
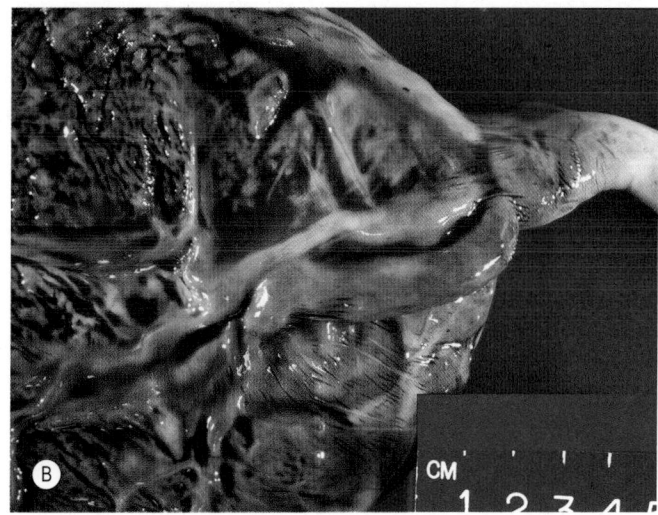

FIGURE 15.12 Abnormal umbilical cord insertion types. (A) Marginal cord insertion associated with hypercoiling and stillbirth. (B) Velamentous cord insertion associated with chorionic plate fetal vascular thrombosis and stillbirth.

the umbilical vessel branches, the chorionic plate vessels, as they splay out onto the chorionic plate surface. In the transition from the protective umbilical cord stroma of Wharton's jelly, vessels remain covered by the superficial stroma of the chorionic plate, and tethered to its deeper layers, thus protecting the vessel walls from the external mechanical forces of compression and tearing. When reporting cord insertion, always include the distance from the placental margin.

There are three types of abnormal cord insertions, which are presented in decreasing order of frequency. A **marginal** or **battledore insertion** is defined as one occurring within 1 cm of the placental disc margin (Fig. 15.12A). A **velamentous** or **membranous insertion** occurs when the umbilical cord inserts into the extraplacental membranes (Fig. 15.12B). A **furcate umbilical cord** demonstrates branching of the umbilical vessels above the chorionic plate, unprotected by Wharton's jelly. All three anomalous insertion types render the umbilical vessels and/or their chorionic plate tributaries more susceptible to compression and tearing, particularly velamentous and furcate insertions. Marginal cord insertions, while rendering umbilical vessels somewhat prone to compression, also increase the likelihood that first generation vessel branches will extend onto the extraplacental membranes, resulting in so-called intramembranous vessels, rather than splaying onto the chorionic plate. The risk of intramembranous vessels also exists with velamentous but not with furcate cord insertions.

Length

Normative values exist for umbilical cord lengths from the midsecond trimester through term.[35] Unlike placental weight norms, which have increased over the past several decades as newborn weights have increased, umbilical cord lengths have remained constant over time. In general, umbilical cord length

is positively correlated with intrauterine fetal movement: reduced activity is associated with shorter cords.[36] It is stated in the obstetrical literature that approximately 32 cm of umbilical cord length is the minimum required at term for uncomplicated fetal descent through the birth canal during the second stage of labor.[37] Shorter cord lengths may result in failure of descent, coupled with restriction of umbilical blood flow due to stretching tension and lumenal collapse. **Short total umbilical cord length** is associated with reduced intrauterine movement, which may be correlated with neonatal hypotonia, and relatively undercoiled umbilical cords. Both cord length and coiling reflect robustness of intrauterine activity. However, it is well to remember that the length of umbilical cord received in the pathology laboratory rarely reflects the entire umbilical cord length, unless the fetus and placenta are received attached by an intact umbilical cord. Thus, true umbilical cord length should be anticipated as longer than the cord length received, with variance depending upon cord segments which may have been retained for umbilical blood pH testing, or retained on the fetal abdomen, or discarded prior to receipt in pathology.

In contrast, **long umbilical cords** are always long for gestational age when compared to normative values, and are made longer if segments are retained prior to receipt in the pathology laboratory. Long umbilical cords are associated with increased fetal movement in utero, which is also correlated with increased cord spiraling. Additionally, long cords are associated with an increased risk of umbilical cord compression due to wrapping around the fetal body, most commonly as nuchal cords. It has been demonstrated clinically that nuchal or other body-wrapped cords are correlated with suboptimal neonatal presentation depending upon the number of cord wrappings around any body part.[38] Ultrasonographically, chronicity of cord wrapping as assessed at regular screening intervals also impacts neonatal presentation, presumptively due to the effects of prolonged, or intermittent and partial, umbilical blood flow restriction.[39, 40] In the second trimester, excessively long umbilical cords may be associated with intrauterine demise, possibly due to the inability of fetal blood pressure to ensure blood propulsion through the cord (personal communication, Dr. Ona Faye-Petersen). Curiously, second trimester demise associated with long, excessively spiraled cords may be recurrent.[41]

Number of vessels

The normal number of umbilical vessels is three: two umbilical arteries, which carry relatively deoxygenated blood from the fetal body to the placenta; and one umbilical vein, which delivers oxygenated blood from the placenta to the fetus. The definitive umbilical vasculature is derived from early embryonic allantoic vessels; a second embryonic vasculature, the vitelline or omphalomesenteric circulation, regresses under normal circumstances by about 6 weeks' pc (post conception). The umbilical vein enters the fetal circulation via the ductus venosus, which delivers oxygen and nutrient-rich blood between the left and quadrate hepatic lobes directly into the inferior vena near the right atrium. The umbilical arteries arise from the anterior branch of the internal iliac arteries to carry oxygen and nutrient-diminished blood back to the placenta. Once extrauterine life and blood flow are established, the umbilical vein is obliterated, forming the ligamentum teres. The umbilical arteries likewise obliterate to form the medial umbilical ligaments (medial umbilical folds), which are paired structures invested within the fascia and peritoneum of the anterior abdominal wall, situated lateral to the midline median umbilical ligament (median umbilical fold; former urachus).

A two-vessel cord represents a **single umbilical artery** (SUA); sometimes remnant smooth muscle fibers of the remotely involuted second umbilical artery are visible microscopically. While single umbilical artery is associated with a number of fetal anomalies (renal in particular) and syndromes, SUA is seen with much greater frequency as an isolated finding in otherwise normal placentas and fetuses. The exception to this statement is in the circumstance of sirenomelia, where somatic and visceral development below the umbilicus is variably deficient or absent. The external phenotype is one of a rudimentary fused and tapered lower extremity, reminiscent of the mermaid sirens from Greek mythology who lured seafarers with their haunting voices. Sirenomelic fetuses usually exhibit a two-vessel cord, comprised of a single artery entering the fetal abdomen centrally and inserting into the abdominal aorta at the level of the celiac trunk, which is absent. The single umbilical artery in sirenomelia thus represents a persistent vitelline circulation (see Ch. 4.2 and Fig. 4.2.4); absence of the allantoic circulation is evidenced by absent internal mesenteric circulation. In contradistinction, occasionally a vitelline vessel remnant remains patent in an otherwise normal three-vessel cord, visible microscopically and rarely on gross examination as a diminutive fourth vessel within the periphery of Wharton jelly.

Coiling; maximum extent (number of coils per 10 cm)

The umbilical cord coils or twists as umbilical vessels lengthen by spiraling around one another; whether arteries spiral around the vein or vice versa is debatable. In general, as gestation proceeds umbilical cord coiling becomes more pronounced on the surface of the umbilical cord. As with umbilical cord length, the extent of umbilical cord coiling is positively correlated with the extent of fetal activity in utero. Cord coiling is not solely determined by fetal activity, however, as evidenced by the observation that coiling is established within the first trimester, though the factor(s) which mediate directionality are not understood. Directionality of cord coiling is defined as follows: if the coil traverses upper left to lower right when the cord is examined vertically, equivalent to the left arm of a 'V', the cord is defined as having a left or counterclockwise spiral. Directionality of umbilical coiling is apparently of no direct clinical significance, despite the fact that left-spiraled cords are seven times more common than right helical cords. Mixed-direction coiling also occurs. Of clear clinical significance, however, are undercoiled and hypercoiled umbilical cords.[42–44] Under normal circumstances, the average value for umbilical cord coiling in uncomplicated live births is approximately 2 coils per 10 cm of cord length.[45] **Undercoiled or hypocoiled cords** (<10th percentile = <0.7 coils/10 cm, Fig. 15.13A) are associated with adverse fetal outcome in circumstances of chronically limited fetal motion in utero (e.g., gastroschisis with very short cord, forms of congenital hypotonia, mechanical movement restriction such as cornual pregnancy) and with other clinicopathologic conditions. **Excessively coiled or hypercoiled cords** (>90th percentile = >3 coils/10 cm, Fig. 15.13B) are also associated with adverse outcomes, including umbilical vascular thrombosis, cord torsion (Fig. 15.13C), fetal growth restriction and stillbirth. Umbilical cord coiling is not always uniform along the length of the cord; it may be greater at the fetal pole than elsewhere,[46] and may reverse direction along the cord length. The most dramatic example of differential coiling is in cases of excessively spiraled nuchal or body-wrapped cords, where the segment of wrapped cord is flat and non-spiraled, in contrast to hypercoiling along the remainder of the cord length (Figs 15.13D, and 15.14). A handy visual guideline to support hypercoiling is to note whether non-contiguous external surfaces of Wharton jelly become apposed to (come into contact with) one another as a result of spiraling; if so, the cord or its segment is likely to be hypercoiled by formal coiling index assessment.

Knots

Umbilical cord knots are divided into true knots and false knots (pseudoknots, varices). **Varices** are much more common than true knots, and represent localized vessel outpouchings due to kinking or ectasia. Varices are confined within Wharton's jelly, and rarely lead to compromised blood flow or thrombosis, despite their sometimes dramatic appearances. **True knots**, on the other hand, reflect an area of cord which has looped upon itself and knotted. All umbilical vessels are present within the

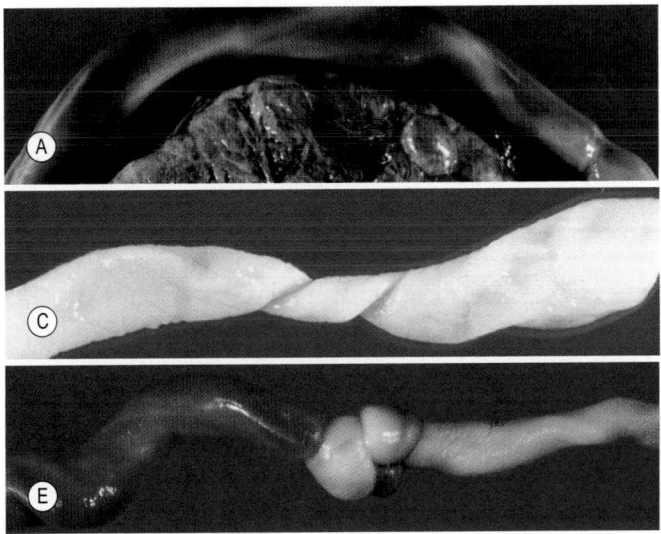

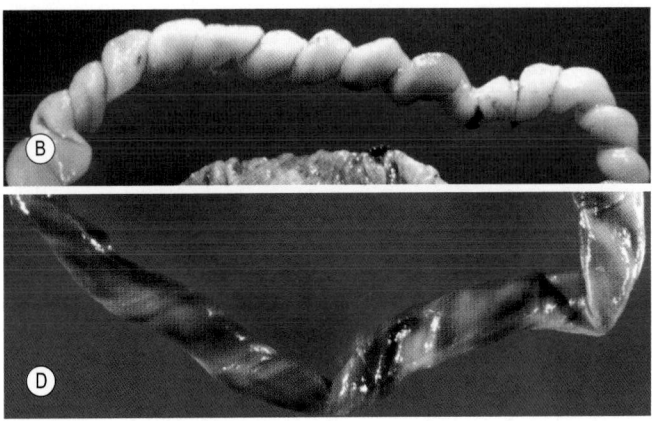

FIGURE 15.13 Abnormal umbilical cord presentations in stillbirth. All were associated with fetal vascular thrombosis except C. (A) Hypocoiled nuchal cord. (B) Hypercoiled cord. (C) Cord torsion. (D) Flat nuchal cord. (E) True cord knot.

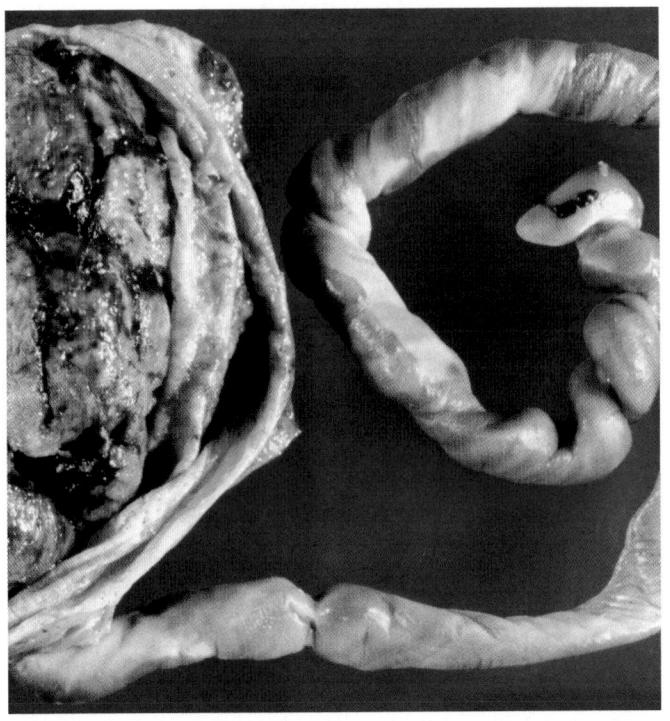

FIGURE 15.14 Regional variation in cord coiling. Flat, uncoiled nuchal/body cord at the placental insertion pole, with adjacent hypercoiling.

knot, and non-contiguous cord surfaces come into contact as a result of knot formation (see Fig. 15.13E). True knots occur as fetal activity loops the umbilical cord; the fetal body must then pass through the loop to create a non-reducible knot. While knots represent regions of increased-angle blood flow, there is usually no apparent adverse outcome at delivery. However, sometimes umbilical cord knots lead to intrauterine demise due to fatal blood flow restriction. When this is the case, secondary pathologic findings reflecting obstructed flow may be present,

increasing diagnostic certainty regarding the mechanism of demise. Potential secondary changes include differential vascular ectasia on opposing sides of the knot; differential discoloration of Wharton's jelly on opposing sides of the knot (Fig. 15.13E); or thrombosis; or marked compression of Wharton's jelly within the knot.

Hue; overall color, discrete discolored lesions

The normal umbilical cord is off-white and semiopaque. Discoloration of Wharton's jelly occurs in a handful of circumstances: with prolonged meconium discharge; with fungal or advanced funisitis; with umbilical vascular thrombosis; and secondary to intrauterine demise.

With **meconium** discharge, the umbilical cord is initially unstained, but assumes a green hue after some hours of meconium exposure; after more prolonged exposure, the umbilical cord may become green-brown to brown, similar to the temporal evolution of meconium discoloration of the extraplacental membranes and chorionic plate.

Peripheral (fungal) funisitis produces one of the few pathognomonic placental lesions: punctate opaque white microabscesses immediately beneath the external cord surface (Fig. 15.15). Advanced funisitis, by contrast, produces more generalized umbilical cord opacity due to the presence of acute inflammation which concentrically surrounds the periphery of one or more umbilical vessels, in a segmental to diffuse distribution along the cord length.

The umbilical vein is the usual site of umbilical vascular thrombosis. When **discoloration** accompanies thrombosis, in addition to vascular ectasia one may see burgundy to brown discoloration in a spiral distribution along the cord length. This observation reflects one of two secondary changes: the extravasation of blood breakdown pigment through the umbilical vascular wall, or altered hue due to tissue non-viability of the thrombosed vessel wall (remember, fetal blood participates in

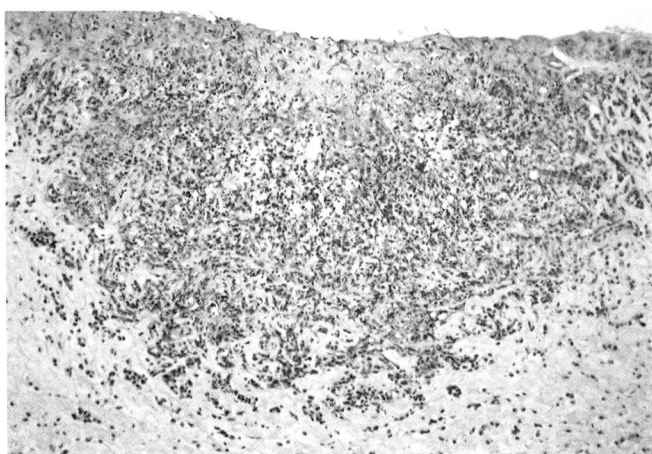

FIGURE 15.15 Peripheral (fungal) funisitis. Microabscess on the surface of Wharton jelly, surrounding superficially invasive candidal hyphae (PAS stain).

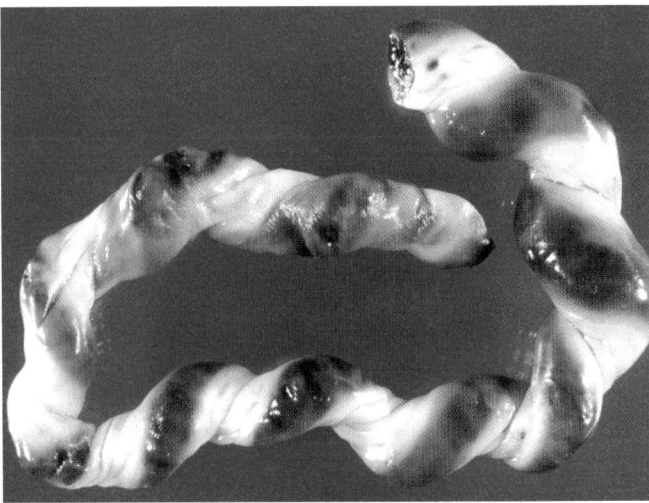

FIGURE 15.16 Spiral umbilical cord discoloration due to umbilical vein thrombosis.

nourishment of tissues adjacent to vascular lumens, including endothelium, vascular smooth muscle, and even the interior of Wharton jelly) (Fig. 16.16).

The principle of umbilical cord discoloration due to tissue non-viability also applies to the umbilical cord in cases of prolonged intrauterine demise before delivery. As the interval between demise and delivery increases, the umbilical cord may assume a progressively darker diffuse red-brown hue. Alteration in umbilical cord color does not always follow in linear fashion the demise-to-delivery interval, however, as has been shown previously.[47]

In general, microscopic evaluation of the umbilical cord is predictably disappointing when attempting to correlate gross discoloration with microscopic pigment deposition. In the latter two circumstances just described, thrombosis and IUFD, non-viable myocytes and stromal cells may be the only microscopically identifiable change. Even with gross meconium staining, meconium-laden Wharton's jelly stromal cells and macrophages are inconspicuous relative to their counterparts in the placental membranes. Meconium-laden stromal cells are most evident in cases of extensively prolonged meconium discharge, when dense meconium uptake appears deep within Wharton jelly. It is in this context that one may see meconium-induced umbilical vascular necrosis, with pigmented stromal macrophages admixed with pyknotic myocytes (Fig. 15.17). This same phenomenon occurs on the chorionic plate with chorionic plate vessels, and is discussed in greater detail below in 'Markers of Intrauterine Stress,' under the heading of 'Meconium.'

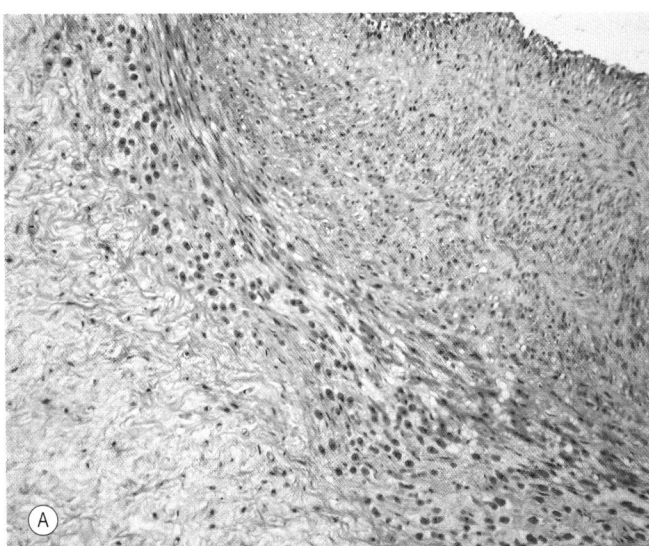

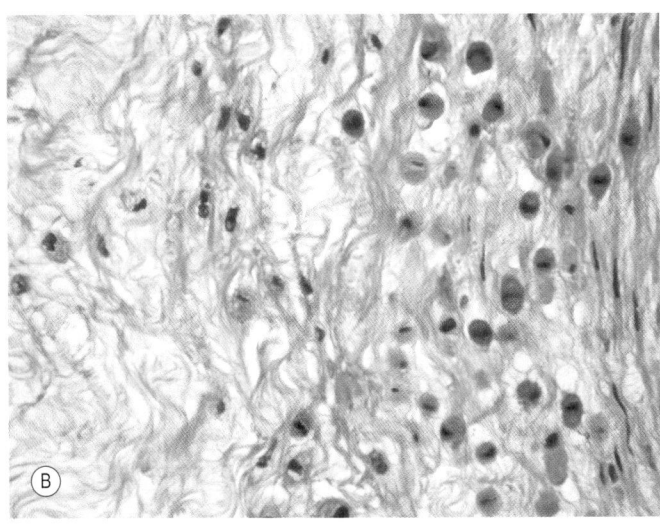

FIGURE 15.17 Meconium vascular necrosis. (A) The external perimeter of umbilical vessel myocytes are rounded and pyknotic. (B) Closer inspection reveals admixed meconium-laden macrophages on the right side of the photograph.

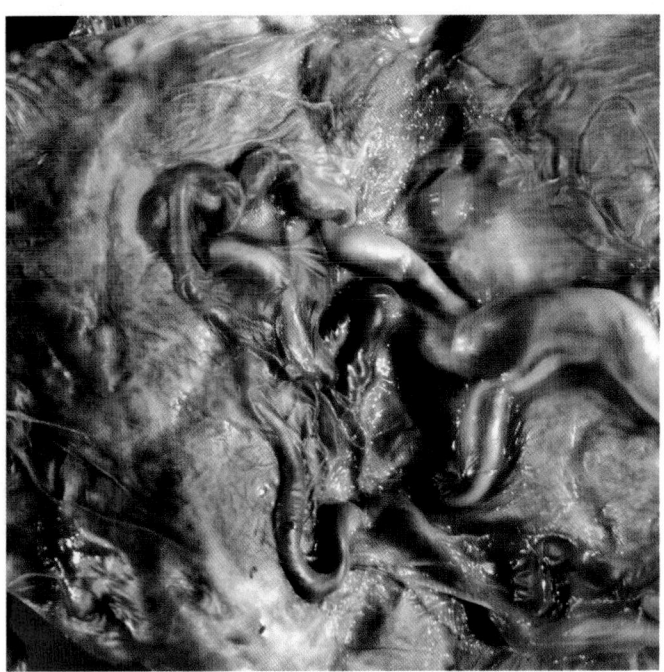

FIGURE 15.18 Thrombosed chorionic plate vessels. Some of the larger tributaries are partially calcified. The fetus was stillborn.

Vessel caliber

Meaningful aberrations of umbilical vessel caliber are identifiable segmentally or diffusely throughout the umbilical vessel length. **Ectasia** typically involves the umbilical vein, and when marked may indicate recent **thrombosis**. Established umbilical thrombosis is firm to palpation in the unfixed state, and blood is immobile when the vessel is compressed. Ectasia and thrombosis typically occur in situations due to non-acute mechanically restricted blood flow, including hypercoiling, true knots, and nuchal or body-wrapped cords. When ectasia, with or without thrombosis, involves umbilical vessels, chorionic plate vessels are also visibly dilated. In fact, these changes are best recognized within chorionic plate vessels, and are most dramatic at the umbilical cord insertion onto the chorionic plate (Fig. 15.18). This specific localization is likely due to the sharp angle produced by the first generation chorionic vessels as they branch off the umbilical cord, leading to angled blood flow under normal conditions. This lowers the threshold for superimposed mechanisms of flow restriction to produce vascular ectasia and thrombosis.

Markedly **hypovolemic** or **avolemic umbilical vessels** are seen with extreme fetal anemia or exsanguination, such as with fetal–maternal hemorrhage and ruptured vasa previa. This pattern of extreme hypo- to avolemia is also visible within chorionic plate vessels, and can be better appreciated there since more vessels are visible for gross observation, and since less stroma invests and obscures chorionic plate vessels relative to umbilical vessels. With lack of normal blood volume, blood vessel caliber narrows and may give the inaccurate gross appearance of obliterated vessel lumens. Usually, there is a mixture of avolemic and hypovolemic vessels, affecting both the arterial and venous

vascular trees. This widespread aberration in luminal diameter separates these pathologic conditions from the variation in vessel caliber one may see under normal circumstances.

Wharton jelly abnormalities

Abnormalities of Wharton's jelly which can be of pathologic significance per se involve narrowing and restriction of the cord: compression, torsion, or decreased hydration of Wharton jelly. Although **umbilical cord edema** may be dramatic, when present it usually accompanies widespread placental edema, and thus serves as a marker for whatever process has led to excess fluid in the extravascular placental and umbilical stroma. The subheading 'Villous Edema' is discussed below in 'Additional Microscopic Pathology by Placental Location.'

Umbilical cord flattening, or compression of Wharton jelly, is due to external mechanical forces, and is most readily seen with tight nuchal or body-wrapped cords, which result in segmental cord flattening in the region of cord compression against the fetal body part (see Fig. 15.13D). The significance of Wharton jelly compression, of course, is the increased risk for pathologic compression of umbilical blood vessels. It is important to note, however, that areas of the umbilical cord may appear flattened without identifiable clinical or pathologic cause. Furthermore, most segments of flat cord are not associated with clearly evident compromised blood flow; thus, the significance of Wharton jelly compression must be taken in the context of other clinical and pathologic findings. Additional mechanisms which may lead to pathologic cord compression include uterine space-occupying lesions such as a large submucosal leiomyoma, cornual pregnancy or midline uterine septum, and non-acute oligo-hydramnios, which renders the umbilical cord more susceptible to compression between the fetal body and uterine wall.

In contrast to umbilical cord compression, which involves a segment of cord, **umbilical cord torsion** refers to a discrete focus of hypertwisted cord, resulting in sharply angulated blood flow (see Fig. 15.13C). The most common location of cord torsion is at the fetal pole, where Wharton jelly is physiologically deficient relative to the remainder of the cord. Whereas hypercoiled umbilical cords exhibit sequential coils of angled flow, umbilical cord torsion may occur in the absence of generalized overcoiling. In cases of stillbirth exhibiting cord torsion without an other-wise identifiable cause of death, opinions are sharply divided regarding the probability that cord torsion can be fatal. In part, this reflects the opinion of some that cord torsion is strictly a postmortem phenomenon. Others reason that since fetal activity ceases at demise, postmortem torsion, presumably the result of fetal motion, is unlikely to occur. For skeptics of the latter opinion evidence of thrombosis, fibrosis, or mineralization in the con-stricted segment can help support antemortem onset of the constriction. Finally, by analogy, since other mechanisms of umbilical blood flow restriction are known to cause stillbirth (hypercoiling, nuchal cords, true knots), it stands to reason that torsion may be included in this group.

Deficiency of Wharton jelly can also refer to physiologically reduced hydration of the umbilical cord stroma leading to an overall **narrow ('thin') umbilical cord**. Narrow umbilical cords, defined as less than 0.8 cm in diameter in the 3rd trimester, are associated with growth-restricted fetuses and small placentas for gestational age. The generalized reduction of Wharton's jelly may in this group of fetuses render the cord more susceptible to external compression anywhere along its length.[48]

Unusual contents (vitelline remnants including vitelline vessels and omphalomesenteric duct structures; urachal remnants; Meckel diverticulum)

Most structures present within Wharton's jelly, other than the umbilical vessels, represent embryonic remnants of no clinical significance. **Vitelline structures** include vascular remnants of the vitelline circulation, which can be single diminutive vessels or multiple minute clustered channels, sometimes referred to as an umbilical or vitelline hemangioma. Curiously, with circumstances which herald an acute fetal inflammatory response, vitelline vessels exhibit diapedesis of fetal neutrophils, attesting to the integrity of the vitelline circulation with the systemic fetal circulation in utero.

The other vitelline (omphalomesenteric) embryologic remnant which may be found as an incidental observation occurs almost always as an epithelial nest in the periphery of Wharton jelly, between the umbilical vessels and the external cord surface. In the usual case, the epithelial cells are undifferentiated, vaguely resembling immature columnar cells clustered in a microscopic nest. In unusual circumstances, intestinal-type omphalomesenteric remnants may be well enough developed to recapitulate small intestinal morphology, replete with mucosa, submucosa, and muscularis propria. In these circumstances, the presence of such well-developed umbilical remnants raises suspicion for equivalently developed in vivo embryologic remnants, namely the presence of Meckel diverticulum (Fig. 15.19). A call to clinicians is warranted.

In contrast to the location of vitelline remnants, **urachal remnants** are positioned centrally, between the paired umbilical arteries. As with vitelline remnants, the epithelial cells are undifferentiated, though there may exist a resemblance to urothelium. Although the presence of a urachal remnant is nearly always an incidental observation, implications exist, albeit uncommonly, for later life. A patent urachal remnant in childhood or adulthood may present as a urachal cyst, manifest by serous drainage from the umbilicus, with or without midline mass effect. More ominously, urachal remnants may prove the source for adult-onset neoplasia, ranging in histologic presentation from urothelial cysts to adenocarcinomas of low malignant potential (so-called borderline tumors) to frank adenocarcinoma, all of mucinous type.[49]

The one clinically significant circumstance in which no umbilical pathology is evident is that of **acute umbilical cord prolapse**. Umbilical cord prolapse occurs during the intrapartum, when the umbilical cord slips past the presenting fetal part, and becomes wedged between the fetal body and uterine wall. This situation occurs before the fetal head or other presenting part is engaged low in the uterus, and following membrane rupture

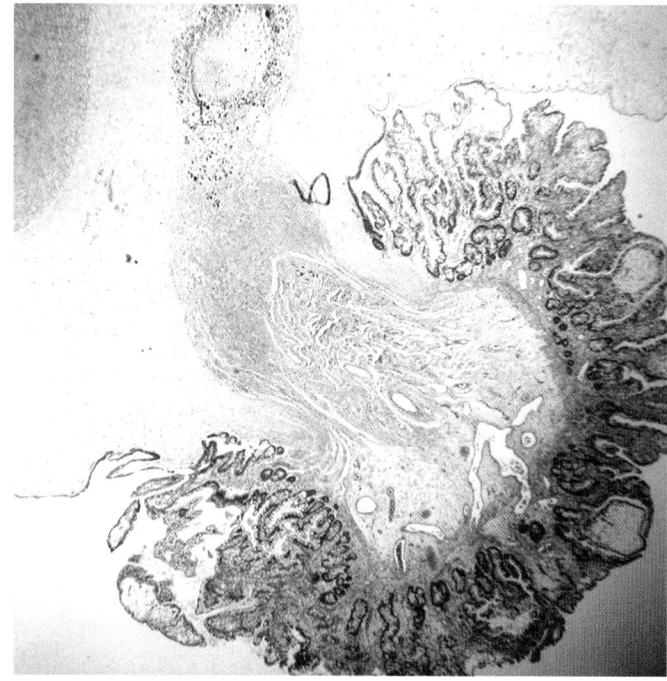

FIGURE 15.19 Well-developed omphalomesenteric duct remnant at the periphery of Wharton jelly. Mucosa, submucosa, and partial muscularis propria are recognizable. The patient may have a Meckel diverticulum as the in vivo component of this omphalomesenteric derivative. (Courtesy of David Genest, MD, formerly of the Division of Women's and Perinatal Pathology, Dept. of Pathology, Brigham and Women's Hospital, Boston, MA.)

when the amount of amniotic fluid is relatively decreased. Because enough room is needed for the cord to slip past the fetal body and into the vagina, umbilical cord prolapse is much more common with preterm premature membrane rupture. Since the umbilical cord carries the entirety of oxygenated blood through the umbilical vein to the fetus, acute cord prolapse is an obstetrical emergency, as fetal death may ensue within minutes of complete umbilical blood flow occlusion. And since cord compression occurs acutely, there is insufficient time for pathologically evident changes to evolve; rarely perivascular bleeding may be present, due to compressive disruption of umbilical vessel integrity.

Amnion and chorion

Placental compartments which include amnion and chorion are the extraplacental membranes and chorionic plate. Moving from the amniotic fluid contact surface inward, discernible layers are as follows: amnion derivatives, the amnion epithelium and amnion stroma; and chorion derivatives deep to the amnion, the chorion stroma and chorion epithelium. Because the amnion and chorion stroma layers become passively apposed to one another once the amniotic cavity fills the uterus, these two stromal layers can be distinguished microscopically as a separation plane, which is most readily seen with membrane edema. When the surface membrane becomes detached from the chorionic plate or extraplacental chorion/decidua, the detached tissue is seen microscopically as composed of amnion epithelium and stroma. This observation is occasionally of clinical significance, such as in cases of chronic amnion rupture leading to oligohydramnios and 'chorion nodosum,' that is, amniotic fluid squames and vellus hairs which become adherent to the neo-surface, the chorionic stroma. The other circumstance in which amnion detachment may be significant is in cases where it may be important to sample the deeper membrane layers, such as to search for decidual arteriopathy. Sampling the detached amnion alone is in this circumstance inadequate, since the extraplacental chorion/decidua is the tissue of interest. Further discussion of membrane abnormalities in this section will be restricted to the extraplacental membranes, unless the same principles also apply to the chorionic plate. Distinct chorionic plate abnormalities are covered as an entry later within this section.

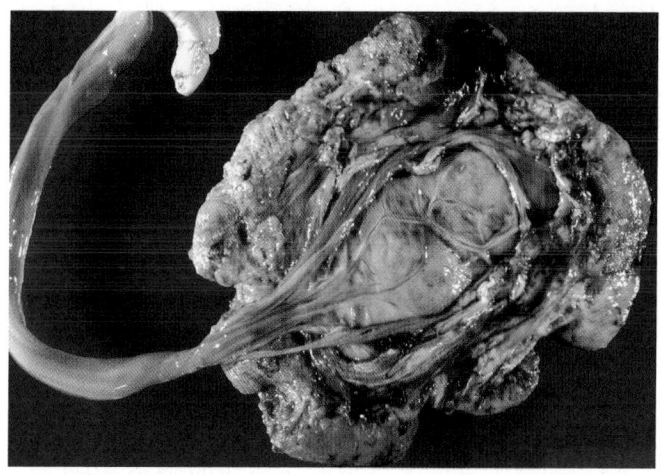

FIGURE 15.20 Circumvallate membrane insertion in a preterm delivery. The membranes are discolored light brown along rim of insertion onto the placental disc due to persistent marginal bleeding, resulting in the pathologic designation of *diffuse chorioamnionic hemosiderosis*.

Extraplacental membranes

In addition to amnion and chorion layers, the extraplacental membranes also contain maternal endometrium, in this location referred to as decidua parietalis or decidua capsularis. The decidua parietalis is the remnant decidual layer which originally covers the implanted blastocyst. As the amniotic cavity expands to obliterate the coelomic cavity, the overlying decidua parietalis comes into contact with the opposing decidual surface of the uterine cavity, the decidua capsularis. Thus, the extraplacental membrane decidua is actually composed of two originally separate layers. This observation is of clinical significance with decidual arteriopathy, where inadequately remodeled spiral arterioles are found in the deep decidua, the decidua capsularis, but not the decidua parietalis. Sampling of the thickest extraplacental membranes thus provides the greatest opportunity to yield histologically abnormal decidual vessels.

Membrane completeness

Notation of whether the extraplacental membranes are complete is useful, in cases where the clinical query of retained products of conception arises in the days and weeks following delivery. **Incomplete membranes** are described as absent, incomplete, or indeterminate, the latter in cases when membranes are received fragmented, precluding evaluation for completeness.

Membrane insertion

Normal membrane insertion onto the placental disc is described as marginal, referring to its insertion at the disc periphery, where the fetal and maternal disc surfaces meet. Abnormal membrane attachments can be partial, involving a portion of the disc circumference, or complete, involving the entire disc perimeter. **Circummarginate** membrane insertion occurs when the extraplacental membranes either lift off or are folded over onto the fetal disc surface internal to the disc perimeter. **Circumvallate** membrane insertion also involves attachment of the extraplacental membranes central to the periphery, but with the additional finding of a macroscopic ridge composed of variable combinations of folded membrane, necrotic decidua, or old organizing blood clot (Fig. 15.20). Most importantly, both circummarginate and circumvallate insertions can be indicative of chronic peripheral placental separation. Since circumvallate insertion is more likely to show significant amounts of old organizing blood clot, it is more frequently associated with adverse pregnancy outcome. The histologic counterpart of chronic peripheral separation is referred to as diffuse chorioamnionic hemosiderosis; its clinical counterpart is chronic abruption/oligohydramnios sequence. In other cases, however, circumvallate membranes are folds without obvious hemorrhage, and circummarginate membranes may be positional as sometimes occurs in diamnionic dichorionic separate twin placenta discs with fused membranes. Microscopic sampling will distinguish circumvallate from circummarginate placentation, and will allow the identification of hemosiderin and/or blood clot associated with diffuse chorioamnionic hemosiderosis. Diffuse chorioamnionic hemosiderosis (DCH) is discussed in more detail below in 'Constellation Disorders.'

Membrane hue, transparency, and texture

The normal extraplacental membrane and chorionic plate surface appearance at delivery is colorless, transparent, smooth, and glistening. Abnormal membrane coloration is most commonly due to meconium (green to brown), chronic abruption (also green to brown), or chorioamnionitis (off-white to tan to light green). Detailed gross and microscopic features of these conditions, and their clinical significance, are discussed under their respective headings. Other circumstances which can lead to membrane discoloration are the accumulation of materials within or beneath the membranes, such as blood, serous fluid, and fibrin.

Intramembranous blood is usually of no clinical significance. It is most commonly seen on the chorionic plate, due to traction on the umbilical cord during the third stage of labor (placental delivery). Uncommonly, intramembranous blood may be pathologic, reflecting transection of fetal surface or intramembranous vessels prior to infant delivery. Because these vessels are major tributaries of umbilical cord vessels, fetal exsanguination may occur within minutes. In these cases, entrapped fetal blood is bright red, and a search adjacent to the intramembranous blood should yield the transected hypovolemic vessel. Intramembranous vessels may occur with marginal or velamentous cord insertions, where one or more umbilical vessel tributaries splay onto the extraplacental membranes rather than the fetal surface. This risk of transection is greatest with vasa previa, when membrane rupture also ruptures intermembranous vessels coursing over the endocervical os. In contrast, fetal surface vessels are much better protected against spontaneous rupture. When vessel integrity is breached in this location, the cause is almost always inadvertently iatrogenic, such as with attempted fetal internal scalp electrode placement.

Retromembranous blood is due to a different mechanism: accumulation of maternal blood beneath the extraplacental membranes. Retromembranous blood may be seen in acute or chronic bleeding, of arterial or venous origin. In cases of acute placental abruption due to arterial bleeding, no additional pathologic findings may be present except accumulated retromembranous blood, thus the diagnosis must be confirmed on clinical grounds. Acute venous bleeding due to marginal placental separation may also deposit retromembranous blood; this condition may lead to preterm delivery. With chronic peripheral separation, it is common to see old retromembranous blood layered between the membranes and more recently deposited blood. In these cases, old blood is visible histologically as palely eosinophilic fragmented red cells; membrane hemosiderin is a common accompaniment.

Subchorionic blood, that is subchorionic hematoma, is not usually visible from the fetal surface of the placental disc. This lesion is addressed with placental disc cut surface lesions.

Intermembranous serous fluid may produce surface nodules comprised of serous fluid accumulated beneath the amnion epithelium known as **amniotic cysts**. Amniotic cysts, produced by sequestered amniotic epithelium transudation, may range in dimension from a few millimeters to several centimeters; they are of no clinical significance.

Subchorionic fibrin is often noted as white plaques deep to the chorionic plate surface. Subchorionic fibrin, as an isolated area of fibrin deposition within the placental disc, is not of clinical significance.

Membrane surface lesions

Materials that may be deposited in utero recently prior to delivery, and are thus removable at placental examination, include freshly passed meconium and recently extravasated blood. Materials found on the amnion surface which are not removable manually include amnion nodosum and squamous metaplasia. **Amnion nodosum** is always clinically and pathologically significant, representing the abnormal accumulation of normal amniotic fluid components on the amnion surface. Amnion nodosum reflects severe prolonged oligohydramnios, irrespective of the mechanism leading to pathologically reduced amniotic fluid. Thus, amnion nodosum is seen in circumstances of prolonged amniotic fluid leakage, that is, prolonged membrane rupture prior to delivery. Amnion nodosum also results from cases of prolonged inadequate amniotic fluid production, delivery, or maintenance. To elaborate, inadequate amniotic fluid production occurs with bilateral renal agenesis; inadequate delivery from urinary outlet obstruction such as due to posterior urethral valves; inadequate maintenance from chronic amnion rupture or preterm premature membrane rupture. Amnion nodosum appears as minute punctate raised off-white opaque lesions which are uniformly distributed on the amnion surface. Microscopically, amnion nodosum is comprised of exfoliated fetal surface skin cells ('squames') and fetal hair (Fig. 15.21A). Sometimes, amnion epithelium resurfaces the nodules of amnion nodosum, which may result in microscopic diagnostic confusion. In diagnostically difficult cases, where amnion nodosum may be confused with squamous metaplasia or reactive amnion epithelium, keratin immunohistochemistry can highlight fetal squames entrapped within nodules of amnion nodosum (Fig. 15.21B).

Squamous metaplasia occurs on the amnion epithelial surface, as does squamous metaplasia elsewhere on epithelial surfaces, specifically in response to direct mechanical or chemical irritation. To date, there has been no correlation between the presence of squamous metaplasia and clinically or pathologically significant circumstances. Squamous metaplasia tends to occur as variably sized plaques around the umbilical cord insertion site. One possible explanation for the evolution of squamous metaplasia is as a consequence of the constant stretching of the periumbilical amnion caused by fetal movements in utero. Metaplastic squamous deposits appear as off-white surface nodules, millimeters in size but larger than the pinpoint uniform and diffusely distributed surface nodules of amnion nodosum. Microscopically, squamous metaplasia appears as stratified squamous epithelium which is frequently keratinized, demonstrating keratohyaline globules (Fig. 15.22).

Abnormal membrane structures

Most abnormal surface structures are discussed elsewhere, including nodular or cystic structures such as yolk sac, serous cyst, subchorionic fibrin, and aberrant fetal vessels. A few membrane lesions remain worthy of special consideration, namely fetus papyraceus and amniotic bands.

Fetus papyraceus refers to the skeletonized embryofetal remnant of a prior multiple gestation following early fetal demise. Historically, fetus papyraceus occurred spontaneously; in current times, selective reduction of one or more multiple gestation fetuses in assisted fertilizations is the most common mechanism leading to fetus papyraceus. When a fetus papyraceus is present,

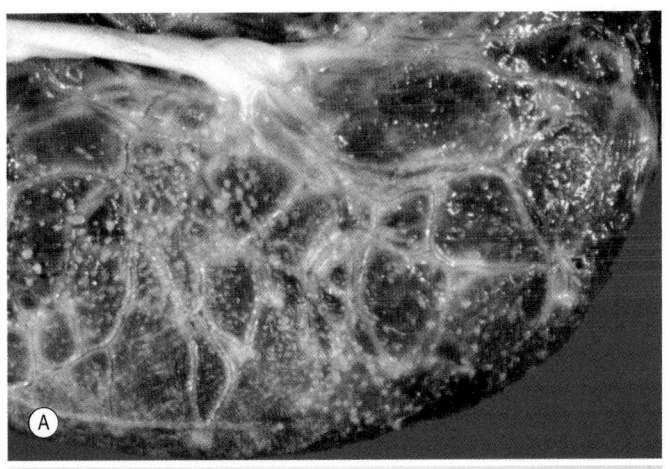

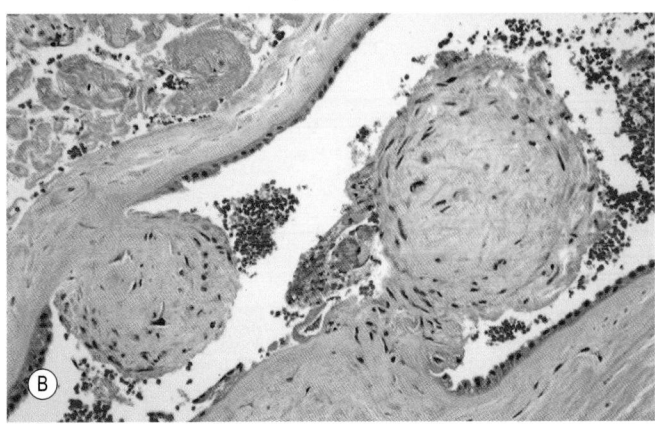

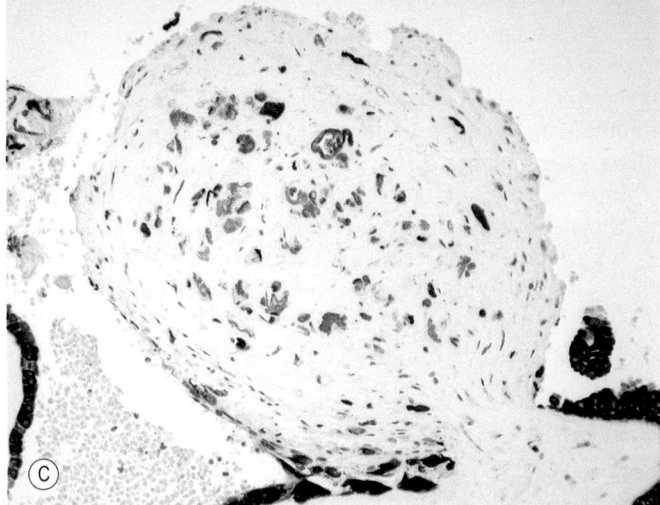

FIGURE 15.21 Amnion nodosum. (A) Innumerable pinpoint fetal surface nodules comprised of (B), fetal squames, vellus hairs, fibrin, and stromal fibroblast ingrowth. (C) Keratin immunohistochemistry highlights entrapped fetal squames.

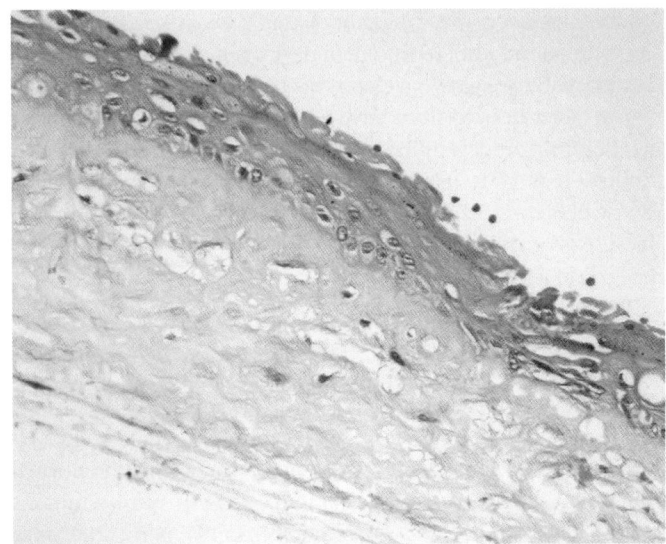

FIGURE 15.22 Squamous metaplasia. The normally unistratified cuboidal amnion epithelium has been stimulated to undergo metaplastic change to a more resilient stratified squamous phenotype; surface keratinization is common.

the extraplacental membranes are characteristically thickened, reflecting involution of the surrounding gestational sac. While the etiology of spontaneous multifetal pregnancy loss is usually not discerned from pathologic evaluation, the gestational age at embryofetal demise after about 8 weeks gestation can be ascertained by measurement of foot length, which remains relatively invariate despite the prolonged interval between demise and delivery.

Amniotic bands (also discussed in Chs 4 and 21) occur when the amnion epithelium and stroma become detached from the deeper chorionic structures of the extraplacental membranes and chorionic plate. Strands of amnion, still attached to the underlying chorion at one pole of the amniotic strips, then float in the amniotic fluid, where they are prone to becoming wrapped around fetal extremities and the umbilical cord. Amniotic bands are also susceptible to being swallowed as the fetus performs the normal intrauterine action of ingesting and inspiring amniotic fluid. The potential deleterious effects of amniotic bands are many. If amniotic bands wrap around still-growing extremities, the resultant ischemic damage to tissues distal to the bands leads to distal hypoplasia or amputation (Fig. 4.2.21B). If amniotic bands are ingested, the tethered bands may cause permanent disruption of the developing fetal face, resulting

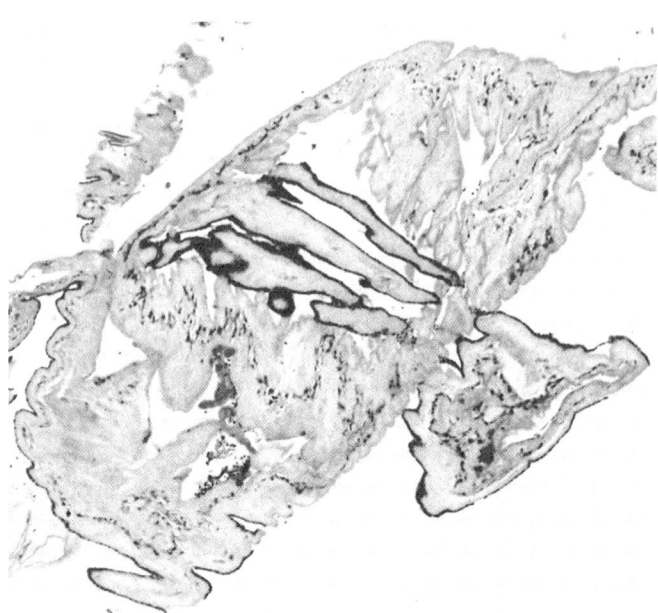

FIGURE 15.23 Amniotic band. This strip of amnion was sampled from a tissue tag adherent to the site of fetal extremity amputation.

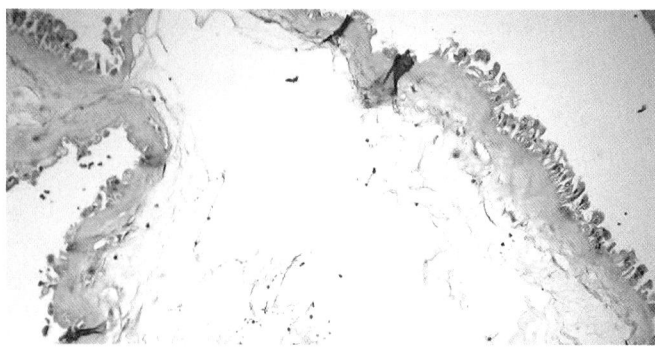

FIGURE 15.24 Reactive amnion epithelium. The normal cuboidal to low columnar amnion demonstrates alteration to a pseudostratified tall columnar phenotype; in this case membrane edema is also present.

in bizarre, asymmetric facial and cranial malformations (Fig. 4.2.25A). If amniotic bands envelop the umbilical cord, fatal umbilical blood flow restriction can lead to fetal demise.

The etiology of amniotic band formation is unknown; the predominant hypothesis has been excessive fetal activity leading to tearing of the amnion surface. Amniotic bands have been identified following invasive procedures which disrupt the integrity of the extraplacental membranes, such as amniocentesis. Why they occur in only a small subset of all patients undergoing such procedures is unknown. When amniotic band sequence is suspected in a malformed fetus, sampling of tissue strands located around disrupted fetal structures should be undertaken. Amniotic bands are confirmed by their histologic appearance, comprised of amnion epithelium and stroma (Fig. 15.23).

Microscopic amnion changes

A few features of amniotic epithelium that are not detectable grossly warrant comment. So-called 'reactive amnion epithelium' occurs when some stimulus, either chemical or mechanical, induces the normally low cuboidal amnion epithelium to alter its phenotype, becoming most commonly tall columnar to pseudostratified (Fig. 15.24). This change may be degenerative in origin, with amnionic epithelial cells partially detaching from the basement membrane, mimicking a columnar phenotype. The amniotic fluid substance which appears to induce the most dramatic amnion changes is meconium. Reactive epithelial changes can also occur with chorioamnionitis, yet the degree of cytologic alteration is generally less dramatic than with meconium. Many times, though, reactive amnion epithelium is present on microscopic examination without identifiable cause. As an isolated finding, this epithelial change is of no clinical significance.

Amnion epithelial necrosis, as with reactive changes, occurs with some frequency. It is most commonly seen with prolonged chorioamnionitis. Meconium can also induce amnion necrosis with prolonged exposure; a close look may identify meconium staining of affected amniocytes. Necrosis may also simply identify the membrane rupture site.

In rare cases, amnion cytoplasmic expansion due to 'bubbly' inclusions may reflect storage material from one of the **inborn errors of metabolism**, or etiologically unrelated, from gastroschisis. For a discussion of placental cell types which may be affected with storage disorders, please see 'Villi' under 'Additional Microscopic Pathology by Placental Location.'

Placental disc: general observations

Weight

As the fetus grows, so too does the placenta. Just as normal weight ranges have been established for fetuses throughout gestation, so too are there normative tables for placental weights, from about 20 weeks' gestation until term.[50, 51] In developed countries, both fetal and placental weights have increased over time, such that normative tables derived from birth weights and placental weights in decades past underestimate normal weight in the twenty-first century. It is thus recommended that more current tables be used when comparing placental specimens to normative values. Because fetal and placental weights have increased in proportion, the ratio of fetal to placental weight has remained stable over time.

Growth-restricted placentas usually occur in pregnancies complicated by fetal growth restriction. As a general statement, because of decreased placental reserve, pathologic lesions in small placentas are more likely to be associated with adverse fetal/neonatal outcome than are placental abnormalities which can be seen in heavy placentas. In chromosomally normal gestations, small placentas commonly result from conditions leading to prolonged reduction in uteroplacental perfusion. Since maternal blood nourishes the placenta as well as the fetus, maternal vascular diseases such as hypertension, preeclampsia, and autoimmune disorders complicated by vascular disease may induce a constellation of pathologic placental changes, such as placental infarction and abruption, in addition to overall diminished placental growth. For a discussion of this constellation of features, please see 'Maternal Vascular Underperfusion' in 'Constellation Disorders' below.

Sometimes placental growth restriction results from maternal vascular underperfusion due not to intrinsic vascular disease but to diminished perfusion of other causes, such as abnormal implantation (cornual pregnancy) or competition for uterine space (multiple gestations, large submucosal leiomyomas).

Heavy placentas occur most commonly with large for gestation fetuses; gestational diabetes predisposes to fetal and placental macrosomia. A heavy placenta per se probably does not adversely affect fetal well-being, although it does present additional tissue mass with increased nutrient demands. Other specific circumstances which lead to heavy placentas include Rh incompatibility, genetic overgrowth syndromes such as Beckwith-Wiedemann syndrome, metabolic storage diseases, molar pregnancy, mesenchymal dysplasia, and mass lesions such as large chorangiomas.

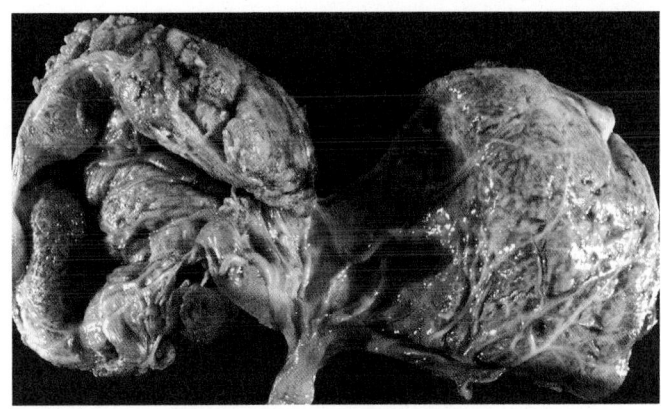

FIGURE 15.25 Bilobate placenta with central velamentous cord insertion. The placenta had implanted over a uterine septum, giving rise to its abnormal shape.

Dimensions (width by maximal thickness)

Placental dimensions are usually recorded on gross examination, although this information is of limited value since placental weight as a measure of placental size is more amenable to comparison with normative tables.

Shape

Normal placental shape is **discoid** or **ovoid**, resulting from fairly uniform outward growth around a normally positioned (central to eccentric) umbilical cord. Aberrations in placental shape usually reflect intrauterine physical constraints on normal radial growth. Abnormal shapes include **bilobate** placentas and placental discs with **accessory (succenturiate) lobes**. The former condition results from early regression of the central disc, leaving two placental lobes of roughly equal size. This occurs in situations where the central disc is implanted over an area of inadequate maternal perfusion, such as a uterine septum or cesarean section scar. Accessory lobes, which may be single or multiple, result from localized peripheral regression of the definitive disc, leaving islands of chorionic villi which may or may not be attached to the main disc by a strip (isthmus) of villous parenchyma. Bilobate discs and accessory lobes may have pathologic consequences when the umbilical cord or large fetal surface vessels traverse the thinned chorionic surface between lobes, rendering these vessels prone to compression, thrombosis, and tearing (Fig. 15.25). A rare abnormality of shape, **placenta membranacea**, results from failed regression of the chorion laeve in early gestation, leading to circumferential persistence of vascularized chorionic villi.

Fetal surface (chorionic plate) observations

Arborization pattern of chorionic plate vessels

Under normal circumstances, the major tributaries of the umbilical vessels, the chorionic plate vessels, splay radially onto the surface of the chorionic plate. In circumstances where the umbilical cord is not received with the placental disc, the umbilical cord insertion can be estimated by tracing the convergence point of these surface vessels. Unusual arborization patterns typically occur as a consequence of abnormal umbilical cord insertion. In marginal or velamentous cord insertions, the vessels preferentially radiate unidirectionally over the chorionic plate surface rather than in a circumferential pattern. Complications can occur when occasional surface vessels follow an intramembranous course, thereby rendering them susceptible to mechanical trauma.

Chorionic plate arteries branch over, and are thus superficial to, the chorionic plate veins. Arteries and veins are paired at their periphery, where they extend downward into the disc to divide into the next generation of stem villous vessels. Thus, for each terminal branch of a chorionic plate artery, there will be in its vicinity a chorionic plate vein. This pairing reflects the segmentation pattern of the fetal vascular tree, resulting in a regionally continuous arterial-to-venous fetal circulation. This physiology is especially significant in twin–twin transfusion, which is covered in Chapter 9.

Chorionic plate vessel caliber and texture

In the fresh state, chorionic plate surface vessels contain uncoagulated burgundy-colored blood. Chorionic plate veins tend to be somewhat more prominent than arteries under normal circumstances, perhaps due to their slightly wider caliber and greater distensibility. There is some variation in the amount of blood present in chorionic plate vessels at delivery; however, on average, blood should be present and movable in virtually all arteries and veins. In circumstances of extreme fetal hypovolemia, such as fetal–maternal hemorrhage and fetal exsanguination, surface vessels are collapsed and virtually bloodless. This condition may be overlooked unless consciously looked for, as the absence of blood is less dramatic than when vessels are markedly distended.

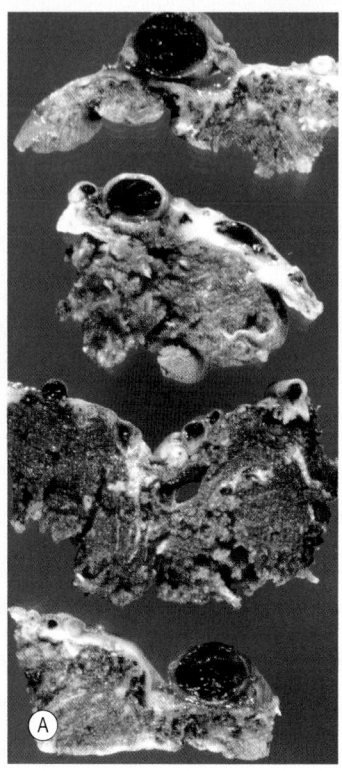

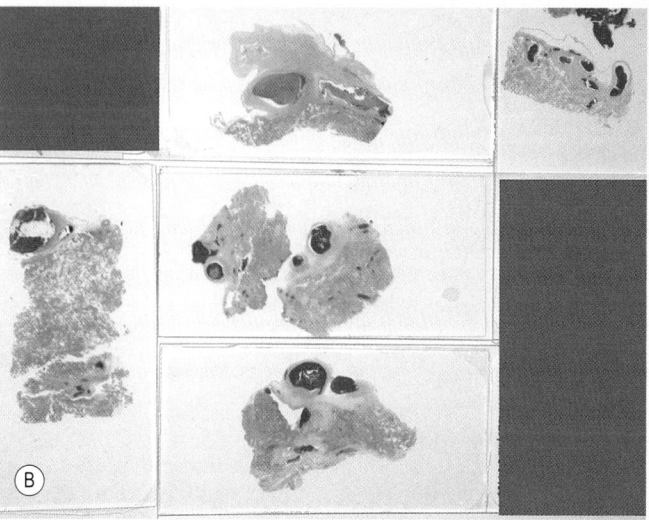

FIGURE 15.26 Chorionic plate thrombosis. Ectatic and thrombosed surface vessels can be appreciated grossly (A) and in slide preparation (B), sometimes without the aid of a microscope.

Pronounced vascular ectasia may indicate thrombosis. Visually, thrombosed surface vessels rise well above the chorionic plate surface, and in the fresh state are distended with non-movable clotted blood. Recent thrombosis is burgundy colored; as the thrombus organizes, white streaks of incorporated fibrin may be seen (Fig. 15.26). In remotely thrombosed vessels the lumen may appear normovolemic or collapsed, with only central dystrophic calcification remaining (Fig. 15.27). Thrombosis is more frequent in chorionic plate veins than arteries, though in some cases both vessel types may be affected.

Hue, opacity, texture, surface lesions

These surface considerations are addressed in the section 'Extraplacental Membranes' above. The one surface lesion which is unique to the chorionic plate is the **yolk sac remnant**, representing the vestige of the once-vital yolk sac. Visible as an off-white or tan elevated plaque a few millimeters in width, and located near the umbilical insertion, it is an occasionally present incidental finding. Microscopically, yolk sac remnants exhibit nodular dystrophic calcification without specific features. Since they are single lesions, they should not be confused with other surface findings such as amnion nodosum or squamous metaplasia.

Subsurface lesions

Subamniotic lesions (amniotic cysts, intramembranous blood) have been covered in the section 'Extraplacental Membranes'

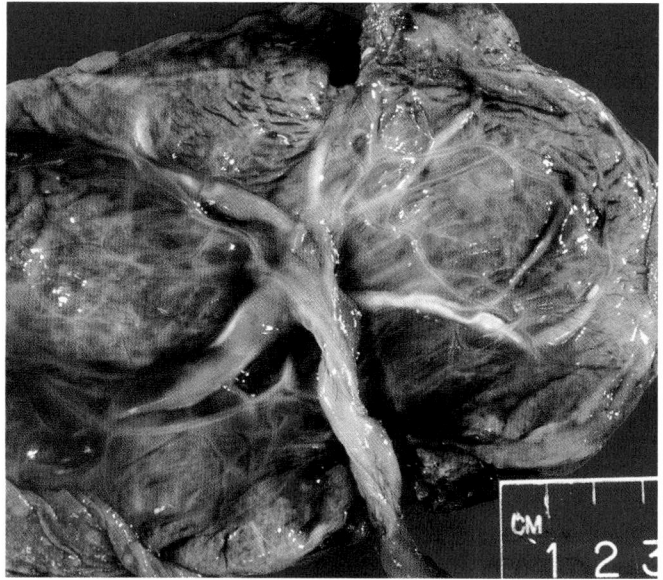

FIGURE 15.27 Calcified and regionally collapsed chorionic plate vessels, due to fetal vascular thrombosis of weeks' duration prior to delivery. Stillborn fetus.

above. Subchorionic lesions, sometimes visible from the fetal surface as discolorations and/or masses, are covered here.

Subchorionic fibrin is frequently observed, as irregular off-white plaques with indistinct borders. Subchorionic fibrin can produce modest elevation of the fetal surface, but does not

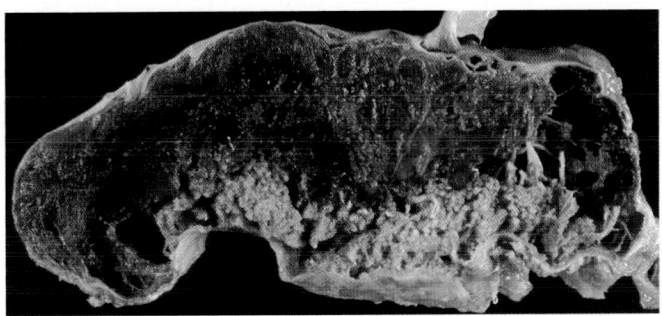

FIGURE 15.28 Massive subchorionic hematoma associated with second trimester stillbirth.

form a discrete surface lesion. Subchorionic fibrin deposits under the chorionic plate, at least in part because of turbulent maternal intervillous flow. This eddying of blood occurs because arterial inflow in this location, being farthest from the uterine arteries, is at lower pressure, and because flow is redirected by contact with the underside of the chorionic plate. Most of the time, subchorionic fibrin is not clinically significant, even when the amount seems impressive on gross examination.

Subchorionic hematoma represents blood accumulation in the subchorionic space. Although the intervillous space is normally blood filled, abnormal accumulations of blood are recognized by the regional expansion of the intervillous space, which results in displacement of villi to accommodate the space-occupying lesion. Subchorionic hematomas, also called Breus' moles when visible as nodules from the chorionic plate surface, can be caused by several mechanisms. A marginal placental abruption may disrupt the integrity of the placental disc edge, allowing blood to dissect into the subchorionic space. Rarely, in patients with heritable thrombophilia, a so-called **massive subchorionic hematoma** may occur, virtually replacing the subchorionic maternal intervillous space (Fig. 15.28).[52] The intitating event in this disorder, at least in some circumstances, might be rupture of a major fetal vessel, which may in part explain the high incidence of intrauterine demise with massive subchorionic hematoma.[53]

Subchorionic chorangioma may produce a nodular fetal surface lesion, if it is several centimeters in size and located subjacent to the chorionic plate. Chorangiomas are discussed below under 'Cut Surface Lesions.'

Maternal surface (decidua basalis) observations

Contour

The normal contour of the intact maternal disc surface, also called the basal plate, is gently convex. The basal plate is divided into cotyledons, which are demarcated by shallow crevices formed from invaginations of the decidua basalis by septal columns. The decidua basalis imparts a smooth surface, which

may be punctuated by pinpoint pits representing the sites of draining maternal vessels. Deviations from the normal contour without secondary lesions are usually due to an anatomic abnormality of the implantation site, such concavity produced by a submucosal leiomyoma. Rarely, the leiomyoma may be delivered with the placenta, causing some diagnostic confusion. If secondary lesions are present, then aberrations in contour are due to some pathologic processes. Concavity of a placental abruption site is due to the combination of a space-occupying retroplacental hematoma and overlying placental infarction, the latter resulting in reduced disc thickness at the abruption site (Fig. 15.29).

Completeness

The completeness of a placenta with an intact maternal surface is easily ascertained. It can be more difficult to determine whether a placenta with a disrupted surface is complete. An attempt to approximate the disrupted surfaces, to see if they reestablish intact cotyledon(s), is most helpful. If, following this maneuver, placental tissue still appears absent, then intactness should be reported as indeterminate or incomplete, depending on the confidence level of the observer. Grossly missing cotyledons, if not present within the specimen container, should raise concern for retained placental fragments and the attendant risk of postpartum hemorrhage.

Adherent blood

It is common to observe some loosely adherent blood on the maternal surface. Whether adherent blood is normal requires assessment of: the amount of blood present, percent of the disc area involved, degree of adherence, degree of organization, and whether secondary placental changes are present. In general, retroplacental blood reflecting normal placental separation during the third stage of labor will have a burgundy color and currant-jelly texture, will be loosely adherent to the disc, will be marginal, will be at most a few millimeters thick, and will not have produced secondary changes such as concavity of the underlying disc. In some circumstances recent marginal and retromembranous hemorrhages of larger size (so-called marginal abruptions) may precipitate labor and thus be clinically significant, particularly in preterm deliveries.[54] These hemorrhages probably reflect rupture of distended marginal uterine veins. The clinical entity of abruptio placenta, on the other hand, is arterial in origin. Pathologic adherent retroplacental blood in abruptio placenta is more likely to manifest the opposite findings, including lamination, organization, firm adherence, more extensive and central disc involvement, and indentation of the underlying disc. In addition, abundant detached clotted and unclotted blood may accompany the placenta within the specimen container. Such detached clots are of particular significance if they show signs of organization and if their contours conform to indentations on the basal surface of the placenta. Placental abruptions occurring just prior to delivery provide the exception to this paradigm, as insufficient time may

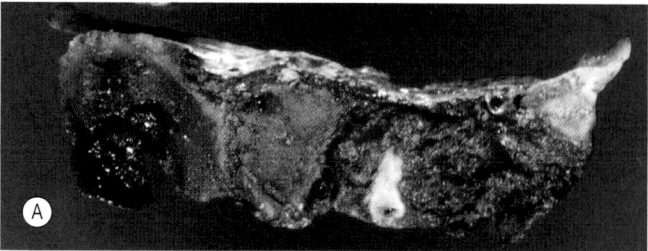

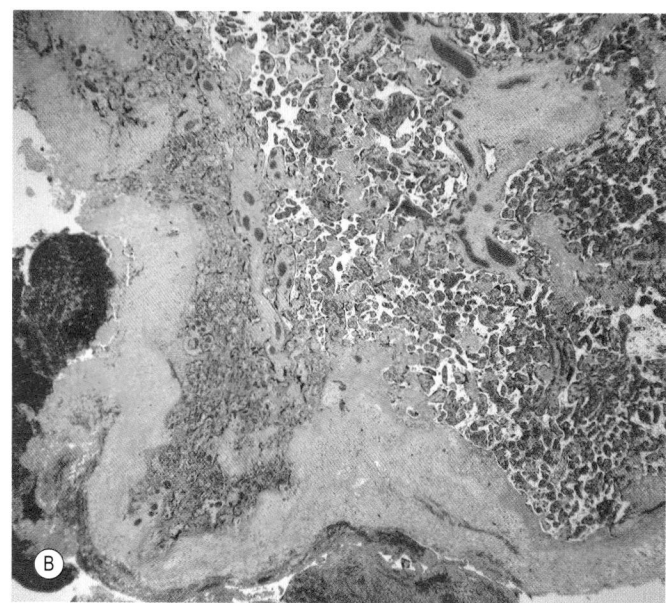

FIGURE 15.29 Acute placental abruption. (A) Recent placental abruption is identified on the left, by the presence of laminated retroplacental blood with overlying recent placental infarction. Concavity results from mass effect of blood plus collapse of the overlying maternal intervillous space. (B) Microscopic equivalent of A.

have elapsed between abruption and delivery for any of the gross characteristic changes to evolve. In this setting, the absence of findings in a strong clinical context supports an acute event.

Calcification

At term, it is normal to see off-white, chalky calcific stippling of the basal plate, which is sometimes erroneously overinterpreted as excessive. If there is an abnormal amount of calcification for gestational age on cut surface then the basal plate will likewise show extensive calcification. In preterm placentas, basal plate calcification is always abnormal, and may signify premature placental 'senescence' due to chronic parenchymal ischemia.

Cut surface observations

Hue

The normal appearance of the cut placenta is gestational age dependent. In the second trimester, the normal placental parenchyma is pale, from tan to pink-red. Yet a uniformly pale parenchyma at term indicates severe fetal anemia and/or hydrops, as the normal term placental cut surface color is deep red to burgundy.

Texture by palpation

The normal cut surface texture is spongy at all stages of gestation. Consolidated or firm areas are always deviations from the norm insofar as by palpation they do not represent typical spongiform villous parenchyma. The following section, on placental lesions, presents a more extensive discussion of palpated and visualized lesions.

Lesions

Consolidated but visually indiscernible red lesions likely represent recent *placental infarcts*. Intermediate-aged infarcts, sometimes referred to as 'organizing' infarcts, assume a progressively firmer and paler appearance with time, and are dull on cut surface. Remote infarcts are off-white and solid. Infarcts do not truly organize in the strict sense, by fibroblastic ingrowth; rather, infarcted villi become progressively more condensed and pink by microscopic examination, losing all hematoxylophilic nuclear detail with time. It is not uncommon to find one or two infarcts in a term placenta; the common ones tend to be basal and/or marginal, wedge-shaped lesions ranging in diameter from millimeters to a few centimeters. The greater the number of infarcts, the larger the size of individual lesions, the more centrally located or transmural the infarcts, and the more temporally heterogeneous, the more likely they are to reflect some form of maternal vascular disease (Fig. 15.30). As a rule of thumb, it is stated that the fetus can tolerate loss of about 50% of functional placental volume, but this figure is modified by how rapidly loss of function occurs and the condition of the remaining tissue. Fetuses can tolerate incremental loss to a greater degree than an acute loss of the same placental volume. Thus, a fetus may survive incremental placental infarcts ultimately involving 70% of the disc, whereas an acute placental abruption involving 30% of the placenta may produce the same severity (but obviously not the same chronicity) of hypoxic stress. On occasion, firm lesions may represent more slowly evolving perivillous fibrin plaques that can be distinguished from infarcts histologically by virtue of the lack of villous collapse (i.e., retention of intervillous space) and the presence of slowly evolving villous ischemic degenerative changes (i.e., villous fibrosis rather than coagulative necrosis (Fig. 15.31).[55]

Laminated lesions usually represent **intervillous thrombi**, whether they are recent and mostly red or older and more off-white. Intervillous thrombi range in size from several millimeters to several centimeters, and can be located virtually anywhere within the villous parenchyma. Intervillous thrombi represent the site of fetal bleeding into the maternal circulation, a process that occurs to some extent in most pregnancies without clinical consequence.[56] The rare circumstance in which intervillous thrombi are of clear pathologic significance is with massive fetal–maternal hemorrhage. In these cases, the intervillous thrombi are often larger or multifocal. Recent red gelatinous to laminated lesions in these cases signify rapid, often fatal, fetal–maternal hemorrhage in which there is little time for the thrombus to organize.

Well-circumscribed red to tan nodules may represent **chorangiomas**, which are capillary hemangiomatous proliferations arising within placental villi, ranging in diameter from a few millimeters to several centimeters. Red chorangiomas contain actively circulating capillary blood, while tan chorangiomas are likely to have undergone ischemic infarction. Rarely, multifocal and broad areas of the placental cut surface will be involved by chorangiomas. This condition, known as **chorangiomatosis**, can lead to fetal congestive heart failure, as increased cardiac output is required to accommodate perfusion within the vastly expanded chorangiomatous capillary network.

Semitranslucent parenchymal cysts are usually **septal cysts**, incidental lesions comprised of clear to red gelatinous fluid microscopically surrounded by trophoblast and fibrin. These lesions represent inclusion cysts formed by nests of intermediate trophoblast from the decidua basalis that become entrapped within the infolding placental septae.

Regions of **perivillous fibrin** have protean gross configurations, based upon variable location, size, and shape. Cut surface appearance is off-white and semiglistening, with the texture of impenetrably hardened custard. The contours are circumscribed but irregular, and individual foci can be millimeters to many centimeters in maximal width. Perivillous fibrin is more accurately termed fibrinoid, since it is largely composed of extracellular matrix proteins secreted by intermediate trophoblast and not just fibrin alone. However, the term perivillous fibrin remains in common usage. A few particular perivillous fibrin distribution patterns bear elaboration. So-called **maternal floor infarction (MFI)** is on cut surface a rind of perivillous fibrin which coats the entire basal plate, varying in thickness from several millimeters to several centimeters. A related lesion, **massive perivillous fibrin deposition (MPFD)**, does not cover the entirety of the basal plate but is notable for irregular extension toward the fetal surface, and may involve a single expanse or multiple regions of the disc (Fig. 15.32).[57] Both MFI and MPFD are associated with intrauterine demise, fetal growth restriction, and lesion recurrence in future pregnancies.[58–63] Recurrence rates, especially with MFI, of 12–78% in various series suggest that maternal factors are essential in pathogenesis. As described above, microscopically perivillous fibrin appears as a homogeneous eosinophilic intervillous material which coats and agglutinates villi. Intervillous cytotrophoblasts are often admixed within the fibrin. Encased villi undergo slow ischemic vascular involution,

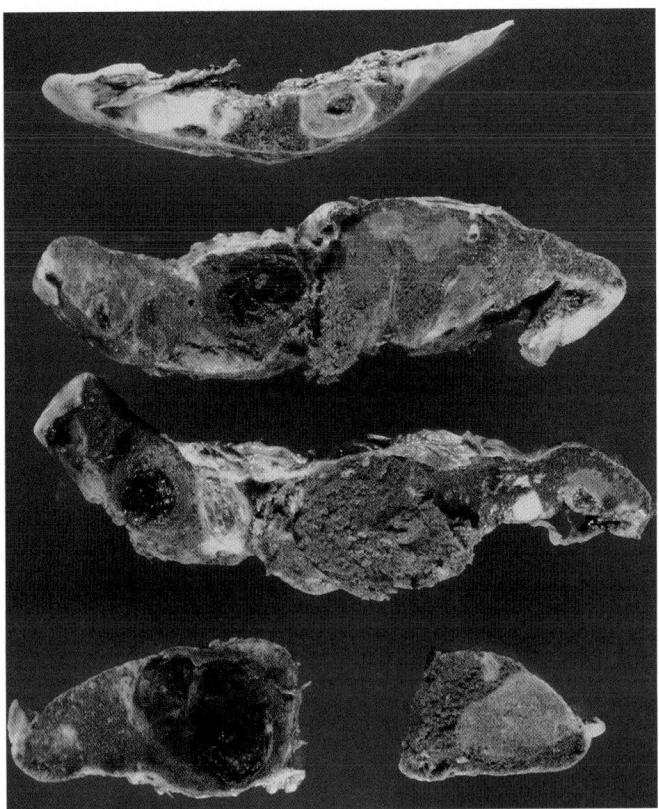

FIGURE 15.30 Multiple temporally heterogeneous infarcts involving the full thickness and breadth of the placental disc. The mother had poorly controlled pregestational insulin-dependent diabetes mellitus.

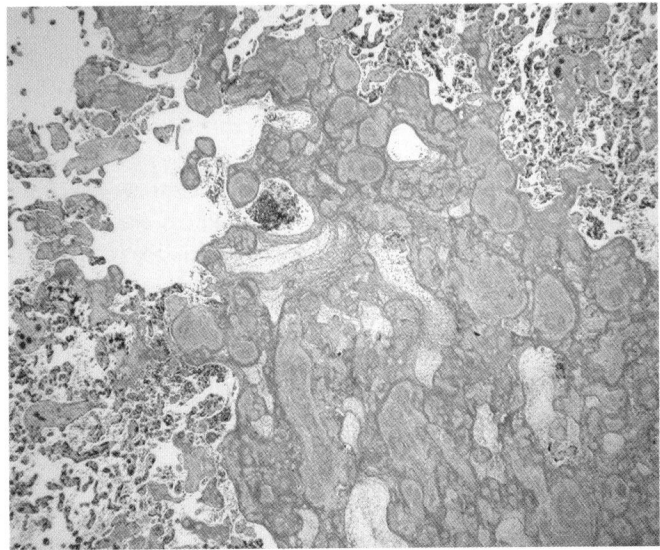

FIGURE 15.31 Microscopic interface between massive perivillous fibrin deposition (MPFD) and uninvolved chorionic villi. Note preservation of the intervillous space in MPFD, in contrast to its collapse with placental infarction.

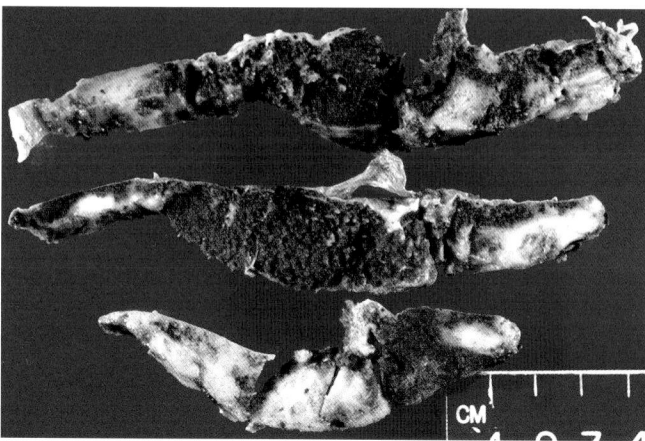

FIGURE 15.32 Sizeable deposits of perivillous fibrin, so-called *massive perivillous fibrin deposition*. The gross appearance of this placenta led the prosector to describe the presence of multiple remote placental infarcts, a common observational error.

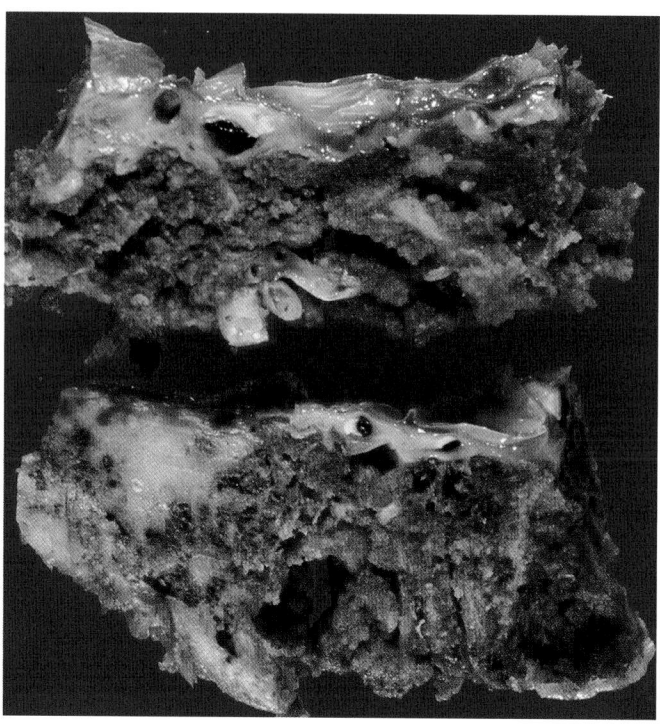

FIGURE 15.33 Wedge-shaped, grossly visible area of avascular villi due to upstream fetal vascular thrombosis. Adjacent to this region are partially calcified chorionic plate thrombi. Both calcification and avascularity attest to chronicity.

although stromal cells remain viable (see Fig. 15.31). Affected villous tissue is rendered incapable of fetal oxygen and nutrient delivery, thus accounting for growth restriction and intrauterine demise in severely affected cases. Deposition of fibrin in the intervillous space is expected in all placentas beyond about 20 weeks; the amount tends to increase with gestational age. Under normal circumstances, fibrin spares the distal villi, depositing in areas of physiologically diminished perfusion, such as the marginal disc and around subchorionic villi. Exaggeration of the amount and extent of intervillous fibrin may be one of several pathologic findings in chronically underperfused placentas; see 'Maternal Vascular Underperfusion' under 'Constellation Disorders' below for details.

Macroscopically visible areas of **avascular villi** are much less common than microscopically detected avascular villous foci. Visible lesions are due to remote cessation of blood flow in large upstream feeding vessels, affecting enough downstream branches to be seen grossly. Lesions are subchorionic, in contrast to the much more common basal placental infarcts (Fig. 15.33). Microscopically, avascular villi appear fibrotic due to increased collagen deposition coincident with vascular involution. Nuclear staining of stromal cells and villous trophoblasts is retained. The clinicopathologic significance of these lesions is discussed in the later section on 'Fetal Thrombotic Vasculopathy.'

To emphasize what has been elaborated upon above, firm, off-white areas may be any number of lesions: older infarcts, organized intervillous thrombi, perivillous fibrin, or regions of avascular villi. Clues on gross inspection to the pathologic significance of a lesion include a combination of lesion size and location. Generally speaking, the larger a lesion, or the more area of the placenta involved by multiple lesions, irrespective of what they represent, the more likely the lesion(s) to be pathologic to fetal well-being.

Additional microscopic pathology by placental location

Intervillous space

Sickled maternal erythrocytes can be identified in the maternal circulation with either sickle cell trait or disease; it is not possible to distinguish between the two pathologically. In contrast, fetal hemoglobin prevents fetal erythrocytes from sickling if the fetus also has sickle cell trait or disease.

Metastatic maternal cancer detected within the intervillous space is rare but well documented. Mothers usually have a known history of primary or metastatic cancer prior to placental evaluation; at times, however, placental metastasis may provide the initial diagnosis of metastatic maternal disease. Please see the entry 'Placental Neoplasia' in 'Specific Topics in Placental Pathology' below for details.

In maternal sepsis, **bacteria** and other hematogenously spread organisms can be seen by special stain in the maternal intervillous space. If the mother is not leukopenic or otherwise immunodeficient, leukocytosis may also be evident.

Villi

Derangements in villous histology associated with chronic uteroplacental underperfusion are covered later; see 'Maternal

Vascular Underperfusion' in 'Constellation Disorders' below. These lesions include: **increased intervillous fibrin, increased syncytial knots, villous agglutination**, and **distal villous hypoplasia**. This constellation of findings is sometimes referred to as 'accelerated villous maturation,' or **Tenney-Parker change**.

Assessment of villous maturation has received much attention in the historical literature, although it is but one feature of many used to assess the quality of uteroplacental perfusion. Villous maturation is gauged relative to gestational age. **Distal villous immaturity**, also known as **delayed villous maturation**, occurs in circumstances of persistent growth of immature intermediate villi, in concert with lack of distal villous maturation. The phenotype of distal villous immaturity includes large terminal villi, diminished syncytiotrophoblast knotting, and villous capillaries more centrally positioned rather than directly apposed to the villous trophoblast. These changes lead to a deficiency of peripheral capillarization with lack of syncytiocapillary (also known as vasculosyncytial) membranes, a finding that is markedly increased in the placentas of stillborns.[64] Distal villous immaturity occurs most commonly with gestational diabetes, probably reflecting increased placental insulin which stimulates continued villous growth. Distal villous immaturity should not be confused with diffuse villous enlargement due to villous edema, or with focal changes due either to physiologic regional variation in villous maturation or continued villous branching.

Villous edema results from excess fluid accumulation in villous stroma, and can be patchy or diffuse. It is rarely an isolated finding, and is most significant not in itself but as a marker of whatever pathologic process has produced the edema. The physiologic mechanisms leading to villous edema are probably diverse and may be multifactorial. Examples include intrauterine fetal heart failure, subacute or chronic fetal anemia, and cytokine-mediated increased villous vascular permeability. Villous edema is commonly seen in the placentas of very low birth weight infants with acute chorioamnionitis, where it is patchily distributed and primarily localized to immature intermediate villi. Global villous hydrops affecting all portions of the villous tree is only seen in severely pathologic conditions, as an accompaniment to fetal hydrops when the mechanism is subacute or chronic, such as with infectious hemolytic/aplastic anemia due to fatal **Parvovirus** infection (Fig. 15.34). Histologically, villous edema appears as clearing of the villous stroma, with distention of villous diameter. Sometimes edema fluid separates the villous stroma from the villous trophoblast membrane, producing a visible cleft in the interspace. Villous edema should be distinguished from the more watery-appearing stroma of immature normal villi, and from the specific cistern formation seen with molar gestations and mesenchymal dysplasia.

Chorangiosis refers to an excess of villous capillary cross-sections, resulting from low-level chronic hypoxia which stimulates capillary proliferation. Absolute capillary numbers per villus are probably not increased; rather, existing capillaries lengthen and become more tortuous, giving the inaccurate impression on cross-section of numerically increased capillaries.

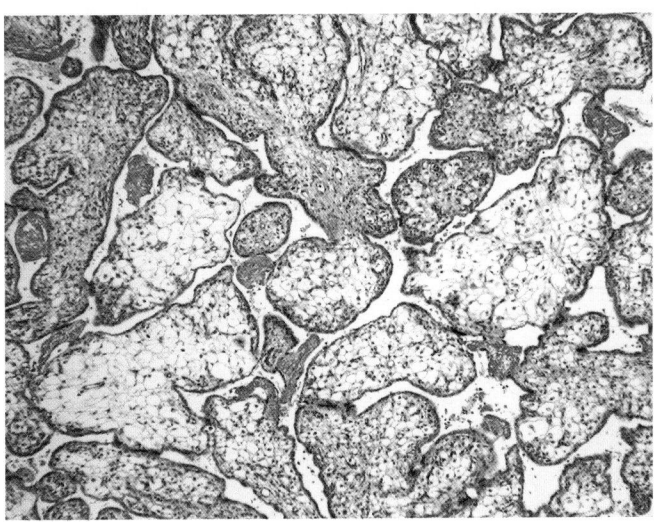

FIGURE 15.34 Late second trimester villous hydrops due to fatal *Parvovirus* infection.

The strict definition of chorangiosis follows the rule of 10s: ten or more capillary cross-sections involving ten or more villi in several different areas of the placenta.[65] Most pathologists reserve the diagnosis for cases that easily meet or exceed minimal definitional criteria. Chorangiosis is not pathologically significant in itself, but as with villous edema serves as a marker lesion for underlying pathophysiology, namely chronic low-level hypoxia or other causes of increased angiogenesis.

Chronic villitis refers to the presence of a mononuclear inflammatory infiltrate of maternal origin targeted specifically to chorionic villi. Chronic villitis is subdivided into so-called non-specific chronic villitis or villitis of unknown etiology (VUE) and specific villitis of infectious origin. **Non-specific chronic villitis** is the more common lesion, accounting for over 90% of all placentas demonstrating chronic villitis. In most cases, non-specific chronic villitis is of no apparent clinical consequence, unless the extent of affected villi is sufficient to critically reduce functional villous volume, or the villous infiltrate spreads into stem villi leading to fetal vascular occlusion (**obliterative fetal vasculopathy**).[66] Extensive non-specific chronic villitis may be associated with intrauterine growth restriction, stillbirth, and an increased risk of recurrence in subsequent pregnancies.[67-70] Stem villus villitis can lead to adverse neurologic outcome.[71] Low-power examination readily identifies affected villi, which appear hematoxylin-rich due to hypercellularity. Higher-power examination reveals a mature lymphohistiocytic villous stromal infiltrate of maternal derivation, variably involving terminal, intermediate, and smaller generation stem villi (Fig. 15.35). Ancillary histologic findings, of no inherent pathologic significance, include aggregation of adjacent affected villi, perivillous fibrin deposition, chronic lymphoplasmacytic deciduitis, and/or chronic lymphoplasmacytic chorioamnionitis. Non-specific chronic villitis represents a maternal immune response to unknown antigen(s), which have been postulated to be fetal, villous, and/or infectious (viral) in origin. *Specific chronic villitis*, on the other hand, is a distinctive

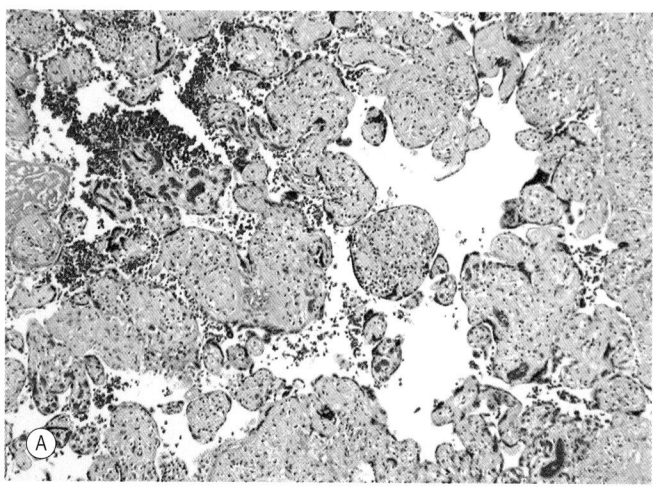

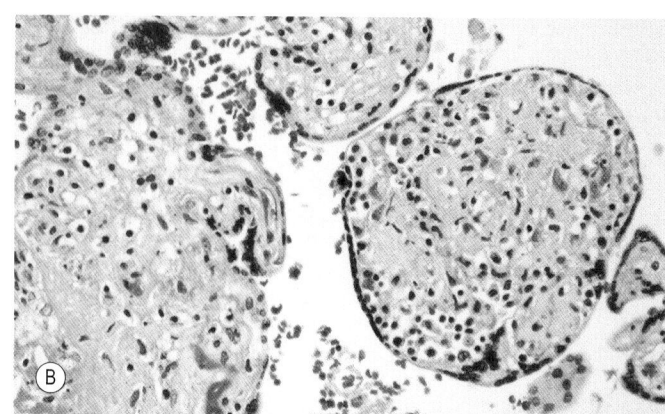

FIGURE 15.35 Villitis of unknown etiology (non-specific chronic villitis). (A) Villi are hypercellular and agglutinated. (B) Closer inspection reveals a lymphohistiocytic villous stromal infiltrate with secondary destruction of villous capillaries (obliterative fetal vasculopathy).

lymphoplasmacytic villitis which is always of infectious etiology. The most common responsible agent by far is *Cytomegalovirus* (CMV) (Fig. 15.36), followed by *Treponema pallidum*, *Herpes simplex* virus (HSV), *Toxoplasma gondii*, and least commonly by *Varicella-Zoster* virus (VZV) and *Trypanosoma cruzi*.[72–77] Identification of plasma cells within villitis requires a search for the causative agent, by light microscopy and, if available, by organism-specific immunohistochemistry. The herpesviruses (CMV, HSV, VZV) infect villous vascular endothelium, while *T. pallidum*, *T. gondii*, and *T. cruzi* infect umbilical, chorioamnionic, and/or villous stromal cells. Common additional histologic features of infectious villitis include villous destruction, stromal karyorrhectic debris, and stromal hemosiderin. Low-power histology is similar to non-specific chronic villitis. Pathologic consequences of specific chronic villitis are largely those attributable to fetal infection, acquired through hematogenous spread from mother to placenta to fetus.

Intravillous hemorrhage refers to the extravasation of fetal blood from villous capillaries into the villous stroma. Intravillous hemorrhage can occur in several circumstances, which are of widely varying significance; thus the cause in a particular case should be elucidated. Intravillous hemorrhage results from the disruption of villous vascular integrity by both pathologic and non-pathologic mechanisms. Sometimes, placentas delivered following Cesarean section will demonstrate areas of basally oriented intravillous hemorrhage, which may result from the sudden alteration of uteroplacental perfusion at the time of uterine incision (T. Boyd, personal observation). In this circumstance, intravillous hemorrhage is an incidental finding. Basally oriented intravillous hemorrhage can also occur with placental abruption, as a result of sudden cessation of intervillous flow. In this case, intravillous hemorrhage may serve as a marker for acute abruption, if retroplacental blood has not had sufficient time to clot prior to delivery. Cesarean section and abruption-associated intravillous hemorrhage are acute events which result in the extravasation of intact red cells, akin to a placental

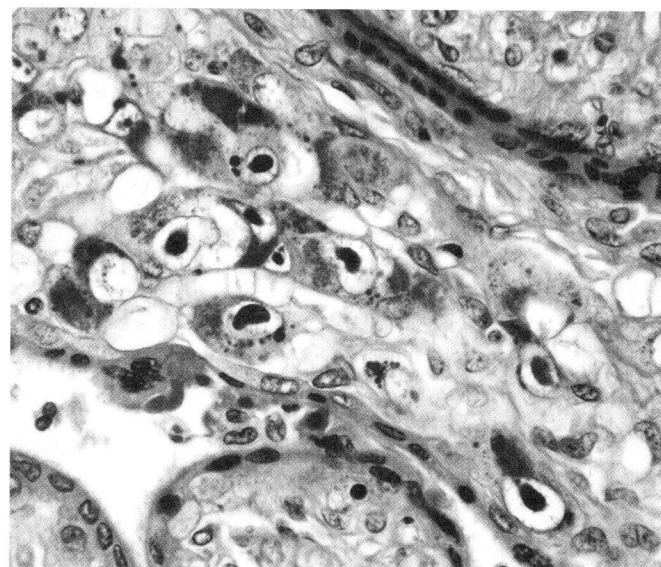

FIGURE 15.36 Early second trimester demise due to *Cytomegalovirus* infection. Villous endothelial cells demonstrate cytomegaly, with impressive nuclear and cytoplasmic viral inclusions. In this case, viral cytopathic effect was extensive, but villitis was minimal. Heavy viral load may have led to rapid fetal demise, eclipsing the time necessary to mount a robust lymphoplasmacytic inflammatory response.

'bruise'. By contrast, in non-acute pathologic conditions, intravillous red cells are fragmented by the process of vascular involution (Fig. 15.37). In the setting of fetal thrombotic vasculopathy (FTV), where upstream chorionic plate or stem villus thrombosis leads to cessation of villous capillary flow, capillary lumen integrity is destroyed, probably due in part to endothelial ischemia and in part to the absence of flow pressure. The histologic result is the gradual disappearance of villous capillaries, beginning with karyorrhexis of capillary-derived nuclei (endothelium, nucleated blood cells), and luminal

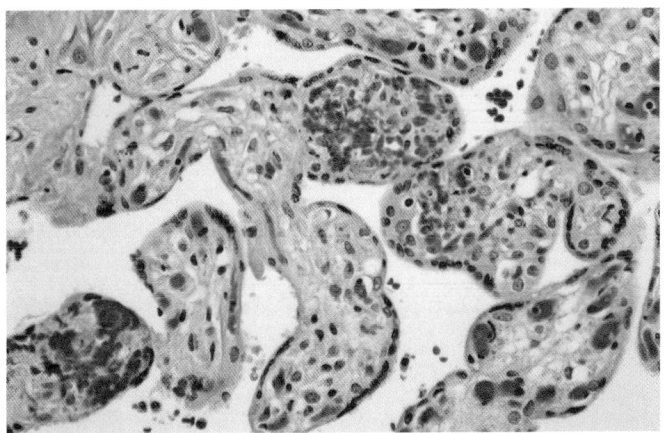

FIGURE 15.37 Intravillous hemorrhage. Erythrocyte fragmentation identifies the cause as cessation of villous vascular flow, in this case due to fetal thrombotic vasculopathy.

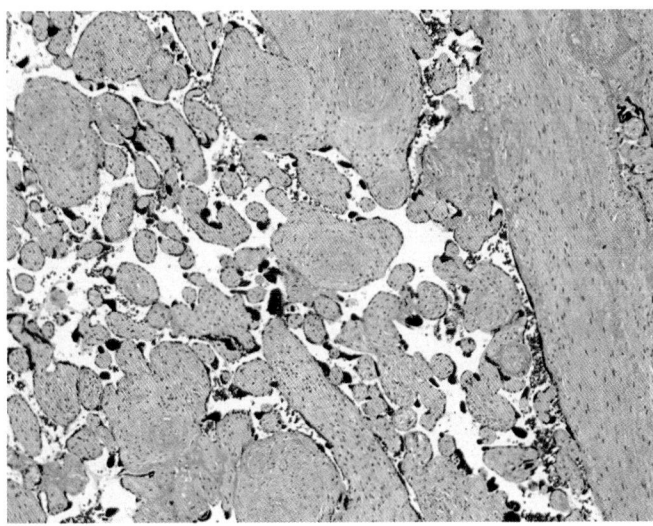

FIGURE 15.39 Temporally uniform advanced villous vascular involution, leading to *avascular villi*. Placenta from a stillborn twin; demise had been documented weeks prior to co-twin's live birth.

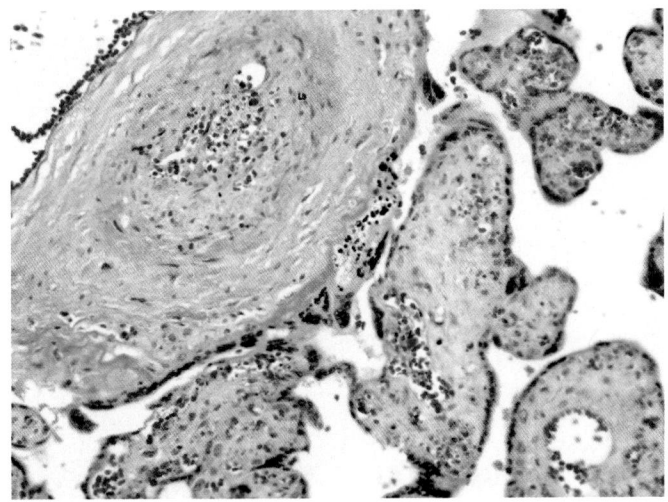

FIGURE 15.38 Red blood cell extravasation and fragmentation accompany obliteration of a muscularized villous vessel lumen by fibroblast ingrowth. As in Fig. 15.37, the histologic appearance of villous-stromal karyorrhexis (previously called hemorrhagic endovasculitis) also reflects cessation of villous vascular flow.

involution with extravasation of fragmented erythrocytes (Fig 15.38); this histologic phenotype in FTV has been termed **villous-stromal karyorrhexis**. The end stage of capillary involution results in **avascular villi** also termed villous fibrosis. This same process occurs in villi following stillbirth (see below), due to the cessation of fetal blood flow throughout the placenta. Histologically, the evolution of villous involution and fibrosis in stillbirth is for the most part temporally uniform, affects the placenta globally, and correlates with the interval between demise and delivery as determined by other parameters (Fig. 15.39).[47, 78, 79] In contrast, villous vascular changes due to fetal thrombotic vasculopathy are regional and temporally heterogeneous with respect to uninvolved villi

and/or other areas of FTV occurring at different time points in utero.

Postmortem changes occur in a fairly stereotypical manner following intrauterine demise, and involve all placental compartments. Vascular changes are probably most readily appreciated. In the umbilical cord, vascular smooth muscle fibers become elongated and attenuated, exhibiting modest nuclear pyknosis and cytoplasmic hypereosinophilia. Muscularized vessels of the chorionic plate and stem villi undergo passive involution until complete luminal fibrosis occurs. Intermediate phase changes include a variable combination of red cell extravasation, modest fibrin deposition, and bland fibroblast luminal ingrowth which may create luminal septation (Fig. 15.40). Passively involuting vessels are not distended. In addition, a mild histologic chorioamnionitis may evolve within the extraplacental membranes over the course of days or weeks following demise, perhaps reflecting a low-grade maternal response to, or superinfection of, devitalized tissues. The key histologic features that identify this as a postmortem change are the mild or 'early' appearance when compared to the more advanced postmortem changes already described, and of course the absence of a concomitant fetal inflammatory response. Postmortem vascular involution may be difficult to discriminate from antemortem vascular pathology associated with fetal thrombotic vasculopathy, particularly in cases where postmortem vascular involution is superimposed on FTV. Please refer to 'Fetal Vascular Thrombosis' in 'Constellation Disorders' below for details.

Histologic changes in villous capillaries or muscularized stem villus vessels involving erythrocyte fragmentation as a component feature, in conjunction with destruction of vascular luminal integrity, have been alternatively described in the literature under the rubric **hemorrhagic endovasculitis** or **HEV**.[80–82] In the authors' opinion, this histopathology does not represent a distinctive disorder, but rather is a component

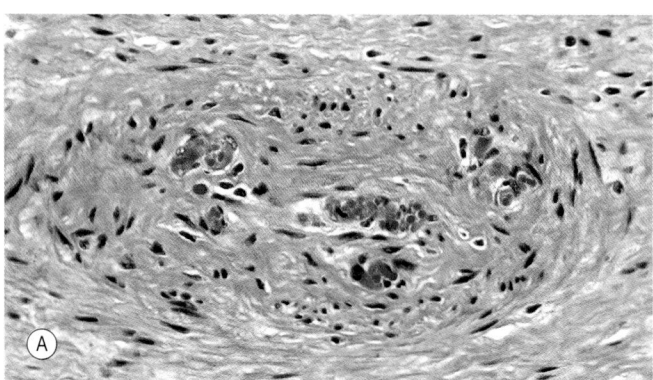

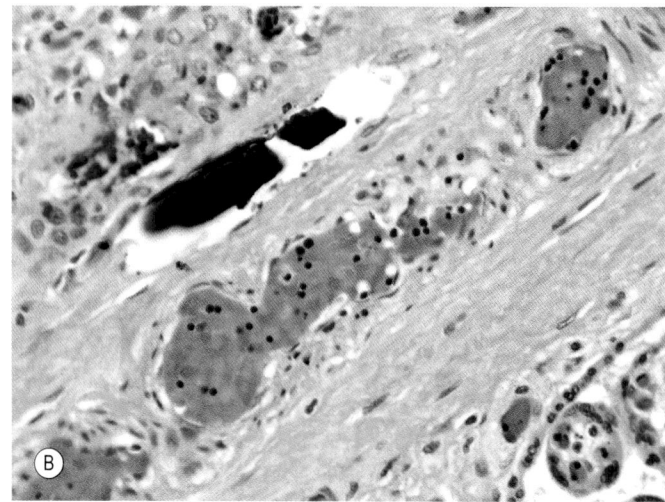

FIGURE 15.40 Postmortem villous vascular involution. (A) Fibroblast ingrowth and (B), luminal septation of non-distended muscularized villous vessels.

feature of villous vascular alterations due to other conditions, most notably fetal thrombotic vasculopathy and postmortem involution. Other conditions in which so-called HEV may appear include chronic villitis, placental infarction, and intervillous thrombi. In the latter two conditions, HEV occurs in adjacent still-viable villi, due to villous blood flow which has been disrupted through damage to neighboring villi within the lesions.

Inborn errors of metabolism that result in the abnormal accumulation of intracellular material are called **storage disorders**. In general, storage disorders are tissue-specific with respect to cell types in which abnormal metabolites accumulate. Thus, not all storage disorders will be evident in any one organ, and the placenta is no exception. The most common storage disorders which are identifiable on placental examination are galactosialodosis and I-cell disease. Other less common conditions are discussed in recent review articles.[83, 84] Placental cell types that accumulate storage material are trophoblasts and villous stromal cells. Storage product of any kind in the placenta appears as clear vacuoles which distend the cytoplasm. Identification of the specific storage material requires the usual ancillary tests, including electron microscopy, molecular genetics, and biochemistry. In families with previously affected pregnancies, antenatal testing can be performed as early as the late first trimester with chorionic villus sampling, or in the early second trimester by amniocentesis.

Mesenchymal dysplasia is a specific derangement in villous stromal development, leading to the placental phenotype of stromal overgrowth, which can be easily confused, grossly and microscopically, with hydatidiform mole.[85, 86] The gross appearance of mesenchymal dysplasia is of massively enlarged and hydropic chorionic villi affecting a proportion of the villous parenchyma (Fig. 15.41). In this respect, the distribution of hydropic villi is similar to partial molar placentas; however, the size of villous enlargement is more like complete hydatidiform

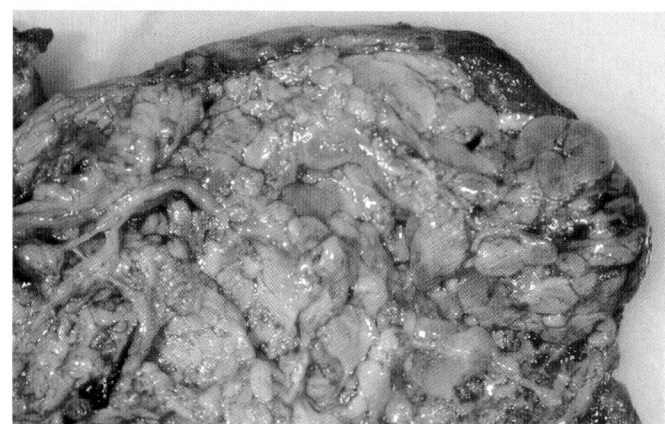

FIGURE 15.41 Mesenchymal dysplasia. Grossly hydropic chorionic villi, mimicking molar gestation. (Courtesy of Jonathan Hecht, MD PhD, Dept. of Pathology, Beth Israel-Deaconess Medical Center, Boston, MA.)

moles. Placentas are heavy for gestational age, usually beyond the 95th percentile. Microscopically, hydropic change occurs in intermediate and tertiary villi, which exhibit central stromal clearing (cistern formation) sharply rimmed by hypercellular villous stroma. Other enlarged but non-hydropic villi exhibit stromal hypercellularity. Affected villi demonstrate reduction in villous capillaries, in absolute number and in vessel caliber (Fig. 15.42). In contrast, chorionic plate and stem villus vessels are ectatic and may exhibit organizing thrombosis. Other placental compartments are not abnormal. There are two clinical considerations in making the diagnosis of mesenchymal dysplasia: to distinguish the lesion from hydatidiform mole, and to raise the possibility of fetal Beckwith-Wiedemann syndrome (BWS), which has been implicated in about half of published cases of mesenchymal dysplasia. Fetal consequences, apart from BWS, include growth restriction and stillbirth.

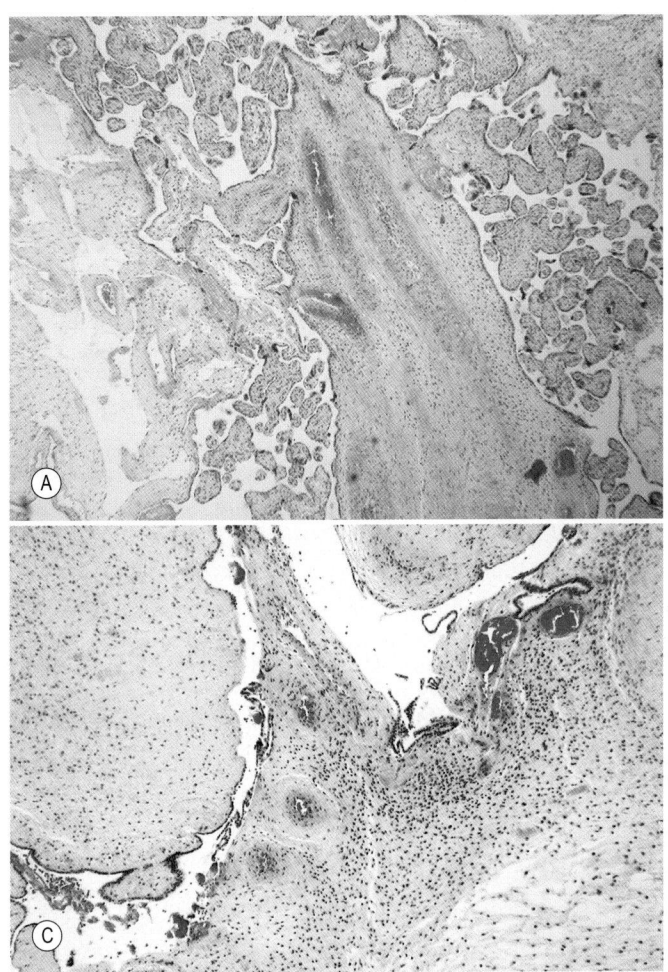

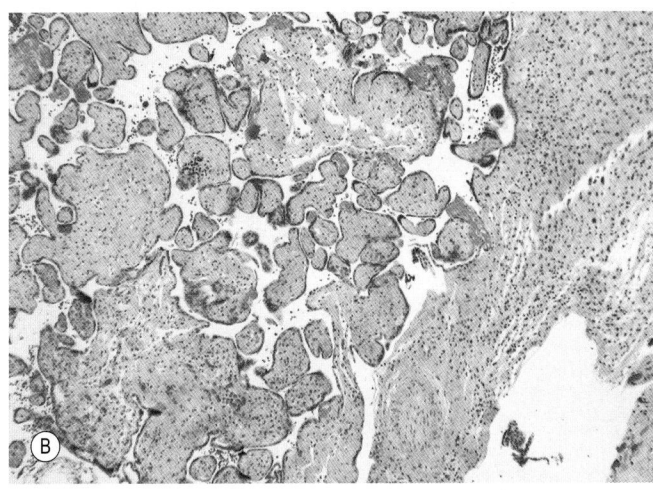

FIGURE 15.42 Mesenchymal dysplasia. Villous enlargement and stromal hypercellularity are readily evident. Also present is stromal clearing leading to bizarre villous cisterns (left side of (A), patchy in (B) and generalized villous hypovascularity in (C).

Basal plate

Microscopic disorders of the basal plate, not identifiable by gross examination, are relatively few.

Placenta accreta refers to abnormal placental implantation on to the uterine wall. When identifiable on placental examination, the lesion is demonstrated at the basal plate. With respect to terminology, **placenta accreta** in specific refers to placental implantation on the myometrial surface; **placenta increta** to placental villi surrounded by myometrium, and **placenta percreta** to placental extension through the uterine wall. The final common pathway of disorders resulting in all types of accreta is deficient endometrium, resulting in placental implanation directly on to myometrium. Under normal circumstances, the endometrium transforms into a thick decidualized lining during pregnancy; it is this layer that, having the weakest tensile strength, cleaves during placental delivery, leaving the superficial layers of decidua attached to the placental base while the generative deeper decidualized endometrium is retained in utero. Factors that lead to placenta accreta are those in which the endometrium is inherently deficient, such as placental implantation in the lower uterine segment (hence the association with placenta previa). More commonly

however, endometrial deficiency is acquired, as with instrumentation during repeated or aggressive curettage. In developed countries, the most common cause of placenta accreta in previous Cesarian section having resulted in a transmural scar devoid of endometrium. The presence of placenta accreta increases the risk of recurrent and potentially more severe accreta in future pregnancies. In some cases recurrent accreta may lead to uncontrollable postpartum hemorrhage, or the inability to separate the placenta from the uterus even after prolonged manual traction, necessitating postpartum hysterectomy. As a point of clarification, the placenta does not "invade" the myometrium in cases of increta and percreta; rather it intersects and splays the myometrium apart to variable degrees. Partial myometrial separation leads to increta, while complete myometrial separation is recognized as percreta. **Placenta accreta**, when identifiable on placental examination in the absence of hysterectomy, is virtually always a microscopic diagnosis. In many cases the placenta is sent to pathology because of abnormal adherence; occasionally, however, placenta accreta is identified independent of clinical suspicion. The microscopic diagnosis rests upon the identification of myometrial fibers in direct contact with placental villi without intervening decidual cells, which in turn is dependent on the adequacy of basal plate sampling (Fig. 15.43). Sometimes,

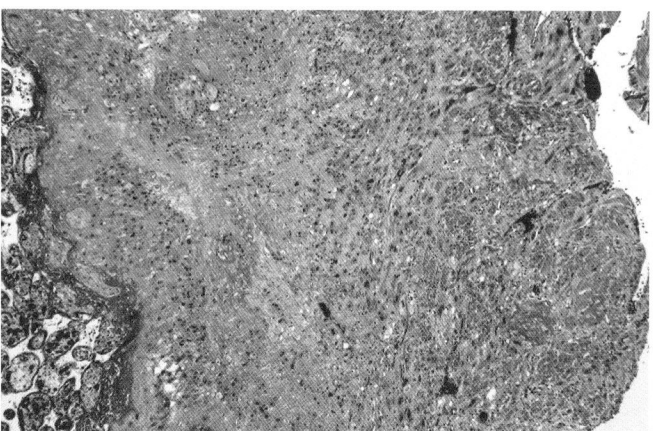

FIGURE 15.43 Placenta accreta. Chorionic villi implanting over myometrium, without intervening decidua. Intervening cells in this case are implantation trophoblasts.

myometrium may be difficult to distinguish from elongated decidual cells; muscle specific actin immunohistochemistry or trichrome stain will assist in distinguishing between the two. Even in the absence of clinically suspected placenta accreta, when a histologic diagnosis of accreta is made a note suggesting that the patient is at risk for recurrent accreta should be considered, recognizing that the clinical consequences of this microscopic finding may not be predictable. As a cautionary note, myometrial cells underlying the normal decidualized basal plate are sometimes seen, particularly following Cesarean section, and are not indicative of accreta.

Decidual arteriopathy is more reliably diagnosed within the decidua capsularis of the extraplacental membranes, since physiologic changes occur within the basal plate arterioles that may mimic arteriopathy. Pathologic vascular alterations associated with intrinsic maternal vascular disease, which may be diagnosed with reasonable confidence in the basal plate, include so-called fibrinoid necrosis of spiral arteries with or without atherosis. Fibrinoid necrosis is defined as the replacement of arterial smooth muscle by uniform hyaline-like acellular material, devoid of cells except when complicated by atherosis, in which case intramural lipid-laden macrophages are present (Fig. 15.44). This histologic lesion is mimicked by luminal fibrin accumulation within normally transformed decidual arterioles. In physiologic vessels, intravascular trophoblasts are identifiable, and the vascular contours appear appropriately distended and patulous (Fig. 15.45). Intramural lipid-laden macrophages, which are diagnostic of *atherosis* and represent unequivocal pathology of maternal vascular disease, are not present in normally transformed basal plate arterioles. Mural hypertrophy of membrane arterioles and muscularized basal plate arteries represent variant decidual arteriopathy phenotypes (Fig. 15.46). Decidual arteriopathy occurs in conditions of intrinsic maternal vascular disease of varying etiologies including pregestational diabetes mellitus, essential hypertension, and autoimmune diseases such as lupus erythematosus and scleroderma, particularly when associated with the lupus anticoagulant. Pregnancy-related maternal vascular disorders of acute onset that can produce histologic decidual vasculopathy include severe preeclampsia, eclampsia, and the HELLP (Hemolysis, Elevated Liver Enzymes and Low Platelets)

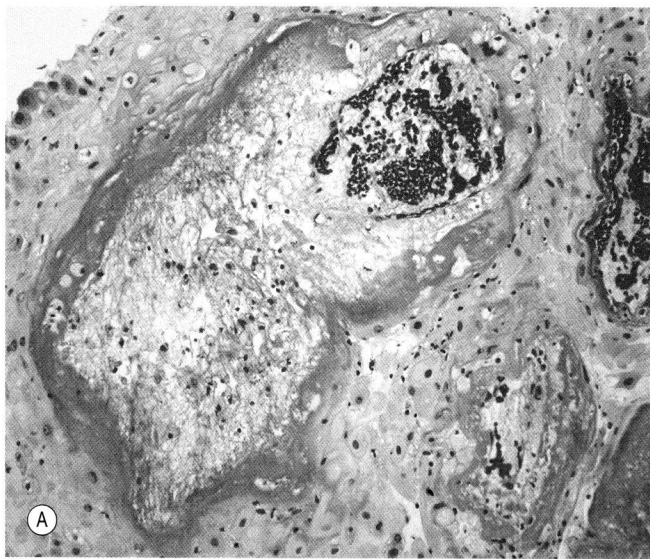

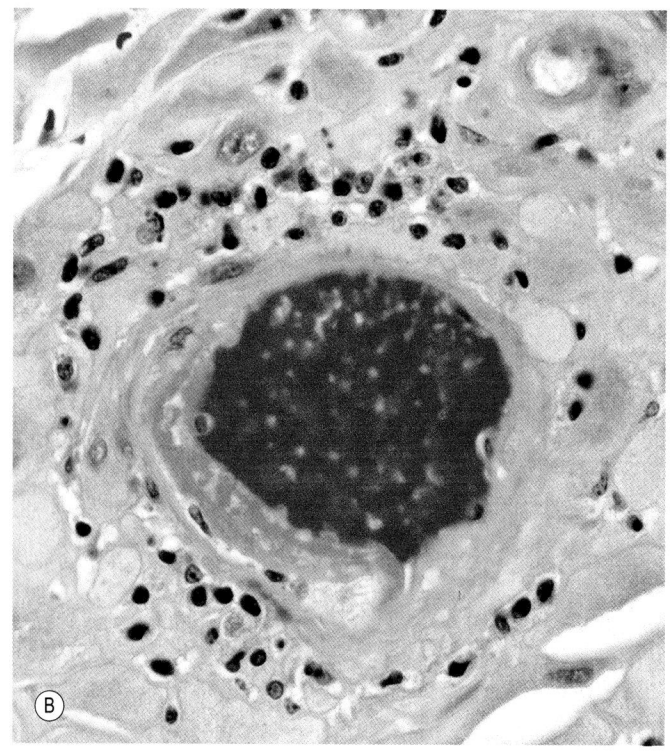

FIGURE 15.44 Decidual arteriopathy. Transmural hyalinized fibrinoid deposition with admixed lipid-laden macrophages ('fibrinoid necrosis' and 'atherosis,' respectively). (A) Near-total luminal obliteration by organizing fibrin deposition, highlighting the thrombogenic nature of this process. (B) Lymphoplasmacytic periarteritis is also present.

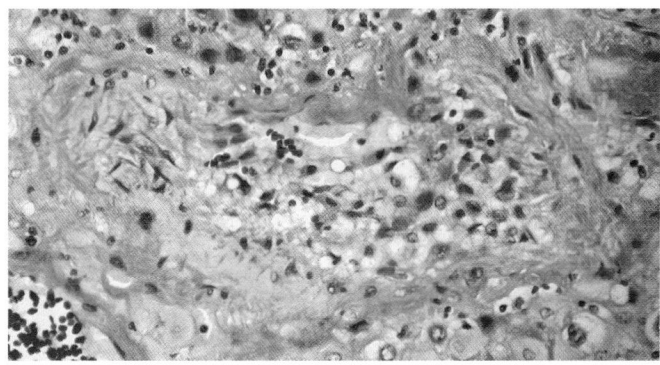

FIGURE 15.45 Normal trophoblast vascular remodeling. Late first trimester decidual artery, with luminal trophoblast plug. Physiologic lumen recanalization and mural remodeling have not yet occurred.

syndrome. Occasionally, acute atherosis will also accompany idiopathic intrauterine growth restriction in the absence of clinical hypertension or other maternal vascular disorders. When decidual arteriopathy is present, the maternal and/or fetal clinical profile is virtually always abnormal, while the converse is not always true, i.e., clinical abnormalities may be striking without overt placental pathology. This apparent disjunct may be partially attributable to patchy evolution of decidual arteriopathy in the extraplacental membranes and basal plate, and to the inherent variability of placental sampling in the absence of a gross pathologic correlate.

The common type of mononuclear inflammation within the decidua basalis is comprised of maternally derived T lymphocytes, and is not clinically significant. However, a few specific

patterns of **chronic deciduitis** warrant mention. Lymphoplasmacytic deciduitis represents a B-lymphocyte derived response to target, but almost always unknown antigens, and is commonly seen in conjunction with non-specific chronic villitis.[87] On occasion, decidual plasma cells may be seen in the absence of chronic villitis. This histologic pattern has been postulated to reflect antibody-mediated response to undisclosed infectious agents and is increased in the placentas of preterm infants where it may sometimes be of etiologic significance.[51, 88] The other pattern of specific basalis chronic inflammation is a lymphocytic decidual perivasculitis, which can be present in association with decidual arteriopathy (see Fig. 15.46B). From a pathologic perspective, no pattern of basalis inflammation is uniquely predictive, since those of potential relevance are typically found in association with other lesions.

Acute deciduitis, when clinically relevant, is also seen in conjunction with active inflammation elsewhere in the placenta. Acute deciduitis accompanies acute chorioamnionitis, representing the extravasation of maternal neutrophils from decidual vessels in response to infection. Retroplacental bleeding may accompany amniotic fluid infection, appearing grossly as a marginal placental abruption. In this context, retroplacental hematoma often results from inflammation-induced disruption of decidual vessels, and should be recognized as a consequence of ascending infection in light of other pathologic findings. This association between marginal bleeding, acute deciduitis, and chorioamnionitis is particularly evident in second trimester extreme preterm deliveries associated with amniotic fluid infection and clinical cervical incompetence (see 'Amniotic Fluid Infection' in 'Constellation Disorders' below). Acute deciduitis can also occur in any condition which interrupts

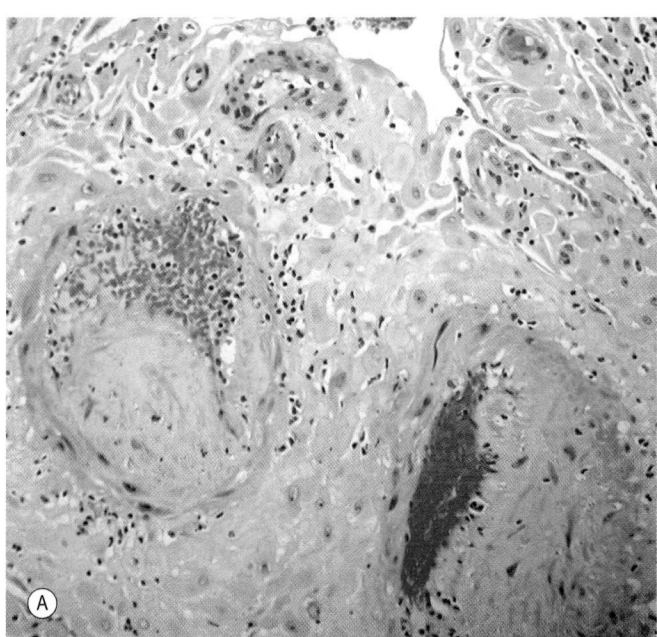

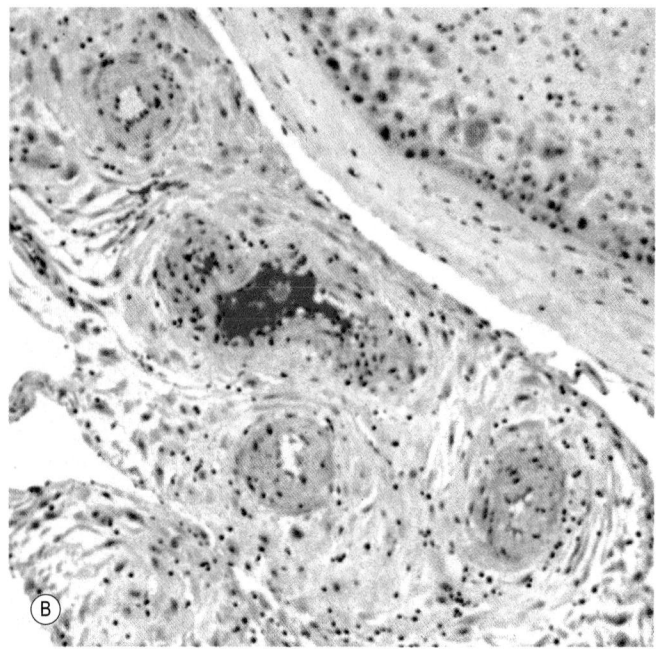

FIGURE 15.46 Mural hypertrophy of decidual arterioles within the extraplacental membranes. (A) In addition, there is marked intimal proliferation, reducing luminal diameter. (B) Note accompanying lymphocytic arteritis and periarteritis.

decidual viability, in which case there are usually accompanying areas of decidual ischemic necrosis (laminar necrosis of membranes), possibly reflecting small vessel occlusive disease.[89]

Specific topics in placental pathology

Maternal disease complicating pregnancy

Late recurrent pregnancy loss is defined for the purposes of this discussion as pregnancy loss after fetal viability has been achieved. Late recurrent loss, much less common than recurrent loss prior to fetal viability, is attributable to various maternal conditions rather than to intrinsic fetal disease. Treatable conditions that can lead to repetitive loss if not recognized include all forms of potentially recurrent, pregnancy-associated or chronic **maternal vascular disease**, such as severe pre-eclampsia, chronic hypertension, diabetes mellitus complicated by diabetic vasculopathy, and certain **autoimmune disorders** (scleroderma, lupus erythematosus). Other maternal disorders which can lead to recurrent loss if untreated include severe forms of **alloimmunity** such as Rh incompatibility and neonatal alloimmune thrombocytopenia. Idiopathic thrombo-inflammatory disorders such as chronic histiocytic intervillositis and maternal floor infarction do not present with maternal signs or symptoms, and thus are not diagnosed until stillbirth. **Uterine anomalies**, such as Müllerian malformations (e.g., uterine septum, bicornuate uterus),[90] submucosal leiomyoma, or uterine hypoplasia due to maternal in utero DES exposure,[91] may lead to recurrent late pregnancy loss, usually due to extreme premature delivery. These disorders are also etiologic in subsets of patients with infertility and early recurrent pregnancy loss, as discussed in 'The First Half of Gestation' above. Occasionally, consequences of abnormal implantation result in later losses due to compromised maternal or fetal blood flow. Cornual or uterine septum implantation and vasa previa in a low-lying placenta are a few examples. In each of these maternal disorders mentioned above, associated placental findings, when present, are as described elsewhere.

Substance use which may have deleterious fetal consequences includes prenatal exposure to alcohol, cigarette smoke, cocaine, and potentially teratogenic medications such as retinoic acid used to treat acne and angiotensin-converting enzymes (ACE inhibitors) used for hypertension. Substances inducing maternal vasoconstriction such as cigarette smoking and cocaine may lead to placental growth restriction and increase the risk of placental abruption. As a general statement, potentially serious or lethal fetal effects of teratogens are not usually reflected in striking placental pathology.

Many self-limited **maternal infections** may adversely affect the fetus. Some of the more common include *Parvovirus B19*, *Cytomegalovirus*, and *Listeria* monocytogenes.[92–97] Placental pathology is described in separate sections on 'Chronic Villitis' and 'Acute Villitis.' Uncommonly, maternal sepsis may lead to stillbirth. If fetal death occurs during active maternal infection, the cause is usually hypoxia from maternal septic shock, in which case placental findings may be restricted to intervillous leukocytosis and fetal normoblastemia.[98] Rarely, intrauterine demise may occur days or weeks following maternal recovery from sepsis. Placental changes, though dramatic, may not be immediately recognizable as secondary to prior maternal infection if demise occurs in the weeks following maternal illness. The intervillous space may be laden with fibrin, in which residual maternal leukocytes are entrapped; their numbers reduce over time. Intervillous fibrin, which prevents access of villi to maternal blood, results in ischemic villous vascular involution, upstream villous vascular thrombosis, and marked nucleated erythroid precursors (T. Boyd, personal observation). Presumably, these findings represent the effects of interrelated factors that pathologically alter the intervillous space, namely, infectious organisms and the inflammatory and/or coagulopathic processes they incite.

Placental neoplasia

Neoplasms identified within the placenta fall into three categories: tumors of placental origin, tumors within the maternal circulation, and tumors within the fetal circulation.

The most common tumor within the placenta by far is the **chorangioma**.[99, 100] Chorangiomas may be macroscopically visible if large enough to reach discrimination to the unaided eye. Grossly, they are firm and pink-red if perfused, or off-white if infarcted. They may occur anywhere within the placental disc, and are usually more-or-less spherical. Microscopically, chorangiomas are equivalent to capillary hemangiomas, comprised of capillary-sized vessels which enlarge contiguous affected villi. Larger, even muscularized feeding and draining vessels may also be scattered throughout the lesion. Chorangiomas are not clinically significant unless they attain a large enough size to result in fetal heart failure, as they demand increased cardiac output to perfuse the increased capillary mass. Rarely, chorangiomas are associated with synchronous neonatal vascular proliferations,[101] prompting speculation that similar growth factor pathways may be implicated.

Incidental **ectopic adrenal tissue** is identified rarely within the placenta. Although of uncertain histogenesis and perhaps non-neoplastic, it is included in this section because of its histologic appearance as a monotonous cellular proliferation.[102] Various pathogenetic mechanisms have been proposed, including embolization from fetus to placenta, monodermal teratoma, and aberrant extraembryonic mesodermal differentiation.[103] **Ectopic hepatic nodules** have also been reported.[104]

Choriocarcinoma is the only malignant tumor of extra-embryonic (placental) origin. Approximately 50% of choriocarcinomas occur following known gestational trophoblastic disease, usually complete hydatidiform moles, and more rarely partial moles. About 25% of choriocarcinomas occur following normal pregnancies, and the remaining 25% occur following spontaneous abortion. The gross appearance will thus depend

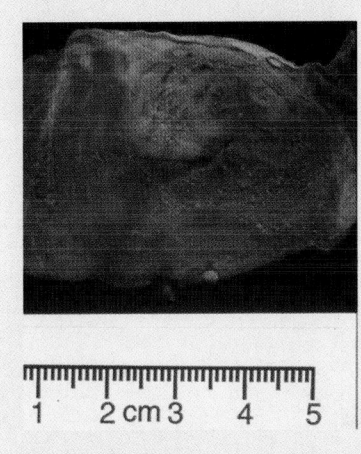

FIGURE 15.47 Placental choriocarcinoma. Nondescript off-white consolidated placental mass. Histology revealed in situ choriocarcinoma in an otherwise unremarkable term placenta. (Courtesy of David Genest, MD, formerly of Women's and Perinatal Pathology, Brigham and Women's Hospital, Boston, MA.)

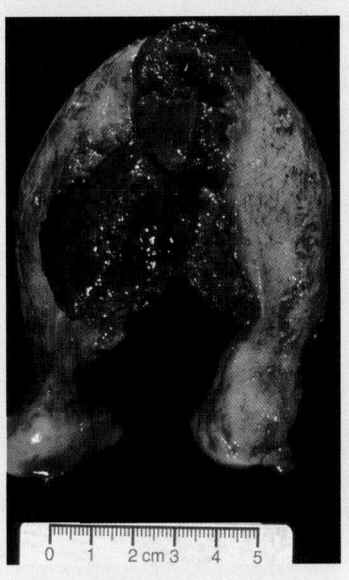

FIGURE 15.48 Choriocarcinoma, hysterectomy. Grossly, tumor is deeply invasive and hemorrhagic. This patient presented with persistent postpartum vaginal bleeding several weeks after an uncomplicated term delivery. (Courtesy of David Genest, MD, formerly of Women's and Perinatal Pathology, Brigham and Women's Hospital, Boston, MA.)

upon the context in which choriocarcinoma is identified. Within the placenta, choriocarcinoma may grossly appear firm and tan or soft and hemorrhagic, depending upon the relative proportions of tumor and blood (Fig. 15.47).[105] Within the uterus, choriocarcinoma is typically a fleshy invasive hemorrhagic tumor (Fig. 15.48). Metastases are hemorrhagic. The microscopic appearance of choriocarcinoma is the same as elsewhere, comprised of markedly atypical mitotically active cytotrophoblast nests surrounded by arcades of atypical syncytiotrophoblast (Fig. 15.49). Tumor cell nests may be difficult to identify against a background of hemorrhage and necrosis. Immunohistochemical staining is strongly positive for hCG, particularly within syncytiotrophoblasts. Neoplastic syncytio- and cytotrophoblasts are also positive for hPL.

Congenital neonatal solid tumors appearing by hematogenous spread within the fetal vasculature of the placenta are rare. **Neuroblastoma** is the most reported tumor, distantly followed by **hepatoblastoma**.[106, 107] Twin-to-twin transmission of congenital neuroblastoma through anastomoses within the monochorionic twin placenta has been described.[108]

Congenital leukemia, though also rare, is evident by extreme hypercellularity, comprised predominantly of blasts, within the fetal vasculature of the placenta. Reported subtypes of congenital leukemia include acute lymphoblastic and acute myelogenous leukemias, including congenital erythroleukemia (FAB M6).[109] More common than true congenital leukemia, though still rare, is **transient myeloproliferative disorder (TMD)**, a self-limited leukemoid disorder acquired congenitally or within the early neonatal period. Cytogenetics demonstrates clonality, in that leukemoid cells are trisomic for chromosome 21 regardless of the fetus' constitutional karyotype. Histologically, TMD is indistinguishable from acute myelogenous leukemia; it is the transient clinical course in the setting of Down syndrome, or rarely in chromosomally normal fetuses,[110] that defines the disorder. An intriguing pathogenetic theory is that TMD may result from 'abnormal prenatal production of placental regulatory hemopoietic factors caused by chromosomal defect(s) confined to placental tissues'.[111]

Malignant maternal tumors metastatic to the placenta include, in decreasing order of frequency, **melanoma, leukemia/lymphoma, breast cancer, lung cancer, sarcomas, gastric cancer, and gynecologic cancers**.[112] As of 2002, about one-third of maternal-to-placental metastases reported in the literature have been due to malignant melanoma (Fig. 15.50); of these cases, about one-fifth have metastasized to the fetus, and almost all fetuses have died.[113]

Both fetal and maternal tumors with placental metastases can lead to intrauterine or neonatal demise. While somatic tumor burden is one obvious cause, the direct effects of placental involvement may also lead to stillbirth. Extensive fetal vascular tumor volume can lead to demise by villous vascular tumor plugging, resulting in fatal hypoxia. Alternatively, fetal blood hyperviscosity due to tumor cellularity may predispose to blood flow stasis, leading to an unusual cause of lethal fetal vascular thrombosis.

Constellation disorders

The following four abnormal intrauterine conditions each exhibit a multitude of pathologic findings which, when present in constellation, define the disorders and the pathologic states from whence they arise.

Amniotic fluid infection

Amniotic fluid infection (AFI) refers to the presence of infectious organisms in the amniotic fluid. Intra-amniotic infection (IAI) is an interchangeable term, used most frequently in the clinical literature. The histologic counterpart of AFI is referred to in general terms as chorioamnionitis, understanding

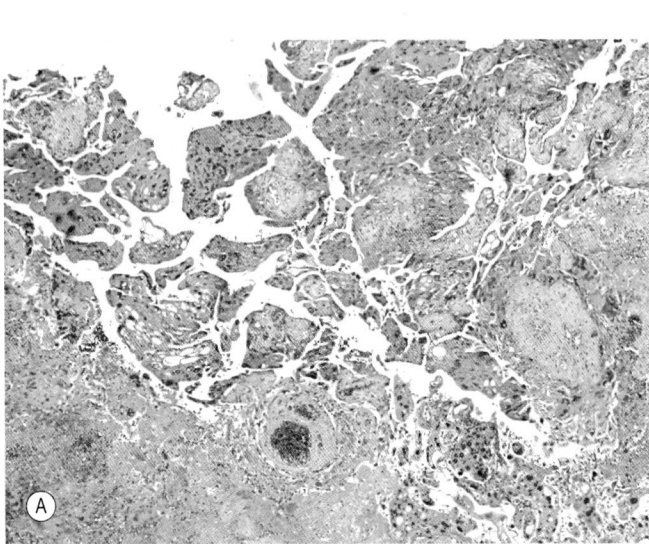
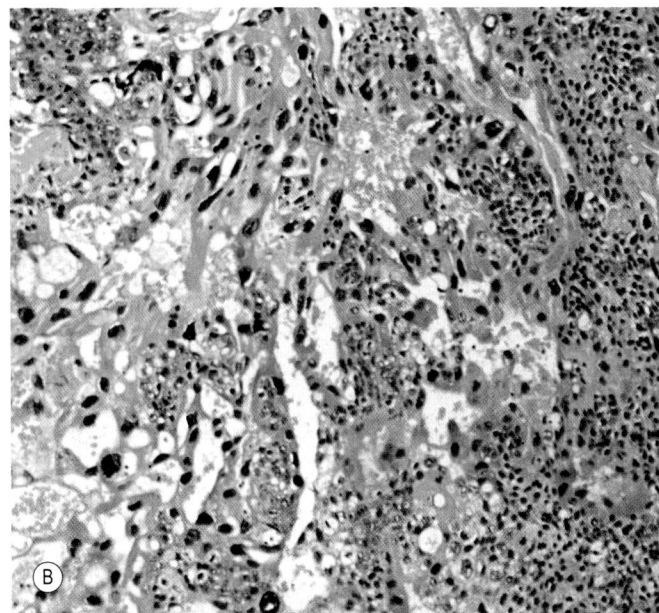

FIGURE 15.49 Placental choriocarcinoma. (A) Microscopic evaluation reveals markedly atypical cyto- and syncytiotrophoblast, best appreciated on higher power (B).

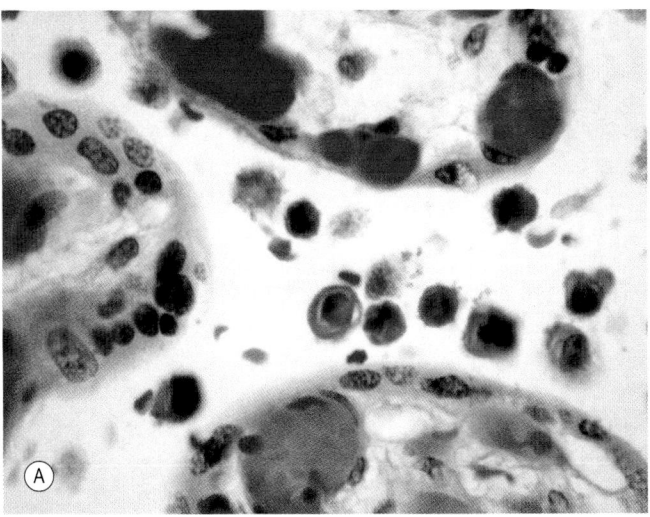
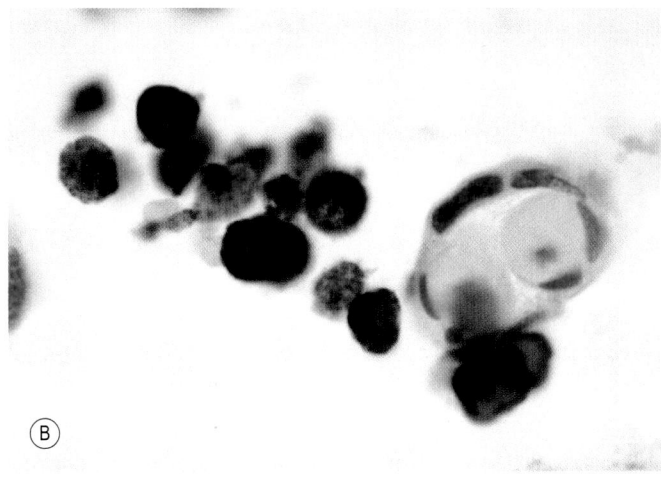

FIGURE 15.50 (A) Discohesive cytologically atypical cells within the maternal intervillous space. (B) Immunohistochemistry positive for HMB-45, supporting the diagnosis of metastatic maternal malignant melanoma. Subsequent maternal clinical evaluation did not reveal the primary lesion (Courtesy Bradley Quade, MD PhD, Division of Women's and Perinatal Pathology, Department of Pathology, Brigham and Women's Hospital, Boston, MA).

that duration and extent of inflammation (stage and grade respectively; vide infra) are not reflected in 'chorioamnionitis' when used as an umbrella designation.

Amniotic fluid infection typically occurs via ascension of infectious organisms from the perineum and/or vagina into the normally sterile uterine cavity. Although this process can occur at any time during gestation, it is rare in the first trimester, and uncommon in the first half of pregnancy except in the clinical context of cervical incompetence. In the previable period

(<24 weeks gestation), amniotic fluid infection usually results in stillbirth. Fetal demise may occur in the intrapartum period due to extreme prematurity and the inability to withstand the physiologic stressors of labor. After viability, labor induced by amniotic fluid infection usually results in live birth. Neonatal outcome depends on a host of factors including gestational age, duration of infection, organism virulence, proper balance between excessive and/or deficient maternal and fetal inflammatory responses, and coincident maternal or fetal disease(s).

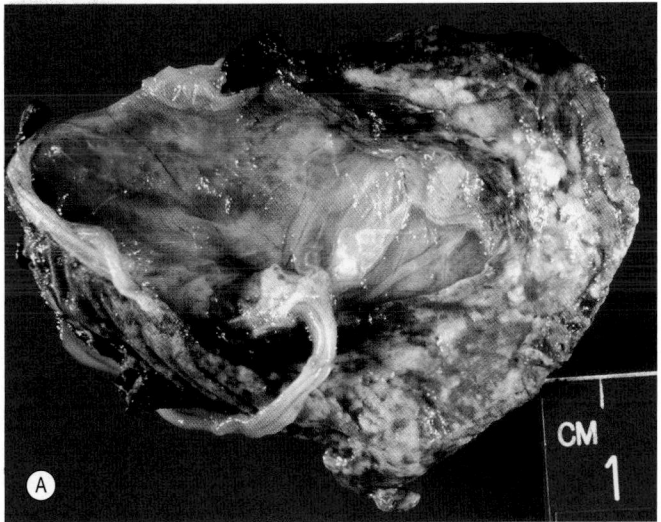
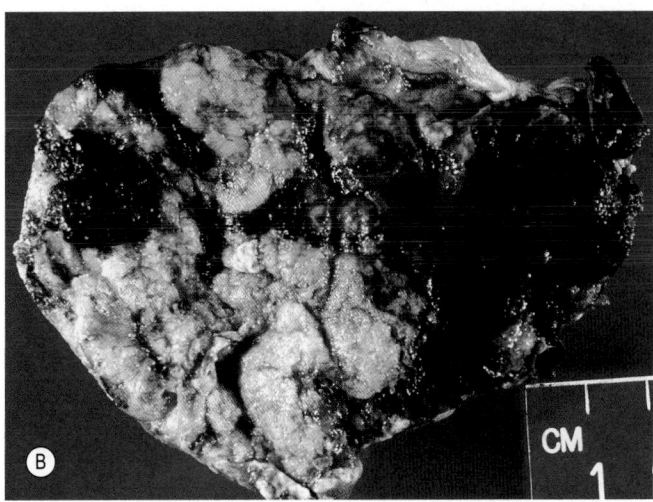

FIGURE 15.51 Amniotic fluid infection (acute chorioamnionitis) in the setting of extreme preterm delivery. (A) Note the opacity of chorionic plate membranes. (B) Associated retroplacental hematoma, due to inflammation-induced disruption of decidual vessel integrity.

Causative organisms are usually commensal (symbiotic) or colonizing (potentially disease-producing) bacteria present within the vaginal canal and/or perineum. Examples of commensal organisms include the normal lactobacillus-predominant vaginal flora, or the anaerobic-predominant vaginal flora that replace lactobacillus (i.e. bacterial vaginosis). Colonizing bacteria include *group B streptococcus*, an organism identified in the vaginal canal of a significant minority of reproductive age women. Less frequently *E. coli* colonize the vagina through fecal contamination. Aerobic bacteria, anaerobic bacteria, and streptococcal strains in addition to group B streptococcus are among the other common agents responsible for ascending amniotic fluid infection. *Fusobacteria*, *Chlamydia trachomatis*, *Ureaplasma urealyticum* and *Mycoplasma* in particular are prevalent in preterm delivery and/or preterm membrane rupture. *Candida albicans*, and rarely other fungi, sometimes cause fungal amniotic fluid infection, though neonatal morbidity rarely results.

Rarely, amniotic fluid infection occurs by direct inoculation of organisms, such as during amniocentesis or manual vaginal examination, in which the instrument or operator's hand is inadvertently contaminated. In these circumstances, causative organisms tend to be of cutaneous origin, such as *Staphylococcus epidermidis*. Other distinctive routes of spread include hematogenous dissemination from oral flora during dental procedures, and local spread from pelvic organs such as the urinary bladder, fallopian tube, or intestine.

Grossly, placentas with well-established chorioamnionitis demonstrate opacity of the extraplacental membranes and chorionic plate, which may be patchy or diffuse. Opacity results from the inability of light to pass through the neutrophilic infiltrate, as occurs can be seen in separated buffy coat of whole blood. Discoloration is usually off-white or tan but may exhibit green or light brown hues, the former due to neutrophil peroxidase, and thus be mistaken grossly for meconium. The degree of amniotic surface discoloration is not always a reliable indicator of chorioamnionitis, as discoloration may be due to other pigments (meconium, hemosiderin); conversely, some placentas with chorioamnionitis are transparent or unpigmented grossly. In general, the more premature the placenta, the more likely it is to be discolored in the presence of chorioamnionitis; this observation may reflect a greater intensity of inflammation at delivery (Fig. 15.51A).

The histologic evolution of amniotic fluid infection follows a stereotypical progression, and includes both maternal and fetal inflammation.[114, 115] The onset of maternal inflammation occurs in two locations: the extraplacental membranes and the chorionic plate. Maternal inflammation generally precedes the fetal inflammatory response, and so will be considered first.

With ascending infection, maternal neutrophils exit maternal decidual vessels to produce acute deciduitis, initially at the placental edge closest to the endocervical os; this may result in so-called marginal abruption due to venous bleeding from marginal 'sinus' veins (Fig. 15.51B). As neutrophils in the decidua continue to migrate via chemotaxis toward the amniotic fluid, **acute deciduitis** evolves into **acute chorionitis**, and then **acute chorioamnionitis,** depending upon the location of neutrophils within the extraplacental membranes. A second initial site of inflammation occurs within the placental disc, as maternal neutrophils derived from intervillous blood accumulate in subchorionic fibrin (so-called Langhan's stria) to produce **acute subchorionitis**. With chemotactic progression, neutrophils migrate through the chorionic plate stroma; this evolution pattern equates to acute chorionitis/chorioamnionitis, although maternally derived chorionic plate inflammation does not have a specific term.

The fetal inflammatory response is also seen at two locations: the umbilical cord and the chorionic plate. Neutrophilic umbilical vascular inflammation is generally termed **umbilical vasculitis**; extension into Wharton's jelly is termed **perivasculitis** or **funisitis** (Fig. 15.52A). Umbilical cord inflammation occurs

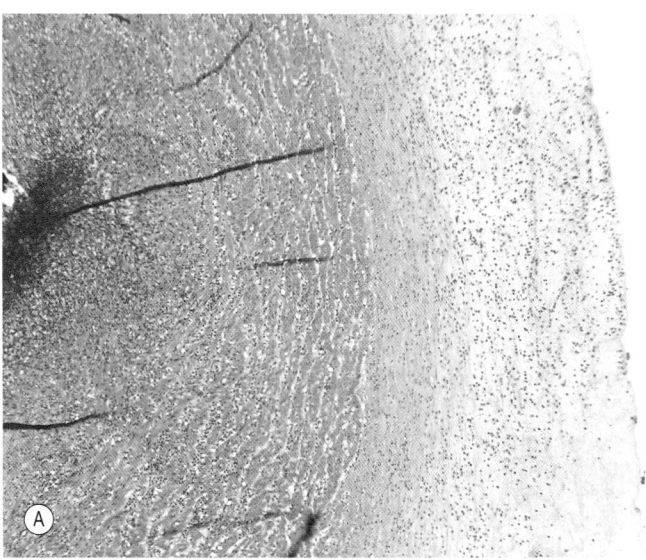
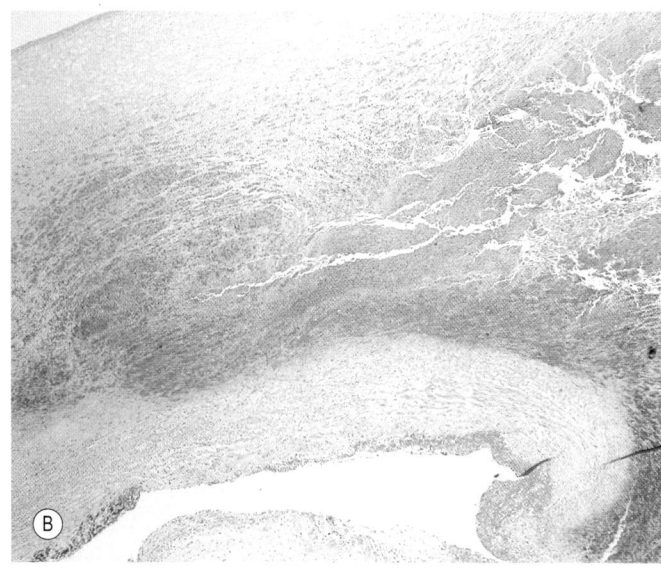

FIGURE 15.52 Active funisitis. (A) Note the presence of neutrophils throughout the umbilical cord cross-section, reflecting a robust fetal inflammatory response to organisms within the amniotic fluid. (B) Necrotizing funisitis, in association with non-occlusive and partially calcified thrombus. The features in B indicate longstanding inflammation.

initially within the muscular wall of the umbilical vein (**phlebitis**); inflammation within one or both arteries (**arteritis**) follows. Like their maternal counterparts, fetal neutrophils migrate toward organisms within the amniotic fluid via chemotaxis; thus, a polarized, centrifugal pattern of neutrophilic inflammation results. Only in advanced stages of the inflammatory response do fetal neutrophils exit umbilical vessels circumferentially, producing rings of neutrophilic debris surrounding vessel walls (**subacute necrotizing funisitis**) (Fig. 15.52B).[116] Within the chorionic plate, this same pattern of polarized inflammation occurs as fetal neutrophils exit chorionic plate vessels nearest the surface of the placental disc. Fetal neutrophilic inflammation within chorionic vessel walls and beyond into the chorionic plate is termed **chorionic vasculitis**. It is the chorionic equivalent of umbilical vasculitis.

Schemata exist for reporting the duration (stage) and intensity (grade) of both maternal and fetal inflammatory responses.[115, 117, 118] Thus, stage 1 maternal inflammation is limited to acute subchorionitis and/or acute chorionitis, stage 2 is chorioamnionitis NOS, and stage 3 is necrotizing chorioamnionitis. Grade 1 chorioamnionitis reflects non-confluent neutrophil inflammation, or "routine" chorioamnionitis. Grade 2 chorioamnionitis refers to confluent neutrophils (>30/hpf) and/or microabscess formation. With respect to the fetal inflammatory response, stage and grade are constructed as follows: stage 1 refers to chorionic vasculitis and/or umbilical phlebitis, stage 2 umbilical arteristis (one or both arteries), and stage 3 advanced funisitis, that may include necrotizing and/or circumferential perivascular inflammation. Grading of the fetal inflammatory response is as with maternal grade: grade 1 is non-confluent, grade 2 is dense, extensive inflammation. Whereas stage is roughly correlated with the length of time amniotic fluid has been present, the data less linearly relate grade to chronicity.

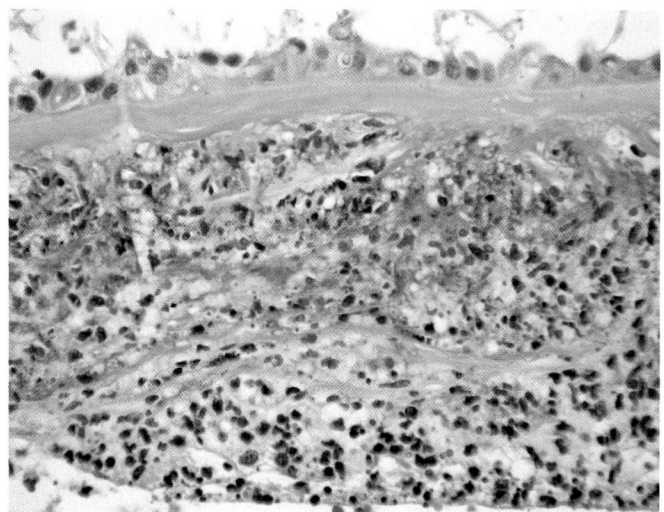

FIGURE 15.53 Acute chorioamnionitis leading to preterm delivery, due to fungal amniotic fluid infection. A few yeast forms are present within reactive amnion epithelium. Neutrophil karryorhexis and stromal degeneration have commenced, producing early necrotizing chorioamnionitis.

With both maternal and fetal inflammation, however, readily identified degenerating (karyorrhectic) neutrophils reflect an interval between the onset of inflammation and delivery of roughly a day or more. Likewise, necrotizing chorioamnionitis and particularly necrotizing funisitis reflect a period of at least a few and possibly several (three or more) days between inflammation and delivery. In these contexts, 'necrotizing' refers to a combination of karryorhectic neutrophilic debris and underlying destruction of inflamed tissues (Fig. 15.53).

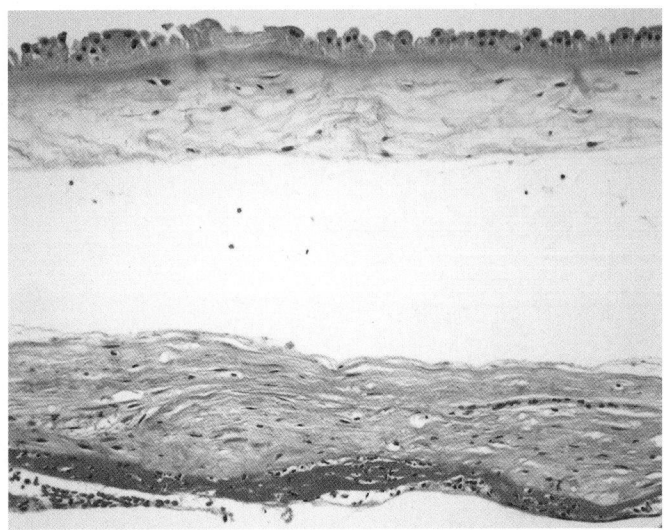

FIGURE 15.54 Early (minimal) acute subchorionitis. This placenta was sent for examination unrelated to clinical concern for amniotic fluid infection. This degree of neutrophilic entrapment within subchorionic fibrin likely resulted from a several hour interval between membrane rupture and delivery, and should not be overinterpreted as indicative of clinically significant infection.

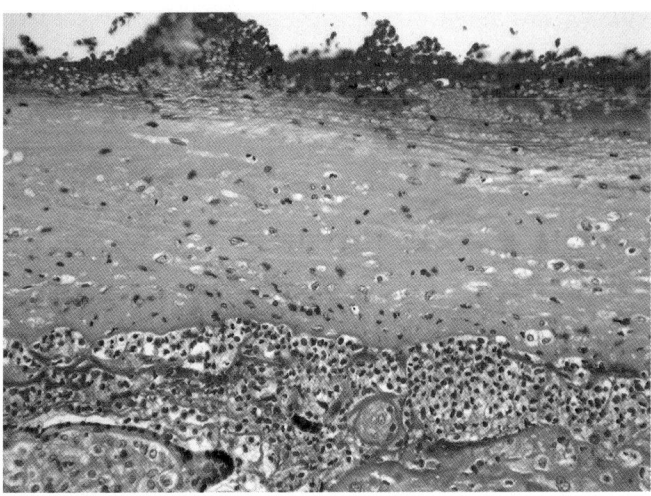

FIGURE 15.55 Intense acute subchorionitis. Neutrophil microabscesses line the subchorionic plate. This pattern is diagnostic of infection, in this case due to *Listeria monocytogenes*.

It is well to emphasize that amniotic fluid infection is not equivalent to fetal infection. Unequivocal fetal infection occurs when organisms from the amniotic fluid incite a tissue-based acute inflammatory response in the lung, producing fetal/neonatal pneumonia, or when organisms gain entry into the systemic fetal circulation, producing fetal bacteremia. Fetal infection evolves following fetal inspiration (breathing) and ingestion (swallowing) of infected amniotic fluid, which leads to the potential but by no means inevitable consequences of pneumonia and/or sepsis. With sepsis, organisms may gain entry into the systemic circulation either through alveolar capillaries or capillaries within the intestinal lamina propria. The histologic presence of a fetal inflammatory response within the placenta (fetal vasculitis) reflects local recognition by fetal neutrophils of infected amniotic fluid; it does not equate to fetal infection. Even the histologic presence of neutrophils in fetal airways or the intestinal lumen is not synonymous with infection; rather, these findings represent fetal inspiration and ingestion, respectively, of amniotic fluid neutrophils. Infectious organisms in alveolar spaces and/or the intestinal lumen evoke a less straightforward interpretation of whether fetal infection is present. However, infectious organisms identified within somatic fetal vessels is diagnostic of bacteremia.

A few specific circumstances of 'chorioamnionitis' warrant elaboration.

1. *Subchorionitis.* Histologic subchorionitis likely evolves within many hours following membrane rupture. Thus, it is fairly common to see neutrophils aligned within subchorionic fibrin in placentas sent for pathologic evaluation for indications other than clinical chorioamnionitis, when membrane rupture precedes delivery by 6 or more hours

(Fig.15.54). The intensity of subchorionic neutrophilic aggregation in this context lies in sharp contrast to acute subchorionitis associated with well-established maternally derived active inflammation elsewhere, be it acute subchorionitis (Fig. 15.55), acute chorioamnionitis, or acute villitis.

2. *Fungal infection.* Fungal funisitis can produce a pathognomonic gross pattern of punctate opaque white lesions near the surface of Wharton jelly, which microscopically represent microabscesses. GMS or PAS stain frequently reveal superficially invasive hyphae to which neutrophils chemotactically respond (see Fig. 15.15).[119,120]

3. *Meconium.* Whether neutrophils respond to meconium, independent of the mechanism inciting meconium release, is controversial. That no clinicopathologic studies exist correlating placental culture results to cases where both meconium and chorioamnionitis are present hampers validation or refutation of the concept. In favor of meconium-induced placentitis are the following observations: meconium aspiration can elicit meconium pneumonitis, a neutrophilic inflammatory pattern histologically similar to infectious pneumonia; and, in cases of meconium-induced umbilical vascular necrosis, intense umbilical vasculitis/funisitis may be present without any extraplacental membrane or chorionic plate inflammation.[121]

Hematogenous placental infection

Less commonly than by the ascending vaginal route, organisms may infect the placenta by hematogenous spread from maternal blood. Mothers may be symptomatic or asymptomatic. Hematogenous infection includes that caused by viruses and protozoa in addition to bacteria, and as a general rule produces specific patterns of placentitis that vary by organism. This lies in contrast to the fairly uniform appearance of amniotic fluid infection, irrespective of causative organism. Organism species responsible for hematogenous placental infection are more restricted than the panoply of species, albeit mainly bacteria, that produce amniotic fluid infection, and include, in the current era, most commonly the following:

Viruses: Cytomegalovirus, Herpes simplex virus, Parvovirus B19;

Protozoa: *Toxoplasma gondii*; and

Bacteria: *Treponema pallidum* (syphilis), *Listeria monocytogenes.*

In contrast to the histologic evolution of ascending infection, hematogenously spread infection often elicits an inflammatory response within the placental disc, resulting in villitis and/or intervillositis. In later stages of inflammation, subchorionitis, chorioamnionitis, and deciduitis may also develop, presumably due to passage of organisms through the placenta and into the amniotic fluid (see Fig. 15.55).

Villitis may be acute or chronic, referring to recruited inflammatory cells rather than the time course of disease. **Acute villitis** is infectious; in florid form, it consists of neutrophil aggregates within the maternal intervillous space, which encroach upon, involve, and in some cases coagulate parenchymal villi in necroinflammatory, fibrin-rich masses. Smaller microabscesses may be found in the center of intervillous neutrophil clusters, or within individually inflamed villi (Fig. 15.56). Fibrin commonly accompanies and, as a cautionary note, may overshadow and thus obscure the neutrophilic infiltrate. *Listeria monocytogenes* is the classic causative organism in cases of acute villitis; other less common organisms include *Campylobacter fetus*, enteric bacilli, and the pathogenic streptococci.[96, 98, 122] Maternal spirochetosis due to *T. pallidum* most commonly causes an acute or mixed acute and chronic villous vasculitis; however, non-syphilitic spirochetes rarely produce the same histologic phenotype (Fig. 15.57).

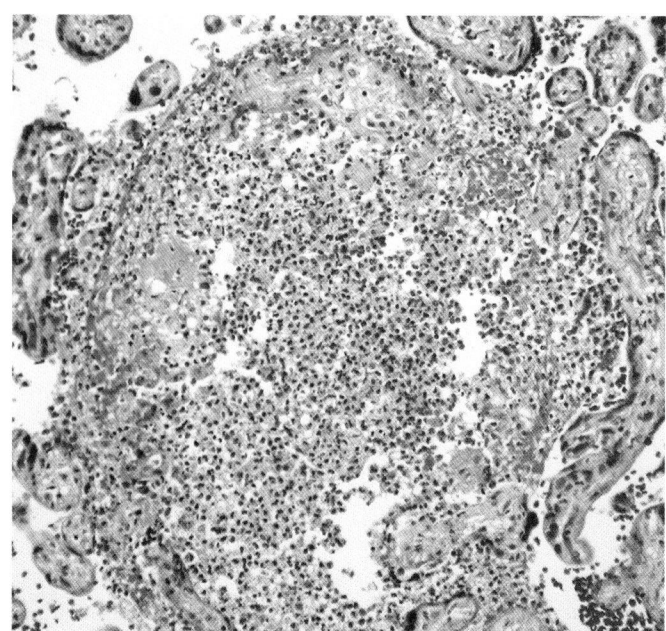

FIGURE 15.56 Acute villitis. In this field, intervillous fibrin is minimal relative to the neutrophilic infiltrate. *Listeria monocytogenes*; same case as Fig. 15.55.

Maternal vascular underperfusion

Pathologic states leading to chronic suboptimal **uteroplacental underperfusion** include many conditions that feature intrinsic maternal vascular disease. These include: chronic hypertension, diabetes mellitus with clinical arteriopathy, HELLP, preeclampsia and eclampsia, and some forms of autoimmunity such as lupus erythematosus and scleroderma. Decidual arteriopathy with or without atherosis, discussed above, may be present within the decidua capsularis and/or decidua basalis. The placenta is

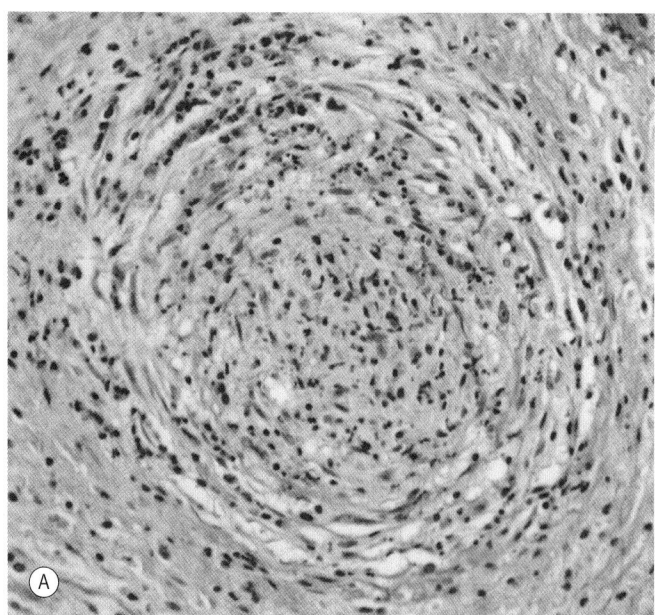

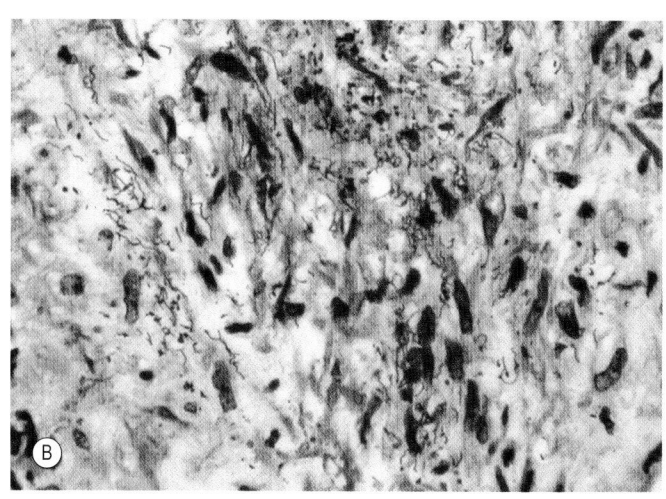

FIGURE 15.57 Obliterative stem villous vasculitis due to maternal spirochetosis (possibly *Borrelia* or *Leptospira* spp.; PCR was negative for *T. pallidum*). (A) Note concentric 'onion skin' appearance of inflammation and fibrosis. (B) Silver (Steiner) stain reveals unequivocal spirochetes. (Courtesy Christopher Crum, MD, Chief, Division of Women's and Perinatal Pathology, Department of Pathology, Brigham and Women's Hospital, Boston, MA).

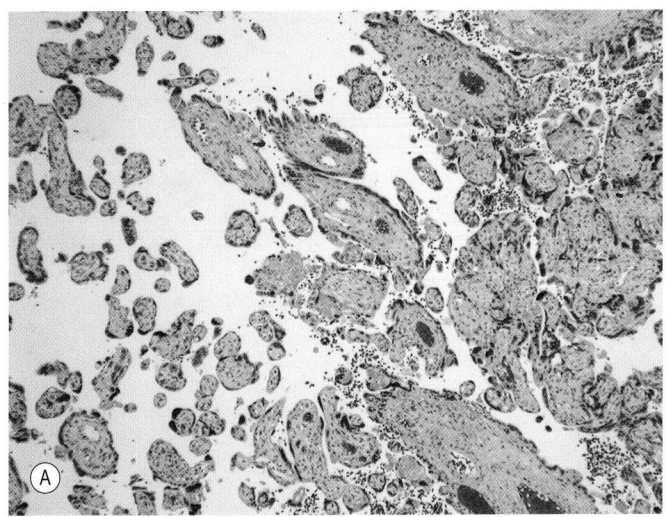
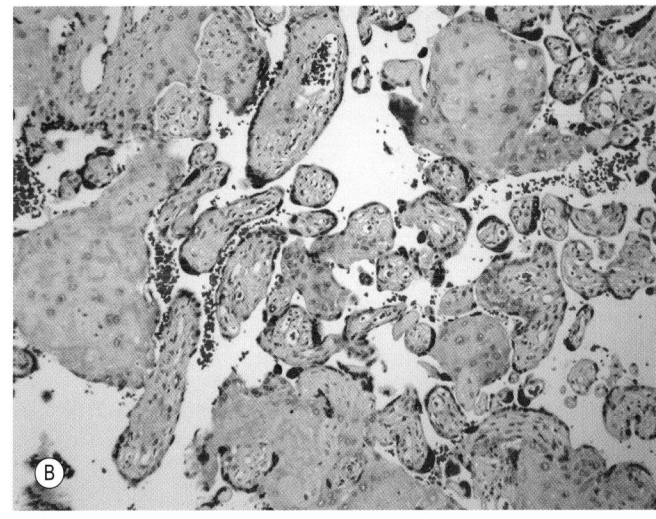

FIGURE 15.58 Maternal vascular underperfusion. A constellation of microscopic villous pathologic features is often present. (A) Distal villous hypoplasia (left side), agglutinated villi (right side) and increased syncytial knots. (B) Increased intervillous fibrin, in which cytotrophoblast proliferation may be prominent.

often small for gestational age, and may exhibit multifocal and temporally heterogeneous infarction and/or abruption. The umbilical cord may be narrow, defined as <0.8 cm in diameter in the third trimester. Microscopically, a number of parenchymal abnormalities may be evident in varying combination, all of which reflect long-term poor perfusion of the villous tree and the intervillous space. Villous abnormalities include increased syncytial knots, distal villous hypoplasia (also called terminal villous deficiency), and agglutinated terminal villi. Intervillous space abnormalities included increased intervillous fibrinoid, often accompanied by proliferation of intervillous intermediate trophoblast (so-called X cells) (Fig. 15.58). Additional abnormalities may be present within the decidua basalis, but are somewhat more subtle and thus more difficult to diagnose confidently. These include increased numbers of multinucleated implantation site trophoblasts ('placental site giant cells') and increased numbers of immature intermediate trophoblasts, reflecting superficial placental implantation.[48, 123] This phenomenon, established early in placentation, may be due to the inability of implantation site trophoblasts to adopt a normally invasive phenotype due to hypoxia from maternal vascular underperfusion. This in turn results in inadequate remodeling of spiral arterioles which further aggravates hypoxia in a self-potentiating 'feed-forward' mechanism of accelerating pathology. One of the most important reasons to recognize placental underperfusion is because many causative maternal conditions are chronic, and thus carry an increased risk for recurrent fetal morbidity and mortality in future pregnancies.

Diffuse chorioamnionic hemosiderosis

Diffuse chorioamnionic hemosiderosis (DCH) is the pathologic equivalent of clinical chronic abruption–oligohydramnios sequence.[124–126] Clinically, patients present with persistent intermittent to continuous bleeding, and eventually oligohydramnios. Preterm delivery is common. Predisposing risk factors include smoking and multiparity. Grossly, the membranes and fetal surface may appear tan to brown, often with a green hue, thus being mistaken for meconium staining. The most striking histologic feature is the presence of hemosiderin-laden stromal macrophages within the extraplacental membranes and chorionic plate, which account for the surface discoloration (Fig. 15.59A). In circumstances where microscopic recognition of macrophage pigment as hemosiderin may be problematic, iron stain is useful (Fig. 15.59B). Other findings that reflect persistent bleeding include circumvallate placentation (see Fig. 15.20) and degenerated blood beneath the extraplacental membranes, around the placental margin, and extending into the subchorionic space (Fig. 15.59A), all representing chronic bleeding from marginal maternal veins ('marginal sinuses').[127] Aside from complications of prematurity, there may also be an increased risk for neurologic impairment in term neonates with placentas exhibiting DCH.[128]

Fetal vascular thrombosis

Thrombosis within the placental fetal vascular tree is probably an underrecognized cause of severe neonatal morbidity, particularly central nervous system injury, and stillbirth. Conditions that predispose to thrombosis follow Virchow's triad of blood hyperviscosity, endothelial damage, and reduced flow. Of these factors, reduction of blood flow velocity through the umbilical cord by a variety of mechanical mechanisms is the most significant factor. Umbilical cord abnormalities that predispose to cord compression include hypercoiling, nuchal or body-wrapping, velamentous or marginal insertion, and narrow cord diameter.[129] Factors of the intrauterine environment that may contribute include oligohydramnios and, rarely, anatomic

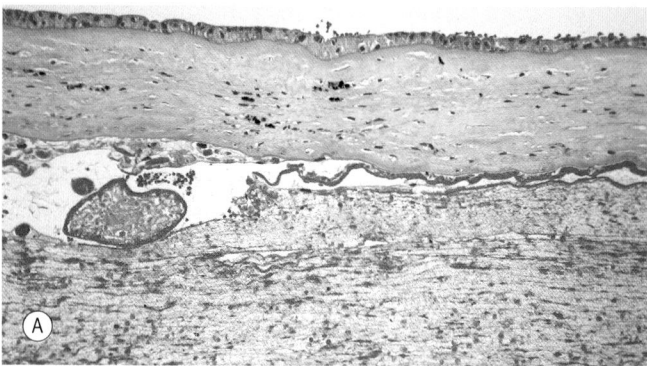
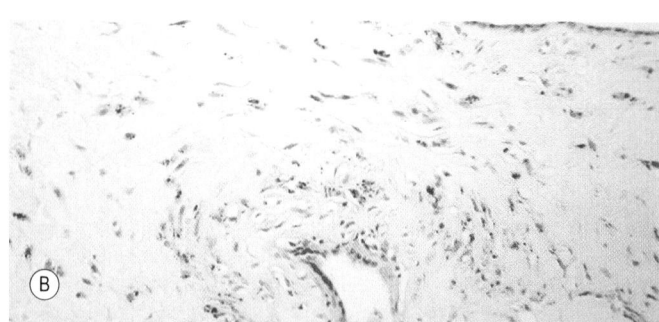

FIGURE 15.59 Diffuse chorionic hemosiderosis. (A) Chorionic plate hemosiderin-laden macrophages and subchorionic hematoma. (B) Iron stain (Prussian blue) highlights chorionic plate and membrane hemosiderin.

anomalies such as uterine septum. These conditions predispose to umbilical cord compression between the fetal body and uterine wall. Less commonly, factors from the other components of Virchow's triad may be operative: hyperviscosity due to heritable coagulopathy, or hypercellularity (e.g., polycythemia, congenital leukemia), or endothelial damage due to preexisting fetal vasculitis. The association between fetal (especially chorionic) vasculitis and thrombosis occurs particularly in preterm deliveries due to amniotic fluid infection (D. Genest, personal communication), perhaps in part because the fetal inflammatory response can be intense in these cases, resulting in a greater degree of inflammation-induced endothelial damage.

In circumstances of reduced umbilical blood flow, the pattern of thrombosis reflects the location of obstruction. Thrombosis is much more commonly observed in chorionic plate and early generation stem villus vessels than in cord vessels, despite the fact that obstruction often occurs within the cord (see Figs 15.18 and 15.26). There are likely at least two reasons for this observation. First, the perpendicular angle taken by cord vessels as they branch onto the chorionic plate creates a physiologic region of turbulent flow, such that further flow reduction may induce preferential thrombosis at this site. Second, there are many more chorionic plate and stem villus vessels sampled during routine placental examination than there are cord vessel sections, suggesting sampling bias may also be a factor (Fig. 15.60). If downstream regions of disrupted blood flow are seen, the usual pattern is regional; clustered villi that show vascular red cell extravasation and fragmentation in earlier lesions, or avascular villi when thrombosis has occurred remotely with respect to delivery. The term employed for this downstream pathology, **fetal thrombotic vasculopathy (FTV)**, is operationally defined as 15 or more affected terminal villi per section.[66] However, from a pathogenetic perspective, unequivocal upstream thrombosis also falls within this rubric. Temporal heterogeneity of placental lesions reflects ongoing thrombosis (Fig. 15.61). Dystrophic calcification within thrombosed fetal vessels indicates the onset of pathologic blood flow restriction remotely (at least weeks) prior to delivery (Fig. 15.62).

There is a second pattern of fetal vascular occlusion, unrelated to umbilical cord obstruction. This occurs with chronic villitis,

which destroys villous vessels within the body of the placental disc, typically affecting terminal, intermediate, and small stem villi. This vasodestructive inflammatory pattern has been coined 'obliterative fetal vasculopathy.'[66] In these cases, erythrocyte extravasation and avascular villi occur in conjunction with chronic villitis (see Fig. 15.35). Villous vessels upstream of affected villi exhibit passive involution, reminiscent of changes that occur following intrauterine demise.

Fetal thrombotic vasculopathy is an important lesion to recognize in medicolegal investigations of unexpected, untoward neonatal outcome, especially neurodevelopmental outcome, since it is evolving as one of the principal placental disorders identified in this context.[71,130,131] As with all obstetrical malpractice claims, cause and timing of fetal stressor(s) is of paramount importance.

Markers of intrauterine stress

Meconium

On close microscopic scrutiny of placentas submitted for pathologic evaluation, for indications other than meconium, and where meconium discoloration is not observed grossly, it is possible to find rare and sometimes faintly pigmented membrane macrophages. Pigment in these circumstances has been variably attributed to prior physiologic meconium discharge, or lipofuscin. It has been hypothesized that minute quantities of meconium can be passed in the final weeks of pregnancy.[132,133] Presumably this physiologic meconium discharge is of such minor amount that amniotic fluid does not appear discolored to the naked eye, and meconium is not detected on gross placental examination. In any event, as an isolated observation these pigment-laden cells should not be overly construed as clinically significant.

Pathologic meconium discharge, on the other hand, meaning meconium discharge of sufficient degree to be recognized clinically and pathologically, is distinct from purported late gestational physiologic meconium release. Under these circumstances, meconium is released in response to intrauterine fetal stress. The

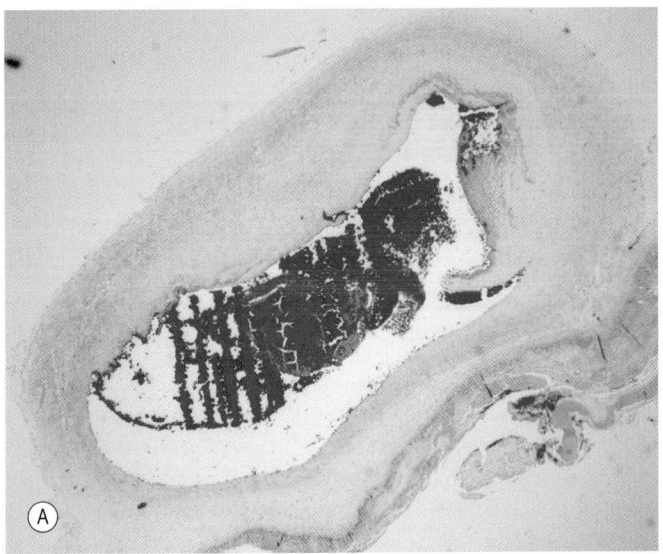

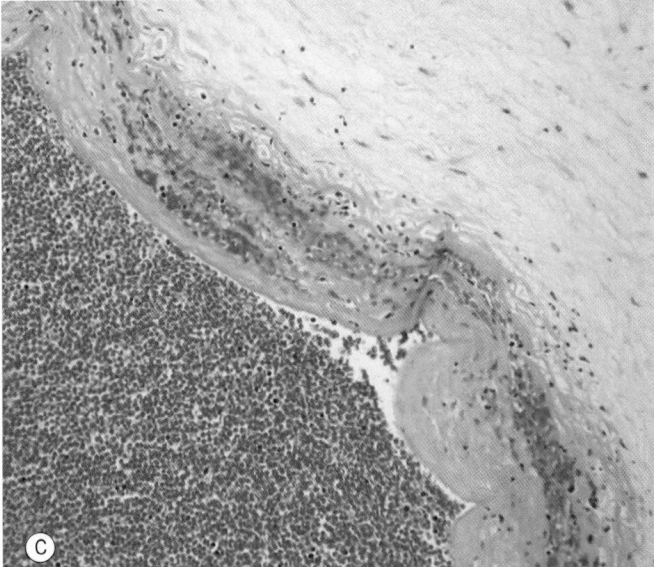

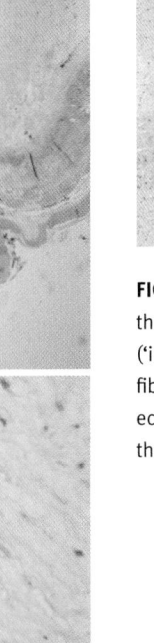

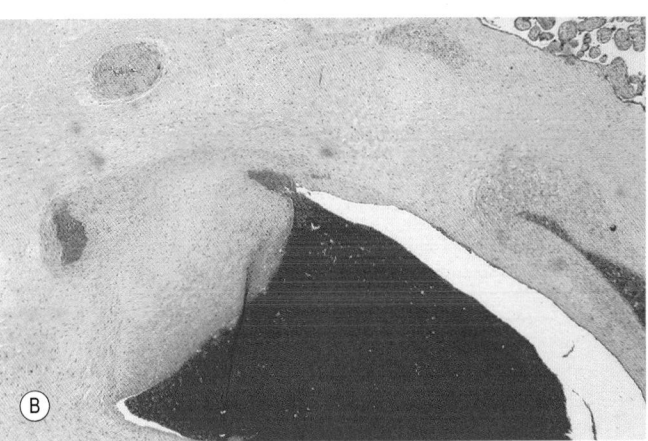

FIGURE 15.60 Fetal vascular thrombosis. (A) Organizing chorionic plate thrombus. (B) Organizing stem villous thrombus, with intimal proliferation ('intimal cushion'). (C) Fairly recent thrombus, demonstrating laminated fibrin and entrapped degenerating red cells. Note the marked vascular ectasia, one of the hallmark features of chorionic plate and stem villus thrombosis.

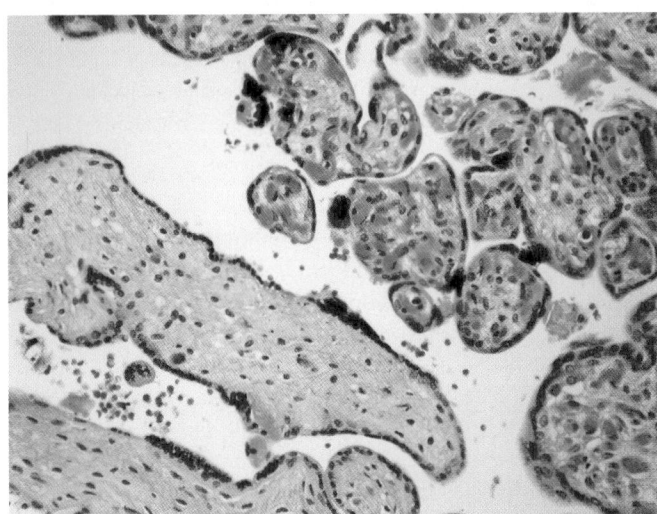

FIGURE 15.61 Avascular villi in fetal thrombotic vasculopathy. Temporal heterogeneity of villous vascular involution supports antenatal/antemortem pathology.

mechanism of antenatal stress may or may not be evident, yet the passage of visible meconium indicates a fetal response to one or more stimuli which exceed physiologic tolerance.

To the naked eye, both clinically and in the laboratory, freshly discharged meconium is green; with the passage of time between meconium release and delivery, on the order of days and longer, the gross appearance of meconium shifts toward shades of brown. As a general statement, meconium density increases in parallel to increasing fetal stress, though factors such as amniotic fluid volume, gestational age (meconium release is uncommon before 32 weeks) and reporter subjectivity can significantly modify the equation. Duration of meconium discharge may in some cases correlate with duration of stress.

Microscopically, meconium appears orange-brown and nonrefractile. Freshly discharged meconium is particulate to globular and amorphous. It is most commonly seen in slide preparations entrapped between layers of extraplacental membranes (Fig. 15.63). With the passage of time, meconium enters the placenta, taken up by stromal macrophages. Meconium-laden macrophages assume a globoid shape as their cytoplasm distends

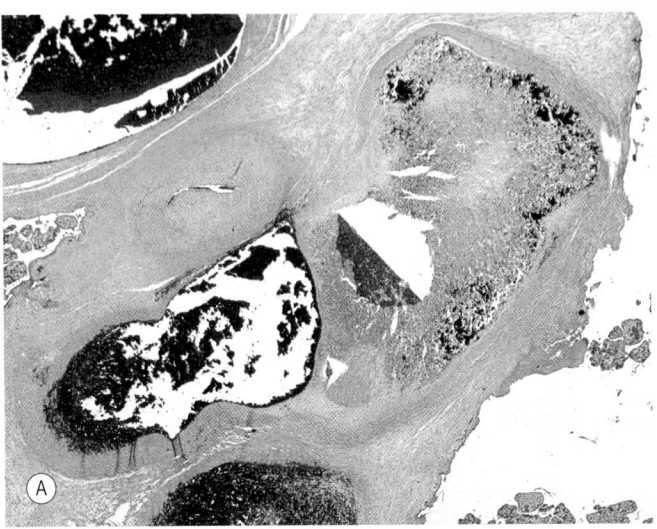
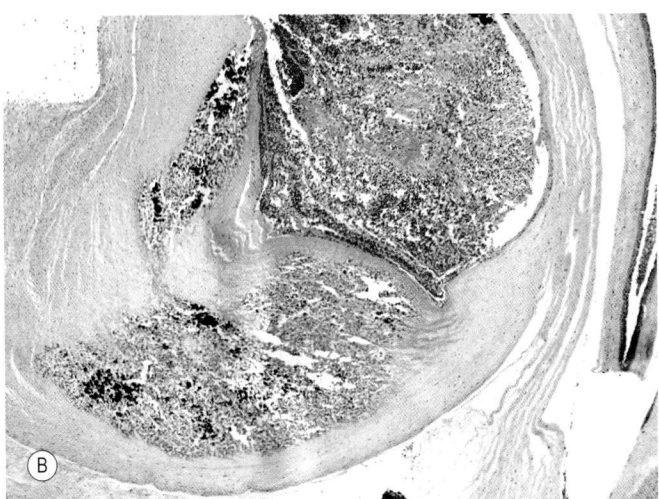

FIGURE 15.62 Fetal thrombotic vasculopathy. Calcified stem villus (A) and chorionic plate (B) thrombi reflect lesion chronicity. Severely growth-restricted neonate with systemic thrombosis (CNS, liver).

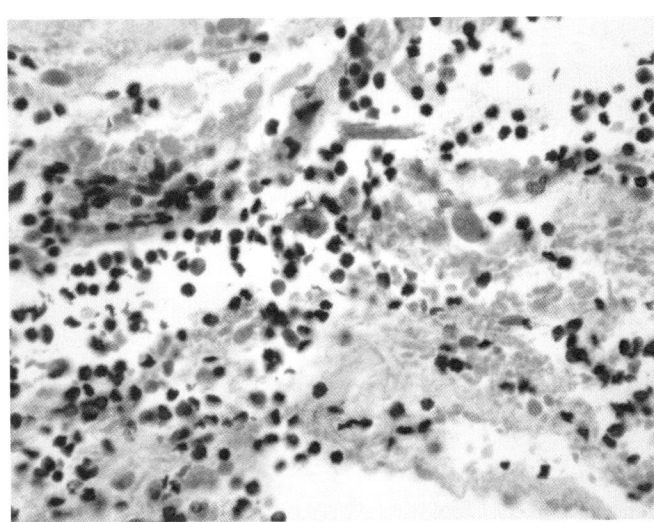

FIGURE 15.63 Meconium entrapped between extraplacental membrane folds. Microscopically, recently discharged meconium is amorphous, globular to finely particulate, and orange-brown.

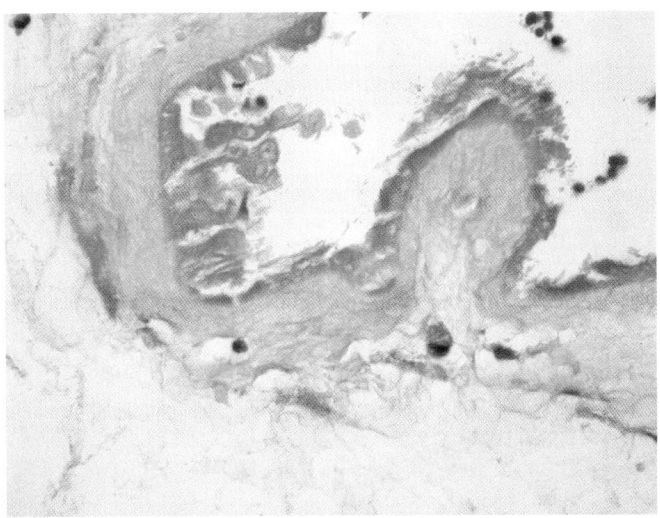

FIGURE 15.64 Meconium-laden macrophage within the amnion stroma. The tinctorial quality of ingested cytoplasmic meconium is similar to its appearance prior to phagocytosis. Note reactive amnion epithelium and membrane edema.

with meconium. Ingested meconium maintains its non-refractile orange-brown hue, and may be globular or evenly distributed within macrophage cytoplasm (Fig. 15.64). Phagocytosed meconium is most easily confused with hemosiderin; hemosiderin-laden macrophages are distinguished by their darker brown and refractile pigment. However, in some cases an iron stain may be needed to distinguish between these two pigments. Meconium-laden macrophages are most readily seen in the extraplacental membranes, but can be found in any location in contact with amniotic fluid, including the chorionic plate, the umbilical cord, and the vessels therein.

As the time interval between meconium discharge and delivery increases, meconium can be seen in progressively

deeper layers of the extraplacental membranes, chorionic plate, and umbilical cord. It is estimated that meconium is taken up into the placenta within about an hour following discharge, remains confined to the amnion/chorion stroma for about three hours after discharge, and begins to appear in the chorion epithelium and decidua capsularis thereafter. One particular consequence of prolonged meconium discharge is its ability to induce fetal vascular necrosis. As meconium traverses deep into Wharton jelly, or into the chorionic plate, meconium macrophages may come into contact with the outer smooth muscle layers of umbilical and chorionic plate vessels. Careful examination of the vessel walls of umbilical cord and/or large chorionic vessels can often reveal meconium-laden histiocytes in these locations. With prolonged exposure to caustic substances within meconium such as bile acids, these myocytes may undergo histologic necrosis, as evidenced by spherical cell contraction, nuclear pyknosis, and eventual myocytolysis (apoptotic cell death).[134, 135] Meconium vascular necrosis is identified, at least in the initial stages of evolution, at the periphery of umbilical vessels or at the surface of chorionic vessels, in areas closest to the amniotic fluid. With time, progressively more of the vascular circumference and vascular thickness undergo apoptotic cell death, as meconium travels deeper into affected sites (see Fig. 15.17).

Meconium-induced vascular necrosis is an independent measure of poor fetal outcome, likely reflecting an adverse intrauterine environment due to two interrelated but distinct mechanisms.[71] First, vascular necrosis leads to vasoconstriction as measured experimentally;[136] this altered vascular tone induces hypoxic fetal stress, in addition to whatever stressor(s) elicited meconium discharge initially. Second, that sufficient meconium was discharged and taken up over a prolonged time to reach umbilical and chorionic vessels may be viewed as a surrogate measure of significant and prolonged intrauterine stress.

Given the significance meconium has been and is afforded in the medicolegal arena, it is important to emphasize that pathologic meconium discharge reflects antenatal fetal stress, but that **stress is not equivalent to injury**. This statement is readily reflected by the fact that intrapartum meconium passage is not rare, occurring in about 10% of term deliveries, whereas untoward neonatal outcome is much less common.[137–139]

As with all pathologic findings that reflect fetal stress, it is the cumulative evidence that leads to pathologic interpretation of **duration** and **intensity** of stress. In a particular clinical context, the **mechanism** of stress may also be revealed or at least supported pathologically. However, it is the clinician's purview, not the pathologist's, to assess injury resulting from stress using clinical parameters, at times in conjunction with pathologic findings. There are exceptions to the principle, such as circumstances where the mechanism of stress is obviously the mechanism of injury, and both are evident on pathologic grounds. In these cases it may be in the pathologist's purview to formulate a definitive opinion regarding cause of stress and injury. Generally speaking, this occurs most readily in stillbirth cases, since the duration and/or intensity of antenatal stresses are of sufficient degree to cause death, and the mechanisms of death are more likely to leave readily identifiable pathologic footprints. Absent dramatic events for which there is compelling pathology, however, the pathologist's expertise lies in determining mechanism, duration, and intensity of antenatal stress. Correlation with injury requires clinical information and expertise which is often beyond the confines of pathologic interpretation.

Nucleated red blood cells

Nucleated erythrocytes are difficult to find in the fetal circulation, including the fetal vasculature within the placenta, after about 12

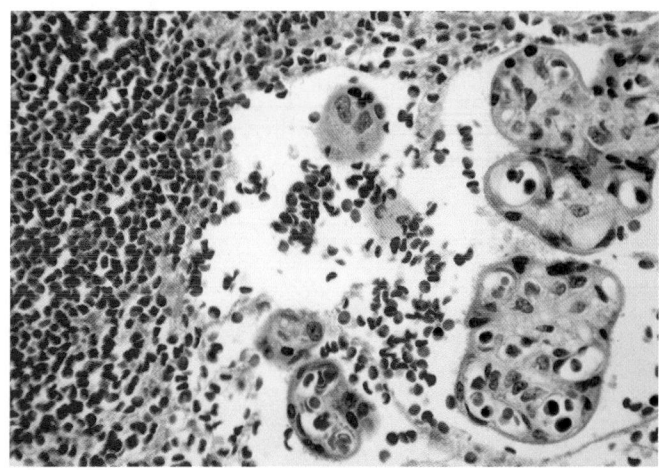

FIGURE 15.65 Marked normoblastemia due to fetal–maternal hemorrhage. Note also normoblasts within the intervillous blood on the left, attesting to fetal origin. Anemic live born, initial hematocrit 11%.

weeks' gestation, when yolk sac red cell production ceases as the fetal liver and later the fetal bone marrow become the primary sites of erythropoiesis. Nucleated red blood cells (NRBCs) are released into the fetal circulation thereafter in response to fetal stress, typically of hypoxic etiology, although other causes such as infection, which may include a component of hypoxic stress, can also elicit normoblastemia (Fig. 15.65). Stillborn fetuses dying from non-hyperacute etiologies characteristically exhibit normoblastemia, the degree of which will depend upon the mechanism, duration, and severity of stress prior to demise.

A small number of preformed nucleated red cells begin to be released into the peripheral circulation, from the liver and perhaps the bone marrow, within a few hours following a hypoxic stimulus (authors' personal observation). The finding of appreciable numbers of NRBCs in the placental circulation likely requires a longer time period on the order of 6–12 hours or more.[140, 141] Should the stimulus be of sufficient duration and intensity, the relative immaturity of red blood cell precursors entering the circulation increases, reflecting not only erythroblast release but also enhanced erythroblast production. Placental erythroblastosis requires severe ongoing hypoxic stress, of at least many days if not weeks in duration, and thus implies an etiology which is likewise ongoing. Alloimmune hemolytic anemia due to Rh incompatibility, and *Parvovirus* infection in the late second trimester, are classic examples (Fig. 15.66).

Postscript and acknowledgement

Despite the relatively long period of time necessary for human gestation, and the myriad of mechanisms by which pregnancy can go awry, there is good news. Considering all gestations that come to term, most babies turn out just fine.[142, 143]

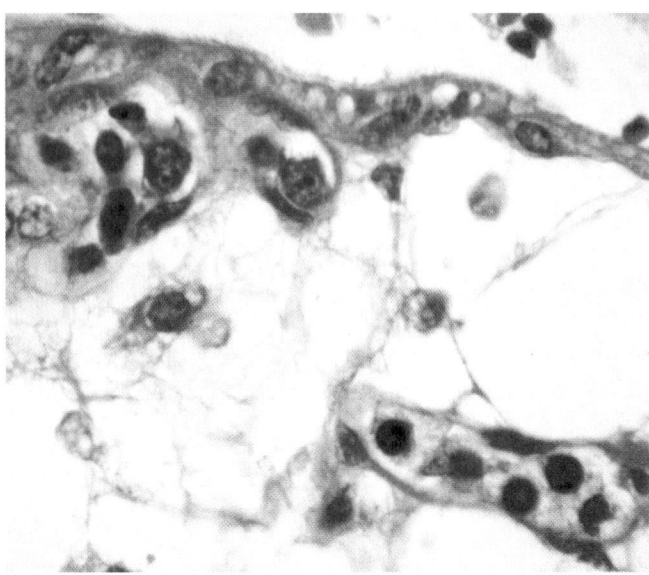

FIGURE 15.66 Erythroblastosis due to fatal *Parvovirus* infection. *Parvovirus* infection is recognizable in erythroblasts by nuclear clearing and enlargement (villous capillaries, top of photograph), and in more mature erythroid precursors by hematoxylin stained homogeneous 'glassy' nuclear inclusions (villous capillary at bottom).

The first author is indebted to the Division of Women's and Perinatal Pathology, Department of Pathology, Brigham and Women's Hospital, Harvard Medical School, Boston, MA; and in particular to former staff members Raymond Redline, M.D. and David Genest, M.D.; for their mentorship in an academic tradition of Perinatal Pathology that began historically under the tutelage of Dr. Shirley Driscoll and continues under Dr. Christopher Crum. Most of the photographs not individually cited are credited to the first author's years of service in Pathology at Baystate Medical Center, Tufts University School of Medicine, Springfield, MA, and her former colleagues to whom she is grateful: Solveig Pflueger, M.D., Ph.D., David Gang, M.D. and Claudia Cosgrove, P.A.

References

Placental origins

1. Boyd JD, Hamilton WJ. The human placenta. Cambridge, UK: W. Heffer and Sons; 1970.
2. Hertig A. Human trophoblast. Springfield, IL: C. C. Thomas; 1968.
3. O'Rahilly R, Muller F. Developmental stages in human embryos. Washington DC: Carnegie Institute of Washington; 1987.
4. Ramsey EM, Donner MW. Placental vasculature and circulation. Philadelphia, PA: WB Saunders; 1980.
5. Castellucci M, Scheper M, Scheffen I, et al. The development of the human placental villous tree. Anat Embryol 1990; 181:117–128.
6. Challier JC, Galtier M, Cortez A, et al. Immunocytological evidence for hematopoiesis in the early human placenta. Placenta 2005; 26:282–288.
7. Li L. Finding the hematopoietic stem cell niche in the placenta. Dev Cell 2005; 8:297–298.

8. Zaragoza MV, Keep D, Genest DR, et al. Early complete hydatidiform moles contain inner cell mass derivatives. Am J Med Genet 1997; 70:273–277.

The first half of gestation: the first trimester and early second trimester

9. Hogge WA, Byrnes AL, Lanasa MC, et al. The clinical use of karyotyping spontaneous abortions. Am J Obstet Gynecol 2003; 189(2):397–400.
10. Redline RW, Zaragoza MV, Hassold T. Prevalence of developmental and inflammatory lesions in non-molar first trimester spontaneous abortions. Hum Pathol 1999; 30:93–100.
11. Redline RW, Hassold T, Zaragoza MV. Prevalence of the partial molar phenotype in triploidy of maternal and paternal origin. Hum Pathol 1998; 28:505–511.
12. Genest DR. The pathology of pregnancy waste. Adv in Pathol and Lab Med 1994; 7:281–312.
13. Genest DR, Boyd T, Roberts D. Fetoplacental histology as a predictor of karyotype: a controlled study of spontaneous first trimester abortions. Hum Pathol 1995; 26:201–209.
14. Smith HO, Kohorn E, Cole LA. Choriocarcinoma and gestational trophoblastic disease. Obstet Gynecol Clin North Am 2005; 32(4): 661–684.
15. Keep D, Zaragoza M, Hassold T, et al. Very early complete hydatidiform mole. Hum Pathol 1996; 27:708–713.
16. Castrillon DH, Sun D, Weremowicz S, et al. Discrimination of complete hydatidiform mole from its mimics by immunohistochemistry of the paternally imprinted gene product p57KIP2. Am J Surg Pathol 2001; 25:1225–1230.
17. Thaker HM, Berlin A, Tycko B, et al. Immunohistochemistry for the imprinted gene product IPL/PHLDA2 for facilitating the differential diagnosis of complete hydatidiform mole. J Reprod Med 2004; 49: 630–636.
18. Ayinde OA, Aimakhu CO, Adeyanju OA, et al. Abdominal pregnancy at the University College Hospital, Ibadan: a ten-year review. Afr J Reprod Health 2005; 9(1):123–127.
19. Badria L, Amarin Z, Jaradat A, et al. Full-term viable abdominal pregnancy: a case report and review. Arch Gynecol Obstet 2003; 268(4):340–342.
20. Goddijin M, Leschot NJ. Genetic aspects of miscarriage. Baillières Best Pract Res Clin Obstet Gynaecol 2000; 14(5):855–865.
21. Brancati F, Mingarelli R, Dallapiccola B. Recurrent triploidy of maternal origin. Eur J Hum Genet 2003; 11(12):972–974.
22. Slim R, Fallahian M, Riviere JB, et al. Evidence of a genetic heterogeneity of familial hydatidiform moles. Placenta 2005; 26(1):5–9.
23. Fisher RA, Hodges MD, Newlands ES. Familial recurrent hydatidiform mole: a review. J Reprod Med 2004; 49(8):595–601.
24. Salim R, Regan L, Woelfer B, et al. A comparative study of the morphology of congenital uterine anomalies in women with and without a history of recurrent first trimester miscarriage. Human Reprod 2003; 18(1):162–166.
25. Nayar R, Lage JM. Placental changes in a first trimester missed abortion in maternal systemic lupus erythematosus with antiphospholipid syndrome: a case report and review of the literature. Hum Pathol 1996; 27:201–206.
26. Boyd TK, Redline RW. Chronic histiocytic intervillositis: a placental lesion associated with recurrent reproductive loss. Hum Pathol 2000; 31:1389–1392.
27. Doss BJ, Greene MF, Hill J, et al. Massive chronic intervillositis associated with recurrent abortions. Hum Pathol 1995; 26:1245–1251.
28. Labarrere C, Mullen E. Fibrinoid and trophoblastic necrosis with massive chronic intervillositis: An extreme variant of villitis of unknown etiology. Am J Reprod Immunol Microbiol 1987; 15:85–91.
29. Nijhuis EWP, van Nort G. Clinicopathological correlations in chronic intervillositis. Pediatr Dev Pathol 1998; 1:457.
30. Ordi J, Ismail MR, Ventura PJ, et al. Massive chronic intervillositis of the placenta associated with malaria infection. Am J Surg Pathol 1998; 22:1006–1011.

31. Valderrama E. Massive chronic intervillositis: Report of three cases. Lab Invest 1992; 66:10P.

32. Jacques SM, Qureshi F. Chronic intervillositis of the placenta. Arch Pathol Lab Med 1993; 117:1032–1035.

The last half of gestation: systematic placental evaluion

33. Langston C, Kaplan C, MacPherson T, et al. Practice guideline for examination of the placenta. Arch Pathol Lab Med 1997; 121:449–476.

34. Boyd TK, Gang DL, Lis G, et al. Normative values for placental weights (N = 15 463): Baystate Medical Center. Mod Pathol 1999; 12:1P.

Pathologic placental findings of clinical significance in mid- to late gestation and their mimics

35. Mills JL, Harley EE, Moessinger AC. Standards for measuring umbilical cord length. Placenta 1983; 4:423–426.

36. Moessinger AC, Blanc WA, Merone PA, et al. Umbilical cord length as an index of fetal activity: experimental study and clinical implications. Pediatr Res 1982; 16:109–112.

37. Gardiner JP. The umbilical cord: normal length; length in cord complications; etiology and frequency of coiling. Surg Gynaecol Obstet 1922; 34:252–256.

38. Spellacy WN, Graven H, Fisch RO. The umbilical cord complications of true knots, nuchal coils and cords around the body. Am J Obstet Gynecol 1966; 94:1136–1142.

39. Clapp JF 3rd, Stepanchak W, Hashimoto K, et al. The natural history of antenatal nuchal cords. Am J Obstet Gynecol 2003; 189:488–493.

40. Clapp JF 3rd, Lopez B, Simonean S. Nuchal cord and neurodevelopmental performance at 1 year. J Soc Gynecol Investig 1999; 6:268–272.

41. Bakotic BW, Boyd T, Poppiti R, et al. Recurrent umbilical cord torsion leading to fetal death in 3 subsequent pregnancies: a case report and review of the literature. Arch Pathol Lab Med 2000; 124(9):1352–1355.

42. Strong TH Jr, Jarles DL, Vega JS, et al. The umbilical coiling index. Am J Obstet Gynecol 1994; 170:29–32.

43. Machin GA, Ackerman J, Gilbert-Barness E. Abnormal umbilical cord coiling is associated with adverse perinatal outcomes. Pediatr Dev Pathol 2000; 3:462–471.

44. Blickstein I, Varon Y, Varon E. Implications of differences in coiling indices at different segments of the umbilical cord. Gynecol Obstet Invest 2001; 52(3):203–206.

45. van Diik CC, Franx A, de Laat MW, et al. The umbilical coiling index in normal pregnancy. J Matern Fetal Neonatal Med 2002; 11(4):280–283.

46. Blickstein I, Varon Y, Varon E. Implications of differences in coiling indices at different segments of the umbilical cord. Gynecol Obstet Invest 2001; 52(3):203–206.

47. Genest DR. Estimating the time of death in stillborn fetuses. 2. Histologic evaluation of the placenta – a study of 71 stillborns. Obstet Gynecol 1992; 80:585–592.

48. Redline RW, Boyd T, Campbell V, et al. Maternal vascular underperfusion: nosology and reproducibility of placental reaction patterns. Pediatr Dev Pathol 2004; 7:237–249.

49. Upadhyay V, Kukkady A. Urachal remnants: an enigma. Eur J Pediatr Surg 2003; 13(6):372–376.

50. Pinar H, Sung CJ, Oyer CE, et al. Reference values for singleton and twin placental weights. Pediatr Pathol Lab Med 1996; 16:901–907.

51. Dy CL, Chari RS, Russell LJ. Updating reference values for placental weights in Northern Alberta. Am J Obstet Gynecol 2004; 190(5):1458–1460.

52. Heller DS, Rush D, Baergen RN. Subchorionic hematoma associated with thrombophilia: report of three cases. Pediatr Dev Pathol 2003; 6:261–264.

53. Shanklin DR, Scott JS. Massive subchorial thrombohaematoma (Breus' mole). Br J Obstet Gynaecol 1975; 82:476–487.

54. Harris BA. Peripheral placental separation: a review. Obstet Gynecol Surv 1988; 43:577–581.

55. Becroft DM, Thompson JM, Mitchell EA. Placental infarcts, intervillous fibrin plaques, and intervillous thrombi: incidences, cooccurrences, and epidemiological associations. Pediatr Dev Pathol 2004; 7:26–34.

56. Kaplan C, Blanc WA, Elias J. Identification of erythrocytes in intervillous thrombi: a study using immunoperoxidase identification of hemoglobins. Hu. Pathol 1982; 13:554–557.

57. Katzman PJ, Genest DR. Maternal floor infarction and massive perivillous fibrin deposition: histological definitions, association with intrauterine fetal growth restriction, and risk of recurrence. Pediatr Dev Pathol 2002; 5:159–164.

58. Andres RL, Kuyper W, Resnik R, et al. The association of maternal floor infarction of the placenta with adverse perinatal outcome. Am J Obstet Gynecol 1990; 163:935–938.

59. Naeye RL. Maternal floor infarction. Hum Pathol 1985; 16:823–828.

60. Clewell WH, Manchester DK. Recurrent maternal floor infarction: a preventable cause of fetal death. Am J Obstet Gynecol 1983; 147:346–347.

61. Vernof KK, Benirschke K, Kephart GM, et al. Maternal floor infarction – relationship to X-cells, major basic protein, and adverse perinatal outcome. Am J Obstet Gynecol 1992; 167:1355–1363.

62. Bendon RW, Hommel AB. Maternal floor infarction in autoimmune disease: Two cases. Pediatr Pathol Lab Med 1996; 16:293–297.

63. Mandsager NT, Bendon RW, Mostello D, et al. Maternal floor infarction of placenta: prenatal diagnosis and clinical significance. Obstet Gynecol 1994; 83:750–754.

Additional microscopic pathology by placental location

64. Stallmach T, Hebisch G, Meier K, et al. Rescue by birth: defective placental maturation and late fetal mortality. Obstetr Gynecol 2001; 97:505–509.

65. Altshuler G. Choriangiosis: An important placental sign of neonatal morbidity and mortality. Arch Pathol Lab Med 1984; 108:71–74.

66. Redline RW, Ariel I, Baergen RN, et al. Fetal vascular obstructive lesions: nosology and reproducibility of placental reaction patterns. Pediat and Devel Pathol 2004; 7:443–452.

67. Redline RW, Abramowsky CR. Clinical and pathologic aspects of recurrent placental villitis. Hum Pathol 1985; 16:727–731.

68. Russell P. Inflammatory lesions of the human placenta. Placenta 1980; 1:227–244.

69. Russell P, Atkinson K, Krishnan L. Recurrent reproductive failure due to severe villitis of unknown etiology. J Reprod Med 1980; 24:93–98.

70. Knox WF, Fox H. Villitis of unknown aetiology: its incidence and significance in placentae from a British population. Placenta 1984; 5:395–402.

71. Redline RW. Severe fetal placental vascular lesions in term infants with neurologic impairment. Am J Obstet Gynecol 2005; 192:452–457.

72. Mostoufi-Zadeh M, Driscoll SG, Biano SA, et al. Placental evidence of cytomegalovirus infection of the fetus and neonate. Arch Pathol Lab Med 1984; 108:403–406.

73. Qureshi F, Jacques SM, Reyes MP. Placental histopathology in syphilis. Hum Pathol 1993; 24:779–784.

74. Heifetz S, Bauman M. Necrotizing funisitis and herpes simplex infection of placental and decidual tissues. Hum Pathol 1994; 25:715–722.

75. Elliott WG. Placental toxoplasmosis: report of a case. Am J Clin Pathol 1970; 53:413–417.

76. Qureshi F, Jacques S. Maternal varicella during pregnancy: correlation of maternal history and fetal outcome with placental histopathology. Hum Pathol 1996; 27:191–195.

77. Bittencourt AL. Congenital Chagas disease. Am J Dis Child 1976; 130:97–103.

78. Genest DR, Williams MA, Greene MF. Estimating the time of death in stillborn fetuses: I. Histologic evaluation of fetal organs; an autopsy study of 150 stillborns. Obstet Gynecol 1992; 80(4):575–584.

79. Genest DR, Singer DB. Estimating the time of death in stillborn fetuses: III. External fetal evaluation; a study of 86 stillborns. Obstet Gynecol 1993; 80(4):593–600.

80. Sander CH. Hemorrhagic endovasculitis and hemorrhagic villitis of the placenta. Arch Pathol Lab Med 1980; 104:371–373.

81. Shen-Schwarz S, MacPherson TA, Mueller-Heubach E. The clinical significance of hemorrhagic endovasculitis of the placenta. 1988; 159:48–51.

82. Sander CM, Gilliland D, Akers C, et al. Livebirths with placental hemorrhagic endovasculitis: interlesional relationships and perinatal outcomes. Arch Pathol Lab Med 2002; 126:157–164.

83. Roberts DJ, Ampola MG, Lage JM. Diagnosis of unsuspected fetal metabolic storage disease by routine placental examination. Pediatr Pathol 1991; 11:647–656.

84. Lake BD, Young EP, Winchester BG. Prenatal diagnosis of lysosomal storage diseases. Brain Pathol 1998; 8:133–149.

85. Ohyama M, Kojyo T, Gotoda H, et al. Mesenchymal dysplasia of the placenta. Pathology Internat 2000; 50:759–764.

86. Jauniaux E, Nicolaides KH, Hustin J. Perinatal features associated with placental mesenchymal dysplasia. Placenta 1997; 18:701–706.

87. Khong TY, Bendon RW, Qureshi F, et al. Chronic deciduitis in the placental basal plate: definition and inter-observer reliability. Hum Pathol 2000; 31:292–295.

88. Goldenberg R, Hauth J, Andrews W. Intrauterine infection and preterm delivery. N Engl J Med 2000; 342:1500–1507.

89. Stanek J, Al-Ahmadie HA. Laminar necrosis of placental membranes: a histologic sign of uteroplacental hypoxia. Pediatr Dev Pathol 2005; 8:34–42. Epub 2005 Feb 8.

Specific topics in placental pathology

90. Saygili-Yilmaz E, Yildiz S, Erman-Akar M, et al. Reproductive outcome of a septate uterus after hysteroscopic metroplasty. Arch Gynecol Obstet 2003; 268(4):289–292.

91. Milhan D. DES exposure: implications for childbearing. Int J Childbirth Educ 1992; 7(4):21–28.

92. Morey AL, Keeling JW, Porter HJ, et al. Clinical and histopathological features of parvovirus B19 infection in the human fetus. Br J Obstet Gynaecol 1992; 99:566–574.

93. Fowler KB, Stagno S, Pass RF. Maternal immunity and prevention of congenital cytomegalovirus infection. JAMA 2003; 289:1008–1011.

94. Watt-Morse ML, Laifer SA, Hill LM. The natural history of fetal cytomegalovirus infection as assessed by serial ultrasound and fetal blood sampling: a case report. Prenat Diagn 1995; 15:567–570.

95. Mascola L, Ewert D, Eller A. Listeriosis: a previously unreported medical complication in women with multiple gestations. Am J Obstet Gynecol 1994; 170:1328–1332.

96. Driscoll SG, Gorbach A, Feldman D. Congenital listeriosis: diagnosis from placental studies. Obstet Gynecol 1962; 20:216–220.

97. Vawter GF. Perinatal listeriosis. Perspect Pediatr Pathol 1981; 6:153–166.

98. Bendon R, Bornstein S, Faye-Petersen O. Two fetal deaths associated with maternal sepsis and with thrombosis of the intervillous space of the placenta. Placenta 1998; 19:385–389.

99. Benirschke K. Recent trends in chorangiomas, especially those of multiple and recurrent chorangiomas. Pediat Devel Pathol 1999; 2:264–269.

100. Ogino S, Redline RW. Villous capillary lesions of the placenta: Distinctions between chorangioma, chorangiomatosis, and chorangiosis. Hum Pathol 2000; 31:945–954.

101. Bakaris S, Karabiber H, Yuksel M, et al. Case of large placental chorioangioma associated with diffuse neonatal hemangiomatosis. Pediatr Dev Pathol 2004; 7:258–261. Epub Mar 17, 2004.

102. Qureshi F, Jacques SM. Adrenocortical heterotropia in the placenta. Pediatr Pathol Lab Med 1995; 15(1):51–56.

103. Guschmann M, Vogel M, Urban M. Adrenal tissue in the placenta: a heterotopia caused by migration and embolism? Placenta 2000; 21(4):427–431.

104. Jacques SM, Qureshi F. Adrenocortical and hepatic nodules within placental tissue. Pediatr Dev Pathol 2003; 6(5):464–466.

105. Mosher R, Genest DR. Primary intraplacental choriocarcinoma: clinical and pathologic features of seven cases (1967–1996) and discussion of the differential diagnosis. J Surg Pathol 1997; 2:83–97.

106. Ohyama M, Kobayashi S, Aida N, et al. Congenital neuroblastoma diagnosed by placental examination. Med Pediatr Oncol 1999; 33(4):430–431.

107. Doss BJ, Vicari J, Jacques SM, et al. Placental involvement in congenital hepatoblastoma. Pediatr Dev Pathol 1998; 1(6):538–542.

108. Boyd TK, Schofield DE. Monozygotic twins concordant for congenital neuroblastoma: a case report and review of the literature. Pediatr Pathol Lab Med 1995; 15(6):931–940.

109. Allan RR, Wadsworth LD, Kalousek DK, et al. Congenital erythroleukemia: a case report with morphological, immunophenotypic, and cytogenetic findings. Am J Hematol 1989 31(2): 114–121.

110. de Tar MW, Dittman W, Gilbert J. Transient myeloproliferative disease of the newborn: case report with placental, cytogenetic, and flow cytometric findings. Hum Pathol 2000; 31(3):396–398.

111. Kalousek DK, Chan KW. Transient myeloproliferative disorder in chromosomally normal newborn infant. Med Pediatr Oncol 1987; 15(1):38–41.

112. Jackisch C, Louwen F, Schwenkhagen A, et al. Lung cancer during pregnancy involving products of conception and a review of the literature. Arch Gynecol Obstet 2003; 268(2):69-–77. Epub Nov 2002.

113. Alexander A, Samlowski WE, Grossman D, et al. Metastatic melanoma in pregnancy: risk of transplacental metastases in the infant. J Clin Oncol 2003; 21(11):79–86.

Constellation disorders

114. Blanc W. Amniotic infection syndrome: pathogenesis, morphology, and significance in circumnatal mortality. Clin Obstet Gynecol 1959; 2:705–734.

115. Redline RW, Faye-Petersen O, Heller D, et al. Amniotic infection syndrome: nosology and reproducibility of placental reaction patterns. Pediatr Dev Pathol 2003; 6:435–448.

116. Navarro C, Blanc WA. Subacute necrotizing funisitis. A variant of cord inflammation with a high rate of perinatal infection. J Pediatr 1974; 85:689–697.

117. van Hoeven KH, Anyaegbunam A, Hochster H, et al. Clinical significance of increasing histologic severity of acute inflammation in the fetal membranes and umbilical cord. Pediatr Pathol Lab Med 1996; 16:731–744.

118. Dexter SC, Pinar H, Malee MP, et al. Outcome of very low birth weight infants with histopathologic chorioamnionitis. Obstet Gynecol 2000; 96:172–177.

119. Qureshi F, Jacques SM, Benson RW, et al. Candida funisitis: A clinicopathologic study of 32 cases. Pediat and Devel Pathol 1998; 1:118–124.

120. Hood IC, DeSa DJ, Whyte RK. The inflammatory response in candidal chorioamnionitis. Hum Pathol 1983; 14:984–990.

121. Burgess AM, Hutchins GM. Inflammation of the lungs, umbilical cord and placenta associated with meconium passage in utero. Review of 123 autopsied cases. Pathol Res Pract 1996; 192:1121–1128.

122. Coid CR, Fox H. Short review: Campylobacters as placental pathogens. Placenta 1983; 4:295–306.

123. Redline RW, Patterson P. Preeclampsia is associated with an excess of proliferative immature intermediate trophoblast. Hum Pathol 1995; 26:594–600.

124. Redline RW, Wilson-Costello D. Chronic peripheral separation of placenta: the significance of diffuse chorioamnionic hemosiderosis. Am J Clin Pathol 1999; 111:804–810.

125. Ohyama M, Itani Y, Yamanaka M, et al. Maternal, neonatal, and placental features associated with diffuse chorioamniotic hemosiderosis, with special reference to neonatal morbidity and mortality. Pediatrics 2004; 113:800–805.

126. Elliott JP, Gilpin B, Strong TH Jr, et al. Chronic abruption-oligohydramnios sequence. J Reprod Med 1998; 43:418–422.

127. Bey M, Dott A, Miller JM. The sonographic diagnosis of circumvallate placenta. Obstet Gynecol 1991; 78:515–517.

128. Redline RW, O'Riordan MA. Placental lesions associated with cerebral palsy and neurologic impairment following term birth. Arch Pathol Lab Med 2000; 124:1785–1791.

129. Redline RW. Clinical and pathological umbilical cord abnormalities in fetal thrombotic vasculopathy. Hum Pathol 2004; 35:1494–1498.

130. Kraus FT, Acheen VI. Fetal thrombotic vasculopathy in the placenta: cerebral thrombi and infarcts, coagulopathies, and cerebral palsy. Hum Pathol 1999; 30:759–769.

131. Leistra-Leistra MJ, Timmer A, van Spronsen FJ, et al. Fetal thrombotic vasculopathy in the placenta: a thrombophilic connection between pregnancy complications and neonatal thrombosis? Placenta 2004; 25: S102–S105.

Markers of intrauterine stress

132. Cifti AO, Tanyel FC. In utero defecation: a new concept. Turk J Pediatr 1998; 40(1):45–53.

133. Cifti AO, Tanyel FC, Karnak I, et al. In-utero defecation: fact or fiction? Eur J Pediatr Surg 1999; 9(6):376–380.

134. Altshuler G, Arizawa M, Molnar-Nadasdy G. Meconium-induced umbilical cord vascular necrosis and ulceration: a potential link between the placenta and poor pregnancy outcome. Obstet Gynecol 1992; 79:760–766.

135. King EL, Redline RW, Smith SD, et al. Myocytes of chorionic vessels from placentas with meconium associated vascular necrosis exhibit apoptotic markers. Hum Pathol 2004; 35:412–417.

136. Altshuler G, Hyde S. Meconium-induced vasocontraction: a potential cause of cerebral and other fetal hypoperfusion and of poor pregnancy outcome. J Child Neurol 1989; 4:137–142.

137. Locatelli A, Regalia AL, Patregnani C, et al. Prognostic value of change in amniotic fluid color during labor. Fetal Diagn Ther 2005; 20(1):5–9.

138. Himmelmann K, Hagberg G, Beckung E, et al. The changing panorama of cerebral palsy in Sweden. IX. Prevalence and origin in the birth-year period 1995–1998. Acta Paediatr 2005; 94(3):287–294.

139. Kabbur PM, Herson VC, Zaremba S, et al. Have the year 2000 neonatal resuscitation guidelines changed the delivery room management or outcome of meconium-stained infants? J Perinatol 2005; 25(11):694–697.

140. Hermansen MC. Nucleated red blood cells in the fetus and newborn. Arch Dis Child Fetal Neonatal Ed 2001; 84:F211–F215.

141. Blackwell SC, Hallak M, Hotra JW, et al. Timing of fetal nucleated red blood cell count elevation in response to acute hypoxia. Biol Neonate 2004; 85:217–220. Epub Dec 23, 2003.

142. Orji EO, Shittu AS, Makinde ON, et al. Effect of prolonged birth spacing on maternal and perinatal outcome. East Afr Med J 2004; 81(8):388–391.

143. Callaway LK, Lust K, McIntyre HD. Pregnancy outcomes in women of very advanced maternal age. Aust NZ J Obstet Gynaecol 2005; 45(1):12–16.

Further reading

Benirschke K, Kaufmann P. Pathology of the human placenta, 4th edn. New York: Springer; 2000.

Faye-Petersen OM, Heller DS, Joshi VV. Handbook of placental pathology, 2nd edn. Abingdon, Oxon UK: Taylor and Francis; 2006.

Kaplan C. Color atlas of gross placental pathology. New York: Igaku-Shoin; 1994.

Kraus FT, Redline R, Gersell DJ, et al. AFIP atlas of nontumor pathology: placental pathology. Washington DC: American Registry of Pathology; 2004.

Perinatal, fetal, and embryonic autopsy

16

Joseph R. Siebert

'*Mortui Vivos Docueran (Let the dead teach the living...)*'

Introduction

The perinatal autopsy has the potential to provide the last and most definitive summary of a life unfortunately shortened. When the autopsy succeeds, a host of individuals benefit, especially parents, other family members, clinical care providers, and at times society at large. Parents will understandably have tremendous grief over their loss and may worry that their baby's problem will recur in future pregnancies; they may also harbor concerns over other aspects of the pregnancy or even their care. Care givers too may have a variety of concerns. Autopsy can provide valuable explanations and sometimes put these issues to rest. The benefits are maximal when collaboration between pathologist and clinician occurs before and after the autopsy, and when findings are relayed to appropriate individuals in an accurate and timely manner.

The major **objectives** of the perinatal autopsy are to evaluate pregnancy and birth, determine gestational age, document growth and development, detect underlying abnormalities (anomaly, infection, metabolic defect, other), evaluate diagnoses and therapy, and determine the cause of death.[1, 2] Consent for autopsy is generally sought by clinical workers and must be requested compassionately and respectfully and be fully informed. In particular, the permit must specify which tissues may be examined and which may be retained. Pathologists must ensure that their work falls within the scope of the autopsy permit, and that all medicolegal requirements are met before an autopsy is conducted. Laws specific to fetal autopsy may vary by state or country, with some requiring permits on fetuses exceeding a given gestational age (e.g. 20 weeks) or body weight (e.g. 350 or 500 g). The prosector needs to understand pertinent regulations and/or adopt a policy of obtaining permission on every autopsy performed, regardless of gestational age or body weight.

The **value** of the perinatal autopsy has been demonstrated in a number of studies.[3–11] Workers have made important contributions to technical aspects of the perinatal autopsy[1, 12–15] and created practice guidelines for both pathologists[3, 13] and clinicians.[16–21]

As the objectives listed above indicate, the approach to the perinatal autopsy differs considerably from that of older individuals. Both maternal health and the intrauterine environment have a large effect upon development and must be evaluated. Many of the diseases encountered in the young differ from those of adulthood; congenital anomalies may be highly complex, but must be recognized and their significance appreciated. The goal of this chapter is then to provide readers with the basic technical skills required to foster a better understanding of perinatal death. For information regarding specific disorders, readers should turn to relevant chapters.

The laboratory environment

The size and intricate nature of specimens dictate a large part of the technical approach to the perinatal autopsy. Tissues must be seen well, and manipulated with relative ease, if pathologic changes are to be identified. Light must be abundant, and a magnifier or dissecting microscope available and ready for use. The prosector should give thought to posture, for years of hunching over tiny bits of tissue will take their toll. It is often possible to sit while working. Ideally, an attendant will be available to help the pathologist, take dictation, answer or make telephone calls, assist with cultures, and so on.

The **dissecting instruments** required for perinatal autopsy are small and delicate, and must be treated with care. Small scissors, forceps, and scalpels will be helpful. Iris scissors or other tools of the eye surgeon are especially appreciated.

Approach to the perinatal autopsy
Use of established protocols

The routine of autopsy performance should not transcend to ritual, but instead, follow a systematic approach that gathers and records all pertinent observations. Samples are available in the literature, or workers may choose to design their own.[19, 22] The **autopsy protocol** should include space for recording specific measurements and norms for particular gestational ages; the use of checklists insures the efficient and complete recording of findings. The document will form the basis for the autopsy report, and to be complete, will also include a list of diagnoses, summary of clinical and autopsy findings, and pertinent discussion of the findings and their relevance to the case. For the sake of cleanliness, an abbreviated form of the protocol, or worksheet, can be used during the autopsy and data transferred to the formalized report afterwards. Seemingly mundane anatomic features must be noted, in order to rule out the host of congenital disorders. Some constitute very basic observations. Is the stomach on the left side? Is the spleen present? Is it single or multiple? Are the kidneys present? Is the diaphragm intact? All of these observations are highly significant.

Weights and measurements

Certain weights and measurements are essential to document growth and development.[1, 23–25] The size and weight of the body and organs vary, primarily with age, and secondarily as a result of disorders of growth and development. These weights and measurements must be ascertained accurately and compared with standard tables (see Tables). In addition to weights and measurements, the gyral pattern of the brain and the histologic evaluation of certain organs (e.g. lung and kidney) are helpful in assessing anatomic maturity.[1, 26]

Weights

Scales accurate to 0.1 g are necessary for perinatal specimens. Electronic versions equipped with a taring feature are highly efficient, as they can be reset quickly between samples. Small fetuses can be weighed on such scales, although a larger scale may be necessary for older infants; it should be checked for accuracy and receive regular maintenance. All major organs should be weighed (i.e. thymus, heart, lungs, liver, spleen,

kidneys, adrenal glands, brain, and placenta) and the data recorded in the autopsy protocol, along with expected values. Care should be taken to remove extraneous tissues and blot organs prior to weighing, in order to reduce the amount of error inherent in such small specimens. It is important for prosectors to follow a method that is identical to published ones, so that weights are directly comparable. For example, the heart should be weighed without descending aorta, liver without gallbladder, and kidneys without ureters.

Measurements

The **crown–heel** (CH) and **crown–rump** (CR) lengths should be determined to the nearest 0.5 cm. Chest and abdominal circumferences are taken at the level of the nipples and umbilicus respectively. Certain internal controls are available for these data. Normally, the CR length in young patients is approximately two-thirds of the CH, and the occipitofrontal, or head, circumference (OFC) and CR length in the neonate do not differ by more than 1.0 cm or so.[27, 28] The normal OFC, chest, and abdominal circumferences decrease progressively in order from superior to inferior. If these relationships deviate substantially from the norm, then explanations must be sought. **Foot length** correlates especially well with gestational age, and should be obtained in every case. The measurement is also of particular value in disrupted fetuses or those with abnormal CH or CR lengths, e.g. anencephaly or skeletal dysplasia (see Tables). Other specialized measurements may be required as indicated: internipple distance, width/length of fontanelles (especially anterior), distance between cranial sutures, lengths of limbs (upper, lower limb, digit).

The metric documentation of changes in the face is often a valuable component of the autopsy. In addition to the usual qualitative evaluation of the eyes and eyelids (size, shape, and orientation), the distances between the **inner canthi** and **outer canthi** can be obtained. From a statistical point of view, these two measurements account for a great deal of the variability and hence descriptive value in facial form.[29] An abnormal increase in inner canthal distance is termed ocular hypertelorism; a decrease is referred to as ocular hypotelorism. These changes are found in a large number of conditions. In addition, measurements like nasal height and width, philtrum height, mouth width, and ear length can be obtained and compared with published norms.[28–32]

Photographs

In addition to metric documentation, recording findings by visual means is also important (Figs 16.1–16.3). The subject of medical photography, and specifically gross specimen photography, has been addressed in numerous publications. The benefits of quality photography, ranging from documentation to research and teaching and even to aiding the process of grieving, have been recognized widely.[33–37] Photographs are not just a part of the idealized or academic autopsy, but are a necessary part of routine examination and as such become part of the medical

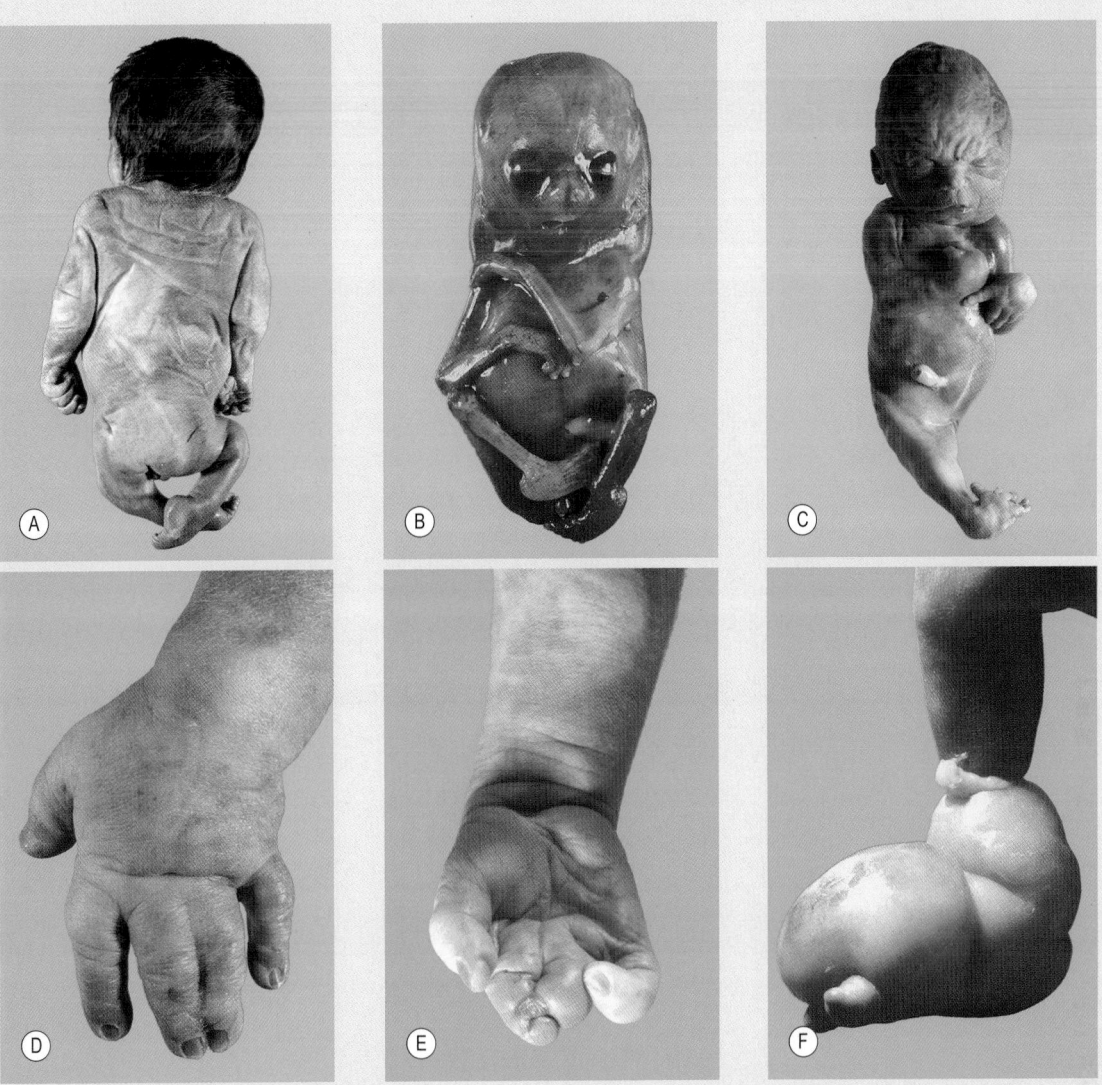

FIGURE 16.1 External examination. (A) Posterior view of the 31-week male fetus of a diabetic mother. Diminution of legs and absent lumbosacral spine confirmed the diagnosis of caudal regression syndrome, a recognized complication of maternal diabetes. (B) Lethal multiple pterygia syndrome occurs on an autosomal recessive basis and was recurrent in the family of this 16-week female fetus. The condition includes severe wasting, multiple pterygia across major joints, nuchal cystic hygroma, and hydrops, evident in this image, and cleft palate, not shown, but present in this fetus. Severe arthrogryposis hampers ultrasonography, making autopsy a highly productive means of examination. In this case, no cause for the musculoskeletal anomalies was found despite a careful immunohistochemical workup. (C) Sirenomelia, changes associated with oligohydramnios, and a number of anomalies of the gastrointestinal and genitourinary systems were diagnosed in this 24-week male fetus. Postmortem radiography provided additional information concerning skeletal anatomy (separate femora and tibiae; fused fibulae; eight phalanges). Dissection and injection of the vascular system showed a persistent vitelline (omphalomesenteric) artery arising from the mid-aorta. This vascular anomaly is thought to incite a vascular steal phenomenon, with subsequent ischemia and production of distal anomalies. (D) Syndactyly of the third and fourth digits is highly suggestive of triploidy, the diagnosis of which was confirmed in this case by flow cytometry and karyotyping. The 35-week male infant died at 34 h of severe congenital heart disease. (E) Amputation of the distal ends of the second, third, and fourth fingers was diagnosed by ultrasonography at 14 weeks and thought to be due to amnion rupture. The male infant was born at term, but no amniotic bands could be identified. (F) In contrast to the case illustrated in Figure 16.1E, constriction and edema of the right lower leg by a prominent amniotic band was dramatic in this 24-week male fetus. The foot and band of amnion would presumably be missing by term, making diagnosis at that time presumptive rather than certain.

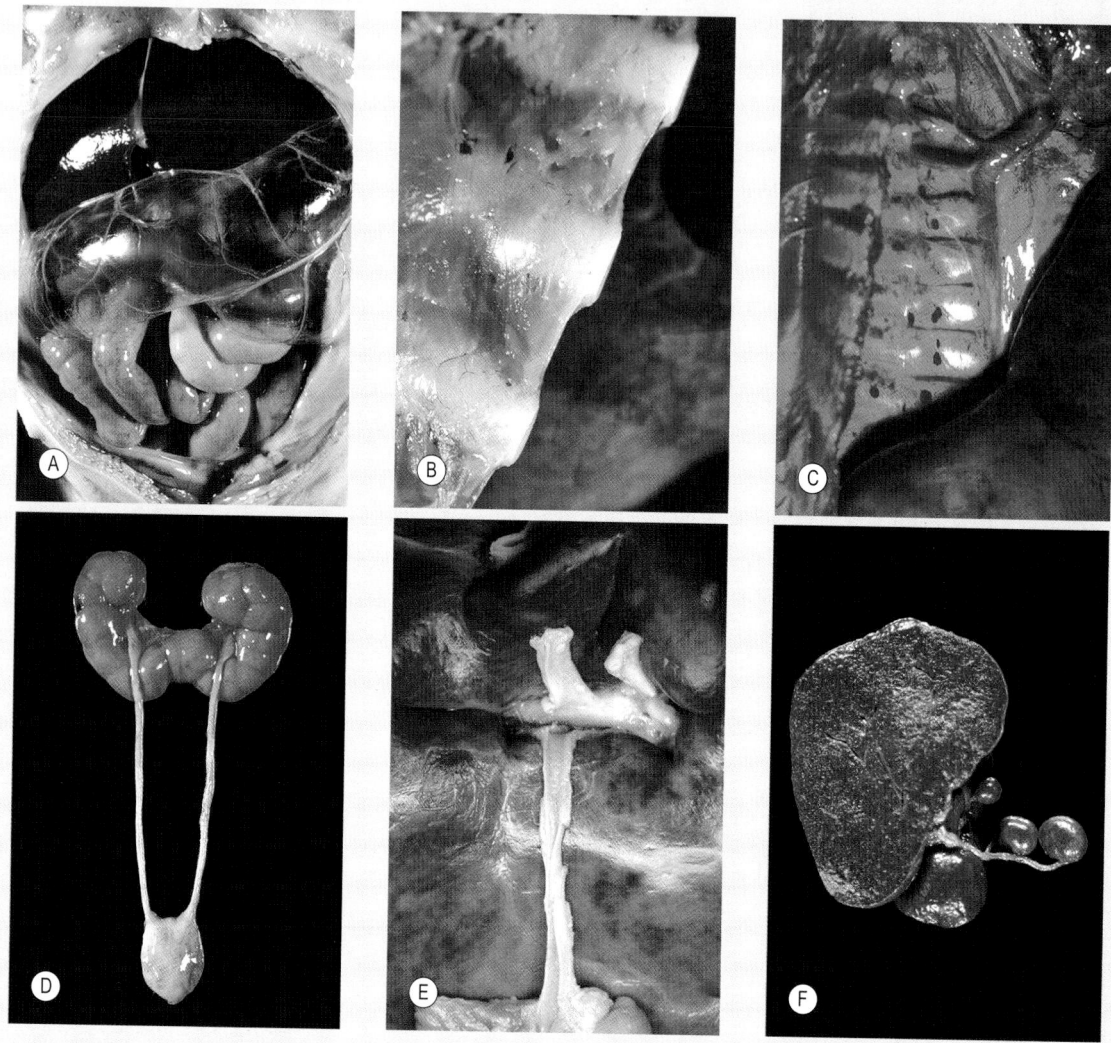

FIGURE 16.2 Examination of viscera. (A) Careful dissection of the abdomen may reveal free gas in the peritoneal cavity. In this case, gas is entrapped by the translucent omentum. The 36-week female infant died of respiratory insufficiency, complicated by interstitial and retroperitoneal emphysema. (B) In fetal and perinatal cases, the chest is easily opened by incising cartilage medial to the costochondral junction. The use of rib cutters is considerably more awkward and creates jagged edges of bone which may injure the prosector. (C) Reflection of the right lung reveals a normal azygos vein on the right posterior chest wall. The vessel is dilated by additional systemic venous blood in cases of absent intrahepatic inferior vena cava. (D) Organ systems are first examined while intact. In this instance, a horseshoe kidney and otherwise normal urinary tract was identified in a 33-week female with trisomy 18. (E) Absent gall bladder. The common bile duct (open) drains directly from the porta hepatis to the duodenum (also open). Portions of the hepatic artery and portal vein are adjacent to the bile duct. (F) Polysplenia is associated with a host of anomalies, including laterality defects and complex congenital heart disease. Note the large spleen and three accessory spleens, with splenic artery.

record. They provide indisputable evidence of findings, assuming they are not altered digitally. (One can establish a chain of custody for image files if this is of concern, as it may be in medicolegal cases.) Photographs are an excellent way of eliciting consultation. The pathologist can, for example, share images of a dysmorphic face with a medical geneticist and gain important, even diagnostic, information. Of course, photographs must be of good technical quality (i.e. properly composed, in focus, correctly lit and exposed). Images obtained for medicolegal purposes must pass the intense scrutiny of the justice system.[38,39] The disadvantages or inadequacies of various imaging techniques have been recognized as well.[40–42]

External examination

Inspection of the external features of the body parallels the physical examination performed in clinical settings. The process

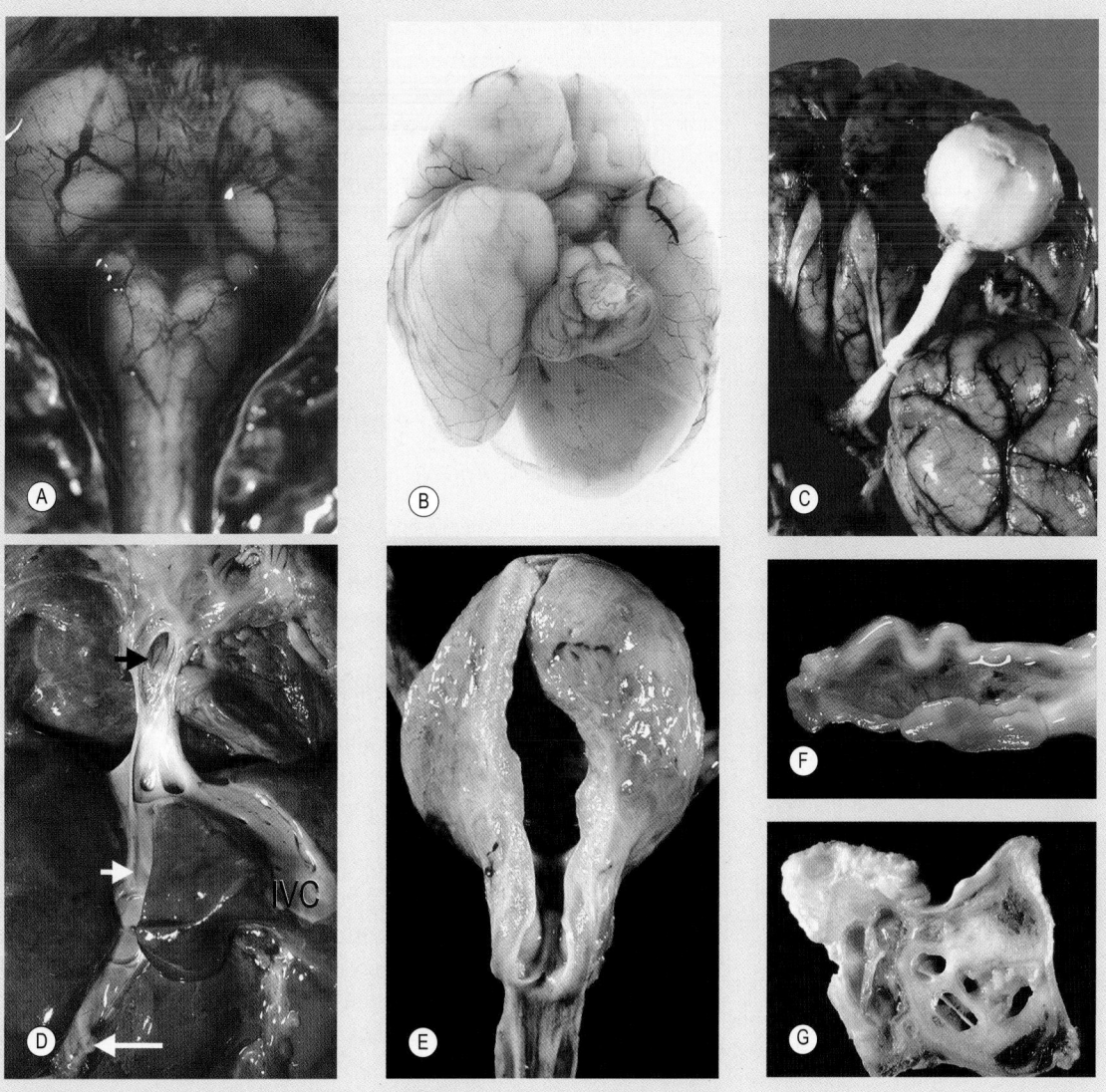

FIGURE 16.3 Special dissections and anatomic features. (A) Posterior in situ view of normal cerebellum, with intact vermis (in midline) and prominent fourth ventricle. This dissection is of great value in fetuses at mid-gestation and beyond, where ultrasound diagnosis can be problematic. The prosector must carefully strip meninges to provide better exposure of the vermis. (B) Basal view of 24-week brain with large medial cyst (porencephaly) involving left parieto-occipital lobe. Placing the brain in water allows delicate cysts to expand, and facilitates both diagnosis and photography. (C) The eyes must be removed in certain cases (see text for method). With care, the globe can be removed intact with the brain, making the entire optic nerve available for examination. (D) Anterior view of heart (opened) and liver (partly sectioned), showing several components of the fetal circulation, i.e. patent foramen ovale (black arrow), patent ductus venosus (short white arrow), umbilical vein (long white arrow), and inferior vena cava (IVC). The gall bladder and porta hepatis are apparent in the lower right portion of the image. Absence of the ductus venosus is a cause of fetal hydrops. (E) Anterior view of the urinary bladder and proximal male urethra, showing dilated ureters, hypertrophy of the bladder wall and neck, and posterior urethral valves. Dissection must be precise, as the proximal urethra lies posterior to the symphysis pubis (see text for method). (F) Close-up view of normal infantile ovary and fallopian tube. The configuration should not be confused with the narrower streak ovary of Turner (45,X) syndrome. (G) Section taken through temporal bone, showing anatomy of the middle and inner ear. Note the exudate filling the inner ear. Such examination may help to identify a route of infection in cases of acute meningitis (see text for method).

is carried out carefully and systematically, as the examiner shifts focus from one end of the body to the other, and from anterior and posterior. Developing and following such a routine insures that no pertinent feature is overlooked (Fig. 16.1). The distribution and severity of maceration are noted. Jaundice is best appreciated in the sclerae, and cyanosis in the vermilion border and fingernail beds. Pitting edema will be noticeable in the dorsal surfaces of the feet and over the shins.

Clinical workers should be asked to keep all **tubes** and **lines** in place and undisturbed if possible. (Sometimes, if parents wish to hold a baby after death, endotracheal and other intrusive implements may be removed at the discretion of the care giver). At autopsy, the placement of each is documented.

Initial incision

Dissection is a skill developed with time and patience. The beginning prosector would do well to follow a few points. One always begins at the beginning, and for the prosector, this means starting the **dissection** at a known point. Should a tangle of anomalous blood vessels appear confusing, for example, one begins with a vessel or other structure that is recognized, perhaps the ascending aorta or even heart, then dissects carefully, identifying structures as the examination moves into unknown territory. This process will be made easier if those tissues lying closest to the prosector are dissected first; then the prosector continues to dissect deeper tissues. Dissection is really a controlled form of destruction, and so one is advised to work in a disciplined fashion, preserving structures wherever possible and separating or discarding tissues only after careful thought. In complex malformations, photographic documentation between each step may be useful. Crush artifact is produced as easily at autopsy as at surgery, and one would do well to grasp connective tissues with the forceps rather than organs themselves.

The **incision** traditionally employed for thoracoabdominal autopsy is Y-shaped. The upper two incisions extend from the anterior aspect of each shoulder to the xiphoid process; the third incision descends from the xiphoid to the symphysis pubis and passes the umbilicus on the left. (In this way, the right-sided umbilical vein is avoided.) Skin covering the chest is reflected upwards with skeletal muscles (i.e. pectoralis major and minor), a process that exposes the clavicles and gives the prosector access to the neck structures. Care must be exercised during this procedure, as the skin, which is especially delicate in the young fetus, can be lacerated ('button-holed'). The prosector must learn to recognize subcutaneous tissues and refrain from incising beyond this plane, as inadvertent lacerations may interfere with postmortem viewing, should that be desired. If skeletal muscles are reflected with the skin, the ribs are much better visualized. For a chest-only autopsy, a wider U-shaped incision will expose the lateral margins of the ribs and maximize exposure.

The abdominal skin is then reflected laterally along the costal margins. As the peritoneal cavity is entered, careful note of free gas or fluid is made (Fig. 16.2A). The umbilical vein should be examined for signs of inflammation, varix, rupture,

or thrombus. It can be opened at this point, or severed at the inner (peritoneal) surface of the umbilicus and preserved for later examination as part of the liver block. The two umbilical arteries are examined and inspected in their entirety; each should sweep anteriorly from its respective common iliac artery to the lateral margin of the urinary bladder, then course toward the umbilicus on either side of the urachus. The arteries and urachus should be examined for patency and the arteries for hemorrhage or thrombosis. Single umbilical artery is an important anomaly and should be documented. Likewise, patent urachus may be associated with a variety of genitourinary anomalies (see Ch. 22).

Internal examination

Peritoneal cavity

The peritoneal cavity is inspected prior to opening the thoracic cavity (in order to maintain the integrity of the respective cavities) and with the body positioned horizontally to preserve natural positions of each organ. The leaves of the **diaphragm** normally arch to the fourth rib or fourth intercostal space bilaterally. Increased intrathoracic pressure or the presence of a mass will depress the diaphragm, while decreased intrathoracic pressure or contents or flaccid diaphragm (seen when the phrenic nerve or musculophrenic branch of the phrenic nerve is transected surgically) is associated with an abnormally high diaphragm.

The position of the liver is documented by measuring the extent to which its lobes extend below the costal margins. Likewise, the position and size of the spleen is noted. The position, caliber, and **rotation** of each component of the gastrointestinal tract are ascertained. The root of the mesentery is fixed to the posterior peritoneal surface at the ligament of Treitz (upper left quadrant) proximally and cecum (lower right quadrant) distally. It is important to document this relationship, as a short or absent mesenteric root is associated with malrotation and possible volvulus. The mesentery itself must be examined for a possible defect, which could accommodate an internal hernia. The adrenal glands and kidneys are usually visible through the translucent peritoneum and should be documented. When the kidneys are absent or low-set, the adrenal glands will assume an oval shape (a feature that can provide an important clue to renal anatomy in the disrupted fetus).

Structures of the pelvic cavity are documented. The height of the urinary bladder above the symphysis pubis affords a quantitative measure of distention. The internal genitalia are inspected; the testes will be undescended in younger fetuses and removed with abdominal contents.

Pleural cavities

Prior to opening the pleural cavities, the possibility of **pneumothorax** should be entertained. This will be suggested by clinical history or the observation of a flattened diaphragm. Free air in the chest may be documented by separating skin from ribs and creating a pocket several millimeters deep, filling it with water, and incising one of the intercostal muscles under water. The egress of air bubbles will indicate the presence of a pneumothorax. Another method is to attach a medium-gauge needle to a syringe containing several cubic centimeters of water (without plunger), and insert the tip of the needle between two ribs anterolaterally on the side in question. Again, air bubbles will appear in the water if a pneumothorax is present. If pneumothorax is unsuspected and neither of these steps is taken, it is still possible to diagnose free air. If the air is under pressure, it will escape noticeably when the chest is incised, creating a sound or causing movement of the rib cage in a manner that may be either subtle or quite distinctive.

The chest is then opened completely by incising chondral cartilages a few millimeters medial to the costochondral junctions (Fig. 16.2B). The scalpel blade can be inserted easily just medial to the head of each clavicle, through the sternoclavicular articulation, and the sternum mobilized. The chest plate (sternum with medial lengths of ribs) is then carefully freed from underlying soft tissues. Rib cutters are unnecessary, but also leave sharp, jagged edges which may injure the prosector.

In rare conditions, e.g. pentalogy of Cantrell, the **pericardium** manifests a defect in the anterior wall. Should the prosector suspect this anomaly, either by clinical history or by observing one of the other more obvious features of the disorder (omphalocele, ectopia cordis, diaphragmatic defect), the lower rib margin and sternum should be reflected very carefully, under full visualization, so that any defect in the pericardium can be identified. Without using such care, the pericardium is likely to be damaged by the dissection, and a true defect overlooked or an artifact misdiagnosed.

Workers traditionally examine the sternum and count ossification centers, which are easily seen when the structure is transilluminated. The number of centers varies widely and should not be used to estimate gestational age.[43] However, the observation offers hints to the progression of the ossification process. In a term infant, the manubrium contains one center and the body of the sternum one to four; sternal ossification centers appear between the gestational weeks 21 and 33.[44]

Upon entering the chest, each cavity should be inspected for fluid. This should be done immediately, as blood may drain from transected vessels into the chest, giving the erroneous impression of hemothorax. If the prosector wishes to obtain a **lung culture**, it is best done at this time. The lung is reflected medially, by one or two fingers placed behind the lung. Care is taken to avoid touching the lateral surface, and the lung is incised under sterile conditions. If the pleural surface has been contaminated, it can be sterilized by searing. A sterile suture removal kit containing scissors and forceps works well for culturing. Areas of consolidation or pleural exudates are indications for culturing, although neither is a common finding in the perinatal period. Each lung is examined carefully, not only for signs of infection, but for developmental changes. The configuration of each should be discerned; this entails counting lobes and recording any variations from normal. Interlobar fissures may be underdeveloped in the young fetus, but from at least mid-gestation on, the right lung should have three lobes and the left two.

The **thymus** can now be examined. Because of the important diagnostic implications for DiGeorge/velocardiofacial and other syndromes, the presence and configuration of the thymus are very important observations to make.[45, 46] The gland should have two symmetric cervical and two thoracic lobes, though the precise configuration varies. Ectopic thymic nodules are sometimes found in the neck, where they can be mistaken for lymph nodes. The thymus is dissected free of its soft tissue attachments, with care given to preserving the underlying left innominate vein. The vessel is easily damaged, even excised, as the thymic attachments are dissected. Absence of this vessel is an important feature of certain forms of congenital heart disease, and in particular, suggests the presence of a left superior vena cava.

Pericardial cavity

The integrity and tension of the pericardium are ascertained and the pericardial cavity opened. Again, the presence of free gas or fluid is determined. Once the pericardium has been opened, and if one desires to obtain blood for culturing, a needle can be inserted into the right atrium under sterile conditions. If the chamber contains clotted blood, changing the position of head or abdomen/legs sometimes yields fluid blood. The surface of pericardium (and epicardium) should be smooth and glistening. Any roughness or fibrinous deposition suggests pericarditis, and either cultures or samples for microscopy should be obtained. Following examination, the pericardial sac is cut away. It may be discarded if normal, as it is seldom altered in the fetus or neonate.

Opening the heart

Two methods for examining the heart at autopsy are described in this section. For additional details and discussion of specific disease entities, readers are advised to see Chapter 23. The heart is best examined in situ, while anatomic relationships with other structures are intact. The prosector must be familiar with **fetal anatomy** of the cardiovascular system, which differs from the older child or adult in several ways (i.e. foramen ovale, ductus arteriosus, ductus venosus, umbilical arteries and vein). Several excellent resources provide additional information on this complex examination.[8, 47, 48] The heart is inspected externally, then internally, in a systematic fashion that follows the movement of blood. The major veins of the chest are identified – azygos (Fig. 16.2C), jugular, left innominate, superior and inferior venae cavae. The pathway and caliber of each is noted. Increased diameters indicate that the vessel is carrying extra blood; explanations for this must be sought. A very large azygos vein, for example, may represent azygos continuation of the inferior vena cava. The pulmonary veins are examined by reflecting the heart to each side. The great arteries and branches are studied; the configuration of the aortic arch is inspected. An indentation on the lateral wall of the aorta at the level of the ductus arteriosus may indicate the presence of a coarctation, which can be confirmed upon opening the aorta. The external configuration of the atria and contours of the ventricles are examined. The left anterior descending coronary artery outlines the position of the interventricular septum and provides a means of comparing the sizes of the ventricles.

Once the external features of the heart are understood, the heart may be opened. In the abnormal heart, this dissection must be performed with extreme care. The prosector must maintain a conservative approach, preserving all tissues until final diagnoses are reached. An incision is made in the superior vena cava and carried inferiorly through the right atrium to end in the upper inferior vena cava. This will permit visualization of the interior of the right atrium and tricuspid annulus. A second cut, made through the tricuspid ring to the apex of the right ventricle following the lateral margin will open the right side of the heart and provide a more complete view of atrium and ventricle. The foramen ovale, with ostium secundum, and orifices of the azygos vein and coronary sinus are identified. The foramen ovale should be patent until about 3 postnatal months; if it is found to be closed in the perinatal period, the diagnosis of premature closure can be made. This is a recognized cause of fetal hydrops and/or hypoplastic left heart syndrome.[48, 49] The adequacy of closure of the septum secundum can be tested by compressing the heart against the vertebrae. This effectively increases pressure in the left atrium, causing the septum primum to bulge slightly upward (to the right) when competent. The configuration of the tricuspid valve, right ventricle, and main pulmonary artery are studied. The endocardium, myocardium, and configuration of trabeculae, pectinate and papillary muscles, and chordae tendineae are examined. The third incision, along the septum from the apex through the pulmonic valve can be extended out the right and left pulmonary arteries to the respective pulmonary hila; the ductus arteriosus is identified and examined at this time.

The left heart is dissected in a manner similar to the right. An incision in the left atrial appendage is carried into one of the left pulmonary veins; a second incision in the free wall of the left ventricle is made along the posterior margin of the interventricular septum to the left ventricular apex. A third incision follows, from the apex to and through the aortic valve. At this point, the coronary arteries may be inspected. The incision can be extended into the ascending aorta, but only if the ascending aorta and main pulmonary artery are separated. Care must be taken to preserve the mitral valve, the anterior leaflet of which sweeps up to the aortic annulus. After opening the left heart, the interior of the left atrium is examined, and pulmonary venous orifices identified; the mitral valve and left ventricle are inspected, followed by examination of the aortic valve and ascending aorta. The aortic arch can be incised and origins of major arteries seen. The distal (aortic) end of the ductus arteriosus is examined and any narrowing in the aorta (coarctation) documented. The descending aorta may be opened, although it is often left until evisceration has been completed. The heart and lungs remain attached throughout this process, to be studied in more detail after evisceration. Circumferences of the four valves and thickness of the ventricular walls are obtained most easily ex situ.

Alternate dissection of the heart

If the heart has been kept intact and fixed by perfusion, **windows** can be cut into the walls of each cardiac chamber, main pulmonary artery, and aorta. The chief advantage of this is that the valves, papillary muscles, and chordae tendineae remain intact, and can be studied from above or below. Windows must be cut carefully and conservatively, beginning near the center of each atrial or ventricular wall or artery. Formalin and remaining blood clots are washed away and windows enlarged as necessary. The heart is then examined systematically in a manner akin to that described above, following the paths of blood flow. A probe and possibly a tiny, flexible LED-style light will be helpful. Specimens prepared in this manner can be preserved in separate containers for future teaching or research purposes. They are especially valuable if accompanied by individual descriptions and diagnoses. If desired, a fine barium powder can be blown or sprayed through the windows, carefully outlining specific structures for radiographic study.

Removing the organs en bloc

After all pertinent information is gained from examining the chest and abdominal cavities and heart, the organs are removed from the body. Ligating the common carotid, subclavian, and common iliac arteries will assist funeral directors with embalming, if that is planned (it is not feasible in the small fetus). Without ligation, the inherent elasticity of vessels causes them to retract into the soft tissues of the neck or shoulders after they are transected. The structures of the neck, chest, abdomen, and pelvis are removed in a single block, a process that is quite easy in the young and preserves important relationships for later inspection.

Some may choose to remove the intestinal tract independent of other viscera. After this, the soft tissues supporting the organs are freed sequentially. It is easier to begin the evisceration from below. The rectum is freed bluntly laterally, then posteriorly by the fingers or gentle spreading action of the scissors. The rectum, vagina in females, and proximal urethra are then transected and these structures mobilized; iliac arteries and veins are severed. The diaphragmatic leaves are incised along the posterolateral body walls to the midline, and kidneys/adrenal glands mobilized. Remaining soft tissues, chiefly peritoneum, are incised, which effectively frees all the abdominal and retroperitoneal structures.

The **neck structures** are brought down next. The soft tissues supporting trachea and esophagus are incised medial to the carotid arteries (care must be taken to avoid lacerating the arteries, an act that will complicate embalming). The esophagus and trachea are freed from below and the dissection carried upwards to the larynx. The airway can be transected in one of two ways. The goal of each method is to preserve the epiglottis for inspection. The most reliable way of preserving the epiglottis is to cut across the airway above the hyoid bone. A slightly simpler way is to incise the thyrohyoid membrane just above the thyroid notch. In this latter approach, care must be taken to position the scalpel blade parallel to and above the epiglottis, to avoid amputating it.

The **tongue** can be removed, but this requires special care and practice to avoid lacerating the skin of the anterior neck or face. The scissors are extended upwards toward the chin, anterior to the larynx, until the genioglossus muscle can be severed. The incisions are then carried laterally, so that the posterior wall of the pharynx is cut. Careful probing with the scissors will reveal any soft tissues that need to be cut before the tongue is completely freed and brought down through the neck. This procedure makes the tongue available for measurement, histologic, or other examination and allows better visualization of the oral cavity.[50] The submaxillary salivary glands may be encountered beneath the mandibular arches and can be sampled if desired.

The chest organs are mobilized last of all, by incising parietal pleura at each side of the aorta and esophagus. The entire organ block can now be lifted from the body and moved to a flat surface for additional examination and dissection.

Removing the brain and spinal cord

The postmortem examination of the brain has been described in numerous publications.[8, 9, 14, 15, 51–53] Before proceeding, the prosector must ensure that the **autopsy permit** includes removal of the brain, for this is arguably the most intrusive part of the entire examination. The scalp, fontanelles, and cranial sutures are examined, the latter by palpation, and changes documented. The decision to culture cerebrospinal fluid is best made prior to incising the scalp (see 'Bacterial culture' below).

The traditional scalp incision extends transversely over the cranial convexity from ear to ear; it is kept behind each ear by a centimeter or so and behind the crown of the head, again by about 1 cm. In this way, the repaired incision can be concealed should a funeral with viewing be desired. Suture lines can be hidden when the patient has hair, but this is often not the case in the very young. A small cap can be placed over the head for viewing, although this is less than optimal. For this reason, it is best to arrange for viewings prior to autopsy.

The initial incision creates anterior and posterior flaps of skin, which are reflected to expose the **calvaria**. The fontanelles, sutures, and galea are examined again, and changes documented as indicated. The calvaria can then be removed by a variety of techniques. A common method is to incise the membranous bone along each of the sutures, sagittal, coronal, and lambdoidal. This effectively mobilizes the frontal and parieto-occipital bones, which can be reflected outward to expose the brain. Another method is to make a circumferential cut through the calvarial bones above the reflected skin, creating a calotte which is removed by cutting the falx cerebri.

After the **brain** has been exposed, it is examined in situ. This step is especially important in cases of severe maceration, where the very act of removing the brain can be destructive. The brain is then removed completely by severing all cranial nerves, vessels, pituitary stalk, tentorium cerebelli, and other portions of dura mater. This is the most delicate part of the procedure and must be done with great care. The head can be tilted back and the brain supported by one hand, while cuts are made with the other; the brain is gently rolled from side to side to facilitate severing nerves, supportive tissues, and finally the cervical spinal cord. Some advocate using the table surface to support the brain as it is removed.

When the brain is particularly fragile, as it will be if young, autolytic, or altered by cystic change (hydranencephaly, porencephaly, large arachnoid cyst), the head can be suspended in a large flat container of water (or saline), and the brain removed essentially under water. The fluid will support the brain, which can then be examined and carefully transferred to formalin. The brain can also be photographed submerged and dramatic images of fully inflated cysts or other tenuous structures obtained (Fig. 16.3B).

After the brain is removed, it is examined on all sides and placed in fixative, usually formalin or a 50:50 mixture of formalin and Bouin fixative. The brain should be supported from below or suspended by the basilar artery to avoid flattening artifact. Ten to 14 days are generally sufficient for fixation, prior to sectioning (see below).

Attention should then be turned to the **cranial base** and **dural sinuses**. The former exhibits a configuration that essentially mirrors the base of the brain, and hence can be very informative, especially when the brain cannot be examined, as may be the case in severe autolysis or fetal disruption.[9, 54] The pituitary gland is removed from the sella turcica by careful teasing; the process may be facilitated by amputating the posterior clinoid processes, which are cartilaginous in the fetus or newborn.

Removal of the vertebral bodies and **spinal cord** proceeds with comparative ease in the fetus or young infant and can be performed with scalpel and stout scissors. The first two steps are as follows: palpate the costovertebral junction, a depression between the head of the ribs and lateral aspect of each vertebral body. Incise this with a scalpel angled at about 45 degrees. This cut will not reach the spinal canal except in the early gestational fetus, where extra care must be taken to avoid lacerating the cord. An intervertebral disc is then incised in the midlumbar region to expose the spinal canal. One blade of a strong scissors is inserted into the canal, and the scalpel cut completed. The prosector must avoid damaging the spinal cord in the process. The anterior portion of the vertebral column can then be dissected free. The spinal cord is mobilized by severing spinal nerves with a scalpel. After the spinal cord is exposed, additional nerves, such as the sciatic plexus, can be identified and sampled if necessary. During manipulation, the spinal cord should be kept straight by mild traction directed inferiorly on the dura mater; if the cord is bent upwards and back upon itself, damage to the cord will ensue. Ideally, the cord is fixed in a straight position. With care, the brain and entire spinal cord can be removed intact, a process that is especially beneficial in the Chiari malformation.

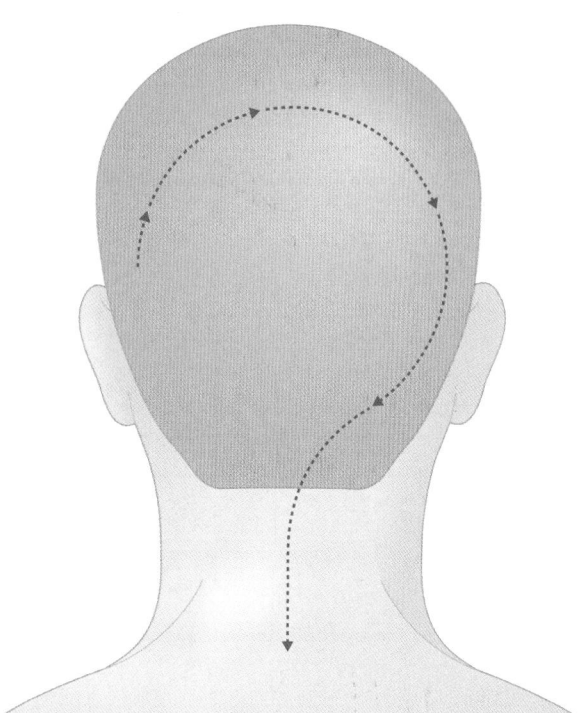

FIGURE 16.4 An alternative to the usual incision, i.e. the straight cut across the top of the forehead extending from a point behind one ear to a point behind the other. This incision is especially useful for opening the head in cases of Arnold-Chiari malformation when one is obliged to inspect carefully the posterior aspect of the brainstem.

Special dissections of the central nervous system and cranium

On occasion, the brain requires greater scrutiny in situ. A prime example is the variety of **posterior fossa anomalies** (Dandy-Walker malformation or variant; mega cisterna magna), which are easily damaged if more traditional methodology is employed. The posterior fossa is best examined in situ by placing the body prone and reflecting the scalp in the usual manner. Two approaches to this dissection have been described. The skin overlying the occiput and upper cervical region can be incised in the midline perpendicular to the standard ear-to-ear incision, then reflected laterally, exposing occiput and cervical vertebrae.[9] Alternatively, a question-mark shaped incision (Fig. 16.4) can be extended across the convexity and then to the midline overlying the cervical spine.[14, 15] Either exposes the posterior calvaria, allowing the lambdoid sutures to be incised and occipital bone and vertebral lamina cut away. In this way, the cerebrum, cerebellum, and upper cervical cord are exposed (Fig. 16.3A). This is a necessary step in the diagnosis of Dandy-Walker or other posterior fossa anomalies.[9, 55] The technique can also be used to inspect the central nervous system for edema[56] or the presence of a Chiari malformation.

In cases of suspected **stenosis of the foramen magnum** (observed in osteochondrodysplasia), the region surrounding the foramen magnum can be removed intact with upper cervical vertebrae. The posterior half of the cranial base must be mobilized, first by transecting the middle cranial fossae with a power saw, then by continuing the dissection subcutaneously and posterolaterally to free the cervical vertebrae.[57]

It is often desirable to remove a **myelomeningocele** or other spinal defect intact with the spinal cord and adjoining vertebrae for further study. An ellipse of skin is incised surrounding the defect and the incision carried deep to the vertebral column. The spinal cord is then dissected free in the usual manner, and the defective portion brought through the incised skin.

In most institutions, examination of the **eyes** is deemed a special procedure which requires informed consent (see also Ch. 39). One or both globes may be removed using either an anterior or posterior approach; with special care, they can be removed intact with optic nerves and brain (Fig. 16.3C). With the anterior approach, the prosector must use care to avoid lacerating the eyelids, which are especially delicate in the fetus. Retractors may be helpful in preventing damage, as extraocular muscles and optic nerve are severed sequentially and the globe gently pulled from the orbit. In the posterior approach (preferred by the author), the brain is first removed, exposing the cranial base. The frontal plates are incised (using scalpel in perinatal cases, followed by strong scissors) and a square of bone about 1.5 cm on a side is removed. The globe and retro-orbital fat pad will be visible. The prosector then places the index finger between the eyelids, effectively retracting them, and exerts gentle upward pressure on the globe, while cutting extraocular muscles, optic nerve, and extraneous soft tissues. By this method, the inner surface of the eyelids can be seen and thus avoided. (For examination and section of the eyeball see chapter 39.)

The **middle ears** may be examined by cutting blocks or wedges of temporal bone. A hand saw may suffice in the young, although the vibrating power saw is required in infants and older individuals. The specimen may be fixed and later sectioned for decalcification and microscopic examination. This approach has been used traditionally to search for otitis media, a possible route of infection in acute meningitis (Fig. 16.3G).

Examination of the brain after fixation

The prosector may wish to consult qualified neuropathologists and/or neuropathologic textbooks before examining brains that are severely malformed or altered by other disorders. However, brains that are not likely to be so altered can be examined in a more routine fashion, one that is very similar to that employed in adult pathology. Perinatal brains are fixed for 1–2 weeks, then rinsed in water, and the cortical surfaces examined. Fixation of autolyzed brains in Bouin helps preserve anatomic integrity of tissues. A comparison of **gyral pattern** with published norms for gestational age is an essential part of this process.[58] In this way, the developmental age can be documented. The leptomeninges, cranial nerves, and superficial arteries (circle of Willis) are inspected. The cerebellum and brain stem are likewise examined.

The cerebrum and cerebellum/brainstem are first separated, by a single flat incision through the midbrain (cerebral peduncles). Each portion of the brain may be weighed separately if desired;

this provides an internal control for development. The cerebrum is cut traditionally in the coronal plane. However, this approach may be modified to correspond with imaging studies, and the brain sectioned in the horizontal or sagittal plane. Multiple cuts are made of 0.5–1.0 cm in thickness. Great care must be taken if the brain is softened. Slices are laid on a flat surface systematically for further examination, photography, and sectioning. The cerebellum and brain stem may be separated or sectioned together, most usually in the horizontal plane.

An important diagnosis in the perinatal period, **ventriculomegaly**, may be difficult to reach (or confirm, if made by prenatal ultrasonography). The brain may be soft, and the shape of ventricles preserved poorly, or the brain may be disrupted. In these instances, the thickness of the cortical mantle can often be determined and compared with published norms.[59] Significant thinning of the mantle occurs in some but not all forms of ventricular dilatation.

At the end of the gross examination of the brain, a series of routine **histologic sections** can be taken; the location of each should be recorded. The following routine sections are recommended: frontal cortex, internal capsule, basal ganglia, wall of lateral ventricle, hippocampus, cerebellum, pons, medulla, spinal cord, pituitary, and choroid plexus. In addition, any pathologic lesion(s) should be sampled.

Additional samples

Once the evisceration has been completed, the body cavities are examined completely. The state of the parietal pleura and peritoneum is inspected and the configuration and number of ribs and vertebrae ascertained. One or more **costochondral junctions** are bisected and then removed for microscopic sampling (each portion should be approximately 1.0 cm in length and contain both cartilaginous and bony portions of rib). The psoas major can be sampled, and other **skeletal muscles** obtained as indicated. A variety of muscles should be examined in cases of central nervous or muscular system disease. Beckwith produced a particularly valuable list of muscles that can be obtained without additional incisions at autopsy.[60] Recommended samples are: temporalis or anterior belly of digastric (V cranial nerve), posterior belly of digastric (VII), sternocleidomastoid (XI), tongue (XII), strap muscles (C1, 2, 3), diaphragm (C3, 4, 5), deltoid (C5, 6), pectoralis minor (C7, 8), intercostals (thoracic levels of spinal nerves), psoas major (L2, 3), quadriceps (L3, 4), obturator internus (L5, S1, 2), and levator ani (S3, 4). Tibialis anterior (L5, S1, 2) and gastrocnemius (S1, 2) are easily sampled, but require additional incisions. Skin can be taken parallel to the chest or abdominal incision, again eliminating the need for additional incisions.

In the male fetus, the **testis** is generally non-descended and identified within the abdominal or pelvic cavity. However, the testis must be removed from the scrotum in the older fetus or newborn. This is accomplished without particular difficulty. The inguinal canal can be entered through the prominent inguinal ring, and then widened by spreading both blades of the scissors. The scrotum is compressed gently, the testis expressed upward through the canal, and soft tissue attachments severed. If necessary, especially in older infants, additional access to the inguinal canal is gained by inserting one blade of the scissors into the inguinal canal and making a firm cut across a lower band of rectus abdominis muscle. The vas deferens can be preserved for later sectioning, if indicated.

Postmortem reconstruction of the body

Reconstruction borders on impossible in the young fetus, whose skin is so delicate that suturing is ineffectual. Removal of the brain disrupts the calvaria and, in the context of thin fetal skin, can be difficult to conceal. However, in the newborn, reconstruction is possible. Skin can be sutured or stapled in the usual fashion. Small wooden implements can be fashioned to replace a long bone, or plaster bandages moistened and molded into any desired shape. In cases requiring extensive dissection, it is advisable to contact the funeral director, explain the necessity of the procedure, and ensure that it will not interfere with family plans.

Dissecting the viscera

In the Rokitansky-style **evisceration**, the organs are removed together, in a 'block'. This has the advantage of preserving vascular and other connections, as well as retroperitoneal structures, which are not readily examined in situ. (The Virchow-style evisceration consists of removing organs one at a time, and may be preferable in certain situations, e.g. when the organs are very large or otherwise encumbered, such as an unwieldy mass.) After evisceration the relationships of organs are again determined, but from a posterior viewpoint rather than anterior. The same rules for dissection apply to the ex situ examination: if dealing with unrecognized structures, begin at the beginning and carry the dissection into unrecognized regions by starting at recognized landmarks; treat the tissue gently; be sure to identify structures prior to proceeding with an irreversible part of the dissection. Weights of the organs are obtained prior to sectioning.

The organ block is positioned on its anterior surface and supported by a smooth surface such as a wet sponge at comfortable height. The block can be oriented in a variety of ways, but placing it in the anatomic position seems most logical and facilitates many aspects of the dissection. Examination begins with the most posterior structures and moves anteriorly, layer by layer. Attention is first directed to the aorta and inferior vena cava. If the prosector has kept proximal portions of the common iliac arteries and veins intact, they will provide orientation for examining the aorta and vena cava. Each is opened, along with major tributaries (and minor tributaries if indicated), then reflected upward or cut away. The diaphragm is reflected and adrenal glands and posterior surfaces of the urinary system exposed and examined; the ureters are inspected again to ensure their presence and identify areas of dilatation, narrowing, or atresia. The adrenal glands are removed; the kidneys are mobilized and removed, intact with vessels, ureters, and urinary bladder if indicated (Fig. 16.2D). The bladder is opened in the anterior midline, and additional cuts made at right angles to the first cut through each ureteral orifice. See 'The male urethra' below for additional discussion.

For optimal inspection, the female genital tract is separated from the urinary bladder and rectum. This is straightforward, as connecting tissues are delicate and planes of dissection obvious in the fetus or young infant. The vagina and uterus are opened in the anterior midline and examined. The endometrium may be hemorrhagic, an effect of maternal hormones; the prosector should understand that the normal fetal and newborn ovary is narrow and elongated (Fig. 16.3F), and should not be confused with the streak ovary of Turner (45,X) syndrome.

The liver is examined next. The umbilical vein remains intact with the liver and can be opened, revealing any pathologic change. By continuing this incision, the intrahepatic portal system is entered and the **ductus venosus** recognized as a thin-walled structure aligned linearly with the umbilical vein and draining to the inferior vena cava (Fig. 16.3D). The gallbladder and structures of the porta hepatis – portal vein, hepatic artery, and common bile duct – are identified and dissected as indicated. These structures must not be overlooked, for they may be altered in a variety of congenital disorders (Fig. 16.2E). A recommended way to identify and open the portal vein is to locate it in the splenic hilum, and follow it as it courses along the posterosuperior margin of the pancreas. After these structures are examined, the spleen is removed and examined. Accessory spleens are seen commonly in young individuals, but the presence of several is indicative of polysplenia (Fig. 16.2F). The gastrointestinal tract is now exposed and ready for examination. The esophagus is opened in the posterior midline while intact with the trachea. In this way, a tracheoesophageal fistula can be identified. After opening, the incision may be carried into the stomach (incising along the greater curvature allows the stomach to be opened flat for photography), or the entire gastrointestinal tract can be separated from the block and mesentery for later opening. The mesentery is examined as necessary (lymph nodes are very small in the fetus and newborn, unless enlarged pathologically). The liver is separated from thoracic viscera by severing the diaphragmatic connections and inferior vena cava.

Attention is turned next to the thoracic block. The right hilum is ascertained to eparterial, the left hyparterial (i.e., with the mainstem bronchus anterior to the right, and posterior to the left pulmonary arteries, respectively). The larynx, trachea, and major bronchi are opened from the posterior aspect, otherwise the organs are examined most easily from an anterior perspective. If abnormalities in heart-lung connections exist, the organs are not separated. After major hilar structures of the lungs have been opened and inspected, attention is turned to the lungs themselves. Lobation and condition of the visceral pleura were presumably ascertained during the in situ examination, but can be examined more thoroughly ex situ. The lungs may then be perfused (see 'Inflation of lungs' below) or sectioned. If the latter is preferred, the lungs are reflected laterally and sectioned from the hilum toward the periphery, parallel to the plane of the bronchi. This technique produces a

logical orientation for the hilar structures and lungs and allows the lungs to be positioned flat for photography.

For additional comments on the dissection of the heart, see 'Opening the infant heart' above and Chapter 23.

Routine microscopic sections

Upon occasion (i.e. metabolic disorders), autopsy should be conducted as soon after death as possible, to obtain and treat tissues optimally. The **'immediate autopsy'** requires planning and coordination, points that have been made previously.[61] More routinely, sections are taken at the time of gross autopsy or a day later. For the sake of efficiency, many take sections at the time of autopsy. This may be the preferred method on very busy perinatal services. However, if tissues are fixed and sectioned the day after autopsy, the increased firmness ensures that more precise sections can be made. This is especially noticeable in autolytic tissues. In many instances, the prosector will wish to submit every major tissue for microscopic examination. However, this is not always indicated, practical, or possible.[62] Tissues may be severely autolyzed or, in the case of fetal disruption, not available for examination. The prosector will need to bring experience and diagnostic or other needs to bear in making such decisions.

Certain developmental differences in the perinatal period require alterations in the routine submission of tissue for microscopic examination. In the lung, concern for hypoplasia dictates examination of both hilar and pleural regions; in small lungs, these areas can be included in the same section. One is advised to section the mid-portion of the adrenal gland, where medulla is more common. Similarly, for the pancreas, more islet tissue is found in the head of the gland. Many examiners strip the capsule when examining the kidney, but this is ill-advised in the young fetus or infant, as the process will dislodge blastema, the presence of which is a reliable indicator of maturity; stripping may also remove nephrogenic rests in older children. Kidney sections should extend through the cortex and medulla, so that one can discern the number of generations of glomeruli and also rule out dysplasia, a feature common to a number of conditions. The larynx is sectioned horizontally, to include thyroid gland and possibly parathyroid gland. In the heart, a section taken through the atrioventricular junction includes diverse tissues, atrium, valve, coronary artery, and ventricle; careful orientation of the section will ensure that endocardium, myocardium, and epicardium appear on the final slide.

At this point, samples of liver and placenta are frozen at −70°. This procedure is routine and makes tissue available for unforeseen tests (see Ch. 19).

Examination of twins or other multiple gestations

The complete autopsy description of a twin must also include a description of the other twin and of the placenta.[63] Pathologists must take care to correlate **twin identification** at autopsy with that assigned clinically, so that analysis and subsequent discussion of findings can occur without confusion. The twin identified as twin A by the obstetrician must also be the pathologist's twin A. The twins (if both are received) must be compared, and done so systematically with regard to external appearance, including size and sex, and concordance or discordance of significant anomalies or other findings. Fetal growth must be assessed in both twins and documented with a full battery of weights and measures. Because fluid shifts (and hence changes in weight) can be both dynamic and pronounced, linear measurements often provide better estimates of fetal age and growth.[63]

The placenta(s) of twin or other multiple gestation pregnancies are examined for configuration, as well as **vascular anastomoses**. It can be helpful to make sketches or label specimens prior to photography; the injection of colored dyes or milk facilitates the identification of abnormal vascular connections.

Some workers report the autopsy findings of both twins in a single report. Others prefer to assign different case numbers, thus keeping tissue and data completely separate, and issue two separate, cross-referenced reports. The latter approach is preferable in our experience.

The reader is referred to Chapters 9 and 15 for more complete discussion of the problems inherent to the products of multiple gestation and their placentas.

Examination of the stillborn fetus

In examining the stillborn fetus, important goals are to establish the cause of death and, if possible, to identify or exclude the presence or role of congenital, infectious, or other disease. Parents often wish to gain an understanding of the time of death, and that can certainly be estimated.[64–66] However, published criteria for **estimating the time of intrauterine demise** are only approximations, a point that workers can verify for themselves in cases where the exact time of death, period of intrauterine retention, and delivery are known [e.g. in cases of pregnancy termination by potassium chloride (KCl) administration-note that KCl markedly accelerates autolysis in these cases].

Examination is hampered by **maceration** of the body and autolysis of viscera, which can vary from mild to very severe. Measurements and weights are obtained in the usual fashion, although weights are decreased by autolysis. The prosector should not be dissuaded by the condition of tissues, and may still find meaningful congenital anomalies. Microscopic examination of autolyzed tissue may still reveal viral inclusions or other information. In the severely autolyzed brain, for example, one may still recognize neurons and possibly achieve some understanding of a process such as arthrogryposis. Skin or viscera are inappropriate for karyotyping in cases of advanced maceration, but placenta can serve this function, as it survives beyond the time of fetal demise.

Examination of the placenta is an important part of the stillborn autopsy and often is contributory to the final diagnosis. The concept of a maternal–fetal–placental unit should be used to explore the many variables.

Examination of the embryo and young fetus
Examination of the chorionic sac

The examination of very young specimens requires specialized knowledge and skills, which have been put forth in several detailed publications, from which the following discussion is drawn (see Ch. 2).[15, 27, 67–69] **Early abortion** specimens may be complete or incomplete. For accurate pathologic evaluation of any early conceptus, all aborted tissues must be examined and thorough obstetric, medical, and family histories reviewed. Menstrual dates are valuable for dating the gestational sac and embryo.[69] Information about drug ingestion (e.g. anticonvulsive medication) or exposure to infection during pregnancy (e.g. rubella) is essential for directing the pathologist's efforts.

Aborted tissue should be submitted fresh, not fixed in formalin, in a sterile, or at least a clean, tightly closed container or bag so that it is not dehydrated.[27] Small specimens should be kept moist with gauze soaked in sterile saline. An early spontaneous abortus is best examined in a large sterile Petri dish, with sterile instruments, under a dissecting microscope. Sterile technique allows the taking of samples for tissue culture and chromosome analysis, if indicated, after the examination under the dissecting microscope is completed. The dissecting microscope should have a camera for photographic documentation.[68] Small embryos are transferred to a smaller dish for further examination. Since embryonic specimens are generally fragile, it is recommended that they be examined floating in saline or after fixation.

An intact **chorionic sac** commonly appears as a fluctuant globular structure in a pear-shaped specimen that represents a decidual cast of the uterine cavity. Smaller intact chorionic sacs may be received free of decidua and surrounded only by blood clots. The surface of a well-developed chorionic sac is usually covered by abundant chorionic villi. Sacs showing abnormal development of amnion, yolk sac, and embryo manifest little or no villous development.[27] After opening the intact chorionic sac, the presence or absence of amniotic sac, yolk sac, body stalk/cord, and embryo are documented. When any of these are present, their size and relationship to the chorionic sac and other structures are recorded.

Villi are observed most efficiently in saline under the dissecting microscope.[70] Normal villi are of uniform diameter, with a symmetric branching appearance and multiple buds along their length. Sparse development and abnormal morphology (swelling, clubbing, and hypoplasia) of chorionic villi are common in early abortion specimens. Villi with swollen tips are described as clubbed, villi with clear vesicles at their end as cystic, and villi with a few buds or thin irregular branches as hypoplastic. Histologically, clubbed and cystic villi are usually hydropic and avascular; hypoplastic villi are fibrotic, with vascular obliteration.

A ruptured chorionic sac has a collapsed wrinkled appearance due to amniotic fluid loss, and the embryo is frequently missing.

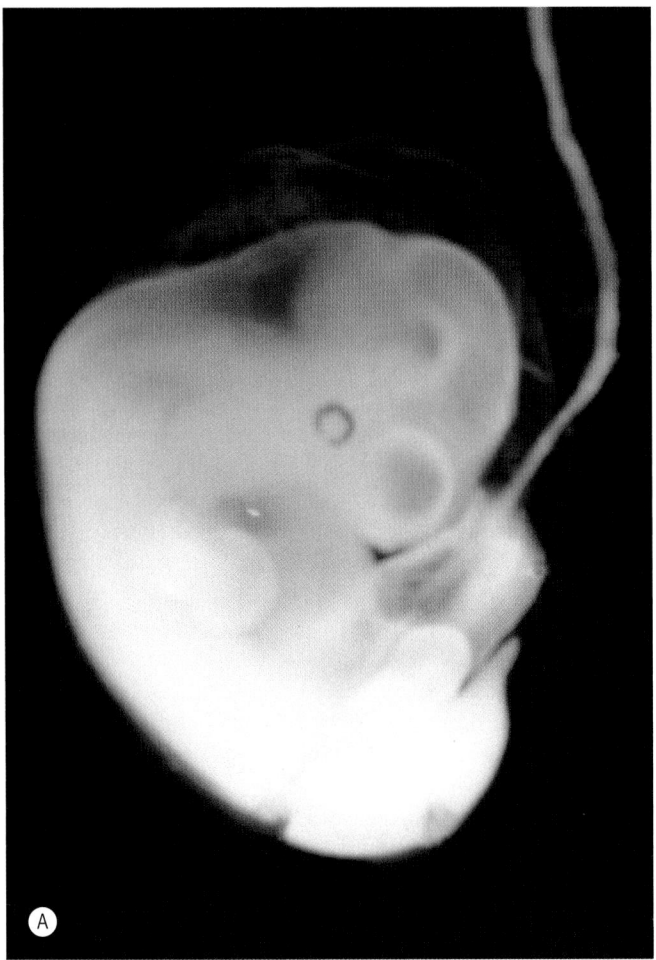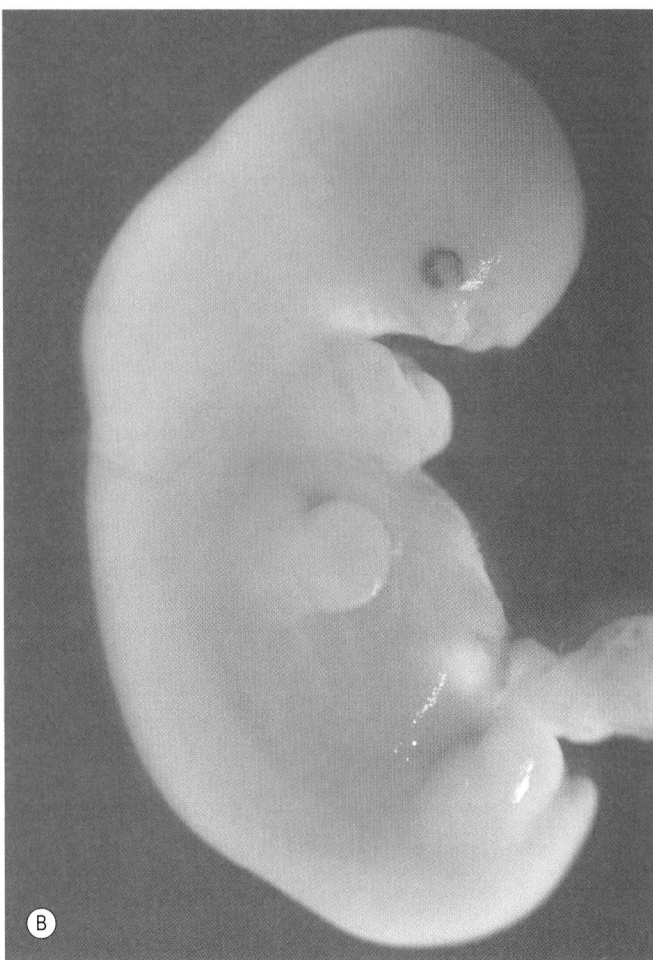

FIGURE 16.5 Stages of late embryonic development. (A) Stage 18 of 23 stages in the Streeter classification system (approximately 44 days post conception).[72] Cervical and lumbar flexures are evident, and finger/toe rays are becoming visible; pigmentation in the margin of the optic cup is obvious.[73] (B) Stage 19 (approximately 48 days post conception). Some straightening in the trunk is evident; the limbs have a forward orientation and the digits are more prominent.[73] The mildly autolytic embryo shows some disruption in the region of the mandible.

A fragmented chorionic sac without detectable embryo can still yield information about embryonic development, but only if the villi are examined histologically. Histologic abnormalities in the chorionic villi relate to the time at which embryogenesis was disturbed. If embryonic death occurred before the embryonic circulation was established in the placental villi, i.e. before the end of the third week, the villi will be avascular and hydropic and have attenuated trophoblast layers. However, if the embryonic circulation was established and then ceased because of embryonic death, increased villous stromal cellularity, followed by fibrosis, and vascular obliteration will be apparent.[71]

Examination of the embryo

The developmental stage of the embryo is determined by the correlation of several external features (Fig. 16.5)[72] and **CR length**.[73] The difference between age by dates and age by physical appearance helps one estimate the length of retention in utero after embryonic death.

CR length correlates with developmental age and should be obtained without straightening the embryo. Since embryos in the third and early fourth weeks are nearly straight, their linear measurement indicates greatest length. In embryos with flexed heads (fifth and sixth weeks of development), however, the CR length is actually a neck–rump measurement. The true CR length can be measured only in older embryos. Length and development can then be compared and developmental age established.

Although CR length is very important for staging normally developing embryos and embryos with focal defects, it is meaningless for staging embryos with growth disorganization, damaged or severely macerated embryos (see Ch. 6). Growth disorganization has been classified previously:[68, 74]

- GD 1: intact, but empty chorionic or amniotic sac without identifiable embryo;

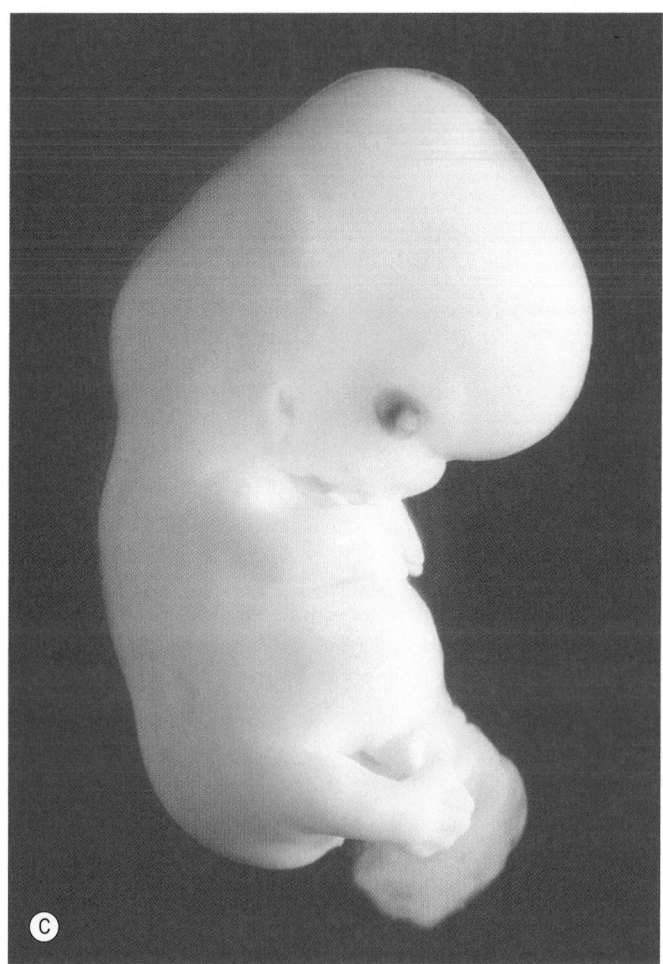

FIGURE 16.5 (cont'd) (C) Stage 20. The elbows are bent and the fingers curve over the cardiac bulge.[73]

- GD 2: solid, but fragmented embryonic tissue (1–4 mm) without discernible cranial–caudal orientation or external features;
- GD 3: smooth, cylindrical embryo (up to 10 mm), with recognizable orientation (due to presence of retinal pigmentation), but no limb buds or other external landmarks;
- GD 4: stunted embryo, with severe distortion of body shape and anatomic features that manifest aberrant size and development.

In instances of growth disorganization, developmental age can be estimated on the basis of external features (hand, eye) or organ development, but malformations often cannot be diagnosed, since maceration can produce focal defects that mimic open neural tube defect or cleft lip.

Examination of the small or disrupted fetus

Late abortion specimens (9 to 18 developmental weeks or 11 to 20 gestational weeks) consist of an identifiable fetus and a placenta, each of which should be examined. Routine exami-

nation of the fetus consists of both external and internal examinations, radiologic examination and karyotyping if indicated, photographic documentation, and histologic examination.[75] Routine weights and measurements are obtained (see Tables). CR length and foot length are the main criterion for establishing developmental age. Tables are also available for determining developmental age from CH length, hand length, or body weight. These may be substituted for CR length when the specimen is incomplete, fragmented, or otherwise abnormal; the measurements can be used in addition to the CR length to verify its accuracy.

A detailed external examination is carried out in the usual fashion. Some facial characteristics of common syndromes, such as trisomy 21 or trisomy 18, may be only partially developed or even absent in previable fetuses. In the examination of the limbs, the length, the number of digits and their position, and the presence or absence of flexion deformities are very important. Care should be taken in this evaluation to avoid assigning importance to artifactual deformities.

Macerated and damaged fetuses should not be ignored, even though they may be distorted. In spite of molding and other deformity, such external malformations as neural tube defect, cleft lip and palate, syndactyly, polydactyly, amputations, and constrictions can be diagnosed. Artifacts produced by maceration in previable fetuses are different from those seen in embryos. Although the external and internal examinations of non-macerated fetuses are usually done with the fetus in a fresh state, macerated fetuses should be fixed before internal dissection, since their tissues are fragile and artifacts may easily be introduced. Smaller fetuses (9–11 weeks) can be examined with the dissecting microscope after sectioning the trunk at 0.5–1 cm intervals.[76] Organ weights for fetuses of 9–20 weeks of developmental age are given in the Tables.

Examination of the brain is feasible only in non-macerated fetuses. The brain is often liquefied in macerated fetuses. Brain tissue should be removed after fixation in situ in 10% formaldehyde or Bouin's fixative. This is by incising or opening the cranium. Artifacts are found frequently in fetuses that are spontaneously aborted or terminated in the second trimester of pregnancy.[77]

When pregnancies are terminated by **dilation and evacuation**, specimens are disrupted, but the degree of disruption varies widely and examination is possible regardless.[78] Tissues are carefully and systematically separated into four categories: blood clot, placenta, body fragments, and visceral fragments. It may be useful to float fragments in saline for ease in separation, and to use a dissecting microscope to examine smaller portions. The prosector's knowledge of anatomic relationships will be especially important in these cases. The thymus, for example, may be intact with heart, adrenal gland attached to kidney, and so on. The cranial base may be examined for abnormalities in the absence of brain tissue. A foot length will help in estimating gestational age. Unfortunately, it is also true that fetal disruption can preclude meaningful pathologic examination, a point that clinicians and parents must appreciate in their own decision making.[79]

TABLE 16.1 CRITERIA FOR ESTIMATING FERTILIZATION AGE DURING THE FETAL PERIOD

Age (weeks)	Crown–rump length (mm)	Foot length (mm)	Fetal weight (g)	Main external characteristics	Microscopic appearance
Previable fetuses					
9	50	7	8	Eyes closing or closed, head more rounded, external genitalia still not distinguishable as male or female, intestines are in umbilical cord	
10	61	9	14	Intestine in abdomen, early fingernail development	Cartilage in trachea
12	87	14	45	Sex distinguishable externally, well-defined neck	Bronchial glands and goblet cells evident
14	120	20	110	Head erect, lower limbs well developed	Prominent duct system in lung
16	140	27	200	Ears stand out from the head	Cartilage in segmental bronchi
18	160	33	320	Vernix caseosa present, early toenail development	
20	190	39	460	Head and body hair (lanugo) visible	Lymphatics present in lung, periarteriolar lymphocytes in spleen, thymic cortex equal to medulla in thickness
22	210	45	630	Skin wrinkled and red	
24	230	50	820	Fingernails present, lean body	
Viable fetuses					
26	250	55	1000	Eyes partially open, eyelashes present	
28	270	59	1300	Eyes open, good head of hair, skin slightly wrinkled	
30	280	63	1700	Toenails present, body filling out, testes descending	
32	300	68	2100	Fingernails reach fingertips, skin pink and smooth	
36	340	79	2900	Body usually plump, lanugo hair almost absent, toenails reach toe tips	
38	360	83	3400	Prominent chest, breasts protrude, testes in scrotum or palpable in inguinal canals, fingernails extend beyond fingertips	

From Gilbert-Barness and Debich-Spicer 2005,[15] with permission and with permission from WB Saunders.

Culture and other studies

The reader is referred to Chapter 19 for a detailed discussion of these topics.

Bacterial cultures

Tissue may be obtained from a variety of regions. **Blood** is most often drawn from the right atrium. To gain sterile access to that chamber, one may open the pericardial cavity and, without touching the surface of the heart, insert a medium gauge needle, and withdraw several cubic centimeters of blood. If the heart has been contaminated, the epicardium can be seared and then needled. If insufficient blood is obtained, the head and/or lower body can be manipulated, with the hope of draining additional blood into the atrium. A **lung** may be cultured,

again under sterile conditions if the pleura is not touched or otherwise contaminated. The **spleen** may also be cultured. Multiple positive cultures provide evidence of sepsis rather than **contamination**.

Cerebrospinal fluid can be obtained by a number of techniques. It can be withdrawn from a lateral ventricle, cisterna magna, or subdural space of the spinal cord. A sterile needle inserted through a lateral margin of the anterior fontanelle and directed toward the inner canthus of the opposite side of the face will permit one to sample the contralateral lateral ventricle. Puncturing the midline skin of the posterior neck will allow the prosector to reach the cisterna magna. These spaces can also be sampled after the calvarial bones have been reflected, but care must be taken to avoid contamination. A straightforward approach is to perform a lumbar puncture, either through dorsal skin, or after evisceration, through one of the intervertebral discs, generally L3 or L4. The latter method is perhaps the easiest, as the

TABLE 16.2 CROWN–RUMP LENGTH AND DEVELOPMENTAL AGE IN PREVIABLE FETUSES

Crown–rump length (mm)	Days after ovulation		Crown–rump length (mm)	Days after ovulation	
30–31	56		98–99	92	
32–34	57		100–101	93	
35–36	58		102–103	94	
37	59	9th week	101	95	14th week
38–39	60		105–106	96	
40–41	61		107–108	97	
42	62		109–110	98	
43–44	63				
45–46	64		111–112	99	
47–48	65		113–114	100	
49	66		115–116	101	
50–51	67	10th week	117–118	102	15th week
52–53	68		119–120	103	
54	69		121–122	104	
55–56	70		123–124	105	
57–58	71		125–126	106	
59–60	72		127–128	107	
61–62	73		129	108	
63–64	74	11th week	130–131	109	16th week
65	75		132–134	110	
66–67	76		135–136	111	
68–69	77		137–138	112	
70–71	78		139	113	
72–73	79		140–141	114	
74	80		142–143	115	
75	81	12th week	144–145	116	17th week
76–78	82		146–147	117	
79–80	83		148–149	118	
81	84		150	119	
82	85		151–152	120	
83–86	86		153	121	
87–89	87		154–155	122	
90–91	88	13th week	156–157	123	18th week
92–93	89		158	124	
94	90		159–160	125	
95–97	91		161–162	126	
			163–164	127	19th week
			165	128	

After McBride et al 1984 and Kalousek et al 1990,[68, 103] with permission.

disc is readily accessible. In any of these instances, overlying skin or disc material must be sterilized prior to obtaining fluid.

Viral cultures

If viral infection is suspected, a small sample of tissue, e.g. lung or spleen, is obtained as soon as the body cavity is opened. If the organ to be cultured has not been contaminated, sterile instruments (a suture removal kit works well) may be used to excise

tissue, which is then placed into sterile transport media. If the surface of the organ in question has been contaminated, it may be effectively sterilized by searing.

Toxicology

Toxicology studies are not routine in perinatal autopsies. When indicated however, blood, urine, stomach contents, bile, and liver may be submitted to the appropriate toxicology laboratory.

TABLE 16.3 TIME OF FIRST APPEARANCE OF CENTERS OF OSSIFICATION

Head	Week	Vertebrae	Week
Mandible	7	Arches	
Occipital bone (squamous portion)	8	All cervical and upper 1st or 2nd dorsal	9
Occipital bone (lateral and basilar portion)	9–10	All dorsal and 1st or 2nd lumbar	10
Superior maxilla	8	Lower lumbar	11
Temporal bone (petrous portion, mastoid and zygoma)	9	Upper sacral	12
Sphenoid (inner lamella of pterygoid process)	9	4th sacral	19–25
Sphenoid (great wings)	10	Bodies	
Sphenoid (lesser wings)	13	From 2nd dorsal to last lumbar	10
Sphenoid (anterior body)	13–14	From lower cervical to upper sacral	11
Nasal bone	10	From upper cervical to lower sacral	12
Frontal bone	9–10	5th sacral	13–28
Bony labyrinth	17–20	1st coccygeal	37–40
Milk teeth (rudiments)	17–28	Structural arrangement	13–16
Hyoid bone (greater cornua)	28–32	Odontoid process of axis	17–20
Body		Costal process	
Clavicle (diaphysis)	7	6th and 7th cervical	21–32
Scapula	8–9	5th cervical	32–36
Ribs		4th, 3rd, 2nd cervical	37–40
5th, 6th, 7th	8–9	Transverse process	
2nd, 3rd, 4th, 8th, 9th, 10th, 11th	9	Cervical and dorsal	21–24
1st	10	Lumbar	25–28
12th (very irregular)	10	**Pelvic girdle**	
Sternum	21–23	Ilium	9
Upper extremity	21–24	Ischium (descending ramus)	16–17
Humerus (diaphysis)	8	Os pubis (horizontal ramus)	21–28
Radius (diaphysis)	8	**Lower extremity**	
Ulna (diaphysis)	8	Femur (diaphysis)	8–9
Phalanges		Femur (distal epiphysis)	35–40
Terminal	9	Tibia (diaphysis)	8–9
Basal 3rd and 2nd	9	Tibia (proximal epiphysis)	40
Basal 4th and 1st	10	Fibula	9
Basal 5th	11–12	Os calcis	21–29
Middle 3rd, 4th, 2nd	12	Astragalus	24–32
Middle 5th	13–16	Cuboid	40
Metacarpals		**Metatarsals**	
2nd and 3rd	9	2nd and 3rd	9
4th, 5th, 1st	10–12	4th, 5th, 1st	10–12
		Phalanges	
		Terminal 1st	9
		Terminal 2nd, 3rd, 4th	10–12
		Terminal 5th	13–14
		Basal 1st, 2nd, 3rd, 4th, 5th	13–14
		Middle 2nd	20–25
		Middle 3rd	21–26
		Middle 4th	29–32
		Middle 5th	33–36

From Potter and Craig 1975,[104] with permission.

TABLE 16.4 CALCULATED VALUES OF LENGTH OF THE EXTREMITIES AT THE CLOSE OF EACH FETAL MONTH, IN MILLIMETERS

Portion of extremity measured	3 Months	4 Months	5 Months	6 Months	7 Months	8 Months	9 Months	10 Months
Length of lower extremity	23.4	59.8	91.0	118.6	143.7	166.8	188.5	208.9
Thigh length (trochanter to knee)	11.5	27.5	41.3	53.5	64.6	74.8	84.4	93.4
Leg length (knee to lateral malleolus)	9.7	26.6	41.1	53.9	65.6	76.4	86.4	95.9
Foot length	4.8	18.4	30.0	40.2	49.6	58.2	66.3	73.8
Length of upper extremity	24.3	58.2	87.2	112.8	136.2	157.7	177.9	196.8
Arm length (acromium to elbow)	10.2	23.6	34.8	44.8	53.8	62.2	70.0	77.3
Forearm length	7.7	18.7	28.1	36.5	44.1	51.1	57.6	63.8
Hand length	3.5	15.6	24.3	32.0	39.1	45.5	51.6	57.2

From Scammon and Calkins 1929,[24] with permission.

TABLE 16.5 CALCULATED VALUES OF EXTERNAL DIMENSIONS OF THE HEAD AT THE CLOSE OF EACH FETAL MONTH, IN MILLIMETERS

Dimensions of head	3 Months	4 Months	5 Months	6 Months	7 Months	8 Months	9 Months	10 Months
Occipitofrontal circumference	60.8	117.9	166.8	210.1	249.6	285.9	319.9	351.9
Occipitofrontal diameter	20.6	40.5	57.6	72.6	86.4	99.0	110.9	122.0
Suboccipitobregmatic circumference	60.3	113.1	158.4	198.5	235.1	268.7	300.2	329.8
Suboccipitobregmatic diameter	20.2	37.1	51.6	64.4	76.1	86.9	96.9	106.4
Suboccipitofrontal circumference	61.0	116.0	163.1	204.8	242.8	277.8	310.6	341.3
Suboccipitofrontal diameter	22.2	40.4	56.0	69.8	82.4	93.9	104.8	114.9
Occipitomental circumference	53.6	106.9	152.6	193.0	229.8	263.7	295.5	325.3
Occipitomental diameter	18.6	38.5	55.6	70.6	84.4	97.0	108.9	120.0
Biparietal diameter	15.5	31.5	45.3	57.5	68.6	78.8	88.4	97.4

From Scammon and Calkins 1929,[24] with permission.

TABLE 16.6 ORGAN WEIGHT IN RELATION TO TOTAL BODY WEIGHT

Organ	Total body weight (g)								
	500–999	1000–1499	1500–1999	2000–2499	2500–2999	3000–3499	3500–3999	4000–4499	≥ 4500
Thyroid	0.8	0.8	0.9	1.1	1.3	1.6	1.7	1.9	2.4
Thymus	2.1	4.3	6.6	8.2	9.3	11.0	12.6	14.3	17.3
Both lungs	18.2	27.1	37.9	43.6	48.9	54.9	58.0	65.8	74.0
Heart	5.8	9.4	12.7	15.5	19.0	21.2	23.4	28.0	36.0
Spleen	1.7	3.4	4.9	7.0	9.1	10.4	12.0	13.6	16.7
Pancreas	1.0	1.4	2.0	2.3	3.0	3.5	4.0	4.6	6.2
Both kidneys	7.1	12.2	16.2	19.9	23.0	25.3	28.5	31.0	33.2
Both adrenals	3.1	3.9	5.0	6.3	8.2	9.8	10.7	12.5	15.1
Brain	108.7	179.5	255.6	307.6	358.7	403.3	420.6	424.1	406.2
Liver	38.8	59.8	76.3	98.1	127.4	155.1	178.1	215.2	275.6

From Gilbert-Barness and Debich-Spicer 2004,[14] with permission.

Workers are advised to contact appropriate specialists prior to obtaining and remitting specimens.

Chromosome analysis

Conditions that warrant **cytogenetics** include congenital malformation, including ambiguous genitalia or dysgenetic gonads; any tiny or macerated fetus with a suspicious finding; nuchal hygroma or significant thickening (> 3 mm); congenital neoplasm, e.g. leukemia or teratoma; recurrent pregnancy loss; and fetus with anomaly suggested by prior ultrasound examination or other study in which an autopsy will not be performed. In other instances, for example stillbirth without pertinent history or abnormal findings, they are probably *not* indicated. This is especially true when a

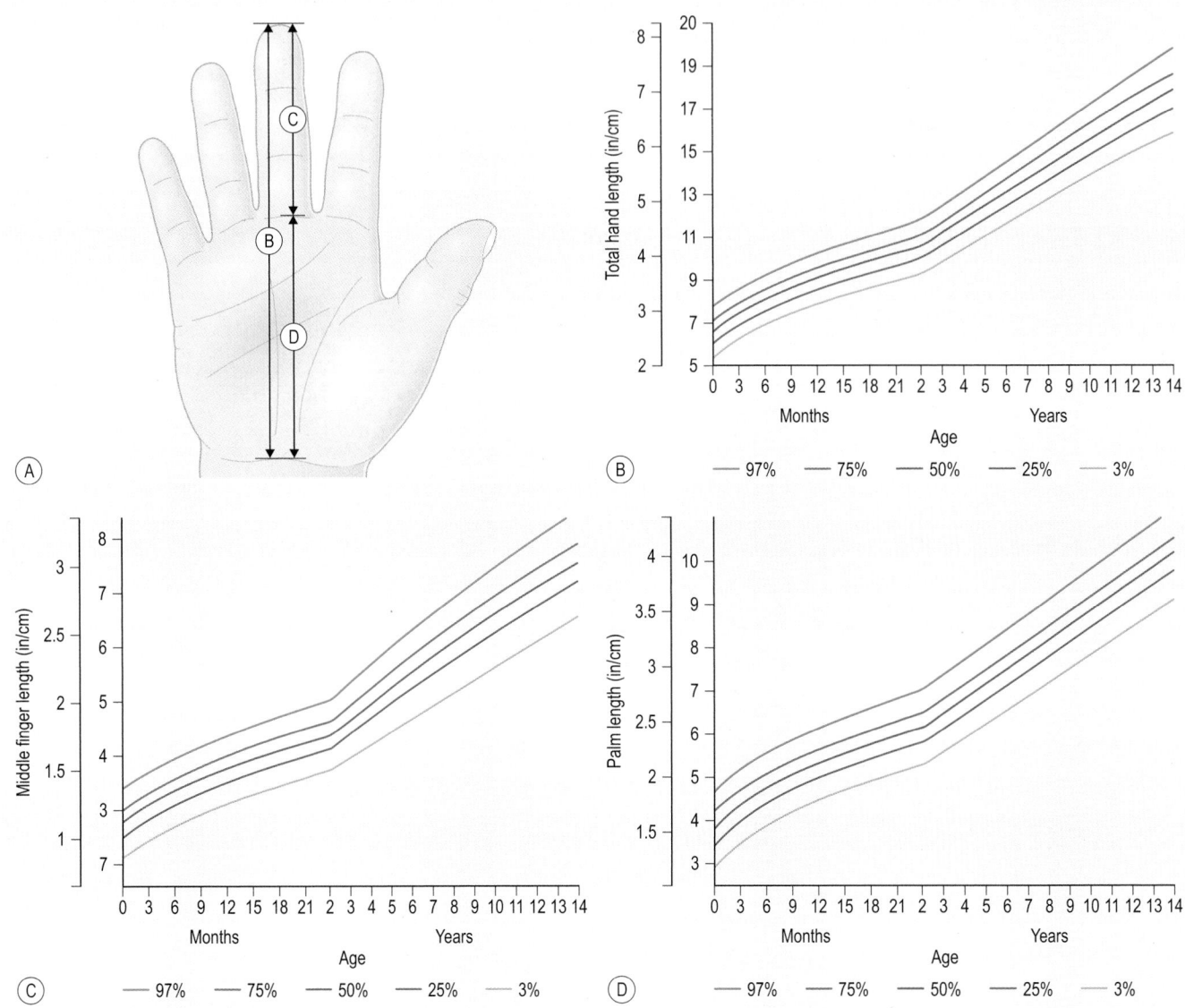

FIGURE 16.6 Hand measurements. (From Feingold and Bossert 1974,[105] with permission.)

thorough autopsy reveals some other explanation for the death, such as perinatal asphyxia, birth trauma, or maternal disease. Tissue for culture should be taken using a sterile procedure, cleaning the skin with either sterile saline or Ringer's lactate. Acetone or alcohol should be avoided, as both destroy cells. Skin, fascia, lung, chorionic villi from the placenta, and cartilage are the best sources for culture. This method may also be used for fibroblast cultures for metabolic and enzyme studies, as well as for electron microscopy. Care must be taken to obtain fetal tissue (from just beneath the chorion), although the possibility of maternal contamination still exists and cannot be excluded if the autopsied patient is female.

Metabolic studies

Fibroblast cultures prepared from autopsy material may be used for metabolic studies. In addition, tissue frozen at −70° C and tissue fixed in glutaraldehyde is usually required. The tissues employed include liver, brain, and occasionally kidney (see Ch. 19).

Specialized procedures

Upon occasion, the perinatal autopsy requires specialized anatomic studies. Each carries its own special demands and requires a

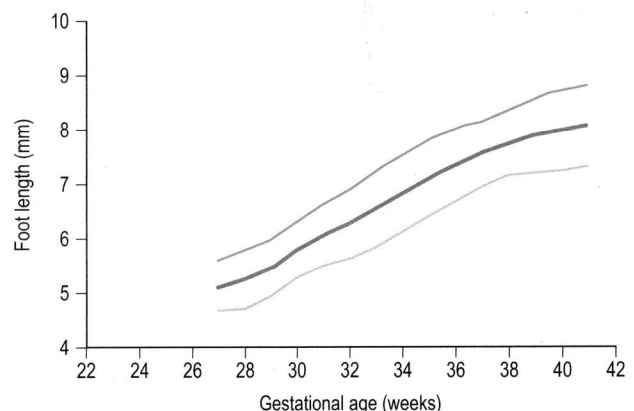

FIGURE 16.7 Foot length by gestational age. (From Merlob et al 1984,[106] with permission.)

TABLE 16.7 HAND AND FOOT LENGTHS CORRELATED WITH DEVELOPMENTAL AGE IN PREVIABLE FETUSES

Developmental age (weeks)	Hand length (mm)	Foot length (mm)
11	10	12
	±2	±2
12	15	17
	±2	±3
13	18	19
	±1	±1
14	19	22
	±1	±2
15	20	25
	±3	±3
16	26	28
	±2	±2
17	27	29
	±3	±4
18	29	33
	±2	±2

After McBride et al 1984 and Kalousek et al 1990,[68, 103] with permission.

certain skill on the part of the prosector. It is suggested, therefore, that workers develop these skills *before* it is necessary to employ them under demanding circumstances.

Postmortem perfusion of tissues or organs

Inflation of the lungs

Inflating one or both lungs with formalin is a popular autopsy technique and has been described by others.[80] The procedure has the advantage of returning the lung to a physiologic state, in which the state of antemortem inflation can be perceived. However, inflation also carries some disadvantages. The inflation should ideally occur at physiologic pressures, which may be difficult to

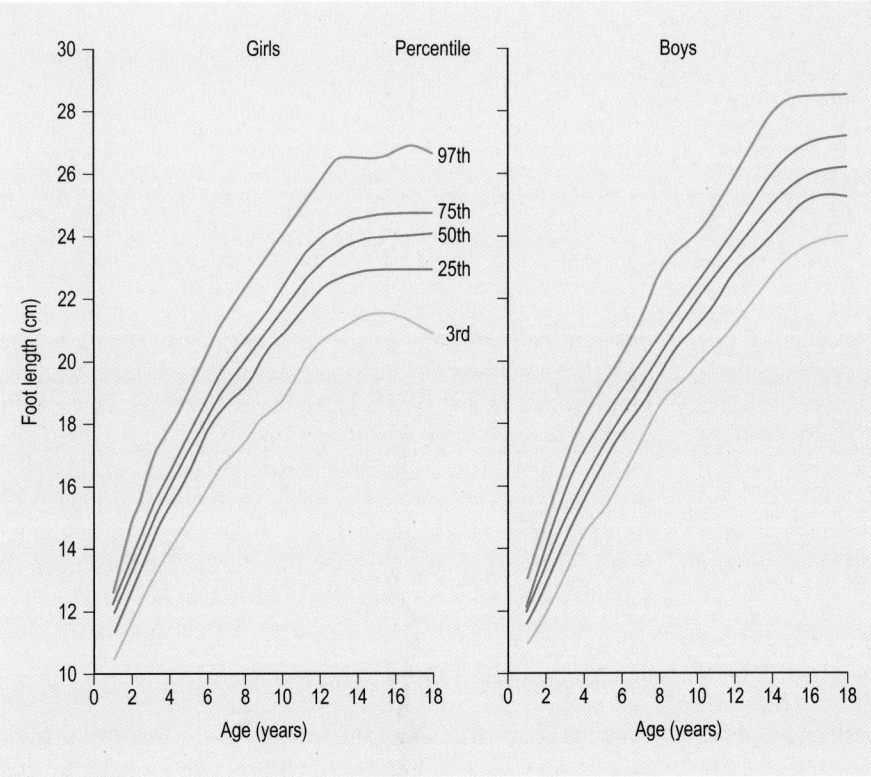

FIGURE 16.8 Mean and percentile values for foot length. (After Blais et al 1956,[107] with permission.)

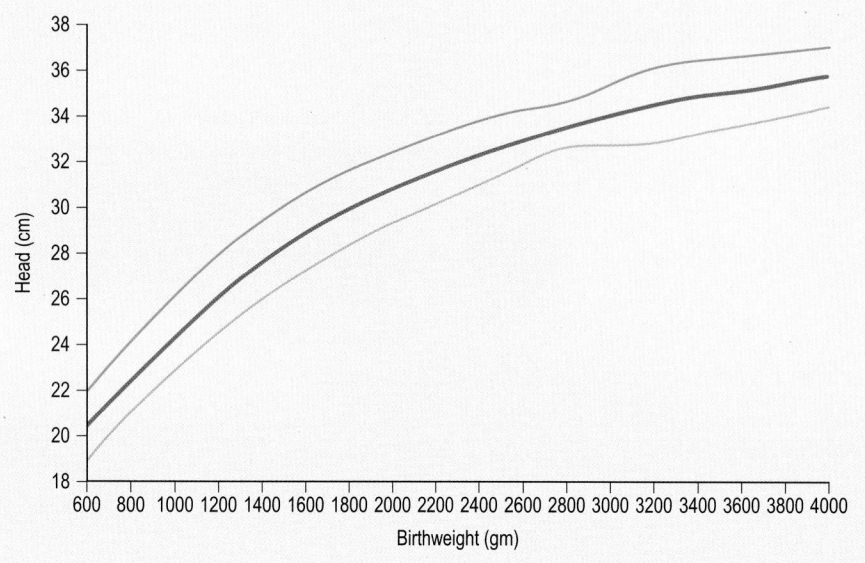

FIGURE 16.9 Head circumference by birth weight (3rd and 97th percentiles). (From Usher and McLean 1969,[108] with permission.)

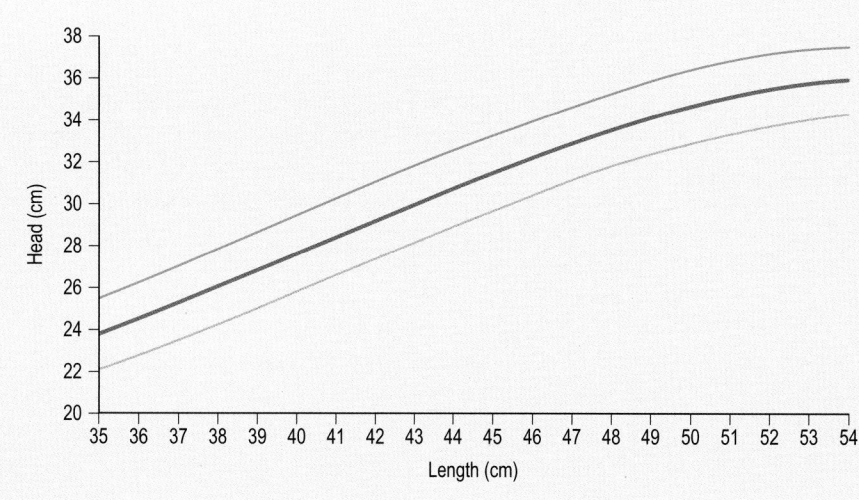

FIGURE 16.10 Head circumference by birth length (3rd and 97th percentiles). (From Usher and McLean 1969,[108] with permission.)

estimate and/or requires a special apparatus to attain. If the perfusion is incomplete, tissue fixation will be incomplete as well. If formalin is injected through the airway, material from the upper airway may be washed into the distal airway artifactually. One solution from this quandary is to perfuse one lung and section one lung.

In perinatal cases, and particularly fetuses in which no lung inflation has ever occurred, slicing the lungs seems like a more efficient use of the prosector's time.

Perfusion-fixation of the heart

From time to time, or especially for research or teaching purposes, it may be desirable to inflate the heart with formalin and fix it in a position that approximates the antemortem configuration. The most facile method for this is to maintain connections with the lungs (which are not sliced), ligate all vessels except the superior or inferior vena cava, and then to perfuse a large amount of formalin through the cardiopulmonary circuit. A small electric pump can be used, or the process can be done manually by syringe. Vessels may be flushed with saline prior to the introduction of formalin. Some advocate using an aqueous solution of sodium citrate, which is purported to dissolve clots.

In situ perfusion and fixation of the brain

If one is concerned about the fragility of the brain in a given case, it is possible to **perfuse the brain** with formalin in situ.

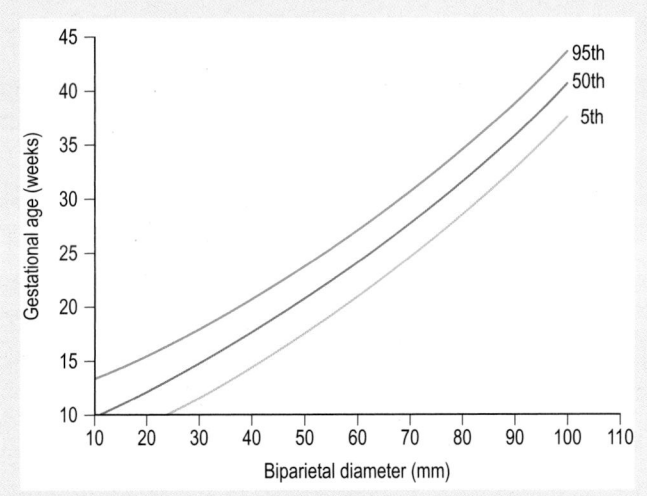

FIGURE 16.11 Relationship between gestational age and biparietal diameter. (From Gilbert-Barness and Debich-Spicer 2004,[14] with permission.)

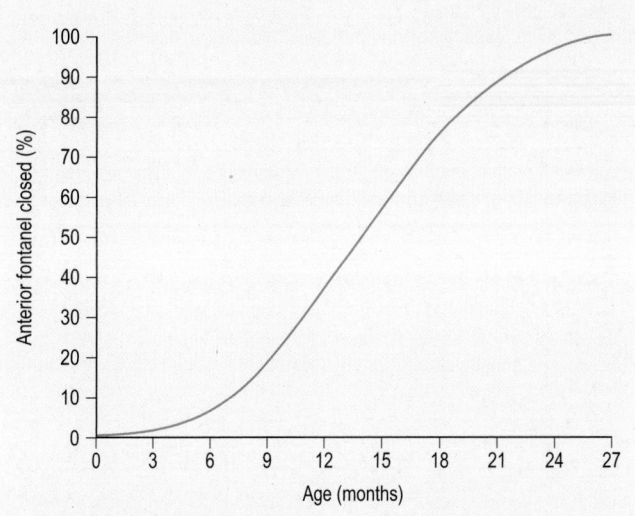

FIGURE 16.12 Percentage of anterior fontanel closed by age (0–24 months). (From Duc and Largo 1986,[109] with permission.)

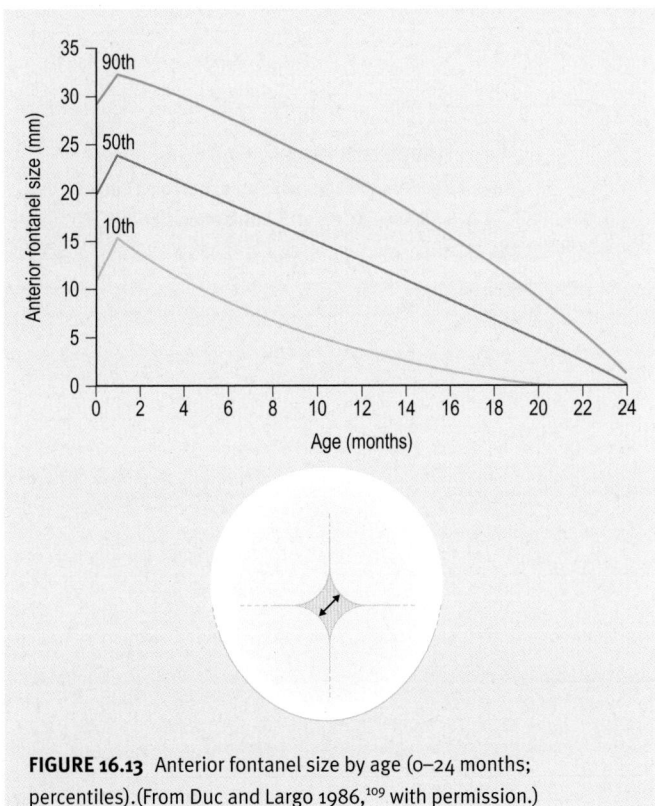

FIGURE 16.13 Anterior fontanel size by age (0–24 months; percentiles).(From Duc and Largo 1986,[109] with permission.)

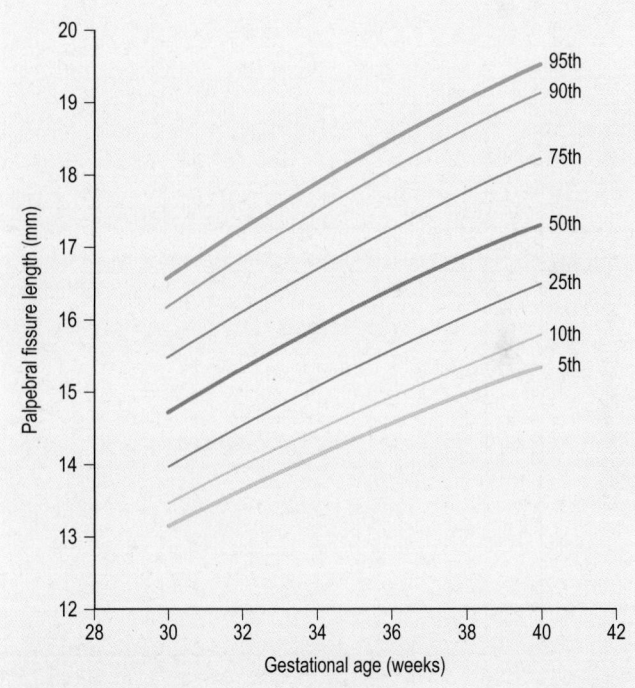

FIGURE 16.14 Palpebral fissure length by menstrual age (percentiles). (From Thomas et al 1987,[110] with permission.)

Fluid may be injected through the common carotid arteries, using a drip bottle or syringe. Using this approach, both the internal and external carotid arteries will be perfused, and both brain and face fixed in the process. Formalin fixation of the face is probably not a concern in perinatal cases, though the advice and consent of a funeral director should be sought

before proceeding thusly in older infants. The internal carotid artery can be cannulated independent of the external carotid, but it is a more difficult process, especially in the young fetus. If an IV-style drip apparatus is employed, it can be run for 30–60 min; if a syringe is used, one can gently perfuse 50–75cc bilaterally.

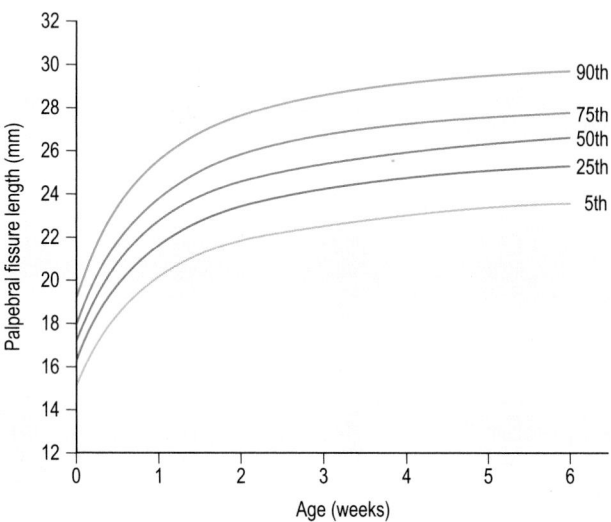

FIGURE 16.15 Palpebral fissure length by age (0–6 years; percentiles). (From Thomas et al 1987,[110] with permission.)

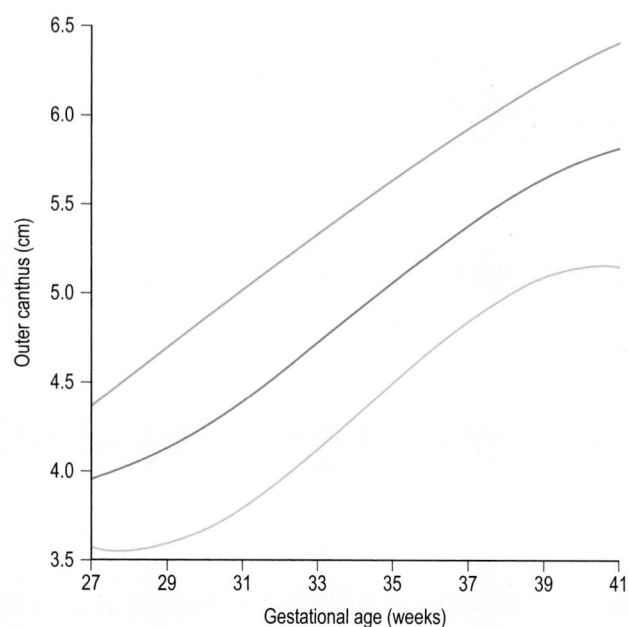

FIGURE 16.16 Outer canthal measurement by gestational age (percentiles). (From Merlob et al 1984,[106] with permission.)

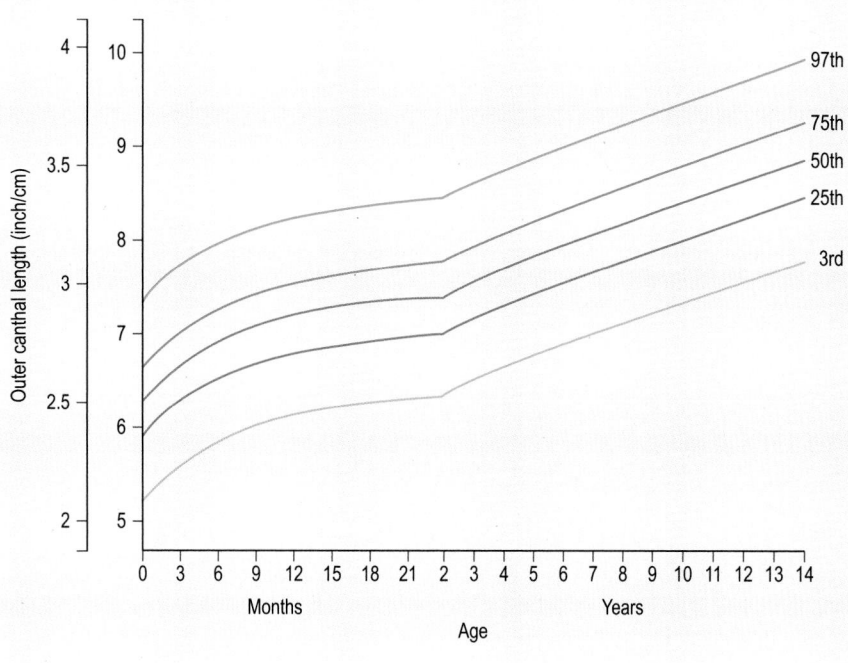

FIGURE 16.17 Outer canthal measurement by age (0–14 years; percentiles). (From Feingold and Bossert 1974,[111] with permission.)

It is also possible to perform a **ventricular tap** and infuse formalin directly into the lateral ventricles. A medium-gauge needle is placed in the lateral corner of the anterior fontanelle and directed toward the inner canthus of the contralateral eye. Fluid is then injected gently.

With any of these techniques, the prosector might then wait 30–60 min before removing the brain. A better approach is to infuse and then refrigerate the body overnight, removing the brain the following day. Fixation tends to be variable and will probably not be reliable in the severely autolytic brain.

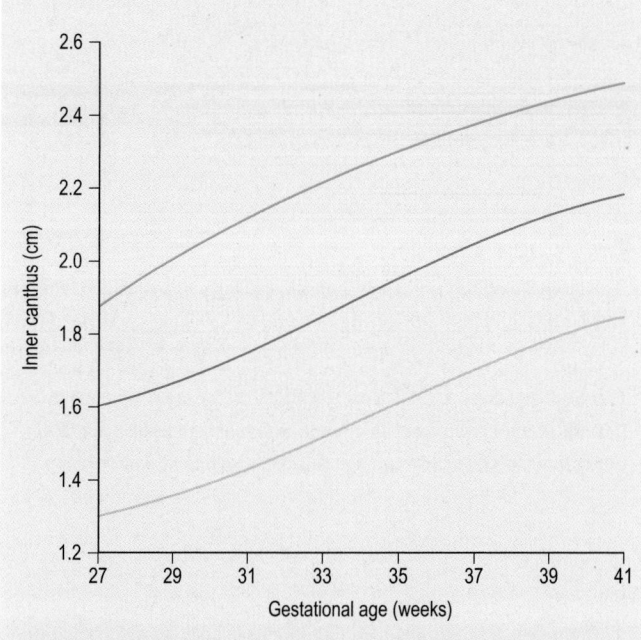

FIGURE 16.18 Inner canthal measurement by gestational age (3rd and 97th percentiles). (From Merlob et al 1984,[106] with permission.)

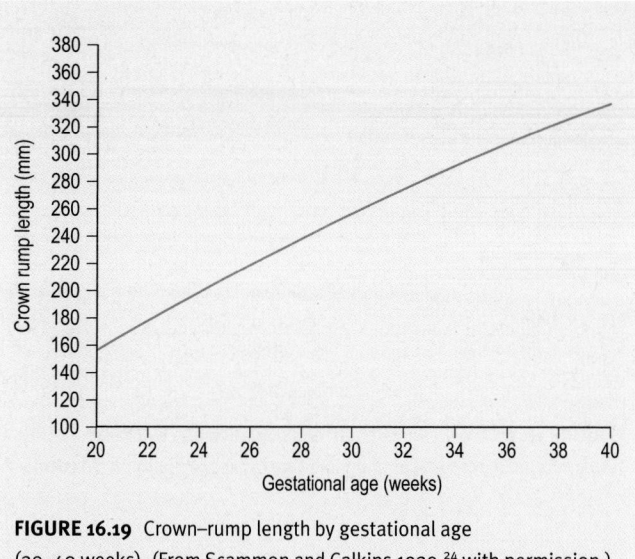

FIGURE 16.19 Crown–rump length by gestational age (20–40 weeks). (From Scammon and Calkins 1929,[24] with permission.)

Other injection studies

The course, configuration, or integrity of a vessel or other hollow structure can be studied by injection of radiopaque and/or colored dye. Such substances can be mixed with gelatin or other hardening material to give the injection a degree of permanence. A number of methods have been published.[81–83] One entails heating 500 mL distilled water, 650 g barium sulfate, 15 g gelatin, and 3 g thymol (a preservative) to 45° C and stirring to achieve a smooth consistency. The material may be stored for up to 1 year, and may be colored if desired. Dyes are also available clinically or commercially.

The consistency of the **dye** must be considered, as some materials may be too fluid or too viscous for their intended use. Injections should be done conservatively, so that only desired structures are perfused and imaged. A series of injections of increasing volume is made, and each injection followed by radiography, in an effort to achieve optimal visualization. Care is also taken to avoid spilling material into the work field.

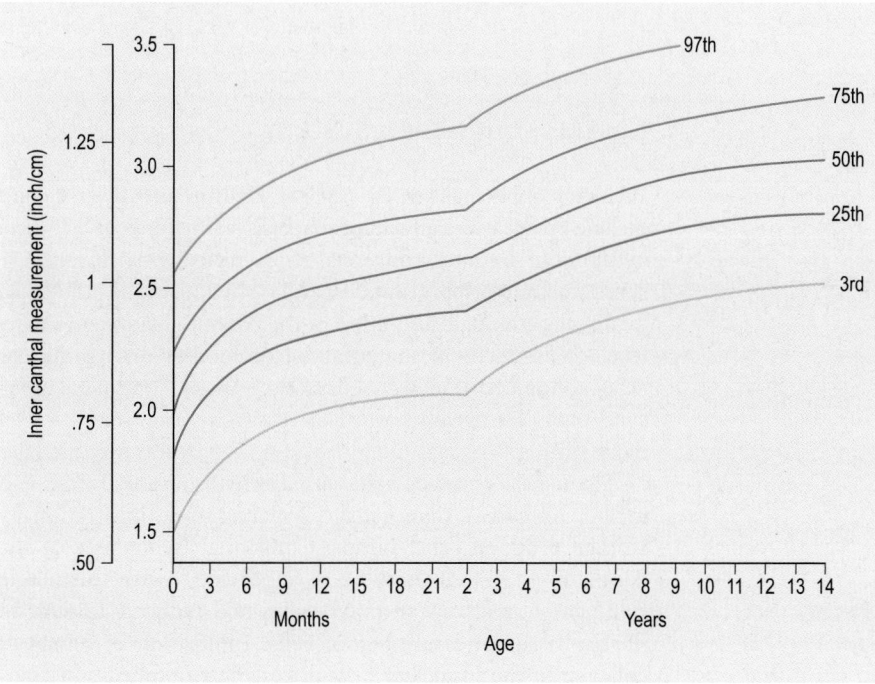

FIGURE 16.20 Inner canthal measurement by age (0–14 years; percentiles). (From Feingold and Bossert 1974,[111] with permission.)

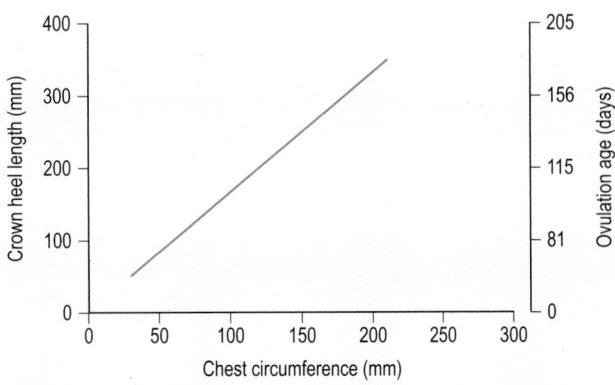

FIGURE 16.21 Crown–heel length and ovulation age by chest circumference. (From Scammon and Calkins 1929,[24] with permission.)

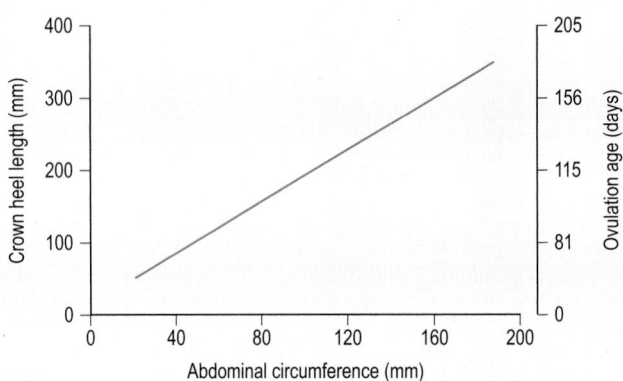

FIGURE 16.22 Crown–heel length and ovulation age by abdominal circumference. (From Scammon and Calkins 1929,[24] with permission.)

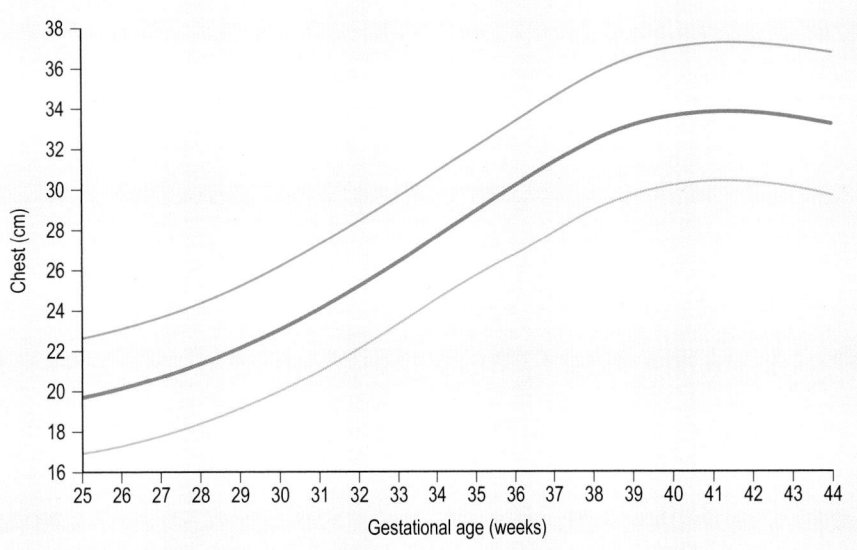

FIGURE 16.23 Chest circumference by gestational age (3rd and 97th percentiles). (From Usher and McLean 1969,[108] with permission.)

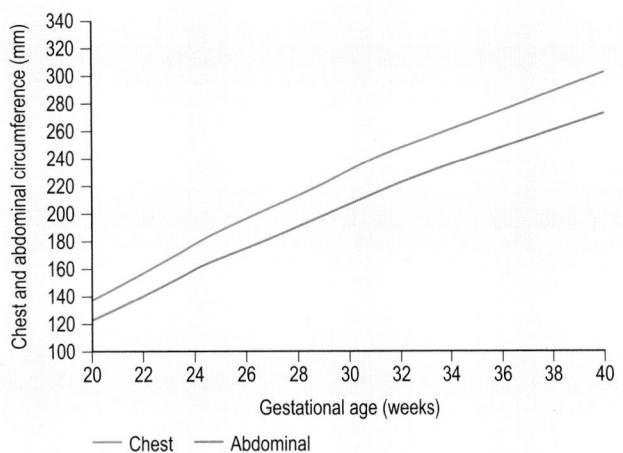

FIGURE 16.24 Chest and abdominal circumferences by gestational age. (From Scammon and Calkins 1929,[24] with permission.)

Cardiac conduction system

Perinatal abnormalities in **cardiac rhythm** are diverse, and include bradycardia or tachycardia, bradyarrhythmia or tachyarrhythmia, atrial flutter, congenital atrioventricular block, long QT syndrome, and ectopic beats.[84] Cardiac rhythm can be influenced by direct pathologic alteration of the conduction system at any level, or indirectly by maternal autoantibodies, arrhythmia, or other condition, or maternal drug exposure.[85–89] Perinatal lupus syndromes are a well known, if relatively rare, cause of fetal dysrhythmia.[90]

Tissue changes associated with dysrhythmia are diverse, and include apoptosis, hemorrhage, inflammation, infiltration by storage products, and tumor. Congenital hypoplasia of the conducting system has been reported,[91] with histologic findings of small SA and AV nodes and reduced amount of fibrous tissue and number of cells. Infiltration of bands of collagen or mononuclear cells or calcification occurs in asso-

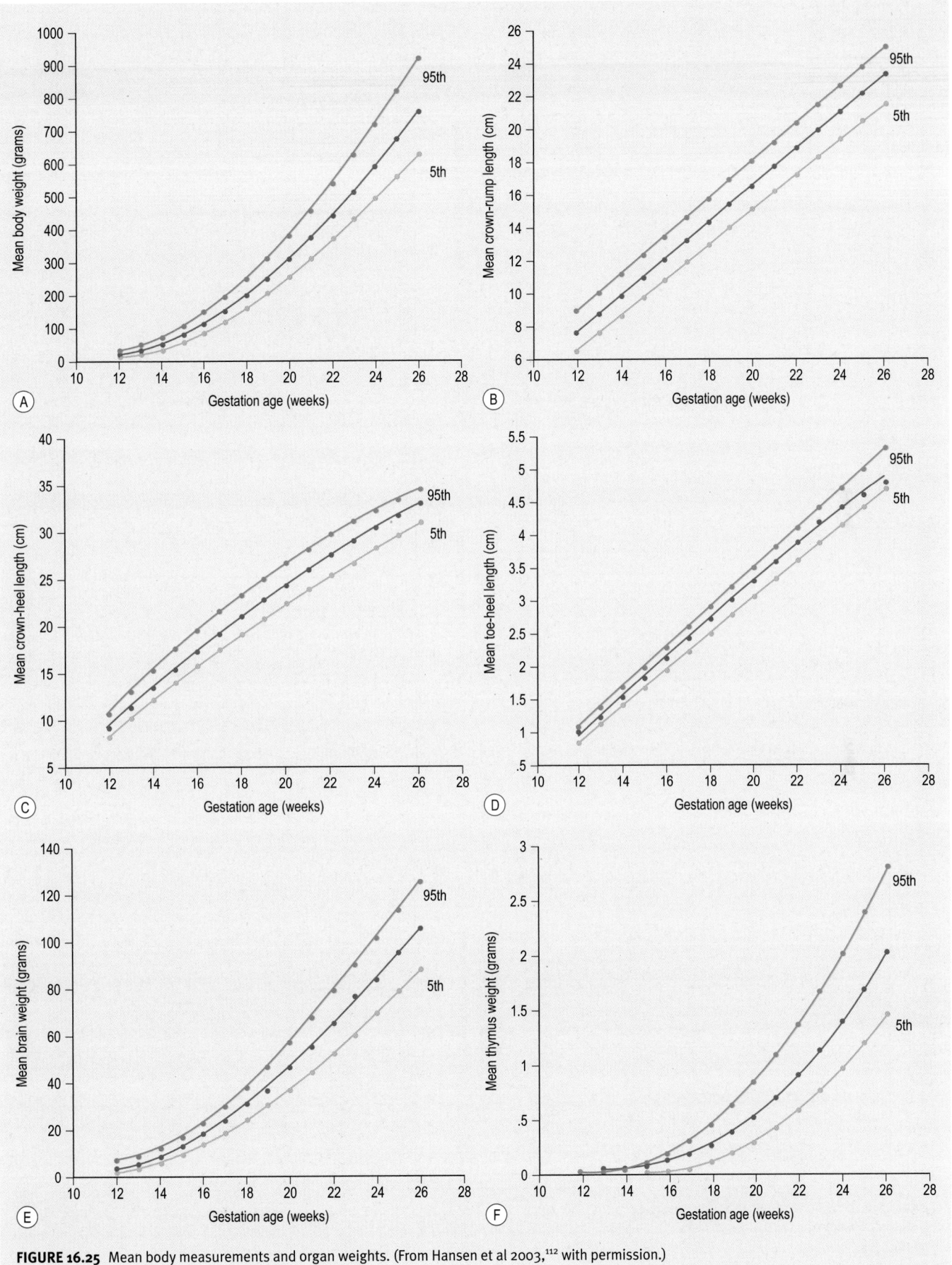

FIGURE 16.25 Mean body measurements and organ weights. (From Hansen et al 2003,[112] with permission.)

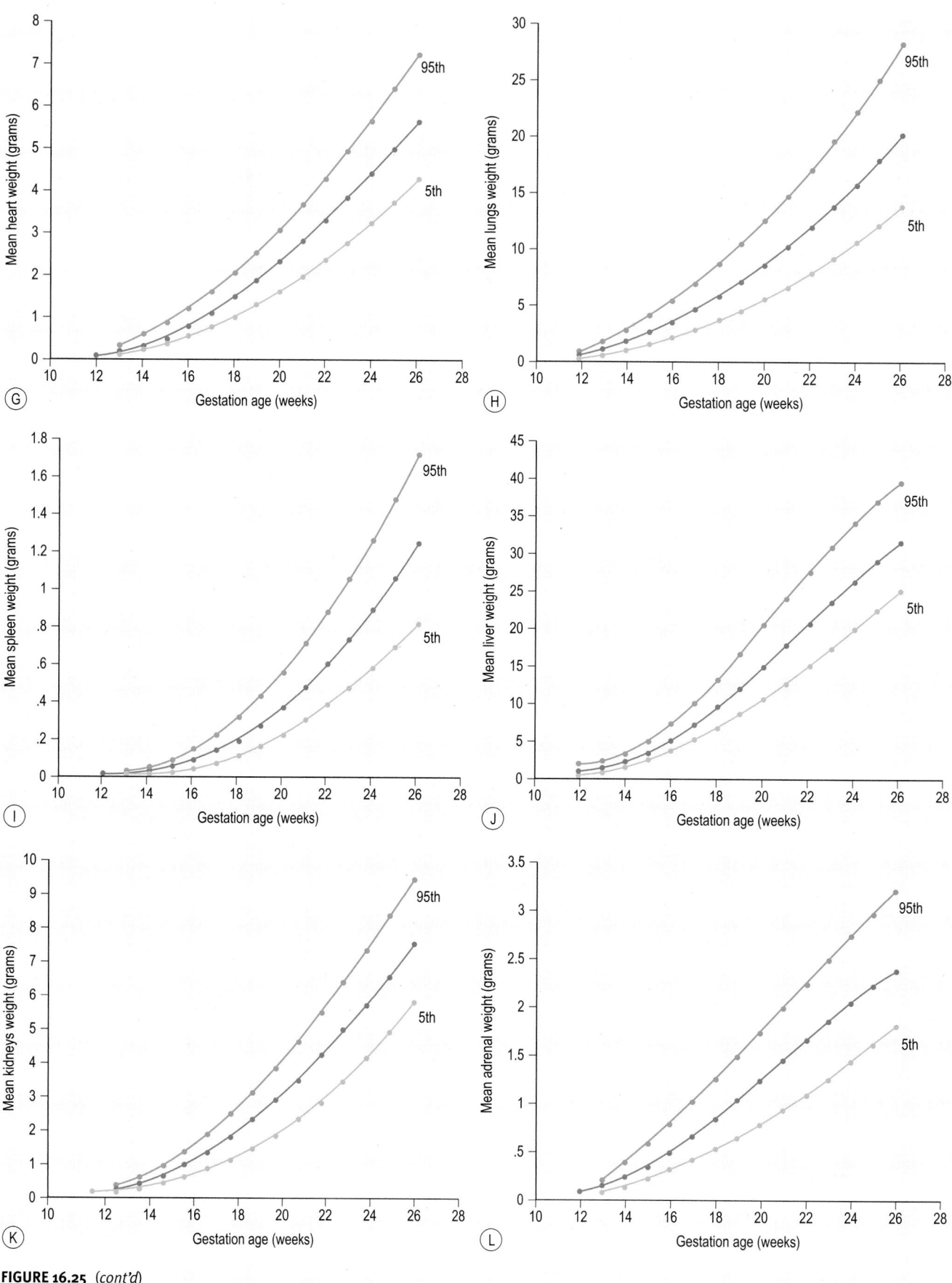

FIGURE 16.25 (cont'd)

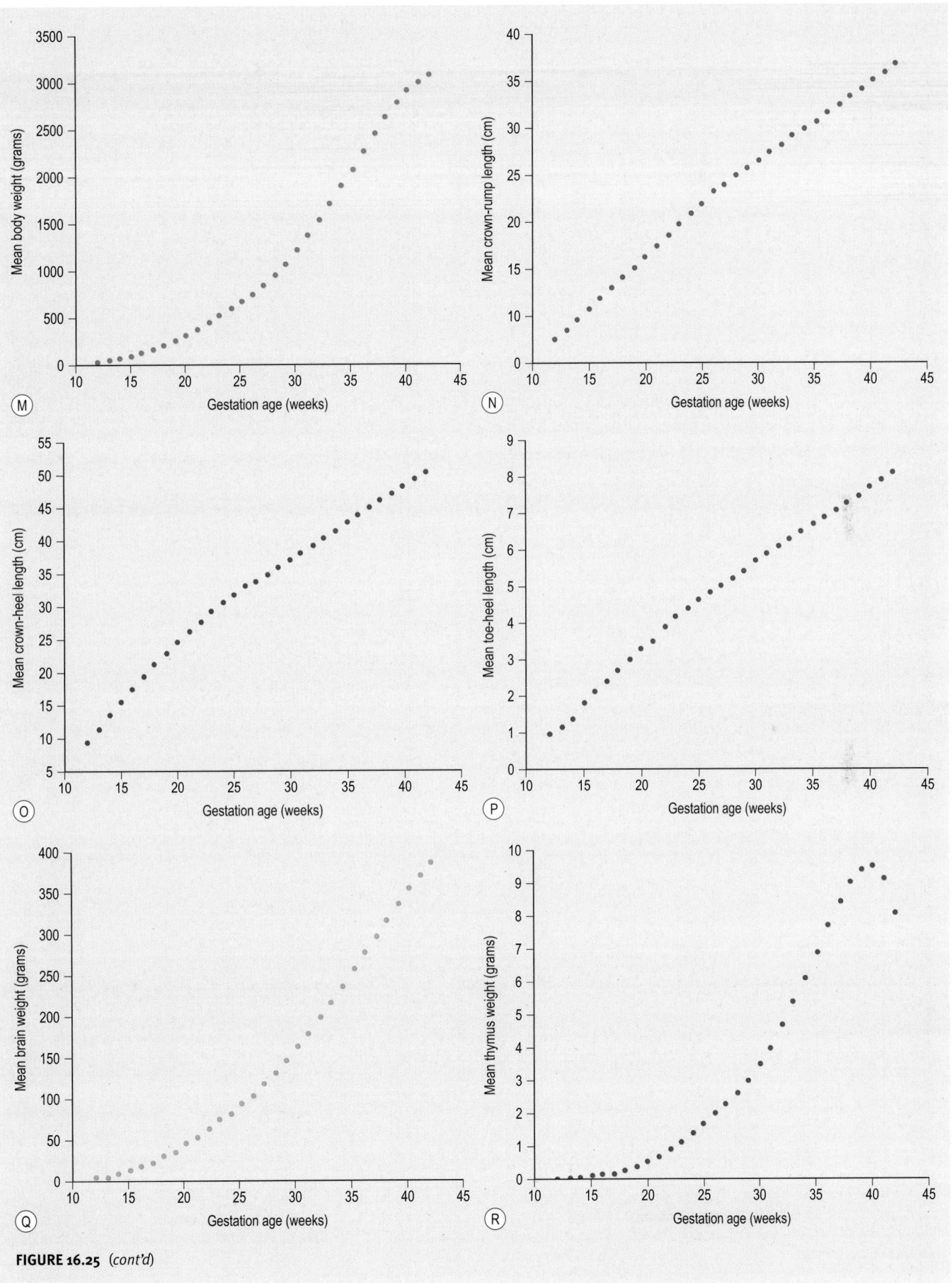

FIGURE 16.25 (cont'd)

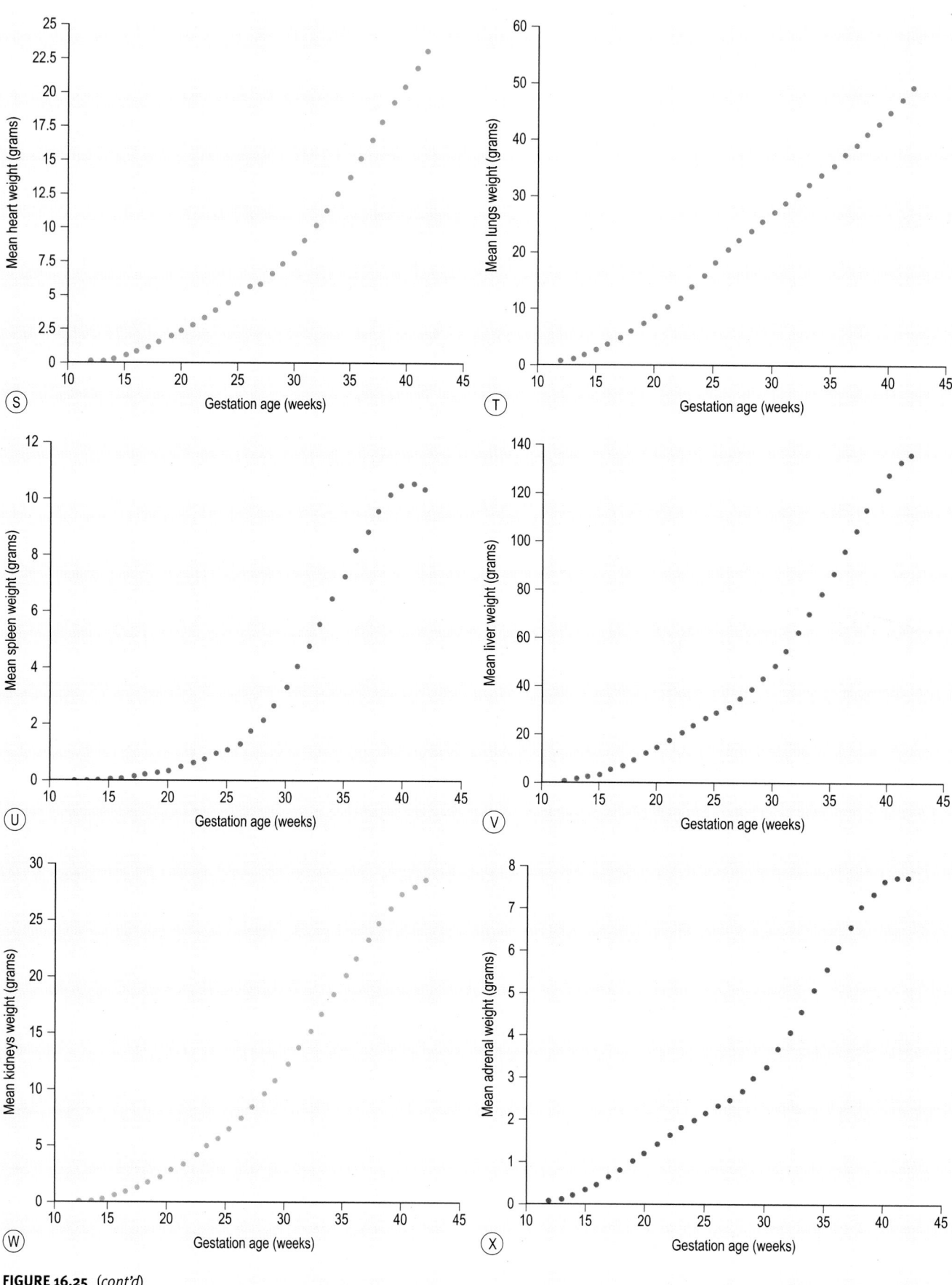

FIGURE 16.25 (*cont'd*)

TABLE 16.8 MEASUREMENTS AND ORGAN WEIGHTS IN CHILDREN

Age	Body length (cm)	Brain (g)	Heart (g)	Right lung (g)	Left lung (g)	Spleen (g)	Liver (g)	Right kidney (g)	Left kidney (g)	Combined adrenals (g)	Thymus (g)	Pancreas (g)
Birth– 3d	49	335	17	21	18	8	78	13	14	–	–	–
3–7 d	49	358	18	24	22	9	96	14	14	–	–	–
1–3 weeks	52	382	19	29	26	10	123	15	15	–	–	–
3–5 weeks	52	413	20	31	27	12	127	16	16	4.9	5.5–8.5	5.7
5–7 weeks	53	422	21	32	28	13	133	19	18	–	–	–
7–9 weeks	55	489	23	32	29	13	136	19	18	4.9	5.0–10.0	7.2
2–3 months	56	516	23	35	30	14	140	20	19	4.9	10.0	8.0
4 months	59	540	27	37	33	16	160	22	21	4.8	9.5	10.0
5 months	61	644	29	38	35	16	188	25	25	5.0	12.5	11.0
6 months	62	660	31	42	39	17	200	26	25	4.9	10.0	11.0
7 months	65	691	34	49	41	19	227	30	30	5.5	11.0	11.0
8 months	65	714	37	52	45	20	254	31	30	5.4	9.0	12.0
9 months	67	750	37	53	47	20	260	31	30	5.4	9.5	15.0
10 months	69	809	39	54	51	22	274	32	31	5.7	20–38	13.5
11 months	70	852	40	59	53	25	277	34	33	6.1	20–38	15.0
12 months	73	925	44	64	57	26	288	36	35	6.2	20–38	14.5
14 months	74	944	45	66	60	26	304	36	35	–	20–38	–
16 months	77	1010	48	72	64	28	331	39	39	–	20–38	–
18 months	78	1042	52	72	65	30	345	40	43	–	20–38	–
20 months	79	1050	56	83	74	30	370	43	44	–	20–38	–
22 months	82	1059	56	80	75	33	380	44	44	–	20–38	–
24 months	84	1064	56	88	76	33	394	47	46	–	20–38	–
3 years	88	1141	59	89	77	37	418	48	49	–	25	–
4 years	99	1191	73	90	85	39	516	58	56	–	25	–
5 years	106	1237	85	107	104	47	596	65	64	–	25	–
6 years	109	1243	94	121	122	58	642	68	67	–	25	–
7 years	113	1263	100	130	123	66	680	69	70	–	25	–
8 years	119	1273	110	150	140	69	736	74	75	–	25	–
9 years	125	1275	115	174	152	73	756	82	83	–	25	–
10 years	130	1290	116	177	166	85	852	92	95	–	25	–
11 years	135	1320	122	201	190	87	909	94	95	–	25	–
12 years	139	1351	124	–	–	93	936	95	96	–	25	–

After Sunderman and Boerner 1969, Coppoletta and Wolbach 1933[119, 113] and Schulz et al 1969,[114] with permission.

ciation with maternal disease such as systemic lupus erythematosus. Immunoglobulin G (IgG) and IgA in the SA and AV nodes, endocardium, or myocardium of the fetal heart reflect an on-going immunologic process. In glycogen storage disease, large, vacuolated, glycogen-positive cells are seen in the conduction system, and can be of sufficient volume to cause grossly visible swelling in the upper reaches of the interventricular septum.[92] In structurally abnormal hearts, the position and course of the conducting system are variable. A basic, though not absolute, tenet is that SA nodal alterations may be encountered in hearts with atrial abnormalities, while AV nodal changes may be seen in aberrant ventricular morphology; septal defects displace adjacent elements of the conducting system.[93] Damage to the conducting system may also occur as a result of cardiac surgery.

Finding morphologic evidence to support arrhythmia as a cause of death may be challenging and requires knowledge of, and a systematic approach to, the **conduction system**. Because microscopic examination is generally extensive, the prosector may wish to photograph the external and internal features of the heart prior to obtaining sections. A number of references provide detailed information on the examination of the conduction system.[93–96]

Components of the system are small, but not infinitesimally so. The fetal AV node is, for example, approximately 8–9 mm long. The SA node is situated at the junction of SVC and right atrium. To examine this node, a tissue block needs to include the medial edge of the cava and lateral margin of the atrial wall; the width of this block should be at least 1 cm. To examine the blood supply of the SA node, the anterolateral walls of the right

TABLE 16.9 MEANS AND STANDARD DEVIATIONS OF WEIGHTS AND MEASUREMENTS OF LIVEBORN INFANTS

Gestation	Body weight (g)	Crown–rump (cm)	Crown–heel (cm)	Toe–heel (cm)	Brain (g)	Thymus (g)	Heart (g)	Lungs (g)	Spleen (g)	Liver (g)	Kidneys (g)	Adrenals (g)	Pancreas (g)
20	381	18.3	25.6	3.6	49	0.8	2.8	11.5	0.7	22.4	3.7	1.8	±0.5
	±104	±2.2	±2.2	±0.7	±15	±2.3	±1.0	±2.9	±0.3	±8.0	±1.3	±1.0	0.5
21	426	19.1	26.7	3.8	57	1	3.2	12.9	0.7	24.1	4.2	2	0.5
	±66	±1.2	±1.7	±0.1	±8	±0.3	±0.4	±2.8	±0.2	±4.2	±0.7	±0.5	
22	473	20	27.8	4	65	1.2	3.5	14.4	0.8	25.4	4.7	2	0.6
	±63	±1.3	1.6	±0.4	±13	±0.3	±0.6	±4.3	±0.4	±5.2	±1.5	±0.6	±0.3
23	524	20.8	28.9	4.2	74	1.4	3.9	15.9	0.8	26.6	5.3	2.1	0.7
	±116	±1.9	±3.0	±0.5	±11	±0.7	±1.3	±4.9	±0.4	±8.0	±1.8	±0.8	±0.4
24	584	21.6	30	4.4	8.3	1.5	4.2	17.4	0.9	28	6	2.2	0.8
	±92	±1.4	±1.7	±0.3	±15	±0.7	±1.0	±5.9	±0.5	±7.1	±1.8	±0.8	±0.5
25	655	22.5	31.1	4.6	94	1.8	4.7	19	1.1	29.7	6.8	2.2	0.9
	±106	±1.6	±2.0	±0.4	±25	±1.2	±1.2	±5.3	±1.6	±9.8	±1.9	±1.4	±0.3
26	739	23.3	32.2	4.8	105	2	5.2	20.6	1.3	32.1	7.6	2.4	1
	±181	±1.9	±2.4	±0.7	±21	±1.1	±1.3	±6.3	±0.7	±10.9	±2.5	±1.1	±0.5
27	836	24.2	33.4	5	118	2.3	5.8	22.1	1.7	35.1	8.6	2.5	1.2
	±197	±2.5	±3.5	±0.5	±21	±1.2	±1.9	±9.7	±1.0	±13.3	±3.0	±1.1	±0.5
28	949	25	34.5	5.2	132	2.6	6.5	23.7	2.1	38.9	9.7	2.7	1.4
	±190	±1.7	±2.3	±0.6	±29	±1.5	±1.9	±10.0	±0.8	±12.6	±12.0	±1.2	±0.5
29	1077	25.9	35.6	5.4	147	3	7.2	25.3	2.6	43.5	10.9	3	1.5
	±449	±2.8	±4.4	±0.8	±49	±1.9	±2.7	±12.6	±0.9	±15.8	±4.4	±1.2	±1.0
30	1219	26.7	36.7	5.7	163	3.5	8.1	26.9	3.3	49.1	12.3	3.3	1.7
	±431	±3.3	±4.2	±0.7	±38	±2.6	±2.6	±20.3	±2.0	±18.8	±8.5	±2.7	±1.0
31	1375	27.6	37.8	5.9	180	4	9	28.5	4	55.4	13.7	3.7	1.8
	±281	±3.8	±3.1	±0.7	±34	±3.4	±2.8	±13.2	±1.2	±17.3	±5.2	±1.3	±0.6
32	1543	28.4	38.9	6.1	198	4.7	10.1	30.2	4.7	62.5	15.2	4.1	2
	±519	±9.5	±5.7	±1.1	±48	±3.6	±4.4	±19.0	±5.4	±30.0	±7.4	±1.7	±0.8
33	1720	29.3	40	6.3	217	5.4	11.2	31.8	5.5	70.3	16.8	4.6	2.1
	±580	±3.3	±3.5	±0.7	±49	±3.2	±4.0	±13.5	±3.5	±25.4	±7.7	±1.5	±0.8
34	1905	30.1	41.1	6.5	237	6.1	12.4	33.5	6.4	78.7	18.5	5.1	2.3
	±625	±4.3	±4.0	±0.6	±53	±3.8	±2.8	±16.5	±3.0	±30.2	±9.3	±2.2	±1.1
35	2093	30.9	42.3	6.7	257	6.9	13.7	35.2	7.2	87.4	20.1	5.6	2.5
	±309	±2.0	±2.9	±0.4	±45	±4.5	±3.6	±20.5	±5.2	±30.6	±10.9	±2.8	±0.6
36	2280	31.8	43.4	6.9	278	7.7	15	36.9	8.1	96.3	21.7	6.1	2.6
	±615	±3.9	±5.9	±1.1	±96	±5.0	±5.1	±17.5	±3.1	±33.7	±6.8	±3.1	±0.7
37	2462	32.6	44.5	7.1	298	8.4	16.4	38.7	8.8	105.1	23.3	6.6	2.8
	±821	±5.0	±7.0	±1.2	±70	±5.6	±5.7	±22.9	±6.4	±33.7	±9.9	±3.3	±0.9
38	2634	33.5	45.6	7.3	318	9	17.7	40.6	9.5	113.5	24.8	7.1	3
	±534	±3.2	±5.1	±0.8	±106	±2.8	±5.4	±17.1	±3.5	±34.7	±7.2	±2.9	±1.1
39	2789	34.3	46.7	7.5	337	9.4	19.1	42.6	10.1	121.3	26.1	7.4	3.3
	±520	±1.9	±4.4	±0.5	±91	±2.5	±2.8	±14.9	±3.5	±39.2	±4.9	±2.5	±0.5
40	2922	35.2	47.8	7.7	356	9.5	20.4	44.6	10.4	127.9	27.3	7.7	3.6
	±450	±2.8	±4.2	±0.8	±79	±5.0	±5.6	±22.7	±3.3	±35.8	±11.5	±3.0	±1.3
41	3025	36	48.9	7.9	372	9.1	21.7	46.8	10.5	133.1	28.1	7.8	3.9
	±600	±3.1	±5.4	±0.8	±65	±4.8	±10.9	±26.2	±4.5	±55.7	±12.7	±2.8	±1.5
42	3091	36.9	50	8.1	387	8.1	22.9	49.1	10.3	136.4	28.7	7.8	4.3
	±617	±2.4	±3.8	±1.1	±61	±3.8	±6.2	±14.6	±3.6	±38.9	±9.7	±3.2	±1.9

Data from Women and Infant's Hospital, Providence, RI

TABLE 16.10 MEANS AND STANDARD DEVIATIONS OF WEIGHTS AND MEASUREMENTS OF STILLBORN INFANTS

Gestation	Body weight (g)	Crown–rump (cm)	Crown–heel (cm)	Toe–heel (cm)	Brain (g)	Thymus (g)	Heart (g)	Lungs (g)	Spleen (g)	Liver (g)	Kidneys (g)	Adrenals (g)	Pancreas (g)
20	313	18.0	24.9	3.3	41	0.4	2.4	7.1	0.3	17	2.7	1.3	0.5
	±139	±2.0	±2.3	±0.6	±24	±0.3	±1.0	±3.0	±1.0	±9	±2.9	±0.6	±0.1
21	353	18.9	26.2	3.5	48	0.5	2.6	7.9	0.4	18	3.1	1.4	0.5
	±125	±4.8	±3.6	±0.6	±18	±0.3	±0.9	±3.8	±0.6	±7	±1.3	±0.7	±0.4
22	398	19.8	27.4	3.8	55	0.6	2.8	8.7	0.5	19	3.5	1.4	0.6
	±117	±9.6	±2.5	±0.4	±15	±0.4	±0.9	±3.1	±0.4	±10	±0.8	±0.6	±0.5
23	450	20.6	28.7	4	64	0.8	3	9.5	0.7	21	4.1	1.5	0.7
	±118	±2.3	±3.3	±0.5	±18	±0.5	±1.4	±5.7	±0.5	±7	±1.7	±0.8	±0.3
24	510	21.5	29.9	4.2	74	0.9	3.3	10.5	0.9	22	4.6	1.5	0.7
	±179	±3.1	±4.3	±0.8	±25	±0.7	±1.8	±5.6	±0.7	±8	±2.4	±0.8	±0.3
25	581	22.3	31.1	4.4	85	1.1	3.7	11.6	1.2	24	5.3	1.6	0.8
	±178	±4.0	±6.5	±0.8	±31	±0.8	±1.3	±4.9	±0.4	±35	±2.4	±0.8	±0.7
26	663	23.2	32.4	4.7	98	1.4	4.2	12.9	1.5	26	6.1	1.7	0.8
	±227	4.1	±5.3	±0.9	±37	±1.4	±2.2	±8.7	±1.1	±16	±3.6	±0.9	±0.7
27	758	24.1	33.6	4.9	112	1.7	4.8	14.4	1.9	29	7	1.9	0.9
	±227	±2.9	±3.2	±1.4	±37	±1.1	±3.6	±9.7	±1.0	±24	±3.1	±1.5	±0.3
28	864	24.9	34.9	5.1	127	2	5.4	16.1	2.3	32	7.9	2.1	1
	±247	±2.2	±5.6	±1.2	±39	±2.1	±2.6	±7.0	±1.1	±32	±2.5	±1.6	±0.3
29	984	25.8	36.1	5.3	143	2.4	6.2	18	2.7	36	9	2.4	1.1
	±511	±4.1	±5.9	±1.2	±57	±2.6	±2.4	±13.6	±2.0	±23	±4.5	±1.2	±1.2
30	1115	26.6	37.3	5.6	160	2.8	7	20.1	3.1	40	10.1	2.7	1.2
	±329	±2.4	±3.6	±0.7	±72	±4.1	±2.8	±8.6	±1.5	±22	±6.0	±1.3	±0.2
31	1259	27.5	38.6	5.8	178	3.2	8	22.5	3.6	46	11.3	3	1.4
	±588	±3.0	±2.7	±0.7	±32	±1.9	±3.1	±10.1	±4.0	±38	±4.1	±1.8	±1.4
32	1413	28.4	39.8	6	196	3.7	9.1	25	4.2	52	12.6	3.5	1.6
	±623	±2.8	±5.4	±0.6	±92	±2.2	±4.1	±10.7	±2.4	±32	±8.0	±1.8	±0.6
33	1578	29.2	41.1	6.2	216	4.3	10.2	27.8	4.7	58	13.9	3.9	1.8
	±254	±3.5	±3.1	±0.4	±51	±1.5	±2.0	±5.8	±2.3	±17	±3.5	±1.4	±0.8
34	1750	30.1	42.3	6.5	236	4.8	11.4	30.7	5.3	66	15.3	4.4	2
	±494	±3.5	±4.3	±0.8	±42	±5.6	±3.2	±15.2	±2.5	±22	±5.1	±1.3	±0.5
35	1930	30.9	43.5	6.7	256	5.4	12.6	33.7	5.9	74	16.7	4.9	2.3
	±865	±3.9	±5.8	±0.9	±70	±3.4	±5.3	±14.3	±6.8	±46	±7.1	±1.9	±0.7
36	2114	31.8	44.8	6.9	277	6.1	13.9	36.7	6.5	82	18.1	5.4	2.6
	±616	±4.0	±7.2	±0.8	±94	±4.1	±5.8	±16.8	±2.9	±36	±6.3	±2.4	±2.6
37	2300	32.7	46	7.2	297	6.7	15.1	39.8	7.2	91	19.4	5.8	2.6
	±647	±5.1	±7.9	±0.9	±69	±3.9	±9.9	±11.1	±6.3	±57	±9.7	±6.2	±3.1
38	2485	33.5	47.3	7.4	317	7.4	16.4	42.9	7.8	100	20.8	6.3	3.2
	579	±2.6	±3.9	±0.8	±83	±6.1	±4.4	±15.7	±5.9	±44	±6.0	±2.1	±1.6
39	2667	34.4	48.5	7.6	337	8.1	17.5	45.8	8.5	109	22	6.7	3.5
	±596	±3.7	±4.9	±0.5	±132	±4.7	±3.9	±15.2	±4.5	±53	±5.8	±5.3	±1.9
40	2842	35.2	49.7	7.8	355	8.9	18.6	48.6	9.2	118	23.1	7	3.9
	±482	±6.4	±3.2	±0.7	±57	±4.3	±12.9	±19.4	±4.1	±49	±8.6	±2.9	±1.7
41	3006	36.1	51	8.1	373	9.6	19.5	51.1	9.9	126	24.1	7.1	4.2
	±761	±3.7	±5.4	±0.8	±141	±5.6	±4.9	±17.0	±4.5	±53	±10.5	±3.0	
42	3156	36.9	52.2	8.3	389	10.4	20.3	53.2	10.6	135	24.9	7.2	4.5
	±678	±2.0	±3.0	±0.5	±36	±5.0	±4.5	±10.1	±3.7	±54	±8.1	±2.9	±2.3

Data from Women and Infant's Hospital, Providence, RI

TABLE 16.11 WEIGHTS AND MEASUREMENTS OF FETUSES OF 8–26 WEEKS' GESTATION (MEAN VALUES)

Gestation (weeks)	Weight (g)*	Crown–heel length (cm) *	Crown–rump length (cm)	Foot length (cm)
8	10	2		
9	11	3		
10	14	4		
11	18	6	4	0.9
12	25	7	6	1.1
13	27	9	7	1.4
14	38	10	8	1.7
15	53	13	9	2.1
16	73	14	10	2.2
17	122	17	12	2.4
18	161	19	13	2.6
19	188	20	14	2.9
20	227	21	15	3.2
21	303	24	16	3.4
22	384	26	18	3.8
24	389	27	19	4.1
26	394	28	20	4.5

After Potter and Craig 1975, [104] with permission.

atrium must be sectioned (the SA nodal artery arises from either the right or left main circumflex coronary artery). The atrial septum contains fibers of the superior and middle preferential pathways, which run between the foramen ovale (fossa ovalis) and tricuspid ring. Because the AV node and bundle branches course through the interventricular septum, examination proceeds most easily if the free walls of the right and left ventricles are removed. The upper septum is then sectioned in multiple transverse planes, which are oriented parallel to the tricuspid ring (or, when viewed from the left, perpendicular to the aortic valve ring).

The skeletal system

Standard radiographic or computed tomography imaging is indicated in any case of skeletal dysplasia, and in fact, some advocate the use of **radiography** in every fetal or perinatal death. The use of a laboratory-based radiographic instrument such as the *Faxitron* is strongly recommended, and provides high quality detail. Newer instruments are now produced to employ a digital format; older ones use film formats such as Porta Pak PPL film (PPL80139639, large) or PPL8015059 (10 × 12 inches) available from Kodak. Placing specimens in a silver nitrate solution for 6–12 h enhances radiologic detail. For a more thorough discussion of skeletal abnormalities, see Chapter 34.

Bony tissue should also be studied grossly and microscopically. The routine microscopic examination of costochondral junction provides a useful way of assessing growth in the fetus or infant. In some forms of dysplasia, the examination of long bones, i.e. femur, rib, or vertebral column, may be diagnostic. The examination of femur will require incising the upper leg and freeing the bone carefully, as the ends are cartilaginous in the fetus or infant. In cases of spondylocostal dysplasia or other conditions that exhibit marked alterations of the chest, the entire rib cage, with vertebral column, can be removed for further study or teaching purposes. In cases requiring extensive dissection, some reconstruction of the body may be desired. Local funeral directors will probably have opinions or desires in this regard (see 'Reconstruction of the body' above.)

The male urethra

In cases of bladder outlet obstruction, the entire urethra must be examined for **posterior urethral valves** or other abnormality (i.e. anterior urethral valves, megaurethra). Valves in the posterior urethra (prostatic and membranous portions, extending from the bladder to the bulb) are considerably more common and located chiefly in the prostatic portion, but valves in the anterior urethra (spongiose portion, from the bulb to the meatus) are also reported.

Dissection is challenging and requires precision, for an erroneous cut may destroy the thin, delicate valve tissue.[9] With care, this procedure is successful in the young fetus. The proximal urethra lies posterior to the symphysis pubis, the midline cartilage of which must be excised to expose the base of the penis. The entire penis can be dissected free at this point, but, in order to preserve penile skin – and the appearance of an intact penis – the

TABLE 16.12 GESTATIONAL AGE AND MEAN ORGAN WEIGHTS AND MEASUREMENTS WITH ONE STANDARD DEVIATION

Gestation age (weeks)	Body weight	SD	n	Crown–rump (cm)	SD	n	Crown–heel (cm)	SD	n	Toe–heel (cm)	SD	n	Brain (g)	SD	n	Thymus	SD	n
12	21	±6.4	8	7.6	±0.6	10	9.3	±1.0	9	1.0	±0.1	11	3.5	±1.5	6	0.01		3
13	31	±10	21	8.7	±0.8	21	11.4	±1.0	16	1.2	±0.1	27	4.6	±1.7	11	0.03	±0.01	9
14	49	±16	18	9.8	±1.1	18	13.5	±1.5	17	1.5	±0.1	18	7.8	±4.1	12	0.05	±0.03	13
15	75	±22	49	10.9	±1.0	43	15.4	±1.4	40	1.8	±0.2	50	12.6	±3.4	31	0.09	±0.05	37
16	108	±25	36	12.0	±1.1	37	17.3	±1.5	36	2.1	±0.2	41	17.5	±3.7	23	0.14	±0.08	27
17	149	±32	50	13.2	±1.1	48	19.2	±1.6	47	2.4	±0.2	53	22.6	±4.7	34	0.18	±0.06	41
18	195	±44	44	14.3	±1.2	47	21.0	±1.6	44	2.7	±0.2	50	29.9	±7.5	40	0.27	±0.10	39
19	248	±46	52	15.4	±1.2	51	22.7	±1.4	44	3.0	±0.1	57	35.2	±6.6	43	0.39	±0.12	41
20	307	±47	66	16.5	±1.2	65	24.4	±1.8	64	3.3	±0.3	67	45.5	±7.2	54	0.53	±0.18	56
21	370	±60	38	17.7	±1.4	36	26.0	±2.1	35	3.6	±0.3	38	53.3	±8.8	33	0.70	±0.26	34
22	438	±74	50	18.8	±1.6	50	27.5	±2.1	50	3.9	±0.3	50	63.5	±10.5	45	0.91	±0.34	45
23	510	±77	39	19.9	±1.3	40	29.0	±1.8	40	4.2	±0.2	40	74.9	±13.5	34	1.14	±0.43	36
24	586	±74	29	21.0	±1.4	30	30.4	±1.4	30	4.4	±0.2	30	81.7	±14.8	28	1.41	±0.48	22
25	665	±104	24	22.1	±1.1	22	31.8	±1.8	24	4.6	±0.2	24	93.6	±12.2	23	1.70	±0.54	17
26	747	±110	13	23.3	±1.1	13	33.1	±1.6	13	4.8	±0.2	13	103.4	±12.9	12	2.04	±0.39	10

Gestation age (weeks)	Heart (g)	SD	n	Lungs (g)	SD	n	Spleen (g)	SD	n	Liver (g)	SD	n	Kidneys (g)	SD	n	Adrenals (g)	SD	n
12	0.15	±0.02	5	0.5	±0.3	7	0.01		3	1.0	±0.4	7	0.16	±0.04	6	0.10	±0.04	6
13	0.2	±0.1	11	1.1	±0.4	12	0.01	±0.01	10	1.4	±0.5	14	0.21	±0.08	13	0.15	±0.04	11
14	0.3	±0.1	15	1.8	±0.7	16	0.03	±0.02	16	2.3	±1.1	15	0.35	±0.11	16	0.22	±0.11	15
15	0.5	±0.2	38	2.6	±0.9	37	0.06	±0.04	38	3.3	±1.2	37	0.61	±0.20	37	0.33	±0.11	38
16	0.8	±0.2	31	3.5	±1.3	33	0.09	±0.05	30	5.0	±1.4	30	0.97	±0.33	32	0.48	±0.19	33
17	1.1	±0.4	39	4.6	±1.5	40	0.14	±0.07	45	7.1	±1.9	39	1.33	±0.46	45	0.65	±0.22	44
18	1.5	±0.4	43	5.8	±2.2	40	0.19	±0.10	44	9.5	±2.5	38	1.75	±0.51	40	0.83	±0.31	43
19	1.9	±0.5	48	7.1	±2.0	45	0.27	±0.11	46	12.1	±3.2	47	2.28	±0.56	46	1.03	±0.34	47
20	2.3	±0.6	61	8.6	±2.6	55	0.36	±0.17	59	14.9	±3.8	56	2.89	±0.63	56	1.23	±0.38	61
21	2.8	±0.6	37	10.2	±3.0	38	0.47	±0.20	34	17.8	±4.1	37	3.46	±0.96	38	1.43	±0.45	37
22	3.3	±0.8	44	11.9	±3.5	43	0.60	±0.18	46	20.7	±4.3	46	4.20	±1.33	44	1.64	±0.48	45
23	3.8	±0.9	39	13.8	±3.8	31	0.73	±0.27	34	23.6	±6.8	36	5.01	±1.16	32	1.83	±0.50	36
24	4.4	±0.9	29	15.8	±5.3	26	0.89	±0.31	27	26.4	±5.9	24	5.66	±1.47	28	2.02	±0.57	25
25	5.0	±1.0	22	18.0	±5.3	18	1.05	±0.25	18	29.1	±4.7	18	6.52	±1.25	22	2.19	±0.54	21
26	5.6	±1.1	11	20.2	±5.4	10	1.24	±0.36	9	31.6	±6.3	11	7.50	±1.60	11	2.35	±0.63	10

From Hansen et al 2003,[112] with permission

muscular penis can be carefully shelled out from the penile sheath, which is then filled with body tissue and closed with sutures. The body of the penis, thus exposed, is removed with bladder, ureters, and kidneys. Following evisceration, the urethra is opened in the midline, from distal to proximal, or serially sectioned (Fig. 16.3E).

Examination of the placenta

Examination of the placenta is a critical part of the fetal and perinatal autopsy. For a complete discussion of this process, the reader is referred to Chapter 15.

The parental conference

Workers must understand that parents and other family members react to the loss of a fetus or newborn in a wide variety of ways and therefore modify their actions accordingly.[97–102] Some parents exhibit a very low affect and seem to accept the loss in almost matter-of-fact manner, appearing, at least outwardly, to care little about the loss. It is unclear if this is really the case, and of course, judging this behavior will not be in anyone's interest. Some may exhibit the opposite behavior, one that is extremely emotional and may require acute counseling by appropriate specialists. Still others respond in an intellectual manner charac-

TABLE 16.13 ORGAN WEIGHTS IN FETUSES FROM 9 TO 20 WEEKS OF DEVELOPMENT

Developmental age (days)	Weight (g)	Crown–rump length (cm)	Brain (g)	Heart (g)	Lungs (g)	Liver (g)	Adrenals (g)	Kidneys (g)	No. of cases
63	11	3	1.2	0.1	0.1	0.2	0.1	0.1	30
67	13	4	1.5	0.2	0.3	0.7	0.1	0.1	27
71	15	6	2.6	0.2	0.4	0.8	0.1	0.1	15
73	20	7	4.3	0.3	0.4	1.1	0.1	0.2	21
76	25	7	4.8	0.4	0.7	1.1	0.2	0.2	14
79	30	8	5.4	0.4	1.0	1.3	0.2	0.2	15
84	35	9	6.2	0.5	1.4	2.0	0.2	0.3	14
89	45	9	7.4	0.5	1.9	2.5	0.4	0.4	22
90	50	10	8.5	0.5	1.9	3.0	0.5	0.5	23
91	60	10	10	0.5	2.5	3.4	0.6	0.6	21
96	80	11	12	0.7	3.0	4.3	0.6	0.8	7
100	90	12	14	0.9	3.0	4.7	0.7	0.9	15
105	100	12	17	1.1	3.9	5.6	0.7	1.4	28
109	125	13	23	1.3	4.1	7.4	0.7	1.4	21
115	150	14	23	1.4	5.3	9.2	0.8	1.4	20
117	175	14	23	1.4	5.6	11	0.8	1.8	27
118	200	15	33	1.7	7.2	12	1.1	2.2	39
124	250	16	39	2.2	9.1	15	1.2	2.7	37
130	300	17	46	2.4	10	17	1.5	3.1	43
133	350	18	54	2.9	11	21	2.0	3.8	31
143	400	18	61	3.4	11	23	2.2	4.2	32

From Gilbert-Barness and Debich-Spicer 2004,[14] with permission.

terized by intense questioning or scrutiny of the literature, often via the Internet. In this latter approach, parents may acquire a large amount of information in short order. The pathologist will need to evaluate the quality of such information, and ensure that it is accurate, reliable, and understood. Some parents may wish to have reports or tissue sent to other laboratories for diagnostic or research purposes and may actually identify and contact these institutions independently. Pathologists should work carefully with all parents, realizing that a combination of grief, intense desire for information, and possibly other factors, including ones that go unexpressed or even unrecognized, drive the process.

As part of their routine care, obstetricians arrange meetings with mothers a few weeks after the delivery. **Autopsy reports** should be made available to clinical colleagues for these conferences. At times it may also be desirable for pathologists to meet with parents. At these conferences pathologists seek to inform parents, in words that they can understand, of the autopsy findings and the implications those findings carry for them, other family members, and any future children. Conferences are arranged following completion of the autopsy report, generally a few weeks after the examination has been conducted. The passage of time also allows parents to recover somewhat from their most intense grief. Pathologists should use great care in making comments about the nature of clinical care, for this is an arena with which the pathologist may not have particular familiarity. In most instances, conflicting interpretations will not benefit the family.

The pathologist would do well to begin the parental conference by expressing regret over the loss and inquiry into the mother's and family's well-being and availability of support systems. It may be possible or necessary to recommend other specialists to follow up on this. The autopsy findings are described next, with attention given to the principal disease,

TABLE 16.14 REGIONAL DEVELOPMENT OF THE CEREBRAL HEMISPHERES

Lobe	Fissures and sulci	Gestational age (weeks)	Gyri	Gestational age (weeks)
Frontal	Interhemispheric fissure	10	Gyrus rectus	16
	Transverse cerebral fissure	10	Insula	18
	Hippocampal sulcus	10	Cingulate gyrus	18
	Callosal sulcus	14	Prerolandic gyrus	24
	Sylvian fissure	14	Superior frontal gyrus	25
	Olfactory sulcus	16	Middle frontal gyrus	27
	Circular sulcus	18	Triangular gyrus	28
	Cingulate sulcus	18	Medial and lateral orbital gyri	28
	Rolandic sulcus	20	Callosomarginal gyrus	28
	Prerolandic sulcus	24	Anterior and posterior orbital gyri	36
	Superior frontal sulcus	25		
	Inferior frontal sulcus	28		
Parietal	Interhemispheric fissure	10	Cingulate gyrus	18
	Transverse cerebral fissure	10	Postrolandic gyrus	25
	Sylvian fissure	14	Superior parietal lobule	26
	Parietooccipital fissure	16	Inferior parietal lobule	26
	Rolandic sulcus	20	Angular gyrus	28
	Postrolandic sulcus	25	Supramarginal gyrus	28
	Interparietal sulcus	26	Paracentral gyri	35
Temporal	Sylvian fissure	14	Superior temporal gyrus	23
	Superior temporal sulcus	23	Parahippocampal gyrus	23
	Collateral sulcus	23	Middle temporal gyrus	26
	Middle temporal sulcus	26	Fusiform gyrus	27
	Inferior temporal sulcus	30	Inferior temporal gyrus	30
			External occipitotemporal gyrus	30
			Transverse temporal gyrus	31
Occipital	Interhemispheric fissure	10	Superior occipital gyri	27
	Calcarine fissure	16	Inferior occipital gyri	27
	Parieto-occipital sulcus	16	Cuneus	27
	Collateral sulcus	23	Lingual gyrus	27
	Lateral occipital sulcus	27	External occipitotemporal gyrus	30

From Gilles et al 1983,[115] with permission.

followed by related and unrelated findings. The pathologist must assess the level of parental understanding, and tailor language to maximize the transfer of information. It will probably be helpful to have illustrations or photographs available, or to make sketches during the conference, in order to explain the findings. Lingering questions should be sought, and final decisions made about organ or tissue retention made, should that be an issue. The conference can end with the invitation to continue the conversation at a later date if the need arises. (See Ch. 7 for additional discussion regarding the special demands of counseling families of stillborn infants.)

Acknowledgements

The author gratefully acknowledges Marie Valdés-Dapena, Dagmar K. Kalousek, and Dale S. Huff, previous authors of this chapter, for their contributions.

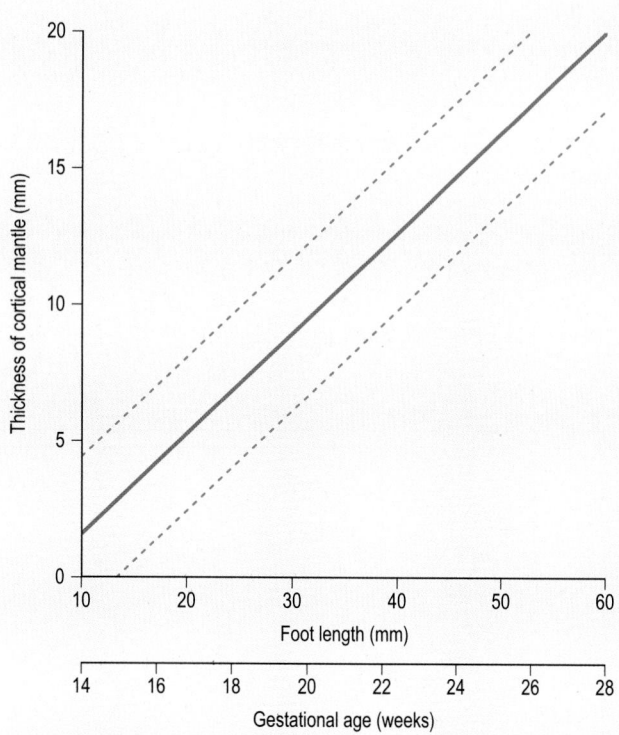

FIGURE 16.26 Cortical mantle thickness. (From Siebert et al 1999,[59] with permission.)

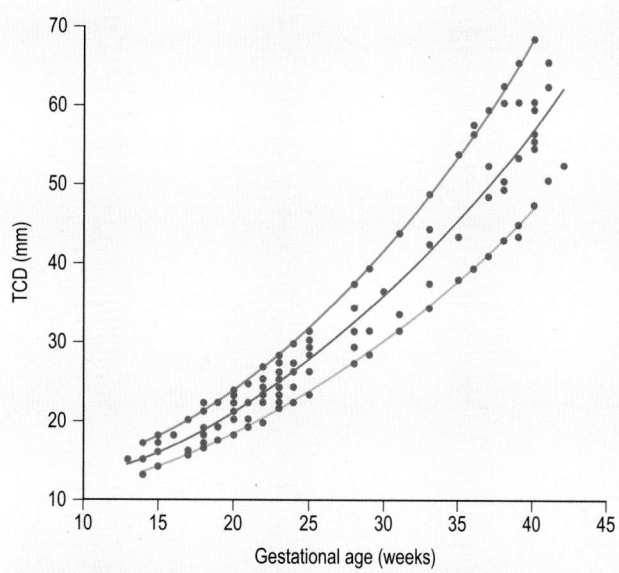

FIGURE 16.27 Mean transverse cerebellar diameter (TCD) with two standard deviations at each gestational age. (From Pinar et al 2002,[116] with permission.)

TABLE 16.15 TIME PERIODS OF EMBRYONIC AND FETAL DEVELOPMENT IN HUMANS

Developmental event	Developmental age (days)
Somites first appear	20
Rostral neuropore closes	24
Caudal neuropore closes	26
Upper limb bud appears*	26–27
Lower limb bud appears *	28–30
Crown–rump length 5 mm	29–30
Paddle-shaped hand plate	31–32
Paddle-shaped foot plate	33–36
Aortopulmonary spiral septum begins	34
Herniation of gut	34
Eye pigment *	34–35
Crown–rump length, 10 mm	37
Ossification begins	40–43
Müllerian duct appears	40
Digital rays, upper extremity *	41–43
Cloaca divided by urorectal septum	43
Testes, histologic differentiation	43
Notches between finger rays	44–46
Digital rays, lower extremity *	44–46
Heart septation complete	46–47
Webbed fingers	49–51
Notches between toe rays	49–51
Free fingers *	52–53
Webbed toes	52–53
Eyelids closed	56–58
Palate closed completely	56–58
Herniation of gut reduced *	60
Urethral groove closed in male	90

* Important landmarks.

From O'Rahilly and Muller 1987[73] and Gilbert-Barness and Debich-Spicer 2004,[14] with permission.

TABLE 16.16 AUTOPSY PROTOCOL

Autopsy protocol

Autopsy # _____

Hospital Chart # _____

Brithweight: _____

Name: _____

Age: _____

Gestational age: _____

Sex: _____

Race: _____

Date and time of admission: _____

Date and time of death: _____

Date and time of autopsy: _____

Autopsy performed by: _____

Protocol:

The body is that of a _____ infant weighting _____ gm. The crown-rump length is _____ cm; time rump-heel, _____ cm. The occipitofrontal circumference is _____ cm, that of the chest is _____ cm, and that of the abdomen is _____ cm. Rigor _____ .

Hypostasis _____ . Icterus _____ .

Cyanosis _____ . Edema _____ .

The pupils are _____

The sclerae are _____

The ears _____

The nose _____

The mouth _____

There is/are _____ needle puncture mark(s) _____

The umbilical cord is _____

The anus is _____

The external genitalia are _____

The skin is _____

Peritoneal cavity:

The peritoneal surface is _____

The peritoneal cavity contains _____

The diaphragm arches to the _____ on the right and to the _____ on the left.

The umbilical vein _____ .

There are _____ umbilical arteries.

The measurements of the liver are as follows: _____ .

The spleen _____

The appendix is in the right lower quadrant. The stomach is _____

The small intestine is _____

The large intestine is _____

The mesenteric lymph nodes are _____

The root of the mesentery _____

TABLE 16.16 AUTOPSY PROTOCOL (*CONT'D*)

Pleural cavities:

The pleural surfaces are _____

_____ .

The right pleural cavity contains _____ .

The left pleural cavity contains _____ .

The lungs occupy _____ of their respective pleural cavities.

Each lung has a normal number of lobes.

Pericardial cavity:

The pericardial surfaces are _____

_____ .

The cavity is free from adhesions and contains _____

_____ .

Cardiovascular system:

Heart: The heart weighs _____ g (normal is _____ g).

The foramen ovale is _____

The ductus arteriosus is _____

The mural and valvular endocardium is _____

The myocardium is _____

The coronary ostia and coronary sinus are in normal position. The great vessels arising from the heart and those arising from the aortic arch do so in normal position.

The measurements of the heart are as follows:

TV _____ , PV _____ , MV _____ , AV _____ ,

RVM _____ , LVM _____ cm.

The thoracic and abdominal aorta _____

_____ .

Respiratory system:

Lungs: The combined weight of the lungs is _____ g (normal is _____ g).

On section _____

_____

The trachea and major bronchi are lined by _____ mucosa; their lumina contain _____

Hematopoietic system:

Spleen: The spleen weighs _____ g (normal is _____ g). The capsule is _____

On section the parenchyma is _____

The malpighian corpuscles are _____

The lymph nodes are _____

Bone marrow is _____

Gastrointestinal system:

The mucosa of the esophagus is _____

and its lumen contains _____ .

The mucosa of the stomach is _____

and its lumen contains _____ .

The mucosa of the small intestine is _____

and its lumen contains _____ .

The length of the small bowel is _____ cm; the large bowel, _____ cm.

The mucosa of the large intestine is _____

and its lumen contains _____ .

Liver: The liver weighs _____ g (normal is _____ g).

The capsule is _____

On section the parenchyma is _____

The sinus intermedius and ductus venosus are _____

_____ .

The bile, which is _____ , is freely expressed from the gallbladder into the duodenum.

TABLE 16.16 AUTOPSY PROTOCOL (*CONT'D*)

Pancreas: The pancreas is tan and coarsely lobulated. On section _____
_____
_____ .

Endocrine system:
Adrenals: The combined weight of the adrenals is _____ g. They are _____
_____
_____ .

The cut surfaces reveal _____
peripheral zones and _____ central zones.

Gennitourinary system:
Kidneys: The combined weight of the kidneys is _____ g (normal is _____ g).
The renal arteries and veins are free from thrombi. _____
surfaces _____
_____ .

On section the cortex and medulla are _____
_____ demarcated. The renal pelves and ureters are lined by _____
Bladder: The mucosa of the bladder is _____
_____ .

The relations at the trigone are normal.
Genitalia: The prostate is small and firm and reveals no gross abrnomalities. The vaginal mucosa is _____ .
The uterus, tubes, and ovaries reveal no gross abnormalities. The uterus and ovaries are of normal size.
Organs of the Neck: The thymus weighs _____ g. The surface is _____
_____ .

The cut surfaces _____ .
The thyroid and larynx reveal no gross abnormalities. The larynx is lined by _____
_____ mucosa and is empty. The submaxillary glands _____
_____
_____ parathyroids are identified. Positions: _____
_____ .

HEAD: The soft tissues of the scalp are _____
_____ . The anterior fontanelle measures _____ cm.
The posterior fontanelle is _____ .
The sutures _____ .
The dura mater is _____ .
The falx cerebri and the tentorium cerebelli are intact. The pia arachnoid is _____
_____ .

There is no subarachnoid hemorrhage nor exudate. The convolutions and sulci are _____ .
The brain is fixed in toto. The dural sinuses are free from thrombi.
The middle ears are _____ .
A segment of the _____ spinal cord is removed by the antnerior approach and reveals no gross
abnormalities.
The pituitary _____ .
Musculoskeletal system:
Bones: The manubrium sternum contains _____ center of ossification.
The _____ , _____ , _____ sternebrae
each contain _____ centers of ossification. The are _____ pairs of
ribs. Two lower costochondral junctions are removed from each side.

TABLE 16.17 SUMMARY OF EMBRYONIC DEVELOPMENT

Crown–rump length (mm)	Days after ovulation	Carnegie stage	Main external features
0.1	0–2	1	Fertilized oocyte
	2–4	2	Morula
	4–6	3	Blastocyst
		4	Bilaminar embryo
0.2–0.4	6–15	5	Bilaminar embryo with primary yolk sac
		6	Trilaminar embryo with primitive streak
0.4–1.0	15–17	7	Trilaminar embryo with notochordal process
1.0–1.5	18–20	8	Primitive pit and notochordal canal formed
1.5–2.0	20–22	9	Deep neural groove; first somites present; heart tubes begin to fuse
2.0–3.0	22–24	10	Neural folds begin to fuse; heart begins to beat; embryo straight; 4–12 pairs of somites
3.0–4.0	24–26	11	Rostral neuropore closing, embryo slightly curved; 13–20 pairs of somites
4.0–5.0	26–30	12	Upper limb buds appear; caudal neuropore closed; tail appearing; 21–29 pairs of somites
5.0–6.0	28–32	13	Four pairs of branchial arches; lower limb buds appear; tail present; 30 or more somites
6.0–7.0	31–35	14	Lens pits and nasal pits visible; optic cups present
7.0–10.0	35–38	15	Hand plates formed; lens vesicles and nasal pits prominent
10.0–12.0	37–42	16	Foot plates formed; nasal pits face ventrally; pigment visible in retina
12.0–14.0	42–44	17	Finger rays appear; auricular hillocks developed; upper lip formed
14.0–17.0	44–48	18	Toe rays and elbow region appear; eyelids forming; ambiguous genital tubercle seen
16.0–20.0	48–51	19	Trunk elongating and straightening; midgut herniation to umbilical cord
20.0–22.0	51–53	20	Fingers distinct but webbed; scalp vascular plexus appears
22.0–24.0	53–54	21	Fingers free and longer; toes still webbed
24.0–28.0	54–56	22	Toes free and longer; eyelids and external ear more developed
28.0–30.0	56–60	23	Head more rounded; fusing eyelids

From Jirasek 1983,[117] Moore and Persaud 1993,[118] O'Rahilly and Muller 1987,[73] and Streeter 1951,[72] with permission.

TABLE 16.18 CONVERSION FACTORS

To convert from	To	Multiply by
Metric to English		
Centimeters (cm)	Inches (US) (in)	0.394
Centimeters (cm)	Feet (US) (ft)	0.033
Square meters (m²)	Square feet (US) (ft)	10.753
Grams (g)	Ounces (avoirdupois) (oz)	0.035
Grams (g)	Pounds (avoirdupois) (lb)	0.002
Kilograms (kg)	Ounces (avoirdupois) (oz)	35.274
Kilograms (kg)	Pounds (avoirdupois) (lb)	2.205
Milliliters (mL)*	Ounces (US fluid) (fl oz)	0.034
Liters (L)	Quarts (UK liquid) (qt)	1.057
Liters (L)	Gallons (US) (gal)	0.264
English to Metric		
Inches (US) (in)	Centimeters (cm)	2.54
Feet (US) (ft)	Centimeters (cm)	30.480
Square feet (US) (ft)	Square meters (m²)	0.093
Ounces (avoirdupois) (oz)	Grams (g)	28.350
Pounds (avoirdupois) (lb)	Grams (g)	453.592
Ounces (avoirdupois) (oz)	Kilograms (kg)	0.02835
Pounds (avoirdupois) (lb)	Kilograms (kg)	0.454
Ounces (US fluid) (fl oz)	Milliliters (mL)*	29.574
Quarts (US liquid) (qt)	Liters (L)	0.946
Gallons (US) (gall)	Liters (L)	3.785
Pressure conversion		
cm H$_2$O	mm Hg	0.760
mm Hg	cm H$_2$O	1.316
	Temperature conversion	
°C	°F	°F = (1.8 × °C) +32
°C	°C	$°C = \dfrac{(°F - 32)}{1.8}$

Concentration conversion for ethyl alcohol:

1000 µg/mL = 100 mg/dL mmol/L = 1.0 promille= 0.1%

*For most purposes, cubic centimeter (cc) is equal to milliliter (mL)
From Ludwig 2002,[81] with permission.

References

Introduction

1. Macpherson TA, Valdes-Dapena M. The perinatal autopsy. In: Wigglesworth JS, Singer D, eds. Perinatal pathology. Philadelphia: WB Saunders; 1988:93–122.
2. Ochs R, Carr RF, Griffin TD, et al. Perinatal autopsies: a challenge for the nonpediatric pathologist, Pathol Ann 1988; 23:235–255.
3. Bove KE. Practice guidelines for autopsy pathology: the perinatal and pediatric autopsy. Autopsy Committee of the College of American Pathologists. Arch Pathol Lab Med 1997; 121:368–376.
4. Boyd PA, Tondi F, Hicks NR, et al. Autopsy after termination of pregnancy for fetal anomaly: retrospective cohort study. Br Med J 2004; 328:137–142.
5. Brodlie M, Laing IA, Keeling JW, et al. Ten years of neonatal autopsies in tertiary referral centre: retrospective study. Br Med J 2002; 324:761–763.
6. Faye-Peterson OM, Guinn DA, Wenstrom KD. Value of perinatal autopsy. Obstet Gynecol 1999; 94:915–920.
7. Gordijn SJ, Erwich JJHM, Khong TY. Value of the perinatal autopsy: critique. Pediatr Devel Pathol 2002; 5:480–488.
8. Langley FA. The perinatal postmortem examination. J Clin Pathol 1971; 24:159–169.
9. Siebert JR, Kapur RP. Congenital anomalies in the fetus: approaches to examination and diagnosis. Path Case Rev 2000; 5:3–13.
10. Michalski ST, Porter J, Pauli RM. Costs and consequences of comprehensive stillbirth assessment. Am J Obstet Gynecol 2002; 186:1027–1034.
11. Newton D, Coffin CM, Clark EB, et al. How the pediatric autopsy yields valuable information in a vertically integrated health care system. Arch Pathol Lab Med 2004; 128:1239–1246.
12. Valdes-Dapena M, Huff D. Perinatal autopsy manual. Washington: Armed Forces Institute of Pathology; 1983.
13. Valdes-Dapena M, Huff D. Guidelines for post mortem reports. Bull Roy Col Pathol 1983; 84:11.
14. Gilbert-Barness E, Debich-Spicer DE. Embryo and fetal pathology: color atlas with ultrasound correlation. Cambridge: Cambridge University Press; 2004.
15. Gilbert-Barness E, Debich-Spicer DE. Handbook of pediatric autopsy pathology. Totowa: Humana Press; 2005.
16. Carey JC. Diagnostic evaluation of the stillborn infant. Clin Obstet Gynecol 1987; 30:342–351.
17. Curry CJR. Pregnancy loss, stillbirth, and neonatal death: a guide for the pediatrician. Pediatr Clin North Am 1992; 39:157–191.
18. Curry CJR, Honore LH. A protocol for the investigation of pregnancy loss. Clin Perinatol 1990; 17:723–742.
19. Mueller RF, Sybert VP, Johnson J, et al. Evaluation of a protocol for post-mortem examination of stillbirths. N Engl J Med 1983; 309:586–590.
20. Pauli RM, Reiser CA. Wisconsin stillbirth service program: II. Analysis of diagnoses and diagnostic categories in the first 1,000 referrals. Am J Med Genet 1994; 50:135–153.
21. Pauli RM, Reiser CA, Lebovitz RM, et al. Wisconsin stillbirth service program: I. Establishment and assessment of a community-based program for etiologic investigation of intrauterine deaths. Am J Med Genet 1994; 50:116–134.

Approach to the perinatal autopsy

22. Wright VJ, Dimmick JE, Kalousek DK. The preliminary investigation (protocol) of the malformed fetus or neonate – or – what to do until the pathologist comes. Birth Defects 1979; 15:93–104.
23. Jones KL, Hanson JW, Smith DW. Palpebral fissure size in newborn infants. J Pediatr 1978; 92:787.
24. Scammon RE, Calkins LA. The development and growth of the external dimensions of the human body in the fetal period. Minneapolis: University of Minnesota Press; 1929.
25. Wigglesworth JS, Singer D. Textbook of fetal and perinatal pathology, 2nd edn. Malden: Blackwell Science; 1998.
26. Chi JG, Dooling EG, Gilles FH. Gyral development of the human brain. Ann Neurol 1977; 1:86–93.
27. Valdes-Dapena M, Kalousek D, Huff D. Perinatal, fetal, and embryonic autopsy. In: Gilbert-Barness E, ed. Potter's pathology of the fetus and infant. St. Louis: Mosby; 1997.
28. Hall JG, Froster-Iskenius UG, Allanson JE. Handbook of normal physical measurements. Oxford: Oxford Medical Publications; 1989.
29. Siebert JR. Prenatal growth of the median face. Am J Med Genet 1986; 25:369–379.
30. Birnholz JC, Farrell EE. Fetal ear length. Pediatrics 1988; 81:555–558.
31. Chambers HM, Knowles SAS, Staples A, et al. Anthropometric measurements in the second trimester fetus. Early Hum Dev 1993; 33:45–45.
32. Guihard-Costa A-M, Menez F, Delezoide AL. Standards for dysmorphological diagnosis in human fetuses. Pediatr Devel Pathol 2003; 6:427–434.
33. Edwards WD. How to photograph pathology specimens for teaching purposes. Bull Pathol Educ 1987; 12:65–69.
34. Primeau RN, Recht CK. Professional bereavement photographs: one aspect of a perinatal bereavement program. J Obstet Gynecol Neonat Nurs 1994; 23:22–25.
35. Sawyer DR. Perinatal bereavement: the photographer's role in infant death. J Biolog Photog 1998; 66:35–37.

36. Vetter JP. The color photography of gross specimens. Pathologist 1984; 78:155–162.

37. Vetter JP. Biomedical photography. Boston: Butterworth-Heinemann; 1992.

38. Krauss TC. Close-up medical photography: Forensic considerations and techniques. In: Wecht C, ed. Legal medicine. Boston: Butterworths; 1989: 93–111.

39. Krauss TC, Warlen SC. The forensic science use of reflective ultraviolet photography. J Forensic Sci 1985; 30:262.

40. Adnot J. Medical photography [letter]. J Dermatol Surg Oncol 1991; 17: 624–625.

41. Alvord EAJ, Siebert JR. Neuropathology: art and science [letter]. J Neuropathol Exp Neurol 1997; 56:1373–1374.

42. Tirrell S, Rutledge JC, Siebert JR. Picture this! Imaging techniques for surgical pathology. J Histotechnol 2004; 27:231–235.

43. Barr M. Sternal variability in normal and abnormal human fetuses. Teratology 1984; 29:17A.

44. Dimmick JE, Kalousek DK. Developmental pathology of the embryo and fetus. Philadelphia: JB Lippincott; 1992.

45. Siebert JR, Graham JMJ, MacDonald C. Pathologic features of the CHARGE association: support for involvement of the neural crest. Teratology 1985; 31:331–336.

46. Conley ME, Beckwith JB, Mancer JF, et al. The spectrum of the DiGeorge syndrome. J Pediatr 1979; 94:883–890.

47. Donnelly WH, Hawkins H. Optimal examination of the normally formed perinatal heart. Hum Pathol 1987; 18:55–60.

48. Sherman FE. An atlas of congenital heart disease. Philadelphia: Lea & Febiger; 1963.

49. Schall SA, Dalldorf FG. Premature closure of the foramen ovale and hypoplasia of the left heart. Int J Cardiol 1984; 5:103–107.

50. Siebert JR. A morphometric study of normal and abnormal fetal to childhood tongue size. Arch Oral Biol 1985; 30:433.

51. Bass T, Bergevin MA, Werner AL, et al. In situ fixation of the neonatal brain and spinal cord. Pediatr Pathol 1993; 13:699–705.

52. Isaacson G. Postmortem examination of infant brains. Arch Pathol Lab Med 1984; 108:80–81.

53. Powers JM. Practice guidelines for autopsy pathology. Autopsy Committee of the College of American Pathologists. Arch Pathol Lab Med 1995; 119:777–783.

54. Siebert JR, Kokich VG, Warkany J, et al. Atelencephalic microcephaly: Craniofacial anatomy and morphologic comparisons with holoprosencephaly and anencephaly. Teratology 1987; 36:279–285.

55. Doherty D, Glass IA, Siebert JR, et al. Successful Joubert syndrome prenatal diagnosis by ultrasound, verified by fetal MRI and confirmed by post-mortem examination: implications. Prenat Diagn 2005; 442–447.

56. Emery JL. The postmortem examination of a baby. In: Mason J, ed. Pediatric forensic medicine and pathology. London: Chapman & Hall; 1989.

57. Knisely AS, Singer DB. A technique for necropsy evaluation of stenosis of the foramen magnum and rostral spinal canal in osteochondrodysplasia. Hum Pathol 1988; 19:1372.

58. Dorovini-Zis K, Dolman CL. Gestational development of the brain. Arch Pathol Lab Med 1977; 101:192–195.

59. Siebert JR, Nyberg DA, Kapur RP. Cerebral mantle thickness: a measurement useful in the anatomic diagnosis of fetal ventriculomegaly. Pediatr Devel Pathol 1999; 2:168–175.

60. Beckwith JB. Sampling of muscle at autopsy in cases of lower motor neuron disease. Am J Clin Path 1964; 42:92–93.

61. Trump BF, Valigorsky JM, Dees JH, et al. The modernization of the autopsy: application of ultrastructural and biochemical methods to human disease. MCV Quarterly 1973; 9:323–333.

62. Siebert JR, Rutledge JC, Kapur RP. Histologic examination in cases of pregnancy termination. Lab Invest 2994; 84:275.

Examination of twins or other multiple gestations

63. Baldwin VJ. Pathology of multiple pregnancy. New York: Springer-Verlag; 1994.

Examination of the stillborn fetus

64. Genest DR. Estimating the time of death in stillborn fetuses. II. Histologic evaluation of the placenta; a study of 71 stillborns. Obstet Gynecol 1992; 80:585–592.

65. Genest DR, Singer DB. Estimating the time of death in stillborn fetuses. III. External fetal examination; a study of 86 stillborns. Obstet Gynecol 1992; 80:593–600.

66. Genest DR, Williams MA, Greene MF. Estimating the time of death in stillborn fetuse. I. Histologic evaluation of fetal organs; an autopsy study of 150 stillborns. Obstet Gynecol 1992; 80:575–584.

Examination of the embryo and young fetus

67. Kalousek DK, Baldwin VJ, Dimmick JE, et al. Embryofetal-perinatal autopsy and placental examination. In: Dimmick J, Kalousek D, eds. Developmental pathology of the embryo and fetus. Philadelphia: JB Lippincott; 1992.

68. Kalousek DK, Fitch N, Paradice BA. Pathology of the human embryo and previable fetus: an atlas. New York; Springer-Verlag; 1990.

69. Kalousek DK, Lau AE, Baldwin VJ. Development of the embryo, fetus, and placenta. In: Dimmick JE, Kalousek DK, eds. Developmental pathology of the embryo and fetus. Philadelphia: JB Lippincott; 1992.

70. Szulman AE. Examination of the early conceptus. Arch Pathol Lab Med 1991; 115:696–700.

71. Rushton DI. Examination of products of conception from previable human pregnancies. J Clin Pathol 1981; 34:819–835.

72. Streeter GL. Developmental horizons in human embryos. Description of age groups XIX, XX, XXI, XXII, and XXIII, being the fifth issue of a survey of the Carnegie Collection (prepared for publication by C.H. Heuser and G.W. Corner). Carnegie Instn Wash Publ 1951; 34:165–196.

73. O'Rahilly R, Muller F. Developmental stages in human embryos. Washington: Carnegie Institution; 1987.

74. Poland BJ, Miller JR, MHarris M, et al. Spontaneous abortion: a study of 1961 women and their conceptuses. Acta Obstet Gynecol Scand 1981; 102(suppl):5–32.

75. Ornoy A, Borochowitz Z, Lachman R, et al. Atlas of fetal skeletal radiology. Chicago: Year Book; 1988.

76. Berry CL. The examination of embryonic and fetal material in diagnostic histopathology laboratories. J Clin Pathol 1980; 33:317–326.

77. Knowles SAS. Examination of products of conception terminated after prenatal investigation. J Clin Pathol 1986; 39:1049–1065.

78. Klatt EC. Pathologic examination of fetal specimens from dilation and evacuation procedures. Am J Clin Pathol 1995; 103:415–418.

79. Siebert JR, Kapur RP, Resta RG, et al. Methods for induced abortion [letter]. Obstet Gynecol 2005; 10:221–222.

Culture and other studies

80. Slavin G, Wright BM. Postmortem inflation and fixation of the lung. Pathol Res Pract 1979; 165:458–459.

81. Ludwig J. Handbook of autopsy practice, 3rd edn. Totowa: Humana Press; 2002.

82. Hales MR, Carrington CB. A pigment gelatin mass for vascular injection. Yale J Biol Med 1971; 43:257–270.

83. Schlesinger MJ. A new radiopaque mass for vascular injection. Lab Invest 1957; 6:1–11.

84. Larmay HJ, Strasburger JF. Differential diagnosis and management of the fetus and newborn with an irregular or abnormal heart rate. Pediatr Clin North Am 2004; 51:1033–1050.

85. Buyon JP, Clancy RM. Maternal autoantibodies and congenital heart block: mediators, markers, and therapeutic approach. Semin Arthritis Rheum 2003; 33:140–154.

86. Gowda RM, Khan IA, Mehta NJ, et al. Cardiac arrhythmias in pregnancy: clinical and therapeutic considerations. Int J Cardiol 2003; 88:129.

87. Kleinman CS, Nehgme RA. Cardiac arrhythmias in the human fetus. Pediatr Cardiol 2004; 25:234–251.

88. Mardirosoff C, Dumont L, Boulvain M, et al. Fetal bradycardia due to intrathecal opioids for labour analgesia: a systematic review. Br J Obstet Gynaecol 2002; 109:274–281.

89. Ristic AD, Maisch B. Cardiac rhythm and conduction disturbances: what is the role of autoimmune mechanisms? Herz 2000; 25:181–188.

90. Buyon JP, Clancy RM. Neonatal lupus syndromes. Curr Opin Rheumatol 2003; 15:535–541.

91. Ho SY, Mortimer G, Anderson RH, et al. Conduction system defects in three perinatal patients with arrhythmia. Br Heart J 1985; 53:158–163.

92. Bharati S, Serratto M, Dubrow I, et al. The conduction system in Pompe's disese. Pediatr Cardiol 1982; 2:25–32.

93. Rosenberg HS, Donnelly WH. The cardiovascular system. In: Wigglesworth J, Singer D, eds. Textbook of fetal and perinatal pathology, 2nd edn. Malden: Blackwell Science; 1998.

94. Bharati S, Lev M. The cardiac conduction system in unexplained sudden death. Mount Kisco: Future Publishing Company; 1990.

95. Davies MJ, Anderson RH, Becker AE. The conduction system of the heart. Boston: Butterworth; 1983.

96. de Sa DJ. Complications of therapy in the prenatal and perinatal period. In: Reed GB, Claireaux AE, Cockburn F, eds. Diseases of the fetus and newborn: pathology, imaging, genetics, and management, 2nd edn. London: Chapman & Hall; 1995.

The parental conference

97. Arnold JA, Gemma PB. A child dies: a portrait of family grief, 2nd edn. Philadelphia: The Charles Press Publishers; 1994.

98. Schiff HS. The bereaved parent. New York: Crown Publishers; 1977.

99. Westberg GE. Good grief: a constructive approach to the problem of loss. Minneapolis: Augsburg Fortress; 1962.

100. Laing IA. Clinical aspects of neonatal death and autopsy. Semin Neonatol 2004; 9:247–254.

101. Snowdon C, Elbourne DR, Garcia JH. Perinatal pathology in the context of a clinical trial: attitudes of bereaved parents. Arch Dis Child Fetal Neonatal Ed 2004; 89:F208.

102. Lyon A. Perinatal autopsy remains the 'gold standard.' Arch Dis Child Fetal Neonatal Ed 2004; 89:F284.

103. McBride ML, Baillie, J, Poland BJ. Growth parameters in normal fetuses. Teratology 1984; 29:185.

104. Potter EL, Craig JM. Pathology of the fetus and infant, 3rd edn. Chicago: Year Book; 1975:15–24.

105. Feingold M, Bossert HW. Normal values for selected physical parameters: an aid to syndrome delineation. Birth Defects Orig Artic Ser 1974; 10:1–16

106. Merlob P, Sivan Y, Reisner SH. Anthropometric measurements of the newborn infant. White Plains: The March of Dimes Birth Defects Foundation, BD:OAS 20(7); 1984.

107. Blais MM, Green WT, Anderson M. Length of the growing foot. Bone Joint Surg 1956; 38(A):998–1001.

108. Usher R, McLean F. Intrauterine growth of liveborn Caucasian infants at sea level: standards obtained from measurements in 7 dimensions of infants born between 25 and 44 weeks of gestation. J Pediatr 1969; 74. 901–910.

109. Duc G, Largo RH. Anterior fontanel: size and closure in term and preterm infants. Pediatrics 1986; 78(5):904–908.

110. Thomas IT, Gaitantzis VA, Frias JL. Palpebral fissure length from 29 weeks gestation to 14 years. J Pediatr 1987; 111(2):267–268.

111. Feingold M, Bossert HW. Normal values for selected physical parameters: an aid to syndrome delineation White Plains: The March of Dimes Birth Defects Foundation, BD:OAS X (13); 1974.

112. Hansen K, Sung CJ, Huang C, et al.Reference values for second trimester fetal and neonatal organ weights and measurements. Pediatr Dev Pathol 2003; 6(2):160–167.

113. Sunderman FW, Boerner F. Normal values in clinical medicine. Philadelphia: WB Sunder; 1949,

114. Schulz DM, Giordano DA, Schulz DH. Weights of organs of fetuses and infants. Arch Pathol 1969; 74:244–350.

115. Gilles FH, Leviton A, Dooling EC. The developing human brain – growth and epidemiologic neuropathology. Boston: John Wright, 1983.

116. Pinar H, Burke SH, Huang CW, et al. Reference values for transverse cerebellar diameter throughout gestation. Pediatr Dev Pathol 2002; 5(5): 489–494.

117. Jirasek JE: Atlas of human prenatal morphogenesis. Boston: Martinus Nijhoff; 1983.

118. Moore KL, Persaud TVN. The developing human: clinically oriented embryology, 5th edn. Philadelphia: WB Saunders; 1993.

119. Coppoletta JM, Wolbach SB. Body length and organ weights of infants and children. Am J Pathol 1933; 9:55–70.

Pediatric forensic pathology

Janice J. Ophoven

'*The beginning of wisdom is found in doubting, by doubting we come to question, and by searching we may come upon the truth.*'
Pierre Abeland

'*We shall draw from the heart of suffering itself the means of inspiration and survival.*'
Sir Winston Churchill

Pediatric forensic pathology is a newly emerging field of pathology that has developed out of the necessity to analyze cases of injury or death in children. These cases include conditions such as sudden unexpected death in infancy (sudden infant death syndrome; SIDS) and childhood (sudden unexplained death syndrome; SUDS), childhood accidents, iatrogenic injury, inflicted injury and neglect, and homicide. The importance of the pediatric pathologist's contributions to this body of knowledge cannot be understated.

Forensic pathology is the subspecialty of pathology that involves the interpretation of findings in living and deceased individuals to render opinions regarding cause and manner of disease, injury or death; the identification of deceased individuals; the significance of clinical findings; correlation of and reconstruction of wounds, wound patterns, wound sequences and timing; and coordination and/or performance of comprehensive medicolegal death investigations.[1] In the USA this process is typically carried out under the auspices of a coroner or medical examiner's office.[2] The forensic pathologist undergoes specialized training to perform death investigations and medicolegal autopsies. The forensic pathologist utilizes scientific and experiential knowledge and techniques to interpret and explain tissue injury (both natural and traumatic). This field contributes to the development of strategies to understand and prevent injury, disease and death, as well as to assist in the determination of fact in courts of law.[1] Published practice guidelines for forensic pathology are currently available from the College of American Pathology and the Royal College of Physicians.[1,3]

The forensic pathologist is responsible for ensuring that a proper medicolegal death investigation is performed during the process of death certification. A comprehensive medicolegal death investigation is a structured process, carried out by trained personnel, to acquire and review the information necessary for a complete investigation including scene investigation, body examination, documentation of materials, as well as collection and proper handling of

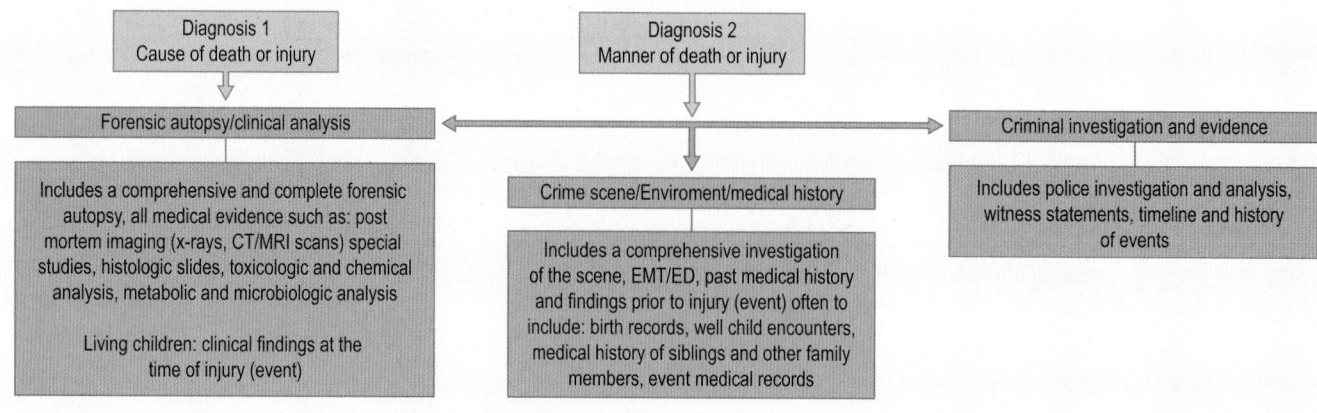

FIGURE 17.1 Elements of a comprehensive forensic analysis. (J Ophoven)

toxicologic specimens and other evidence, and collection and analysis of other medical or historical information.

The diagnosis of cause and manner of death is determined through the use of accepted scientific methods and procedures following a complete and thorough investigation (Fig. 17.1). The possibility of suspicious injuries or medicolegal questions may not appear until the autopsy procedure has begun. If necessary, the final opinions must be deferred until the process is complete in order to prevent misguided or misinformed inquiry. Because the process of death investigation is a multidisciplinary process, many states have prepared guidelines for infant death investigation available at minimal to no cost.[4]

The circumstances under which a death is reported to the medical examiner or coroner vary by locality. In most instances a physician, police officer, paramedic, or hospital nursing supervisor reports the death (Box 17.1). Familiarity with local regulations regarding reporting is especially important for the pathologist. **All sudden or unexpected deaths, all child deaths outside the hospital, deaths in the emergency room**, and all deaths that may be due entirely, or in part, to any factor other than natural disease must be reported. Examples of reporting requirements include, but are not limited to:

- unnatural deaths including violent deaths (homicidal, suicidal, or accidental);
- deaths under suspicious circumstances;
- deaths associated with burns or chemical, electrical, or radiation injury;
- deaths that occur during, in association with, or as a result of diagnostic, therapeutic, or anesthetic procedures;
- unexpected deaths of persons not disabled by disease and of persons notwithstanding a history of underlying disease;
- possible threat to public health;
- deaths in which a fracture of a major bone (femur, humerus, tibia etc.) has occurred within the past 6 months;
- deaths occurring outside a licensed health care facility;
- deaths occurring in an emergency department;

- deaths of persons arriving at an emergency department 'dead on arrival';
- deaths due to neglect;
- stillbirths of 20 weeks' or longer gestation unattended by a physician;
- deaths of children < 1 year of age that are suspected to be due to SIDS;
- deaths of unborn or newborn infants in which there has been maternal use or exposure to unprescribed controlled substances;
- deaths in a family or child care facility with a previous infant death or near death; and
- any unexpected or unexplained death of an infant or child. This includes children with handicaps or potentially life-limiting disease that have not been pre-reported or registered with hospice.[4]

When there is doubt as to whether a death is a coroner or medical examiner's case, the death should be reported.

Frequently overlooked are the deaths of those who succumb to complications of violent injuries months or even years after the event. Children left in a vegetative state after serious injuries from child abuse may die years later from infectious or neurologic complications. In these cases the manner of death is still homicide and the proper authorities must complete the death investigation. Establishing a relationship between the hospital-based pathologist and the medical examiner or coroner, prior to the need for cooperation, will go far towards meeting the goals of both disciplines. The hospital-based pathologist can have an important role in education and establishing policies and procedures within the hospital to ensure proper handling of medicolegal cases. In many jurisdictions, those pathologists with a special interest in forensics have provided consultative services or even formal affiliations with local medical examiners. The role of the pediatric pathologist in forensic matters is expansive and most certainly will increase with community expectations (Box 17.2).

- Patients who are expected to die at home may be registered with an official hospice program and in some jurisdictions may be reported prior to death. Once death occurs, it should be reported.

- Include all relevant information when reporting death to include name, address, age, sex, race, next-of-kin, history summary, physical findings, name of last attending physician, and other pertinent data.

- After completing the investigation, the coroner or medical examiner's office decides jurisdiction of the case. When jurisdiction is assumed, the coroner or medical examiner signs the death certificate.

- The coroner or medical examiner's office will reserve the right to accept or decline jurisdiction.

- In cases in which the coroner or medical examiner is likely to accept jurisdiction, clothing or effects should not be removed, nor should the body be handled, the scene altered, or a postmortem examination performed except by authorization. When a child dies in the emergency room or shortly after admission to the hospital, preservation of the clothing, medical evidence, and witness statements, as well as documentation of wounds prior to resuscitation and/or therapeutic alteration are critical, and should be released to the investigating agency without delay.

- Do not release body to anyone other than the appropriate personnel without authorization.

- Contact the coroner or medical examiner's office *before* harvesting any organs or tissues for donation. Pressure to release organs for transplantation must be balanced with adequate death investigation. In some circumstances the investigation can be coordinated with the donation procedures, but this must be decided on a case-by-case basis, and the decision should be left with the coroner or medical examiner.

- When case jurisdiction by the coroner or medical examiner is inevitable, defer discussion with the next-of-kin regarding consent for autopsy. In circumstances that may later result in criminal charges, all communication regarding autopsy or investigation results should be released through the coroner or medical examiner.

Many pediatric forensic cases result in physicians testifying to facts before the court. Because of physicians' special training and expertise, many fact witnesses or participants in the care of the child will also be called upon to render opinions as expert witnesses due to their specialized training and expertise. An expert witness is a witness who has particular knowledge of the subject about which he is called upon to testify and who is permitted to assist the jury in understanding information outside their common knowledge. The legal definition of expert opinion is beyond the scope of this chapter, however, it is critical that any clinician providing testimony ensures that the information provided is scientific, evidence-based and unbiased.[5, 6] Despite the tragedy of serious injury and death

from possible inflicted injury, the overriding duty of the physician is to the court, not as an advocate to a party, the parents, or the child.[7] The pathologist/clinician untrained or inexperienced in forensic pathology should be especially careful to avoid rendering medicolegal opinions outside of expertise, especially concerning cause, manner, and timing of injury or death in infants and children. As society places more demands upon the legal system in matters of childhood deaths, increasing expertise on the part of medical practitioners will be required.

Cause, mechanism, and manner of death – general principles

The primary responsibility of the forensic medicolegal system is to establish for public record the cause, mechanism, and manner of death. These terms must be clearly defined and understood to ensure proper medicolegal interpretation as well as to appropriately certify the death certificate.

The **cause of death** is the disease or injury responsible for initiating the chain of physiologic events resulting in death. The **proximate cause** of death is the disease or injury that initiates an uninterrupted series of events terminating in death (the event that leads to death). The **immediate cause** of death is the reasonable or foreseeable complication of the initiating disease or injury (what killed the individual at a particular time and place).[8] The **mechanism of death**, on the other hand, refers to the physiologic derangement or biochemical disturbance produced by the cause of death that is incompatible with life. On the typical death certificate the mechanism is listed first, followed by the cause.

The **manner of death** refers to the circumstances in which the death occurred and how that cause of death came to be. In the circumstance of a childhood death this diagnosis is typically made after full analysis of autopsy findings, complete medical history, scene investigation (when appropriate), witness statements, and other investigative materials as needed. Determination of manner of death distinguishes the medicolegal system from private medical practice. The supervising or attending physician is responsible for signing the death certificate in obvious natural deaths. The coroner or medical examiner is responsible for signing all others. There are five manners of death in most US jurisdictions: natural, accident, suicide, homicide, and undetermined (Table 17.1).[9]

Therapeutic misadventure or accident (therapeutic complication) is a term used to describe circumstances of death in which the deceased has suffered an unexpected and fatal complication of medical or surgical procedures.[10, 11] Generally, these include deaths that occur during, in association with, or as the result of diagnostic, therapeutic, or anesthetic procedures; deaths that occur unexpectedly during, with, or as a result of medical procedures; deaths alleged to have been caused by malpractice; and deaths suspected to be due to prescribed drugs or toxins. Cooper[12] reviews investigation of deaths occurring

BOX 17.2 ROLE OF PEDIATRIC PATHOLOGIST IN FORENSIC MEDICINE

Surgical pathology

  Intraoperative consultation and differential diagnoses

  Documentation and chain of custody

  Child abuse reporting

Autopsy pathology

  Perinatal deaths

  SIDS program support

  Organ donation

  Traumatic deaths with prolonged hospitalization

  Sudden unexpected deaths in hospitalized children

  Iatrogenic injury

  Therapeutic misadventures/accidents

  Death certification

Laboratory medicine

  Infectious disease

  Sexual assault laboratory interpretation

  Toxicology and chemistry

  Analysis of chronic nutritional deprivation

  Coagulation analysis reporting

Perinatology

  Cause and manner of death

  Time of injury or death

  Medicolegal issues

Birth and death certificates

  Standardized protocols

  Placenta examination

  Evaluation of the abandoned infant

Clinical care

  Diagnostic assessment

  Documentation of injuries

  Ambulatory medicine

  Pattern of injury

  Education and research

  Sexual assault team

Child physical and sexual abuse programs

  Forensic evaluations

  Liaison between medical–legal–social specialties

  Participation in criminal investigation and analysis

  Educational resource – pathology of injury

  Clinical research

Medical education and research

  Pediatric and pathology residency programs

  State mortality review programs

  Continuing education for law enforcement and legal professionals

Expert testimony

TABLE 17.1 MANNER OF DEATH

Natural	Death due solely or nearly totally to disease, prematurity or aging
Accident	Death resulting from an injury or poisoning where there is little or no evidence of intent to cause harm or death. The death was unforeseen, inadvertent or otherwise unintentional
Suicide	Death resulting from an injury or poisoning that is the result of an intentional, self-inflicted act where the anticipated or expected result is self-harm or death
Homicide	Death of an individual as the result of the volitional act of another to cause fear, harm, or death. The circumstances may be either lawful or unlawful
Undetermined	Classification of death where information pointing to one manner of death is no more compelling than one or more other manners of death following thorough consideration of all available information

After Hanzlick et al 2001,[9] with permission.

during invasive medical and surgical procedures and recommends the investigation of death relating to medical care or procedure should aim to answer these questions:

- Did the medical intervention contribute to or cause the death? If yes, how?
- Did natural disease or pre-existing conditions contribute to or cause the death? If yes, how?
- Was the preoperative assessment or care appropriate and was the intervention indicated?
- Was the medical care before, during, and after the intervention adequate?

There are no specific criteria available for the designation of treatment-related mortality or therapeutic accident and the process varies between clinicians, hospitals, and countries. When identified, therapeutic accidents must be reported to the coroner or medical examiner's office for investigation. The assignment of **therapeutic misadventure** or **therapeutic accident** as the manner of death is a sophisticated forensic determination best left to persons with extensive experience (see also sudden death).

The decision to accept a case for investigation or jurisdiction varies among coroners and medical examiners, sometimes within the same office. In cases where there may be concerns about negligence, the hospital-based autopsy pathologist should seriously consider the possible perception of conflict of interest. In these circumstances it is advisable to refer the autopsy to an independent facility.

In any death, it is important to analyze clinical history, but in the circumstance of mortality associated with medical care, it may be critical to review the full history and medical record prior to beginning postmortem examination whenever possible. All medical paraphernalia should be left in situ prior to examination, especially vascular lines, and nasogastric and endotracheal tubes. Location and tip sites should be identified. Although the interpretation of postmortem cultures can be problematic, specimens should be collected and submitted whenever appropriate. If toxicologic concerns are present, careful collection, site location, and specimen handling is necessary. Literature review and consultation with relevant clinical experts regarding the nature and relative risk of the intervention before making a determination of therapeutic accident is recommended. This author makes it a habit to discuss the case with clinicians involved in the case before and after the postmortem examination to identify key questions and concerns and to clarify any potential misunderstandings.

Iatrogenic injury is generally defined as injury that is the result of an unfavorable response to medical treatment, or that is induced by the therapeutic effort itself. Reported examples of iatrogenic injury include scalded skin syndrome secondary to infected circumcision, vascular injuries secondary to catheterization or blood sampling,[13] esophageal perforation, chronic upper airway complications, complications of pharmaceuticals, etc. Woods et al[14] reviewed adverse events and preventable adverse events in children. The data suggested that approximately 70 000 hospitalized children experienced an adverse event each year. Unfortunately, iatrogenic injury is not an infrequent complication in children subjected to critical care in the neonatal and postneonatal period.[15] These problems can result in severe morbidity or mortality. **Iatrogenic diseases** and **complications of perinatal or critical care** constitute a substantial component of the pathologic lesions discovered at autopsy in children who have been provided intensive care. The role of these complications as an extension of the underlying disease process must be distinguished from a true accident (see Ch. 13).

Similarly, the distinction between natural disease and obstetric accidents must be carefully considered. If there is any question, the medical examiner should be notified. Morbidity and mortality from trauma in the prenatal or intrapartum period should be interpreted using standard forensic principles.

The private practitioner typically signs death certificates only when the manner of death is related to natural causes with the exception death from SIDS. The manner of death in these patients is traditionally labeled 'natural causes' despite the fact that the cause and mechanism of death are unknown. All SIDS cases should be referred to the coroner or medical examiner for complete investigation. If there is a possibility that the death is not due to natural causes, the medical examiner or coroner

must be notified at the time of death or as soon as practicable thereafter.

Forensic issues in the pediatric autopsy

Just as the pediatric autopsy has specific techniques and procedures, so does the forensic postmortem examination (Box 17.3). The objectives of the medicolegal autopsy and the hospital autopsy are very different, and therefore the protocols and reports of the two procedures are traditionally very different.[8, 16–18] When the autopsy is conducted by the hospital-based pediatric pathologist, an awareness of basic forensic concepts is imperative in order to document and preserve the medical facts and evidence for future analysis if a potential medicolegal issue arises. Essentials of the forensic autopsy are available in excellent reviews[1, 19] as are guidelines and protocols for the pediatric forensic examination[20, 21] Special autopsy checklists for non-accidental injury (NAI), possible metabolic disorders,[4] (Table 17.2) possible sepsis, and poisoning (Box 17.4) are available and can be used in appropriate cases.[20, 22–27] **The International Standardized Autopsy Protocol** is a detailed and comprehensive guideline that serves as a good educational

---

BOX 17.3 FUNDAMENTAL ASPECTS OF THE MEDICOLEGAL AUTOPSY

Investigation of the death scene (home or incident site)

Investigation of the death scene (body)

Event and past medical history

Chain of evidence

Radiologic examination

Trace evidence

Autopsy procedures

Specimen collection (toxicologic analyses, vitreous chemistry, etc.)

Sexual assault exam

External trace evidence

External examination

External evidence of therapy

External evidence of injury

Internal evidence of therapy

Internal evidence of injury

Internal examination

Special procedures or consultations

Documentation

Histopathologic examination

Interpretation and document preparation

TABLE 17.2 AUTOPSY CHECKLIST FOR POSSIBLE METABOLIC DISORDERS

Specimen	Storage recommendations
Urine	−70°C in 1 mL aliquots for amino acid and organic acid analysis
	Note: urine may be squeezed from the diaper if otherwise clean
Blood	EDTA blood stored as whole blood
	Heparinized blood – centrifuge promptly and store separately in 1 mL aliquots of packed cells and plasma. Store at −70°C (preferred) or at −20°C
	DNA cards for metabolic screen and/or DNA typing
	Serum: Allow blood to clot, centrifuge, pipette off and store serum in an acid-washed tube. Store at −70°C (preferred) or at −20°C
Vitreous	Send for electrolyte, urea, nitrogen, creatinine and glucose analysis. Long-term storage at −70°C (preferred) or at −20°C
Skin or pericardium	Clean skin with alcohol and place a 3.0 × 3.0 mm piece in a sterile tissue transport media for fibroblast culture. Store at −70°C if immediate culture is not available
	Note: Fibroblast may grow up to nine days after death, however for accurate tissue enzyme analysis specimens should be taken within several hours of death
Other tissues: brain, heart, kidney, liver, skeletal muscle, adrenal gland	1 mm tissue cubes place in 4% glutaraldehyde for electron microscopy 10 cm × 1 cm² blocks snap frozen in liquid nitrogen and stored at −70°C
	1 mm cubes quenched in liquid nitrogen and stored at −70°C for enzyme histochemistry
	1 cm tissue cubes of heart, liver, brain, muscle, adrenal gland, and kidney quenched in liquid nitrogen and stored at −70°C and stained with Oil red O
	5 g of spleen fresh or stored at −70°C for DNA analysis
	Note: Both MCAD and LCAD enzymes within the liver have been stable for up to 100 h if the body is refrigerated, and for at least 5 years if tissues are maintained at −70°C.

EDTA, Ethylenediaminetetraacetic acid; LCAD, long-chain acyl-CoA dehydrogenase deficiency; MCAD, medium-chain acyl-CoA dehydrogenase deficiency.
After Byard 2004,[20] with permission.

BOX 17.4 AUTOPSY CHECKLIST FOR POSSIBLE POISONING

Specimen sampling (*routine)

*Blood: Cardiac (for screening only) and peripheral (for quantification)

*Gastric aliquot (measure total volume)

*Urine

*Vitreous humor

*Liver

Brain

Fecal material

*Bile

Kidney

Skeletal muscle

Hair and nails

---

tool for the academic documentation of autopsy examination and findings in sudden infant death.[28] Many states have developed comprehensive infant death investigation guidelines.[4] Individuals who have responsibility for infant autopsies should be familiar with forensic postmortem guidelines before initiating the postmortem examination.

The medicolegal autopsy report is a document that will be used by law enforcement and others and should contain complete and precise descriptions of the observations made. Standardized autopsy language, content and report templates,[29] many available electronically, allow for more uniform reporting of autopsy information. It is important to be familiar with the procedures and materials for preservation of evidence, how to obtain access to the criminal laboratory resources and support personnel, as well as how to contact individuals with special expertise. In the emerging world of Internet communications, access to specialty organizations and list services can provide special expertise even to the remotest of locations.

Infant death investigation requires careful coordination of the many disciplines participating in health care delivery, emergency response, law enforcement, and forensic medicolegal analysis.[4, 30–32] Continuing education and multidisciplinary programs have emphasized the roles and responsibilities to the investigative process for paramedics, emergency and critical care personnel as participants in the investigative process. In many children's hospitals the child abuse program has taken the role of coordinating the investigative process. This can work well only if the participants are able to function in a neutral, diagnostic role; not as advocates for the criminal process. In the ideal circumstance, the members of the investigative teams have established relationships and understand the nature of the various roles and responsibilities. In many jurisdictions the participants

BOX 17.5 DEATH SCENE INVESTIGATION

Home or incident site

Geographic location

Comparison to other neighboring dwellings

Appearance of dwelling

   State of repair

   Degree of cleanliness

   State and appropriateness of furnishings

   Dangerous environmental conditions

   Presence of paints, solvents, or other chemicals

   Presence of rodent or insect infestation

   Interior and exterior ambient temperature

Weather conditions (when appropriate: room and outdoor temperature)

Nature and quality of clothing

Amount and type of available food

Condition and appearance of siblings

Behavior of parents and others present

Presence of paraphernalia suggestive of drug abuse

Condition and safety of electric and plumbing fixtures

Scald cases

   Water temperature at faucet

   Water temperature at water heater

   Heights of tubs, sinks, and fixtures

Photographs, measurements, and drawings of the general and specific scene

Fall cases

   Surface impacted: surface and base

   Footing or evidence of tripping

   Height and location of fall

   Witnesses – including children

Body

Terminal position

   Was it moved or altered?

   Pattern of lividity

   Presence of rigor mortis

   Co-sleeping placement found

   Evaluate and when possible measure body and room temperature

Hygiene

Apparent state of health

Resuscitation attempted

   Type and extent, duration

   Equipment used

   Response

Attire, bedding surface, pillows

Toys or objects near body

Presence of purge or exudates, frank blood on bedding, face, clothes

Trauma

Odors

Obtain evidence

   Stains

   Blood

   Medications

   Objects

   Documentation

   Photograph

   Sketch

are not in real time communication and availability of information may proceed piecemeal. It is therefore critical to maintain ongoing collaboration to ensure that all parties understand their roles and responsibilities. The autopsy pathologist is ultimately responsible to ensure that the necessary information is available before final diagnoses and opinions are released.

Communication with law enforcement to provide additional information, scene visits, and scene reenactment or witness inquiry can be essential in answering the ultimate question of cause and manner of death. Details required for a thorough death investigation are extensive and must be coordinated by experienced personnel (Box 17.5). The role of the forensic pathologist in providing ongoing training and education cannot be underestimated.

Pediatric forensic death investigation

The pediatric forensic autopsy should begin with investigation of the death scene(s). Scene investigation will be required in all cases of SIDS and cases of unexpected deaths of children where trauma or inflicted injury may be a consideration. Scene investigation should start where the body is initially discovered. In child abuse cases, there may be several 'scenes' including where the injuries reportedly took place, the site to which the body was moved, transport vehicles, the hospital or emergency department where the child was initially examined, and the facility where the death occurred. Trace evidence, scene information and events may be important from many or all of these loci as well as the victim's and (when known) the suspect's clothing.

TABLE 17.3 HISTORY

Medical history	General and recent state of health
	Medications
	Physician and hospital records
	Prenatal records
	Birth records analysis: complications, assisted delivery
	Growth and development analysis
	Growth rate charts (OFC, weight and length)
	Developmental level of child
	Well child, urgent care, ED encounters
	Insurance reports
Family history	Family size and structure
	Age distribution of siblings
	Socioeconomic conditions
	Recent change or stressors
	Medical background of parents
	Medical background of siblings
Other	Welfare, police, and child protection records
	School records (when appropriate)
Postmortem	Statements
	Parent or guardian observations and explanation
	Siblings and other witnesses
	Investigative reports
	Police/Fire/Rescue
	Paramedic
	CPS documents and consultations
	Others as available

CPS; Child protective services; ED, emergency department; OFC, occipital–frontal circumference.

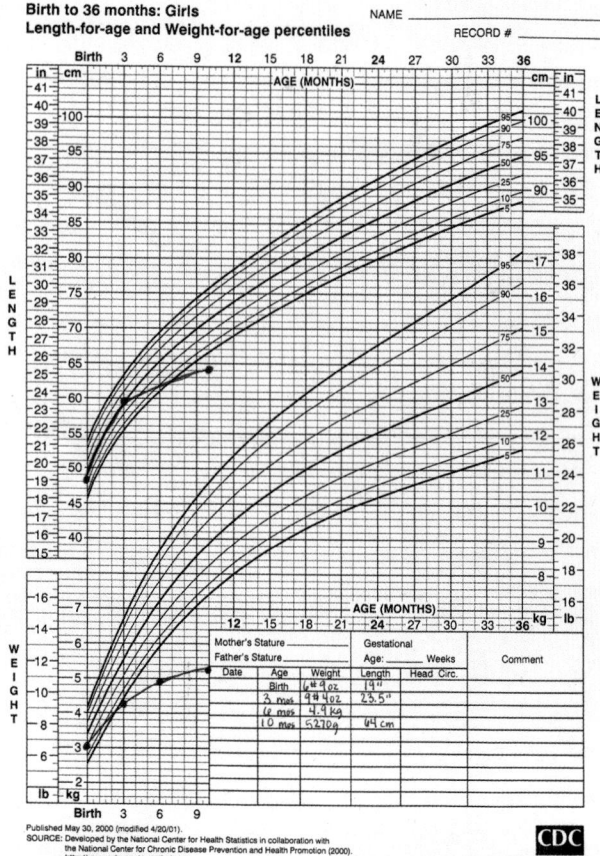

FIGURE 17.2 Growth curve demonstrating failure to thrive.

In some circumstances the scene of the fatal event is not immediately accessible. This includes cases in which the child is brought to the emergency room (ER) before the pronouncement of death and often before the full extent of the problem is known or 'foul play' is suspected. In these instances **the child is the death scene** and the physical evidence admitted with and on the child must be completely documented and protected from contamination. If possible, the deceased child should be handled minimally in the ER to preserve physical evidence.

Any items can constitute physical evidence. It is most important that nothing be moved or touched at the scene before investigators arrive. If evidence must be secured or removed, it is imperative that the individuals handling the materials document the location, appearance, and condition as well as the date, times, and chain of custody. Proper handling of specimens includes placing and sealing damp articles in clean, dry, labeled paper bags to avoid mildew and contamination. Photographs are valuable in tracking and supporting the reconstruction of evidence and events.

An adequate history documenting the circumstances surrounding the death is of vital importance (Table 17.3). Although complete information may not be obtainable before the autopsy, considerable effort must be made to procure the entire history before cause and manner of death are determined. In the young infant (< 12 months) detailed analysis of birth records, medical encounters and details of recent hospitalizations may be necessary to assess the condition of the child prior to death. These documents may demonstrate a pattern of medical inattention, slowing or abnormal growth (Fig. 17.2), indications of chronic illness, or significant pre-existing injury.

The postmortem examination

The forensic autopsy protocol includes radiology, external examination, photography, internal examination, histopathology examination, and other special studies. Other important facets of the examination include detailed collection of evidence and clothing inventory and description.

Appropriate **radiologic** examination is necessary in cases of sudden unexpected death (Table 17.4). The skeletal survey is a necessary adjunct to the pediatric forensic autopsy to identify the presence of pre-existing or unknown traumatic injury, to identify and assist in diagnosis of disease, and to guide the appropriate

TABLE 17.4 SUGGESTED RADIOGRAPHIC VIEWS TO CONFIRM CHILD ABUSE AT POSTMORTEM EXAMINATION[119]

Appendicular skeleton – anterior-posterior (AP)	Humeri Forearms Femurs Lower legs Hands (oblique PA) and feet are not routinely indicated
Axial skeleton	Thorax (AP and lateral) Pelvis (AP: including mid and lower spine) Lumbar spine (lateral) Cervical spine (lateral) Skull (frontal and lateral)
Extremity joints (individual AP)	Right and left shoulder, elbow, wrist, hip, knee, and ankle
Other	Radiographic examination during course of autopsy may provide additional documentation (e.g. removal of ribs, high-detail radiography for metaphyseal fractures)
Technique	High resolution High contrast Screen/film speed not to exceed 200 low kV peak (bone technique) Single emulsion or special film-screen combination

TABLE 17.5 DOCUMENTATION AND REPORT PREPARATION

Photography	High quality digital/35 mm color transparencies Appropriate color balance Light source without distortion (flash or flood) Ruler present in all fields of view Identifying tag in all photographs Entire body and all surfaces including face Wounds photographed before and after cleaning Gaping wounds (incised or stab) photographed open and artificially closed with transparent tape Scalp hair shaved as indicated (save hair) Injuries photographed with anatomic landmarks Magnification capabilities for necessary details (macro-type lens)

Autopsy protocol	Report contains information regarding conduct of procedure, to include:
	    Name of deceased, birth date
	    Case number
	    Name of facility
	    Name of pathologist
	    Name(s) of person(s) assisting
	    Name(s) of all persons in attendance
	    Time and date of death or when found
	    Time and date of autopsy
	    Identification: how the decedent is identified
	    List external injuries (when absent, none noted)
	    List internal injuries
	Report written clearly in language understandable by lay personnel
	Injuries listed clearly
	Pertinent negatives documented
	List specimens and site of collection
	Include reports of any special studies:
	Neuropathology, odontology, crime laboratory
	Pathologic diagnoses

Analysis and documentation of additional materials reviewed	Analysis of medical history Radiologist report and X-rays Toxicologic reports Laboratory analyses Investigative reports
Interpretation	Traditionally the forensic autopsy report interpretation is limited to cause and manner of death

gross and histologic sampling of injury.[33] The 'babygram' or one-shot radiographic image is not an acceptable replacement for the technically appropriate skeletal survey. When the technology is available the preferred technique is high-detail radiography with histopathologic correlation.[34] Postmortem magnetic resonance imaging (MRI) and computed tomography (CT) imagery can be utilized when premortem studies are not available or are inadequate for documentation of neck/spinal injuries, as well as to assist in delineating brain injuries in suspected child abuse.[35] If adequate premortem studies are available, they need not be repeated postmortem.

In the **external examination**, confirmation of the child's identification, evidence of therapy, and the presence of all injuries must be detailed (Box 17.6). External soft tissue injuries must be handled appropriately, especially in case of possible inflicted injuries. The use of body charts and diagrams are often helpful adjuncts for review by investigative personnel. For documentation of injuries, defining the location of the lesion using the following three parameters is recommended:

- number of inches or centimeters from the top of the head or above the sole of the foot;
- number of inches or centimeters to the right or left of the anterior or posterior midline; and
- number of inches or centimeters from a well-established landmark such as the nipple in the prepubertal child or male, sternal notch,

umbilicus, acromion, external auditory canal, angle of the jaw, or appropriate reference joint (for injuries to extremities).

As injuries evolve or the body is dissected for postmortem examination, evidence can be lost that is irretrievable. Therefore, adequate **photography** (Table 17.5) is critical in documenting injury and is often used for review by other

BOX 17.6 EXTERNAL EXAMINATION OF THE BODY

Evidence of injury

Careful examination of all body areas

    Scalp – shave hair when necessary

    Nape of neck

    Surface of hands/between fingers

    Soles of feet

    Back and buttocks

    All body orifices and genitalia

    Conjunctiva, inner eyelids

    Inner surfaces of oral cavity/frenulum

    Incisions into suspicious soft tissue areas

Use of diagrammatic sketches

Description of recent, healing, and healed injuries

Location of injuries in relation to anatomic landmarks (measured)

Measured dimensions of injuries and/or lesions (× 3 axes)

Examination for pattern

Description of color

Use of standardized descriptors or language

Photograph with identifier and ruler; all injuries

Incision of lividity to confirm absence of bruising

Excision of wounds in toto when appropriate

Representative sampling of wounds, bruises, and fractures

External evidence of therapy

Evidence of resuscitation (CPR)

Catalog and describe therapeutic paraphernalia

Site or location

    Indwelling vascular lines

    Chest tubes

    Catheters

    Venipuncture marks

    Tape marks

    Therapeutically induced trauma

Confirm identification

If unknown, obtain footprints

    If decomposed, forensic odontology specimens, forensic entomology, radiologic analysis, and anthropologic analysis may be indicated

Clothing examination and description

Catalog and describe general appearance of clothing and personal items

Describe and document tears and stains with collection of trace evidence

Collection of evidence

Sexual assault examination when indicated: Oral, rectal, anal, skin, and clothing

Bite mark evidence

Blood – toxicology

Vitreous humor – postmortem chemistry

Infectious culture

Hairs, fibers, or other trace evidence

Sampling of traumatic injuries for histopathology

External examination: general

Calculate child's age

    To nearest $1/2$ month < age 3 years

    To nearest 1 month > 3 years

Record weight

    To nearest 1–2 oz or ~50 g < 2 years

    To nearest 1 lb or 0.5 kg > 2 years

    Estimation of degree of dehydration must be included

Record length

    To nearest $1/2$ inch or 1 cm

    Estimation of degree of shortening due to postmortem contracture or change

Record OFC

    To nearest $1/2$ inch or 1 cm

Plot weight, height, OFC, and 'weight for height' on standard curves (www.cdc.gov/growthcharts)

Comparison of growth and development with normal values and previous records

Assessment of state of nutrition

Assessment and description of postmortem changes

    Livor

    Rigor

    Body temperature

    General state of hygiene

    Presence and characteristics of decomposition

    Presence of animal/insect activity

CPR, Cardiopulmonary resuscitation; OFC, occipital–frontal circumference.

experts and for display in court.[36, 37] Forensic photography requires high quality photographs with adequate light source and appropriate identification with a ruler in the photo. Efforts should be made to reduce the background materials and the field should be clean for courtroom viewing. Photographic documentation should be coordinated by local law enforcement rather than using inexperienced staff or inadequate equipment.

Subcutaneous fat measurement usually performed at umbilicus

Estimated urinary volume

Contents of gastrointestinal tract described

Collection, measurement, and preservation of gastric contents when appropriate

Careful examination of clavicle and ribcage (skeletal examination)

Measurement of volume of body cavity fluids, weight of blood clots when appropriate

Orderly examination and documentation of normal findings

Appropriate organ weights and measurements using quality controlled equipment and procedure

Careful stripping and preservation of dura

Careful internal dissection of neck organs (after removal of brain and chest organs)

Posterior neck dissection, when appropriate

Internal evidence of injury

Internal evidence of disease

Internal evidence of therapy

In circumstances of possible bite mark injuries, the American Board of Forensic Odontology (ABFO) has published guidelines for preservation and analysis of evidence.[38] A forensically trained odontologist should be consulted before the lesions are disturbed.

A careful, thorough **internal examination** (Box 17.7) for forensic purposes begins with standard pediatric autopsy procedures. Organ weights and measures must be compared to expected weights for age and body size. Meticulous documentation of internal injury, evidence of therapy, and disease is essential. Additional measurements, organ dissections, and special studies are performed as indicated (Table 17.6). Pertinent negatives should be listed in the autopsy protocol.

Prior to the internal dissection, materials for toxicology or chemistry testing must be collected. There are no specific requirements, however, if there is not an adequate premortem sample for electrolyte testing, sampling of vitreous fluid must be seriously considered. In the event of no anatomic cause of death, this important diagnostic test may be vital. In the event of significant postmortem decomposition, liver and spleen can be preserved for toxicologic analysis. Many laboratories routinely preserve liver specimens for toxicologic evaluation as needed.

Histopathology examination consists of sampling and viewing routine microscopic sections of viscera as well as sections from visceral and soft tissue abnormalities and injuries. The pediatric pathologist routinely collects a complete sampling of appropriate tissue sections. Unfortunately there are no uniformly accepted guidelines for postmortem histology in childhood. Sampling of traumatic injuries; sampling routine organs with and without pathology; and appropriate fixation and sampling of brain, brainstem and spinal cord are mandatory in any case of sudden traumatic death that could involve inflicted injury and in any case that is yet unexplained following autopsy. Special dissection may be indicated in sexual assault, history of fall, cases with possible deep tissue contusions, premortem or postmortem diagnosis of occult fractures etc. Fractures and injuries must be sampled and examined histologically when there is suspicion of abuse. Often overlooked is the bone sampling of the skull fracture.

Consultation with physician experts is a regular and expected part of clinical practice. Similarly, in the forensic autopsy it is commonplace to consult with a number of available experts in fields such as neuropathology, radiology, forensic odontology, anthropology, cardiac pathology, etc. Special testing and consultation should be considered at the beginning of the autopsy to ensure the proper approaches, prioritization, and preparation for special studies and proper collection and handling of materials for special consultation. In the unusual childhood injury or death, it is better to pend or defer a diagnosis or death certificate while consultation proceeds rather than render what may be an incorrect diagnosis. Neuropathology examination using industry specific sampling and processing is expected in children who die with brain injuries.[38] Cardiac pathology consultation in certain unexplained sudden deaths is available for the pathologist with less experience in special myocardial conduction dissection. The metabolic autopsy can and should be initiated in children with clinical indications (Table 17.2).

Unfortunately there are numerous examples of cases going to trial for criminal charges of homicide with poor quality or no autopsy photographs, inadequate central nervous system (CNS) examination in fatal brain injury cases, inadequate assessment of the presence or absence of tissue vital reaction – all of which may be required to answer critical mediocolegal questions.

Chain of custody is the procedure established to verify the possession of an object from the time it is collected until it is offered into evidence in court. Typically the police laboratory is given the responsibility of ensuring the appropriate handling of trace evidence as it is passed from one individual to another for processing, storage, or transfer to law enforcement or crime laboratory personnel. Each piece of trace evidence (including any laboratory specimens used in a possible criminal investigation) should be labeled with victim's name, date and time of collection, type of specimen, identifying number or code, and initials of the person who obtained the specimen. Proper closure with evidence tape secures the specimen. The specimen may be directly transferred to a law enforcement officer, a locked container, or another area of restricted access. A document identifying all individuals receiving the specimen, personally logged with time and date of transfer, must be included.

Pitfalls in pediatric forensic investigations are listed in Box 17.8.[40]

TABLE 17.6 SPECIAL STUDIES

Postmortem chemistry	Vitreous humor: collect and analyze electrolytes and other chemistries
	Serum and CSF: obtain as indicated
Microbiology/Virology	Lung, blood, spleen, nasopharyngeal swabs, CSF for culture or rapid antigen testing when appropriate
Toxicology	Blood, urine, bile, liver, gastric contents, other tissues as indicated
Bite mark analysis	Recovery of serologic specimens before contamination can occur
	Forensic odontology examination prior to any disruption of wound
	Black and white and color photography
	Impression castings when appropriate
DNA	Collect and appropriately retain blood sample for potential DNA typing
	All cases
Postmortem retinal photography/ Removal of eyes in young infants and children	When appropriate
Neuropathology	When head trauma is suspected, brain, brainstem and spinal cord should be examined only after complete fixation
Blood and body fluids	Specimens preserved for special analysis by forensic laboratory, as indicated (e.g. antigen testing or DNA analysis)
Metabolic assays and testing (MCAD, long QT)	When appropriate
Histopathology	Routine
	Special studies
	Iron morphometry – lung – possible suffocation
	Iron and trichrome – wound healing, subdural hemorrhage
	β-amyloid precursor protein (β APP) – head trauma analysis
Sexual assault examination	
Cardiac pathology examination	
Postmortem special diagnostic imaging	

NOTE: Retain liver, gastric contents, bile in all sudden, unexpected, unexplained death

BAPP, β-amyloid precursor protein; CSF, cerebrospinal fluid; MCAD, medium-chain acyl-CoA dehydrogenase deficiency. Iron staining, e.g., Turnbull blue.

Postmortem changes[41]

Appropriate interpretation of postmortem changes is crucial in pediatric death investigation.[42–44] Many children die before paramedics arrive and are subsequently transported to hospitals where they are pronounced dead. Since a complete and adequate assessment is not made in the field before transport, it is critical that specific physical changes be noted in the ER and again at the postmortem examination. Basic postmortem changes or findings should be considered and documented: algor mortis, livor mortis, rigor mortis, gastric content, evidence and extent of postmortem decomposition, postmortem artifact, and artifacts of medical intervention or body handling. With this data, a better assessment of the **postmortem interval** becomes more likely. Approximate time or range of time of death can be vitally important in determining the appropriateness of the history provided should the death be due to other than natural causes. *The Estimation of the Time Since Death in the Early Postmortem Period* is an excellent reference that provides current scientific principles and analytical tools for interpreting time of death.[45]

Algor mortis

Algor mortis can simply be defined as postmortem cooling of the body. The rate of cooling is affected by a wide variety of factors such as ambient temperature, conductive surfaces in contact with the body, body posture, body size, clothing, body fat, air flow across the body, premortem conditions such as hyper- or hypothermia, and humidity. Infants and children cool more quickly because the heat gradient from the body core is steeper.[45]

Typically, little cooling takes place during the first hour after death; in fact, the core temperature may rise. One method commonly used to estimate the postmortem interval is that the body cools at approximately 1–1.5°C per hour for the first 6 to 12 hours. Studies using this methodology have been demonstrated to be highly inaccurate.[46] The rate of cooling slows as the body approaches the ambient environmental temperature. As a general rule internal organ temperatures generally reach ambient temperature within 18–24 hours.

Temperature recording of the internal organs, prior to autopsy, is best approximated via deep auditory canal, rectum, deep nostril, or small incision with thermometer probe

BOX 17.8 PITFALLS IN PEDIATRIC FORENSIC PATHOLOGY[40]

- Incomplete or absent scene investigation
- Improper postmortem interval assessment
- Inadequate or incomplete medical records
- Incomplete pre-autopsy study
- Inadequate or incomplete autopsy documentation (description, photography, special studies)
- Inadequate gross autopsy examination
- Incomplete microscopic examination
- Incomplete laboratory studies
- Failure to document and differentiate artifacts
- Failure to give appropriate importance and significance to findings
- Over interpretation of circumstances or conditions beyond that which is scientifically supportable, especially if the interpretation exceeds the expertise of the examiner
- Taking an adversarial or advocacy role in the investigative proceedings, rather than functioning as a neutral interpreter of scientific fact. Use of inflammatory or biased language jeopardizing the scientific content of the findings.
- Failure to obtain consultation in areas of inexperience before rendering opinions or suggesting further action. Several kinds of consultants who must be available in children's autopsies in which death related to injury or neglect are considerations include: pathologist experienced in forensic pathology (preferably board certified), pediatric pathologist, pediatric radiologist, neuropathologist, pediatrician and pediatric subspecialists, cardiac pathologist, forensic odontologist, forensic anthropologist

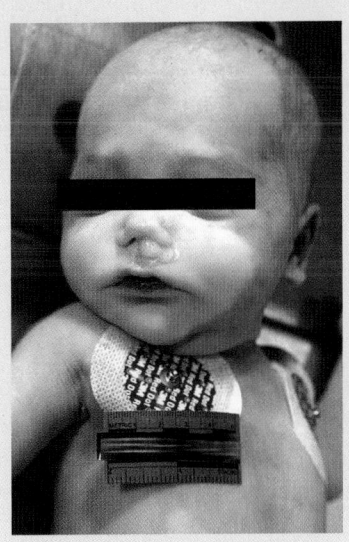

FIGURE 17.3 Dependent livor mortis with pressure sparing of compressed facial tissue.

introduced into the liver parenchyma. The temperature assessment based on feeling the body has little value in the determination of postmortem interval. It would be ideal to document ambient room or environment temperatures as well as deep nasal or external auditory temperature in all cases.

Interpretation of body temperature must take into account the available information regarding the circumstances of death and environmental temperatures. For instance, in children, rapid antemortem temperature instability and cooling can occur during resuscitation, especially in circumstances associated with severe shock. Heat stress or injury may affect postmortem body temperatures.

Livor mortis

Livor mortis (hypostasis, lividity) is the purple discoloration of the skin and organs that develops about the dependent portions of the body after death. It is the direct result of blood settling or pooling into capillaries that dilate after circulation stops. Livor mortis is typically absent where the weight of the body against a supporting object (i.e. mattress, diaper, bedclothes) has compressed the capillaries and inhibits them from filling with blood (Fig. 17.3). Livor mortis also occurs internally, most typically in lungs and bowel loops and should not be confused with visceral bruising or injury. Livor mortis pattern can be useful in determining the terminal position of the body in identifying discrepancies in the historical account of death.

The onset of **livor mortis begins at death** with the cessation of circulation. It can be observed in the dependent tissues within the first hour postmortem. Livor mortis is typically well developed within 4–6 hours with its **peak expected at 8–12 hours**. After 8–12 hours livor mortis becomes fixed, referring to failure of the discoloration to blanch with pressure. This fixation is a result of a number of factors, including the congealing of fat and jelled blood that obstructs the capillaries, leakage of blood into the tissues, and hemolysis. Livor mortis will occur with change of body position indefinitely until the body tissues become discolored from tissue hemolysis with early postmortem decomposition.[44] The traditional pathology assessment of color and degree of fixation of livor mortis does not have significant application in determining time of death.

The color of livor mortis may provide clues to cause of death. **Deep purple livor** is often seen in **asphyxial deaths**, whereas **bright cherry livor** is characteristic of **carbon monoxide poisoning, cyanide poisoning,** or a death in **ice water or snow**. Brown livor mortis is characteristic of methemoglobinemia. The *absence* of livor can be observed in cases of severe anemia or exsanguination. Livor may also be absent externally in drowning when the body remains submerged for a number of hours. A special form of livor known as **Tardieu spots, confluent petechial hemorrhage** that represents leakage of blood from congested capillaries, can be frequently seen in **asphyxial deaths associated with venous congestion as well as some circumstances of dependent livor mortis**.

Differentiation of a bruise from livor mortis can be difficult and cannot always be accomplished by external observation.

To distinguish a bruise from livor mortis, incise the area. Incision into a bruise will display blood enmeshed into the tissue and upon microscopic examination will often reveal vital reaction or fibrin deposition. If the discoloration is due to livor mortis, the blood will leak from the tissue and can be wiped away, leaving the tissue essentially unstained; microscopically there will be no vital reaction or fibrin deposition.

Rigor mortis

Rigor mortis is stiffness or rigidity of the muscles that is the consequence of postmortem muscle contraction. With onset of rigor, muscles no longer respond to electrical or chemical stimuli. The process is not completely understood but coincides with the loss of adenosine triphosphate (ATP) from muscle cells with simultaneous increase in lactic acid.

At the time of somatic death, the muscles begin a three-phase process. Initially, they remain flaccid and receptive to electrical or chemical stimuli. Muscle (such as patellar) reflexes may be elicited for a short period postmortem. Next, the muscles develop the rigidity described as rigor mortis; and finally, the rigidity relents coincident to the onset of putrefaction. After rigor relents, it will not reform.

Rigor mortis can first be observed in the short-fiber muscle groups. These include the eyelids and muscles of mastication. The shoulders, arms, and lastly the bulky leg muscles follow these muscle groups. Rigor may also be observed as cutis anserina (goose bumps) as it develops in the erector pili muscles.

The variation in the development of rigor limits its usefulness in determining the postmortem interval. The onset and subsequent development of rigor is influenced by external and internal factors that include the state of health, fever, convulsions, strenuous physical activity immediately preceding death, effects of poison, and elevated environmental temperatures. It can be significantly delayed by rapid cooling of the body. Freezing of the body may postpone the onset of rigor, which will occur when the tissues are thawed.

The development of rigor in children is typically more rapid than in adults. Complete rigor has been observed in SIDS victims within 2 hours of having been put to bed. Rigor may also be poorly or incompletely developed in infants and in circumstances of decreased muscle mass, such as in severe malnutrition or chronic disease state. The relenting of rigor mortis also occurs more quickly in infants.

Krompecher et al[47] have proposed a standardized measurement of cadaveric rigidity. Using this technique the following observations are reported:

- If there is an increase in muscle rigidity under observation, the postmortem interval is < 5 hours.
- If there is a decrease in muscle rigidity under observation, the postmortem interval is no less than 7 hours.
- If the rigidity has completely relented the postmortem interval is ≥ 24 hours.

Rigor preserves the posture of the body at the time of death, assuming that the body was not moved. It is therefore critical that the death scene investigator observe and evaluate the state of rigor mortis before manipulating the body.

Gastric contents

Examination of gastric contents is a routine part of the forensic examination. Presence of food and the degree of digestion can be important in piecing together the nature and content of the last meal or meals. Gastric contents should be preserved in any case where toxicology or poisoning is considered. The factors that affect gastric emptying are numerous and unpredictable thus, the presence or absence of gastric emptying should not be considered in assessing time of death.

Postmortem decomposition

Postmortem decomposition takes two separate forms: **autolysis** and **putrefaction**. Autolysis refers to fermentative processes that occur without the participation of bacteria. Histologically, these processes involve the disintegration of cellular structures. Biochemically, this corresponds to a loss of orderly metabolism. Resistance to autolysis varies from organ to organ and also from thorax to abdomen, the latter being much more susceptible. Autolysis occurs very early in enzyme-producing organs, such as the pancreas and adrenals, and occurs last in the reproductive organs. Factors that can accelerate autolysis include body and environmental temperature (most pronounced at 37–40°C) and hepatic atrophy leading to metabolic disturbances. The autolytic process also varies between individuals. Because of this variability, its use in establishing the postmortem interval is limited, and any attempt to do so must include knowledge of the environmental conditions.

Putrefaction is tissue degeneration and breakdown due to bacteria and fermentation. After death, the bacteria of the gastrointestinal (GI) tract invade the vascular system, spreading through the body, producing putrefactive change. Putrefaction is influenced by internal (i.e. presence of bacteria) and external (i.e. humidity and ambient temperature) factors that affect the process in an unpredictable manner. The sequence of events is not consistent, but generally the initial observation is greenish discoloration of the lower abdomen followed by greenish discoloration of the head, neck, shoulders; swelling of the face; and marbling (greenish black discoloration along blood vessels). Generalized bloating, skin slippage, and hair slippage follow. The process may be accelerated in the presence of traumatic injury and/or increased ambient temperature. There is no definitive approach to assessing time since death based on putrefaction because so many variables can be involved (Fig. 17.4).

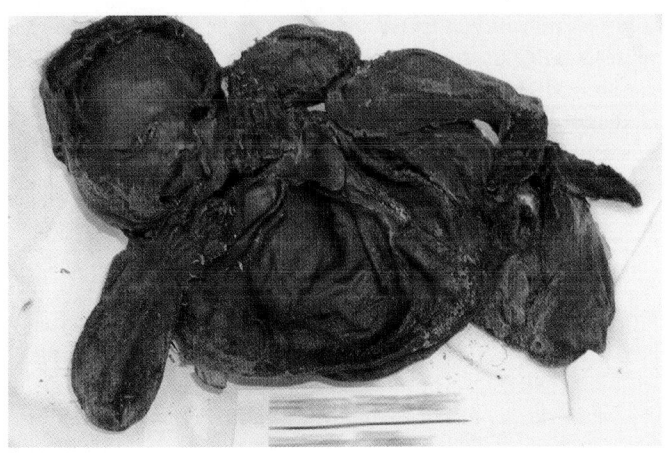

FIGURE 17.4 Advanced decomposition in an abandoned infant with mummification.

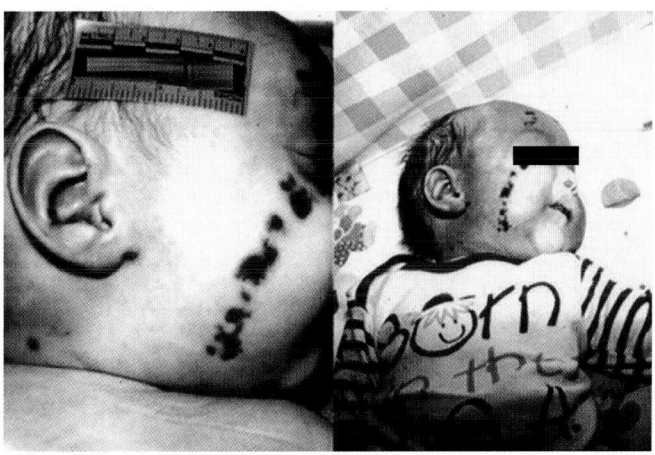

FIGURE 17.5 Facial lesions due to postmortem insect activity.

Maceration

When a fetus dies in an intact amniotic sac, decomposition (maceration) begins immediately.[48] As the amniotic sac does not normally contain bacteria the decomposition typically is not putrefactive. Rapid loss of tone and tissue softening occurs. Early changes are most obvious in the skin and are characterized by delamination of the epidermis from the dermis. This provides the appearance of **skin slippage,** which typically occurs in the last trimester. Earlier in gestation the skin is less differentiated and more adherent to the underlying connective tissue. Fluid accumulation between the epidermis and dermis forms **bullae,** which generally rupture during birth and give the appearance of large-scale peeling of skin. As the red blood cells hemolyze, the skin develops a reddish discoloration and eventually muscles, connective tissue, viscera, and the umbilical cord develop a uniform similarity of color. Hemolyzed blood and fluids collect in the peritoneal and pleural cavities. It is important to distinguish the postmortem changes of maceration from those of putrefaction in the abandoned infant.

Timing of injury and death in the stillborn infant is a question that frequently arises in the perinatal autopsy. Pattern of injury, vital reaction, placenta, umbilical cord, and infant examination as well as careful clinical review must be a part of the diagnostic process. Genest and colleagues reviewed factors to be considered in determining the timing of death in the stillborn infant from the external examination and histologic examination of fetal tissues and placenta (Table 17.7).[49–51]

Postmortem artifact and injury

Postmortem artifacts and injuries can also complicate interpretation of the examination. These include desiccation, the appearance of trauma caused by insects or animals and traumatic injuries occurring postmortem (Fig. 17.5). Artifacts induced by freezing of tissues, such as those seen in the frozen body of a concealed newborn, must not be confused with intrauterine maceration. Careful photographic documentation of the body at various times in the investigative process can assist the analysis of postmortem artifacts. It is also important to note that early putrefactive changes can occur ante mortem when life is supported for a protracted period.

Postmortem chemistries

Laboratory chemical analysis may provide a cause of death, assist in interpreting autopsy findings, and assist in determining the approximate postmortem interval.[52] In children and infants, blood of sufficient quantity is typically obtained at autopsy after the body cavity has been opened. At that time, blood can be obtained from a number of sources. Blind cardiac puncture should never be attempted, as contamination may occur should the needle be advanced into the trachea or esophagus. Blood to be analyzed should be placed in appropriate sterile tubes. Blood to be held for further analysis should be separated and the serum frozen. Hemolyzed blood may still be useful for many determinations and should not be discarded. Urine is easily obtained and should be preserved.

Postmortem **vitreous chemistries** are especially useful and should be a part of the standard pediatric autopsy.[53–56] The interpretation of postmortem chemistries requires an understanding of how the various fluids are affected by postmortem changes.[57] The chemical composition of vitreous humor is more stable postmortem than either blood or cerebrospinal fluid (CSF) and reflects antemortem plasma concentrations of sodium, chloride, and urea nitrogen.[58] Coe[59] identified that high or low values of vitreous sodium and chloride, high vitreous urea nitrogen determinations and elevated vitreous glucose values accurately reflect antemortem physiologic abnormalities. The fall of glucose post mortem may be both rapid and severe, invalidating the use of vitreous glucose to determine antemortem hypoglycemia. Postmortem vitreous fluid obtained after embalming will still provide accurate results.[60]

TABLE 17.7 STILLBIRTH: DETERMINATION OF POSTMORTEM INTERVAL[49–51]

Histologic features in stillborn examination	
Good predictors of death-to-delivery interval	
Kidney: loss of tubular nuclear basophilia*	4 h
Liver: loss of hepatocyte nuclear basophilia	24 h
Myocardium: inner half loss of basophilia	24 h
Myocardium: outer half loss of nuclear basophilia	48 h
Bronchus: loss of epithelial nuclear basophilia	96 h
GI tract: maximal loss of nuclear basophilia	96 h
Adrenal: maximal loss of nuclear basophilia	1 week
Trachea: chondrocyte loss of nuclear basophilia	1 week
Kidney: maximal loss of nuclear basophilia	> 4 weeks
Examination of placenta in determination of time of death	
Histologic features in placenta examination	
Good predictors of death-to-delivery interval	
Intravascular karyorrhexis	6 h
Stem vessel luminal abnormalities	
Multifocal (10–25% of stem villi)	48 h
Extensive (> 25% stem villi)	14 days
Extensive villous fibrosis	14 days
Examination of stillborn in determination of time of death	
External fetal examination in the stillborn	
Good predictors of death-to-delivery interval	
Desquamation 1 cm	6 h
Cord discoloration (brown or red)	6 h
Desquamation face, back, or abdomen	12 h
Desquamation 5% of body	18 h
Desquamation 2 or more of 11 zones	18 h
Skin color brown or tan	24 h
Moderate or severe desquamation	24 h
Mummification (any)	2 weeks

*Loss of nuclear basophilia means at least 1% of nuclei are totally pink; the presence of nuclear basophilia means all nuclei are partially blue.

Gentle aspiration of the clear fluid from the globe of the eye can be performed utilizing a 3 mL syringe with a 20-gauge needle, inserted into the globe near the outer canthus. At least 1 mL of vitreous can be obtained from each globe even in the newborn infant. The fluid sample can be run on a regular chemistry analyzer. As in any other area of clinical chemistry, the important factors to record are sample time, sample source, method of acquisition, analytic methodology, and normal values. Vitreous electrolytes may be the only clue to cause of death in some cases of sudden death in infancy.

Glucose

Postmortem serum glucose is notoriously unreliable and should not be utilized. Postmortem glycolysis decreases the serum glucose, and elevation of the levels from normal can be seen when stress is noted in the terminal event. Vitreous humor is not significantly affected by terminal stress, and the value is representative of the overall physiologic state before death. An elevated vitreous glucose level with the presence of ketones is diagnostic of diabetic ketoacidosis. Interpretation of low postmortem glucose as evidence of antemortem hypoglycemia is controversial.

Lactic acid

Sturner and colleagues studied the postmortem values of vitreous lactic acid for 102 children dying from a variety of causes, including SIDS.[61] The lowest average values were seen in asphyxial deaths (137–151 mg/dL); the highest value was seen in SIDS with secondary findings (221 mg/dL). Sturner and colleagues concluded that decreased lactic acid values combined with history, circumstances, and autopsy findings may aid in distinguishing a SIDS death from death by asphyxia. This test is not part of the routine postmortem analysis.

Nitrogen retention

Urea and creatinine remain stable after death in both the vitreous humor and CSF. Vitreous urea nitrogen is also interpretable after embalming. Elevated urea nitrogen in combination with an electrolyte imbalance is diagnostic of antemortem dehydration. Because creatinine is less subject to variation from antemortem prerenal conditions, both analyses should be performed if renal disease may be implicated in the proximate cause of death.

Electrolytes

Sodium and **chloride** levels decrease erratically in blood after death. In the vitreous humor, both remain relatively stable in the early postmortem period but decline with increased postmortem interval. Vitreous sodium values in the early postmortem period reflect antemortem serum levels, whereas vitreous chloride levels run generally slightly higher (about 120 mEq/L) than blood.

Serum **calcium** levels obtained very shortly after death reflect the antemortem values; however, they increase as time passes. The vitreous calcium level remains stable until frank decomposition commences, at which point it increases.

Vitreous electrolyte abnormalities

Vitreous **potassium** values increase linearly during the postmortem interval. It can be used as an adjunct in estimating the postmortem interval by obtaining the vitreous from one eye and then from the other eye several hours later. By plotting the increase against the known interval, the time of death may be estimated. Two important points to consider are:

- the values are greatly affected by temperature and are of little value when the body begins decomposition; and
- vitreous values are valid only when obtained from an intact globe – an additional specimen cannot later be obtained from the same globe and be considered valid.

The use of vitreous potassium has not been established as a reliable method of estimating the postmortem interval in children, and levels cannot be used to diagnosis antemortem hypo- or hyperkalemia. Vitreous potassium when evaluated in conjunction with other vitreous electrolytes can be useful for assessing the amount of postmortem change that may be reflected by those results.

Coe described four patterns of postmortem vitreous electrolyte abnormalities[62]:

- dehydration pattern (**hypertonic pattern**) characterized by increased vitreous sodium and chloride with a moderate elevation in urea nitrogen;
- **uremic pattern,** with increased vitreous urea nitrogen and creatinine without a substantial increase in sodium and chloride;
- low-salt pattern (**hypotonic pattern**), which shows decreased vitreous sodium and chloride levels with relatively low potassium values (< 15 mEq/L); and
- **decomposition pattern,** which shows low vitreous sodium and chloride values with concomitant high vitreous potassium value (> 20 mEq/L)

Protein

Total serum protein and electrophoresis determination, serum immunoglobulins, serum hemoglobin electrophoresis, and serologic studies are a reliable reflection of the antemortem state.[62–65] Some proteins found routinely in the plasma are not identifiable in vitreous, and negative values in those circumstances cannot be interpreted.

Enzymes

Enzymatic quantitation is highly erratic in all sites with the exception of **cholinesterase,** which remains stable during the postmortem period.[66] Assessment of the hepatic glycogen may reflect the premortem state of the individual with normal glycogen stores in infants with 'truly' sudden death, without sustained premortem stress or with abnormality of the stress response.[67]

Hormones

Cortisol levels in blood reflect the premortem state and remain stable for approximately 18 hours.[68] **Catecholamines** tend to rise rapidly in blood and reflect premortem stress. **Thyroid** levels fall slightly with the postmortem interval, while thyroid-stimulating hormone levels remain relatively stable,[69] although care must be exercised in over interpretation of low values.[70] Initial studies were promising in finding elevated levels of triiodothyronine in children dying with SIDS,[71] but this was subsequently determined to be most likely a postmortem change.[72]

Melatonin levels have been shown to be significantly lower in the SIDS population. Sturner's group studied the melatonin levels of infants dying at night.[73] Their results indicated lower melatonin levels than in infants dying of other causes. The implication of this study suggests that infants dying from SIDS may have an abnormal circadian rhythm.

Postmortem metabolic screening is recommended in all sudden unexpected deaths in infants and newborns. It is estimated that as many as 3–6% of sudden unexpected death in infancy are due to inherited disorder of fatty acid metabolism.[74] Many forensic offices submit dried filter paper specimens to the state-screening laboratory for multianalytic screening. Chace et al[75] analyzed 7058 filter-paper specimens for acylcarnitine and amino acid profiles by tandem mass spectrometry. Specialized interpretation was undertaken to identify disorders of fatty acid, organic acid, and amino acid metabolism. Probable metabolic disorders were reflected in 66 cases.

Cases where a metabolic disorder is suspected from autopsy findings or antemortem clinical history should receive a metabolic autopsy.[4, 76] Most laboratories at children's hospitals have identified reference laboratories for specific analysis or DNA probe studies. One such reference laboratory is the Biochemical Genetics Laboratory at the Mayo Clinic. Specific analysis, such as prolonged QT interval should be submitted to select laboratories with ongoing research experience.

Toxicology[77]

Heavy metal analysis[78] and postmortem drug or toxicologic screening can play a critical role in evaluating unexplained illness or unexpected death in children. Identification of reliable toxicology or criminal laboratories available to the hospital-based pathologist or through local law enforcement agencies will facilitate the appropriate use of these resources.

Serious errors in interpretation can occur if there is not proper understanding of the limitations of postmortem drug measurements, toxicologic sampling and handling. Unfortunately the drug(s) involved and their pharmacokinetic properties are frequently not available at the time of autopsy. Postmortem change and ischemia leads to tissue deterioration that can affect the pharmacokinetic and distribution behavior of some drugs. When measuring and interpreting drug concentrations after death the effect of postmortem pharmacokinetics may not reflect the true antemortem drug concentration.[79] Cardiac blood or blood aspirated from intravenous catheter will reflect significantly different values than peripheral blood. Because of challenges in collecting peripheral blood in newborn and young infants the probability of contamination is high. It is far better to be cautious, identify the specimen and the exact site from which the specimen is collected and preserve more than necessary rather than be left with data that cannot be interpreted[78] (Box 17.9).

Blood or specimens must be properly stored at low temperatures –40°C for days; –70°C preffered for longer periods) in the presence of proper preservatives.

Wounds[81–83]

Excellent discussions of the basic forensic principles of mechanical trauma are available.[82, 84–86] Mechanical force applied to any living tissue can produce a wound. Newton's Second Law governs wound mechanics: **force = mass × acceleration**. The wound-producing capacity or kinetic energy of an object is determined by mass (M) and velocity (V): Kinetic $E = MV^2/2$. Understanding tissue injury requires an understanding of injury tolerance thresholds and injury mechanics.[87–90] The nature of the damage inflicted reflects the amount of force transmitted to the tissue, the rate of application of force to the tissues, the surface area to which the force is applied, and the particular characteristics of the targeted tissue.[85]

In recent years biomechanical science and experimental models have contributed to the understanding of wound mechanics especially in cases of traumatic brain injury. **Biomechanics** is the application of mechanics to biological systems. **Mechanics** is defined as the consequences of the application of forces and couples (a set of equal, parallel and oppositely directed forces) to one object or a system of objects (solid, liquid or gas). Theory of **impact** and the mechanics of **energy transfer** under conditions of impact are complex concepts, and yet the principles must be a part of forensic wound analysis.[90]

Mechanical trauma can take many forms. Blows to the body transmit force to the underlying organs and tissues until the force is dissipated. Two of the most important factors in the development of a pattern are the **rigidity of the offending object** and the **presence of bone or organ** beneath the skin that localizes the force to one area. Absence of a visible cutaneous injury does not mean that the body did not receive a blow to the area. The absence of abdominal wall bruises in the child sustaining fatal visceral trauma frequently misleads the inexperienced examiner, both in suspecting or identifying the injury and interpreting its

cause. Clothing and hair can also dissipate force, diminishing the chance of developing a pattern injury. Infants can receive serious blunt force trauma to the head without external evidence of injury.

Most cutaneous injuries in childhood are a combination of abrasions and contusions. Bruises are less likely than abrasions to be specific, although they may reflect the area involved in contact with low-energy forces and may outline the offending object in higher-energy forces.

Distortion of the patterns can also result from swelling and healing. Therefore, early documentation of injuries and appropriately timed follow-up observations are necessary. Children with trauma suspicious for inflicted injury should have all injuries carefully documented as soon as feasible. The usual hospital note is inadequate for this purpose and photographic documentation from experienced technicians should be obtained.

Pattern of injury

Simply stated, 'pattern of injury' refers to a combination or distribution of external and/or internal trauma that suggests a causative mechanism or sequence of events. The principle of identifying a pattern of injury applies whether it is caused by accidental injury, criminal assault, or self-inflicted harm. Examples of pattern injury are the pattern of bruises and fingernail marks imparted from throttling in manual strangulation, imprints of instruments or surfaces, and abrasion pattern from shoe or carpet. Common pattern injuries in child abuse include facial slap marks, buttocks bruising from corporal punishment (Fig. 17.6), grab marks to the ears. Grab marks on the lateral upper arms or chest may be observed in abused infants. Blows with rigid objects may depress the skin in such a way as to force blood and lymph laterally, rupturing vessels and outlining the object (railroad track pattern). Common things produce common injuries: railroad track injuries from cord straps (Fig. 17.7); patterned oval contusions from knuckles or fingertips. A thorough understanding of pattern of injury has wide application in child abuse detection. Awareness of the common patterns of both accidental and non-accidental injury, relative to the developmental age of the victim, is crucial to accurate diagnostic interpretation.

Defense wounds are pattern injuries sustained in an attempt to ward off harm. These wounds typically are seen on the parts of the body that victims would interpose between themselves and the assailant, especially the back of hands, forearms, elbows, and shoulders. In children who have been the victim of physical abuse, clustering of fingernail marks or bruises may be seen on the forearms or backs of hands as they attempt to shield their face and head (Fig. 17.8). Clusters of bruises on the extensor surfaces of the lateral shoulders, forearms, and hands, often in a symmetric pattern, may indicate an attempt to shield the face from pummeling blows. Fingernail marks may be observed in young victims of suffocation from their own efforts to free their airway. Bruising of the upper legs and inner thighs may be observed in sexual assault victims.

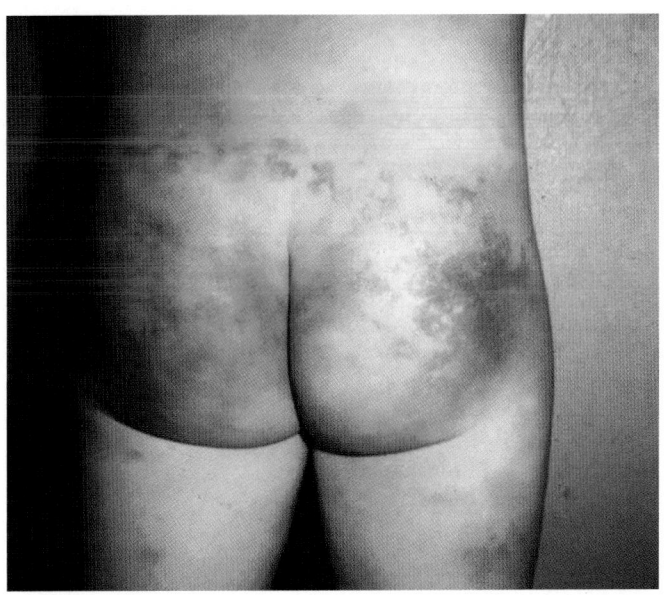

FIGURE 17.6 Bruises due to corporal punishment.

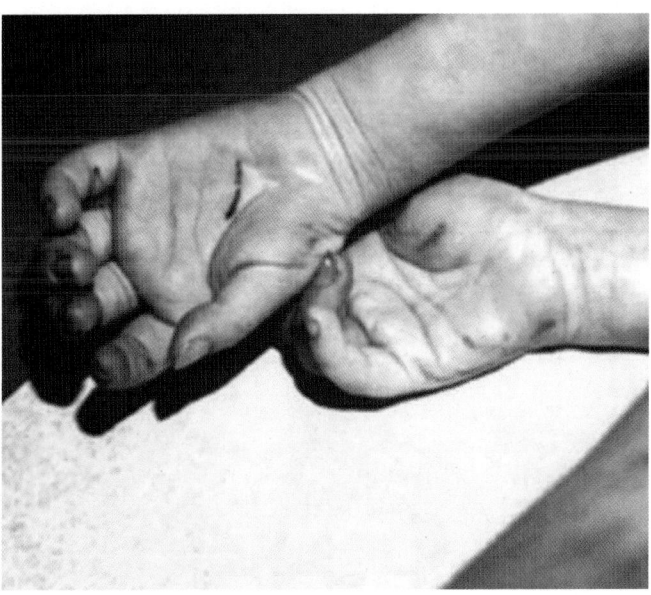

FIGURE 17.8 Palmar defense wounds in fatal child abuse.

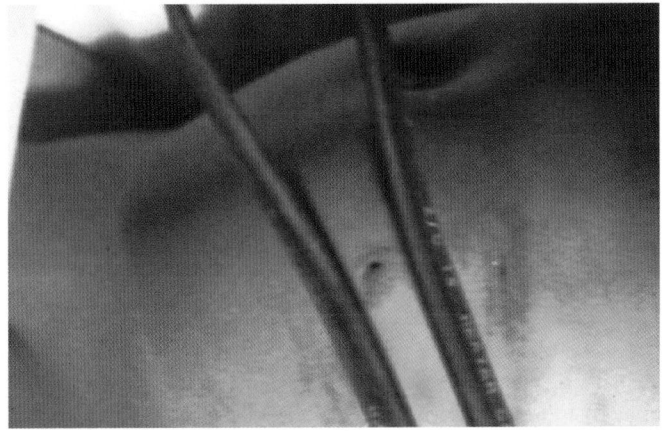

FIGURE 17.7 Pattern injury caused by electrical cord with railroad track bruises.

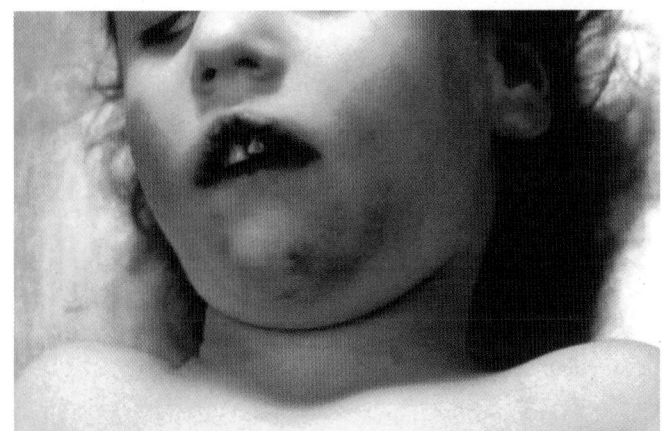

FIGURE 17.9 Facial bruises due to cardiopulmonary resuscitation with mask.

Cardiopulmonary resuscitation (CPR)-related artifacts in pediatric rescue, even medically trivial soft tissue injuries, especially of the face and neck, can have forensic significance. Leadbeater[91] and Darok[92] have extensively reviewed injuries associated with CPR. Even with the performance of competent CPR, injuries can result, especially if resuscitation is prolonged. Injuries to the face, mouth, airway, thoracic cage, intrathoracic organs, and abdominal viscera have been observed (Fig. 17.9). Medically significant injuries include hepatic laceration, gastric rupture, diaphragmatic contusions and tears, rib fractures, pulmonary contusions, and cardiac injury. Bush et al[93] estimates the incidence of medically significant injuries from CPR in children at approximately 3%. Kaplan and Fossum[94] describe facial injuries in nine infants subjected to CPR, and suggest techniques for effective investigation and interpretation of these injuries. Serious or life-threatening injuries are uncommon complications of clinical efforts to support the airway or resuscitate, but injuries are reported.[95, 96] Although the likelihood of serious injury is low, the possibility of inadvertent injury must be considered. Because significant injuries are rare following CPR in childhood, possibility of abuse should be appropriately evaluated.[97, 98] The author reviewed a case of a 5-month-old infant who received adult-type CPR from her frantic grandmother in full straddle position with double-handed chest compressions. Findings included posterior left rib fractures and pericardial tamponade with right atrial injury (Fig. 17.10).

Abrasions

Abrasions (scrape, scratch, graze) are injuries to the skin caused by contact with a rough surface or object with sufficient force to scrape away the superficial skin layers by friction, crushing, or

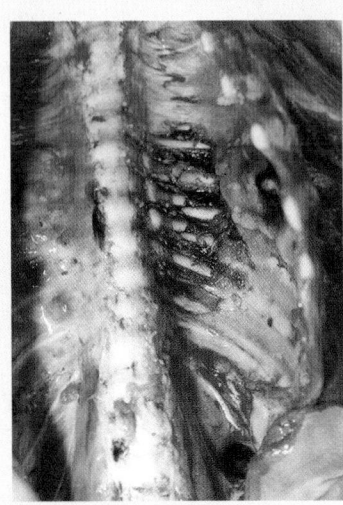

FIGURE 17.10 Fractured ribs caused by untrained cardiopulmonary resuscitation on a young infant.

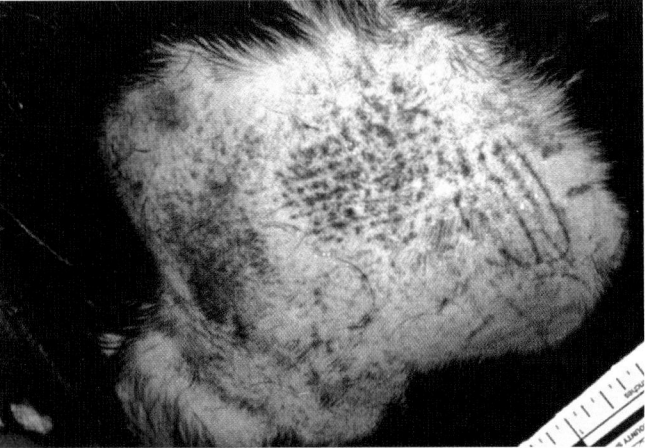

FIGURE 17.11 Scalp abrasion showing pattern of impact surface.

grinding (Fig. 17.11). Abrasion patterns frequently observed in accidental and non-accidental trauma in childhood include pavement abrasions, scalp wounds from blunt trauma and falls, fingernail scratches, bite marks, imprint abrasions from blunt trauma, ligature marks, and rope burns. Close examination of an abrasion, especially in sliding injuries, may show partially detached sheets of epidermal cells 'rolled up' on themselves on the distal end of the wound – small tags or fringes of skin at the finishing edge. Recognizing a pattern in the epidermal defects may occasionally identify the nature of the abrading object, as with teeth marks and fingernail scratches. Abrasions also indicate the exact point of contact and can reflect the degree of force imparted. In many circumstances it is possible to distinguish a direct impact abrasion from one resulting from a sliding motion. These principles are especially important in child pedestrian–motor vehicle accident reconstruction.

It is important to note that abrasions tend to dry and darken after death and can be **confused with a burn** by the inexperienced observer. Postmortem pressure marks or postmortem abrasions should be distinguished from antemortem abrasion injuries. Over interpretation may lead to an unnecessarily extensive investigation in an otherwise straightforward case.

Bruises (contusions)[81, 99, 100]

Contusion, ecchymosis, and bruise are interchangeable terms referring to leakage of blood into tissue due to rupture of small vessels. **Hematoma** is a term commonly used to denote a collection of blood in tissue. Escaping blood within tissue flows along traumatic or natural cleavage lines and the area becomes discolored. The characteristics or appearance of a bruise is influenced by a number of factors including age and health of the individual, skin color, bleeding tendency, presence of certain drugs, force and location of injury, and depth and extent of subcutaneous extravasation.

It is not possible to determine with accuracy the degree of force that causes any particular bruise. Examination of a contusion cannot reveal the direction in which the force was applied, nor can it indicate whether the moving body struck the object or vice versa. A bruise does not always indicate the exact point of impact and frequently is much larger than the actual surface area impacted. If an abrasion injury is present along with a bruise, a point of impact usually can be identified. The size of a bruise does not reflect the size of the offending object but is more related to the characteristics of the tissue (such as toughness or elasticity, vascularity, and density), time elapsed since injury, and the relative location of the blood within the layers of skin and deeper soft tissues.

In some circumstances a bruise may indicate the characteristics of the offending object, such as the parallel configuration of bruising (railroad tracks) caused by a hanger or a rod-like object. Pattern injuries involving contusions can be an important part of the determination of inflicted injury. Unless a bruise carries the clear imprint of the instrument or there are multiple bruises of uniform shape, few bruise patterns can be used to reach conclusions of diagnostic significance regarding details of the injury.

The location of bruises may also be of forensic importance. Bruising may be accentuated in the presence of loose, vascular skin and fat. An excellent example is the periorbital area, where the tissue is vascular and loose over the skull and facial bone. Black eyes can result from settling of blood into the soft tissues of the periorbital region from blows to the head at some distance from the eye.

Differentiating inflicted bruises from bruises sustained from everyday play and accidents is a crucial diagnosis. However, the evidence base to perform this process has not been clearly defined.[101] Maguire et al[102] performed a systematic review of literature pertaining to patterns of bruises in children to distinguish 'abuse from non-abuse.' Their findings conclude that bruises in non-mobile infants, over soft tissue areas (e.g. abdomen), bruises that carry the imprint of an implement, and multiple bruises of uniform shape are suspicious for abuse.

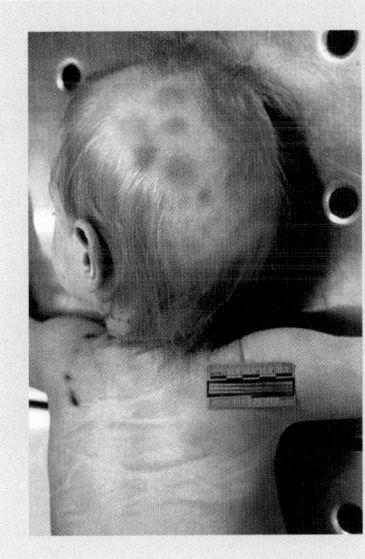

FIGURE 17.12 Multiple head bruises in fatal child abuse.

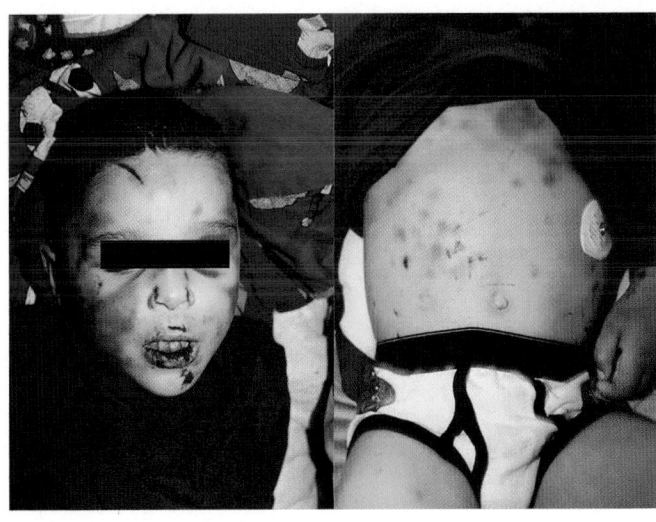

FIGURE 17.13 Bruises and injuries to face and torso in fatal child abuse.

Accidental bruises associated with normal childhood development are small and increase in number with age. Accidental bruises are more often observed over bony prominences on the front of the body and forehead.[103] The prevalence, numbers and location of bruises appear to be directly linked to motor developmental ability. Infants who do not walk or move about are unlikely to sustain unexplained bruises.[103, 104] The mean number of bruises in cases of child abuse is higher than in cases of accidental bruising. The most common inflicted injury is head contusions. A common feature in the abused children is clustering of bruises, or evidence of bruises of uniform shape (Fig. 17.12).

Multiple bruises of various stages, bruising in areas of the body atypical for the child's developmental level, and severe bruising without reasonable explanation are strongly suggestive of non-accidental trauma or rough handling. **Black eyes, bruises over the jaw,** and **injuries to the cheeks, trunk, genitals, and thighs** are suspicious for **abuse** (Fig. 17.13).[105]

Significant blows that injure underlying anatomy may not leave an external bruise. This is especially true of blows to the abdomen, where there is no firm underlying ventral structure to support the impact sufficient to rupture vessels within the skin and subcutaneous tissue. However, a forceful blow with sufficient energy to compress internal organs against the vertebral column may cause mortal injury.

Maguire et al[106] performed a systematic review of methods and reliability of clinical assessment of the ages of bruises in children. Their analysis concludes that any color can be observed in a bruise at any time before its resolution and clinical assessment of the age of a bruise in vivo or from a photograph cannot be accurately performed.[107] Color can be a reflection of depth, size, thickness, and overall skin coloring. Even on the same individual, two different bruises acquired at the same time can appear differently in color. The differences can be related to the amount of blood present, the location on the body, and the relative position of the hemorrhage within the layers of skin and subcutaneous tissue.

A bruise may not be immediately evident, at times taking several hours to develop. Changes first observed may include erythema and swelling. It is advisable to photograph, document and reevaluate bruises over several hours. Review of injuries after completion of the internal postmortem examination, after drainage of blood from the tissues, or the day after autopsy, may allow for better delineation of lesions. Improper photographic documentation and sampling can lead to serious problems with interpretation. Vogeley et al[108] reports enhancement of visualization of subtle bruises with the use of wood lamp illumination and describes a method for digital photography of bruises visualized in this manner. Vanezis[100, 107] provides excellent in-depth reviews of documentation, aging and interpretation of bruises at autopsy. Key points and recommendations include:

- Verify that the discolored area is in fact a bruise.
- Identify a pattern when possible.
- Identify site of injury and whether it is located over bone.
- Describe color, shape, size, site, and presence or absence of healing.
- Assess the distribution and number of bruises.
- Identify presence or absence of congestion or vascularity at bruise site.
- Describe related injuries.
- Identify presence of natural disease or constitutional factors that may contribute to bruising.

At postmortem examination all, or appropriately representative, bruises should be carefully incised (Fig. 17.14) and microscopic sections taken in order to identify presence and character of vital reaction. This is especially important if time of injury and manner of death are a concern. If contusions are present in multiple tissue layers in the scalp, all affected areas must be included in the histologic analysis. Iron and trichrome stains can reveal unexpected evidence of vital reaction and should be used liberally.

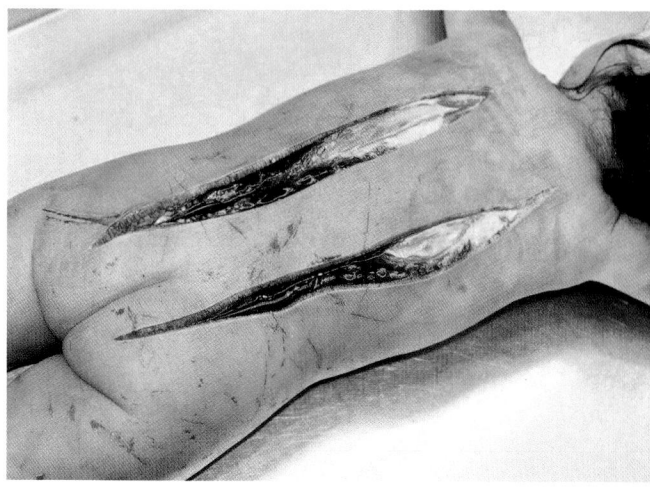

FIGURE 17.14 Autopsy technique of examining and confirming soft tissue injuries.

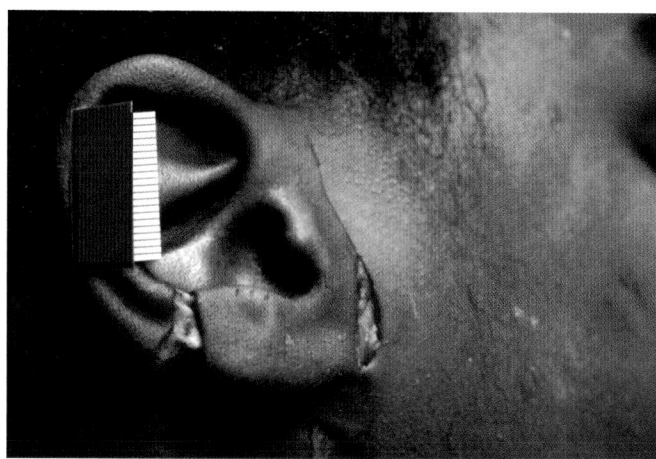

FIGURE 17.15 Incision wounds.

Distinction between bruises that occur before or after death may be impossible when the injuries are inflicted just before, during, or within a short time of death. Especially problematic can be interpretation of soft tissue hemorrhage in the neck tissues.

Lacerations

The term **laceration** is often improperly confused with cuts or incised wounds. Lacerations are actually splits or tears in the skin produced by blunt trauma causing tissue shearing or excessive stretching. This may be caused by impact from a blunt instrument with force exceeding the skin's elasticity. A laceration typically involves the skin over a bony prominence, such as the hand, head, knee, or elbow. Because of the forceful disruption of the tissue, one of the characteristics of a laceration is tissue bridges composed of stronger, more elastic elements of the tissue, nerves, and small blood vessels traversing the defect. The edges of a laceration usually have an irregular, rough appearance, and, if the result of an impact, the adjacent skin may show an abraded and/or bruised margin.

Lacerations are often seen in crush injuries applied over a relatively small area. Compression of hollow, fluid-containing viscera may result in laceration of the wall or frank perforation. Crush injuries to the abdomen delivered by blunt trauma may result in laceration of the internal organs without external signs of trauma.

Lacerations resulting from an oblique application of force can result in linear or curved tears. If curved, the **convexity of the laceration will face the direction of the force.** Lacerations that result from **directly applied or multidirectional forces** are more typically **linear or stellate**.

At the time of examination it is important to describe the wound and photograph with a scale as near to the defect as possible. Measurements of the wound gaping and apposed

should always be made and photographs taken. This information may help identify the type of impact surface or object.

Incisions

Incisions are wounds caused by sharp instruments that cleanly separate tissue structures. Incisional wounds are typically longer than deep (Fig. 17.15). The wound may tail off to a shallower depth at one end and may be quite irregular if the damaged skin is not taut or if rotational forces are applied, either by the victim twisting or by the assailant's motion. It is not usual to see bruising inflicted with an incised wound. Incisions show **well-defined margins without bridging** and may present in various patterns. These may range from a surgical appearance caused by an extremely sharp instrument to a clefted appearance caused by a chopping injury from an instrument such as a hatchet. It may be possible to identify the characteristics of the instrument by examining the wound.

Incisional wounds are not typical in classic child abuse, but this pattern of injury may be important in interpreting wounds in cases of child murder and infanticide.

Stab wounds

Stab wounds occur when a relatively sharp object penetrates the body. Compared with an incision, they are typically **much deeper than wide,** are much more dangerous to internal structures and blood loss is often much greater internally than externally. Stab wounds are infrequently found in classic child abuse, but appropriate use of the terminology to describe therapeutic wounds or suspicious injuries is important.

Stab wounds may vary in appearance from person to person, or at different body points, because of the elasticity of the skin. The cleavage lines of the skin (Langer lines) also distort a wound and give it a gaping appearance. Determination of the length of a weapon can rarely be made by examining the wound, since depth of the wound is more a product of the force applied behind the weapon than of its length.

Stab wounds often reflect characteristics of the causative instrument. These wounds generally do not have an abraded margin, unless the weapon has an expanding cross-sectional area. The wound itself often has an elliptic appearance if produced by a knife. Double-edged knife wound margins come to a point at either focus; a single-edged knife creates a wound with one sharp end, while the other edge may have a squared-off appearance and may display slight abrasion. Round objects such as a screwdriver may produce a wound defect very similar to a bullet wound. Stab wounds into visceral organs such as the liver or kidney may also provide a template of the weapon.

Before examination of a wound, **reapproximating the margins with clear cellophane tape** may provide valuable information. Photographing the wound before dissection is also important and should include a scale. Probing of the wound should be done with caution to avoid producing artifactual trauma. Physicians may use penetrating injuries as sites for chest tubes or may surgically extend the wound to provide exposure to the underlying structures. Careful documentation of such instances is very important to the later forensic examination. Competent documentation of the measurements and appearance of the wound will prove invaluable for future medicolegal interpretation even if wound characteristics have been obliterated due to antemortem probing or repair.

Skeletal injuries

Forces that interrupt the uniform state of motion or rest of the body are most likely to damage the least plastic tissue, the bony skeleton. Fractures can provide information as to the nature of the traumatic event or the object that may have produced the injury, especially when this examination is combined with observation of other trauma. Because of potential lever effect in transmitting energy in skeletal trauma, it may be difficult to determine the amount of force applied in any particular fracture. In interpreting these injuries, such factors as the details of the event, body position, momentum of the body, and pathologic anomalies must be considered.

Fractures of the skull may indicate, to varying degrees, the direction of the applied force, and perhaps the direction from which the blow was struck. The skull may also provide a partial mold of the offending object, for example, a hammer may produce crescent-shaped defects or may simply punch out a circular defect if the vector is nearly perpendicular to the bone.

The propensity of a bone to fracture varies with the age of the individual and the bone involved. Because of the increased pliability of the infant skull, **complex fractures in infants are observed only in severe trauma.**[89] In the very young, an impact to the skull may produce only a momentary deformity. The 'ping-pong' fracture, a deformity similar to that left on a ping-pong ball that has been depressed and popped back out, is unique to this age group.

The finding of **multiple bony injuries** of varied ages in the otherwise normal child is suspicious for child abuse**.** A combination of radiographic techniques and repeat examinations is frequently necessary to accurately delineate the extent and timing of multiple injuries (repeat radiographs, radionucleotide imaging, CT scan).

Vital reaction and timing of injury

Determination of when an injury occurred is often an important part of the forensic analysis. The forensic implications of the time interval from the moment of injury to the time of death are obvious. Vital reaction is the tissue response to injury, which may or may not be visible to the naked eye, manifested in histologic and/or histochemical change. Changes can vary from person to person depending on the nature of the injury, presence of shock, extent of damage, location on the body and type of tissue injured, age of the individual, previous state of health, nature of underlying illness, and presence of infection.[109] It should be noted, that only approximations can be drawn from the examination of a wound for vital reaction. The determination of the interval between injury and death is imprecise, even by the most experienced pathologists.

Visual examination of bruises and other injuries must be interpreted cautiously. Nikolic et al[110] studied postmortem bleeding from large vessel injury. Bleeding into tissues can occur after death and cannot in and of itself be a determination of evidence of a 'beating heart'. Absence of blood also does not mean that the injury is necessarily postmortem.

The evolution of injury is unpredictable; however a few guidelines are helpful in assessing timing of injury. **Erythema** can occur within minutes of injury and may last for several hours (Fig. 17.16). **Tissue swelling, coloration or settling of a bruise, absence of scab formation** (by about 24 hours in small wounds), or beginning epithelialization (about 36 hours) may indicate antemortem injury with varying reliability. Careful antemortem observation and photographic documentation of the visual changes of the wounds can be invaluable in supporting the diagnosis of acute injury.

The first reliable microscopic sign of vital reaction is leukocytic infiltration (Fig. 17.17). **Margination** of a few polymorphonuclear neutrophil leukocytes (PMNs) at the periphery of a lesion may not constitute a vital reaction. The timing of a distinct **leukocytic infiltration** is controversial, but the earliest expected time interval is 4–8 hours after injury. At 8–12 hours PMNs, macrophages, and activated fibroblasts may be detected in a distinct peripheral wound zone. **Monocytes** are seldom seen infiltrating the wound less than 12 hours after injury (Table 17.8). **Mitotic activity** can be observed in fibroblasts by 15 hours and **fibroblastic infiltration** of the wound by 2–4 days.[111] In some circumstances, **necrosis** is apparent within the connective tissue at the center of the wound by 36 hours, **vascularized granulation tissue** can be observed by 3 days, **hemosiderin deposition** develops by 2 or 3 days, and **collagen fibers** may be observed by

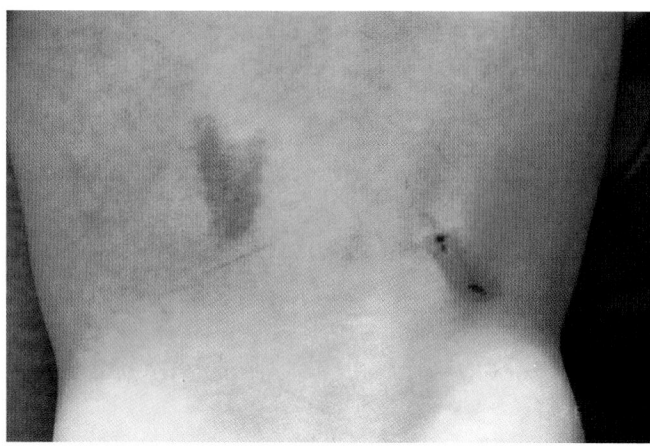

FIGURE 17.16 Erythema and abrasion from fingernail scratches.

4–6 days. In small wounds, **scar formation** may be evident by 1 week.

The lack of histologic vital reaction is *not* diagnostic of postmortem injury, as predictable histologic evidence of reaction to injury may not be observed for hours or even days after injury. In serial tests on surgical wounds, Bednar[112] demonstrated that fibroblastic proliferation in the corium was predominant in infants; in adults, rapid regeneration of the epidermis was more apparent. Because of its effect on healing, if infection is present in the tissues, interpretation of the vital changes is difficult. The presence of a distinct fibrin network, especially at the margin of a hemorrhage, points to the hemorrhage occurring before death, if other vital reactions are present. Examination of the wound for elastic fibers may be useful in assessing the timing of hemorrhage. Vital reaction processes will continue as long as there is perfusion and cellular viability. Therefore it is imperative to include history of

resuscitation (including length if prolonged) and duration of life support.

Certain types of vital reaction have particular importance in pediatric forensic analysis:

- neomembrane formation in the subdural space in the analysis of traumatic brain injury;
- development of respirator brain;
- evidence and characteristics of axonal injury in the brain;
- acute, subacute or chronic vital reaction in soft tissue and visceral injuries;
- radiographic and histologic evidence in the dating of fractures; and
- vital reaction at the umbilical stump in the abandoned newborn.

Aging of brain contusions may be fairly accurate when based on the microscopic patterns of neuronal and glial injuries, granulocytic response, vascular changes, and presence of fat and hemosiderin within tissue macrophages.

Histochemical analysis is dependent on immediate analysis, which is not feasible in most forensic cases and is limited to laboratories experienced with the procedures and limitations of interpretation. The obvious drawback to any enzyme methodology is the unknown time intervals and the sometimes unavoidable problems in obtaining timely and appropriately handled tissues. For this reason, the histochemical analysis is not routinely used in standard forensic evaluation. Two zones can be distinguished histochemically around an antemortem wound.[113] The wound periphery shows an increase in enzyme activity as little as 1 h after the injury. In the most immediate wound vicinity, tissue exhibits a progressive loss of enzyme activity at 1–4 hours after injury, an early sign of imminent necrosis.

Special histochemical stains have been available to the pathologist for decades. Gram stains, iron and trichrome, silver and periodic acid-Schiff stains for fungus, and special stains for mycobacterium are useful in documenting infectious agents in tissue. Iron stains allow for the identification of hemosiderin-

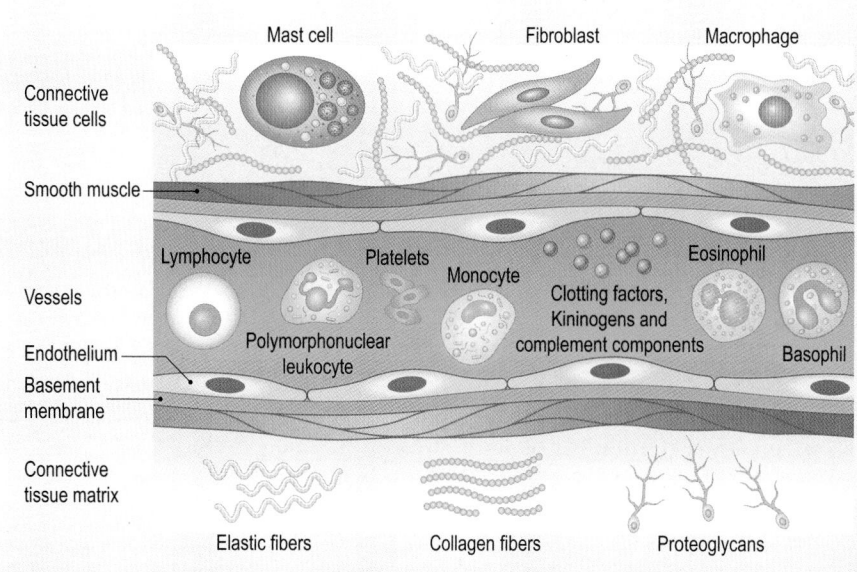

FIGURE 17.17 Components of acute and chronic inflammation responses: circulating cells and proteins, cells of blood vessels, and cells and proteins of the extracellular matrix. (With permission from Elsevier.)

TABLE 17.8 HISTOLOGY SCHEMA – TIMING OF INJURY[100, 101, 106, 107]

Time interval	Histology	Cellular appearance
< 4 h	No distinct signs of inflammation No distinction between ante- and postmortem skin wound PMNs appear within 15–30 min	PMNs; Last up to months
4–12 h	PMNs, macrophages, and fibroblasts form distinct peripheral wound zone at 8–12 h Imminent necrosis in central zone	PMN more frequent than macrophages (ratio 5:1)
12–48 h	PMN to macrophage ratio falls to 0.4:1 with an increase in the relative number of macrophages Less than 16 h 'newer' fibrin stains yellow with Martius scarlet blue After 16 h older fibrin stains bright red Cut edge of epidermis shows cytoplasmic processes 24–48 h: epidermis migrates from the incised edge towards the center of the wound 32 h and after, necrosis is apparent in the central wound zone 48 h: macrophages reach maximum concentration in peripheral zone	Macrophage/PMN ratio at 16–24 h, routinely seen at > 11 days, latest up to months
2–4 days	2–4 days: fibroblasts migrate from connective tissue to wound periphery 3 days: (migrating keratinocytes) Epithelialization of small wounds and abrasions complete; thereafter regenerated epidermis becomes highly stratified and thicker than the normal surrounding epidermis 3–4 days: capillary buds appear	Migration earliest 2 days, routine at > 9 days Lipophage, erythrophages, Siderophages/hemosiderin, and granulation tissue earliest at 3 days; latest up to months
4–8 days	Re-epithelialization complete 4 days: first new collagen fibers seen 4–5 days: profuse in-growth of new capillaries; capillaries continue to proliferate until 8th day 6 days: lymphocytes reach maximum concentration in wound periphery	5 to more than 21 days
8–12 days	Hematoidin, and lymphocyte-infiltrates Decrease in number of inflammatory cells, fibroblasts, and capillaries; increase in the number and size of collagen fibers	Earliest 8 days; latest months
More than 12 days	12 days: regression of cellular activity in both epidermis and dermis. Vascularity of dermis diminishes. Collagen fibers restored. Epithelium shows stainable basement membrane. 14 days: fibroplasia reaches its peak. Thereafter there is a gradual shrinkage and maturation of connective tissue in the wound	

PMNs, Polymorphonuclear neutrophil leukocytes.

positive cells and trichrome stains provide better detail in a healing wound (Fig. 17.18). Newer techniques are available such as immunoperoxidase for β-amyloid precursor protein associated with axonal injury as well as other antibodies that allow for identification of certain cell types in tissue. There are no hard and fast rules for when special stains should be performed. As in any other area of medicine, it is a combination of experience and curiosity that usually guides the decision.

Causes of injury[114–116]

Injuries comprise **42% of all deaths in children 1–4 years of age**.[117] Although the overall childhood mortality rate has decreased substantially over the last three decades, almost all of the decline is attributable to a decrease in deaths from natural causes.[118] Children less than 1 year of age have the highest rate of accidental injury-related deaths, at a rate more than twice that of all other children.[119] Suffocation is the second leading cause of death in children < 1 year of age. Each year approximately 20 000 children and teenagers die as a result of injury.

Tomashek and colleagues[120] summarize trends in postneonatal mortality (PNM) attributable to injury in the USA from 1988 to 1998. Overall PNM (deaths 28 days to 364 days) attributable to injury decreased. During this period 12 209 postneonatal deaths were attributed to injury for an average of 1110 deaths per year. Nearly half of the unintentional injuries were a form of asphyxia and motor vehicle crash-related deaths. The proportion of PNM attributable to accidental injuries decreased

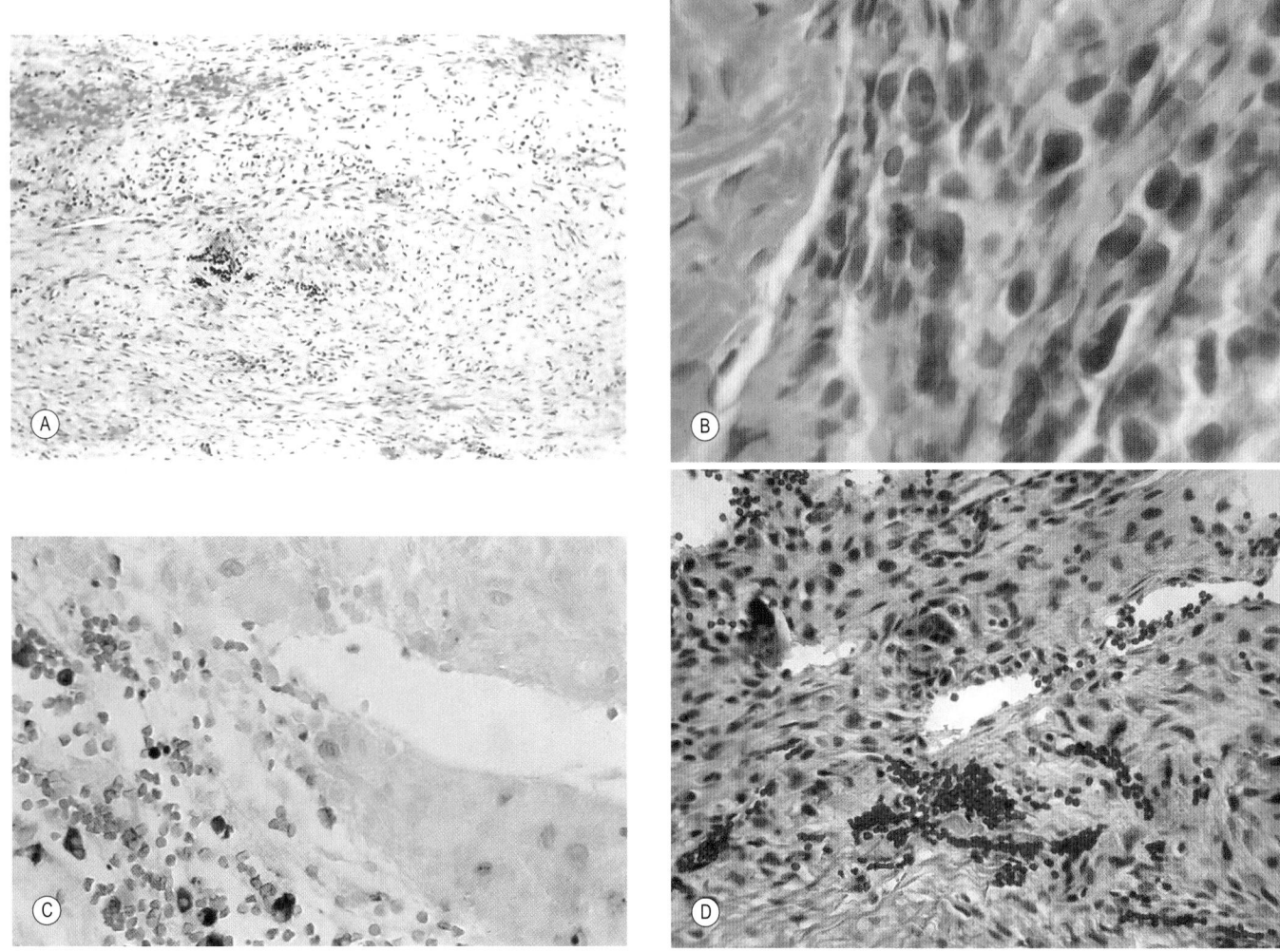

FIGURE 17.18 Vital reaction. (A) Hematoxylin and eosin stain showing established soft tissue reaction (× 100). (B) Hemosiderin deposits in dural macrophages (× 400). (C) Positive tissue iron stain (× 100). (D) Trichrome stain demonstrating established vital reaction (× 100).

from 74.6 to 66.2%. Rates of all types of accidental injuries decreased with the exception of mechanical suffocation which increased. Hessol and Fuentes-Afflick[121] analyzed ethnic disparities in infant mortality. After adjusting for maternal and infant factors, black women had a higher PNM risk and Latin women a lower PNM risk than white women. In addition, they found that unmarried women, while demonstrating significantly decreased risk of neonatal death, had a significantly higher risk of PNM. Malloy[122] reported no significant increase in PNM rate for aspiration, asphyxia, or respiratory failure for years 1991–1996 coincident with the introduction of the 'Back to sleep campaign' for prevention of SIDS. The proportion of PNM contribution by SIDS declined from 37.1% in 1991 to 28.8% in 1996. There was a significant increase in the PNM risk for suffocation in bed or cradle. Corey and co-workers[123] reported an 11-year autopsy review of accidental infant deaths. The causes of death included asphyxia in mechanically unsafe sleeping environments (the largest group), overlying, drowning, scald burns, plastic bag suffocation, house fires, motor vehicle collisions, aspiration of foreign bodies, hypothermia, blunt head trauma, and alcohol toxicity.

Agran et al[124] analyzed Californian hospital discharges and death certificates to identify age and external causes of injury (e-codes) for children younger than 4 years of age. There were a total of 23 173 injuries, 636 of which resulted in death. The leading major causes of injury in descending order were falls, poisoning, transportation, foreign body and fires/burns. Falls exceeded poisoning by a factor of two. In 3-month intervals during the first year of life the leading causes of injury varied (Fig. 17.19):

- 0–2 months – falls from height;
- 3–5 months – battering;
- 6–8 months – falls from furniture;
- 9–11 months – non-airway foreign body;
- falls from stairs peaked at age 6–8 months and 9–11 months.

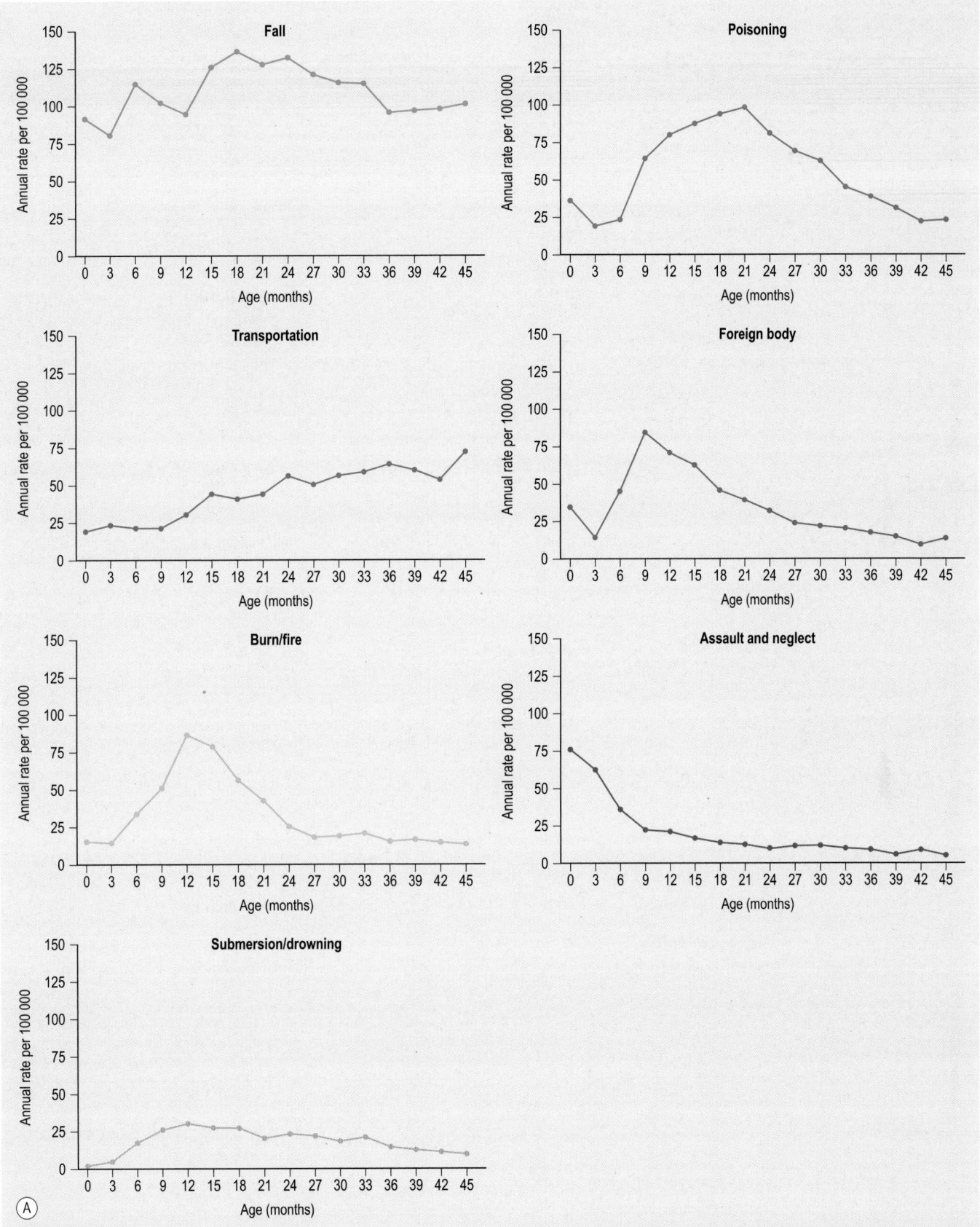

FIGURE 17.19 (A) Annual rate of injury hospitalization and death per 100 000 population by major category of injury and 3-month age intervals, 0–4 years, California 1996–1998.

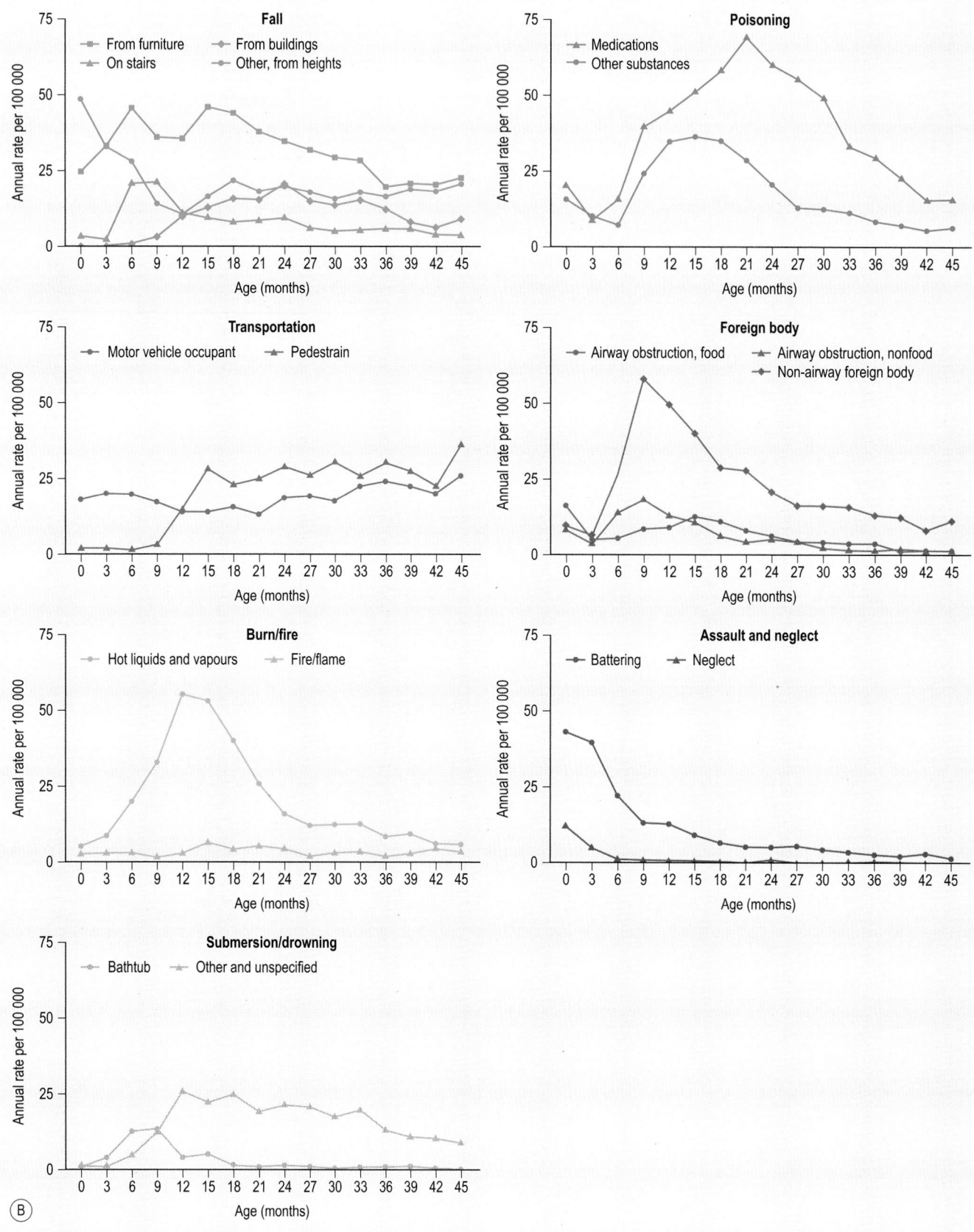

FIGURE 17.19 (*cont'd*) (B) Annual rate of injury hospitalization and death per 100 000 population by specific category of injury and 3-month age intervals, 0–4 years, California 1996–1998. (With permission from the American Academy of Pediatrics.)

Transportation injuries

Injuries due to transportation include passenger, pedestrian, and other motorized and non-motorized vehicles. Most automobile injuries in children are passenger injuries. The child passenger injury rate is 2.5 times the pedestrian rate in the USA.[117] Infants are twice as likely as older children to be killed while riding in an automobile. Karwacki and Baker[125] analyzed a series of 89 fatalities in children less than 15 years of age for the years 1973–1977. Children under 1 year of age were overrepresented, constituting 15% of the fatalities despite accounting for only 2% of the number involved in accidents. The occupant death rate for children in crashes was 6.4/1000 for children under 1 year of age and 1.0/1000 for those over 1 year. Most of the children (about 97%) were not restrained properly and 55% were seated in the front of the vehicle. Head injuries were most common in children under 2 years of age. Karwacki and Baker suggested that the predominance of head injuries in the very young was related to anatomic differences. In a similar analysis, Baker[126] demonstrated the highest death rate was in children under 6 months of age (9.0/100 000), with an especially high risk at 2 to 3 months, and decreasing mortality with increasing age.

Motor vehicle crash injuries patterns are related to four mechanisms of action and result from impact between:

- vehicle and the other impacted object;
- unrestrained occupant and the interior of the vehicle;
- occupant's organs and the enclosing body wall or cavity (skull, chest wall, pelvis); and
- occupant and loose objects in the vehicle.

Agran and colleagues examined the mechanism of injury in crash and non-crash motor vehicle occupant injuries in children.[127, 128] In a multiple-year study, they determined that 10–12% of the injuries occurred from a **non-crash event,** i.e. an injury-producing accident in which there is no collision with a fixed object or another vehicle. These included sudden stops, turns, swerves, sudden accelerations, and opening the doors of the moving vehicle. The analysis also revealed a high-risk pattern in non-crash falls or ejections: **ejection of the unrestrained child** after falling against or opening an unlocked door. When both crash and non-crash injuries (82 non-crash, 466 crash) were compared, the severity of injury score was highest in victims who were ejected from the vehicle. Non-crash events produced injury by ejection in 45% of the victims; 5% of the children in crash events were injured in this manner.

In recent years biomechanical analysis of motor vehicle injuries led to improved safety measures for transporting young infants. Air bag deployment represents a recognized fatal threat to infants and children. When the airbag inflates it is literally an explosive force comparable to a collision at 300 km/h.[129] Two injury types have been diagnosed:

- crush injury to the skull in infants; and
- cranial and cervical spine trauma in older children traveling restrained or improperly restrained in front passenger seat.[130]

Airbag-related deaths and serious injuries to children have led to recommendations for rear seat, rear facing infant car seats.

Falls

A fall can be defined as a sudden, often unexpected change under the influence of gravity causing the individual to impact a surface or object. Falls are common in childhood and seldom cause serious injury, although serious injury is possible.[131] The Avon Longitudinal Study of Parents and Children[132] study conducted at the University of Bristol reviewed 11 466 postal questionnaires describing accidents from birth to 6 months. In 2554 children, 3357 falls were reported; 53% from furniture, 12% fell while being carried. Only 14% reported visible injury, of which 97% involved the head. Serious injury was reported in 21 falls resulting in concussion or fracture. Agran et al[124] analyzed a cohort of 23 173 injuries in children < 4 years of age:

- Falls were the leading cause of injury for all age groups, and the rate was nearly twice that of the second leading cause, poisoning.
- Falls from furniture represented the leading cause of falls for all age groups 3 months and older, peaking at 6–8 months and 15–17 months.
- Other falls from height represented the leading cause for falls in the 0–2-month age group that decreased with age. Many of these falls were from being dropped by an older sibling.[133]
- Falls from stairs peaked at 6–8 months and 9–11 months.
- Falls from buildings peaked at 24–26 months.
- Falls from playground equipment were greater at 18–20 months and peaked at 39–41 months.

Murray et al[131] demonstrated in a retrospective review of pediatric patients, that falls less than 15 feet had a higher incidence of intracranial injuries and fewer extremity fractures than patients who fell more than 15 feet. Kim et al[134] reported four fatalities from 'low-level falls' none of which showed 'stigmata' or concerns regarding child abuse. Minor skull fractures can occur from falls from 3 to 5 1/2 feet. Severe accidental skull fractures can result from falls downstairs and from falls greater than 6 feet. Reichelderfer et al[135] demonstrated that serious head injuries in playgrounds could occur when the impact exceeds 50 G. A fall of only 3 inches to concrete can generate 100 to 200 G.

Falls from furniture, dropped infants or falls with infants are frequently reported as the cause of head trauma in childhood. **Accidental falls and drops from relatively short vertical distances can produce skull fractures and even brain injury.**[136] When fractures occur, they are **often simple linear fractures** without associated neurologic severe symptoms, complications, or sequelae.[137–140] Fractures of the skull in young children that are more extensive or complex and involve brain injury and/or neurologic symptoms and sequelae should be investigated for possible child abuse.

Falls from upper bunk beds can result in significant injuries from falls during sleep as well as play.[141] The spectrum of injuries associated with falls from beds has been reported by Macgregor[142] and Belechri.[143] Both report an over-representation of brain injuries, fractures, lacerations, soft tissue injuries, and injuries requiring hospitalization.

Chiaviello et al[144] reviews **infant walker** injuries from the University of Virginia Pediatric Emergency Room. The series included infants as young as 3 months. Injuries predominately involved the head and neck (97%) and involved stairways in many (71%). Significant injuries occurred in 19 of 65 (29%) including skull fracture, contusion, intracranial hemorrhage, full thickness burns, C-spine fracture and deaths. Stoffman and colleagues[145] reviewed medical records of children less than 24 months seen in the ER for head trauma. Infant walkers were involved in 42% of the injuries in children under 12 months of age. All the walker-related injuries involved stairs. More than 75% of injuries were related to falls down stairs. While most injuries were minor, 10% of walker injuries resulted in skull fracture.[146] In 1999, an estimated 8800 children younger than 15 months were treated in US emergency departments for walker-related injuries.

Stairway related injuries were the subject of another study by Chiaviello and associates[147] at the University of Virginia. Although the majority of injuries were minor, significant injuries did occur, predominately to head and neck. Serious injuries occurred in 15 of 69 participants (22%) including concussion, skull fractures, cerebral contusion, subdural hematoma, and C-2 fracture.

The distance of fall sufficient to cause brain injury is a topic of significant controversy. Each case must be subjected to forensic evaluation that considers the biomechanical and medical evidence. There is no question that infants can sustain skull fractures from passive low-level fall.[148] Wilkins[149] provides an excellent commentary on the variables that can affect injury severity for any given fall. These may include:

- distance fallen;
- nature of the surface on to which the child falls;
- forwards or sideways protective reflexes (there is no backwards protective reflex or righting reflex);
- whether a fall is in some way broken;
- whether the child propelled itself (momentum);
- mass of body and head;
- proportion of the kinetic energy absorbed in deforming the skull, the brain or the rest of the body and in compressing the ground;
- part of the body that hits the ground first;
- whether or not some kinetic energy is dissipated in causing fractures;
- whether the contact with the ground is focal or diffuse (is the fall on a point or flat surface); and
- secondary brain injury (hypoxic/ischemic encephalopathy).

To better understand the risk of injury from fall the forensic analysis must include:

- measurement of maximum fall height;
- consideration of site(s) of body impact;
- knowledge or inspection of the impact surface;
- understanding of biomechanical principles such as impact or impulse loading and injury tolerances;
- detailed description or reenactment of the fall;

- evaluation or consideration of pre-existing conditions or traumatic injuries (i.e. chronic subdural effusion; hydrocephalus)
- consideration of the unique characteristics of the infant skull – flexibility, thickness, elasticity; [26, 89, 135, 136, 148, 150, 151] and
- interpretation of findings in light of literature observations and controversies.

Asphyxia[152, 153]

Asphyxia is the leading cause of accidental death in children under 1 year of age.[154] Asphyxia generally refers to: inadequate intake of oxygen, interference with the oxygenation of blood, or cessation of effective respiration. For purpose of this discussion, asphyxia will refer to mechanical interference with breathing or acute airway obstruction, not the entire spectrum of hypoxia (i.e. carbon monoxide or cyanide poisoning). The essential process of asphyxia is interference with effective respiration. The result is hypoxia or anoxia, reduction of blood and tissue oxygen tension, cyanosis from accumulation of reduced hemoglobin, and accumulation of body carbon dioxide. In the neurologically intact individual, hypoxia and increased carbon dioxide stimulate the respiratory center and initiate the struggle to breathe. As the process continues, cyanosis deepens, veins may become engorged, and showers of petechial hemorrhages occasionally appear on the skin, conjunctiva, surface of the lungs, and heart. Eventually, consciousness is lost, convulsions may occur, and terminal vomiting is common. Typically the process takes about 2–3 minutes to unconsciousness and within 4–5 minutes to cause death.

Asphyxia can result under a variety of circumstances (Fig. 17.20):

- Traumatic asphyxia – interference with effective respiration due to external chest compression.
- Positional asphyxia – interference with respiration due to the position of the body.
- Unsafe sleeping[155, 156] – occurs when an infant's body or face is compressed by soft bedding, improper use of pillows, improper placement in swing, infant seat, or broken crib.
- Wedging – occurs when an infant's body or face is compressed within a narrow space resulting in interference with chest wall movements or obstruction of the airway.[157]
- Strangulation (neck compression) – interference of respiration by applying pressure to the neck using hands, ligature, or object.
- Choking (airway obstruction from foreign body) – interference with respiration from internal obstruction of movement of the air into lungs.
- Overlaying – the accidental suffocation by a sleeping adult.
- Hanging (suspended by body weight) – ligature strangulation in which force applied to the neck is derived from the weight of the body.
- Suffocation (nose and mouth occlusion) – interference with respiration due to external interference with movement of oxygen into the lungs.

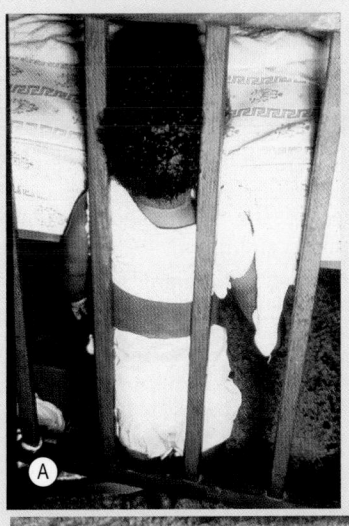

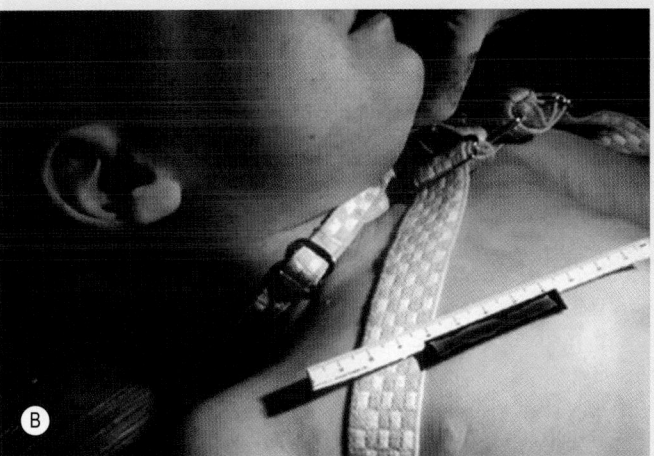

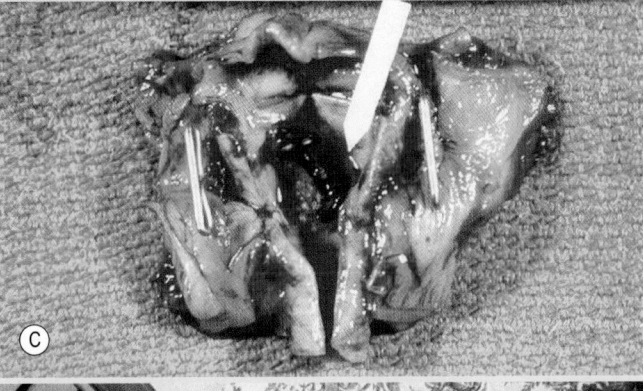

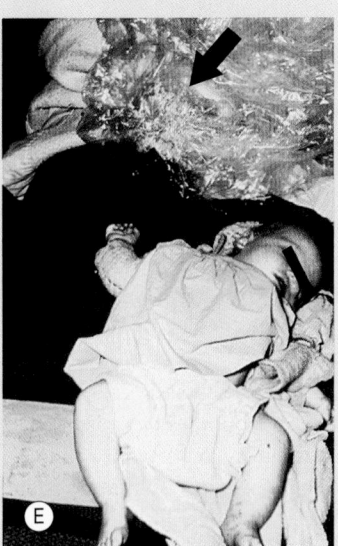

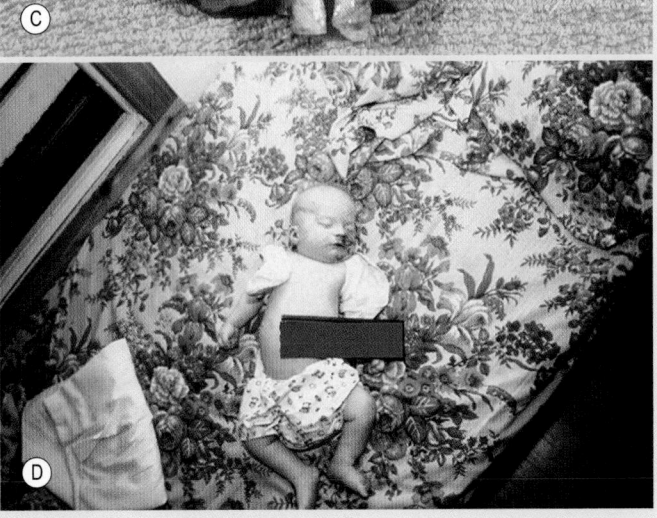

FIGURE 17.20
(A) Accidental asphyxia due to wedging. (B) Accidental ligature strangulation with child restraint. (C) Accidental asphyxial choking in an infant. (D) Accidental asphyxial death in an infant from overlaying. (E) Accidental asphyxia suffocation from plastic wrap, arrow shows vomitus.

- Homicidal suffocation – any of the above forms committed with the intent to kill.

Findings in asphyxial deaths may include facial petechiae, impressions of clothing or ligature marks, bruising or abrasions from wedging.

Choking on food/foreign objects and **unsafe sleeping circumstances** are the two greatest contributors to asphyxial death in childhood.[158–162] Severely disabled children have an increased risk of accidental asphyxia.[163] Accidental suffocation of an infant by a sleeping adult has been associated and reported with sleeping on polystyrene-filled cushions.[164, 165] Gilbert-Barness and colleagues reviewed 52 sudden deaths in infants of 2–9 months of age, emphasizing the risks to infants from waterbeds and soft bedding.[165] Other unsafe sleeping circumstances include v-shaped pillows, waterbeds, and mesh-sided cots.[116] Drabo and Dannenberg[166] reviewed US Consumer Safety Commission's Death Certificate files to evaluate information about infant products and patterns of suffocation. The most frequent cause of suffocation was wedging (bed or mattress and wall) and oronasal obstruction by a plastic bag. Patterns of suffocation were significantly related to age group. Drabo and Dannenberg concluded that suffocation hazards are not well recognized by care givers and that bed sharing and use of adult beds should be discouraged. Mitchell and others[167] have observed that children accustomed to supine sleep are at increased risk for sudden death in a prone position. Unsafe sleep practices such as position and unsafe sleeping surface increase the risk of sudden infant death.[164, 166, 168] Merchant et al[169] have observed that preterm and term newborn infants placed in car seats demonstrate reduced oxygen saturation levels especially if the infant remains in the seat for more than 20 minutes (preterm) or 60 minutes (full term).

Overlaying is the term applied to the accidental death by smothering caused by a larger person sleeping on top of an infant. Collins[157] reviewed a 15-year experience with childhood deaths in overlaying and wedging. Thogmartin et al[170] observed an association between unexplained infant deaths, and bed sharing, regardless of the sleep position of the infant. Blair et al[171] identified a particularly high risk of sudden deaths associated with infant sharing sofa with an adult during sleep. Risk factors for overlaying include fatigue, intoxication and sedation, in rare circumstances maternal sleeping during breastfeeding, and sleeping on sofa or recliner. This author has seen a dramatic increase in deaths attributed to unsafe sleeping or overlaying. Jurisdictions with aggressive and well-trained death investigators are uncovering increasing numbers of children dying in unsafe sleeping conditions. Although multiple unexplained deaths of siblings should be investigated as possible homicide, this author has experienced mothers with two separate fatalities of babies that eventually were determined to be combinations of unsafe sleeping and SIDS.

A wide range of conditions or diseases can cause fatal asphyxia. Undetected congenital anomalies can result in acute upper airway obstruction. This author reported a young infant dying suddenly with striking congenital subglottic stenosis. Byard and Taskos[152] provide a review of conditions associated with natural death with upper airway obstruction.

In most cases of infantile asphyxia, autopsy findings are non-specific and there are no specific diagnostic signs or criteria.[153] The postmortem appearance of an individual who has died from asphyxia may show intense venous congestion and cyanosis with pronounced lividity, petechial hemorrhages, pulmonary congestion and edema, and fluidity of the blood. Autopsy findings that have been observed in asphyxial deaths include:

- cutaneous petechiae;
- intrathoracic petechiae;
- focal intra-alveolar hemorrhage;
- oral nasal blood;
- increased intra-alveolar siderophages;
- alveolar overexpansion and rupture;
- pulmonary congestion with swelling of pneumocytes;
- microthrombosis;
- leukocyte margination in pulmonary microvasculature;
- collapse of bronchi; and
- perivascular, cuff-like edema around larger and medium-sized pulmonary branches.

Jaffe[172] reviews the pathogenesis of **petechial hemorrhage**. Their pathologic significance was first recognized in the literature by Tardieu in 1855.

The finding of petechiae is not diagnostic of a specific condition and has been reported in various conditions such as hypoxia due to suffocation or strangulation, positional asphyxia, Valsalva pressure, postmortem lividity, SIDS, scurvy, septicemia, disseminated intervascular coagulopathy (DIC), primary thrombocytopenia, fat embolism, and mechanical disruption due to blunt impacts.[173]

Moore and Byard[174] report the pathologic findings in hanging and wedging deaths in childhood. Petechial hemorrhages were found on the face in all the hanging deaths (eight of eight), whereas intrathoracic petechiae were identified in only two of the eight cases.

Petechiae are small extravasations of blood resulting from capillary hemorrhage. Petechial hemorrhages are most numerous where the capillaries are least supported, such as subconjunctival tissues, under pleural and pericardial membranes, and anywhere the degree of congestion is sufficient (brain, lungs, mucous membranes, eardrum). They can occur in all organs but receive particular notice when present in skin. Petechial hemorrhage involving the head is thought to be the product of mechanical vascular phenomena: specifically impaired venous return with increased venous pressure in the presence of continued arterial input. These circumstances can occur in asphyxial or natural conditions. An interesting observation is the *absence* or rare petechial hemorrhages of the thymus in cases of asphyxia due to overlaying.

Delmonte and Capelozzi[175] have identified morphologic variants in an analysis of lungs in asphyxial deaths (suffocation, strangulation, drowning, and aspiration). Pulmonary hemorrhage has been reported in acute asphyxia. The differential diagnosis of pulmonary hemorrhage is considerable but the finding at sudden death is cause for concern. Yukawa[176] studied pulmonary hemorrhage using digital image analysis and suggests that a moderate degree of pulmonary parenchymal hemorrhage may be an indication of airway obstruction for a significant period of time and suggests that diagnosis of SIDS in these circumstances may be inappropriate. The Center for Disease Control has published an excellent review of acute idiopathic pulmonary hemorrhage in infants with recommendations for investigation and surveillance.[177]

Recent literature has suggested that routine evaluation of pulmonary hemosiderin in sudden infant death is warranted.[178] Hanzlick and Delaney[179] have provided a semiquantitative method for scoring pulmonary hemosiderin and report the results in 59 infant deaths (Fig. 17.21). The scoring system uses three reviewers and Prussian blue-stained sections examined at 10× with an iron score from 0 (no stainable iron) to 4 (prominent stainable iron throughout the section). Scores can range from 0 to 48. Mean scores were 6. In five of six infants dying from conditions other than SIDS the score was 12 or higher, more than twice the mean. One of the high scoring infants died with asphyxia. This study group suggests that scores of 16 or greater may be a marker for cause of death other than SIDS.[180] Schluckebier et al[181] used a similar scoring system and also found low numbers of siderophages in all SIDS cases. High numbers of pulmonary siderophages were seen in five, all of

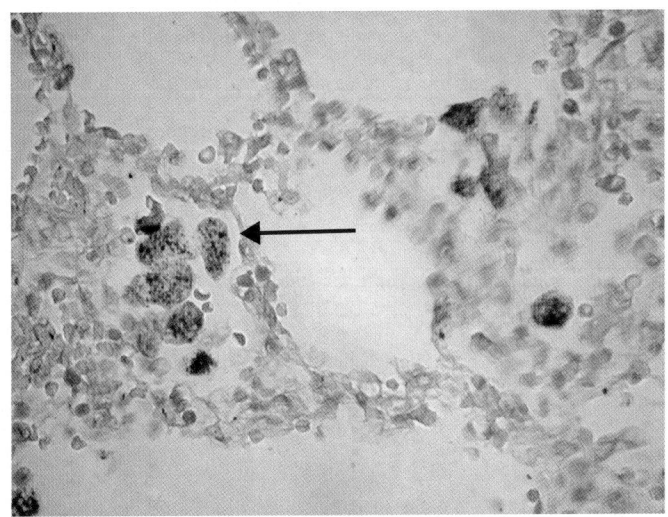

FIGURE 17.21 Pulmonary siderophages in homicidal suffocation.

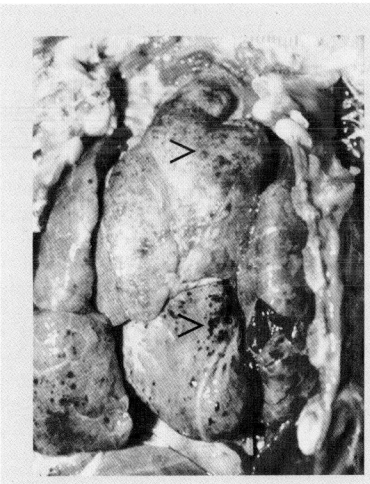

FIGURE 17.22
Intrathoracic petechiae found in 3-month-old infant; cause of death, sudden infant death syndrome.

which were suspicious deaths including a case of repeated suffocations and intentional homicide. Milroy[182] also reports a case of repeated suffocation and death with intra-alveolar hemosiderin. At the October 2004 Pediatric Pathology Society interim meeting Hanzlick concluded that:

- siderophages may be considered increased if focal abundant siderophages exist within most or all low power fields;
- the average number of siderophages per 20 high power fields exceeds 100;
- when siderophages are increased further investigation is warranted;
- when siderophages are increased the diagnosis of SIDS should be avoided;
- when siderophages are increased asphyxia should be considered;
- it is a good idea to stain for siderophages routinely in infant deaths;
- siderophages mean some sort of hemorrhage at least 2 days prior.

Scene investigation can be of critical importance in diagnosing asphyxia[156] (Table 17.9). Identification of the circumstances or manner of asphyxial death may be very difficult if the death scene is altered, investigation is incomplete, or the circumstances of the asphyxia are non-accidental. Krous et al[183] noted the importance of oronasal blood in sudden infant death. Careful scene investigation and autopsy can frequently distinguish between serosanguinous purge and frank blood. Oronasal blood observed prior to CPR may be an important indication of accidental or inflicted suffocation.

Sudden infant death syndrome (see also Ch. 18)

With the advent of the international 'back to sleep' campaign the occurrence of SIDS has decreased. SIDS is still a leading cause of infant death and occurs in infants found supine.[184] Evidence of chronic hypoxemia in utero has been suggested by finding elevated levels of fetal hemoglobin and in the liver, increased intramedullary hematopoiesis in the liver of SIDS victims.[185-188] The epidemiology of SIDS has remained constant despite recent decrease in overall incidence of SIDS in many countries:[189]

- characteristic age distribution (4–16 weeks);
- higher incidence in male, low birth weight and shorter gestation babies;
- history of neonatal problems at delivery;
- young maternal age;
- higher parity;
- infants of single mothers;
- multiple births;
- prone sleeping; and
- maternal smoking

Gross and microscopic findings in SIDS remain a constant:

- normal appearing infant with good nutritional status;
- intrathoracic petechial hemorrhages with emphasis on thymic petechiae (Fig. 17.22);
- heavy congested lungs;
- liquid blood;
- clenched hands;
- empty bladder;
- milk in stomach; and
- focal non-specific inflammation in upper airways

Krous et al[190] have studied characteristics of intrathoracic petechiae in SIDS victims with specific reference to sleep position. They found that neither age nor face down position was not associated with greater severity of thymic petechiae. Risse and Weiler[191] examined thymic petechial hemorrhages in SIDS victims and found that thymic petechiae are found in the majority of SIDS infants – both those with and those without a history of CPR. They also found that in non-SIDS (without extrinsic suffocation), hemorrhage pattern was different from SIDS victims in that the hemorrhages were of different sizes and irregularly distributed over the cortex and medulla.[192] Infants suffering from extrinsic suffocation have revealed much less pronounced thymic petechiae than SIDS victims.[192]

TABLE 17.9 INVESTIGATIVE CONSIDERATIONS IN POSSIBLE ASPHYXIAL DEATHS

Scene investigation	Examination of death scene
	Meticulous scene investigation and documentation of sleep conditions (bed, crib, couch, by experienced investigator)
	Inquiry of the caregiver if the body was moved or the scene altered
	Ideally the bedding and sleep surface should be carefully handled and taken for evidence processing. Presence of bright red blood on the infant, at the scene or on the parent clothing is a *red flag*
	Room temperature and description of infant swaddling must be detailed
	Competent assessment of infant core temperature at the scene (as soon as feasible)
	Careful examination at scene (when feasible) for presence of blood in nose or mouth
	Careful documentation, optimally video re-enactment of event (infant position when placed and when found)
	Details of individuals present: who placed and who found the infant
	Details of activities of daily living in the infant for the week prior to death
	Details of resuscitative efforts and duration
	Documentation by law enforcement when history of co-sleeping is elicited
History	Medications and prescriptions
	Assessment of growth and development pattern
	Review of pregnancy birth records
	Review of all medical encounters
	Review and documentation of known SIDS risk factors
	Detailed analysis of prior mortalities and when necessary reconsideration of original findings
Autopsy	Full body radiographs
	Appropriate photographic documentation of any injuries
	Careful examination and collection of trace evidence (fragments of lint or material)
	Complete autopsy to include infectious, metabolic, toxicologic analysis
	Collection and analysis of postmortem chemistries (vitreous or CSF)
	Magnification and otoscopic examination of oronasal tissues for subtle trauma or hemorrhage
	Careful inspection and documentation of cutaneous petechiae or injury
	Careful dissection of gastroesophageal tissues for detection of swallowed blood
	Careful dissection of airway for detection of aspirated blood (airway or stomach)
	Documentation of location, nature and distribution of intrathoracic petechial hemorrhage
	Evaluation of pulmonary aeration, congestion, alveolar overdistention or alveolar rupture
	Documentation and distribution of any gross pulmonary hemorrhage
	Histologic sampling of pertinent injuries to include histologic and morphometric examination of lung tissue for hemorrhage and presence of iron stained macrophages
	Careful and accurate documentation of OFC, length, weight
	Collection of appropriate specimens for special testing (prolonged QT, special metabolic)
	Special consideration in cases of multiple sudden unexpected deaths

CSF, Cerebrospinal fluid; OFC, occipital–frontal circumference; SIDS, sudden infant death syndrome.

Distinction between SIDS and accidental or homicidal asphyxia is a problem that forensic pathologists must address in all unexplained deaths in infancy. Within the last decade several cases of serially suffocated infants have been documented. There has been increased sensitivity as well as suspicion in cases of multiple sudden deaths in infancy or early childhood.[193] Multiple unexplained deaths do not in and of themselves mean homicide. However it is also now clear that the most common cause of multiple unexplained deaths in infancy is homicide. SIDS is not genetic or hereditary. Recurrence of sudden infant death in a family or reports of 'simultaneous SIDS' should precipitate comprehensive investigation for unsafe sleeping or possible intentional suffocation. Ladham et al[194] review a case of simultaneous SIDS as well as cases in twins. While the diagnosis of SIDS remains controversial for some, the unique and recurring circumstances of the fatalities and autopsy findings in these infants have not changed significantly over the years. Updates to the medical literature continue to assist in refining and improving the investigation, family resources, education, and ongoing research in the field. Excellent reviews are available.[195–201]

Drowning[202, 203]

The World Health Organization defines drowning as the process of experiencing respiratory impairment from submersion/immersion in liquid. Drowning is a complex form of hypoxia, involving not only asphyxia but also hydrostatic and osmotic effects of inhaled fluid in alveoli.[204-206] In most cases, death by drowning is due to inhalation of variable amounts of fluid. Drowning is the second leading accidental cause of death in childhood. Around 40–50% of all drownings and near-drownings occur in the 0–4 years age group, with toddlers (1–2 years) at greatest risk.[207]

Recommended guidelines for uniform reporting of data from drowning, 'The Utstein Style', were created and published as an advisory statement by an international consensus conference in 2003.[208] Recommendations include:

- Discontinue the use of the term secondary drowning or near drowning.
- Clarify that wet drowning implies aspiration of liquid; dry drowning implies no aspiration.
- Active and passive drowning should be replaced with witnessed and unwitnessed event.
- Precipitating events such as injury or medical condition should be recognized such as seizure, unconsciousness, trauma, pre-existing illness or condition.
- Immersion implies covered in water.
- Submersion implies the entire body, including airway is underwater.
- A time criterion is defined as the period of time between two events.
- Outcomes or types of morbidity should be identified such as:
  - brain death due to hypoxic or ischemic brain injury;
  - acute respiratory distress syndrome;
  - multisystem organ failure;
  - sepsis syndrome.
- Carefully document drowning characteristics:
  - was the event witnessed?
  - describe the body of water involved;
  - when was loss of consciousness noted?
  - was there pre-EMS (emergency medical services) resuscitation?
  - time EMS was called;
  - initial EMS vital signs (pupillary reaction, temperature, blood pressure, oxygen saturation);
  - time EMS resuscitation initiated;
  - neurologic status at the scene;
  - water temperature (when appropriate);
  - estimated time of submersion;
  - presence or absence of cyanosis;
  - method(s) of CPR used.

The family bathtub is the second most common site for childhood drowning and the most common site of infant drowning.[209] Saxena and Ang discussed the importance of careful neuropathologic examination in bathtub-related deaths to look for anatomic lesions.[210] The majority of drowning cases in young infants and children reflects lapse in adult supervision.

Non-accidental immersion must also be considered in immersion injuries in childhood.[211] Inflicted submersions may account for as many as 38% of bathtub events in children less than 5 years of age. The child victims of non-accidental

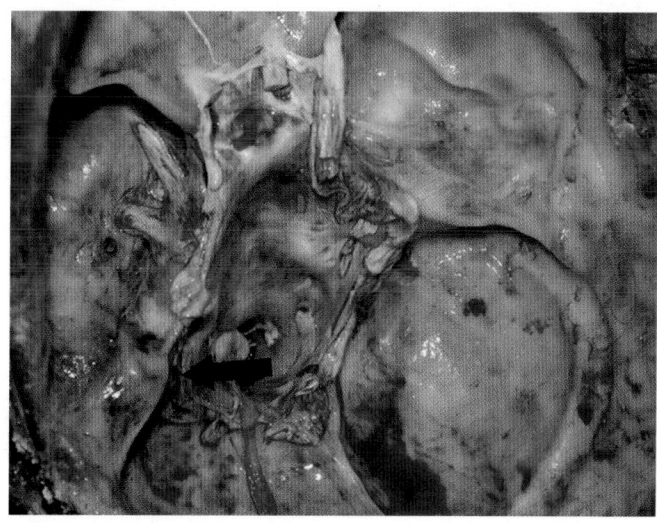

FIGURE 17.23 Hemorrhage of the petrous bone found in a child who drowned, see arrow.

immersion are frequently slightly older, are often handicapped, and may be the oldest child of a small sibship. These events may also occur at unusual times of day. Findings of post-immersion syndrome changes in the lungs and cerebral edema suggested to Griest and Zumwalt[212] that there may have been a delay in obtaining medical attention. Nixon and Pearn[213, 214] and Griest and Zumwalt[212] contend that deliberate immersion is not considered as frequently as it should be in pediatric cases because of the absence of specific traumatic injuries. Successful investigation of these very difficult cases requires cooperation between the investigative agencies and the pathologist as well as a complete death investigation.

Bucket immersion fatalities appear to be a risk for a specific age group (8–15 months).[215] These children are old enough to pull themselves to the edge of a pail but lack the motor skills and balance to extricate themselves if they fall in. Hot tub drownings are of particular interest because of the high temperatures and presence of **Pseudomonas sp.**, which makes these cases different from other immersion deaths.[216] Case reports of near drowning and fatalities in neonates delivered into water raises concern regarding the risk of delivery under water.[217]

There are no reliable tests that permit the unequivocal diagnosis of drowning, although the literature contains descriptions of typical postmortem findings in drowning victims. Diagnosis is made based on the circumstances of death. Postmortem findings may include: white or hemorrhagic foam in trachea and bronchi; water in stomach; overinflation of the lungs; non-specific brain swelling; hemorrhage in petrous or mastoid bones[218] (Fig. 17.23); pulmonary edema and hemorrhage; and alveolar distention with thinning of septa 'emphysema aquosum'. Development of subdural blood and other forms of intracerebral hemorrhage can occur following a drowning or near drowning event.[219] In cases of children suffering severe anoxic injury the mechanism of intracranial hemorrhage may be related to cerebral reperfusion.[220, 221]

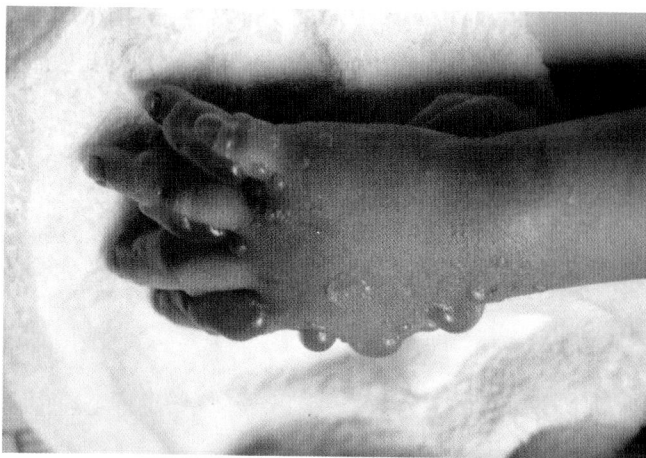

FIGURE 17.24 Stocking glove scald pattern in an infant; hand was dipped under hot tap water.

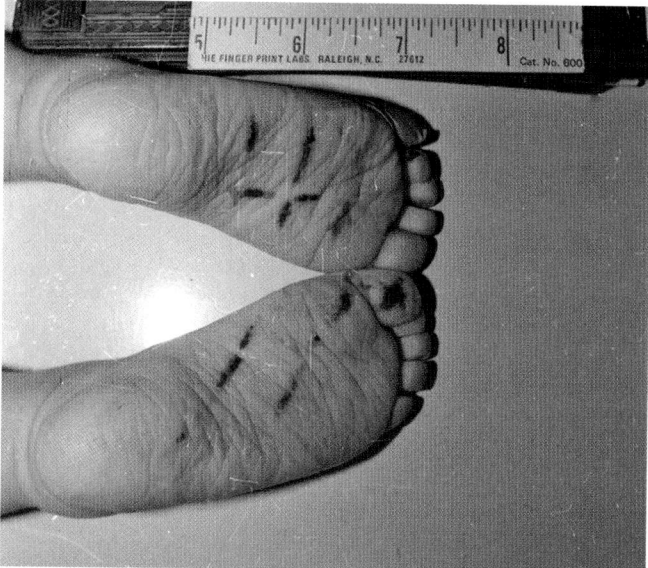

FIGURE 17.25 Contact burn; feet placed on hot heater grid.

Burns[222–224]

Thermal injury, or damage to tissue from the application of heat, occurs under a variety of conditions and can be categorized by type of injury or type of agent:

- scald (Fig. 17.24);
- contact (Fig. 17.25);
- flame;
- electrical;
- friction;
- chemical; and
- radiant.

The depth of a burn injury is a function of the temperature of the burn agent, the duration of exposure, and the thickness of the skin involved.[230] Because relative skin thickness is reduced in children, especially infants, they are more susceptible to shorter exposure times and lower temperatures.

A total of 70–90% of childhood burns occurs in the home. **House fires** cause 92% of all accidental burn- and fire-related deaths in children and are a major cause of death in black children aged 1–9 years.[225] The origins of the fires include cigarette lighters (20%), electrical malfunctions (18%), and playing with matches (8%).

Death due to fires requires a multidisciplinary investigative team. The forensic pathologist's responsibility includes identification of the victim and determination of cause of death. In infants and small children killed in a conflagration, identification may be especially challenging. In the event of severe thermal trauma carefully examine the airway, esophagus and stomach for evidence of soot or smoke inhalation. Its presence suggests respiration after onset of the fire. Inhalation of hot vapors can leave evidence of burning in the nasal and oral passages, upper airway, and esophagus. Experience with artifacts of thermal injury to the body is important to distinguish thermal fractures and heat hematomas from antemortem injury. Carbon monoxide determination is a routine analysis and can be run emergently during the postmortem examination.

Smoke inhalation injury may account for as many as 75% of fire-related deaths in the USA. However the percentage of children who experience respiratory symptoms after burns is significantly less than adults.[226] Fire in closed spaces increases the risk of smoke inhalation and exposure to polyurethane, wool, and silk increases risk of cyanide gas production. The damaging effect of smoke can result from three mechanisms:[227]

- thermal injury to oropharynx and airway;
- asphyxia from decreased oxygen, carbon monoxide production, the effect of cyanide gas, and production of methemoglobin; and
- pulmonary irritation resulting in direct tissue injury, airway clogging from debris, acute bronchospasm and inflammation.

Carbon monoxide toxicity is reportedly the leading cause of death by poisoning for all age groups in the USA. Neonates and fetus-in-utero are more vulnerable to carbon monoxide exposure due to the natural left shift of the dissociation curve of fetal hemoglobin. Carbon monoxide is formed as a byproduct of burning carbon compounds. Jaffe[228] discusses the complex pathogenicity of carbon monoxide on tissue and points out that injury does not result from reduction of oxygen capacity alone. Carbon monoxide has a greater affinity for the hemoglobin molecule than oxygen. Carbon monoxide exposure also results in a left shift of the oxygen saturation curve. The principal toxicity is due to cellular hypoxia. Carbon monoxide also binds to cardiac myoglobin resulting in myocardial depression and hypotension.[229]

Scald injuries represent about 40% of thermal injuries in children who receive medical attention, and about 75% of burn injuries in children less than 4 years of age. Scald injuries are usually described as spill or splash versus immersion type burns. Most of the accidental injuries result from incidents in the kitchen, but many also result from inappropriately hot tap water used in bathing. The rapidity of scalding injury increases drastically above 127°F. At 127°F full thickness burns can occur in adults in 1 minute.[231] At 130°F, full-thickness burns can occur in 30 seconds, and at 150°F in 2 seconds. At temperatures greater than 140°F, children can receive burns in one-quarter the time as an adult.[232] Feldman[233] reported a survey of hot water temperature settings in Seattle homes, showing that 80% of the homes had unsafe water temperatures set at greater than 130° F (average temperature 142°F). Comfortable bathing temperature for infants is about 101°F. Maximum water heater settings between 120 and 130°F are recommended. When investigating a scald injury, review on-site hot water testing data. Run the water in full position, hot only, for 3 to 5 minutes and measure with a reliable thermometer. Stevens[234] also recommends determining the volume produced per minute and temperature of contained water in the tub to assess relative heat loss.

Although tap-water burns are a relatively small percentage of all scald burns, Feldman and colleagues found them to be the most common abusive scald burns.[233] Showers and Garrison[235] studied 139 burn abuse patients, demonstrating that contact burns were the most common, occurring in 53% of cases (a third of which were cigarette burns), followed in frequency by immersion burns. However, scald burns resulted in two-thirds of the admissions to hospital.

When a scald injury occurs, there may be an interval in which the damaged nerve endings are relatively insensitive and the child may stop crying. The child may be crying prior to hot water exposure, so the severity of the injury may not be immediately appreciable. Feldman and colleagues[233] point out the special risk to handicapped children from scald injuries, both the risk from deliberate injury and the increased risk of accidental scalds secondary to limited communication skills and/or diminished sensation.

Scald injuries tend to produce three patterns of injury: spatters and splashes, immersion lines, and contact or protection patterns. **Spill or splash injuries** occur when hot liquids fall from a height onto the skin of the victim. The natural tendency of liquid to flow downward, cooling as it flows, produces a deeper burn in the upper aspect of the injury. The wound has irregular margins and a non-uniform depth. Depth becomes shallower as the fluid progresses toward the gravity-dependent portion of the body generating an arrowhead pattern. Liquid falling or projected in air may assume a round, spherical shape, and when impacts skin, results in a round injury. Clothing tends to diffuse the liquid and may offer a relative protection or lesser degree of burn. Spatters and splashes tend to be located on the face, hands, forearms, and feet.

Non-accidental burn injuries incurred during punishment or toilet training typically result in burns to the hands, feet, and buttocks. Immersion burns commonly result in a sharp line of demarcation separating normal from injured skin (Fig. 17.26). Air trapped in body creases or clothing or escaping from the mouth may protect the immersed skin. Maximal flexion of body may prevent hot liquid from contact with the skin, generating a flexion or striped configuration pattern. This pattern is usually seen anterior to the hip area or on the lower abdomen. Hot water when exposed to a cold surface will exchange heat rapidly. Contact with the bottom or sides of the tub or sink may generate a region of protected skin within a

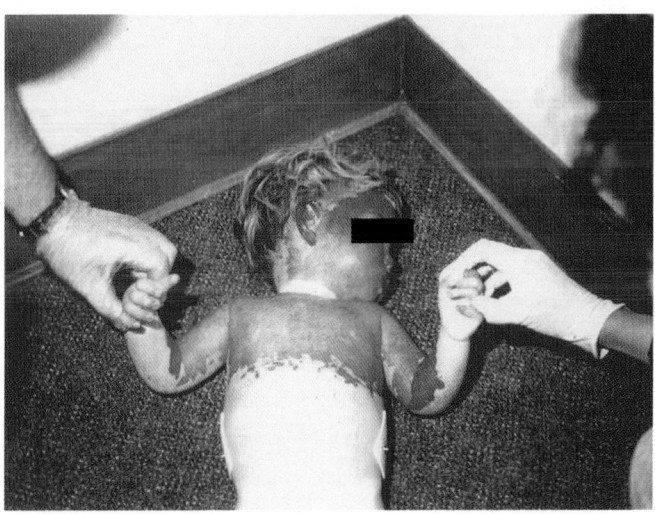

FIGURE 17.26 Infant immersed in bath water.

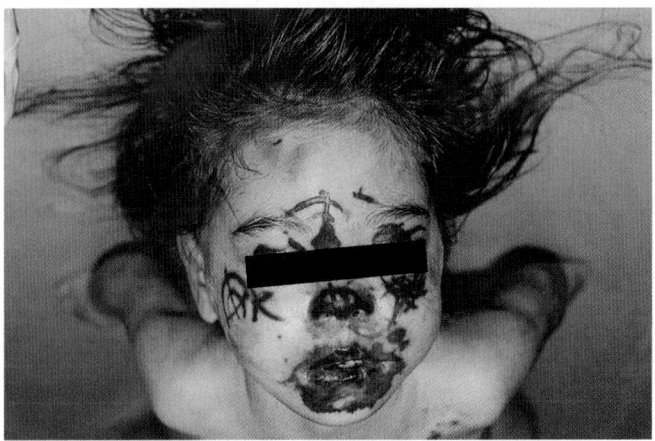

FIGURE 17.27 Pattern burn injury; burns to the mouth were caused by a hot liquid heated in the microwave; the remainder of the burns were postmortem and caused by contact with hairdryer head.

region of severely burned tissue, producing a 'hole-of-the-donut' pattern. Careful inspection of the burn pattern and distribution may enable the examiner to reconstruct the body position at the time of the burn.

Inflicted contact burns may leave evidence of the shape of the object. Electric hair dryers have a striking pattern (Fig. 17.27). Alexander[236] described two patients with unique **non-accidental microwave oven burns**. The pattern of microwave injury reflects the relative water content of the tissue components, with greater damage to skin and muscle than to adipose tissues.

Child abuse burns, particularly scalds, are a significant part of the spectrum of non-accidental injury (NAI). Jenny[224] summarizes burn injuries in children as well as skin conditions confused with abusive burns. In a nationwide survey of abused children, approximately 10% sustained burns. Although the true incidence of child abuse by burning is unknown, epidemiologic surveys[237] report that 6–28% of childhood burn victims were injured deliberately. The mortality rate of non-

BOX 17.10 CRITERIA SUGGESTING NON-ACCIDENTAL BURN INJURY[231–239]

History and social information

Inadequate supervision of child at time of injury

Unexplained delay between time of injury and first attempt to obtain medical attention

Account of accident not compatible with age and abilities of child

Differing historical accounts of burn

Inappropriate or lack of parental concern

Responsible adults alleging there were no witnesses to event; child was just discovered to be burned

Unrelated adult or relatives seeking medical care

Injury attributed to action of a sibling or other child

Burn attributed to child

Child with poor record of preventive and acute health care

Child with previous history of serious injury, or prior hospitalization for 'accidental trauma'

Inappropriate behavior manifested by child: excessively withdrawn, submissive, or over polite; does not cry during painful procedures

Poor parent–child relationship

No medical caregiver identified for child

Severe environmental stress, especially in a single-parent family

Inappropriate expectations of child by parent

Family previously known to protective services agencies

Common physical findings

History of burn incompatible with physical findings

Burn incompatible with developmental age of child

Burn depth uniform

Full-thickness burn

Areas other than front of body

'Mirror image' burns of extremities

Scalded hands or feet, often symmetric (glove-stocking pattern) with sharp demarcation lines, suggesting forcible immersion

Localized burns to perineum, genitalia, and buttocks

Burns to palms or soles

Multiple burns, suggesting more than one event

Cigarette-type burns, circular appearance, frequently clustered, often involving hands and forearms, present in normally clothed areas, scalp, bottom of feet

Deep contact burn imprints with crisp margins of entire burn surface; clear imprint of burned object

Excessive splash burns above primary impact site, suggesting fluid thrown

Sparing of body surfaces that would be expected with given history

Presence of spared areas within burn suggesting forced immersion

Burns assessed as older than historical account

Evidence of neglect of injury, infection; and/or generalized neglect

Unrelated hematomas, lacerations, fingernail marks and scars

Unsuspected fractures on skeletal survey

---

accidental burns approaches 30%, while death occurs in only about 2% of accidentally burned children. Abuse should be a major diagnostic consideration in any child with burns (Box 17.10). Hight and colleagues[238] emphasized the need to recognize intentionally inflicted injuries, citing the high repeat injury rate (30–70%) and mortality (30–40%) of these children once returned to their original environment.

Purdue and associates[239] studied 678 children admitted to the burn unit at Parkland Memorial Hospital. A total of 71 of the patients (10.5%) were diagnosed with deliberately inflicted burns. The mean age of these children was 1.8 years and the mean burn size comprised 13.5% body surface area. Tap-water scald was the most frequent cause of injury, with an immersion pattern present in 59% (six patients demonstrated a forced immersion pattern). Overall 14 of the children had associated non-burn trauma, and four died. Compared with children accidentally burned, the abused children had a significantly higher mortality rate, longer length of stay, and younger age. All the deaths occurred in children under 10 months of age while no children with accidental scald burns died. The mortality of infants less than 1 year was 19% in the abused group and 0% in the accidental group when inhalation injury was excluded. Tap-water scalds comprised 83.0% of the scald injuries in the abused

population and 15.7% in the accident population. No full-thickness tap-water scalds occurred in the accident population. Simultaneous deep scald burns of the buttocks, the perineum, and both feet were interpreted as pathognomonic of deliberate injury, and no accidental scalds demonstrated this pattern.

Caustics (acid and base agents) can cause significant tissue damage on contact. These injuries typically fall into either chemical burn or corrosive ingestion categories. The severity of the injury is related to a number of factors including pH of the agent, concentration of the agent, duration of contact time, volume of the offending agent, and the physical form of the agent.[240, 241]

Distinguishing healed or healing burn scars with scars from impetigo or infected bug bites may not be easy. This is especially difficult in situations with poor photography. Careful evaluation of the location, measurement, and history of skin infections in family members must be documented.

Electrical injury[242]

Electrical injury occurs to skin or internal organs from exposure to electrical current. In the USA electrical injuries cause approximately 1000 deaths and 20 000 visits to emergency department annually.[243]

Electrical injuries can affect the body in a variety of ways:
- nervous system (most commonly affected);
- cardiac and vascular injury;
- tissue thermal injury – arc, contact, flash or thermal burns;[244] and
- respiratory arrest.

Electrical injuries can result from a number of mechanisms: contact burns (deep coagulative necrosis), localized arc burns, non-contact flash burns, flame-type thermal burns, and injuries resulting from sustained muscle contraction. Electrical injuries should be viewed and managed as multisystem injuries. Low voltage injuries (110–440 V) are most common, accounting for more than 60% of injuries, commonly resulting from chewing on electrical cords or sticking objects into electrical outlets. Electrical injuries to children represent approximately 20% of all low voltage injuries. The severity of electrical injury depends on three factors: resistance of the skin and internal body structures, alternating current (AC) vs direct current (DC) (polarity), and duration of the stimulus. AC is significantly more dangerous than DC because of the tetanic muscle contractions the current can generate. Ohm's law states that the current flow (amperes) is equal to the potential difference (voltage) divided by the resistance (ohms). Skin resistance, a major factor in determining the amount of current flow, is affected by age, skin thickness, and water content. The skin resistance of a newborn infant is extremely low because of the high water content and thin stratum corneum. Contact with water also reduces skin resistance; hence, the severe mouth burns of a toddler in contact with the electrical cord. **Bathtub electrocutions** are a special risk to children under 5 years of age, typically resulting from exposure to hairdryers (about 60%).[245]

Environmental injuries

Environmental injuries or accidents for purposes of this discussion will refer to injuries or death due to affects of external conditions. Although the forensic pathologist has many circumstances to consider, those that are most likely to affect infants and children are:
- conditions that cause heat stress-hyperthermia;
- conditions that cause cold stress-hypothermia; and
- altitude sickness

Hyperthermia[240–242]

Heat related illness involves a continuum of clinical syndromes ranging from heat syncope to heat stroke. Heat stroke occurs when the body is unable to rid itself of excess heat, resulting in a rapid rise in core body temperature which poses an immediate medical emergency. Non-exertional, or classic heat stroke, can develop over a period of days in infants and young children and can also occur quickly in exposure to a hot environment, such as a child left unattended in a vehicle. Exertional heatstroke generally occurs in young individuals who engage in strenuous exercise for prolonged time in a hot environment.

Abnormal elevation of body temperature (pyrexia) can result from one of two mechanisms: fever or hyperthermia. In hyperthermia, defined as **core body temperature greater than 40°C,** thermal control mechanisms fail with heat production exceeding heat dissipation. In fever, the hypothalamic thermal set point rises and thermal control mechanisms raise the body temperature. The preoptic area of the anterior hypothalamus controls thermoregulation. Various clinical disorders can disrupt thermoregulatory homeostasis, with consequent hyperthermia. These include increased heat production, decreased heat dissipation, and hypothalamic insult. Whether the stimulus is fever or hyperthermia, autonomic and somatic nerve activation is the final pathway to pyrexia resulting in increased muscle tone, decreased sweating, and increased cutaneous vasoconstriction.[249, 250] Numerous exogenous agents can cause severe hyperthermia. Because salicylates uncouple oxidative phosphorylation in skeletal muscle, hyperthermia is seen in children with severe aspirin toxicity.[246] At core body temperatures above 40.5°C (104.9°F) oxidative phosphorylation becomes uncoupled and cellular enzymes fail. Cells that are most sensitive to increased body temperature are vascular endothelium, hepatocytes, and neural tissue.

Infants are at risk for heat illness because of inefficient sweating, higher metabolic rate and inability to care for themselves or control their environment. Infants have difficulty regulating body temperature because of a relatively diminished layer of insulating fat, small size, and high ratio of skin surface to body weight.[251] Infantile thermoregulatory mechanisms are less effective and may be inadvertently or carelessly undermined by the caretaking adult. Bolton et al[252] present an excellent theoretical model to understand thermal balance in infancy and its possible association with circumstances of sudden death. The risk to young children and infants in poorly ventilated rooms or closed automobiles is well recognized.[253, 254] Children with an impaired sweating mechanism are also at special risk. These include those with cystic fibrosis, congenital anhidrosis, and quadriplegia.

Krous et al[267] reviewed the circumstances, pathologic changes and manner of death in environmental hyperthermia in infants and young children. A total of 19 cases of heat-related deaths were reviewed in children aged between 53 days and 9 years. Children left unattended in vehicles were older in average age than children who died in bed. Hepatocellular necrosis and DIC were observed in victims who survived 6 hours or more. The most consistent postmortem finding was intrathoracic petechiae.

Examination of heat death requires careful investigation because the histologic effects of heat on organs alone cannot prove death by heat injury (Table 17.10).[268, 269] The investigation must include:
- measurement of environment at scene (as well as the maximum possible temperature for that location during the time of concern);
- description of clothing;

TABLE 17.10 AUTOPSY FINDINGS IN HYPERTHERMIA

Brain	Generalized hyperemia, fine macular hemorrhages in cerebral medulla, cerebral edema, extravasation in pia and arachnoid, paraventricular focal necrosis, degenerative changes of cortical neurons, signs of shock
Lungs	Severe vascular congestion, focal edema and hemorrhage, interstitial edema, subpleural hemorrhages, signs of shock
Liver	Focal hepatocellular necrosis, hepatocellular swelling, signs of shock
Kidney	Congestion, interstitial edema, signs of shock
Cardiac muscle	Interstitial edema, focal myocardial necrosis
Adrenal gland	Interstitial edema, focal epithelial necrosis, decreased lipids in outer cortex
Spleen	Perifollicular hemorrhages in spleen and abdominal lymph nodes
Petechial hemorrhage	Pleura, pericardium, endocardium, thymus[130]

- description of bedding and how the child was wrapped or placed;
- location and characteristics of heat vents, space heaters or other sources of radiant heat;
- history regarding recent fluid intake and output;
- presence or absence of preexisting condition or illness that could affect fluid balance; and
- assessment of prior growth and weight against postmortem findings.

In cases where the measured antemortem body temperature at the time of collapse was = 40.6°C (= 105°F), the cause of death should be certified as heat stroke or hyperthermia. Deaths may also be certified as heat stroke or hyperthermia with lower body temperatures when cooling has been attempted prior to arrival at the hospital and/or with a clinical history of mental status changes and elevated liver and muscle enzymes. In cases where the antemortem body temperature cannot be established the environmental diagnosis should be listed as the cause of death or as a significant contributing condition.[270]

Donoghue et al[270] published criteria for the diagnosis of heat related deaths. The National Association of Medical Examiners Ad Hoc Committee on the Definition of Heat-Related Fatalities recommends the following definition of 'heat-related death': a death in which exposure to high ambient temperature either caused the death or significantly contributed to it. The committee recommends that the diagnosis of heat-related death be based on a history of exposure to high ambient temperature and the reasonable exclusion of other causes of hyperthermia. Diagnosis may be established from the circumstances surrounding the death, investigative reports concerning environmental temperature, and/or measured antemortem body temperature at the time of collapse.

In reviews of infants dying in circumstances suggestive of **heat stroke,** similar clinical and pathologic features were observed: sudden onset, fever, convulsions, shock, hepatorenal disturbance, acidosis, diarrhea, and DIC.[271, 272] A cutaneous manifestation of heatstroke is hemorrhagic diathesis. Laboratory findings in heatstroke reflect multisystem organ damage. These include: leukocytosis, hemoconcentration, thrombocytopenia, findings consistent with DIC [increased partial thromboplastin time (PTT), decreased fibrinogen, increased fibrin split products], renal abnormalities, abnormalities of hepatic function, metabolic abnormalities such as respiratory alkalosis due to direct CNS stimulation, hypophosphatemia, hypocalcemia, hypomagnesemia, elevated creatine phosphokinase and hypoglycemia.[245] Autopsy findings revealed cerebral edema, focal necrosis and fatty change of the hepatocytes, dilation of the renal tubules, and (in some cases) unusual changes of the intestinal villi.

Bacon[258] identified the narrow age range (2–10 months) of children when death or encephalopathy was attributed to overheating and suggested that this age range may reflect a time of increased **thermoregulatory instability**. Heat production in proportion to surface area, the cause of this instability, reaches a maximum by about 5 months of age, while **the ability to lose heat by sweating develops slowly over the first year of life**. Rutter and Hull[259] examined the response of full-term infants to increasing increments of heat in the environment. As the infants approached the point of sweating, the authors made a number of observations: spontaneous activity ceased, the skin reddened, and the child assumed a sun-bathing posture. Newborns did not increase evaporative water loss until the ambient temperature reached 34°C, older infants perspired at lower temperatures, infants perspired readily at 1 day of age; thereby suggesting that postnatal and gestational age influenced the environmental temperature at which sweating was observed. Stanton[255] also observed that infants cried in response to cold but remained passive when the ambient temperature was raised. Gozal and colleagues[260] reported a 6-month-old infant who developed cyanosis and central hypoventilation associated with environmentally induced hyperthermia from **overwrapping** (temperature 41.2°C). Bass and colleagues[261] studied the effects of temperature and oxygenation and concluded that cells are more heat sensitive under conditions of anoxia.

Hemorrhagic shock with encephalopathy syndrome (HSES) describes a condition characterized by abrupt onset of hyperpyrexia, shock, encephalopathy, diarrhea, and DIC with renal and hepatic failure in previously healthy infants.[262] Non-ketotic hypoglycemia has also been documented in some cases. The etiology of HSES is unknown, however, hyperpyrexia appears to play a central role in the pathogenesis.[263] Coma, recurrent seizures, and brain edema are the most common cause of morbidity and mortality. Brain findings demonstrate cerebral edema with white matter petechial hemorrhages.[264] Basal ganglia and cerebellum are relatively spared. CT scans display diffuse areas of low density in the cerebral cortex with intraventricular and parenchymal hemorrhages. MRI reveals hemorrhagic cortical lesions.[265] The median time for abnormal laboratory values peak between 1.2 and 1.4 days.[266]

Overheating or heat stress may be overlooked in the analysis of sudden, unexpected death in infancy. Stanton[255] reviewed a series of SIDS deaths and observed similar non-specific intestinal changes in 8 of 33, with none of 12 patients dying of chronic or congenital conditions showing these changes. On the other hand, Schurs-Masters et al[256] conducted an epidemiologic study of heat stress and the incidence of SIDS. They failed to find a relationship between excessively elevated environmental temperatures and the incidence of SIDS. Elabbassi et al[257] demonstrated that under consistent environmental conditions there is no association between body position and body overheating.

Hypothermia[267–273]

Hypothermia, defined as **body temperature less than 35°C,** is a more frequently recognized contributing factor in childhood death.[273–275] Hypothermia is classified as accidental or unintentional (as in cardiopulmonary bypass) and primary or secondary. Accidental hypothermia is defined as an unintentional decline in core temperature below 35°C (95°F). Primary hypothermia results from accidental exposure to cold. Secondary hypothermia occurs when the presence of a disease state causes a failure of thermoregulation. Although no precise figures are known for temperatures potentially dangerous to life, Saukko and Knight[276] suggest that air temperature below 10°C (50°F) is low enough to cause hypothermia in vulnerable persons. Factors such as breeze, wind, and damp conditions of clothing can aggravate the rate of cooling.

Hypothermia can result from decreased heat production from a variety of mechanisms:

- hormone deficiency, severe malnutrition, hypoglycemia, or neuromuscular inefficiencies as seen in the extremes of age;[277]
- increased heat loss such as accidental hypothermia, vasodilation from pharmacologic or toxicologic causes, erythrodermas (e.g. burns) that decrease the body's ability to preserve heat, or iatrogenic etiologies; and
- impaired thermoregulation which is typically related to hypothalamic failure.

Children have reduced thermoregulatory capacity and have physical limitations regarding the availability of corrective actions when exposed to temperature extremes. Infants are especially vulnerable due to the high surface to body weight ratios, with highest risk to the newborn in the first weeks after birth.

In patients found dead of exposure the principal finding is low core temperature. Body core temperatures 10–15°F lower than normal are associated with decreased tissue oxygenation and increased risk for cardiac arrhythmias. When body core temperature falls below 32°C there is decreased level of consciousness and decrease of respiratory rate, pulse and blood pressure. Recovery is rare at less than 26°C (78.8°F.) Immersion hypothermia causes loss of body heat at a significantly higher

rate than does exposure to the same temperature in dry cold air. Humans are able to maintain and retain body heat balance in water at 22°C, with survival time decreased sharply in water less than 16°C.

Spontaneous hypothermia followed by delayed hyperthermia is not uncommon after resuscitation from cardiac arrest in children. Hickey et al[280] report this observation in resuscitated adults as well. Desai and Srikandan[281] report a child with severe hypothermia secondary to ibuprofen. Complications of active external rewarming can result in 'core temperature drop' which results from rapid return of cold peripheral blood to the heart. 'Rewarming acidosis' results from pooled lactic acid joining the central circulation. Peripheral vasodilation may cause venous pooling and 'rewarming shock'.[281]

Profound hypothermia can mimic death and controversy surrounds criteria for death in a hypothermic patient. Severe bradycardia with absent pulse and respirations, severe shock, and reduced brainwaves may give the appearance of death using minor criteria at low body core temperature (less than 86°F). Recent cases have shown that children who rapidly become hypothermic, usually after ice water submersion, may have a very prolonged period for salvage. Determination of death should not be made until the victim, carefully returned to normal core temperature, still fails to re-establish signs of life.

Findings at autopsy are varied and non-specific for hypothermia (Box 17.11). The body may show patches of pink–brown discoloration typically over extensor surfaces and joints. Internally acute gastric erosions, pulmonary edema, less frequently pancreatitis, and perivascular brain hemorrhage especially the wall of the third ventricle have been observed. Coe[52, 57, 59] reported that elevated vitreous glucose in the postmortem examination may be a reflection of significantly elevated blood glucose in patients treated for hypothermia.

For investigative purposes, a thermocouple or non-clinical thermometer is preferred for environmental and core body temperature documentation.

BOX 17.11 AUTOPSY FINDINGS IN HYPOTHERMIA[268, 276]

Pink lividity and internal tissues

Coarse macular hemorrhages of gastric and intestinal mucosa

Gastric or intestinal erosions, Wischnevsky ulcers

Pancreatic (fat) necrosis from autodigestion

Multiorgan infarcts

Intrapulmonary hemorrhages in majority of children

Depletion of hepatic glycogen

Fatty degeneration of renal proximal tubular epithelium

Subpleural and subpericardial hemorrhage

Lipid depletion of adrenals and brown fat in infants

Muscle hemorrhage in body core, especially iliopsoas muscle

Altitude sickness

Moderate altitude sickness is defined as illness associated with altitudes of 8000–10 000 feet (2400–3000 m) and **high altitude sickness** is defined as illness associated with attitudes of 10 000–18 000 feet (3000–5500 m) above sea level. Altitude sickness includes acute mountain sickness (AMS), high altitude cerebral edema (HACE), and high altitude pulmonary edema (HAPE).[282] AMS typically presents at greater than 2500 meters and is characterized by headache, anoxia, vomiting, fatigue or insomnia.[282, 283] Presenting symptoms in children less than 3 years of age may be non-specific and difficult to distinguish from changes due to travel. Symptoms usually begin 4–12 hours after ascent. HACE, usually preceded by AMS, consists of ataxia, behavioral changes, hallucinations, confusion, disorientation, decreased level of consciousness, focal neurologic signs, and coma. HAPE, also often preceded by AMS, is caused by altitude hypoxia and is characterized by dyspnea, exercise intolerance, cough and hemoptysis, tachycardia, tachypnea, cyanosis, and fever. Although comprehensive studies of the incidence of altitude sickness are not available, the following observations have been documented by the International Society for Mountain Medicine Consensus Committee[284] regarding children at altitude:

- The incidence of AMS in children appears to be the same as adults.
- The nature and incidence of HAPE may differ between children who visit high altitude and those who reside at high altitude and return (reascend) from low or sea level travel. Children who reside at high altitude have a higher risk of reascent HAPE.

Risk factors for acute altitude illness in children include:

- rate of ascent;
- absolute altitude;
- exertion;
- length of altitude exposure;
- cold (temperature);
- preceding viral infection;
- perinatal pulmonary hypertension;
- congenital heart disease especially unilateral absence of pulmonary artery or patent ductus arteriosus;
- individual variations in susceptibility; and
- reascent to altitude.

Age and health of the child and duration of exposure to altitude may add theoretical concerns to risk of exposure to altitude in children. There is no data on safe absolute altitude for ascent in children. Healthy children are at risk for HAPE, especially following rapid ascent.[285] Children have a similar occurrence rate of HACE as adults.[286]

It is unclear from the literature whether exposure to altitude increases risk of SIDS. However, Kohlendorfer et al[287] identified altitude of residence as a significant risk predictor of SIDS in combination with prone sleeping position.

Poisoning[288]

Toxicology is the study of the mechanisms by which chemicals produce adverse effects on cells and organisms. Poison is a term that applies to a substance that when introduced to the body produces a toxic or harmful consequence. This usually results from action that impairs or prevents normal metabolic processes. Busy emergency departments and poison control centers successfully manage most toxic ingestions in children.

There are more than one million unintentional poisonings among children less than 3 years of age reported annually to poison control centers in the USA.[289] The most toxic exposures reported in children are due to commercial products, pharmaceuticals, and natural toxins (plants) available in the home. These agents include analgesics (acetaminophen,[290] aspirin, ibuprofen, narcotics), cleaning agents, plants, cough and cold preparations,[291] vitamins, alcohols, hydrocarbons (gasoline), lead, and carbon monoxide.[292, 293] Child-resistant packaging and locks, more effective management of poisoning by regional control centers, and overall prioritization of educational efforts directed at prevention are contributing factors to a decrease in poisoning deaths in childhood. Some issues still in need of attention include the increasing problem of alcohol poisoning in children;[295] narcotic abuse and accidental deaths in children;[289] adverse therapeutic drug reactions;[296–299] poor packaging of household containers; and chronic lead poisoning, especially in new immigrant populations.[300] Childhood poisoning is an important cause of morbidity and mortality especially in developing countries.[301, 302]

Michael and Sztajnkrycer[289] have identified nine common agents that may result in catastrophic consequences at low or even 'one-pill' doses in children:

- calcium channel agonists;
- camphor;
- clonidine and the imidazolines;
- cyclic antidepressants;
- opioids and opiates;
- Lomotil;
- salicylates;
- sulfonyl ureas; and
- toxic alcohols (methanol, ethylene glycol, isopropanol).

Iatrogenic poisoning or medication errors occur with improperly prescribed, improperly administered, or idiosyncratic reactions to drugs ordered under medical supervision. These events are under-reported as they are not typically referred to poison control centers.

Infant botulism has surpassed the prevalence of food-borne and wound botulism in the USA.[303] As of 1996 the Centers for Disease Control and Prevention (CDC) had documented over 1500 cases and it is estimated that as many as 250 cases a year may go unrecognized. Soil and honey contamination are the two recognized sources of botulinum spores in infants.

Risks to children exposed to drugs and alcohol are well recognized. Cases of babysitters exposing children in their charge to marijuana and alcohol have been reported.[307, 334] Intentional drug use in children as young as 6 years and poisoning of infants by young siblings have been reported. When any drug ingestion is considered, a full drug screen should be performed to rule out multiple drug exposure.[305]

Infants can be exposed to drugs through mother's milk, passive inhalation, and other environmental exposure. Alternative medicine and home remedies can result in serious intoxication. This author evaluated a young child inadvertently poisoned with salt as the consequence of a traditional medicine treatment.

Intentional poisoning as a form of child abuse is now well recognized, but is fortunately uncommon.[303] Fatal and non-fatal injury from the deliberate intoxication of young children with therapeutic drugs, drugs and substances of abuse, salt, and water have been reported.[304–311] Hickson and co-workers[312] report nine infants who experienced apparent acute life-threatening events (ALTE) that occurred as the result of poisoning by a caretaker. Rivenes et al[313] report a case of intentional caffeine poisoning in a 5-week-old infant and Morrow[314] reports fatal caffeine intoxication in a 13-month-old. Both cases had associated physical findings of inflicted trauma. Perez et al[315] report a 5-week-old with intentional opiate intoxication.

Recurrent poisoning from a variety of substances has been reported with child abuse from fabricated illness (see Munchausen syndrome by proxy; MSBP).[316] A series of infants dying suddenly and unexpectedly with negative autopsy identified Benadryl in the postmortem samples. The determination of cause of death due to intentional poisoning was made, in the absence of signs and symptoms of intoxication. [317]

Failure to suspect intentional poisoning results in failure to detect and intervene. The diagnosis of intentional poisoning requires a high index of suspicion in children with unexpected and unexplained illness. Absence of any clear cause of death may suggest possible drug ingestion. Any time a child is admitted with possible non-accidental trauma, blood and urine should be collected for drug screening. Routine collection of the proper specimens for appropriate toxicologic analysis in sudden death in infants is also recommended.[318] Armstrong et al[319] report a case of fatal oxycodone levels in a 2-year-old. Routine hospital drug screens would not identify this intoxication because oxycodone is not routinely screened unless requested. Evaluation of signs and symptoms and selection of specific drugs for quantification may be indicated if poisoning is suspected.

There are excellent review articles that address the complexities and problems associated with postmortem changes and pharmacokinetics and their interpretation.[320, 321] Unless the examiner is experienced in postmortem interpretation and knowledgeable regarding binding and redistributive properties of drugs, extreme caution must be exercised when interpreting postmortem drug concentrations. Identification of a drug or exogenous chemical in body fluids and tissues only indicates exposure to the drug or compound. A number of artifacts occur postmortem that affect concentration of drugs in specimens: blood composition changes after death; many drugs are unstable in biological samples, and postmortem diffusion of drugs proceeds from sites of high concentrations in major organs (lungs, liver, cardiac muscle and stomach).[311] Drug concentrations vary in the same individual between samples taken from different sites. Cardiac blood is frequently used for drug screening; unfortunately, it is not an acceptable source for quantification or interpretation of premortem drug levels.

The best estimate of antemortem drug concentrations is achieved by collecting blood as soon as possible and at sites away from the mediastinum and abdomen. Femoral blood is recommended but even at this site there is no way to verify that the values reflect levels at the time of death.

Intrauterine injury/birth trauma

The forensic analysis of peripartum and intrauterine injuries requires access to information from maternal, fetal, and placental sources. The gestational development and inter-relationships between fetus and mother supported by the placenta are complex and change dramatically as the pregnancy proceeds. Adverse physical and chemical conditions will affect the developing fetus differently depending on the stage and characteristics of exposure. Injuries from intrauterine drug exposure, prenatal trauma, intrapartum or birth trauma can result in injuries that may not be detected at delivery. Although birth trauma accounts for very few neonatal deaths, injuries resulting from birth still occur (estimated at 6–8 injuries/1000 live births). Laroia[322] summarizes the spectrum of birth injuries including the patterns of soft tissue injuries most frequently associated with birth.

Trauma affects 6–7% of pregnancies in the USA and is the leading cause of non-obstetric maternal mortality.[323] Motor vehicle crashes, domestic violence and falls are the most common causes of maternal injury. Fetal mortality after trauma is significant. Weiss et al [324] summarize the spectrum of fetal deaths related to maternal injury in 240 traumatic fetal injury cases (an incidence of 3.7 fetal deaths/100 000 live births). Ali et al[323] report predictors of fetal mortality in pregnant trauma patients: injury severity score, blood loss, abruptio placenta and presence of DIC. Minor trauma during pregnancy is associated with significant increase in risk for fetal morbidity and mortality. Dobo et al[325] estimate that 12% of pregnant patients with minor trauma have ensuing pregnancy complications.

There are many forensic issues to consider when assessing birth injury and death which include:
- overall well-being of the fetus as reflected by growth for gestational age (appropriate, small, or large for gestational age);
- presence or absence of abnormalities of placentation;
- assessment of timing of injury;
- presence or absence of inflammation;
- determination of time of death;
- presence or absence of serious or lethal malformation;
- analysis of risk factors in pregnancy (e.g. smoking, drug use, trauma);
- analysis of prenatal care and complications; and
- presence or absence of birth injuries.

Birth trauma can be defined as injuries due to avoidable or unavoidable mechanical forces affecting an infant during labor and delivery. Birth injury is thought to affect 2–7/1000 live births, but the majority of cases do not result in mortality (5–8/100 000 live births). Factors commonly associated with birth injuries include:[322]

- primigravida;
- oligohydramnios;
- macrosomia (> 4000 g);
- very low birth weight or prematurity;
- certain congenital anomalies (spinal dysraphism);
- large fetal head;
- cephalopelvic disproportion;
- abnormal fetal presentation;
- difficult delivery;
- prolonged or rapid labor;
- instrument deliveries (use of vacuum extractor or forceps); and
- versions or extractions.

  Birth injuries can include:
- soft tissue injuries;
- fractures (skull, clavicle, long bone, ribs);
- cranial injuries;
- spinal and spinal cord injuries;
- peripheral nerve injuries; and
- visceral injuries (liver, spleen, adrenal).

Intracranial injury is the most common important birth injury and is generally thought to be related to excessive molding of the head or sudden pressure changes in head shape. Fatal birth injuries typically involve intracranial hemorrhage. Hemorrhage may arise from tears within the dura, rupture of vessels, or trauma to the brain substance resulting in contusion or tears with intraventricular or intraparenchymal hemorrhage. Intracranial birth injuries typically present as symptoms of apnea and seizures.[326] The most common intracranial injury is subdural hemorrhage (SDH). Hayashi et al[327] reviewed 48 cases of neonatal SDH secondary to birth trauma and developed a classification based on the extent and location of the hemorrhage. SDH has previously been considered to be a traumatic injury resulting from a difficult or complicated delivery. Chamnanvanakij et al[328] reviewed a serious of SDH in full-term infants and found that SDH is an infrequent but potentially serious problem. SDH was associated with normal spontaneous vaginal delivery and with assisted forceps delivery. Acute SDH has also been reported following caesarean section delivery.[329] The clinical signs and symptoms attributed to the SDH was most often a subtle clinical problem.

Cerebral infarction or perinatal stroke is a more common occurrence than past estimates have suggested. Stroke syndrome may be difficult to recognize and presentation in the neonatal period is more frequently recognized than those that occur prenatally. Included in the risk factors for cerebral infarction in the neonate are: intrapartum trauma; trauma to the mother; and prenatal substance abuse; as well as numerous maternal, fetal, and neonatal conditions; and placental disorders.[330] Infants with perinatal stroke may be asymptomatic in the neonatal period and present with overt problems days to months after an asymptomatic prenatal and peripartum period. The analysis of stroke requires comprehensive evaluation of maternal, fetal, and neonatal findings.[330–332] MRI scans are the preferred neuroimaging tests with special attention to vascular circulation. Ultrasound is not a sensitive indicator of perinatal stroke.[331, 333]

Intrauterine drug exposure and neonatal deaths in cases of maternal drug use continues to be a forensic challenge. Determination of the role of illicit drugs in abruptio placenta, premature delivery, intrauterine growth retardation, and intrauterine stroke are a few of the not infrequent questions posed to the examining pathologist.

Children born to substance abusers have a variety of problems including high potential for neglected pregnancy, prenatal exposure to drugs, medical and obstetric complications, intravenously transmitted disease, premature birth and stillbirth, fetal addiction and withdrawal, intrauterine growth retardation, postnatal mortality, failure to thrive, SIDS, infectious diseases, neurobehavioral problems, fetal alcohol syndrome, effects of passive inhalation of crack cocaine, as well as the potential risks of abuse, neglect, and accidental death.[335–337] The number of children born each year exposed to intrauterine drugs and/or alcohol is estimated to be between 550 000 and 750 000.

The deleterious effects of maternal alcohol consumption have been recognized for decades. Fetal alcohol spectrum disorder affects 1/750–1000 live births with at least 5000 infants with fetal alcohol syndrome born in the USA each year[338] and continues to be a leading cause of mental retardation.[339, 340] Because the placenta is permeable to ethanol, maternal blood alcohol becomes the fetus's blood alcohol. The fetus has no alcohol dehydrogenase and the fetal alcohol levels persist as the maternal level diminishes. Physical and postmortem findings in these children suggest that alcohol affects the developing fetus by reducing the number of cells and normal cellular migration, especially in brain tissue.[341]

The syndrome of neonatal narcotic withdrawal is well documented.[342] Onset of labor with abruptio placenta has immediately followed intravenous use of cocaine. The rate of spontaneous abortion in pregnant women using cocaine is high, and exposed infants are at increased risk for congenital anomalies, intracranial hemorrhage, cerebral infarction, and perinatal mortality.[343, 344] Volpe[345] summarized the mechanisms of action and deleterious effects of cocaine on the developing infant. Infants exposed to the drug in utero show significant depression of interactive behavior,[345] and prenatal exposure to drugs is a significant risk factor for SIDS.[339, 340] Phencyclidine (PCP) has been identified in cord blood of newborns and in breast milk. In a study of 200 randomly selected patients in labor and delivery at Los Angeles, University of Southern California Women's Hospital, PCP was detected in 12% of cord blood samples and 8.43% of maternal samples.[348]

The concept of fetal abuse and neglect continues to evolve.[349, 350] How do we effectively protect the child at risk without jeopardizing the personal freedom of the mother?[351] The courts do recognize the rights of a viable fetus to a healthy existence.[352] Some jurisdictions have accepted a child born with fetal alcohol syndrome as prima facie evidence of child abuse; others have used positive cord blood toxicology for street drugs as evidence of abuse (furnishing drugs to a minor) in order to protect the infant. MacMahon[353] reports the long-term follow-up of in utero exposed infants whose mothers were reported to child protective services.

Child abuse and neglect[354]

In 1946, John Caffey identified a pattern of multiple long bone fractures and subdural hematomas[355] that was later identified as a pattern of NAI.[356, 357] Despite the attention child abuse and neglect has received since Caffey's landmark publication, historical interest in this problem has dated from early history.[358–360]

In the last 25 years the definitions of child abuse have undergone remarkable transformation. Community investment in legal, social, and medical expertise is substantial. In some larger cities there are multidisciplinary centers for the evaluation and documentation of child abuse affiliated with children's hospitals. Controversies have also arisen within the medical community regarding the characteristics of inflicted injuries. These include the theory and dynamics of shaken infant syndrome, injuries from short falls, Munchausen syndrome by proxy (MSBP), serial suffocations in infancy, the role of biomechanical analysis, and evidence-based medicine. Most of the debate centers on the interpretation of injuries and how they came to be, rather than on the physical evidence.

Physicians now routinely consider child abuse as a part of the differential diagnosis when a child presents gravely ill or with traumatic injuries. At one time the professional responsibility to report abuse or suspected abuse was discretionary. Today, suspected abuse must be reported to police or child protection authorities; failure to report often carries legal sanctions.

While the actual incidence of child abuse has not been accurately determined, the National Child Abuse and Neglect Data System (NCANDS) estimates that 896 000 children (12.3/1000) were victims of abuse or neglect in 2002.[361] Olesen and colleagues report an incidence of maltreatment necessitating hospital therapy in 26.8/100 000 children under 15 years of age.[362] In children under 1 year of age, abuse ranks second only to SIDS as the cause of death beyond the newborn period. For children over 1 year of age, abuse ranks second only to accidents. NCANDS reports an estimated 1400 child fatalities due to abuse in 2002.[361] The rate of abuse and neglect fatalities increased slightly in 2002 (from 1.96/100 000 to 1.98/100 000 children), which may reflect changes in reporting procedures rather than an increase in abusive events.

Preschool children represent 28% of the childhood population but sustain 74% of abuse-related fatalities.[363] More than 50% of abused children are under 3 years of age, and approximately 25% are more than 1 year old. Infants less than 1 year account for 41% of fatalities.[361] Overpeck et al[364] provide an analysis of risk factors for infant homicide in the USA. The study included 2776 homicides occurring between 1983 and 1991 and showed that half the homicides occurred by the fourth month of life associated with very young mothers with history of previous births.

There is no specific profile of the perpetrator in fatal child abuse. The relationship of the perpetrator changes with the age of the injured child. Both male and female perpetrators are frequently young, immature, socially isolated, members of the lower socioeconomic stratum, often victims of abuse themselves, and experiencing recent family stress.

Factors that should be considered when evaluating an injured child include:
- nature and character of injuries
- feasibility and analysis of the reported event(s)
- age and development of the child
- evidence of significant physical or medical neglect
- unreasonable delay in seeking medical attention
- presence of previous significant or suspicious injuries in child or siblings
- significant changes in explanation of events or the history that doesn't match the clinical findings
- overall health and well-being of the child and siblings
- presence of multiple unexplained injuries
- witnessed or acknowledged inflicted injuries
- presence of documented domestic violence
- presence of documented substance abuse

Strait et al[365] provide an excellent tool for evaluating humeral fractures in children less than 3 years of age without obvious etiology that can serve as an excellent baseline for analysis of a variety of childhood injuries. Analytical findings have been categorized as follows:
- abuse
  - definite abuse
  - likely abuse
- indeterminate
  - questionable abuse
  - unknown cause
- not abuse
  - likely accident
  - definite accident

Wissow[366] published a summary of current issues and the approach to childhood abuse and neglect. Southall et al[367] suggest that protection of children from ill treatment might be enhanced if the abuse were classified by apparent motive and degree rather than by type of injury.

Definitions

The Child Abuse Prevention and Treatment Act (P.L. 93-247) defines abuse and neglect as 'the physical or mental injury, sexual abuse, negligent treatment, or maltreatment of a child under the age of 18 by a person responsible for the child's welfare under circumstances which indicate that the child's health or welfare is harmed or threatened thereby'. Simply stated, abuse is the harm or threatened harm to a child's welfare and/or well-being, which occurs through non-accidental physical or mental injury. The National Center on Child Abuse and Neglect defines the various forms of abuse and neglect.[363] The legal definition of abuse and neglect varies by state, some of which provide exemptions for religious beliefs, corporal punishment, cultural practices, and poverty. The National Adoption Information Clearinghouse provides statutory summaries by state.[368] Their criteria include:

- Abuse – premeditated ill treatment undertaken for gain by disturbed, dangerous, and manipulative individuals.
- Active ill treatment – impulsively undertaken because of socioeconomic pressures; lack of education, resources, and support; or mental illness.
- Universal mild ill treatment – behavior undertaken by normal caring parents in all societies.
- Neglect – 'unintentional' failure to supply the child's needs.

Corporal punishment has been and currently is a legal method for disciplining children in many communities. In some states corporal punishment is legal in the home as well as in the school. The distinction between corporal punishment and abuse can be very difficult. Sweden banned corporal punishment in 1979 and many European countries have followed.

The presentation of child abuse[23, 369–372]

The literature regarding child abuse is vast and presents a full spectrum of ideas, opinions, and analyses of clinical findings.[26, 27, 83] Children present with abuse and/or neglect under a variety of circumstances (Box 17.12). Child abuse can present obviously, as in the battered child, or covertly, as in the child victimized by factitious illness (Munchausen syndrome by proxy MSBP). Injury itself cannot be the determining element. Each case requires a careful and unbiased forensic analysis of the injury, prior medical history, environment, and evaluation of the event before final diagnosis of cause and circumstance of injury or death can be rendered (Fig. 17.28). As in any field of medicine, impressions and differential diagnosis should be formulated and, if necessary, further evaluation or testing performed to verify the final diagnosis. **Differential diagnosis** is the process of determining those diseases or conditions that would be consistent with the current clinical circumstances or findings.

Neglect is a general term applied to a form of maltreatment that reflects failure to provide age appropriate care to an infant or child. It encompasses the failure to utilize or access food and water and provide for the well-being of the growing child. Polanksy et al[373] define child neglect as 'a condition in which the caretaker responsible for the child either deliberately or by extraordinary inattentiveness, permits the child to experience avoidable present suffering and/or fails to provide one or more of the ingredients generally deemed essential for developing a person physical, intellectual, and emotional capacities'. Polansky et al describe neglect in the context of the characteristic of the mother:

- impulse-ridden
- apathetic futile
- mothers suffering from reactive depression
- mentally retarded
- psychotic

Neglect can also be described by motive or by consequence:

- malnutrition
- physical violence
- failure to protect or rescue
- medical neglect

BOX 17.12   PATTERNS OF INJURY IN CHILD ABUSE AND NEGLECT

Physical trauma

   Excessive soft tissue in injuries reflecting rough handling

   Pattern of soft tissue injuries reflecting corporal punishment

   Soft tissue associated with intentional cruelty

   Burns – acute or aged

   Single fractures

   Multiple fractures, acute

   Multiple fractures of varying ages

   Traumatic head injuries without brain damage

   Traumatic head injury with brain damage, single event

   Traumatic head injury with brain damage, multiple events

   Visceral trauma

   Spinal cord injury

   Sexual injury

Special conditions

   Poisoning

   Medical neglect

   Caloric deprivation

   Failure to protect from dangerous environmental conditions

   Munchausen syndrome by proxy – fictitious or induced medical injury

   Serial homicide – suffocation of infants and young children

   Abandoned newborns

   Battered child syndrome with torture

   Children who kill children

   Intrauterine abuse and neglect

   Deaths due to community violence

Evaluation of the domestic circumstances and the caregivers' capacities must be considered before determination of preventable neglect is made. For further information, the US Department of Health and Human Services has published a detailed manual for the definition, analysis, and interpretation of child neglect.[374]

Many who review childhood fatalities are acutely aware of the uncertain distinction between 'accidental death' as an act of God and 'accidental death' from flagrant inattention to reasonable protection. Most accidental deaths in childhood fall somewhere in between, but in cases in which flagrant or willful inattention results in serious harm or death, the component of neglect should be recognized and should be documented on the death certificate. In addition to accurately classifying childhood deaths, this will aid social and legal agencies in further investigation and perhaps protection of surviving siblings. Classic examples of this form of neglect include children overlaying by

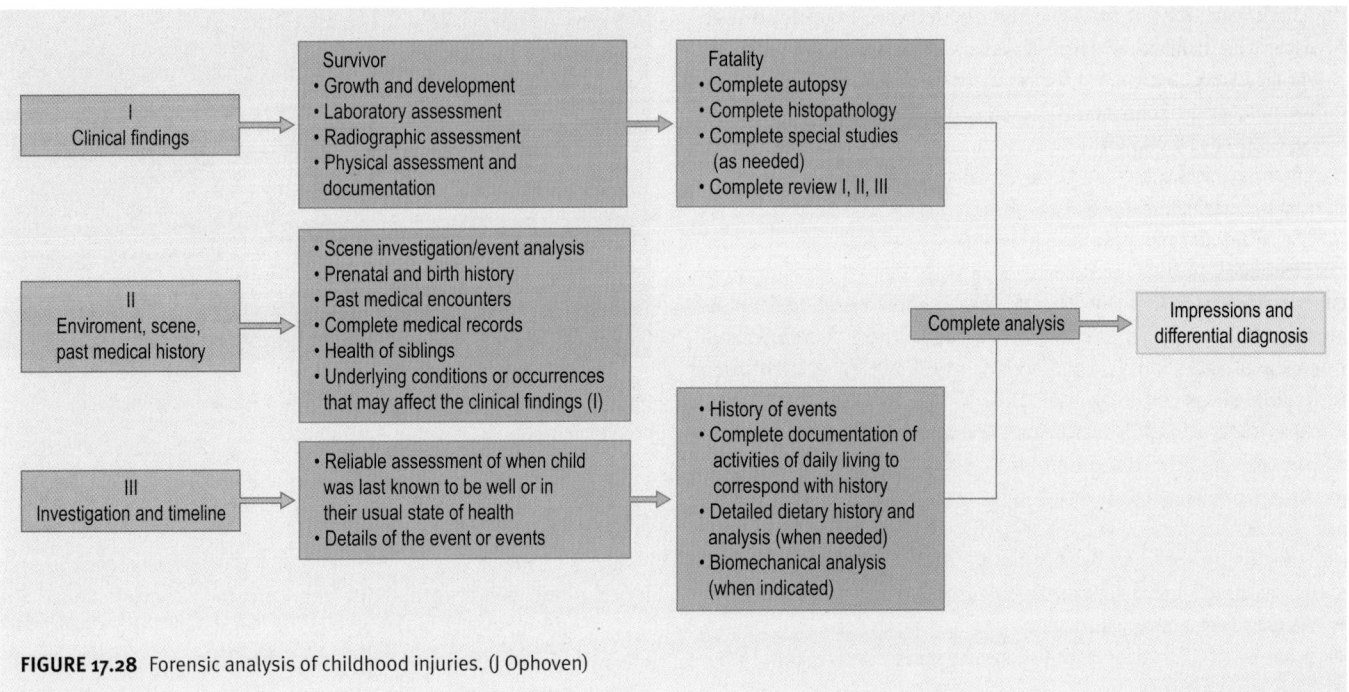

FIGURE 17.28 Forensic analysis of childhood injuries. (J Ophoven)

an intoxicated parent, fire deaths of young children left unattended, and motor vehicle fatalities with an intoxicated parent driver.

Medical neglect refers to the failure to provide appropriate health care for a child although financially able to do so. Failure to obtain timely medical intervention on behalf of a child in one's care may result from a number of factors including lack of sufficient experience/ability to perceive severity, misinformation, cultural or religious factors, fear, and willful neglect. Any time a child is deprived of reasonable access to necessary and timely care, a form of neglect is present, even if the neglect is culturally or legally sanctioned. An example of such a situation includes the Southeast Asian community's cultural reluctance to provide immunization, and religious sects intentionally withholding acute medical intervention. For the forensic pathologist, the presence of medical neglect can be an important factor in the determination of the manner of death in the presence of natural disease.

Religiously-motivated medical neglect The US Supreme Court ruled that 'the right to practice religion freely does not include the liberty to expose the community or the child to communicable disease, or the latter to ill health or death'. [Prince v Massachusetts 321 U.S. 158(1944)]. Despite this ruling nearly all states have exemptions in both the juvenile and criminal codes. Asser and Swan[375] published a review of 113 child fatalities focusing on religiously motivated medical neglect from 1975 to 1995. Of the 98 children with non-cancerous conditions 92 would have had an excellent prognosis with standard medical care. Ridgway[376] presents a summary of court-mediated disputes between physicians and families and points out the scarcity of legal opinions on the matter.

Malnutrition and dehydration The ability to properly access and utilize food and water is a basic function of health and well being of the growing and developing child. A disruption in these processes and the consequent injury or death raises important and complex forensic questions. The terminology, evaluation, diagnosis, and complications of malnutrition and dehydration are not uniformly applied and this problem can complicate matters even further.

- Undernutrition or undernourishment – Intake of an insufficient quantity of food.
- Malnutrition – intake of inadequate quality of food.
- Starvation – death due to malnutrition.
- Wasting – acute or subacute malnutrition (weight for length abnormal).
- Stunting – small for age with proportional weight for length.
- Emaciation or cachexia – extreme leanness due to malnutrition or disease.
- Kwashiorkor – refers to 'sickness of weaning' and reflects inadequate intake of protein with fair to normal caloric intake (weight for length may be normal or only minimally low).
- Marasmus – body wasting due to inadequate intake of protein and calories (weight for length usually less than 70% expected).
- Protein energy malnutrition[378] – deficiency in weight/growth due to deficiency of protein intake includes both marasmus and kwashiorkor.
- Micronutrient deficiencies – such as rickets or scurvy.
- Anorexia – refusal to eat, loss of appetite.

Failure to Thrive (FTT) defines the physical state of a child with interrupted growth. A suggested working definition is a weight deviation downward from the true percentile (typically achieved between 4 and 8 weeks of age) crossing two or more percentile lines on the growth curve and persisting for more than 1 month. FTT is traditionally divided into organic (due to disease) and functional (non-disease). Functional FTT can be categorized as accidental (ignorance, poverty, breastfeeding failure) or non-accidental. The causes are numerous and the circumstances of growth failure typically reflect more than one condition or variable. A detailed discussion of FTT and its diagnosis exceeds the purpose of the chapter. Excellent reviews on the subject are available.[378–380]

The accusation of intentional or non-accidental maltreatment is a circumstance that must be addressed applying good forensic analysis. FTT must be carefully investigated before accusations of intentional injury or criminal actions are made, especially when it occurs in the challenged family. Calculations of caloric requirements, careful and detailed dietary history, evaluation of mental health, documentation of physical injuries, and examination of neonatal and subsequent medical encounters are some of the necessary categories of data. Growth can be assessed using a variety of parameters such as:[381, 382]

- height for age and weight for age compared to mean for age
- weight for height measurement
- centimeters of growth/year in children greater than 2 years
- body mass index
- Waterlow and Gomez classifications (analyzing height and weight data to assess nutritional/malnutritional status of children)

This author has participated in the evaluation of cases involving accusations of 'intentional starvation' that in fact were explained by breastfeeding failure, prolonged use of the BRAT diet [B: bananas R: rice (or other starchy food) A: applesauce T: toast] following an episode of diarrhea, and misuse of Enfamil AR for severe neonatal gastroesophageal reflux disease.

Laboratory analysis of functional FTT can play a critical role in defining the nature of malnutrition. Verification and calculation of the character and degree of dehydration in the determination of caloric deficit is also important. Infants suffering from malnutrition may present with acute deterioration. This typically results from acute infection due to immunosuppression and/or complications of dehydration due to weakness and inanition. At a minimum the forensic analysis must include detailed growth curve analysis from birth (height, weight, occipital–frontal circumference); acid base status with serum osmolality; urinalysis; protein profile to include albumin, prealbumin, transferrin and total protein analysis;[377] hepatic enzymes; glucose; ketones; renal function studies; and bone age. In the case of a deceased infant without hospitalization, vitreous chemistry analysis of electrolytes and protein analysis is advised.

FTT due to inadequate caloric intake is a complex problem and may be due to fundamental difficulties within the parent–child relationship.[384] Infants and children adapt to inadequate calorie intake with both physiologic and behavioral responses.[385, 386] Gremse[387] and Tolia[388] describe a subset of infants who have received long-term critical care from extreme prematurity or neonatal complications who present with serious challenges to adequate nutrition because of feeding aversions and avoidance.

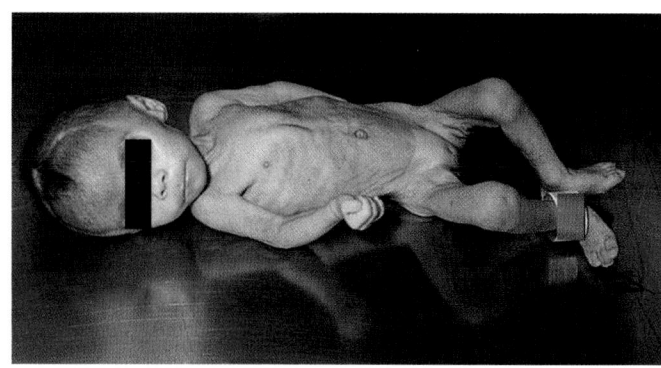

FIGURE 17.29 Starvation and dehydration: breastfeeding failure in premature twin.

Starvation[383] (Fig. 17 29)

Inadequate food intake is the most common cause of malnutrition world wide especially in developing countries. Starvation can result from **willful withholding** of adequate food; **unintentional dietary deprivation,** as seen with an impaired parent or well-intentioned but inadequate diet;[390, 391] or **cultural neglect** in the economically deprived populations of developed countries or epidemic starvation in Third World countries. International death from malnutrition and preventable infectious disease are estimated at 40 000 children per day. Fatal starvation is a rare cause of death in developed countries. Chronic illness is the major contributing cause of nutritional deficiencies in developed countries.[389]

Studies by Taitz and King[394] show that 26% of 269 abused children demonstrated impaired growth (71 of 269). Also, 10 of 11 children exhibited catch-up growth when placed in foster care, whereas only 4 of 28 children who remained in the home did so. Significant wasting, as seen in chronic malnutrition, was found in a study of abused children among urban poor, suggesting that the growth of abused children differs significantly from the growth of children who are not abused.[393] The cause of growth failure in abused and neglected children is still an unanswered question. The dramatic catch-up growth displayed by these children when placed in a nurturing environment, the basis on which the diagnosis of functional FTT is based, suggests that a combination of factors is at play. The fact that a child gains weight following hospitalization must not be interpreted as diagnostic of NAI. Nutritional factors and endocrine disturbances, as well as environmental factors of failed maternal attachment and parental anger and hostility, are all proposed.[394]

Infants who fail to thrive secondary to maternal deprivation may have some of the following characteristics:[395, 396]

- less than third percentile for height and weight on standard growth curves
- withdrawal, lethargy, or apathy
- retarded motor, social, and language development
- autoerotic behavior
- delayed skeletal maturation, usually commensurate with abnormal height age

- retained growth hormone responsiveness[398]
- regained appetite and weight gain when removed from home
- presence of physical abuse is unusual

Fatalities associated with malnutrition due to starvation often will reflect findings common in other abuse and neglect situations (Box 17.13).

Analyzing deaths due to starvation or malnutrition, requires expert knowledge and comprehensive death investigation and analysis, and is further complicated by the fact that death is usually the consequence of general debility. The forensic pathologist will often be asked to estimate the nature and duration of starvation. Even in advanced stages of starvation, death may be sudden and unexpected. Madea[382] demonstrates the application of various classifications of malnutrition. Malnourished children suffer from depression of the immune system, and death is commonly the result of infection. Davis et al[398] and Meade and Brissie[399] report cases of homicidal starvation and point out the importance of adequate investigation of previous growth and development as well as the need for careful caloric and fluid intake calculations in the death investigation.[398–400] Investigation of the severely starved child should include a detailed nutritional interview and scene or environmental investigation.

Dehydration and sodium imbalance

Infants and young children commonly present with conditions that place them at risk for dehydration or volume depletion. Whitehead et al[401] reviewed 37 fatal dehydration deaths autopsied at Adelaide Children's Hospital over a 33 year period. Causative factors included gastroenteritis, high environmental temperatures, neglect (failure to thrive), mental retardation, congenital adrenal hyperplasia, and unsuspected cystic fibrosis. Vitreous humor electrolytes and immunoassay for rotavirus were important diagnostic adjuncts. The forensic analysis of the seriously ill or deceased infant requires an understanding of abnormalities of fluid and acid–base balance. (Krous HF, Hypernatremic Dehydration, Failure to Thrive, Starvation and Neglect in Children presented at Pediatric Forensic Issues conference, San Diego, 1998.)

Definitions:

- Dehydration – a physiologic disturbance affecting water and salt losses.
- Volume depletion – refers to intravascular depletion of fluid.
- Isonatremic volume depletion – indicates that water and solute (specifically sodium) are lost in proportionate quantities (serum sodium within normal range).
- Hypernatremic dehydration – volume depletion with excess free water loss (increased plasma osmolarity).
- Hyponatremic dehydration – plasma volume contraction with free water excess.

> **BOX 17.13 FATAL MALNUTRITION: INDICATORS AND AUTOPSY FINDINGS**
>
> Indicators of neglect/starvation
>
> Clinical history and autopsy negative for organic failure to thrive
>
> Obvious chronic wasting inconsistent with an acute illness
>
> Deteriorated appearance that should have indicated need for medical attention
>
> Unkempt appearance with or without other signs of physical abuse
>
> History inconsistent with medical facts
>
> History of oral intake unrealistic or inconsistent with facts
>
> Evidence of environmental neglect
>
> Failure to provide reasonable health care or attention to medical needs; occasionally evasive behavior toward health care providers and/or child protection workers
>
> Documented prior concern raised by other observers, relatives
>
> Child singled out for neglect
>
> Autopsy findings associated with fatal malnutrition [383]
>
> Cachexia
>
> Dehydration
>
> Diffuse loss of deep and subcutaneous fat
>
> Thin, dry, fissured skin, often with associated cutaneous findings of neglect
>
> Atrophic organs
>
> Stress atrophy of thymus
>
> Empty or near-empty stomach and intestine with thinned walls
>
> Dilated gallbladder
>
> Gelatinoid atrophy of fat and brown fat transformation
>
> Alterations in hepatic fat content with starvation pigment deposition
>
> Gastric erosions
>
> Non-specific degenerative changes of skeletal and myocardial muscle fibers
>
> Dry or impacted stool
>
> Frequent evidence of immune deficiency with infection as the terminal event
>
> Kwashiorkor is associated with salt tissue edema, skin lesions, hepatomegaly and red hair (reflecting hypoalbuminuria)
>
> Evidence of growth failure
>
> Heterogeneous renal changes

- Inappropriate ADH (antidiuretic hormone) – the most common cause of isovolemic hyponatremia in childhood is hyponatremia and hypo-osmolality resulting from action of ADH despite normal or increased plasma volume.[402]
- Diabetes insipidus (DI) – condition caused by excess urine production that occurs when the amount of ADH is less than

normal (central DI) or when the kidneys response to ADH is defective (nephrogenic DI).[404]

- Cerebral salt wasting – the development of excessive renal salt loss (natriuresis) and subsequent hyponatremic dehydration in patients with intracranial disease.
- Osmolarity – is the measure of solute concentration in a fixed solvent volume:

    Calculate serum osmolarity = 2[Na$^+$] + Glucose/18 + Bun/2.8 + other osmolarities.

- Salt poisoning – ingestion of excessive salt.

Common causes of dehydration in young infants are vomiting, diarrhea and increased insensible water loss. Infants can become dehydrated much more quickly than older children and adults because of their higher metabolic rate, increased body surface to mass index, and higher relative water content in tissue (75% of body weight in term neonates, 90% in 23 week preterm neonates, and 70% in infants).[404, 405] Young infants have decreased capacity to concentrate and dilute urine in response to changes in intravascular volume. Sudden changes in weight may not reflect changes in intravascular volume and detection of skin and mucosa are not sensitive indicators of hydration in infants.[405]

Analysis of the fluid and acid base status of the critically ill or deceased child is a necessary part of the investigation. Details of recent intake and output, environmental stresses such as excessive heat, recent illness that can increase insensible fluid losses (e.g. fever) or actual losses such as diarrhea, vomiting, illness or injury, medications, and iatrogenic injury with fluid therapy. Laboratory studies should be examined from the admission specimens, perimortem specimens and vitreous, in the event of a fatality. The specific studies should include:

- electrolytes – premortem (PrM) and postmortem vitreous (V)
- blood gases – PrM
- blood urea nitrogen and creatinine – PrM,V
- glucose – PrM
- plasma – PrM
- urine specific gravity – PrM

Derangements in plasma sodium levels

Sodium metabolism can become deranged in many disease states. Mild hyper- and hyponatremia are not uncommon in the hospitalized patient. Excellent reviews have been published summarizing cause, clinical manifestations and treatment of hyponatremia, hypernatremia and life-threatening acid–base problems.[406–411] Significant complications of hyper- and hyponatremia are often reflected in to CNS dysfunction. Rapid correction of hyponatremia has been associated with central pontine myelinolysis and rapid hypernatremic rehydration can result in intracerebral and subarachnoid hemorrhage (SAH) and edema. Lantz et al from the Departments of Pathology and Ophthalmology at Wake Forest University report a case of fatal hyponatremia with cerebral edema and seizures with peripheral retinal hemorrhage (RH). Unexpected CNS complications of hyponatremia may be observed in patients on intravenous fluids.

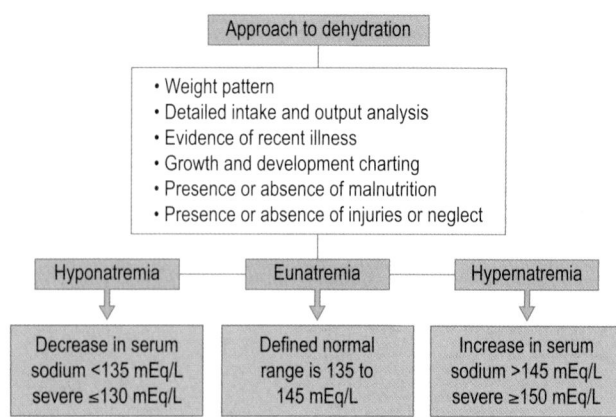

FIGURE 17.30 Evaluation of dehydration. (J Ophoven)

West and Harding[412] report an infant with neonatal seizures due to maternal water intoxication. Arieff and Kronlund[413] report a case of fatal child abuse due to forced water intoxication in three children. This author reported a young child with failure to thrive and coma due to forced water intoxication.[414]

Hypernatremia and hyponatremia are terms that reflect the level of salt in the body tissues, not necessarily the level of dehydration (Figs 17.30–17.32). Kaplan et al[415] discuss acute fatal hypernatremic dehydration in breastfed infants due to lactation failure. Hypernatremia can be associated with evidence of head trauma.[416] Significant hypernatremia carries high morbidity and mortality especially during treatment. Distinguishing hypernatremic dehydration from salt poisoning or salt overload is a rare but serious clinical and forensic question.[417]

Investigation of possible salt and volume depletion conditions should be carefully investigated in all sudden unexpected deaths. Some pathologists may be reluctant to sample vitreous in order to preserve the eyes for ophthalmic examination, but, in the absence of head trauma it is always advisable to sample the vitreous. In the author's experience, unanticipated hypernatremia has been discovered only after vitreous chemistry analysis in several cases. Analysis becomes more difficult if the history includes the possibility of complications of hypernatremia dehydration or salt poisoning with associated cerebral hemorrhage. It is the author's practice that if the plasma sodium level exceeds 175 mEq/L, exogenous salt intoxication should be considered.

Clinical findings of injury and trauma

Cutaneous trauma and soft tissue injuries

Soft tissue injuries are the most common presenting complaint in childhood trauma. Facial and neck trauma occurs frequently in children but serious injuries are uncommon. Banks and Merlino[418] summarize minor oral injuries in children. Serious facial trauma is not normally the consequence of childhood

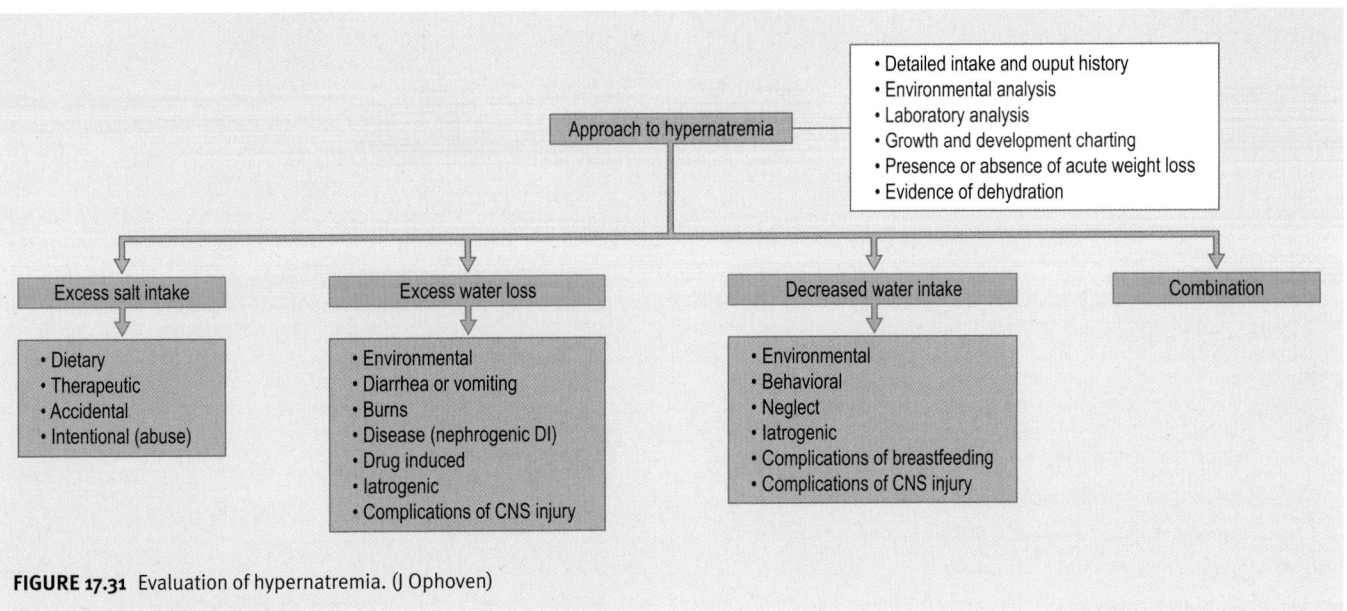

FIGURE 17.31 Evaluation of hypernatremia. (J Ophoven)

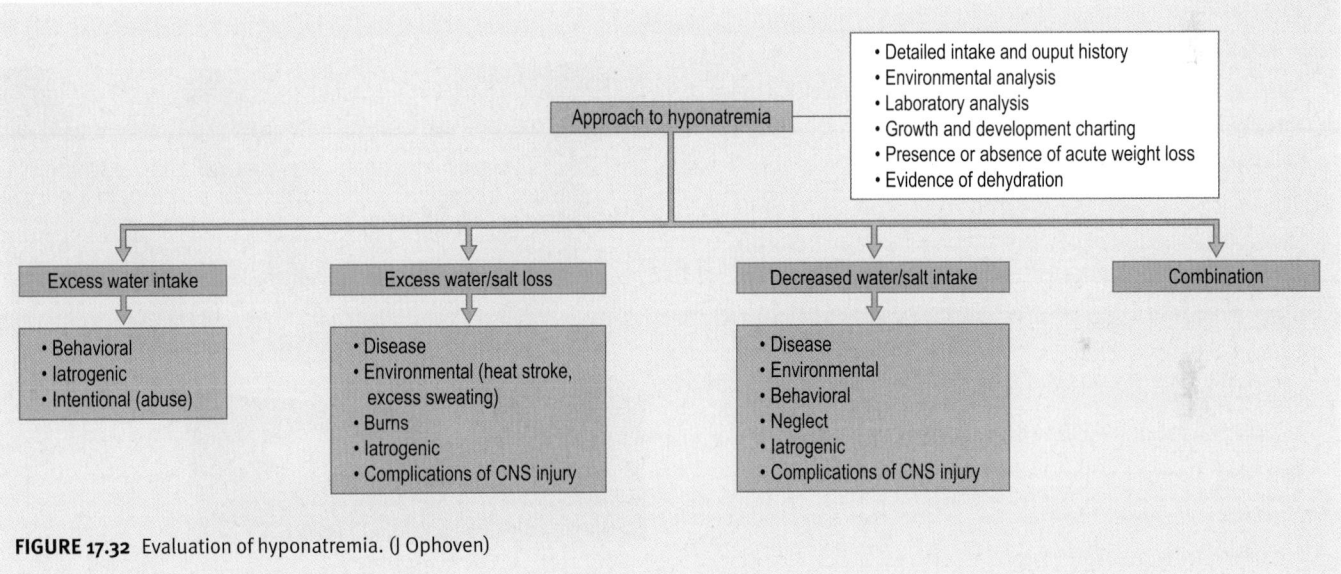

FIGURE 17.32 Evaluation of hyponatremia. (J Ophoven)

play. Oral facial trauma was found in 49% of 260 cases of child abuse seen during a 5-year period at the Children's Hospital Medical Center, Boston. An additional 16% of the cases involved head trauma, making the total percentage of head and facial trauma 65%.[419] Patterns of oral facial injury may be observed in physical and sexual abuse[420] (Box 17.14). Although auricular hematoma or trauma to the auricle can be the result of childhood play, injuries of this nature to the young infant are highly suspicious.

Cutaneous trauma in various forms is the most common finding in physical abuse of children and is often the first indication that abuse should be suspected.[42, 422] Jenny[224] provides an excellent review of how cutaneous injuries can manifest in childhood, the nature of inflicted trauma, and the differential diagnosis of skin lesions confused with inflicted trauma. Bruising is the most frequent sign of external trauma in the general pediatric examination. Often it is associated with normal, play-induced injuries consistent with developmental age. Common sites for bruises include the anterior lower legs, knees, and elbows, as well as the forehead in the toddler. Tumbling accidents can produce multiple bruises but are usually associated over bony prominences. Most falls produce a single bruise on a single surface. **Multiple bruises on multiple body planes should be suspicious for an abuse pattern**. Bruises suggestive of assault are seen about the chest, lower back, buttocks, genitals and inner thighs, upper arms, and face (cheek, earlobe, upper lip and frenulum) (Figs 17.33 and 17.34). Assault bruises are often of varying ages, suggesting chronic

Facial injuries

    Hand injuries due to slapping or grabbing by fingers

    Pattern injuries reflecting blow with instrument such as a belt

    Bites

    Perioral bruises due to gagging

    Burns

    Fractures of facial/jaw bones

Eye injuries

Ear injuries

    Pinch or grab marks to auricle

    Soft tissue lacerations from pulling ears

    Cauliflower ear, tympanic membrane perforations

Injuries to teeth

    Traumatized or avulsed teeth

    Discolored teeth indicating repeated trauma

    Multiple healed fractures of tooth roots

Injuries to mouth

    Pattern injury/petechiae – erythema to soft and hard palate suggesting sexual misuse

    Sexually transmitted disease

    Burns resembling instrument/scalding liquids or toxic chemicals

    Marks indicating blunt trauma from instrument or finger, especially on palate, vestibule, and floor of mouth

    Detached labial or lingual frenulum indicating blunt trauma

Neck injuries[421, 561]

    Rope or restraint marks

    Abrasions and contusions reflecting choking injury

    Vocal cord injuries

Scalp injuries

    Contusions reflecting blunt trauma

    Pattern injuries reflecting blow with an instrument

    Lacerations and abrasions

    Traumatic alopecia – hair pulling may result in massive subgaleal bleeding

    Subgaleal hemorrhage – may be sufficient in caliber to cause hypovolemic shock

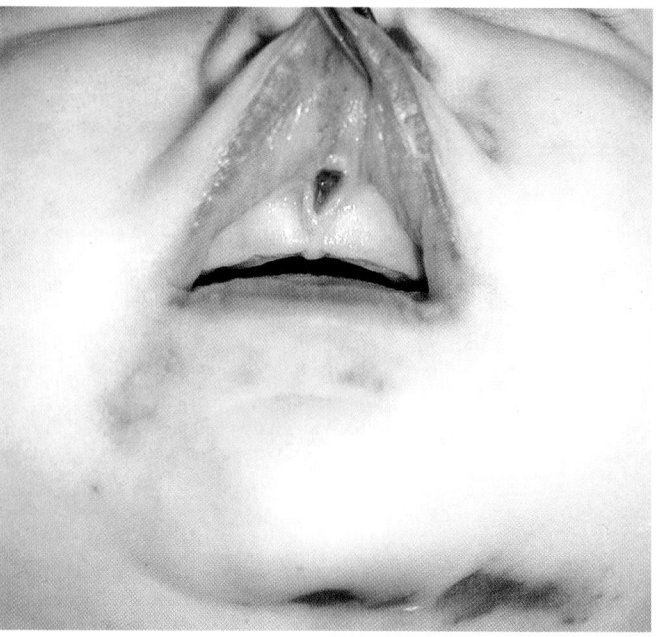

FIGURE 17.33 Frenulum tear

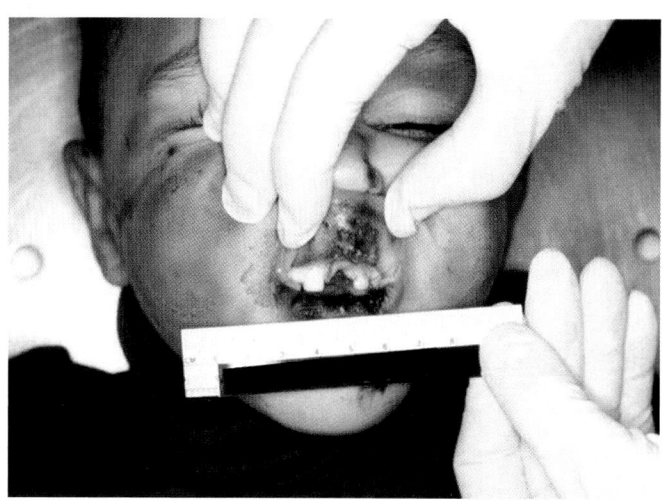

FIGURE 17.34 Labial contusion, frenulum tear and acute tooth evulsion.

abuse, and symmetric bruises are rarely accidental, especially those about the face (Fig. 17.35). Bruises in the premobile child should be suspicious for inflicted injuries but are not pathognomonic of inflicted trauma. McMahon et al[423] reviewed case records of 371 children suspected of suffering inflicted trauma. Soft tissue injuries were found in 92% of cases (341 chidren) with ecchymoses identified most commonly (62% –

555 of 892 soft tissue injuries). Very few of the injuries showed an identifiable pattern. Of the 44 children in the series aged 9 months or less the findings included:

- An average of only one soft tissue injury.
- A total of 30 had soft tissue injury involving the head or face.
- Seven had burn injury.
- This age group was the most seriously injured (two suffered fatal injuries; 45% also had fracture).

Labbe and Caouette[424] suggest that physicians pay special attention to any bruise in children less than 9 months of age, and to bruises with uncommon characteristics (unusual locations; greater than or equal to 15 injuries, and injuries other than bruises, abrasions or scratches). Maguire et al[425] recommend special attention to bruises in non-mobile infants, over soft tissue areas

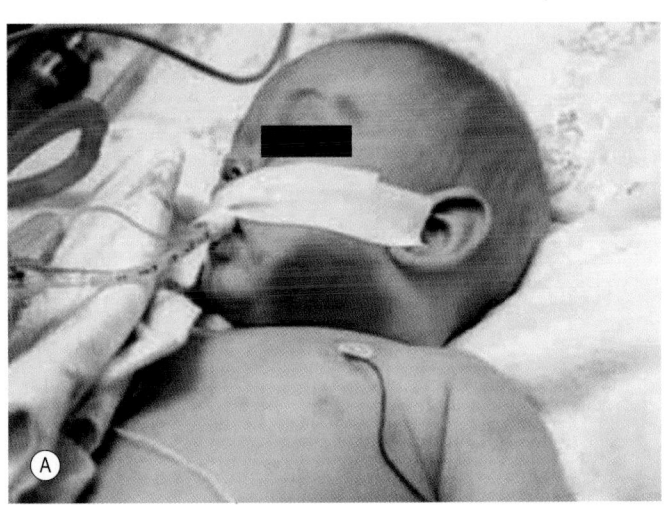 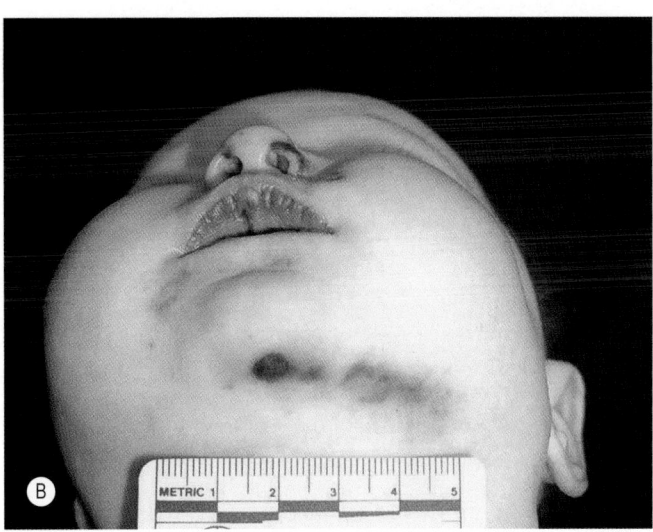

FIGURE 17.35 (A), (B) Facial injuries in fatal child abuse.

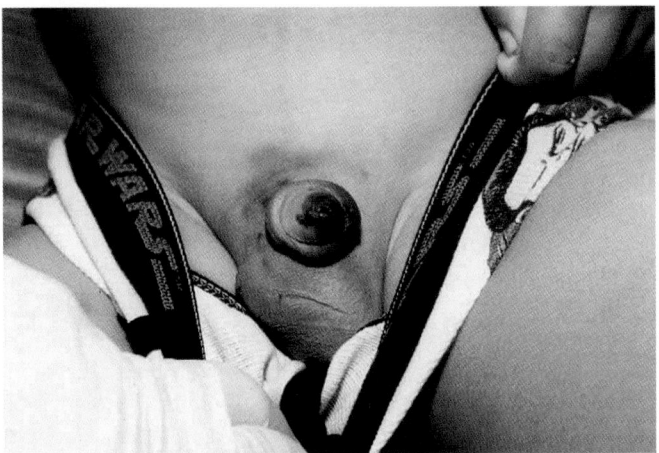

FIGURE 17.36 Pinch bruise to the genitals.

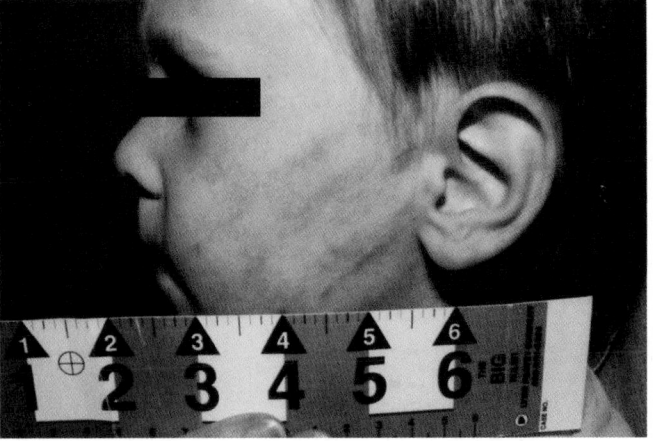

FIGURE 17. 37 Slap injury to the face with imprint of finger marks.

(cheeks or abdomen), bruises that carry the imprint of an implement, and multiple bruises of uniform shape. Carpenter[103] studied bruises in babies less than 9 months of age and verified the prevalence at 12.5%. Numbers of bruises increased with increasing mobility and were typically observed over bony prominences.

Children presenting with soft tissue injuries associated with inflicted trauma can exhibit a variety of abnormalities:

- multiple acute contusions
- massive single impact
- evidence of repeated injuries with scarring
- cigarette burns
- bed/pressure sores
- chemical burns from unattended diapers
- associated evidence of abuse and neglect and/or poor nutrition
- patterns consistent with corporal punishment

Patterned bruises often provide a clue to the mechanism of injury. **Gripping** often leaves either round or oblong patterns and may include fingernail imprints or abrasions. These injuries are typically seen around the face, upper arms, and thorax. Circular bruises, particularly if there is an unbruised area across the center providing a clamshell appearance, may indicate **pinching**. Pinch bruises found on the ears, especially bilaterally, and on the glans penis (Fig. 17.36) are suspicious for abuse pattern. Pattern erythema, petechial hemorrhages, and/or ecchymoses delineating the shape of the hand are pathognomonic of **slap marks**. Slapping can leave a handprint type of pattern, or, as is often the case in facial slapping, the predominant pattern is of the four fingers (Fig. 17.37). Parallel patterns are suggestive of trauma inflicted by a belt, strap, switch, looped cord, or buckle. These patterns often approximate the width of the object. **Bizarre marks** should be carefully examined for tell-tale patterns, e.g. hairbrush, ring imprint, choke collar, restraint or gag injuries, or curling iron contact burns. Special attention should be paid to any adult **bite marks**.[426, 427] (Fig. 17.38). In the author's experience, adult bite marks are always suspicious, and careful

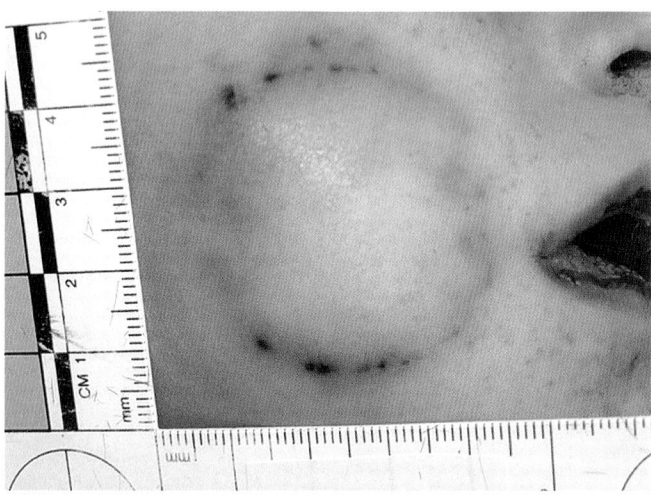

FIGURE 17.38 Adult bite mark to the cheek.

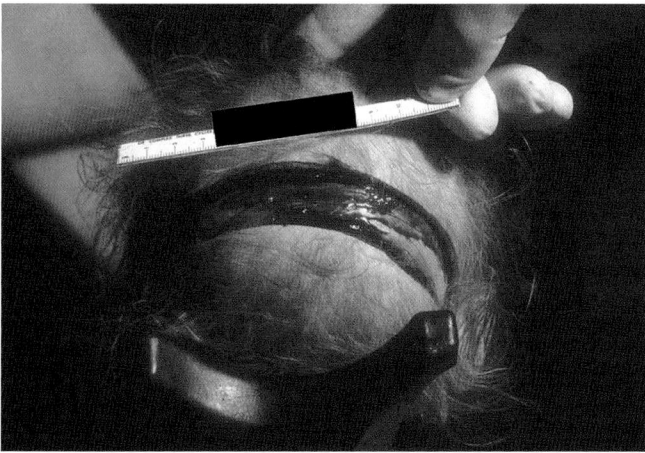

FIGURE 17.39 Subgaleal hemorrhage.

investigation should be conducted. Any child death with a pattern injury suggesting adult bite marks should be treated and investigated as possible homicide and the proper investigative authorities contacted before initiating the autopsy. Care must be taken to prevent contamination of the lesions (e.g., to prevent removal of epithelial cells from a bite).

Serious blunt traumatic injuries may be sustained with no external evidence of trauma. Areas less susceptible to external signs of bruising include the scalp and the abdomen, where the external trauma, if present, rarely reflects the severity of the underlying injury. Extensive subgaleal hemorrhage in a small infant may produce sufficient hypovolemia to cause death without any external marks or wounds to delineate the impact point (Fig. 17.39). Darkly pigmented skin may also mask the area of bruising and requires very careful evaluation.

Areas most commonly involved with blunt trauma are the head, abdomen, buttocks, thighs, chest, and upper arms. In children who die in circumstances suspicious for abuse, careful incision into the deep soft tissues at these sites is an important

adjunct to the complete autopsy. In addition, an inspection of the mouth should never be overlooked. This should include the frenulum.

Downes et al[428] studied the prevalence and distribution of petechiae in well babies. They concluded that many well babies have petechial spots and recommend that this observation not to be interpreted in and of itself as a pathologic finding.

When external trauma is observed and the history provided appears dubious, or when abuse is suspected, an examination of the internal systems is indicated, including a radiographic survey of the body and CT scan.

Skeletal injuries[429, 430]

Fractures are a common bone injury in child abuse and in accidental injury. Fracture refers to a break in the continuity of a bone or a part of the mineralized bone structure due to physical force. Fractures can result from impact, rotation, binding, or other mechanical forces applied to a normal bone or trivial injury in unhealthy bone. The incidence of pediatric fractures increases with age with fracture rates similar for boys and girls in younger children.[431] The actual incidence of skeletal injuries in the abused child is unknown.

The process of bone formation (ontogenesis) involves three main steps:
- production of extracellular organic matrix (osteoid)
- mineralization of the matrix to form bone
- bone remodeling by resorption and formation

In the growing bone the cartilage cells in the epiphyseal growth plate proliferate in orderly columns. This area of the bone is relatively unprotected during growth and thus more vulnerable to injury in infants and young children. When skeletal maturity is achieved the cartilage growth ceases and the epiphysis fuses with the bone shaft. Bone developing from a fibrous membrane is a process known as intramembranous ossification. The cranial bones of the skull are flat membranous bones. Bones formed from endochondral ossification are produced by bone replacing hyaline cartilage.

The periosteum is strong in young bone and often remains partially or completely intact with fracture. Over time infants' bones increase in thickness and become less flexible and more resistant to stress. Children exhibit very different fracture patterns than adults because of the varying amounts of cartilage in immature bone and the thick periosteum. Physeal injuries are specific to the immature bone because they involve the open growth plate.

The effect of a simple fracture force on bone is to disrupt the bone cortex and bony trabeculae; lift or tear the periosteum; and tear periosteal, endosteal and Haversian blood vessels. This results in local hemorrhage between the bone fragments, elevation of periosteum, and variable extension of blood into adjacent soft tissues (Fig. 17.40). Cells at the fracture site undergo necrosis due to direct trauma as well as secondary ischemia. The progress of the cellular vital reaction at the injury site results in organization of blood clot, connective tissue

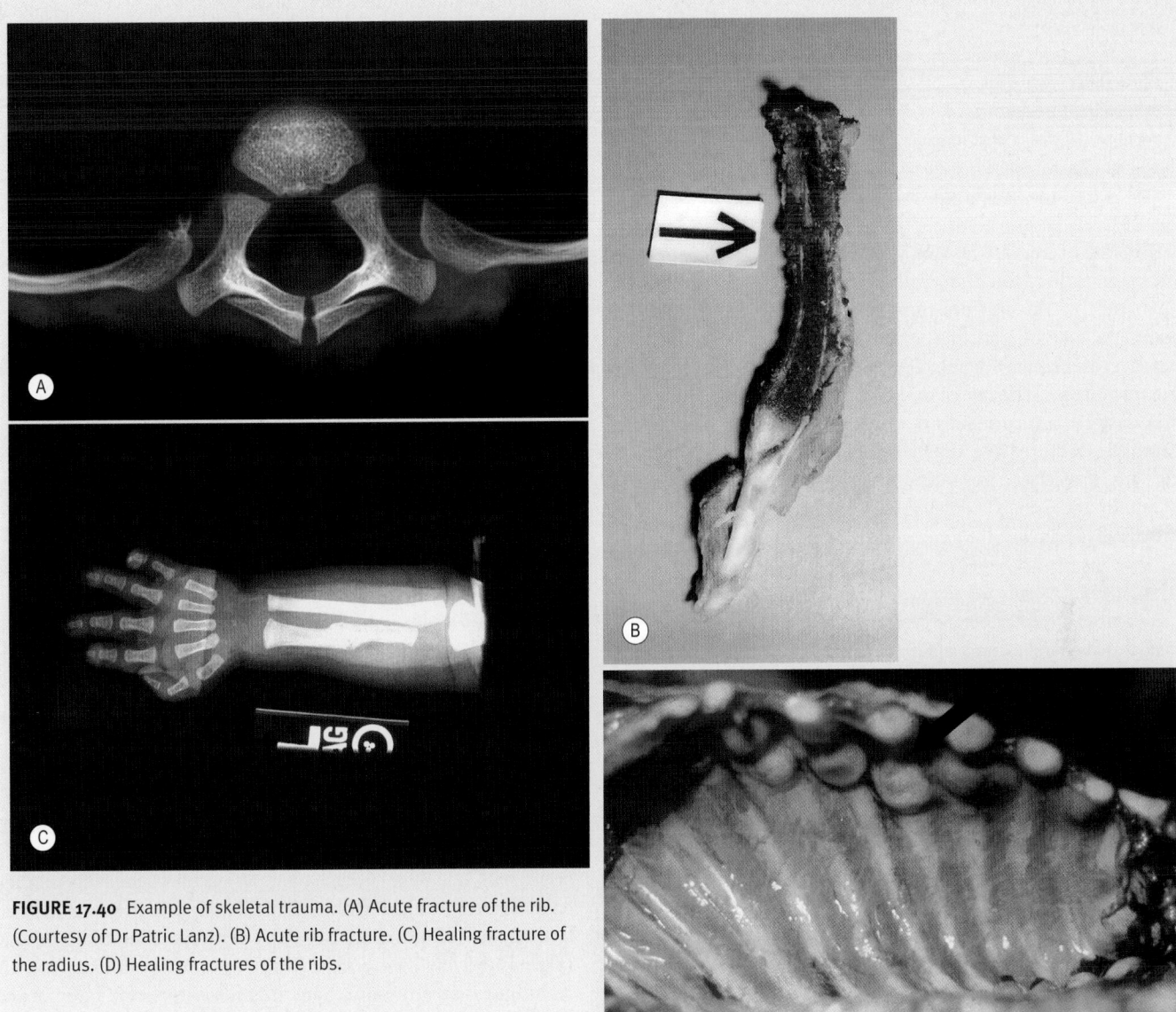

FIGURE 17.40 Example of skeletal trauma. (A) Acute fracture of the rib. (Courtesy of Dr Patric Lanz). (B) Acute rib fracture. (C) Healing fracture of the radius. (D) Healing fractures of the ribs.

migration, neovascular channels, and eventual development of granulation tissue. Bone repair occurs endosteally (internal) and subperiosteally (external). The repair process is traditionally viewed in three arbitrary stages:[430]

- organization of the hematoma with formation of granulation tissue
- formation of primitive or woven bone around the fracture bridging the bone fragments (primitive callus)
- replacement of callus by routine lamellar bone and bony union (secondary callus)

Bone remodeling will continue over subsequent weeks and months.

Considering the importance of fracture dating there is remarkably little scientific evidence to allow accurate radiographic determination of the age of bony injuries.[432] Although the dating of fractures is very inexact, some guidelines can be used. Prosser et al[433] conducted a systemic review of the literature to define the evidence for radiologic dating of fractures in the context of child protection. They concluded that dating of fractures is inexact and that most radiologists date fractures subjectively. The literature provides little consistent data to act as a resource. The authors point out the urgent need for research in this area. Islam et al[434] studied a series of 707 radiographs of forearm fractures in 141 patients. They concluded that there is wide variation in the appearance and duration of the radiographic signs of bone healing. Their results are summarized as follows:

- 85% of fractures showed marginal sclerosis at fracture margin 5 weeks after injury
- 62% of fractures showed widening of the fracture up to 6 weeks post injury

- 100% of fractures showed periosteal reaction at 4 weeks post injury
- 10% of fractures showed periosteal reaction separable from cortex at 7 weeks
- 90% of fractures showed density greater than or equal to adjacent cortex at 10 weeks post injury
- 100% of fractures showed calcific callus at 4 weeks post injury
- 50% of fractures had fracture callus less dense than adjacent cortex 8–10 weeks post fracture

The rate of fracture healing is affected by many factors: type and magnitude of force, strength of the bone, severity of injury, the nature of the fracture, degree of vascular injury, type of treatment, age of patient, hormonal and nutritional factors, presence or absence of infection, and presence or absence of systemic disease. The rate of healing of physeal injuries is thought to be faster than cancellous or cortical bone. **Vital reaction to traumatic fracture** has a 'timetable' of histologic phases of healing that are predictable regardless of the mechanism of injury. O'Connor and Cohen[432] detail these histologic stages of healing:

- Stage of induction – the time between injury and the appearance of new bone.
- Stage of soft callus – development of internal and external callus as evidenced by proliferating osteoblasts, deposition of new bone, neovascular and maturing fibrous tissue.
- Stage of hard callus – deposition of lamellar bone with bridging of the fracture site, diminished inflammation and granulation tissue.
- Stage of remodeling – return of original configuration of cortex and medullary cavity.

Analysis of any radiographic abnormality includes verification of its nature and character. The term 'possible' fracture can rapidly develop a life of its own in the context of child abuse. Identification of normal variants and conditions that can be confused with abusive injuries has been well reviewed by Kleinman et al[435] and others.[436–442] Some of these conditions include:

- normal variants
- birth trauma
- accidental injury
- metabolic bone disease (prematurity, rickets, vitamin C and copper deficiency)
- congenital skeletal dysplasia (osteogenesis imperfecta)
- infection (congenital syphilis, osteomyelitis)
- toxicity or drug affect (vitamin A, methotrexate, chronic steroid therapy)
- congenital insensitivity to pain

Postmortem radiography in unexpected deaths in infancy is an established tool for identifying occult trauma and is considered routine in many autopsy protocols in infant deaths. Technical quality is critical and access to high-resolution detail to guide histologic sampling is a reasonable goal.[33, 443]

When performing forensic analysis of fractures in childhood a number of questions need to be answered, including the following:

- Is the historical account of the injury appropriate?
- Was medical care promptly sought?
- Is there evidence of old fractures and are they accounted for?
- Are other injuries of varying ages present?

- Is the patient often seen for injuries?
- Does the injury fall into the pattern of typical abuse injuries?
- Are there predisposing factors or conditions that increase risk for 'fragile' bones?

A number of **patterns of skeletal injuries** or abnormalities are encountered in young infants with some frequency in the evaluation of possible child abuse.[444–446] Fracture patterns that occur commonly in all ages include:

- diaphyseal fractures
- linear skull fractures
- subperiosteal new bone formation
- clavicular fractures

Fracture patterns that are most common in infants less than one year are rib, metaphyseal, diaphyseal and linear skull fractures. Fracture patterns that are commonly attributed to child abuse include:

- metaphyseal fractures
- rib fractures
- scapular fractures
- vertebral fractures
- multiple/bilateral fractures especially of differing ages
- complex skull fractures
- digital fracture in the non-ambulatory infant

The most common fractures in abused children are diaphyseal fractures. In infancy skull fractures, rib fractures and metaphyseal injuries predominate; after 1 year of age, long bone fractures are the most common skeletal injury in abuse.[446]

Periosteal new bone formation is a non specific finding and may be due to infections, metabolic disorders such as Caffey disease, vitamin A intoxication, scurvy or rickets, leukemia, or myelodysplasia. It can also be due to trauma – either birth, accidental, or abuse. Physiologic periosteal changes in infancy have been confused with inflicted injury and are a normal finding in young infants aged 1–4 months. This radiographic finding typically involves the femur, humerus, and tibia.[447]

Subperiosteal hemorrhage lifts the osteogenic layer of the periosteum. A variety of forces can cause this phenomenon, including difficult breech deliveries, twisting, and direct blows. Subperiosteal hemorrhage is a frequent finding in abused infants.[448] X-ray results often are initially negative after injury, and a radionucleotide scan may provide earlier detection. Usually the perichondral attachments are preserved, which results in the maximum hemorrhage thickness along the diaphysis with tapering toward the epiphysis. When this type of injury is severe, it manifests clinically as soft tissue swelling.

The **metaphyseal injuries** described by Caffey[355] have been the subject of numerous publications. This finding is highly suspect for child abuse or rough handling in the otherwise normal child and should trigger a child abuse investigation. Caffey initially described the injury as stripping of the periosteum resulting in an avulsion of a portion of bone at the site of the tightest periosteal attachment. Kleinman and colleagues[449, 450] combined in-depth pre- and postmortem radiographs with histopathologic analysis of the metaphyseal lesion in abused infants. Metaphyseal lesions, both radiographically and histologically, are planar, not circumferential. The basic alteration is a subepiphyseal

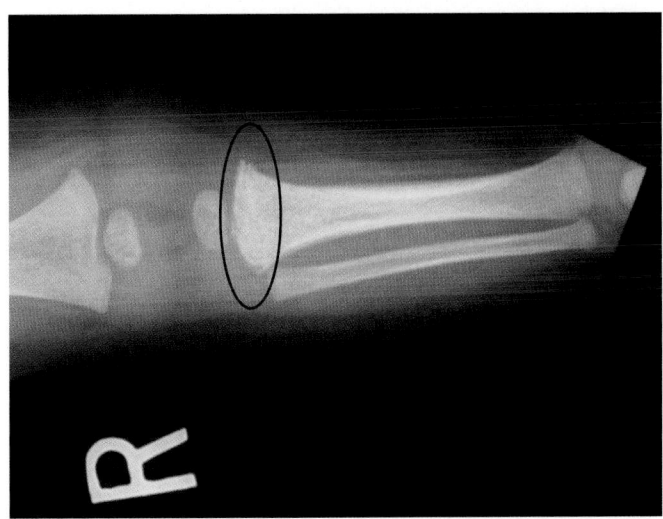

FIGURE 17.41 Metaphyseal fractures of the proximal tibia.

planar series of microfractures through the most immature portion of the metaphyseal bone, the primary spongiosa (Fig. 17.41).[451] The fracture results in the isolation of a mineralized disc of bone of various sizes. Metaphyseal–epiphyseal fractures require biomechanical forces that deliver planar shearing forces that result in subphyseal microfractures.[452] Metaphyseal fractures, though suspicious for child abuse, can be seen in the absence of abuse.

Kleinman describes the most effective methods to remove, prepare, and study postmortem bone specimens using high-resolution radiography in combination with histologic examination to identify the metaphyseal lesions.[453] In some instances the radiographic picture is not confirmed at postmortem examination. A number of factors affect the radiographic appearance of these lesions, including the projection, the shape of the specific metaphysis involved, and the age and degree of healing of the wound. The author recommends postmortem histologic examination of all radiographically suspicious bony injuries in cases of possible homicide. Caution is still required before concluding that the injuries are absolute evidence of intentional injury until the analysis/investigation is complete.

Long bone fractures

Diaphyseal fractures are often seen in association with child abuse.[454] The two most common sites of long bone fractures are the femur and the humerus. Scherl et al[455] evaluated 207 children less than age 6 with non-pathologic diaphyseal fractures of the femur. A total of 76 cases were investigated for abuse. Fractures were more often transverse in both accidental and investigated cases. The author's conclusion suggests that type of fracture is not predictive of accidents or inflicted injury. Thomas et al[456] discuss the challenge of distinguishing abusive long bone fractures in young children and identify factors that might be useful in distinguishing accident from abuse. Criteria suggestive of abuse include serious injury without appropriate history, suspicious delay in reporting injury, and multiple or healing unexplained fractures. Strait et al[365] have enhanced the criteria into a useful tool for various abusive injuries.

Beals and Tufts, utilizing 22 years of data from the University of Oregon Health Sciences Center, found 80 fracture episodes in 79 children.[457] With the range limited to less than 4 years of age, two peaks of incidence were identified, the first in early infancy and the second just before age 3. In the latter population, 30% of the fractures were found to be due to child abuse; in those under 1 year old, child abuse was the most common cause. Most of the fractures were in the mid-diaphysis with approximately a quarter in the distal third. Thomas et al[456] published a series of long bone fractures in young child and created a case classification to assist in the analysis of accidental versus inflicted etiology. These criteria have been applied to case evaluation in femur and humerus fractures.[458] The majority of abuse related femur fractures of the long bones occur in infants less than 1 year old.[459]

Humerus fractures are frequent injuries in childhood, both from inflicted and accidental etiology. Strait et al[365] discuss the challenges of diagnosing humeral injury in young children when the etiology is not obvious. Their discussion and criteria are useful in any case of single event injuries in children. **Humeral fractures** are often bilateral, resulting from shaking, pulling, or twisting, and the proximal metaphyseal fracture is the most common. Distal humeral epiphyseal separation is difficult to recognize and can easily be confused with a dislocation. This type of injury is often associated with birth trauma or trauma in infancy. The cause of a 'punched-out' defect in the distal humeral metaphysis is unclear. It may result from avulsion of the anterior capsular attachment and can easily be confused with osteomyelitis. Shaft injuries tend to be either oblique or spiral; however, transverse fractures can occur as the result of a direct blow. The majority of humeral fractures in children are accidental, but in all children less than 15 months, abuse should be considered.[365]

Fractures of the forearm involving the radius and ulna are common in abused children and represent 10–20% of abuse-related fractures. Transverse fractures of the shaft are common and there is typically marked soft tissue swelling. Torus fractures, commonly known as 'buckle' fractures, are the most common accidental fracture of the distal radius and ulna. Proximal fractures of the radius and ulna are very rare in both accidental and abuse circumstances.

The hands are frequently overlooked in the skeletal survey. The two most common injuries are metacarpal fractures and fracture dislocations.

In the lower extremity, tibial metaphyseal fractures are most common predominate, with distal metaphyseal fractures and are often related to abuse.[460] Tibial diaphyseal fractures occur less frequently and are often due to torsional stress of the newly ambulating toddler. Fractures of the fibula are rarely seen in this age group, regardless of the mechanism of trauma.

Fractures of the feet are very uncommon. When present, they typically involve the metatarsals. Usually very little history is provided and this type of injury has a high suspicion for abuse. Fractures of the pelvis are also very uncommonly observed in child abuse but have been reported. This may be due, in part, to the fact that the area is often overlooked during survey.

Bony thoracic trauma involves the ribs, clavicle, scapula, and sternum.

Rib fractures[461, 462] are rare in healthy infants, and their presence in the absence of metabolic bone disease strongly suggests abuse. The incidence of rib fractures in abused patients varies from 5 to 27%. Peak incidence of rib fractures as a result of abuse is in infants younger than 1 year of age. Fractures are often occult, do not display external trauma, and rarely involve intrathoracic parenchymal injury. The ribcage in the child is quite resilient, since costal cartilages are not calcified. An impact to the rib can dissipate the imparted energy by the flexibility of the cartilage. Most abuse-related rib fractures are related to side–side (posteromedial fractures) or anteroposterior compression (anterior, mid-axillary fractures).[463] Rib fractures are frequently bilateral, often involving multiple ribs with the fracture located posteriorly. In younger infants the assumed mechanism of fracture is anteroposterior compression, whereas in older children fractures can result at the site of a direct blow. Anterior fractures usually occur at the costochondral junction and are the metaphyseal equivalent with injury at the cartilage growth plate. Fractures of the first rib are rare and in the otherwise normal child are highly suspicious for inflicted injury. Before rib fractures or any other fractures can be attributed to abuse, causes such as accident, prematurity, intrauterine immobilization, birth injury, metabolic disorders, chronic disease or steroid effect, and bone dysplasias, or conditions that can affect bone strength or integrity must be ruled out. Rib fractures following chest physiotherapy for pulmonary toilet in neonates as well as for bronchiolitis or pneumonia in infancy have been reported.[464, 465]

Rib fractures from CPR are a common occurence in adults. The risk of rib fractures from CPR in infants and children is more controversial. Because anterior-posterior compression is involved, details of the procedure should be verified.

Feldman and Brever[466] studied the incidence of rib fractures in children with emphasis on children receiving CPR, comparing the results with rib fractures associated with child abuse. Despite varying degrees of skill in administering CPR, no rib fractures were identified in the non-abuse population. Leadbetter reviews injuries in childhood related to resuscitation.[90] Included in his analysis was review of seven publications regarding rib fractures and CPR. Two of the reports found no CPR related fractures and four of the reports include young infants without evidence of abuse who suffered rib fractures associated with resuscitation.

An acute rib fracture site is often invisible and does not become apparent until callus formation is well under way. Posterior rib fractures are notoriously difficult to identify in the acute phase.[467] Rib fractures may be identified by radionuclide scans but must be radiographically confirmed. Follow-up radiographs may be indicated. The author has experience with a number of cases with premortem diagnosis of multiple fractures including the skull that were not verified with further review or autopsy examination.

Zumwalt and Fanizza-Orphanos[468] reviewed the postmortem examination of rib fractures in fatal child abuse. Key points of their review include:

- Soft tissue hemorrhage can be observed for 3–4 weeks after injury.
- Size of callus does not correlate with age of injury.
- Fractures of long bones in children generally require 8–10 weeks to unite solidly.
- On cut section the central portion of periosteal callus contains significant proportions of cartilage.
- Marrow is replaced by fibroblastic elements in the early days and weeks of healing.
- The medullary canal is eventually replaced by usual bone marrow elements.
- Clinical fractures in small children heal at an accelerated rate.
- Cellular proliferation from both periosteal and medullary cellular elements is evident histologically within a few days after fracture.
- Cellular granulation tissue (callus) can be seen in 5–7 days in mature bone.
- New bone appears histologically within 5–10 days and continues for weeks to months.
- Radiographic evidence of callus has been observed at 5 days following birth trauma.

Clavicle fractures are common childhood fractures, with the mid shaft the most frequently affected area. Clavicular fractures are observed in 2–6% of abused patients. The history is important, as this fracture is very difficult to differentiate from birth trauma.

Fractures of the sternum or scapula are rare and suggest abuse when there is a lack of plausible explanation. Both require a massive amount of direct force. The acromion is the most often injured and may easily be overlooked.

The incidence of **spinal fractures** in abuse is not known. Most involve the vertebral body, typically with a compression deformity.[469] This type of trauma may lead to herniation of the disc into the vertebral body, resulting in anterosuperior notching. Approximately two-thirds of patients with abuse-induced spinal trauma are under 3 years of age, and more than 50% are under 1 year of age. The injury may often be occult or may appear as an accentuated kyphosis and can involve the spinal cord. The most common cause of such injuries is thought to be **hyperflexion/extension**. Other, more infrequent injuries are posterior spinous fractures, injury of the posterior ligamentous complex, and fracture of the C2 pedicle.

The analysis of the otherwise healthy child with multiple healing fractures, although distressing, is usually a straight-forward process. The problems arise when a child presents with a single injury/fracture. The characteristics of the fracture itself are seldom sufficient to assure certain diagnostic criteria for abuse. Kenney[438] presents an excellent discussion and guidelines. Similar challenges confront the analysis of the infant with fractures and a history of significant prematurity in the newborn period with risk factors for metabolic bone disease, or osteopenia of prematurity.[436, 440, 470] These include a history of prolonged total parenteral nutrition, diuretic therapy, bronchopulmonary dysplasia, and steroid treatment. Multiple fractures in the presence of these conditions may be impossible to differentiate from inflicted injury.

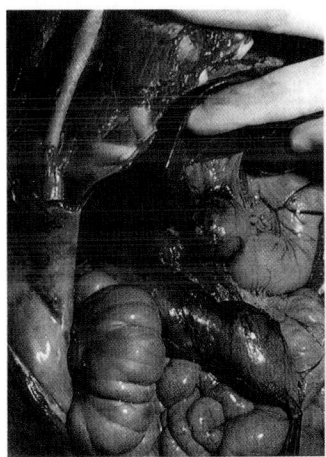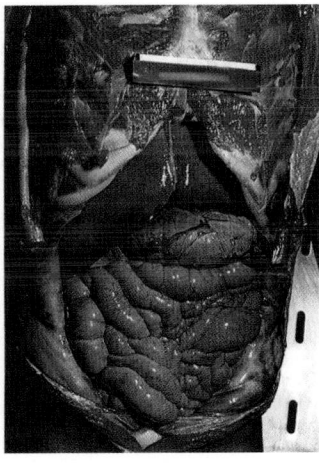

FIGURE 17.42 Inflicted abdominal trauma with contusions and peritonitis.

Visceral trauma[116, 471–473]

Visceral injuries in infants and children are rare, but when they occur in the absence of significant traumatic event (such as traffic accident or severe fall) the etiology is frequently determined to be non-accidental trauma. Despite significant internal injury, visceral injuries may not produce the type of signs and symptoms that prompt immediate medical attention resulting in serious and often fatal delay in medical treatment.[474–476]

As a blunt force is applied to the body surface, deformation results in inward displacement and energy transfer through the tissues. The rate and magnitude of distortion are the major determinates of the resulting nature and severity of internal injury. Cooper and Taylor[472] review the biophysics of blunt force injury to the chest and abdomen. Slow velocity of compression (> 20–50 milliseconds) is unlikely to cause injury. Rapid compression (< 5 milliseconds) may produce severe damage even with minimal compression (3–4 inches). Injury is a reflection of tissue mechanical failure, body cavity wave propagation and crush injury. Waves of force can occur as stress waves (compression), shock waves (such as in explosions) or shear waves (transverse waves of longer duration and low velocity).[116] Indirect injury can be the result of:[472]

- a synchronous motion of adjunct structures
- stretching at sites of attachment
- collision of viscera with stiff structures

Bowel injuries may also result from creation of a pressure differential across the bowel wall at a distance from the impact site.

Abdominal injuries are the second most common cause of death in fatal child abuse. The true incidence of abuse-induced trauma to the viscera is not known. What *is* known is that most often the mechanism is due to crushing or compressive impacts associated with blunt trauma. Causes in this category include punches with a clenched fist, kicks, or rapid deceleration after impact with an immovable surface. The most common blunt abdominal injuries are lacerations and ruptures of hollow and solid viscera (i.e. bowel, mesentery, liver, spleen, kidneys, and

pancreas) (Fig. 17.42).[477–479] Non-accidental internal injuries are usually located below the diaphragm. Cobb and associates summarized the findings in 12 cases of intestinal perforation from blunt trauma.[480] Child abuse was the cause in eight, motor vehicle accidents in four. The delay in seeking treatment was considerably longer in the abused children.

Blows to the abdomen frequently involve the intestinal wall, and deceleration or shearing forces produce injury at the mesenteric attachments. Kleinman[481] describes several injury mechanisms. Sudden increased intraluminal pressure occurs when the viscus impacted is located directly over or under the spine, pelvis, or thorax and subjected to decelerating or shearing forces at the mesenteric attachments. Sequelae include duodenal perforation and intramural intestinal hematoma.[482, 483] These injuries frequently result in seromuscular tearing of the intestinal wall and contusion and laceration of the mesenteric attachments. As the bowel wall becomes devitalized, perforation and subsequent peritonitis may follow the original injury by hours or even days. Many of these children have received repeated blows to the abdomen over time, and careful examination and microscopic sampling of the abdominal contents has revealed extensive fibrosis confirming subacute or remote injury. One of the most frequent mechanisms of fatal injuries in inflicted childhood trauma is occult abdominal trauma with unattended **intestinal perforation**.[480, 484]

Small bowel or mesenteric injury often occurs with blunt force abdominal trauma. Motor vehicle accidents, child abuse, falls from height, sports and even Heimlich maneuvers have been implicated in small bowel/mesenteric injury. The pathophysiology of injury to small bowel and mesentery was first offered in 1890 by Motz and remains a reasonable approach to understanding the mechanisms of injury:[485]

- crush injury resulting from impact of a stationary object on the anterior abdominal wall catching a loop between and the spin or solid organ
- shearing forces of the bowel and mesentery at fixed points of attachment
- burst injury caused by increased intraluminal pressure

Bowel injuries may result in self-limiting hematomas, secondary perforations due to venous necrosis, or frank perforations. Proximal jejunum and duodenum account for approximately 90% of small bowel injuries in child abuse.[471] Mesenteric injuries may cause significant hemorrhage or later result in devascularization of bowel. **Chylous ascites** has been reported in association with abuse, most likely explained on the basis of mesenteric trauma.

Signs and symptoms of peritoneal irritation may be subtle in the young infant. This may be complicated by use of antibiotics for what is thought to be otitis or upper respiratory infection. External physical stigmata of injury (i.e. abdominal bruising) are the exception, and the child's condition may remain undiagnosed even under medical care, especially if they are unconscious on presentation. Case and Nandire[486] report a child with gastric laceration due to blunt trauma from child abuse, and Sujka and colleagues[487] describe a 3-week-old child presenting with acute scrotal swelling as the first evidence of intra-abdominal trauma from battering.

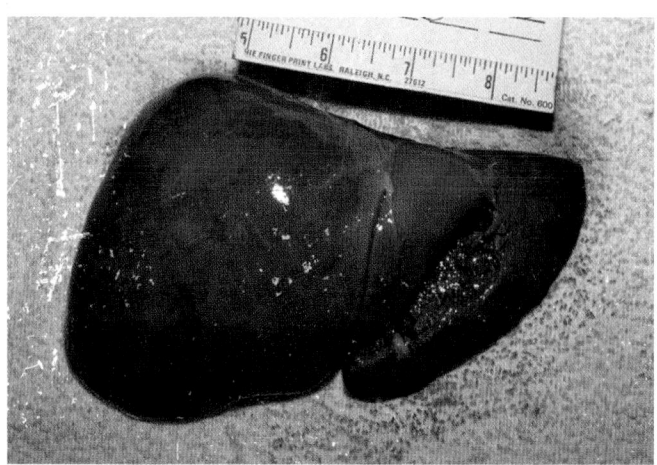

FIGURE 17.43 Laceration of the liver due to blunt force trauma to the abdomen.

As a consequence of the difficulty in diagnosing occult visceral trauma many emergency department professionals are adding CT scans of the chest and abdomen to the evaluation of children presenting with possible head trauma. Detailed imaging allows for better understanding of the character of traumatic intra-abdominal abnormalities. These include: free intraperitoneal air, free retroperitoneal air, extraluminal oral contrast material, free intraperitoneal fluid, bowel wall defect, bowel wall thickening, mesenteric stranding, fluid at the mesenteric root, focal hematoma, active hemorrhage, and mesenteric pseudoaneurysm. Strouse et al[488] provides an excellent clinical/CT scan correlation of bowel and mesenteric trauma in children. Hanks et al[489] points out the utility of the CT scan in delineating the extent of intra-abdominal injuries following blunt force trauma.

Timing the injury or establishing the age of injuries can be challenging in children with inflicted injuries to the abdomen. It is important that available tissues be collected for careful histologic examination during laparotomy to assist in determining the age of inflammatory or traumatic lesions. Surgeons need to be alerted to this task and to coordinate with the surgical pathologist when necessary. When assessing the timing of onset of symptoms careful and detailed evaluation of activities of daily living and subtle variations in eating and bowel habits should be sought.

Hepatic contusions are probably more common than recognized, as they are typically not diagnosed in the absence of significant bleeding or hepatic failure. The spectrum of causes of hepatic injury in children differs from adults and is typically more severe. Isolated hepatic trauma is more common in childhood. Blunt hepatic injury can result in relatively minor sub/capsular hematoma to massive disruption or transection of liver (Fig. 17.43). Similarly signs and symptoms may be absent, mild, slow deterioration, or catastrophic hemorrhage and shock. A grading system for hepatic injury has proved useful for clinical management and may be a useful observation at postmortem examination for

research classification. Vascular instability is a significant prognostic indicator. Careful dissection and documentation of arterial and hepatic venous disruption may assist in the analysis of survival time post injury.

Pancreatic injury occurs in up to 10% of pediatric blunt abdominal trauma. Pancreatitis and pancreatic pseudocysts in infants and children are most often the result of trauma. Delayed diagnosis is unfortunately common.[490] **Pancreatic pseudocysts,** which may present occultly and in the absence of a pancreatitis history, should be assumed to be post-traumatic.[491–493]

Traumatic injuries to the kidneys are extremely rare in association with child abuse, but acute renal failure resulting from rhabdomyolysis and myoglobinuria has been reported.[494]

Diagnosing **duodenal trauma** once had to be restricted to a radiographic upper GI series; however, sonography has proved quite effective.[495] In children presenting with unexplained GI symptoms (vomiting and dehydration along with elevated amylase and white blood cell count) sonography has detected the injury. The appearance of the classic bowel lesion is a central echogenic core representing compressed mucosa and a thick sonolucent halo representing thickened bowel wall due to edema, hemorrhage, or neoplasm. In the variety of cases, the lesions have appeared predominantly hypoechoic to echoic. Cases combining both may be due to lesions of varying ages. More than 75% of patients with such lesions have associated ascites.

Birth trauma can result in intra-abdominal injuries and usually involve rupture or subcapsular hemorrhage into the liver, spleen, or adrenal. Uhing[496] summarizes three potential mechanisms for intra-abdominal injuries following birth:
- direct trauma
- compression of the chest against the surface of the spleen or liver
- chest compression that leads to tearing of the ligamentous insertions of the liver or spleen

Discussion of traumatic visceral injuries must also include the patterns of injury that occur following appropriate and suboptimal use of restraints. Solid and hollow visceral injuries have been linked to seat belts. Current literature emphasizes the importance of age appropriate seating position and restraint use to minimize risk of injury to infants and children.[497, 498] Children restrained in a suboptimal fashion are more likely to suffer injuries to hollow viscous.[499]

Thoracic trauma in the young infant most often results in injury to the chest cage. However, thoracic injuries account for approximately 14% of pediatric trauma related deaths and are second only to head injuries as the leading cause of death from blunt force trauma.[500–502] Etiology of thoracic injuries is most commonly traffic accidents, falls, and abuse. Thoracic injuries from child abuse are thought to be due to direct impact. Pulmonary contusion is the most commonly observed intra-thoracic injury in childhood trauma.[503] Traumatic asphyxia is a unique and unusual form of injury that results from prolonged compression of the chest wall with resulting airway occlusion and retrograde high pressure in the superior vena cava. These patients demonstrate characteristic cervical/facial cyanosis, vascular congestion, subconjunctival hemorrhage, and diffuse petechiae. Vascular trauma can lead to vasospasm or thrombosis with devastating ischemic consequences in any location.

Pathology of head injuries in infancy[26, 484, 504–506]

Head injury is the most frequent cause of traumatic death in the pediatric population, comprising between 50 and 80% of all trauma related deaths each year.[507] Motor vehicle accidents are the most common cause of traumatic brain injury (TBI) in children age 0–4 years followed by inflicted injuries, pedestrian injuries and falls. In children aged 0–2 years falls and traffic accidents are the most common causes of TBI.[508] McClelland et al have reported that head injury is the leading cause of death in child abuse.[509] McClelland also estimates that most severe TBI in children less than 1 year is due to abuse and that approximately 10% of all traumatic injuries in children less than 5 years of age will have a non-accidental cause. Keenan et al[510] studied 152 cases of traumatic brain injury in children 2 years or younger. Around 53% of the cases were identified as victims of inflicted injury with a higher incidence occurring during infancy than the second year. Billmire and Myers[511] conducted a retrospective review of all medical records and CT scans of children less than 1 year of age with head injury admitted to Children's Hospital Medical Center, Cincinnati, over a 2-year period. Here 64% of all head injuries, excluding uncomplicated skull fracture, were interpreted as due to child abuse. The true incidence of non-accidental head trauma in childhood is not precisely known. What is known is children suffer serious and fatal brain injuries from accidents and inflicted trauma.

The forensic pathologist is often in a key position to ensure complete collection of and thorough examination of the necessary elements for medicolegal analysis of TBI in an infant. Questions routinely posed to the forensic analyst are:

- Are the findings due to traumatic injury?
- How did this happen or how could this have happened? (type and cause of injury)
- When did the injury take place?
- Could a specific event or 'accident' have caused the injury or injuries?
- Is there more than one episode of injury?
- What do the medical findings tell about the injury or death of the child?

It is imperative that questions are answered only after the necessary evidence and information has been collected and evaluated.

Biomechanics of head injury[88–90, 507, 512]

TBI is caused by one of two mechanisms:
- Impulse loading – head moves as a result of motion imparted to some other part of the body.

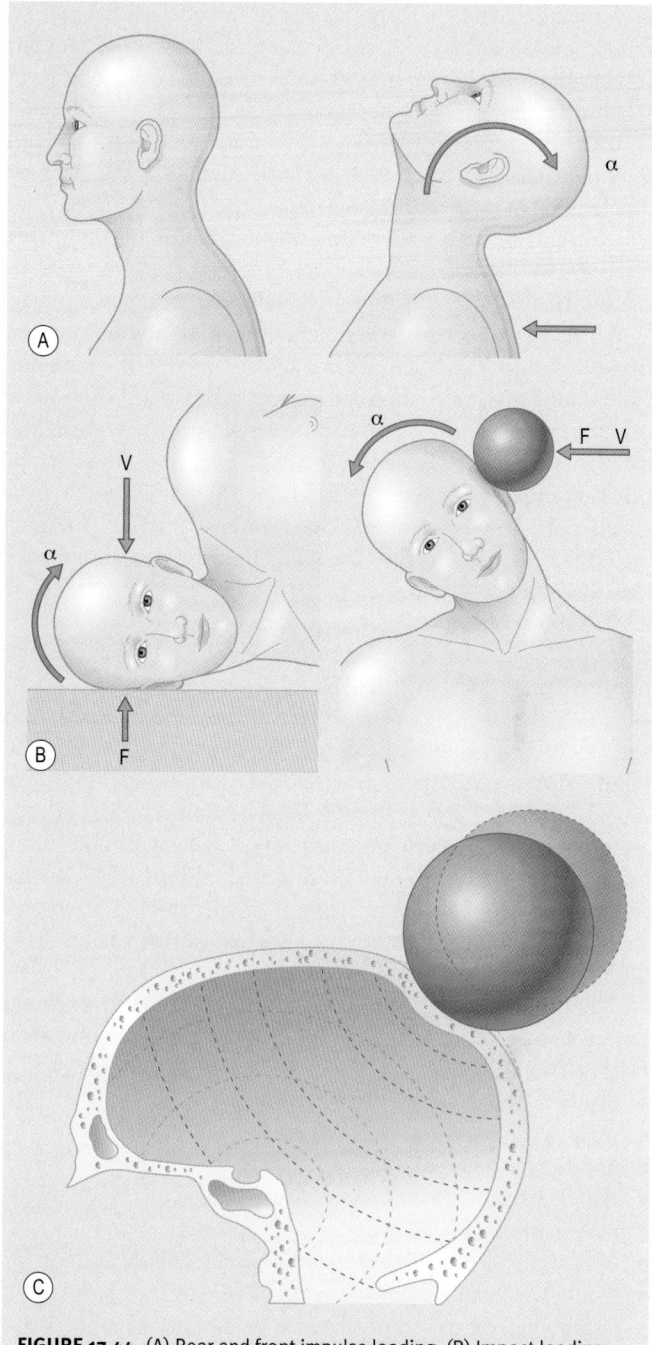

FIGURE 17.44 (A) Rear and front impulse loading. (B) Impact loading with a fixed and moving object. (C) Contact phenomenon and wave propagation in impact to the head. (With permission from Lippincott.)

- Impact loading – head either strikes a stationary object or is struck by a moving object (Fig. 17.44).

These mechanisms are completely distinct and have totally different consequences. Impulse loading will cause the head to rotate on the cervical spine (translational motion, rotational motion, and a combination of both). With such motion, the skull moves at a different rate than the brain because they are not rigidly connected. Primary injuries from impulse loading may include SDH, hematoma, and traumatic axonal injury. Injury tolerances have been estimated for linear and angular acceleration in children. Impact is the collision of two objects at a rate sufficient to cause observable effects. Significant impact typically produces a contact injury (scalp contusion or skull fracture), followed by translational and angular acceleration or deceleration of the brain. During impact (i.e. from a fall) the skull will stop and the brain will continue to move within the skull. This can result in traumatic axonal injury, diffuse axonal injury (DAI), subdural hematoma, and intracerebral hemorrhage.

In order to understand head injury in childhood it is critical that one understands the differences between TBI in infants and in adults. The structural properties of the infant skull (ease of deformation and decreased threshold to fracture) and the mechanical properties of the infant brain are different from those of an older child or adult. In the preterm child the skull consists of a fibrous membrane that ossifies by intramembranous ossification. In early infancy the skull bones are thin and pliable, and the inner and outer table can hardly be distinguished. A distinct inner table usually does not become apparent until about 2 years of age. The intracranial fossae are shallower and the non-myelinated infant brain has a softer texture. The infant skull is highly flexible owing to the relative lack of ossification and open fontanelles and sutures. The skull does not become tightly closed until approximately 3–4 years of age and does not completely approach adult biomechanics until puberty, although by age 5–6 years the differences are small. The child's brain does not achieve adult size and weight until about 5 years of age. Age-dependent properties of the developing brain and skull affect injury thresholds. Different sized brains have different injury thresholds.

The mechanism of injury in infant head trauma (in general as well as with inflicted injury) appears to relate to a number of factors:[504]

- highly deformable skull
- suture patency
- high head to body ratio
- thin skull bones
- more elastic spinal column
- immature skeletal joints and vulnerable craniocervical junction
- reduced neck muscle tone
- largely unmyelinated brain substance
- distinct biomechanical properties
- differences in infant brain physiology
  - differences in arterial blood pressure and cerebral blood flow
  - increased basal reactivity and metabolic rate.

Margulies and Thibault[89] compared the mechanical properties of infant and adult skulls and found significant variation in the failure stress of the skull of the neonate, the young infant, and the adult, with the resistance to fracture for an adult 11 times greater than for newborn. Failure is a stress or strain that does not allow a return to the normal physical state. Ommaya et al[507] found that adult brains were more vulnerable to angular velocity and acceleration than the infant brain which required higher levels of angular acceleration to cause similar injury. The newborn and infant skull can be characterized as elastic interlocking plates capable of resisting compression and shear (TBI), but incapable of transmitting bending (fractures) across the sutures or fontanelles.

In very basic terms, injury to the head is a factor of stress (force per unit area) and strain [change in length per unit reference length (elongation, compression, deformation, shear, bending, torsion)] or by load deformation. To cause scalp contusion or laceration; to fracture the skull; to produce subarachnoid or subdural hemorrhage; to cause subdural hematoma; to cause cerebral concussion; to produce DAI the stress must exceed the strength and injury threshold of the material.

Impact loading of the infant head produces potentially damaging levels of strain within the entire structure. Deformation, rather than acceleration, appears to be the critical factor. When an infant skull hits an unyielding surface the tendency is for the skull to deform, with larger cranial shape change than in adults, resulting in diffuse brain distortion. The deformation of the skull in infants can produce large strains throughout the brain without skull fracture. Impulse loading may also result in strains of the brain, but in these conditions there is minimal or no deformation of the skull.

In recent years biomechanical analysis and research has added substantially to the body of knowledge, and understanding of the complex nature of brain injury. Collaboration between biomechanical engineers, physicians, and researchers will provide continued developments in the understanding of childhood head injury.

Presentation of head injury (Fig 17.45)

The major pathologies encountered in childhood head trauma include subdural hematoma, cerebral edema, hypoxia, hypoxic-ischemic injury, and, less commonly, subarachnoid hemorrhage. There are significant differences of opinion regarding the analysis, interpretation, and diagnosis of traumatic brain injury in infants (Table 17.11). Divisions or 'schools of thought' have resulted in heated debate within the medical community. Eventually medical evidence and scientific principles will answer the questions.[136, 454]

Skull fracture

Skull fractures are relatively common in childhood head injury. Fractures occur when the elastic limits of the skull are exceeded by the impacting force and indicate direct impact of the head with a solid object. Patterns of fractures to the infant skull are similar to the adult with some variations due to immaturity.[26] In infants, if the impact is broad and of sufficient force, the entire skull is deformed.[89] If the impact site is small, as in missile injuries, no deformation may result. The inner table breaks before the outer table during deformation, and the lines of stress radiate in a curvilinear pattern outward from the impact site. Fractures occur along the stress lines and may have a radiating or concentric appearance reflecting the surface force.

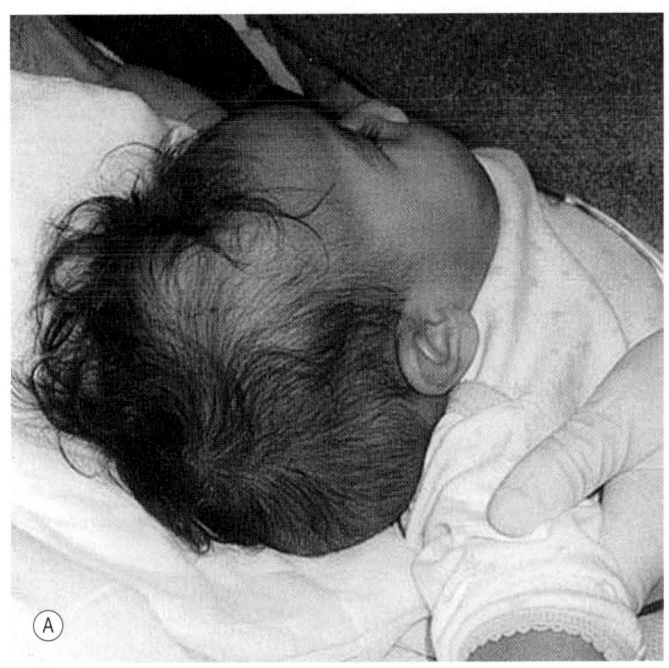

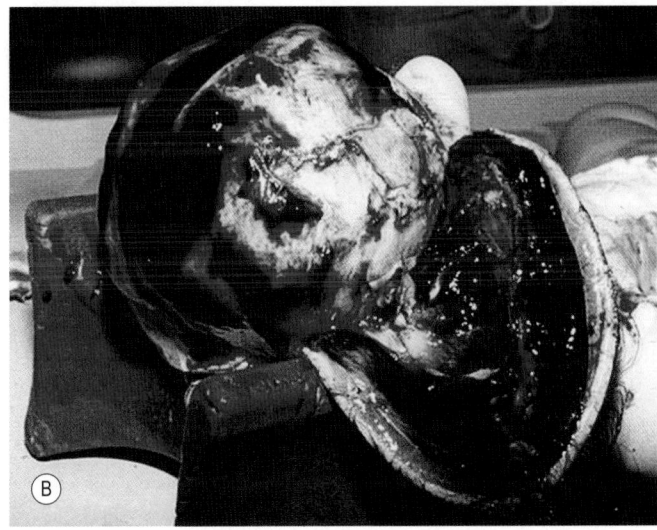

FIGURE 17.45 Fatal blunt force head trauma. (A) Child presenting awake and screaming with obvious soft tissue swelling. (B) Infant had massive eggshell fracture to skull and unrelenting cerebral edema.

TABLE 17.11 HEAD TRAUMA: CONTROVERSIES (SEE ALSO PAGES 804–805)

Position A	New considerations	Position B
– Any age child can be shaken with sufficient force to cause: Traumatic axonal injury Subdural hematoma Retinal hemorrhage – This action will result in immediate and obvious symptoms. If lethal, the occurrence was shortly before medical attention or authorities notified – Short falls do not cause serious head injury in infancy – Severe retinal hemorrhage is pathognomonic of rotational injury or abuse due to shaking in infancy	– Small infants may be at increased risk for brainstem injury from shaking – Hypoxic injury may cause intradural/subdural hemorrhages	– Shaking alone cannot produce sufficient biomechanical force even in the very small infant to cause: Subdural hemorrhage Traumatic axonal injury Retinal hemorrhage – Abusive head trauma is due to impact loading forces typically due to blunt force injury. Severe impact may occur without obvious external signs. Serious head injury in infants and children can present with occult signs and symptoms. – Retinal hemorrhage can be an indicator of severe head trauma, but the mechanism cannot be determined by their presence

Skull fractures can be defined as follows (Fig. 17.46):

- Linear – usually caused by impact of moving head against solid object. Linear fractures are often observed in simple falls.
- Basilar – most occur from impacts to the occiput, sides, or front of head. Basilar fractures are often caused by a fall against an unyielding surface, inflicted blows with objects, and accidental and intentional falls from heights.
- Depressed – typically result from impact with moving object. A circle or plate of calvarium gets 'punched' out into the intracranial shape and may retain the shape of the offending object. Findings may include lacerated dura, subdural and/or epidural bleeding, and brain contusion. Depressed skull fractures reportedly account for 7–11% of children admitted to the hospital and 15–22% of children with skull fractures.[513]
- Comminuted (simple or multiple) – these are similar to depressed fractures and may occur at the site of impact with wide areas of fragmentation. Associated brain injures are common and morbidity and mortality rates are high.
- Diastatic ('bursting') – fracture line involves separation of one or more of the cranial sutures and is characterized by a widely diastatic (> 4 mm) skull fracture and may be associated with acute extracranial cerebral herniation beneath unbroken scalp.[514] Findings often include epidural hemorrhage, lacerated dura, and severe brain damage. Infants with cranial burst fracture can present with hemorrhagic shock and CT scan typically shows marked soft tissue swelling.
- Expressed, stellate, multiple, contrecoup – combination of fractures.

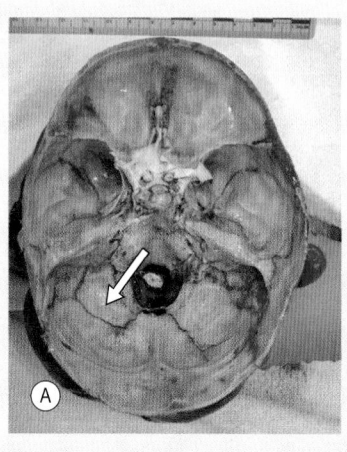 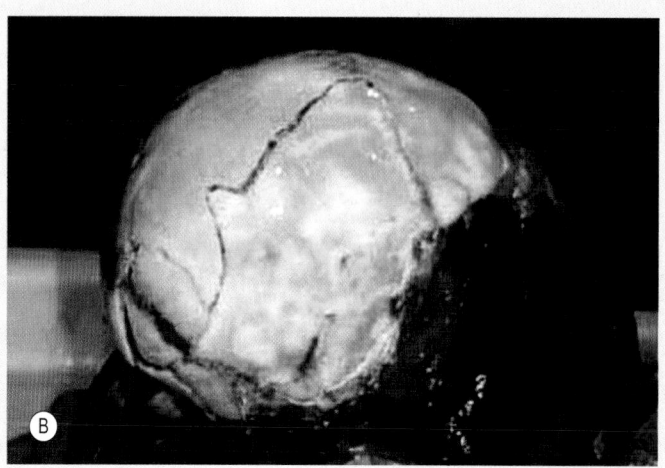

FIGURE 17.46 Skull fractures in fatal child abuse. (A) Basilar. (B) Eggshell.

Observations about childhood skull fractures include:

- Fracture lines tend to end at sutures.
- An infant dropped on the vertex may show bilateral fracture lines along the parietal boss.
- A blow or fall on the top of the head can result in horizontal crack running posterior from the front parietal suture.
- Bilateral fractures can be the result of a single or more than one blow.
- Suture diastasis can occur with or without fractures.
- Massive skull fractures can occur with little or no resultant brain injury.
- No pattern of skull fracture is diagnostic of abuse.[515]
- Soft tissue swelling over the acute fracture site is often observed (Fig. 17.47) but may be absent even in the presence of acute fracture.
- CT scans and scintigraphy are often unreliable in evaluating presence or absence of skull fracture. Traditional skull series remains the best method to identify skull fractures.

Greenes and Schutzman[516] reviewed a series of 101 patients less than 2 years of age with isolated skull fracture in the absence of intracranial injury. Falls were the most common reported mechanism (89%) and many falls were less than 3 feet (18%). Non-accidental trauma was suspected in only 10 patients. A total of 72 patients had clinical signs of potential serious head injury (loss of consciousness, seizures, vomiting, lethargy, irritability, depressed mental status, focal neurologic findings). Most subjects (91%) had single skull fractures, but 9% suffered multiple fractures. Of those with multiple fractures, non-accidental trauma was considered in two cases, and three of the falls were relatively innocuous. Linear fractures were observed in 78 patients and 22 patients had depressed fractures. Six of the subjects with depressed skull fractures fell less than 3 feet and had no evaluation for non-accidental trauma.

Leventhal et al[445] analyzed fractures in children less than 3 years of age to identify patterns of accidental and inflicted injury. They noted 104 skull fractures in 94 children; 75 in those less than 12 months of age. The majority of both accidental and inflicted injuries were linear fractures involving the parietal bones. Small

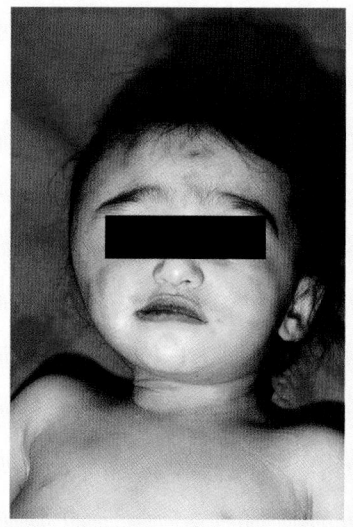

FIGURE 17.47 Soft tissue swelling over fracture site.

numbers of parieto-occipital fractures (attributed to abuse) and frontal fractures (determined to be accidental) were observed.

Dating skull fractures is difficult because of the unique relationship of the calvarium to the galea and the dura. Typical callus formation, useful in dating fractures in other anatomic sites, does not occur in this location. Fracture lines may be evident weeks or months after the injury, with only **relative sharpness** of the fracture edges useful for evaluation.

In the postmortem examination of an infant or child with suspicious head injury, histologic sampling of the skull fracture (as well as any injuries in possible NAI) is strongly recommended.

Parenchymal brain injury – diffuse axonal injury[506, 517–522]

Parenchymal brain injuries are ultimately the cause of death in one form or another in the majority of abusive head trauma fatalities. However, the nature of the initial injuries, secondary consequences, presence or absence of pre-existing injuries or conditions, and prolongation of life support can make the forensic interpretation of parenchymal injuries difficult and, at times, impossible. Parenchymal injury can include focal hemorrhage and tears of parenchyma, microscopic vascular injury, venous thrombosis, cerebral infarction due to vascular trauma or secondary injury, a variety of axonal injury and patterns, anoxic neuronal injury, acute and chronic vital reaction, reperfusion alterations and vascular changes, cystic transformation associated with encephalomalacia and brain atrophy, metabolic encephalopathy arising from hormone abnormalities and cellular hypoglycemia, and finally the deteriorating brain pathology associated with life support following brain death.

Medana and Esiri[517] reviewed the evidence for axonal damage and correlation with neurologic outcome in a variety of diverse human CNS disorders including head and spinal cord trauma. Diffuse traumatic axonal injury has been observed in adults with head trauma resulting from road traffic accidents, falls from a height, assaults, and sports injuries. Damage to axons is an almost universal finding in mild, moderate and severe head trauma with outcomes ranging from mild concussion to coma to death. Traumatic axonal injury may be focal or diffuse including the brainstem. The degree of axonal stretch determines the changes in axolemma permeability through development of mechanical defects in the membrane. These injuries result in changes in permeability and onset of increase in osmotic pressure at the cellular level.

Increasing application of immunohistochemistry staining for β-amyloid precursor protein (BAPP) has allowed for identification and evaluation of axonal injuries. The rounded eosinophilic axon 'retraction' balls have classically been identified, as early as 12–15 h following injury in the adult. Vowles and co-workers[523] demonstrate that diffuse axonal injury typified by retraction balls and axonal swellings may occur in early infancy in the same way as that described in adults. The time frame for appearance of axonal balls for the infant brain is unknown. Accumulation of microglial cells can be documented with CD68 and typically shows increased numbers within 36 h and clustering by 2 weeks to several months.[506] Graham et al[524] presents a review of axonal pathology with BAPP immunohistochemistry (Figs 17.48 and 17.49). Their findings confirm that proper interpretation of these stains requires sufficient sampling (n = 15), processing using standardized protocols and at times mapping using anatomic diagrams. They conclude that random sampling of a small number of sections may lead to misinterpretation. Reichard et al[522] studied 28 cases of NAI fatalities and conclude that BAPP aids in the documentation of NAI CNS injury in children.

When DAI occurs in children more than 1 year old the pattern is similar to that seen in adults. However in recent studies by Geddes and others,[519–521] DAI was rare in infants less than 1 year old. Around 84% had global hypoxic damage and only 2 of 37 had traumatic axonal injury (both had severe contact head injuries with skull fractures). They concluded that either the non-myelinated axons of the infant brain are less

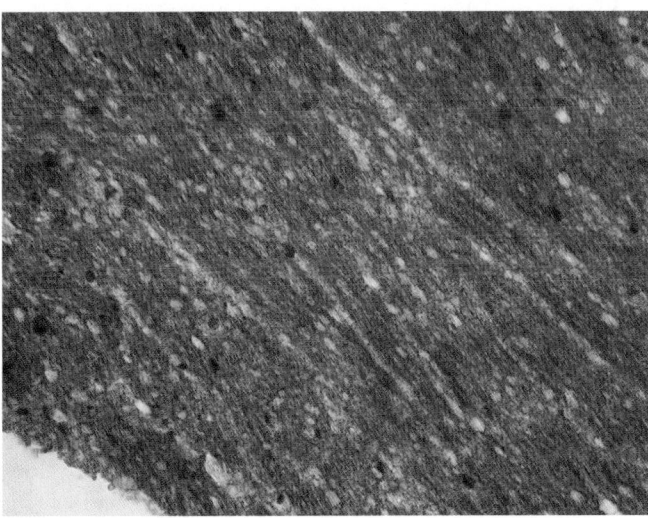

FIGURE 17.48 β-amyloid precursor protein staining showing hypoxic axonal injury pattern, white matter (× 10).

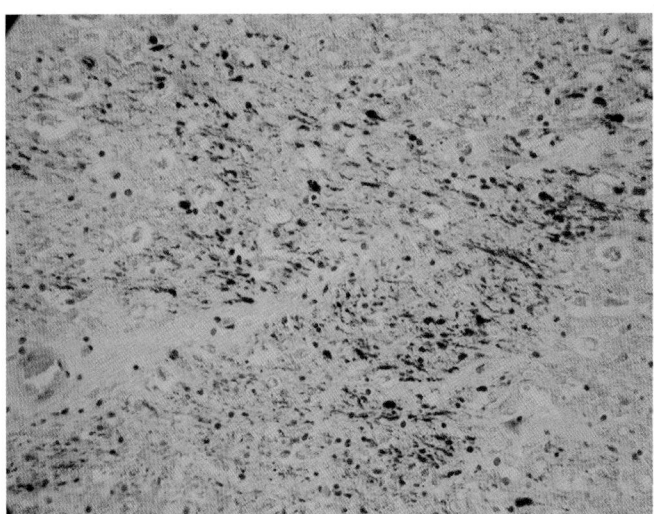

FIGURE 17.49 β-amyloid precursor protein stain showing traumatic axonal injury pattern (× 10).

susceptible to damage during impulse loading, or in shaking type injuries the brain in not exposed to forces necessary to cause traumatic DAI. Axonal pathology was associated with brain swelling and raised intracranial pressure and was predominantly vascular in nature. Herniation of the brainstem through the foramen magnum (either as a result of deformation or during secondary brain swelling) may cause focal traumatic axonal injury mimicking 'shaking'/hyperextension.

Pittella and Gusmao[525] examined a series of 120 fatalities from road traffic incidents with specific emphasis on diffuse vascular injury (DVI) and its relationship to DAI. DVI is the pathologic finding of multiple small hemorrhagic lesions of traumatic origin. DVI is not as well understood as patients with this finding usually die within 24 h. Because both DVI and DAI are associated with acceleration injuries they theorized that

DVI should be associated with DAI. Their results showed a relationship between DVI and DAI suggesting that the findings represent a pathologic spectrum rather than distinct entities. DVI was identified macroscopically and was more apparent microscopically. Lesions were located predominantly in white matter of frontal and temporal poles, in and adjacent to thalamus and brainstem. This author's experience has been that DVI is rare in NAI but the pattern and location are similar to this series.

Cerebral trauma in the young infant may produce radiographic lesions including contusions, hematoma, traumatic clefts and focal lesions at the gray–white junction consistent with shearing injury. *Contusional hemorrhages* are typically small in brain-injured children and are characterized by high-density foci on CT. They are most frequently found along the cerebral convexities (frontal and parasagittal) and are the consequence of contact forces or impact. The position of cerebral contusions is usually related to the site of impact. Furthermore, they are frequently associated with other cerebral injuries. Deep contusions may also occur, especially in the corpus callosum and thalamus, and uncommonly in the posterior fossa. Grossly visible contusional tears in the white matter and microscopically visible tears in the outer cortex parallel to the brain surface are uncommon in childhood head trauma but are observed.[526] This is in contrast to the hemorrhagic contusions typically seen in adults. Lindenberg and Freytag[527] studied 16 infants with this unique pattern of contusional tears. Predilection areas for the white matter tears were the orbital and temporal lobes and the first frontal convolutions, and for cortical tears the crests of the convolutions of the cerebral convexities.

Hausmann[528] reviewed the morphologic changes of cortical contusions in human brain injury and lists criteria for estimating age of cortical contusions following traumatic brain injury evaluating:

- cortical hemorrhages
- inflammatory cellular response
- macrophage – microglial reaction
- reactive gliosis

Earlier changes associated with cortical contusions are hemorrhage and microscopic signs of neuronal degeneration. Infant red blood cells can be observed months following injury. This is followed by local cellular reaction. Immunohistochemical analysis of leukocyte subtypes has demonstrated early arrival of neutrophils (CDIS) followed by different subtypes 1–4 days after injury (VCA, UCHL-1, CD3). Microglial phagocytic cells, reactive astroglial cells, neovascularization and glial scar occur over time at the injury site.

Subdural hemorrhage/hematoma[529–534]

SDH is a common injury in child abuse (Fig. 17.50). Incidence of SDH in infants less than 1 year old is estimated at 24/100 000. Lonergan and Baker[484] provide a comprehensive review of SDH findings in non-accidental childhood head injury. Traumatic subdural bleeding implies damage to the bridging veins that

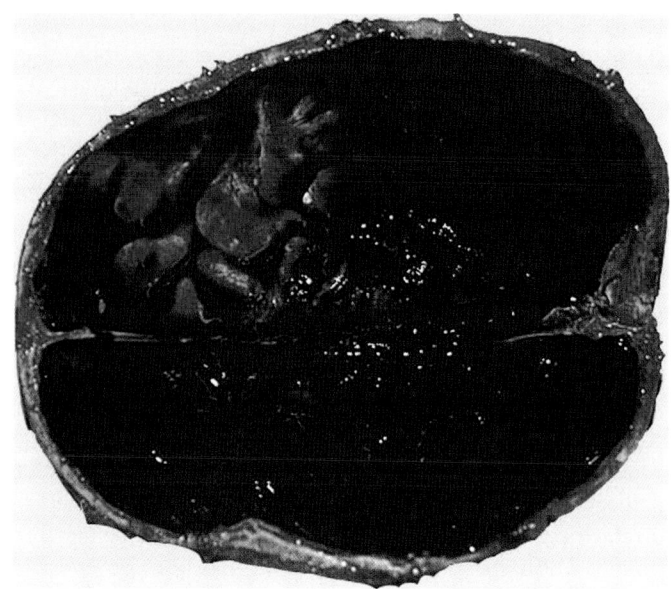

FIGURE 17.50 Subdural hemorrhage in fatal blunt force trauma to the head.

traverse the subdural space. The most frequently involved veins are those draining to the sagittal sinus, and the earliest accumulations are typically interhemispheric. Large extradural (epidural) extracerebral hematomas are uncommon in infants and children with fatal head injuries because of the normal firm adherence of the dura mater to the skull. Subdural hemorrhage in young infants is more typically a thin layer of blood over the hemispheres or within the interhemispheric fissure. Massive space-occupying subdural hemorrhages sufficient to compress the underlying brain substance are less common. Subdural blood is a frequent finding in fatal head injuries in childhood. In the presence of significant space occupying SDH with shift of the midline, vascular impairment can lead to stroke or unilateral cerebral infarction. Traumatic ischemic stroke can also result from extracranial or intracranial arterial dissection.

Acute subdural hematoma, an injury assumed to be less than 3 days old, is a common presenting feature in head trauma in childhood (Fig. 17.51). Subacute subdural is an arbitrarily assigned age between acute and chronic and is usually considered to be 5–10 days of age or more. An acute SDH shows relatively no reactive histologic changes. As the vital reaction proceeds, early changes include leukocytic infiltration, hemosiderin deposits, neovascularization and collagen generation. Onset of reactive changes can vary but early changes may be seen within 24–48 h.

Vinchon et al[533] reports a series of infants under 24 months of age with SDH due to traffic accidents reported on the day of trauma. In 7 of 18 patients, subdural collection was evident on day of trauma, in three of these seven the collection was already hypodense. Three of the 18 patients presented with RHs.

Re-bleeding of subdural hematoma can occur.[535, 536] Radiologic clues for re-bleed of pre-existing SDH are well recognized. An important radiologic finding for diagnosis of re-bleed is the presence of a clear interface of SDH separating an inner hyperdense and outer hypodense SDH.[507]

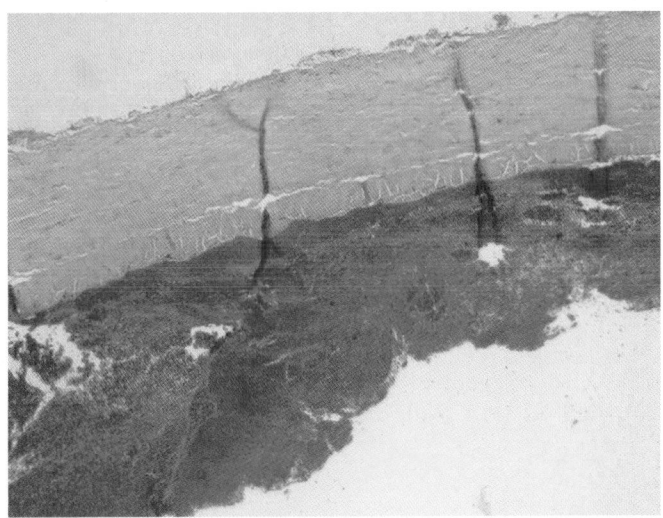

FIGURE 17.51 Acute subdural hemorrhage (× 2.5).

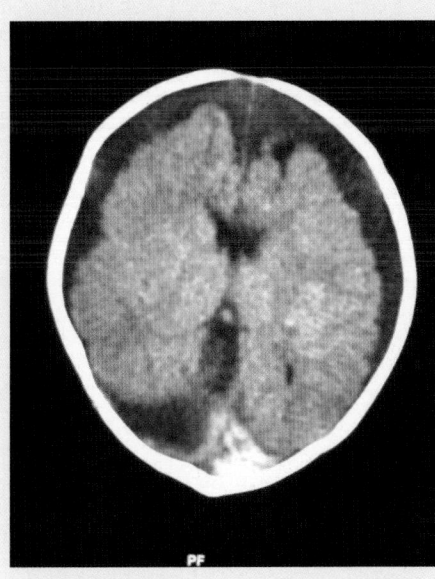

FIGURE 17.52 A 2-month-old infant with a 6 week history of vomiting and lethargy; computed tomography scan showed large supra and infra tentorial subdural hematoma with blood of varying ages.

Radiographic analysis of head trauma and the evolution of injuries can be helpful in forensic analysis. Jaspan et al[537] propose a protocol for neuroimaging in possible non-accidental head injury in childhood. CT scans are the principal tool for identifying the presence of acute or subacute hemorrhage, other collections, edema, skull fractures and scalp injury (Fig. 17.52). MRI scan with spectroscopy, if performed early enough in the clinical course, may be useful in estimating the age of subdural blood and detail parenchymal injuries. Acute and subacute clotted blood (3 h to 7–10 days) may appear high density. Hyperacute 'unclotted hemorrhage' (less than 3 h), very chronic (more than 10 days), and non-hemorrhagic collections (subdural effusions or hygroma) appear hypodense or isodense with CSF. Hyperacute or very acute hematomas are characteristically mixed density subdural hematomas that typically develop under two conditions:

- active bleeding source
- presence of a coagulopathy

Dias et al[458] point out the importance of careful and sequential radiographic analysis of the head injured infant. Vinchon[533, 534] reviews the role of imaging and its potential contribution to timing of injury in a series of traumatic SDH in infants following a motor vehicle accident. Review of the imaging studies with a radiologist experienced in pediatric neuroimaging can be helpful in the forensic analysis.

The diagnosis of SDH does not in and of itself mean an abusive traumatic etiology. Differential diagnoses include:

- accidental trauma
- birth trauma
- coagulopathy
- infection (meningitis)
- congenital metabolic abnormalities
- cortical vein or sinus thrombosis
- minor injury with pre-existing intracranial pathology

Kelly and Hayes[531] reviewed children presenting with SDH and RH over a 10-year period; 41 deemed NAI and 23 accidental. The mortality in the NAI group was higher. Accidental injury determination was directly linked to history of trauma; in contrast many NAI had a vague history.

When subdural hemorrhage is examined at postmortem examination, it is important to document the size, location, extent, and volume and to obtain microscopic sections of dura and clot. Careful examination of all the tissue layers, with appropriate documentation and microscopic sampling, is imperative. The location, size, color, and microscopic appearance of any hemorrhages may provide invaluable information about the nature and mechanism of the injury (Fig. 17.53). It is important to identify and document evidence of previous bleeding in the dura and subdural space. Postmortem diagnostic imaging can be performed and may be an important tool in the forensic analysis and may direct the autopsy toward subtle abnormalities.[538] The author has used postmortem MRI scan in locating upper spinal cord injury in a homicide investigation.

Chronic subdural[539–542] (Fig. 17.54)

Chronic (>10 days) or mixed subdural collections are a relatively common complication of head injury in infancy and are not an uncommon finding on initial scans. Hwang and Kim[541] reviewed infantile head injury with special reference to the development of chronic subdural hematoma.

The histopathology of subdural membranes in infancy and adults are similar. Over time a thick fibroblastic outer layer containing proliferating vascular channels is formed. The thinner inner membrane formed adjacent to the arachnoid has been examined ultrastructurally by Yamashima.[542] Histologic studies have shown that vascularized membranes form around organizing subdural hematomas (Fig. 17.55). Small blood vessels can bleed into the hematoma cavity. Subdural hygromas refers to leakage of CSF from tears in the arachnoid membrane. McLone and Gutierrez[543] have studied the ultrastructure of subdural

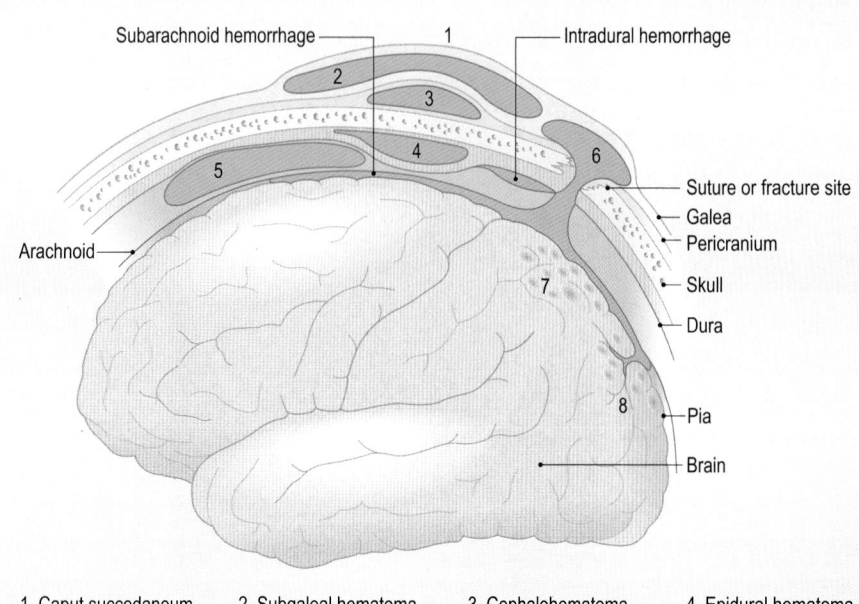

Subarachnoid hemorrhage — 1 — Intradural hemorrhage

Suture or fracture site
Galea
Pericranium
Skull
Dura
Arachnoid →
Pia
Brain

1, Caput succedaneum	2, Subgaleal hematoma	3, Cephalohematoma	4, Epidural hematoma
5, Subdural hematoma	6, Leptomeningeal cyst	7, Cerebral contusion	8, Cerebral laceration

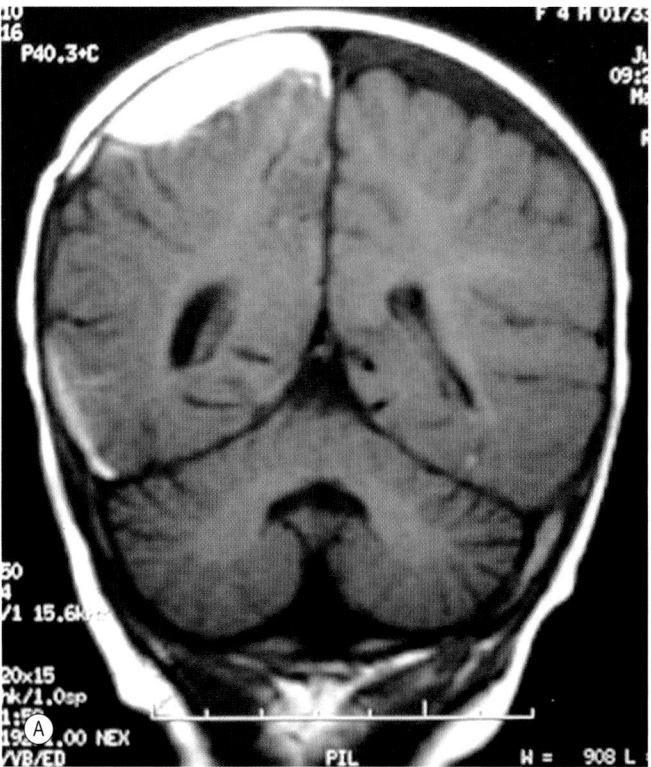

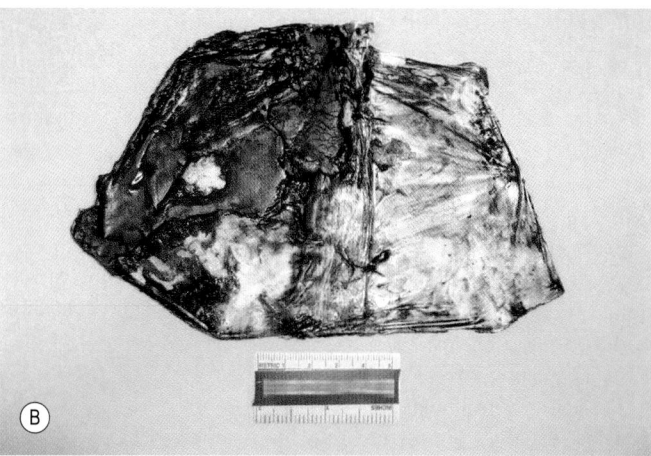

FIGURE 17.54 Chronic subdural. (A) Magnetic resonance imaging of the head demonstrating acute and chronic subdural hemorrhage (B) Dura with adherent subdural blood.

membranes in infants. Capillary fragility within the membranes is one of the major causes of repeated hemorrhage within subdurals and their secondary gradual progression.[540] Leestma's table of histology findings in the development of the dural membrane is useful in assessing the characteristics of vital reaction in the subdural space[530, 544] (Table 17.12).

Complications of chronic subdural hematoma may be the precipitating event in childhood head injury. Clinical signs and symptoms of chronic subdural can be silent despite significant fluid volume. Plunkett[540] reported a series of pediatric chronic SDH; presenting symptoms included macrocephaly, anorexia, lethargy and seizures. Careful analysis of medical records and investigation should document and evaluate failure to thrive, abnormal head growth, and any unexplained signs and symptoms that may have heralded TBI. In the young infant, birth and postpartum records should be evaluated for possible undetected birth injury. In the event of a fatality involving TBI, neuropathology

TABLE 17.12 AGING AND DATING OF HEMATOMAS

Interval	Clot	Dural side	Arachnoid side
24 h	Intact RBCs	Thin layer fibrin	Thin layer fibrin
36 h	Intact RBCs	Early fibroblastic activity	Thin layer fibrin
4 days	Loss of RBC sharp contour and variability of staining	2–4 layers of fibroblasts	Thin layer fibrin
5 days	Loss of RBC sharp contour and variability of staining	3–5 layers of fibroblasts. First siderophages appear at edges	Thin layer fibrin
7–8 days	Laked RBCs, clot liquefies, fibroblasts enter clot	12–14 layers of fibroblasts; neomembrane visible grossly when clot scraped away	Thin layer fibrin
11 days	Broken up into islands by capillaries and fibroblasts and thick strands of fibrin	Fibroblasts migrate around the edges of the clot	Siderophages are visible on arachnoid side
15–17 days	Most original RBCs lysed. Capillary formation obvious	Membrane to dural thickness	Variably thin, earliest complete neomembrane. Clot may be completely enveloped
18–26 days	Clot completely liquefied. Larger vessels permeate	Membrane same thickness as dura. Siderophages in membranes	Membrane up to dural thickness. Siderophages in membranes
27–36 days	Large capillaries	Well-formed membrane	Well-formed membrane
1–3 months	Giant capillaries secondary bleeding and fresh RBCs	Hyalinization of membranes, less cellular, more collagen	Hyalinization of membranes, less cellular, more collagen. Nearly thickness of dura
3–6 months	No original RBCs and only focal rebleeding	Hyalinized neomembrane	Hyalinized neomembrane
> 1 year	No RBCs	Resembles dura	Resembles dura

RBCs, Red blood cells. (From Leestma JE[530], with permission)

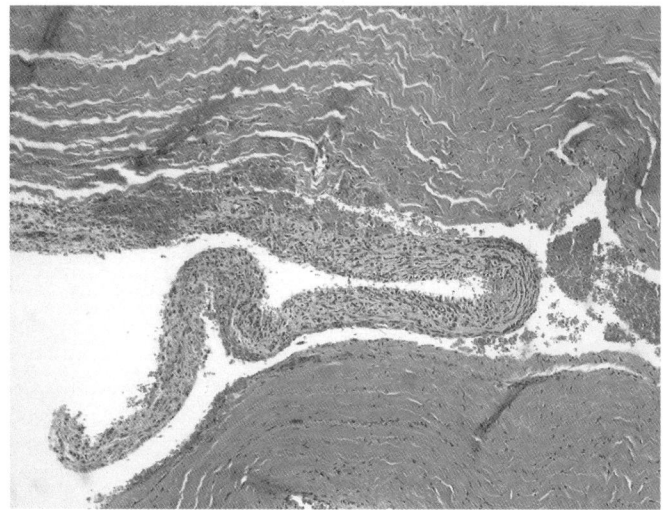

FIGURE 17.55 Neomembrane development on the dura; chronic injury (× 2.5).

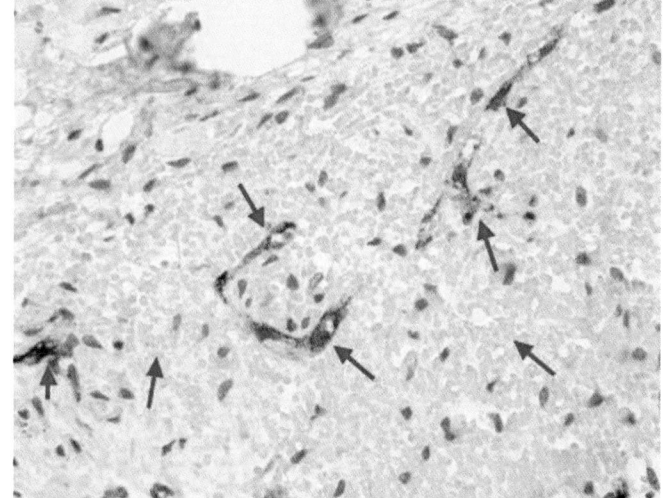

FIGURE 17.56 The factor VIII stain for blood vessels shows brand new delicate blood vessel formation (angiogenesis) within an area of subdural hemorrhage (× 40). (Courtesy of Dr Roscoe Akinson.)

consultation is often of assistance in interpreting the CNS findings (Fig. 17.56).

Hydrocephalus and subdural hemorrhage

The presence of SDH in an infant with hydrocephalus must be interpreted very carefully. The clinical finding of excessive rate of head enlargement in a child less than 2 years is the hallmark of hydrocephalus. Progressive enlargement of the head at a rate greater than predicted for normal growth requires further evaluation. Hydrocephalus is not an unusual condition in infancy especially with increasing survivals with premature infants with intraventricular hemorrhage. Lorch et al[545] reports the prevalence of 'benign' extra axial fluid in infant survivors of intensive care with macrocephaly. This occurrence is associated with increased risk of developmental delay and cerebral palsy. In children born prematurely, onset of symptoms may be delayed for days to weeks.[546]

Papasian and Frim[547] examined the forces necessary to cause SDH in an infant with external hydrocephalus, suggesting increased risk for SDH from minor head trauma. Their findings indicate that the same force caused veins to stretch proportionately more and veins would be more likely to fail with widened extra-axial space.

External hydrocephalus has been associated with subdural hematoma in infancy and the occurrences of the hematomas have been associated with minor trauma.[546–552] Piatt reports a case of a 4-month-old infant presenting seizures found to have SDH, bilateral RH, macrocephaly and external hydrocephalus.[553]

Subarachnoid hemorrhage

The prevalence of SAH in child abuse is unclear, but is commonly seen at autopsy. SAH occurs in 25–75% of head trauma victims and results from a variety of factors, including contusional or white matter tears that extend to the surface, tears of major vessels, and parenchymal injuries that extend to the ventricles. SAH is not in and of itself specific for abuse.

Secondary injuries

Following TBI the damage to the brain from direct disruption of the brain tissues is termed primary brain injury. The ensuing altered hemodynamic respiratory function and cellular derangement is termed secondary injury. TBI results in complex physiologic responses that involve post-traumatic ischemia, energy failure, excitotoxicity, mitochondrial failure, oxidative stress, inflammation and secondary brain swelling, and neuronal death.[554]

Hypoxic ischemic change with **cerebral edema** is one of the most common sequelae in infant TBI, and is more common than in adults. Cerebral edema can be focal or diffuse and is usually associated with diminished gray–white matter differentiation. A significant percentage of fatal head injuries in infants are the result of increased intracranial pressure and secondary hypoxic-ischemic injury. Cerebral edema is a common manifestation of significant head trauma in childhood.

Post-traumatic apnea is associated with radiologic evidence of brain swelling, an early indicator of hypoxic brain damage. Infants who present in coma with apnea and diffuse brain swelling/hypoxic ischemic injury have a high mortality rate. Kemp et al[555] reviews the association of apnea, brain swelling and non-accidental head injury. As the brain swells the cerebral vascular supply can be further compromised by increased intracranial pressure.

Geddes[519, 520] and others have demonstrated that a frequent abnormality in brain-injured infants is hypoxic brain damage. Geddes et al sampled dural membranes in infants less than 5 months of age with severe hypoxic brain injury and found microscopic intradural and subdural blood.

Stroke in childhood denotes the sudden onset of focal neurologic deficit due to interruption of blood flow to a part of the nervous system. Because intracerebral hemorrhage can be the consequence of and not the cause of cerebral infarction, careful analysis for possible cause should be taken. Rivkin and Volpe[556] provide an excellent summary of strokes in childhood. The incidence of stroke in childhood is estimated at 2.5/100 000. Causes of stroke in childhood are different from those in adulthood, but the etiology is not determined in up to 30% of cases. Ischemic injury results from three mechanisms: embolism, thrombosis, or decreased systemic perfusion. Cerebral ischemia is the final pathway leading to brain injury regardless of mechanism. Focal injury can result from pressure extended by blood mass effect as well as hemorrhage related ischemia. Primary SAH can result from hypoxic-ischemic brain insult. In neonates, focal seizures are the most common clinical feature of stroke. In the early period following infarction, the affected cerebral territory may not be well visualized by CT scan. Diffuse weighted MRI is a better method to evaluate infarction in the first hours after the event.

Other secondary injuries that must be considered include metabolic chaos, physiologic instability, brain death, multisystem organ failure, status epilepticus, surgical intervention, prolonged critical care/life support, iatrogenic injury, pneumonia, septicemia, effects of pharmaceuticals.

Neck injuries[557–561]

Spinal injuries are not common in child abuse and children represent 5% or less of spinal injuries. Spinal cord injuries have been reported in child abuse as isolated injuries and as part of a multi-injury spectrum. Zimmerman[562] reviewed the literature regarding abuse-related cervical spine injuries and described children with cervical, thoracic, and lumbar cord injuries many without fracture. Lustrin et al[558] published an extensive review of radiographic anatomy variants and trauma in the pediatric cervical spine. Schwartz et al[563] reviewed pediatric cervical spine injuries sustained in falls from heights of less than 5 feet. The eight children ranged from 9 to 68 months. All eight of the children had clinical evidence of injury on history or physical examination.

Jaffe et al[564] developed a clinical algorithm for early identification and management of cervical spine injury in childhood trauma victims. Atlanto-occipital distraction injuries are the most common neck injuries in children and occur more frequently in children than adults. Associated cranial subdural hematomas have been reported in association with these injuries.[451] Ruge et al[565] found a significantly high proportion of children less than 3 years old with C1–C2 level injury. These injuries are typically caused by hyperextension or flexion injuries to the neck. The occipito-cervical complex (O_c–C_2 complex) functions as a single unit that facilitates movement of the head on the spine. The special vulnerability in this area is related to the absence of substantial stabilizing structures in the

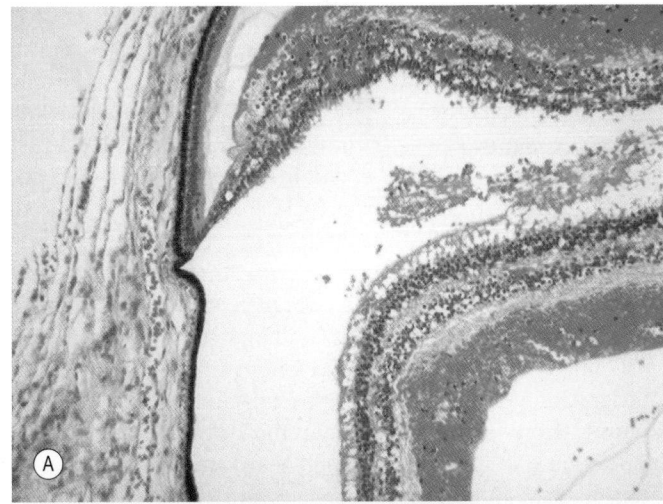

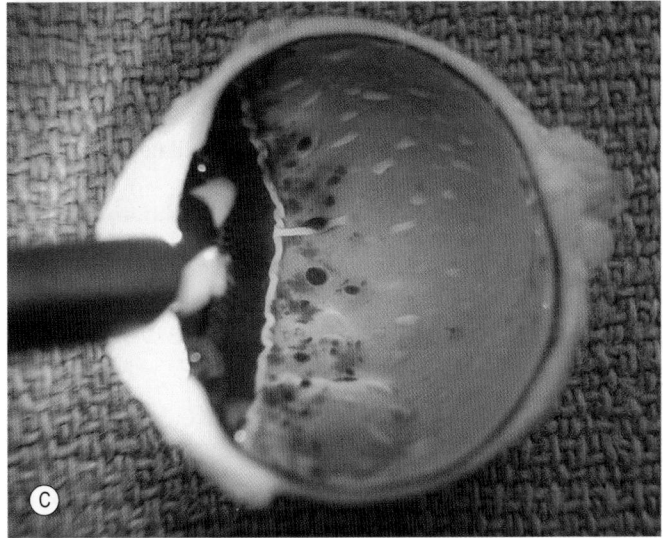

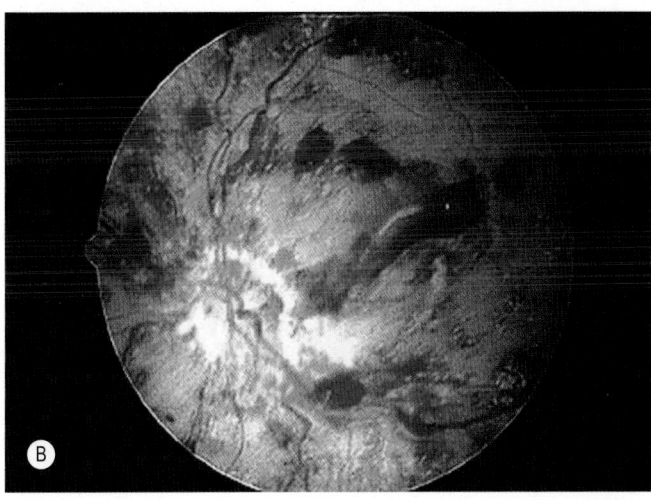

FIGURE 17.57 Retinal hemorrhage. (A) Histological slide showing retinal hemorrhage. (Hematoxylin and eosin; × 2.5.) (B) Retinal hemorrhage demonstrated, funduscopic photography. (C) Peripheral retinal hemorrhages at autopsy.

- vulnerable growth zone at the vertebral growth plate
- shallow cervical facet joints

Retinal hemorrhage[568–570] (Fig. 17.57)

RH is a clinical and pathologic finding that continues to elude clear explanation. The mechanism of occurrence of RH is not well understood and the literature does not suggest that the presence of RH with or without SDH in and of itself is diagnostic of inflicted injury.[571] The association of RH with traumatic brain injury has been considered an important diagnostic adjunct in the diagnosis of the abused infant, however it is also well recognized that RH can occur in a variety of circumstances. These include: retinopathy of prematurity, severe hypertension, external hydrocephalus,[553] carbon monoxide poisoning, meningitis, septicemia, CPR, viral infections, accidental and non-accidental trauma, metabolic disorders, central venous thrombosis, clotting disorders and blood dyscrasias, Terson syndrome, osteogenesis imperfecta and Ehler-Danlos syndrome, and elevated intracranial pressure. Intraretinal hemorrhages are a common finding at birth and typically resolve by 4–6 weeks. The incidence is higher for vacuum assisted deliveries and lowest for cesarean section.[572] RHs and SDH have also been documented in intrapartum stillbirth and cesarean section deliveries. In the absence of premortem retinal folds or retinoschisis, the cause of RH cannot be limited to traumatic injury.

RHs are the result of bleeding within the retina. RHs may be vitreous, pre-retinal, intraretinal or subretinal. They may involve one or more layers of the retina and may be unilateral or bilateral. Superficial nerve fiber intraretinal hemorrhage is often described as flame or splinter shaped; deeper RHs are termed dot or blood hemorrhages. Morphology of the RH is determined by the anatomy of the location of the hemorrhage

area. Diagnosis is typically made by MRI scan since plain radiographs and CT scans frequently do not show these injuries.

SCIWORA (spinal cord injury without radiographic abnormality) is a unique injury to children under 8 years of age. Traumatic myelopathy without demonstrated vertebral injury accounts for many childhood spinal cord injuries (ranging from 13 to 66% in reported cases).[566] Cases have been reported of children suffering traumatic myelopathy falling backwards off a bed, a 3-year old who tripped and fell, a 2-year old who somersaulted off a couch etc.[567] Pang[566] studied 55 children with SCIWORA age 6 months–16 years. Of these 10 had upper cervical, 33 had lower cervical, and 12 had thoracic spinal cord injuries. All but one of the children with severe injuries (22) were less than 8 years old. There are factors relating to the spine in the young child that predispose to SCIWORA:[559]

- ligamentous laxity
- relatively large and heavy heads
- immature cervical musculature
- anterior wedging of vertebral bodies
- underdeveloped uncinate process

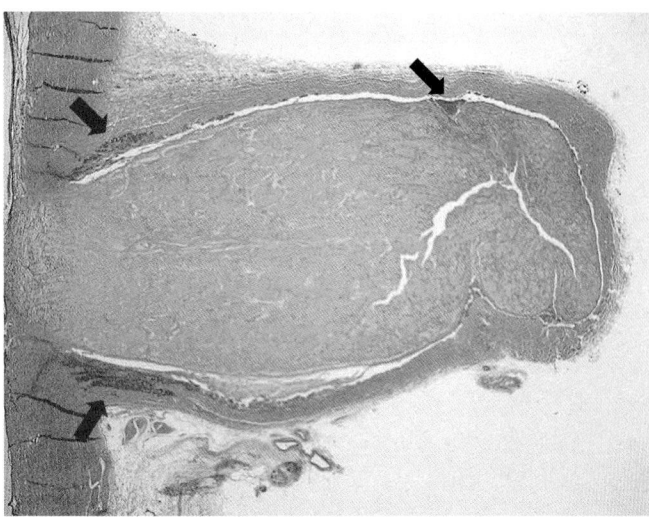

FIGURE 17.58 Optic nerve sheath hemorrhage (× 2.5).

not the cause. (GGW Adams, Forensic science, Evidence based medicine and the 'shaken baby syndrome' presented at AAFS Dallas, February 2004.)

The mechanism of traumatic RH is unknown and the pattern of hemorrhages seen in children can vary widely. Recent case analysis, literature reviews, neuropathologic research, biomechanical applications, and clinical experience have resulted in a reorientation of the original theories regarding the finding of RHs and the 'whiplash shaken infant'. Suggested mechanisms for the pathogenesis of RH in abusive head trauma include:

- increased intrathoracic pressure
  - Purtscher's retinopathy
  - CPR
- increased intracranial pressure
- increased central retinal venous pressure
- hypoxia
- vitreoretinal traction
- fragility of the infant vascular system and susceptibility to abrupt pressure changes

The most common ocular changes in traumatic head injury are SDH of the optic nerve sheath and RH involving all layers of the retina (Fig. 17.58). Most of these hemorrhages clear with time, but macular scarring and vitreous organization as the consequence of child abuse is well recognized. The most common cause of permanent loss of vision in head injured child is irreversible injury to the visual pathways. Gilliland and Luthert[573] review ocular pathology, histopathology and RH specifically, as it relates to suspected non-accidental injury. The paper reviews the current literature, the importance of postmortem examination of the eye with emphasis on documentation of ocular pathology, current controversies, and possible bias regarding interpretation of ocular findings in the brain-injured infant.

RH associated with TBI is predominately located at the far retinal periphery and posterior pole with relative sparing of the equatorial/post equatorial zone. The hemorrhage frequently is confluent and is described as having a 'red velvety' appearance and may contain Roth spots (white centers). RHs are commonly superficial (nerve fiber layer) or severe (all layers) with white centers composed of fibrin-platelet aggregates. Vitreous hemorrhage can be diffuse or localized (subhyaloid – between vitreal and retinal). Perimacular folds and retinoschisis refer to hemorrhage below the internal limiting membrane. Hemorrhagic retinal detachment is hemorrhage beneath the photoreceptor layer. There does appear to be a correlation between the severity of the RH and the severity of the head injury.

Controversies and ambiguities persist in the interpretation of RH. Although the presence of perimacular folds and schisis cavities (from splitting of the retinal layers) is found in association with inflicted childhood neurotrauma, they have also been reported in accidental trauma[574] and Terson syndrome.[575] Presence of retinal iron may reflect pre-existing injury, however iron-positive staining can occur as early as 2 days after injury.

The evaluation of potential abusive head injury typically includes routine ophthalmologic examination with pupillary dilation in suspicious cases. The decision to dilate the pupils in the face of serious head injury must be cautiously made. The description of RH should accurately detail location, type, and degree.

Postmortem examination of the nervous system in cases of head trauma[39]

The examination and documentation of the pattern of injuries in fatal child abuse in infants and children less than 2 years of age must be systematically established. The importance of this principle is obvious but there are few established guidelines for the optimal examination. Judkins et al[39] provides a comprehensive technical communication for the examination of the nervous system in the suspected infant victim of abuse. These guidelines recommend: posterior dissection of the neck and spinal cord; careful examination of scalp (Fig. 17.59), skull, and dura with dural stripping from calvarium and skull base; in situ documentation and examination of corpus callosum; removal of brain and spinal cord in continuity; fixation of brain, spinal cord, blood clots and eyes prior to examination; and proper selection of tissue for histologic examination (Box 17.15). Careful neck dissection should be performed at autopsy to identify soft tissue bleeding especially in the paraspinal muscles. Presence of extradural or spinal epidural blood is not well understood and in the absence of soft tissue injury should be interpreted with caution. Brainstem injury is very unusual and is associated with traumatic disruption of the craniocervical junction. Geddes[504] recommends a mid sagittal cut through the brainstem specifically at the ponto-medullary junction if this injury is suspected.

At postmortem examination in any case of suspected non-accidental trauma, removal of the eyes and histologic examination is commonly performed. Green[576] provides the Sheffield processing schedule for postmortem examination of the eyes.

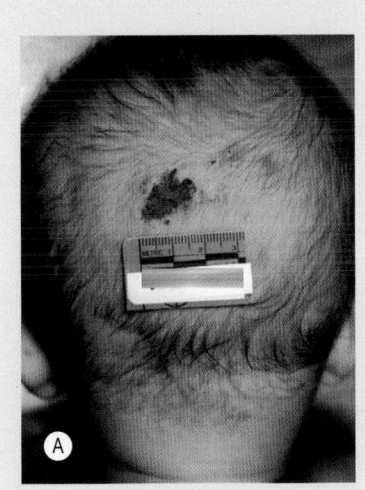 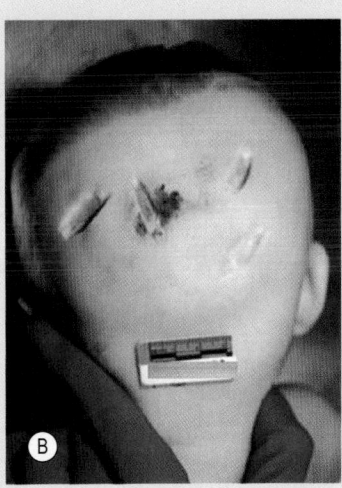 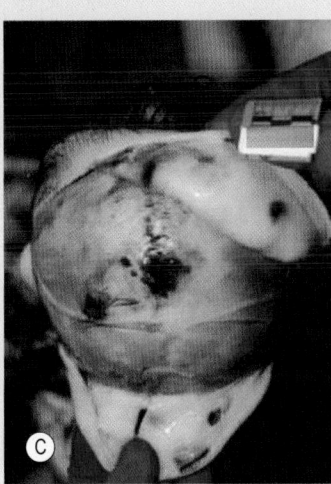

FIGURE 17.59
Documentation of traumatic injuries at postmortem. (A) Occipital scalp abrasion. (B) Injuries sampled after scalp is shaved. (C) Subgaleal contusion at impact site.

BOX 17.15 HEAD TRAUMA: HISTOPATHOLOGY SECTIONS

- Superior frontal gyrus
- Gyrus rectus
- Centrum ovale, anterior
- Corpus callosum through genu, anterior midbody and splenium
- Motor cortex at genu of internal capsule
- Section of palladium, anterior thalamus
- Section of putamen and insular cortex
- Thalamus at posterior limb of internal capsule
- Parietal cortex at posterior limb of internal capsule
- Hippocampus
- Calcarine cortex
- Transverse section, midbrain
- Sagittal section cerebellar vernier
- Dentate nucleus
- Rostral pons
- Mid pons at middle cerebellar peduncle
- Medulla: mid and caudal
- Junction of medulla and spinal cord
- Spinal cord including nerve roots and dura
- Both eyes with optic nerves and dura
- Dura with subdural and/or epidural clots

Parsons and Start[577] review autopsy techniques for identifying ophthalmic pathology. The paper reviews various techniques for dissection, fixation of ocular tissues, and orientation and preparation for histologic examination of tissue sections. The authors recommend suspending the eyes upside down from a corkboard. Orienting the eye using the superior oblique muscle can assist in differentiating right from left at cutting. Two parallel cuts 1 mm below the limbus superiorly and above the limbus inferiorly, processing the entire center block, avoids the disruption of cutting through the lens until the section is into paraffin block. Gilliland and Folberg[578] describe a method for postmortem examination to correlate with antemortem clinical findings by performing a coronal section through the pars plana just anterior to the ora serrata. Decision to preserve both eyes should be made only if vitreous chemistries are not a potential critical diagnostic element. Patrick Lantz and co-workers at Wake Forest University at Winston Salem NC utilize a methodology for postmortem fundus examination and photography to identify presence and distribution of RH prior to removal. This allows for selection of vitreous sampling as well as verification of RH. Amberg and Pollak[579] report a method for endoscopic fundal photography. They describe funduscopic findings in different patterns in craniocerebral trauma, traumatic asphyxia, and decompression sickness.

The patterns of histologic abnormality in fatal TBI in infancy vary widely. Hypoxic axonal injury patterns are frequently identified and only rarely are traumatic axonal abnormalities present. Immunohistochemistry staining for amyloid precursor protein may be helpful to exclude or identify patterns of axonal injury. Interpretation must be correlated with gross findings and neuroanatomy. Interpretation of special stains should be conservative until more is understood about infant postmortem findings. Timing of injury is often a focus of the forensic autopsy and there are several publications detailing clinical findings useful in determining age of injury.[542, 580, 581]

The examining pathologist is responsible for identifying which cases require additional consultation prior to final diagnosis. The complexity and serious consequences involved in criminal charges should suggest consultation with neuroradiology, neuropathology, ophthalmic pathology and/or biomechanical experts when appropriate.

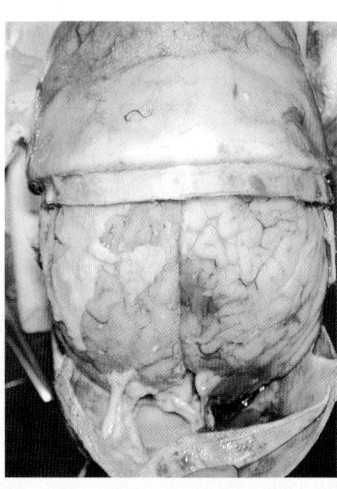

FIGURE 17.60 *Citrobacter* meningitis in 5-week infant.

Mimics[224, 582–586] (Fig. 17.60)

Plunkett, Bandek and Barnes presented an overview of natural conditions that can mimic head trauma in infancy and childhood at the American Society of Neuroradiology in June 2004. These cases included vascular malformations, CNS infection, hemophagocytic lymphohistiocytosis,[587] glutaric acidemia type 1 deficiency,[588] and cortical venous thrombosis/sagittal sinus thrombosis. Although uncommon in childhood, cerebral vein and sinus thrombosis can be a lethal complication of infection, vascular injury following invasive procedure, trauma, dehydration, or prothrombotic conditions.[589–591] Rutty et al[592] report a case of fatal late onset hemorrhagic disease of the newborn (vitamin K deficiency) in a 9-week-old infant initially mistaken for child abuse. Conditions such as von Willebrand disease have resulted in intracranial hemorrhage. Infantile scurvy, Barlow disease (vitamin C deficiency), has been recognized for many decades as a cause of RH, SDH, and bone abnormalities.

False accusation of child abuse can have horrendous consequences for the families involved. The final diagnosis of child abuse rests on a combination of physical findings, history, and investigation of the circumstances of injury or death. The decision regarding whether or not the history makes sense must be made in a context of neutral interpretation of the medical facts as well as knowledge and experience. Knowledge of patterns of abuse, diseases, or conditions that simulate abuse[593–621] and of postmortem changes is important, and accurate interpretation should be left to those individuals with sufficient experience and training to do so. All categories of injury that have been attributed to child abuse have reported mimics or 'pseudoabuse'. These include bone, cutaneous, head, and sexual variants. Extensive reviews of mimics of child abuse are available.[582, 584] The process of evaluation and diagnosis of childhood diseases and conditions includes the careful formation of differential diagnosis. When the differential includes child abuse, investigation must reasonably exclude conditions that can be confused with inflicted injury (Box 17.16).

BOX 17.16 HEAD TRAUMA: MIMICS[584–586]

- Accidental trauma
- Non-traumatic coma
- Birth related injuries
- Spectrum of stroke in infancy
- Complications of prematurity
- Cortical venous thrombosis
- Pre-existing conditions or abnormalities unknown such as the foreign born adoptee
- Anoxia
- Certain nutritional or metabolic disorders – glutaric aciduria type 1, osteogenesis imperfecta, vitamin C deficiency (scurvy)
- Benign external hydrocephaly
- Coagulation disorders, e.g. von Willebrand disease
- Vascular malformations
- Infections
- Hemophagocytic lymphohistiocytosis
- Complications of hypernatremic dehydration
- Complications of hyponatremic dehydration

Whiplash shaken infant (shaken baby syndrome, shaken impact)

In 1974, John Caffey described a form of inflicted traumatic brain injury that he hypothesized involved vigorous manual shaking of infants by the extremities or shoulders, with 'whiplash-induced' intracranial and intraocular bleeding but without external signs of head trauma. The association of **subdural hematoma, retinal hemorrhage, and increased intracranial pressure** has been a diagnostic enigma since it was first described. Because the events are unwitnessed except by the perpetrator, the mechanism of injury has been the source of much speculation. Rotational forces, hyperextension–flexion, angular acceleration–deceleration injury with tearing of the bridging veins have been included as potential mechanisms.

Children presenting with probable inflicted head injury in the late 1980s and 1990s were frequently given the diagnosis of whiplash shaken infant or shaken baby syndrome (SBS). Duhaime and colleagues[622] reviewed 48 cases suspicious for the whiplash shaken infant syndrome seen at the Children's Hospital of Philadelphia between 1978 and 1985. Autopsy findings in 13 patients were analyzed, and findings consistent with blunt impact injury were seen in all 13. This discovery led to a model of injury from which the authors concluded that shaking alone, in an otherwise healthy infant, is unlikely to cause this pattern of injury. At that time, injuries were thought to be caused by a combination of impact with acceleration–deceleration injury and the term shaken impact syndrome was adopted. Over the last 5 years substantial concerns regarding the validity of some of the theories and beliefs regarding shaken baby syndrome have arisen.[136, 624–626] The nature of these concerns include:

- timing of injury and onset of symptoms in the brain-injured infant
- radiographic and pathologic diagnostic criteria for traumatic axonal injury
- biomechanical potential of severe shaking to produce RH and SDH
- interpretation of RH and its association with SBS
- identification and interpretation of pre-existing conditions and injuries
- theoretical mechanisms of injury in accidental and abusive head trauma
- forensic analysis, opinions, terminology, and established scientific evidence and their role in expert testimony regarding SBS and abusive head trauma
- standardization of autopsy criteria for documentation and evaluation of the CNS in brain-injured infants

Leestma[626] conducted a comprehensive review of the English language literature of brain injury in admittedly shaken infants. Out of 324 reports of child abuse published between 1969 and 2001 with detailed case information, 54 cases were identified in which someone admitted shaking the infant. Only 11 of 54 of admittedly shaken infants showed no sign of impact. Leestma concludes that the very small number of identified cases does not allow for valid statistical verification of the common assumptions associated with SBS.

Historical questions and controversies

Significant controversy and debate has emerged regarding the potential for injury in household falls and accidents (Table 17.11).[627] There has been considerable change in the approach to childhood injuries in the past 5–10 years. Awareness of the role of inflicted trauma has added significant knowledge and resources to the investigation of serious injuries in infancy. Included in these resources are increasing contributions from the field of biomechanics.[87, 628, 629]

Ommaya et al[507] identified several ambiguous or unsupported assumptions regarding adult and pediatric head injury that appear in the literature. These assumptions are often used as the basis for a diagnosis of abuse without clinical validation or supporting biomechanical analysis:

- Low falls (< 4 feet) are not likely to cause skull fractures, acute SDH or brain injury in infants.
- Traumatic retinoschisis in NAI is caused directly by repetitive shaking.
- Acute and relatively asymptomatic SDH cannot result in a lucid interval in a patient who later dies.
- Time for onset of signs and symptoms of severe traumatic brain injury is always brief.

It is imperative that the forensic pathologist analyzing cases of fatal head injury in the child understand that these assumptions are not supported by the biomechanical literature and evidence.

Biomechanical studies have demonstrated that the head accelerations generated by shaking are below the thresholds for traumatic diffuse axonal injury, SDH, hematoma, and even concussion. If one could shake an infant or child vigorously enough to cause such traumatic brain injury, significant injury would also be found in the neck region, including the craniocervical junction. At this time the current literature and biomechanical studies have not verified that shaking can generate forces that exceed injury thresholds for traumatic brain injury in infants and children.[507, 622, 630]

Approach to head trauma – accident vs inflicted injury

There are no pathognomonic clinical features that when viewed in isolation allow for distinction between accident or non-accidental traumatic brain injury in infancy.[631] Therefore diagnosis is based on evaluation of background information, clinical history, clinical course to recovery or death, and awareness of the variability of presenting signs and symptoms (Boxes 17.17 and 17.18) Every case requires open unbiased analysis and opinions must be based on evidence. Biomechanical analysis may be necessary before diagnosis of inflicted injury is made.

The author's experience in this area provides the following recommendations and cautions (Box 17.19):

- Most simple falls result in little or no injury, but some falls do cause injury.[136, 632]
- Infant skulls and brains are different than older children and the effect of biomechanical principles must be understood and applied to case analysis.[89]
- Pre-existing injuries affect nature and character of presenting signs and symptoms of head injury.

BOX 17.17 HEAD TRAUMA: PRESENTATION/SIGNS AND SYMPTOMS

- Undetected/unnoticed/unknown
- History of nausea and vomiting, 'flu-like syndrome', gastroenteritis
- History of failure to thrive – sudden onset, chronic
- Evidence of abnormal head growth
- Evidence of abnormal development or setbacks
- Presentation with seizures
- Presentation with signs and symptoms of acute injury (< 72 h)
- Presentation with signs and symptoms of hyperacute injury, 'lights out injury'
- Presentation with sudden apnea, following hours/days of progressive deterioration
- Found deceased
- Any of the above with evidence of multiple injuries

- Evidence of hypoxia: acid–base abnormalities
- Evidence of hyper- or hyponatremia
- Evidence of growth failure, acute or chronic
- Evidence of dehydration
- Evidence of coagulopathy
- Evidence of multisystem organ failure

- The forensic pathologist should participate in a comprehensive analysis of medical, clinical and investigative evidence in any case of suspected fatal abusive head trauma
- Inflicted injuries must be considered and investigated in any child presenting with brain and or spinal cord injury
- Understanding of biomechanical principles is necessary before rendering opinion regarding feasibility or non-feasibility of accidental injuries
- The role of the pathologist is to guide a complete and unbiased investigation prior to determining manner of death
- Timing of injury requires a complex forensic analysis and is unique for each case
- Final diagnoses may require significant time and special consultation to complete
- The role of 'pre-existing' or co-existing conditions with head trauma in infancy is not routinely considered in literature on shaken baby syndrome (SBS)
- Acute subdural, subarachnoid hemorrhage, cerebral edema and retinal hemorrhages are very common in apparently abusive traumatic head injuries
- The infant skull is uniquely vulnerable to deforming impact. Impact appears to be the defining variable
- Impacts may be more difficult to detect in very young babies
- Delays can occur between injury and onset of symptoms
- The pathogenesis or mechanism of injury in traumatic retinal hemorrhage is not well understood
- Possible 'true' shaken baby cases are uncommon and may reflect injury to brainstem
- Despite the physical resilience of infants and children falls can seriously injure and kill
- Young children are especially vulnerable to upper cervical spinal cord injuries without evidence of radiographic abnormality, but are rare in isolation
- Unattended young infants can and have been seriously injured by other children
- The prevailing views of SBS and its causality remain controversial

- Incomplete examination can result in misdiagnosis or misinterpretation of the findings.
- Premature judgment prior to complete forensic analysis can compound the tragedy of childhood injury and death.
- Difference of expert opinion should be collegial and must provide an opportunity for improvement in knowledge.

Plunkett[632] reviewed 18 fall-related fatalities in the US Consumer Product Safety Data Base, 1988–1999. Falls were 0.6–3 m in children aged from 12 months to 13 years. His conclusions include:

- Every fall is a complex event and there should be a biomechanical analysis if the injury seems inconsistent with the story.
- RH can occur in the presence of increased intracranial pressure or venous obstruction.
- Traumatic axonal injury is unlikely to occur from a low-velocity impact.
- Cerebral vascular thrombosis or dissection must be considered with delayed deterioration and especially in the presence of cerebral infarct or unusually distributed cerebral edema.
- A fall from less than 3 m can cause fatal head injury.

There is no question that the majority of innocuous falls do not produce serious injury in otherwise healthy children.[633–635] However, falls can and do cause serious injuries as is well documented in the literature pertaining to playground injures.[135] In the obviously abused child, the history of a fall must raise suspicion and trigger an investigation. However, in the circumstance of a reported fall, the biomechanics, injury pattern, and other variables must be considered before determination of inflicted injury is considered.

Neonaticide, infanticide, abandoned newborn, and stillbirth[636–645]

The history of infanticide/neonaticide traces back to ancient times and is a fascinating reflection of cultural attitudes toward gender and the value of the child in society.[646, 647] Stillbirth is defined as the death of an infant, at a legally specified gestational age (typically 28 weeks) that after complete delivery from the mother's body does not breathe or show signs of life. The World Health Organization defines stillbirth as death of a fetus before complete expulsion or extraction from the mother, irrespective of the gestational age.[643] Neonaticide is defined as the killing of a newly born infant (less than 24 h of life) following live birth. The neonatal period extends for the first 30 days, but for these cases the term is applied to babies killed at birth or shortly thereafter.

Between 1979 and 1990 the author participated in the investigation of over 20 cases of abandoned newborns from the immediate vicinity of Minnesota and Wisconsin. These cases demonstrate some striking similarities (Box 17.20). In the subsequent years cases from across the country have been included in the series. Remarkable similarities in maternal characteristics continue to be observed.

BOX 17.20 ABANDONED INFANT COMMON FEATURES IN MOTHERS

Immature mother, often passive affect

Relatively inexperienced sexually; promiscuity rare

Average intelligence

None deny understanding of basic sex education principles

Many have completed school courses including conception, birth process, and parent responsibilities

Mother frequently still lives with parents

No apparent chemical dependency

Apparently 'successful' in concealing pregnancy from friends, often boyfriend and parents

Pregnancy interpreted as weight gain

All initially claim child was born dead; appeared dead

None had made any arrangements for birth

Majority admitted they knew they were pregnant

None called for assistance during labor and delivery

Child is frequently delivered into high-risk circumstance/location

All concealed infant's body and placenta

Majority obtained postpartum medical care

History or presence of mental health problems; depression

Assessment

The killing of a newborn by its mother is a very special problem for the forensic and pediatric pathologist, and unfortunately an all too frequent one[648-650] (see checklist in appendix). The problems facing the forensic pathologist in cases of abandoned newborns are unique and require understanding of the complexities of perinatal and placental pathology as well as the forensic issues specific to cases of this nature. The pathologic findings in these infants are usually non-specific especially if cause and time of death are uncertain. The forensic pathologist must address numerous questions when analyzing cases of potential infanticide:

- Are there recognized risks for infant morbidity and mortality present pre partum?
- Could this pre- or peripartum condition(s) contribute to the death of this infant?
- Was the fetus known to be developing normally by examination?
- Was the infant viable?
- Was the infant born alive?
- Is a cause of death evident?

Not all newborn infants found dead, even in highly suspicious or concealed circumstances, are victims of infanticide. The incidence of stillbirth, even in developed countries is estimated at 1 in 200 pregnancies and, as such, is over five times more common than SIDS. Among the known risks of stillbirth are poor obstetric history, advanced gestational age, nulliparity, smoking and obesity.[645] More than 50% of all stillbirths despite complete placental examination and autopsy remain unexplained. Determination of live birth or stillbirth may not be possible if there are no independent witnesses. Stillbirth cannot be excluded in the majority of cases.

Pregnancy outcomes require that complex inter-related maternal–fetal–placental systems culminate successfully at the time of birth. Some of these factors include:

- successful and healthy maturation of infant to term
- sufficient health of the mother to support the pregnancy to term
- adequacy of the placenta to support appropriate growth and development of infant to term
- adequacy of the placenta to support the fetus through labor and delivery
- absence of significant serious life-threatening stress to infant during labor and delivery
- absence of life-threatening or mortal anomalies in the infant
- absence of serious birth injuries
- delivery of the infant into a clinically safe environment
- evidence or proof of life or survival following labor and delivery

A number of key issues must be considered when assessing cases of found or abandoned infants:

- identification of the infant
- gestational age
- infant growth and development
- placental exam and findings
- viability
- determination of live birth
- presence of intrauterine stress
- presence of natural disease or anomalies
- trauma – birth, inflicted or post mortem
- cause of death, mechanism of death
- maternal factors and health
- location and circumstance of concealing body
- presence or absence of postmortem change

In evaluating these cases, a determination of viability must be made. Outside of an intensive care unit setting, this is usually felt to be approximately 28 weeks' gestation. After viability is established, the consideration of factors in the determination of live birth must be made. This is a multifactorial determination. If determination of live birth is made, a cause of death must be assigned.

The challenge of establishing 'live birth' is a factor unique to the evaluation of the abandoned infant. 'Live birth' is a legal consideration and the definition can vary by jurisdiction or country. An autopsy cannot determine whether the heart was beating after delivery. Robinson and Lucas[653] defined live birth as a child that has breathed with its own lungs and established independent circulation. Practically this implies aeration of the lungs with first breath(s) and a heartbeat. Findings considered proof of life are:

- witnessed live birth
- food or extrauterine material in the stomach
- inflammatory changes (vital reaction) at the umbilical stump
- environmental or trace evidence that verifies survival after expulsion

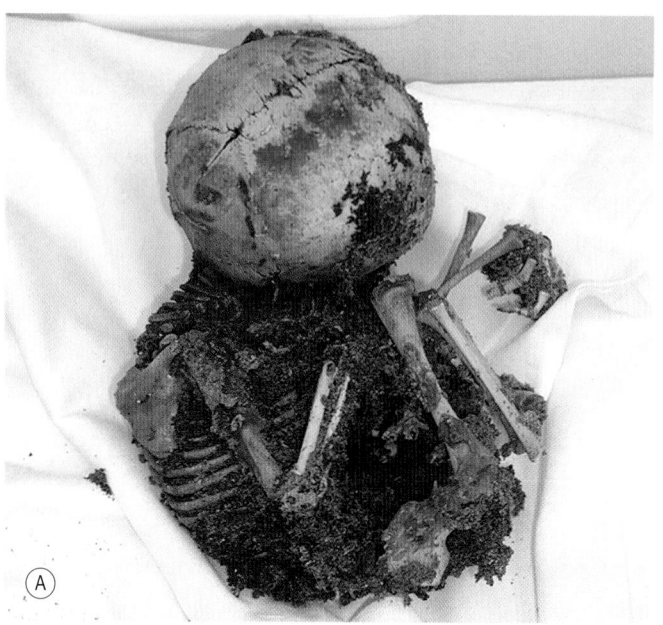

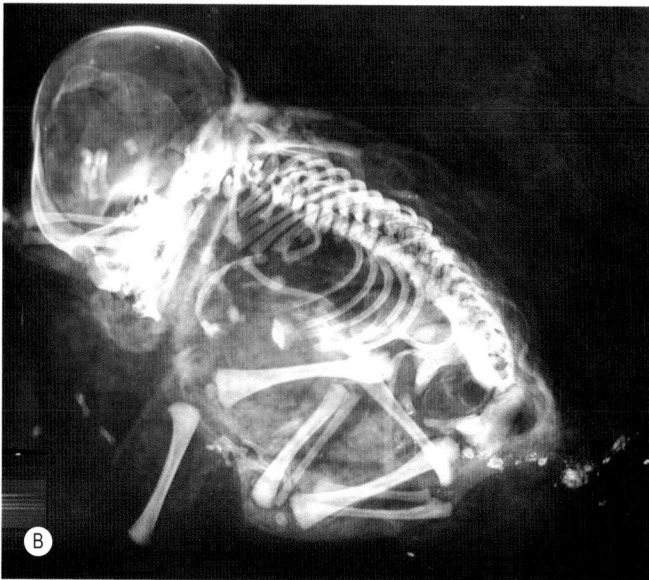

FIGURE 17.61 Infanticide/abandoned baby. (A) Skeletal remains. (B) Radiograph.

Pulmonary interstitial emphysema has been suggested as an indicator of live birth, but this author has not found this determination to be helpful.[653] In some circumstances the appearance of the body, distribution of livor, position of rigor, skin color, and trace evidence suggest that the infant was live-born. This aspect of the examination may also provide evidence to support or deny the mother's story.

Investigation

Even though determination of live birth and viability will be performed at the autopsy table, the scene of every abandoned infant case must be treated as a homicide. It is important to have a crime lab process the scene and videotape and photograph the scene. Careful evaluation and documentation of circumstances that could have caused postmortem injury should be noted. If the scene is out of doors, every effort must be made to attempt to find where the actual delivery occurred so that this site can also be treated as part of the crime scene.

Different communities have reflected different methods of disposal of abandoned infants. In the USA abandoned newborns are frequently placed in plastic bags somewhere in the residence, in Japan coin-operated railway lockers are common. Search warrants may be necessary to retain the rest of the garbage that is within a dumpster or dump site. This author investigated three infants in varying stages of decomposition that had been packaged and moved with the mother over a 30-year period from residence to residence (Fig. 17.61).

Forensic investigation of these cases necessitates careful documentation and laboratory analysis to confirm identity/maternity, documentation of evidence to establish live birth, verification of viability, and, when possible, determination of cause of death. Pathologists and pediatric pathologists are frequently asked to participate in the evaluation and medicolegal action in these cases of abandoned infants. Knowledge of and experience with all the important factors in these cases is requisite to prevent inappropriate prosecution, or failure of appropriate prosecution because of unnecessary controversy or misinterpretation of evidence.

Extensive clinical information should be obtained including prenatal records if available. Depending upon the age of the mother, school records may be pertinent; training in CPR, and IQ tests may be important. Any records regarding family difficulties and/or problems also need to be obtained. An examination by an obstetrician/gynecologist should be performed on the mother. As is the routine in any homicide investigation, interview with witnesses is a critical element in the case analysis. The individual responsible for interviewing mother needs to work closely with the investigating pathologist to ensure complete and accurate fact finding.

Autopsy

These cases should be treated as potential homicides and a forensic pathologist should perform the autopsy. Full body radiographs and extensive photographs should be obtained, documenting any injuries and criteria for gestational age estimation. Multiple measurements, including crown–heel length, occipital–frontal circumference, nipple line circumference, umbilical line circumference, and foot length should be obtained. Body weight on a reliable scale should be obtained. Markers of maturity should be assessed such as presence of lanugo, distribution of vernix caseosa, nipple bud development, skin development, ear cartilage development, external genitalia

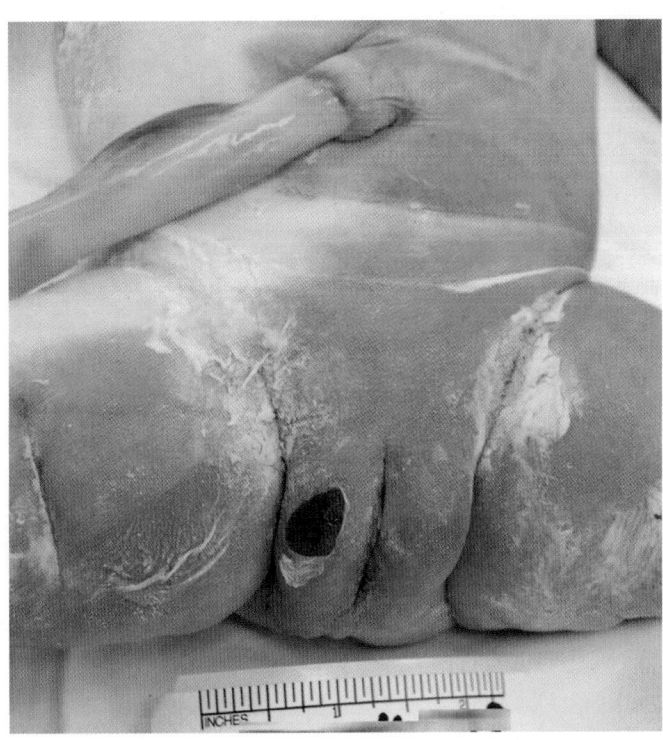

FIGURE 17.62 Abandoned infant. Skin slippage in early decomposition.

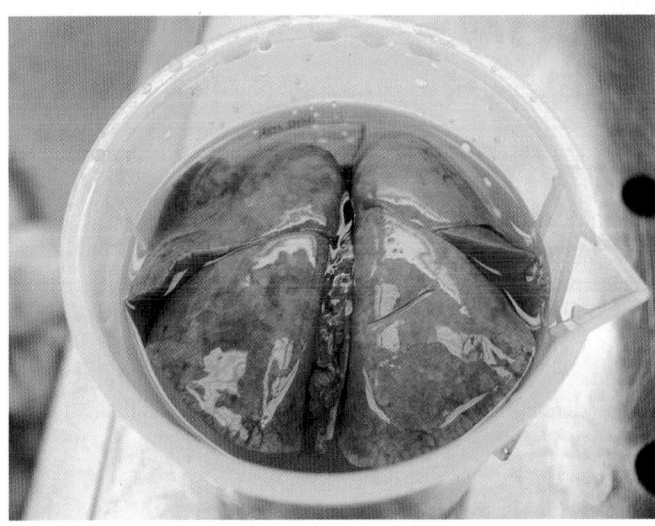

FIGURE 17.63 Lung block float test.

development, fingernail and toenail length, creases on the plantar surfaces of the feet, and general body appearance. Assessment of intrauterine growth and development must be performed.

The placenta, membranes, and umbilical cord should be examined. Aggressive efforts must be made to obtain the placenta for examination for placental abnormalities reflecting abnormal placentation, umbilical cord and fetal membranes, chronic placental insufficiency, passage of meconium in utero, and chorioamnionitis. A section should be obtained at the junction of the umbilical cord with the abdominal wall. A second section of umbilical cord should be obtained distal to the abdominal wall. These should be examined microscopically for the presence or absence of funisitis and also for a vital reaction.

Any evidence of congenital anomalies should be detailed. The patency of the choanal passages should be checked. The oral airway should be examined for evidence of obstruction. Signs of distress should be evaluated. These include intrathoracic petechiae, intra-alveolar hemorrhage and aspirated amniotic debris. Evidence of meconium staining should be noted. Evidence of post-birth passage of meconium should also be looked for. Presence or absence of rigor mortis and livor mortis should be assessed. Presence of postmortem decomposition or maceration should be detailed and documented (Fig. 17.62). The internal examination should include assessment for congenital malformations, injuries, and evidence of infection.

Gastric contents should be carefully evaluated. The presence of foreign material may confirm live birth. The presence or absence of air within the GI tract should be noted.

The gross appearance of the lungs should be documented, noting atelectasis, partial atelectasis, or inflated lungs. Material present within the airway should be examined. Swammerdam suggested in 1667 that fetal lungs will float on water after respiration has taken place. The 'float test' to assess aeration was first applied to a case of suspected infanticide by Johann Scheyer in 1683. The lungs, trachea and bronchi, and heart should be removed en bloc and placed in water or formalin. If the tissue floats (provided that putrefaction and a history of CPR are absent), the test is positive (Fig. 17.63). The float test is not a reliable indicator of independent breaths and thus cannot be interpreted as proof-of-life. Air can be taken into the GI tract and lungs prior to delivery. Each lung should be tested separately as well as sections from each lobe. Section of liver should also be 'floated' as a control to assist in verifying absence of significant postmortem bacterial gas. Any evidence of postmortem decomposition negates the interpretation of the float test. The gross and microscopic aeration pattern must be carefully examined and documented. A radiographic pulmonary and intestinal gas pattern is part of the standard autopsy in these patients, but neither is diagnostic. Pulmonary edema foam and middle ear aeration are findings to be considered when appropriate.

The presence or absence of head trauma should be detailed. The presence or absence of subgaleal hemorrhage and periventricular hemorrhage, recent or remote, should be noted (subgaleal hemorrhage may be seen in stillborn deliveries).

A complete microscopic examination should be performed. Special attention should be given to pulmonary histology with notation of expansion pattern, aspiration of amniotic contents, presence of intrauterine infection, pulmonary hemorrhage, postmortem gas pattern, and relative degree of alveolar expansion verses aeration of terminal and respiratory bronchioles. Specimen should be obtained for toxicologic analysis and DNA testing. Microbiologic cultures, if appropriate, should be obtained. Hair samples should be obtained.

The documentation of an overt act against the infant with obvious cause of death is the exception in the abandoned infant. Instances of neglect, or 'acts of omission', specifically 'failure to rescue' such that the infant could not survive are more frequently the case. This includes postural/asphyxial and hypothermic conditions of birth into a toilet,[653, 654] failure to properly secure the umbilical stump, and lack of availability of life support in an unattended delivery. Marks, abrasions, focal hemorrhage may take place during the extraction process and may not indicate inflicted injury. The infant's body can also be damaged after death especially if moved. Careful case investigations have documented the cause of death as exposure (overt act) when the evidence supports the abandonment of the child while still alive. Care should be exercised in interpreting facial petechiae in the newborn as evidence of inflicted asphyxia. Facial petechiae are a common/normal finding in newborns. Precipitous delivery is reportedly common in these cases and places the infant at risk for intracranial trauma/hemorrhage.

Gestationally non-viable infants can be born alive in unattended circumstances, and frequently are. The maturity of the infant is the primary factor in assessing viability, often defined at 28 weeks' postconceptual age. Careful, complete, and specialized pathologic examination should be performed in all cases when the circumstances and manner of death are unclear. In some jurisdictions, all infant deaths at more than 20 weeks' gestation unattended by a physician must be reported to the medical examiner.

The presence of natural disease that may have interfered with the infant's ability to sustain extrauterine existence, the presence of signs of intrapartum stress or asphyxia, or serious complicating placental abnormalities must be clearly identified. The assessment of intrauterine growth and development must be performed by an experienced pathologist to render an opinion of appropriateness for gestational age, evidence of abnormal presentation during delivery, and pertinent placental factors.[655] Pediatric and/or perinatal pathologist can be important resources in the assessment of these cases.

The obvious question in these cases is the why. Spinelli[639] reviews 16 cases of neonaticide with psychiatric evaluation of the mothers. She reports striking similarities among many of the women evaluated. The common findings include depersonalization, dissociative hallucinations and intermittent amnesia at delivery. Each of the women showed passive affect and child-like demeanor.

Sexual abuse in infancy and childhood[582, 656–659]

The incidence of childhood sexual abuse is not precisely known but is estimated to be 100 000–500 000 cases per year, representing 10–20% of confirmed cases of child abuse. As awareness of the problem and regional resources to deal with this multifaceted problem develop, the role of the hospital

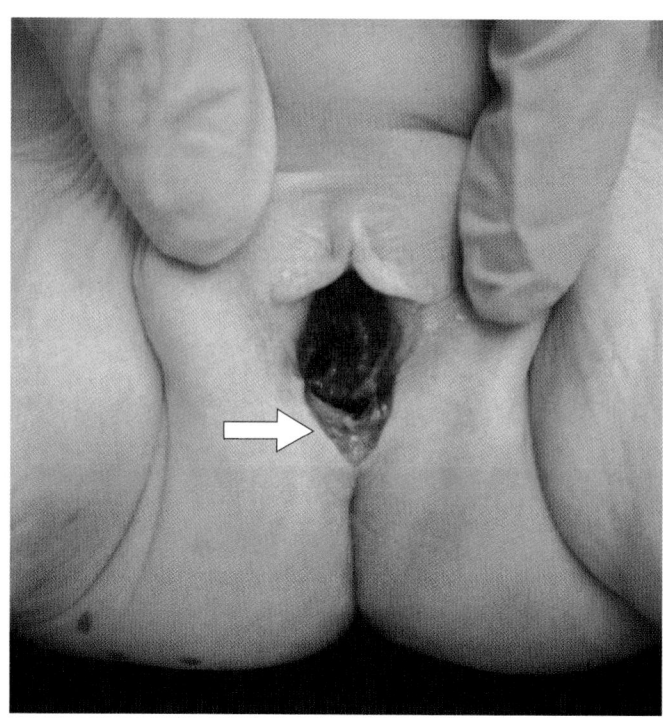

FIGURE 17.64 Sexual trauma. Healing perineal laceration following penile penetration in a 5-month infant.

pathologist and pediatric pathologist will certainly expand to include expertise in this area. The pathology of child sexual abuse, physical diagnosis, laboratory diagnosis, and microbiologic analysis are beyond the scope of this chapter. Any individual involved in evaluating childhood deaths or who has laboratory responsibilities when victims of suspected abuse are evaluated should be familiar with basic pathologic findings and documentation techniques, as well as assault examination laboratory procedures and protocols.

Medical evidence of sexual misuse can be divided into three main categories: physical trauma, evidence of ejaculate, and sexually transmitted disease. For the examining clinician or pathologist the investigation and diagnosis of 'sexual assault' in the young infant is less problematic than in the toddler and older child. In the infant the diagnosis is dictated by the medical evidence (Fig. 17.64).

There is remarkable paucity of scientific literature regarding sexual injury and genital anatomy in the infant. Berenson[660] has described the appearance of the newborn hymen and determined that lateral and ventral clefts, tags, and intravaginal ridges were a normal finding. She followed up her initial observations with a longitudinal study to evaluate changes in hymenal morphology over the first year of life.[661] Annular hymen was the most common configuration in the newborn and at 1 year. Crescentic hymen was not observed in newborns. Inferior clefts between 4 and 8 o'clock were not seen at birth or 1 year. Change in configuration was observed over time in 24 of 55 infants. The most striking finding was the decrease in amount of hymenal tissue over time. Additional observations included the occurrence of labial adhesions, especially with history of candida infection. Berenson et al[662, 663] has published on the evaluation and interpretation in prepubertal girls. They utilized a method for photographing hymenal morphology that uses grid photography and standardized magnification and focal lengths.[664] This kind of documentation is the exception, and in most cases the medical evidence is inadequate for evaluation. McCann and associates at UC. Davis[660–669] and Myhre et al[668, 669] in Norway have contributed extensively to the body of knowledge regarding the wide variations of normal in perianal and genital findings in childhood. In young infants still influenced by maternal estrogen the hymen may appear thicker and has been described with a 'waxy' appearance. When the hormonal influences wanes, the hymen becomes very thin, the hymenal orifice smooth and translucent and sensitive to touch. The mucous membranes of the vagina are thin, friable and demonstrate decreased resistance to trauma and infection.

Evaluating and characterizing the presence or absence of anogenital trauma should utilize basic principles of clinical description. This includes using scientifically applicable terminology, understanding of normal anatomy and variations, understanding of the body's response to injury, understanding vital reaction, basic histology and pathology, understanding the nature, character and causation of anogenital trauma in infancy, and understanding the effects of trauma on tissue. Description or characterization of injuries or abnormalities to the genitals should reflect the same pathologic terminology applied to injuries in other parts of the body: laceration, contusion, abrasion, erythema, edema, scar tissue, etc.

Tissues in the anogenital area of the infant in diaper can rapidly become irritated by fecal material, diaper rash, infantile candidiasis, etc. Soiling following a bout of gastroenteritis can leave infant tissue more fragile and inflamed. Venous congestion, hemorrhoids and other sequelae of chronic constipation can easily be confused with trauma if a complete history is not available. Siegfried and Frasier[670] review anogenital skin diseases in childhood and emphasize the spectrum of disorders in the differential diagnosis. Concerns should be raised any time there is presence of pathologic discharge, bleeding in the diaper, evidence of frank anogenital trauma of any nature in the infant.

Unfortunately the young infant can and is the victim of devastating sexual injury and the tissue damage can be massive. More frequently than not, the infant with serious penetrating sexual injuries will have serious additional injuries to the torso or head and neck.

Postmortem evaluation of the infant with possible sexual misuse requires careful dissection (Fig. 17.65) and documentation of external and internal trauma. Examination of the tissue planes in a specimen that includes bladder, vagina, uterus, and anorectal tissues is recommended.

The anus muscles relax following death frequently allowing visualization of the inner anal mucosa[671] (Fig. 17.66). The irregular margin between the delicate keratinized anal tissue and the unkeratinized mucosa (the anal verge) has not infrequently been interpreted as 'lacerations' by emergency

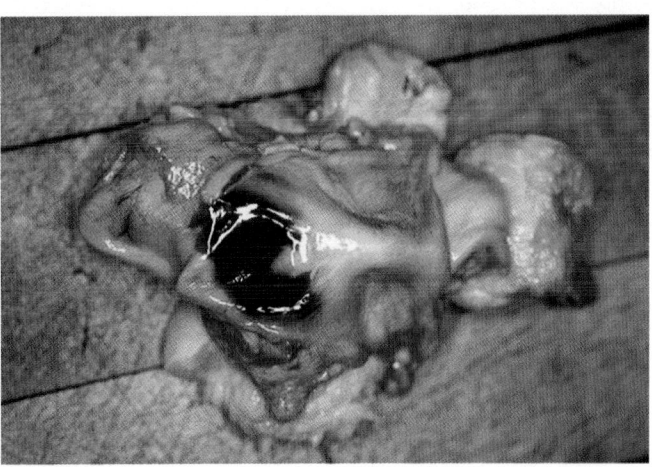

FIGURE 17.65 Dissected block of infant female genitalia in suspected sexual assault.

department personnel. Once the possibility of sexual violence is associated with an infant's death the machinery of law enforcement necessarily begins. If the examiner is inexperienced, it would be better to verify the concern immediately rather than subject the caregivers to the additional burden of interrogation that these accusations bring. This author has experience with as many as 10 cases of infant deaths where the diagnosis of anal injury or penetration was reversed after the tissue was examined microscopically.

Analysis of specimens for the presence or absence of ejaculate (acid phosphatase, prostate specific antibody, sperm and sperm motility) is typically performed by local crime labs and is recommended in children presenting < 72 h after reported sexual contact. Forensic evidence should also be collected in any suspicious fatality or when there is bleeding or acute injury.[672] Interpretation of the findings is usually straightforward – positive or negative. Standardized kits are available in most emergency rooms or medical examiners facilities.

The diagnosis of sexually transmitted disease (STD) in a prepubertal child should initiate an evaluation for sexual abuse.[673] Once vertical or horizontal transmission has been excluded, some STDs may indicate sexual misuse. Jain[674] reviews the evaluation for STD in the pediatric patient. Infections associated with STD are: gonorrhea, chlamydia, syphilis, genital herpes, anogenital warts, trichomoniasis, human immunodeficiency virus (HIV), hepatitis B or C virus, bacterial vaginosis, genital mycoplasmata, and molluscum contagiosum. Diagnosis of sexually transmitted disease in a young infant is suspicious for sexual contact but not diagnostic.

Sudden unexpected death in infancy and homicide

The sudden unexpected and unexplained death of the infant < 1 year continues to be the number one circumstance of death

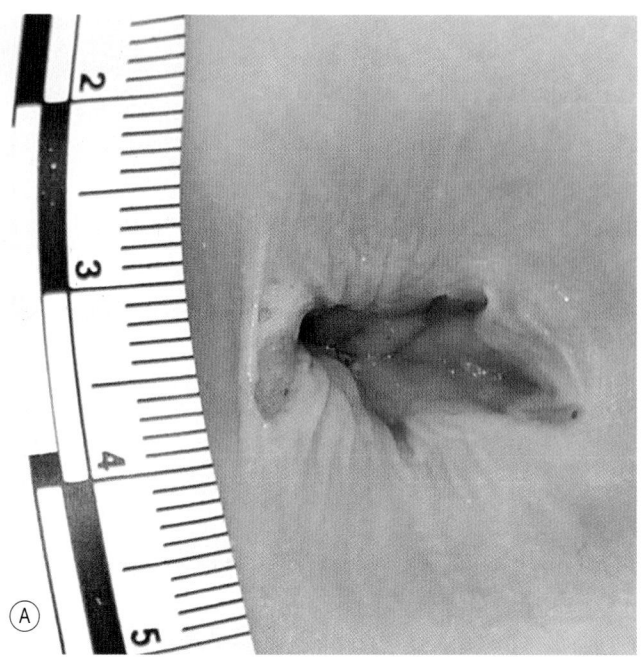

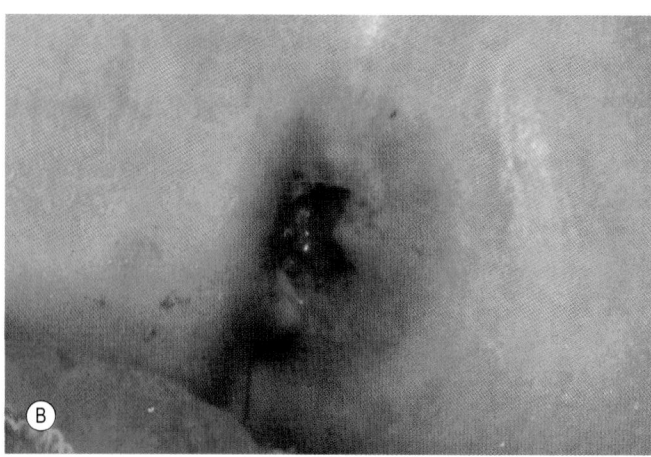

FIGURE 17.66 (A) Normal infant anus with exposure of internal mucosa at postmortem. Note irregular margin can be mistaken for lacerations. (B) Postmortem findings of acute sexual penetration, anus.

TABLE 17.13 POSTNEONATAL (28 DAYS–11 MONTHS) MORTALITY (PNM) STATISTICS FOR THE YEAR 2000[126]

Cause	No. per 100 000 live births
1. Sudden infant death syndrome	57.1
2. Congenital malformations, deformations and chromosomal abnormalities	39.4
3. Accidents	19.4
4. Disease of the circulatory system	10.1
5. Assault (homicide)	7.6
6. Septicemia	6.8
7. Influenza and pneumonia	6.4
8. Chronic respiratory disease	6.0
9. Gastritis, duodenitis, and non-infective enteritis and colitis	5.4
10. Malignant neoplasms	2.0
Overall morality rate	228.1

in the postnatal period (Table 17.13). Sudden unexpected death in childhood can be divided into two major categories: traumatic and non-traumatic, and then classified as explained and unexplained. SIDS is the most common form of postnatal and unexplained non-traumatic sudden death in infancy presenting to the forensic community. Cote et al[675] reviewed sudden unexpected deaths in infancy and found the most common non-SIDS diagnosis was infection followed by cardiac pathology. They also found a higher incidence of non-SIDS diagnoses at centers with expertise in pediatric pathology. Parham et al[676] reviewed 439 sudden deaths in children aged from 1 day to 19 years and used four anatomic categories or case types.

- previously undiagnosed condition of medical significance
- previously undiagnosed condition without medical significance
- previously undiagnosed condition with uncertain medical significance
- findings expected for a previously diagnosed medical condition

Mitchell et al[677] analyzed the stages of investigation of 60 sudden infant deaths to evaluate the relative contribution of the elements of the process to final determination of cause of death. Scene investigation (2 of 43), radiographic examination (2 of 11), external examination (2 of 60), histology (7 of 60), and microbiological examination (3 of 58) provided positive findings. These results gave alternative diagnoses to SIDS in 25% of the cases.

The approach to investigation and analysis of sudden infant death has been extensively reviewed in the literature.[184–201] The forensic examination of an unexpected death requires analysis of more than findings at autopsy. Negative autopsy following metabolic, toxicologic, chemical and radiologic studies leaves the pathologist with a challenging differential diagnosis:

- **Natural causes** – masked infection, prolonged QT interval, undetected metabolic disease, SIDS.
- **Accident** – asphyxia, suffocation, overlaying, unsafe sleeping conditions, undetected poisoning, undetected hypo- or hyperthermia.
- **Homicide** – inflicted respiratory compromise, covert child abuse.
- **Undetermined** – findings are not conclusive to exclude two of the above.

Sudden death from natural causes in infancy is most commonly related to infectious or cardiac mechanisms, although any disorder that can become lethal to a child may do so suddenly.[678, 679] Byard provides an excellent review and pathology reference to the natural conditions that can result in sudden death in childhood.[680] Burchfield and Rawlings[681] described 10 apparently healthy infants in the normal newborn nursery found by caregivers to be limp, apneic, and requiring resuscitation. All the infants were full term and appropriate for gestational age. Prenatal or perinatal complications were present in 9 of the 10 infants. Five of the infants died. No anatomic cause of death was identified in all four of the infants autopsied. Evaluation of the five survivors failed to determine a cause for the episodes. Careful postmortem examination and case investigation should be performed in all such cases.[682]

Homicide and unexplained deaths[192, 683]

In the last 10–15 years a number of families have presented with serial events of sudden unexpected and apparently unexplained deaths of multiple siblings, specifically very young infants and rarely toddlers. As would be expected, the findings at autopsy were inconclusive in the majority of cases. Similarly, the investigative process for many of these families did not include the comprehensive and sophisticated features and techniques that accompany today's homicide investigations. That does not preclude the necessity to initiate comprehensive homicide investigations when suspicions are raised even if it is many years later.

The diagnosis of serial killing cannot be based on statistics or probabilities. However, careful evaluation of the case material, witness statements, medical records and law enforcement investigations in conjunction with absence of heritable or explainable cause of death, allows for certification in some cases of homicidal asphyxia. Oehmichen[684] reports a case of successive killing of three siblings, 1 year, 2.5 months and 3 years. Petechial hemorrhages were found in all three infants. The 3-year-old was determined to be homicide and following conviction for smothering, the mother acknowledged killing the other infants in the same manner. Unfortunately there is no definitive method to make the distinction from medical criteria alone, especially in the circumstance of an isolated event or single fatality.

Infant homicide has been estimated to account for 10% of sudden unexplained infant deaths.[685] In a study of 81 covert infant non-natural deaths, 77% had a history of apparent life threatening event (ALTE) and 48% had been hospitalized within 1 week preceding the death.[198] At autopsy 43% of the infants were found with frank blood within or around the nose or mouth. Careful attention and documentation of blood at the scene, oronasal, tracheal, esophageal/gastric swallowed blood as well as description of nature and distribution of pulmonary hemorrhage is necessary in investigation of possible asphyxia due to suffocation. Only recently has the observation of pulmonary hemorrhage, oronasal blood and increased pulmonary siderophages been an adjunct to the pathology review of possible homicidal suffocation (see asphyxia section).

The CDC convened a study group to recommend case severity classification and identification criteria for acute idiopathic pulmonary hemorrhage in infancy. Different pathophysiologic processes are associated with pulmonary hemorrhage and were divided into four pathophysiologic processes:

- conditions of bleeding into normal tissue sites with mechanical disruption causing bleeding (intentional suffocation, mitral valve disease)
- vascular inflammation/vascular malformation
- coagulopathy
- neonatal and general differential diagnoses associated with pulmonary hemorrhage

Presence of increased pulmonary siderocytes in children with history of recurrent ALTE or apnea should raise suspicion of inflicted suffocation. Multiple soft tissue and conjunctival petechiae although not diagnostic should raise concern for circumstances of raised capillary pressure and hypoxia. Carpenter et al[686] reviews repeat sudden unexpected infant death. Child abuse was not uncommon, but cause of death in the subsequent case or cases was in most cases natural.

Apparent life-threatening events

ALTE are episodes during which the child is observed to be limp, cyanotic or pale and apneic. Repeat imposed upper airway obstruction events will present to medical attention as ALTE. The differential diagnosis of ALTE can be extensive. In circumstances where there is recurrent ALTE following negative work-up for gastroesophageal reflux disease, epilepsy, central apnea, etc., inflicted or episodic incomplete suffocation must be considered. Covert video surveillance (CVS) has proved invaluable in identifying children at risk for inflicted apnea.[687] Samuels et al[688] studied 157 patients referred for evaluation of recurrent ALTE. Final diagnosis was reached in 77 of 157: 18 of the infants suffered deliberate suffocation, 10 suffered hypoxia from epileptic seizures, 7 were associated with fabricated history and data, and 40 from acute hypoxia of respiratory origin, and two were associated with changes in peripheral perfusion and skin color without hypoxemia. Three of the patients subsequently died suddenly and unexpectedly. This author participated in the investigation of two children with recurrent inflicted apnea in which the younger child was killed 2 weeks after extensive hospitalization. Disbelief in the possibility of intentional suffocation by the attending physician resulted in termination of attempts to investigate and protect the children.

In some jurisdictions the autopsy pathologist is only contracted to perform the autopsy; the remainder of the analysis and death certification is performed by other individuals. Under these conditions, without access to and participation in the investigative process the pathologist has no choice but to certify the cause of death or manner as undetermined. That does not mean that the death is not a homicide.

It is important to note that sudden unexpected death in the presence of chronic disease still requires careful evaluation.[689] Buehler and colleagues[690] reported the arrest of a nurse employed in the cardiology service of a children's hospital who was accused of overdosing four patients with digoxin over a

3 month period. Buchino et al[691] reviews the sudden unexpected death of hospitalized children. The authors provide a useful classification by circumstance:

- Natural – includes pulmonary emboli, acute cerebral edema in diabetic ketoacidosis, cardiac arrhythmia.
- Failure to monitor – usually in a child not recognized to be seriously ill.
- Therapeutic misadventure – medication errors, device failure or malfunction, complications of vascular catheter.
- Suicide
- Homicide - classification into three categories:
  - euthanasia
  - covert intentional death in the context of MSBP
  - mental instability.

Sudden unexpected deaths in hospital should always be reported to the coroner/medical examiner. Kamerling et al[692] report a case of intentional tracheal extubation by the child's mother. Fortunately rare, cases of this nature emphasize the need to evaluate each case on its own merit without presuming that an underlying chronic illness is the explanation for an unexpected death.

Munchausen syndrome by proxy[27, 693, 694]

'I made a balloon of such extensive dimension, that an account of the silk it contained would exceed all credibility........on the 30th of September, when the college of physicians chose their annual officers, and dined sumptuously together, I filled my balloon, brought it over the dome of their building, clapped the sling round the golden ball at the top, fastening the other end of it to the balloon, and immediately ascending with the whole college to an immense height, where I kept them upwards of three months......It is a well known fact that during the three months the college was suspended in the air, and therefore incapable of attending their patients, no deaths happened, except a few.......If the apothecaries had not been very active during the above time, half the undertakers, in all probability, would have been bankrupt.'

From the Adventures of Baron Munchausen (Rasper, 1936)

Baron Karl von Munchausen served as a mercenary cavalry officer in the hire of the Czar of Russia during the Russo-Turkish war. He retired to his estate in 1760 and amused friends and local tavern dwellers by telling extraordinary tales of his prowess as a soldier and sportsman. Munchausen syndrome was first defined in 1951[695] in an effort to characterize a unique group of patients who travel from hospital to hospital, fabricating stories of ill health and willing to subject themselves to needless surgery.

Meadow[697] coined the phrase Munchausen by proxy to describe the circumstances in which parents cause harm to their children by falsifying stories, fabricating evidence, or even inflicting illness or injury. The perpetrator is most often the mother, who is frequently described as intelligent, often medically astute or from a health care background, pleasant, cooperative, generally appreciative of good medical care, and appearing to flourish in the hospital environment. The most vulnerable and those with the highest mortality are the infants and very young children. Victims are often subjected to numerous and prolonged hospitalizations and repeated painful and costly diagnostic procedures. In this author's experience, one such child had been hospitalized over 200 times. Morbidity and mortality rates are much greater than was first apparent – estimated in one series to be as high as 10%.[697–699] The victims reportedly range from a few weeks to 21 years in age. Personal experience with children covertly abused by an 'apparently caring' parent suggests that the prevalence is vastly underestimated. There is an increasing association with SIDS, near-miss SIDS, recurrent SIDS, and conditions of fabricated illness.[687, 700, 701] The most common presenting complaints have been bleeding, seizures, CNS depression, apnea, vomiting, diarrhea, fever, and rash.[702]

The essential features of the condition have been summarized by Rosenberg:[693]

- production of a spurious or genuine illness in a child by a caregiver
- repetitive visits to medical attention for assessment, investigation and treatment
- complete absence of symptoms and signs or dramatic improvement or resolution of the illness in the absence of the offending parent
- denial by the perpetrator of the cause of the illness
- significant mortality rate

Over the years much of the public and media focus has been on the 'motivation' of the perpetrator and the unique name often applied to this form of child abuse. Whatever it is called, caregivers, most frequently mothers, fabricate signs and symptoms of disease. This process may be as simple as exaggerating benign symptoms to actually inflicting injury or poisoning children to mortal illness or death. Many of the perpetrators enjoy the attention or publicity that they receive for their child's condition. One such mother was named 'mother of the year' at the national level.

There is a similar form of animal abuse where pet owners create illness and injuries in their animals.

Meadow suggests five consequences of this form of abuse:

- unnecessary, harmful, painful, examinations and treatments;
- abusive actions by the perpetrator can induce genuine disease in the child;
- the child may die as a consequence of the actions;
- the child may develop chronic invalidism; and
- the victim may go on to develop Munchausen syndrome as an adult or perpetrate the abuse in their children.

There is probably no problem or condition that cannot be fabricated or produced as part of the spectrum of abuse. Review of the recent literature reveals reports of injured children in numerous countries and in most if not all medical specialties. Rosenberg[693] presents an exhaustive list of presenting signs and symptoms and diagnoses. Some of these include complications of central venous catheterization,[703] factitious immunodeficiency,[704] cystic fibrosis,[705] familial Munchausen disorder,[706] outpatient Munchausen by proxy – the allergic form,[707, 708] and numerous forms of chemical- and drug-induced symptoms in the context of Munchausen by proxy. Cases include: intentionally induced premature labor and delivery at 26 weeks' gestation, injection of feces and gasoline, fabrication of cystic fibrosis with falsified sweat tests, placement on the liver and small bowel transplant list, fabricated sexual abuse,[709] salt poisoning, anticoagulant poisoning, factitious urethral stones, factitious Crohn disease, fabricated seizure disorder and more. Emergency room physicians may have significant exposure to children subjected to this kind of abuse. The child may present with life-threatening conditions.[710]

Sutphen and Saulsbury reported two patients with Munchausen by proxy resulting from chronic ipecac ingestion.[711] Both patients had intractable vomiting and diarrhea. One showed clinical and laboratory evidence of skeletal and cardiac myopathy. In cases of ipecac poisoning, myopathy results in proximal muscle weakness stemming from a direct toxic effect of emetine on the muscle fiber. The weakness may persist long after ipecac has been discontinued but is usually reversible. The most serious consequences are from cardiac myopathy, again due primarily to the emetine. After a single dose of ipecac, peak serum levels are achieved within 30 min, detectable in the urine 20–40 min after ingestion. Traces of the drug may be detectable for 20–40 days. Before the correct diagnosis was made, the children were subjected to extensive and invasive diagnostic procedures. Multiple reports of abuse by ipecac have appeared in the literature,[712, 713] including a fatality from cardiomyopathy.[714]

Polymicrobial infections in children with and without a diagnosis of immunodeficiency is a troublesome presentation of the disorder.[715, 716] In the author's experience, these children have been subjected to numerous and prolonged hospitalizations and repeated painful and costly diagnostic procedures.

The story of Bryk[717] reveals the true nature of source of the perpetrators of this 'secret' violence against silent victims. She was subjected to covert and repeated musculoskeletal trauma that left her with draining wounds contaminated with potting soil, remarkable soft tissue and skeletal injuries and even fractures inflicted during one of her many hospitalizations.

Because this form of child abuse frequently involves active participation by medical professionals, super specialization and care fragmentation can make it easier for the perpetrator to manipulate the system.[709, 718] This author was involved with a case of two grade school children who confounded the school system for years with increasing medical demands and complexities placed on school officials. The children were labeled by their mothers with polyarthritic juvenile rheumatoid arthritis, chronic asthma, epilepsy, sleep disorders, autism, and childhood depression among other diagnoses. Evaluation of medical records revealed no 'medical home' responsible for the diagnoses and no medical records or laboratory data supporting the diagnoses.

One of the extremes of this kind of abuse is the serial and intentional suffocation of infants and children. This author has participated in the investigation of eight families with 35 serially killed infants initially diagnosed as natural disease or SIDS.

Meadow[719] reported a mortality rate of 33% in a series of 27 infants repeatedly suffocated by their mother, with 18 previous deaths in 33 older siblings (mortality rate 55%). Galvin et al[720] have provided a recent update on the MSBP form of child abuse, with special focus on the infants presenting with SIDS/ALTE. These authors suggest that fabricated illness should routinely be considered in the differential diagnosis of ALTE.

Court video surveillance (CVS) has been a definitive diagnostic tool in this form of child abuse.[721] Viewing these tapes has also been an important adjunct to skeptical medical providers and the public to understanding and verifying the harm these children suffer. CVS of children suspected of MSBP may be the best confirmatory mechanism in some cases,[722] especially those involving 'apneic' episodes or ALTE.[715, 716] In this author's experience, a 'caring' father was videotaped smashing his 10-month-old daughter's face into the hospital bed with the full weight of his body until her fighting ceased (over 60 s). Hall et al[721] summarizes 41 cases of child and families admitted to CVS units at Scottish Rite Children's Medical Center in Atlanta GA. CVS was used to make the diagnosis of MSBP in 13 of 23 and supported the diagnosis in 5 of 23. The methods of injury included suffocation, injection of body fluids, administration of medications and burns.

The diagnosis of fabricated illness child abuse begins with suspicion. Rosenberg provides a series of diagnostic criteria to assist in the process.[693] When investigating cases of this nature, it is imperative to assemble a multidisciplinary team and develop a method to protect the child. Often it will require recruiting an independent pediatrician to re-evaluate the medical history and supervise the child's health care. Law enforcement must be alerted and prepared to take action to protect if the diagnosis is confirmed.[687] Experienced participants in investigation of these cases strongly recommend against confrontation or any alert regarding this diagnosis by inexperienced medical personnel unless law enforcement is present and prepared to act. If alerted or suspicious, perpetrators have been known to harm the children in the hospital, remove them against medical advice and resort to lethal consequences to 'prove' their child is ill. An additional problem is the occurrence of flight of the family to another facility or even community and beginning the process again.

The role of the pathologist in unraveling the process cannot be emphasized too strongly. Laboratory investigation of the presenting complaints is a common thread in nearly every case. When chemical abuse is suspected as part of the symptoms in MSBP common drug monitoring techniques can be used to establish the diagnosis.[725]

Death investigation and autopsy of children who have died with suspicions of inflicted medical conditions require a comprehensive forensic analysis. In the case of a child where the abuse is in the context of fabricated illness or medical abuse the analysis is even more challenging. These children are often frequent visitors to specialty children's hospital and the hospital pathologist may hold the key to diagnosis. Assembling the necessary materials is time consuming and frequently requires multiple jurisdictions to evaluate the medical conditions of all siblings and ideally the parents, surviving or deceased.

Calendaring the family medical encounters has often identified a profile or pattern of hospital admissions that can lead to diagnosis. Routine toxicology screens should not be relied on to identify the offending agents. Vitreous or cerebrospinal fluid electrolytes should be routine in any found dead child, but is imperative in these cases. These are cases that may require exhaustive review and consultation for the relatively inexperienced examiners.

Acknowledgements

To John I Coe for providing a lifetime of mentoring.

To Boyd Stevens for introducing me to principles of forensic science in children.

To Kara Rahimi for her attention to the details of this manuscript.

Most importantly to my sister and work partner Judy Olein, who through her dedicated efforts and support made this chapter possible.

Dedication

To the little ones from whose suffering comes understanding

References

Pediatric forensic pathology

1. Randall BB, Fierro MF, Froede RC. Practice guideline for forensic pathology. Arch Pathol Lab Med 1998; 122:1056–1064.
2. Hanzlick R, Combs D. Medical examiner and coroner systems. JAMA 1998; 279:870–874.
3. The Royal College of Pathologists. Code of practice and performance standards for forensic pathologists. Online. Available: http://www.rcpath.org 2004.
4. Minnesota Department of Health Division of Family Health Maternal and Child Health Section. Infant death investigation guidelines: to investigate sudden, unexplained deaths of infants 0–24 months of age. Saint Paul: MDH; 2002.
5. Barnes PD. Ethical issues in imaging nonaccidental injury: child abuse. Top Magn Reson Imaging 2002; 13(2):85–94.
6. Williams C. The role of the expert witness. Arch Dis Child 2002; 87:267–268.
7. David TJ. Avoidable pitfalls when writing medical reports for court proceedings in cases of suspected child abuse. Arch Dis Child 2004; 89:799–804.

Cause, mechanism, and manner of death–general principles

8. Wright RK, Wetli CV. A guide to the forensic autopsy – conceptual aspects. Pathol Ann 1981; 16(2):273–288.
9. Hanzlick R, Hunsacker III JC, Davis G. A guide for manner of death classification. 1st edn. St Louis: NAME; 2001.
10. Macer K. Death resulting from paediatric surgery and anesthesia. In: Mason JK, ed. Paediatric forensic medicine and pathology. London: Chapman and Hall; 1989:317–337.

11. Murphy GK. Therapeutic misadventure: an 11-year study from a metropolitan coroner's office. Am J Forensic Med Pathol 1986; 7:115–119.
12. Cooper PN. The investigation of deaths occurring during and after invasive medical and surgical procedures. In: Rutty GN, ed. Essentials of autopsy practice. London: Springer; 2001:159–173.
13. Edirisinghe NK. Iatrogenic vascular lesions: surgical perspective. Online. Available: http://www.emedicine.com/ped/topic2886.htm
14. Woods D, Thomas E, Holl J, et al. Adverse events and preventable adverse events in children. Pediatrics 2005; 115(1):155–160.
15. Metzker A, Brenner S, Merlob P. Iatrogenic cutaneous injuries in the neonate. Arch Dermatol 1999; 135:697–703.

Forensic issues in the pediatric autopsy

16. Hirsch CS. Medicolegal autopsy: practical perspectives. In: Curran WI, McGarry AL, Petty CS, eds. Modern legal medicine, psychiatry, and forensic medicine. Philadelphia: FA Davis; 1980:129–138.
17. Spitz WU. The medicolegal autopsy. Hum Pathol 1980; 11:105–112.
18. Bove KE. Practice guidelines for autopsy pathology. Arch Pathol Lab Med 1997; 121:368–376.
19. Saukko P, Knight B. The forensic autopsy. In: Saukko P, Knight B, eds. Knight's forensic pathology. 3rd edn. London: Arnold; 2004:1–51.
20. Byard RW. Appendices V, VI, VII, VIII. In: Byard RW, ed. Sudden death in infancy and childhood and adolescence. 2nd edn. Cambridge: Cambridge University Press; 2004:612–617.
21. Guidelines for autopsy investigation in post-neonatal infant deaths or sudden unexpected deaths in infancy. RCPath September 2002. Online. Available: http://www.recpath.org
22. Task Force for the study of non-accidental injuries and child deaths. Protocol for child death autopsies. Springfield: Illinois Department of Children and Family Services 1986:1–20.
23. Zumwalt RE, Hirsch CS. Pathology of fatal child abuse and neglect. In: Helfer RE, Kempe RS, eds. The battered child, Chicago: University of Chicago Press; 1987:247–285.
24. Norman MG, Newman DE. Postmortem examination of the abused child: pathological, radiographic and legal aspects. Perspect Pediatr Pathol 1984; 8:313–343.
25. Knight B. The autopsy in the non-accidental injury syndrome. In Mason JK, ed. Paediatric forensic medicine and pathology. London: Chapman and Hall; 1989:2269–2287.
26. Saukko P, Knight B. Fatal child abuse. In: Saukko P, Knight B, eds. Knight's forensic pathology. 3rd edn. London: Arnold; 2004:461–479.
27. Byard RW, Cohle SD. Homicide and suicide. In: Byard RW, ed. Sudden death in infancy and childhood and adolescence. 2nd edn. Cambridge: Cambridge University Press; 2004:77–163.
28. Krous HR, Byard RW. Appendix 1: International standardized autopsy protocol for sudden unexpected infant death. In: Byard RW, Krouse HR, eds. Sudden infant death syndrome. London: Arnold; 2001:319–333.
29. Hanzlick RL. The autopsy lexicon: suggested heading for the autopsy report. Arch Pathol Lab Med 2000; 124:594–603.
30. Wagner GN. Crime scene investigation in child-abuse cases. Am J Forensic Med Pathol 1986; 7:94–99.
31. New Mexico Office of the Medical Investigator. Scene investigator's guidelines. Albuqurque. 2002. Online. Available: http://www.thename.org/index.php?option=com_docman&task=doc_download&gid=63&Itemid=26.
32. Wilson C, Cutfield W, Christodolou J. Metabolic disease, guidelines for investigating. Paediatric Clinical Guidelines 2001. Online. Available: *http://www.starship.org.nz*

The postmortem examination

33. Kleinman PK. Postmortem imaging. In: Kleinman PK, ed. Diagnostic imaging of child abuse. 2nd edn. St. Louis: Mosby; 1998:242–246.
34. McGraw EP, Pless JE, Pennington DJ, et al. Post mortem radiography after unexpected death in neonates, infants, and children: should imaging be routine? AJR Am J Roentgenol 2002; 178:1517–1521.

35. Hart BL, Dudley MH, Zumwalt RE. Post mortem cranial MRI and autopsy correlation in suspected child abuse. Am J Forensic Med Pathol 1996; 17(3):217–224.

36. Ricci LR. Photodocumentation of the abused child. In: Reece RM, Ludwig S, eds. Child abuse: medical diagnosis and management. 2nd edn. Philadelphia: Lippincott Williams & Wilkins; 2001:385–404.

37. US Department of Justice Office of Justice Programs. Photo documentation in the investigation of child abuse, March 2000. Online. Available: http://www.ncjrs.gov/html/ojjdp/portable_guides/photodoc/

38. American Board of Forensic Odontology. ABFO Bitemark Guidelines. Online. Available: http://www.forensicdentistryonline.org/Forensic_pages_1/bitemark_guidelines.htm

39. Judkins AR, Hood IG, Mirchandani HG, et al. Rationale and technique for examination of nervous system in suspected infant victims of abuse. Am J Forensic Med Pathol 2004; 25:29–32.

40. Sturner WQ. Common errors in forensic pediatric pathology. Am J Forensic Med Pathol 1998; 19(4):317–320.

Postmortem changes

41. Rutty GN. Post mortem changes and artifacts. In: Rutty GN, ed. Essentials of autopsy practice, volume 1. London: Springer; 2001:63–95.

42. Madea B, Henssge C. Timing of death. In: Payne-James J, Busuttil A, Smock W, eds. Forensic medicine: clinical and pathological aspects. London: Greenwich Medical Media; 2003:91–114.

43. Saukko P, Knight B. The pathophysiology of death. In: Saukko P, Knight B, eds. Knight's forensic pathology. 3rd edn. London: Arnold; 2004:52–97.

44. Knight B, Nokes L. Temperature-based methods I. In: Knight B, ed. The estimation of the time since death in the early postmortem period. 2nd edn. London: Arnold; 2002:3–42.

45. Knight B. The estimation of the time since death in the early postmortem period. 2nd edn. London: Arnold; 2002

46. James W, Knight B. Errors in estimating time since death. Med Sci Law 1965; 5:111–116.

47. Krompecher T. Rigor mortis: estimation of the time since death by evaluation of cadaveric rigidity. In: Knight B, ed. The estimation of the time since death in the early postmortem period. 2nd edn. London: Arnold; 2002:144–160.

48. Wigglesworth JS. The macerated stillborn fetus. In: Livosi VA, ed. Perinatal pathology. Philadelphia: WB Saunders; 1996:78–80.

49. Genest DR, Williams MA, Grene MF. Estimating the time of death in stillborn fetuses: I. Histologic evaluation of fetal organs; an autopsy study of 150 stillborns. Obstet Gynecol 1992; 80:575–584.

50. Genest DR. Estimating the time of death in stillborn fetuses: II. Histologic evaluation of the placenta; a study of 71 stillborns. Obstet Gynecol 1992; 80:585–592.

51. Genest DR, Singer DB. Estimating the time of death in stillborn fetuses: III. External fetal examination; a study of 86 stillborns. Obstet Gynecol 1992; 80:593–600.

52. Coe JI. Postmortem chemistry of blood, CSF, and vitreous humor. In: Tedeschi CG, Eckert WG, Tedeschi LG, eds. Forensic medicine: a study in trauma and environmental hazards. Philadelphia: WB Saunders; 1977:1033–1060.

53. Huser CJ, Smialek JE. Diagnosis of sudden death in infants due to dehydration. J Forensic Med Pathol 1986; 7:278–282.

54. Blumenfeld TA, Mantell CH, Catherman RL, et al. Postmortem vitreous humor chemistry in sudden infant death syndrome and other causes of death in childhood. Am J Clin Pathol 1979; 71:219–223.

55. Sturner WQ, Dempsey J. Sudden infant death: chemical analysis of vitreous humor. J Forensic Sci 1973; 18:12–19.

56. Coe JI. Postmortem chemistry update: emphasis on forensic application. Am J Forensic Med Pathol 1993; 14(2):91–117.

57. Coe JI. Post-mortem biochemistry of blood and vitreous humor in paediatric practice. In Mason JK, ed. Paediatric forensic medicine and pathology. London: Chapman and Hall; 1989:191–203.

58. Gagajewski A, Murakami MM, Kloss J, et al. Measurement of chemical analytes in vitreous humor: stability and precision studies. J Forensic Sci 2004; 49(2):1–4.

59. Coe JI. Postmortem chemistries on human vitreous humor. Am J Clin Pathol 1969; 51(6):741–750.

60. Coe JI. Comparative postmortem chemistries of vitreous humor before and after embalming. J Forensic Sci 1976; 21(3):583–586.

61. Sturner WQ, Sullivan A, Suzuki K. Lactic acid concentrations in vitreous humor: their use in asphyxial deaths in children. J Forensic Sci 1983; 28:222–230.

62. Coe JI. Comparison of antemortem and postmortem serum proteins. Bull Bell Museum Pathobiol 1973; 2:40–42.

63. Robinson DM, Kellenberger RE. Comparison of electrophoretic analysis of antemortem and postmortem sera. Am J Clin Pathol 1962; 38:371–377.

64. Brazinsky JH, Kellenberger RE. Comparison of immunoglobulin analyses of antemortem and postmortem sera. Am J Clin Pathol 1970; 54:622–624.

65. McCormick GM. Nonanatomic postmortem techniques: postmortem serology. J Forensic Sci 1972; 17:57–62.

66. Petty CS, Lovel MP, Moore EJ. Organic phosphorus insecticides and postmortem blood cholinesterase levels. J Forensic Sci 1958; 3:226–237.

67. Vawter GF, McGraw CA. A hepatic metabolic profile in sudden infant death (SIDS). Forensic Sci Int 1986; 30:93–98.

68. Finlayson NB. Blood cortisol levels in infants and adults: a postmortem study. J Pediatr 1965; 67:284–292.

69. Coe JI. Postmortem values of thyroxine and thyroid stimulating hormone. J Forensic Sci 1973; 18:20–24.

70. Bonnell HL. Antemortem chemical hypothyroxinemia. J Forensic Sci 1983; 28:242–248.

71. Chacon MS, Tildon JT. Elevated levels of tri-iodothyronine in victims of SID. J Pediatr 1981; 99:758–760.

72. Schwarz EH, Chasalow FI, Erickson MM, et al. Elevation of postmortem triiodothyronine in SIDS and in infants who died of other causes: a marker of previous health. J Pediatr 1983; 102:200–205.

73. Sturner WQ, Lynch HJ, et al. Melatonin levels in body fluids of SIDS infants. Abstract of paper presented at the XIth International Association of Forensic Science, Vancouver, British Columbia, Canada, 1987.

74. Borg RG, Martin SK, Rinnaldo P. Biochemical diagnosis of fatty acid oxidation disorders by metabolite analysis of postmortem liver. Human Pathol 1994; 25:735–741.

75. Chace DH, DiPerna JC, Mitchell BL. Electrospray tandem mass spectrometry for analysis of acylcarnitines in dried postmortem blood specimens collected at autopsy from infants with unexplained cause of death. Clin Chem 2001; 47(7):116–1182.

76. Callum W, Cutfield W, Christodolou J. Metabolic disease, guidelines for investigating Online. Available: http://www.starship.org.nz

77. Baselt RC. Disposition of toxic drugs and chemicals in man. 5th edn. Foster City: Chemical Toxicology Institute; 2000.

78. Mittleman RE, Steele B, Moskowitz L. Postmortem vitreous humor in fatal acute iron poisoning. J Forensic Sci 1982; 27:955–957.

79. Sherpher MF, Lake KD, Kamps MA. Postmortem changes and pharmacokinetics: review of the literature and case report. Ann Pharmacother 1992; 510–514.

80. Drummer O, Forrest AR, Goldberger B, et al. Forensic science in the dock. BMJ 2004; 329:636–637.

Wounds

81. Saukko P, Knight B. The pathology of wounds. In: Saukko P, Knight B, eds. Knight's forensic pathology. 3rd edn. London: Arnold; 2004:136–173.

82. Robinson S. The examination of the adult victim of assault. In: Mason JK, Purdue BN, eds. The pathology of trauma. 3rd edn. London: Arnold; 2000:141–154.

83. Wynne J. The physical and emotional abuse of children. In: Payne-James J, Busuttil A, Smock W eds. Forensic medicine: clinical and pathological aspects. London: Greenwich Medical Media; 2003:471–485.

84. Fisher RS. History of forensic pathology. In: Spitz WU, Fisher RS, eds. Medicolegal investigation of death. 2nd edn. Springfield: Charles C Thomas; 1980.

85. Hirsch CS, Zumwalt RE. Forensic pathology. In: Damjanov I, Linder J, eds. Anderson's pathology. 10th edn. St Louis: Mosby-Year; 1996.

86. Simpson K, Knight B. Forensic medicine. 9th edn. London: Edward Arnold; 1985:48–70.

87. Goldsmith W, Plunkett J. A biomechanical analysis of the causes of traumatic brain injury in infants and children. Am J Forensic Med Pathol 2004; 25(2):89–100.

88. McLean AJ, Anderson RW. Biomechanics of closed head injury. In: Reilly R, Bullock R eds. Head injury. London: Chapman and Hall; 1997:25–37.

89. Margulies SS, Thibault KL. Infant skull and suture properties: measurements and implications for mechanics of pediatric brain injury. J Biomechan Eng 2000; 122:364–371.

90. Goldsmith W. Impact: the theory and physical behaviour of colliding solids. Minneola: Dover; 2001.

91. Leadbeatter S. Resuscitation injuries. In: Rutty GN, ed. Essentials of autopsy practice. London: Springer; 2001:43–62.

92. Darok M. Injuries resulting from resuscitation procedures. In: Tsokos M, ed. Forensic pathology reviews. Vol. 1. Totowa: Humana Press; 2004:293–303.

93. Bush CM, Jones JS, Cohle SD, et al. Pediatric injuries from cardio-pulmonary resuscitation. Ann Emerg Med 1996; 28(10):40–44.

94. Kaplan JA, Fossum RM. Patterns of facial resuscitation injury in infancy. Am J Forensic Med 1994; 15:187–191.

95. Weber S. Traumatic complications of airway management. Anesthesiol Clin North Am 2002; 20(3):503–512.

96. Tcherveniakov A, Tchalakov P, Tcherveniakov P. Traumatic and iatrogenic lesions of the trachea and bronchi. Eur J Cardiothorac Surg 2001; 19:19–24.

97. Ryan MP, Young SJ, Wells DL. Do resuscitation attempts in children who die, cause injury? Emerg Med J 2003; 20:10–12.

98. Spevak MR, Kleinman PK, Belanger PL, et al. Cardiopulmonary resuscitation and rib fractures in infants: a postmortem radiologic–pathologic study. JAMA 1994; 272(8):617–618.

99. DiMaio DJ, DiMaio VJ. Wounds due to blunt trauma. In: DiMaio DJ, DiMaio VJ, eds. Forensic pathology. New York: Elsevier; 1989:87–107.

100. Vanezis P. Bruising: concepts of ageing and interpretation. In: Rutty GN. Essentials of Autopsy Practice. London: Springer; 2001:221–240.

101. Schwartz AJ, Ricci L. How accurately can bruises be aged in abused children? Literature review and synthesis. Pediatrics 1996; 97(2):254–257.

102. Maguire S, Mann MK, Seibert J, et al. Are there patterns of bruising in childhood which are diagnostic or suggestive of abuse? A systematic review. Arch Dis Child 2005; 90:182–186.

103. Carpenter RF. The prevalence and distribution of bruising in babies. Arch Dis Child 1999; 80:363–366.

104. Sugar NF, Taylor JA, Feldman KW. Bruises in infants and toddlers. Arch Pediatr Adolesc Med 1999; 153(4):399–403.

105. Pascoe JM, Hildebrandt TM. Patterns of skin injury in nonaccidental and accidental injury. Pediatrics 1979; 64:245–247.

106. Maguire S, Mann MK, Seibert J, et al. Can you age bruises accurately in children? A systematic review. Arch Dis Child 2005; 90:187–189.

107. Vanezis P. Interpreting bruises at necropsy. J Clin Pathol 2001; 54:348–355.

108. Vogeley E, Clyde Pierce M, Bertocci G. Experience with wood lamp illumination and digital photography in the documentation of bruises on human skin. Arch Pediatr Adoles Med 2002; 156:265–268.

Vital reaction and timing of injury

109. Loberg EM, Torvik A. Brain contusions: the time sequence of the histologic changes. Med Sci Law 1989; 29:109–115.

110. Nikolic S, Atanasijevic T, Micic J, et al. Amount of postmortem bleeding – an experimental autopsy study. Am J Forensic Med Pathol 2004; 25 (1):20–22.

111. Raekallio J. Timing of the wound. In: Tedeschi CG, Eckert WG, Tedeschi LG, eds. Forensic medicine: a study in trauma and environmental hazards. Vol 1. Philadelphia: WB Saunders; 1977; 22–28.

112. Bednar B. Skin wound healing (an electronoptic study). Cesk Patol 1976; 12:67–71.

113. Wilson EF. Estimation of age of cutaneous contusions in child abuse. Pediatrics 1977; 60:750–752.

Causes of injury

114. National Center for Health Statistics, Centers for Disease Control and Prevention. Report to the nation: trends in unintentional childhood injury mortality, 1987–2000. Online. Available: http://www.usa.safekids.org/content_documents/nskw03_report.pdf.

115. Sanchez JI, Paides CN. Childhood trauma: now and in the new millennium. Surg Clin North 1999; 79(6):1503–1535.

116. Byard RW, Cohle SD. Accidents. In: Byard RW, ed. Sudden death in infancy and childhood and adolescence. 2nd edn. Cambridge: Cambridge University Press; 2004:11–73.

117. National Center for Health Statistics. Vital statistics for the US, 1984. Hyattsville: US Department of Health and Human Services; 1987.

118. Rivara FP. Traumatic deaths of children in the United States: currently available prevention strategies. Pediatrics 1985; 75:456–462.

119. American Academy of Pediatrics. Diagnostic imaging of child abuse. Pediatrics 2000; 105(6):1345–1348.

120. Tomashek KM, Hsia J, Iyasy S. Trends in postneonatal mortality attributable to injury, United States, 1988–1998. Pediatrics 2003; 111:1219–1225.

121. Hessol NA, Fuentes-Afflick E. Ethnic differences in neonatal and post-neonatal mortality. Pediatrics 2005; 115:44–51.

122. Malloy MH. Trends in postneonatal aspiration deaths and reclassification of sudden infant death syndrome: impact of the 'back to sleep' program. Pediatrics 2002; 109:661–665.

123. Corey TS, McCloud LC, Nichols GR, et al. Infant deaths due to unintentional injury: an 11 year autopsy review. Am J Dis Child 1992; 146:968–971.

124. Agran PF, Anderson C, Winn D, et al. Rates of pediatric injuries by 3-month intervals for children 0 to 3 years of age. Pediatrics 2003; 111(6):683–692.

125. Karwacki JJ, Baker SP. Children in motor vehicles – never too young to die. JAMA 1979; 242:2848–2851.

126. Baker SP. Motor vehicle occupant deaths in young children. Pediatrics 1979; 64:860–861.

127. Agran PA, Dunkle DE. Motor vehicle occupant injuries to children in crash and noncrash events. Pediatrics 1982; 70:993–996.

128. Agran PF, Dunkle DE, Winn DG. Motor vehicle childhood injuries caused by noncrash falls and ejections. JAMA 1985; 253:2530–2533.

129. Howard AW. Automobile restraints for children: a review for clinicians. CMAJ 2002; 167(7):769–773.

130. Marshall KW, Koch BL, Egelhoff JC. Air bag-related death and serious injuries in children: injury patterns and imaging findings. Am J Neuroradiol 1998; 19:1599–1607.

131. Makoroff K. Pediatric head injury from falls. Cincinnati Children's Hospital. Online. Available: http://www.cincinnatichildrens.org/svc/prog/child-abuse/tools/falls.htm

132. Warrington SA, Wright CM, ALSPAC Study Team. Accidents and resulting injuries in premobile infants: data from the ALSPAC study. Arch Dis Child 2001; 85:104–107.

133. Murray JA, Chen D, Velmahos GC, et al. Pediatric falls: is height a predictor of injury and outcome? Am Surg 2000; 66(9):863–865.

134. Kim KA, Wang MY, Griffith PM, et al. Analysis of pediatric head injury from falls. Neurosurg Focus 2000; 8(1): article 3.

135. Reichelderfer TE, Overback A, Greensher J. Unsafe playgrounds. Pediatrics 1979; 64:962–963.

136. Denton S, Mileusnic D. Delayed sudden death in an infant following an accidental fall: a case report with review of the literature. Am J Forensic Med Pathol 2003; 24(4):371–376.

137. Fingerhut LA, Kleinman JC. Injury fatalities among young children. Public Health Rep 1988; 103:399–405.

138. Grcevic N. Topography and pathogenic mechanisms of the lesion in 'inner cerebral trauma'. Rad Yug Acad Sci 1982; 402:265–331.

139. Hahn YS, Raimondi AJ, McClone DC, et al. Traumatic mechanisms of head injury in child abuse. Childs Brain 1983; 10:229–241.

140. Hobbs CJ. Skull fracture and the diagnosis of abuse. Arch Dis Child 1984; 59:246–252.

141. Mayr JM, Seebacher U, Lawrenz K, et al. Bunk beds – a still underestimated risk for accidents in childhood? Eur J Pediatr 2000; 159(6):440–443.

142. Macgregor DM. Injuries associated with falls from beds. Inj Prev 2000; 6:291–292.

143. Belechri M, Petridou E, Trichopoulos D. Bunk versus conventional beds: a comparative assessment of fall injury risk. J Epidemiol Community Health 2002; 56:413–417.

144. Chiaviello CT, Christoph RA, Bond GR. Infant walker-related injuries: a prospective study of severity and incidence. Pediatrics 1994; 93(6): 974–976.

145. Stoffman JM, Bass MJ, Fox AM. Head injuries related to the use of baby walkers. Can Med Assoc J 1984; 131:573–575.

146. Smith AG, Bowman MJ, Luria JW. Babywalker-related injuries continue despite warning labels and public education. Pediatrics 1997; 100(2).

147. Chiaviello CT, Christoph RA, Bond GR. Stairway-related injuries in children. Pediatrics 1994; 94(5):679–681.

148. Weber W. On the biomechanical fragility of the infant skull. Z Rechtsmed 1985; 94:93–101.

149. Wilkins, B. Head injury: abuse or accident? Arch Dis Child 1997; 76(5):393–396.

150. Reiber GD. Fatal falls in childhood. How far must children fall to sustain fatal head injury? Report of cases and review of the literature. Am J Forensic Med Pathol 1993; 14:201–207.

151. Hall JR, Reyes HM, Horvat M, et al. The mortality of childhood falls. J Trauma 1989; 29:1273–1275.

152. Byard RW, Tsokos M. Infant and early childhood asphyxial deaths. In: Tsokos M ed. Forensic pathology reviews. Vol. 2. Totowa: Humana Press; 2004:101–123.

153. Saukko P, Knight B. Suffocation and 'asphyxia' and fatal pressure on the neck. In: Saukko P, Knight B. Knight's forensic pathology. 3rd edn. London: Arnold; 2004:352–394.

154. Baker SP, Fisher FS. Childhood asphyxiation by choking or suffocation. JAMA 1980; 244:1343–1346.

155. Scheers NJ, Rutherford GW, Kemp JS. Where should infants sleep? A comparison of risk for suffocation of infants sleeping in cribs, adult beds, and other sleeping locations. Pediatrics 2003; 112(4):883–889.

156. Byard RW. Hazardous infant and early childhood sleeping environments and death scene examination. J Clin Forensic Med 1996; 3(3):115–122.

157. Collins KA. Death by overlaying and wedging. Am J Forensic Med Pathol 2001; 22(2):155–159.

158. Sturner WQ, Spruill FG, Smith RA, et al. Accidental asphyxial deaths involving infants and young children. J Forensic Sci 1976; 21:483–487.

159. Smialek MD, Smialek PZ, Spita WN. Accidental bed deaths in infants due to unsafe sleeping conditions. Clin Pediatr 1977; 16:1031–1036.

160. Rothman BF, Boeckman CR. Foreign bodies in the larynx and tracheo-bronchial tree of children: a review of 225 cases. Ann Otol Rhinol Laryngol 1980; 89: 434–436.

161. Stallings CS, Baker SP. Childhood asphyxiation by food: a national analysis and overview. JAMA 1984; 251:2231–2235.

162. Mittleman RE. Fatal choking in infants and children. Am J Forensic Med Pathol 1987; 5:201–210.

163. Amanuel B, Byard RW. Accidental asphyxia in bed in severely disabled children. J Paediatr Child Health 2000; 36(1):66–68.

164. Kemp JS, Unger B, Wilkins D, et al. Unsafe sleep practices and an analysis of bedsharing among infants dying suddenly and unexpectedly: results of a four-year, population-based, death-scene investigation study of sudden infant death syndrome and related deaths. Pediatrics 2000; 106(3):41–48.

165. Gilbert-Barness E, Hegstrand L, Chandra S, et al. Hazards of mattresses, beds and bedding in deaths of infants. Am J Forensic Med Pathol 1991; 12:27–32.

166. Drago DA, Dannenberg AL. Infant mechanical suffocation deaths in the United States 1980–1997. Pediatrics 1999; 103(5):59–66.

167. Mitchell EA, Thach BT, Thompson JM, et al. Changing infants' sleep position increases risk of sudden infant death syndrome. Arch Pediatr Adolesc Med 1999; 153:1136–1141.

168. Scheers NJ, Dayton CM, Kemp JS. Sudden infant death with external airways covered: case-comparison study of 206 deaths in the United States. Arch Pediatr Adolesc Med 1998; 152:540–547.

169. Merchant JR, Worwa C, Porter S, et al. Respiratory instability of term and near-term healthy newborn infants in car safety seats. Pediatrics 2001; 108(3):647–652.

170. Thogmartin JR, Siebert CF, Pellan WA. Sleep position and bed-sharing in sudden infant deaths: an examination of autopsy findings. J Pediatr 2001; 138(2):212–217.

171. Blair PS, Fleming PJ, Smith IJ, et al. Babies sleeping with parents: case-control study of factors influencing the risk of the sudden infant death syndrome. BMJ 1999; 319(4):1457–1462.

172. Jaffe FA. Petechial hemorrhages – a review of pathogenesis. Am J Forensic Med Pathol 1994; 15(3):203–307.

173. Ely SF, Hirsch CS. Asphyxial deaths and petechiae: a review. J Forensic Sci 2000; 45(6):1274–1277.

174. Moore L, Byard RW. Pathological findings in hanging and wedging deaths in infants and young children. Am J Forensic Med Pathol 1993; 14:296–302.

175. Delmonte C, Capelozzi VL. Morphologic determinants of asphyxia in lungs. Am J Forensic Med Pathol 2001; 22:139–149.

176. Yukawa N, Carter N, Rutty G, et al. Intra-alveolar haemorrhage in sudden infant death syndrome: a cause for concern? J Clin Pathol 1999; 52(8): 581–587.

177. Centers for Disease Control and Prevention. Acute idiopathic pulmonary hemorrhage among infants. MMWR Morbidity and Mortality Weekly Report 2004; 53(RR-2).

178. Jackson CM, Gilliland MGF. Frequency of pulmonary hemosiderosis in eastern North Carolina. Am J Forensic Med Pathol 2000; 21(1):36–38.

179. Hanzlick R, Delaney K. Pulmonary hemosiderin in deceased infants: baseline data for further study of infant mortality. Am J Forensic Med Pathol 2000; 21(4):319–322.

180. Delaney K, Hanzlick R, Wolfe M. Pulmonary macrophage counts in deceased infants: baseline data for further study of infant mortality. Am J Forensic Med Pathol 2000; 21(4):315–318.

181. Schluckebier DA, Cool CD, Henry TE, et al. Pulmonary siderophages and unexpected infant death. Am J Forensic Med Pathol 2002; 23(4):360–363.

182. Milroy CM. Munchausen syndrome by proxy and intra-alveolar haemosiderin. Int J Legal Med 1999; 112(5):309–312.

183. Krous HF, Nadeau JM, Byard RW, et al. Oronasal blood in sudden infant death. Am J Forensic Med Pathol 2001; 22(4):346–351.

184. Byard RW, Krous HF. Diagnostic and mediocolegal problems with sudden infant death syndrome. In: Tsokos M ed. Forensic pathology reviews. Vol. 1. Totowa: Humana Press; 2004:189–198.

185. Guilian GG, Gilbert EF, Moss RL. Elevated fetal hemoglobin levels in sudden infant death syndrome. N Engl J Med 1987; 316:1122–1126.

186. Gilbert-Barness E, Kenison K, Carver J. Fetal hemoglobin and sudden infant death syndrome. Arch Pathol Lab Med 1993; 117:177–179.

187. Fagan DG, Lancashire RJ, Walker A, et al. Determinants of fetal hemoglobin in newborn infants. Arch Dis Child 1995; 72:F111–114.

188. Byard RW, Cote A, Praud JP, et al. Fetal hemoglobin synthesis determined by Y-mRNA/Y-mRNA + B-mRNA quantitation in infants at risk for sudden infant death syndrome being monitored at home for apnea. Pediatrics 2003; 112:285–288.

189. Leach CEA, Blair PS, Fleming PJ, et al. Epidemiology of SIDS and explained sudden infant deaths. Pediatrics 1999; 104:43–52.

190. Krous HF. Intrathoracic petechiae in sudden infant death syndrome: relationship to face position when found. Pediatr Dev Pathol 2001; 4:160–166.

191. Risse M, Weiler G. Resuscitation measures and petechial thymus hemorrhages in sudden infant death. Z Rechtsmed 1990; 103(3):207–212.

192. Risse M, Weiler G. Differential diagnosis SIDS/non-SIDS on the basis of histological findings of petechial thymus hemorrhages. Forensic Sci Int 1989; 34(1):1–7.

193. Firstman R, Talen J. The death of innocents. New York: Bantam; 1997.

194. Ladham S, Koehler SA, Shakir A, et al. Simultaneous sudden infant death syndrome: a case report. Am J Forensic Med Pathol 2001; 22(1):33–37.

195. Beckwith JB. Defining the sudden infant death syndrome. Arch Pediatr Adolesc Med 2003; 157:286–290.

196. Rognum TO, Arnestad M, Bajanowski T, et al. Consensus of diagnostic criteria for the exclusion of SIDS. Nordisk Rettsmedisin NR 2003; 3/4: 62–73.

197. Sadler DW. The value of a thorough protocol in the investigation of sudden infant deaths. J Clin Pathol 1998; 51(9):689–694.

198. Carolan PL. Sudden infant death syndrome. Online. Available:http://www.emedicine.com/ped/topic2171.htm

199. Byard RW, Krous HF. Sudden infant death syndrome. New York: Oxford University Press; 2001.

200. Byard RW, Cohle SD. Sudden infant death syndrome. In: Byard RW, ed. Sudden death in infancy and childhood and adolescence. 2nd edn. Cambridge: Cambridge University Press; 2004:491–575.

201. Valdes-Dapena M, McFeeley PA, Hoffman HJ, et al. Histopathology atlas for the sudden infant death syndrome. Washington: Armed Forces Institute of Pathology; 1993.

202. Saukko P, Knight B. Immersion deaths. In: Saukko P, Knight B, eds. Knight's forensic pathology. 3rd edn. London: Arnold; 2004:395–411.

203. Golden FS, Tipton MJ, Scott RC. Immersion, near-drowning and drowning. Br J Anaesth 1997; 79:214–225.

204. Sarniak AP, Vohra MP. Near-drowning: fresh, salt, and cold water immersion. Clin Sports Med 1986; 5:33–46.

205. Pearn J. Pathophysiology of drowning. Med J Aust 1985; 142:586–588.

206. Modell JH. Current concepts: drowning. N Engl J Med 1993; 328:253–256.

207. Spyker DA. Submersion injury: epidemiology, prevention and management. Pediatr Clin North Am 1985; 32:113–115.

208. Idris AH, Berg RA, Bierens J, et al. Recommended guidelines for uniform reporting of data from drowning: the 'utstein style.' Circulation 2003; 108:2565–2574.

209. Pearn JH, Brown J, Wong R, et al. Bathtub drownings: report of seven cases. Pediatrics 1979; 64:68–70.

210. Saxena A, Ang LC. Epilepsy and bathtub drowning: important neuropathological observations. Am J Forensic Med Pathol 1993; 14:125–129.

211. Feldman KW. Immersion injury in child abuse and neglect. In: Reece RM. Ludwig S, eds. Child abuse: medical diagnosis and management. 2nd edn. Philadelphia: Lippincott Williams & Wilkins; 2001:443–452.

212. Griest KJ, Zumwalt RE. Child abuse by drowning. Pediatrics 1989; 83:41–46.

213. Nixon J, Pearn J. Non-accidental immersion in bathwater: another aspect of child abuse. Br Med J 1977; 1:271–272.

214. Nixon J, Pearn J. Non-accidental immersion in the bath: another extension to the syndrome of child abuse and neglect. Child Abuse Negl 1977; 1:445–446.

215. Scott PH, Eigen H. Immersion accidents involving pails of water in the home. J Pediatr 1980; 96:282–284.

216. Tron VA, Baldwin VJ, Pirie GE. Hot tub drownings. Pediatrics 1985; 75:789–799.

217. Nguyen S, Kuschel C, Teele R, et al. Water birth – a near-drowning experience. Pediatrics 2002; 110:411–413.

218. Kaga K, Nitou T, Suzuki JI, et al. Temporal bone pathology findings due to drowning. Rev Laryngol Otol Rhinol 1999; 120(1):27–29.

219. Mizushima H, Hanakawa K, Kobayashi N, et al. Acute subdural hematoma due to near-drowning. Neurol Med Chir (Tokyo) 1999; 39:752–755.

220. Dubowitz DJ, Bluml S, Arcinue E, et al. MR of hypoxic encephalopathy in children after near drowning: correlation with quantitative proton MR spectroscopy and clinical outcome. Am J Neuroradiol 1998; 19:1617–1627.

221. Volpe JJ. Hypoxic-ischemic encephalopathy: biochemical and physiological aspects. In: Neurology of the newborn. 3rd edn. Philadelphia: Saunders; 1991:211–259.

222. Saukko P, Knight B. Burns and scalds. In: Saukko P, Knight B, eds. Knight's forensic pathology. 3rd edn. London: Arnold; 2004:312–325.

223. Settle JA. Burns. In: Mason JK, Purdue BN, eds. The pathology of trauma. 3rd edn. London: Arnold; 2000:211–229.

224. Jenny C. Cutaneous manifestations of child abuse. In: Reece RM, Ludwig S, eds. Child abuse: medical diagnosis and management. 2nd edn. Philadelphia: Lippincott Williams & Wilkins; 2001:23–45.

225. Waller AE, Baker SP, Szocka A. Childhood injury deaths: national analysis and geographic variations. Am J Public Health 1989; 79:310–315.

226. Nazarian EB, Connolly H. Inhalation injury. E-Medicine. Online. Available: http://www.emedicine.com/ped/topic1189.htm

227. Lafferty KA. Smoke inhalation. E-Medicine. Online. Available: http://www.emedicine.com/emerg/topic538.htm

228. Jaffe FA. Pathogenicity of carbon monoxide. Am J Forensic Med Pathol 1997; 18(4):406–410.

229. Lucchesi M, Shochat G. Toxicity, carbon monoxide. E-Medicine. Online. Available: http://www.emedicine.com/ped/topic315.htm

230. Moritz AR, Henriques FC. Studies of thermal injury: the relative importance of time and temperature in the causation of cutaneous burns. Am J Pathol 1947; 23:695–720.

231. Feldman KW. Child abuse by burning. In: Helfer RE, Kempe RS, eds. The battered child. 4th edn. Chicago: University of Chicago Press; 1987:197–213.

232. Feldman KW. Help needed on hot water burns. Pediatrics 1983; 71:145–146.

233. Feldman KW, Schaller RT, Feldman JA, et al. Tap water scald burns in children. Pediatrics 1978; 62:1–7.

234. Stevens BG. Medico-legal aspects of child abuse, mini-course materials. Society for Pediatric Pathology; 1984.

235. Showers J, Garrison KM. Burn abuse: a four year study. J Trauma 1988; 28:1581–1583.

236. Alexander AC, Surrell JA, Cohle SD. Microwave oven burns to children: an unusual manifestation of child abuse. Pediatrics 1987; 79(2): 255–260.

237. Watkins AH, Gagan RJ, Cupoli JM. Child abuse by burning. J Fla Med Assoc 1985; 72:497–502.

238. Hight DW, Bakalar HR, Lloyd JR. Inflicted burns in children – recognition and treatment. JAMA 1979; 242:517–520.

239. Purdue GF, Hunt JL, Prescott PR. Child abuse by burning – an index of suspicion. J Trauma 1988; 28:221–224.

240. Cox R, Brooks J. Burns, chemical. Online. Available:http://www.emedicine.com/emerg/topic73.htm

241. Kardon E. Toxicity, caustic ingestions. Online. Available:http://www.emedicine.com/emerg/topic86.htm

242. Koumbourlis AC. Electrical injuries. Crit Care Med 2002; 30(11 Suppl): S424–430.

243. Hostetler MA. Burns, electrical. E-Medicine. Online. Available: http://www.emedicine.com/ped/topic2734.htm

244. Wright RK. Electrical Injuries. E-Medicine. Online. Available: http://www.emedicine.com/emerg/topic162.htm

245. Budnick LD. Bathtub-related electrocutions in the United States, 1979–1982. JAMA 1984; 252:918–920.

246. Simon HB. Hyperthermia, fever, and fever of undetermined origin. Mechem CC. Temperature-related emergencies. Sci Am Med 2000; XXIV:1–11

248. Kunihiro A, Foster J. Heat exhaustion and heatstroke. E-Medicine. Online. Avaiable: http://www.emedicine.com/emerg/topic236.htm

249. Schwarz MN, Simon HB. Pathophysiology of fever and fever of unknown origin. Sci Am 1989; 7(XXIV):1–12.

250. Robinson MD, Seward PN. Heat injury in children. Pediatr Emerg Care 1987; 3:114–117.

251. LeBlanc MH. The physics of thermal exchange between infants and their environment. Med Instrumentation 1987; 21:11–15.

252. Bolton DPB, Nelson EAS, Taylor BJ, et al. Thermal balance in infants. J Appl Physiol 1996; 80(6):2234–2242.

253. King K, Vance JC. Heat stress in motor vehicles: a problem in infancy. Pediatrics 1981; 68:579–582.

254. Zumwalt RE, Petty CS, Holman W. Temperatures in closed automobiles in hot weather. Forensic Sci Gazette 1976; 7:7–8.

255. Stanton AN. Is overheating a factor in some unexpected infant deaths? Lancet 1980; 1(8177):1054–1057.

256. Scheers-Masters JR, Schootman M, Thach BT. Heat stress and sudden infant death syndrome incidence: a United States population epidemiologic study. Pediatrics 2004; 113:586–592.

257. Elabbassi EB, Bach V, Makki M, et al. Assessment of dry heat exchanges in newborns: influence of body position and clothing in SIDS. J Appl Physiol 2001; 91:51–56.

258. Bacon CJ. Overheating in infancy. Arch Dis Child 1983; 58:673–674.

259. Rutter N, Hull D. Response of term babies to a warm environment. Arch Dis Child 1979; 54:178–183.

260. Gozal D, Colin AA, et al. Environmental overheating as a cause of transient respiratory chemoreceptor dysfunction in an infant. Pediatrics 1988; 82:738–740.

261. Bass H, Moore JL, Coakley WT. Lethality in mammalian cells due to hyperthermia under oxic and hypoxic conditions. Int J Radiat Biol 1978; 33:57–67.

262. Levin M, Hjelm M, Kay JD, et al. Haemorrhagic shock and encephalopathy: a new syndrome with a high mortality in young children. Lancet; 2983(ii):64–67.

263. Little D, Wilkins B. Hemorrhagic shock and encephalopathy syndrome: an unusual cause of sudden death in children. Am J Forensic Med Pathol 1997; 18(1):79–83.

264. Chaves-Carballo E, Montes JE, Nelson WB, et al. Hemorrhagic shock and encephalopathy – clinical definition of a catastrophic syndrome in infants. Am J Dis Child 1990 Oct; 144(10):1079–1082.

265. Thebaud B, Husson B, Navelet Y, et al. Haemorrhagic shock and encephalopathy syndrome: neurological course and predictors of outcomes. Intensive Care Med 1999; 25(3):293–299.

266. Jardine DS, Bratton SL. Using characteristic changes in laboratory values to assist in the diagnosis of hemorrhagic shock and encephalopathy syndrome. Pediatrics 1995; 96:1126–1131.

267. Krous HF, Naduea JM, Fukumoto RI, et al. Environmental l hyperthermic infant and early childhood death. Am J Forensic Med Pathol 2001; 22(4):374–382.

268. Janssen W. Forensic histopathology. Berlin: Springer-Verlag; 1984:258–260.

269. Tedeschi CG. Systemic and localized hyperthermic injury. In: Tedeschi CG, Eckert WG, Tedeschi LG, eds. Forensic medicine, a study in trauma and environmental hazards. Vol 1. Philadelphia: WB Saunders; 1977: 701–723.

270. Donoghue RE, Graham MA, Jentzen JM, et al. Criteria for the diagnosis of heat-related deaths: National Association of Medical Examiners: position paper. Am J Forensic Med Pathol 1997; 18(1):11–14.

271. Bacon C, Scott D, Jones P. Heatstroke in well-wrapped infants. Lancet 1979; 1(8113):442–425.

272. Bacon CJ, Bellman MH. Heatstroke as a possible cause of encephalopathy in infants. Br Med J 1983; 287:328.

273. Fitzgerald FT, Jessop C. Accidental hypothermia: a report of 22 cases and review of the literature. Adv Intern Med 1982; 27:127–150.

274. Savides EP, Hoffbrand BI. Hypothermia, thrombosis, and acute pancreatitis. Br Med J 1974; 1:614.

275. Hirvonen J. Systemic and local effects of hypothermia. In: Tedeschi CG, Eckert WG, Tedeschi LG, eds. Forensic medicine, a study in trauma and environmental hazards. Vol 1. Philadelphia: WB Saunders; 1977: 758–774.

276. Saukko P, Knight B. Neglect, starvation and hypothermia. In: Saukko P, Knight B, eds. Knight's forensic pathology. 3rd edn. London: Arnold; 2004:412–420.

277. Decker W, Li J. Hypothermia. E-Medicine. Online. Available: http://www.emedicine.com. 08/14/2001

278. Phillips TG. Hypothermia. E-Medicine. Online. Available: http://www.emedicine.com. 10/19/2001

279. Mallet ML. Pathophysiology of accidental hypothermia. Q J Med 2002; 95:775–785.

280. Hickey RW, Kochanek PM, Kerimer H, et al. Hypothermia and hyperthermia in children after resuscitation from cardiac arrest. Pediatrics 2000; 106:118–112.

281. Desai PR, Sriskandan S. Hypothermia in a child secondary to ibuprofen. Arch Dis Child 2003; 88:87–88.

282. Kuo DC, Jerrard DA. Environmental insults: smoke inhalation, submersion, diving, and high altitude. Emerg Med Clin North Am 2003; 21(2):475–497.

283. Roach RC, Bartsch P, Oelz O, et al. Lake Louise AMS Scoring consensus Committee. The Lake Louise acute mountain sickness scoring system. In: Sutton JR, Houston CS, Coates G, eds. Hypoxia and molecular medicine. Burlington VT: Queen City Press; 1993:272–274.

284. Pollard AJ, Niermeyer S, Barry P, et al. ISMM Consensus Statement. Children at high altitude: an international consensus statement by an ad hoc committee of the international society for mountain medicine, March 12, 2001. Online. Available: http://www.ismmed.org/ISMM_Children_at_Altitude.htm

285. Duster MC. Pulmonary hypertension, high altitude. E-Medicine. Online. Available: http://www.emedicine.com/ped/topic2783.htm

286. Dietz TE. Altitude sickness – cerebral syndromes. E-Medicine. Online. Available: http://www.emedicine.com/emerg/topic22.htm

287. Kohlendorfer U, Kiechl S, Sperl W. Living at high altitude and risk of sudden infant death syndrome. Arch Dis Child 1998; 79:506–509.

288. Baselt RC. Disposition of toxic drugs and chemicals in man. 5th edn. Foster City: Chemical Toxicology Institute; 2000.

289. Michael JG, Sztajnkrycer MD. Deadly pediatric poisons: nine common agents that kill at low doses. Emerg Med Clin North Am 2004; 22:1019–1050.

290. Miles FK, Kamath R, Dorney SFA, et al. Accidental paracetamol overdosing and fulminant hepatic failure in children. Med J Aust 1999; 171:472–475.

291. Boland DM, Rein J, Lew EO, et al. Case report: fatal cold medication intoxication in an infant. J Anal Toxicol 2003; 27(7):523–526.

292. Kirk MA, Tomaszewski C, Kulig K. Poisoning in children. In: Reisdorf EJ, Roberts MR, Wiegenstein JG, eds. Pediatric emergency medicine. Philadelphia: WB Saunders; 1993.

293. Woolf AD. Poisoning in children and adolescents. Pediatr Rev 1993; 14:411–422.

294. Regan FA, Samuels MS, Hite SA. Ethanol ingestion in children. JAMA 1979; 242:2787–2788.

295. Densen-Gerber J. Forensic pathology of drug related child abuse. In: Legal medicine annual. New York: Appleton-Century-Croft; 1979:135–147.

296. Mullick FG, Drake DM, Irey NS. Morphologic changes in adverse drug reactions in infants and children. Hum Pathol 1977; 8:361–378.

297. Mullick FG. Adverse effects of drugs and toxins in the pediatric age group. Forensic Sci Int 1986; 30:155–161.

298. Whyte J, Greenan E. Drug usage and adverse drug reactions in paediatric patients. Acta Paediatr Scand 1977; 66:767–775.

299. Mullick FG. Adverse drug reactions in the pediatric age group. Annual course in pediatric pathology. Washington: Armed Forces Institute of Pathology; 1994.

300. Brody DJ. Blood lead levels in the US population: phase II of the Third National Health and Nutrition Examination Survey (NAHANES III, 1988 to 1991). JAMA 1994; 272:277–283.

301. World Health Organization. Environmental toxic exposures and poisoning in children. Online. Available: http://www.mindfully.org/Health/Children-Exposures-Poisoning-WHO11oct01.htm

302. Gupta SK, Peshin SS, Srivastava A, et al. A study of childhood poisoning at national poisons information centre, All India Institute of Medical Science, New Delhi. J Occup Health 2003; 45:191–196.

303. Bays J, Feldman KW. Child abuse by poisoning. In: Reece RM. Ludwig S, eds. Child abuse: medical diagnosis and management. 2nd edn. Philadelphia: Lippincott Williams & Wilkins; 2001:405–441.

304. Rogers D. Non-accidental poisoning: an extended syndrome of child abuse. Br Med J 1976; 1:793–796.

305. Watson JBG, Davies JM, Hunter JLP. Nonaccidental poisoning in childhood. Arch Dis Child 1979; 54:143–144.

306. Lorber J, Reckless JPD, Watson JB. Nonaccidental poisoning: the elusive diagnosis. Arch Dis Child 1980; 55:643–647.

307. Shnaps Y, Frand M, Roten Y, et al. The chemically abused child. Pediatrics 1981; 68:119–121.

308. Dine MS, McGovern ME. Intentional poisoning of children – an overlooked category of child abuse: report of seven cases and review of the literature. Pediatrics 1982; 70:32–35.

309. Case MES, Short CD, Polkis A. Intoxication by aspirin and alcohol in a child. Am J Forensic Med Pathol 1983; 4:149–151.

310. Tilelli JA, Ophoven JP. Hyponatremic seizures as a presenting symptom of child abuse. Forensic Sci Int 1986; 30:213–217.

311. Buchta R. Deliberate intoxication of young children and pets with drugs: a survey of an adolescent population in a private practice. Am J Dis Child 1988; 142:701–702.

312. Hickson GB, Altemeier WA, Martin ED, et al. Parental administration of chemical agents: a cause of apparent life-threatening events. Pediatrics 1989; 83:772–776.

313. Rivenes SM, Bakerman PR, Miller MB. Intentional caffeine poisoning in an infant. Pediatrics 1997; 99(5):736–737.

314. Morrow PL. Caffeine toxicity: a case of child abuse by drug ingestion. J Forensic Sci 1987; 32:1801–1805.

315. Perez A, Scribano PV. An intentional opiate intoxication of an infant: when medical toxicology and child maltreatment services merge. Pediatr Emerg Care 2004; 2(11):769–772.

316. Valentine JL, Schexnayder S, Jones JG, et al. Clinical and toxicological findings in two young siblings and autopsy findings in one sibling with multiple hospital admissions resulting in death: evidence suggesting Munchausen syndrome by proxy. Am J Forensic Med Pathol 1997; 18(3):276–281.

317. Baker C, Kadish H, Schunk JE. Evaluation of pediatric cervical spine injuries. Am J Emerg Med 1999; 17:230–234.

318. Giroud C, Mangin P. Drug assay and interpretation of results. In: Payne-James J, Busuttil A, Smock W eds. Forensic medicine: clinical and pathological aspects. London: Greenwich Medical Media; 2003:609–621.

319. Armstrong EJ, Jenkins AJ, Sebrosky GF, et al. An unusual fatality in a child due to oxycodone. Am J Forensic Med Pathol 2004; 25(4):338–341.

320. Shepherd MF, Lake KD, Kamps MA. Postmortem changes and pharmacokinetics: review of the literature and case report. Ann Pharmacother 1992; 26:510–514.

321. Richardson T. Pitfalls in forensic toxicology. Ann Clin Biochem 2000; 37:20–44.

322. Laroia N. Birth Trauma. Online. Available:http://www.emedicine.com/ped/topic2836.htm

323. Ali J. Predictors of fetal mortality in pregnant trauma patients. J Trauma 1997; 42(5):782–785.

324. Weiss HB, Songer TJ, Fabio A. Fetal deaths related to maternal injury. JAMA 2001; 286(15):1863–1868.

325. Dobo SM, Johnson VS. Office management of trauma: evaluation and care of the pregnant patient with minor trauma. Emergenza 2000:1–24.

326. Pollina J, Dias MS, Li V, et al. Cranial birth injuries in term newborn infants. Pediatr Neurosurg 2001; 35(3):113–119.

327. Hayashi T, Hashimoto T, Fukuda S, et al. Neonatal subdural hematoma secondary to birth injury. Child Nerv Syst 1987; 3:23–29.

328. Chamnanvanakij S, Rollins N, Perlman JM. Subdural hematoma in term infants. Pediatr Neurol 2002; 26(4):301–304.

329. Haase R, Jursaw I, Nagel F, et al. Acute subdural hematoma after caesarean section: a case report. Pediatr Crit Care Med 2003:4(2):246–248.

330. Scher MS, Wiznitzer M, Bangert BA. Cerebral infarctions in the fetus and neonate: maternal-placental-fetal considerations. Clin Perinatol 2002; 29:693–724.

331. Nelson KB, Lynch JK. Stroke in newborn infants. Lancet 2004; 3:150–158.

332. Ozduman K, Pober BR, Barnes P, et al. Fetal stroke. J Pediatr Neurol 2004; 30(3):151–162.

333. Golomb MR, Dick PT, MacGregor DL, et al. Cranial ultrasonography has a low sensitivity for detecting arterial ischemic stroke in term neonates. J Child Neurol 2003:18:98–103.

334. Schwartz R, Peary P, Mistretta D. Intoxication of young children with marijuana: a form of amusement for 'pot'-smoking teenage girls. Am J Dis Child 1986; 140:326.

335. Deren S. Children of substance abusers: a review of the literature. J Subst Abuse Treat 1986; 3:77–94.

336. Larson E. Intoxication in utero. In: Mason JK, ed. Paediatric forensic medicine and pathology. London: Chapman and Hall; 1989:37–47.

337. Tomison AM. Child maltreatment and substance abuse. National Child Protection Clearing House. Online. Available: http://www.aifs.gov.au/nch/discussion2.html#defs

338. California Fetal Alcohol Spectrum Organization. Online. Available:http://www.calfas.org/fasdfacts.htm

339. Streissguth AP, Clarren SK, Jones KL. A natural history of the fetal alcohol syndrome – a 10-year follow-up of 11 patients. Alcohol Health Res World 1985; 2(8446):85–91.

340. Kruse J. Alcohol use during pregnancy. Am Fam Physician 1984; 29:199–203.

341. Webb S, Hocjberg MS, Sher MR. Fetal alcohol syndrome: report of case. JAMA 1988; 116:196–198.

342. Deren S. Children of substance abusers: a review of the literature. J Subst Abuse Treat 1986; 3:77–94.

343. Finnegan LP. The effects of narcotics and alcohol on pregnancy and the newborn. Ann N Y Acad Sci 1981; 362:136–157.

344. Cregler LL, Mark H. Medical complications of cocaine abuse. N Engl J Med 1986; 315:1495–1500.

345. Volpe JJ. Mechanisms of disease: effect of cocaine use on the fetus. N Engl J Med 1992; 327:399–407.

346. Chasnoff IJ, Burns WJ, Schnoll SH. Cocaine use in pregnancy. N Engl J Med 1985; 313:666–669.

347. Chavez CJ, Ostrea EM, Stryker JC. Sudden infant death syndrome among infants of drug-dependent mothers. J Pediatr 1979; 95:407–409.

348. Kautman KR, Petrucha RA, Pitts FN Jr, et al. Phencyclidine in umbilical cord blood: preliminary data. Am J Psychiatry 1983; 140:450–452.

349. Landwirth J. Fetal abuse and neglect: an emerging controversy. Pediatrics 1987; 79:508–514.

350. Shaw MW. Conditional prospective rights of the fetus. J Leg Med 1984; 5:63–116.

351. Nelson LJ, Milliken N. Compelled medical treatment of women-life, liberty, and law in conflict. JAMA 1988; 259:1060–1066.

352. Camissa SM, Ziontz N. Beyond the right to life – the right to health. Leg Med 1987; 1:179–199.

353. MacMahon JR. Perinatal substance abuse: the impact of reporting infants to child protective services. Pediatrics 1997; 100(5):E1.

354. Golden MH, Samuels MP, Southall DP. How to distinguish between neglect and deprivational abuse. Arch Dis Child 2003; 88:105–107.

355. Caffey J. Multiple fractures of long bones in infants suffering from subdural hematoma. AJR Am J Roentgenol 1946; 56:163–173.

356. Silverman FN. The roentgen manifestation of unrecognized skeletal trauma in infants. AJR Am J Roentgenol 1952; 69:413–427.

357. Kempe CH, Silverman FN, Steele BF, et al. The battered child syndrome. JAMA 1962; 181:17–24.

358. Knight B. The history of child abuse. Forensic Sci Int 1986; 30:135–141.

359. Radbill SX. Children in a world of violence: a history of child abuse. In: Helfer RE, Kempe RS, eds. The battered child. 4th edn. Chicago: The University of Chicago Press; 1987:3–22.

360. Lynch MA. Child abuse before Kempe: an historical literature review. Child Abuse Negl 1985; 9:7–15.

361. National Clearinghouse on Child Abuse and Neglect. Child abuse and neglect fatalities: statistics and interventions. 2004. Online. Available: http://nccanch.acf.hhs.gov

362. Olesen T, Egeblad M, et al. Somatic manifestations of children suspected of having been maltreated. Acta Paediatr Scand 1988; 77:154–160.

363. Sedlak AJ, Broadhurst DD. Executive Summary of the Third National Incidence Study of Child Abuse and Neglect. 1996. Online. Available: http://nccanch.acf.hhs.gov/pubs/statisinfo/nis3.cfm.

364. Overpeck MD, Brenner RA, Trumble AC, et al. Risk factors for infant homicide in the United States. N Engl J Med 1998; 339:1211–1216.

365. Strait RT, Siegel RM, Shapiro RA. Humeral fractures without obvious etiologies in children less than 3 years of age: when is it abuse? Pediatrics 1995; 96(4):667–671.

366. Wissow LS. Child abuse and neglect – review article. N Engl J Med 1995; 332(21):1425–1431

367. Southall DP, Samuels MP, Golden MH. Classification of child abuse by motive and degree rather than type of injury. Arch Dis Child 2003; 88:101–104.

368. National Clearinghouse on Child Abuse and Neglect. 2003 Child abuse and neglect state statute series statutes-at-a-glance: definitions of child abuse and neglect. Online. Available: http://nccanch.acf.hhs.gov

369. Gothard TW, Runyan DK, Hadler JL. The diagnosis and evaluation of child maltreatment. J Emerg Med 1985; 3:181–194.

370. Norman MG, Smialek JE, Newman DE, et al. The postmortem examination on the abused child. Perspect Pediatr Pathol 1984; 8:313–343.

371. Reece RM, Grodin MA. Recognition of nonaccidental injury. Pediatr Clin North Am 1985; 32:41–60.

372. Schmitt BD. The child with nonaccidental trauma. In: Helfer RE, Kempe RS, eds. The battered child. 4th ed. Chicago: University of Chicago Press; 1981:178–196.

373. Polansky NA, Chalmers MA, Buttenwieser EW, et al. Damaged parents: an anatomy of child neglect. Chicago: University of Chicago Press; 1981.

374. US Department of Health and Human Serivces, Gaudin. Child neglect: a guide for intervention. User manual series 1993. Online. Avaiable: http://www.nccanch.acf.hhs.gov/pubs/ usermanuals/neglect/neglectb.cfm

375. Asser SM, Swan R. Child fatalities from religion-motivated medical neglect. Pediatrics 1998; 101:625–629.

376. Ridgway D. Court-mediated disputes between physicians and families over the medical care of children. Arch Pediatr Adolesc Med 2004; 158:891–896.

377. Lin A, Santoro D. Protein-energy malnutrition. Online. Available: http://www.emedicine.com/derm/topic797.htm

378. Gahagan S, Holmes R. A stepwise approach to evaluation of under-nutrition and failure to thrive. Pediatr Clin North Am 1998; 45(1):169–187.

379. Schwartz D. Failure to thrive: an old nemesis in the new millennium. Pediatr Rev 2000; 21(8):257–264.

380. Kane ML. Pediatric failure to thrive. Clin Fam Pract 2003; 5(2):293–311.

381. Kumar S, Olson DL, Schwenk WF. Malnutrition in the pediatric population. Dis Month 2002; 48(11):703–712.

382. Madea B. Death as a result of starvation: diagnostic criteria. In: Tsokos M, ed. Forensic pathology reviews. Vol 2. Totowa: Humana Press:3–23.

383. Beck FK. Prealbumin: a marker for nutritional evaluation. Am Fam Physician 2002; 65(8):1575–1578.

384. Chatoor I, Ganiban J, Colin V, et al. Attachment and feeding problems: a reexamination of nonorganic failure to thrive and attachment insecurity. J Am Acad Child Adolesc Psychiatry 1998; 37(11):1217–1224.

385. Shetty PS. Adaptation to low energy intakes: the responses and limits to low intakes in infants, children and adults. Eur J Clin Nutr 1999; 53 (suppl 1):S14–33.

386. Marchini G, Persson B, Berggren V, et al. Hunger behaviour contributes to early nutritional homeostasis. Acta Paediatr 1998; 87(6):671–675.

387. Gremse DA. Characterization of failure to imbibe in infants. Clin Pediatr (Phila) 1998; 37(5):305–309.

388. Tolia V. Very early onset nonorganic failure to thrive in infants. J Pediatr Gastroenterol Nutr 1995; 20(1):73–80.

389. Grigsby DG. Malnutrition. Online. Available: http://www.emedicine.com/ped/topic1360.htm

390. Carvalho NF, Kenney RD, Carrington PH, et al. Severe nutritional deficiencies in toddlers resulting from health food milk alternatives. Pediatrics 2001; 107(4):46–52.

391. Pugliese MR, Blumberg DL, Hludzinski J, et al. Nutritional rickets in suburbia. J Am Coll Nutr 1998; 17(6):637–641.

392. Taitz LS, King M. Growth patterns in child abuse. Acta Paediatr Scand 1988 (suppl); 343:62–72.

393. Karp RJ, Scholl TO, Decker E, et al. Growth of abused children-contrasted with the non-abused in an urban poor community. Clin Pediatr 1989; 28:317–320.

394. Taitz LS, King JM. A profile of abuse. Arch Dis Child 1988; 63:1026–1031.

395. Kempe RS, Goldbloom RB. Malnutrition and growth retardation ('failure to thrive') in the context of child abuse and neglect. In: Helfer RE, Kempe RS, eds. The battered child, 4th edn. Chicago: University of Chicago Press; 1987:312–335.

396. Kleinman PK. Miscellaneous forms of abuse and neglect. In: Kleinman PK, ed. Diagnostic imaging of child abuse, Baltimore: Williams & Wilkins; 1987:201–212.

397. Sills RH. Failure to thrive: the role of the clinical laboratory evaluation. Am J Dis Child 1978; 132:967–969.

398. Davis JH, Rao VJ, Valdes-Dapena M. A forensic science approach to a starved child. J Forensic Sci 1984; 29:663–669.

399. Meade JL, Brissie RM. Infanticide by starvation: calculation of caloric deficit to determine degree of deprivation. J Forensic Sci 1985; 30:1263–1268.

400. Nagao M, Maeno Y, Koyama H, et al. Estimation of caloric deficit in a fatal case of starvation resulting from child neglect. J Forensic Sci 2004; 49(5):1–4.

401. Whitehead FJ, Couper RTL, Moore L, et al. Dehydration deaths in infants and young children. Am J Forensic Med Pathol 1996; 17(1):73–78.

402. Pascual-y-Baralt JF. Syndrome of inappropriate antidiuretic hormone secretion. Online. Available: http://www.emedicine.com/PED/topic2190.htm

403. Cooperman M. Diabetes insipidus. Online. Available: http://www.emedicine.com/med.topic543.htm.

404. Egland AG. Pediatrics, dehydration. Online. Available: http://www.emedicine.com/EMERG/topic372.htm

405. Ambalavanan N. Fluid, electrolyte, and nutrition management of the newborn. Online. Available: http://www.emedicine.com/ped/topic2554.htm

406. Adrogue HJ, Madias NE. Hyponatremia. N Engl J Med 2000; 342(21): 1581–1589.

407. Adrogue HJ, Madias NE. Hypernatremia. N Engl J Med 2000; 342(20): 1493–1499.

408. Adrogue HF, Madias NE. Medical progress: management of life-threatening acid–base disorders. New Engl J Med 1998; 388(1):26–34 and 338(2):107–111.

409. Sterns RH. Renal function and disorder of water and sodium balance. Nephrology 2003:1–19.

410. Vellaichamy M. Hyponatremia. Online. Available: http://www.emedicine.com/PED/topic1124.htm

411. Vellaichamy M. Hypernatremia. Online. Available:http://www.emedicine.com/ped/topic1082.htm

412. West CR, Harding JE. Maternal water intoxication as a cause of neonatal seizures. J Paediatr Child Health 2004; 40:709–710.

413. Arieff AI, Kronlund BA. Fatal child abuse by forced water intoxication. Pediatrics 1999; 103(6):1292–1295.

414. Tilleli J, Ophoven J. Hyponatremic seizures as a presenting symptom of child abuse. Forensic Sci Int 1986; 30:213–217.

415. Kaplan JA, Siegler RW, Schmunk GA. Fatal hypernatremic dehydration in exclusively breast-fed newborn infants due to maternal lactation failure. Am J Forensic Med Pathol 1998; 19(1):19–22.

416. Corey-Handy T, Hanzlick R, Shields LB, et al. Hypernatremia and subdural hematoma in the pediatric age group: is there a causal relationship? J Forensic Sci 1999; 44(6):1114–1118.

417. Coulthard MG, Haycock GB. Distinguishing between salt poisoning and hypernatremic dehydration in children. BMJ 2003; 326(7381):157–160.

Clinical findings of injury and trauma

418. Banks K, Merlino PG. Minor oral injuries in children. Mt Sinai J Med 1998; 65(5–6):333–342.

419. Becker DB, Needleman HL, Kotelchuck M. Child abuse and dentistry: orofacial trauma and its recognition by dentists. J Am Dent Assoc 1978; 97:24–28.

420. Christian CW, Mouden LD. Maxillofacial, neck, and dental manifestations of child abuse. In: Reece RM. Ludwig S, eds. Child abuse: medical diagnosis and management. 2nd edn. Philadelphia: Lippincott Williams & Wilkins; 2001:109–122.

421. Ellerstein NS. The cutaneous manifestations of child abuse and neglect. Am J Dis Child 1976; 133:906–909.

422. Raimer BG, Raimer SS, Hebeler JR. Cutaneous signs of child abuse. J Am Acad Dermatol 1981:5:203–214.

423. McMahon P, Grossman W, Gaffney M, et al. Soft-tissue injury as an indication of child abuse. J Bone Joint Surg Am 1995; 77-A(8):1179–1183.

424. Labbe J, Caouette G. Recent skin injuries in normal children. Pediatrics 2001; 108(2):271–276.

425. Maguire S, Mann MD, Sibert A, et al. Are there patterns of bruising in childhood which are diagnostic or suggestive of abuse? A systematic review. Arch Dis Child 2005; 90:182–186.

426. Whittaker DK. The dentist's role in non-accidental injury cases. In: Mason JK, ed. Paediatric forensic medicine and pathology. London: Chapman and Hall; 1989:115–130.

427. Levine L. Bite marks in child abuse. In: Sanger RE, Bross DC, eds. Clinical management of child abuse and neglect: a guide for the dental professional. Chicago: Quintessence; 1984:53–59.

428. Downes AJ, Crossland DS, Mellon AF. Prevalence and distribution of petechiae in well babies. Arch Dis Child 2002; 86:291–292.

429. Huurman WW, Ginsburg GM. Musculoskeletal injury in children. Pediatr Rev 1997; 18(12):429–440.

430. Mellors RC. Fractures. In: Bone. Online. Available: http://www.edcenter.med.cornell.edu/CUMC_PathNotes/Skeletal/Bone_05.html

431. Lyons RA, Delahunty AM, Kraus D, et al. Children's fractures: a population based study. BMJ 1999; 5:129–132.

432. O'Connor JF, Cohen J. Dating fractures. In: Kleinman PK, ed. Diagnostic imaging in child abuse. 2nd edn. Baltimore: Mosby; 1998:168–177.

433. Prosser I, Maguire S, Harrison SK, et al. How old is this fracture? Radiologic dating of fractures in children: a systematic review. AJR Am J Roentgenol 2005; 184:1282–1286.

434. Islam O, Soboleski D, Symons S, et al. Development and duration of radiographic signs of bone healing in children. AJR Am J Roentgenol 2000; 175:75–78.

435. Kleinman PK, ed. Diagnostic imaging in child abuse 2nd edn. Baltimore: Mosby; 1998:178–236.

436. Rauch F, Glorieux FH. Osteogenesis imperfecta. Lancet 2004; 363:1377–1385.

437. Heird WC. Vitamin deficiencies and excesses. In: Behrman, ed. Nelson textbook of pediatrics. 17th edn. Philadelphia: Saunders; 2003:177–190.

438. Kenney IJ. Doubt, difficulties, and practicalities in the diagnosis of non-accidental injury: a personal view. Imaging 2001; 13:295–301.

439. Rauch F, Schoenau E. Skeletal development in premature infants: a review of bone physiology beyond nutritional aspects. Arch Dis Child, Fetal Neonatal Ed 2002; 86:82–85.

440. Miller ME. The bone disease of preterm birth: a biomechanical perspective. Pediatr Res 2003; 53(1):10–15.

441. van Staa TP, Leufkens HG, Abenhaim L, et al. Oral corticosteroids and fracture risk: relationship to daily and cumulative doses. Rheumatology 2000; 39:1383–1389.

442. van Staa TP, Cooper C, Leufkens HGM, et al. Children and the risk of fractures caused by oral corticosteroids. J Bone Miner Res 2003; 18(5):913–918

443. McGraw, Pless JE, Pennington DJ, et al. Postmortem radiography after unexpected death in neonates, infants, and children: should imaging be routine? AJR Am J Roentgenol 2002; 178:1517–1521.

444. Bandyopadhyay S, Yen K. Non-accidental fractures in child maltreatment syndrome. Clin Pediatr Emerg Med 2002; 3(2):145–152.

445. Leventhal JM, Thomas SA, Rosenfield NS, et al. Fractures in young children: distinguishing child abuse from unintentional injuries. Am J Dis Child 1993; 147:87–92.

446. Nimkin K, Kleinman PK. Imaging of child abuse. Radiol Clin North Am 2001; 39(4):843–864.

447. Plunkett J, Plunkett M. Physiologic periosteal changes in infancy. Am J Forensic Med Pathol 2000; 21(3):213–216.

448. Tufts E, Blank E, Dickerson D. Periosteal thickening as a manifestation of trauma in infancy. Child Abuse Negl 1982:6:359–364.

449. Kleinman PK, Marks SC, Blackbourne R. The metaphyseal lesion in abused infants. AJR Am J Roentgenol 1986; 146:895–905.

450. Kleinman PK, Blackbourne BD, Marks SC, et al. Radiologic contributions to the investigation and prosecution of cases of fatal infant abuse. N Engl J Med 1989; 320:507–511.

451. Sun PP, Poffenbarger GJ, Durhan S, et al. Spectrum of occipitoatlantoaxial injury in young children. J Neurosurg (Spine 1) 2000; 93:28–39.

452. Cooperman DR, Merten DF. Skeletal manifestations of child abuse. In: Reece RM, ed. Child abuse: medical diagnosis and treatment. 2nd edn. Philadelphia: Lippincott Williams & Wilkins; 1994:123–156.

453. Kleinman PK. The postmortem examination. In: Kleinman PK, ed. Diagnostic imaging in child abuse. Baltimore: Williams & Wilkins; 1987:213–219.

454. Worlock P, Stower M, Barbor P. Patterns of fractures in accidental and nonaccidental injury in children. Br Med J 1986; 293:100–102.

455. Scherl SA, Lively N, Russinoff S, et al. Accidental and nonaccidental femur fractures in children. Clin Orthop Relat Res 2000; 376:96–105.

456. Thomas SA, Rosenfield NS, Leventhal JM, et al. Long-bone fractures in young children: distinguishing accidental injuries from child abuse. Pediatrics 1991; 88(3):471–476.

457. Beals RK, Tufts E. Fractured femur in infancy: the role of child abuse. J Pediatr Orthop 1983; 3:583–586.

458. Dias MS, Backstrom J, Falk M, et al. Serial radiography in the infant shaken impact syndrome. Pediatr Neurosurg 1998; 29:77–85.

459. Schwend RM, Werth C, Johnston A. Femur shaft fractures in toddlers and young children: rarely from child abuse. J Pediatr Orthop 2000; 20(4):475–481.

460. Mellick LB, Reesor K, et al. Tibial fractures of young children. Pediatr Emerg Care 1988; 4:97–101.

461. Bulloch B, Schubert, Brophy PD, et al. Cause and clinical characteristics of rib fractures in infants. Pediatrics 2000; 105:48–52.

462. Glass RBJ, Norton KI, Mitre SA, et al. Pediatric ribs: a spectrum of abnormalities. RadioGraphics 2002; 22:87–104.

463. Kleinman PK. Bony thoracic trauma. In: Kleinman PK, ed. Diagnostic imaging of child abuse. Baltimore: Williams & Wilkins; 1987:67–89.

464. Chalumeau M, Foix-L' Helias L, Scheimnamm P, et al. Rib fractures after chest physiotherapy for bronchiolitis or pneumonia in infants. Pediatr Radiol 2002; 32:644–647.

465. Williams AN, Sunderland R. Neonatal shaken baby syndrome: an aetiological view from Down Under. Arch Dis Child Fetal Neonatal Ed 2002; 86:F29–F30.

466. Feldman KW, Brever DK. Cardiopulmonary resuscitation and rib fractures. Pediatrics 1984; 73:339–342.

467. Kleinman PK, Marks SC, Adams VI, et al. Factors affecting visualization of posterior rib fractures in abused infants. AJR Am J Roentgenol 1988; 150:635–638.

468. Zumwalt RE, Fanizza-Orphanos AM. Dating of healing rib fractures in fatal child abuse. Adv Pathol 1990; 3:193–205.

469. Kleinman PK. Spinal trauma. In: Kleinman PK, ed. Diagnostic imaging in child abuse. 2nd edn. Baltimore: Mosby; 1998:149–167.

470. Faerk J, Peitersen B, Petersen S, et al. Bone mineralization in premature infants cannot be predicted from serus alkaline phosphatase or serum phosphate. Arch Dis Child Fetal Neonatal Ed 2002; 87:133–136.

471. Kleinman PK. Visceral trauma. In: Kleinman PK, ed. Diagnostic imaging in child abuse 2nd edn. Baltimore: Mosby; 1998:248–284.

472. Cooper GJ, Taylor DEM. Biophysical impact injury to the chest and abdomen. J Royal Army Medical Corps 1989; 135:58–67.

473. Ludwig S. Visceral injury manifestations of child abuse. In: Reece RM, Ludwig S, eds. Child abuse: medical diagnosis and management. 2nd edn. Philadelphia: Lippincott Williams & Wilkins; 2001:157–175.

474. Blaivas M, Sierzenski P, Theodoro D. Significant hemoperitoneum in blunt trauma victims with normal vital signs and clinical examination. Am J Emerg Med 2002; 20(3):218–221.

475. Ozturk H, Onen A, Otcu S, et al. Diagnostic delay increases morbidity in children with gastrointestinal perforation from blunt abdominal trauma. Surg Today 2003; 33:178–182.

476. Niederee MH, Byrnes MC, Helmer SD, et al. Delay in diagnosis of hollow viscus injuries: effect on outcome. Am Surg 2003; 69:293–299.

477. Ng CS, Hall CM, Shaw DG. The range of visceral manifestations of non-accidental injury. Arch Dis Child 1997; 77:167–174.

478. Gaines BA, Ford HR. Abdominal and pelvic trauma in children. Critical Care Med 2002; 30(11):S461–463.

479. Nance ML. Abdominal trauma. Online. Available: http://www.emedicine.com/ped/topic3045.htm

480. Cobb ML, Vonocur CD, Wagner CW, et al. Intestinal perforation due to blunt trauma in children in an era of increased nonoperative treatment. J Trauma 1986:26:461–463.

481. Kleinman PK. Occult nonskeletal trauma in the battered child. Radiology 1981:141:393–396.

482. Gaines BA, Schultz BS, Morrison K, et al. Duodenal injuries in children: beware of child abuse. J Pediatr Surg 2004; 39(4):600–602.

483. Champion MP, Richards CA, Boddy SA, et al. Duodenal perforation: a diagnostic pitfall in non-accidental injury. Arch Dis Child 2002; 87(5): 432–433.

484. Lonergan GJ, Baker AM, Morey MK, et al. Child abuse: radiologic-pathologic correlation. RadioGraphics 2003; 23:811–845.

485. Wilson RF, Walt AJ. Injury to the stomach and small bowel. In: Wilson FR, Walt AJ, eds. Management of trauma, pitfalls and practice. 2nd edn. Baltimore: Williams & Wilkins; 1996:497–509.

486. Case ME, Nandire R. Laceration of the stomach by blunt trauma in a child: a case of child abuse. J Forensic Sci 1983; 28:496–501.

487. Sujka SK, Jewett TC, Karp MP. Acute scrotal swelling – first evidence of intraabdominal injury in a battered child. J Pediatr Surg 1988; 23:380.

488. Strouse PJ, Close BJ, Marshall KW, et al. CT of bowel and mesenteric trauma in children. RadioGraphics 1999; 19:1237–1250.

489. Hanks PW, Brody JM. Blunt injury to mesentery and small bowel: CT evaluation. Radiol Clin North Am 2003; 41:1171–1182.

490. Gilchrist JA, Broadley PS, Shawis RN. Pancreatic trauma in a child. Emerg Med J 2001; 18:146.

491. Slovis Tl, Berdon WE, Haller JO, et al. Pancreatitis and the battered child syndrome: report of two cases with skeletal involvement. AJR Ther Nucl Med 1975; 125(2):456–461.

492. Tam PKH, Saing H, Irving IM, et al. Acute pancreatitis in children. J Pediatr Surg 1985; 20:58–60.

493. Ziegler DW, Long JA, et al. Pancreatitis in childhood: experience with 49 patients. Ann Surg 1988; 207:257–261.

494. Schwengel D, Ludwig S. Rhabdomyolysis and myoglobinuria as manifestation of child abuse. Pediatr Emerg Care 1985; 1:194–197.

495. Orel SG, Nussbaum AR, Sheth S, et al. Duodenal hematoma in child abuse: sonographic detection. AJR Am J Roentgenol 1988; 151:147–149.

496. Uhing MR. Management of birth injuries. Clin Perinatol 2005; 32:19–38.

497. Durbin DR, Chen I, Smith R, et al. Effects of seating position and appropriate restraint use on the risk of injury to children in motor vehicle crashes. Pediatrics 2005; 115(3):305–309.

498. Braver ER, Whitefield R, Ferguson SA. Seating positions and children's risk of dying in motor vehicle crashes. Inj Prev 1998; 4:181–187.

499. Lutz N, Arbogast KB, Cornejo RA, et al. Suboptimal restraint affects the pattern of abdominal injuries in children involved in motor vehicle crashes. J Pediatr Surg 2003; 38:919–923.

500. Holmes JF, Sokolove PE, Brant WE, et al. A clinical decision rule for identifying children with thoracic injuries after blunt torso trauma. Ann Emerg Med 2002; 39(5):492–499.

501. Westra SJ, Wallace EC. Imaging evaluation of pediatric chest trauma. Radiol Clin North Am 2005; 43:267–281.

502. Bliss D, Silen M. Pediatric thoracic trauma. Crit Care Med 2002; 30(11):S409–415.

503. Balci AE. Blunt thoracic trauma in children: review of 137 cases. Eur J Cardiothorac Surg 2004; 26(2):387–392.

Pathology of head injuries in infancy

504. Geddes J. Pediatric head injury. Online. Available: http://brainpath. medsch.ucla.edu/isnpress/devopdfs/23%20geddes.pdf

505. DiMaio DJ, DiMaio VJ. Neonaticide, infanticide, and child homicide. In: DiMaio DJ, DiMaio VJ, eds. Forensic pathology. New York: Elsevier; 1989:299–326.

506. Whitwell HL. Head injury. In: Rutty GN, ed. Essentials of autopsy practice. London: Springer; 2001:175–198.

507. Ommaya AK, Goldsmith W, Thibault L. Biomechanics and neuropathology of adult and paediatric head injury. Br J Neurosurg 2002; 10(3):220–242.

508. Miura FK, Plese JP, Ciquini O, et al. Depressed skull fractures in children under 2 years of age. Retrospective study of 43 cases. Arq Neuropsiquiatr 1995; 53(3-B):644–648.

509. McClelland CQ, Rekate H, Kaufman B, et al. Cerebral injury in child abuse: a changing profile. Childs Brain 1980; 7:225–235.

510. Keenan, HT, Runyon DK, Marshall SW. A population-based study of inflicted traumatic brain injury in young children. JAMA 2003; 290(5):621–626.

511. Billmire ME, Myers PA. Serious head injury in infants: accident or abuse? Pediatrics 1985; 75:340–342.

512. Bandak FA. Impact traumatic brain injury: a mechanical perspective. In: Oehmichen M, Konig HG, eds. Neurotraumatology: biomechanic aspects, cytologic and molecular mechanics. Luckeck: Schmidt-Ronchild; 1997; 59–83.

513. Ersahin Y, Mutluer S, Mirzai H, et al. Pediatric depressed skull fractures: analysis of 530 cases. Childs Nerv Syst 1996; 12(6):323–331.

514. Ellis TS, Vezina G, Donahue DJ. Acute identification of cranial burst fracture: comparison between CT and MR imaging findings. Am J Neuroradiol 2000; 21:795–801.

515. Glass RBJ, Fernbach SK, Norton KI, et al. The infant skull: a vault of information. RadioGraphics 2004; 24(3):507–522.

516. Greenes DS, Schutzman SA. Infants with isolated skull fracture: what are their clinical characteristics, and do they require hospitalization? Ann Emerg Med 1997; 30(3):253–259.

517. Medana IM, Esiri MM. Axonal damage: a key predictor of outcome in human CNS disease. Brain 2003; 126:515–530.

518. Adams JH, Graham DI, Gennarelli TA. Contemporary neuropathological considerations regarding brain damage in head injury. In: Becker DR, Povlishock JT, eds. Central nervous system trauma status report. Bethesda: National Institute of Neurological and Communicative Disorders and Stroke, National Institute of Health; 1985:65–77.

519. Geddes JR, Hackshaw AK, Vowles GH, et al. Neuropathology of inflicted head injury in children. I. Patterns of brain damage. Brain 2001; 124:1290–1298.

520. Geddes JF, Vowles GH, Hackshaw AK, et al. Neuropathology of inflicted head injury in children. II. Microscopic brain injury in infants. Brain 2001; 124:1299–1406.

521. Geddes JF, Whitwell HL, Graham DI. Traumatic axonal injury: practical issues for diagnosis in medicolegal cases. Neuropathol Appl Neurobiol 2000; 26:105–116.

522. Reichard RR, White SL, Hladik CL, et al. β-amyloid precursor protein staining of non-accidental central nervous system injury in pediatric autopsies. J Neurotrauma 2003; 20(4):347–355.

523. Vowles GH, Scholtz CL, Cameron JM. Diffuse axonal injury in early infancy. J Clin Pathol 1987; 40:185–189.

524. Graham DI, Smith C, Reichard R, et al. Trials and tribulations of using β-amyloid precursor protein immunohistochemistry to evaluate traumatic brain injury in adults. Forensic Sci Int 2004; 146:89–96.

525. Pittella JE, Gusmao SN. Diffuse vascular injury in fatal road traffic accident victims: its relationship to diffuse axonal injury. J Forensic Sci 2003; 48(3):626–630.

526. Calder IM, Hill I, Scholtz CL. Primary brain trauma in non-accidental injury. J Clin Pathol 1984; 37:1095–1100.

527. Lindenberg R, Freytag E. Morphology of brain lesions from early blunt trauma in early infancy. Arch Pathol 1969; 87:298–305.

528. Hausmann R. Timing of cortical contusions in human brain injury. In: Tsokos M, ed. Forensic pathology reviews. Vol. 1. Totowa: Humana Press; 2004:53–75.

529. Howard MA, Bell BA, Uttley D. The pathophysiology of infant subdural haematomas. Br J Neurosurg 1993:7:355–365.

530. Leestma JE. Table 1. Aging and dating of hematomas. In: Leestma JE, ed. Forensic Neuropathology. New York: Raven Press. 1988:216.

531. Kelly P, Hayes I. Infantile subdural haematoma in Auckland, New Zealand: 1988–1998. N Z Med J 2004; 117(1201):U1047.

532. Fung ELS, Sung RY, Nelson EA, et al. Unexplained subdural hematoma in young children: is it always child abuse? Pediatr Int 2002; 44:37–42.

533. Vinchon M, Noizet O, Defoort-Dhellemmes S, et al. Infantile subdural hematomas due to traffic accidents. Pediatr Neurosurg 2002; 37:245–253.

534. Vinchon M, Noule N, Tchofo PJ, et al. Imaging of head injuries in infants: temporal correlates and forensic implications for the diagnosis of child abuse. J Neurosurg (Pediatrics 2) 2004; 101:44–52.

535. Usinski R. Shaken baby syndrome: fundamental questions. Brit J Neurosurg 2002; 16:217–219.

536. Hymel KP, Jenny C, Block RW. Intracranial hemorrhage and rebleeding insuspected victims of abusive head trauma: addressing the forensic controversies. Child Maltreat 2002; 7(4):329–348.

537. Jaspan T, Griffiths PD, McConachie NS, et al. Neuroimaging for non-accidental head injury in childhood: a proposed protocol. Clin Radiol 2003; 58:44–53.

538. Hart BL, Dudley MH, Zumwalt RE. Postmortem cranial MRI and autopsy correlation in suspected child abuse. Am J Forensic Med Pathol 1996:17(3):217–224.

539. Swift DM, McBride L. Chronic subdural hematoma in children. Neurosurg Clin North Am 2000; 11(3):439–446.

540. Plunkett J. Pediatric chronic subdural hematoma: a retrospective comparative analysis. Pediatr Neurosurg 1992; 18:266–271.

541. Hwang SK, Kim SL. Infantile head injury with special reference to the development of chronic subdural hematoma. Childs Nerv Syst 2000; 16:591–594.

542. Yamashima T. The inner membrane of chronic subdural hematomas. Neurosurg Clin North Am 2000; 11(3):413–424.

543. McLone DG, Gutierrez FA. Ultrastructure of subdural membranes of children. Concepts Pediatr Neurosurg 1981; 1:174–187.

544. Leestma JE, Kirkpatrick JB, eds. Forensic neuropathology. New York: Raven Press; 1988: 216 pp.

545. Lorch SA, D'Agostino J, Zimmerman R, et al. 'Benign' extra-axial fluid in survivors of neonatal intensive care. Arch Pediatr Adolesc Med 2004; 158:178–182.

546. Luerssen TG, Sutton LN, Bruce DA, et al. Posttraumatic hydrocephalus in the neonate and infant. In: Raimondi AJ, Choux M, DiRocco C, eds. Head injuries in the newborn and infant. New York: Springer-Verlag; 1986:241–256.

547. Papasian NC, Frim DM. A theoretical model of benign external hydrocephalus that predicts a predisposition towards extra-axial hemorrhage after minor head trauma. Pediatr Neurosurg 2000; 33:188–193.

548. Garton HJL, Piatt JH. Hydrocephalus. Pediatr Clin North Am 2004; 51:305–325.

549. Pittman T. Significance of a subdural hematoma in a child with external hydrocephalus. Pediatr Neurosurg 2003; 39:57–59.

550. Ravid S, Maytal J. External hydrocephalus: a probable cause for subdural hematoma in infancy. Pediatr Neurol 2003; 28:139–141.

551. Dickerman RD, McConathy WJ, Lustrin E, et al. Rapid neurological deterioration associated with minor head trauma in chronic hydrocephalus. Childs Nerv Syst 2003; 19:249–251.

552. Azais M, Echenne B. Idiopathic pericerebral effusions of infancy (external hydrocephaly). Ann Pediatr (Paris) 1992; 39(9):550–558.

553. Piatt JH. A pitfall in the diagnosis of child abuse: external hydrocephalus, subdural hematoma, and retinal hemorrhages. Neurosurg Focus 1999; 7(4).

554. Bayir H, Kochanek PM, Clark RSB. Traumatic brain injury in infants and children: mechanisms of secondary damage and treatment in the intensive care unit. Crit Care Clin 2003:19:529–549.

555. Kemp AM, Stoodley N, Cobley C, et al. Apnoea and brain swelling in non-accidental head injury. Arch Dis Child 2003; l88:472–476.

556. Rivkin MJ, Volpe JJ. Strokes in children. Pediatr Rev 1996; 17(8):265–278.

Neck injuries

557. Deliganis AV, Baxter AB, Hanson JA, et al. Radiologic spectrum of craniocervical distraction injuries. RadioGraphics 2000; 20:S237–S250.

558. Lustrin ES, Karakas SP, Ortiz AO, et al. Pediatric cervical spine: normal anatomy, variants, and trauma. RadioGraphics 2003; 23:539–560.

559. Dias MS. Traumatic brain and spinal cord injury. Pediatr Clin North Am 2004; 51:271–303.

560. Hall DE, Boydston WL. Pediatric neck injuries. Pediatr Rev 1999; 20(1): 13–19.

561. Proctor MR. Spinal cord injuries. Critical Care Med 2002; 30(11):S489–499.

562. Zimmerman S. Cervical spine trauma in child abuse. Online. Available: http://www.cincinnatichildrens.org/svc/prog/child-abuse/tools/cervical-spine.htm

563. Schwartz GR, Wright SW, Fein JA, et al. Pediatric cervical spine injury sustained in falls from low heights. Ann Emerg Med 1997; 30(3).

564. Jaffe DM, Binns H, Radkowski MA. Developing a clinical algorithm for early management of cervical spine injury in child trauma victims. Ann Emerg Med 1987; 16(3):270–276.

565. Ruge JR, Sinson GP, McLone DG, et al. Pediatric spinal injury: the very young. J Neurosurg 1988; 68:25–30.

566. Pang D. Spinal cord injury without radiographic abnormality (SCIWORA). In: Pang D, ed. Disorders of the pediatric spine. New York: Raven Press; 1995:509–516.

567. Ergun A, Oder W. Pediatric care report of spinal cord injury without radiographic abnormality (SCIWORA): case report and literature review. Spinal Cord 2003; 41:249–253.

568. Adams G, Ainsworth J, Butler L, et al. Update from the ophthalmology child abuse working party: Royal College Ophthalmologists. Eye 2004; 18:795–798.

569. Makoroff K. Review of retinal hemorrhages. Online. Available: http://www.cincinnatichildrens.org/svc/prog/child-abuse/tools.retinalhemorrhage.htm

570. Kaur B, Taylor D. Fundus hemorrhages in infancy. Surv Ophthalmol 1992; 37(1):1–17.

571. Gilliland MGF, Folberg R, Hayreh SS. Age of retinal hemorrhages by iron detection: an animal model. Am J Forensic Med Pathol 2005; 26(1):1–4.

572. Emerson MV, Pieramici DJ, Stoessel KM, et al. Incidence and rate of disappearance of retinal hemorrhage in newborns. Ophthalmology 2001; 108:36–39.

573. Gilliland MG, Luthert P. Why do histology on retinal haemorrhages in suspected non-accidental injury? Histopathology 2003; 43:592–602.

574. Lantz PE, Sinal SH, Stanton CA, et al. Perimacular retinal folds from childhood head trauma. BMJ 2004; 328:754–756.

575. Medele RJ, Stummer W, Mueller AR, et al. Terson's syndrome in subarachnoid hemorrhage and severe brain injury accompanied by acutely raised intracranial pressure. J Neurosurg 1998; 88:851–854.

576. Green MA. Investigation of unexpected child death. In: Rutty GN. Essentials of autopsy practice. London: Springer; 2001:110–113.

577. Parsons MA, Start RD. Necropsy techniques in ophthalmic pathology. J Clin Pathol 2001; 54:417–427.

578. Gilliland MG, Folberg R. Retinal hemorrhages: replicating the clinician's view of the eye. Forensic Sci Int 1992; 56(1):77–80.

579. Amberg R, Pollak S. Postmortem endoscopy of the ocular fundus: a valuable tool in forensic postmortem practice. Forensic Sci Int 2001; 124:157–162.

580. Anderson R, Opeskin K. Timing of early changes in brain trauma. Am J Forensic Med Pathol 1998; 19(1):1–9.

581. Durham SR, Raghupathi R, Helfaer M, et al. Age-related differences in acute physiologic response to focal traumatic brain injury in piglets. Pediatr Neurosurg 2000; 33:76–82.

582. Bays J. Conditions mistaken for child sexual abuse. In: Reece RM, Ludwig S, eds. Child abuse: medical diagnosis and management. 2nd edn. Philadelphia: Lippincott Williams & Wilkins; 2001:287–306.

583. Evans MJ. Mimics of non-accidental injury in children. In: Rutty GN. Essentials of autopsy practice. London: Springer; 2001:121–142.

584. Bays J. Conditions mistaken for child physical abuse. In: Reece RM, Ludwig S, eds. Child abuse: medical diagnosis and management. 2nd edn. Philadelphia: Lippincott Williams & Wilkins; 2001:177–206.

585. Stewart GM, Rosenberg NM. Conditions mistaken for child abuse: Part 1. Pediatr Emerg Care 1996; 12 (2):116–121.

586. Stewart GM, Rosenberg NM. Conditions mistaken for child abuse: Part 2. Pediatr Emerg Care 1996; 12 (3):217–221.

587. Rooms L, Fitzgerald N, McClain KL. Hemophagocytic lymphohistiocytosis masquerading as child abuse: presentation of three cases and review of central nervous system findings in hemophagocytic lymphohistiocytosis. Pediatrics 2003; 11(5):636–640.

588. Hartley LM, Khwaja OS, Verity CM. Glutaric aciduria type I and nonaccidental head injury. Pediatrics 2001; 107(1):174–175.

589. Stam J. Thrombosis of the cerebral veins and sinuses. N Engl J Med 2005; 352(17):1791–1798.

590. Sebire G, Tabarki B, Saunders DE, et al. Cerebral venous sinus thrombosis in children: risk factors, presentation, diagnosis and outcome. Brain 2005; 128:477–489.

591. Lancon JA, Killough KR, Tibbs RE, et al. Spontaneous dural sinus thrombosis in children. Pediatr Neurosurg 1999; 30:23–29.

592. Rutty GN, Smith CM, Malia RG. Late-form hemorrhagic disease of the newborn: a fatal case report with illustration of investigations that may assist in avoiding the mistaken diagnosis of child abuse. Am J Forensic Med Pathol 1999; 20(1):48–51.

593. Wheeler DM, Hobbs CJ. Mistakes in diagnosing non-accidental injuries: 10 years' experience. Br Med J 1988; 296:1233–1236.

594. Saulsbury FT, Hayden GF. Skin conditions simulating child abuse. Pediatr Emerg Care 1985; 1:147–150.

595. Waskerwitz S, Christoffel KK, Hauger S. Hypersensitivity vasculitis presenting as suspected child abuse: case report and literature review. Pediatrics 1981; 67:283–284.

596. Brown J, Melinkovich P. Schönlein-Henoch purpura misdiagnosed as child abuse. JAMA 1986; 256:617–618.

597. Alper J, Holmes LB, Mihm MC Jr. Birth marks with medical significance: nevocullular nevi, sebaceous nevi, and multiple café au lait spots. J Pediatr 1979; 95:696–700.

598. Sekula SA, Tschen JA, Duffy JO. Epidermal nevus misinterpreted as child abuse. Cutis 1986; 3714:276–278.

599. O'Hare AE, Eden OB. Bleeding disorders and non-accidental injury. Arch Dis Child 1984; 59:860–864.

600. Kirschner RH, Stein RA. The mistaken diagnosis of child abuse – a form of medical abuse? Am J Dis Child 1985; 139:873–875.

601. Guarnaschelli J, Lee J, Pitts FW. 'Fallen fontanelle' (caida de Mollera) – a variant of the battered child syndrome. JAMA 1972; 222:1545–1546.

602. Yeatman GW, Dang VV. Cao G10 (coin rubbing) – Vietnamese attitudes toward health care. JAMA 1980; 244(24):2748–2749.

603. Schmitt BD, Gray JD, Britton HL. Car seat burns in infants: avoiding confusion with inflicted burns. Pediatrics 1978; 62:607–609.

604. Nunez AE, Taff ML. A chemical burn simulating child abuse. Am J Forensic Med Pathol 1985; 6:181–185.

605. Horodniceanu C, Grünebaum M, Volovitz B, et al. Unusual bone involvement in congenital syphilis mimicking the battered child syndrome. Pediatr Radiol 1978; 7:232–234.

606. Fiser RH, Kaplan J, Holder JC. Congenital syphilis mimicking the battered child syndrome. How does one tell them apart? Clin Pediatr 1972; 11:305–307.

607. Asnes RS, Wisotsky DH. Cupping lesions simulating child abuse. J Pediatr 1981; 99:267–268.

608. Owen SM, Durst RD. Ehlers-Danlos syndrome simulating child abuse. Arch Dermatol 1984; 120:97–101.

609. Winship IM, Winship WS. Epidermolysis bullosa misdiagnosed as child abuse. S Afr Med J 1988; 73:369–370.

610. Adler R, Kane-Nussen B. Erythema multiforme: confusion with child battering syndrome. Pediatrics 1983; 72:718–720.

611. Jenny C, Kirby P, Fuquay D. Genital lichen sclerosus mistaken for child sexual abuse. Pediatrics 1981; 83:597–599.

612. Shaw JCL. Copper deficiency and non-accidental injury. Arch Dis Child 1988; 63:448–455.

613. Carty H. Brittle or battered. Arch Dis Child 1988; 63:350–352.

614. Smialek JE. Significance of mongolian spots. J Pediatr 1980; 97:504–505.

615. Asnes RS. Buttock bruises: mongolian spots (letter). Pediatrics 1984; 74:321.

616. Reinhart MA, Ruhs H. Moxibustion – another traumatic folk remedy. Clin Pediatr 1985; 24:58–59.

617. Paterson CR. Osteogenesis imperfecta in the differential diagnosis of child abuse. BMJ 1989; 299(6713):1451–1454.

618. Copeland AR. A case of panhypogammaglobulinemia masquerading as child abuse. J Forensic Sci 1988; 33:1493–1496.

619. Dannaker CJ, Glover RA, Goltz RW. Phytophotodermatitis – a mystery case report. Clin Pediatr 1988; 27:289–290.

620. Coffman K, Boyce WT, Hansen RC. Phytophotodermatitis simulating child abuse. Am J Dis Child 1985; 139:239–240.

621. Levin AV, Selbst SM. Vulvar hemangioma simulating child abuse. Clin Pediatr 1988; 27:213–215.

622. Duhaime AC, Gennarelli TA, Thibault LE, et al. The shaken baby syndrome: a clinical, pathological, and biomechanical study. J Neurosurg 1987; 66:409–415.

623. Prange MT, Coats B, Duhaime AC, et al. Anthropomorphic simulations of falls, shakes, and inflicted impacts in infants. J Neurosurg 2003; 99:143–150.

624. Donohoe M. Evidence-based medicine and shaken baby syndrome. Part I: literature review, 1966–1998. Am J Forensic Med Pathol 2003; 24:239–242.

625. Nashelsky MB, Dix JD. The time interval between lethal infant shaking and onset of symptoms: a review of the shaken baby syndrome literature. Am J Forensic Med Pathol 1995; 16(2):154–157.

626. Leestma JE. Case analysis of brain-injured admittedly shaken infants: 54 cases, 1969–2001. Am J Forensic Med Pathol 2005; 26(2):1–14.

627. Reiber GD. Fatal falls in childhood. How far must children fall to sustain fatal head injury? Report of cases and review of the literature. Am J Forensic Med Pathol 1993; 14:201–207.

628. Hymel KP, Bandak FA, Partington MD, et al. Abusive head trauma? A biomechanics-based approach. Child Maltreat 1998; 3(2):116–128.

629. Prange MT, Coats B, Duhaime AC, et al. Anthropomorphic simulations of falls, shakes, and inflicted impacts in infants. J Neurosurg 2003; 99:143–150.

630. Smith SL, Andrus PK, Gleason DD, et al. Infant rat model of the shaken baby syndrome: preliminary characterization and evidence for the role of free radicals in cortical hemorrhaging and progressive neuronal degeneration. J Neurotrauma 1998; 15:693–705.

631. Stoodley N. Neuroimaging in non-accidental head injury: if, when, why and how. Clin Radiol 2005; 60:22–30.

632. Plunkett J. Fatal pediatric head injuries caused by short distance falls. Am J Forensic Med Pathol 2001; 22(1):1–12.

633. Helfer RE, Slovis TL, Black M. Injuries resulting when small children fall out of bed. Pediatrics 1977; 60:533–535.

634. Duhaime AC, Alario AJ, Lewander WJ. Head injury in very young children: mechanisms, injury types and ophthalmologic findings in 100 hospitalized patients younger than 2 years of age. Pediatrics 1992; 90:179–185.

635. Kirschner RH, Wilson H. Fatal child abuse: the pathologist's perspective. In: Reece RM, ed. Child abuse: medical diagnosis and treatment. Philadelphia: Lea and Febiger; 1994:517–543.

Neonaticide, infanticide, abandoned newborn, and stillbirth

636. British Columbia Reproductive Care Program. Perinatal Mortality Guideline 5: Investigation and Assessment of Stillbirths. May 2000. Online. Available: http://www.rcp.gov.bc.ca/guidelines.htm.

637. Saukko P, Knight B. Infanticide and stillbirth. In: Saukko P, Knight B, eds. Knight's forensic pathology. 3rd edn. London: Arnold; 2004:439–450.

638. Byard RW. Medicolegal problems with neonaticide. In: Tsokos M, ed. Forensic pathology reviews. Vol.1. Totowa: Humana Press; 2004:171–185.

639. Spinelli MG. A systematic investigation of 16 cases of neonaticide. Am J Psychiatry 2001; 158(5):811–813.

640. Herman-Giddens ME, Smioth JB, Mittal M, et al. Newborns killed or left to die by a parent: a population based study. JAMA 2003; 289(11):1425–1429.

641. Froede RC, Henry TE. The identification of the dead, abandoned baby. In: Mason JK, ed. Paediatric forensic medicine and pathology. London: Chapman and Hall; 1989:85–99.

642. Bowen DA. Concealment of birth, child destruction and infanticide. In: Mason JK, ed. Paediatric forensic medicine and pathology. London: Chapman and Hall; 1989:178–190.

643. Caracostea G. Systematic review on the incidence/prevalence of stillbirths. Online. Available: http://www.gfmer.ch/Endo/Course2003/Stillbirths.htm.

644. Magee JF. Investigation of stillbirth. Pediatr Dev Pathol 2001; 4:1–22.

645. Smith GCS, Crossley JA, Aitken DA, et al. First-trimester placentation and the risk of antepartum stillbirth. JAMA 2004; 292(18):2249–2254.

646. Radbill SX. A history of child abuse and infanticide. In: Kempe CH, Helfer RE, eds. The battered child. 2nd edn. Chicago: The University of Chicago Press; 1974:3–21.

647. Behlmer GK. Deadly motherhood: infanticide and medical opinion in mid-victorian England. J Hist Med Allied Sci 1979; 34:403–427.

648. Saunders E. Neonaticides following 'secret' pregnancies: seven case reports. Public Health Rep 1989; 104(4):368–372.

649. Resnick PJ. Murder of the newborn: a psychiatric review of neonaticide. Am J Psychiatry 1970; 126(10):1414–1420.

650. Funayama M, Sagisaka K. Consecutive infanticides in Japan. Am J Forensic Med Pathol 1988; 9:9–11.

651. Robinson AE, Lucas BGB. Gradwohl's legal medicine. 3rd edn. Chicago: Year Book; 1976:256–258.

652. Lavezzi WA, Keough KM, Der'Ohannesian P, et al. The use of pulmonary interstitial emphysema as an indicator of live birth. Am J Forensic Med Pathol 2003; 24(1):87–91.

653. Mitchell EK, Davis JH. Spontaneous births into toilets. J Forensic Sci 1984; 29:591–596.

654. Shiono H, Maya A. Medicolegal aspects of infanticide in Hokkaido district, Japan. Am J Forensic Med Pathol 1986; 7:104–106.

655. Ito Y, Tsuda R, Kimura H. Diagnostic value of the placenta in medicolegal practice. Forensic Sci Int 1989; 40:79–84.

Sexual abuse in infancy and childhood

656. Finkel MA, DeJong AR. Medical findings in child sexual abuse. In: Reece RM, Ludwig S, eds. Child abuse: medical diagnosis and management. 2nd edn. Philadelphia: Lippincott Williams & Wilkins; 2001:207–286.

657. Giardino AP. Child abuse and neglect: sexual abuse. Online. Available: http://www.emedicine.com/topic2649.htm

658. McCann JJ. The anatomy of child and adolescent sexual abuse: a CD-ROM atlas/reference. Available at: http://www.intercorpinc.com/aboutauth.html

659. California Office of Criminal Justice Planning. California medical protocol for examination of sexual assault and child sexual abuse victims. 2001. Online. Available: http://www.ucdmc.ucdavis.edu/medtrng/domain/pdfs/oes%20forms/oes%20923-950%20Protocol.pdf

660. Berenson AB. Appearance of the hymen at birth and one year of age: a longitudinal study. Pediatrics 1993; 91(4):820–825.

661. Berenson AB. A longitudinal study of hymenal morphology in the first 3 years of life. Pediatrics 1995; 95(4):490–496.

662. Berenson AB, Chacko MR, Wiemann CM, et al. Use of hymenal measurements in the diagnosis of previous penetration. Pediatrics 2002; 109(2):228–235.

663. Berenson AB, Chacko MR, Wiemann CM, et al. A case-control study of anatomic changes resulting from sexual abuse. Am J Obstet Gynecol 2000; 182(4):820–831.

664. Berenson AB, Grady JJ. A longitudinal study of hymenal development from 3 to 9 years of age. J Pediatr 2002; 140:600–607.

665. McCann J, Wells R, Simon M, et al. Genital findings in prepubertal girls selected fro nonabuse: a descriptive study. Pediatrics 1990; 86:428–439.

666. McCann J, Voris J, Simon M, et al. Perianal findings in prepubertal children selected for nonabuse: a descriptive study. Child Abuse Negl 1989; 13:179–193.

667. McCann J, Voris J. Perianal injuries resulting from sexual abuse: a longitudinal study. Pediatrics 1993; 91(2):390–397.

668. Myhre AK, Berntzen K, Bratlid D. Genital anatomy in non-abused preschool girls. Acta Paediatrica 2003; 92(12):1453–1462.

669. Myhre AK, Bemtzen K, Bratlid D. Perianal anatomy in non-abused preschool children. Acta Paediatr 2001; 90(11):1321–1328.

670. Siegfried EC, Frasier LD. Anogenital skin diseases of childhood. Pediatr Ann 1997; 26(5):321–331.

671. McCann J, Reay D, Siebert J, et al. Postmortem perianal findings in children. Am J Forensic Med Pathol 1996; 17(4):289–298.

672. Christian CW, Lavelle JM, DeJong AR, et al. Forensic evidence findings in prepubertal victims of sexual assault. Pediatrics 2000; 106(1):100–104.

673. Centers for Disease Control and Prevention. Sexually transmitted diseases treatment guidelines 2002. MMWR Morbidity and Mortality Weekly Report 2002; 51 (RR-6):1–80.

674. Jain N. Sexually transmitted diseases in the pediatric patient. B C Med J 2004; 46(3):133–138.

Sudden unexpected death in infancy and homicide

675. Cote A, Russo P, Michaud J. Sudden unexpected deaths in infancy: what are the causes? J Pediatr 1999; 135(4):437–443.

676. Parham DM, Savell VH, Kokes CP, et al. Incidence of autopsy findings in unexpected deaths of children and adolescents. Pediatr Dev Pathol 2003; 6:142–155.

677. Mitchell E, Krous HF, Donald T, et al. An analysis of the usefulness of specific stages in the pathologic investigation of sudden infant death. Am J Forensic Med Pathol 2000; 21(4):395–400.

678. McNamara DG. Special problems in infants, children and young adults, including postoperative sudden death: summary. J Am Coll Cardiol 1985; 5:138B–140B.

679. Ackermann DM, Edwards WD. Sudden death as the initial manifestation of primary pulmonary hypertension: report of 4 cases. J Forensic Med Pathol 1987; 8:97–102.

680. Byard RW. Sudden death in infancy, childhood, and adolescence. 2nd edn. Cambridge; Cambridge University Press; 2004.

681. Burchfield DJ, Rawlings J. Sudden deaths and apparent life-threatening events in hospitalized neonates presumed to be healthy. Am J Dis Child 1991; 45:1319–1322.

682. Huser CJ, Smialek JE. Diagnosis of sudden death in infants due to acute dehydration. Am J Forensic Med Pathol 1986; 7:278–282.

Homicide and unexplained deaths

683. Byard RW, Beal SM. Munchausen syndrome by proxy: repetitive infantile apnoea and homicide. J Paediatr Child Health 1993; 29:77–79.

684. Oehmichen M. Petechiae of the baby's skin as differentiation symptom of infanticide versus SIDS. J Forensic Sci 2000; 45(3):602–607.

685. Levene S, Bacon CJ. Sudden unexpected death and covert homicide in infancy. Arch Dis Child 2000; 89:443–447.

686. Carpenter RG, Waite A, Coombs RC, et al. Repeat sudden unexpected and unexplained infant deaths: natural or unnatural? Lancet 2005; 365:29–35.

Acute life-threatening events

687. Southall DP, Plunkett MCB, Banks MW, et al. Covert video recordings of life-threatening child abuse: lessons for child protection. Pediatrics 1987; 100(5):735–760.

688. Samuels MP, Poets CF, Noyes JP. Diagnosis and management after life threatening events in infants and young children who received cardiopulmonary resuscitation. BMJ 1993; 306(6876):489–492.

689. Istre GR, Gustafson TL, Baron RC, et al. A mysterious cluster of deaths and cardiopulmonary arrests in a pediatric intensive care unit. N Engl J Med 1985; 313:205–211.

690. Buehler JW, Smith LE, et al. Unexplained deaths in a children's hospital: an epidemiologic assessment. N Engl J Med 1985; 313:211–216.

691. Buchino JJ, Corey TS, Montgomery V. Sudden unexpected death in hospitalized children. J Pediatr 2002; 140(4):461–465.

692. Kamerling LB, Black XA, Fiser RT. Munchausen syndrome by proxy in the pediatric intensive care unit: an unusual mechanism. Pediatr Crit Care Med 2002; 3(3):305–307.

Munchausen syndrome by proxy

693. Rosenberg DA. Munchausen syndrome by proxy. In: Reece RM, Ludwig S, eds. Child abuse: medical diagnosis and management. 2nd edn. Philadelphia: Lippincott Williams & Wilkins; 2001:363–383.

694. Abdulhamid I. Munchausen syndrome by proxy. Online. Available:http://www.emedicine.com/ped/topic2742.htm

695. Asher R. Munchausen's syndrome, Lancet 1951; 1:339–341.

696. Meadow R. Munchausen syndrome by proxy: the hinterland of child abuse. Lancet 1977; 2:343–345.

697. Meadow R. Munchausen syndrome by proxy. Arch Dis Child 1982; 57:92–98.

698. Meadow R. Management of Munchausen syndrome by proxy. Arch Dis Child 1985; 60:385–393.

699. Jones JG, Butler HL. Munchausen syndrome by proxy. Child Abuse Negl 1986; 10:33–44.

700. Geelhoed GC, Pemberton PJ. SIDS, seizures or esophageal reflux? Another manifestation of Munchausen syndrome by proxy. Med J Aust 1985; 143:357–358.

701. Truman TL, Ayoub CC. Considering suffocatory abuse and Munchausen by proxy in the evaluation of children experiencing apparent life-threatening events and sudden infant death syndrome. Child Maltreat 2002; 7(2):138–148.

702. Sullivan CA, Francis GL, Bain MW, et al. Munchausen syndrome by proxy: 1990. A portent for problems. Clin Pediatr 1991; 30:112–116.

703. Malatak JJ, Wiener ES, Gartner JC, et al. Munchausen syndrome by proxy: complication of central venous catheterization. Pediatrics 1985; 75:523–525.

704. Kohl S, Pickering LK, Dupree E. Child abuse presenting as immuno-deficiency disease. J Pediatr 1978; 93:466–468.

705. Orenstein DM, Wasserman AL. Munchausen syndrome by proxy simulating cystic fibrosis. Pediatrics 1986; 78:621–624.

706. Pickford E, Buchanan N, McLaughlin S. Munchausen syndrome by proxy: a family anthology. Med J Aust 1988; 148:646–650.

707. Guandolo VL. Munchausen syndrome by proxy: an outpatient challenge. Pediatrics 1985; 75:526–530.

708. Warner JO, Hathaway MJ. Allergic form of Meadow's syndrome (Munchausen by proxy). Arch Dis Child 1984; 59:151–156.

709. Perman, CM. Diagnosing the truth: determining physician liability in cases involving munchausen syndrome by proxy. J Urban Contemporary Law 1998; 54(267):267–290.

710. Mason JD. Munchausen syndrome by proxy. Online. Available: http://www.emedicine.com/emerg/topic830.htm

711. Sutphen JL, Saulsbury FT: Intentional ipecac poisoning: Munchausen syndrome by proxy. Pediatrics 1988; 82:453–456.

712. McClung HJ, Murray R, Braden NJ, et al. Intentional ipecac poisoning in children. Am J Dis Child 1988; 142:637–639.

713. Feldman KW, Christopher DM, Opheim KB. Munchausen syndrome/bulimia by proxy: ipecac as a toxin in child abuse. Child Abuse Negl 1989; 13:257–261.

714. Day L, Kelly C. Fatal cardiomyopathy: suspected child abuse by chronic ipecac administration. Vet Hum Toxicol 1989; 1:255–257.

715. Amir J. Polymicrobial bacteremia and child abuse (letter). Am J Dis Child 1989; 143:444.

716. Halsey NA, Frentz JM, et al. Recurrent nosocomial polymicrobial sepsis secondary to child abuse. Lancet 2:558, 1983.

717. Bryk M, Siegel PT. My mother caused my illness: the story of a survivor of Munchausen by proxy syndrome. Pediatrics 1997; 100(1):1–7.

718. Jureidini JN, Shafer AT, Donald TG. 'Munchausen by proxy syndrome': not only pathological parenting but also problematic doctoring? Med J Aust 2003; 178(3):130–132.

719. Meadow R. Suffocation, recurrent apnea, and sudden infant death. J Pediatr 1990; 117(3):351–357.

720. Galvin HK, Newton AW, Vandeven AM. Update on Munchausen syndrome by proxy. Curr Opin Pediatr 2005; 17:252–257.

721. Hall DE, Eubanks L, Meyyazhagan S, et al. Evaluation of covert video surveillance in the diagnosis of Munchausen syndrome by proxy: lessons from 41 cases. Pediatrics 2000; 105:1305–1312.

722. Williams C, Bevan VT. The secret observation of children in hospital. Lancet 1988; 1:780–781.

723. Rosen C, Frost JD. Two siblings with recurrent cardiorespiratory arrest: Munchausen by proxy or child abuse? Pediatrics 1983; 71:715–720.

724. Southall DP, Stebbens VA, et al. Apnoeic episodes induced by smothering: two cases identified by covert video surveillance. Br Med J 1987; 1:1637–1641.

725. Mahesh VK, Stern HP, et al. Application of pharmacokinetics in the diagnosis of chemical abuse in Munchausen syndrome by proxy. Clin Pediatr 1988; 27:243–246.

Sudden death in infants

18

PART 1   *Enid Gilbert-Barness*

Sudden and unexpected death in infants

Then came there two women, that were harlots, unto the king, and stood before him. And the one woman said, 'O my lord, I and this woman dwell in one house; and I was delivered of a child with her in the house. And it came to pass the third day after that I was delivered, that this woman was delivered also; and we were together; there was no stranger with us in the house, save we two in the house. And this woman's child died in the night; because she overlaid it.'   1 Kings 3.16-19

The sudden and unexpected death of an apparently healthy baby is a tragedy for parents, grandparents, and siblings – and for the pediatrician. At the same time these deaths are challenges for forensic and pediatric pathologists. The pediatric or forensic pathologist or the coroner responsible for the death investigation, including the autopsy, is required to serve not only the family (with honesty and compassion) but the law. The differential diagnosis of sudden death in infants can be challenging and complex and includes Sudden Infant Death Syndrome (SIDS). A distinction is made between sudden death occurring in an infant and sudden infant death syndrome. The two are not synonymous. Infants may die suddenly and unexpectedly from a variety of causes. Only after a thorough autopsy, death scene investigation, and review of clinical history can one legitimately sign out the death as sudden infant death syndrome. Even after this due diligence, approximately 85% of cases of sudden death in infants (including SIDS) are left unexplained; the other 15% comprise a variety of explained medical disorders, including accidental and non-accidental trauma and overlay.

The sudden infant death syndrome
The old definition

In 1989, the National Institute of Child Health and Human Development (NICHD) convened a group to consider redefining the sudden infant death syndrome.[1] The entity had originally been both named and officially defined in 1969 at the Second International Conference on Causes of Sudden Death in Infants.[2] The second definition is the following: 'The sudden death of an infant under one year of age which remains unexplained after a thorough case investigation, including performance of a complete autopsy, **examination of the death scene, and review of the clinical history**.'[3]

New general definition of SIDS

SIDS is now defined as sudden, unexpected death of an infant <1 year of age, with onset of the fatal episode apparently occurring during sleep, that remains unexplained after a thorough death scene investigation, including performance of a complete autopsy and review of the circumstances of death and the clinical history.[3] Therefore, SIDS is essentially a diagnosis of exclusion to be used when other possibilities, including metabolic disorders, have been ruled out. Most SIDS deaths occur between 1 and 4 months of age. African-American babies are two to three times more likely to die from SIDS than white babies and American Indian babies are three times more susceptible. More males than females are affected.[2]

An expert panel of pediatricians, pediatric pathologists, and forensic pathologists agreed upon the following definitions and subclassification.[2]

- Category IA SIDS: classic features of SIDS present and completely documented
  Category IA includes infant deaths that meet the requirements of the general definition and also all of the following requirements.
  - Clinical
    - More than 21 days and <9 months of age.
    - Normal clinical history, including term pregnancy (gestational age of = 37 weeks).
    - Normal growth and development.
    - No similar deaths among siblings, close genetic relatives (uncles, aunts, or first-degree cousins), or other infants in the custody of the same caregiver.
  - Circumstances of death
    - Investigation of the various scenes where incidents leading to death might have occurred and determination that they do not provide an explanation for the death.
    - Found in a safe sleeping environment, with no evidence of accidental death.
  - Autopsy
    - Absence of potentially fatal pathologic findings. Minor respiratory system inflammatory infiltrates are acceptable; intrathoracic petechial hemorrhage is a supportive but not obligatory or diagnostic finding.
    - No evidence of unexplained trauma, abuse, neglect, or unintentional injury.
    - No evidence of substantial thymic stress effect (thymic weight of <15 g and/or moderate/severe cortical lymphocyte depletion). Occasional 'starry sky' macrophages or minor cortical depletion is acceptable.
    - Negative results of toxicologic, microbiologic, radiologic vitreous chemistry, and metabolic screening studies.
- Category IB SIDS: classic features of SIDS present but incompletely documented
  Category IB includes infant deaths that meet the requirements of the general definition and also meet all of the criteria for category 1A except that investigation of the various scenes where incidents leading to death might have occurred was not performed and/or one of the following analyses was not performed: toxicologic, microbiologic, radiologic, vitreous chemistry, or metabolic screening studies.
- Category II SIDS
  Category II includes infant deaths that meet category I criteria except for one of the following:

- Clinical
  - Age range outside that of category IA or B (i.e., 0–21 days or 270 days [9 months] through first birthday).
  - Similar deaths among siblings, close relatives, or other infants in the custody of the same caregiver that are not considered suspect for infanticide or recognized genetic disorders.
  - Neonatal or perinatal conditions (for example, those resulting from preterm birth) that have resolved by the time of death.
- Circumstances of death
  - Mechanical asphyxia or suffocation caused by overlaying not determined with certainty.
- Autopsy
  - Abnormal growth and development not thought to have contributed to death.
  - Marked inflammatory changes or abnormalities not sufficient to be unequivocal cause of death.
- Unclassified Sudden Infant Death
  The unclassified category includes deaths that do not meet the criteria for category I or II SIDS, but for which alternative diagnoses of natural or unnatural conditions are equivocal, including cases for which autopsies were not performed.
- Post-*resuscitation* cases
  Infants found in extremis who are resuscitated and later die ('temporarily interrupted SIDS') may be included in the aforementioned categories, depending on the fulfillment of relevant criteria.

While there is some concern that the 'cutoff point' in the NICHD definition is 1 year of age, SIDS is primarily a phenomenon of early infancy with 85% occurring between 2 and 4 months. The findings at autopsy in infants after accidental or inflicted asphyxia are often minimal.[6–10]

The term 'SIDS' remains, therefore, one of exclusion and should not be used if there is evidence of possible accidental asphyxia, inflicted injuries, or significant organic diseases.

The two new elements in the definition of SIDS, death scene investigation and review of clinical history, were added because since 1988 coroners and medical examiners have become aware that the pathologist frequently has not been informed of, nor has discovered some critical element or circumstance at the scene. For example, the baby's head may have become wedged in the space between the mattress and the crib side so that the infant's nose, having been pressed into the mattress, was occluded resulting in asphyxiation. In such a situation a diagnosis of SIDS might be made if it were established on the basis of the autopsy alone.

Furthermore, and particularly in recent years, there have been several highly publicized instances of so-called **Munchausen syndrome by proxy** wherein a mother repeatedly semisuffocates her baby and then takes the infant to the emergency room, claiming each time that the baby has suffered an apneic attack. Eventually, after a series of such incidents, the mother causes the baby's death by suffocation and claims that it was due to SIDS. Apparently, this is an abnormal psychological mechanism whereby the mother satisfies her need for attention.[9] Because it now appears that SIDS is probably not genetically controlled, medical examiners should be cautious in attributing the second or third apparent crib death in a family to SIDS and should instead initiate an investigation into the likelihood of filicide (homicide by a parent) or a metabolic disease.

There are still many unresolved cases wherein the history, investigation, and autopsy reveal information that places the death outside the category of SIDS but does not explain the cause of death. Examples of the latter are **suspected** cases of abuse, neglect, or accidental suffocation; cases with episodes of vomiting or diarrhea during the 24 hours before death without pathologic evidence of infection or dehydration; cases in which the information regarding death is not reliable; and cases in which the autopsy findings are not sufficient to explain death, such as mild bronchopneumonia and maternal drug abuse.[1]

Collaboration between SIDS International and the NICHD in the United States resulted in the formulation of an International Standardized Autopsy Protocol (ISAP).[12,13] This protocol has been endorsed by both the Society for Pediatric Pathology (SPP) and the National Association of Medical Examiners (NAME). At around the same time, a formal death scene investigation protocol, entitled 'Sudden Unexplained Infant Death Investigation Report Form' (SUIDIRF), was prepared by the Centers for Disease Control and Prevention.[14, 15]

External examination, radiology, internal examination, histology, microbiology, toxicology, electrolyte, and metabolic and genetic studies have all contributed to significantly increased accuracy in diagnosis.[16–18]

If a pathologist is not able to attend the scene, police crime scene/physical investigation officers may be able to take video recordings and/or photographs which should be reviewed by the pathologist.

In Meadow's report of 42 cases of infant homicide misdiagnosed as SIDS, it is likely that variable standards were applied to investigations and autopsy procedures.[19] It has been stated that 'investigations into the pathology and circumstances of sudden infant death are often scanty and inexpert' with significant omissions being documented when cases were audited.[20,21] These reports clearly demonstrate the need for higher standards in the investigation of infant deaths.

If there are multiple infant deaths in one family, homicide should be seriously considered. Rare inherited metabolic or cardiac diseases should also be vigorously pursued. The dictum that the first death is SIDS, the second death is 'undetermined,' and the third death is automatically 'homicide' cannot be supported, unless all other causes of death have been ruled out, since inflicted trauma and a metabolic disease are some of many possibilities.

Although a SIDS death occurring in an infant who has suffered significant apneic episodes must remain a possibility, it is mandatory to consider both underlying organic illness and inflicted suffocation. As noted above, the presence of oronasal blood may be an important marker suggesting inflicted suffocation.[22–24] Possible causes of apparent life-threatening events are listed in Box 18.1.1.

BOX 18.1.1 POSSIBLE CAUSES OF APPARENT LIFE-THREATENING EVENTS

Cardiovascular
 Congenital malformation
 Myocarditis
 Cardiomyopathy
 Arrhythmia
 Vascular ring

Respiratory
 Upper airway obstruction
 Congenital alveolar hypoventilation
 Infections

Central nervous system
 Epilepsy
 Tumors
 Trauma
 Shaking
 Infections

Gastrointestinal
 Gastroesophageal reflux/aspiration
 Pyloric stenosis

Metabolic and endocrine
 Hypoglycemia
 Hyponatremia
 Hypocalcemia
 Hypothyroidism
 Carnitine deficiency
 Fructosemia
 Reye syndrome
 Leigh syndrome

Infectious
 Septicemia

Mechanical
 Accidental smothering
 Munchausen syndrome by proxy

Miscellaneous
 Anemia
 Hypothermia

Idiopathic

Adapted from Byard and Krous.[8]

Epidemiology

Sudden, unexplained infant death is the third leading cause of infant mortality in the United States. The US birth rate per 1000 is 14.1. The number of SIDS deaths is 2234 or 8.1% of all total infant deaths recorded in the year 2001. This does not, however, reflect any influence that may become evident with a change in sleeping position. Rates of SIDS have been rapidly declining in recent years. However, they remain disproportionately higher among black infants than among white infants. The number of infant deaths in the United States in 2001 was 27 568 and the infant mortality rate was 6.8 per 1000 live births. The SIDS death rate in 2001 for white infants is 7.8%; for black infants it is 8.8% of all total causes of death. SIDS is the leading cause of death for postnatal (28 days to 11 months) infants in the US and the third leading cause of death in infants under 1 year of age.[25] The incidence of SIDS has decreased from 110.5/100 000 live births in 1990 to 47.2/100 000 in 1998 in Calfornia.[26] With the introduction of the 'Back to Sleep' campaign by the American Academy of Pediatrics in 1992, the incidence of SIDS has decreased by almost 50%.[27]

Approximately 2000 babies die from SIDS in the US every year. It is currently believed that SIDS results when the baby's body has difficulty regulating blood pressure, temperature, breathing, and/or a combination of these due to an underlying vulnerability or developmental problem. When stressed by environmental factors such as sleeping in the prone position, these babies can die from SIDS.[28]

SIDS deaths are rare in Asian communities and are more common in indigenous and African-American populations.[29-33] Among American Indians, SIDS rates have been consistently higher than among white infants, except in Oklahoma where birth weights are similar to white infants.[33-36] Although it may be emotionally painful for the family, a death scene investigation will help shed light on the cause of death by providing a detailed record of the location and circumstances of the death. Therefore, the investigator must attempt to learn as much as possible about the events leading up to the death, even to the very moment that death occurred.[37]

Fewer diagnoses of SIDS are now being made on the basis of autopsy reports and death scene investigations. As these practices become more standardized, the reported prevalence of SIDS may change[37] and true SIDS as a cause of death should be relatively rare.

The NICHD epidemiologic study

Around 1980, the US NICHD undertook to gather epidemiologic data concerning a group of SIDS cases in the United States representing approximately 10% of all deaths of infants under 1 year of age and to compare those babies with a control group of twice the number of healthy, living infants from the same geographic areas.[38-40] The original intent had been to study 1000 babies who died from SIDS and 2000 babies in control groups in six geographic areas.

A single panel of three pathologists examined all microscopic slides and reviewed all other information about each case that the original medical examiner had, including the circumstances of death, toxicologic studies, and microbiologic studies. Data used for the study were garnered from only 757 cases of SIDS and double that number in two control groups, i.e., control group A matched for age only and control group B matched for age, race, and birth weight. A series of studies based on those data has been published since the project was completed.[38-40]

Age of the infant

The original, official definition of SIDS published in 1969 made no mention of age except for its inclusion of the word *infant*, which according to pediatric usage means 'a baby up to 1 year old.'[2] However, an unofficial policy pervaded pediatric forensic practice; many practitioners avoided using the term for the sudden, inexplicable death of an infant less than 1 month of age, presumably in an effort to avoid confusion of neonatal SIDS cases with other recognized causes of neonatal mortality.

In 1989, the working group concluded that any specific designation of a lower age limit would be both arbitrary and unwarranted. Thus, the definition currently embraces all infant deaths of this nature down to and including the day of birth. At least one publication is devoted to the existence of this neonatal component.[41] Nevertheless, a diagnosis of SIDS for infants younger than 1 month and older than 6 months should be made with caution and only after all possible causes are excluded, particularly metabolic diseases. Eighty-five percent of deaths from SIDS occur between 2 and 4 months of age, and 95% occur under 6 months of age. The hiatus for SIDS under 1 month of age may be explained by the effectiveness of gasping during the first month and not thereafter.[42]

Rates of occurrence

SIDS rates vary from country to country. They are exceedingly low in Japan and China. They also differ according to ethnicity.

In recent years, a sudden and striking diminution has occurred in the numbers and rates of SIDS in certain countries.[26,43,44] This drop in rates and numbers has been particularly dramatic in New Zealand where previously rates had been among the highest in the world. For example, previously in Dunedin, at the southernmost tip of the country, the rates were about four times those in the United States.[45]

Following initiation of national campaigns in these countries for the prevention of SIDS, the rates in Australia,[43] New Zealand,[45] and in parts of Great Britain[44,46] dramatically decreased. Their prevention programs included recommendations regarding mothers not smoking during pregnancy, abandonment of the prone sleeping position for the infant, abandonment of overwrapping the baby, and abandonment of co-sleeping. Reductions in SIDS rates have also been achieved by these same means in a number of countries including Holland and Norway and in King's County, Washington, in the United States.[47] A case-control study, sponsored by the NICHD conducted in the Chicago area has reported on the risk of SIDS and the role of the sleep environment.[47]

Ethnicity

In the early 1960s, data from Philadelphia showed that the rate of SIDS among black infants was four times higher than that among white infants.[49] The supposition was that the difference in SIDS rates somehow reflected economic disadvantages among black people. Since then, many studies have confirmed that economic factors do make a significant difference. However, it appears that sociocultural issues also play a part.

In 1990, investigators in Chicago found that the rate of SIDS among Mexican-Americans living in Chicago was lower than that for white infants, despite the Mexican families being much poorer.[50] Shortly thereafter, a similar survey in Miami revealed the same phenomenon. The rate of SIDS was appreciably lower among the Cuban population (then constituting roughly 48% of the population) than among the non-Hispanic white population even though the former were not as well-to-do as the latter.[51]

At least five strata of vulnerability occur in the United States. The highest rate is among certain tribes of Native Americans.[31] The black race is the next most susceptible, followed by whites, then Hispanics; Asians have the lowest rate.[52]

A study among Native Americans in the State of Washington showed their SIDS rate to be three times that of white infants in the area.[33] However, further analysis of the data showed that after adjustment had been made for the mother's age, marital status, parity, and cigarette smoking during pregnancy, their unusually high rate was due to the prevalence of certain recognized risk factors, at least some of which, in turn, were related to socioeconomic status.

A smaller study in South Dakota showed the rate of SIDS among the Indians to be 3.95 times that of white infants. However, the rate declined to only 2.51 when adjusted for maternal education and the trimester in which prenatal care had begun.[31]

A 1990 report from Birmingham, England, detailed a pattern similar to that in the United States with a rate of only 1.18 among Asians and 5.25 among Afro-Caribbeans.[53] These authors, too, concluded that sociocultural differences are probably the most important underlying factors.

Recurrence in families

The risk of recurrence of SIDS in a family is between 13 per 1000[54] and less than 1 per 1000 live births.[55] Irgens and colleagues of Norway, for example, report that the risk for all infants in that country is 1.3 per 1000 live births, but for subsequent children in a family that has experienced SIDS it is approximately 5.0.[56] The lack of concordance in twins is against the likelihood that SIDS is a genetic disorder.

The apparent increased incidence in siblings is probably due to inclusion of other disorders, including some genetic diseases, and other risk factors that may be repeated in subsequent pregnancies,[54] such as sleeping habits.

Monitoring Home monitoring of infants has not been effective in reducing either morbidity or mortality.[57] Monitoring is not considered necessary for infants with only one sibling SIDS death.[57]

Differential diagnosis: SIDS versus child abuse

One of the most difficult problems currently facing coroners and medical examiners in relation to SIDS is that of

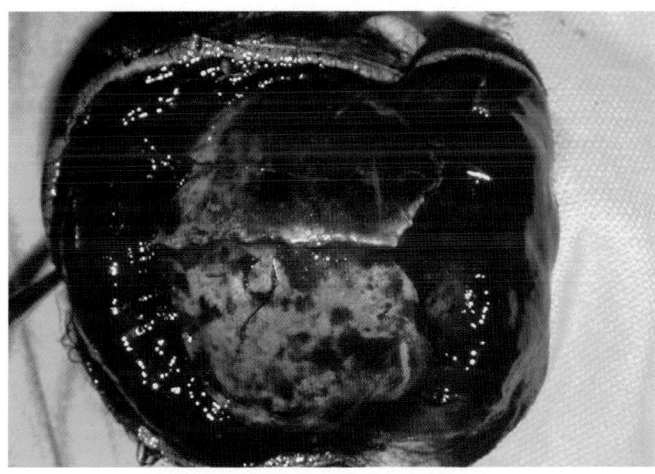

FIGURE 18.1.1 This infant suffered bilateral subdural hematomas with a fractured skull as a result of abuse.

differentiating cases of SIDS from those infant deaths that are the result of child abuse. The principal basis for that difficulty is the virtual **impossibility of distinguishing SIDS at autopsy from suffocation with a soft object. Postmortem findings in the two are virtually identical**. Hence, ultimately, differentiation is based on the circumstances of death and the family's medical history, especially in regard to previous deaths of the same, unexpected sort among siblings.

In the United States the number of recurrences is not expected to exceed 2% of all subsequent siblings in that family. If a forensic pathologist cannot explain the most recent – or any – of a set or series of infant deaths in a family, the most recent case is usually designated 'undetermined.' Confidential inquiries related to sudden infant death by Emery and Taylor,[58] uncovered cases of deaths from child abuse that had been attributed to SIDS.

Physical abuse is usually evident in those instances. When an infant's death is due to subdural hematoma (Fig. 18.1.1) or massive hemorrhage into the abdomen or around the spinal cord (Fig. 18.1.2) and abdominal organs (Fig. 18.1.3), there can be no doubt that trauma was the cause. However, suffocation with a soft object (e.g., the cupped hand of an adult) is virtually impossible to prove by postmortem examination of the body.[59]

So-called **shaken baby syndrome** may be difficult to diagnose. Although hemorrhage into the retina and/or optic nerve is frequently present, it is not pathognomonic because these hemorrhages can be created during other forms of stress, such as vigorous attempts at resuscitation.[60–62] Goetting and Sowa[61] reported the results of a prospective study of 20 children who had experienced cardiopulmonary resuscitation terminally. Five of those deaths were due to SIDS, seven to sepsis, three to near-drowning, three to asthma, two to poisoning, and one each to asphyxiation and aspiration. Two of the 20 (10%) had retinal hemorrhages; one died as a result of near-drowning and the other of SIDS.

In the Munchausen syndrome by proxy[63,64] all the infants died in the presence of the mother only. Meadow[63] published a series of 27 such cases from 27 different families. Eighteen of

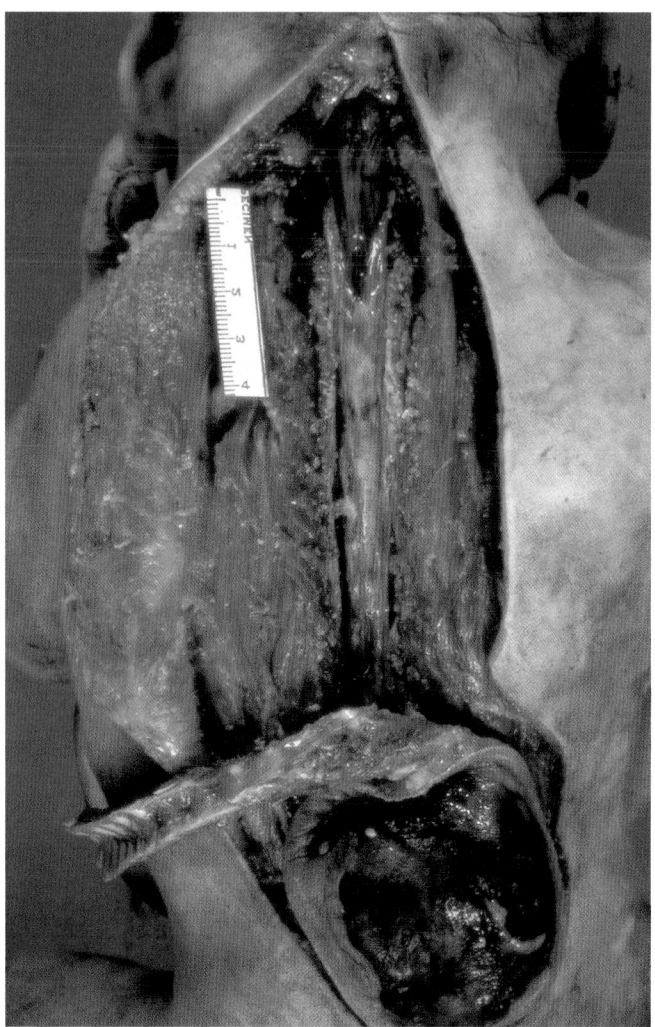

FIGURE 18.1.2 Hidden evidence of abuse is apparent here in the hemorrhage deep into the (pigmented) skin, subcutaneous tissues of the back, and around the spinal cord.

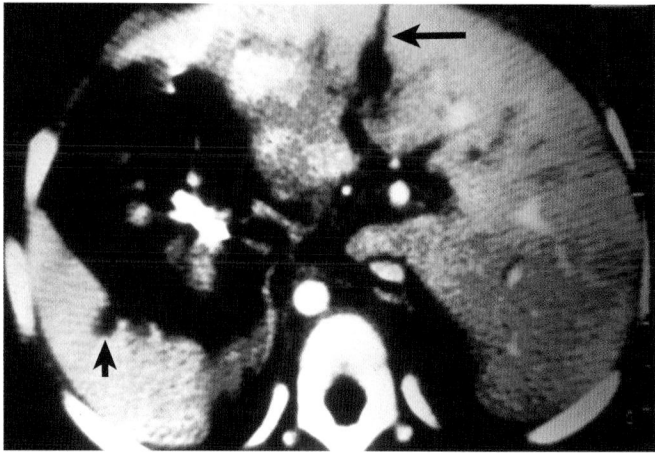

FIGURE 18.1.3 Liver subcapsular hemorrhage. The infant had been kicked in the abdomen with no external evidence of injury.

those children were still alive – one had brain damage – and nine were dead. Twenty-four were reported to have had prior episodes. Eighteen had older siblings who had died suddenly and unexpectedly in early life. Most of them also had recurrent, apparently life-threatening episodes. The majority of those had been certified as SIDS, but it is probable that they, too, were suffocated. Several cases of sudden infant death in a family or under the care of a child care provider have later been disclosed as homicide.[65]

Newlands and Emery[66] searched the Child Protection Register for children with siblings who died of SIDS in southern Derbyshire, England. Confidential inquiries into all child deaths and registered deaths from SIDS were made over 4 years, from 1984 to 1988. From a cohort of 288 children, one in 30 on the register had a sibling whose death was registered as caused by SIDS. Suffocation of these infants appeared to be most likely. That child abuse by suffocation is an important factor in one in ten SIDS deaths has been reported by Emery and Taylor.[58] The

Sheffield Intervention Program has been effective in the prevention of such deaths.[67, 68]

Bed-related deaths and the prone sleeping position

Infants may die unexpectedly in the prone position.[69, 70] Provocative experimental studies by Emery and Thornton[71] in 1968 used the cadavers of infants between the ages of 6 and 9 weeks who had been found dead in their cribs. They measured resistance to the flow of air pumped through the upper respiratory tract when the body of the infant was placed face down on a pillow. If the pillow was damp, as may occur from the moisture of respiration or vomitus, the mean increase in pressure was 235%.[71]

An exceptionally low rate of sudden infant death has been observed in Asian countries, with an incidence of 0.04 per 1000 live births.[72] In Asian cultures, the supine sleeping position is almost universal.

Beal[73] and others observed the incidence of SIDS in New Zealand to be increased among the Maoris, who almost invariably used the prone position for their babies. The researchers recommended avoidance of that position. That recommendation resulted in a decrease of over 50% in the SIDS rate among infants in Australia.

Infants who sleep face down and who have been exposed to cigarette smoke during pregnancy and in infancy have significantly higher rates of SIDS than those sleeping in the supine position. Infants who sleep on their sides have an increased risk of SIDS due to rolling on to their abdomens during sleep.[74] A higher risk of SIDS exists in infants who have been put to sleep prone for the first time, so-called unaccustomed prone,[75, 76] and it is estimated that in approximately 15% of cases suspected to be SIDS, the autopsy identifies another cause of death, such as a disease or genetic disorder, as well as unintentional injury or unnatural death.[36]

No increase in deaths due to aspiration of gastric contents has been reported since routine back sleeping has been adopted. On the contrary, significant aspiration occurs instead in infants who sleep face down.[77]

Prone sleeping involves many potential problems including diaphragmatic splinting/fatigue, rebreathing of carbon dioxide, reflex, decreased vasomotor tone with tachycardia, blunting of arousal responses, upper airway obstruction from soft bedding, and overheating.[78]

The three major risk factors for sudden infant death in Great Britain, Australia, and New Zealand were the prone sleeping position, maternal smoking, and lack of breast feeding. Among those, the prone position was the most significant.[79, 80] All three factors were independent but appeared to account for 79% of deaths.[80] In Avon, publicity recommending the supine sleeping position resulted in a decrease in the incidence of SIDS from 3.5 per 1000 live births to 1.7 per 1000.[81] The overall incidence of SIDS in England has fallen from 2.5 to 0.7 per 1000 live births.[46] In King's County, Washington State, in the United States, a striking decrease of 52% occurred over a period of 8 months following the publication of an article in the *Seattle Times* advising against the prone position for sleeping infants.[14, 47] In England, a decrease in SIDS incidence from 2.5 to 0.7 per 1000 live births has resulted from recommendations for the supine sleeping position.[46] The dramatic decrease in sudden infant deaths in New Zealand may be attributed not only to the change in sleeping position but also to the advice against the use of sheepskin as a sleeping surface for infants.[82] A case-control study from Tasmania[83] found that SIDS was significantly associated with sleeping in the prone position (odds ratio 4:5). The strength of the association increased still further if the infant slept on a natural fiber mattress, was swaddled at bedtime, slept in a heated room, or had been ill recently.

Infants in the prone position on thick, soft, cushiony surfaces (e.g., lamb's wool [sheepskin rugs], certain sofa cushions filled with synthetic material, and bean bags) may rebreathe their own expired air, high in carbon dioxide. In the face straight-down position and/or with bedclothes against the face, studies have confirmed the high risk of either airway obstruction or CO_2 rebreathing.[84] In any circumstance in which the infant cannot continue to lift and hold the head out of a dangerous 'sunken in' state, the infant may suffocate.[85] So compelling has been the evidence for SIDS risk and the prone sleeping position that the American Academy of Pediatrics (AAP) has endorsed the recommendation for the supine position for infants during sleep.[86] Because of the dangers of certain types of mattresses and bedding, Emery designed a mattress with a thin polyurethane base with an overlying corrugated open-cell foam pad covered by a flame-retardant washable polyester netting through which the infant can easily breathe.[87] This is used in Great Britain.

Other mechanisms of sudden death in a prone position include asphyxia caused by respiratory obstruction and backward displacement of the mandible. The high cephalad position of the cervical structures in the young infant with close apposition of the soft palate and the back of the tongue may enhance the possibility of airway obstruction.[88] With growth and development, at 5–6 months of age, adequate space is established between the soft palate and tongue above, and the larynx below. Furthermore, Emery emphasized the possibility of respiratory obstruction in infants when the nose is compressed in a mattress or bedding. Infants up to about 4 months of age are obligate nasal breathers. The compression of the soft nasal cartilage precludes the infant's ability to breathe and may result in an asphyxial death. At 5–6 months of age the mouth breathing reflex is established. In the prone position, the blood supply to the brain stem may be compromised by extension of the neck. The assumption that if vomiting or regurgitation should occur in an intact infant, aspiration would occur in the supine position is without documentation,[89, 90] and the incidence of death due to aspiration in that position has actually decreased.[91]

The implication of restrictive clothing and hyperthermia should also be evaluated in cases of sudden infant death, particularly in the prone sleeping position.[92] Overheating is more significant in infants who are sleeping in the prone position.[93–98] Soft pillows and mattresses may also increase the risk of infant death in the prone position,[99–103] possibly associated with airway occlusion or hyperthermia. The prone position may reduce the infant's ability to lose heat from the face when exposed to heat stress.[91] In addition, when infants sleep prone, the risk of death may be increased by the residua of recent illness or by excess heat in the room.[83, 104] Thermal stress and carbon dioxide rebreathing are not mutually exclusive, as hyperpnea secondary to rebreathing increases heat production and potential heat stress is presumably associated with an increased carbon dioxide production. Rebreathing of warmed expired air also reduces respiratory heat exchange and enhances thermal stress. Rebreathing of expired air has been implicated in 25% of presumed SIDS-related deaths by Kemp and Thach.[104]

Although the lateral position for sleeping has also been recommended, positioning infants on their sides may not be as safe as the supine position. Mitchell[105] noted the relatively unstable nature of the lateral position, which may result in the infant rolling over into the prone position; lividities may help ascertain this position.

Even when the sleeping surface is not markedly compressible, an infant whose **physiologic capacity to respond appropriately** to a challenge, such as an elevated carbon dioxide level, might die if there is failure to lift and turn the head, a response of which most newborn infants are capable. This may explain why a compromised infant may die in the prone position (with nose down) even on a surface not perceived to be particularly dangerous.

The exact position of the baby's face at the time of death, the surface on which the infant is found, whether the baby was lying prone, and whether the face and nose were pressed **into** the surface of a soft mattress, pillow, or soft bedding should be ascertained in any case of sudden infant death in the prone position.

For infants asleep on waterbeds at the time of death, the following information should be ascertained: the filling and tenseness of the mattress and whether free-floating or baffled; whether the infant's head could create a sinkhole in the mattress;[87, 106, 107] and whether the infant's head was **trapped** between the mattress and the bed frame.[103] The hazards of mattresses, beds (particularly waterbeds), and bedding have been reported in a series of 52 sudden deaths in infants in which 20 resulted from suffocation due to the design of the mattress or bedding.[103, 108]

If the infant is discovered some appreciable time after death, the pattern of livor mortis will usually be of help in establishing which part of the infant's face was compressed when death occurred.

In light of present understanding the pathologist must consider the following:

1. The nature of **the surface** on which the baby was resting, i.e., was it soft and compressible? Could it have been indented by the weight of the baby's head? Would it have caused obstruction of the airway because it was non-porous, or had the infant's nose been 'trapped' in it?
2. The position of the **baby's nose**. Was it straight down into that surface so that either occlusion or re-breathing was inevitable?

The US Consumer Product Safety Commission in 1995 after a 2-year intense investigation has concluded that at least 30% of SIDS deaths each year are most likely caused by suffocation.[87] In these cases, the cause and manner of death are best certified as asphyxia – accident.

A correlation between the use of conjugate *Haemophilus influenzae* B vaccine in infants starting at 2 months of age and the reduction in the number of SIDS cases in the United States has been made.[109]

Co-sleeping

For purposes of this discussion, 'co-sleeping' means an adult sleeping with an infant in the same bed, sofa, pallet, chair, etc; not merely sleeping in the same room.

Co-sleeping has been discussed as a cause of crib death since biblical times. It is often said that the first recorded case appears in the Old Testament, in the Book of Kings. Solomon is forced to decide which of two mothers is the real parent of an infant who 'died in the night because she overlaid it.'[110] The presumption was that the mother of the dead baby had suffocated her child by unconsciously lying on him or her, and thus causing asphyxiation during sleep. Overlying except when a parent has taken drugs or alcohol is rare, compared with co-sleeping in a number of societies including Asian societies.[111] The question of the effects of co-sleeping is still controversial. Mosco et al. maintains that co-sleeping, which has a long evolutionary history, prevents death by the mother's unconscious moving and breathing through the night that stimulate the baby's breathing.[112] Some (especially forensic) pathologists are convinced that even an undrugged mother could conceivably lie on her new baby and thus asphyxiate it. An excellent, thorough review of this subject has been published.[113, 114] Co-sleeping is not always intentional. A breast-feeding mother with large,

pendulous breasts may nurse on the sofa or in a chair and fall asleep unintentionally and the infant may suffocate accidentally. Some medical examiners or coroners may still be reluctant to consider overlay as a cause of death to spare the family feelings. However, if the circumstances cannot rule it out and the remainder of the investigation, autopsy, and clinical history provide no alternative answers, it is a disservice to the family and to possible future infants of that family, to ignore it.

Bedsharing Bedsharing has certain well-recognized risks.[115] One of the most dangerous situations predisposing to smothering occurs when an infant is placed between parents on a soft mattress and covered by blankets. Large parents, especially when intoxicated, sedated, or fatigued, increase the risk of overlaying.[116, 117]

Maternal cigarette smoking

In 1993, a large, nationwide, case-control study of maternal cigarette smoking and its impact on the risk for SIDS was published.[118] The study groups comprised 485 infants whose deaths were from SIDS and 1800 babies born of non-smoking mothers. These investigators discovered that the infants of mothers who smoked during pregnancy had a risk of succumbing to SIDS that was 4.09 times higher than that of the babies of non-smoking mothers; infants exposed to tobacco smoke also have impaired arousal.[119]

Infants of mothers who smoked **after** their pregnancy also had an increased risk that was dose-related. Smoking by the infants' fathers did not increase their risk if the mothers were non-smokers. In the NICHD study, maternal cigarette smoking (of all the risk factors) proved to have the strongest statistical association with SIDS.[39]

Both intrauterine and postpregnancy exposure of the infant – whether black or white – are associated with an increased risk for SIDS.[120] Furthermore, the combined exposure of maternal smoking during and after pregnancy is more dangerous than either one of those exposures alone.

DTP immunization

In the NICHD study it became apparent that, overall, infants with SIDS were **less** likely than infants in the control group to have received **any** DTP immunization.[121] Only 39.8% of infants with SIDS had received one or more DTP immunizations compared with 55% of infants in a control group A and 53.2% of those in control group B.

Only 1.8% infants with SIDS died **within 24 hours** of having had the DTP immunization compared with 5.0% of infants in control group A and 2.2% in control group B. SIDS is less common in infants who had been immunized.[122] In South Australia, when the age of first immunization was dropped from 3 to 2 months, there was no fall in the median or average age of SIDS infants, as would be expected if the two events were causally related.[123] The findings suggest that DTP immunization is not a significant factor in the causation of SIDS.

Metabolic disorders and SIDS: MCAD deficiency

At least 12 fatty acid oxidation disorders as well as other metabolic disorders are known to be responsible for cases of sudden and unexpected death in infancy (Box 18.1.2).[124–126] Of these, medium-chain acyl-CoA dehydrogenase (MCAD) deficiency is the most common. The postmortem diagnosis of inborn metabolic disorders in sudden death victims is important for genetic counseling and for the evaluation of siblings who may be at risk. The diagnosis of fatty acid oxidation disorders may be suspected from the presence of a fatty liver at autopsy; this may be overlooked. A diagnosis of MCAD deficiency can be established by molecular analysis in frozen or fixed tissues.[127,128] Postmortem testing for other disorders in solid tissues is not available at the molecular level.

A postmortem screening method for fatty acid oxidation disorders by the simultaneous measurement of C_8 to C_{20} fatty acids, glucose, lactate, and other metabolites from the methanol wash of a pellet obtained by ultracentrifugation of liver homogenate has been developed. *Cis*-4-decanoic acid was present in five confirmed cases with MCAD deficiency and in one case with glutaric aciduria type II and was absent in 97 of 100 randomly chosen sudden death cases, at least 81 of which were diagnosed as SIDS. In this series, C_{14} to C_{18} monounsaturated fatty acids were significantly elevated in the one examined case affected with long-chain acyl-CoA dehydrogenase (LCAD) deficiency. The metabolite profiles in two cases with carnitine uptake deficiency were less informative, but they shared with all the other disease controls a very low glucose concentration, a finding compatible with premortem hypoglycemia. It has been recommended that all infants who die suddenly and unexpectedly should be appropriately investigated for a metabolic disorder as part of the routine autopsy procedure.[129] However, the MCAD gene mutation is rare. In two separate investigations involving thousands of cases (with controls), one based in Los Angeles and the other in Quebec, the frequency of this gene mutation was the same, approximately 0.56 per thousand live births in both.[130,131] Other studies have shown different results.[129] In the living child the clinical manifestations of MCAD deficiency range in severity from no signs or symptoms to the so-called apparently life-threatening episodes (ALTEs). New technologies, such as electrospray ionization tandem mass spectrometry, have revolutionized the investigation of metabolic disease at postmortem, allowing the identification of a wide range of such diseases in minute quantities of blood, plasma, and bile.[132]

Pathologic physiology

Airway obstruction

In the early 1970s there was considerable discussion of the likelihood that upper airway obstruction was the cause of crib death. Proponents of that theory believed that the typical intrathoracic petechiae (present in about 80% of autopsies on infants with SIDS) was the result of increased negative pressure within the thoracic cavity, induced directly by inhalation against an obstruction. However, intrathoracic petechiae are characteristic of autopsies in cases of placental abruption, and in that setting the fetus has often succumbed before ever having had the opportunity to breathe. Hence, the specific cause of these petechiae in the pleura and pericardium in SIDS is not known.

Idiopathic central apnea

Steinschneider[133] reported five infants in one family who were diagnosed as SIDS. He then proposed that idiopathic, spontaneous, central apnea was a major cause of SIDS and on this basis apnea monitors were introduced. Twenty-three years later the mother confessed to smothering the infants with a pillow because their screaming made her feel useless.[134] Southall and colleagues[135] showed prospectively that not 1 of 27 infants who eventually succumbed to SIDS had abnormal pneumograms, which were performed when these infants were about 6 weeks of age.

In 1985, the American Academy of Pediatrics concluded that apnea monitors should be prescribed for babies only when the infant in question had experienced an ALTE. The Academy specifically **did not recommend** its use in subsequent siblings, depending on the judgment of individual pediatricians.[136, 137]

Bradycardia

In 1991 and 1994, Kelly et al.[138] and Meny and colleagues,[139] respectively, published their experience in regard to six infants

Male gender

2–4 months old

Premature

Low birth weight

High birth order

Multiple births

Short interpregnancy interval

Poor prenatal care

Lower socioeconomic status family

Young parents

Low level of maternal education

Maternal drug use

Winter months

Prone sleeping position[‡]

Exposure to cigarette smoke (during and after pregnancy)[‡]

Overheating

Adapted from Byard and Cohle.[1]
[‡] Major risk factors

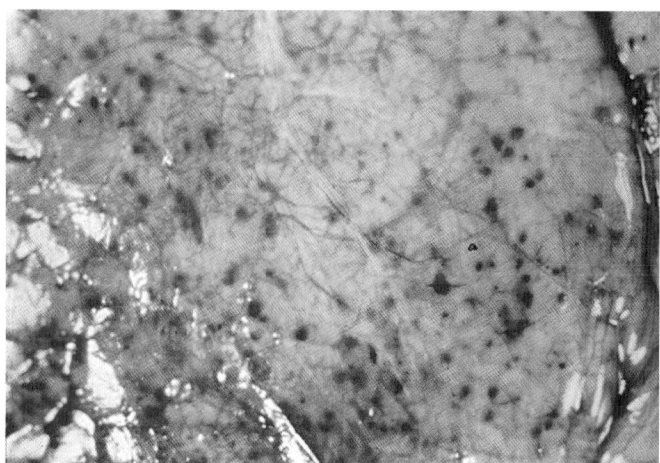

FIGURE 18.1.4 Thymic petechiae. Anterior and posterior aspects of the thymus show clearly many pinpoint hemorrhages scattered all over the thymus; they are numerous in cut sections as well.

(of 1067) who died suddenly and unexpectedly. Five of the infants were on memory-equipped cardiorespiratory monitors, and one was on a respiratory monitor with an alarm log. All six were born prematurely. On the basis of the autopsies, three of the deaths were ascribed to SIDS and three to bronchopulmonary dysplasia. In all six records **bradycardia** was the dominant feature, rather than central apnea. Bradycardia was preceded by tachycardia in two of the infants. Five of the babies died within 20 minutes of the initial event. Bradycardia was the most significant feature in all six records, but its etiology remains unknown. Whether either hypoxemia or obstructive apnea played any role in these events is also undetermined. Improved technology in the form of cardiorespiratory monitors that provide data on a hard copy has been developed and introduced in the last few years. Some babies will die despite the correct use of the most sophisticated cardiorespiratory monitors. In all these cases, death was preceded by several minutes of worsening bradycardia. All of this highlights the **limitations** of the current clinical use of home monitors, especially those designed to monitor respiration only.

Risk factors versus prediction

Features associated with an increased risk of sudden infant death syndrome are shown in Box 18.1.3. Programs are presently being designed for the prevention of SIDS. For example, maternal cigarette smoking during pregnancy, mater-

nal anemia, and prone sleeping should be avoided. Being a Native American is known to be a so-called risk factor for SIDS. **Premature babies** have a higher risk than do full-term babies. However, it is most important to distinguish between **risk factors** such as these and **prediction of SIDS**. It should be emphasized that approximately 75% of infants with SIDS had no risk factors. However, some potential risk factors should not be overlooked. In a recent study, the level of fetal hemoglobin (HbF) in hemolysates of infants who died from SIDS were found to be markedly increased.[140]

Gross and microscopic autopsy findings

The typical SIDS infant has a normal nutritional status. Findings at autopsy are characteristic. These include petechial hemorrhages of the thymus gland, visceral pleura, and epicardium. In the typical autopsy of a death from SIDS no disease process that accounts for death is found. There may be very little pathologic alteration in any of the organs that is detectable by ordinary means. Nevertheless, certain lesions are commonly encountered.[141] These are said to be classic findings or typical of SIDS and include thymic (Fig. 18.1.4), pleural, and epicardial petechiae, pulmonary congestion (Fig. 18.1.5), and pulmonary edema.

The etiology of intrathoracic petechiae has been debated, with suggestions that they result from upper airway obstruction or terminal gasping.[142–148] Petechiae may arise from increased negative intrathoracic pressure due to agonal gasping.

Thymic petechiae, for example, were recorded as being present, either grossly or microscopically, in 63% of the SIDS cases in the NICHD study. This does not indicate that petechiae are either **diagnostic** of SIDS or even **necessary** for the diagnosis. The same lesions were present in 38% of the controls and were absent in 37 of the SIDS cases.

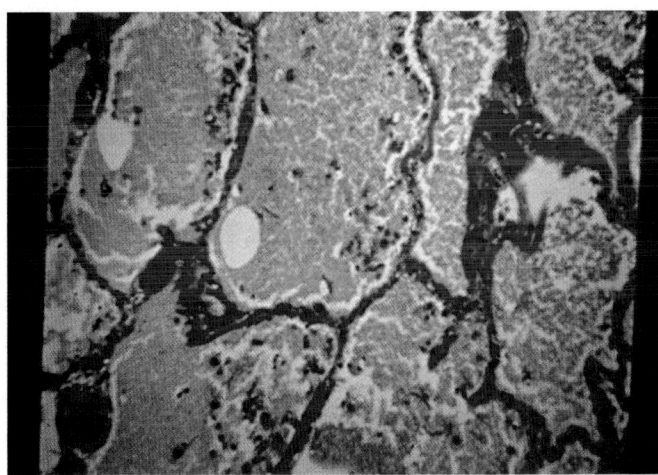

FIGURE 18.1.5 Pulmonary congestion. All of the capillaries in these alveolar walls are dilated and engorged.

Mucosal oral and nasal secretions are commonly observed in SIDS cases. In the absence of prior cardiopulmonary resuscitation, bloody secretion should raise the possibility of accidental or inflicted suffocation.[22]

Pulmonary congestion and edema are common findings and are interpreted as evidence of terminal left ventricular failure. Hemosiderin in the lungs may indicate previous trauma or asphyxial episodes.[149–151]

Central nervous system in SIDS

Many investigators believe that the central nervous system (CNS) is fundamental to the pathogenesis of SIDS or at least to a considerable number of those deaths. Neuropathologists have explored the possibility that the suspected alterations in CNS function in those babies may be reflected in morphologic changes visible by light or electron microscopy.

Several groups have reported morphologic changes in the brains of affected infants, especially in the brain stem and in the medulla. Prominent among the morphologic changes reported are the following:

Astrogliosis;[152–154]

Delayed myelination;[155]

Delayed 'pruning' (or maturation) of dendritic branches;[156,157]

Megalencephaly;[155,158]

Encephalomalacia involving white matter;[159]

Changes in the vagus nerve;[160,161] and

Hypoplasia of the arcuate nucleus.[162]

In a small number of cases, Filiano and Kinney[162] found **hypoplasia of the arcuate nucleus** near the ventral surface of the medulla in infants with SIDS. This nucleus is believed to facilitate chemosensitivity to carbon dioxide and/or hydrogen ions. In a meticulous review of microscopic sections from 41 infants with SIDS and 27 infants in a control group, those investigators found two victims of SIDS who had isolated

hypoplasia of the arcuate nucleus.[162] It has been postulated that this hypoplasia may lead to death by way of 'dyssynergy' between cerebellar coordination of ventilation and autonomic–chemosensory–arousal integration during sleep and hypercarbia in a particularly critical period of infant development. Further studies by Kinney et al.[163] have identified decreased muscarinic receptor binding in the arcuate nucleus (a site of cardiorespiratory control). Alterations in the myelination of the vagus nerve suggest a generalized developmental delay. Neuropathological studies have provided support for central defects with abnormalities in the medullary serotonergic network and arcuate nucleus.[164–168] Increased numbers of SIDS deaths between 2 and 4 months of age would be in keeping with underlying neurological defects being exposed during a time when control of arousal cycles and autonomic function is undergoing considerable modification.

Increased numbers of neuronal dendritic spines and gliosis of the brainstem have been proposed as a marker for previous hypoxic damage in certain infants who die of SIDS.[169, 170]

The QT prolongation could be dangerous in babies and a possible cause of their fatal arrhythmia[171, 172] but solid evidence of its occurrence is still controversial. The capricious nature of episodic QT prolongation documented in human infants poses difficulties in demonstrating lethal cardiac electrical instability.[173]

In 1998, Schwartz et al.,[174] in their 19-year prospective study, performed follow-up electrocardiograms in an unselected population of over 33 000 infants, finding that congenital prolongation of the QT interval accounts for a portion of the crib death cases. However, Schwartz et al. admitted that the long QT syndrome can account for only a fraction of the crib death cases, and precise quantification of this fraction remains difficult despite the data obtained from their large epidemiologic study.[174, 175] Guntheroth and Spiers[176] state that submitting all the infants and newborns to an electrocardiogram screening would be an ineffectual waste of medical resources and it would cruelly alarm thousands of parents.

Viskin et al.[177] recommend genetic screening in every case of probable long QT syndrome, but state that a positive result will confirm the diagnosis and that, however, no mutations are found in many patients with a definite diagnosis of long QT syndrome, so a negative result is not very helpful.

Prolongation of QT intervals on electrocardiographic analysis, in two cases in Arkansas, were found to have sodium channel mutations associated with prolonged QT interval.

Hypoxemia

Many of the abnormalities found in SIDS may be related to hypoxemia as first suggested by Naeye.[178, 179]

In addition to the studies of Naeye[180, 181] and colleagues of brain stem abnormalities and delay in myelination in some cases, there appears to be other evidence of hypoxemia in SIDS. Elevated levels of **fetal hemoglobin** (Fig. 18.1.6)[140, 182, 183] as well as increased extramedullary hematopoiesis (Fig. 18.1.7) in the liver have been found in some autopsy cases of SIDS as compared with age-matched autopsy and live control groups.[184–188] Bard and

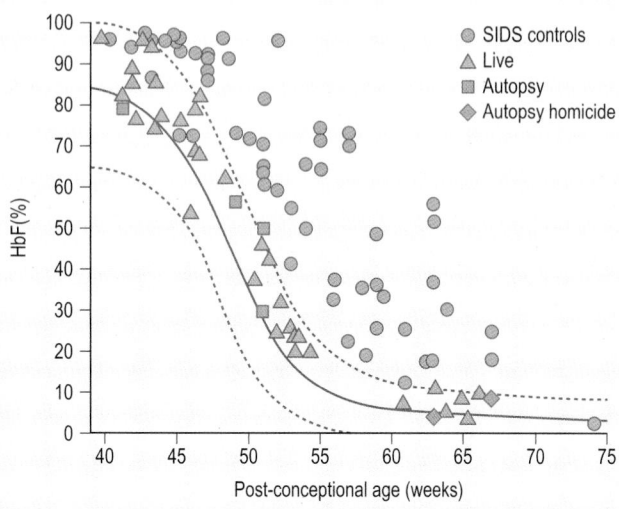

FIGURE 18.1.6 Graph showing elevated fetal hemoglobin levels in SIDS compared with live and autopsy controls. The solid line denotes the calculated mean value for the normal decline in HbF and the broken lines ± 2 standard deviations. (From Giulian G, Gilbert EF, Moss R. Elevated fetal hemoglobin levels in sudden infant death syndrome. 1987; N Eng J Med 316:1122.)

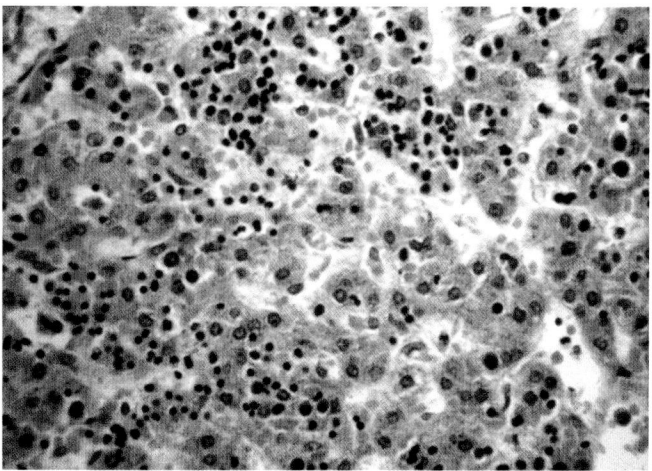

FIGURE 18.1.7 Microscopic section of liver in SIDS showing extramedullary hematopoiesis.

colleagues[187] related increased fetal hemoglobin synthesis to hypoxemia. In addition, Rognum and Saugstad[189] found high levels of hypoxanthine in the vitreous humor of the eye and the urine in some cases of SIDS.

Although the population with SIDS is heterogeneous, the results of these studies suggest that some victims experience subtle functional abnormalities before death that could reflect a chronic hypoxemia with increased fetal hemoglobin and respiratory and cardiac instability during sleep that may precede death (Fig. 18.1.8).

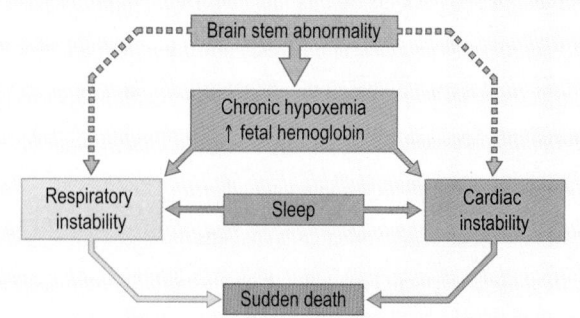

FIGURE 18.1.8 Proposed mechanism for chronic hypoxemia in sudden infant death syndrome.

The possible preventative effect of pacifiers on SIDS has been conducted by meta-analysis.[190] The use of pacifiers may be a strategy to further reduce the risk of SIDS.

Summary

Current evidence suggests that the roots of SIDS are to be found in intrauterine life. Many infants with SIDS appear to be subtly different from normal, in both structure and function, beginning in intrauterine life. A few things can be done to **prevent** the susceptible infant from succumbing to sudden death. It appears that the supine or lateral sleeping position is likely to prevent some instances of sudden death. Other factors should be addressed during pregnancy, including cigarette smoking and drug abuse, and mothers should be encouraged to breast feed. However, co-sleeping and bedsharing should be discouraged. Deaths that are clearly due to asphyxia from suffocation should be designated as such and should not be reported as SIDS. When it is not possible to differentiate the two, the designation **sudden undetermined** death is preferable.

No individual or combined pathologic findings are diagnostic of SIDS. Sudden, unexplained infant deaths may be due to various intrauterine, environmental factors.[191–193] These include abnormalities in the brainstem due to prematurity hypoxia, environmental stress including prone sleeping, smoke exposure,[194, 195] and an unsafe sleeping environment. Genetic factors may also be implicated that include the serotonin transporter gene,[196, 197] genes pertinent to autonomic nervous control,[198] and genes related to dysgenesis of the testes.[199] The pathologist should pursue evidence of such when conducting postmortem investigation.

References

The sudden infant death syndrome

1. Willinger M, James LS, Catz D. Defining the sudden infant death syndrome (SIDS). Deliberations of an expert panel convened by the National Institute of Child Health and Human Development. Pediatr Pathol 1991; 11:677.

2. Krous HF, Beckwith JB, Byard RW, et al. Sudden infant death syndrome and unclassified sudden infant deaths: a definitional and diagnostic approach. Pediatrics 2004; 114:234–238.

3. Bergman AB, Beckwith JB, Ray CG, eds. Proceedings of the Second International Conference on Causes of Sudden Deaths in Infants. Seattle: University of Washington Press; 1970.

4. National Institute of Child Health and Development. Sudden infant death syndrome fact sheet. April 1997.

5. Moore L, Byard RW. Pathological findings in hanging and wedging deaths in infants and young children. Am J Forensic Med Pathol 1993; 14:296–302.

6. Byard RW. Hazardous infant and early childhood sleeping environments and death scene examination. J Clin Forensic Med 1996; 3:115–122.

7. Byard RW, Donald T, Chivell W. Non-lethal and subtle inflicted injury and unexpected infant death. J Law Med 1999; 7:47.

8. Byard RW, Krous HF. Suffocation, shaking and SIDS – can we tell the difference? J Paediatr Child Health 1999; 35:432–433.

9. Byard RW, Beal SM. Munchausen syndrome by proxy: repetitive infantile apnoea and homicide. J Paediatr Child Health 1993; 29:77–79.

10. Krous HF. An international standardized autopsy protocol for sudden unexpected infant death. In: Rognum PO, ed. Sudden infant death syndrome: new trends in the nineties. Oslo: University of Scandinavia Press; 1995:75–89.

11. Meadow R. Suffocation, recurrent apnea, and sudden infant death. J Pediatr 1990; 117:351.

12. Krous HA; An international standardized autopsy protocol for sudden unexpected infant death. In: Rognum TO, ed. Sudden infant death syndrome: new trends in the nineties. Oslo: Scandinavian University Press; 1995:81–95.

13. Krous HF, Byard RW. International standardized autopsy protocol for sudden unexpected infant death. Appendix I. In: Byard RW, Krous HF, eds. Sudden infant death syndrome: problems, progress and possibilities. London: Arnold; 2001:319–333.

14. Centers for Disease Control and Prevention (CDC). Guidelines for death scene investigation of sudden unexplained infant deaths. Recommendations of the interagency panel on sudden infant death syndrome. MMWR 1996; 45:1–22.

15. Byard RW, Krous HF, eds. Sudden unexplained infant death investigation report form (SUIDIRF). Appendix II. In: Byard RW, Krous HF, eds. Sudden infant death syndrome: problems, progress and possibilities. Arnold; London: 2001; 334–347.

16. Mitchell E, Krous HF, Donald T, et al. An analysis of the usefulness of specific stages in the pathological investigation of sudden infant death. Am J Forensic Med Pathol 2000; 21:395–400.

17. Berry J, Allibone E, McKeever P, et al. The pathology study: the contribution of ancillary pathology tests to the investigation of unexpected infant death. In: Fleming P, Blair P, Bacon C, et al., eds. Sudden unexpected deaths in infancy: The CESDI SUDI Studies 1993–1996. London: The Stationary Office; 2000:97–112.

18. Arnestad M, Vege A, Rognum TO. Evaluation of diagnostic tools applied in the examination of sudden unexpected deaths in infancy and early childhood. Forensic Sci Int 2002; 125:262–268.

19. Meadow R. Unnatural sudden infant death. Arch Dis Child 1999; 80:7–14.

20. Bacon CJ. Cot deaths after CESDI. Arch Dis Child 1997; 76:171–173.

21. Anonymous. Unexplained deaths in infancy. Lancet 1999; 353:161.

22. Krous HF, Nadeau JM, Byard RW, et al. Oronasal blood in sudden infant death. Am J Forensic Med Pathol 2001; 22:346–351.

23. Meadow R. Suffocation, recurrent apnea, and sudden infant death. J Pediatr 1990; 117:351–357.

24. Becroft DM, Thompson JM, Mitchell EA. Nasal and intrapulmonary haemorrhage in sudden infant death syndrome. Arch Dis Child 2001; 85:116–120.

25. National Vital Statistics Report: 529, Nov 7, 2003.

26. Bayard RW, Krous HF. Sudden infant death syndrome: overview and update. Pediatr Dev Pathol 2003; 6:112–127.

27. Daley KC. Update on sudden infant death syndrome. Curr Opin Pediatr 2004; 16:227–232.

28. Lee NNY, Chan YF, Davies DP, et al. Sudden infant death syndrome in Hong Kong: confirmation of low incidence. Br Med J 1989; 298:721.

29. Alessandri LM, Read AW, Burton PR, et al. An analysis of sudden infant death syndrome in aboriginal infants. Early Hum Dev 1996; 45:235–244.

30. Adams MM. The descriptive epidemiology of sudden infant deaths among natives and whites in Alaska. Am J Epidemiol 1985; 122:636–643.

31. Oyen N, Bulterys, Welty TK, et al. Sudden unexplained infant deaths among American Indians and whites in North and South Dakota. Paediatr Perinatal Epidemiol 1990; 4:175–183.

32. Mitchell EA, Stewart AW, Scragg R, et al. Ethnic differences in mortality from sudden infant death syndrome in New Zealand. Br Med J 1993; 306:13–16.

33. Irwin KL, Mannino S, Daling J. Sudden infant death syndrome in Washington state: why are Native American infants at greater risk than white infants? J Pediatr 1992; 121:242–247.

34. Bulterys M. High incidence of sudden infant death syndrome among northern Indians and Alaska natives compared with southwestern Indians: possible role of smoking. J Community Health 1990; 15:185–194.

35. Blok JH. The incidence of sudden infant death syndrome in North Carolina's cities and counties:1972–1974. Am J Public Health 1978; 68:367–372.

36. Kaplan DW, Bauman AE, Krous HF. Epidemiology of sudden infant death syndrome in American Indians. Pediatrics 1984; 74:1041–1046.

37. US Department of Health and Human Services, What is SIDS? Pamphlet, 2004.

38. Hoffman HJ, Damus K, Hillman L. Adverse reproductive factors and the sudden infant death syndrome. In: Harper RM, Hoffman HJ, eds. Sudden infant death syndrome: risk factors and basic mechanisms. New York: PMA Publishing; 1988.

39. Hoffman HJ, Damus K, Hillman L, et al. Risk factors for SIDS: results of the National Institute of Child Health and Human Development SIDS Cooperative Epidemiologic Study. Ann NY Acad Sci 1988; 533:13.

40. Hoffman HJ, Hillman SH. Epidemiology of the sudden infant death syndrome: maternal, neonatal, and postnatal risk factors. Clin Perinatol 1992; 19:717.

41. Polberger S, Svenningsen SW. Early neonatal sudden infant death and near death of full term infants in maternity wards. Acta Paediatr Scand 1985; 74:861.

42. Guntheroth WG, Kawabori I. Hypoxic apnea and gasping. J Clin Invest 1975; 56:1371.

43. Beal SM, Finch CF. An overview of retrospective case-control studies investigating the relationship between prone sleeping position and SIDS. J Paediatr Child Health 1991; 27:334.

44. Fleming PJ, Gilbert R, Azaz Y. Interaction between bedding and sleeping position in the sudden infant death syndrome: a population based case-control study. Br Med J 1990; 301:85.

45. Mitchell EA, Brunt JM, Everard C. Reduction in mortality from sudden infant death syndrome in New Zealand: 1986–1992, Arch Dis Child 1994; 70:291.

46. Halliday H. Irish-American Pediatric Society Meeting, Burlington, Vt., Sept. 1995.

47. Hauck FR, Herman SM, Donovan M, et al. Sleep environment and the risk of sudden infant death syndrome in an urban population: the Chicago infant mortality study. Pediatrics 2003; 111:469.

48. Spiers PS, Guntheroth WG. Recommendations to avoid the prone sleeping position and recent statistics for sudden infant death syndrome in the United States. Arch Pediatr Adolesc Med 1994; 148:141.

49. Valdes-Dapena M. Sudden and unexpected death in infants: the scope of our ignorance. Pediatr Clin North Am 1963; 10:693.

50. Black L, David RJ, Brouillette RT. Effects of birth weight and ethnicity on incidence of sudden infant death syndrome. J Pediatr 1986; 108:209.

51. Copeland AR. Sudden infant death syndrome (SIDS): the Metropolitan Dade County experience, 1979–1983, Med Sci Law 1987; 27:283.

52. Grether JK, Schulman J, Croen LA. Sudden infant death syndrome among Asians in California. J Pediatr 1990; 116:525.

53. Kyle D, Sunderland R, Stonehouse M. Ethnic differences in incidence of sudden infant death syndrome in Birmingham. Arch Dis Child 1990; 65:830.

54. Guntheroth WG, Lohmann R, Spiers PS. Risk of sudden infant death syndrome in subsequent siblings. J Pediatr 1990; 116:520.

55. Beal SM. Siblings of sudden infant death syndrome victims. Siblings of sudden infant death syndrome victims. Clin Perinatol 1992; 19:839.

56. Irgens LM, Oyen N, Skjaerven R. Recurrence of sudden infant death syndrome among siblings. Acta Paediatr 1993; 82(Suppl)389:23.

57. Poets CF. The role of monitoring. In: Byard RW, Krous HF, eds. Sudden infant death syndrome: problems, progress and possibilities. London: Arnold; 2001:243–257.

58. Emery JL, Taylor EM. Investigation of SIDS (Letter). N Engl J Med 1986; 315:1676.

59. Werne J, Garrow I. Sudden death in infants allegedly due to mechanical suffocation. Am J Publ Hlth 1947; 37:674.

60. Bacon CJ, Sayer GC, Howe KW. Extensive retinal hemorrhages in infancy: an innocent cause. Br Med J 1978; 1:281.

61. Goetting MG, Sowa B. Retinal hemorrhage after cardiopulmonary resuscitation in children: an etiologic evaluation. Pediatrics 1990; 85:585.

62. Kanter RK. Retinal hemorrhage after cardiopulmonary resuscitation or child abuse. J Pediatr 108:430. 1986;

63. Meadow R. Munchausen syndrome by proxy. Arch Dis Child 1982; 52:92.

64. Galvin HK, Newton AW, Vandeven AM. Update on Munchausen syndrome by proxy. Curr Opin Pediatr 2005; 17:252–257.

65. Bjerklie D, Taylor E, Tippit S. When is crib death a cover for murder? Time 1994; 11 April:63.

66. Newlands M, Emery JL. Child abuse and cot deaths. Child Abuse Negl 1991; 15:275.

67. Carpenter RG, Gardner A, Jepson M, et al. Prevention of unexpected infant death: evaluation of the first seven years of the Sheffield Intervention Program. Lancet 1983; 1:723.

68. Taylor EM, Emery JL. Two-year study of the causes of post-perinatal infant deaths classified in terms of preventability. Arch Dis Child 1982; 57:668.

69. Adelson L, Kinney ER. Sudden and unexpected death in infancy and childhood. Pediatrics 1956; 17:663.

70. Carpenter RG, Shaddick CW. Role of infection, suffocation, and bottle-feeding in cot death. Br J Prev Soc Med 1965; 19:1.

71. Emery JL, Thornton JA. Effects of obstruction to respiration in infants, with particular reference to mattresses, pillows and their coverings. Br Med J 1968; 3:209.

72. Davies DP. Cot death in Hong Kong: a rare problem? Lancet 1985; 2:1346.

73. Beal SM. Sudden infant death syndrome: epidemiological comparisons between South Australia and communities with a different incidence. Aust Paediatr J 1986; 22(Suppl1):13–16

74. Skragg RKR, Mitchell EA. Side sleeping position and bed sharing in the sudden infant death syndrome. Ann Med 1998; 30:345-349.

75. Oyen N, Markestad T, Skjaerven R, et al. Combined effect of sleeping position and prenatal risk factors in sudden infant death syndrome: The Nordic Epidemiological SIDS study. Pediatrics 1997; 100:613–621.

76. Mitchell EA, Thach B, Thompson J, et al. Changing infants' sleep position increases risk of sudden infant death syndrome. Arch Pediatr Adolsec Med 1999; 153:1136–1141.

77. Byard RW, Beal SW. Fatal gastric aspiration and sleeping position in infancy and early childhood. J Paediatr Child Health 2000; 36:403–405.

78. Stanley FJ, Byard RW. The association between the prone sleeping position and SIDS: an editorial overview. J Paediatr Child Health 1991; 27:325–328.

79. Dwyer T, Ponsonby A-LB, Newman NM, et al. Prospective cohort study of prone sleeping position and sudden infant death syndrome. Lancet 1991; 337:1244.

80. Mitchell EA, Scragg R, Stewart AW, et al. Results from the first year of the New Zealand cot death study. NZ Med J 1991; 104:71.

81. Wigfield RE, Fleming PJ, Berry PJ, et al. Can the fall in Avon's sudden infant death rate be explained by changes in sleeping position? Br Med J 1992; 304:282.

82. Gilbert-Barness EF, Barness LA. Sudden infant death syndrome: is it a cause of death? Arch Pathol Lab Med 1993; 117:1246.

83. Ponsonby A-LB, Dwyer T, Gibbons LE, et al. Factors potentiating the risk of sudden infant death syndrome associated with the prone position. N Engl J Med 1993; 329:377.

84. Waters KA, Gonzales AV, Jean C, et al. Consequences of the prone sleep position in normal infants. Pediatr Res 1995; 37:396A.

85. Chiodina BA, Thach BT. Impaired ventilation in infants sleeping face down: potential significance for the sudden infant death syndrome. J Pediatr 1993; 123:686.

86. American Academy of Pediatrics Task Force: Infant positioning and SIDS. Pediatr 1992; 89:1120.

87. Emery JL. Towards safer cot mattresses. Health Visitor 1990; 63:157.

88. Gilbert-Barness E, Barness LA. Sudden infant death: a reappraisal. Contemp Pediatr 1995; 12:88.

89. Holt KS. Early motor development, posturally induced variations. J Pediatr 1960; 57:571.

90. Engelberts AC, de Jonge GA. Choice of sleeping position for infants: possible association with cot death. Arch Dis Child 1990; 65:462.

91. De Jonge GA. Written communication to Guntheroth WG. In: Guntheroth WG, Spiers PS. Sleeping prone and the risk of sudden infant death syndrome. JAMA 1992; 267:2359.

92. Nelson EA, Taylor BJ, Weatherall IL. Sleeping position and infant bedding may predispose to hyperthermia and the sudden infant death syndrome. Lancet 1989; 1:199–201.

93. Gilbert R, Rudd P, Berry PJ, et al. Combined effect of infection and heavy wrapping on the risk of sudden unexpected infant death. Arch Dis Child 1992. 67:171–177.

94. Fleming PJ, Blair PS, Bacon C, et al. Environment of infants during sleep and the risk of sudden infant death syndrome: results of 1993–1995 case-control study for confidential inquiry into stillbirths and deaths in infancy. Br Med J 1996; 313:191–195.

95. Wailoo MP, Peterson SA, Whitaker H. Disturbed nights and 3–4 month old infants: the effects of feeding and thermal environment. Arch Dis Child 1990; 65:499–501.

96. Kleeman WJ, Schlaud M, Poets CF, et al. Hyperthermia in sudden infant death. Int J Legal Med 1996; 109:139–142.

97. Williams SM, Taylor BJ, Mitchell EA. New Zealand Cot Death Study Group. Sudden infant death syndrome: insulation from bedding and clothing and its effect modifiers. Int J Epidemol 1996; 25:366–375.

98. Ponsonby A-L, Dwyer T, Gibbons LE, et al. Thermal environment and sudden infant death syndrome; case-control study. Br Med J 1992; 304:277–282.

99. Ponsonby A-L, Dwyer T, Kasl SV, et al. The Tasmanian SIDS Case-Control Study: univariable and multivariable risk factor analysis. Paediatr Perinatal Epidemiol 1995; 9:256–272.

100. Kemp JS, Nelson VE, Thach BT. Physical properties of bedding that may increase risk of sudden infant death syndrome in prone-sleeping infants. Pediatr Res 1994; 36:7–11.

101. Mitchell EA, Scragg L, Clements M. Soft cot mattresses and the sudden infant death syndrome. NZ Med J 1996; 109:206–207.

102. Kemp JS, Livne M, White DK, et al. Softness and the potential to cause rebreathing: differences in bedding used by infants at high risk and low risk for sudden infant death syndrome. J Pediatr 1998; 132:234–239.

103. Gilbert-Barness E, Hegstrand L, Chandra S, et al. Hazards of mattresses, beds and bedding in deaths of infants. Am J Forensic Med Pathol 1991; 12:27–32.

104. Kemp JS, Thach BT: A sleep position-dependent mechanism for infant death on sheepskins. Am J Dis Child 1993; 147:642.

105. Mitchell EA. Cot death: should the prone position be discouraged?, J Paediatr Child Health 1991; 27:319.

106. Gilbert-Barness E, Barness LA. Cause of death: SIDS or something else? Contemp Pediatr 1992; 9:13.

107. Ramanathan R, Chandra S, Gilbert-Barness E, et al. Sudden infant death syndrome and water beds (letter to the editor). N Engl J Med 1988; 318: 1700.

108. Gilbert-Barness E: More on sudden infant death syndrome and water beds (letter to the editor). N Engl J Med 1988; 319:1415.

109. Septkowitz S. Sudden infant death syndrome and *Hemophilus influenzae* infection. Arch Pediatr Adolesc Med 1994; 148:1109.

110. The Bible, 1 Kings 3.16-28.

111. McKenna JJ, Mosko S. Evolution and infant sleep: an experimental study. Acta Paediatr 1993; 82(Suppl):389.

112. Mosko S, McKenna JJ, Dickel M. Parent–infant co-sleeping: the appropriate context for the study of infant sleep and implications for sudden infant death syndrome (SIDS) research. J Behav Med 1993; 16:589.

113. Thoman EB, Anders TF, Sadeh A. Infant sleep research and ecological validity. Sleep 1993; 16(3):272.

114. McKenna JJ, Thoman EB, Anders TF. Infant–parent co-sleeping in an evolutionary perspective: implications for understanding infant sleep development and the sudden infant death syndrome (a review). Sleep 1993; 16:263.

115. Hauck FR. Changing epidemiology. In: Byard RW, Krous HF, eds. Sudden infant death syndrome: problems, progress and possibilities. London: Arnold; 2001:31–57.

116. Byard RW. Is co-sleeping in infancy a desirable or dangerous practice? J Paediatr Child Health 1994; 30:198–199.

117. Byard RW, Hilton J. Overlaying, accidental suffocation and sudden infant death. J SIDS Infant Mort 1997; 2:161–165.

118. Mitchell EA, Ford RP, Stewart AM. Smoking and the sudden infant death syndrome. Pediatrics 1993; 91:893.

119. Horne RSC, Ferens D, Watts AM, et al. Effects of maternal tobacco smoking, sleeping position, and sleep state on arousal in healthy term infants. Arch Dis Child Fetal Neonatal 2002; 87:F100–F105.

120. Schoendorf KC. Relationship of SIDS to maternal smoking during and after pregnancy. Pediatr 1992; 90:905.

121. Hoffman JH, Hunter JC, Damus K, et al. Diphtheria-tetanus-pertussis immunization and sudden infant death. Results of the National Institute of Child Health and Human Development Cooperative Epidemiologic Study of Sudden Infant Death Syndrome risk factors. Pediatr 1987; 79:598.

122. Beal SM. The rise and fall of several theories. In: Byard RW, Krous HF, eds. Sudden infant death syndrome: problems, progress and possibilities. London: Arnold; 2001:236–242.

123. Beal SM. SIDS and immunization (Letter). Med J Aust 1990; 153:135–136.

124. Anon. Sudden infant death and inherited disorders of fat oxidation [editorial]. Lancet 1986; 2:1073.

125. Harpey JP, Charpentier C, Paturneau-Jouas M. Sudden infant death and inherited disorders of fatty acid β-oxidation. Biol Neonate 1990; 58(Suppl):70.

126. Pollitt RJ. Defects in mitochondrial fatty acid oxidation: clinical presentations and their role in sudden infant death. Paediatr Paedol 1993; 38:13.

127. Bennett MJ, Hale DE, Coates PM, et al. Postmortem recognition of fatty acid oxidation disorders. Pediatr Pathol 1991; 11:365.

128. Bennett MJ, Pollitt RJ, Talz LS, et al. Medium-chain acyl-CoA dehydrogenase deficiency: a useful diagnosis five years after death. Clin Chem 1990; 36:1695.

129. Bennett MJ, Powell MT. Metabolic disease and sudden, unexpected death in infancy. Hum Pathol 1994; 25:744.

130. Arens R, Gozal D, Jain K. Prevalence of medium-chain acyl-coenzyme A dehydrogenase (MCAD) in the sudden infant death syndrome. J Pediatr 1993; 122:715.

131. Lemieux B, Giguere R, Cyr D. Screening urine of 3-week-old newborns: lack of association between sudden infant death syndrome and some metabolic disorders. Pediatrics 1993; 91:986.

132. Olpin SE. The metabolic investigation of sudden infant death. Ann Clin Biochem 2004; 41 (pt 4):282–293.

133. Steinschneider AL. Prolonged apnea and the sudden infant death syndrome: clinical and laboratory observations. Pediatrics 1972; 50:646.

134. 'A housewife is convicted of murdering her five children,' New York Times, 22 April 1995.

135. Southall DP, Richards JM, de Swite M. Identification of infants destined to die unexpectedly during infancy: evaluation of predictive importance of prolonged apnea and disorders of cardiac rhythm or conduction. Br Med J (Clin Res) 1983; 286:1092.

136. Little GA, Ariagno RB, Beckwith B. American Academy of Pediatrics Task Force on Prolonged Infantile Apnea: Prolonged Infantile Apnea: 1985. Pediatrics 1985; 76:129.

137. Anon. National Institute of Health Consensus Development Conference on Infantile Apnea and Home Monitoring. Pediatr 1987; 79:292.

138. Kelly DH, Pathak A, Meny R. Sudden severe bradycardia in infancy. Pediatr Pulmonol 199110:199.;

139. Meny R, Carroll J, Carbone T. Cardiorespiratory recordings from infants dying suddenly and unexpectedly. Pediatrics 1994; 93:44.

140. Byard RW, Cote A, Praud JP, et al. Fetal hemoglobin synthesis determined by Y-mRNA/Y-mRNA + B-mRNA quantitation in infants at risk for sudden infant death syndrome being monitored at home for apnea. Pediatrics 2003; 112:4:285–288.

141. Valdés-Dapena M, McFeeley PA, Hoffmann HJ, et al. Histopathology atlas for the sudden infant death syndrome. Washington, DC: Armed Forces Institute of Pathology; 1993.

142. Krous HF, Nadeau JM, Silva PD, et al. Intrathoracic petechiae in sudden infant death syndrome: relationship to face position when found. Pediatr Dev Pathol 2001; 4:160–164.

143. Krous HF. The microscopic distribution of intrathoracic petechiae in sudden infant death syndrome. Arch Pathol Lab Med 1984; 108:77–79.

144. Krous HF, Jordan J. A necropsy study of distribution of petechiae in non-sudden infant death syndrome. Arch Pathol Lab Med 1984; 108:75–76.

145. Byard RW, Krous HF. Petechial hemorrhages and unexpected infant deaths. Legal Med 1999; 1:193–197.

146. Beckwith JB. Intrathoracic petechial hemorrhages: a clue to the mechanism of death in sudden infant death syndrome? Ann NY Acad Sci 1988; 533:37–47.

147. Poets CF, Meny RG, Chobanian MR, et al. Gasping and other cardio-respiratory patterns during sudden infant deaths. Pediatr Res 1999; 45:350–354.

148. Beckwith J. Observations on the pathologic anatomy of SIDS. Seattle: University of Wasington Press; 1970.

149. Byard RW, Stewart WA, Telfer S, et al. Assessment of pulmonary and intrathymic hemosiderin deposition in sudden infant death syndrome. Pediatr Pathol Lab Med 1997; 17:275–282.

150. Milroy CM. Munchausen syndrome by proxy and intraalveolar haemo-siderin. Int J Legal Med 1999; 112:309–312.

151. Becroft DM, Lockett BK. Intra-alveolar pulmonary siderophages in sudden infant death: a marker for previous imposed suffocation. Pathology 1997; 29:60–63.

152. Bruce K, Becker LE. Quantitation of medullary astrogliosis in sudden infant death syndrome. Pediatr Neurosurg 1991; 17:74–92.

153. Kinney HC, Burger PC, Harrell FE. Reactive gliosis in the medulla oblongata of victims of the sudden infant death syndrome. Pediatrics 1983; 72:181.

154. Takashima S, Armstrong D, Becker LE. Cerebral hypoperfusion in the sudden infant death syndrome? Brain stem gliosis and vasculature. Ann Neurol 1978; 4:257.

155. Kinney HC, Filiano JJ, Harper RM. The neuropathology of the sudden infant death syndrome: a review. J Neuropathol Exp Neurol 1992; 51: 115.

156. Quattrochi JJ, Baba N, Liss L. Sudden infant death syndrome (SIDS): a preliminary study of reticular dendritic spines in infants with SIDS. Brain Res 1980; 181:245.

157. Quattrochi JJ, McBride PT, Yates AJ. Brainstem immaturity in sudden infant death syndrome: a quantitative rapid Golgi study of dendritic spines in 95 infants. Brain Res 1985; 325:39.

158. Shaw CM, Siebert JR, Haas JE. Megalencephaly in sudden infant death syndrome. J Child Neurol 1984; 4:39.

159. Takashima S, Armstrong D, Becker LE. Cerebral white matter lesions in sudden infant death syndrome. Pediatrics 1978; 62:115.

160. Becker LE, Zhang W, Pereyra PM. Delayed maturation of the vagus nerve in SIDS. Acta Neuropathol (Berl) 1993; 86:617.

161. Sachis PN, Armstrong DL, Becker LE. The vagus nerve and SIDS: a morphometric study. J Pediatr 1981; 98:278.

162. Filiano JJ, Kinney HC. Arcuate nucleus hypoplasia in the sudden infant death syndrome. J Neuropathol Exp Neurol 1992; 51:394.

163. Kinney HC, Filiano JJ, Sleaper CA, et al. Decreased muscarinic receptor binding in the arcuate nucleus in sudden infant death syndrome. Science 1995; 269:1446.

164. Kinney HC, Filiano JJ. Brain research in SIDS. In: Byarw RW, Krouse HF, eds. Sudden infant death syndrome: problems, progress and possibilities. London: Arnold; 2001:118–137.

165. Panigrahy A, Filiano J, Sleeper LA, et al. Decreased serotonergic receptor binding in rhombic lip-derived regions of the medulla oblongata in the sudden infant death syndrome. J Neuropathol Exp Neurol 2000; 59: 377–384.

166. Nachmanoff DB, Panigrahy A, Filiano JJ, et al. Brainstem 3H-nicotine receptor binding in the sudden infant death syndrome. J Neuropathol Exp Neurol 1998; 57:1018–1025.

167. Kinney HC, Filiano JJ, Assman SF, et al. Tritiated-naloxone binding to brainstem opioid receptors in the sudden infant death syndrome. J Auton Nerv Syst 1998; 69:156–163.

168. Panigrahy A, Filiano JJ, Sleeper LA, et al. Decreased kainate receptor binding in the arcuate nucleus of the sudden infant death syndrome. J Neuropathol Exp Neurol 1997; 56:1253–1261.

169. Becker LE. Neural maturational delay as a link in the chain of events leading to SIDS. Can J Neurolog Sci 1990; 17:361–371.

170. Becker LE, Takashima S. Chronic hypoventilation and development of brainstem gliosis. Neuropediatriacs 1985; 16:19–23.

171. Guntheroth WG. The QT interval and sudden infant death syndrome. Circulation 1982; 66:502–504.

172. Southall DP, Arrowsmith WA, Stebbins V, et al. QT interval measurements before sudden infant death syndrome. Arch Ds Child 1986; 61: 327–333.

173. James TN. Long reflections on the QT interval: the sixth annual Gordon K. Moe lecture. J Cardiovasc Electrophysiol 1996; 7:738–759.

174. Schwartz PJ, Stramba-Badiale M, Segantini A, et al. Prolongation of the QT interval and the sudden infant death syndrome. N Engl J Med 1998; 338:1709–1714.

175. Schwartz PJ, Priori S, Dumaine R, et al. Brief report: a molecular link between the sudden infant death syndrome and the long QT syndrome. N Engl J Med 2000; 343:262–267.

176. Guntheroth WG, Spiers PS. Prolongation of the QT interval and the sudden infant death syndrome. N Engl J Med 1998; 339:1161–1163.

177. Viskin S, Fish R, Roth A, et al. QT or not QT? N Engl J Med 2000; 343: 352–356.

178. Naeye RL. Hypoxia and the sudden infant death syndrome. Science 1974; 186:857.

179. Naeye RL, Ladis B, Drage JS. Sudden infant death syndrome: a prospective study. Am J Dis Child 1976; 130:1207.

180. Naeye RL, Localio AR. Determining the time before death when ischemia and hypoxemia initiated cerebral palsy. Obstet Gynecol 1995; 86:713–719.

181. Naeye RL, Lin HM. Determining when hypoxemia–ischemia damaged fetal brains. Am J Obstet Gynecol 2001; 184:217–224.

182. Fagan DG, Lancashire RJ, Walker A, et al. Determinants of fetal hemoglobin in newborn infants. Arch Dis Child 1995; 72:F111.

183. Guilian GG, Gilbert EF, Moss RL, Elevated fetal hemoglobin levels in sudden infant death syndrome, N Engl J Med 1987; 316:1122.

184. Gilbert-Barness E, Kenison K, Carver J. Fetal hemoglobin and sudden infant death syndrome. Arch Pathol Lab Med 1993; 117:177.

185. Gilbert-Barness EF, Kenison K, Giulian G, et al. Extramedullary hematopoiesis in the liver in sudden infant death syndrome. Arch Pathol Lab Med 1991; 115:226.

186. Gilbert-Barness E, Valdes-Dapena M, Steinschneider A, et al. Hepatic erythropoiesis in sudden infant death syndrome. Ped Path 1992; 12:481.

187. Bard H, Fouron JC, Prosmanne J, et al. Effect of hypoxemia on fetal hemoglobin synthesis during late gestation. Pediatr Res 1992; 31:483.

188. Fagan DG, Walker A. Hemoglobin F levels in sudden infant death. Br J Haematol 1992; 82:422.

189. Rognum TO, Saugstad OD. Hypoxanthine levels in vitreous humor: evidence of hypoxia in most infants who died of sudden infant death syndrome. Pediatrics 1991; 87:306.

190. Zotter H, Keble R, Kurz R, et al. Pacifier use and sudden infant death syndrome: should health professionals recommend pacifier use based on present knowledge? Wien Kin Wochenscher 2002; 114:791–794.

191. Kinney HC, Filiano JJ, White WF. Medullary serotonergic network deficiency in the sudden infant death syndrome: review of a 15-year study of a single dataset. J Neuropathol Exp Neurol 2001; 60(3):228–247.

192. Gunetheroth WG, Spiers PS. The triple risk hypotheses in sudden infant death syndrome. Pediatrics 2002; 110(5):E64.

193. Filiano JJ, Kinney HC. A perspective on neuropathologic findings in victims of the sudden infant death syndrome: the triple-risk model. Biol Neonata 1994; 65(3–4):194–197.

194. DiFranza JR, Aligne CA, Weitzman M. Prenatal and postnatal environmental tobacco smoke exposure and children's health. Pediatrics; 113(4Suppl):1007–1015. 2004

195. Parsiow PM, Cranage SM, Adamson TM, et al. Arousal and ventilatory responses to hypoxia in sleeping infants: effects of maternal smoking. Respir Physiol Neurobiol 2004; 140(1):77–87.

196. Richerson GB. Serotonergic neurons as carbon dioxide sensors that maintain pH homeostasis. Nat Rev Neurosci, 2004; 6:449–461.

197. Weese-Mayer De, Zhou L, Berry-Kravis EM, et al. Related articles. Links association of the serotonin transporter gene with sudden infant death syndrome: a haplotype analysis. Am J Med Genet 2003; 122A(3):238–245.

198. Weese-Mayer DE, Berry-Kravis EM, Zhou L, et al. Sudden infant death syndrome: case-control frequency differences at genes pertinent to early autonomic nervous system embryologic development. Pediatr Res 2004; 56(3):391–395.

199. Puffenberger EG, HU-Lince D, Parod JM, et al. Mapping of sudden infant death with dysgenesis of the testes syndrome (SIDDT) by a SNP genome scan and identification of TSPYL loss of function. Proc Natl Acad Sci USA 2004; 101(32):11689–11694. Epub July 23, 2004.

PART 2   *Richard L. Naeye*

Mechanism of the sudden infant death syndrome

'And I said to the man who stood at the gate of the year: "Give me a light that I
may tread safely into the unknown."
And he replied:
"Go out into the darkness and put your hand into the Hand of God. That shall be
to you better than light and safe than a known way."   Minnie Louise Haskins 1875–1957

The sudden infant death syndrome (SIDS) is the designation for infant deaths in the first year of life that are sudden, unexpected, and unexplained. The number of such deaths has decreased in recent years because of widespread recognition that sleeping in the prone position and exposure to cigarette smoke predispose to the deaths. Whether other preventable causes of the deaths can be identified remains to be seen. In the interim a multitude of **genetic, developmental** and **environmental** risk factors and disorders are being identified as causes of the deaths. Identifying the cause of death in a single victim can range from simple to complex and requires the integration of information from many different sources. At least three factors are present in most of the deaths:

- the child is at a vulnerable stage of development;
- a predisposing genetic factor exists;[1]
- a trigger event is present.

These trigger factors include infection in addition to a child's sleeping position and cigarette smoking in the household.

In the past most SIDS investigations were conducted with only limited integration of readily available information. They covered a narrow spectrum of findings designated to support or refute a single theory about what caused the deaths. As a consequence, most investigators could only speculate on how their observations might relate to the findings of others. A seminal event in SIDS research has been the shift from strictly environmental or single organ malfunction to more complex causes of the deaths. Still other studies are finding a sibship aggregation and other evidence of a death's genetic origin.[1]

The malfunctions that lead to SIDS can take place at many different levels. Some appear to originate in brain dysfunctions that disappear as children grow older. Multiple pathways can be involved in the death sequence. Included are pulmonary hypoventilation, a failure to arouse from central apnea, and an inability to reverse a cardiac arrhythmia or to stop a seizure. Some victims have had dysfunctions which only appeared when a child was stressed. Testing may eventually identify some of these dysfunctions as delays in the development of control mechanism for vital respiratory, cardiovascular, or neuromuscular functions. Whatever the malfunction, it usually self-corrects if the infant survives the first year of life. For example, in one study analyses of home cardiorespiratory recordings from 24 children deemed at risk for SIDS disclosed the presence of a unique pattern of complex, closely spaced hypoxic gasps followed by ineffective autoresuscitation that disappeared as they grew older.[2]

Hypoxemia

Hypoxemia appears to be part of several common final pathways to SIDS. Over 80% of the victims of SIDS have increased levels of hypoxanthine in the vitreous humor, a well-recognized consequence of severe, sustained hypoxemia before death.[3] This finding indicates that these victims of SIDS did not die suddenly. In other studies victims of SIDS have had high lactic acid levels in the vitreous humor, another marker of antecedent hypoxemia.[4] In such cases blood flow through the child's circulation must have continued for a time after breathing became seriously impaired or ceased. Evidence of acute or chronic hypoxemia is shown in Boxes 18.2.1[4–10] and 18.2.2.[11–20]

Elevated or normal numbers of lymphocytes and normoblasts in the infant's blood can sometimes be used to determine the time that severe hypoxemia began before death. The time that these two types of cells enter an infant's blood in large numbers is an accurate indicator of the time that severe hypoxemia began.[21] Lymphocyte counts increase to more than 10 000/mL and nucleated red blood cells to more than 2000/mL within 2 h of the start of severe hypoxemia. If the hypoxemia persists or recurs after a period of being absent, normoblast numbers remain elevated but not lymphocyte numbers.

BOX 18.2.1 EVIDENCE OF RECENT, ACUTE HYPOXEMIA IN VICTIMS OF SIDS

Demonstrated by transcutaneous oxygen monitors before death[5]

Increased numbers of lymphocytes in the peripheral blood[6]

Increased numbers of normoblasts in the peripheral blood[6]

Elevated levels of hypoxanthine in the vitreous humor[4]

Elevated levels of lactic acid in the vitreous humor[4]

Elevated blood levels of cortisol[7]

Large numbers of petechiae on the surfaces of thoracic organs[8, 9, 10]

BOX 18.2.2 EVIDENCE OF CHRONIC HYPOXEMIA IN VICTIMS OF SIDS

Elevated blood levels of fetal hemoglobin[11–14]

Normoblast hyperplasia in the bone marrow[15]

Increased hepatic erythropoiesis[16–18]

Abnormal retention of brown fat around abdominal organs[16, 19]

Increased numbers of neuroendocrine cells in the epithelial lining of the airways[20]

BOX 18.2.3 BRAIN AND OTHER NERVOUS SYSTEM ABNORMALITIES IN VICTIMS OF SIDS

Abnormal proliferation of astroglial fibers in the brainstem[23–26]

Subcortical and periventricular leukomalacia[27]

Slow dendritic maturation in the brainstem[28]

Hypomyelination of brainstem respirator control centers[15, 29]

Neuronal deficit in 12th cranial nerve nucleus[15]

Hypomyelination of the vagus nerve[30]

BOX 18.2.4 CARDIAC ABNORMALITIES THAT PRECEDED DEATH IN SIDS VICTIMS

Bradycardia (sometimes preceded by tachycardia)[31]

Impaired cardiac repolarization[32]

Multifocal atrial tachycardia[33]

Short RR interval on electrocardiogram during rapid eye movement sleep[34]

Prolonged QT interval on electrocardiogram[35]

Also identified have been abnormalities in arousal responses and cardiac autonomic controls during sleep–wake processes. Following these discoveries, a whole series of anatomic studies have revealed specific structural abnormalities in midbrain arousal pathways in some SIDS victims.[22]

Failure to arouse from a prolonged apneic episode

Short periods of apnea are normal in early infancy, but episodes that last more than 20 s are abnormal. The most unambiguous postmortem marker for this mode of death would probably be easily recognized damage or maldevelopment in the victims' brainstem centers that control breathing. It might seem that this diagnostic requirement could often be met because abnormalities are present in the brainstems of many victims of SIDS. These findings are shown in Box 18.2.3.[23–30]

Cardiac arrhythmias

A variety of cardiac arrhythmias have been recorded in infants who become victims of SIDS (Box 18.2.4).[3–5, 31–35] There are also multiple, widely recognized tissue and laboratory markers for repeat episodes of acute hypoxemia in

many victims of SIDS (Box 18.2.4). This hypoxemia is probably the usual cause of the cardiac arrhythmias in victims of SIDS but this issue is not fully resolved.[5, 36] Hypoxemia of several origins can precede the arrhythmias.[8, 37] For example, bradycardia can precede or develop simultaneously with central apnea and can occur as single or repeat episodes of varying length.[31]

Brain dysfunction

There is much indirect evidence that most currently unexplained cases of SIDS had their origin in brain dysfunction that adversely affected cardiopulmonary functions and perhaps sleep–waking states. The first evidence for this is epidemiologic. Around 90% of deaths from SIDS occur between 2 weeks and 6 months of age, a period when the brain is undergoing rapid developmental changes in its structure, biochemical composition, and functions. At 6 months of age a relatively stable configuration is achieved for brain-controlled cardiopulmonary function and sleep–waking patterns.[38] Most victims of SIDS die when they are presumably asleep or in transition between sleeping and waking, so reaching this relatively stable sleep–waking pattern may explain the rapid decline in the frequency of SIDS after 6 months of age.

There is evidence that several of the abnormalities are the consequence of hypoxemia. These include a delay in the myelination of some areas of the brain, brainstem gliosis in a pattern that would be expected to be produced by chronic hypoxemia, and a slower than normal remodeling of dendrites, a process that normally takes place both before and after birth.[15, 39–41] The remodeling of dendrites takes the form of a pruning back of overabundant spines as synaptic connections are established. **Delayed myelination** is present in the brains of many victims of SIDS, and in the brains of infants without SIDS who were exposed to two major risk factors of SIDS – namely, maternal cigarette smoking during pregnancy and sustained hypoxemia prior to death (Box 18.2.3). None of the brain abnormalities associated with SIDS is present in all of the victims. This is probably another indication of the heterogeneity of the initiating mechanisms responsible for SIDS.

Some of the final SIDS pathways to death may long continue to be unexplained because of their complex causes and the absence of the needed skills and resources to identify the multiple links in the fatal chain of events. Identifying these pathways can also be delayed by the need of legal authorities to look for evidences of neglect or abuse. Whatever the chain of events, the explanation of each death should have strong supporting evidence. Such evidence may require a detailed review of the child's behavior, development, and medical records.

Other studies have found evidence that some SIDS victims possessed inherent weaknesses which only became evident when the infant was subjected to stress. Many of these malfunctions now appear to be manifestations of the uneven maturation of control systems that self-correct if the infant survives the first year of life. For example, in one study analyses of home cardiorespiratory recordings from 24 children deemed at risk for SIDS disclosed the presence of a unique pattern of complex, closely spaced hypoxic gasps followed by ineffective autoresuscitation.[2] They in turn were associated with abnormalities in both arousal responses and cardiac autonomic controls during sleep–wake processes. Following these discoveries, a whole series of anatomic studies revealed specific structural abnormalities in midbrain arousal pathways in some SIDS victims.[22] Testing may eventually be able to identify such impairments or delays in the development of needed control systems.

Markers that may precede final pathways to SIDS

Risks include the disorders that episodically reduce blood flow from the uterus to the placenta – namely, maternal cigarette smoking, third trimester decreases in maternal diastolic blood pressure to values less than 60 mm Hg, the use of **cocaine** or **amphetamines** during pregnancy, and twin pregnancies.[42–45] **Fetal hemoglobin** has been found in the blood of many victims of SIDS, evidence of predeath hypoxemia[12–14] in addition to SIDS. **Maternal cigarette smoking** during pregnancy and pregnancy with twins also increase the levels of fetal hemoglobin in the blood of neonates.[46]

Genetic origins

Inherited metabolic disorders account for a small but significant number of sudden unexplained deaths in the first year of life. For example, inherited disorders of fatty acid oxidation can closely mimic SIDS. Attention has long been focused on central cardiorespiratory control systems. For example, the long QT syndrome has been identified in some children who subsequently became SIDS victims.[47]

Infections, their relationship to SIDS

The seasonal distribution of SIDS suggests a link with infections. Such evidence includes:
- a high incidence of concurrent respiratory infections
- a high frequency of nicotine use in the child's household
- a protective role for breastfeeding.

Identified in SIDS victims have been enteroviruses, adenoviruses, Epstein-Barr viruses, parvoviruses and other infectious agents.[48]

Placental infection

Finally, raised maternal serum levels of α-fetoprotein during the second trimester of pregnancy is a marker of placental dysfunction and reportedly a risk predictor for SIDS.[49]

REFERENCES

Mechanism of the sudden infant death syndrome

1. Oyen N, Skjaerven R, Irgens LM, et al. Population-based recurrence risk of sudden infant death syndrome compared with other infant and fetal deaths. Am J Epidemiol 1996; 144:300–305.
2. Sridhar R, Thach RT, Kelly DH, et al. Characterization of successful and failed autoresuscitation in human infants, including those dying of SIDS. Ped Pulmonol 2003; 35:113–122.

Hypoxemia

3. Rognum TO, Saugstad OD. Hypoxanthine levels in vitreous humor: evidence of hypoxia in most infants who die of sudden infant death syndrome. Pediatrics 1991; 87:306–310.
4. Sturner WQ, Sullivan A, Suzuki K. Lactic acid concentrations in vitreous humor: their use in asphyxial deaths in children. J Forensic Sci 1983; 28:222–230.
5. Poets CF, Samuels MP, Noyes JP, et al. Home monitoring of transcutaneous oxygen tension in the early detection of hypoxemia in infants and young children. Arch Dis Child 1991; 66:676–682.
6. Naeye RL, Localio AR. Establishing the time when hypoxia initiated cerebral palsy, Proceedings of the 5th Fukuoka International Symposium on Perinatal Medicine 1996:95–1007.
7. Naeya RL, Fisher R, Rubin HR, et al. Selected hormone levels in victims of the sudden infant death syndrome. Pediatrics 1980; 65:1134–1136.

8. Guntheroth WG. Crib death, the sudden infant death syndrome. 2nd edn. New York: Futura; 1989:195–225.

9. Valdes-Dapena MA. The sudden infant death syndrome: pathologic finding. In: Hunt CE, ed. Clinics in perinatology: apnea and SIDS. Philadelphia: WB Saunders; 1992:701.

10. Guntheroth WG. The significance of pulmonary petechiae in crib death. Pediatrics 1973; 52:601–603.

11. Giulian GG, Gilbert EF, Moss RL. Elevated fetal hemoglobin levels in sudden infant death syndrome. N Engl J Med 1987; 316:1122–1126.

12. Gilbert-Barness EF, Kenison K. Fetal hemoglobin levels in SIDS. N Engl J Med 1990; 323:1281–1282.

13. Fagan DG, Walker A. Haemoglobin F levels in sudden infant deaths. Br J Haematol 1992; 82:422–430.

14. Gilbert-Barness EF, Kenison K, Carver J. Fetal hemoglobin and sudden infant death syndrome. Arch Pathol Lab Med 1993; 117:177–179.

15. Naeye RL, Olsson JM, Combs JW. New brainstem and bone marrow abnormalities in victims of sudden infant death syndrome. J Perinatol 1989; 9:180–183.

16. Naeye RL. Hypoxia and the sudden infant death syndrome. Science 1974; 186:837–838.

17. Valdes-Dapena MA, Gillane MM, Ross D, et al. Extramedullary hematopoiesis in the liver in sudden infant death syndrome. Arch Pathol Lab Med 1979; 103:513–515.

18. Gilbert-Barness EF, Kenison K, Giulian G, et al. Extramedullary hematopoiesis in the liver in sudden infant death syndrome. Arch Pathol Lab Med 1991; 115:226–229.

19. Valdes-Dapena MA, Gillane MM, Catherman R. Brown fat retention in sudden infant death syndrome. Arch Pathol Lab Med 1976; 100:547–549.

20. Gillan JE, Curan C, O'Reilly E, et al. Abnormal patterns of pulmonary neuroendocrine cells in victims of sudden infant death syndrome. Pediatrics 1989; 84:828–834.

21. Olpin SE. The metabolic investigation of sudden infant death. Ann of Clin Biochem 2004; 41:282–293.

22. Sawaguchi T, Patricia F, Kadhim H, et al. The correlation between ubiquitin in the brainstem and sleep apnea in SIDS victims. Early Human Develop 2003; 75(suppl):S75–97.

Failure to arouse from a prolonged apneic episode

23. Becker LE, Takashima S. Chronic hypoventilation and development of brainstem gliosis. Neuropediatrics 1985; 16:19–23.

24. Quattrochhi JJ, McBride PT, Yates AJ. Brainstem immaturity in sudden infant death syndrome: a quantitative rapid Golgi study of dendritic spines in 95 infants. Brain Res 1985; 325:39–48.

25. Takashima S, Becker LE. Developmental abnormalities of medullary respiratory centers in sudden infant death syndrome. Exp Neurol 1985; 90:580–587.

26. Becker LE. Neural maturational delay as a link in the chain of events leading to SIDS. Can J Neurol Sci 1990; 17:361–371.

27. Naeye RL, Ladis B, Drage JS. Sudden infant death syndrome: a prospective study. Am J Dis Child 1976; 130:1207–1210.

28. Takashima S, Mito T. Neuronal development in the medullary reticular formation in sudden infant death in premature infants. Neuropediatrics 1985; 16:76–79.

29. Takashima S, Becker LE. Delayed dendritic development of catecholaminergic neurons in the ventrolateral medulla of children who died of sudden infant death syndrome. Neuropediatrics 1991; 22:97–99.

30. Sachis PN, Armstrong DL, Becker LED, et al. The vagus nerve and sudden infant death syndrome: a morphometric study. J Pediatr 1981; 98:278–280.

Cardiac arrhythmias

31. Meny RG, Carroll JL, Carbone MT, et al. Cardiorespiratory recordings from infants dying suddenly and unexpectedly at home. Pediatrics 1994; 93:44–49.

32. Sadeh D, Shannon DC, Abboud S, et al. Altered cardiac repolarization in some victims of sudden infant death syndrome. N Engl J Med 1987; 317:1501–1505.

33. Yeager SB, Houghen TJ, Levy AM. Sudden death in infants with chaotic atrial rhythms. Am J Dis Child 1984; 138:689–692.

34. Weinstein SL, Steinschneider A. QT_c and RR intervals in victims of the sudden infant death syndrome. Am J Dis Child 1985; 139:987–990.

35. Schwartz PJ, Montemerlo M, Facchini M. The QT interval throughout the first 6 months of life: a prospective study. Circulation 1982; 66:496–501.

36. Freed GE, Steinschneider A, Glassman M, et al. Sudden infant death syndrome and an understanding of selected clinical issues. Pediatr Clin North Am 1994; 41:967–990.

37. Hunt CE, Broillette RT. Sudden infant death syndrome. 1987 Perspective. J Pediatr 1987; 110:669–678.

Brain dysfunction

38. Kinney HC, Filiano JJ, Harper RM. The neuropathology of the sudden infant death syndrome: a review. J Neuropathol Exp Neurol 1992; 51:115–126.

39. Takashima S, Armstrong D, Becker LE, et al. Cerebral white matter lesions in sudden infant death syndrome. Pediatrics 1978; 62:155–159.

40. Kinney HC, Brody BA, Finkelstein DM, et al. Delayed central nervous system myelination in the sudden infant death syndrome. J Neuropathol Exp Neurol 1991; 50:29–48.

41. Carey EM, Foster PC. The activity of 2?3?-cyclic nucleotide 3′-phosphohydrolase in the corpus callosum, subcortical white matter, and spinal cord in infants dying of the sudden infant death syndrome. J Neurochem 1984; 42:924–929.

Markers that may precede final pathways to SIDS

42. Hoffman HJ, Hillman KS. Epidemiology of the sudden infant death syndrome: maternal, neonatal and postneonatal risk factors. In: Hunt ED, ed. Clinics in perinatology: apnea and SIDS. Philadelphia: WB Saunders; 1992:717–737.

43. Hoffman HJ, Damus K, Hillman K, et al. Risk factors for SIDS: results of the National Institute of Child Health and Human Development SIDS Cooperative Epidemiological Study. Ann N Y Acad Sci 1988; 533: 13–30.

44. Naeye RL, Landis B, Darage JS. Sudden infant death syndrome, a prospective study. Am J Dis Child 1976; 130:1207–1210.

45. Naeye RL. Sudden infant death syndrome: is the confusion ending? Mod Pathol 1988; 1:169–174.

46. Fagan DG, Lancashire RJ, Walker A, et al. Determinants of fetal hemoglobin in newborn infants. Arch Dis Child 1995; 72:F111–F114.

Genetic origins

47. Miller TE, Estrella E, et al. Recurrent third-trimester fetal loss and maternal mosaicism for long QT syndrome. Circulation 2004; 109:3029–3034.

Infections, their relationship to SIDS

48. Dettmeyer R, Basner A, Schlamann M, et al. Role of virus-induced myocardial infections in sudden infant death syndrome: a prospective postmortem study. Ped Res 2004; 55:947–952.

Placental infection

49. Smith GC, Wood AM, Pell JP, et al. Second trimester maternal serum levels of α-fetoprotein and the subsequent risk of SIDS. N Eng J Med 2004; 351:978–986

PART 3   *Enid Gilbert-Barness*

Sudden explained death in infants

'The Moving Finger writes; and, having writ,
Moves on: nor all your Piety nor Wit Shall lure it back to cancel half a Line,
Nor all your Tears wash out a Word of it.'   Rubaiyat by Omar Khayyam

Differential diagnosis of unexpected infant death due to natural diseases is shown in Box 18.3.1. Approximately 15% of sudden death in infants can be explained after the performance of a complete autopsy. These explained deaths, although in the minority, are of great importance for a number of reasons. In some instances, only the complete autopsy will reveal the evidence of death due to abuse. However, it is not only the law that is served; either at the time of death or at some later time, the parents eventually need and should be supplied with an explanation for their infant's sudden demise. Often they are unable to bring their mourning to a close without that knowledge. Furthermore, in some instances, the diseases to which babies suddenly succumb are genetically controlled; necropsy may provide the family with their first awareness of that fact. One of the best examples of that is tuberous sclerosis, which so often manifests in the infant by way of sudden death as a result of rhabdomyomas of the heart. That disease is inherited as an autosomal dominant and diagnosis is, therefore, of the utmost importance to families.

The list of recognizable conditions that comprise this category is long. Only the more common entities are presented here, and they are arranged according to the anatomic site of the mortal lesion (Box 18.3.2).

Cardiovascular causes[1]

Cardiac pathologic features are frequent when the child is witnessed to be awake at the time of sudden death.[2]

Myocarditis

Myocarditis is one of the most common identifiable causes of sudden infant death and it is almost always perceived for the first time in examination of the microscopic sections. Because the etiology is usually viral, the inflammatory cells are uniformly lymphocytes. Although bacteria and fungi may also cause inflammation of infant heart muscle, they do so only rarely.[3] In babies in the first year of life the coxsackie virus, especially group B3, and *Toxoplasma gondii* are often the agents involved.[4]

Coxsackie B myocarditis is most prevalent in summer and early autumn and most often affects the infant in the first month of life. The onset of the disease is sudden. The infant may have an elevated or subnormal temperature. Some infants recover completely, but for others the course may be rapidly fatal. It is this group that presents as apparent sudden infant death syndrome (SIDS).[5,6]

At autopsy, the heart may be enlarged and/or heavy. There may be petechiae in the epicardium and myocardium. However, upon gross inspection the heart often appears entirely normal. The first obvious pathologic feature seen upon histologic inspection is the many lymphocytes between muscle fibers. The lymphocytes may be accompanied by histiocytes and plasma cells. Necrosis of individual myocardial fibers is also present and in some cases prominent.[6]

Lesions are common in organs other than the heart, including liver, lung, kidney, and nervous system. In slightly more than half of the cases, myocarditis is accompanied by meningoencephalitis, which may be mild.

Congenital aortic stenosis

Stenosis of the aortic valve may occur as a solitary lesion or in association with other cardiac malformations. The valve may be extremely small and the opening merely a slit (Fig. 18.3.1). There is a male predominance. In cases of moderate (rather than severe) stenosis of the aortic valve, the mitral valve may be patent and of normal morphology, but the endocardium of the left ventricle is usually sclerotic. Secondary endocardial sclerosis and papillary muscle necrosis may also occur, and the left ventricle is enlarged. Infants with this lesion are apt to die within the first 3 weeks of life.[7-12]

BOX 18.3.1 DIFFERENTIAL DIAGNOSIS OF UNEXPECTED INFANT DEATH DUE TO NATURAL DISEASES

Vascular

Coronary artery abnormalities: anomalous coronary arteries, aplasia/hypoplasia, idiopathic arterial calcinosis, coronary arteritis (Kawasaki disease)

Aortic abnormalities: supravalvular stenosis, coarctation, William syndrome, DiGeorge syndrome

Venous abnormalities: total anomalous pulmonary venous drainage

Vascular malformations

Pulmonary hypertension

Miscellaneous: fibromuscular dysplasia, thromboembolism

Cardiac

Congenital cardiac defects (before and after surgery)

Cardiomyopathies

Tumors

Conduction defects – long QT interval

Infections

Miscellaneous: endocardial fibroelastosis

Respiratory

Upper airway obstruction

Bronchopulmonary dysplasia

Infections

Miscellaneous: massive pulmonary hemorrhage, tension pneumothorax

Central nervous system

Epilepsy

Hemorrhage: bleeding diatheses, vascular malformations

Tumors

Metabolic disorders

Infections

Miscellaneous: tuberous sclerosis

Gastrointestinal

Intestinal obstruction: intussusception, volvulus

Intestinal perforation

Gastroesophageal reflux/aspiration

Late-presenting congenital diaphragmatic hernia

Infections: gastroenteritis

Miscellaneous: cystic fibrosis, malnutrition

Genitourinary

Primary renal disease: pyelonephritis, glomerulonephritis

Urinary tract obstruction

Wilms tumor

Endocrine

Congenital adrenal hyperplasia

Hematologic

Bleeding diatheses

Malignancies: lymphoma, leukemia

Hemoglobinopathies: sickle cell disease

Anemia

Miscellaneous: infections, polycythemia, splenic disorders

Metabolic

Fatty acid oxidation defects: acyl-CoA dehydrogenase deficiencies (medium-chain and long-chain acyl-CoA dehydrogenase)

Reye syndrome

Carbohydrate disorders: glycogen storage diseases

Organic acid disorders

Infectious

Cardiovascular: myocarditis

Respiratory: acute bronchopneumonia

Central nervous system: meningitis, encephalitis

Gastrointestinal: gastroenteritis, botulism

Genitourinary: pyelonephritis

Generalized: septicemia, endotoxemia

Miscellaneous

Chromosomal disorders: trisomy 21

Skeletal disorders: achondroplasia

Connective tissue disorders: Marfan syndrome, Ehlers-Danlos syndrome type IV

Idiopathic

Sudden infant death syndrome

Endocardial sclerosis (endocardial fibroelastosis)

The process is recognized most often in the left ventricle, although it does occur elsewhere in the heart (Fig. 18.3.2). It is often overlooked when the prosector fails to inspect the color of the endocardium because the lesion is often subtle. When in doubt, the best way to be certain is to compare the lining of the left ventricle with that of the right in the same heart because the color of the two should be identical. If endocardial sclerosis is present, the prosector can easily discern a clear difference between the two chambers.[13, 14]

This lesion may be missed in examining microscopic sections of the heart because the **thickness of the endocardium**

Cardiovascular
  Myocarditis (usually viral)
  Congenital heart disease
  Congenital aortic valvular stenosis
  Endocardial fibroelastosis
  Anomalous origin of the left coronary artery
  Cardiomyopathy
  Rhabdomyoma (in tuberous sclerosis)

Respiratory
  Bronchopneumonia
  Bronchiolitis

Gastrointestinal tract
  Dehydration with fluid and electrolyte imbalance (usually due to diarrhea)

Dehydration in cystic fibrosis (with overheating)

Adrenal insufficiency

children with this lesion die suddenly, within the first few months of life, and it is an important part of the differential diagnosis of SIDS. Most cases are sporadic; a few are familial. The lesion is almost never seen in stillborns or newborns.[3]

Anomalous origin of the left coronary artery

This condition may be a cause of sudden death and may result in extensive infarction of the wall of the left ventricle.[15]

Hypertrophic cardiomyopathy

The heart of an infant with this form of cardiomyopathy is both larger and heavier than expected for the age. The histologic appearance is a composite of features with marked hypertrophy of individual myocardial cells that have enlarged hyperchromatic nuclei. This marked hypertrophy may cause compression bridging of coronary arteries, especially the left anterior descending branch, with resultant myocardial ischemia.[16] Multiple forms of familial hypertrophic cardiomyopathy exist, with autosomal dominant [e.g. HCM (MIM192600)] and autosomal recessive [HCM8 (MIM608751)] transmission.

may not be inspected in reviewing these routine sections. One important microscopic feature of the lesion is that it is not only the lining of the chamber that is thickened. There are many **extensions** of dense connective tissue that continue into the underlying myocardium for a considerable distance, in long, slender, tapered bands. It is thought that these extensions further embarrass left ventricular function, i.e. contraction and dilatation of the chamber by 'splinting' the muscle.

The etiology of this lesion is unknown. Some have suggested that it may be caused by intrauterine viral infection. Most often,

Tuberous sclerosis with cardiac rhabdomyomas

Individual rhabdomyomas do occur as hamartomas within the hearts of infants, in which case they present as subendocardial

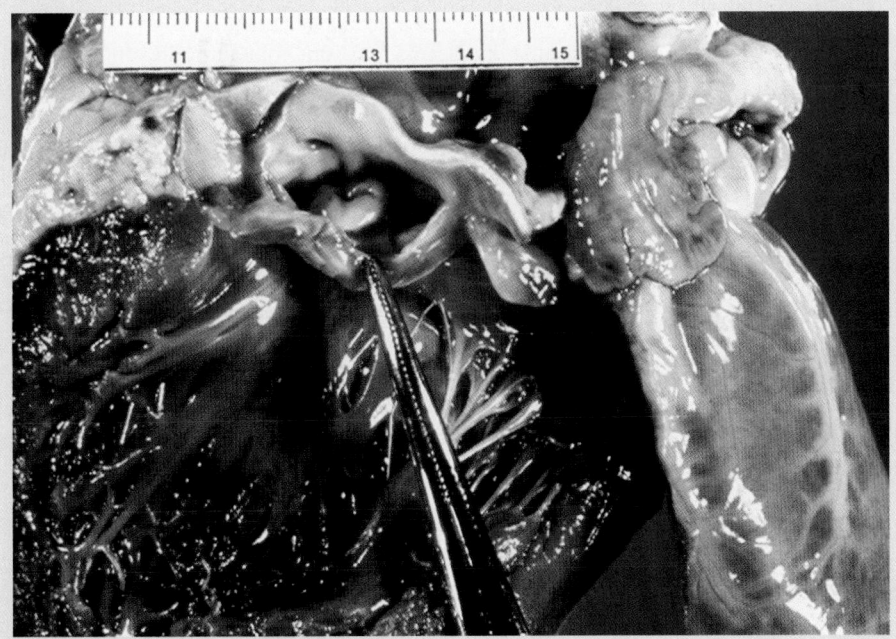

FIGURE 18.3.1 Congenital aortic valve seen from above, markedly stenotic (almost atretic).

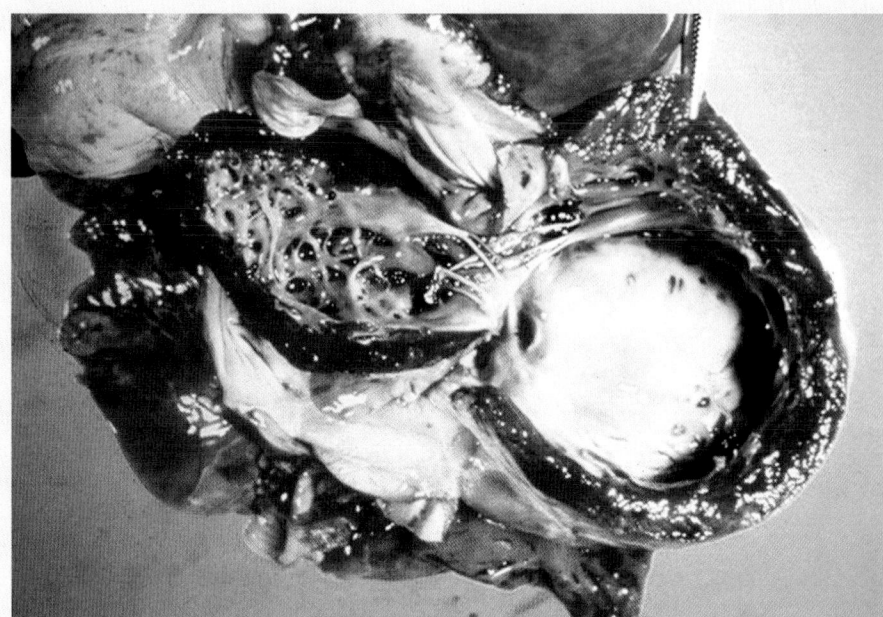

FIGURE 18.3.2 Endocardial sclerosis. The endocardium of the entire left ventricle is thickened, opaque, and white. Note the characteristic globular shape of the left ventricle.

masses, expanding the wall and the adjacent chamber. These single masses are not associated with other congenital cardiac abnormalities.

The multiple rhabdomyomas of the heart in tuberous sclerosis may be a cause for sudden, unexpected death in infants. Presumably, one or more of the hamartomas cause death by inducing fatal arrhythmia because of their close proximity to the conduction system.

Upon gross inspection the rhabdomyomas are seen scattered at random about the wall of the heart. They range from microscopic size to 2 cm in diameter. They are sharply demarcated and strikingly paler than surrounding myocardium (Fig. 18.3.3). Upon microscopic inspection they are seen to consist of many large, vacuolated, clear myocardial cells, the cytoplasm of which is filled with glycogen. In some, dark strands of cytoplasm are stretched out radially from central nuclei, across the pale glycogen to the cell walls. These are called **spider cells** and are characteristic of the lesion and unique to it.[1, 17–19]

The conduction system in sudden infant deaths

No significant morphologic alterations have been found in the cardiac conduction system in SIDS.[20]

Disturbances in rhythmogenic function due to abnormal cardiac Na^+/K^+ channels can result in familial forms of sudden infant death. The genes *KCNQ1* (MIM607542), *HERG* (MIM152427), *SCN5A* (MIM600163), *KCNE1* (MIM176261), *KCNE2* (MIM603796) and *LQT1* (MIM192500) are all involved in cardiac Na^+/K^+ channels, and their mutations can result in the long QT syndrome or other dysrhythmias and cause sudden cardiac death. These mutations are all autosomal dominant; they have an electrophysiologic phenotype, but do not alter cardiac morphology.

Respiratory causes

Bronchopneumonia

Pneumonia in infants is bronchopneumonia. In infants less than 1 year of age true lobar type of pneumonia is very rare. Bronchopneumonia, like SIDS, occurs most commonly in late winter and early spring when respiratory infections are at their peak. In non-SIDS sudden deaths it is often preceded by an episode of viral upper respiratory infection, as is the case with SIDS. Males are affected more often than are females.

The clinical features of the disease are variable in babies. A mild upper respiratory infection with a stuffy nose, fretfulness, and a diminished appetite for several days usually precedes the onset of death from pneumonia. The illness is characterized by an abrupt onset of fever, apprehension, and respiratory distress. Cough is unusual. Physical examination of the chest is seldom helpful.

At autopsy, although pneumonia is sometimes evident on gross inspection of the lungs, it is characteristically difficult or impossible to diagnose initially, probably because all infant lungs are firm. The fact that they feel uniformly solid is likely attributable to the relative abundance of elastic tissue. The lungs collapse spontaneously after the death of the infant when

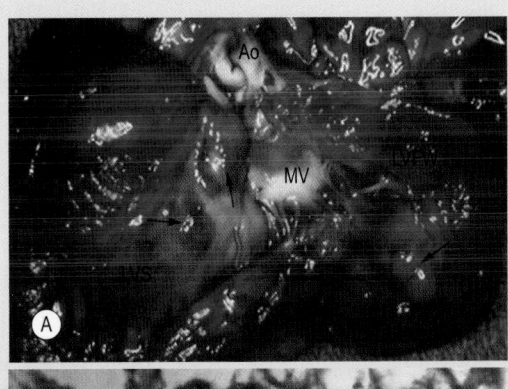

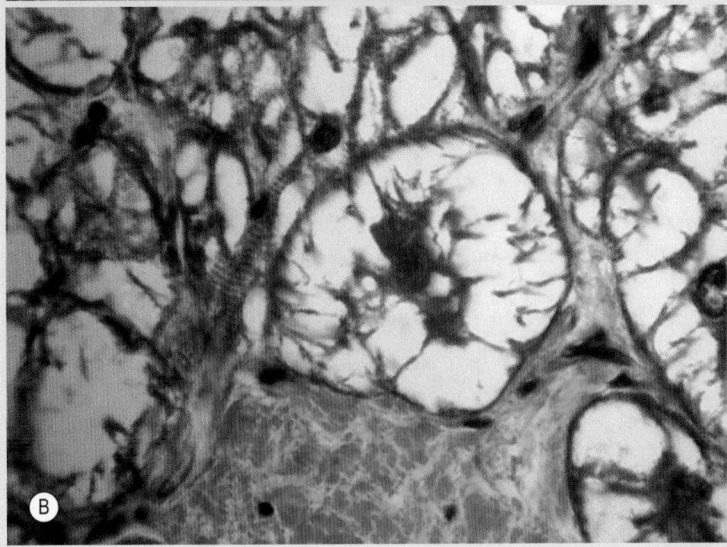

FIGURE 18.3.3 (A) One of the many rhabdomyomas (arrows) in this heart is apparent on the cut surface. The lesion is sharply demarcated (the shape of a finger) and paler than surrounding myocardium. (MV, mitral valve; LVFW, left ventricular free wall; Ao, aorta) (B) Microscopic appearance of a cardiac rhabdomyoma. Individual myocardial fibers are markedly enlarged and most bear single, large, clear vacuoles.

respiration ceases. Hence, even when pneumonia is present in the lungs (Figs 18.3.4 and 18.3.5) of an infant who has died suddenly and unexpectedly, it is often not diagnosed on gross inspection.[21] At least one section of each lobe, therefore, should be submitted routinely for microscopic examination. If there is little exudate, it is probable that pneumonia represents only an incidental finding and is not the cause of death.[1] When in doubt, correlation of the culture from the histologic appearance of the culture site can be helpful.

Bronchiolitis

Bronchiolitis in infants is viral.[22] Respiratory syncytial virus is responsible for more than half of the cases; other agents include parainfluenza 3 virus, mycoplasma, and some adenoviruses. It is common in infants in the first 2 years of life; the peak incidence is at about 6 months of age. Like SIDS, it is most prevalent in the winter and early spring.

Early symptoms are a mild upper respiratory infection with serous nasal discharge and sneezing. After a few days of fever a diminished appetite may occur, followed by respiratory distress with a wheezy cough, dyspnea, and irritability.[1, 23]

Histopathologically, the disease is characterized by thickening of the bronchiolar walls, the result of edema and abundant

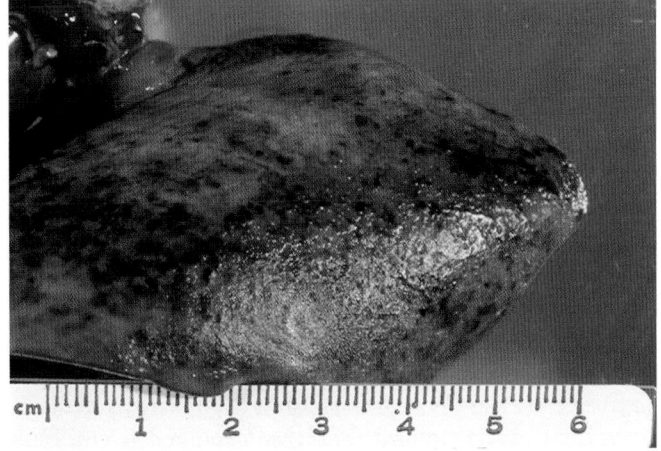

FIGURE 18.3.4 Gross appearance of consolidated lung with petechial hemorrhages on the pleural surfaces in infant with pneumonia.

mononuclear inflammatory cell infiltrate (Fig. 18.3.6). There may be mucus and inflammatory cells in the lumina of small airways. Especially in infants, these slender airways may be critically narrowed by even minor thickening of the wall. Nevertheless, the mortality in bronchiolitis is minimal, being no more than 1%.

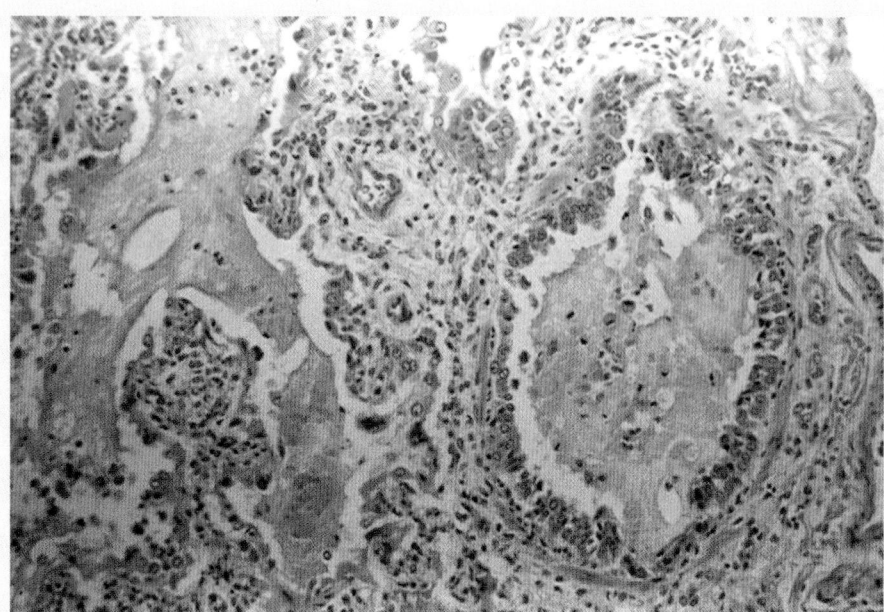

FIGURE 18.3.5 Bacterial pneumonia in an infant (high magnification). Many of the open air spaces are filled with purulent exudate.

Dehydration secondary to diarrhea with fluid and electrolyte imbalance

Infants, especially those in the first year of life, are susceptible to fluid loss with electrolyte imbalance. To compound that difficulty, they quickly become gravely dehydrated and may die as a result of either protracted vomiting or diarrhea.[23, 24]

Parents often do not realize the gravity of vomiting and diarrhea in their infant. Consequently, they may postpone consultation with a physician until their infant is moribund.[25]

At autopsy, the diagnosis of dehydration is best made before the body is opened by carefully examining it and obtaining vitreous humor for biochemical determinations. In dehydration, the eyes are sunken. If the body has not yet been refrigerated, the skin can be tested by pinching a fold that remains 'tented' or raised, confirming the presence of dehydration. Two features of the internal examination may be of help, an empty stomach or an empty colon.

Examination of microscopic sections in cases of acute gastroenteritis may not be helpful. However, if diarrhea has been protracted and accompanied by malabsorption, and in some cases of starvation, there may be characteristic microscopic features in the mucosa of the small bowel with ablation of villi.[24, 25]

Fluid and electrolyte imbalance in cystic fibrosis

Occasionally, an infant – almost always Caucasian – is brought into the emergency room moribund or already dead, and only when microscopic sections are examined is it apparent that the baby has succumbed to excessive sodium and fluid loss as a consequence of cystic fibrosis of the pancreas.[24, 25] Usually, inspissated mucous secretion is noted in the mucosal glands of the small and large bowels (Figs 18.3.7 and 18.3.8). Plugs of similar pink-staining secretion also appear in dilated pancreatic acini (Fig. 18.3.9).

Adrenal insufficiency

Infants with hypoplastic adrenal glands may die suddenly and unexpectedly in an Addisonian crisis.[26]

Tumors

Tumors are rare but a significant cause of sudden infant death in infancy and early childhood. Those most frequently related to sudden unexpected death are cardiac tumors and brain tumors; other malignant and vascular tumors are less frequently implicated.[27–32]

Other causes of sudden death in infants

A full autopsy dissection in an infant must include the upper aerodigestive tract since intrinsic lesions, e.g. lingual

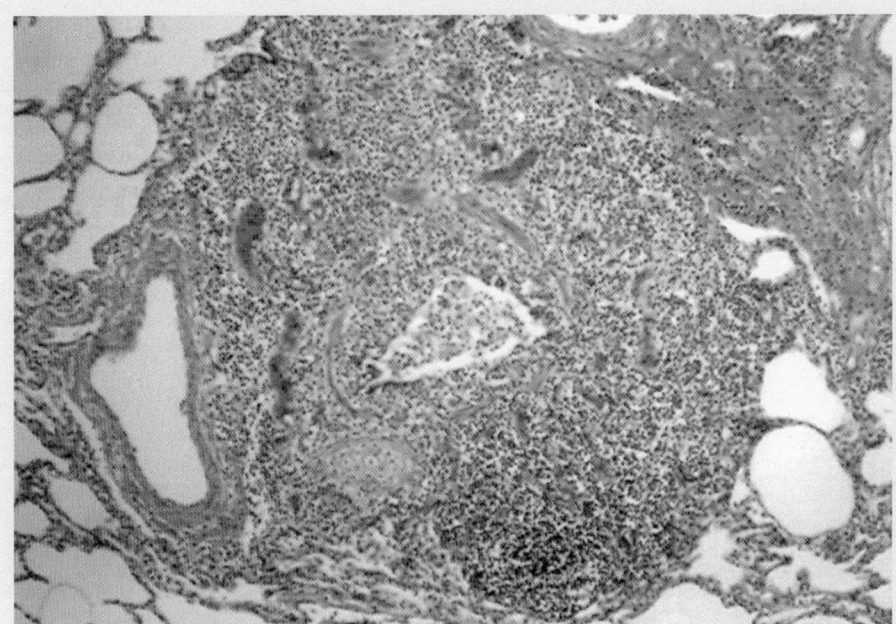

FIGURE 18.3.6 Bronchiolitis. In the center of the field is a small bronchiole the wall of which is five to six times the normal thickness, made so by a heavy and dense accumulation of lymphocytes.

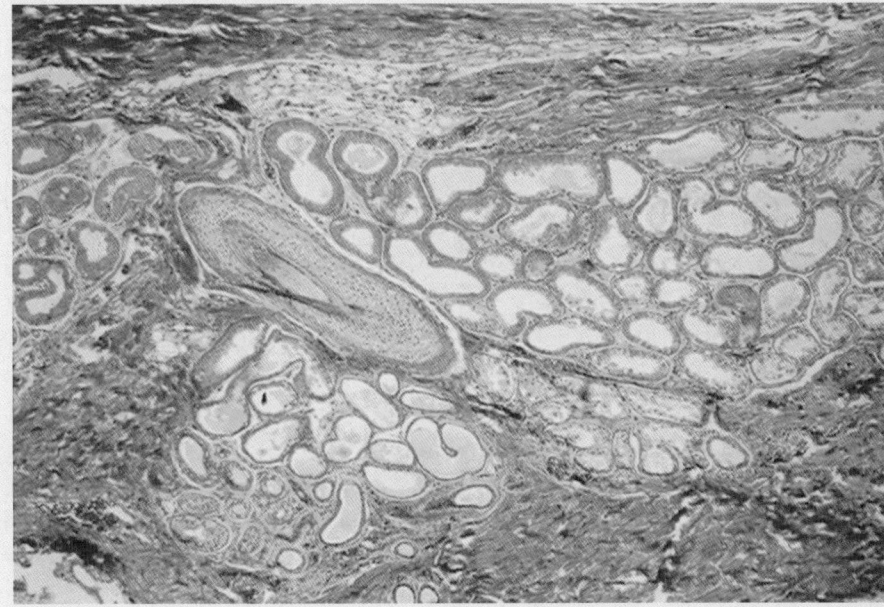

FIGURE 18.3.7 Section of duodenum from an infant with cystic fibrosis (high magnification). Brunner glands are dilated and filled with inspissated pink-staining proteinaceous secretion.

thyroglossal duct cysts and hemangiomas, may results in sudden airway compromise. Obstruction from foreign bodies within the airway or esophagus may also cause respiratory compromise.[33]

Bleeding may occur spontaneously from vascular malformations or from tumors. Spontaneous hemorrhage may be the first indication of an underlying coagulopathy. Less common causes of unexpected death in infants include intestinal obstruction from volvulus or intussusception, or mediastinal shift from a late-presenting congenital diaphragmatic hernia.[34]

Accidental death due to a dangerous sleeping environment may only be obvious after the scene has been carefully examined. Autopsy findings may be either subtle or not present at all.[35, 36] Inflicted suffocation may escape detection even after a scene examination and autopsy have been conducted. Poisoning with rare organic toxins may also present diagnostic difficulties even after usual toxicologic screening has been performed.[37]

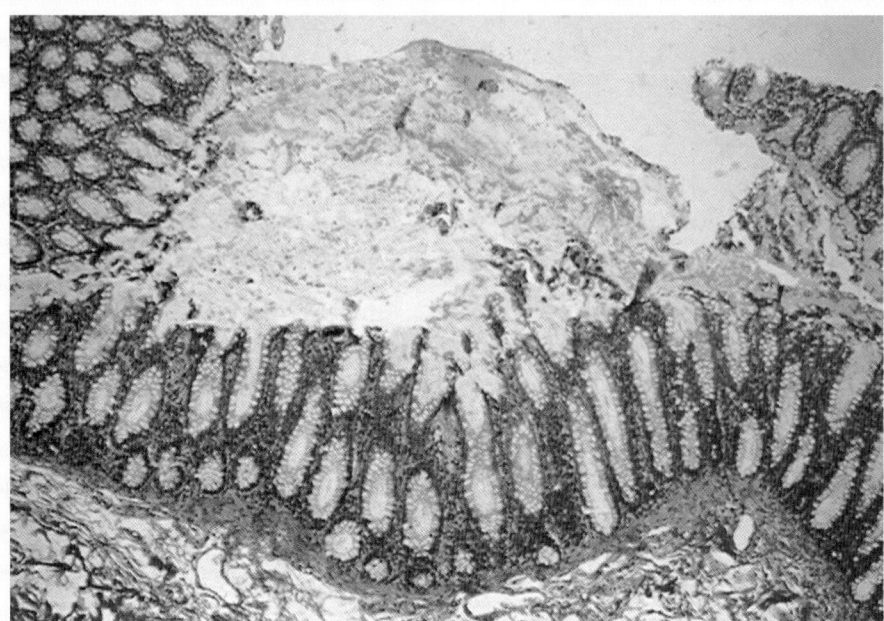

FIGURE 18.3.8 Dilated glands of the colonic mucosa in this infant with cystic fibrosis. They, too, contain dark pink-staining plugs of inspissated mucus.

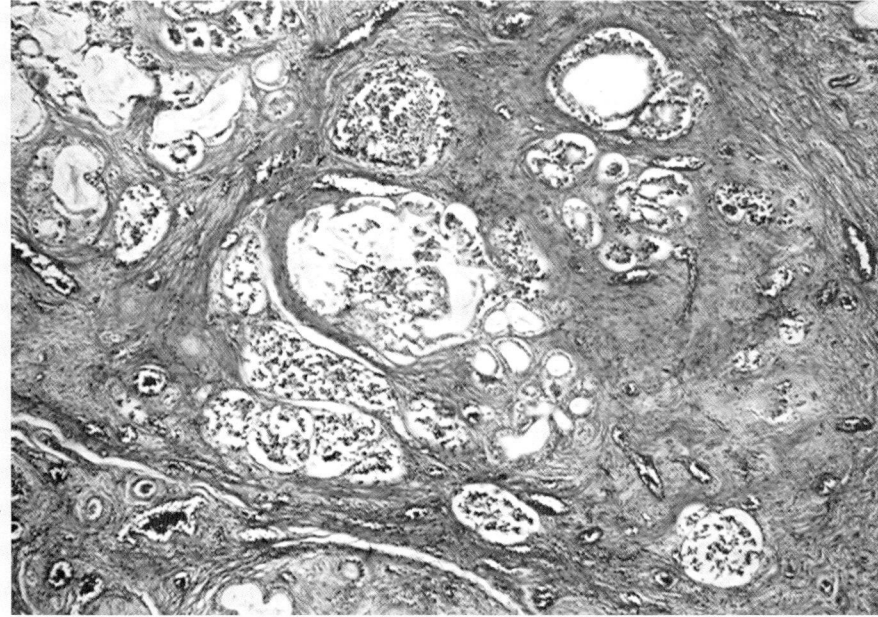

FIGURE 18.3.9 Section of pancreas from an infant with cystic fibrosis. There is fibrosis and the small ducts in the center of the image are abnormally dilated. Often, at high magnification, dilated acini can be found as well, also filled with pink-staining secretion.

References

Cardiovascular causes

1. Liberthson RR. Sudden death from cardiac causes in children and young adults. N Eng J Med 1996; 334:1039–1044.
2. Dancea A, Cote A, Roblicek C, et al. Cardiac pathology in sudden unexpected infant death. J Pediatr 2002; 141:336–342.

Myocarditis

3. Arey JB. Malformations of the endocardium, myocardium, and pericardium. In: Arey JB, ed. Cardiovascular pathology in infants and children. Philadelphia: WB Saunders; 1994.
4. Fechner RE, Smith MG, Middlekamp JN. Coxsackie B virus infection of the newborn. Am J Pathol 1963; 42:493–505.
5. Hosier DM, Newton WA. Serious Coxsackie infection in infants and children. Myocarditis, meningoencephalitis, and hepatitis. AMA J Dis Child 1958; 97(3):251–267.

6. Valdés-Dapena MA, McFeeley PA, Hoffman HJ. Histopathology atlas of the sudden infant death syndrome. Washington: Armed Forces Institute of Pathology; 1993.

Congenital aortic stenosis

7. Arey JB. Malformations of the valvular, supravalvular, and infravalvular regions. In: Arey JB, ed. Cardiovascular pathology in infants and children. Philadelphia: WB Saunders; 1984.
8. Becker AE, Anderson RH. Pathology of congenital heart disease. London: Butterworths; 1981.
9. Campbell M, Kauntze R. Congenital aortic valvular stenosis. Br Heart J 1953; 15:179–194.
10. Doyle EF, Arumugham P, Lara E. Sudden death in young patients with congenital aortic stenosis. Pediatrics 1974; 53:481–489.
11. Ongley PA, Nadas AS, Paul MH. Aortic stenosis in infants and children. Pediatrics 1958; 21:207–221.
12. Patterson K, Donnelly WH, Dehner LP. The cardiovascular system. In: Stocker JT, Dehner LP, eds. Pediatric pathology. Philadelphia: JB Lippincott; 1992.

Endocardial sclerosis

13. Kelly J, Andersen DH. Congenital endocardial fibroelastosis. II. A clinical and pathological investigation of those cases without associated cardiac malformations including a report of two familial instances. Pediatrics 1956; 18:539–555.
14. McKinney B. Endocardial fibroelastosis. In: McKinney B, ed. Pathology of the cardiomyopathies. London: Butterworths; 1994.

Enomolous origin of the left coronary artery

15. Lev M. Congenitally malformed hearts. Springfield: Charles C. Thomas; 1953.

Hypertrophic cardiomyopathy

16. McKenna WJ, Deanfield JE. Hypertrophic cardiomyopathy. An important cause of sudden death. Arch Dis Child 1984; 59:971–975.

Tuberous sclerosis with cardiac rhabdomyomas

17. Arey JB. Tumors of the heart and pericardium. In: Arey JB, ed. Cardiovascular pathology in infants and children. Philadelphia: WB Saunders; 1984.
18. McAllister HA, Fenoglio JJ. Tumors of the cardiovascular system. Fascicle 15. In: Atlas of tumor pathology. 2nd series. Washington: Armed Forces Institute of Pathology; 1978.
19. Potter EL, Craig JM. Pathology of the fetus and the infant. 3rd edn. Chicago: Year Book Medical Publishers; 1975.

The conduction system in sudden infant deaths

20. Bajanowski T, Ortmann C, Teige K, et al. Pathological changes of the heart in sudden infant death. Int J Legal Med 2003; 117:193–203.

Bronchopneumonia

21. Valdés-Dapena MA. The pathology of the sudden infant death syndrome. Am J Pathol 1982; 106:118–131.

Bronchiolitis

22. Aherne W, Bird T, Court SD. Pathological changes in virus infections of the lower respiratory tract in children. J Clin Pathol 1970; 23:7–18.

Dehydration secondary to diarrhea with fluid and electrolyte imbalance

23. Darrow DC, Pratt EL, Flett J. Disturbances of water and electrolytes in infantile diarrhea. Pediatrics 1949; 3:129–156.

Fluid and electrolyte imbalance in cystic fibrosis

24. Finberg L. Dehydration in infants and children. N Engl J Med 1967; 276:458–460.
25. Finberg L. Hypernatremic (hypertonic) dehydration in infants. N Engl J Med 1973; 289:196–198.

Adrenal insufficiency

26. Russell MA, Opitz JM, Visekul C, Gilbert EF. Sudden infant death due to congenital adrenal hypoplasia. Arch Pathol Lab Med 1977; 101:168–169.

Tumors

27. Mohammed W, Murphy A. Cardiac fibroma presenting as sudden death in a six-month-old infant. West Indian Med J 1997; 46:28–29.
28. Matturri L, Ottaviani G, Rossi L. Sudden and unexpected infant death due to an hemangioendothelioma located in the medulla oblongata. Adv Clin Pathol 1999; 3:29–33.
29. Gleckman AM, Smith TW. Sudden unexpected death from primary posterior fossa tumors. Am J Forensic Med Pathol 1998; 19:303–308.
30. Isaacs H Jr. Tumors of the newborn and infant. St Louis: Mosby-Yearbook; 1991.
31. Perrot LJ. Malignant hemangioendothelioma: a case of sudden unexpected death in infancy. Am J Forensic Med Pathol 1997; 18:96–99.
32. Krous HF, Chadwick AE, Isaacs H Jr. Tumors associated with sudden infant childhood death. Pediatr Dev Pathol 2005; 8:20–25.

Other causes of sudden death in infants

33. Byard RW. Mechanisms of unexpected death in infants and young children following foreign body ingestion. J Forensic Sci 1996; 41:438–441.
34. Byard RW, Cohle SD. Sudden death in infancy, childhood and adolescence. Cambridge: Cambridge University Press; 1994.
35. Byard RW. Hazardous infant and early childhood sleeping environment and death scene examination. J Clin Forensic Med 1996; 3:115–122.
36. Byard RW, Beal S, Blackbourne B, et al. Specific dangers associated with infants sleeping on sofas. J Paediatr Child Health 2001; 37:476–478.
37. Byard RW, James RA, Felgate P. Detecting organic toxins in possible fatal poisonings – a diagnostic problem. J Clin Forensic Med 2002; 9:85–88.

Use of ancillary tests in perinatal pathology

19

Raj P. Kapur

'*....Think! How the hell are you gonna think and hit at the same time?*'   Yogi Berra

Introduction

In perinatal pathology, many anatomic diagnoses are established by careful gross examination and microscopic studies. In other instances, these traditional approaches lead one to suspect one or more condition, but definitive diagnosis is not possible without additional testing. In this regard, a very important part of the initial examination is to collect and preserve appropriate samples for ancillary tests, and then to use special studies judiciously with a clear understanding of how the results will contribute to diagnosis, counseling, or the management of future pregnancies.

One approach is to collect and save a myriad of different specimens from every case, hoping to cover all potential studies that might be needed later. In general, this technique of 'global' sampling is impractical, if for no other reason than the daunting resources needed for specimen storage. Alternatively, an effort could be made during the gross examination to predict what will be required for each case, and only obtain samples for those tests. The unfortunate risk with this 'targeted' strategy is that important diagnostic considerations may be overlooked initially or arise from data that emerge later (e.g. pertinent family history, microscopic findings, novel genetic tests). An ideal practice probably lies between these two extremes.

In this chapter, a compromise between the global and targeted approaches is advocated. According to this protocol, pieces of liver and placenta are saved frozen from every case, and other types of special tissue handling are done only when indicated. The goals of this chapter are to review some of the common types of ancillary testing and discuss their indications and tissue requirements. It should become clear that many of these tests can be accomplished with frozen liver or placenta and, therefore, do not require any deviation from the base protocol. **The key** is to learn to recognize those situations in which other types of tissue handling are required. For this reason the chapter ends with a simple algorithm that can be applied at the time of gross examination to anticipate and use most of the ancillary tests relevant to fetal pathology.

Routine storage of frozen liver and placenta

In addition to detailed gross descriptions, high quality photographs and other imaging methods (e.g. radiographs, sketches) when indicated (see Ch. 16), procurement of a frozen tissue sample is an important component of the perinatal pathology examination. Frozen tissue provides a source of DNA, RNA (much less stable than DNA), proteins, and other molecules that may be used in a variety of ways (Table 19.1).

TABLE 19.1 POTENTIAL USES OF FROZEN TISSUE SAMPLES

Use	Constituent*	Example
Electrophoresis	Hemoglobin	Thalassemia
Western blot	Viral protein	Human immunodeficiency virus
HPLC	Amino acids	Glutaric acidemia
GC-MS	Cholesterol	Smith-Lemli-Opitz syndrome
Enzyme assay	Enzyme activity	Glycogen storage disease
Southern blot/PCR	DNA	Mutational or linkage analysis
Comparative genomic hybridization	DNA	Confined placental aneuploidy
RT-PCR	RNA	Mutational analysis

*The stability of some of these constituents varies and may be affected significantly by autolysis.
HPLC, High-pressure liquid chromatography; GC-MS, gas chromatographic mass spectroscopy; PCR, polymerase chain reaction; RT, reverse transcriptase.

Because of dramatic technical and diagnostic advances in molecular genetics, the practice of routinely freezing tissue has become commonplace. Each month, new associations are established between congenital phenotypes and mutations in specific genes. The pace of these new discoveries is awe-inspiring and difficult to monitor. In parallel with these discoveries exists the potential to perform **mutational analysis** on a DNA sample from an affected fetus (or its placenta). Molecular diagnosis of a particular mutation can have profound implications beyond confirmation of a clinical diagnosis. In many cases, it is technically possible to test parents or other relatives to identify carriers of a given mutation. The results of such tests can be used to provide accurate estimates for recurrence in subsequent pregnancies and to perform prenatal diagnosis in some instances.

The following history illustrates the benefits of frozen tissue for the counseling and management of a hereditary disorder. The index case was a term infant that survived for 1 h with severe respiratory distress. Autopsy demonstrated gross and histopathologic changes diagnostic of autosomal recessive polycystic kidney disease (Fig. 19.1A–C).[1] At the time of autopsy, a liver sample was frozen. When the mother became pregnant again, the gene for this disorder had been mapped, but not identified. However, it was possible for a reference laboratory to perform linkage analysis using DNA extracted from a chorionic villous sample, the sibling's frozen liver, and DNA from the parents. These studies established a 95% likelihood that the second fetus was affected and the pregnancy was electively terminated at 20 weeks' gestation. Although prenatal ultrasonographic studies were inconclusive prior to termination, microanatomic studies of the fetal kidney and liver confirmed recurrent autosomal recessive syndrome (Fig. 19.1D–F).

Given that numerous specific genes have been implicated in specific disorders, it is impossible to expect a pathologist to know the availability of every genetic test at the time of fetal examination. Furthermore, novel genetic tests may become available months to years after a case is evaluated, but at a time when family members are still interested. The pathologist can best serve the patient by freezing tissues at the time of autopsy and saving them, so that appropriate testing can be solicited if desired. In many instances, request for the tissue will come from geneticists or genetic counselors, who integrate the anatomic pathology results with other clinical information from the family.

Unfortunately, the limited availability of specific tests can be frustrating for patients and pathologist. Many molecular diagnostic studies that can be done to exclude/confirm specific genetic defects have been developed in research laboratories, which either do not function as reference laboratories or do so on a highly restricted basis. A useful source of **information about genetic testing** and laboratories that can perform specific molecular tests is **GeneTests**™ (http://www.genetests.org), an on-line testing resource that includes a genetics laboratory directory, a resource list of genetics clinics, an introduction to genetics counseling and testing concepts, and up-to-date reviews of various genetic disorders. The information provided at this site is free.

Mutational analysis is only one of many ancillary tests that can be performed with frozen tissues. In principle, any fetal tissue is a suitable source of DNA that might be used for this purpose. We advocate storage of liver and placenta for several reasons. In contrast with skin or many connective tissues, a relatively high density of nuclei is present in the fetal liver with relatively little extracellular matrix. Hence, the concentration of DNA in hepatic extracts is high. Hematopoietic cells contribute significantly to the density of nuclei in fetal liver, so mRNA or protein extracts will include hematopoietic (e.g. hemoglobin) and hepatocellular gene products, which may have diagnostic utility of their own. In addition, many metabolic disorders are due to deficiency of enzymes that are found in the liver and some can be confirmed by enzymatic assays of non-autolyzed liver tissue. Frozen placental samples are particularly valuable when the fetus is autolyzed and the integrity of nuclei acids or proteins in other fetal tissues is poor. Maternal perfusion of the intervillous space maintains the viability of fetal cells in the placenta long after the fetus has died. However, analyses of placenta must be interpreted cautiously, recognizing that a sample may be contaminated by maternal cells. To minimize the latter possibility, a relatively shallow excision of placenta should be obtained from the fetal surface (see Ch. 16).

Apart from tests that can be performed on frozen liver or placenta, certain tissues require **special handling**. The remainder of this chapter focuses on these procedures, the tests for which they are needed, and their indications.

Tissue culture

Some diagnoses are confirmed most efficiently by culturing fetal cells (Table 19.2). Such cultures are established by dissociating

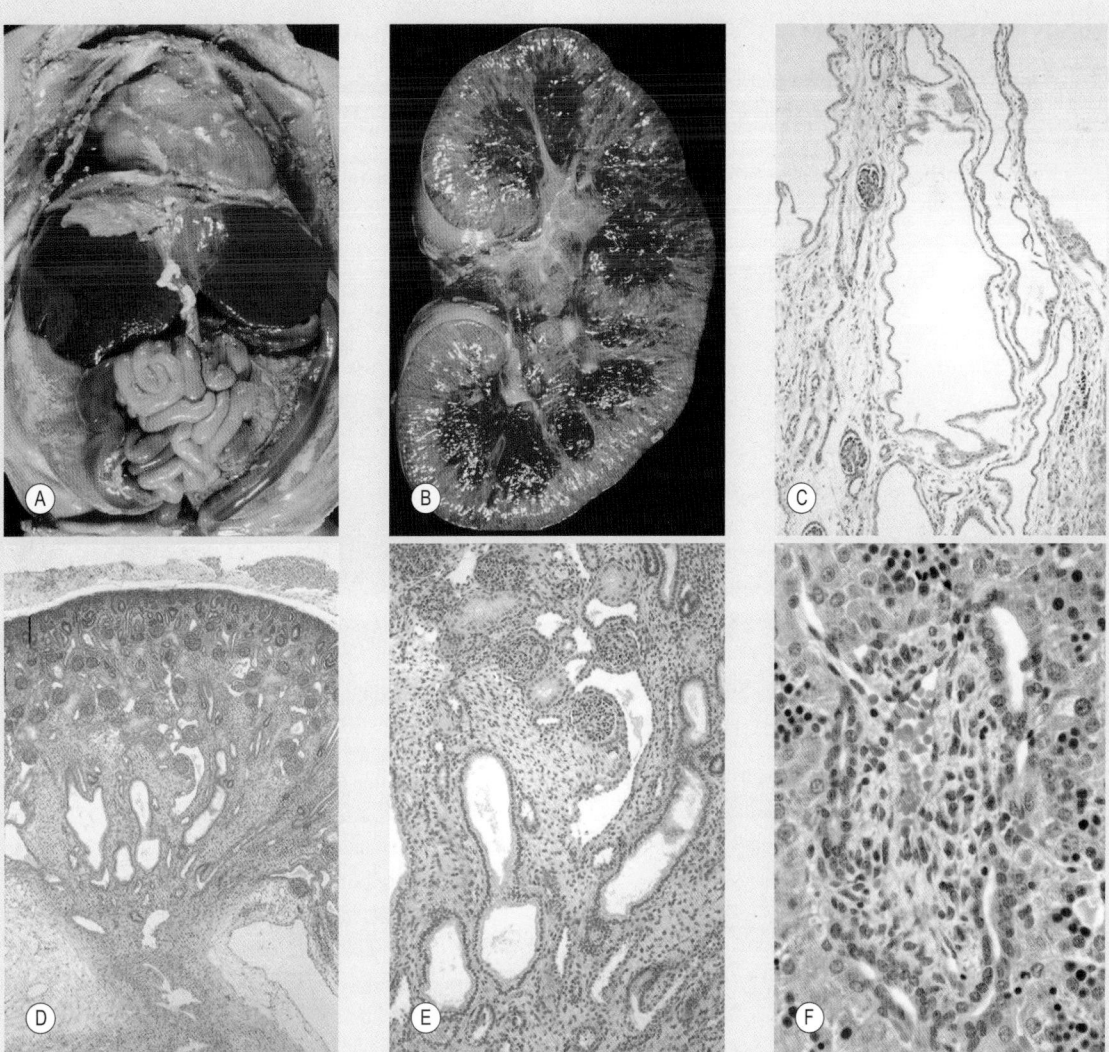

FIGURE 19.1 Practical value of frozen tissue samples. (A) Internal organs of full-term infant with massive nephromegaly. (B) The cut surface of the unfixed kidney shows medullary cysts and prominent radial markings that correspond histologically (C) to cystically dilated collecting ducts characteristic of autosomal recessive polycystic kidney disease. The sibling of A was electively aborted at 20 weeks' gestation after molecular genetic studies, using DNA from the frozen liver sample, indicated a 95% chance that he would have the disease. Although neither the gross findings nor a prenatal ultrasound were diagnostic, histologic studies of the kidney (D,E) and liver (F) demonstrate abnormal dilatation of renal collecting ducts and early biliary dysgenesis, which confirm the molecular diagnosis. (From Kapur[1] with permission.)

tissue to form a single cell suspension, which is plated in an appropriate medium. Although most protocols incorporate antibiotics into the medium, microbial contamination, particularly fungi, can compromise these studies. The likelihood of contamination is less if samples are collected at the beginning of the internal examination. Epidermal, oral, pulmonary, or gastrointestinal tissues are excluded, and sterile instruments are used to procure the sample. Usually, fibroblasts are the heartiest fetal cells; they adhere readily to plastic tissue culture substrates and outgrow other cell types in a tissue sample. For this reason, almost any fetal tissue will suffice, but connective tissue-rich sites (e.g. muscle and surrounding fascia) work well. Typically, we incise the abdomen and use sterile instruments to sample abdominal wall connective tissue away from the site of the incision. Samples are placed in serum-free tissue culture medium and transported immediately to the tissue culture facility.

Obviously, viable cells are necessary for successful growth in vitro. Even after death, viable cells persist for hours to days, depending on how the body is stored. As the need for cell culture is often apparent at delivery, obstetricians or other personnel should be trained to obtain appropriate samples. The likelihood of successful culture of fetal fibroblasts declines much faster in utero after demise, as opposed to a refrigerated non-macerated fetus. When the fetus is autolyzed, cultures of placental tissue should be attempted as they sometimes yield viable fibroblasts.

TABLE 19.2 DIAGNOSES THAT CAN BE ESTABLISHED FROM FIBROBLAST CULTURES AND THEIR ASSOCIATED FINDINGS*

Diagnostic consideration	Fetal findings	Appropriate test
Chromosomal disorder	At least one major malformation History of multiple spontaneous abortions Moderate or severe intrauterine growth restriction (possible confined placental mosaicism)	Cytogenetics
Fanconi anemia	Radial ray reduction defect +/– VACTERL association-like features	Chromosomal breakage studies Somatic cell hybridization-complementation studies
Roberts syndrome	Limb reduction defects and cleft lip/palate	C-banded karyotype with attention to centromere 'puffing' and anaphase 'lag'
Lysosomal storage disease	Unexplained non-immune hydrops	Enzyme activity assays

*These tests can also be performed on amniocytes, which may be obtained prenatally.

VACTERL association (V, vertebral anomalies; A, anal atresia; C, cardiac anomalies; TE, tracheoesophageal fistula or esophageal atresia; R, renal/urinary anomalies; and L, limb defect)

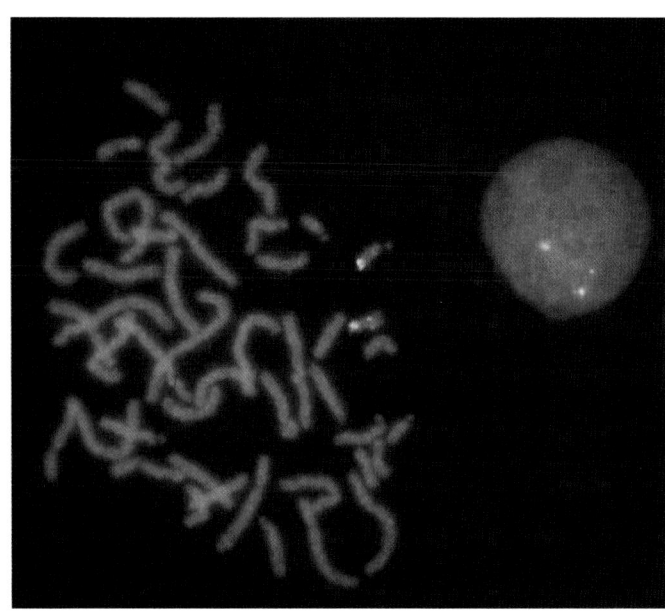

FIGURE 19.2 Fluorescence in situ hybridization is used to confirm a 22q11.2 deletion in a patient with velocardiofacial syndrome (VCFS)/DiGeorge syndrome. The fluorescence photomicrograph includes a metaphase chromosomal spread and adjacent interphase nucleus (right). The two green signals in each cell are produced by a probe to a subtelomeric portion of chromosome 22, which is intact in most patients with VCFS/DiGeorge syndrome. This probe positively identifies each member of the chromosome 22 pair. The red signals emanate from a probe that hybridizes to the region deleted in most patients with VCFS/DiGeorge syndrome. Two red signals are expected in each nucleus of a normal individual, but only one red signal is present in the nuclei of this affected individual. The combined red and green signals that are associated with the metaphase chromosomes demonstrate deletion of the VCFS/DiGeorge (red) locus from one member of the chromosome 22 pair. (Photograph provided by Kent Opheim.)

Traditional cytogenetics

One of the most common reasons for culturing cells is for **karyotype** analysis. The spectrum of chromosomal defects that can be resolved by this technique and the phenotypes associated with some of the more common chromosomal disorders are discussed in Chapter 5. The laboratory procedure required to obtain a comprehensive karyotype is labor intensive and expensive. Clinical guidelines for cytogenetic testing are not universally accepted. Virtually all authorities agree that chromosomal studies are needed for individuals with multiple malformations or minor anomalies that suggest a particular chromosomal disorder (e.g. trisomy 21). However, less consensus exists regarding isolated malformations, certain congenital neoplasms, early spontaneous pregnancy loss, non-dysmorphic intrauterine growth restriction, or spontaneous fetal demise. The liberal criteria presented in Chapter 16 encompass most autopsy cases, including those with one or more major malformation.

In some instances, alternatives to traditional cytogenetics may be considered either because fibroblast cultures were not or could not be established. Two of the most useful techniques are fluorescence in situ hybridization (FISH) and comparative genomic hybridization (CGH).

Fluorescence in situ hybridization

FISH is a method by which the integrity, number, and sometimes the chromosomal location of specific DNA sequences can be determined.[2] A fluorescently labeled probe, which binds specifically to a genomic target of interest, is applied to interphase or metaphase preparations from the patient (Fig. 19.2). **Interphase** studies resolve how many loci in a nucleus contain the complementary DNA sequence, but generally do not indicate its chromosomal location. Interphase nuclei can be obtained from touch preparations (including those derived from frozen tissue samples), cell cultures, or tissue sections. The latter are technically more difficult to process and interpret, in part because many of the nuclei are not intact. **Metaphase** studies require cell culture, but will resolve some types of chromosomal rearrangements (e.g. translocations) of the locus in question that cannot be assessed with interphase nuclei.

Because FISH targets specific sequences, the procedure is not a screening approach, like traditional cytogenetics or

TABLE 19.3 SELECTIVE DISORDERS THAT CAN BE CONFIRMED BY FLUORESCENCE IN SITU HYBRIDIZATION (FISH)

Disorder	FISH probe
Common trisomies (+13, +18, +21)	Chromosome-specific locus
Monosomy X	Chromosome-specific locus
Velocardiofacial / DiGeorge syndrome	22q11.2; 10p13-14
N-MYC amplification in neuroblastoma	N-MYC
Sex chromosome rearrangements or deletions with sexual ambiguity	X- and Y-chromosome-specific probes; SRY
XX/XY or 45, X/46, XY chimerism	X- and Y-chromosome-specific probes
Subtelomeric rearrangements	Chromosome arm-specific subtelomere

TABLE 19.4 PHENOTYPIC FEATURES OF VELOCARDIOFACIAL SYNDROME (CONFIRMED 22q11.2 DELETION)

	Percentage of affected individuals
Cardiovascular	74
Tetralogy of Fallot	22
Interrupted aortic arch	15
Ventricular septal defect	13
Truncus arteriosus	7
Vascular ring	5
Other	14
Normal	26
Palatal	34
Submucosal cleft palate	16
Overt cleft palate	11
Bifid uvula	5
Cleft lip and palate	2
No structural defect*	66
Other	
Polydactyly or other extremity	21
Vertebral	19
Rib	19
Renal or other genitourinary	31

*Includes velopharyngeal incompetence.

From McDonald-McGinn et al 2003,[3] and references therein, McDonald-McGinn et al 1999,[4] and Ming et al 1997[5]

comparative genomic hybridization (see below). FISH is used to test a specific hypothesis about a particular portion of the genome. It can be used to identify particular aneuploidies (e.g. trisomy 18) because chromosome specific probes are available that recognize centromeric sequences. Rapid screens for common trisomies (+13, +18, +21) and monosomy X are now available in many laboratories, which apply multiple interphase FISH probes in parallel or in combination with spectrally distinct fluorophores. Examples of conditions that can be confirmed by FISH are listed in Table 19.3.

The indications for most of the FISH studies listed in Table 19.3 are obvious. Testing for **velocardiofacial syndrome (VCFS)/DiGeorge syndrome** is less straightforward, because the phenotype is highly variable and encompasses some fairly common types of human malformation (Table 19.4).[3–5] VCFS is an autosomal dominant disorder that is incompletely penetrant. Approximately 95% of patients with this condition harbor a deletion in chromosome 22q11.2, which can be detected by FISH analysis. Very rare patients with a similar pattern of malformations carry deletions of chromosome 10p13-14, which can also be resolved by FISH.[6] The combination of cleft palate and cardiac outflow tract malformation, with or without anomalies in other organ systems should prompt consideration of VCFS and FISH studies for 22q11.2 deletion. It is less clear whether to perform such test for patients with isolated cardiac or palatal defects and a negative family history. As the yield from FISH studies is particularly high for tetralogy of Fallot, truncus arteriosus, and interrupted aortic arch, testing is usually pursued in such cases, even in the absence of other anomalies.

One application of FISH is to identify **subtelomeric chromosomal rearrangements**.[2] Unbalanced gain or loss of loci near the ends of chromosomes have been reported in 3–9% of individuals with moderate to severe mental retardation with or without associated dysmorphic features.[7,8] The incidence of subtelomeric rearrangements is not known for malformed fetuses or infants whose mental abilities cannot be assessed, but subtelomeric rearrangements have been detected by FISH studies of fetuses with multiple congenital malformations and no resolvable karyotype abnormalities in traditional G-banded

preparations.[9,10] Subtelomeric studies require cell culture and metaphase chromosome preparations. At this time, most laboratories do not perform subtelomeric FISH analysis as part of the routine cytogenetic evaluation of a dysmorphic fetus or infant.

Comparative genomic hybridization

CGH is a very useful method to screen for the loss or gain of particular chromosomal regions. The procedure involves mixing equimolar amounts of a patient's DNA with control DNA from a normal individual (Fig. 19.3). Prior to mixing, both the control and patient DNA samples are fragmented and labeled with different color fluorophores (typically red and green). The control and patient DNA fragments compete with each other as the mixture is hybridized to metaphase chromosomes from a normal individual. A computer imaging system captures fluorescent images of the metaphase spread and color-codes those areas where the control and patient DNA samples show unequal amounts of hybridization. Chromosomal loci with a 1.5-fold excess of patient DNA hybridization are trisomic and those with a 0.5-fold patient DNA are monosomic. In contrast to traditional FISH, CGH is a screening procedure that evaluates the entire genome for relatively large zones of trisomy or monosomy. However, CGH will not resolve small deletions that could be detected if one used appropriate probes and FISH.

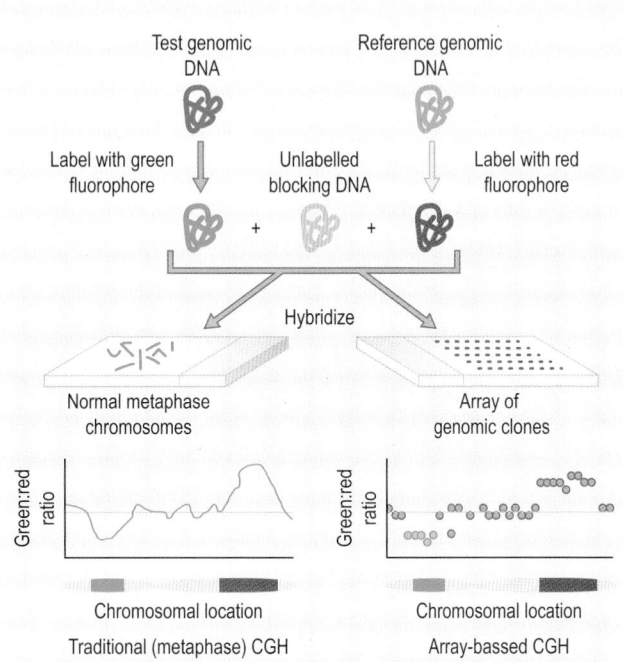

Test genomic
DNA

Reference genomic
DNA

Label with green
fluorophore

Unlabelled
blocking DNA

Label with red
fluorophore

Hybridize

Normal metaphase
chromosomes

Array of
genomic clones

Green:red ratio

Green:red ratio

Chromosomal location

Chromosomal location

Traditional (metaphase) CGH

Array-bassed CGH

FIGURE 19.3 Traditional and array-based comparative genomic hybridization (CGH). Both types of CGH begin with equimolar amounts of DNA from the patient and a reference sample (normal individual). Each is labeled with a different fluorophore and the labeled DNAs are mixed with unlabeled DNA to suppress non-specific hybridization. In this example, the patient's DNA is labeled with a green fluorophore and the reference DNA is red. Traditional CGH entails hybridization of the mixture to normal metaphase chromosomes. Chromosomal loci, which are overrepresented in the patient's genome (e.g. duplications), exhibit greater green fluorescence, whereas deleted areas appear redder. Computer imaging can detect these differences and map the positions of putative deletions or duplications along individual chromosomes. Array-based CGH is based upon similar principles, except that the mixture of patient and reference DNA is hybridized to a defined set of genomic clones that represent distinct chromosomal loci. Again, the relative amount of green and red fluorescent signal will distinguish clones that correspond to normal, duplicated, or deleted regions in the patient's genome. Array-based CGH can resolve alterations of much smaller loci than traditional CGH.

A great advantage of CGH is that it can be conducted with DNA extracted from frozen tissue or even fixed, embedded, archival samples. Despite the potential value of conventional CGH, it is not available in many laboratories, and it is likely to be replaced by array-based CGH in the near future.

Array-based comparative genomic hybridization

A new type of CGH is emerging which promises to combine sensitive detection of even small deletions or duplications with low cost and rapid turn-around time.[11, 12] In array-based CGH, equimolar mixtures of fluorescently labeled patient and control DNA fragments are hybridized to a microarray of cloned DNA fragments that represent the entire human genome (Fig. 19.3). Just as with metaphase-based CGH, trisomy or monosomy for portions of the patient's genome produce measurable differences in the ratios of fluorescent signals emitted from genomic clones that correspond to the duplicated or deleted sites. Since the chromosomal location and genetic content of each fragment in the array is known, this method defines duplicated or deleted regions with much finer resolution than traditional cytogenetics or metaphase-based CGH. Despite an inability to detect balanced rearrangements, array-based CGH is likely to replace more costly and labor-intensive karyotype analysis in many clinical applications (e.g. routine prenatal screening).

Cytogenetic breakage studies

Cytogenetic breakage studies are conducted with cell cultures that are treated with clastogenic agents to expose defects in DNA repair.[13] The latter manifest as increased chromosomal breaks and abnormal sister chromatid exchanges relative to normal cells cultured under similar conditions.[14] An experienced cytogenetics laboratory is important for these studies because interpretation of breakage studies can be difficult and may require control cells from the same site (e.g. fetal fibroblasts), as opposed to postnatal leukocytes, which are used in many laboratories.[15] A less time-consuming alternative to cytogenetic chromosomal breakage studies has been developed based on flow cytometric analysis of cell cycle progression after exposure to DNA cross-linking agents.[16–19] This technique has mostly been applied to rapidly dividing hematopoietic cells, and may not be as useful with solid tissue samples.

At present, cytogenetic breakage studies are the most sensitive method to confirm the diagnosis of **Fanconi anemia**, a pleiotropic, autosomal recessive condition in which limb abnormalities are a common feature.[19] More than 50% of Fanconi anemia patients have radial ray defects (e.g. radial aplasia, hypoplastic thumb), which may be unilateral or bilateral.[19, 20] A wide variety of other anomalies are also observed in Fanconi anemia, many of which are features of the VACTERL association (V, vertebral anomalies; A, anal atresia; C, cardiac anomalies; TE, tracheoesophageal fistula or esophageal atresia; R, renal/urinary anomalies; and L, limb defect) (see Ch. 3). Established indices for Fanconi testing in perinatal pathology have not been established, although the phenotypic spectrum of Fanconi anemia is so broad that chromosomal breakage studies could be justified in many fetuses with VACTERL-like findings and no limb defects. At a minimum, it seems reasonable to evaluate those individuals with unexplained radial ray reduction defects with or without other findings of Fanconi anemia. In addition, recurrent VACTERL in siblings may warrant studies to exclude Fanconi anemia.

Fanconi anemia is a multigene disorder.[19, 21] At this time, 11 different 'complementation groups' have been defined and the

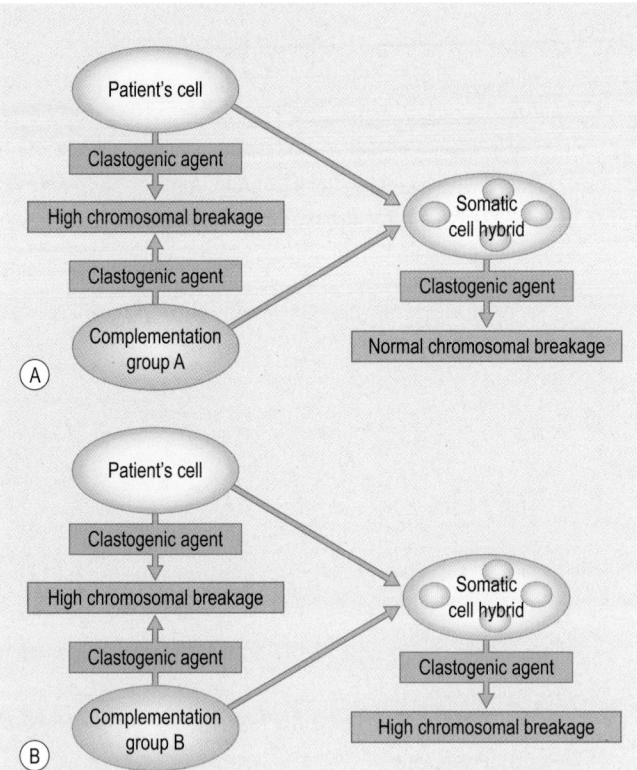

FIGURE 19.4 Complementation group testing in Fanconi anemia by somatic cell hybridization. To determine a patient's complementation group, the patient's cells are fused with cells from established complementation groups and the resulting somatic cell hybrids are tested for chromosomal breakage. (A) When fused with cells from a different complementation group, the latter compensate for the recessive defect in the patient's cells and restore a normal rate of chromosome breakage. (B) When fused with cells from the same complementation group, the recessive defect and high chromosomal breakage rate remain.

specific genes responsible for many of these groups have been identified. A patient's complementation group is determined by fusing his/her cells with cells of established complementation groups and examining chromosomal breakage in the somatic cell hybrids (Fig. 19.4). The patient belongs in the complementation group that fails to rescue the breakage phenotype in these cell fusion assays. Most of the genes that are disrupted in patients with Fanconi syndrome encode proteins that mediate DNA repair. Mutational analysis of one or more of these genes is a potential alternative to complementation studies, but is less efficient and will miss cases of Fanconi anemia due to complementation groups for which mutational analysis is not yet possible. Novel techniques have been introduced to replace somatic cell hybridization for complementation group determination, but at present these are only available for select complementation groups.

Roberts syndrome is another syndrome characterized by limb abnormalities, growth restriction, and unusual cytogenetic findings.[22, 23] The limb defects range from mild reduction anomalies to 'seal-limb' (severely shortened arms and forearms) malformations. Usually all four extremities are affected. Facial clefts are also common. Chromosomes from affected patients exhibit a variety of abnormal appearances including repulsion of heterochromatic regions ('puffing') near centromeres, particularly of chromosomes 1, 9, and 16, splaying of the short arms of the acrocentrics and of the distal Y, and irregularly distributed chromosomes during anaphase.[24–26] Some of these features are optimally resolved with staining techniques that differ from routine cytogenetics. Therefore, cytogenetic confirmation of Roberts syndrome, like Fanconi anemia, requires viable cells and specific instructions to the laboratory to search for the characteristic features. Roberts syndrome is autosomal recessive. Based on complementation assays of chromosomal morphology in somatic cell hybrids, only one complementation group has been identified to date.[27, 28] Mutations in the ESCO2 gene were recently identified as a cause for Roberts syndrome, so that mutational analysis may be an alternative to breakage studies in the near future.[29, 30]

Biochemical tests

Most **metabolic disorders** are neither recognized prenatally nor associated with in utero or perinatal lethality (see Ch. 12). An infant or child with one of these conditions is typically evaluated by a clinical specialist, who orders appropriate laboratory tests to arrive at a specific diagnosis. A small subset of metabolic diseases is associated with malformations or other phenotypic features (Table 19.5).[31–38] In these instances, enzyme analyses or metabolite measurements in fetal blood, amniotic fluid, or urine may be diagnostic, and should be encouraged if the diagnosis is suspected prenatally. Sometimes consequences of the primary disease lead to perinatal demise or elective pregnancy termination before a diagnosis has been established. In principle, some specific metabolic defects may be confirmed from postmortem samples, including frozen liver samples, but the potential impact of postmortem changes on the outcome of many of the relevant assays is unknown. Therefore, when the gross findings suggest a metabolic defect, it is prudent to determine whether prenatal specimens are available and, if not, procure tissue for fibroblast culture.

Many of the phenotypes shown in Table 19.5 are fairly distinct and encountered rarely, so that procurement of special samples for metabolic diagnosis is not a frequent occurrence at autopsy. One potential exception is **non-immune hydrops fetalis (NIHF)**, a common fetal finding with numerous potential etiologies, including many lysosomal storage disorders (Table 19.6 and Ch. 11).[31, 39] The reported prevalence of lysosomal storage diseases among fetuses with NIHF ranges from 0.5 to 15%.[39–42] The highest rates are based on comprehensive biochemical testing of a relatively small series of patients, in which selection bias may be a factor. On the other

TABLE 19.5 METABOLIC DISORDERS CHARACTERIZED BY FETAL ANOMALIES

Disorder	Most useful gross findings	Other findings
Glutaric aciduria type II[32]	Enlarged cystic kidneys[33]	Cardiac malformations
	Irregular cerebral gyri[34]	Dysmorphic facies
Pyruvate dehydrogenase deficiency[35]	Agenesis of the corpus callosum	Facial dysmorphism (long philtrum, upturned nose, wide nasal bridge, frontal bossing)
		Microcephaly
Zellweger syndrome[36]	Multicystic kidneys (subcapsular)	Dysmorphic facies
	Irregular cerebral gyri	Postnatal cirrhosis (late infancy)
	Stippled cartilage	
Rhizomelic chondrodysplasia punctata[36]	Stippled cartilage	
	Short humeri and femurs	
	White matter hypoplasia	
	Dysmorphic facies ('chipmunk cheeks')	
	Cataracts	
Congenital adrenal hyperplasia[37]	Ambiguous genitalia	
	Enlarged and sometimes brown adrenals	
Smith-Lemli-Opitz syndrome (7-dihydroxy-cholesterol dehydrogenase deficiency)	Syndactyly of second and third toes	Congenital heart malformation
	Hypospadias	Renal malformations
	Microcephaly	Postaxial polydactyly
	Dysmorphic brain	
Lysosomal storage disease[31]	Hydrops fetalis	Multiple arthrogryposes
	Hepatosplenomegaly	Ichthyosis
Muscle phosphorylase deficiency (glycogen storage disease, type V)[38]	Multiple arthrogryposes	

TABLE 19.6 LYSOSOMAL STORAGE DISEASE THAT CAN PRESENT AS NON-IMMUNE HYDROPS FETALIS

Hydrops is common	Hydrops is uncommon
Mucopolysaccharidosis, type VII	Mucopolysaccharidosis, type IV
GM$_1$ gangliosidosis	Mucolipidosis I
Infantile sialic acid storage disease	Mucolipidosis II
	Farber disease
	Gaucher disease
	Niemann-Pick A
	Niemann-Pick C
	Wolman disease
	Multiple sulfatase deficiency

After Wraith 2002.[31]

common, it may be impractical to perform such studies for every case. The gross examination of a hydropic fetus may reveal other causes, but seldom suggests specifically a metabolic basis. In contrast, microscopic studies of the placenta or other organs may reveal vacuolated cells or other cytological changes that require further investigation.[43, 44] In assessing the cost–benefit issues, the following are recommended. For all fetuses with NIHF, if the gross examination fails to reveal a specific etiology, either verify that appropriate prenatal samples are available or establish fibroblast cultures to test for lysosomal storage disease. Reserve enzymatic studies for those cases with microscopic changes suggestive of a storage disease, parental consanguinity, or a history of multiple pregnancy losses (particularly recurrent hydrops). In some of these instances, fibroblast cultures are required for cytogenetics, as well. Electron microscopy (see below) can be useful[43, 44] but adds significantly to the cost. It is often compromised by fetal autolysis, and is not as sensitive or specific as enzymatic testing.

hand, studies that reported lower rates include many fetuses with unexplained NIHF that were not formally tested for lysosomal storage disease.

Since most forms of **lysosomal storage disease** are autosomal recessive, the diagnostic implications for future pregnancies are extremely important. However, enzymatic studies to exclude each of the lysosomal storage diseases that have been associated with NIHF are expensive. Because unexplained NIHF is so

Frozen section histochemistry

Histochemical study of frozen tissue sections is used by pathologists in a variety of contexts, including immune-complex disorders, intestinal dysmotility, and various myopathies. In perinatal pathology, the primary role for such preparations is to evaluate for possible **myopathies**. The latter should be suspected if a fetus shows stigmata of in utero dyskinesia such as multiple contractures, pterygia, and polyhydramnios (see Ch. 35). For such cases, a comprehensive examination of skeletal muscle includes routine histology, frozen-section histochemistry, and electron microscopy. In addition, skeletal muscle is frozen and stored for possible biochemical studies.[45] The battery of histochemical stains used routinely by most muscle pathologists is discussed in Chapter 35. If myopathy is a diagnostic consideration, it is important to acquire tissue for histochemistry and electron microscopy as soon as possible after demise, as even an hour of autolysis will compromise studies. Methods for handling biopsies to ensure appropriate fixation and minimize freeze artifact are described elsewhere.[45] For liveborn infants, muscle biopsy (prior to expected demise) may be justified when a myopathy is strongly suspected. Growth plates of bones in autopsies of osteochondral dysplasias should be sampled and frozen, to allow western blotting.

Electron microscopy

Ultrastructural data are helpful in certain situations (e.g. myopathies, glomerulopathies, mitochondrial or storage disorders). In these instances, the need for electron microscopy should be anticipated prior to demise, so that tissue can be obtained and fixed as soon as possible after demise, thereby avoiding artifacts introduced by autolysis.

Flow cytometry

Flow cytometry is seldom applied in perinatal pathology, but is particularly useful in two contexts. First, the patient with congenital leukemia, who is often hydropic at birth and may have circulating blasts. Immunophenotypic characterization of viable blasts obtained from marrow or peripheral blood is used to define the type of leukemia.

Suspected **triploidy** (or tetraploidy) is the other clinical situation in which flow cytometry helps to establish the diagnosis.[46] As discussed in Chapter 5, triploidy produces two distinctly different phenotypes, depending upon whether the extra chromosomal content is maternally or paternally derived.[47, 48] When either phenotype is observed, ploidy analysis of dissociated fetal or placental cells will confirm or exclude the diagnosis. Although it is possible to perform ploidy studies with fixed tissue, it is simpler to use fresh tissue. Cytogenetics or comparative genomic hybridization can also establish the diagnosis, but flow cytometry is less expensive and much quicker. If placental tissue is used for flow cytometric evaluation, the presence of maternal cells provides a convenient internal diploid

standard, but may also lead to confusion about diploid/triploid mosaicism (Fig. 19.5).

Microbiological and viral cultures

Microbial or viral cultures are occasionally useful in the practice of perinatal pathology. It is appropriate to submit tissue for bacterial cultures from an infant who died with signs of acute infection. For several reasons, such cultures are less valuable in the context of fetal demise. The pattern of placental and/or fetal inflammation usually establishes the general diagnosis of **bacterial infection**; cultures most often yield an enteric or genitourinary commensal organism[49] and identification of a specific bacterium does not impact significantly on counseling, management, or treatment. Group B streptococcal (GBS) infection is sometimes cited as a significant pathogen,[50] in part because of the potential for recurrence in subsequent pregnancies. However, the importance of isolating GBS from an isolated case of chorioamnionitis, with or without fetal inflammation, is debatable, particularly in populations where maternal screening for GBS and prophylactic antibiotic treatment are part of routine prenatal care.[51] Infections produced by *Listeria monocytogenes* and *Treponema pallidum* are suggested by certain fetal and/or placental findings (see Ch. 11), and can be confirmed in paraffin sections with special histologic stains. Many fungi can be identified in the same manner, although specific identification is facilitated with cultures. Gross findings that suggest intrauterine fungal or *Listeria* infection are microabscesses in the placenta villi, membranes, or cord, which often appear as discrete pale soft plaques or nodules.

Although the fetus is susceptible to many types of **viral infection** that can lead to intrauterine or perinatal demise, some of these pathogens (e.g. herpes virus, cytomegalovirus) produce specific cytopathologic changes that obviate the need for culture. In addition, polymerase chain reaction (PCR) and/or specific immunohistochemical reagents can be used with paraffin sections to confirm many types of viral infection. A search for enteroviruses and/or other viruses that do not produce diagnostic histologic changes is warranted for infants with suggestive antemortem symptoms (e.g. myocarditis and rash). In addition, enteroviruses and possibly other viruses may be responsible for some cases of otherwise unexplained perinatal morbidity and mortality.[49] Some of the data to support this hypothesis are immunohistochemical and in situ PCR-based studies of placental tissue from symptomatic neonates and controls. In one such investigation, enteroviral infection was found 23/60 (38%) of placentas from cases of severe neonatal morbidity or mortality.[52] Placental histopathology was not helpful in discriminating these cases, but when performed, viral serology or postmortem tissue cultures confirmed the diagnoses. While these results need to be validated, they raise concern that enteroviral infection is under-recognized in many pathology practices. If the data are reproduced by other studies, they suggest that placental immunohistochemistry, serology, in

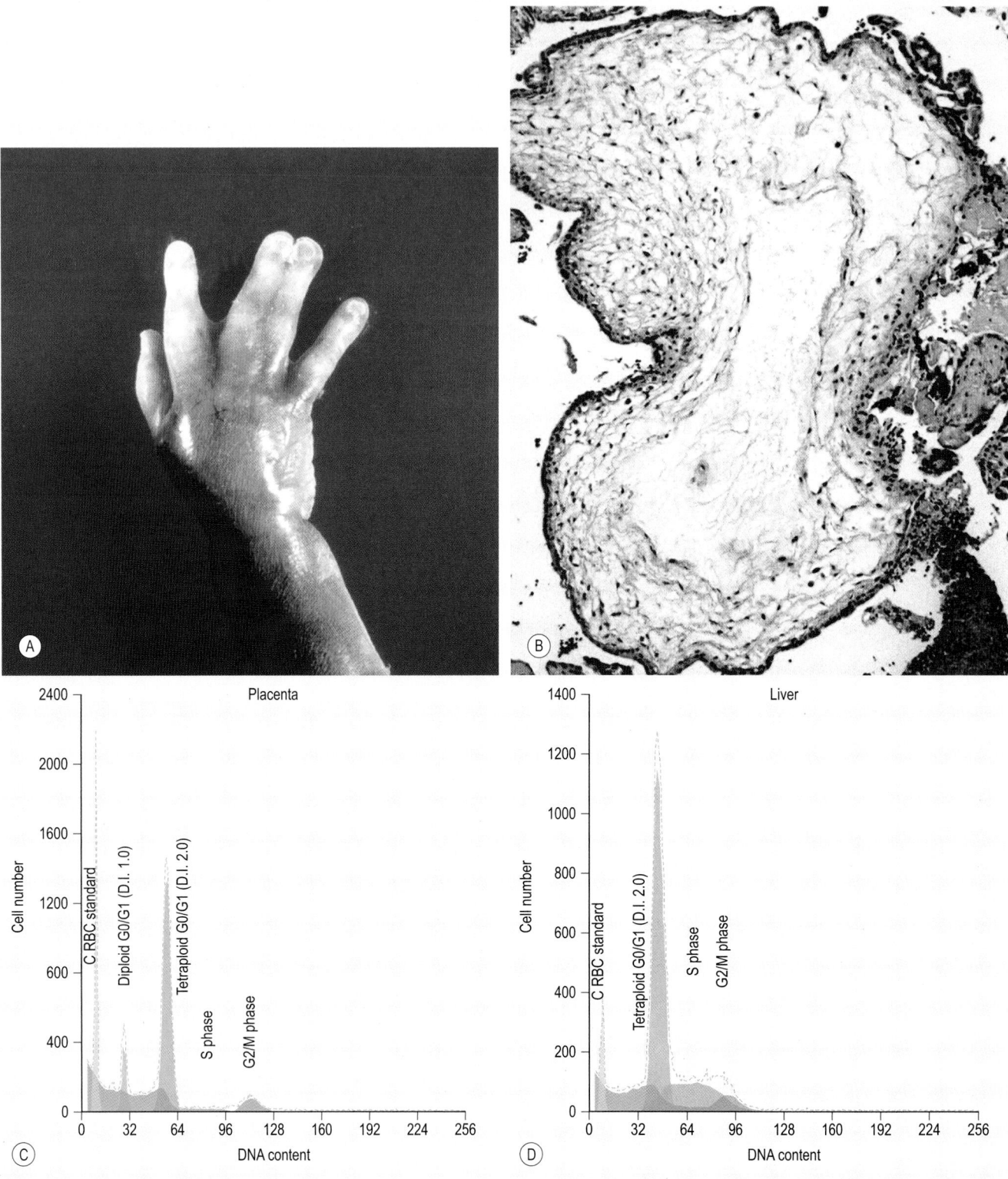

FIGURE 19.5 Diagnosis of triploidy or tetraploidy by flow cytometric DNA quantitation. Certain phenotypic features like III–IV syndactyly (A) and partial molar placental anatomy (B) suggest the diagnosis of triploidy or tetraploidy. (C) Flow cytometric analysis of the placenta indicates that almost 90% of the cells contain a tetraploid DNA content, and only 10% (which may represent maternal cells) are diploid. (D) Analysis of fetal liver from the same case yields a pure tetraploid cell population. The peaks labeled 'C RBC Standard' in C and D represent the DNA content of chicken red blood cells, which are used to calibrate the assay.

FOR EVERY FETAL CASE

Detailed Gross Description and Detailed Records (written, radiographic, photographic)

Frozen Sample of Liver and Placenta

AND IF THE PHENOTYPE

includes ≥ 1 major malformation	THEN	Unfixed fetal and/or placental tissue for cytogenetics
suggests triploidy	THEN	Fresh fetal or placental tissue for flow cytometry
suggests VCFS/DiGeorge	THEN	Fetal and/or placental cytogenetics and fluorescence in situ hybridization
suggests hypokinesia	THEN	EM-fixed and frozen skeletal muscle for histochemistry, if specimen is very fresh
suggests Fanconi anemia or Roberts syndrome	THEN	Culture fetal and/or placental tissues for cytogenetics and chromosomal breakage studies
is unexplained fetal hydrops	THEN	Culture fetal and/or placental tissues for cytogenetics and possible lysosomal enzyme studies
is idiopathic moderate-to-severe growth retardation and mother does not smoke or have chronic hypertension*	THEN	Fetal and placental cytogenetics to exclude confined placental mosaicism

* Pregnancy induced hypertension does not abrogate the need for these studies. EM, Electron microscopy; VCFS, velocardiofacial syndrome.

examination discussed in Chapter 16, which include careful review of the medical record to identify specific diagnostic concerns, pertinent family history, pregnancy history, method of termination, and any completed or pending laboratory test results. Knowledge of the latter may avoid redundant tests and/or may establish the existence of important tissue samples (e.g. amniocyte cultures) that may be used for additional tests depending on the gross findings. The goal is to anticipate all appropriate tests with minimal wasted resources. In some cases (e.g. lysosomal storage diseases), this may require that tissues are procured and frozen or cultured, but not used unless later parts of the examination (e.g. histopathology) suggest or exclude particular diagnoses.

References

Routine storage of frozen liver and placenta

1. Kapur RP. Practicing pediatric pathology without a microscope. Mod Pathol 2001;14:229–235.

Fluorescence in situ hybridization

2. Tsuchiya KD, Opheim KE. The use of fluorescence in situ hybridization in diagnosing pediatric disorders. J Histotechnol 2004; 27:259–264.
3. McDonald-McGinn DM, Emanuel BS, Zackai EH. 22q11.2 deletion syndrome. In: GeneReviews at GeneTests: Medical Genetics Information Resource (database online). Copyright, University of Washington, Seattle. 1997–2006. Available at http://www.genetests.org. Accessed January 31, 2006.
4. McDonald-McGinn DM, Kirschner R, Goldmuntz E, et al. The Philadelphia story: the 22q11.2 deletion: report on 250 patients. Genet Couns 1999; 10:11–24.
5. Ming JE, McDonald-McGinn DM, Megerian TE, et al. Skeletal anomalies and deformities in patients with deletions of 22q11.2. Am J Med Genet 1997; 72:210–215.
6. Berend SA, Spikes AS, Kashork CD, et al. Dual-probe fluorescence in situ hybridization assay for detecting deletions associated with VCFS/DiGeorge syndrome I and DiGeorge syndrome II loci. Am J Med Genet 2000; 91:313–317.
7. Knight SJ, Regan R, Nicod A, et al. Subtle chromosomal rearrangements in children with unexplained mental retardation. Lancet 1999; 354: 1676–1681.
8. Bocian E, Helias-Rodzewicz Z, Suchenek K, et al. Subtelomeric rearrangements: results from FISH studies in 84 families with idiopathic mental retardation. Med Sci Monit 2004; 10:CR143–151.
9. Brackley KJ, Kilby MD, Morton J, et al. A case of recurrent congenital fetal anomalies associated with a familial subtelomeric translocation. Prenat Diagn 1999; 19:570–574.
10. Schellberg R, Schwanitz G, Gravinghoff L, et al. New trends in chromosomal investigation in children with cardiovascular malformations. Cardiol Young 2004; 14:622–629.

Array-based comparative genomic hybridization

11. Snijders AM, Pinkel D, Albertson DG. Current status and future prospects of array-based comparative genomic hybridization. Brief Funct Genomic Proteomic 2003; 2:37–45.
12. Mantripragada KK, Buckley PG, de Stahl TD, et al. Genomic microarrays in the spotlight. Trends Genet 2004; 20:87–94.

situ PCR, or other techniques may be used to diagnose viral infections, eliminating the need for postmortem viral cultures.

Algorithm for use of ancillary tests in perinatal pathology

Many of the principles and assumptions put forth in this chapter lead to an algorithm for ancillary testing that can be used at the time of gross examination (Box 19.1). Application of this approach ensures that tissue has been obtained and handled appropriately for most types of perinatal pathology cases. It should be integrated with the methods for gross autopsy

Cytogenetic breakage studies

13. Auerbach AD, Wolman SR. Susceptibility of Fanconi's anaemia fibroblasts to chromosome damage by carcinogens. Nature 1976; 261:494–496.

14. Latt SA, Stetten G, Jeurgens LA, et al. Induction by alkylating agents of sister chromatid exchange and chromatid breaks in Fanconi's anemia. Proc Natl Acad Sci U S A 1975; 72:4066–4070.

15. Auerbach AD, Sagi M, Adler B. Fanconi anemia: prenatal diagnosis in 30 fetuses at risk. Pediatrics 1985; 76:794–800.

16. Schindler D, Kubbies M, Hoehn H, et al. Presymptomatic diagnosis of Fanconi's anemia. Lancet 1985; 1:937.

17. Seyschab H, Friedl R, Sun Y, et al. Comparative evaluation of diepoxybutane sensitivity and cell cycle blockage in the diagnosis of Fanconi anemia. Blood 1995; 85:2233–2237.

18. Berger R, Le Coniat M, Gendron MC. Fanconi anemia. Chromosomal breakage and cell cycle studies. Cancer Genet Cytogenet 1993; 69:13–16.

19. Tischkowitz M, Dokal I. Fanconi anaemia and leukaemia – clinical and molecular aspects. Br J Haematol 2004; 126:176–191.

20. Giampietro PF, Adler-Brecher B, Verlander PC, et al. The need for more accurate and timely diagnosis in Fanconi anemia: a report from the International Fanconi Anemia Registry. Pediatrics 1993; 91:1116–1120.

21. Rahman N, Ashworth A. A new gene on the X involved in Fanconi anemia. Nat Genet 2004; 36:1142–113.

22. Van den Berg DJ, Francke U. Roberts syndrome: a review of 100 cases and a new rating system for severity. Am J Med Genet 1993; 47:1104–1123.

23. Sinha AK, Verma RS, Mani VJ. Clinical heterogeneity of skeletal dysplasia in Roberts syndrome: a review. Hum Hered 1994; 44:121–126.

24. Jabs EW, Tuck-Muller CM, Cusano R, et al. Studies of mitotic and centromeric abnormalities in Roberts syndrome: implications for a defect in the mitotic mechanism. Chromosoma 1991; 100:251–261.

25. Tomkins DJ, Sisken JE. Abnormalities in the cell-division cycle in Roberts syndrome fibroblasts: a cellular basis for the phenotypic characteristics. Am J Hum Genet 1984; 36:1332–1340.

26. Van den Berg DJ, Francke U. Sensitivity of Roberts syndrome cells to γ radiation, mitomycin C, and protein synthesis inhibitors. Somat Cell Mol Genet 1993; 19:377–392.

27. Allingham-Hawkins DJ, Tomkins DJ. Heterogeneity in Roberts syndrome. Am J Med Genet 1995; 55:188–194.

28. McDaniel LD, Prueitt R, Probst LC, et al. Novel assay for Roberts syndrome assigns variable phenotypes to one complementation group. Am J Med Genet 2000; 93:223–229.

29. Vega H, Waisfisz Q, Gordillo M, et al. Roberts syndrome is caused by mutations in *ESCO2*, a human homolog of yeast *ECO1* that is essential for the establishment of sister chromatid cohesion. Nature Genet 2005; 37:468–470.

30. Schule B, Oviedo A, Johnston K, et al. Inactivating mutations in ESCO2 cause SC phocomelia and Roberts syndrome: no phenotype–genotype correlation. Am J Hum Genet 2005; 77:1117–1128.

Biochemical tests

31. Wraith JE. Lysosomal disorders. Semin Neonatol 2002; 7:75–83.

32. Frerman RE, Goodman SI. Defects of electron transfer flavoprotein and electron transfer flavoprotein-ubiquinone oxidoreductase: glutaric acidemia type II. In: Scriver CR, Beaudet AL, Valle D, et al, eds. The metabolic & molecular basis of inherited disease. 8th edn. New York: McGraw-Hill; 2001:2357–2365.

33. Bohm N, Uy J, Keissling M, et al. Multiple acyl CoA dehydrogenation deficiency (glutaric aciduria type II), congenital polycystic kidneys, and symmetric warty degeneration of the cerebral cortex in two newborn brothers. II. Morphology and pathogenesis. Eur J Pediatr 1982; 139:60–65.

34. Hoganson G, Berlow S, Gilbert EG, et al. Glutaric acidemia type II and flavin-dependent enzymes in morphogenesis. Birth Defects Orig Art Ser 1987; 23:65–74.

35. Robinson BH. Lactic acidemia: disorders of pyruvate carboxylase and pyruvate dehydrogenase. In: Scriver CR, Beaudet AL, Valle D, et al, eds. The metabolic and molecular basis of inherited disease. 8th edn. New York: McGraw-Hill; 2001:2275–2295.

36. Gilbert-Barness E, Barness LA. Metabolic diseases: foundations of clinical management, genetics, and pathology. South Natick: Eaton Publishing; 2000:889pp.

37. White PC. Congenital adrenal hyperplasias. Best Pract Res Clin Endocrinol Metab 2001; 15:17–41.

38. Dimauro S, Andreu AL, Bruno C, et al. Myophosphorylase deficiency (glycogenosis type V; McArdle disease). Curr Mol Med 2002; 2:189–186.

39. Burin MG, Scholz AP, Gus R, et al. Investigation of lysosomal storage diseases in non-immune hydrops fetalis. Prenat Diagn 2004; 24:653–657.

40. Machin GA. Hydrops revisited: literature review of 1414 cases published in the 1980s. Am J Med Genet 1989; 34:366–390.

41. Kattner E, Schafer A, Harzer K. Hydrops fetalis: manifestation in lysosomal storage diseases including Farber disease. Eur J Pediatr 1997; 156:292–295.

42. Piraud M, Froissart R, Mandon G, et al. Amniotic fluid for screening of lysosomal storage diseases presenting in utero (mainly as non-immune hydrops fetalis). Clin Chim Acta 1996; 248:143–155.

43. Nelson J, Kenny B, O'Hara D, et al. Foamy changes of placental cells in probable β glucuronidase deficiency associated with hydrops fetalis. J Clin Pathol 1993; 46:370–371.

44. Soma H, Yamada K, Osawa H, et al. Identification of Gaucher cells in the chorionic villi associated with recurrent hydrops fetalis. Placenta 2000; 21:412–416.

Frozen section histochemistry

45. Patterson K. Pediatric muscle biopsies: new insights (and new dilemmas). J Histotechnol 2004; 27:245–257.

Flow cytometry

46. Sunde L, Mogensen B, Olsen S, et al. Flow cytometric DNA analyses of 105 fresh hydatidiform moles, with correlations to prognosis. Anal Cell Pathol 1996; 12:99–114.

47. Daniel A, Wu Z, Bennetts B, et al. Karyotype, phenotype, and parental origin in 19 cases of triploidy. Prenat Diagn 2001; 21:1034–1048.

48. McFadden DE, Kalousek DK. Two different phenotypes of fetuses with chromosomal triploidy: correlation with parental origin of the extra haploid set. Am J Med Genet 1991; 38:535–538.

Microbiological and viral cultures

49. Goldenberg RL, Thompson BS. The infectious origins of stillbirth. Am J Obstet Gynecol 2003; 189:861–873.

50. McDonald HM, Chambers HM. Intrauterine infection and spontaneous midgestation abortion: is the spectrum of microorganisms similar to that in preterm labor? Inf Dis Obstet Gynecol 2000; 8:220–227.

51. Gibbs RS, Schrag S, Schuchat A. Perinatal infections due to group B streptococci. Obstet Gynecol 2004; 104:1062–1076.

52. Satosar A, Ramirez NC, Bartholomew D, et al. Histologic correlates of viral and bacterial infection of the placenta associated with severe morbidity and mortality in the newborn. Hum Pathol 2004; 35:536–545.

Major anomalies of external anatomy or in-situ relationships

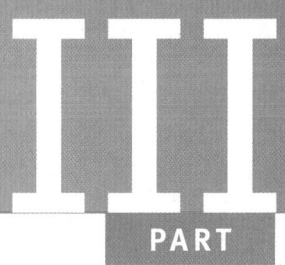

III
PART

Craniofacial abnormalities

20

M. Michael Cohen Jr.

"Faces together with their associated structures allow us to speak and smile; sigh and kiss; smell, touch, chew, and swallow; cry out in pain; and convey a world of feelings and emotions through facial expression."

National Institute of Dental and Craniofacial Research, 2000

Craniofacial embryology

Neurulation

The neural tube is formed by fusion of the neural folds. The process of neurulation is complex and involves proliferation of neuroblasts or matrix cells, development of the neuroepithelium and surface ectoderm, formation of the neural plate median hinge point, apical constriction of neuroepithelial cells, and expansion of the mesoderm and extracellular matrices. At the beginning of the third week, the neural plate appears, followed by elevation of the neural folds. With further development, fusion of the neural folds forms the neural tube with anterior and posterior neuropores (Fig. 20.1). Closure of the anterior neuropore occurs at the 18–20 somite stage and closure of the posterior neuropore at the 25 somite stage.[1, 2]

During the fourth week, the cephalic end of the neural tube develops three primary brain vesicles: the forebrain (prosencephalon), midbrain (mesencephalon), and hindbrain (rhombencephalon). As these vesicles appear, the neural tube bends ventrally, forming a cervical flexure located in the midbrain region. At the beginning of the sixth week, the prosencephalon has become subdivided into an anterior part (telencephalon), two lateral bulges (cerebral hemispheres), and a posterior part (diencephalon with outgrowth of the optic stalks). The rhom-

bencephalon becomes subdivided into an anterior part (metencephalon) and posterior part (myelencephalon).[3]

The face

Neural crest cells play an integral part in facial morphogenesis. Just before the neural folds fuse to form the neural tube, neuroectodermal cells adjacent to the neural plate migrate into the facial region, where they form the skeletal and connective tissue of the face: bone cartilage, fibrous connective tissue, and all dental tissues except enamel. Thus, facial mesenchyme is of neural crest origin. Vascular endothelium and skeletal muscle, however, are of mesodermal origin. Table 20.1 summarizes the origin of some craniofacial components.[3–9]

By the end of the fourth week, the maxillary swellings appear lateral to, and mandibular swellings caudal to, the stomodeum. Above, the frontal prominence forms ventral to the prosencephalon. Nasal placodes arise as thickenings on either side of the frontal prominence. During the fifth week, a horseshoe-shaped ridge, consisting of medial and lateral nasal swellings, surrounds each nasal placode. As mesenchyme elevates the ridges, the nasal pits form (Fig. 20.2). By the sixth week, with continued growth of the maxillary swellings, the nasal and maxillary swellings become separated by deep furrows.[3, 6–9]

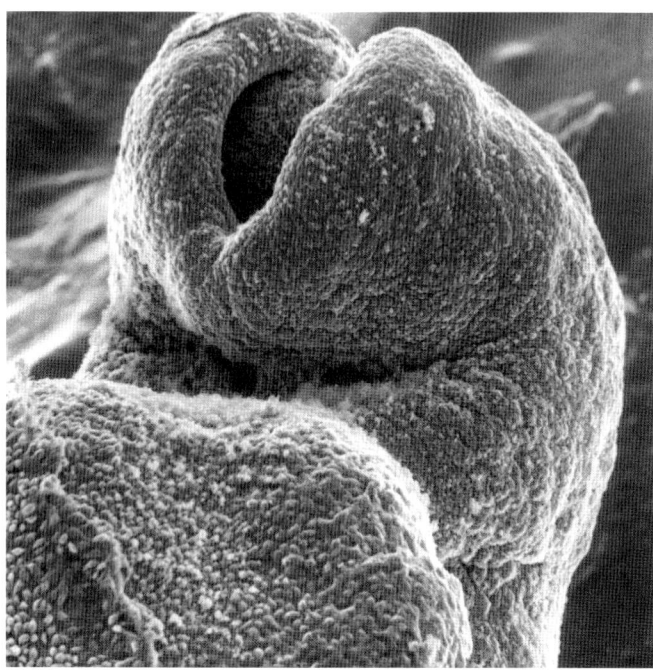

FIGURE 20.1 Scanning electron microscopy image of human closing anterior neuropore. (Courtesy of J. E. Jirásek, Prague.)

TABLE 20.1 ORIGIN OF SOME CRANIOFACIAL COMPONENTS

Neural crest origin	Mesodermal origin
Facial connective tissue	Facial muscles
Facial bones	Endothelial lining of blood vessels
Facial sutures	Chondrocranium
Frontal bone	Parietal bones
Metopic suture	Coronal suture
Sagittal suture	Lambdoid suture
Nasal capsule	Temporal bones except squama
Temporal squama	Occipital bone (somites plus squama)
From Cohen 2005.[4]	

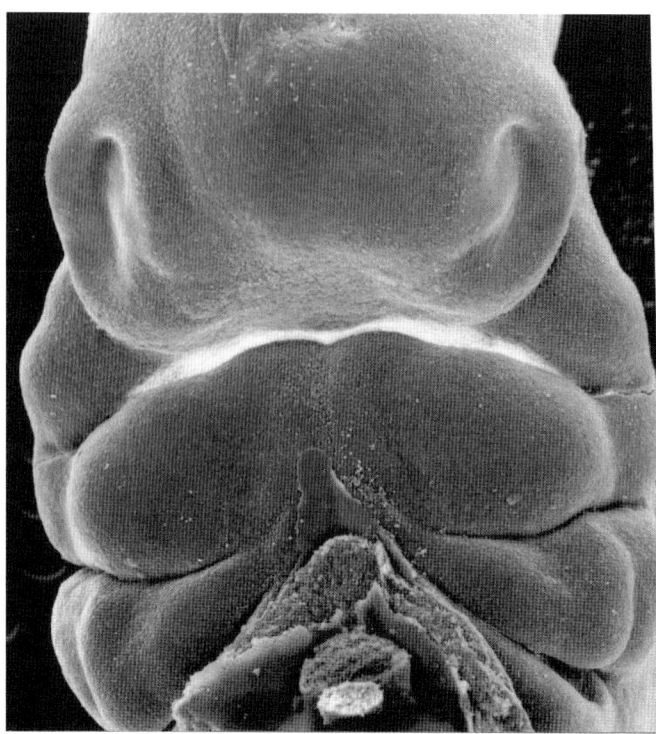

FIGURE 20.2 Scanning electron microscopy image of the face of a 5-week-old embryo. Note the olfactory pits developing on the lateral portion of the frontonasal prominence. (Courtesy of K. Sulik, Chapel Hill, North Carolina.)

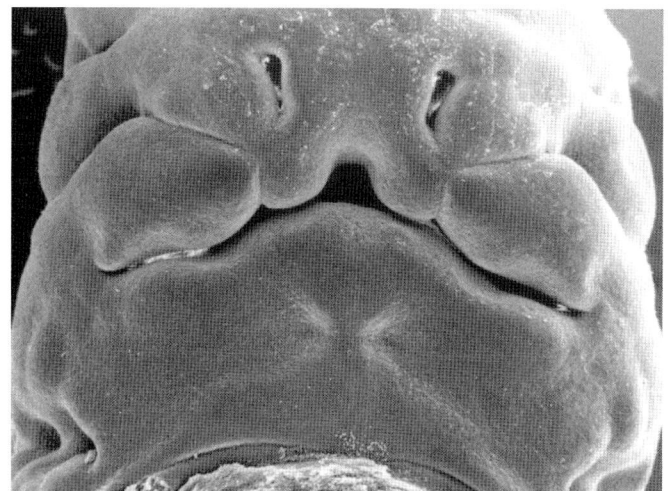

FIGURE 20.3 Scanning electron microscopy of a 6-week-old embryo. During the sixth and seventh weeks, maxillary swellings fuse with medial nasal swellings, and the medial nasal swellings merge with each other. The upper lip is still incompletely formed at the sixth week. (Courtesy of K. Sulik, Chapel Hill, North Carolina.)

During the sixth and seventh weeks, the maxillary swellings fuse with the medial nasal swellings and both medial nasal swellings merge with each other (Fig. 20.3). The deep furrow separating the lateral nasal swelling and the maxillary swelling, the nasolacrimal groove, develops a solid epithelial cord that detaches from the overlying ectoderm in the furrow. After canalization of the cord, the nasolacrimal duct forms and widens at its upper end to create the lacrimal sac. After detachment of the cord, the lateral nasal and maxillary swellings merge to form the alae of the nose.[3, 6–9]

The fusion of the medial nasal swellings with the maxillary swellings and the merging of the medial nasal swellings with each other produce the primary palate or intermaxillary segment, which is composed of three parts:

- a labial component that later forms the philtrum;
- a medial section, the future dental arch containing the four maxillary incisor teeth; and
- a triangular palatal component extending posteriorly to the incisive foramen.[3, 6–9]

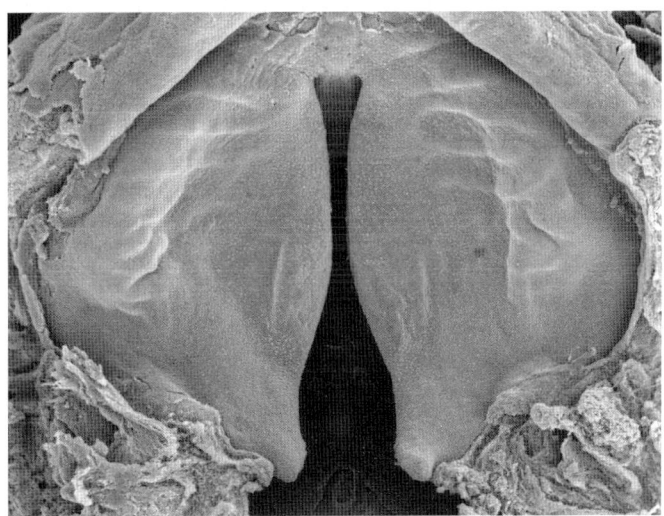

FIGURE 20.4 Scanning electron microscopy of the secondary palate in a 53-day-old embryo. Fusion with the primary palate has occurred. The dating is based on post-fertilization crown-rump length in contrast to the dating in the text, which is based on the LMP. (Courtesy of L. Russell, Chapel Hill, North Carolina.)

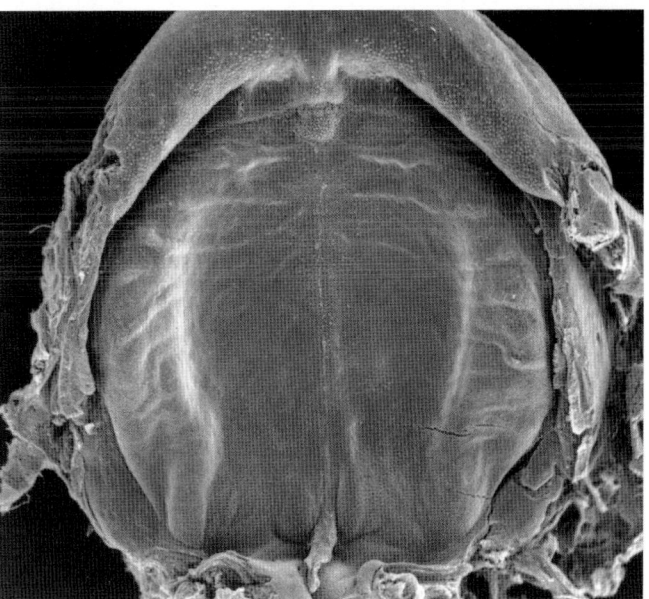

FIGURE 20.5 At 59 days, complete fusion of the secondary palate has occurred. The dating is based on post-fertilization crown-rump length in contrast to the dating in the text, which is based on the LMP. (Courtesy of L. Russell, Chapel Hill, North Carolina.) (Courtesy of L. Russell, Chapel Hill, North Carolina.)

The definitive (secondary) palate is formed from two medial shelf-like outgrowths of the maxillary swellings. These are the vertical palatine shelves, which appear during the sixth week and elevate to a horizontal position during the seventh week (Fig. 20.4). The shelves fuse with the triangular portion of the intermaxillary segment and fuse with each other by programmed cell death of the medial edges, allowing mesenchyme to join in the midline. Complete fusion occurs by the tenth week (Fig. 20.5). The soft palate and uvula form by merging.[3, 6, 8–10]

Pharyngeal arches

The pharyngeal arches appear during the fourth and fifth weeks of development. Deep pharyngeal clefts separate the bars of mesenchyme. Accompanying the arches and externally located clefts, the pharyngeal pouches appear along the lateral walls of the pharyngeal portion of the gut. The maxillary and mandibular swellings develop from the first (mandibular) arch.[11, 12] The pharyngeal arches and their nerves, muscles, cartilages, bones, ligaments, and pharyngeal pouches are summarized in Table 20.2.

The ears develop from six mesenchymal proliferations, the auricular hillocks, three on each side of the first pharyngeal cleft. The definitive auricle results from fusion of the hillocks. With development of the mandible, the ears, which initially form in the lower neck region, ascend to the sides of the head at the level of the eyes.[13]

The second pharyngeal arch grows down over the third and fourth arches, leaving a space that becomes the cervical sinus. The inferior parathyroid gland and thymus arise from the third pharyngeal pouch. The superior parathyroid gland arises from the fourth pharyngeal pouch. The ultimobranchial body arises from the sixth pouch.[11]

Molecular correlates of pharyngeal arch development

Cranial neural crest, originating at the dorsal margin of the neural tube, migrates and populates the pharyngeal arches. Other embryonic germ layers (ectoderm, endoderm, and mesoderm) are involved in pharyngeal arch development. *Otx2* and *Gbx2* determine the midbrain–hindbrain boundary at the isthmus, where Fgf8 acts to suppress Hox gene expression, and together with other factors acting locally, permit the mandibular arch to develop. However, positive Hox gene expression is essential for the developing hyoid arch. Bmp4 causes neural crest cell death at two points, segregating three separate streams of neural crest migration into the pharyngeal arches. Despite the many genes that direct neural crest migration into the pharyngeal arches, the neural crest itself is also an intrinsic source of molecular information that varies between species.[14–18]

Cranial neural crest

The cranial neural crest originates at the dorsal margin of the neural tube. *Wnt* is necessary and sufficient for the induction of neural crest. In the absence of *Wnt* signaling, neural crest cells are not generated.[19] ErbB4, which is expressed in the neural ectoderm, is necessary for neural crest cell migration.[20, 21]

The developing hindbrain is subdivided into cell-lineage restricted units – the rhombomeres. Neural crest cells from rhombomeres 1 and 2 together with caudal midbrain-derived crest cells populate the first (mandibular) arch. Crest cells from

TABLE 20.2 PHARYNGEAL ARCHES

Pharyngeal arches	Nerves	Muscles derived from somitomeres	Skeletal, cartilaginous, and ligamentous structures of neural crest origin	Pharyngeal pouches of endodermal origin
First (mandibular)	Trigeminal (V)	Mastication (temporalis, masseter, medial and lateral pterygoids), mylohyoid, anterior belly of digastric, tensor palatini, tensor tympani	Meckel's cartilage, sphenomandibular ligament, malleus, incus	Eustachian tubes
Second (hyoid)	Facial (VII)	Facial expression (buccinator, auricularis, frontalis, orbicularis oculi, orbicularis oris), posterior belly of digastric, stylohyoid, stapedius	Styloid process, stapes, stylohyoid ligament, lesser cornua of hyoid, upper portion of body of hyoid	Palatine tonsils
Third	Glossopharyngeal (IX)	Stylopharyngeus	Greater cornua of hyoid, lower portion of body of hyoid	Thymus, inferior parathyroid glands
Fourth	Superior laryngeal branch and recurrent laryngeal branch of vagus (X)	Levator veli palatini, pharyngeal constrictors	Laryngeal cartilages	Superior parathyroid glands
Sixth				Ultimobranchial body

From Cohen 2005.[4]

rhombomere 4 populate the second (hyoid) arch. Rhombomeres 6 and 7 contribute to the third, fourth, and sixth pharyngeal arches.[14, 22] Rhombomeres 3 and 5 are depleted of neural crest production, which allows three distinct streams of crest cells to migrate into the pharyngeal arches[14] (*vide supra*).

Although rhombomeres 3 and 5 produce some crest cells, the majority die by apoptosis caused by Bmp4. Decreased Msx2 expression is also found in the apoptotic cells, but Bmp4 plays the pivotal role. Territories opposite rhombomeres 3 and 5 express Sema3A, which also inhibits crest cell migration as does mesenchyme adjacent to these segments. Bmp receptors and their transducers are present in the other rhombomeric crest as well, but they are antagonized by Noggin, thus restricting Bmp4-mediated apoptosis.[14, 15, 23–25]

Rhombomeric *Hox* gene identity

Each rhombomere has a unique *Hox* gene identity. *Hoxa2* is expressed up to the rhombomere 1–2 boundary and *Hoxb2* is expressed up to the rhombomere 2–3 boundary. However, no *Hox* gene expression is found in neural crest anterior to rhombomere 3. Thus, rhombomere 1 and 2 derived crest, which populates the first pharyngeal (mandibular) arch, has no *Hox* gene expression. The midbrain–hindbrain boundary, known as the isthmus, expresses Fgf8, which suppresses Hox expression in delaminating crest from rhombomere 1. Other factors, acting more locally, probably downregulate Hoxa2 expression in deliminating crest from rhombomere 2.[16, 18, 26–28]

Hoxa2 is essential for second pharyngeal (hyoid) arch development. If *Hoxa2* is knocked out, rhombomere 4 crest in the hyoid skeletal identity is lost and replaced by mandibular skeletal patterning. On the other hand, if Hoxa2 is overexpressed in rhombomeres 1 and 2, mandibular skeletal patterning is lost in the mandibular arch and replaced by hyoid skeletal patterning.[29–32]

Endoderm, ectoderm, and mesoderm

The order of embryonic germ layers – endoderm, ectoderm, and mesoderm – reflects their relative importance in patterning pharyngeal arch development. In the pharyngeal pouches, the endoderm bulges out and contacts the ectoderm. At these points, ectoderm and endoderm remain in close contact and expand along the proximal-distal axis, separating the pharyngeal arches. A number of genes are expressed in the endoderm: Bmp7 at the posterior endodermal margin of the pharyngeal pouches; Fgf8 in the anterior endoderm of the pharyngeal pouches; Pax1 in the proximal endoderm of the pharyngeal pouches; and Shh in the early posterior endoderm of the second pharyngeal pouch and, later, in the posterior endoderm of the third pharyngeal pouch.[14, 33]

Jaw patterning signals come from the anterior endoderm, which underlies the neural tube and adjacent paraxial mesoderm between the anterior tip of the embryo and rhombomere 2. If the endoderm under the anterior midbrain is removed, Meckel's cartilage is lost in the lower jaw. Endoderm is not only required

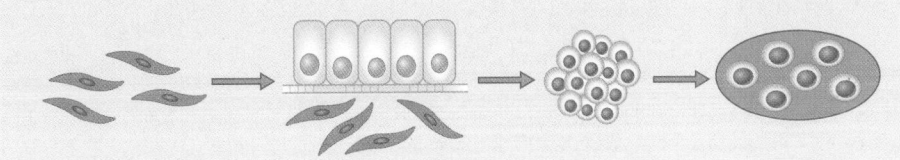

FIGURE 20.6 Epithelial–mesenchymal interaction resulting in condensation and differentiation. (Modified from Hall and Miyake 1995.[37])

for skeletal differentiation but also for skeletal orientation relative to the body axis.[22, 34] Endoderm also induces epibranchial placodes. Furthermore, endoderm is regionalized, forming the thyroid, parathyroids, and thymus.[14]

A zone of frontonasal ectoderm regulates patterning and growth of the face. A molecular boundary has been identified by Fgf8- and Shh-juxtaposed domains, which presage the initial site of frontonasal outgrowth.[35] Vascular endothelial cores and skeletal muscles in the pharyngeal arches are of mesodermal origin.

Intrinsic neural crest patterning

Thus far, the roles of various factors in directing patterning of cranial neural crest in the pharyngeal arches have been emphasized. However, intrinsic neural crest patterning also occurs, and is species specific. For example, in birds, when neural crest cells that participate in beak morphogenesis are exchanged between two species, crest itself determines beak form; quail neural crest cells produce quail beaks in duck hosts and duck neural crest cells produce duck bills in quail hosts. Therefore, cranial neural crest cells are capable of generating interspecific variation.[17]

Craniofacial skeletal development

Skeletogenesis and chondrogenesis result from a sequence of events involving epithelial–mesenchymal interaction, condensation, and differentiation (Fig. 20.6, Table 20.3). The connection between epithelial–mesenchymal interaction is a close one in the skeletogenesis of the craniofacial region, whereas it is less close in the developing skeleton of the limbs.[36–38]

Condensations are aggregations of cells that result from epithelial–mesenchymal interactions and lead to chondrogenesis and osteogenesis. In chondrogenesis, condensation triggers prechondrogenic differentiation. In contrast, with osteogenesis, epithelial–mesenchymal interaction initiates preosteoblastic differentiation before condensation. Preosteoblasts then condense, become osteoblasts, and deposit bone matrix.[36–38]

Calvarial and sutural initiation

The neurocranium is divided into a calvarial component of flat bones which have intramembranous bone formation, and a cranial base component, which arises from endochondral bone formation. The sides and roof of the skull arise as membranous ossification characterized by needle-like bone spicules that radiate peripherally. At the margins of the frontal, parietal, and occipital bones, presumptive sutures and fontanels appear. Facial sutures, the metopic suture, and the sagittal suture are of neural crest origin.[5] The coronal and lambdoid sutures are of mesodermal origin[39, 40] (Table 20.1).

Sutures develop initially by a wedge-shaped proliferation of cells at the periphery of the extending bone fields – the osteogenic front. Osteogenic fronts appear to govern morphogenetic determination of sutural architecture. They approximate each other in one of two ways. They may overlap each other, forming a beveled suture, or they may approximate each other in the same plane with an intervening zone of immature fibrous connective tissue, which leads to an end-to-end type of suture[41, 42] (Fig. 20.7A–D).

End-to-end sutures, such as the sagittal and metopic, are formed in the midline.[43, 44] Midline initiation may be of the end-to-end type because the biomechanical forces on either side of the initiating suture are likely to be equal in magnitude. In contrast, sutures away from the midline, such as the coronal and frontozygomatic, have biomechanical forces of unequal magnitude acting on them and hence are of the overlapping, beveled type.[39, 40]

Development of cranial and facial sutures

At birth, areas where cranial sutures will develop permit adjustive overlap of the calvarial bones as the human head becomes compressed during passage through the birth canal. The resultant molding normalizes during the first week of life by cranial re-expansion and widening of the sutural areas. Engineering structural analysis has shown that the fetal parietal bones are capable of deforming under load distributions typical of those found during normal labor.[45] Thus, molding is a combination of displacement of the cranial bones as well as their intrinsic deformation.

As cranial sutures develop further during infancy, cranial adjustment to the expanding brain takes place by bone deposition at the sutural margins while the sutures proper remain patent. Changes in the regional curvature of the calvarial bones also occur[39, 40] (Fig. 20.7F–G).

Cranial and facial sutures develop differently.[46] Facial bones have fibrous periosteal capsules surrounding them that are fully established by week 17 in utero. In contrast, cranial bones

TABLE 20.3 MAJOR CLASSES OF GENES AND GENE PRODUCTS ASSOCIATED WITH SKELETOGENIC CONDENSATIONS, THEIR FUNCTIONS, AND THEIR STAGES OF ACTION

Gene/gene product	Function	Stage
Growth factors		
BMPs	Regulate *Hox* genes (*Hoxa2, Hoxd11, Pax2*) in response to *Shh*	Growth
	Regulates Msx1, Msx2	Transition to differentiation
FGF2	Regulates N-CAM	Initiation, proliferation, growth
TGFβ	Regulates fibronectin	Initiation
Cell surface, cell adhesion, and extracellular matrix molecules		
Fibronectin	Extracellular glycoprotein regulated by TGFβ regulates N-CAM	Initiation, proliferation
N-cadherin	Cell adhesion molecule	Adhesion
N-CAM	Cell adhesion molecule regulated by FN, *Prx1, Prx2*, and FGF	Initiation, adhesion
Noggin	Secreted protein that binds to and inactivates *BMP2, BMP4, BMP7*	Slows or stops growth
Syndecan	Receptor that binds to tenascin; binds to fibronectin to inactivate N-CAM	Sets boundary
Tenascin	Extracellular glycoprotein that binds to syndecan	Stops condensation growth, sets boundary
Hox genes		
Hoxa2	Regulated by BMPs, downregulates *Runx2*	Sets boundary, growth, prevents differentiation
Hoxa13	Alters adhesive properties	Adhesion
Hoxd11	Regulated by BMP	Proliferation, growth
Hoxd11-13	Transcriptional activation	Transition to differentiation
Transcription factors		
Runx2	Transcriptional activating protein inhibited by *Hoxa2* (a) and regulated by BMP7 and vitamin D_3 (b)	Differentiation of chondroblasts (a) and switches cells into osteoblastic pathway (b)
CFKH1	Chicken forkhead-helix transcription factor that regulates TGFβ and interacts with *Smad* transcription factors	Initiation, proliferation
MFH1	Mesenchymal transcription factor	Proliferation
Pax1, Pax9	Encode nuclear transcription factors, regulated by *BMP7*	Growth
Prx1, Prx2	Upstream regulation of N-CAM	Initiation
Scleraxis	Basic helix-loop-helix protein	Proliferation
Sox9	Regulates *Col2α1*	Proliferation

After Hall and Miyake 2000.[38]

develop in a preformed continuous fibrous membrane, the ectomeninx, and do not develop fibrous capsules until after birth. Thus, the more mature fibrous periosteal layers of the fetal facial sutures may be a more effective barrier against osseous fusion than the as yet immature, unlayered, cranial sutures.[47]

Cranial and facial sutures differ in other respects. Except for the midpalatal suture, facial sutures do not fuse before the seventh to eighth decades.[43, 48] In contrast, cranial sutures close relatively early in adult life. Forces are transmitted from the mandible via the facial bones to the cranial vault. Thus, it would be advantageous for facial sutures to remain patent for life. For all practical purposes, they do.[39, 40]

Molecular correlates of craniofacial embryology

Many genes are expressed in craniofacial development including, among others, *Fgf8, Fgfr2, Shh, Ptch, Gli1, Gli2, Gli3, Bmp2, Bmp4, Bmp7, Msx1, Msx2, Twist, Dlx1, Dlx2, Dlx3, Dlx5*, and *Dlx6*.[4] These and other genes together with their expression patterns are summarized in Table 20.4.

Types of anomalies

Malformations, deformations, and disruptions

Most anomalies observed at birth can be sorted into one of three basic categories – malformations, deformations, or disruptions (Figs 20.8–20.10). There are practical reasons for distinguishing these because the clinical implications of each category are different.[49]

A malformation may be defined as a morphologic defect of an organ, part of an organ, or a larger area of the body resulting from an intrinsically abnormal developmental process. Anencephaly and cleft lip-palate serve as examples. Malformations may be relatively simple or complex. The later the defect is

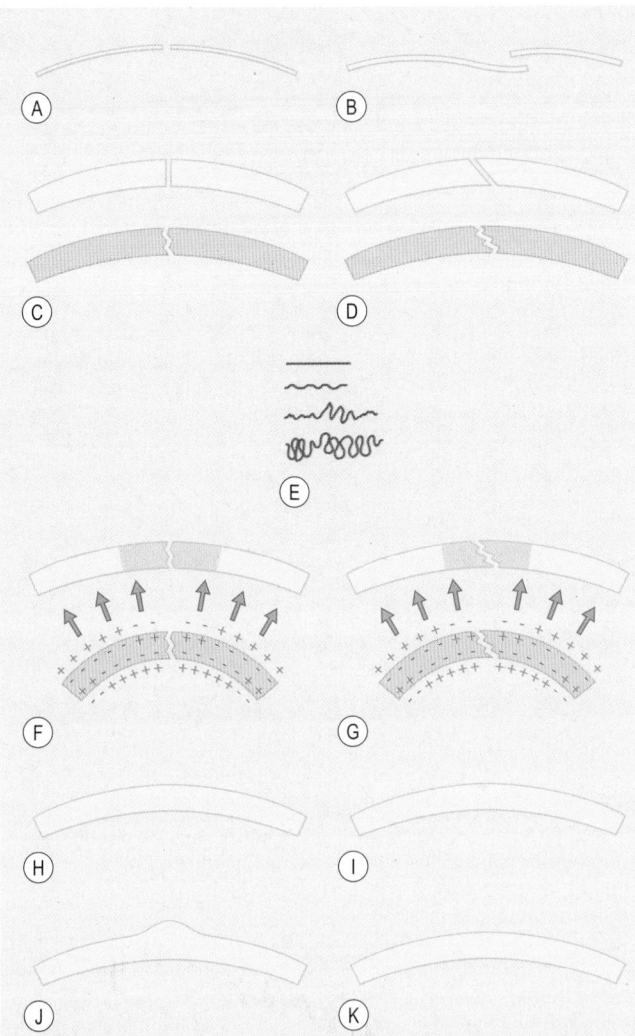

FIGURE 20.7 Diagram of sutural changes. Left: column (A, C, F, H, J) represents midline sutures (sagittal, metopic). Right: column (B, D, G, I, K) represents non-midline sutures (e.g. coronal). (A) End-to-end sutural initiation. (B) Overlapping sutural initiation. (C) Development of interdigitations in midline suture. (D) Development of interdigitations in overlapping suture. (E) Development of interdigitations from straight to slightly interdigitated to interdigitated to very interdigitated. (F) Changes in shape of calvarial bones with brain expansion. Also note bone deposition (diagonal lines) at sutural margins. (G) Changes in shape of calvarial bones with brain expansion. Also note bone deposition (diagonal lines) at non-midline sutural margins. (H) Normal closure of midline suture. (I) Normal closure of non-midline suture. (J) Craniosynostosis of midline suture (sagittal, metopic) showing ridging. (K) Craniosynostosis of non-midline suture without significant ridging (e.g. coronal suture). (Modified from Cohen 1993.[39])

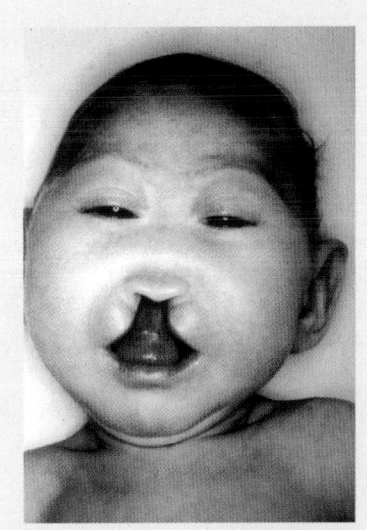

FIGURE 20.8
Malformation. Median cleft lip. Note failure of proper formation of the nose, hypertelorism, and microcephaly. Associated with alobar holoprosencephaly. (Courtesy of A. Richieri-Costa, Bauru, Brazil.)

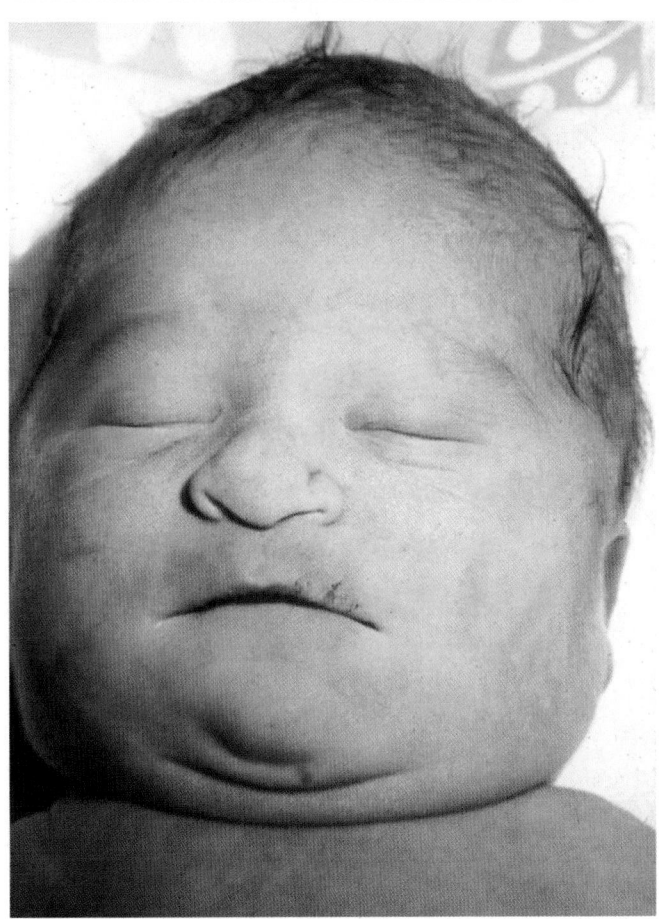

FIGURE 20.9 Deformation. Potter-type face resulting from oligohydramnios. (From Cohen 1997.[49])

initiated, the simpler the malformation. Malformations initiated earlier during organogenesis tend to have more far-reaching consequences.[49]

A deformation may be defined as an abnormal form or position of a part of the body caused by non-disruptive mechanical forces. Examples of deformities include some forms of torticollis, deformational plagiocephaly, and some forms of mandibular asymmetry. Deformations arise most frequently during late fetal life. Since the most common cause is intrauterine molding by mechanical forces, the musculoskeletal system is usually affected. The most important factor contributing to deformations is lack of fetal movement, whatever the cause.

TABLE 20.4 GENES EXPRESSED IN CRANIOFACIAL DEVELOPMENT

Genes	Expression
Homeobox	
Hoxa2	Identifies rhombomere 4 neural crest migrating to hyoid arch
Hoxb2	Expressed up to rhombomere 2-3 boundary
Gastrulation brain homeobox	
Gbx2	Midbrain-hindbrain boundary (isthmus)
Orthodentical-related homeobox	
Otx1	Hindbrain
Otx2	Forebrain, midbrain, isthmic organizer at the midbrain–hindbrain boundary
Muscle-segment homeobox	
Msx1	Osteogenic fronts of calvarial sutures; mesenchyme of maxillary and mandibular prominences
Msx2	Osteogenic fronts of calvarial sutures; mesenchyme of maxillary and mandibular prominences
Paired (aristaless)-like homeobox	
Alx3	Mesenchymal condensations of mandibular and hyoid arches
Alx4	Mesenchymal condensations of skull, hair, and teeth
Paired-box	
Pax1	Pharyngeal pouches; thymus; parathyroids; eustachian tubes; tonsils; ultimobranchial body
Pax2	Midbrain-hindbrain junction; optic stalk
Pax3	Dorsal neural tube; neural crest; thymus; parathyroids; tongue muscles
Pax6	Ocular development
Pax7	Neural crest; skeletal muscles; lateral nasal prominence
Pax8	Thyroid development
Pax9	Neural crest; pharyngeal pouches; thymus; parathyroids; eustachian tubes; tonsils; ultimobranchial body; tooth development
Sonic hedgehog	
Shh	Notochord; floorplate; ventromedial midbrain; ventral forebrain; epithelium of frontal prominence; maxillary prominence; oral epithelium of mandibular prominence; hyoid arch endoderm
Patched	
Ptch1	Epithelial cells adjacent to Shh-expressing cells; mesenchymal cells surrounding epidermal prominence
Ptch2	Co-expressed in epithelium with Shh
Semaphorins	
Sema3A	Inhibits neural crest migration from rhombomeres 3 and 5
Neuregulin receptors	
ErbB4	Neuroectoderm; essential for neural crest cell migration
Gli family	
Gli1	Ventral neural tube; pharyngeal arch mesenchyme
Gli2	Posterior neural tube; pharyngeal arch mesenchyme
Gli3	Posterior neural tube; pharyngeal arch mesenchyme
Wnt family	
Wnt	Neural crest induction
Wnt5a	Maxillary and mandibular prominences
Wnt11	Maxillary prominence
Fibroblast growth factors	
Fgf2	Osteogenic fronts of calvarial sutures
Fgf4	Osteogenic fronts of calvarial sutures; anterior half of mandibular and hyoid arches
Fgf8	Midbrain-hindbrain boundary (isthmus); suppresses Hox expression in delaminating crest from rhombomere 1; ectoderm of maxillary and mandibular prominences
Fgf10	Maxillary mesenchyme; rostral mandibular mesenchyme; and hyoid arch core mesenchyme
Fibroblast growth factor receptors	
Fgfr1	Osteogenic fronts of calvarial sutures; all facial prominences
Fgfr2	Osteogenic fronts of calvarial sutures; ectoderm of maxillary and mandibular prominences
Fgfr3	Osteogenic fronts of calvarial sutures; brain; frontal prominence; maxillary prominence; lateral nasal prominence
Basic helix-loop-helix	
Twist	Head mesenchyme, including osteogenic fronts of calvarial sutures and all facial prominences; branchial arches

TABLE 20.4 GENES EXPRESSED IN CRANIOFACIAL DEVELOPMENT (CONT'D)

Genes	Expression
Runx family	
Runx2	Osteogenesis involving membrane and endochondral bone
Collagens	
COL1A1	Bone of craniofacial skeleton
COL2A1	Cartilage of cranial base and nasal capsule
Alkaline phosphatase	
ALPL	Calcification of craniofacial skeleton
Osteocalcin	
BGLAP	Craniofacial skeleton
Nel-like	
Nell1	Cranial intramembranous bones
Efrins	
Efnb1	Frontonasal neural crest
Bone morphogenetic proteins	
Bmp2	Osteogenic fronts of calvarial sutures; mesenchyme of lateral region of mandibular arch; tooth formation
Bmp4	Selective apoptosis of neural crest cells from rhombomeres 3 and 5; osteogenic fronts of calvarial sutures; epithelium of medial ends of maxillary and mandibular prominences; tooth formation
Bmp7	Entire epithelium covering maxillary and mandibular prominences; tooth formation
Bmp antagonist	
Nog	Neural tube; calvarial sutures; cartilage condensations; frontonasal epithelium
Transforming growth factor β	
Tgfb1	Calvarial sutures
Tgfb2	Calvarial sutures; mesenchyme of secondary palate
Tgfb3	Calvarial sutures; medial edge epithelium of palatal shelves
Retinoids	
RALDH2	Frontonasal area
RALDH3	Nasal placode
Goosecoid	
Gsc	Posterior portion of mandibular arch; anterior portion of hyoid arch
Forkhead	
FOXE1	Oronasal membrane, palate, hair shaft, thyroid, epiglottis
Endothelin	
ET1	Epithelium of facial prominences; mesodermal bone of mandibular arch
EDNRA	Hindbrain normal crest; mesenchyme of facial prominences
ECE1	Mesenchyme of facial prominences
Distal-less related	
Dlx1	Mesenchyme of proximal and distal regions of mandibular and hyoid arches
Dlx2	Mandibular arch; distal region of hyoid arch
Dlx3	Distal tips of first and second arch mesenchyme
Dlx5	Distal mesenchyme of first and second arches
Dlx6	Distal mesenchyme of first and second arches

From Cohen 2005.[4]

Deformations may result from mechanical, malformational, or functional causes.[49]

First pregnancies tend to be associated with unstretched uterine and abdominal muscles, which may result in uteroplacental insufficiency and, in turn, may lead to oligohydramnios. Breech presentation is common since the uterus is too compressed to allow the fetus to rotate into the cephalic position. Uterine constraints on fetal movement allow mild but persistent extrinsic forces to deform the fetus.[49]

During the first few days after birth, infants with deformities can usually be folded into their atypical prenatal postures. Radiographically, the close correspondence between the abnormal posture of the fetus before delivery and the posture of the infant after birth has been observed repeatedly. Such posture

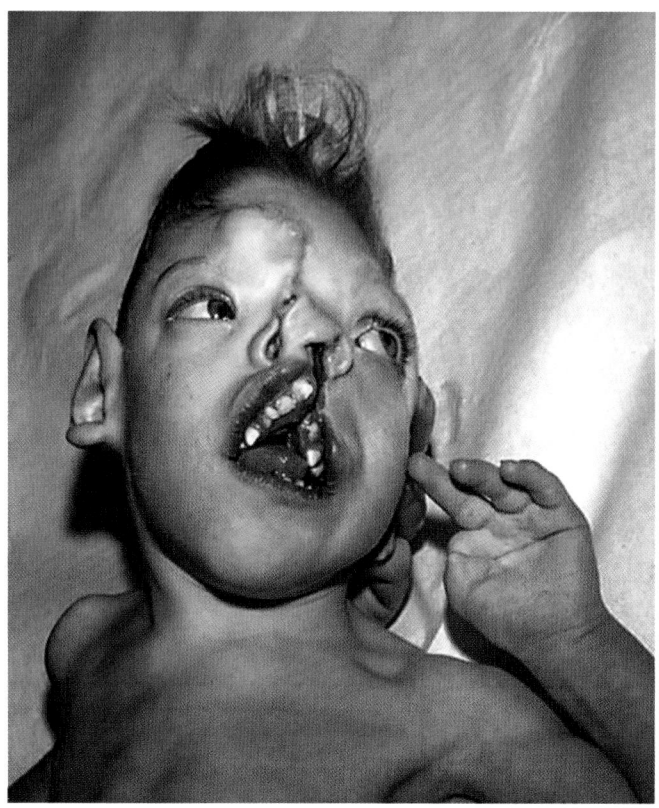

FIGURE 20.10 Disruption from amniotic bands, affecting the face, hands, and cranium. (From Cohen 1997.[49])

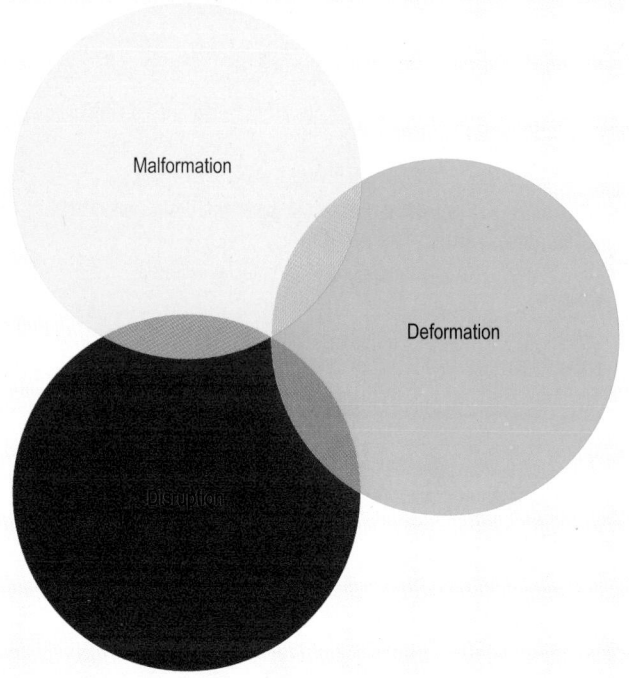

FIGURE 20.11 Venn diagram showing interrelationships between malformations, deformations, and disruptions. (Modified from Cohen 1997.[49])

has been termed the position of comfort. For example, a mandibular deformation may result from sharply lateroflexed position of the head with the shoulder pressed against the mandible for a long period of time late during intrauterine life.[49]

A disruption is a morphologic defect of an organ, part of an organ, or a larger region of the body resulting from a breakdown of, or interference with, an originally normal developmental process. In some cases, amnionic bands can produce dramatic consequences, such as asymmetric encephaloceles, bizarre facial clefting, and limb amputations.[49]

Interrelationships

It should be recognized that although the distinctions between the three types of anomalies – malformations, deformations, and disruptions – are useful for clinical purposes, particularly in the newborn period (Fig. 20.11, Table 20.5), the three classes of anomalies are interrelated in some instances during growth after birth. For example, cleft lip-palate, a malformation, develops secondary facial deformation during postnatal growth.[49]

Malformations can also result in deformations appearing at birth, such as bilateral renal agenesis, producing oligohydramnios and the facial and limb deformities of Potter sequence. Some anomalies, such as Robin sequence, may be malformational or deformational, depending on the initiating factor – intrinsic mandibular hypoplasia (malformational) or extrinsic mandibular constraint (deformational).[49]

TABLE 20.5 GENERAL COMPARISON OF MALFORMATIONS, DEFORMATIONS, AND DISRUPTIONS

Features	Malformations	Deformations	Disruptions
Time of occurrence	Embryonic	Fetal	Embryonic/fetal
Level of disturbance	Organ	Region	Area
Perinatal mortality	+	–	+
Clinical variability of any given anomaly	Moderate	Mild	Extreme
Multiple causes of any given anomaly	Very frequent	Less common	Less common
Spontaneous correction	–	+	–
Correction by posture	–	+	–
Correction by surgery	+	±	+
Relative recurrence rate	Higher	Lower	Extremely low
Approximately frequency in newborns	2–3%	1–2%	1–2%

From Cohen 1997.[49]

Orofacial clefting

Various types of cleft lip and cleft palate are shown in Figures 20.12–20.14.

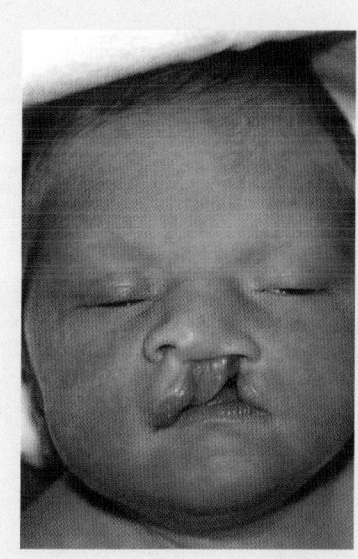

FIGURE 20.12 Unilateral cleft lip and palate. (From Cohen 2005.[4])

Embryonic basis of orofacial clefting

Exact timing and positioning of facial prominences during embryonic development are critical. Any alteration may result in a cleft lip. Genetic or environmental factors (or both) that inhibit the flow of neural crest cells or decrease their numbers may affect their masses so that contact between the facial prominences is inadequate or impossible. The epithelium that covers the mesenchyme may not undergo programmed cell death, so that fusion cannot take place. Any change in the position of the nasal placodes or abnormal directional growth of the facial prominences may result in cleft lip.[6, 7]

Clefts of the lip and palate occur together in approximately 45% of cases. It has been suggested that the tip of the tongue becomes wedged in the labial cleft, thus not allowing the tongue to drop, which would inhibit palatal contact and fusion. This explanation is probably simplistic. It seems more likely that a reduction in the size of the labial maxillary prominences and the palatine process of the maxillary prominences is a more reasonable explanation.[6, 7] Cleft palate may result from defective growth of the palatal shelves, failure of elevation of the shelves, failure of fusion of the shelves, or post-fusion rupture of the shelves. In some instances, micrognathia is a contributing factor that may inhibit elevation of the palatine shelves, as for example, in Robin sequence.[7]

Causes of cleft lip and cleft palate

Cleft lip with or without cleft palate is etiologically distinct from isolated cleft palate. In a patient with cleft lip with or without cleft palate, if another family member is affected, he or she will have either isolated cleft lip or cleft lip together with cleft palate but not isolated cleft palate alone. Similarly, if a patient has isolated cleft palate, another affected family member can have only isolated cleft palate. There are two exceptions. First, in genetic isolates that are inbred, both types may occur by chance. Second, in many genetic syndromes with orofacial clefting, both types may be found. For example, in the autosomal dominantly inherited van der Woude syndrome, in which orofacial clefting is found together with lip pits, patients may have cleft lip, cleft lip-palate, or isolated cleft palate.[50, 51]

Much evidence supports the view that genetic factors are associated with orofacial clefting. In twins with cleft-lip palate, concordance is far greater in monozygotic twins (40%) than in dizygotic twins (4.2%). In twins with isolated cleft palate, concordance is also higher in monozygotic twins (35%) than in dizygotic twins (7.8%).[52]

Many clefts occur sporadically. In some families, however, more than one individual is affected. In a few large families, Mendelian inheritance has been established.[6, 7] Thus, orofacial clefting is heterogeneous and variation in liability is probably determined by a number of major genes, minor genes, environmental factors, and a developmental threshold.[53] Two alternative hypotheses for orofacial clefting have been advanced. One is the multifactorial threshold model. The other involves a

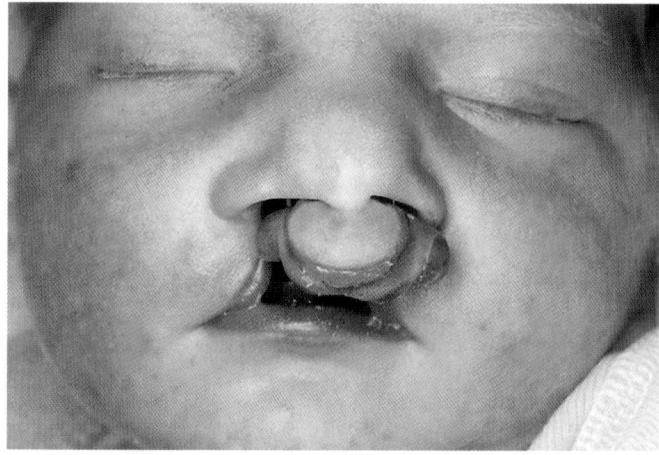

FIGURE 20.13 Bilateral cleft lip. (From Cohen 2005.[4])

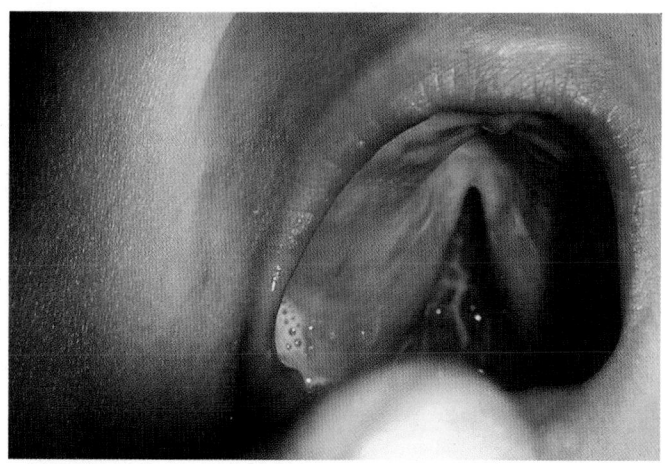

FIGURE 20.14 V-shaped cleft palate. (From Cohen 2005.[4])

TABLE 20.6 CANDIDATE GENES FOR ISOLATED CLEFT LIP AND/OR PALATE*

MSX1	Muscle segment homeobox 1	4p16.1
MSX2	Muscle segment homeobox 2	5q34–q35
IRF6	Interferon regulatory factor 6	1q32–q41
FGFR1	Fibroblast growth factor receptor 1	8p12
PTCH	Patched	9q22.3
PVRL1	Poliovirus receptor-like 1	1q25–q31
PVRL2	Poliovirus receptor-like 2	19q13.2–q13.4
PRDM16	PR domain-containing protein 16	1p36.3
JAG2	Jagged 2	14q32
TBX10	T-box 10	11q13.1–q13.2
TBX22	T-box 22	Xq12–q21
TGFB3	Transforming growth factor β 3	14q24
LHX8	Lim homeobox gene 8	4q25–q31
SATB2	Special AT-rich sequence-binding protein 2	2q33
SKI1	Skinny hedgehog 1	1q32

In the aggregate, these mutations explain about 5% of isolated cases with an additional 10–15% of cases explained by variations surrounding the IRF6 gene.[71] Some of these gene mutations can result in other disorders. For example, mutations in PTCH usually cause nevoid basal cell carcinoma syndrome, isolated basal cell carcinoma, and rarely holoprosencephaly.
Modified from Murray 2004.[71]

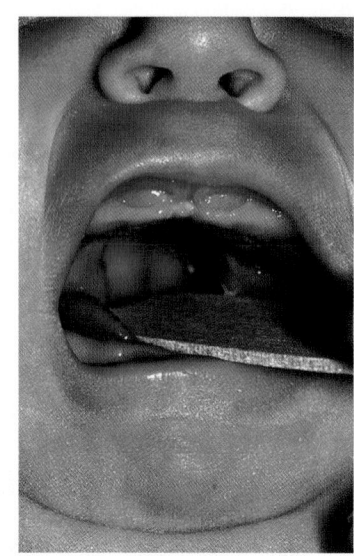

FIGURE 20.15 Robin sequence. U-shaped cleft palate. (From Cohen 1997.[49])

single major gene with reduced penetrance. Both theories have their proponents.[7]

Many candidate genes for orofacial clefting have been suggested by allelic association and by linkage analysis.[52, 54–63] Some syndromes in which specific gene mutations have been identified include, among others, van der Woude syndrome (IRF6),[64] popliteal pterygium syndrome (IRF6),[64] EEC syndrome (TP63),[65, 66] Hay-Wells syndrome (TP63),[67] autosomal recessive cleft palate/ectodermal dysplasia (PVRL1),[68] hypodontia/clefting (MSX1),[69] and cleft palate/ankyloglossia (TBX22).[70] Candidate genes for isolated cleft lip and/or palate are summarized in Table 20.6. In the aggregate, these mutations explain about 5% of isolated cases with an additional 10–15% of cases explained by variations surrounding the IRF6 gene.[71]

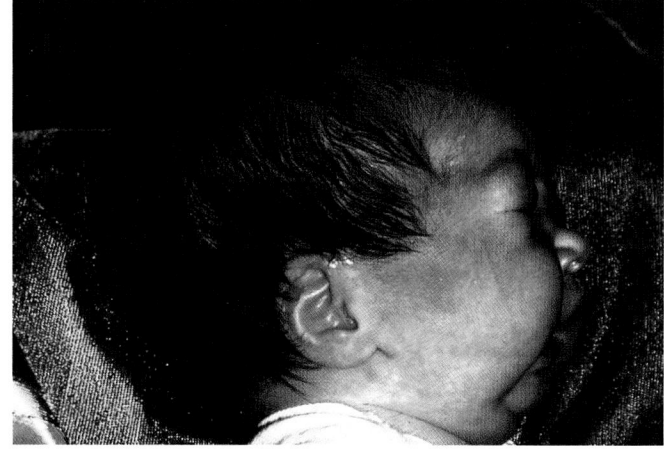

FIGURE 20.16 Robin sequence. Micrognathia. Same infant as in Figure 20.15. (From Cohen 1997.[49])

Robin sequence and Robin complexes

Robin sequence is commonly defined as cleft palate, micrognathia, and glossoptosis (Figs 20.15–20.18). However, Robin sequence has been defined in different ways by using different criteria.[72, 73] In Table 20.7, various criteria for Robin sequence are summarized. Definitions I–IV are clearly Robin sequence, but definition V is non-Robin in type. The cleft palate is V-shaped and, by polysomnography, some respiratory compromise is evident. The mandible is normal or may be slightly small subjectively but impossible to be certain. Thus, at the interface, it is not always possible to distinguish between Robin sequence and ordinary cleft palate.[50, 74, 75]

TABLE 20.7 DEFINING ROBIN SEQUENCE USING DIFFERENT CRITERIA

Definition	Mandibular deficiency	Cleft palate	Upper airway obstruction
I	+	+(U)	+
II	+	+(U or V)	+
III	+	+(U)	–
IV	+	±(U or V)	±
V (non-Robin)	–*	+(V)	+

U, U-shaped cleft palate; V, V-shaped cleft palate.
*Mandible is normal, but may be slightly small subjectively and impossible to be certain
Modified from Cohen 1991,[74] and 2001.[75]

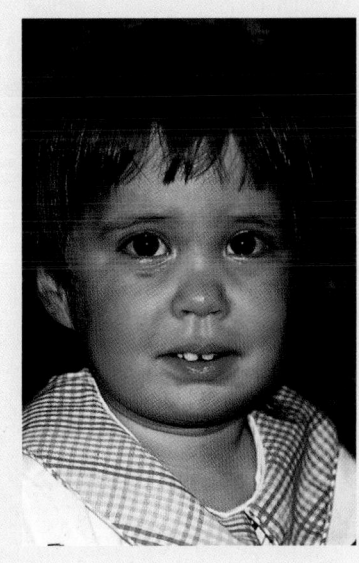

FIGURE 20.17 Robin sequence. Catch-up growth of mandible. Compare with Figure 20.16. (From Cohen 1997.[49])

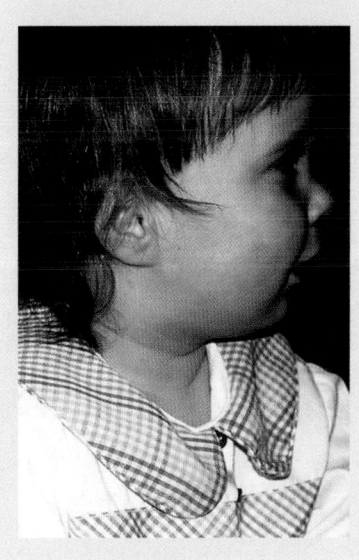

FIGURE 20.18 Robin sequence. Catch-up growth. Same child as in Figure 20.17. Compare with Figure 20.16. (From Cohen 1997.[49])

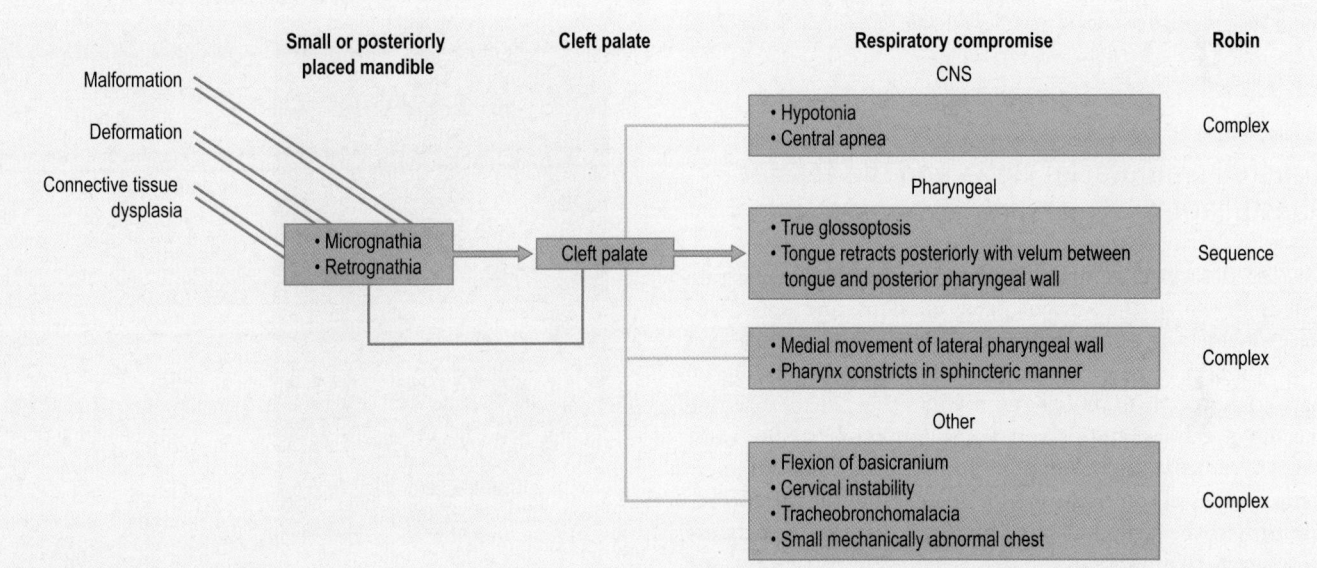

FIGURE 20.19 Robin sequence and complexes. Double lines indicate general causes: malformation, deformation, or connective tissue dysplasia. Thick arrows indicate Robin sequence. Thin lines show all possible ways that the Robin sequence can occur. (Modified from Cohen 1999.[74])

Because of etiologic, pathogenetic, and phenotypic differences, Robin sequence or Robin complexes of various types can occur.[74, 75] These changes are shown in Figure 20.19.

A distinction is made between micrognathia and retrognathia (Fig. 20.19). Micrognathia refers to size, retrognathia to position. In Treacher Collins syndrome, the mandible is short.[76, 77] In deletion 22q11 syndrome, the mandible is essentially normal in size but retrognathic in position because the cranial base angle is larger than normal.[78] Most Robin conditions are micrognathic or retrognathic, but not usually both together (microretrognathia).[49, 74, 75]

Different Robin complexes are exemplified by del(22q11) syndrome and spondyloepiphyseal dysplasia congenita. In del(22q11) syndrome, retrognathia, caused by an obtuse cranial base angle, and cleft palate, either submucous or true, are found. The flat cranial base angle and retrognathia do not contribute to pharyngeal obstruction, which results, in fact, from hypotonia.[78] Robin sequence does not occur. Rather, in this form of Robin complex, all of the manifestations are causally, but not sequentially, related.[74]

An example of multiple mechanisms of respiratory compromise can be found in spondyloepiphyseal dysplasia congenita: small mechanically abnormal chest, tracheobronchomalacia, and/or central apnea due to cervical or medullary compression caused by cervical instability.[79] Another possibility is upper respiratory obstruction based on Robin sequence.

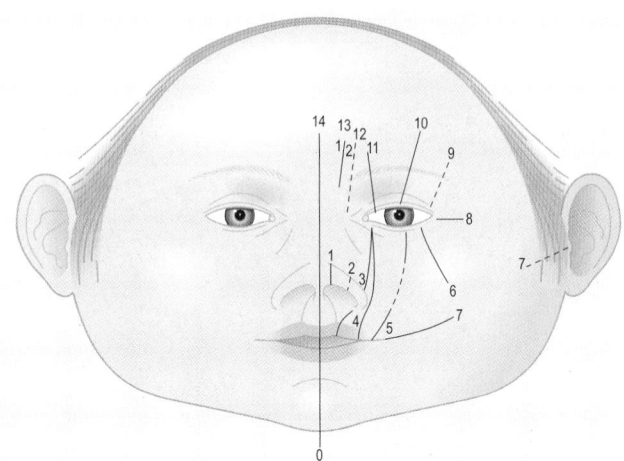

FIGURE 20.20 Tessier craniofacial clefting system. Soft tissue clefts. Dotted lines represent uncertain localization or uncertain clefting. Note that northbound cranial line has a different number than its counterpart southbound facial line. This system is descriptive and anatomic and avoids etiologic and/or pathogenetic speculating. For example, the cause of a No. 10 cleft may be different from the cause of a No. 4 cleft. (Modified from Tessier 1976.[80])

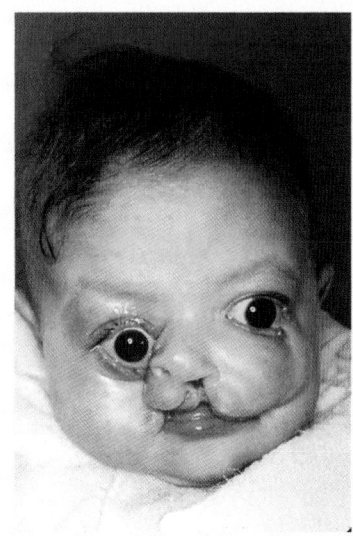

FIGURE 20.21 Multiple clefts. Cleft lip-palate with Tessier No. 6 cleft on left side and No. 4 cleft on right side. (Courtesy of A. Richieri-Costa, Bauru, Brazil.)

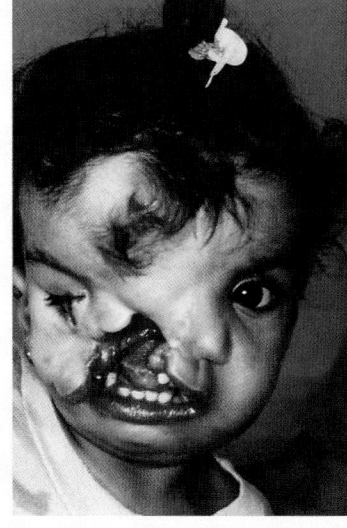

FIGURE 20.22 Complex clefting. Hairline indicator points to cleft area. CT scan showed anterior cranium bifidum occultum and gap in sphenoid bone. (Courtesy of A. Richieri-Costa, Bauru, Brazil.)

Unusual craniofacial clefts and the Tessier classification

Tessier[80] described an anatomic and descriptive classification system in which the various types of bony and soft-tissue defects, which he called clefts, are situated along definite axes with numbers assigned to the sites of clefting, depending on their relationships to the sagittal midline (Fig. 20.20). Clefting may involve bone and/or soft tissue but rarely to the same extent. From the sagittal midline to the infraorbital foramen, abnormalities of soft tissue predominate. From the infraorbital foramen to the temporal bone, however, osseous defects are more severe than those of soft tissue, a notable exception being the ear. Clefts through the orbit use the lower eyelid as an equator. Cleft numbered lines may be either northbound (cranial) or southbound (facial). Cranial numbered lines have facial numbered counterparts, yet these numbers are different to avoid the implication that they necessarily have the same etiopathogenesis. Thus, the Tessier classification permits description of both the location and the extent of unusual facial clefts. Several different types of Tessier clefts may occur in the same patient (Fig. 20.21).

In some instances, overlying soft tissue defects predict the possibility of underlying bony clefts. Elsewhere, I have referred to such features (e.g. colobomatous notching of the upper or lower eyelids or the nostrils or interruption of the eyelashes or the eyebrows) as Tessier signs.[49] Also included in this category are hairline indicators that may point to the cleft[81] (Fig. 20.22).

The causes of most Tessier clefts are unknown. The overwhelming majority occur sporadically. One exception is Treacher Collins syndrome, which is autosomal dominantly inherited. Some Tessier clefts are malformations that can be explained by faulty embryogenesis. Others represent disruptions, however, such as those associated with amniotic bands.[49]

Anencephaly

Anencephaly is characterized by an open neural tube in the cephalic region, with an exposed mass of degenerating neural tissue on the skull floor. The cranial vault is absent, producing characteristic bulging of the eyes and absence of the neck (Figs 20.23 and 20.24). Both the membranous neurocranium and the chondrocranium are grossly malformed.

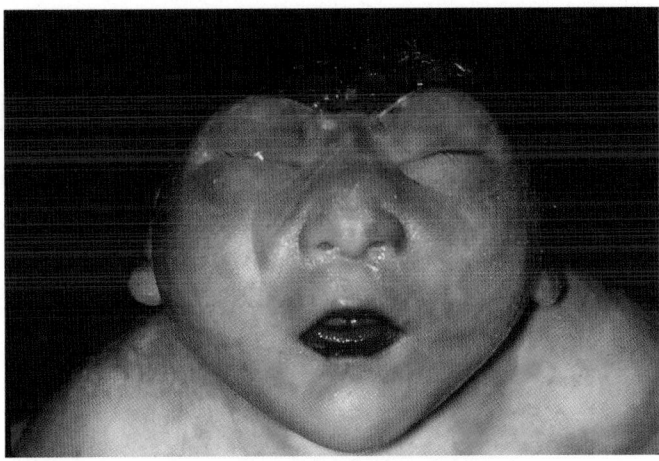

FIGURE 20.23 Anencephaly. Frontal view. (From Cohen 2002.[83])

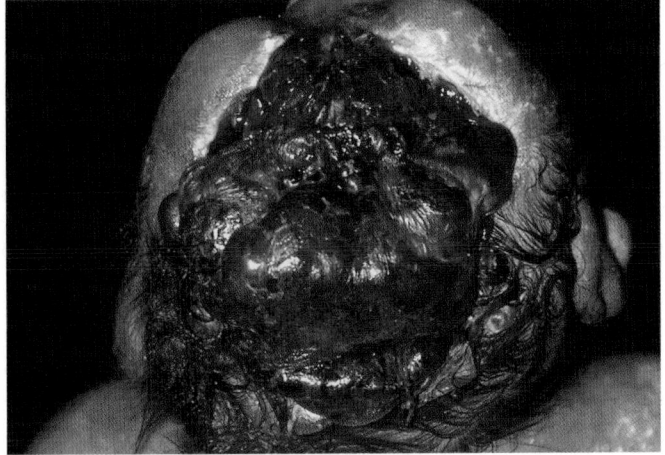

FIGURE 20.24 Anencephaly. Superior view. (From Cohen 2002.[83])

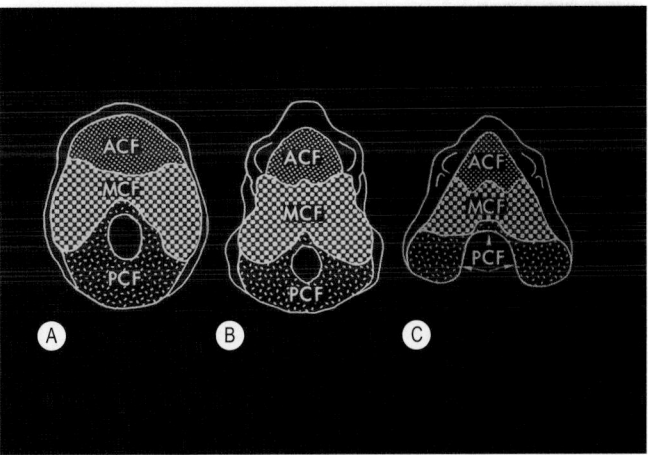

FIGURE 20.25 Anencephaly. Schematic drawing of the bones of the cranial base of a normal fetus (A), a fetus with meroacrania (B), and a fetus with holoacrania (C). Note the anteroposterior position of the lesser wings of the sphenoid and the reduced transverse dimension of the greater wings of the sphenoid (b and c) relative to normal (A). The more anterior position of the lateral end of the petrous portion of the temporal bone is also evident in anencephaly. In holoacrania, supraoccipital components are not united and are widely divergent (C). ACF, anterior cranial fossa; MCF, middle cranial fossa; PCF, posterior cranial fossa. (From Fields et al 1978.[84])

Anencephaly is classified anatomically as meroacrania if the defect does not involve the foramen magnum, holoacrania if the defect extends through the foramen magnum (Fig. 20.25), and holoacrania with rachischisis if spina bifida accompanies anencephaly.[82–84]

Cephaloceles

A cephalocele is a herniation of the brain or meninges through a defect in the skull. Although encephalocele is the term used most commonly for all such lesions, cranium bifidum and cephalocele more properly describe the spectrum of malformations that includes both encephaloceles and cranial meningoceles.[7, 85, 86]

Encephaloceles can be classified as occipital, parietal, or anterior. Further anterior subdivision includes visible ones (sincipital) and not directly visible ones (basal). About 75% of all encephaloceles occur in the occipital region.[87] Although encephaloceles are usually found in the midline (Fig. 20.26), those found in some cases of amniotic band disruption may be placed asymmetrically.

The pathogenesis is unclear. A focal cerebral 'blowout' has been proposed. Possibly a point of least resistance caused by early cerebrospinal fluid pressure might be involved. It has often been assumed that the underlying anomaly is cranium bifidum. Different developmental sites in the midline have been noted, including the occipital fissure, supraocciput, sagittal suture, and metopic suture. The high frequency of hydrocephalus in occipital encephaloceles has been attributed to a disturbance in cerebrospinal fluid dynamics caused by entrapped brain tissue.[86, 87]

Frontonasal dysplasia

Median bony clefting of the frontal or frontonasal region is common in severe instances of frontonasal 'dysplasia' (Fig. 20.27). If the nasal capsule fails to develop properly, the primitive brain vesicle fills the space normally occupied by the capsule, producing anterior cranium bifidum, a morphokinetic arrest in the position of the eyes, and lack of elevation of the nasal tip. Frank encephalocele in the midline can produce the same type of morphokinetic arrest found in frontonasal dysplasia. Less commonly, frontal teratoma, lipoma, hamartoma, intracranial cyst, or intrinsic cartilaginous defect affecting the nasal capsule can produce hypertelorism.[85, 88, 89]

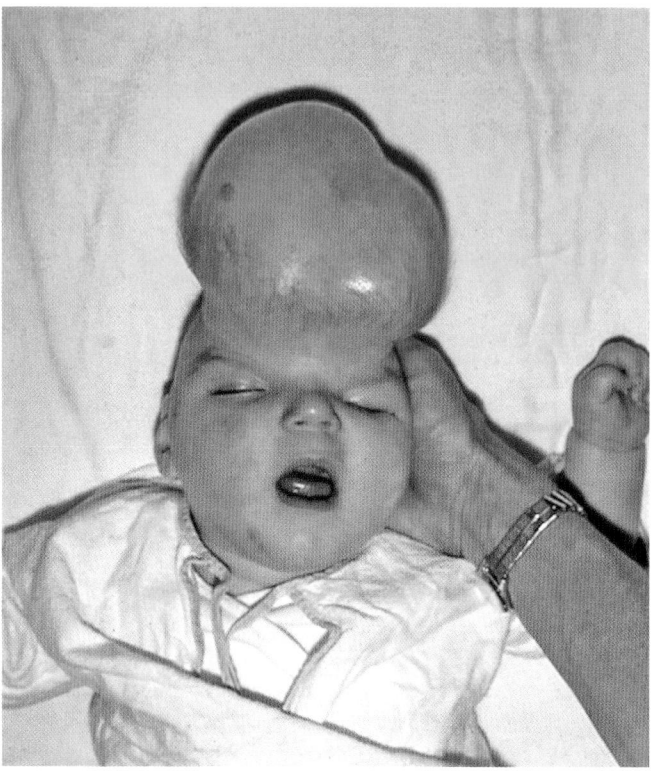

FIGURE 20.26 Interparietal encephalocele overlapping into the superior portion of the metopic suture. Note ocular hypertelorism. (From Cohen and Lemire 1982.[85])

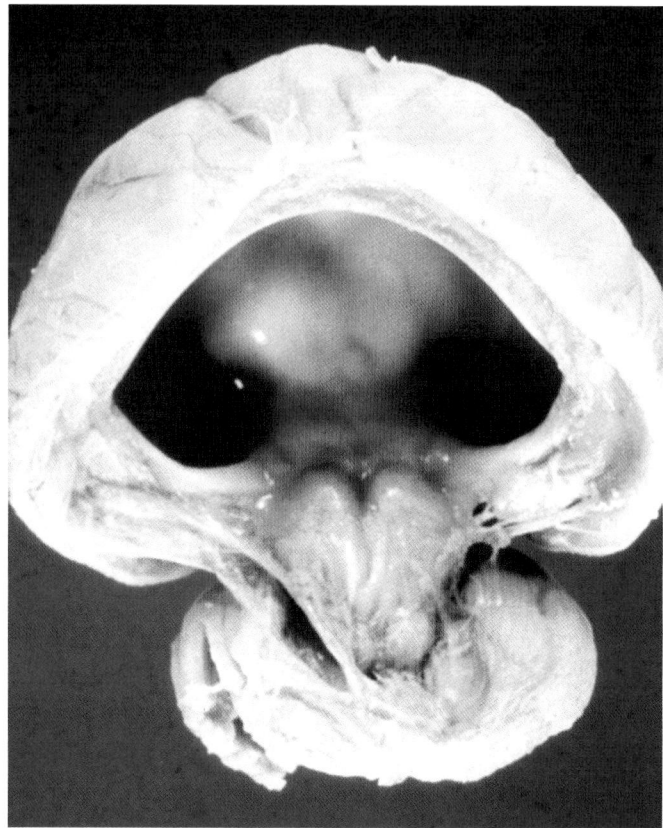

FIGURE 20.28 Alobar holoprosencephaly. (From Pettersen 1976.[90])

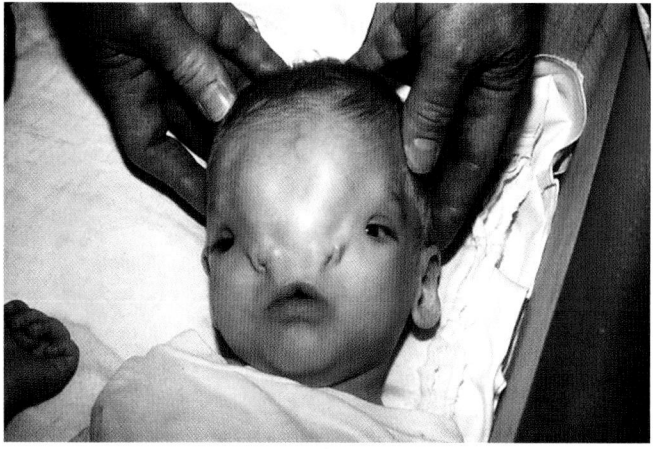

FIGURE 20.27 Frontonasal 'dysplasia'. (From Cohen et al 1971.[88])

Holoprosencephaly

Central nervous system

Holoprosencephaly is a developmental field defect of impaired midline cleavage of the embryonic forebrain. In alobar holoprosencephaly[90] (Fig. 20.28), the prosencephalon fails to cleave sagittally into cerebral hemispheres, transversely into telencephalon and diencephalon, and horizontally into olfactory tracts and bulbs.* Holoprosencephaly may be graded into alobar,

semilobar, and lobar types. Although the classic definition is unambiguous, problems are encountered at the less severe end of the phenotypic spectrum. The classic anatomic definition of holoprosencephaly and the variable definitions used in genetics are both valid and depend on the context in which they are used.[91]

Face

In a classic article, DeMyer et al[92] discussed a graded series of facial anomalies that occur with holoprosencephaly (Figs 20.29–20.32, see also Fig. 20.8). The face predicts the brain approximately 80% of the time. The other 20% of the time, the facial changes are not diagnostic.[93, 94] In cyclopia, the most extreme variant, a single median eye with varying degrees of doubling of the intrinsic ocular structures is associated with arrhinia and usually with proboscis formation. In ethmocephaly,

---

* Although 'cleave' is the commonly used term, no splitting actually occurs. In the sagittal plane, budding of the telencephalic vesicles takes place. In the transverse plane, 'cleavage' is an arbitrary designation given to regions. In the horizontal plane, budding of the olfactory tracts takes place.[91]

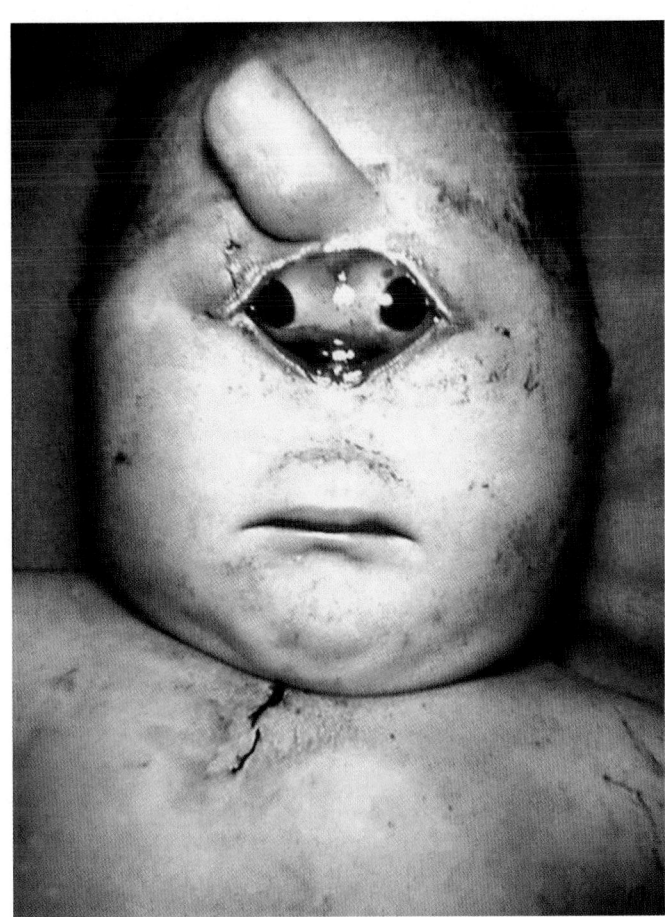

FIGURE 20.29 Cyclopia. (From Cohen et al 1971.[95])

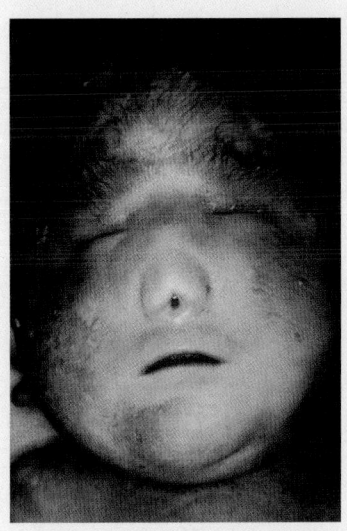

FIGURE 20.31
Cebocephaly. (From
Cohen et al 1971.[95])

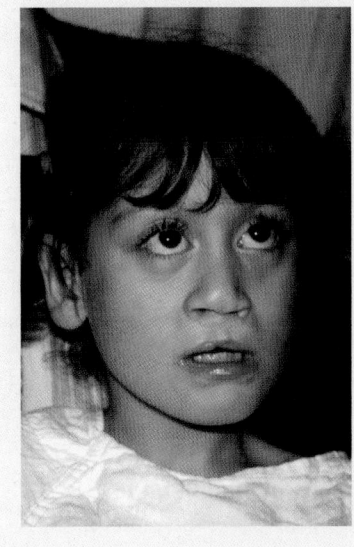

FIGURE 20.32 Ocular
hypotelorism and
repaired cleft lip in a girl
with lobar
holoprosencephaly. (From
Cohen et al 1971.[95])

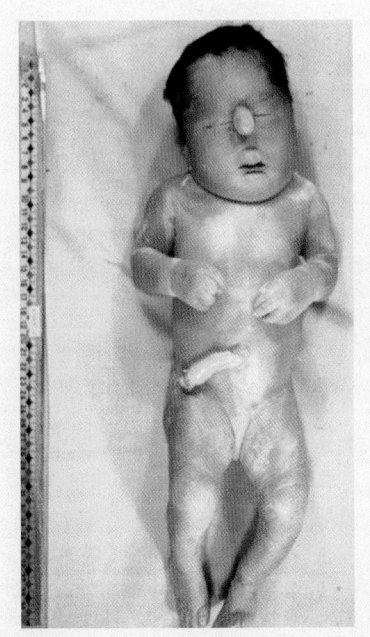

FIGURE 20.30
Ethmocephaly. (From
Cohen et al 1971.[95])

two separate hypoteloric eyes are associated with arhinia and proboscis formation. In cebocephaly, hypotelorism is associated with a blind-ended, single-nostril nose. With median cleft lip, hypotelorism is associated with a flat nose and a median cleft because of agenesis of the primary palate. Less severe facial anomalies may include hypotelorism or hypertelorism, lateral cleft lip, or iris coloboma or any combination of these features.[95, 96]

Numerous mild malformations have been found in holoprosencephaly.[96–102] Single maxillary central incisor [93, 96, 98] and, much less commonly, absence of the nasal septal cartilage[100] can be useful markers in autosomal dominant holoprosencephaly. Other identified defects have included stenosis of the nasal aperture,[97] absence of the labial frenum,[101] and absence of the philtral ridges.[102]

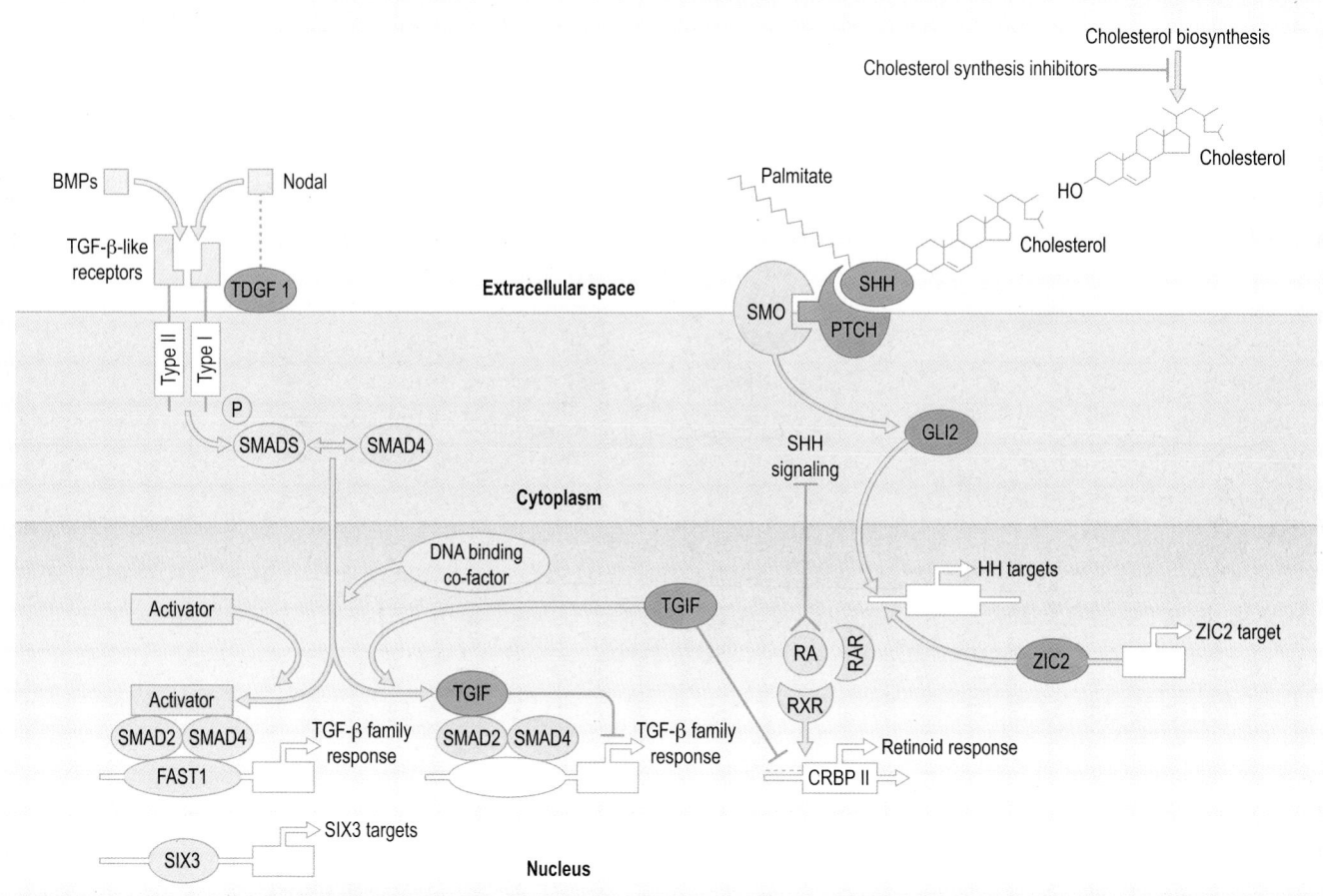

FIGURE 20.33 Mutations for holoprosencephaly in orange: *SHH, PTCH, GLI2, ZIC2, TGIF, TDGF1, FAST1*, and *SIX3*. Another mutation *DHCR7*, involving 7-dehydrocholesterol reductase deficiency, is one of the cholesterol synthesis inhibitors (upper right). Because various pathways are linked to the sonic hedgehog signaling network, the mutations are interrelated. *SHH, PTCH*, and *GLI2* are within the network itself. *ZIC2* and *GLI2* are related: GLI proteins are translocated to cell nuclei by coexpressed ZIC proteins. *TDGF1, TGIF*, and *FAST1* involve Nodal/TGF β signaling. *SIX3* has not been linked to any of these interrelated pathways to date. (From Muenke and Beachy 2001.[111] Modified and updated through the courtesy of M. Muenke, Bethesda.)

Causes of holoprosencephaly

Human holoprosencephaly is etiologically heterogeneous and pathogenetically variable. Identifiable genetic causes account for about 15–20% of all cases of holoprosencephaly.[103–105] Monogenic inheritance has been reported, including autosomal dominant inheritance with wide expressivity and incomplete penetrance,[106, 107] autosomal recessive inheritance,[95, 108] and X-linked inheritance.[109, 110]

Because various pathways are linked to the sonic hedgehog (SHH) signaling network, the mutations are interrelated[111] (Fig. 20.33). *SHH*,[112–115] *PTCH*,[116] and *GLI2*[117] are within the sonic hedgehog signaling network itself. *DHCR7*[118–121] involves 7-dehydrocholesterol reductase in cholesterol biosynthesis. *ZIC2*[122, 123] and *GLI2* are related; Gli proteins are translocated to cell nuclei by coexpressed Zic proteins.[124, 125] *TDGF1*,[126] *TGIF*,[127] and *FAST1*[128] involve *Nodal/TGFβ* signaling. *SIX3*[129]

has not been linked to any of these interrelated pathways to date.

Teratogenic causes of holoprosencephaly are also known. About 1–2% of newborn infants of mothers with diabetes have holoprosencephaly.[130] Holoprosencephaly may also be seen on occasion with fetal alcohol syndrome and retinoic acid embryopathy.[131]

Craniosynostosis

The term craniostenosis is used to indicate premature fusion of one or more sutures. Technically, craniosynostosis is the process of premature sutural fusion, craniostenosis the result. Actually, the terms have been used interchangeably, and craniosynostosis is replacing craniostenosis as the more common term.[132]

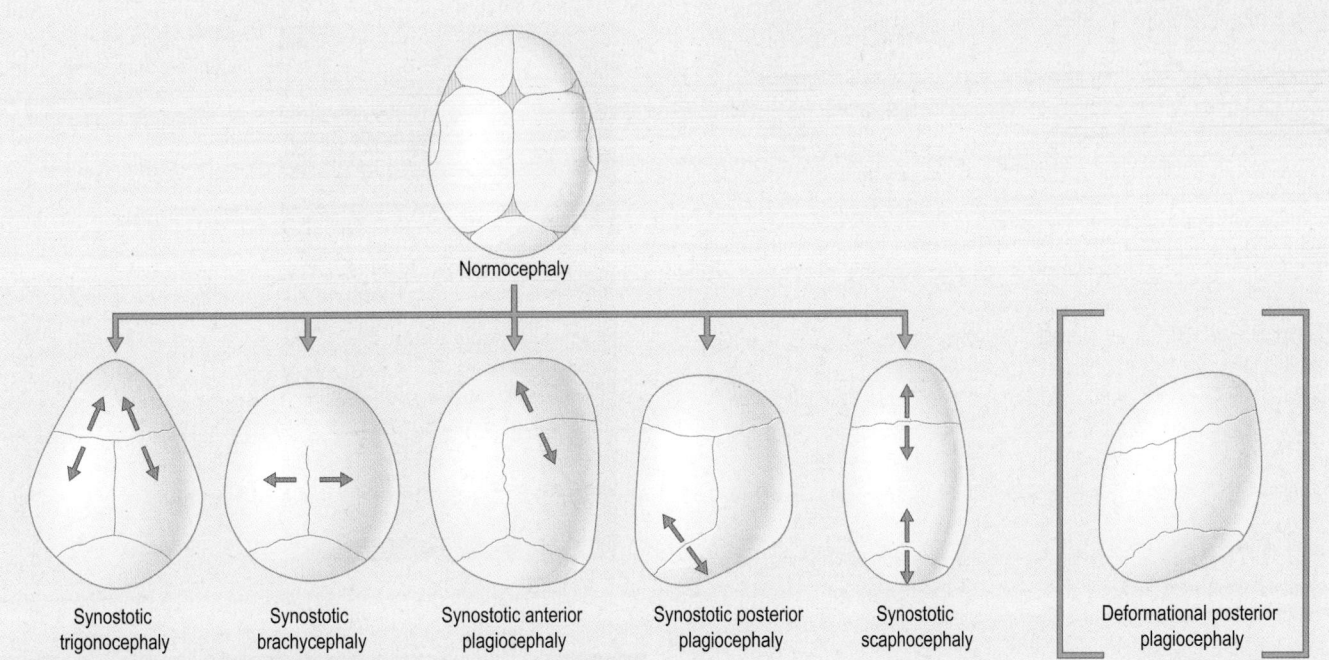

Normocephaly

Synostotic trigonocephaly · Synostotic brachycephaly · Synostotic anterior plagiocephaly · Synostotic posterior plagiocephaly · Synostotic scaphocephaly · Deformational posterior plagiocephaly

FIGURE 20.34 In synostotic scaphocephaly, the sagittal suture is prematurely synostosed. In synostotic brachycephaly and synostotic anterior plagiocephaly, the coronal suture is closed either bilaterally or unilaterally. In synostotic trigonocephaly, the metopic suture is prematurely closed. In the rarely occurring synostotic posterior plagiocephaly, the lambdoid suture is closed unilaterally. This condition is frequently confused with deformational posterior plagiocephaly (bracketed) in which all the sutures are patent. The degree of alteration in cranial shape depends on the timing of synostosis. It may be congenital or develop during infancy, resulting in less severe cranial distortion. Furthermore, cranial shape can be modified when two or more sutures are involved. This figure specifically uses the adjective *synostotic* to describe the cranial shape because brachycephaly, dolichocephaly, and trigonocephaly are known to occur *without* synostosis. (Modified from Cohen and MacLean 2000.[132])

Head shape depends on which sutures are prematurely synostosed (Fig. 20.34), the order in which they synostose, and the timing at which they synostose. Craniosynostosis may be of prenatal or perinatal onset or may occur during infancy or childhood. The earlier synostosis occurs, the more dramatic the effect on subsequent cranial growth and development. The later synostosis occurs, the less the effect on cranial growth and development. Synostosed skulls with minimal dysmorphism have been observed.[132]

Large neurosurgical services generate a characteristic pattern of sutural involvement. Sagittal synostosis is the most common type, occurring more frequently in males than in females. Coronal synostosis is less common than sagittal synostosis; females slightly predominate or, in some surveys, males and females have the same frequency. Multiple synostoses of various types are less common than coronal synostosis. Both metopic and lambdoid synostosis occur with low frequency.[132]

In sagittal synostosis, calvarial midline ridging usually occurs in the posterior half. Coronal synostosis may be bilateral, resulting in brachycephaly, or unilateral, resulting in synostotic frontal plagiocephaly. Metopic ridging is common during infancy and childhood and is not associated with craniosynostosis. Such trigonocephaly self-corrects with time, resulting in a normal cosmetic appearance.[132]

Plagiocephaly

Plagiocephaly is defined as an asymmetric skull. Well-known types include synostotic anterior plagiocephaly (unilateral coronal synostosis), synostotic posterior plagiocephaly (unilateral lambdoid synostosis), deformational anterior plagiocephaly, and deformational posterior plagiocephaly. Of these, deformational posterior plagiocephaly is common and lambdoid synostosis is rare[132] (Table 20.8).

Deformational posterior plagiocephaly, caused by intrauterine factors such as hypotonia, fetal positioning, and prematurity, can produce asymmetric flattening of the occiput that becomes favored by infants sleeping on their backs, which exaggerates the plagiocephaly. This type of plagiocephaly has increased dramatically since the 1992 recommendation of the American Academy of Pediatrics for supine infant sleeping to reduce the risk of sudden infant death syndrome (SIDS).[132]

Craniosynostosis syndromes

Crouzon syndrome is characterized by craniosynostosis, maxillary hypoplasia, shallow orbits, and ocular proptosis (Figs 20.35

TABLE 20.8 TYPES OF PLAGIOCEPHALY

Types of sutures	Synostosed	Relative frequencies
Synostotic anterior plagiocephaly	Unilateral coronal	Less common than bilateral coronal synostosis
	Unilateral frontosphenoidal*	Very rare
	Unilateral frontozygomatic*	Very rare
Synostotic posterior plagiocephaly	Unilateral lambdoid	Rare
Deformational anterior plagiocephaly	No sutures synostosed	Formerly common; now uncommon
Deformational posterior plagiocephaly	No sutures synostosed	Common

*These have been reported in the absence of unilateral coronal synostosis.
After Cohen and MacLean 2000.[132]

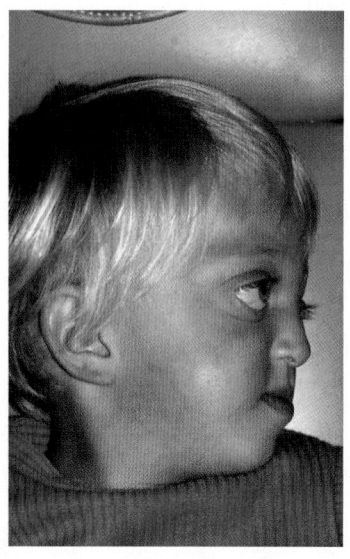

FIGURE 20.36 Crouzon syndrome. Side view.

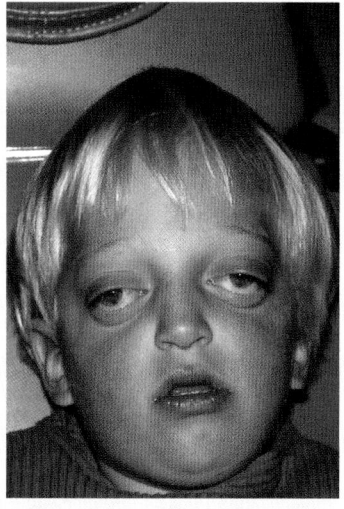

FIGURE 20.35 Crouzon syndrome. Frontal view.

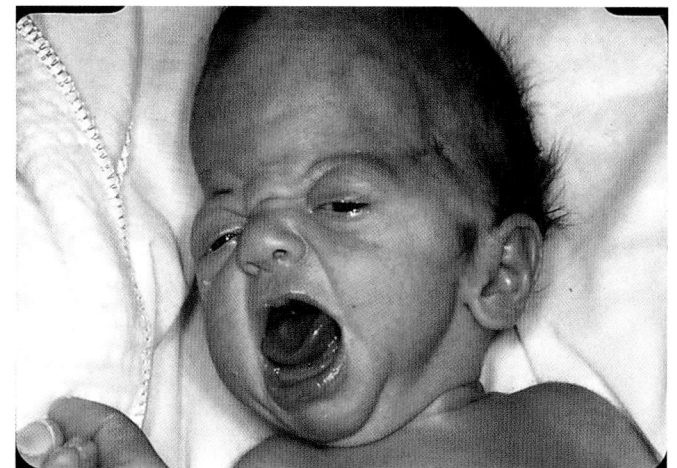

FIGURE 20.37 Apert syndrome. (From Cohen and Kreiborg 1993.[133])

and 20.36). Inheritance is autosomal dominant, with 67% of cases being familial and 33% being sporadic.[132]

Apert syndrome is characterized by craniosynostosis, midface hypoplasia, and symmetric syndactyly of the hands and feet (Figs 20.37 and 20.38). The facial phenotype is variable from mild to severe. Inheritance is autosomal dominant, with most cases representing new mutations.[132, 133]

In Apert syndrome infants, a wide midline calvarial defect is present, extending from the glabella to the posterior fontanel (Figs 20.39 and 20.40). Bony islands, beginning anywhere within the defect, form and coalesce, resulting in complete obliteration of the defect during the first 2 years of life (Figs 20.41 and 20.42). No proper sagittal or metopic suture ever forms. Although the coronal suture is closed at birth, the anterolateral fontanels are abnormally large and both the lambdoid and

squamosal sutures are patent. Characteristics of suture default zones and suture formation are summarized in Table 20.9. Sutural interdigitations never form at the calvarial bony edges of the midline defect. Therefore, the term *craniosynostosis* does not describe the eventual bony obliteration that takes place. In Apert syndrome, sutures fail to form *ab initio* in the midline defect, resulting in a suture default zone. Thus, the appropriate term is *sutural agenesis*, not *craniosynostosis*.[132, 134, 135]

Classic Pfeiffer syndrome (type 1) is likely to be compatible with life and normal or near-normal intelligence in most cases; mild mental deficiency occurs in others. Autosomal dominant families have been recorded.[132]

Type 2 Pfeiffer syndrome is characterized by cloverleaf skull; severe ocular proptosis; often severe central nervous system involvement such as hydrocephalus; elbow ankylosis/synostosis;

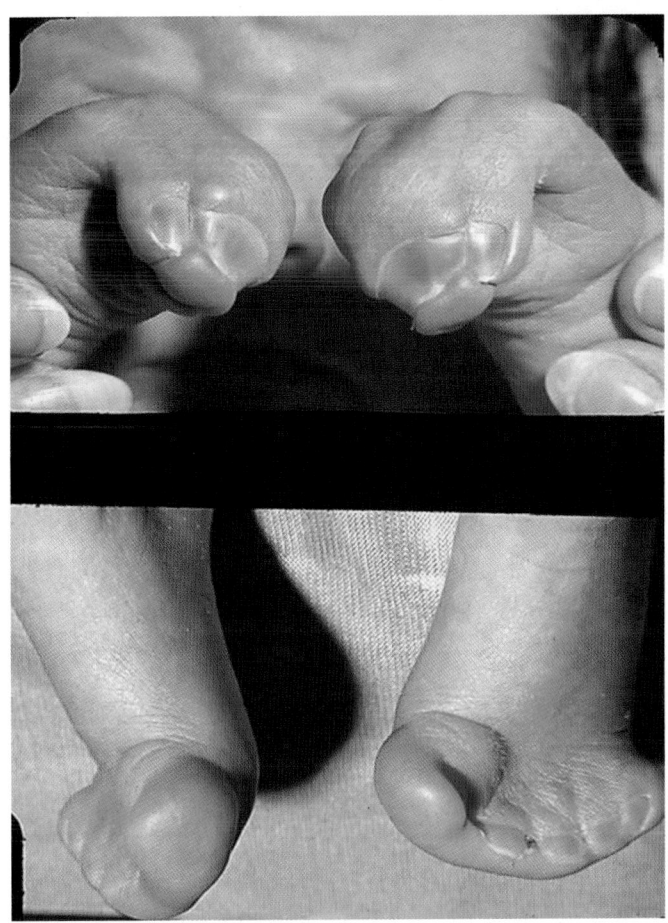

FIGURE 20.38 Apert syndrome. Symmetric syndactyly of hands and feet. (From Cohen and Kreiborg 1993.[133])

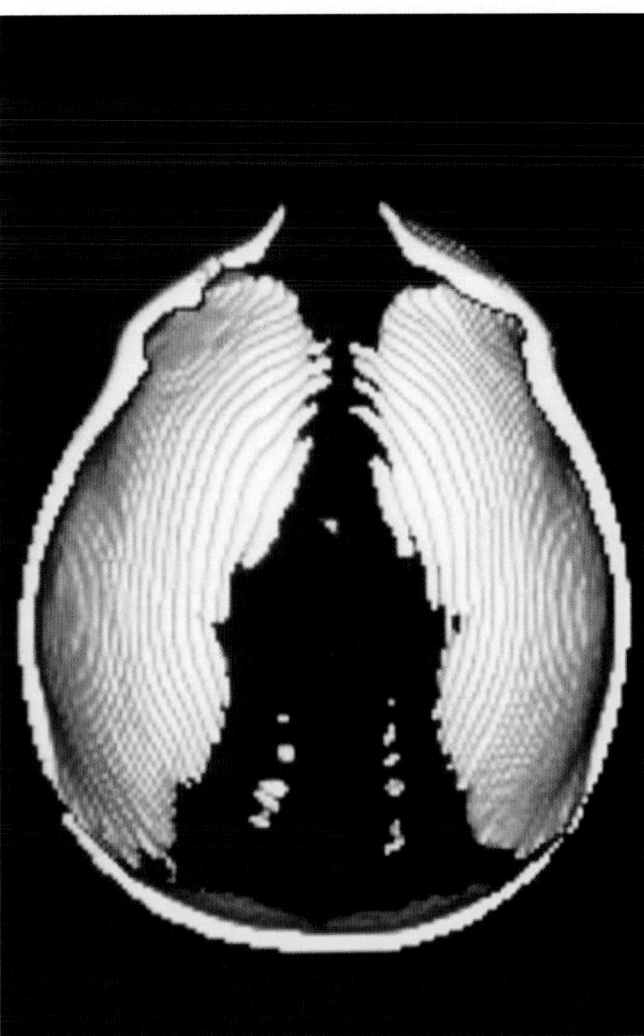

FIGURE 20.39 Three-dimensional reconstruction of computed tomography scans in a 1-month-old infant with Apert syndrome. Endocranial view of cranium showing midline defect extending from the frontal bone to the posterior fontanel area. (From Kreiborg et al 1993.[135])

TABLE 20.9 SUTURES AND SUTURE ZONES IN APERT SYNDROME

Region	Characteristics
Metopic below glabella	Suture formation
Metopic above glabella	Suture default zone; part of midline calvarial defect; closure by coalescence of bony islands
Sagittal	Suture default zone; part of midline calvarial defect; closure by coalescence of bony islands
Coronal	Suture formation; prematurely synostosed at birth
Lambdoid	Suture formation; true Wormian bones on occasion
Squamosal	Suture formation
Sphenotemporal	Suture formation

From Cohen and Kreiborg 1996.[134]

broad thumbs and great toes; and a clustering of unusual low-frequency anomalies (Figs 20.43–20.45). All known cases have been sporadic. No classic type 1 pedigree has shown enough variability of expression to include a Pfeiffer cloverleaf case within the pedigree.[132]

Type 3 Pfeiffer syndrome is similar to type 2 but lacks cloverleaf skull. Hallmarks include severe ocular proptosis, shallow orbits, and marked shortening of the anterior cranial base. A clustering of unusual low-frequency anomalies that are frequently inconsistent from case to case can be found with type 3 as well as with type 2. To date, type 3 cases have been sporadic. Although the three clinical subtypes suggest prognostic trends, they do not have genetic or nosologic status as separate entities; clinical overlap can occur.[132]

In Muenke syndrome, unilateral or bilateral coronal synostosis is found (Fig. 20.46), although a small percentage of patients have macrocephaly. A variety of other anomalies may be present, such as brachydactyly, thimble-like middle phalanges, and, on occasion, broad halluces. Developmental delay has been noted in 37% of affected individuals.[132]

Features of thanatophoric dysplasia include marked shortening of the extremities with numerous skin folds, relatively normal

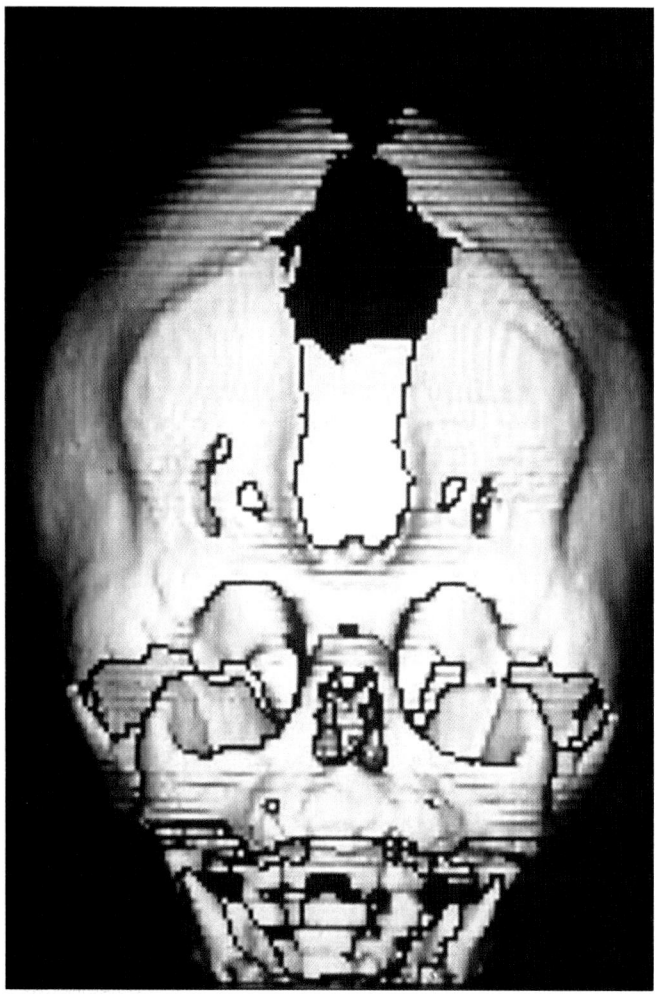

FIGURE 20.40 Three-dimensional reconstruction of computed tomography scans in a 1-month-old infant with Apert syndrome. Frontal view showing extensive midline calvarial defect and unusually large anterolateral fontanels extending into the orbits. (From Kreiborg et al 1993.[135])

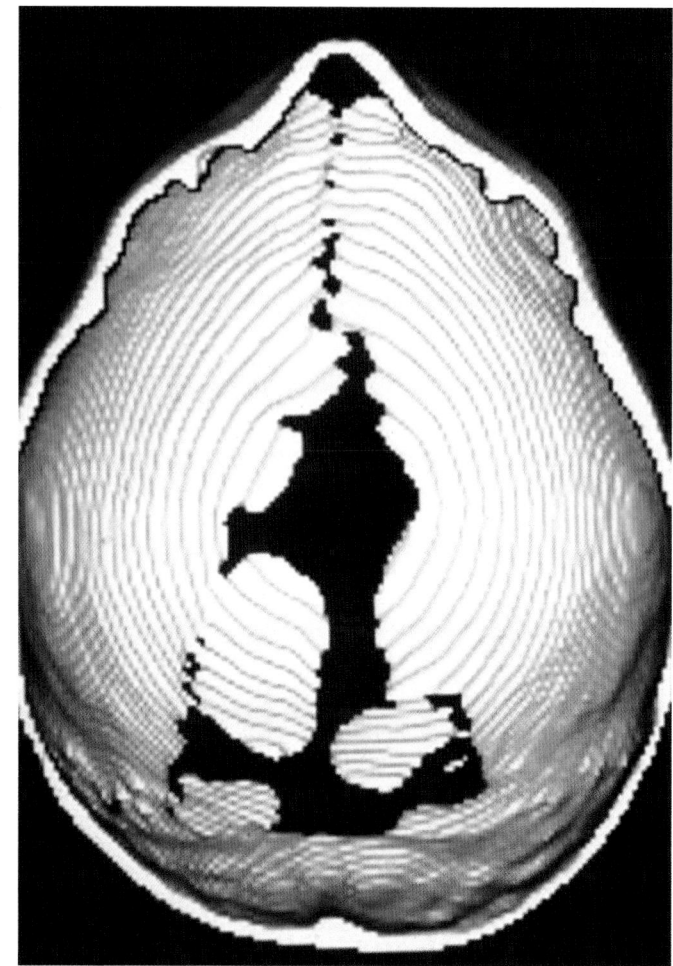

FIGURE 20.41 Three-dimensional reconstruction of computed tomography scans from an 8-month-old infant with Apert syndrome. Endocranial view showing islands of bone coalescing in posterior region. Gap in the frontal bone is now bridged. Same patient as shown in Figure 20.39. (From Kreiborg et al 1993.[135])

trunk length, narrow thorax, disproportionately large head, frontal bossing, protruding eyes, low nasal bridge, and, less commonly, cloverleaf skull (Figs 20.47 and 20.48). Type 1 and type 2 thanatophoric dysplasia are distinguished by their skeletal features. In type 1, the long tubular bones, particularly the femurs, are curved and the vertebral bodies are flat. In type 2, the femurs are straight, the vertebral bodies are not as flat as in type 1, and craniosynostosis is very common. In type 1, 27.6% have craniosynostosis and cloverleaf skull accounts for 3.4% of cases. In type 2, 93% have craniosynostosis and cloverleaf skull accounts for 53% of cases.[132]

Etiologic heterogeneity and pathogenetic variability

Craniosynostosis is etiologically heterogeneous and pathogenetically variable. Overall, 8% of all craniosynostosis pedigrees

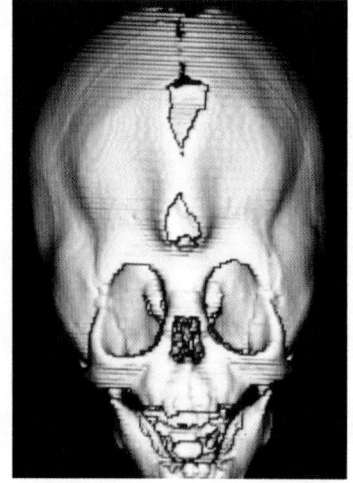

FIGURE 20.42 Three-dimensional reconstruction of computed tomography scans from an 8-month-old infant with Apert syndrome. Frontal view showing bridging of gap in frontal bone. Same patient as shown in Figure 20.40. (From Kreiborg et al 1993.[135])

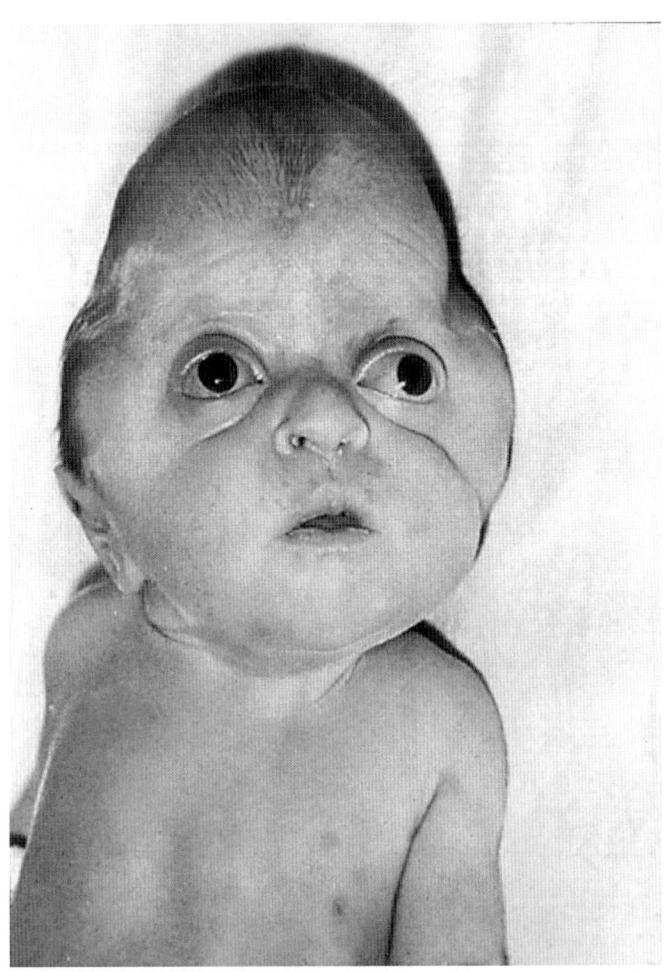

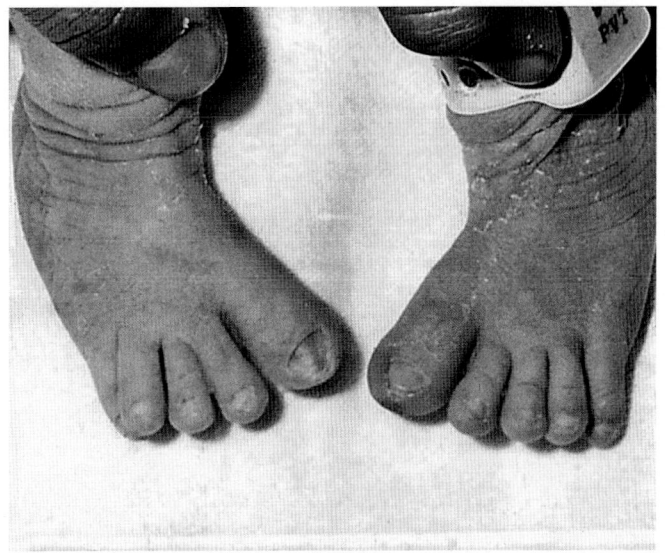

FIGURE 20.45 Type 2 Pfeiffer syndrome showing broad, medially deviated halluces and partial soft tissue syndactyly of the right second and third toes. (Courtesy of A.P. Eaton, Cincinnati, Ohio.)

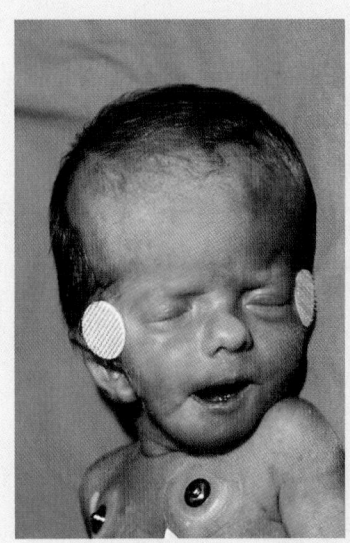

FIGURE 20.46 Muenke syndrome. Coronal synostosis and low nasal bridge.

FIGURE 20.43 Type 2 Pfeiffer syndrome with cloverleaf skull. (Courtesy of A.P. Eaton, Cincinnati, Ohio.)

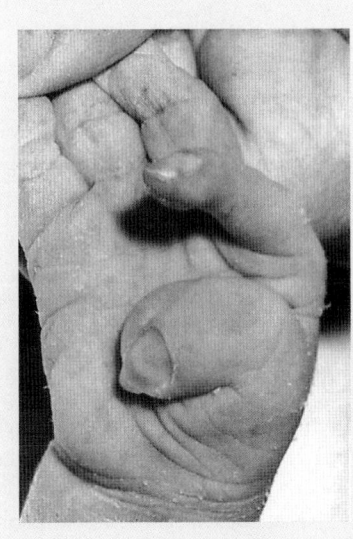

FIGURE 20.44 Type 2 Pfeiffer syndrome showing broad thumb. Also present was coalescence of the first and second metacarpals of the second finger. (Courtesy of A.P. Eaton, Cincinnati, Ohio.)

are familial (n = 725 pedigrees). Evidence generally supports autosomal dominant inheritance. For coronal synostosis, 14.4% of pedigrees are familial (n = 180 pedigrees); for sagittal synostosis, 6% of pedigrees are familial (n = 366 pedigrees); and for metopic synostosis, 5.6% of pedigrees are familial (n = 179 pedigrees).[136–138] Although some pedigrees show synostosis of a specific suture, such as the coronal, sagittal, or metopic suture, other pedigrees may show fusion of different sutures in affected relatives of the same family. Many syndromes have been identified, and well over 100 are known.[132]

Different chromosomal aberrations have been associated with craniosynostosis. In some conditions, craniosynostosis is common [e.g. dup(3q), del(7p), del(9p), and del(11q)], and in

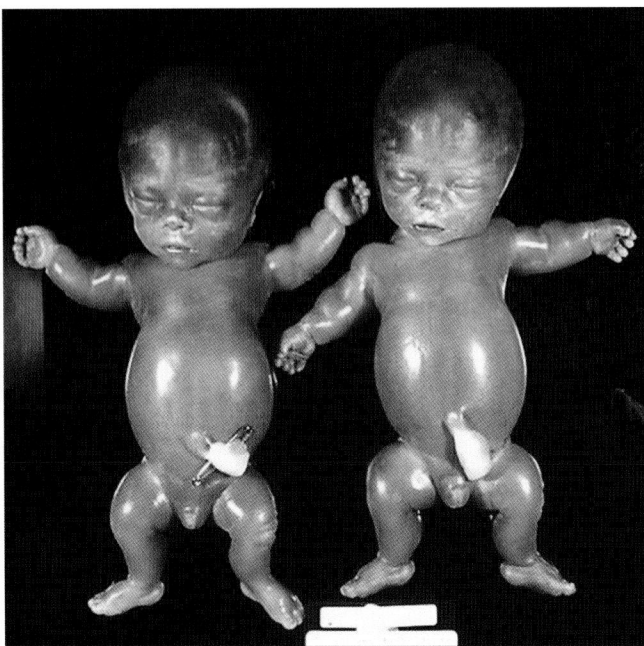

FIGURE 20.47 Identical twins with type I thanatophoric dysplasia. Disproportionately large head, bell-shaped chest, and micromelia. (From Cohen and MacLean 2000.[132])

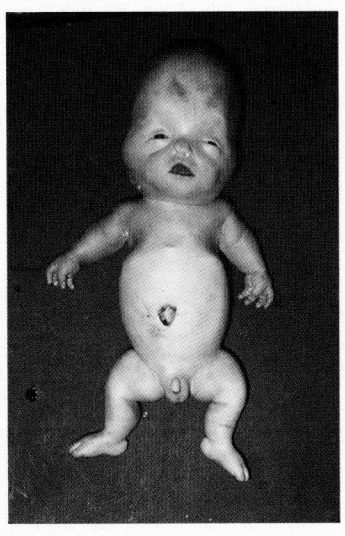

FIGURE 20.48 Type II thanatophoric dysplasia. Cloverleaf skull, bell-shaped chest, and micromelia. (From Cohen and MacLean 2000.[132])

TABLE 20.10 CONDITIONS WITH SECONDARY CRANIOSYNOSTOSIS

Metabolic disorders
   Hyperthyroidism
   Rickets (various forms)
Mucopolysaccharidoses and related disorders
   Hurler syndrome
   Morquio syndrome
   β-Glucuronidase deficiency
   Mucolipidosis III
   α-D-mannosidase deficiency
Hematologic disorders
   Thalassemia
   Sickle cell anemia
   Polycythemia vera
   Congenital hemolytic icterus
Teratogens
   Diphenylhydantoin
   Retinoids
   Valproate
   Aminopterin
   Fluconazole
   Cyclophosphamide
Malformations
   Holoprosencephaly
   Microcephaly
   Encephalocele
Iatrogenic disorders
   Hydrocephalus with shunt

From Cohen and MacLean 2000.[132]

in humans is indirect; it is more compelling for sagittal synostosis than for coronal or metopic synostosis. [132]

Mutations in craniosynostosis syndromes

Mutations have been identified in *FGFRs, TWIST, MSX2, EFNB1, EFNA4, POR,* and *ALPL.* Most mutations are found in FGFR2, although there are several in *FGFR3* and two in *FGFR1*[139–142] (Fig. 20.49, Table 20.10).

Mutations identified on *FGFRs* may be located extracellularly or intracellularly. Almost all nucleotide changes are of the missense or splice-site types. Occasionally, small inframe insertions and deletions are recorded. *FGFR* mutations involve gain of function. They may create or destroy cysteine residues, leaving an unpaired cysteine that can produce intermolecular disulfide bonding and constitutive receptor activation. Accentuated ligand binding, resulting in gain of function, characterizes mutations in the linker region of *FGFR1* (Pfeiffer syndrome), *FGFR2* (Apert syndrome), and *FGFR3* (Muenke syndrome). All human FGFR mutations known to date allow early human development to proceed normally but interfere with later development, particularly of bone. When mesen-

others, craniosynostosis is an unusual occurrence [e.g. dup(5p), del(6)(q22.2-q23.1), del(8q), and dup(15q)].[132]

Primary craniosynostosis is common and includes single- and multiple-suture synostosis – for example, coronal synostosis or coronal and sagittal synostosis. Examples of secondary synostosis include hyperthyroidism and Hurler syndrome. Conditions with secondary synostosis are listed in Table 20.10. They include six teratogens that are associated with occasional cases of craniosynostosis.[132]

Koskinen-Moffett et al[47] provided evidence for prenatal head constraint as a cause of craniosynostosis in mice. The evidence

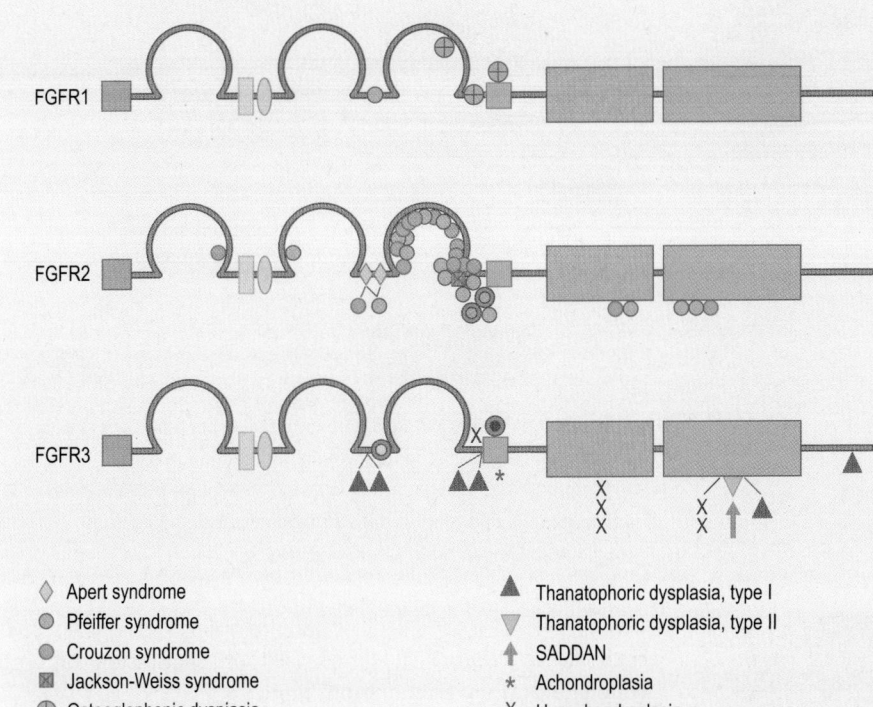

FIGURE 20.49 Most mutations for major craniosynostosis syndromes are on *FGFR2*, with several on *FGFR3* and two on *FGFR1*. Note the mutations for short-limb skeletal dysplasias (achondroplasia, hypochondroplasia, thanatophoric dysplasia type I, and thanatophoric dysplasia type II) on *FGFR3*. Hatched square, signal peptide; solid oblong, acid box; solid oval, CAM homology domain; solid square, transmembrane domain; long solid oblongs, kinase domains 1 and 2. Three loops from left to right are immunoglobulin-like domains (IgI, IgII, IgIII). For clarity, only a few of the many mutations for Crouzon syndrome and Pfeiffer syndrome are shown on *FGFR2*. (Modified from Cohen and MacLean 2000.[132])

◇ Apert syndrome
◎ Pfeiffer syndrome
◯ Crouzon syndrome
⊠ Jackson-Weiss syndrome
⊕ Osteoglophonic dyspiasia
◎ Beare-Stevenson cutis gyrata syndrome

▲ Thanatophoric dysplasia, type I
▽ Thanatophoric dysplasia, type II
⬆ SADDAN
* Achondroplasia
X Hypochondroplasia
◉ Crouzonodermoskeletal syndrome
◎ Muenke syndrome

TABLE 20.11 GENES BEARING KNOWN MUTATIONS FOR CRANIOSYNOSTOSIS

FGFR1	Pfeiffer syndrome
FGFR2	Apert syndrome
	Pfeiffer syndrome
	Crouzon syndrome
	Jackson-Weiss syndrome
	Beare-Stevenson cutis gyrata syndrome
	Non-classifiable and variable craniosynostosis
FGFR3	Thanatophoric dysplasia, type I
	Thanatophoric dysplasia, type II
	Crouzonodermoskeletal syndrome
	Muenke syndrome
TWIST	Saethre-Chotzen syndrome
MSX2	Boston type craniosynostosis
EFNB1	Craniofrontonasal syndrome
EFNB4	Non-syndromal coronal synostosis
POR	Antley-Bixler syndrome
ALPL	Hypophosphatasia, particularly infantile type

After Cohen and MacLean 2000.[132]

chyme is converted to bone, the molecular crosstalk is highly complex and only partially understood.[139]

Other gene mutations for craniosynostosis are also known (Table 20.11). In Saethre-Chotzen syndrome, *TWIST* mutations may be of the nonsense, missense, insertion, or deletion type and

may be found outside or within the coding region. Most mutations truncate the *TWIST* protein, resulting in haploinsufficiency.[132, 143] Boston-type craniosynostosis results from a heterozygous gain-of-function mutation in *MSX2*.[144–146] Craniofrontonasal syndrome is caused by heterozygous loss-of-function mutations in *EFNB1*.[147] Craniosynostosis may be observed in hypophosphatasia, particularly the infantile type. The disorder is caused by mutations in *ALPL*. [148] *EFNA4* mutations rarely cause non-syndromal coronal synostosis. *POR* mutations have caused some cases of Antley-Bixler syndrome.

Cleidocranial dysplasia

Cleidocranial dysplasia is an autosomal dominant skeletal disorder characterized by short stature, brachycephaly, delayed closure of fontanels and sutures, Wormian bones, midface hypoplasia, unerupted teeth, supernumerary permanent teeth, aplasia or hypoplasia of the clavicles, and other skeletal anomalies, such as hypoplastic iliac wings and brachydactyly[149–151] (Figs 20.50 and 20.51).

Cleidocranial dysplasia is caused by mutations in *RUNX2*. These mutations result in haploinsufficiency and may be of the deletion, insertion, missense, or nonsense types.[152] *RUNX2* is the master gene for bone (Fig. 20.52). In the mouse, cleidocranial dysplasia is caused when one allele is suppressed (*Runx2*[+/−]). The null mutant, in which *Runx2* is suppressed at

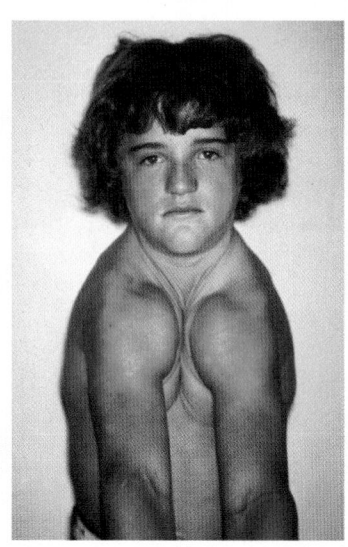

FIGURE 20.50
Cleidocranial dysplasia. Brachycephaly and absent clavicles, permitting approximation of the shoulders in the midline. (From Cohen 2000.[149])

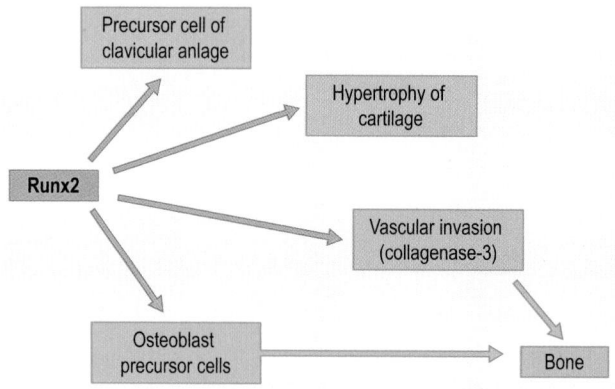

FIGURE 20.52 *Runx2* controls differentiation of precursor cells into osteoblasts, regulates chondrocyte differentiation towards hypertrophy, may cause vascular invasion of cartilage by regulating collagenase-3, and controls differentiation of precursor cells of clavicular anlage. (Modified from Mundlos 1999.[151])

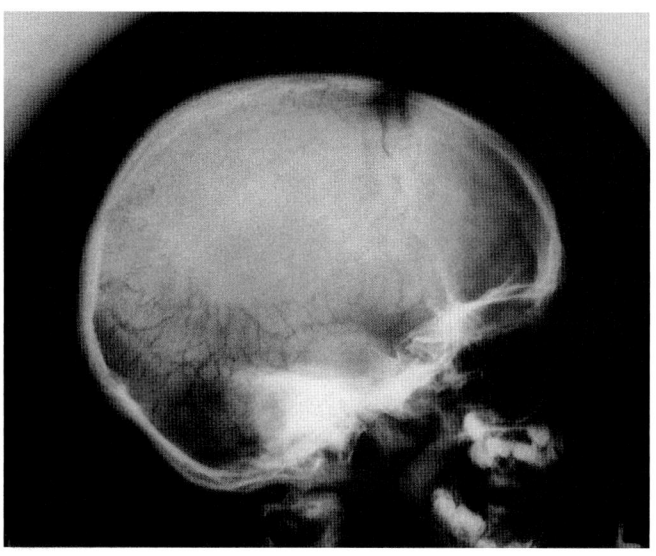

FIGURE 20.51 Cleidocranial dysplasia. Patent anterior fontanel and Wormian bones. (From Cohen 2000.[149])

both alleles (*Runx2⁻/⁻*), shows lack of ossification of both endochondral and membranous bone.[151]

Branchial arch syndromes

Branchial arch syndromes comprise an etiologically heterogeneous group of disorders. The best known of these are hemifacial microsomia, its variant, Goldenhar syndrome, and Treacher Collins syndrome. Some branchial arch syndromes are summarized in Table 20.12.[105]

Hemifacial microsomia

Hemifacial microsomia affects aural, oral, and mandibular growth. The disorder may be mild or severe, and involvement is

TABLE 20.12 SOME BRANCHIAL ARCH SYNDROMES

Syndrome	Major features	Chromosome	Gene
Hemifacial microsomia, Goldenhar syndrome	Hypoplasia and asymmetry involving mandible and ear, usually unilateral; if bilateral, more severe on one side; may be associated with various anomalies especially of the eyes (epibulbar dermoids), cardiovascular malformations, skeletal defects (especially vertebral) and CNS anomalies	?	?
Treacher Collins syndrome	Bilateral zygomatic hypoplasia, down- slanting palpebral fissures, malformed ears, micrognathia	5q32-q33.1	TCOF1
Townes-Brock syndrome	Dysplastic ears, ear tags, sensorineural deafness, bifid or supernumerary finger-like thumbs, hypoplastic kidneys, anal stenosis	16q12.1	SALL1
Branchio-oto-renal (BOR) syndrome	Cup-shaped ears, preauricular pits, branchial cleft fistulas, mixed deafness renal anomalies	8q13.3	EYA1

From Cohen, 2002.[105]

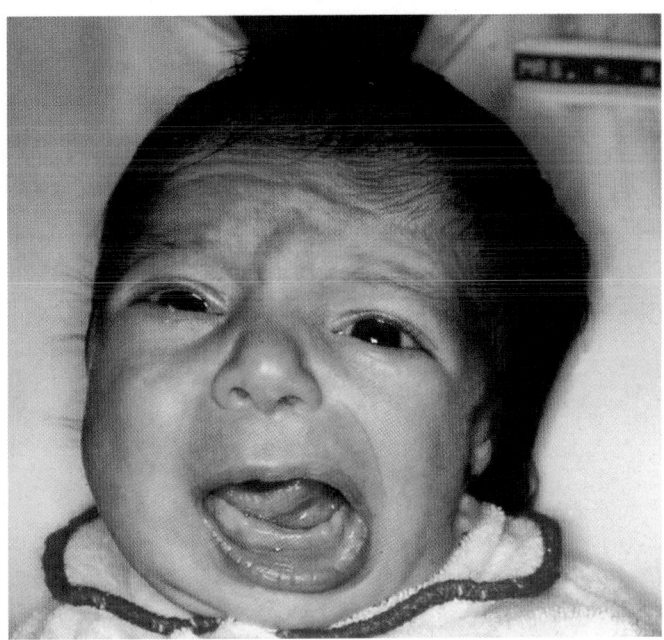

FIGURE 20.53 Hemifacial microsomia.

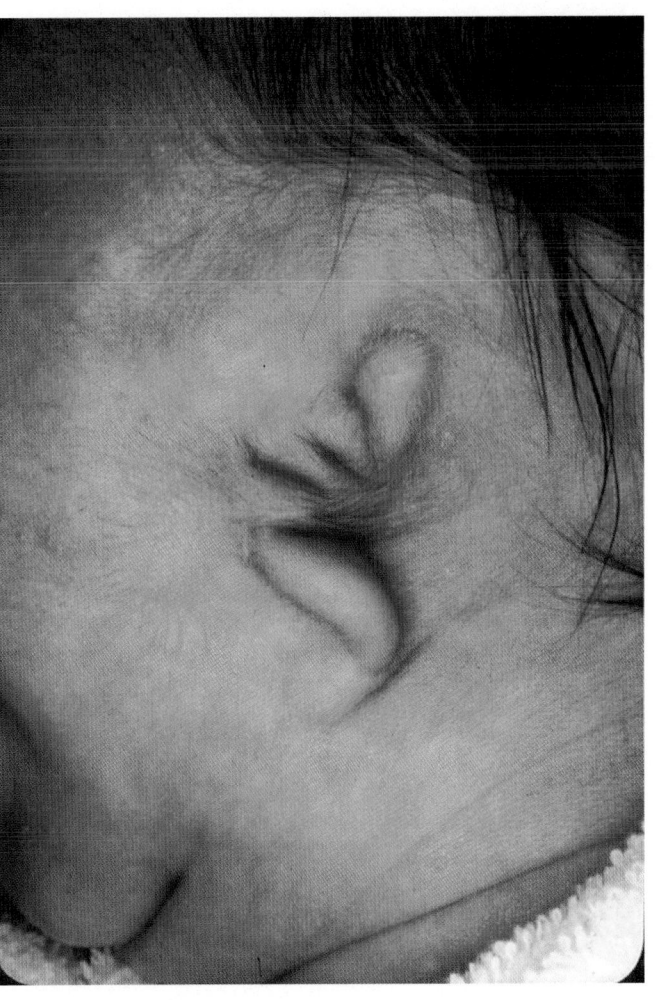

FIGURE 20.54 Hemifacial microsomia.

limited to one side of the face in most cases (Figs 20.53 and 20.54), but bilateral involvement, with more severe expression on one side, is also known to occur. There is a 3:2 predilection for right-sided involvement. A variant of hemifacial microsomia, Goldenhar syndrome, consists of epibulbar dermoids and vertebral anomalies. Terms such as 'first arch syndrome', 'first and second branchial arch syndrome', and 'hemifacial microsomia' impart the erroneous impression that involvement is limited to the face when, in fact, cardiac, renal, skeletal, and central nervous system anomalies may occur as well.[153]

Treacher Collins syndrome

Treacher Collins syndrome consists of bilateral zygomatic hypoplasia, downslanting palpebral fissures, malformed ears, and micrognathia (Fig. 20.55). Inheritance is autosomal dominant, and expressivity varies. The syndrome maps to 5q32-q33.1, and mutations in the *TCOF1* gene are of the nonsense, insertion, deletion, or splice-site types. The introduction of premature termination codons into the reading frame indicates haploinsufficiency.[154–156]

Vascular tumors and malformations

Mulliken and Glowacki[157] and Mulliken[158, 159] made a distinction between hemangiomas and vascular malformations based on cellular kinetics and clinical behavior (Table 20.13). Hemangiomas have endothelial hyperplasia with rapid postnatal growth followed by slow involution. In contrast, vascular malformations are characterized by flat endothelium, and growth of

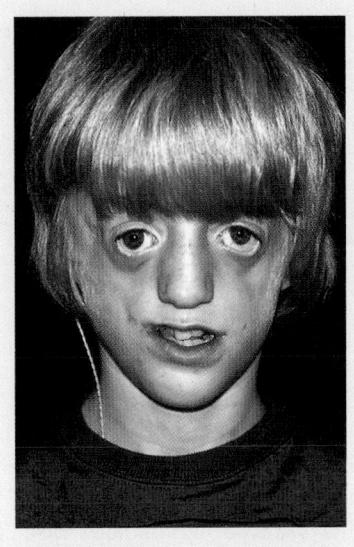

FIGURE 20.55 Treacher Collins syndrome. (From Cohen 1997.[49])

TABLE 20.13 MULLIKEN CLASSIFICATION

	Hemangioma	Vascular malformation
Presentation	Usually not present at birth	Always present at birth but may not be apparent in some cases
Female:male ratio	3:1 (higher in some series)	1:1
Cellular criteria	Endothelial hyperplasia	Flat endothelium
Course	Rapid postnatal growth followed by slow involution	Growth is commensurate with the child's growth

After Mulliken and Gowacki 1982.[157]

TABLE 20.14 BIOLOGICAL CLASSIFICATION OF VASCULAR MARKINGS

Hemangioma	Malformation
	Single channel
Proliferating phase	Capillary (CM)
Involuting phase	Lymphatic (LM)
	Venous (VM)
	Multiple channels
	CLM
	CVM
	CLVM
	LVM

After Mulliken 1993.[158]

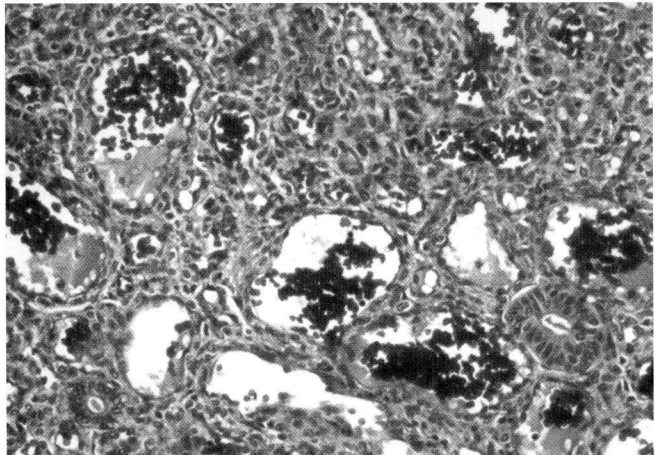

FIGURE 20.56 Histopathology of a hemangioma. (From Cohen 2005.[164])

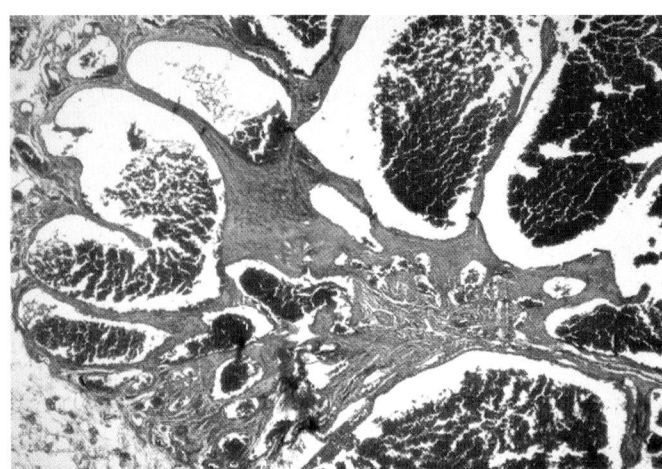

FIGURE 20.57 Histopathology of a vascular malformation. Channels filled with erythrocytes. (From Cohen 2005.[164])

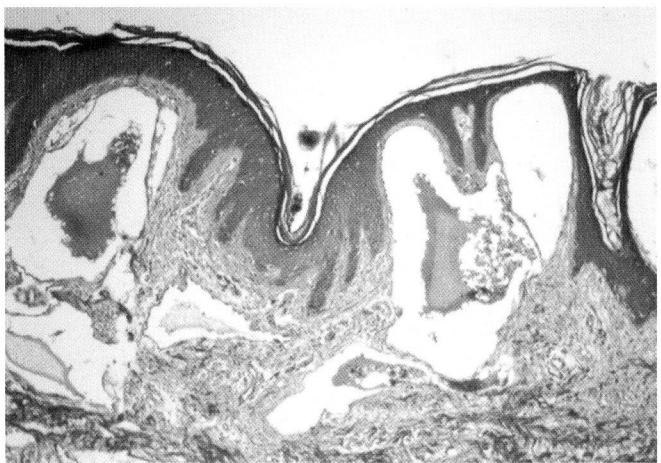

FIGURE 20.58 Histopathology of a lymphatic malformation. (From Cohen 2005.[164])

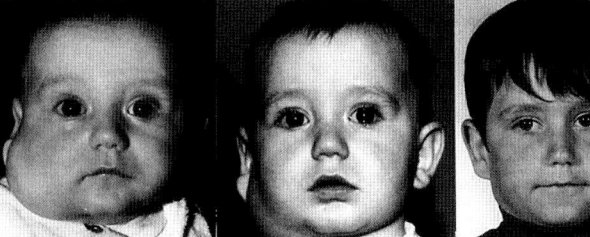

FIGURE 20.59 Proliferation and involution of a hemangioma with no surgical intervention. Left: a 3-month-old boy with a right parotid hemangioma. Note impingement on the ear and extension onto neck. Center: same child at 12 months of age with early signs of involution. Right: same child at 6 years of age showing total resolution of parotid hemangioma, but with excess wrinkling of the skin. (From Williams 1975.[165])

the lesion is commensurate with growth of the child. In vascular malformations, a single type of channel anomaly may predominate, or multiple channel anomalies of various types may occur (Table 20.14, Figs 20.56–20.65).

Mulliken[158] noted that the 'standard' terminology used for vascular lesions has led to confusion, improper diagnosis, illogical treatment, and misdirected research efforts (Fig. 20.66). The

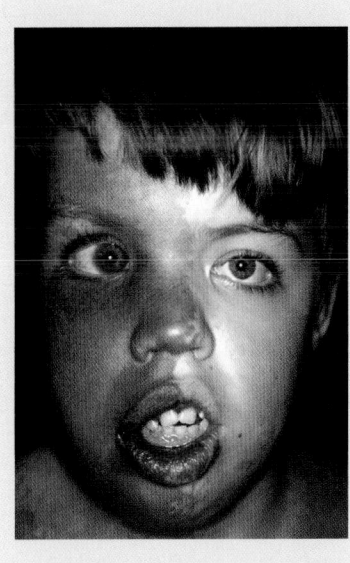

FIGURE 20.60 Sturge-Weber syndrome. (From Cohen 2005.[164])

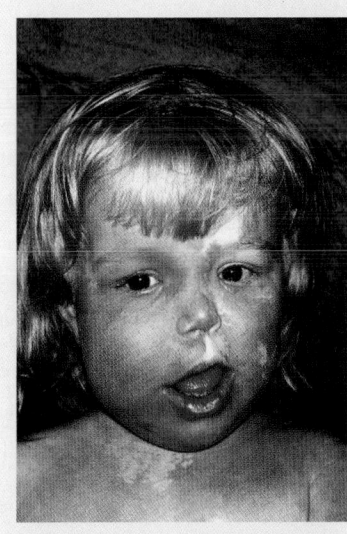

FIGURE 20.62 Sturge-Weber syndrome. Bilateral facial involvement with extension of the capillary malformation to the neck, upper chest, arms, and legs. (From Cohen 2005.[163])

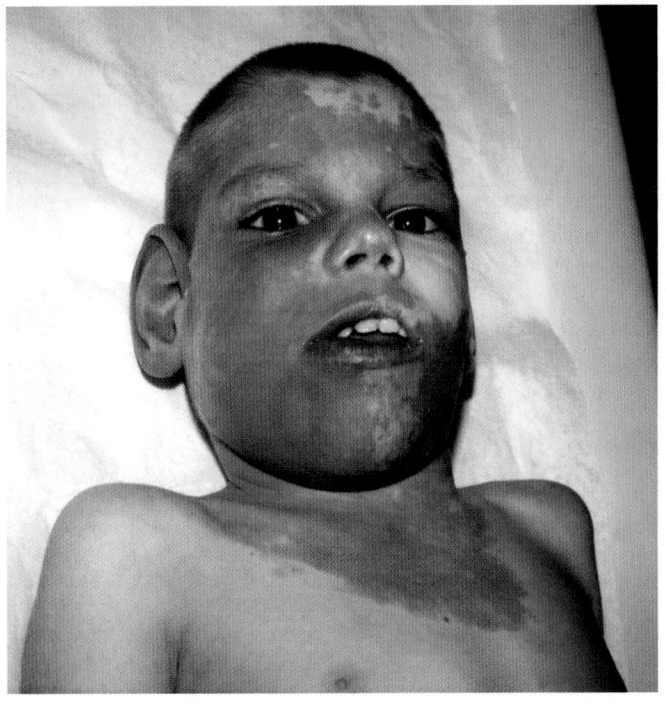

FIGURE 20.61 Sturge-Weber syndrome. Bilateral involvement with extension of the capillary malformation onto the neck and chest. (From Cohen 2005.[163])

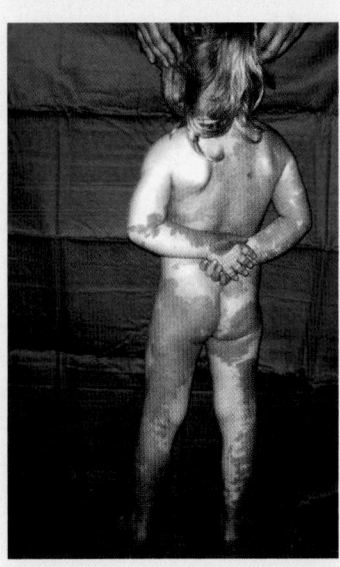

FIGURE 20.63 Sturge-Weber syndrome. Same patient as shown in Figure 20.62. Extension of the capillary malformation to the back, buttocks, arms, and legs. (From Cohen 2005.[163])

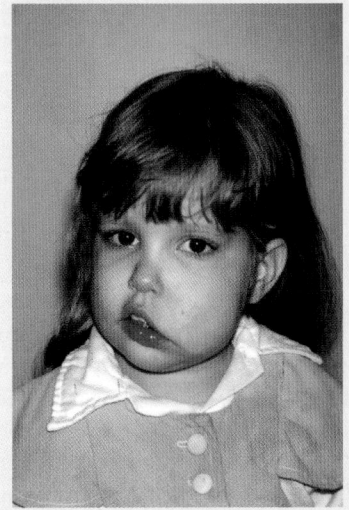

FIGURE 20.64 Lymphatic malformation of the face. (From Cohen 2005.[164])

Mulliken classification (Table 20.13), which is based on the clinical behavior and cellular characteristics of vascular lesions, is considered state-of-the-art in the field of vascular anomalies and was accepted by the International Society for the Study of Vascular Anomalies in the 1996 workshop meeting in Rome.[160]

Burns et al[161] indicated that by clinical and cellular criteria, vascular birthmarks can be classified as hemangiomas, malformations, or macular stains. Because infantile hemangiomas

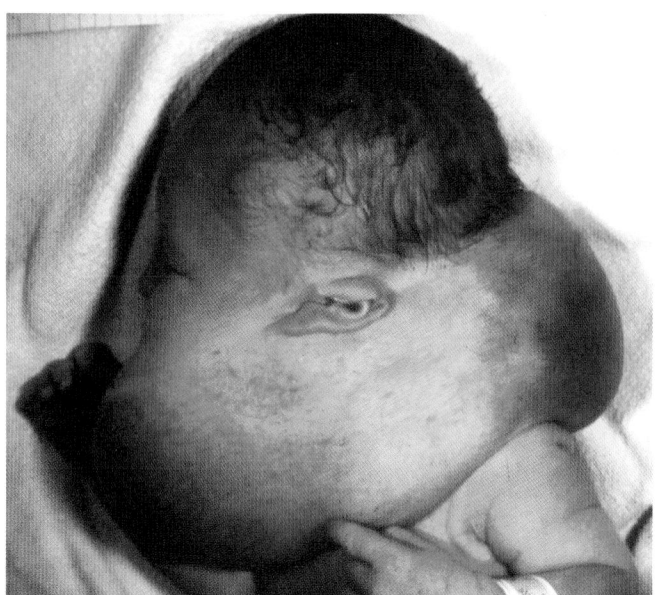

FIGURE 20.65 Large lymphatic malformation of the neck. (From Cohen 2005.[164])

TABLE 20.15 FEATURES OF KLIPPEL-TRENAUNAY, PARKES WEBER, AND STURGE-WEBER SYNDROMES

Syndromes	Vascular malformations	Clinical considerations
Klippel-Trenaunay syndrome	Slow flow, combined vascular malformation (capillary, lymphatic, and venous)	Involves limb(s) and/or trunk
Parkes Weber syndrome	Fast flow, combined vascular malformation (capillary, rarely lymphatic, arterial and venous)	Involves upper/lower limbs
Sturge-Weber syndrome	Slow flow, capillary malformation	Involves leptomeninges with or without choroid and V1 or V1–V2. Capillary malformation can occur elsewhere on body.

From Cohen et al 2002.[163]

References

Craniofacial embryology

1. Nakatsu T, Shiota K. Neurulation in the human embryo revisited. Congenital Anomalies 2000; 40:93–98.
2. Nakatsu T, Uwabe C, Shiota K. Neural tube closure in humans initiates at multiple sites: evidence from human embryos and implications for the pathogenesis of neural tube defects. Anat Embryol (Berl) 2000; 201:455–466.
3. Langman J. Medical embryology. Baltimore: Williams & Wilkins, 1963.
4. Cohen MM Jr. Perspectives on the face. New York: Oxford University Press, 2005.
5. Jiang X, Iseki S, Maxson RE, Sucov HM, Morriss-Kay GM. Tissue origins and interactions in the mammalian skull vault. Dev Biol 2002; 241:106–116.
6. Gorlin RJ, Cohen MM Jr. The orofacial region. In: Wigglesworth JS, Singer DB, eds. Textbook of fetal and perinatal pathology. 2nd edn. Malden: Blackwell Science; 1988:732–778.
7. Gorlin RJ, Cohen MM Jr, Hennekam RCM. Syndromes of the head and neck. 4th edn. New York: Oxford University Press; 2001.
8. Johnston MC, Sulik KK. Embryology of the head and neck. In: Serafin D, Georiade NG, eds. Pediatric plastic surgery. St Louis: CV Mosby; 1984: 184–215.
9. Sulik KK, Schoenwolf GC. Highlights of craniofacial morphogenesis in mammalian embryos as revealed by scanning electron microscopy. Scan Electron Microsc 1985; 4:1735–1752.
10. Ferguson MWJ. Palate development. Development 1988; 103 (suppl):41–60.
11. Larsen WJ. Human embryology. New York: Churchill Livingstone, 1993.
12. Sulik KK. Craniofacial embryology and dysmorphogenesis. In: Siebert JR, Cohen MM Jr, Sulik KK, Shaw CM, Lemire RJ, eds. Holoprosencephaly: an overview and atlas of cases. New York: Wiley-Liss; 1990; 59–98.
13. Sulik KK, Cotanche DA. Embryology of the ear. In: Gorlin RJ, Toriello HV, Cohen MM Jr, eds. Hereditary hearing loss and its syndromes . New York: Oxford University Press; 1995:22–42.
14. Graham A. Development of the pharyngeal arches. Am J Med Genet 2003; 119A:251–256.
15. Graham A, Francis-West P, Brickell P, Lumsden A. The signalling molecule BMP4 mediates apoptosis in the rhombencephalic neural crest. Nature 1994; 372:684–686.
16. Helms JA, Schneider RA. Cranial skeletal biology. Nature 2003; 423: 326–331.

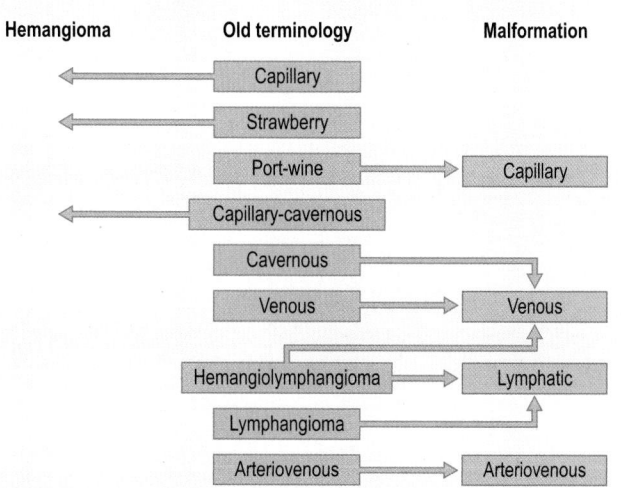

FIGURE 20.66 Confusion resulting from 'standard' terminology of vascular lesions. (Modified from Mulliken 1993.[158])

occur in 10–12% of normal infants by one year of age and macular stains are found in about 40% of normal newborns, the authors queried whether either of these are pathogenetically related in the syndromes in which they have been described. True hemangiomas occur only rarely in malformation syndromes, but vascular malformations are common. Clinical conditions such as Klippel-Trenaunay syndrome, Parkes Weber syndrome, and Sturge-Weber syndrome have vascular malformations, not hemangiomas[162–165] (Table 20.15).

17. Schneider RA, Helms JA. The cellular and molecular origins of beak morphology. Science 2003; 299:565–568.

18. Trainor PA, Ariza-McNaughton L, Krumlauf R. Role of the isthmus and FGFs in resolving the paradox of neural crest plasticity and prepatterning. Science 2002; 295:1288–1291.

19. García-Castro MI, Marcelle C, Bronner-Fraser M. Ectodermal Wnt function as a neural crest inducer. Science 2002; 297:848–851.

20. Gassmann M, Casagranda F, Orioli D, Simon H, Lai C, Rüdiger K, Lemke G. Aberrant neural and cardiac development in mice lacking the ErbB4 neuregulin receptor. Nature 1995; 378:390–394.

21. Golding JP, Trainor P, Krumlauf R, Gassmann M. Defects in pathfinding by cranial neural crest cells in mice lacking the neuregulin receptor ErbB4. Nat Cell Biol 2000; 2:103–109.

22. Chambers D, McGonnell IM. Neural crest: facing the facts of head development. Trends Genet 2002; 296:381–384.

23. Eickholt BJ, Mackenzie SL, Graham A, Walsh FS, Doherty P. Evidence for collapsin-1 functioning in the control of neural crest migration in both trunk and hindbrain regions. Development 1999; 126:2181–2189.

24. Farlie PG, Kerr R, Thomas P, Symes T, Minichello J, Hearn CJ, Newgreen D. A paraxial exclusion zone creates patterned cranial neural crest cell outgrowth adjacent to rhombomeres 3 and 5. Dev Biol 1999; 213:70–84.

25. Graham A, Smith A. Patterning of the pharyngeal arches. BioEssays 2001; 23:54–61.

26. Mason I, Chambers D, Shamin H, Walsh J, Irving C. Regulation and function of FGF8 in patterning of midbrain and anterior hindbrain. Biochem Cell Biol 2000; 78:577–584.

27. Trainor PA, Krumlauf R. Hox genes, neural crest cells and branchial arch patterning. Curr Opin Cell Biol 2001; 13:698–705.

28. Trainor PA, Krumlauf R. Patterning the cranial neural crest: hindbrain segmentation and Hox gene plasticity. Nat Rev Neurosci 2000; 1:116–124.

29. Gedron-Maguire M, Mallo M, Zhang M, Gridley T. Hoxa-2 mutant mice exhibit homeotic transformation of skeletal elements derived from cranial neural crest. Cell 1993; 75:1317–1331.

30. Grammatopoulos GA, Bell E, Toole L, Lumsden A, Tucker AS. Homeotic transformation of branchial arch identity after Hoxa-2 overexpression. Development 2000; 127:5355–5365.

31. Pasqualetti M, Ori M, Nardi I, Rijli FM. Ectopic Hoxa2 induction after neural crest migration results in homeosis of jaw elements in *Xenopus*. Development 2000; 127:5367–5378.

32. Rijli FM, Mark M, Lakkaraju S, Dierich A, Dolle P. A homeotic transformation is generated in the rostral branchial region of the head by disruption of Hoxa-2, which acts as a selector gene. Cell 1993; 75: 1333–1349.

33. Veitch E, Begbie J, Schilling TG, Smith MM, Graham A. Pharyngeal arch patterning in the absence of neural crest. Curr Biol 1999; 9: 1481–1484.

34. Couly G, Creuzet S, Bennaceur S, Vincent C, Le Douarin NM. Interactions between Hox-negative cephalic neural crest cells and the foregut endoderm in patterning the facial skeleton in the vertebrate head. Development 2002; 129:1061–1073.

35. Hu D, Marcucio RS, Helms JA. A zone of frontonasal ectoderm regulates patterning and growth in the face. Development 2003; 130:1749–1758.

36. Hall BK, Miyake T. The membranous skeleton: The role of cell condensations in vertebrate skeletogenesis. Anat Embryol 1992; 186:107–124.

37. Hall BK, Miyake T. Divide, accumulate, differentiate: cell condensation in skeletal development revisited. Int J Dev Biol 1995; 39:881–893.

38. Hall BK, Miyake T. All for one and one for all: condensations and the initiation of skeletal development. BioEssays 2000; 22:138–147.

39. Cohen MM Jr. Sutural biology and the correlates of craniosynostosis. Am J Med Genet 1993; 47:581–616.

40. Cohen MM Jr. Sutural biology. In: Cohen MM Jr, MacLean RE, eds. Craniosynostosis, diagnosis, evaluation, and management. 2nd edn. New York: Oxford University Press; 2000:11–23.

41. Furtwangler JA, Hall SH, Koskinen-Moffett LK. Sutural morphogenesis in the mouse calvaria: The role of apoptosis. Acta Anat 1985; 124:74–80.

42. Johansen V, Hall SH. Morphogenesis of the mouse coronal suture. Acta Anat 1982; 114:58–67.

43. Kokich VG. Age changes in the human frontozygomatic suture. Am J Orthodont 1976; 69:411–430.

44. Koskinen L. Adaptive sutures: changes after unilateral masticatory muscle resection in rats: a microscopic study. Proc Finn Dent Soc 1977; 73(suppl 10–11)3–80.

45. McPherson GK, Kriewall TJ. Fetal head molding: an investigation utilizing a finite element model of the fetal parietal bone. J Biomech 1980; 13:17–26.

46. Pritchard JJ, Scott JH, Girgis FG. The structure and development of cranial and facial sutures. J Anat 1956; 90:73–86.

47. Koskinen-Moffett LK, Moffett BC Jr, Graham JM Jr. Cranial synostosis and intra-uterine compression: A developmental study of human sutures. In: Dixon AD, Sarnat BG, eds. Factors and mechanisms influencing bone growth. New York: Alan R. Liss; 1982:365–378.

48. Miroue M, Rosenberg L. The human facial sutures: a morphologic and histologic study of age changes from 20 to 95 years. MSD Thesis, University of Washington, 1975.

Types of anomalies

49. Cohen MM Jr. The child with multiple birth defects. 2nd edn. New York: Oxford University Press; 1997.

Orofacial clefting

50. Cohen MM Jr. Syndromes with cleft lip and cleft palate. Cleft Palate J 1978; 15:306–328.

51. Cohen MM Jr. Etiology and pathogenesis of orofacial clefting. Oral Maxillofac Surg Clin North Am 2000; 12:379–397.

52. Wyszynski DF, Beaty TH, Maestri NE. Genetics of nonsyndromic oral clefts revisited. Cleft Palate-Craniofac J 1996; 33:406–417.

53. Fraser FC. Liability, thresholds, malformations, and syndromes. Am J Med Genet 1996; 66:75–76.

54. Brewer CM, Leek JP, Green AJ, Holloway S, Bonthron DT, Markham AF, Fitzpatrick DR. A locus for isolated cleft palate, located on human chromosome 2q32. Am J Hum Genet 1999; 65:387–396.

55. Lidral AC, Romitti PA, Basart AM, Doetschman T, Leysens NJ, Daack-Hirsch S, Semina EV, Johnson LR, Machida J, Burds A, Parnell TJ, Rubinstein JL, Murray JC. Association of MSX1 and TGFB3 with nonsyndromic clefting in humans. Am J Hum Genet 1998; 63:557–568.

56. Mitchell LE, Healey SC, Chenevix-Trench G. Evidence for an association between nonsyndromic cleft lip with or without cleft palate and a gene located on the long arm of chromosome 4. Am J Hum Genet 1995; 57: 1130–1136.

57. Murray JC. Face facts: genes, environment, and clefts. Am J Hum Genet 1995; 57:227–232.

58. Qiu M, Bulfone A, Ghattas I, Meneses JJ, Christensen L, Sharpe PE, Presley PT, Presley R. Role of the Dix homeobox genes in proximodistal patterning of the branchial arches: Mutations of Dix-1 and Dix-2 alter morphogenesis of proximal skeletal and soft tissue structures derived from the first and second arches. Dev Biol 1997; 185:165–184.

59. Qiu M, Bulfone A, Martinez S, Meneses JJ, Shimamura K, Pedersen RA, Rubinstein JL. Null mutation of Dix-2 results in abnormal morphogenesis of proximal first and second branchial arch derivatives and abnormal differentiation in the forebrain. Genes Dev 1995; 9:2523–2538.

60. Scapoli L, Pezzetti F, Carinci F, Martinelli M, Carinci P, Tognon M. Evidence of linkage to 6p23 and genetic heterogeneity in nonsyndromic cleft lip with or without cleft palate. Genomics 1997; 43:216–220.

61. Sertié AL, Sousa AV, Steman S, Pavanello RC, Passos-Bueno MR. Linkage analysis in a large Brazilian family with van der Woude syndrome suggests the existence of a susceptibility locus for cleft palate at 17p11.2–11.1. Am J Hum Genet 1999; 65:433–440.

62. Shaw D, Ray A, Marazita M. Further evidence of a relationship between the retinoic acid receptor α locus and nonsyndromic cleft lip with or without cleft palate (CL ± P). Am J Hum Genet 1993; 53:1156–1157.

63. Stein J, Mulliken JB, Stal S, Grasser DL, Malcolm S, Winter R, Blanton SH, Amos C, Seemanová E, Hecht JT. Nonsyndromic cleft lip with or without

cleft palate: Evidence of linkage to BCL3 in 17 multigeneration families. Am J Hum Genet 1995; 57:257–272.

64. Kondo S, Schutte BC, Richardson RJ, Bijork BC, Knight AS, Watanabe Y, Howrd E, Ferreira de Lima RLL, Daack-Hirsch S, Sander A, McDonald-McGinn DM, Zackai EH, Lammer EJ, Aylsworth AS, Ardinge HH, Lidral AC, Pober BR, Moreno L, Arcos-Burgos M, Valencia C, Houdayer C, Bahuau M, Moretti-Forreira D, Richieri-Costa A, Dixon MJ, Murray JC. Mutations in IRF6 cause van der Woude and popliteal pterygium syndromes. Nat Genet 2002; 32:285–289.

65. Barrow LL, van Bokhaven H, Daack-Hirsch S, Andersen T, van Beersum SEC, Gorlin R, Murray JC. Analysis of the p63 gene in classical EEC syndrome, related syndromes, and non-syndromic orofacial clefts. J Med Genet 2002; 39:559–566.

66. Celli J, Duijf P, Hamel BCJ, Bamshad M, Kramer B, Smits APT, Newbury Ecob R, Hennekam RCM, Van Buggenhout G, van Haeringen A, Woods CG, van Essen AJ, de Waal R, Vriend G, Habar DA, Yang A, McKeon F, Brunner HG, van Bokhoven H. Heterozygous germline mutations in the p53 homolog p63 are the cause of EEC syndrome. Cell 1999; 99:143–153.

67. McGrath JA, Duijf PHG, Doetsch V, Irvine AD, de Waal R, Van Molkot KRJ, Wesagowit V, Kelly A, Atherton DJ, Griffiths WAD, Orlow SJ, van Haeringen A, Ausems MGEM, Yang A, McKeon F, Barnshad MA, Brunner HG, Hamel BCJ, van Bokhoven H. Hay-Wells syndrome is caused by heterozygous missense mutations in the SAM domain of p63. Hum Mol Genet 2001; 10:221–229.

68. Suzuki K, Hu D, Bustos T, Zlotagora J, Richieri-Costa A, Helms JA, Spritz RA. Mutations of PVRL1, encoding a cell–cell adhesion molecule/herpesvirus receptor, in cleft lip/palate-ectodermal dysplasia. Nat Genet 2000; 25:427–430.

69. van den Boogaard M-JH, Dorland M, Beemer FA, Ploos van Amstel HK. MSX1 mutation is associated with orofacial clefting and tooth agenesis in humans. Nat Genet 2000; 24:342–343.

70. Marçano ACB, Doudney K, Braybrook C, Squires R, Patton MA, Lees MM, Richieri-Costa A, Lidral AC, Murray JC, Moore GE, Stanier P. TBX22 mutations are a frequent cause of cleft palate. J Med Genet 2004; 41:68–74.

71. Murray JC. Candidate gene resequencing identifies gene variants in isolated cleft lip and palate. 25th Annual David W. Smith Workshop on Malformations and Morphogenesis, Snowbird Ski and Summer Resort, Utah, August 18–21, 2004.

72. Shprintzen RJ. Pierre Robin, micrognathia, and airway obstruction: the dependency of treatment on accurate diagnosis. Int Anesthesiol Clin 1988; 26:64–71.

73. Shprintzen RJ. The implications of the diagnosis of Robin sequence. Cleft Palate-Craniofac J 1992; 29:205–209.

74. Cohen MM Jr. Robin sequence and Robin complexes: Causal heterogeneity and pathogenetic/phenotypic variability. Am J Med Genet 1999; 84:311–315.

75. Cohen MM Jr. Interface between Robin sequence and ordinary cleft palate. Am J Med Genet 2001; 101:288.

76. Kreiborg S, Cohen MM Jr. Syndrome delineation and growth in orofacial clefting and craniosynostosis. In: Turvey TA, Vig VKL, Fonseca RJ, eds. Facial clefts and craniosynostosis: principles and management. Philadelphia: WB Saunders; 1996:57–75.

77. Pruzansky S. Not all dwarfed mandibles are alike. Birth Defects 1969; 5(2):120–129.

78. Arvystas M, Shprintzen RJ. Craniofacial morphology in the velocardiofacial syndrome. J Craniofac Genet Dev Biol 1984; 4:39–45.

79. Harding CO, Green CG, Perloff WH. Respiratory complications in children with spondyloepiphyseal dysplasia congenita. Pediatr Pulmonol 1990; 9:49–54.

80. Tessier P. Anatomical classifications of facial, cranio-facial and laterofacial clefts. J Max-Fac Surg 1976; 4:69–92.

81. Moore MH, David DJ, Cooter RD. Hairline indicators of craniofacial clefts. Plast Reconstr Surg 1988; 82:589–593.

Anencephaly

82. Lemire RJ, Beckwith JB, Warkany J. Anencephaly. New York: Raven Press, 1978.

83. Cohen MM Jr. Malformations of the craniofacial region: evolutionary, embryonic, genetic, and clinical perspectives. Am J Med Genet 2002; 115:245–268.

84. Fields HW Jr, Metzner L, Garol JD, Kokich VG. The craniofacial skeleton in anencephalic human fetuses. 1. Cranial floor. Teratology 1978; 17: 57–65.

Cephaloceles

85. Cohen MM Jr, Lemire RJ. Syndromes with cephaloceles. Teratology 1982; 25:161–172.

86. Hunter AGW. Brain and spinal cord. In: Stevenson RE, Hall JG, Goodman RM, eds. Human malformations and related anomalies. Vol. 2. New York: Oxford University Press; 1993:109–137.

87. Warkany J, Lemire RJ, Cohen MM Jr. mental retardation and congenital malformations of the central nervous system. Chicago: Year Book; 1981.

Frontonasal dysplasia

88. Cohen MM Jr, Sedano HO, Gorlin RJ, Jirasek JE. Frontonasal dysplasia (median cleft face syndrome): comments on etiology and pathogenesis. Birth Defects 1971; 7(7):117–119.

89. Guion-Almeida M-L, Richieri-Costa A, Saavedra D, Cohen MM Jr. Frontonasal dysplasia: analysis of 21 cases and literature review. Int J Oral Maxillofac Surg 1996; 25:91–97.

Holoprosencephaly

90. Pettersen JC. An anatomical study of two cases of cebocephaly. In: Bosma JR Jr, ed. Development of the basicranium. Publication No. (NIH) 76-989. Bethesda: US Department of Health, Education; 1981:240–265.

91. Cohen MM Jr. On the definition of holoprosencephaly. Am J Med Genet 2001; 103:183–187.

92. DeMyer WE, Zeman W, Palmer CG. The face predicts the brain: Diagnostic significance of median facial anomalies for holoprosencephaly (arrhinencephaly). Pediatrics 1964; 34:256–263.

93. Cohen MM Jr. Perspectives on holoprosencephaly. Part III. Spectra, distinctions, continuities, and discontinuities. Am J Med Genet 1989; 34:271–288.

94. DeMyer WE. Holoprosencephaly (cyclopia-arhinencephaly). In: Vinken PJ, Bruyn GW, eds. Handbook of clinical neurology. Amsterdam: North Holland Publishing; 1977: 431–478.

95. Cohen MM Jr, Jirasek JE, Guzman RT, Gorlin RJ, Peterson MQ. Holoprosencephaly and facial dysmorphia: Nosology, etiology and pathogenesis. Birth Defects 1971; 7(7):125–135.

96. Cohen MM Jr, Sulik KK. Perspectives on holoprosencephaly. Part II. Central nervous system, craniofacial anatomy, syndrome commentary, diagnostic approach, and experimental studies. J Craniofac Genet Dev Biol 1992; 12: 196–244.

97. Aylsworth AS, Hicks RPB, Drake AF. New observations in HPE: support for the hypothesis that congenital nasal pyriform aperture stenosis (CNPAS) is a phenotype at the mild end of the holoprosencephaly spectrum. 15th David W. Smith Workshop on Malformations and Morphogenesis. Tampa, Florida, August 4–9, 1994.

98. Berry SA, Pierpoint ME, Gorlin RJ. Single central incisor in familial holoprosencephaly. J Pediatr 1984; 104:877–880.

99. Gurrieri F, Trask BJ, van den Engh G, Krawss CM, Schinzel A, Pettenati MJ, Schindler D. Physical mapping of the holoprosencephaly critical region on chromosome 7q36. Nat Genet 1993; 3:247–251.

100. Hennekam RCM, Van Noort G, de la Fuente FA, Norbruis OF. Agenesis of the nasal septal cartilage: Another sign in autosomal dominant holoprosencephaly. Am J Med Genet 1991; 39:121–122.

101. Martin RA, Jones KL. Absence of the superior labial frenulum in holoprosencephaly: a new diagnostic sign. J Pediatr 1998; 133:151–153.

102. Martin RA, Jones KL, Benirshke K. Absence of the lateral philtral ridges: a clue to the structural basis of the philtrum. Am J Med Genet 1996; 65:117–123.

103. Cohen MM Jr. SHH and holoprosencephaly. In: Epstein CJ, Erickson RP, Wynshaw-Boris A, eds. Inborn errors of development. New York: Oxford University Press; 2004:240–248.

104. Cohen MM Jr. The hedgehog signaling network. Am J Med Genet A 2003; 123(1):5–28.

105. Cohen MM Jr. Craniofacial disorders. In: Rimoin DL, Connor JM, Pyeritz RE, Korf BR, eds. Emery and Rimoin's principles and practice of medical genetics. 4th edn. Vol. 3. London: Churchill Livingstone; 2002:3689–3727.

106. Benke PJ, Cohen MM Jr. Recurrence of holoprosencephaly in families with a positive history. Clin Genet 1983; 24:324–328.

107. Cohen MM Jr. Perspectives on holoprosencephaly. Part I. Epidemiology, genetics, and syndromology. Teratology 1989; 40:211–235.

108. Cohen MM Jr, Gorlin RJ. Genetic considerations in a sibship of cyclopia and clefts. Birth Defects Orig Art Ser V(2) 1969; 5(2):113–118.

109. Hockey A, Crowhurst J, Cullity G. Microcephaly, holoprosencephaly, hypokinesia: Second report of a new syndrome. Prenatal Diagn 1988; 8: 683–686.

110. Morse RP, Rawnsley E, Sargent SK, Graham JM Jr. Prenatal diagnosis of a new syndrome: Holoprosencephaly with hypokinesia. Prenatal Diagn 1987; 7:631–638.

111. Muenke M, Beachy PA. Holoprosencephaly. In: Scriver CR, Beaudet AL, Sly WS, Valle D, Childs B, Kinzler KW, Vogelstain B, eds. The metabolic and molecular bases of inherited disease. 8th edn. New York: McGraw-Hill; 2001; 6203–6230.

112. Belloni E, Muenke M, Roessler E. Identification of *Sonic Hedgehog* as a candidate gene responsible for holoprosencephaly. Nat Genet 1996; 14: 353–356.

113. Nanni L, Ming JE, Bocian M, Steinhaus K, Bianchi DW, Die-Smulders C, Gianotti A, Imaizumi K, Jones KL, Campo MD, Martin RA, Meinecke P, Pierpont MEM, Robin NH, Young ID, Roessler E, Muenke M. The mutational spectrum of the *Sonic Hedgehog* gene in holoprosencephaly: *SHH* mutations cause a significant proportion of autosomal dominant holoprosencephaly. Hum Mol Genet 1999; 8:2479–2488.

114. Roessler E, Belloni E, Gaudenz K, Jay P, Berta P, Scherer SW, Tsui L-C, Muenke M. Mutations in the human *Sonic Hedgehog* gene cause holoprosencephaly. Nat Genet 1996; 14:357–360.

115. Roessler E, Belloni E, Gaudenz K, Vargus F, Scherer SW, Tsui L-C, Muenke M. Mutations in the C-terminal domain of *Sonic Hedgehog* cause holoprosencephaly. Hum Mol Genet 1997; 6:1847–1853.

116. Ming JE, Kaupas ME, Roessler E, Brunner HG, Golabi M, Stratton RF, Sujansky E, Bale SJ, Muenke M. Mutations in *Patched-1*, the receptor for Sonic Hedgehog, are associated with holoprosencephaly. Hum Genet 2002; 110:297–301.

117. Roessler E, Du Y, Mullor JL, Casas E, Allen WP, Ellis I, Gillessen-Kaesbach G, Roeder E, Ming JE, Ruizi Altaba A. Loss-of-function mutations in the human GLI2 gene cause holoprosencephaly and familial pan-hyopituitarism. 52nd Annual Meeting of the American Society of Human Genetics, Baltimore, Maryland. October 15–19 2002; Abstract 132:190.

118. Kelley RI, Roessler E, Hennekam RCM, Fledman GL, Kogaki K, Jones MC, Palumbos JC, Muenke M. Holoprosencephaly in RSH/Smith-Lemli-Opitz syndrome: does abnormal cholesterol metabolism affect the function of *Sonic Hedgehog*? Am J Med Genet 1996; 66:478–484.

119. Wassif CA, Maslen C, Kachilele-Linjewile S, Lin D, Linck TM, Connor WE, Steiner RD, Porter FD. Mutations in the human *sterol Δ^7-reductase* gene at 11q12-13 cause Smith-Lemli-Opitz syndrome. Am J Hum Genet 1998; 63:55–62.

120. Witsch-Baumgartner M, Fitzky BU, Ogorelkova M, Kraft HG, Moebius FF, Glossmann H, Seedorf U, Gillessen-Kaesbach G, Hoffmann GF, Clayon P. Mutational spectrum in the Δ^7-*sterol reductase* gene and genotype-phenotype correlation in 84 patients with Smith-Lemli-Opitz syndrome. Am J Hum Genet 2000; 66:402–412.

121. Yu H, Lee M-H, Starck L, Elias ER, Irons M, Salen G, Patel SB, Tint GS. Spectrum of $\Delta 7$-*dehydrocholesterol reductase* mutations in patients with the Smith-Lemli-Opitz (RSH) syndrome. Hum Mol Genet 2000; 9:1385–1391.

122. Brown LY, Odent S, David V, Blayau M, Dubourg C, Apacik C, Delgado MA, Hall BD, Reynolds JF, Sommer A, Wieczorek D, Brown SA, Muenke M. Holoprosencephaly due to mutations in ZIC2: Alanine tract expansion

mutations may be caused by parental somatic recombination. Hum Mol Genet 2001; 10:791–796.

123. Brown SA, Warburton D, Brown LY, Yu C-Y, Roeder ER, Stengel-Rutkowski S, Hennekam REM, Meunke M. Holoprosencephaly due to mutations in *ZIC2*, a homologue of *Drosophila odd-paired*. Nat Genet 1998; 20:180–183.

124. Brewster R, Lee J, Ruiz i Altaba A. Gli/Zic factors pattern the neural plate by defining domains of cell differentiation. Nature 1998; 393:579–583.

125. Koyabu Y, Nakata K, Mizugishi K, Aruga J, Mikoshiba K. Physical and functional interactions between Zic and Gli proteins. J Biol Chem 2001; 276:6889–6892.

126. de la Cruz JM, Bamford RN, Burdine RD, Roessler E, Barkovich AJ, Donnai D, Schier AF, Muenke M. A loss-of-function mutation in the CPC domain of *TDGF1* is associated with human forebrain defects. Hum Genet 2002; 110:422–428.

127. Gripp KW, Wotton D, Edwards MC, Roessler E, Adès L, Meinecke P, Richieri-Costa A, Zackai EH, Massagué J, Muenke M. Mutations in *TGIF* cause holoprosencephaly and link NODAL signalling to human neural axis determination. Nat Genet 2000; 25:205–208.

128. Ouspenskaia MV, Karkera JD, Roessler E, Shen MM, Goldmunts E, Bowers P, Towbin J, Belmont J, Muenke M. Role of *FAST1* gene in the development of holoprosencephaly (HPE) and congenital cardiac malformations in humans. 52nd Annual Meeting of the American Society of Human Genetics, Baltimore, Maryland. October 15–19 2002; Abstract 822:313.

129. Wallis DE, Roessler E, Hehr U, Nanni L, Wiltshire T, Richieri-Costa A, Gillessen-Kaesbach G, Zackai EH, Romens J, Muenke M. Mutations in the homeodomain of the human *SIX3* gene cause holoprosencephaly. Nat Genet 1999; 22:196–198.

130. Barr M Jr, Hanson JW, Currey K, Sharp S, Toriello H, Schmickel RD, Wilson GN. Holoprosencephaly in infants of diabetic mothers. J Pediatr 1983; 102:565–568.

131. Cohen MM Jr, Shiota K. Teratogenesis of holoprosencephaly. Am J Med Genet 2002; 109:1–15.

Craniosynostosis

132. Cohen MM Jr, MacLean RE. Craniosynostosis: diagnosis, evaluation and management. 2nd edn. New York: Oxford University Press; 2000.

133. Cohen MM Jr, Kreiborg S. An updated pediatric perspective on the Apert syndrome. Am J Dis Child 1993; 147:989–993.

134. Cohen MM Jr, Kreiborg S. Suture formation, premature sutural fusion, and suture default zones in Apert syndrome. Am J Med Genet 1996; 62:339–344.

135. Kreiborg S, Marsh JL, Cohen MM Jr, Liversage M, Pedersen H, Skovby F, Børgesen SE, Vannier MW. The calvaria and cranial base in Apert and Crouzon syndromes: A three-dimensional CT analysis. J Craniomaxillofac Surg 1993; 21:181–188.

136. Lajeunie E, Le Merrer M, Bonaïti-Pellie C, Marchac D, Renier D. Genetic study of nonsyndromic coronal craniosynostosis. Am J Med Genet 1995; 55:500–504.

137. Lajeunie E, Le Merrer M, Bonaïti-Pellie C, Marchac D, Renier D. Genetic study of scaphocephaly. Am J Med Genet 1996; 62:282–285.

138. Lajeunie E, Arnaud E, Le Merrer M, Cinalli G, Marchac D, Renier D. Syndromal and nonsyndromal primary trigonocephaly: Analysis of a series of 237 patients. Am J Med Genet 1988; 75:211–215.

139. Cohen MM Jr. FGFs/FGFRs and associated disorders. In: Epstein CJ, Erickson RP, Wynshaw-Boris A, eds. Inborn errors of development. New York: Oxford University Press; 2004:380–400.

140. Oldridge M, Lunt PW, Zackai EH, McDonald-McGinn DM, Muenke M, Moloney DM, Twigg SRF, Heath JK, Howard TD, Hoganson G, Gagnon DM, Jabs EW, Wilkie AOM. Genotype-phenotype correlations for nucleotide substitutions in the IgII-IgIII linker of FGFR2. Hum Mol Genet 1997; 6:137–143.

141. Wilkie AOM, Slaney SF, Oldridge M, Poole MD, Ashworth GJ, Hockley AD, Hayward RD, David DJ, Pulleyn LJ, Rutland P, Malcom S,

Winter RM, Reardon W. Apert syndrome results from localized mutations of *FGFR2* and is allelic with Crouzon syndrome. Nat Genet 1995; 9:165–172.

142. Wilkie AOM, Wall SA. Craniosynostosis: novel insights into pathogenesis and treatment. Curr Opin Neurol 1996; 9:146–152.

143. Cohen ME, Paznekas WA, Francis, MK, Jabs EW. Effect of human *TWIST* mutations in Saethre-Chotzen syndrome on TWIST protein dimerization. American Society of Human Genetics, 49th Annual Meeting, San Francisco, California, October 19–23, 1999.

144. Jabs EW, Müller U, Li X, Ma I, Luo W, Haworth IS, Kisak I, Sparkes R, Warman ML, Mulliken JB, Snead ML, Maxson R. A mutation in the homeodomain of the human *MSX2* gene in a family affected with autosomal dominant craniosynostosis. Cell 1993; 75:443–450.

145. Müller U, Warman ML, Mulliken JB, Weber JL. Assignment of a gene locus involved in craniosynostosis to chromosome 5qter. Hum Mol Genet 1993; 2:119–122.

146. Warman ML, Mulliken JB, Hayward PG, Müller U. Newly recognized autosomal dominant disorder with craniosynostosis. Am J Med Genet 1993; 46:444–449.

147. Twigg SRF, Kan R, Babbs C, Bochukova EG, Robertson SP, Wall SA, Morriss-Kay GM, Wilkie AOM. Mutations of ephrin-B1 (*EFNB1*), a marker of tissue boundary formation, cause craniofrontonasal syndrome. PNAS 2004; 101:8652–8657.

148. OMIM (Online Mendelian Inheritance in Man), 2004.

Cleidocranial dysplasia

149. Cohen MM Jr. Merging the old skeletal biology with the new. II. Molecular aspects of bone formation and bone growth. J Craniofac Genet Dev Biol 2000; 20:94–106.

150. Cohen MM Jr. *RUNX* genes, neoplasia, and cleidocranial dysplasia. Am J Med Genet 2001; 104–108.

151. Mundlos S. Cleidocranial dysplasia: clinical and molecular genetics. J Med Genet 1999; 36:177–182.

152. Mundlos A, Otto F, Mundlos C, Mulliken JB, Aylsworth AS, Albright S, Lindhout D, Cole WG, Henn W, Knoll JHM, Owen MJ, Mertelsmann R, Zabel BU Olsen BR. Mutations involving the transcription factor CBFA1 cause cleidocranial dysplasia. Cell 1997; 89:773–779.

Branchial arch syndromes

153. Cohen MM Jr, Rollnick BR, Kaye CL. Oculoauriculovertebral spectrum: an updated critique. Cleft Palate J 1989; 26:276–286.

154. Edwards SJ, Gladwin AJ, Dixon MJ. The mutational spectrum in Treacher Collins syndrome reveals a predominance of mutations that create a premature termination codon. Am J Hum Genet 1997; 60:515–524.

155. Gladwin AJ, Dixon J, Loftus SK, Edwards S, Wasmuth JJ, Hennekam RCM, Dixon MJ. Treacher Collins syndrome may result from insertion, deletion, or splicing mutations, which introduce a termination codon into the gene. Hum Mol Genet 1996; 5:1533–1538.

156. Treacher Collins Syndrome Collaborative Group. Positional cloning of a gene involved in the pathogenesis of Treacher Collins syndrome. Nat Genet 1996; 12:130–136.

Vascular tumors and malformations

157. Mulliken JB, Glowacki J. Hemangiomas and vascular malformations in infants and children: A classification based on endothelial characteristics. Plast Reconstr Surg 1982; 69:412–422.

158. Mulliken JB. Cutaneous vascular anomalies. Semin Vasc Surg 1993; 6:204–218.

159. Mulliken JB. Vascular anomalies. In: Aston SJ, Beasley RW, Thorne CHM, eds. Grabb and Smith's plastic surgery. 5th edn. Philadelphia: Lippincott-Raven; 1997:191.

160. Enjolras O, Mulliken JB. Vascular tumors and vascular malformations. Adv Dermatol 1998; 13:375–423.

161. Burns AJ, Kaplan LC, Mulliken JB. Is there an association between hemangioma and syndromes with dysmorphic features? Pediatrics 1991; 88:1257–1267.

162. Cohen MM Jr. Vasculogenesis, angiogenesis, hemangiomas, and vascular malformations. Am J Med Genet 2002; 108:265–274.

163. Cohen MM Jr, Neri G, Weksberg R. Overgrowth syndromes. New York: Oxford University Press; 2002.

164. Cohen MM Jr. Vascular update: Morphogenesis, tumors, malformations, and molecular dimensions. Am J Med Genet 2006; 140A:2013–2038.

165. Williams HB. Hemangiomas of the parotid gland in children. Plast Reconstr Surg 1975; 56:29–34.

Disorders of the anterior thoracic and abdominal walls

21

Luc L. Oligny

No man is an Island, entire of itself; every man is a piece of the Continent, a part of the main; if a clod be washed away by the sea, Europe is the less, as well as if a promontory were, as well as if a manor of thy friends or of thine own were; any man's death diminishes me, because I am involved in Mankind; And therefore never send to know for whom the bell tolls; It tolls for thee. John Donne Devotions XVII

Folding of the embryo (fourth week)

At the end of the 3rd week post conception (pc),* the embryo is a flat structure formed of three layers, the ectoblast, mesoblast and endoblast. At this stage, the heart and future brain are rostral to the future mouth, the buccopharyngeal membrane (Fig. 21.1A). During the 4th week, this tridermic disk undergoes **cephalocaudal and lateral folding,** due to asymmetric growth and increased amniotic fluid pressure (Fig. 21.1B–D). Folding proceeds simultaneously from cranial, caudal, and lateral extremities, centering on the site of the future umbilical ring. Folding is complete by day 28, and results in the outer surface of the embryo being covered by ectoblast except at the level of the umbilical ring, while the endoblast forms a central tube spanning the length of the embryo. At the end of the 4th week, the final 'brain–mouth–heart' topography is established.

---

*Unless otherwise specified, all developmental landmarks mentioned in this chapter are calculated from the time of conception. Gestational age can be calculated by adding two weeks to the pc age.

Normal development of the anterior thoracic wall

The cephalic fold generates the primordium of the thorax and of the epigastric portion of the abdominal wall. During the 6th week, the dorsolateral mesoderm infiltrates the lateral and anterior body wall. Extensions of the lateral vertebral processes (of somitic origin) accompany this mesodermal extension, forming the future ribs.[1]

The **septum transversum** develops during the 4th week, as a mesodermal bridge between the pericardial cavity and the yolk sac (Fig. 21.1B2–D2). Its cranial portion becomes covered by pericardium and pleura, and the liver grows towards and into its dorsocaudal portion. The septum transversum generates most of the **diaphragm.**[1]

The dorsolateral mesoderm separates into three layers, the external and the internal intercostal muscles, and an innermost layer, the transverse thoracic muscle, which probably contributes to the formation of the diaphragm, in conjunction with the septum transversum. These three layers are all formed by the middle of the 7th week.[2]

In the anterior thoracic region, two longitudinal parallel bands of mesenchyme condense in the cephalocaudal axis and chondrify during the 6th week, forming the **sternal bands**

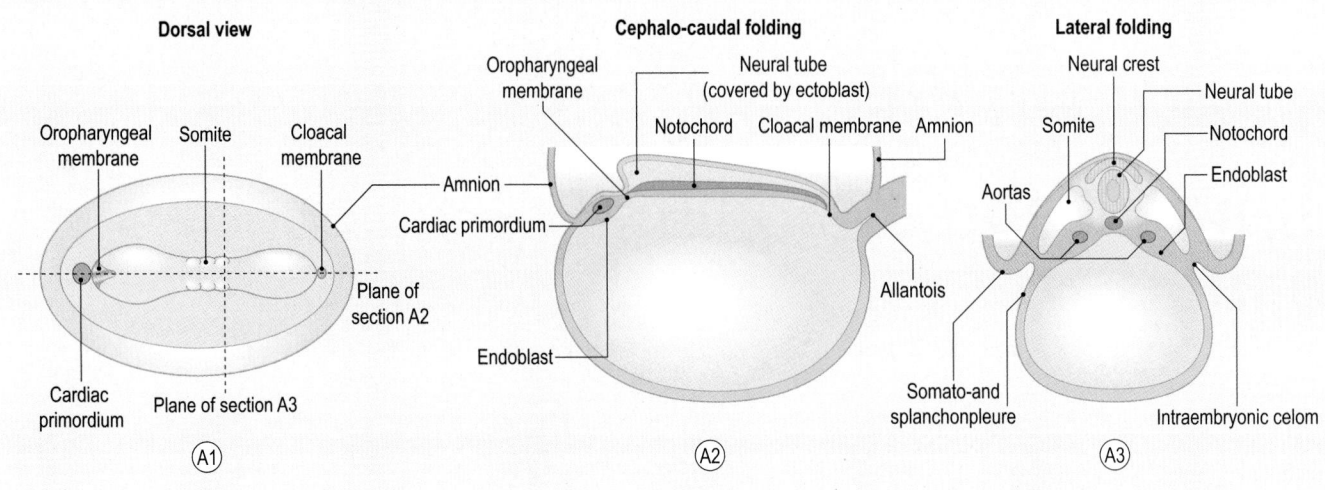

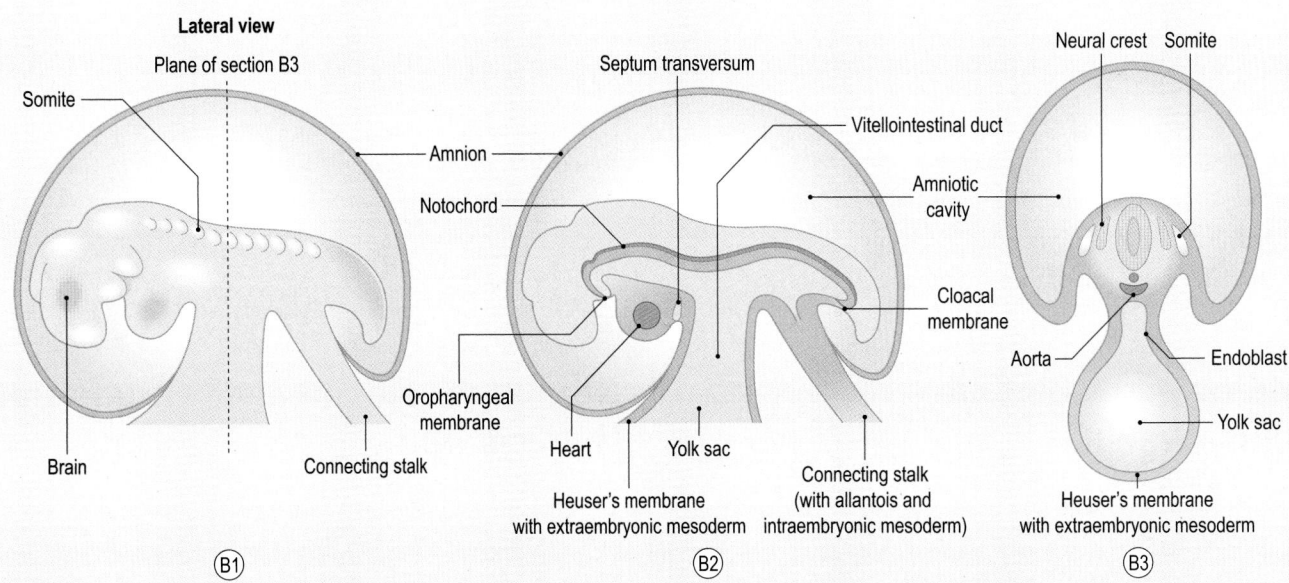

FIGURE 21.1 Development of the embryo during the 4th week post conception. Diagrams A2 and B2 represent, respectively, a longitudinal and a transverse section of the embryo, in the planes indicated on A. Diagrams A through D correspond to approximately 22, 24, 26, and 28 days. The growth of the amniotic cavity is responsible for the lateral folding, whereas the caudocephalic fold is caused by a faster growth of the dorsal surface compared to the ventral plane. (From Essentiel d'embryologie humaine et principes d'embryogenèse moléculaire, © Luc L. Oligny, 2005. Used with permission.)

(Fig. 21.2A). Meanwhile, the paraxial mesoderm generates the **ribs,** which grow out from the thoracic vertebrae, and curve lateromedially towards the sternal bands. Like all bones, the ribs are initially made of cartilage which subsequently ossifies. During the 7th week, the two sternal bands start to fuse at their cephalic ends, and fusion then extends caudally to form the **sternum** (Fig. 21.2B). The cephalocaudal fusion is completed by the 10th week. Ossification of the sternum begins in the 7th month, and progresses until after puberty.[2]

During the 6th week, two lateral ectodermic ridges develop between the upper and lower limb buds, forming the **milk lines** (also called **milk ridges** or **lines of Spence**) which span between the superior-most portion of the axillae to the upper inner thighs (Fig. 21.3A). These lines involute after only a few days, except at the level of the upper chest where the **breast or mammary primordia** form by the 50th day pc (Fig. 21.3B); note that in humans, chronology of breast development is quite variable. Between the 10th and 19th week, only the nipple

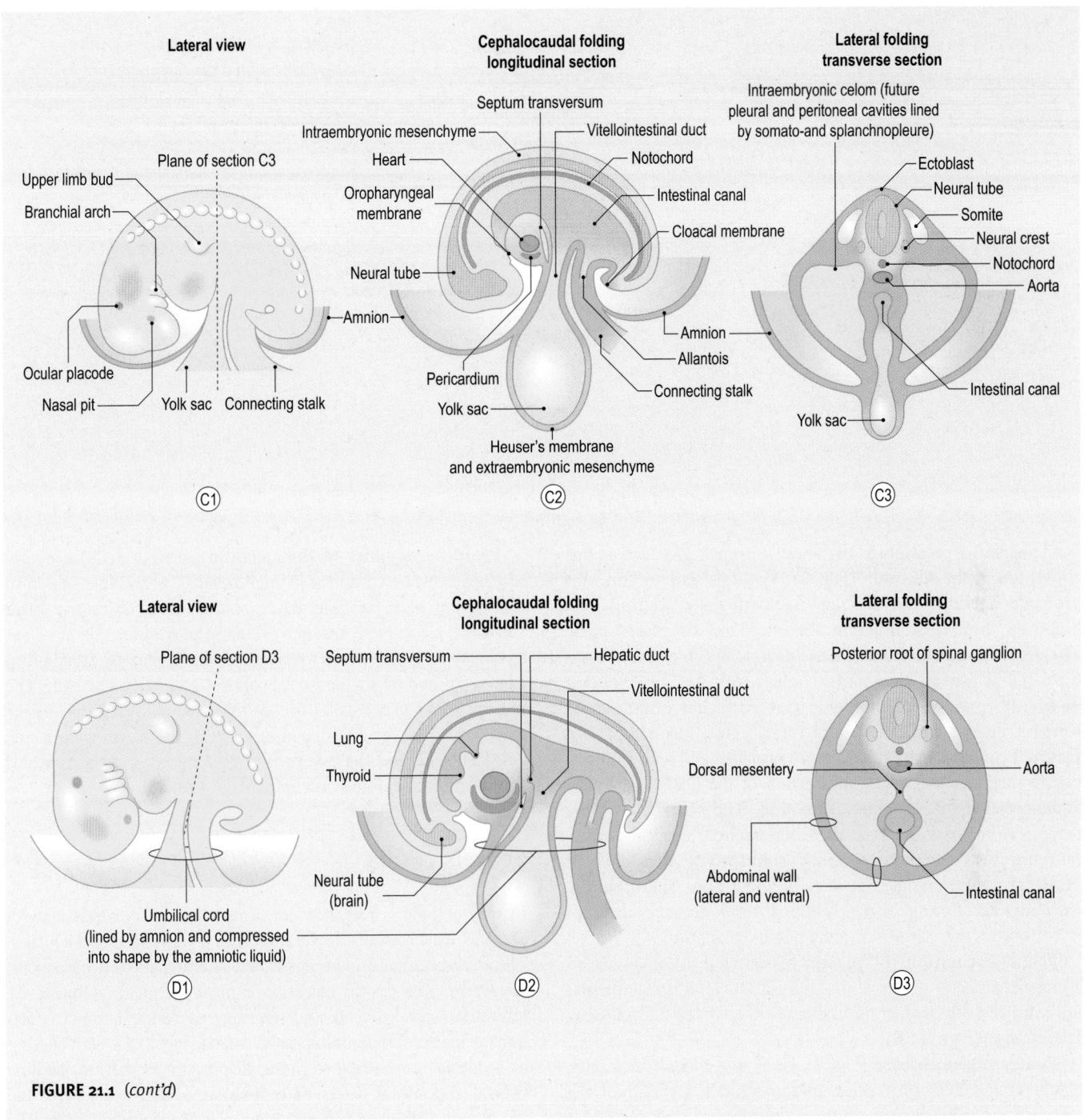

FIGURE 21.1 *(cont'd)*

precursors, the **primary buds,** are evident, not much larger than hair follicles. Between the 19th and 23rd weeks, the basal cells of the primary buds grow within the dermis and subcutaneous mesenchymal tissue, producing 16–24 cords of cells (the **secondary epithelial outgrowths**) which will generate the lactiferous ducts. Near term, the secondary outgrowths have repeatedly branched and become fully canalized; the glands may be secretory due to complex fetal, placental, and maternal endocrine interplay. A morphologic and molecular characterization of human breast development, with special emphasis on the epithelial–myoepithelial–stromal interactions involved, has been reviewed by Jolicoeur.[3,4]

Congenital chest abnormalities
Abnormalities of the sternum

Pectus excavatum (or **funnel chest,** Fig. 21.4A,B) results from an abnormal sternum which is displaced dorsally, leading to a

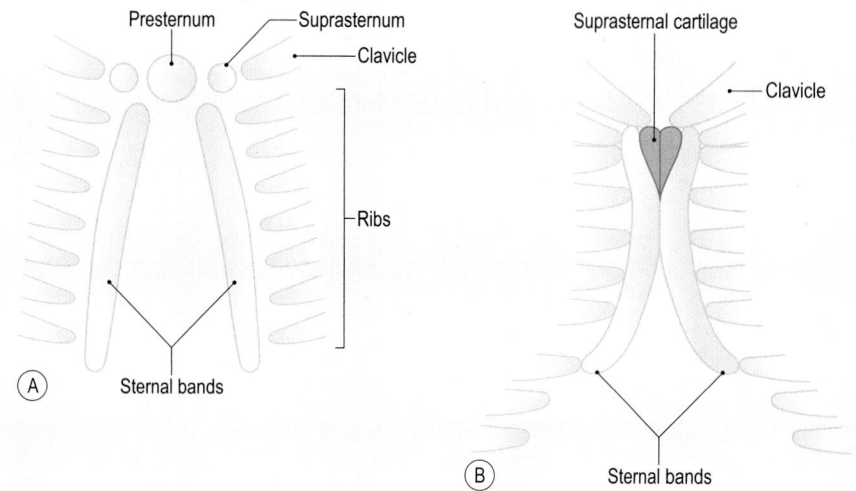

FIGURE 21.2 Development of the sternum. (A) Mesenchymal stage, 6th week. The two paired lateral sternal bands arise independently. (B) Cartilaginous stage, 9th week. The sternal bands have fused with one another and with the suprasternal cartilage medially, and with the ribs laterally. (From Essentiel d'embryologie humaine et principes d'embryogenèse moléculaire, © Luc L. Oligny, 2005. Used with permission.)

cone-shaped depression of the chest, the apex of which is just above the xiphi sternum (Fig. 21.5A). The 3rd to 8th ribs protrude laterally and are depressed medially, leading to a hollowed chest, a protuberant abdomen and a rounded back. The depression may be symmetric or not, and in extreme cases the xiphoid process may be in contact with the spine. Pectus excavatum may or not be evident at birth, but progressively worsens during childhood, and rarely cause respiratory and cardiac problems (e.g., mitral valve prolapse and arrhythmias) due to displacement and compression of the heart and lungs, and restricted diaphragmatic function. The severity of these complications may increase after adolescence. Surgical correction improves the hemodynamic status.[2] The **incidence** of pectus excavatum ranges between 0.1 and 0.4 per 1000 children, with **boys** accounting for nearly 80% of cases. Pectus excavatum is 5–10 times more common than pectus carinatum.

Pectus carinatum (or **pigeon breast,** Fig. 21.4C,D) is an abnormal anterior protrusion of the chest wall. It is usually first noted in the 6th year, progressing with age, especially during adolescence (Fig. 21.5B).

Pouter pigeon breast (Fig; 21.4E,F) is a mixed deformity, characterized by a protrusion of the cephalic portion of the sternum and a depression of the caudal sternum (Fig. 21.5C).

The **pathogenesis** of pectus excavatum and carinatum is not clear, but two mechanical factors are clearly involved: overgrowth of the ribs, and pull of the diaphragm.[2] Although generally sporadic, the isolated form of pectus excavatum can be transmitted in an autosomal dominant fashion (the pectus excavatum syndrome, MIM 169300); pectus excavatum can occur in more than 100 syndromes (e.g., Pierre Robin sequence with pectus excavatum and rib and scapular anomalies, MIM 602196; pectus excavatum, macrocephaly, short stature and dysplastic nails syndrome, MIM 600399). Likewise, pectus carinatum can be familial, being part of more than 70 syndromes, including collagenopathies.

Fusion anomalies of the sternum (sternal clefts) are very rare, and can be complete or incomplete. Incomplete fusion of the sternal bars (see Fig. 21.2) results in an inferiorly **bifid sternum;** a complete absence of fusion of the sternal bars gives rise to **two independent sternums,** each normally attached to ribs, separated by a wide gap of soft tissues covered by skin. The majority of sternal clefts are sporadic, but syndromic forms exist (e.g., the giant congenital aortic aneurysm syndrome, MIM 604622; and the cavernous hemangiomas of the face and supraumbilical raphe syndrome, MIM 140850).

Ectopia cordis

In true ectopia cordis, the sternum is at least partially clefted, and the heart lies outside the chest wall (eventration of the heart). Associated cardiac and other visceral malformations are frequent; interventricular septal defects are most frequent, followed by interatrial septal defects and tetralogy of Fallot. Ectopia cordis may be part of the **pentalogy of Cantrell** (Fig. 21.6), with clefting or agenesis of the distal sternum, diaphragmatic hernia, midline ventral abdominal defect or omphalocele, and a defect of the apical pericardium causing its communication with the peritoneal cavity. The five 'diagnostic' criteria are only found in 60% of cases; the remainder present only four of these criteria, yet they share the same pathogenesis, i.e., an abnormal development of the septum transversum during the 4th week pc. In rare families, the pentalogy of Cantrell has an X-linked recessive transmission, being part of the **thoracoabdominal syndrome** (MIM 313850). It is also found in trisomy 18, albeit rarely.[5]

Ectopia cordis is classified according to the location of the heart: (1) 3% are **cervical,** with the heart displaced in the neck; (2) 64% are **thoracic,** with the heart lying anterior to the sternum; (3) 18% are **thoracoabdominal** with the heart located between the thorax and abdomen (see pentalogy of Cantrell,

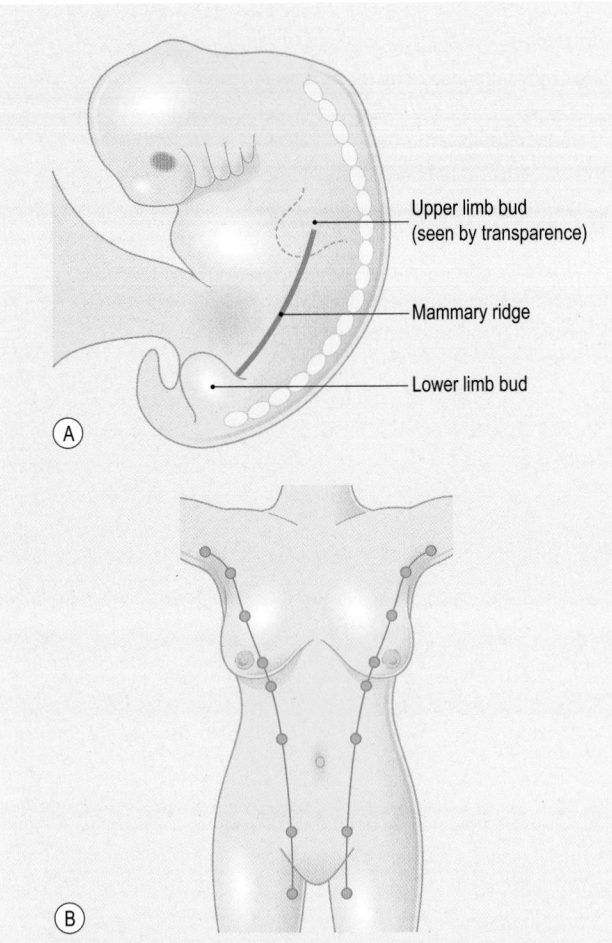

FIGURE 21.3 The milk line. (A). Mammary ridge in a 6-week embryo, arising immediately caudal to the upper limb bud, and extending to the lower limb bud. (B) Sketch of the mammary line in women (in pink), arising from the axillae and extending to the inner thighs. Ectopic nipples and breasts may develop anywhere along this line; most common sites shown in red. (From Essentiel d'embryologie humaine et principes d'embryogenèse moléculaire, © Luc L. Oligny, 2005. Used with permission.)

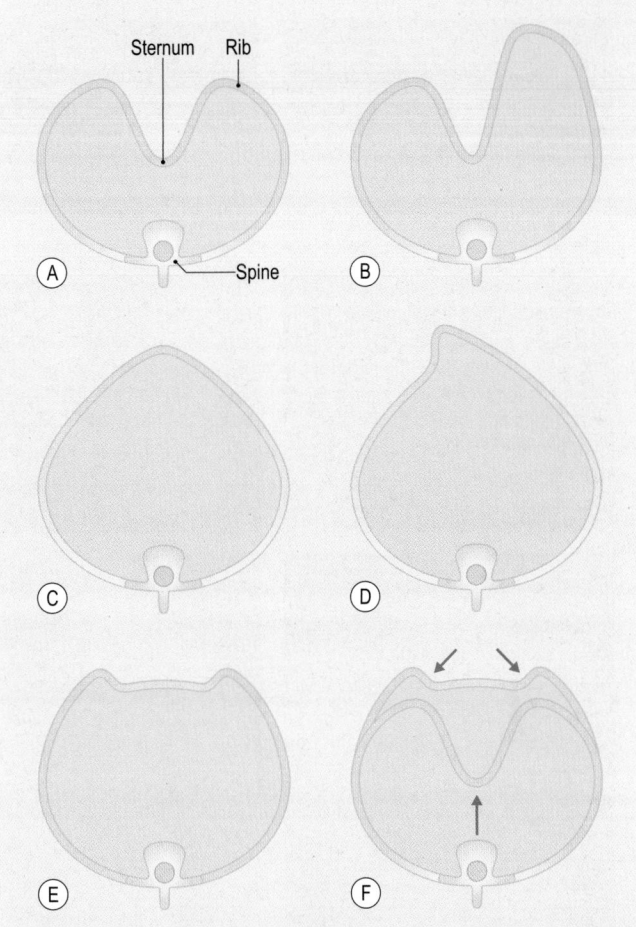

FIGURE 21.4 Diagrammatic representation of chest deformities represented in cross sections. (A and B) Symmetric and asymmetric pectus excavatum. (C and D) Symmetric and asymmetric pectus carinatum. (E) Bilateral protrusion of the ribs, with midline depression of the sternum. (F) Mixed deformity, with bilateral chondromanubrial protrusions (black arrows) and a midline gladiolar depression (red arrow); note that two levels of cross-section are shown on the same diagram. (Figures redrawn and adapted from Skandalakis and Gray.[2])

above); and (4) 15% are **abdominal,** the heart lying within the abdominal cavity.[2] Cervical and thoracic ectopias may occur without an associated sternal cleft. A body wall fusion defect extending to the umbilicus, and cardiac malformations, are generally present in thoracoabdominal ectopia. The heart is uncovered in 40% of cases, covered with a serous membrane in 30%, and covered by skin in 30%.[2] Mortality is high, especially in the cervical form and when associated with severe malformations of the heart and/or other systems.

Ectopia cordis is thought to be secondary to an abnormal cephalic folding of the embryo (4th week; see Fig. 21.1A–C), at least in some cases; the sternal cleft likely results from the primary cardiac eventration. Ectopia cordis must be differentiated from

the amnion rupture sequence and the limb body wall complex (see below).

Abnormalities of the clavicles

Clavicular hypoplasia/aplasia presents with sloped or rounded, narrow shoulders and a long neck; the extreme hypermobility of the shoulders allows painless approximation in the anterior midline. Palpation and X-rays confirm the diagnosis. The defect is only rarely unilateral, and affects both males and females. Syndromic forms must be excluded (e.g., the autosomal dominant forms of cleidocranial dysplasias, MIM 119600 and 168500; the

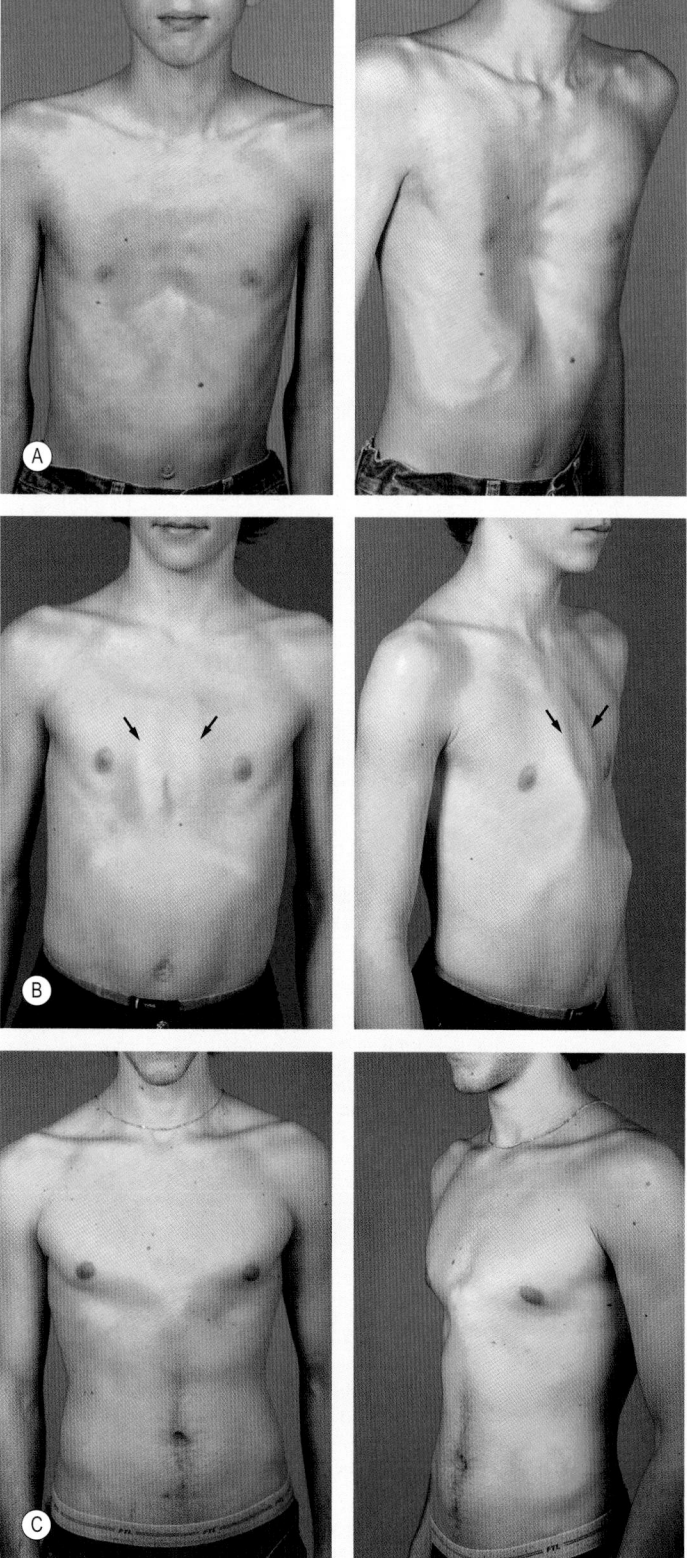

FIGURE 21.5 Pectus excavatum and carinatum. (A1 and A2) Twelve-year-old boy with the most frequent form of pectus excavatum: the thorax is symmetric, with a depression in the inferior portion of the sternum. (B1 and B2) Thirteen-year-old boy with pectus carinatum. Bilateral depressions are seen laterally to the cartilage (arrows) of the costochondral junction which is bilaterally hypertrophic; the sternum projects anteriorly. (C1 and C2) Twenty-year-old with a mixed deformity, the superior portion of the sternum being depressed while the inferior portion is elevated. (Pictures courtesy of Dr. Dickens St-Vil.)

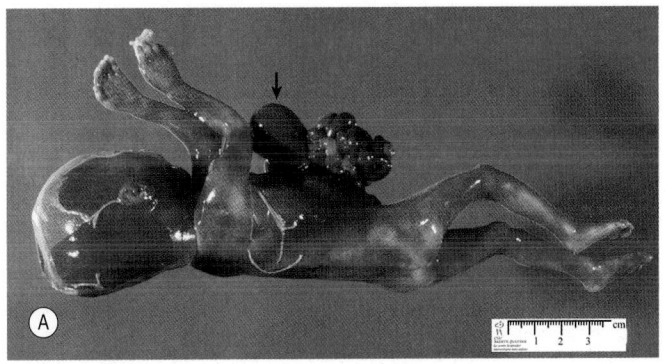
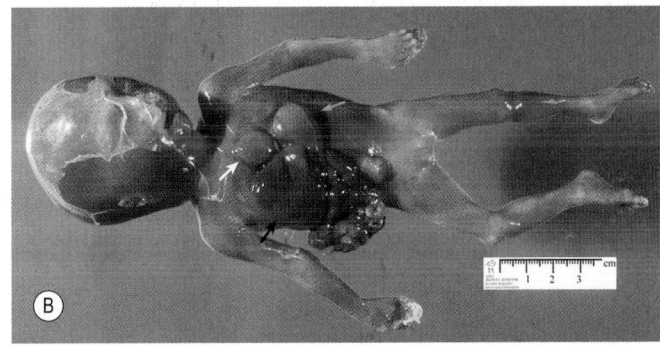

FIGURE 21.6 (A and B) Pentalogy of Cantrell in a female fetus of 18 weeks' gestation weighing 195 g. In addition to the ectopia cordis (white arrow), a gastroschisis is present, with exteriorization of the liver (black arrows), intestines and stomach (green arrow). A left diaphragmatic hernia was also found (not shown).

autosomal recessive form of cleidocranial dysplasia, MIM 216330; karyotypic anomalies such as partial trisomy 11q and trisomy 20p).[6]

In **clavicular pseudarthrosis,** the middle segment of the clavicle fails to develop and is often replaced by fibrous tissue, while the extremities are generally enlarged. It is usually asymptomatic. The majority are right-sided; 10% are bilateral. When left-sided, it may be associated with dextrocardia. Most cases are sporadic, but syndromic autosomal dominant (e.g., Kabuki syndrome, MIM 147920) and X-linked transmission (e.g., craniofrontonasal syndrome, MIM 304110) are known.

The **clavicle can be abnormally shaped** (broad or thick, thin or gracile, laterally hooked) in many syndromes.

Abnormalities of the ribs

The **ribs** at the level of the **sternal costochondral junctions** can be malformed, deformed, absent, or show fusion defects. These anomalies may be isolated or associated with soft tissue anomalies.

Rib malformations may be associated with other skeletal and soft tissue abnormalities. Absent, fused, and supernumerary ribs are relatively frequent, and generally represent incidental radiological findings, but may be associated with paradoxic movements of the chest, arrhythmias, and respiratory problems. Geographic variations are important, with rib anomalies found in 0.15–3.4% of individuals in the United States, and in 10.4% of Samoans.[6] Morphologic abnormalities **can be syndromic** (e.g., rickets, collagenopathies such as osteogenesis imperfecta (Fig. 21.7), lysosomopathies, basal cell carcinoma syndrome, multiple pterygium syndrome, etc.).

The incidence of cervical ribs is 1% in females and 0.4% in males. **Cervical ribs** generally arise from the 7th cervical vertebra; more cephalic cervical ribs are less common. The majority are asymptomatic, most are bilateral but not usually symmetrical. Rarely, they present due to **compression** of the subclavian artery, of somatic branches of the brachial plexus, and/or of sympathetic nerves, but compression by the hypertrophied anterior scalene may be more problematic, since not all cases of such compressions have an associated cervical rib.[6] Most

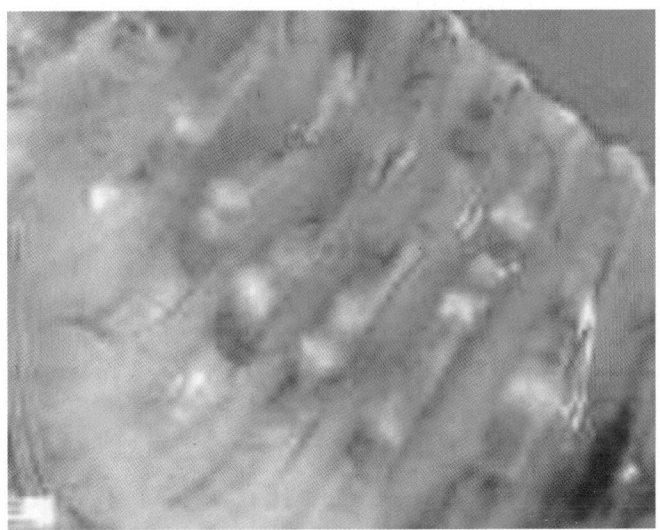

FIGURE 21.7 Ribs with multiple fractures due to osteogenesis imperfecta in a fetus of 20 weeks' gestational age.

cases are sporadic, but some cases have an autosomal dominant transmission with variable expressivity and reduced penetrance (MIM 117900). Cervical ribs can also be syndromic (e.g., Simpson-Golabi-Behmel, MIM 312870, described in more detail in Overgrowth Syndromes, Ch. 41; cervical ribs with Sprengel anomaly, anal atresia and urethral obstruction, MIM 601389; basal cell nevus syndrome, MIM 109400; Noonan syndrome, MIM 163950; HOX-D4 syndrome associated with a susceptibility to acute lymphoblastic leukemia, MIM 142981).

Poland syndrome

Poland syndrome (MIM 173800) is rare, with an incidence of 1 in 7000 to 1 in 100 000 live births,[7] and is characterized by a **unilateral absence or hypoplasia of the pectoralis muscle,** most frequently involving the sternocostal portion of the pectoralis major (Fig. 21.8). A variable degree of ipsilateral hand and digit anomalies is found,[8] including syndactyly and/or brachydactyly

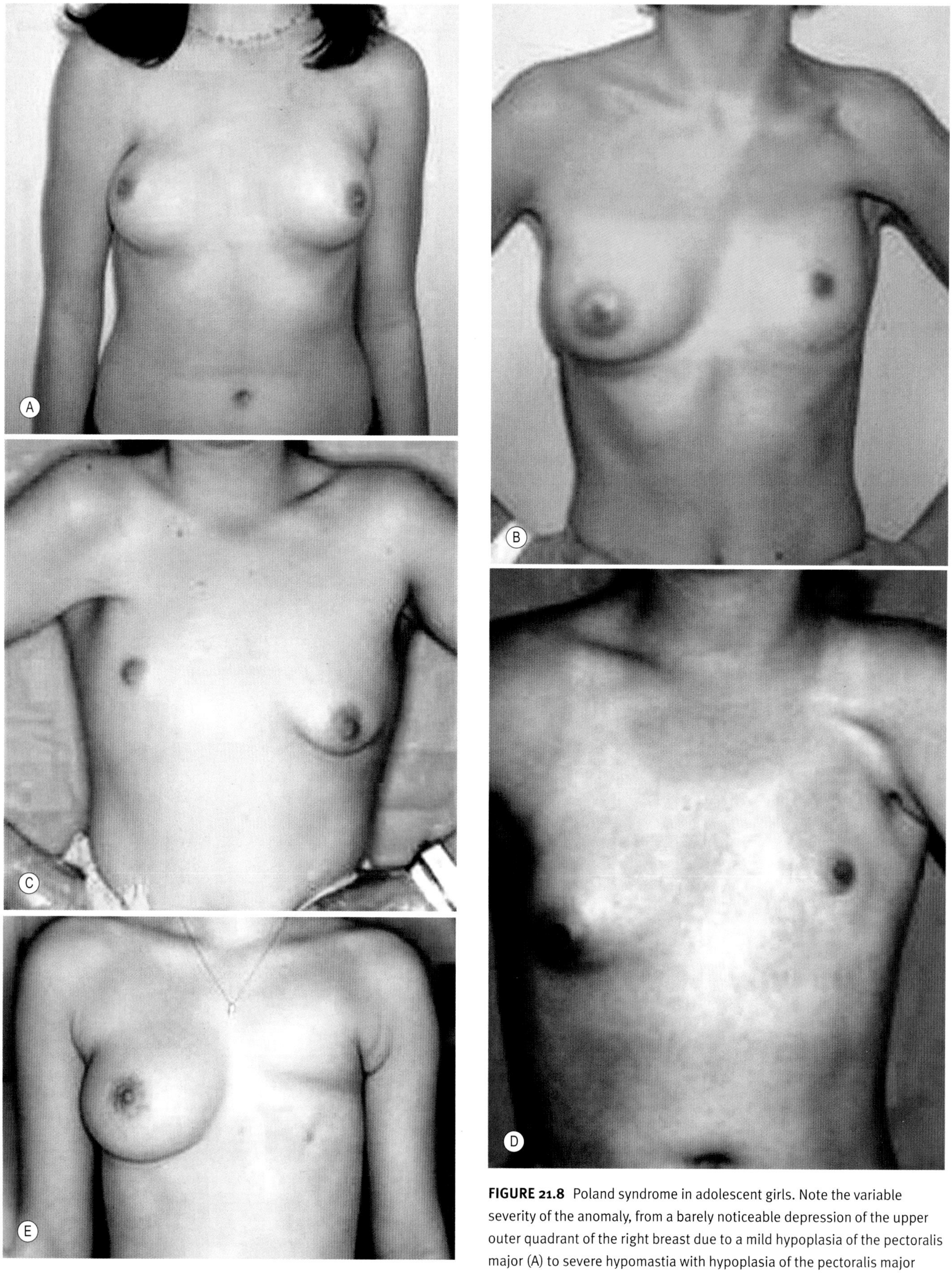

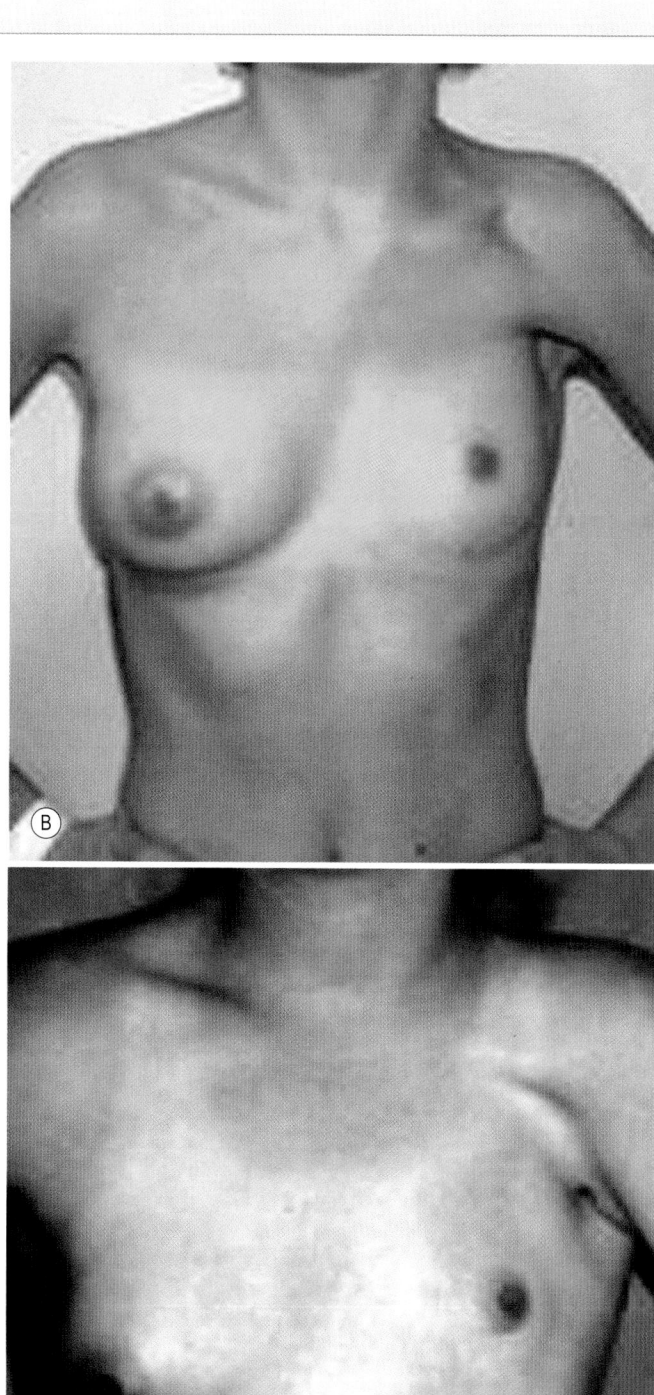

FIGURE 21.8 Poland syndrome in adolescent girls. Note the variable severity of the anomaly, from a barely noticeable depression of the upper outer quadrant of the right breast due to a mild hypoplasia of the pectoralis major (A) to severe hypomastia with hypoplasia of the pectoralis major muscle (E). (Courtesy of Dr. Louise Caouette-Laberge.)

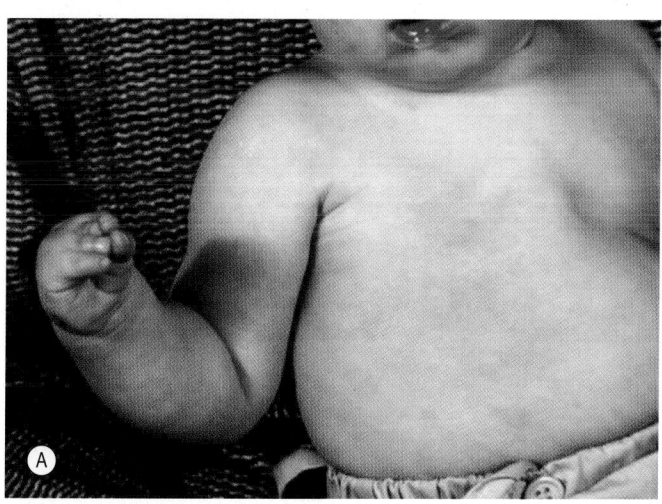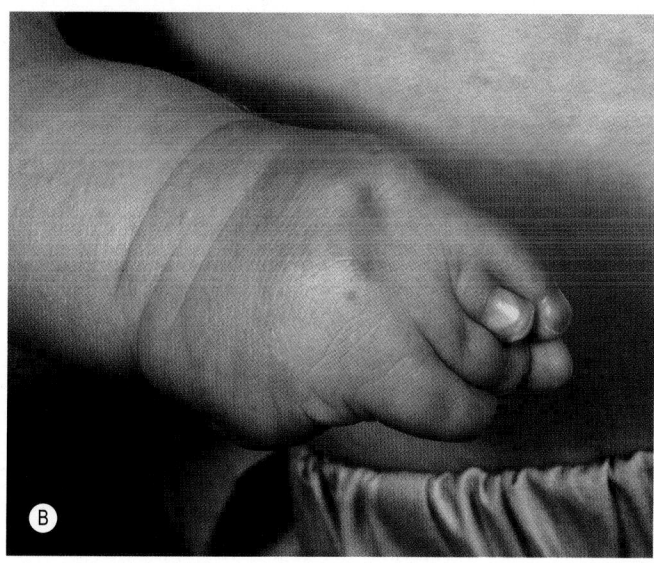

FIGURE 21.9 (A) One-year-old child with Poland syndrome, showing digital anomalies and amastia. (B) Close-up of hand, showing brachysyndactyly. (Courtesy of Dr. Louise Caouette-Laberge.)

(Fig. 21.9). Familial cases with an autosomal pattern of transmission have been reported, but the condition is overwhelmingly sporadic.[8] McGillivray and Lowry[8] have reported 44 cases of Poland syndrome, 40 of whom had abnormal digits; patients with normal digits probably could be diagnosed as having a unilateral thoracic wall aplasia (see below), but most authors argue that unilateral thoracic wall aplasia is part of the Poland syndrome spectrum.[2,9]

Rare families have been reported in which Poland syndrome is associated with a **unilateral gluteal hypoplasia and a brachysyndactyly of the toes** in other family members, highlighting the link between these two syndromes; it has thus been proposed that this form of gluteal hypoplasia is the lower limb equivalent of the Poland syndrome.[10–12] **Bilateral Poland syndrome** is best classified as a thoracic dysplasia.[13,14] The Poland-Moebius syndrome combines Poland syndrome with Moebius syndrome (MIM 157900, i.e., a dysplasia, aplasia, or atrophy of the facial and abducens nerves).

The **pathogenesis** of Poland syndrome may involve an abnormal embryonic development between the 6th and 7th weeks, affecting the subclavian arteries, the vertebral arteries, and/or their branches (the '**subclavian artery supply disruption sequence**').[15] This would explain the occasional association between Poland syndrome and athelia, scapular anomalies, hemivertebrae, hypoplastic or fused ribs, shortening of the radius and ulna, and dextroposition of the heart.

Poland syndrome is reported to be associated with **leukemia,** sarcomas, and breast adenocarcinoma, but these associations may be tenuous.[7,16–19]

'**Unilateral thoracic wall aplasia**' is characterized by the absence of costal cartilage and ipsilateral pectoral muscles; one half of cases are associated with nipple hypoplasia or agenesis. The 3rd and 4th ribs are always involved, and the defect may involve the 1st to the 5th ribs. It is rare, affects mostly males and two-thirds of reported cases involve the right thorax. The axillary hair of the affected side is displaced down the arm. It is thought that the failure of the ribs to fuse with the sternum prevents the pectoralis major and minor from migrating and fusing with their normal attachment sites. This condition is likely part of the Poland syndrome spectrum (MIM 173800).

Jeune's thoracic dystrophy

Jeune et al. described the asphyxiating thoracic dystrophy syndrome[20] (MIM 208500), characterized by a long, narrow, and very small thorax with extreme pulmonary hypoplasia; it is often lethal in infancy. Survivors may develop hepatic dysfunction (polycystic liver disease with hepatic fibrosis and bile duct proliferation), pancreatic fibrosis from pancreatic cysts, and renal failure from chronic nephritis and renal cysts. It results from an autosomal recessive form of chondrodysplasia which maps to 15q13, but the gene is not known.

Congenital abnormalities of the breast

Amastia (absence of breast), **hypomastia** (hypoplastic breast tissue associated with a nipple) and **athelia** (breast tissue devoid of nipple) are rare, and may be **syndromic,** reflecting an **abnormal epithelio-stromal induction**[3] (e.g., Poland syndrome, MIM 173800; amastia, bilateral, with ureteral triplication and dysmorphism syndrome, MIM 104350; ectodermal dysplasia, trichoodontoonychial type, MIM 129510; ectodermal dysplasia 1-anhydrotic type, MIM 305100; AREDYLD syndrome, MIM 207780; scalp-ear-nipple syndrome, MIM 181270; breasts and nipples, absence of syndrome, MIM 113700; choanal atresia syndrome, MIM 608911; and renal tubular dysgenesis syndrome, MIM 267430).

Approximately half of amastia and athelia cases are bilateral, and in unilateral cases there is no right or left predisposition.[2] Conceptually, amastia can result from an absence of formation of the mammary ridge, or from involution of the normal mammary primordia.

The origin of ectopic breasts and nipples is not elucidated. **Polymastia** (supernumerary breast with glandular tissue, with/without nipple or areola) and **polythelia** (supernumerary nipple and/or areola) are divided into **accessory** breasts, when lying within the milk line (see Fig. 21.3), and **ectopic** breasts. The origin of ectopic breasts and nipples is not elucidated. In approximately 60–65% of cases, a single supernumerary breast is present; 30% have two supernumerary breasts, 4% have three, and 2% have four. Eight supernumerary breasts have been reported in one man, and one woman has been found to have ten.[2] In Caucasian women, 95% of accessory breasts arise just below the normal breast, whereas in Japanese women and men, respectively, 95% and 60% are found above the normal breast. Accessory breasts may come to medical attention during pregnancy. Ectopic breasts are extremely rare, and have been reported (in decreasing order of frequency) on the back, dorsolateral thigh, flank and hip, face (cheek and ear), shoulder, neck, and buttock.[2] Athelia is frequent in ectopic breasts.

The estimated **incidence** of supernumerary breasts is approximately 1%. **Ethnic and geographic variations** are known, with a reported **incidence** of 4% in Japan.[2, 21] In a prospective German study, Schmidt found supernumerary breasts in 28 of his 502 patient cohort (5.6%); 20 patients were males, 8 females.[21] **Familial cases** with an autosomal dominant transmission occur (supernumerary nipples – including polymastia – syndrome, MIM 163700). Accessory nipples can also be encountered in a variety of syndromes (e.g., the autosomal recessive postaxial acrofacial dysostosis, MIM 263750; the Pallister-Killian syndrome resulting from a tetrasomy 12p; and cancer-predisposing syndromes such as the X-linked recessive Simpson-Golabi-Behmel syndrome type 1, MIM 312870, and the autosomal dominant Ruvalcaba-Myhre syndrome, MIM 153480).

Urinary tract anomalies have been reported in 23–27% of Hungarian and Israeli children **with supernumerary nipples.** Urbani and Betti also found this association: urinary tract anomalies (adult dominant polycystic kidney disease, unilateral renal agenesis, cystic renal dysplasia, familial renal cysts, and congenital stenosis of the pyeloureteral junction) were present in 7.53% of individuals with polythelia versus 0.68% in patients with normal breast development ($p<0.001$).[22] The fact that Grotto et al. could find no such association probably reflects ethnic or population-based variations.[23] Nevertheless, as this association is reported by many independent authors, and since weak associations are reported between supernumerary nipples and many other malformations and diseases (e.g., hypertension, cardiac malformations and conduction defects, vertebral malformations, etc.), the significance and evaluation of such patients constitutes a clinical challenge. No tests other than a

good physical examination with careful abdominal palpation are indicated for patients not originating from areas of high risk for concomitant urinary tract malformations.[6]

Histologically, supernumerary breasts recapitulate normal nipples and/or areola, with or without associated glandular tissue. Smooth muscle is present in this genital-type skin. Accessory breast tissue within the vulva is rare, and may show a predilection for malignant transformation, possibly due to an abnormal epithelio-stromal induction/interaction.[4]

Breast pathology in children

Fibroadenomas are the most common breast neoplasm of adolescent females, accounting for 75–90% of all unilateral breast masses in this age group. They may reach upward of 8 cm in size, but when large or rapidly growing, a **benign phyllodes tumor** or a **cystosarcoma phyllodes** must be ruled out.[24–27] Although breast cancer is extremely rare in children and adolescents, **all breast masses require a tissue-based diagnosis** (either through a fine needle aspiration or an open biopsy).

Virginal breast hyperplasia (macromastia) is a rapid, massive, and permanent increase in the size of one or both breasts, starting at the time of onset of puberty, but sometimes as late as 19 years of age. This condition is rare, may be bilateral, and may recur post reduction mammoplasty. Histologically, the lesions are generally composed mostly of adipose and connective tissue. Rarely, the histology is characterized by a florid epithelial hyperplasia; such lesions may recur, requiring iterative bilateral reduction mammoplasty (Fig. 21.10).[6, 28–33] A **hormonal effect is postulated,** possibly an increased sensitivity to estrogens and/or progesterone by the mammary adipocytes, fibroblasts, and/or epithelial cells.

Breast hypertrophy can be caused by certain pharmaceutical agents (e.g., D-penicillamine and bucillamine)[34–38] and may be syndromic (e.g., Cowden disease, MIM 158350). Men and women with Cowden disease are also at increased risk of developing breast cancer, generally after 30 years of age.[39–41]

An **autosomal dominant** form of **benign florid nipple papillomatosis** mimicking Paget's disease of the nipple has been reported (MIM 167950).[42]

Gynecomastia occurs in 60–70% of adolescent boys, is bilateral in 75% of cases, and generally consists of a 1–3 cm tender subareolar nodule that usually regresses within 1 year. It ranges from a barely detectable nodule to a breast the size and shape of that of a woman's. **Histologically,** it is characterized by a mild ductal hyperplasia without lobules in an abundant adipose tissue stroma (Fig. 21.11A,B),[43] albeit rare cases have associated lobules in otherwise normal males (Fig. 21.11C,D).[44] A hormonal effect is postulated, as gynecomastia is induced in men treated with estrogens,[45] and the condition reverts with tamoxifen.[46] Isolated **familial forms** are known, with autosomal dominant (hereditary gynecomastia syndrome, MIM 139300) and X-linked (familial gynecomastia syndrome, MIM 306500) transmission. Gynecomastia may also result from **hypogonadism,** of which **Klinefelter's**

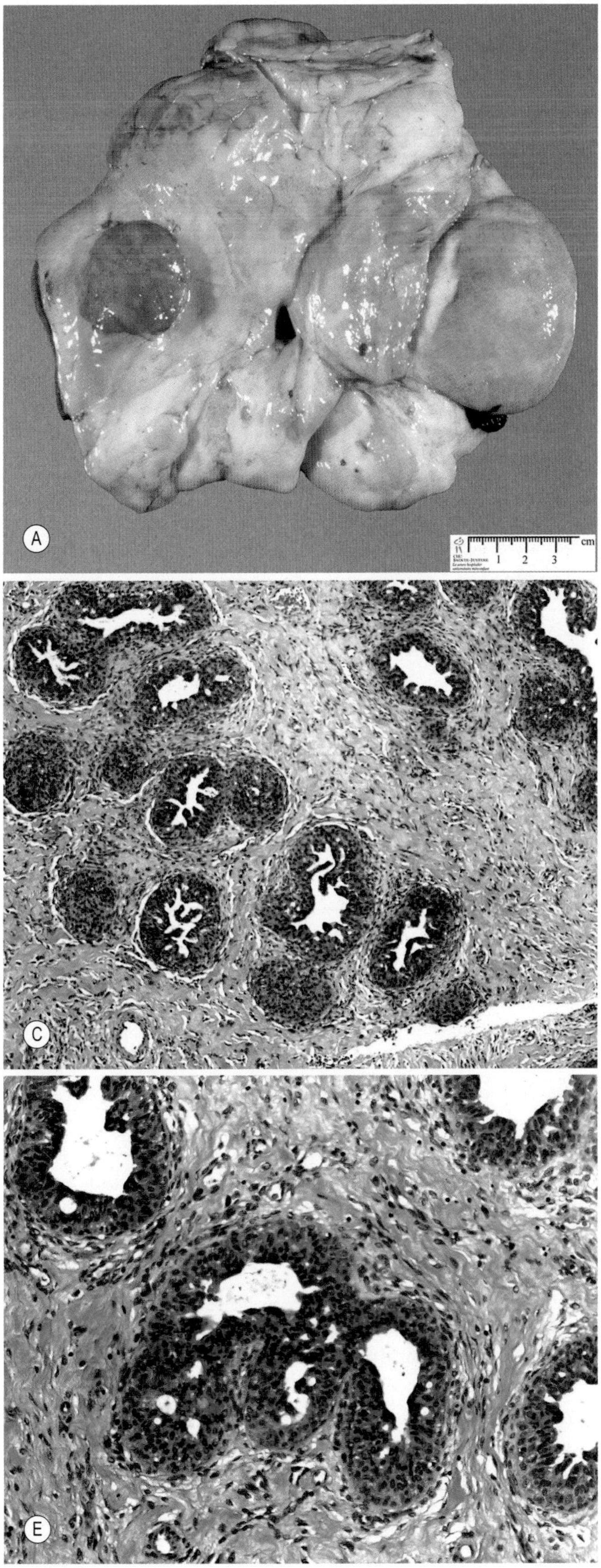

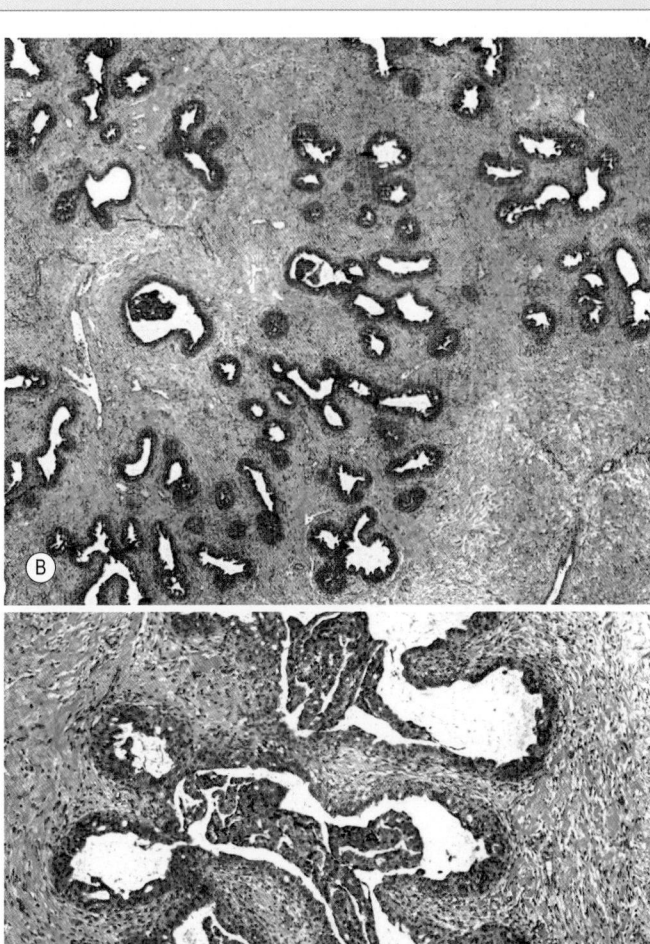

FIGURE 21.10 Juvenile mammary hyperplasia. (A) Bilateral reduction mastectomy in an 11-year-old girl; 1700 g of tissue was resected from each breast, after more than 2,000g had been resected from the left breast the previous year. Although mammary hyperplasia generally involves mostly stromal tissue, this case shows the glandular tissue to be hyperplastic. (B through E) The hyperplasia is focally complex, with apocrine metaplasia. HPS, original magnifications of 25×, 100×, 100×, and 200×, respectively.

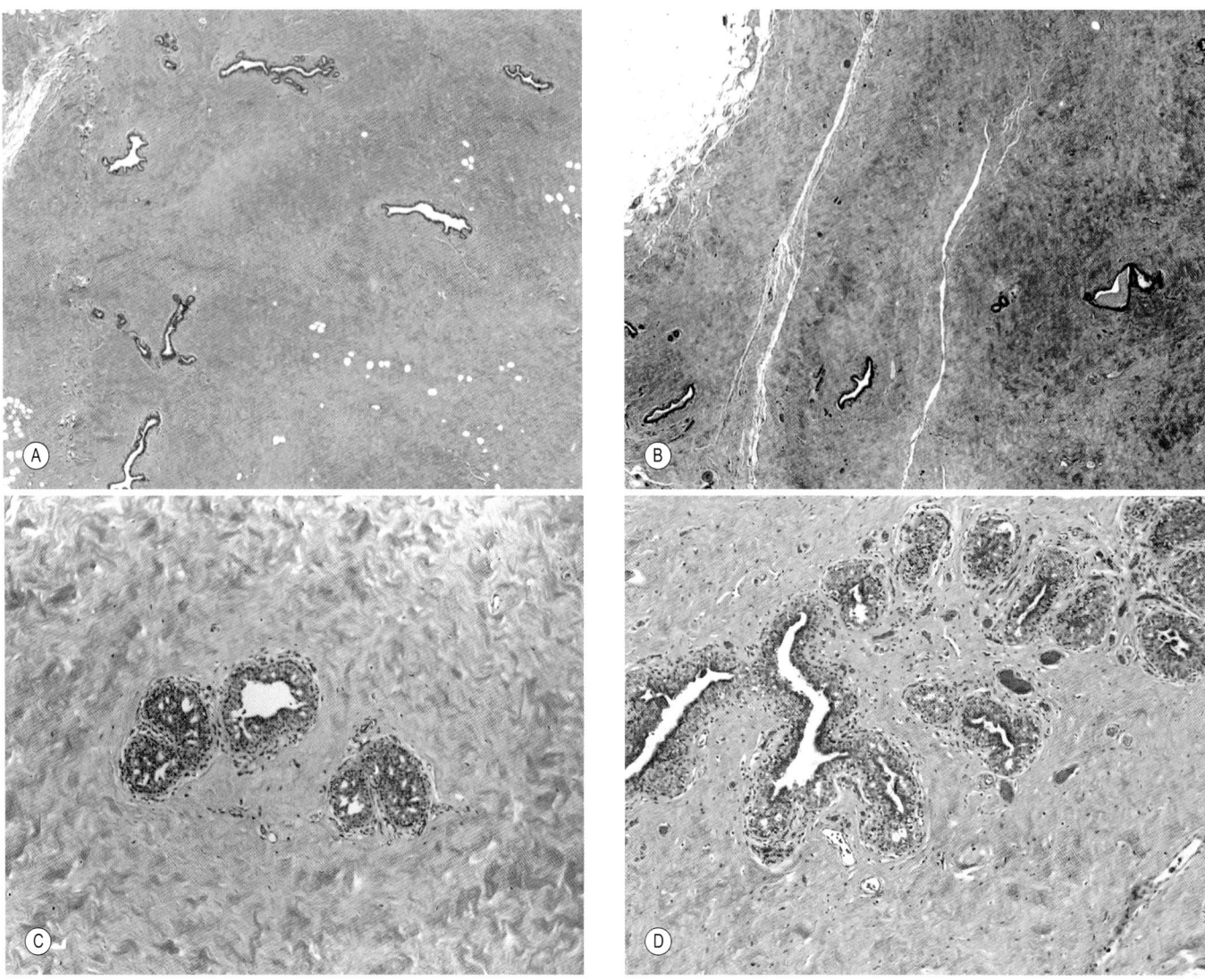

FIGURE 21.11 Gynecomastia. (A and B) Typical histological appearance in boys, 14 and 17 years old, respectively. Note that only ducts are present, without accompanying lobules, and that the abundant stroma is very fibrous. (C and D) Lobules were seen focally in the breast of the 17-year-old, with hyperplastic features. HPS. Original magnification: A and B: 25×; C and D: 100×.

syndrome (47,XXY) is the most frequent cause. Other conditions associated with testicular failure and gynecomastia include Kallmann syndrome 1 (MIM 308700); Kennedy syndrome (MIM 313200); the aromatase gynecomastia syndrome (MIM 107910) resulting from a mutation of *CYP19A1*, which is one of the cytochrome P450 genes; and Reifenstein syndrome (MIM 312300) which affects the androgen receptor. The **differential diagnosis** of gynecomastia includes more than 40 syndromes (e.g., Peutz-Jeghers syndrome, MIM 175200; Wilson-Turner X-linked mental retardation syndrome, MIM 309585, etc.), and a multitude of drugs (e.g., anabolic steroids, estrogen-like substances, testosterone-inhibiting substances, heroin, cannabis, spironolactone, etc.)[6] **Treatment** of isolated non-syndromic forms is by mastectomy, whereas syndromic and drug-induced forms must be treated accordingly.

Exposure to **radiation** between 1500 and 2000 rads prior to puberty can impair breast development; exposure to more than 3000 rads can arrest breast growth, and lead to breast **hypoplasia and fibrosis.** When possible, radiotherapy should spare the nipple–areola complex in children and young adults, to avoid these complications and the risk of developing a **secondary mammary adenocarcinoma.**[6, 47, 48]

Normal development of the anterior abdominal wall

The abdominal wall forms through the folding of the embryo. As in the thorax, the primitive wall is somatopleure, i.e., ectoderm and mesoderm, devoid of muscular, neural and vascular differentiation. During the 6th week, the somatopleure is bilaterally invaded dorsolaterally and then anteromedially by sheets of somitic mesoderm; the abdominal wall closes when these sheets reach the midline, where they form the right and left **rectus abdominis muscles.** Laterally, by the 7th week, these two sheets separate into three muscle layers: (1) the outer layer forms the **external oblique muscle** ventrally and the **serratus** dorsally; (2) the inner layer forms the **internal oblique** and the **musculus transversus;** and (3) the inner layer generates the **musculus transversus abdominis.**

During the 7th week, the somatopleure of the **infraumbilical region** is initially invaded by mesoderm of primitive streak origin, which closes the abdominal wall between the phallus and the body stalk, forming part of the musculature of the bladder (see Back and Perineum, Ch. 22). Subsequently, mesoderm of paraxial origin invades the infraumbilical body wall.

Angiogenesis starts in the extraembryonic mesoderm of the yolk sac on day 14; intraembryonic angiogenesis begins 2 days later. Shortly thereafter, these two vascular systems merge at the level of the connecting stalk, eventually to form the two umbilical arteries and the umbilical vein which are surrounded by a myxoid mesenchyme, Wharton's jelly.

During folding of the embryo (starting on day 22), the connecting stalk (containing the allantois and blood vessels) is pushed against the secondary yolk sac by the increasing amniotic fluid pressure; these structures fuse and become surrounded by amnion, forming the **umbilical cord** (see Fig. 21.1A–D).

In the neonate, the cord attaches onto the abdominal wall at the level of the **umbilical ring,** composed partly by the right and left medial umbilical ligaments (i.e., the obliterated umbilical arteries). In 75% of individuals, the **round ligament** (i.e., the obliterated umbilical vein) attaches onto the urachus, closing off the ring. Furthermore, a transverse **umbilical fascia** covers the entire surface of the ring in 35% of individuals, and covers it partly in 45% of individuals. Hence, the round ligament fails to close the umbilical ring in 25% of individuals, and the umbilical fascia fails to grow over the ring in 20% of individuals (i.e., approximately 5% of individuals have neither the round ligament nor the umbilical fascia closing their umbilical ring).[2]

Between the 6th and the 10th weeks, there is a **physiological intestinal herniation** within the umbilical cord through the umbilical ring. This physiologic herniation contains exclusively loops of intestine, which return into the abdominal cavity during the 10th week.[49] Between the 5th and 8th weeks, the **vitellointestinal duct** (or **omphalomesenteric duct** or **vitelline duct,** see Fig 21.1B–D) normally resorbs,[50] or else a Meckel's diverticulum is present (see below).

Congenital abdominal wall abnormalities

Defects of the abdominal wall and of the umbilicus associated with **malformations of the cloaca and urinary tract** (e.g., the prune belly syndrome, vesical exstrophy, urachal cysts and fistulas) are discussed in Chapter 22.

Abnormalities of the umbilical region

Umbilical granulomas are by far the most common umbilical lesion of infancy, representing an infection, generally bacterial, of the umbilical stump after its separation from the abdominal skin. Such granulomas are solid and red, with a soft, velvety appearance without an associated fistulous tract, yet they can drain small amounts of serous or serosanguinous liquid. They develop within the first few weeks of life, and should not be congenital.[51]

Syndromic umbilical abnormalities exist, warranting a more than cursory examination of this structure.[6] For example, in Aarskog syndrome (MIM 100050), the umbilicus is protruding or pouting; in Rieger syndrome (MIM 180500), it is broad, prominent, with redundant periumbilical skin; in Robinow syndrome (MIM 180700), it is cephalically placed, broad, poorly epithelialized, and scarred; it is low-set in achondroplasia (MIM 100800), and omphaloceles are a component of many syndromes (e.g., Beckwith-Wiedemann syndrome, MIM 130650).

Umbilical hernias are covered by skin; they result from an abnormally large umbilical ring which may have a diameter upwards of 4 cm, associated with a failure of the abdominis recti to approximate after reduction of the physiologic intestinal hernia. They are often associated with an abnormal attachment of the round ligament onto the ring and a lack of closure of the ring by the fascia umbilicalis. Approximately 5% of individuals have neither the round ligament nor the umbilical fascia closing their umbilical ring, accounting for **direct umbilical hernias. Indirect umbilical hernias** are said to occur when the round ligament fails to close the ring, and the ring is partly covered by the umbilical fascia.[2] Umbilical hernias have an incidence range of 4–20% in Caucasian infants and have been reported to be as high as 32–40% in black infants.[2, 6] Such hernias are more frequent in low birth weight neonates, with an incidence of 84% in infants weighing less than 1500 g, and of 21% in those with birth weights greater than 2500 g. Spontaneous regression occurs by 5–6 years of age in 80–95% of hernias less than 1 cm in diameter, and in more than 55% of larger ones; those which have not regressed by 6 years of age are unlikely to do so subsequently, and may require surgical closure. Defects of the linea alba and diastasis recti may accompany umbilical hernias.

In **omphaloceles** (also called **exomphalos** or **amnioceles**), the viscera herniate into the umbilical cord through a widened umbilical ring (Fig. 21.12). The viscera are covered by amnion and peritoneum, with a minimal amount of Wharton's jelly between these two epithelia which may even be fused. Omphaloceles can be classified as small and giant. Meckel's diverticulum and segments of ileum can be inadvertently traumatized during the clamping of the cord, or inadvertently resected during the closure of omphaloceles.[2]

Small omphaloceles usually contain only a few loops of intestines; the umbilical ring is enlarged but normally placed, and the

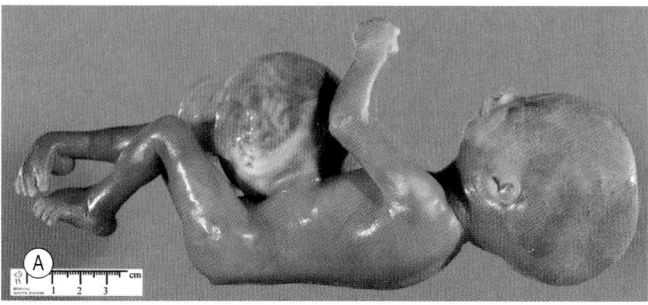

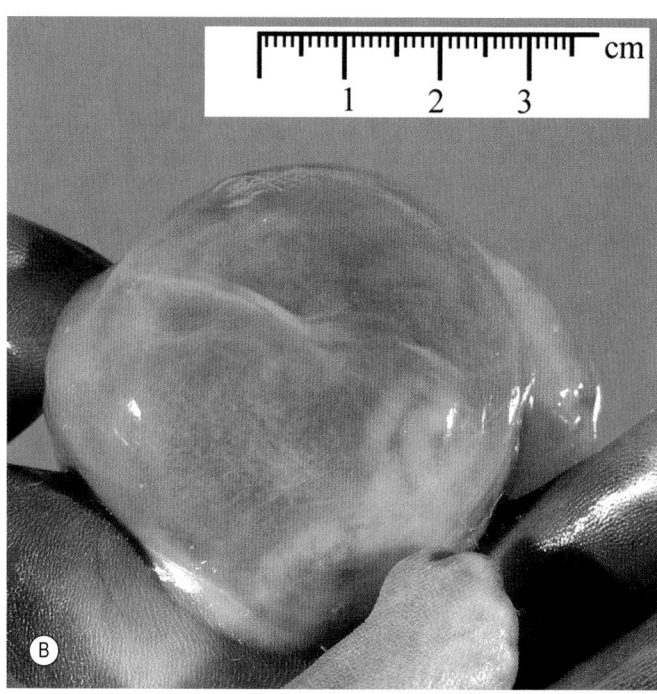

FIGURE 21.12 (A) Omphalocele in a fetus of 21 weeks' gestational age (viewed from the left). Amnion covers most of the viscera; the omphalocele contains the liver which can be seen at the level of the elbow, and most of the other abdominal viscera. The umbilical cord inserts in the inferior portion of the hernial sac. (B) Same fetus, viewed from the right; the liver and bowel loops are seen through the sac. (From www.humpath.com, courtesy of Dr. Jean-Christophe Fournet.)

umbilical cord inserts into the apex of the hernial sac. Small omphaloceles probably result from a failure of the physiologic intestinal hernia to reduce spontaneously during the 10th week.[49]

Giant omphaloceles are defined as having a diameter >5 cm at the level of the umbilical wall. The abdominal wall superior to the umbilicus does not fuse due to an abnormal dorsoventral growth of the somitic myoblasts, which fail to reach the midline bilaterally; the abdominal musculature comprising the upper portion of the umbilical ring is thus deficient, producing a weakness above the umbilical cord. In extreme cases, the ensuing abdominal wall defect may measure up to 15 cm in diameter. In giant omphaloceles, the sac generally contains most or all of the intestine and stomach, frequently with a large portion of the liver, spleen, bladder, uterus, and ovaries, and the cord inserts onto the inferior border of the sac. The thin hernial sac of large omphaloceles may rupture, exposing the viscera to the amniotic liquid; such conditions must be distinguished from gastroschisis (see below).

Omphaloceles may result from an arrest of the progression of the amnioectodermal junction toward the umbilicus. Intra-embryonic mesoderm cannot migrate through this amniotic tissue, preventing its maturation into mature body wall. The covering remains an avascular thin membrane of amnion and extraembryonic mesoderm, which easily stretches when subjected to the increasing intra-abdominal pressure, giving rise to the amniocele.

The **incidence** of omphaloceles is 2.5 in 10 000 live births, and they are twice as frequent in stillbirths. An **abnormal karyotype** is found in half of prenatally diagnosed omphaloceles; trisomy 18 is the most frequent cause, and triploidy, +13, +21, Turner and

Klinefelter's syndromes have been reported. Only 75% of infants with omphaloceles are liveborn, reflecting a high intrauterine mortality rate; a karyotypic anomaly is also present in half of liveborn infants with an omphalocele. Omphaloceles are associated with a major malformation in 40–88% of cases, including cardiac (50%), neural tube (40%), and central nervous system defects; the amnion rupture sequence must be considered in the differential diagnosis. Omphaloceles are frequent in **Beckwith-Wiedemann** syndrome (MIM 130650), presumably because the associated visceromegaly prevents the normal return of the intestines into the abdomen.

Syndromic forms must be excluded. Omphaloceles can have an autosomal dominant (e.g., the omphalocele syndrome, MIM 164750; Shprintzen omphalocele syndrome, MIM 182210), an autosomal recessive (e.g., the lethal form of omphalocele-cleft palate syndrome, MIM 258320) and an X-linked transmission (e.g., omphalocele syndrome, MIM 310980); OMIM lists 58 syndromes associated with omphaloceles. Furthermore, geographic variations are known, and the condition is considered to be multifactorial.

Postnatal complications of isolated large omphaloceles include peritonitis as the protective amnion withers when exposed to air, large abdominal wall defects may impede respiration, and visceral necrosis may occur when the surgical closure generates too much intra-abdominal pressure. **Morbidity and mortality** remain high, and are correlated with the **size of the defect** and the **associated anomalies.**[52]

In **gastroschisis,** the defect is lateral to the umbilical ring, and both the ring and cord are normal. The protruding viscera are not encased in a sac, but rather embedded within a gelatinous mass. It has an overall incidence of 1 in 10 000 live births, but the incidence

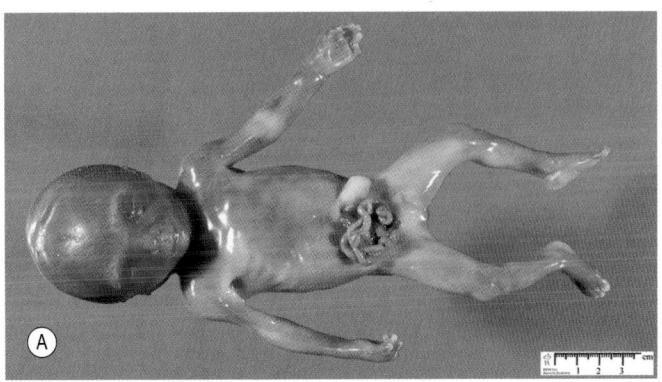

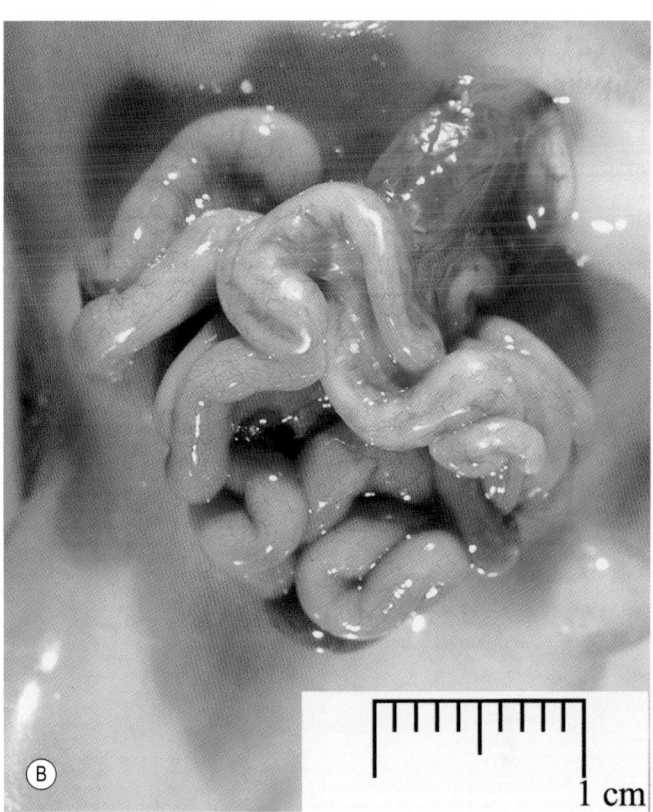

FIGURE 21.13 (A) Gastroschisis in a fetus of 20 weeks' gestational age. As is most frequent in gastroschisis, the abdominal rupture site is to the right of the umbilical cord and the liver does not extrude through the defect. (B) Higher magnification of the matted viscera focally covered by fibrin. (From www.humpath.com, courtesy of Dr. Jean-Christophe Fournet.)

is 7 per 10 000 in mothers less than 20 years of age; it occurs only rarely in mothers older than 25 years of age.[2,6] Gastroschisis is more frequently right-sided, and may extend into the vesical region. Only 10% of patients with gastroschisis die in utero.

In normal embryos, by day 28, the right and left umbilical veins drain the placenta, connecting stalk and abdominal wall. At 33 days, the right umbilical vein has entirely atrophied, except for the short segment draining into the inferior vena cava. This vessel's nutritive function is taken over by the right and left vitelline (omphalomesenteric) arteries. Subsequently, the left vitelline artery atrophies, and the right vitelline artery becomes the superior mesenteric artery.[49,53]

An **abnormal vascular development,** such as a premature atrophy or an abnormal persistence of the right umbilical vein, or a **vascular accident,** such as a disruption of the right umbilical artery, would result in hypoxia of the right-sided abdominal wall, and explain the prevalence of right-sided gastroschisis (Fig. 21.13).[53] Such accidents are thought to occur between the 3rd and 8th weeks pc, but gastroschisis in early embryos is rarely reported, suggesting that herniation through the defect results from stretching of the weakened body wall by the increasing intra-abdominal pressure.[2,6]

A **vascular etiology** is supported by the fact that gastroschisis is associated with: (1) **vasoconstrictors,** such as cocaine and ephedrine used in decongestants; (2) **cyclooxygenase inhibitors** such as aspirin and ibuprofen; and (3) **cigarette smoking.** Indeed, all these factors cause fetal hypoxia, and are associated with bowel atresia and stenosis. The fact that associated anomalies (e.g., renal agenesis, porencephaly, and atresia of the gall-

bladder) are also related to hypoxic insults further supports the vascular accident hypothesis.[2,6,54–59]

For **genetic counseling, omphaloceles,** which are often syndromic and lethal, must be differentiated from *gastroschisis*, which are generally isolated anomalies, viable in ≈85% of cases, and usually sporadic with an empiric recurrence risk of 3.5% (Table 21.1). The amniotic rupture sequence must be included in the differential diagnosis.

Meckel's diverticulum is twice as common in males, and results from a failure of the omphalomesenteric (vitelline) duct (see Fig. 21.1B–D) to resorb by the 8th week. It is present in up to 3% of live births, measures up to 3 inches (8 cm), is usually located 3 feet (100 cm) proximal to the ileocecal valve, and less than 3% are symptomatic (the 'rule of 3s'). The term Meckel's diverticulum encompasses **omphalomesenteric fistulas** and **sinuses, enteric cysts, fibrous bands connecting the small bowel to the umbilicus, and intussusceptions at the umbilicus.** Completely patent fistulas are very rare, and present as a bright red, mucosa-covered nodule seen in the umbilicus after sloughing of the cord, through which feces may leak. Partially patent fistulas attached to the distal ileum by a stenosed fibrous band are more common, and may drain mucous in the umbilicus. Vitelline cysts or enterocysts refer to cysts formed by incomplete stricture/apoptosis of the intermediate segment of omphalomesenteric duct.

The mucosa of Meckel's diverticulum contains acid-secreting gastric epithelium in 30–50% of cases, which may cause ulceration of the adjacent ileal mucosa, most frequently leading to chronic painless bleeding; perforation and peritonitis

TABLE 21.1 DISTINGUISHING CRITERIA BETWEEN OMPHALOCELE AND GASTROSCHISIS

Omphalocele	Gastroschisis
Defect covered by amnion and peritoneum (but may rupture)	Viscera exteriorized
Umbilical cord and ring in continuity with defect	Defect lateral to umbilical cord and ring, generally right-sided
Bowel normally developed	Bowel matted; atresia and stenosis common
Liver present in large defects	Liver remains intra-abdominal
Often syndromic	Generally isolated defect, except for intestinal stenosis or atresia
α-fetoprotein (AFP) normal or slightly elevated	AFP markedly elevated (7-fold increase, on average)
50% aneuploidy	Karyotype generally normal
Mothers older than 35 years	Mothers younger than 25 years
Frequent in spontaneous abortions	Generally does not result in intrauterine death
Recurrence depends on associated syndrome	Recurrence rate of 3.5%

simulating appendicitis may occur. The mucosa may also contain ectopic pancreas. Obstruction, ileal intussusception with the diverticulum as the lead-point, and volvulus are less common causes of presentation. Less than 3% of all Meckel's diverticulae come to medical attention, half before 24 months of age.

Intussusception at the umbilicus is a prolapse of the ileum through the fully patent omphalomesenteric duct, leading to an everted intestine with an exteriorized mucosal surface. When large, it is often T-shaped, with two umbilical stomata leading to the proximal and distal intestine.[2]

The inguinal region
Normal development

In **males**, the **internal inguinal ring** closes after descent of the testis into the scrotum through the **processus vaginalis** during the 7th to 9th gestational month; the processus initially closes at the level of the internal inguinal ring, then just above the testis. Finally, the canal enclosed by these two constrictions becomes atretic. The obliterated canal forms a fibrous band, while the scrotal segment of this canal remains lined by mesothelium; this offshoot of the peritoneal cavity, the fluid-filled **tunica vaginalis,** lies around the anterior portion of the testis (Fig. 21.14A).[2]

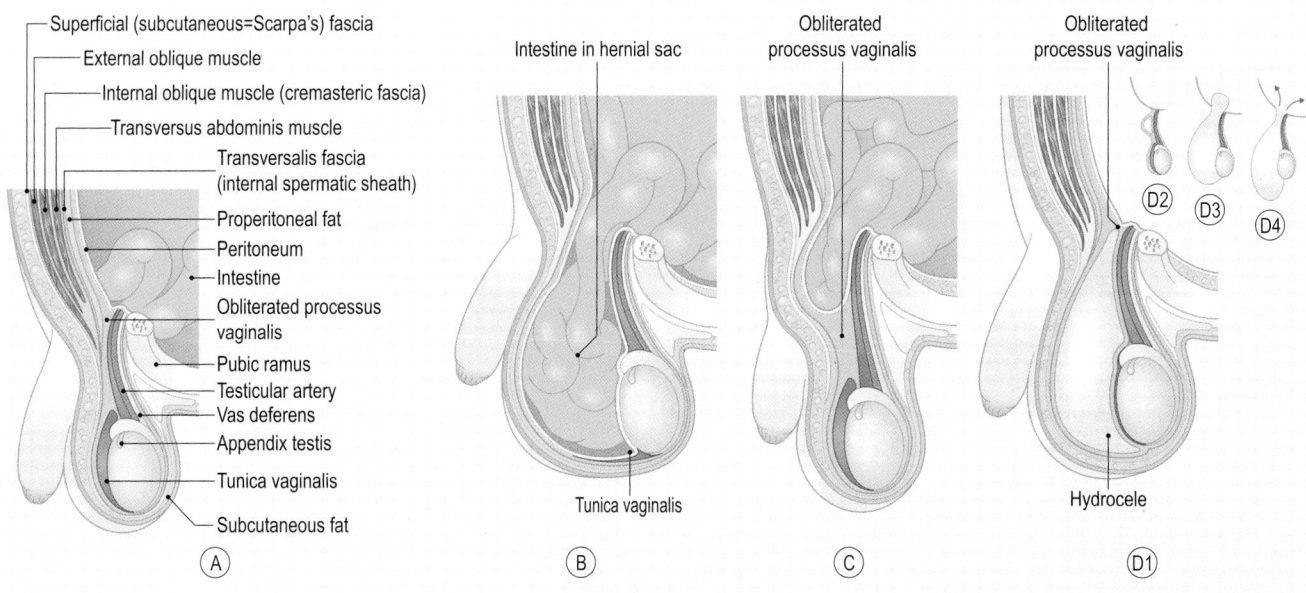

FIGURE 21.14 (A) Normal anatomy of the inguinal sac: the processus vaginalis is completely obliterated. (B) Congenital inguinal hernia, due to a lack of closure of the processus vaginalis. The testis may be in the scrotum, as shown, or be in the abdomen or inguinal canal. (C) Indirect hernia within the blind peritoneal sac, resulting from an incomplete obliteration of the proximal portion of the processus vaginalis. (D) Hydroceles can be of four types: D1, the processus vaginalis is only obliterated at the level of the inguinal ring, resulting in an accumulation of fluid in the distal processus and in the tunica vaginalis; D2, cystic dilatation of the superior portion of the processus vaginalis, not communicating with the tunica vaginalis nor with the peritoneal cavity; D3, hydrocele of the infantile type, bulging into the peritoneal cavity; D4, communicating hydrocele, temporarily reduced by gentle pressure. (Figures redrawn and adapted from Skandalakis and Gray.[2])

In *females*, the **processus vaginalis** corresponds to the **canal of Nuck,** which opens into the **labium majorum,** the homologue of the scrotum. The processus vaginalis is smaller in females than it is in males, and obliterates earlier, i.e., during the 7th week.[2]

Inguinal hernia and hydrocele

Failure of obliteration of the processus vaginalis results in a peritoneal diverticulum through which viscera can herniate (Fig. 21.14B,C), and into which fluid can accumulate to form a hydrocele (Fig. 21.14 D).

In **women,** indirect inguinal hernias are exclusively acquired, because the female fetus has no persisting tunica vaginalis; hence, the congenital form cannot exist. These inguinal hernias rarely extend all the way to the labium majorum, but rather generally remain within the inguinal region. In girls, the ovary and fallopian tube are the most frequently encountered structures within the hernial sac, and the uterus is sometimes herniated in adult women.

In **men,** failure of the processus vaginalis to close throughout its length results in a diverticulum through which abdominal viscera can reach the scrotum. These **indirect inguinal hernias** are referred to as **congenital,** despite the fact that herniation may only occur postnatally (Fig. 21.14B). Such hernias most often result from failure of the processus vaginalis to close after descent of the testis; they are thus lined by the **tunica vaginalis.** Closure of the processus vaginalis is dependent on descent of the testis into the scrotum, explaining the association of indirect inguinal hernias with **cryptorchidism** and **prematurity.** In both males and females, 60%, of indirect inguinal hernias are right-sided, 10% bilateral, and 30% left-sided. The predominance of indirect inguinal hernias on the right side may be related to the fact that the right testis descends after the left. **Incarceration** occurs in 2%.

Meconium within the hernial sac indicates a **meconium peritonitis,** due to a rupture of the bowel wall; such ruptures generally occur in utero, and are generally asymptomatic but may lead to bowel adhesions.[60–62] Meconium periorchitis tends to present in the neonatal period or during infancy, as a hemiscrotal indurated red painful mass suspicious for cancer.[63,64] Histologically, these lesions are inflammatory and may be calcified (Fig. 21.15).

Despite early **orchidopexy,** unilateral **cryptorchidism** is associated with a 9% risk of **infertility;** in bilateral cases, the risk is 54%.[65,66] The risk of **malignancy** in cryptorchid testes post orchidopexy is increased 4–10 fold, whether orchidopexy is performed or not.[67,68]

During orchidopexy, the **appendix testis** (or hydatid of Morgagni) is routinely resected, to prevent subsequent torsion. The appendix testis is a vestige of the cranial end of the müllerian duct; insufficient concentrations of AMH (anti-müllerian hormone) at this level fails to stimulate its involution. The appendix testis is a minute, oval, sessile structure located on the upper pole of the testis, just inferior to the epididymal head.[69] In prepubertal boys, torsion of the appendix testis is as frequent as

torsion of normally descended testes, and is frequently misdiagnosed.[70] Clinically, both these conditions are generally very painful. Torsion of the appendix testis initially reveals an edematous and congested stroma (Fig. 21.16); subsequently, hemorrhagic infarction develops.

Acquired indirect inguinal hernias result from a failure of the upper portion of the processus vaginalis to close, leaving a blind peritoneal sac (the **funicular process**) in continuity with the peritoneal cavity. Acquired indirect hernias are thus lined by peritoneum rather than by tunica vaginalis (see Fig. 21.14C).

In **males,** the hernial sac of both congenital and acquired indirect inguinal hernias contains peritoneal fluid; ileum is the most commonly herniated viscera. **Littre's hernia** refers to the presence of a Meckel's diverticulum within the hernial sac.

Hydroceles (see Fig. 21.14D1) result from a lack of closure of the lower portion of the processus vaginalis while its superior portion closes normally, leading to an accumulation of liquid around the testis and spermatic cord. **Funicular (or cystic) hydroceles** (see Fig. 21.14D2) are fluid-filled cavities lying anterior to the spermatic cord, which do not communicate with the abdominal cavity nor with the tunica vaginalis; they are also called **hydroceles of the spermatic cord.** In **abdominoscrotal hydroceles** (see Fig. 21.14D3), the cyst bulges within the abdominal cavity; this form is also called **infantile hydroceles,** despite the fact that it may present after infancy. In **congenital (or communicating) hydroceles** (see Fig. 21.14D4), a small opening is present at the level of the superior portion of the processus vaginalis, allowing fluid to re-accumulate after the sac is emptied by gentle pressure.[2]

Direct inguinal hernias result from a defect of the abdominal wall between the deep epigastric artery and the edge of the rectus muscle. They account for nearly 4% of all inguinal hernias.

Amnion rupture sequence and limb body wall complex

The amniotic cavity is generated by epiblastic cells (and possibly from cytotrophoblastic cells as well) which differentiate into amnioblasts during the 2nd week pc; the amniotic cavity enlarges relative to the extraembryonic coelomic cavity, until the amnion fuses with the chorionic plate by 12 weeks pc (Fig. 21.17). Failure of the amnionic membrane to fuse with the chorionic plate causes these membranes to dehisce, forming strips of membranes floating within the amnionic cavity, where they can wrap around fetal parts or be swallowed by the fetus.

Kalousek et al. divide the amnion defects into the limb body wall complex (LBWC), caused by an early defect of the amniotic sac, and the amnion rupture sequence (ARS) caused by amniotic bands.[49] In both the LBWC and the ARS, the membranes devoid of amnion become leaky, accounting for the **oligohydramnios** and associated amnion nodosum and Potter's sequence.

The **limb body wall complex** (LBWC, or ADAM – amnionic deformity, adhesion and mutilation complex – or amnionic

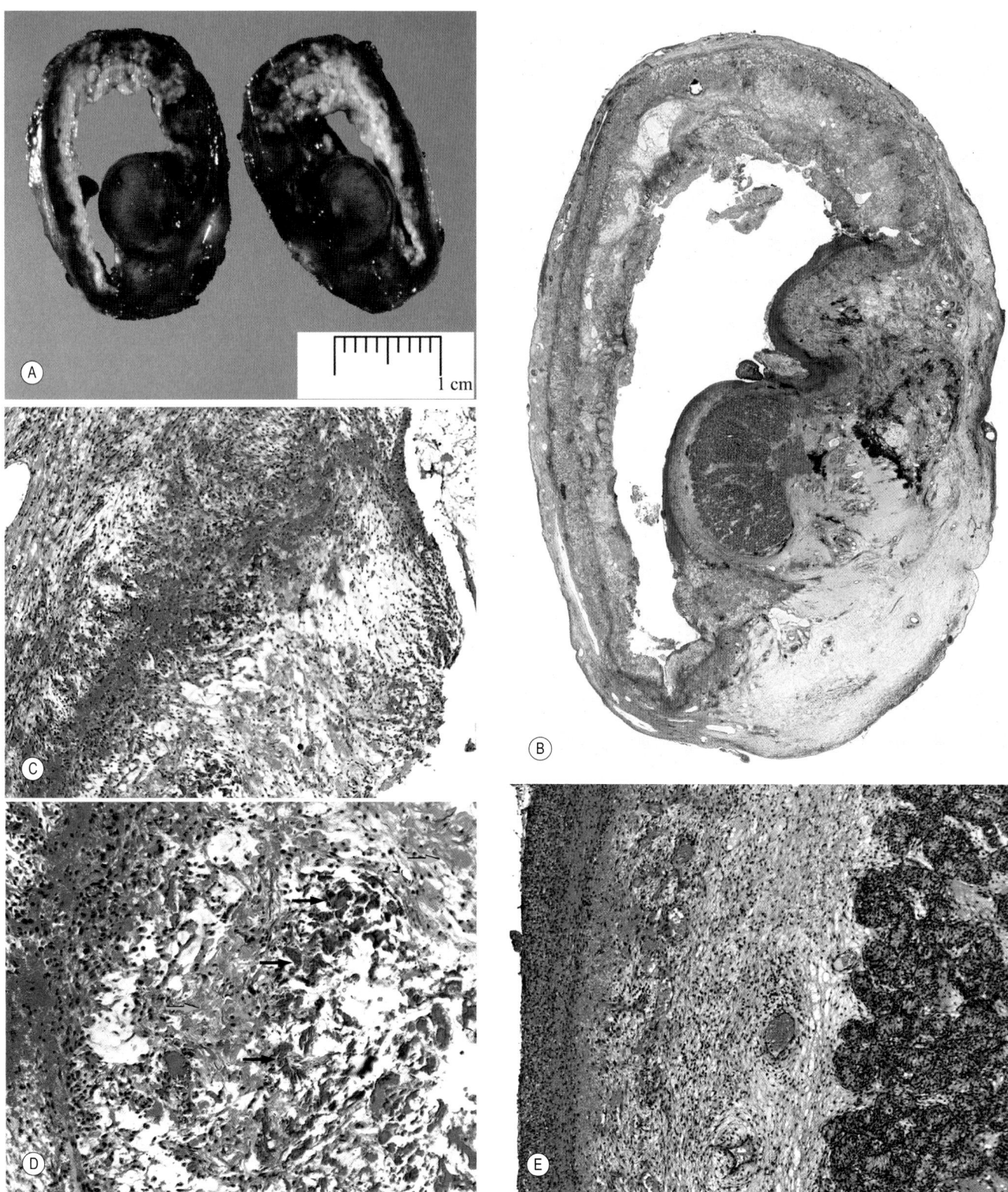

FIGURE 21.15 Meconium periorchitis in an 8-day-old boy, presenting as an enflamed, red, firm and tender lesion involving the right hemiscrotum. (A) The tunica vaginalis is greenish, fibrinous, and the cut surface was gritty. A calcified nodule was present in the distal extremity of the hernial sac (not shown). A portion of testis, 0.8 cm in diameter, is adherent to the sac. (B) Whole mount of HPS-stained section. (C and D) Tunica vaginalis with granulation tissue originating from the mesothelial lining. Numerous calcifications (black arrows) are seen admixed with the meconium (green arrows). (C and D) Tunica vaginalis with granulation tissue originating from the mesothelial lining. Numerous calcifications (black arrows) are seen admixed with meconium (green arrows). HPS, original magnification: 100× and 200× (E) Tunica albuginea with marked acute inflammatory exudate, and early granulation tissue seen in this field. Meconium and calcifications were also present on the tunica focally. HPS, original magnification: 100×.

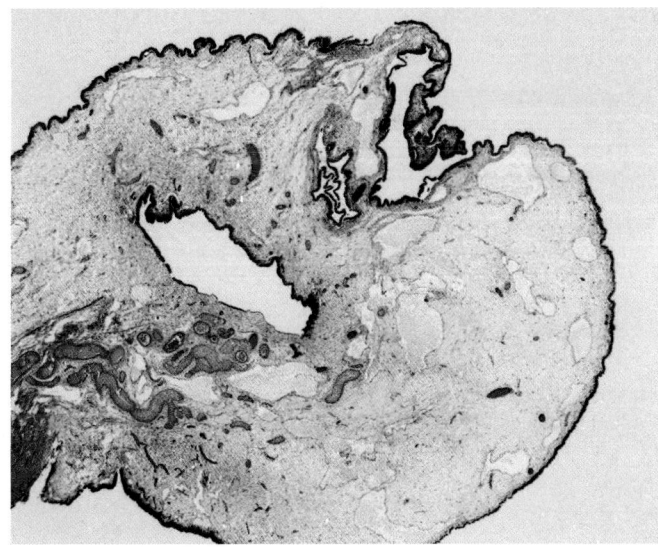

FIGURE 21.16 Appendix testis resected for torsion. Note the markedly edematous stroma as well as the dilated lymphatic and blood vessels. HPS, original magnification: 25×.

band disruption complex, or amnionic adhesion malformation syndrome) is a rare, severe congenital defect defined as a combination of at least two of the following three defects (Fig. 21.18): (1) thoraco- or thoracoabdominoschisis, often with eventration of viscera; (2) exencephaly or encephalocele with or without facial clefts; and (3) limb defects.[71, 72] In normal development, by the end of the first month pc, the amnion and chorion are separated by a thin layer of extraembryonic coelom, and the amnion is tightly apposed to the body stalk. The extraembryonic coelomic cavity will then resorb through the expansion of the amniotic cavity, allowing the amnion to fuse with the chorionic plate (Fig. 21.19). It is likely that the initiating event of LBWC occurs at this stage, i.e., before the amnion and chorion fuse, between the 3rd and 6th weeks pc. The ensuing rupture thus affects not only the development of the body stalk, resulting in an **extremely short or non-existing umbilical cord,** but also of the amnion, and of internal viscera through a vascular disruption.[49] The traction exerted by the short cord also explains the frequent association of LBWC with scoliosis (77% of cases), while vascular disruptions probably explain the diaphragmatic hypoplasia/aplasia (95%).

In Van Allen and colleague's series of 25 cases, 24 had associated internal structural defects, 18 secondary to the vascular

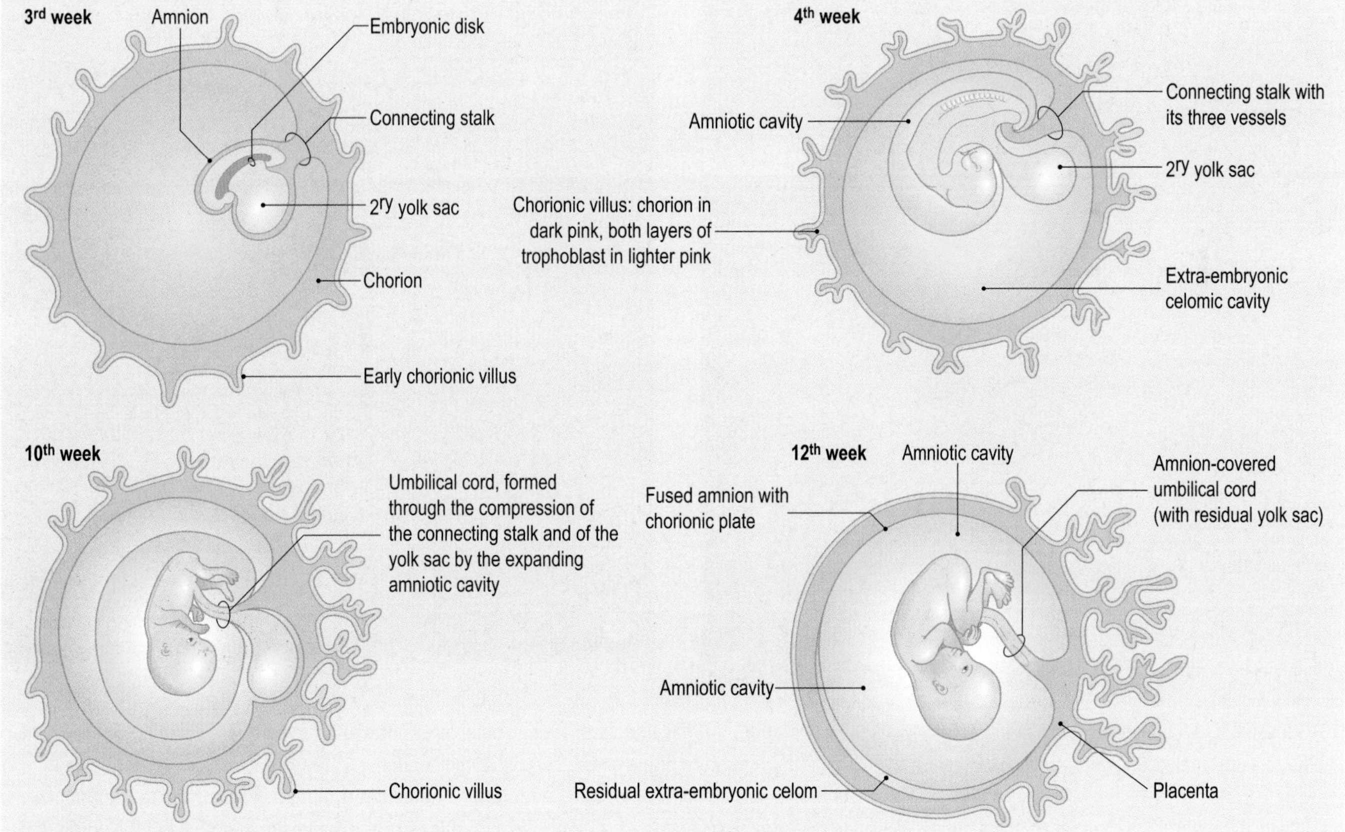

FIGURE 21.17 Development of the amnion relative to the extraembryonic coelom, with formation of the umbilical cord. At 12 weeks post conception, the amnion has expanded to replace most or all the coelomic cavity, and has fused with the chorionic plate. (From Essentiel d'embryologie humaine et principes d'embryogenèse moléculaire, © Luc L. Oligny, 2005. Used with permission.)

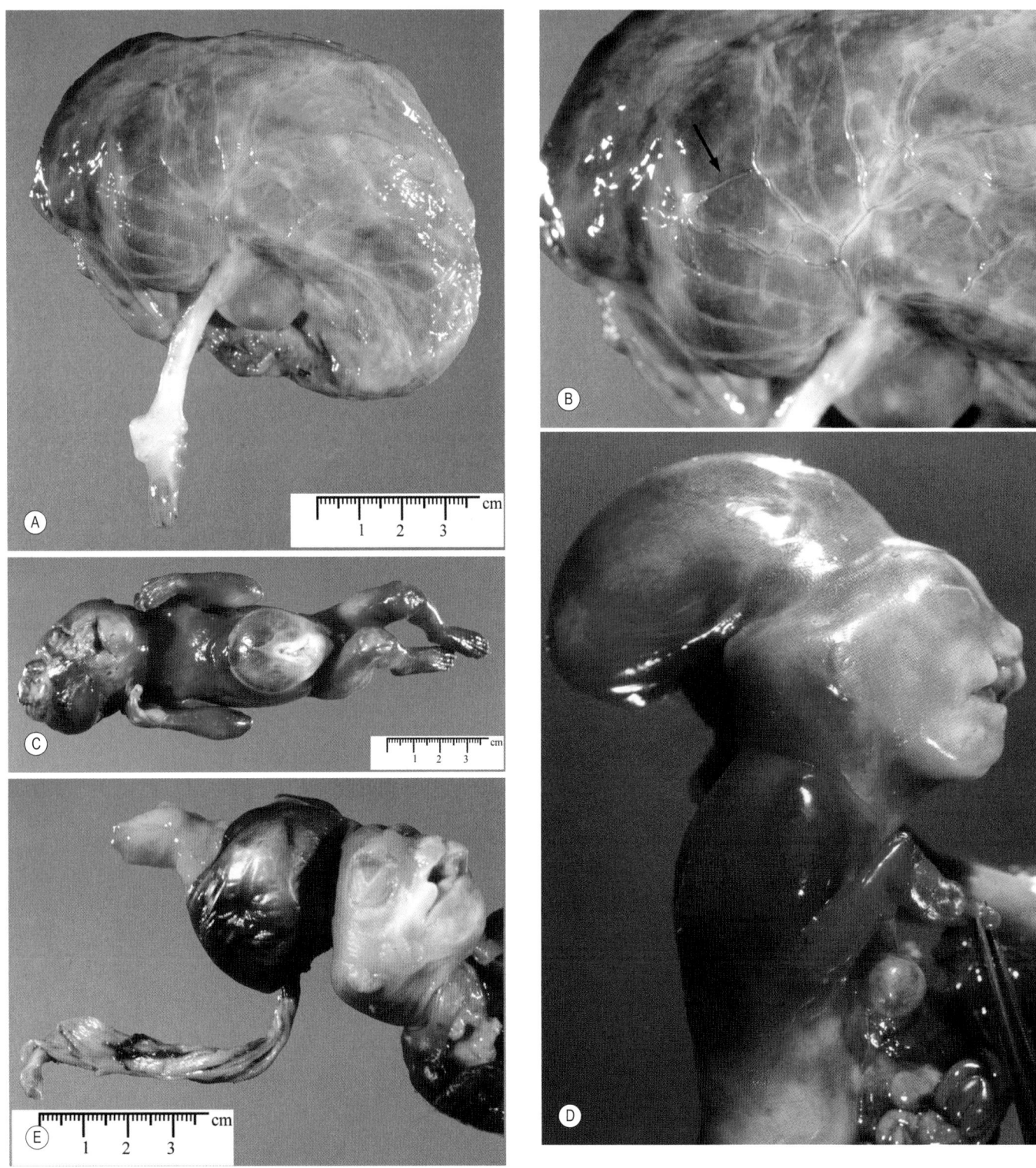

FIGURE 21.18 Limb body wall complex in a fetus of 19 weeks' gestation. (A) Placenta, with amnion completely lifted off the chorionic plate and wrapped around the extremely short cord. (B) Close-up view, showing an amnionic membrane on the surface of the chorionic plate (arrow). (C) The fetus shows characteristic changes of limb body wall complex, with encephalocele/acrania, a facial cleft, amputation of the fingers of the left hand, and an omphalocele within which the heart was herniated (the ectopia cordis and diaphragmatic hernia are not apparent on this picture). The flexion deformity of the wrists and knees is explained by the oligohydramnios which results from the amnionic rupture. (D and E) Fetus of 19 weeks' gestation with exencephaly, facial clefts, abnormal right hand, and exteriorized viscera.

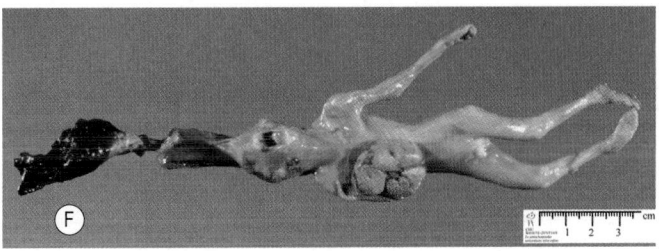

FIGURE 21.18 (*cont'd*) (F) Fetus of 16 weeks' gestation with acrania due to fusion of the head to the chorion of the membranes, resulting in anencephaly. The right hand is amputated, as are the digits of the left hand. The toes are fused bilaterally, and there is eventration of the viscera.

disruption. They found no association between the side and location of the body wall defect and the side of affected limbs, internal and cranial defects. In 85% of cases, there was evidence for persistence of the extraembryonic coelom, which might explain the presence of associated amniotic bands in 40% of cases, and 85% showed persistence of the ectodermal–amnion margin, with the amnion in continuity with the skin of the body wall defect. Their data support a vascular disruption during 4–6 weeks' gestation as an etiology for LBWC, with persistence and loss of existing tissues, persistence of embryonic structures, and secondary deformations.[72] Limb damage was found in 24 of the 25 cases (96%), and was thought to be secondary to a disruption of the embryonic vessels surrounding the tissue (84% of those 25 cases), to amniotic bands or adhesions (16%), and deformation versus hemorrhage (44%; some fetuses had more than one pathogenetic mechanism causing their limb defects).[71] Absent external genitalia and abnormal internal genitalia are frequent (3 of 4 cases reported by Colpaert et al., whose findings also support an abnormal body stalk as the primary anomaly).[73] The LBWC relatively frequently causes ectopia cordis.[49, 72, 73]

The LBWC is rare (incidence of 0.33 per 1000 live births), and **generally sporadic,** but familial cases are reported. Such cases were associated with **smoking** of cigarettes and of marijuana, and with **alcohol;** Luehr et al. recommend abstinence as well as ultrasonographic evaluations of subsequent pregnancies.[74]

The insult in **amnionic rupture sequence** (ARS) probably occurs later than in the LBWC, when the body wall and neural tubes have closed. The nature of the defect depends on two factors: (1) the location of the amniotic bands, which attach to or wrap around the fetus, and (2) on their interference with normal development, as amniotic bands can cause malformations, deformations, or disruptions.

Kalousek and colleagues have reported that the incidence of ARS is much higher in previable spontaneous abortions than in term fetuses (1/56 versus 1/2500), indicating that most cases of ARS are spontaneously aborted, especially when the amnionic bands occur early during development of the embryo or fetus.[49, 75] When neural tube defects (anencephaly or encephalocele) or irregular facial clefts are present, the bands which interfered with the normal sequence of development likely occurred prior to the 40th day pc; disruptions and deformations of structures that had developed normally, such as amputation of digits and/or limbs, pseudosyndactyly and umbilical cord constriction (a frequent cause of fetal death in ARS) indicate a later occurence.[49] The malformations caused by ARS must be distinguished from those that may be found in a syndromic setting, since ARS is sporadic and does not recur, except in the rare cases associated with collagen defects.[49, 76] Distinguishing features are that **clefts do not follow anatomic lines of closure** (e.g., in facial clefts), lesions are not symmetrical, and the amnionic surface of the placenta may be necrotic or absent, with mild reactive, granulation tissue-like changes in the underlying chorion (Fig. 21.20).[75]

Dedication

The profoundness of sorrow does not correlate with the duration of our attachment to a loved one; Vanessa died of cancer at the age of 37, within 6 months of her arrival in Montreal, 3 months after diagnosis. In that very short time, she has deeply touched every member of the department, with her smile and *joie de vivre*. She is painfully missed by all of us who had the privilege of her kindness. This chapter is dedicated to her memory, to the memory of everyone whose life was cut short before its time, and to all who lose a child, with a special attention to Vanessa's parents, Mabel and Gunter. We who delve in pediatrics see many such individuals – may our work and humanity help those who survive their children and loved ones. I also wish to pay tribute to all who invest themselves, body and soul, so that their hard work, teaching, insightful studies and experiments can bring knowledge in order to prevent such human tragedies.

Acknowledgement

The author is grateful to Dr Salam Yazbeck, for critically reviewing this manuscript. Mr. Stéphane Dedelis, our medical photographer, has taken most of the pictures included in this text, and brightened most of the others. Dr. Lynda Abed has been of invaluable help in tracking them down. I thank them for their unrelenting enthusiasm.

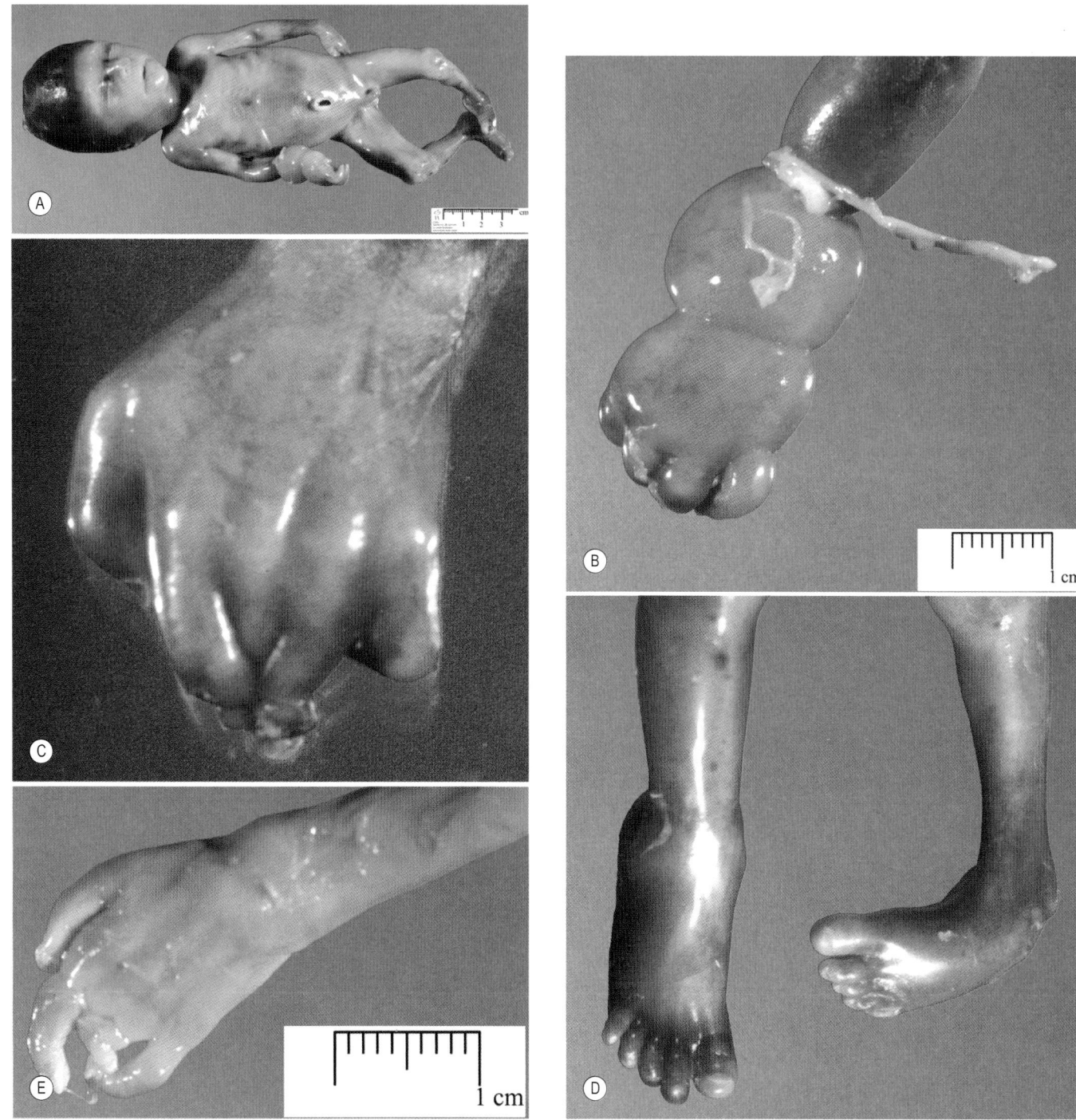

FIGURE 21.19 (A) Amnionic rupture sequence in a fetus of 25 weeks' gestation, with amputation of the right thumb, and constriction of the right wrist. (B) The right forearm is constricted by amnionic membranes, resulting in near-strangulation of the distal limb; the right thumb is amputated. (C) The fingers of the left hand are amputated and fused. (D) The equinovarus results from the oligohydramnios. (E and F) Amnionic rupture sequence of another fetus, of 21 weeks' gestation; note very fine bands of amnion attached to the amputated fingers.

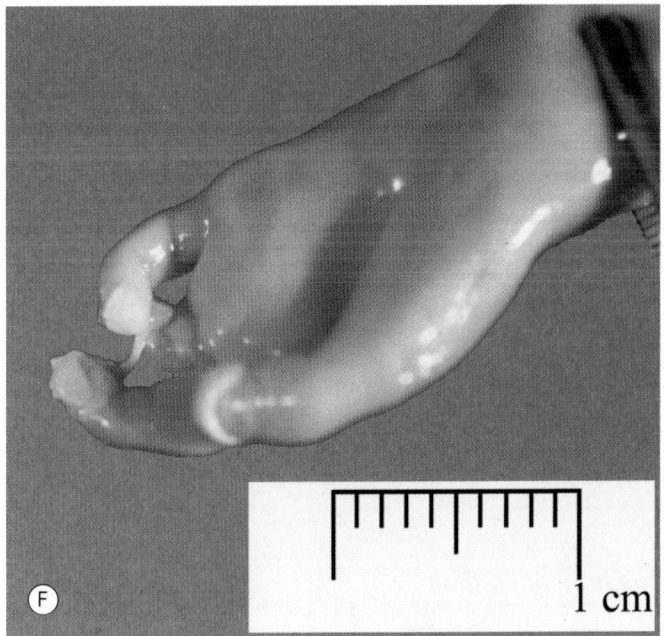

FIGURE 21.19 *(cont'd)* (E and F) Amnionic rupture sequence of another fetus, of 21 weeks' gestation; note very fine bands of amnion attached to the amputated fingers.

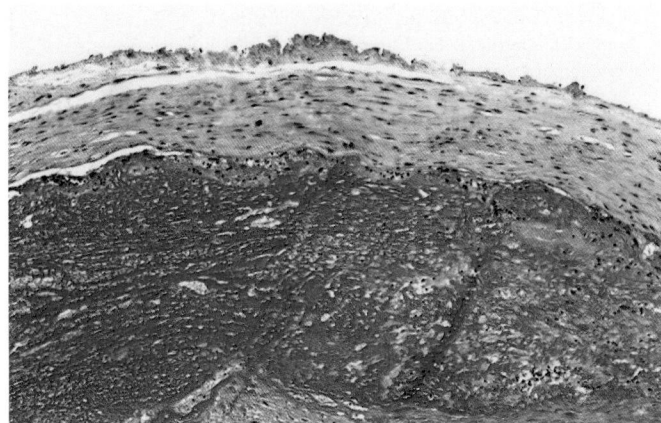

FIGURE 21.20 Placental membranes in amnionic rupture sequence. The membranes are devoid of amnion, and the surface is fibrinous. The chorion is hypercellular, indicating reactive changes rather than an artifactitious stripping of the amnion. HPS, original magnification: 100×.

In memoriam

Dr. Vanessa (Gabriela) Dorn, pediatric pathologist
Born in Argentina, May 28th, 1967
Died in Montreal, November 5th, 2004

References

Normal development of the anterior thoracic wall

1. O'Rahilly R, Müller F. Human embryology and teratology, 3rd edn. New York: Wiley-Liss; 2001.
2. Skandalakis JE, Gray SW. Embryology for surgeons the embryological basis for the treatment of congenital anomalies, 2nd edn. Baltimore: Williams & Wilkins; 1994.
3. Jolicoeur F, Gaboury LA, Oligny LL. Basal cells of second trimester fetal breasts: immunohistochemical study of myoepithelial precursors. Pediatr Dev Pathol 2003; 6:398–413.
4. Jolicoeur F. Intrauterine breast development and the mammary myoepithelial lineage. J Mammary Gland Biol Neoplasia 2005; 10:199–210.

Congenital chest abnormalities

5. Fox JE, Gloster ES, Mirchandani R. Trisomy 18 with Cantrell pentalogy in a stillborn infant. Am J Med Genet 1988; 31:391–394.
6. Stevenson RE, Hall JG, Goodman RM. Human malformations and related anomalies. New York: Oxford University Press; 1993.
7. Fokin AA, Robicsek F. Poland's syndrome revisited. Ann Thorac Surg 2002; 74:2218–2225.
8. McGillivray BC, Lowry RB. Poland syndrome in British Columbia: incidence and reproductive experience of affected persons. Am J Med Genet 1977; 1:65–74.
9. Fraser FC, Ronen GM, O'Leary E. Pectoralis major defect and Poland sequence in second cousins: extension of the Poland sequence spectrum. Am J Med Genet 1989; 33:468–470.
10. Corona-Rivera JR, Corona-Rivera A, Totsuka-Sutto SE, et al. Corroboration of the lower extremity counterpart of the Poland sequence. Clin Genet 1997; 51:257–259.
11. Parano E, Falsaperla R, Pavone V, et al. Intrafamilial phenotypic heterogeneity of the Poland complex: a case report. Neuropediatrics 1995; 26:217–219.
12. Riccardi VM. Unilateral gluteal hypoplasia and brachysyndactyly: lower extremity counterpart of the Poland anomaly. Pediatrics 1978; 61:653–654.
13. Maroteaux P, Le MM. Bilateral Poland anomaly versus thoracic dysplasia. Am J Med Genet 1998; 80:538–539.
14. Shipkov CD, Anastassov YK. Bilateral Poland anomaly: does it exist? Am J Med Genet A 2003; 118:101.
15. Bavinck JN, Weaver DD. Subclavian artery supply disruption sequence: hypothesis of a vascular etiology for Poland, Klippel-Feil, and Mobius anomalies. Am J Med Genet 1986; 23:903–918.
16. Shaham D, Ramu N, Bar-Ziv J. Leiomyosarcoma in Poland's syndrome. A case report. Acta Radiol 1992; 33:444–446.
17. Athale UH, Warrier R. Poland's syndrome and Wilms' tumor: an unusual association. Med Pediatr Oncol 1998; 30:67–68.
18. Esquembre C, Ferris J, Verdeguer A, et al. Poland syndrome and leukaemia. Eur J Pediatr 1987; 146:444.
19. Gilman PA, Miller RW. No link between Poland syndrome and leukemia? Am J Dis Child 1982; 136:176.
20. Jeune M, Beraud C, Carron R. Dystrophie thoracique asphyxiante de caractère familial. Arch Fr Pediatr 1955; 12:886–891.
21. Schmidt H. Supernumerary nipples: prevalence, size, sex and side predilection – a prospective clinical study. Eur J Pediatr 1998; 157:821–823.
22. Urbani CE, Betti R. Accessory mammary tissue associated with congenital and hereditary nephrourinary malformations. Int J Dermatol 1996; 35:349–352.
23. Grotto I, Browner-Elhanan K, Mimouni D, et al. Occurrence of supernumerary nipples in children with kidney and urinary tract malformations. Pediatr Dermatol 2001; 18:291–294.
24. Yilmaz M, Vayvada H, Menderes A, et al. Reduction mammoplasty for phyllodes tumor causing asymmetry in an adolescent female. Breast J 2003; 9:426–427.
25. Martino A, Zamparelli M, Santinelli A, et al. Unusual clinical presentation of a rare case of phyllodes tumor of the breast in an adolescent girl. J Pediatr Surg 2001; 36:941–943.

26. Rajan PB, Cranor ML, Rosen PP. Cystosarcoma phyllodes in adolescent girls and young women: a study of 45 patients. Am J Surg Pathol 1998; 22:64–69.

27. Leveque J, Meunier B, Wattier E, et al. Malignant cystosarcomas phyllodes of the breast in adolescent females. Eur J Obstet Gynecol Reprod Biol 1994; 54:197–203.

28. Agaoglu G, Ozgur F, Erk Y. Unilateral virginal breast hypertrophy. Ann Plast Surg 2000; 45:451–453.

29. O'Hare PM, Frieden IJ. Virginal breast hypertrophy. Pediatr Dermatol 2000; 17:277–281.

30. Khan A, Mohammed-Emamdee R, Lalla R, et al. Massive virginal breast hypertrophy. West Indian Med J 2000; 49:181–182.

31. Netscher DT, Mosharrafa AM, Laucirica R. Massive asymmetric virginal breast hypertrophy. South Med J 1996; 89:434–437.

32. Kucukaydin M, Kurtoglu S, Okur H, et al. Virginal hypertrophy. Case report. Turk J Pediatr 1994; 36:243–248.

33. Hollingsworth DR, Archer R. Massive virginal breast hypertrophy at puberty. Am J Dis Child 1973; 125:293–295.

34. Scott EH. Hypertrophy of the breast, possibly related to medication: a case report. S Afr Med J 1970; 44:449–450.

35. Sakai Y, Wakamatsu S, Ono K, et al. Gigantomastia induced by bucillamine. Ann Plast Surg 2002; 49:193–195.

36. Craig HR. Penicillamine induced mammary hyperplasia: report of a case and review of the literature. J Rheumatol 1988; 15:1294–1297.

37. Thew DC, Stewart IM. D penicillamine and breast enlargement. Ann Rheum Dis 1980; 39:200.

38. Desai SN. Sudden gigantism of breasts: drug induced? Br J Plast Surg 1973; 26:371–372.

39. Sabate JM, Gomez A, Torrubia S, et al. Evaluation of breast involvement in relation to Cowden syndrome: a radiological and clinicopathological study of patients with PTEN germ-line mutations. Eur Radiol 2005.

40. Kelly P. Hereditary breast cancer considering Cowden syndrome: a case study. Cancer Nurs 2003; 26:370–375.

41. Fackenthal JD, Marsh DJ, Richardson AL, et al. Male breast cancer in Cowden syndrome patients with germline PTEN mutations. J Med Genet 2001; 38:159–164.

42. Mandelbaum I. Familial florid papillomatosis of the nipple. Ann Surg 1972; 175:254–256.

43. Sirtori C, Veronesi U. Gynecomastia: a review of 218 cases. Cancer 1957; 10:645–654.

44. Haibach H, Rosenholtz MJ. Prepubertal gynecomastia with lobules and acini: a case report and review of the literature. Am J Clin Pathol 1983; 80:252–255.

45. Prezioso D, Piccirillo G, Galasso R, et al. Gynecomastia due to hormone therapy for advanced prostate cancer: a report of ten surgically treated cases and a review of treatment options. Tumori 2004; 90:410–415.

46. Derman O, Kanbur NO, Tokur TE. The effect of tamoxifen on sex hormone binding globulin in adolescents with pubertal gynecomastia. J Pediatr Endocrinol Metab 2004; 17:1115–1119.

47. Patlas M, McCready D, Kulkarni S, et al. Synchronous development of breast cancer and chest wall fibrosarcoma after previous mantle radiation for Hodgkin's disease. Eur Radiol 2005; 15:2018–2020.

48. Helzlsouer KJ, Harris EL, Parshad R, et al. Familial clustering of breast cancer: possible interaction between DNA repair proficiency and radiation exposure in the development of breast cancer. Int J Cancer 1995; 64:14–17.

Normal development of the anterior abdominal wall

49. Kalousek DK, Fitch N, Paradice BA. Pathology of the human embryo and previable fetus: an atlas. New York: Springer-Verlag; 1990.

50. Larsen WJ, Sherman LS, Potter SS, et al. Human embryology, 3rd edn. New York: Churchill Livingstone; 2001.

Congenital abdominal wall abnormalities

51. Meltzer DI. A newborn with an umbilical mass. Am Fam Physician 2005; 71:1590–1592.

52. Wilson RD, Johnson MP. Congenital abdominal wall defects: an update. Fetal Diagn Ther 2004; 19:385–398.

53. deVries PA. The pathogenesis of gastroschisis and omphalocele. J Pediatr Surg 1980; 15:245–251.

54. Torfs CP, Katz EA, Bateson TF, et al. Maternal medications and environmental exposures as risk factors for gastroschisis. Teratology 1996; 54:84–92.

55. Van Allen MI, Smith DW. Vascular pathogenesis of gastroschisis. J Pediatr 1981; 98:662–663.

56. Hoyme HE, Higginbottom MC, Jones KL. The vascular pathogenesis of gastroschisis: intrauterine interruption of the omphalomesenteric artery. J Pediatr 1981; 98:228–231.

57. Torfs CP, Velie EM, Oechsli FW, et al. A population-based study of gastroschisis: demographic, pregnancy, and lifestyle risk factors. Teratology 1994; 50:44–53.

58. Werler MM, Sheehan JE, Mitchell AA. Association of vasoconstrictive exposures with risks of gastroschisis and small intestinal atresia. Epidemiology 2003; 14:349–354.

59. Drongowski RA, Smith RK Jr, Coran AG, et al. Contribution of demographic and environmental factors to the etiology of gastroschisis: a hypothesis. Fetal Diagn Ther 1991; 6:14–27.

The inguinal region

60. Ekinci S, Karnak I, Akcoren Z, et al. Inguinal hernia as a rare manifestation of meconium peritonitis: report of a case. Surg Today 2002; 32:758–760.

61. Moore TC. Internal hernia with high jejunal obstruction in infancy due to adhesions from antenatal meconium peritonitis. J Pediatr Surg 1973; 8:971–972.

62. Tow A, Hurwitt ES, Wolff JA. Meconium peritonitis due to incarcerated mesenteric hernia: recovery following operation for intrauterine rupture of intestine. Am J Dis Child 1954; 87:192–203.

63. Herman TE, Siegel MJ. Meconium periorchitis. J Perinatol 2004; 24:188–190.

64. Williams HJ, Abernethy LJ, Losty PD, et al. Meconium periorchitis – a rare cause of a paratesticular mass. Pediatr Radiol 2004; 34:421–423.

65. Cortes D, Thorup J, Lindenberg S, et al. Infertility despite surgery for cryptorchidism in childhood can be classified by patients with normal or elevated follicle-stimulating hormone and identified at orchidopexy. BJU Int 2003; 91:670–674.

66. Lee PA, O'Leary LA, Songer NJ, et al. Paternity after cryptorchidism: lack of correlation with age at orchidopexy. Br J Urol 1995; 75:704–707.

67. Moller H, Prener A, Skakkebaek NE. Testicular cancer, cryptorchidism, inguinal hernia, testicular atrophy, and genital malformations: case-control studies in Denmark. Cancer Causes Control 1996; 7:264–274.

68. Abratt RP, Reddi VB, Sarembock LA. Testicular cancer and cryptorchidism. Br J Urol 1992; 70:656–659.

69. Gray H, Williams PL, Bannister LH. Gray's anatomy: the anatomical basis of medicine and surgery, 38th edn. New York: Churchill Livingstone; 1995.

70. Williamson RC. Torsion of the testis and allied conditions. Br J Surg 1976; 63:465–476.

Amnion rupture second sequence and limb body wall complex

71. Van Allen MI, Curry C, Walden CE, et al. Limb body wall complex: II. Limb and spine defects. Am J Med Genet 1987; 28:549–565.

72. Van Allen MI, Curry C, Gallagher L. Limb body wall complex: I. Pathogenesis. Am J Med Genet 1987; 28: 529–548.

73. Colpaert C, Bogers J, Hertveldt K, et al. Limb-body wall complex: 4 new cases illustrating the importance of examining placenta and umbilical cord. Pathol Res Pract 2000; 196:783–790.

74. Luehr B, Lipsett J, Quinlivan JA. Limb-body wall complex: a case series. J Matern Fetal Neonatal Med 2002; 12:132–137.

75. Kalousek DK, Bamforth S. Amnion rupture sequence in previable fetuses. Am J Med Genet 1988; 31:63–73.

76. Young ID, Lindenbaum RH, Thompson EM, et al. Amniotic bands in connective tissue disorders. Arch Dis Child 1985; 60:1061–1063.

Back and perineum

22

Joseph R. Siebert   Raj P. Kapur

'In all things of nature there is something of the marvelous.'   Aristotle (384–322 BC)

Normal development

Gastrulation and patterning caudal mesodermal derivatives

All of the major developmental defects of the back and perineum that are discussed in this chapter involve midline embryonic derivatives. These axial structures are derived in part from mesoderm that arises during gastrulation from two organizing centers, the primitive streak and the caudal eminence. The **primitive streak** is a dorsal longitudinal furrow that appears at the caudal end of the embryonic disc during the second week of gestation and persists until closure of the caudal neuropore (approximately 24 days post-fertilization).[1] Morphologically, the primitive streak forms the first reference point for the left–right and rostral–caudal axes. Functionally, the streak serves as the site of primary gastrulation, where epiblast-derived mesodermal cells undergo an epithelial-to-mesenchymal transformation, ingress, and distribute to much of the embryo and extraembryonic tissues. The **caudal eminence** or tail bud is a condensation of mesenchyme located caudal to the posterior neuropore, between the primitive streak and cloacal membrane.[2] As the primitive streak disappears and after closure of the posterior neural tube, the caudal eminence is a site of secondary gastrulation and neurulation, where mesodermal and neural cells are produced and contribute to the spinal cord, sacrum, and other midline structures at the caudal end of the embryo (Fig. 22.1). Examination of human embryos suggests that the caudal eminence may contribute to post-cloacal gut epithelium,[2] in contrast with avian models.[3]

Fate mapping and other experimental manipulations demonstrate the destination and eventual differentiation of many mesodermal cells that are specified as they pass through the primitive streak. The process of specification is dynamic and involves intercellular signals in the vicinity of the organizing center, which undergo genetically choreographed changes through the period of gastrulation.[4] The dynamic nature of this process causes early mesodermal émigrés from the primitive streak to be programmed differently from later derivatives. This phenomenon is clearly reflected by the nested patterns of HOX gene expression that are established during gastrulation and persist in overlapping mesodermal populations thereafter (discussed in Ch. 1).

Early populations of **mesoderm** to depart from the anterior end of the primitive streak migrate to the rostral end of the embryo, where they contribute to the cranial base.[5] More caudal embryonic mesoderm gives rise to bone, cartilage, muscle, vascular endothelium, stroma, and some parenchymal derivatives in the genitourinary tract and other connective tissues. As the primitive streak regresses, the mesoderm just rostral to the primitive streak and lateral to the notochord condenses into presomitic, intermediate, and lateral plate populations. More rostrally, the paraxial mesoderm on each side of the midline consists of evenly spaced blocks of condensed and epithelialized presomitic mesoderm, termed **somites**. These border the notochord and produce segmented tissues such as vertebral bodies, neural arches, intervertebral discs, ribs, and associated musculature. Somite formation from presomitic mesoderm is critical to the normal segmental organization plan of the human

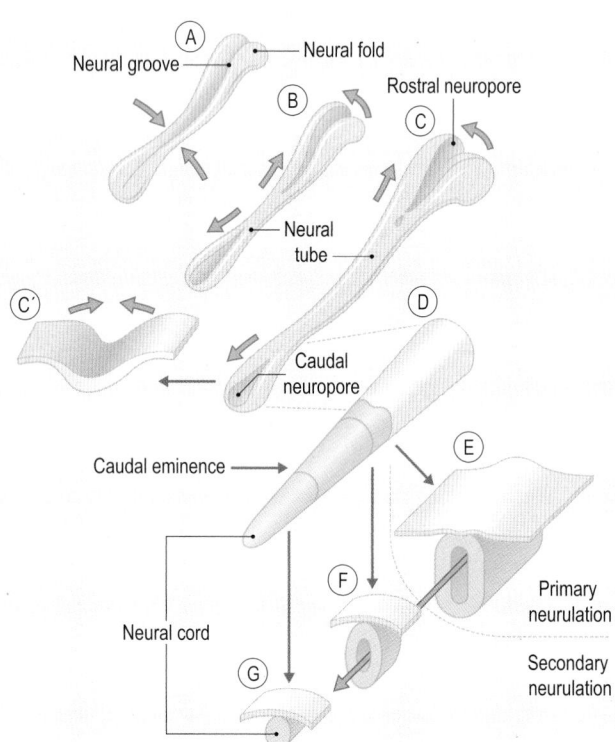

FIGURE 22.1 Development of neural tube. (A) and (B) Beginning of fusion of neural folds at about 22 days. (C) Rostral and caudal neuropores close at approximately 24 and 26 days respectively. (D)–(G) Neural tube caudal to site of caudal neuropore (depression) forms by secondary neurulation (blue) beneath intact surface ectoderm. (From O'Rahilly and Müller 1992,[1] with permission.)

body. Experimental data suggest that proper segmentation begins with the spatially and temporally coordinated expression of specific genes in presomitic mesoderm, based on a 'segmentation clock' that is governed by rhythmic oscillation of specific mRNAs.[6–8] Disruption of the finely tuned molecular signals that govern the segmentation clock are likely to delete, add, or incorrectly specify presomitic mesodermal populations, thereby affecting the gross anatomy of entire body segments.

Individual somites are subdivided into anterior–posterior, medial–lateral, and dorsal–ventral populations of cells that have distinctively different developmental fates. Each vertebral body is derived from the posterior portion of one somite and the anterior portion of the next most caudal somite. The axons of motor nerves and the neural crest cells that form dorsal root ganglia and Schwann cells preferentially invade the cranial half-segment of each somite. Similarly, ribs and neural arches are formed from the caudal half somites.

Human embryos contain 38 or 39 somites.[1] Somites 1–28 are formed from paraxial mesoderm that is produced during primary gastrulation from the primitive streak.[9] More caudal somites arise from mesoderm generated during secondary gastrulation from the tail bud. Studies of avian embryos suggest

that the boundary between these mesodermal populations probably lies within the fifth lumbar vertebra, so that the entire sacrum is a product of secondary gastrulation.[3]

Neurulation

Primary **neurulation**, the conversion of the neural plate into a cylindrical tube, occurs between the second and fourth weeks after fertilization.[1] It is a complicated process that depends on cellular events intrinsic to the neural plate epithelium, as well as forces applied by movement and proliferation of cells in adjacent mesenchyme.[10] Actual closure of the neural tube is accomplished through apposition and adhesion of the dorsal–lateral aspects of the neural plate epithelium and simultaneous fusion of the overlying ectoderm. Three sites of primary closure have been observed in human embryos.[11] The site closest to the caudal neural tube is located at the cervical level and propagates bidirectionally to encompass the posterior neuropore about 28 days after conception. Eventually, the closed neural tube and overlying ectoderm are pushed apart by somite-derived mesodermal cells, which form neural arches of the spine and surrounding soft tissues.

Primary neurulation shapes the brain, spinal cord, and overlying epidermis from the anterior forebrain to the rostral sacrum. Formation of the neural tube caudal to this level occurs by secondary neurulation.[12] Mesenchymal cells at the rostral end of the caudal eminence condense and merge with the adjacent end of the posterior neural tube. Central cavities form spontaneously within the condensed mesenchyme and establish continuity with the lumen of the neural tube, thereby extending the length of the neural tube under an intact epidermal surface.

Primary neurulation requires closure of an initially open neural tube, the lumen of which is exposed to the amniotic cavity. In contrast, secondary neurulation takes place beneath the epidermis. This fundamental difference correlates with the observation that open neural tube defects do not extend into the caudal sacrum, whereas tethered cord, lipomas, and other closed neural tube defects are common in the terminal sacral region.[10] The pluripotent nature of the caudal eminence also explains the location and frequency of congenital sacrococcygeal teratomas.

The neurenteric canal

The neurenteric canal is an important transient landmark in the **gastrulation** stage embryo.[2] This midline passage passes through the full thickness of the embryonic disc to connect the amniotic cavity with the yolk sac. It incorporates the notochordal canal, appears in the earliest stages of gastrulation, and persists until the end of primary gastrulation. The dorsal orifice of the neurenteric canal is located in the rostral end of the primitive streak and its lumen makes a right-angle turn to course rostrally within the notochord, with a long ventral opening into the yolk sac. The caudal eminence forms just posterior to the neurenteric canal. Given its location and course, maldevelopment of the neurenteric canal has been invoked to explain a variety of malformations (e.g. neurenteric cysts) in which neuro-ectodermal and gut derivatives are intimately involved.

Hindgut and perineal development

The **hindgut** is lined by endoderm and surrounding mesoderm that arise during primary and secondary gastrulation. Toward the end of primary gastrulation, the embryo converts from a discoid structure to a cylindrical shape via the combination of head, lateral, and tail folds. The latter rotates the caudal embryo through approximately ninety degrees and displaces the connecting stalk from a position parallel to the caudal end of the embryonic disc to an orientation perpendicular to the ventral abdominal wall (Fig. 21.1). These movements compress the yolk sac and create a blind-ended hindgut 'pocket' in the caudal endoderm. Derivatives of the hindgut include the descending colon, rectum, urinary bladder, urethra, and lower vagina.

The terminal portion of the hindgut, distal to the intra-embryonic coelom, is the **cloaca**. The cloaca communicates with the allantois, an endodermal diverticulum in the connecting stalk, via the urachus. Embryologically, the urachus results from involution of the allantois. The allantois extends initially as a diverticulum of the yolk sac into the connecting stalk. It has limited function – blood cells are formed in its wall (part of the yolk sac) and its blood supply persists as umbilical arteries and vein[13]. The extraembryonic portion of the allantois disappears during the second month of gestation, or persists as a tiny fibrous cord in the umbilical cord. The intracoelomic portion of the allantois involutes completely by the third month of gestation. The urachus remains patent until the fifth month and thereafter persists as the medial umbilical ligament.

The cloaca is partitioned into the rectum and urogenital sinus by a coronal sheet of mesoderm, the **urorectal septum**.[14, 15] The urogenital sinus gives rise to the bladder and lower vagina. The urorectal septum develops through a complex series of mesodermal movements and associated endodermal folds. Although older embryologic studies emphasize active downward mesodermal invasion and elongation of the urorectal septum between the rectum and urogenital sinus, more recent studies emphasize lateral ingrowth of mesoderm to form the septum and relatively little disproportionate growth of the septum relative to adjacent structures.

The ventral portion of the cloaca, immediately caudal to the urachus, is invested with mesoderm. This tissue persists to form the anterior bladder wall and muscles and bones of the overlying inferior abdomen and pelvis. More caudally, the cloacal wall is a two-layered membrane (**cloacal membrane**) that is composed of endoderm and ectoderm, without intervening mesoderm.[16] The cloacal membrane degenerates to form cutaneous orifices of the bladder, rectum, and vagina. Normally, partitioning of the cloaca begins at 4 weeks and is complete by 8 weeks.

Development of the **urethra**, particularly in the male, is complicated and somewhat controversial.[17–19] Contemporary models suggest that the urethral epithelium is derived from an extended portion of the cloacal endoderm that is shaped by proliferation and migration of adjacent mesoderm. This relationship accounts for the association of epispadias and exstrophy. In males, the process involves proximal-to-distal fusion of the endodermal–ectodermal boundary of urethral folds along the inferior surface of the penis.

Malformations of the spine and paraspinal tissues

Spinal rachischisis

Rachischisis is a defect in the spinal column. These bony lesions are generally midline and more common posteriorly than anteriorly. Skin and subcutaneous soft tissue that normally cover the spine may be intact (spina bifida occulta) or absent with posterior rachischisis (spina bifida aperta). Discontinuity of vertebral neural arches allows herniation of spinal meninges, or exposes spinal cord to the external environment. Ventral rachischisis is rarer. Such lesions may be recognized radiographically as midline clefts in vertebral bodies. Ventral defects sometimes act as conduits for fistulae between the central nervous system and the gastrointestinal (GI) tract or prevertebral tumors including teratomas (see the following discussion of Currarino syndrome). The pathogenesis of rachischisis and the pathology of associated central nervous system findings are discussed more fully in Chapter 36.

Congenital scoliosis

Congenital scoliosis can result from **mechanical forces** in utero that deform the spinal column or incite malformation of one or more vertebra, either of which causes the spine to deviate. Sources of deformation include external factors (e.g. oligo-hydramnios, uterine fibroids, amniotic bands) or neuromuscular deficits that result in asymmetric tension on the left and right sides of the spine. Primary vertebral malformations may affect any portion of the vertebral column. Unless a number of vertebrae are involved, the severity of scoliosis at birth is usually subtle and progresses as a child grows. Radiographically-defined types of dysplastic vertebrae include hemivertebrae, unsegmented bars, wedge vertebrae, block vertebrae, and mixed anomalies.[20] When dysplastic vertebrae are identified, malformations of other organs may be found in 44% of patients.[21, 22]

Spondylothoracic dysplasia

Dysplasia of **thoracic vertebrae** is often associated with fusion, branching, ectopia, or agenesis of adjacent ribs. The term spondylothoracic dysostosis (STD) was introduced to refer to patients with symmetric fusion of the ribs at the costo-vertebral

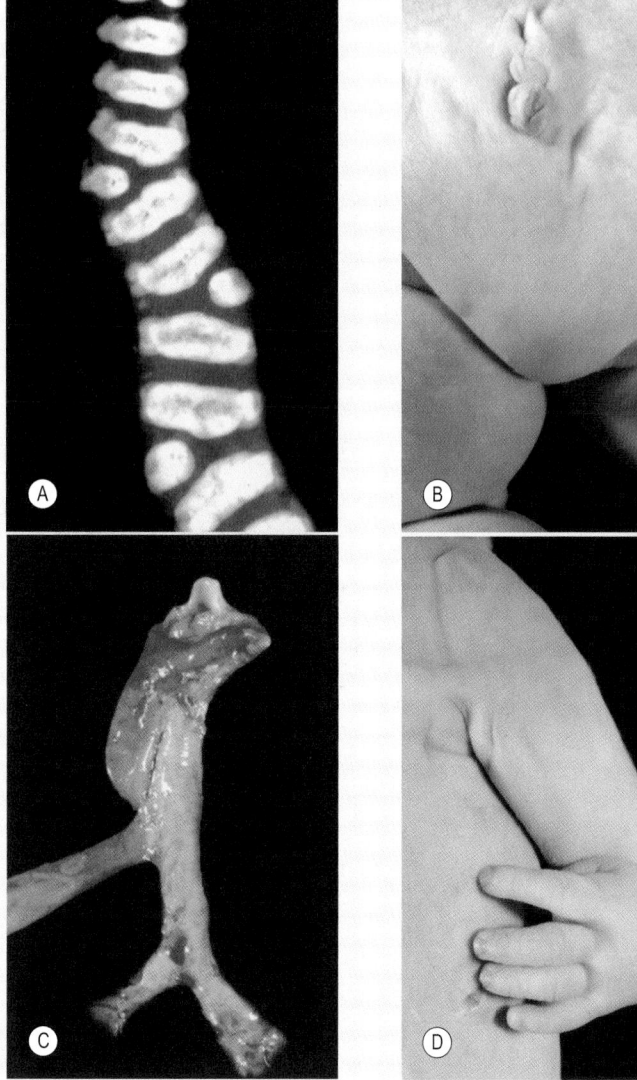

FIGURE 22.2 VATER/VACTERL association.
(A) Anteroposterior radiograph of thoracic hemivertebrae.
(B) Posterior view of infant, showing caudal appendage and absent gluteal folds (rare in VATER/VACTERL association), with imperforate anus. (C) Posterior view of larynx and trachea, showing atresia of proximal esophagus and tracheoesophageal fistula arising at mid trachea. (D) Radial agenesis is associated with characteristic deviation of wrist and hand. The thumb (present in this case) is often absent in radial agenesis.

junctions, as opposed to spondylocostal dysostosis (SCD), in which asymmetric bizarre rib and vertebral alterations (fusion, broadening, bifid) are present, but the costo-vertebral junction is intact.[23] The thoracic skeleton has a 'crab-like' appearance in STD, due to crowding of the posterior elements with dispersion more anteriorly. Jarcho-Levin syndrome is a diagnosis that has been used inconsistently to refer to one, both, or subtypes of these conditions, and some authorities avoid the eponym to prevent confusion.[24]

Both STD and SCD are associated with malformations in many other organ systems. Genetic analysis of both disorders is consistent with autosomal recessive inheritance, despite the fact that autosomal dominant inheritance has been postulated for some cases of STD.[24] Mutations in the δ-like 3 (*DLL3*) gene on chromosome 19 have been found in patients with SCD,[25] but this gene has not been linked to the spondylothoracic phenotype.[24] *DLL3* encodes a ligand for the receptor NOTCH, which is involved in many aspects of embryogenesis including

somitogenesis.[26] The axial defects observed in humans with *DLL3* mutations correlate well with the expression patterns of DELTA and NOTCH in paraxial mesoderm, as well as other organ systems. The gene responsible for STD is unknown, but linkage has been established to chromosome 2q32.1.[24]

VACTERL association

The acronym VACTERL is used to describe the statistical association of vertebral, anal, cardiac, tracheoesophageal, renal and limb anomalies, which occurs more frequently together than predicted by their individual incidences (Fig. 22.2). Although rare examples of familial recurrence have been reported,[27] the association is usually considered sporadic and cause(s) is/are unknown. The broad array of phenotypic changes can complicate diagnosis (Table 22.1).[28–30] A diagnosis of VACTERL is acceptable if anomalies in three or more of the organ

TABLE 22.1 MALFORMATIONS OBSERVED IN VACTERL ASSOCIATION

Vertebral	Scoliosis, kyphosis, lordosis, hemivertebrae, segmentation defects, fused vertebrae, sacral agenesis
Anal	Atresia or stenosis
Cardiac	Atrial septal defect, ventricular septal defect, other cardiac defect
Tracheal	Tracheoesophageal fistula (with atresia or stenosis of esophagus), tracheal stenosis
Esophageal	Atresia or stenosis
Renal	Agenesis, cystic dysplasia, horseshoe kidneys, ectopic/supernumerary kidneys, ureteral anomaly
Radial/Limb	Hypoplastic or absent radii, syndactyly, polydactyly, absent or hypoplastic thumbs
Other	Short stature, rib anomaly, wide cranial sutures, ear anomaly, hypoplasia or agenesis of lung, laryngeal anomalies, hypoplastic stomach or other anomaly, cleft palate, small penis, exstrophy of cloaca

After Botto et al 2003,[28] Dunn et al 1986,[29] and Weaver et al 1984.[30]

systems indicated by the acronym are present and no other recognizable pattern of human malformation exists.[28] Some of the common defects observed in the VACTERL association include vertebral and perineal anomalies, particularly dysplastic or absent vertebrae and anal atresia. Hydrocephalus occurs in a subset of VACTERL patients, as a distinct association (VACTERL-H), which may be an X-linked condition.[31]

Depending on the malformations that exist in an individual patient, other syndromes must be considered in the differential diagnosis. One of the most important entities to exclude is Fanconi anemia, a multigenic autosomal recessive disorder with pleiotropic manifestations that overlap considerably with VACTERL. A diagnosis of Fanconi anemia can be confirmed by chromosomal breakage studies (see Ch. 19), which should be considered, particularly when radial ray reduction defects are present. Several teratogens have been associated with VACTERL (i.e. dibenzepin, levostatin, lead, adriamycin, the latter in rats), but workers have not identified any consistent pattern among these substances.[32, 33] Maternal diabetes is also a recognized risk factor for this association.[34] Sonographic findings of radial aplasia and small or flattened stomach within the context of polyhydramnios (suggestive of esophageal fistula or atresia) suggest the diagnosis of VACTERL.[35] Although the cause of VACTERL association is unknown, it has been speculated that the underlying mechanism involves disruption of the sonic hedgehog (*SHH*) signal transduction pathway.[36, 37] This hypothesis is based on the VACTERL-like phenotypes of various mouse models in which genes that encode components of this molecular pathway have been mutated. To date, no consistent mutations have been observed in homologues of these genes in human VACTERL patients. However, VACTERL association occurs in many patients with distal chromosome 13q deletions,[38] and has been reported with less frequency with other chromosomal alterations.

Neurenteric cysts and fistulae

Neurenteric (or neuroenteric) cysts are rare, **congenital cysts** found in contact with the central nervous system and lined by gastrointestinal (GI) mucosa. Neurenteric cysts and fistulae comprise a group of closed (i.e., skin-covered) or occult spinal dysraphisms that usually present without mass effect. They can be viewed primarily as intraspinal extramedullary lesions. They are often connected to thoracic or abdominal structures, generally derivatives of the primitive gut, by fibrous strands, fistulae, or vertebral clefts.

Neurenteric cysts have been referred to by a wide variety of terms, including NE cyst, enteric or enterogenous cyst, endodermal cyst, cyst of foregut origin, gastrocytoma, teratomatous cyst or tumor, split notochord syndrome, NE canal remnant, and dorsal enteric fistula.[39–41] Neurenteric cysts are rare, having been described less than 30 times in the pediatric literature.[42] This observation may be influenced by the fact that many cases are diagnosed in adulthood. Neurenteric cysts comprise approximately 0.7–1.3% of all spinal tumors and have a male:female ratio of 1.5–3:1.[40, 43] Fistulae are considerably less common than isolated cysts, but little is known about them from an epidemiologic point of view.

Surgical biopsy, excision, or complete autopsy examination reveal cysts with smooth, opalescent surfaces composed of fibrous tissue and lined by ciliated or non-ciliated, simple or pseudostratified cuboidal or columnar epithelium that often produces mucin.[39, 44] Such epithelium can resemble that of the respiratory or GI tract.[41] However, cysts with more respiratory-appearing epithelium are more aptly termed bronchogenic cysts; as such, they may contain cartilage and are thought to arise from remnants of the primitive respiratory system, in a manner akin to neurenteric cysts.[39] Neurenteric cysts react with antibodies to cytokeratin, epithelial membrane antigen, and carcinoembryonic antigen.[45] By electron microscopy, the columnar epithelial cells that line these cysts are associated with basal lamina and apical junctional complexes.[46]

Cysts may be found at any level in the spinal cord, but the most common sites are lower cervical (54%), upper thoracic (21%), and thoracolumbar (15–18%); lumbosacral cysts occur least frequently.[47] Cysts generally lie within the spinal canal and ventral to the spinal cord, although, with enlargement, they can extend lateral or posterior to the spinal cord. In one review, 83% of cases were intradural extramedullary, 14% were intramedullary, and 3% were extradural.[48] A small number may be located within the vertebra.[49] Because of the differential growth of the vertebral column and spinal cord, defects in vertebral bodies may be found several segments below the cyst.[39] In one instance, the thoracic spinal cord was found to herniate into a mediastinal neurenteric cyst.[50] Extraspinal cysts are found most often in the posterior mediastinum or, less often, the abdomen, and associated with anterior defects of the vertebrae.[40, 51] Cysts involving the posterior fossa are very rare, but have been reported.[52] Neurenteric cysts occur as part of **split notochord syndrome**, which is associated with vertebral anomalies (anterior or posterior spina bifida, butterfly vertebrae, or hemivertebrae) and at times intestinal duplication.[42, 53–55] Fistulae consist of fibrous strands or patent channels; open vertebral clefts, when large, permit herniation of viscera to subcutaneous regions of the back.

Pathogenesis is not understood entirely, but several hypotheses have been advanced. One is that islands of endodermal tissue are displaced and come into contact with and adherent to neuroectoderm during the third week of embryonic life. Ordinarily, during this period, mesoderm begins to develop, separating endoderm and ectoderm. The notochord detaches from the endoderm and the neurenteric canal (canal of Kovalevsky) is open (day 18–21), allowing transitory contact of endoderm and neuroectoderm. Differential growth of the embryo is thought to close this canal under normal conditions.[53] Persistence of the neurenteric canal and developing adhesions may result in cyst or fistula formation and other notochordal pathology, particularly split notochord. A neurenteric fistula occurs when the canal persists, traversing an anterior defect in the spine; if the canal (i.e. fistulous tract) is interrupted, an isolated neurenteric cyst results. A second explanation for persistence of the neurenteric canal is overdistention of the neural tube.[56] After neural tube closure, at 4 weeks, an abnormally expanded neural tube could rupture, producing a focal lesion such as neurenteric cyst or sinus, or more widespread neural tube defect. Finally, focal vascular disruption has been suggested as a possible mechanism.[57] None of these hypotheses explains all cases. Exact causes for these aberrations remain to be discovered.

Associated conditions include dermal sinuses, split cord malformations, tight filum terminale, persistent terminal ventricle, and filar and intradural lipomas.[58, 59] Other central nervous system lesions include lipomeningomyelocele,[60] meningomyelocele, or meningocele,[61] and diastematomyelia.[62] Vertebral anomalies are common, and of course requisite in cases of neurenteric fistula. At least two instances of neurenteric cyst in association with Klippel-Feil syndrome have been reported.[45, 63] Cysts may also be found in the GI tract or the bowel may be duplicated.[64] In one study, 69% of patients with neurenteric cysts showed cutaneous stigmata, including hirsutism (hypertrichosis), subcutaneous mass, flat capillary hemangioma, dermal sinus, and pedunculated mass.[58] Although lesions are congenital, cases often present in the first two decades of life or even later.[40] Cysts may recur if surgical resection is incomplete.[65] Shunting of the cyst cavity to the subarachnoid space may help prevent recurrence.[40] Meningitis or epidural abscess may occur, and recur, especially within the context of neurenteric fistula.[42, 64]

Cloacal anomalies

Many variations of cloacal and anorectal anomalies are encountered owing to the complexity of normal development of the urorectal septum and coordination with anal and urogenital membrane rupture in the embryo (Fig. 22.3).[66] The nomenclature can be confusing because terms like 'female pseudohermaphroditism', 'cloacal dysgenesis', 'cloacal dysgenesis sequence', 'persistent cloaca', 'urorectal septum malformation sequence', 'vesicoileal fistula', and 'vesicointestinal fistula' are used inconsistently in the literature and clinic. Subtle differences exist in the application of some of these terms, and an accepted classification of anomalies does not yet exist.[67] 'Cloacal dysgenesis' or 'agenesis of the cloacal membrane', for example, are seemingly broad terms, that some authors restrict to relatively specific changes, namely internal cloacal anomalies without any perineal opening.[68–70] In the sections that follow, an effort is made to define diagnostic terms and use them consistently.

Persistent cloaca

Persistent cloaca is a severe form of anorectal anomaly. It is defined most broadly as any type of persistent connection between bladder, rectum, and/or vagina. Persistent cloaca has traditionally been viewed as an anomaly occurring solely in females, based primarily on arbitrary taxonomic criteria, as opposed to embryogenic principles. The cloaca is found in both sexes. In affected females, the terminal portions of the rectum, vagina, and urinary tract all empty into a common cloacal pouch with a single, or less often absent, perineal opening. In males, the rectum and bladder are usually connected by a fistula and the anus is imperforate. Descriptions of male examples of persistent cloaca have been variably referred to as partial urorectal septum malformation sequence[71] or cloacal dysgenesis sequence.[68, 69, 72] Furthermore, restricting the diagnosis to females has presumably caused a substantial degree of ascertainment bias in previous studies.[71]

Varied anatomic associations with persistent cloaca result in part from variations in the fusion of urorectal septum and, in females, upon the course of development taken by the müllerian ducts after they make contact with the primitive cloaca. Abnormal relationships (fistulas, atresias) between the cloacal derivatives and adjacent organs are common. The confluence of genital, urinary, and intestinal tracts may be low (near the perineum), intermediate, or high, the latter posing the greatest difficulty to surgeons.[73] Labia vary from open to fused; the clitoris likewise varies in configuration and size and may communicate with the cloaca. The vagina, or vaginas, are generally thin-walled, dilated, and may contain calcified material or other debris.[74] The urethra may be stenotic, atretic, elongated, or patulous. Ureters may drain ectopically, or be stenotic or absent; vesicoureteral reflux is common. The kidneys may be hypoplastic, malrotated, ectopic, or fused, and may show features of obstructive dysplasia including cysts. Some have classified the cloaca as vaginal or urethral, depending upon the appearance and nature of communication.[75] This has physiologic significance, in that the more narrow the opening, the less urine or meconium can escape. Sphincter musculature may be rudimentary. The coccyx and sacrum may also be abnormal, for reasons that are not entirely understood.

In the male, persistent cloaca is associated with ambiguous genitalia, split or absent penis, bifid scrotum, hypospadias, penoscrotal transposition, and cryptorchidism. Kidneys may be absent, dysplastic, or hydronephrotic. The duplication and/or schism of external genitalia, especially in males, has given rise

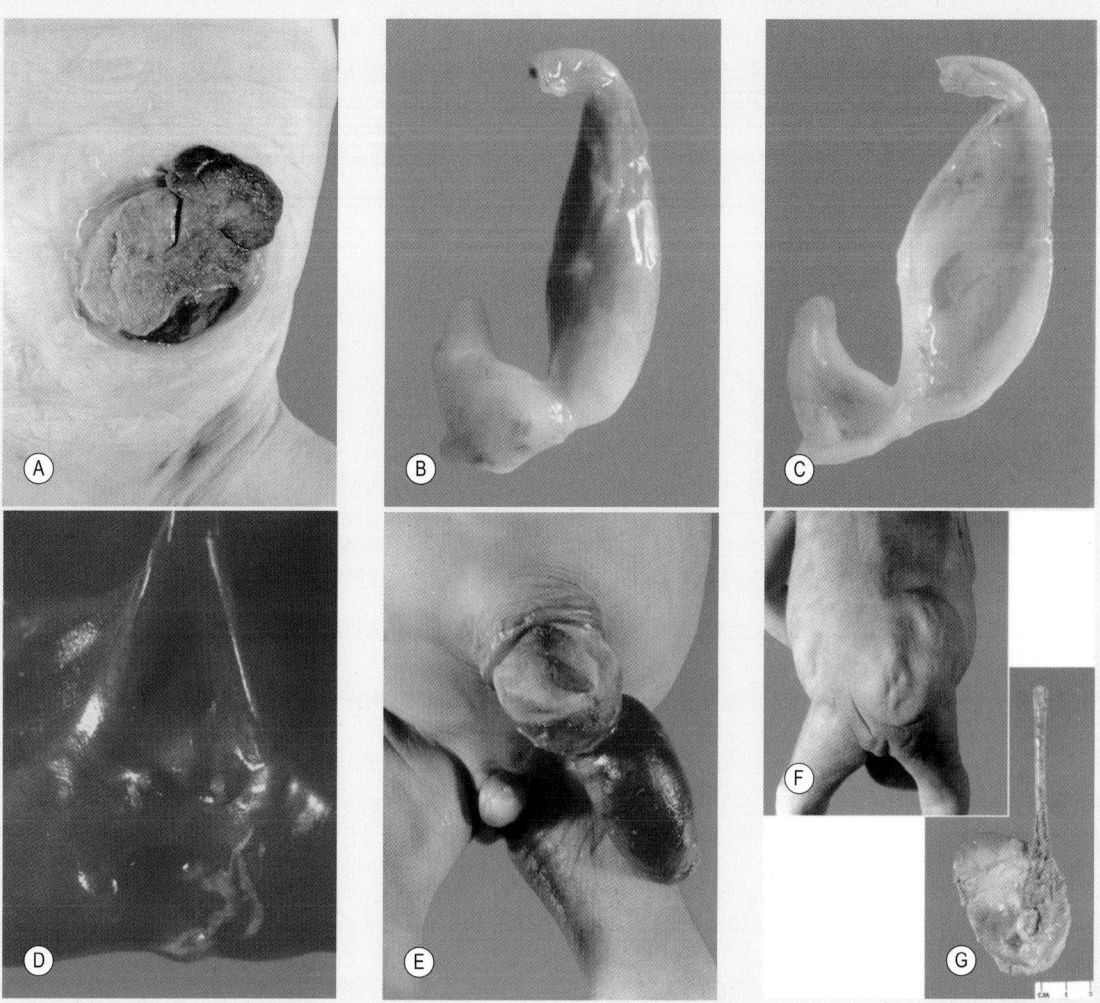

FIGURE 22.3 Anomalies of cloacal development. (A) Superior vesical fissure, with umbilical hernia, from 10-day-old male with trisomy 18. (B) Autopsy specimen, showing urinary bladder (left) and distended rectum (right) from 20-week male fetus; the anus was imperforate. (C) Hemisected bladder and rectum from (B) showing rectovesical fistula. (D) Bladder exstrophy in 20-week female fetus with trisomy 21; fetus suffered intrauterine demise. (E) Cloacal exstrophy with prolapsed ileum in 11-day-old female (46,XX) with ambiguous genitalia and imperforate anus; a monozygotic twin also had cloacal exstrophy.[66] (F) Back of patient illustrated in (E) with cloaca, imperforate anus, and myelocystocele, visible as large, irregular, subcutaneous swelling. (G) Ex situ view of spinal cord with myelocystocele from patient shown in (E) and (F). (From Siebert et al 2005,[214] with permission.)

to complex gender issues, compelling some workers to opt for a female sex assignment when reconstruction does not seem possible. Reports of this relatively rare group of patients have been largely anecdotal, and so this approach continues to receive needed scrutiny.

Ultrasound findings suggestive of persistent cloaca include cystic mass in the pelvic midline, transient ascites, and possible colonic dilatation or hydronephrosis.[76] The early (i.e. first/second trimester) appearance of ascites occurs by retrograde flow of urine through the fallopian tubes.[77,78] This is more likely to occur within the context of narrowed perineal opening and/or elongated, urethra-like cloaca, either of which limit the outflow of urine.[74] Retrograde flow ceases at or around 26 weeks, possibly as the

tubes become irritated by contact with meconium and urine and then obstructed. Subsequent accumulation of urine may then lead to hydrocolpos and hydronephrosis. Repeat paracentesis has been used to placate the ongoing accumulation of ascitic fluid and development of hydronephrosis.[79]

Persistent cloaca is thought to result from incomplete septation of the embryonic cloaca by the urorectal septum. The association of talipes, scoliosis, or other deformities suggests that intrauterine constraint, perhaps with amnion involvement, may also play a role.[80] Classic illustrations of the 4–6-week embryo show the hindgut and tail located very close to amniotic folds (Fig. 21.1), the adhesion of which could conceivably compress or tether the embryo as it elongates and straightens. This view is supported by the association of congenital limb deficiencies or obvious amputations in some patients with cloacal exstrophy,[81] although the possibility of another form of caudal vascular disruption cannot be excluded. Some deformations associated with persistent cloaca probably result from oligohydramnios.

Exstrophy of the bladder

Exstrophy of the urinary bladder is a condition wherein the anterior wall of the bladder and overlying ventral body wall are defective, and the bladder lumen is exposed inferior to the umbilicus. Bladder mucosa is composed of columnar and squamous epithelium, with glandular structures in the submucosa, which is prominent and interlaced with abundant fibrous tissue; smooth muscle layers are reduced in size.[82] Postnatally, irritants produce acute and chronic inflammation. The defect may extend to the umbilicus (which itself can be displaced inferiorly) and involve the dorsal aspect of the penis (epispadias); in females, the result may be bifid clitoris (female epispadias). At the lateral margins of the defect, the bladder mucosa is in continuity with epidermis. The term 'exstrophy–epispadias complex' is used by many to encompass the spectrum from isolated epispadias to severe cloacal exstrophy. Diastasis of the symphysis pubis and rectus abdominis muscles may also occur. The urinary tract may be normal, or altered by unilateral renal agenesis, horseshoe kidney, or megaureter. Associations with other anomalies occur less frequently than with cloacal exstrophy, but include rotational abnormalities of pelvic bones, scoliosis, sacral agenesis, and hindgut duplications.

The epidemiology of bladder exstrophy is sufficiently different from cloacal exstrophy, compelling some to consider them separate entities.[83] The incidence of bladder exstrophy is several times greater than that of cloacal exstrophy, having been estimated at 1:10 000 to 1:50 000 live births.[84] The male:female ratio is skewed, variably reported as 2.3:1 to as high as 6:1.[85, 86] The familial occurrence is relatively rare, but the recurrence risk in families is low, about 1 in 100. This figure is, however, 500 times that of the general population.[85, 87]

Etiology is not known with certainty, but seems to be heterogeneous. Most cases appear to be sporadic, but autosomal dominant inheritance has been described.[88] Recessive inheritance has also been implied, as one known proband was the result of a consanguineous union.[89] Exstrophy of the bladder occurs in mono- or dizygotic twins, and may be concordant or discordant.[83, 86] Like many malformations, the frequency is higher in monozygotic twins.[90]

Pathogenesis is not understood completely, but midline defects in both bladder and abdominal wall appear to result from incomplete closure by mesoderm. The mechanism responsible for bladder exstrophy has been postulated in different ways, as an over-development of the cloacal membrane that prevents the ingrowth of mesoderm, or as premature rupture of the cloacal membrane itself.[91, 92] Damage to the cloacal membrane is thought to occur earlier in cases of cloacal exstrophy than bladder exstrophy.[83] Other suggestions include caudal maldevelopment of

genital tubercles that interferes with closure of the cloacal membrane, or abnormal insertion of the body stalk, with subsequent interference with mesodermal migration.[93] This latter mechanism would seem especially plausible in cases manifesting inferior displacement of the umbilicus. Patients with exstrophy are at risk for the development of neoplasia, several decades after birth, particularly adenocarcinoma, but also squamous cell carcinomas or, rarely, rhabdomyosarcoma or transitional cell carcinoma.[94-96] These can develop in the bladder, sites of urinary-intestinal anastomoses, or the colon.[97, 98]

Morphologic variants of bladder exstrophy include superior or inferior vesical fistula or fissure; closed exstrophy (bifid bladder, possibly with vesicointestinal fistula, thought to represent a secondary repair following cloacal membrane rupture); pseudoexstrophy (mesodermally deficient, but formed cloacal membrane that leads to ventral weakening of bladder with ventral bulge that resembles a hernia); 'duplicate' exstrophy (partial fusion of superior vesicle fistula with abdominal wall, with subsequent trapping and exposing of a portion of bladder mucosa); and variations in the extent of penile epispadias.[99]

Exstrophy of the cloaca

In the years since its original publication, some debate has ensued over whether the term 'exstrophy' applies primarily to exstrophy of the bladder or cloaca. The question has importance, as the two anomalies differ not only anatomically and embryologically, but epidemiologically as well.[83] Carey has opted for limiting the designation to exstrophy of the cloaca.[100]

In **cloacal exstrophy** (also referred to as 'exstrophia splanchnica'), the anterior wall of a persistent cloaca is absent, along with the corresponding overlying portion of the abdominal wall.[101, 102] The pubic bones diverge, each receiving the insertion of separate rectus abdominis muscles. The exteriorized cloaca appears as two sheets of bladder mucosa, each with a ureteral orifice and separated from one another by exposed bowel mucosa with two openings. The upper communicates with the terminal ileum, which frequently prolapses to form an elongated tube, while the lower orifice communicates with a blind-ended segment of colon, generally with imperforate anus. The appendix is frequently duplicated. In males, epispadias is a constant finding and the penis is often bifid or duplicated. The scrotum is absent and the testes are undescended. In females, the vagina is septate, the uterus is duplicated, and the external genitalia are absent. Paired vaginal orifices are present in the exposed cloacal surface.

In cloacal exstrophy, as in persistent cloaca, phenotypic variability is recognized. An expanded phenotype for cloacal exstrophy has been designated **OEIS** (**o**mphalocele, **e**xstrophy, **i**mperforate anus, **s**pinal anomaly).[103] The omphalocele may be large (containing bowel and liver) or small; spinal defects include myelomeningocele and myelocystocele (Fig. 22.3). OEIS is usually sporadic, although familial recurrence of OEIS has been reported. '**Covered exstrophy**' describes secondary closure of the abdominal wall defect after formation of an

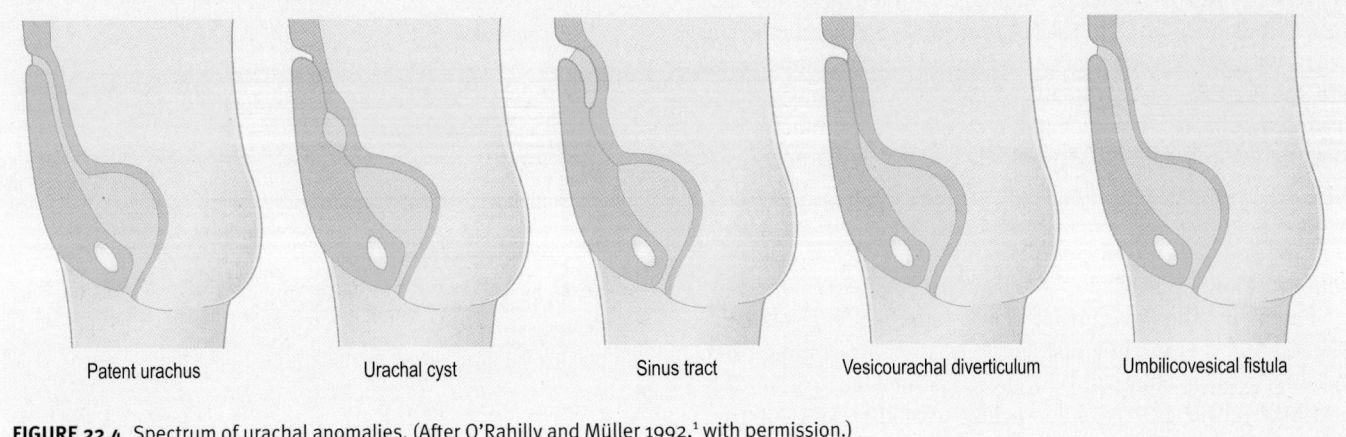

| Patent urachus | Urachal cyst | Sinus tract | Vesicourachal diverticulum | Umbilicovesical fistula |

FIGURE 22.4 Spectrum of urachal anomalies. (After O'Rahilly and Müller 1992,[1] with permission.)

exstrophy. The umbilicus is low set and the lower abdominal wall is paper-thin. Epispadias and some degree of pubic separation are usual. Rarely, a modified cloaca persists and intestine, urinary tract, and vagina all open to the exterior through a single orifice. The urethra or rectum may empty into the vagina, or the lower end of the vagina may communicate with either of these structures. Rarely, the urethra opens into a vagina with a closed external orifice. Flow of urine into the vagina ordinarily causes extreme distention, not only of this structure but also of the uterine corpus. If the vagina opens into the urethra or rectum or if a fold of perineum grows forward and hides the orifices of both the vagina and the urethra, as it does in some forms of female pseudohermaphroditism, a misdiagnosis of absent vagina may be made.

Causes of cloacal exstrophy remain unclear, but are probably heterogeneous. The presence of anomalies in twins is sometimes discordant,[104] which excludes simple genetic or teratogenic mechanisms. Cloacal exstrophy has been produced in the laboratory, but the number of successful models is few and confined mostly to chicks and a few mammalian species. The relative paucity of models of cloacal exstrophy suggests that most teratogens may not affect cloacal membrane development.

The pathogenesis of cloacal exstrophy is not fully understood. A popular view is that exstrophy develops from early rupture of the cloacal membrane, with accompanying incomplete descent of the urorectal septum.[105] Early rupture could cause or result from incomplete investment of parts of the cloacal membrane by mesoderm that form the anterior abdominal muscles and pubic bones.[106] Another view is that the cloacal membrane is abnormally large and/or non-conducive to mesodermal invasion.[92, 107] The contribution of the urorectal septum is unclear, with debate persisting over whether its growth is active or passive.[108–110]

These views may also be incomplete, in that delayed rupture of the cloacal membrane has been documented ultrasonographically between 18 and 26 weeks.[111–113] Differences in the magnitude or timing of membrane rupture or mesodermal invasion may be responsible for these variations.[90, 93] Variation in the degree of abdominal wall closure is recognized. Infrequently, the cloacal membrane has been observed by ultrasonography to persist until the second trimester, only to undergo delayed rupture, producing cloacal exstrophy.[111, 113]

Urachal anomalies

Although not a cloacal anomaly per se, the urachus and cloaca are related developmentally and topographically. The **urachus** is normally invested in umbilicovesical fascia and suspended from the ventral abdominal wall by its own mesentery, the mesourachis.[114, 115] The urachus is bounded laterally by the umbilical arteries (lateral umbilical ligaments after closure) and extends from the inner, peritoneal surface of the umbilicus to the dome of the bladder. Microscopically, a cross-section of urachus reveals an outer muscular layer that may be fully formed, irregular, or absent and a medial vascular layer; when patent, an inner layer consists of transitional or cuboidal epithelium.[115]

Urachal anomalies are most often diagnosed clinically or incidentally at autopsy. A patent urachus is diagnosed easily, for example, in the newborn by the presence of urine escaping from the umbilicus. However, the average age of diagnosis in one series of 45 patients was 4 years, with ages ranging from 1 day to 20 years.[116] A variety of significant complications can arise from urachal anomalies. Sites of infection may be contained within layers of abdominal fasciae, or may spread into the peritoneal cavity; calculus may be observed. In severe cases, infection may result in bladder rupture[117] or lead to death.[118] Large perforated urachal cysts may harbor loops of bowel and lead to strangulation.[119, 120]

The terminology used to describe urachal remnants depends upon the location of patent segments with respect to body wall and bladder (Fig. 22.4). **Urachal cysts** occur when one or more isolated segments of the urachus remain patent. Urachal remnants, cystic or otherwise, exhibit transitional (urinary) or possibly cuboidal epithelium, in contrast to the columnar (intestinal) epithelium of vitelline remnants. Without epithelium, they are termed pseudocysts (although infected cysts may also lose their epithelium). Urachal cysts are often asymptomatic, but when enlarged, can present as abdominal masses. **Sinus tracts** are patent, elongated segments of distal urachus, and are also asymptomatic, becoming apparent chiefly when draining from infection. **Vesicourachal diverticula** occur when a portion of urachus in contact with the bladder remains patent. **Umbilico-vesical fistula** results when the urachus is congenitally absent and the dome of the bladder communicates directly with the umbilicus and exterior.

Patent urachus or urachal cyst is rare. Incidence statistics suggest that they are identified, or at least reported, more often in autopsy series than clinical ones. The incidence at autopsy has been given as 1:7610 for patent urachus and 1:5000 for urachal cysts.[121] The incidence of patent urachus is variably reported, between 1 in 108 000 and 3 in over a million births; the incidence of other urachal anomalies is considerably less. Patent urachus and urachal cysts appear to occur twice as frequently in males, although this ratio is not borne out in all studies. The recurrence risk appears to be very low, although familial cases of urachal sinus are recognized.[122] Additional anomalies are identified in nearly 50% of patients, and include urinary or GI anomalies, omphalocele, and myelomeningocele.[123] Urachal anomalies are seen with increased frequency in individuals with prune belly syndrome, and a patent urachus can, in fact, provide an escape for urine and thus protect the system from excessive distention.[124–126] Cystic masses in the umbilical cord close to the body wall are associated with lethal aneuploidy or other congenital anomalies.[127, 128] Persistent urachal remnants are associated infrequently with the development of neoplasia, which may be benign or malignant, the latter composed chiefly of mucinous adenocarcinoma.[129, 130]

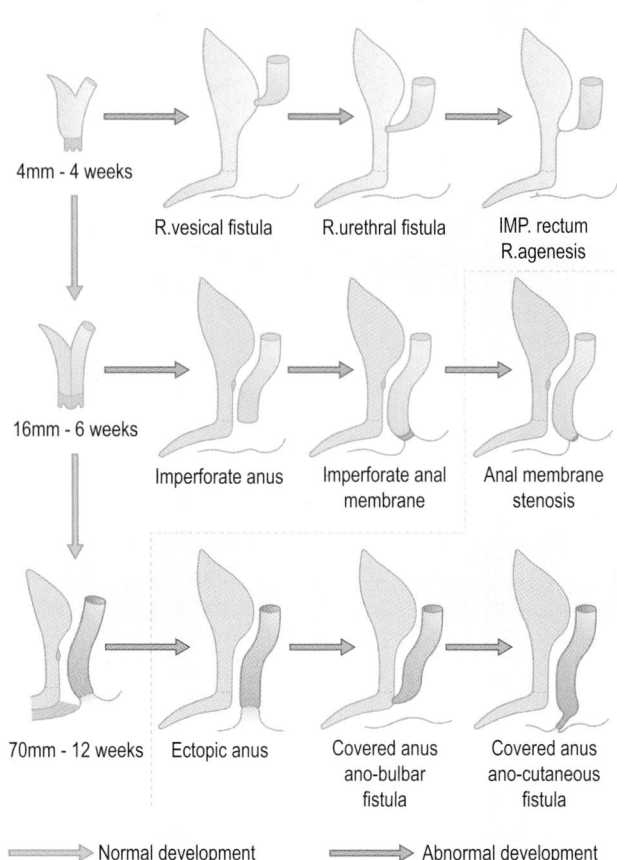

FIGURE 22.5 Anomalies of the male rectum and anus. Normal and abnormal development are shown for the embryonic and early fetal stages. Imp: Imperforate; R: recto- or rectal. (From Stephens 1963,[138] with permission.)

Anorectal malformations

Anorectal anomalies result from improper septation of the cloaca and may or may not involve the urinary bladder or internal genitalia (Figs 22.5 and 22.6). This group of anomalies includes anal stenosis and imperforate anus. **Anal stenosis** refers to a narrow anal canal that may impede defecation. Narrowing may be subtle, and diagnosis aided by published norms.[131, 132] **Imperforate anus** is a skin-covered malformation that interrupts the continuity of the rectal lumen and exterior. With either anal stenosis or imperforate anus, a variety of associated internal rectal malformations can exist. Fistulous connections may be to the urinary bladder, urethra, penoscrotal region, or vagina, which are all regarded as variants of persistent cloaca (discussed earlier). The associated rectal anomalies are classified by their relationship to the levator (puborectal) muscle, which normally forms a sling around the distal rectum. Low defects are atretic/fistulous at or below the level of the levator; high defects are above it. Low abnormalities (anal stenosis; covered anus) are thought to arise from defective formation of the anal pit. High abnormalities (anorectal agenesis; rectal atresia) are more serious

(i.e. greater risk of long-term problems, most notably incontinence), are more difficult to repair, and are more often associated with additional anomalies. Intermediate forms also exist (rectovestibular or rectovestibular urethral fistula; rectovaginal fistula; anal agenesis without fistula), though they are often classified as cloacal anomalies.[133]

Anorectal anomalies occur in approximately 1 of every 5000 births. They present in over 30 varieties, many of which include imperforate anus.[133] Minor anomalies of the anus occur in about 1 of 500 births. Care must be taken to distinguish variants of **normal structures**, such as accessory raphes or even postmortem contraction of skin and anal dilatation, from signs of abuse.[132]

The **etiology** of anorectal malformation is unknown, but is probably heterogeneous. Familial occurrences have been suggestive of X-linked recessive, autosomal recessive, or autosomal dominant inheritance.[134, 135] Teratogenic exposure has been documented, in the sense that imperforate anus is recognized as a complication of maternal diabetes. New information suggests that defects in SHH signaling may be responsible for hindgut malformations, at least in GLI2 and GLI3 deficient

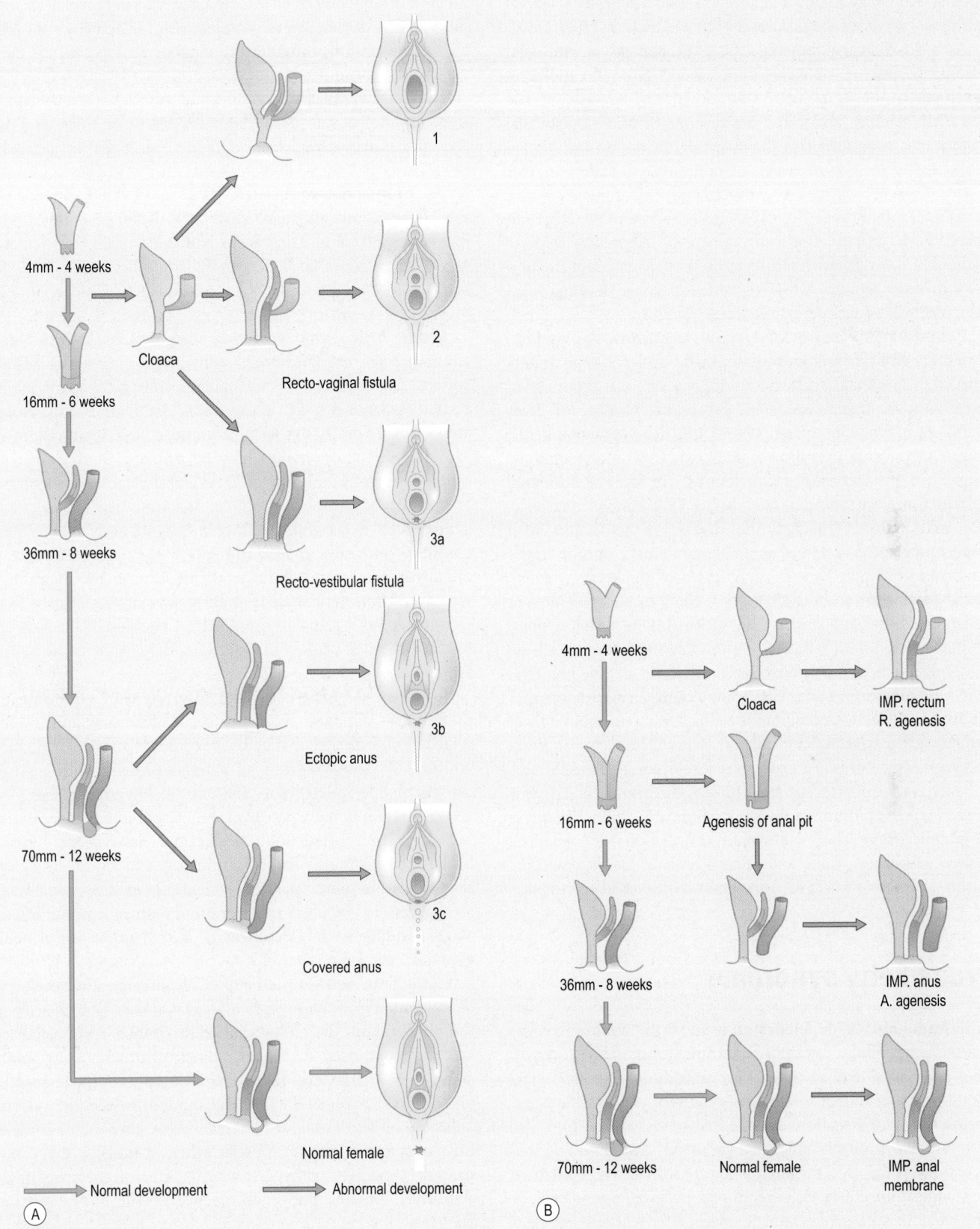

FIGURE 22.6 Anomalies of the female rectum and anus. Normal and abnormal development are shown for the embryonic and early fetal stages. Both communicating and non-communicating forms are depicted. (After Stephens 1963,[138] with permission.)

mice.[136] Anorectal malformations are associated with several chromosomal syndromes: cat-eye, 13q-, and trisomy 18.[137]

As with cloacal anomalies, the **pathogenesis** of anorectal lesions is not completely understood. Normal anorectal development depends upon the downward growth of the urorectal septum and later perforation of the dorsal anal membrane, invagination of the proctodeum, and fusion of anal tubercles by the eighth week of gestation. Variation in this process leads to anal stenosis, covered anus (incomplete rupture of the anal membrane), or anal agenesis (failure of the cloaca to descend and proctodeum to invaginate).[138] Anorectal agenesis is thought to originate from regression of the hindgut beyond the urorectal septum, while rectal atresia may develop from even more excessive regression of the hindgut.[1]

Congenital anomalies of kidneys, cardiovascular system, vertebrae, and pelvic bones are found in up to 50% of infants with high anorectal malformations, but are less common in lower anal malformations. This substantial number of cases manifests as syndromes, associations, and developmental fields, and requires careful syndromic diagnosis.[137] GI malformations consist of tracheoesophageal lesions (in 10%), duodenal obstruction from annular pancreas, Ladd's bands, or atresia, and malrotation; Hirschsprung disease is associated with imperforate anus. Vertebral anomalies are most common in the lumbosacral region (one-third of cases of imperforate anus). Spinal dysraphism is related to the type of anorectal lesion: 46% of patients with dysraphism have high lesions, 17% have low ones. The association with tethered cord and syringohydromyelia are recognized. Currarino triad consists of sacral defect, presacral mass, and imperforate anus (see below). Genitourinary anomalies are also recognized. Vesicoureteric reflux is found in about 60% of patients with anorectal malformation. Renal agenesis or dysplasia and vaginal or uterine anomalies are found; some 35% of female patients with imperforate anus have a bicornuate uterus, for example. Less common is the association with vaginal agenesis or duplication. The widespread association of anorectal malformations with other anomalies is probably best exemplified by the VATER or VACTERL association, as discussed previously.

Prune belly syndrome

Abdominal muscle deficiency or 'prune belly' syndrome is the triad of congenitally-deficient abdominal musculature, urinary tract anomalies, and, in males, cryptorchidism (Fig. 22.7). The condition has also been termed Eagle-Barrett syndrome, urethral obstruction malformation complex, or triad syndrome.[139] The first case was probably published in 1839;[140] several additional reports are available in the older literature (JB Beckwith, personal communication, 2002). Osler reported an affected 6-year-old boy and cited instances of dramatic megacystis without apparent urethral obstruction by Parker in 1895 and Guthrie in 1896;[141] several other classic works also contain case reports.[142-144]

Phenotypes vary, and cases of **incomplete, partial, or pseudo prune belly syndrome** are recognized. Abdominal muscles or the renal system are often affected, but may be normal, in some cases.[145, 146] Around 3% of patients with prune belly syndrome are female, and may manifest normal or atretic urethras and a variety of genitourinary anomalies.[147, 148]

Familial hypoplasia of abdominal muscles without urinary tract anomalies has been reported, but it is unclear if this condition is part of the prune belly spectrum.[149] The incidence has been given as 1 in 35 000–50 000 births.[150] In one substantial review of infants born between 1983 and 1989, incidence was similar, at 3.2/100,000 live births.[151] Of the 60 cases reported in that series, 50 were male; blacks had three times the incidence of whites. Some 60% died, usually in the first week, and 70% had an associated anomaly. Approximately 5% of patients are monozygotic twins with an unaffected co-twin.[146]

Prune belly syndrome may be associated with other anomalies or even syndromes. Some three-quarters of affected patients have additional abnormalities, most often involving the cardiac, pulmonary, GI (malrotation, malfixation, imperforate anus), renal (cystic dysplasia), or musculoskeletal systems.[146] Musculoskeletal anomalies may be primary (limb deficiency, talipes deformity, hip dysplasia, vertebral defects) or secondary (renal osteodystrophy, scoliosis, pectus deformities).[152] In prune belly syndrome, pulmonary hypoplasia is the most common anomaly, and is thought to be a consequence of oligohydramnios and abdominal pressure on the diaphragm. An association with reduction anomalies of the legs has been recognized, and pressure exerted on the external iliac arteries by the distended urinary bladder suggested as the cause of limb anomalies.[153, 154]

In male and female patients with prune belly syndrome and pulmonary stenosis, sensory neural deafness, and mental retardation, inheritance may be autosomal recessive or possibly X-linked.[155] Another group of patients presents with enlarged urinary bladder, microcolon, and intestinal hypoperistalsis.[156, 157] GI obstruction in these patients is functional, and bladder outlets are free of obstruction; abdominal laxity and hydroureteronephrosis also occur. Familial cases follow an autosomal recessive inheritance pattern.[158] Smooth muscle changes are recognized, i.e. vacuolar degeneration, reduced smooth muscle actin, and alterations in contractile and cytoskeleton proteins; ganglion cells are present.[159-161]

In the fetus with prune belly syndrome, the **abdomen** may be expanded and tense, with taut, glassy skin (Fig. 22.7A). In the older infant, the abdominal wall is more likely collapsed, lax, and composed of loose folds of dramatically wrinkled skin (Fig. 22.7B). Careful dissection reveals complete absence or variably hypoplastic rectus abdominis and/or external oblique, internal oblique, or transverse abdominis muscles. Microscopically, skeletal muscle, when identified, may show secondary atrophy or hypertrophy.[162] Ischemic necrosis of the abdominal muscles, presumably a direct result of pressure, has been described in four patients with prune belly syndrome.[163]

The **kidneys** are usually hydronephrotic, with clubbed calices and elongated infundibula. Renal dysplasia is common, often asymmetric, and may be accompanied by cyst formation. Nephrocalcinosis may be diffuse and visible by routine

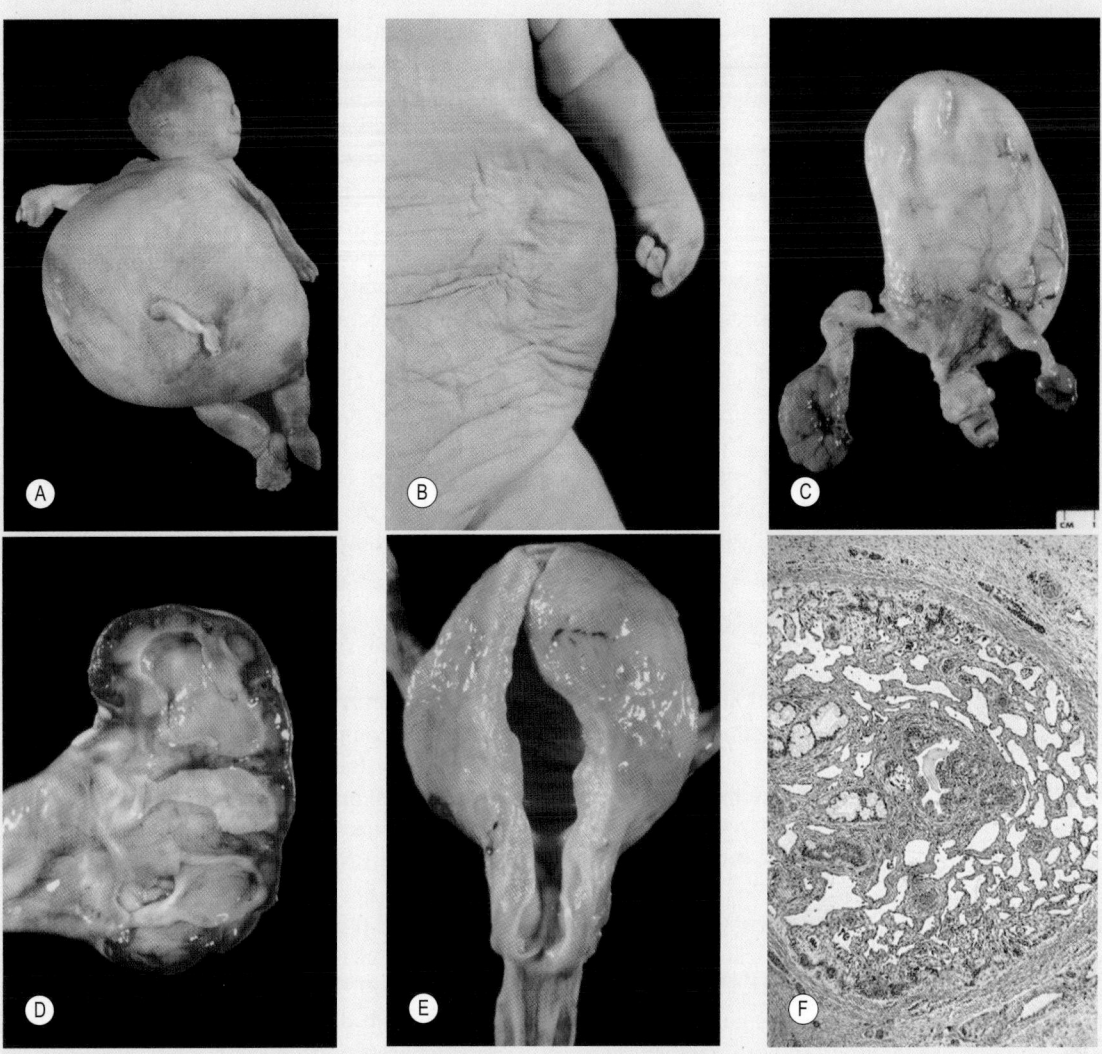

FIGURE 22.7 Prune belly syndrome. (A) This 32-week male fetus was born by caesarean section with marked distention of the abdomen, an early manifestation of prune belly syndrome, and pronounced ascites. The thoracic cage was markedly deformed by the distended abdomen and the lungs were severely hypoplastic. Microscopically, the urinary system showed bilateral multicystic renal dysplasia; the urethra consisted of a single, hypoplastic lumen that extended the length of the penis and clusters of multiple dysplastic urethral lumina that may have been manifestations of recanalization [shown in (F)]. The infant died minutes after birth; clinicians reported that abdominal muscles and diaphragm were so thin that the heart could be seen beating through the body wall. (B) Close-up view of abdomen of 3-month-old male infant, showing prominent wrinkling of the skin, which is characteristic of prune belly syndrome. Massive ascites was diagnosed prenatally and the fetus was delivered by caesarean section at 33 weeks. Posterior urethral valves were resected at 1 month, but the baby died at 3 months of pulmonary hypoplasia and bronchopulmonary dysplasia. (C) Urinary system, with pronounced megacystis. The specimen was from an 18-week male fetus diagnosed with pronounced ascites and distended abdomen (early prune belly syndrome). Distention of the urinary bladder was presumably due to outlet obstruction, although careful examination (including sectioning of the membranous urethra) revealed no specific lesion. Failure to identify a cause of obstruction occurs commonly; it is possible that megacystis results from a physiologic obstruction due to abnormal posture, with kinking of the urethra. An edematous penis and bilateral hydroureter and hydronephrosis are evident. Note the disparity in size of kidneys, also a common finding in prune belly syndrome. Microscopically, kidneys exhibited distorted renal architecture, tubular atrophy, focal fibrosis, and multifocal areas of calcification. (D) Sectioned kidney of infant with prune belly syndrome and posterior urethral valves [illustrated in (E)], showing pronounced distention of the collecting system and ureter. (E) Anterior view of opened urinary bladder and urethra, showing posterior urethral valves. Both ureters were dilated, the left kidney was atrophic, and the right was hydronephrotic [shown in (D)]. (F) Cross-section of urethra showing multiple lumina from 32-week male fetus with early prune belly syndrome [shown in (A)]. It is unclear whether this change is primary or represents the secondary recanalization of a previously atretic urethra. (Hematoxylin and eosin.)

radiography; calcification may extend into ureters and bladder mucosa. The urinary bladder may be distended and relatively thin-walled, without trabeculae, or collapsed and thick-walled. The bladder neck and trigone are widened and ureteral orifices prominent. The dome of the bladder may be adherent to the umbilicus, and exhibit a prominent diverticulum, thought to be a urachal remnant. This area may rupture resulting in the accumulation of urine within the abdomen.[164] The ureters are generally dilated irregularly and follow a tortuous course. Microscopically, muscle fibers may be focally or totally absent in the bladder and ureters, and replaced by fibrous tissue.[165] No clear-cut orientation of circular or longitudinal fibers is recognized. Attenuation of smooth muscle elements may be more pronounced in the lower third of the ureters, but this finding is variable.[166]

The urethra must be examined carefully for the presence of atresia, a rare anomaly, and for more common **posterior urethral valves** (Fig. 22.7E). These are very delicate and easily destroyed by the prosector, as they lie in the prostatic portion of the urethra, immediately dorsal to the symphysis pubis. A technique for dissecting the male urethra has been published.[167] The prosector may choose to open the urethra longitudinally, to facilitate gross examination, or forego this procedure and section the unopened urethra for subsequent microscopic examination. Duplicated, overriding urethral lumens connected by a narrow channel have been described and attributed to urethral kinking.[168] Megaurethra has been reported in some cases. Microscopy may reveal a single dilated, angulated lumen.[164] Multiple urethral lumina may also be seen, the formation of which is unclear and may be a primary change or represent secondary recanalization of a urethra that is, or was, atretic. Penile erectile tissue may be partially or completely absent. The **prostate gland** is hypoplastic in most cases of prune belly syndrome, with limited development of glandular elements and smooth muscle.[169] The possible significance of this finding is reviewed below.

The undescended testis in prune belly syndrome resembles other **cryptorchid testes** in a number of ways. Fetuses exhibit marked Leydig cell hyperplasia.[170] Young men exhibit only Sertoli cells in undescended testes, and boys have no spermatogonia.[171, 172] Segmental atresia of the vas deferens has been reported in one patient with high intra-abdominal testis. In one study, germ cells were atypical, with large nuclei and prominent nucleoli; alkaline phosphatase staining was intensely localized to the cytoplasmic membrane, and similar to intratubular germ cell neoplasia.[173] Long-term follow-up for the development of testicular neoplasia is recommended; retroperitoneal germ cell tumor, teratoma, and testicular seminoma have been diagnosed in survivors.[174–176]

Despite multiple descriptions and reviews, its pathogenesis remains incompletely understood. **Etiology** may be heterogeneous. Mechanical factors, genetic or chromosomal components, teratogens, and infectious agents have been implicated, although few of these have been positively shown to cause prune belly syndrome. Mechanical factors have been implicated most often and are discussed below. Infrequently, prune belly syndrome has been associated with chromosomal changes.

Reports include an interstitial deletion of 6q,[177] trisomy 18,[164] and mosaicism for monosomy 16 (45,XY,-16/46,XY), the latter change in two siblings.[178] The majority of cases have a normal karyotype. This does not rule out a genetic effect entirely, of course, and other familial cases have been reported.[179, 180] One mother exposed to Tigan™ (trimethobenzamide) and Bendectin™ (a preparation of doxylamine succinate and a vitamin supplement) gave birth to monozygotic twins discordant for prune belly syndrome.[181] However, discordance weakens the teratogenic hypothesis in this case. An unspecified teratogenic effect upon somatic mesoderm has been suggested by other workers,[147] as has viral illness early in gestation.[182]

It has not always been clear whether the changes in abdominal musculature or the renal system are primary or secondary. In earlier studies, workers suggested that abdominal muscle maldevelopment is primary[183] and some have placed prune belly syndrome into the category of body wall dysplasia.[106] More recent investigations, however, suggest that this change is, in many cases, secondary to **megacystis** or fetal ascites.[184, 185] A number of workers have suggested that an anatomic obstruction that prohibits the egress of urine from the urinary bladder is central. Obstruction could be due to posterior urethral valves, urethral diaphragm, urethral stenosis, atresia, or multiple lumina; or, the bladder neck could be incompetent, forming a flap-like valve.

Severe prenatal distention of the urinary bladder most often follows urethral or 'bladder-outlet' obstruction, which itself can be due to posterior urethral valves or urethral diverticula, hypoplasia, atresia, or other less common urethral abnormalities, such as polyps, syringoceles, or scaphoid changes.[186] By this mechanism, hypoplasia of abdominal muscles is thought to develop secondary to the pressure exerted by a dilated, hypertrophied urinary bladder.[185, 187] Testicular descent is presumably impeded by the distended urinary bladder,[187] decreased intra-abdominal pressure,[178] or both. Abdominal muscles are formed by the end of the ninth week, before the urinary bladder is able to exert significant pressure,[188] so any effect would have to occur later. Also arguing against a pressure effect, at least in every case, is the observation that many cases of enlarged kidneys or bladder or distended abdomen from other causes (i.e. severe hepatomegaly) occur without abdominal muscle deficiency.[188]

Some have suggested that the variability in urologic findings argues against a simple mechanical cause of prune belly syndrome. Ureters, for example, may exhibit areas that are normal, constricted, or dilated.[165] One possibility is that the development of both abdominal muscles and urinary tract are affected simultaneously. This would have to occur early in fetal life, prior to the ninth week.[188] Prune belly syndrome could represent a true mesenchymal defect, with faulty differentiation or migration of lateral somite mesoderm. Increased apoptosis of the body wall placode could limit the amount of mesoderm available for migration and differentiation, the result being reduced abdominal musculature and a thin body wall.[106] These possibilities have been used to explain the concomitant appearance of anomalies of abdominal muscles and the renal system, or other systems, for example, musculoskeletal. The discordant appearance of prune belly syndrome in one of monozygotic twins has been used to postulate unequal division of the embryo, which might provide the affected twin with insufficient mesenchyme for the developing abdominal wall and urinary tract.[189]

Pathogenesis could also stem from faulty development of urogenital sinus mesenchyme, which forms the prostate, urinary bladder, internal sphincter, prostatic urethra, and membranous urethra. Prostatic anomalies have been implicated as a cause of urethral obstruction. However, it remains unclear whether prostatic anomalies are primary[169] or secondary.[139, 184] Some believe that prostatic dysplasia develops secondary to pressures produced by an excessively dilated urinary bladder.[139] Some studies have suggested that impairing the flow of urine prenatally results in the deregulation of renal precursor cell turnover and expression of growth and transcription factor genes, the outcome being renal dysplasia.[190]

Another mechanism that could be responsible for prune belly syndrome is severe ascites.[191] This may develop from prenatal rupture of an overdistended urinary bladder or, less frequently, from cardiac failure in twins. One case, severe ascites and prune belly syndrome, has been recognized in the pump twin of a case of twin–twin transfusion.[192]

Caudal dysgenesis

As with cloacal dysgenesis and related anomalies, the literature regarding caudal dysgenesis contains complicated nosology with conflicting, and seemingly arbitrary, use of various terms. In this text, the term 'caudal dysgenesis' is used to refer to a heterogeneous group of anomalies characterized by major malformations of caudal midline embryonic derivatives including skeletal, cutaneous, and or visceral structures derived from terminal somites. The latter can be broadly divided into two groups, caudal duplication and caudal dysplasia, depending respectively on whether the anomalies suggest addition or loss of somite derivatives.

Caudal duplication

Duplication of multiple organs or other structures in the caudal region has been described by a variety of terms, including partial twinning and caudal duplication. In severe forms, the genitourinary and distal intestinal tracts, anus, and lumbosacral spine and pelvis are each duplicated (Fig. 22.8). In duplicated cloaca, the urinary bladder and distal colon/rectum are doubled and accompanied by paired ani, genitalia, and urethra, with prominent diastasis of pubic bones; duplication of exstrophied bladders has also been reported.[193]

The hindgut is altered most often, ending blindly or in a fistulous connection to bladder or vagina.[194] The GI tract may, however, be duplicated at any level throughout its course.[195] The

legs or individual leg bones may be duplicated or even triplicated.[196–198] Omphalocele is sometimes present.[199–201] A number of case reports have highlighted single structures, organs, or organ systems, for example penile, Müllerian, colonic, or cloacal duplication.[199, 202–206] It is unclear if these represent examples of caudal duplication, and some may reflect the particular interests of investigators. Nonetheless, the inclusive term 'caudal duplication syndrome' appears justified, especially for severe cases.

Duplications of the intestinal tract are estimated to occur in one of every 4000–5000 births.[207, 208] Isolated duplication occurs less frequently.[205, 209] More often, GI duplication is associated with vertebral and genitourinary anomalies.[199, 205] The association of duplicated appendix with anomalies of the cloaca is not understood. Duplication of the vermiform appendix is itself rare, and observed in about 1 of 12 500 patients.[210] Duplication of the cloaca is an even rarer subset.

The pathogenesis of caudal duplication appears to be multifactorial and involves replication of the caudal eminence. The caudal eminence, or tail bud in non-mammalian embryos, is a secondary organizing center that appears 3 weeks after conception as a mesenchymal condensation between the primitive streak and cloacal membrane, which serves as primary organizing center.[2] After the primitive streak disappears, the caudal eminence gives rise to ectodermal, mesodermal, and endodermal derivatives, including the hindgut, sacrum, terminal spinal cord, urinary bladder, and other soft tissues of the pelvic cavity. During the later stages of gastrulation, the caudal eminence functions as a developmental field that is modulated by a number of factors, including homeobox genes, for example *HLXB9*, and retinoic acid receptors.[8, 212, 213] Partial twinning, possibly by means of duplication of the caudal eminence, or blighted conjoined twinning are mechanisms proposed for some cases of caudal duplication.[67, 202, 205, 213, 214]

Genetic, pharmacologic, or physical manipulations that disrupt the caudal eminence produce a variety of malformations, including cloacal anomalies.[215] Teratogenic effects of exogenous retinoic acid include lower-body and limb duplications in experimental animals.[216] Simple implantation of a multipore filter induces duplication in the chick cloaca.[92] This latter observation suggests that other disruptions, i.e. the presence of fibrous remnants of the neurenteric canal or a pelvic mass, might divide the notochord and affect the hindgut either primarily or through secondary, inductive means.[200] Genetic mechanisms also appear to be involved in the pathogenesis of duplication, although the finding of monozygotic human twins discordant for caudal duplication argues against a consistent genetic etiology.[217] Two mutations in mice, disorganization and fused, are associated with duplication of caudal structures.[217] The human homologue of the gene responsible for fused is *AXIN1*, but mutations in this gene, which maps to 16p, have not been identified in humans with caudal duplication to date.

Because the anomalies of caudal duplication are usually confined to the caudal region, extrapelvic anomalies are seldom seen.[217] Congenital heart disease and unilateral radial aplasia have each been recognized in cases of caudal duplication and colonic

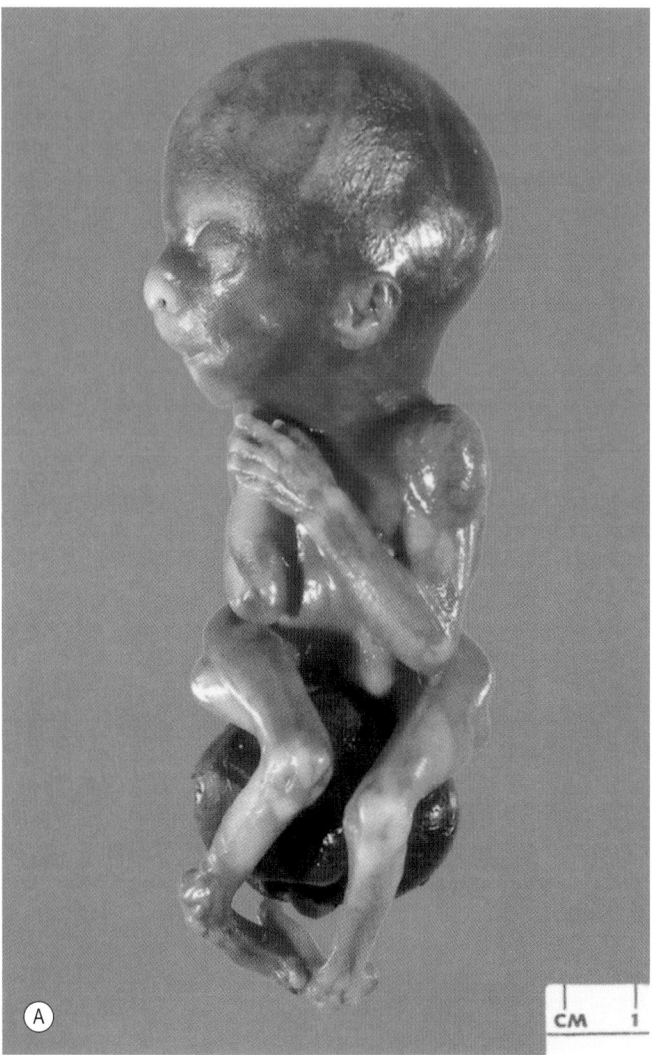
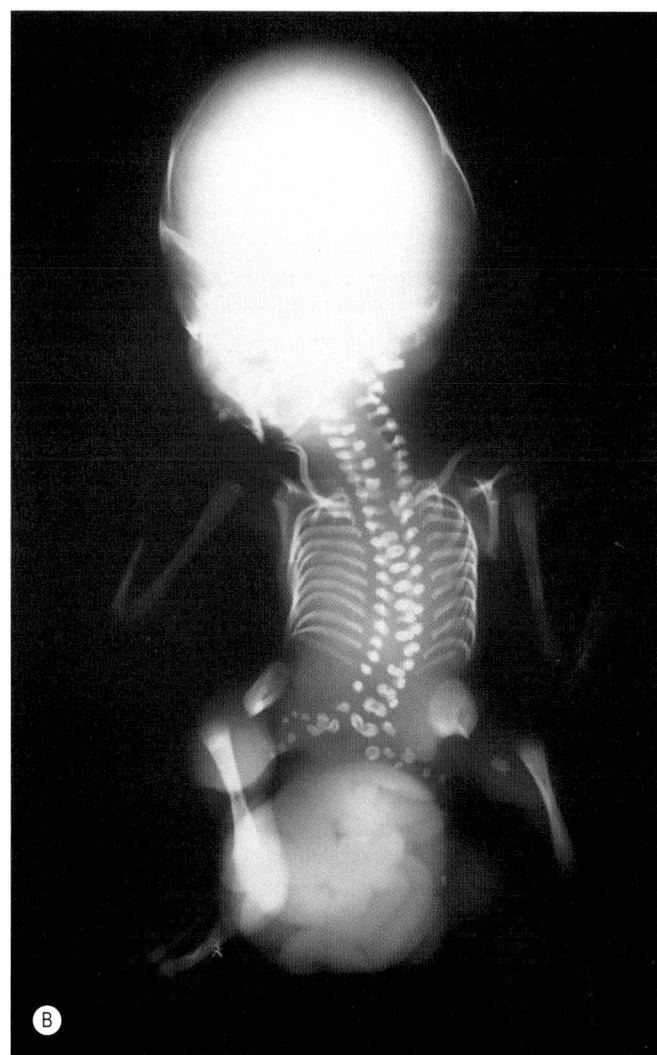

FIGURE 22.8 Caudal duplication. (A) 19-week female fetus with uncovered omphalocele. Liver is extruded, pelvis widened, and limbs deformed. Several exteriorized viscera, including stomach, intestinal tract, and spleen, are posterior to the liver. (B) Radiograph shows scoliosis, hemivertebrae at cervical, thoracic, and lumbar levels, widely separated sacral elements (associated with large myelomeningocele), omphalocele, and splayed pelvic bones.

duplication respectively, but explanations for pathogenesis have not been forthcoming.[202, 205]

Treatment is complex, depending upon the number of altered structures and severity of involvement. Bladder and colonic drainage are critical issues, as is the repair of omphalocele, exstrophy, fistulae, and open spinal defects.[218, 219] A variety of orthopedic and other genitourinary procedures may be required. Inflammation, erosion, or ulceration of the GI tract and irritative voiding or recurrent urinary tract infection are additional complications; the former can mimic other conditions, e.g. Crohn's disease.[195]

Caudal dysplasia

As a type of caudal duplication, the dysplasia group includes a broad spectrum of anomalies, ranging from partial sacral

dysgenesis to complete agenesis of the sacrum and lower extremities. Caudal dysplasia syndrome occurs in isolation or in association with more rostral defects. Maternal diabetes, family history, and monozygotic twinning are established risk factors for some forms of caudal dysplasia, but the underlying pathogenesis of this family of anomalies is not understood and, in some instances, controversial.

Sacral dysgenesis

Sacral dysgenesis manifests as dysplasia, hypoplasia, or absence of sacral vertebra. The sacrum is derived from the medial–ventral portions of somites 30–35, which form a series of ossification centers that are initially visualized as radiographic opacities by 14 weeks' gestation. At term, radiographs of the sacrum demonstrate partial or complete sacral agenesis, with varying deficiency of

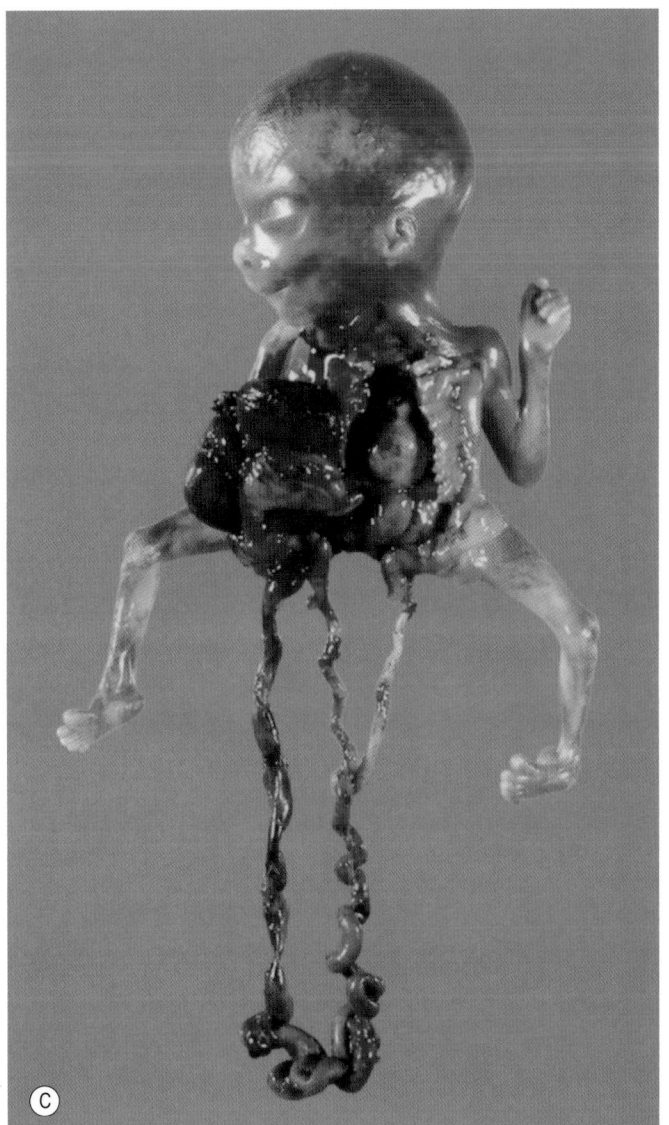

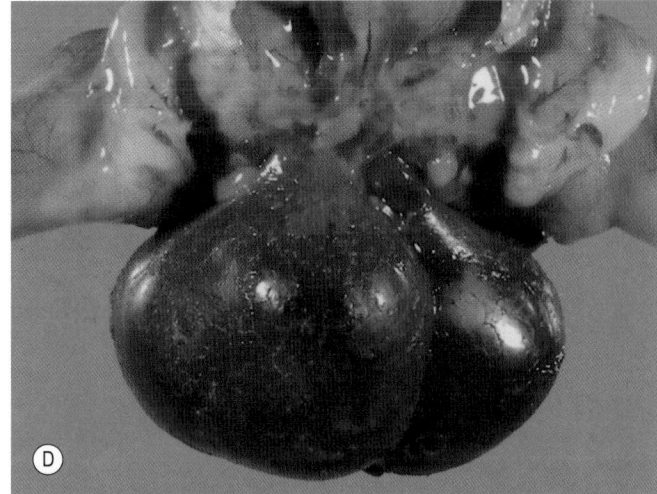

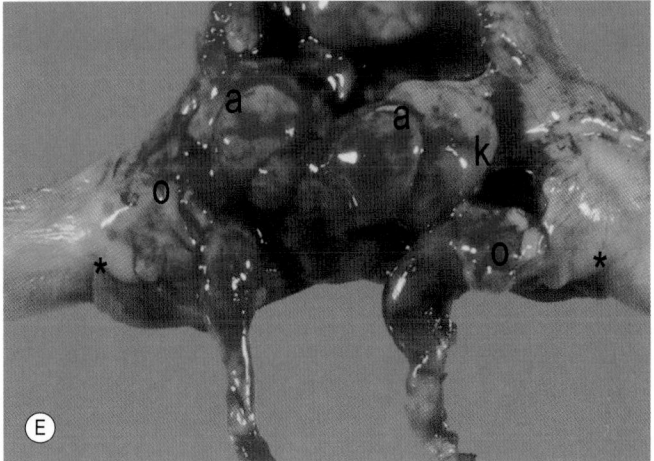

FIGURE 22.8 (*cont'd*) (C) Duplicated colons each lead to a separate and atretic anus. (D) Extruded liver and separated pelvic bones. (E) Abdominal and pelvic structures; duplicated external genitalia (*) and colons are visible, as are two ovaries (o), adrenal glands (a), and left kidney (k). (From Siebert et al 2005,[214] with permission.)

lumbar and coccygeal vertebrae (Fig. 22.9). Although minor asymmetry in sacral ossification centers is normal, marked asymmetry or absence of these vertebral bodies are hallmarks of sacral dysgenesis. Frequently, more rostral lumbar vertebrae are also affected.

Sacral agenesis refers to absence of most or all of the sacrum.[220] However, even complete sacral agenesis can be difficult to appreciate by external gross inspection.[221] In some individuals, an overlying skin defect is a clue to inspect the sacrum more carefully. Similarly, internal anomalies such as congenital pelvic cysts or imperforate anus should prompt thorough evaluation of the sacrum. Complete agenesis results in a fluctuant defect between the iliac bones that can usually be detected in older fetuses by palpation, highlighting the importance of tactile examination of the entire spine. Identification of partial sacral

agenesis in a small fetus is even more difficult and may require radiologic studies.

Sacral agenesis is often associated with malformations of the terminal spinal cord and/or spinal nerves, such as tethering, syrinx, or diastematomyelia (see Ch. 36). Bladder dysfunction and neurologically-induced orthopedic anomalies of the lower extremities are common in older children.[221]

Sacral dysgenesis frequently occurs in the context of other anomalies including the VACTERL association and symmelia (see below). Duncan et al described a 'sacral dysgenesis association' (SDA) to call attention to skeletal, renal, and central nervous system defects that often coexist with sacral dysgenesis.[222] The pattern of anomalies observed in SDA differs from VACTERL and symmelia, in which sacral dysgenesis is accompanied by malformations in many more organ systems.

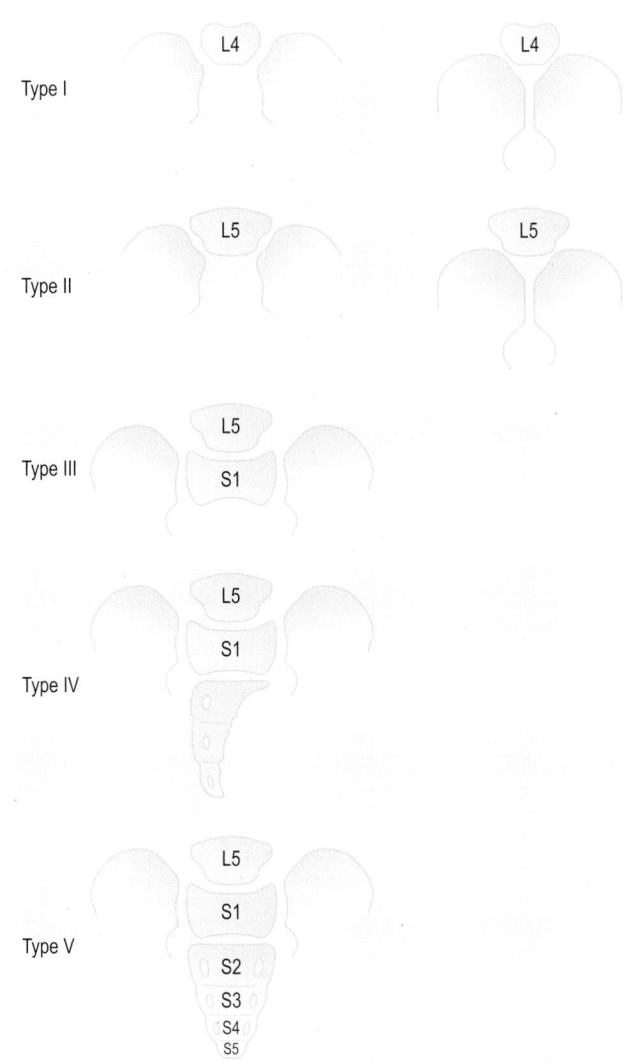

FIGURE 22.9 Varieties of sacral dysgenesis. Type I, Sacral agenesis, with altered transverse pelvic diameter and variable lumbar deficiency. Type II, Sacral agenesis, aberrant pelvic diameter, and normal lumbar vertebrae. Type III, Variable agenesis or hypoplasia of more caudal sacral vertebrae. Type IV, Hemivertebrae (hemisacrum), commonly associated with Currarino syndrome. Type V, Agenesis of coccyx. (After Martucciello et al 2004,[220] with permission.)

Although the etiologies of SDA, VACTERL, and symmelia are unknown, each has different clinical associations, which may be helpful in genetic counseling and pathogenetic investigation.

Currarino syndrome

Currarino syndrome (also referred to as Currarino triad or hereditary sacral agenesis) is an autosomal dominant disorder.[220, 223] As originally described, the syndrome included three features: **partial sacral agenesis, a presacral tumor, and an anorectal malformation**. The sacral defect in these patients is less severe than observed in many other types of sacral agenesis, such as those associated with maternal diabetes or VACTERL association. Currarino syndrome most commonly spares S1 and half of the remaining sacrum. The latter projects inferiorly and has a radiographic appearance termed the 'scimitar sign', in reference to its curved tapering contours. The presacral mass may be an anterior meningocele, enteric cyst, or presacral teratoma. Many patients present with signs of bowel obstruction, due to a primary rectal malformation, external compression by the presacral mass, or a tethered spinal cord. Genitourinary tract malformations (e.g. horseshoe kidney, duplicated ureter, and bicornuate uterus) are occasionally present.

Most, if not all, cases of Currarino syndrome are due to mutations in the *HLXB9* gene.[224] This gene encodes a homeobox-containing transcription factor, the function of which is unclear. Currarino syndrome appears to be caused by haploinsufficiency for *HLXB9*, with near complete penetrance of at least radiologic defects in the sacra of family members who carry *HLXB9* mutations.

Sacral dysgenesis with lower extremity anomalies/symmelia (sirenomelia)

More severe forms of caudal regression are characterized by sacral dysgenesis and coexistent external anomalies of the lower extremities and perineum. The latter include cloacal defects (e.g. exstrophy, anal atresia), malformed and/or malpositioned genitalia, and reduction and/or 'fusion' of the lower extremities. Although several theories exist to explain this combination of defects, most invoke a defect during blastogenesis (see Ch. 3), which reduces the amount of caudal mesoderm derived from the caudal eminence during the fourth week of gestation.[215, 225] This mesoderm forms the caudal somites, which contribute to pelvic, somatic, and visceral organs, including all the axial structures (sacrum, perineum, anus, etc.) that separate the lower extremities. Experimental manipulations that eliminate caudal mesoderm in animal models produce caudal regression anomalies similar to those observed in humans.[215]

A broad range of lower limb defects has been observed in fetuses with sacral dysgenesis. Milder phenotypes include unilateral or bilateral hypoplasia of skeletal elements. More severe anomalies are characterized by loss of the midline separation between the lower extremities, usually with absence, 'fusion', or hypoplasia of skeletal elements and associated soft tissues (symmelia).[226] In such instances, a single caudal extremity is present which projects from the caudal midline and contains variable, but usually bilaterally symmetric skeletal elements. One common phenotype of the single appendage is a broad limb with two femurs and a symmetric wide foot (sympodia), with more than five digits and a dorsal surface that faces posteriorly. Resemblance of such limbs to the mythical caudal anatomy of mermaids or sirens led to the terms 'mermaid syndrome' and 'sirenomelia', which are used to refer to this condition. The phenotypic spectrum of symmelia is actually much broader, including more severe reduction defects in which the single rudimentary lower extremities may consist of a simple fleshy appendage attached to the perineum.

The term 'fused' is frequently used to describe the appearance of the lower extremities in many forms of caudal regression syndrome. However, it is generally accepted that the malformations result from insufficient separation of the primary limb fields, as opposed to fusion of previously separate limb buds. Support for this model derives from various animal models of teratogen-induced caudal regression and anatomic studies of human embryos.[225, 227]

The estimated incidence of **symmelia** is 1/60 000.[226] It occurs 150–250 times more frequently in monozygous twins than in dizygotic twins or singleton pregnancies. Concordant symmelia in twins has not been reported, although co-twins of symmelic fetuses have been observed with other malformations, including cloacal exstrophy. These and other observations suggest that monozygotic twinning is a teratogenic process, which may affect the caudal embryo through a variety of proposed mechanisms.[228–231]

Maternal diabetes is generally cited as another risk factor for symmelia (2–4% of cases), although some have questioned the validity of the association.[232] A variety of experimental studies with animal models support a relationship between maternal diabetes and caudal regression syndrome and demonstrate that similar anomalies can be induced by exposing embryos during late blastogenesis to a variety of teratogens (e.g. cadmium, ochratoxin-A).[215, 227] Among the latter, retinoic acid is particularly effective; interestingly, the teratogenic effect of retinoids is enhanced in diabetic rodents, suggesting that multiple factors may contribute to the pathogenesis of these anomalies.[227, 233]

Symmelia is virtually always associated with bilateral renal agenesis, imperforate anus, and malformed or absent external genitalia.[226] In addition, a characteristic vascular malformation is present: a single umbilical artery that arises directly from the abdominal aorta, in place of the normal paired branches of the iliac arteries. This aberrant arterial anatomy is thought to represent persistence of one of the vitelline arteries, which dominate the extraembryonic circulation early in blastogenesis and normally regress with development of the chorioallantoic vessels. The anomalous umbilical artery in symmelia usually originates from the aorta proximal to the renal arteries and is comparable in caliber to the thoracic aorta. Distal to its origin, the remainder of the aorta and its systemic and visceral branches are hypoplastic. At autopsy, these alterations in the circulatory system can be documented by careful dissection, but are also nicely demonstrated by postmortem angiography.

Padmanabhan recognized six hypotheses that have been put forth to explain the pathogenesis of symmelia.[227]

- Lateral compression – abnormal amniotic folds compress the caudal end of the embryo, impair development of the pelvis, and prevent proper rotation of the limbs.
- Deficient caudal mesoderm – failure of the caudal eminence to produce a full complement of somites, which are needed caudally for successful fission of the hindlimb fields.
- Defective tissue interactions – accelerated differentiation of chordomesoderm due to or as a cause of abnormal cell signaling between primary germ layers.[234]
- Vascular steal – impaired development of caudal embryonic structures due to vascular insufficiency caused by a persistent vitelline–umbilical circulation.
- Overdistention of the neural tube – mechanical interference with caudal development due to primary swelling of the adjacent neural tube.
- Combination of one or more of the above.

An element in each theory is deficient or defective development of caudal mesoderm, which may be a genuine point of convergence for heterogeneous etiologies. The fact that multiple different teratogens and at least one autosomal recessive mutation[235] can produce symmelia in experimental animals suggests that the caudal mesoderm is vulnerable to diverse types of insults and that more than one of the pathogenetic hypotheses may be correct for specific etiologies.

Symmelia is invariably lethal due to renal agenesis and pulmonary hypoplasia. Symmelia is considered to be a sporadic human condition with little risk of recurrence. The *sirenomelic* mutant mouse model indicates that symmelia can result from heritable mutations, although no such examples have been reported in humans. Although severe oligohydramnios may limit the resolution of prenatal ultrasound studies, convergent femoral bones that persistently lie side-by-side is a valuable diagnostic finding.

References

Normal development

1. O'Rahilly R, Müller F. Human embryology & teratology, New York: Wiley-Liss; 1992.
2. Müller F, O'Rahilly R. The primitive streak, the caudal eminence and related structures in staged human embryos. Cells Tissues Organs 2004; 177:2–20.
3. Catala M, Teillet M-A, Le Douarin NM. Organization and development of the tail bud analyzed with the quail-chick chimera system. Mech Dev 1995; 51:51–65.
4. Forlani S, Lawson KA, Deschamps J. Acquisition of Hox codes during gastrulation and axial elongation in the mouse embryo. Development 2003; 130:3807–3819.
5. Gilbert SF. Developmental biology. 7th edn. Sunderland: Sinauer Associates; 2003.
6. Aulehla A, Herrmann BG. Segmentation in vertebrates: clock and gradient finally joined. Genes Dev 2004; 18:2060–2067.
7. Giudicelli F, Lewis J. The vertebrate segmentation clock. Curr Opin Genet Dev 2004; 14:407–414.
8. Pourquie O. The chick embryo: a leading model in somitogenesis studies. Mech Dev 2004; 121:1069–1079.
9. Christ B, Huang R, Wilting J. The development of the avian vertebral column. Anat Embryol 2000; 202:179–194.
10. Copp AJ, Greene NDE, Murdoch JN. The genetic basis of mammalian neurulation. Nature Rev Genet 2003; 4:784–793.
11. Nakatsu T, Uwabe C, Shiota K. Neural tube closure in humans initiates at multiple sites: evidence from human embryos and implications for the pathogenesis of neural tube defects. Anat Embryol 2000; 201:455–456.

12. Saitsu H, Yamada S, Uwabe C, et al. Development of the posterior neural tube in human embryos. Anat Embryol 2004 (Berl) 209:101–117.

13. Moore KL, Persaud TVN. The developing human: clinically oriented embryology. 6th edn. Philadelphia: WB Saunders; 1998.

14. Rogers DS, Paidas CN, Morreale RF, et al. Septation of the anorectal and genitourinary tracts in the human embryo: crucial role of the catenoidal shape of the urorectal sulcus. Teratology 2002; 66:144–152.

15. Hynes PJ, Fraher JP. The development of the male genitourinary system. I. The origin of the urorectal septum and the formation of the perineum. Br J Plast Surg 2004; 57:27–36.

16. Penington EC, Hutson JM. The cloacal plate: the missing link in anorectal and urogenital development. BJU Int 2002; 89:726–732.

17. Hynes PJ, Fraher JP. The development of the male genitourinary system: III. The formation of the spongiose and glandar urethra. Br Assoc Plast Surg 2004; 57:203–214.

18. Hynes PJ, Fraher JP. The development of the male genitourinary system: II. The origin and formation of the urethral plate. Br Assoc Plast Surg 2004; 57:112–121.

19. Penington EC, Hutson JM. The urethral plate – does it grow into the genital tubercle or within it? Br J Urol Int 2002; 89:733–739.

Malformations of the spine and paraspinal tissues

20. McEwen GD, Conway JJ, Miller WT. Congenital scoliosis with a unilateral bar. Radiology 1968; 90:711–715.

21. Mohanty S, Kumar N. Patterns of presentation of congenital scoliosis. J Orthop Surg (Hong Kong) 2000; 8:33–37.

22. Zelop CM, Pretorius DH, Benacerraf BR. Fetal hemivertebrae: associated anomalies, significance, and outcome. Obstet Gynecol 1993; 81:412–416.

23. Solomon L, Jimenez RB, Reiner L. Spondylothoracic dysplasia: report of two cases and review of the literature. Arch Pathol Lab Med 1978; 102:201–205.

24. Cornier AS, Ramirez N, Carlo S, et al. Controversies surrounding Jarcho-Levin syndrome. Curr Opin Pediatr 2003; 15:614–620.

25. Bulman MP, Kusumi K, Fraylling TM, et al. Mutations in the human δ homologue, DLL3, cause axial skeletal defects in spondylocostal dysostosis. Nat Genet 2000; 24:438–441.

26. Dunwoodie SL, Clements M, Sparrow DB, et al. Axial skeletal defects caused by mutation in the spondylocostal dysplasia/pudgy gene Dll3 are associated with disruption of the segmentation clock within the presomitic mesoderm. Development 2002; 129:1795–1806.

27. Nezarti MM, McLeod DR. VACTERL manifestations in two generations of a family. Am J Med Genet 1999; 82:40–42.

28. Botto LD, Khoury MJ, Mastroiacovo P, et al. The spectrum of congenital anomalies of the VATER association: an international study. J Med Genet 1997; 71:8–15.

29. Dunn I, Williams M, Appleyard J. London Dysmorphology Database. In: Winter R, Baraitser M, eds. 1.0.0 edn. Bushey: London Medical Databases Ltd; 2003.

30. Weaver DD, Mapstone CL, Yu P-L. The VATER association. Analysis of 46 patients. Am J Dis Child 1986; 140:225–229.

31. Lomas FE, Dahlstrom JE, Ford JH. VACTERL with hydrocephalus: family with X-linked VACTERL-H. Am J Med Genet 1998; 76:74–78.

32. Merei J, Hasthorpe S, Farmer P, et al. Visceral anomalies in prenatally adriamycin-exposed rat fetuses: a model for the VATER association. Pediatr Surg Int 1999; 15:11–16.

33. Merlob P, Naor N. Drug-induced VATER association: is dibenzepin a possible cause? J Med Genet 1994; 31:423.

34. Loffredo CA, Wilson PD, Ferencz C. Maternal diabetes: an independent risk factor for major cardiovascular malformations with increased mortality of affected infants. Teratology 2001; 64:98–106.

35. Tongsong T, Wanapirak C, Piyamongkol W, et al. Prenatal sonographic diagnosis of VATER association. J Clin Ultrasound 1999; 27:378–384.

36. Arsic D, Qi BQ, Beasley SW. Hedgehog in the human: a possible explanation for the VATER association. J Paediatr Child Health 2002; 38:117–121.

37. Kim JH, Kim PCW, Hui C-C. The VACTERL association: lessons from the Sonic hedgehog pathway. Clin Genet 2001; 59:306–315.

38. Walsh LE, Vance GH, Weaver DD. Distal 13q deletion syndrome and the VACTERL association: case report, literature review, and possible implications. Am J Med Genet 2001; 98:137–144.

39. Burger PC, Scheithauer BW, Vogel FS. Surgical pathology of the nervous system and its coverings. 4th edn. New York; Churchill Livingstone; 2002.

40. Ergun R, Akdemir G, Gezici AR, et al. Craniocervical neurenteric cyst without associated abnormalities. Pediatr Neurosurg 2000; 32:95–99.

41. Lemire R, Loeser J, Leech R, et al. Normal and abnormal development of the human nervous system. Hagerstown: Harper & Row; 1975.

42. Darwish B, Stanley TV, Wickremesekera A, et al. Presacral neuroenteric fistula in a newborn presenting with an epidural abscess: case report and review of the literature. Pediatrics 2004; 114:527–531.

43. Palma L, Di Lorenzo N. Spinal endodermal cysts without associated vertebral or other congenital abnormalities. Acta Neurochir 1976; 33:283–300.

44. Wilkins RH, Odom GL. Spinal intradural cyst tumours of the spine and spinal cord. II. Amsterdam: North-Holland; 1976.

45. Whiting DM, Chou SM, Lanzieri CF, et al. Cervical neurenteric cyst associated with Klippel-Feil syndrome: a case report and review of the literature, Clin Neuropathol 1991; 10:285–290.

46. Matsushina T, Fukui M, Egami H. Epithelial cells in a so-called intraspinal neurenteric cyst: a light and electron microscopic study. Surg Neurol 1985; 24:656–660.

47. Lippman CR, Arginteanu M, Purohit D. Intramedullary neurenteric cysts of the spine. Case report and review of the literature. J Neurosurg 2001; 94:305–309.

48. Agnoli AL, Laun A, Schonmayr R. Enterogenous intraspinal cysts. J Neurosurg 1984; 16:834–840.

49. Arai Y, Yamauchi Y, Tsuji T. Spinal neurenteric cyst. Report of two cases and review of forty-one cases reported in Japan. Spine 1992; 17:1421–1424.

50. Aydin K, Sencer S, Barman A, et al. Spinal cord herniation into a mediastinal neurenteric cyst: CT and MRI findings. Br J Radiol 2003; 76:132–134.

51. Keyaki A, Hirano A, Llena JF. Differential diagnosis and origin of epithelial cyst in the central nervous system. Report of seven cases and review of the literature. Brain Nerve 1989; 41:411–418.

52. Eynon-Lewis NJ, Kitchen N, Scaravilli F, et al. Neurenteric cyst of the cerebellopontine angle: case report. Neurosurgery 1998; 42:655–658.

53. Bentley JF, Smith JR. Developmental posterior enteric remnants and spinal malformations. The split notochord syndrome. Arch Dis Child 1960; 35:76–86.

54. Brooks BS, Duvall ER, El Gammal T, et al. Neuroimaging features of neurenteric cysts: analysis of nine cases and review of the literature. AJNR Am J Neuroradiol 1993; 14:735–746.

55. Feller AH, Sternberg H. The notochord and its genesis. Virchows Arch 1929; 272:613–640.

56. Gardner WJ. Hypothesis: overdistension of the neural tube may cause anomalies of non-neural organs. Teratology 1980; 22:229–238.

57. Stevenson R, Kelly JC, Aylsworth AS, et al. Vascular basis for neural tube defects. A hypothesis. Pediatrics 1987; 80:102–106.

58. Rauzzino MJ, Tubbs RS, Alexander E, et al. Spinal neurenteric cysts and their relation to more common aspects of occult spinal dysraphism, Neurosurg Focus 2001; 10:1–10.

59. Tortori-Donati P, Rossi A, Biancheri R, et al. Magnetic resonance imaging of spinal dysraphism, Top Magn Reson Imaging 2001; 12:375–409.

60. Kumar R, Jain R, Rao K, et al. Intraspinal neurenteric cysts – report of three paediatric cases. Child Nerv Syst 2001; 17:584–588.

61. Ebisu T, Odake G, Fujimoto M, et al. Neurenteric cysts with meningomyelocele or meningocele. Split notochord syndrome. Child Nerv Syst 1990; 6:465–467.

62. Rossi A, Cama A, Piatelli G, et al. Spinal dysraphism: MR imaging rationale. J Neuroradiol 2004; 31:3–24.

63. Gumerlock MK, Spollen LE, Nelson MJ, et al. Cervical neurenteric fistula causing recurrent meningitis in Klippel-Feil sequence: case report and literature review. Pediatr Infect Dis J 1991; 10:532–535.

64. Alrabeeah A, Gillis DA, Giacomantonio M, et al. Neurenteric cysts – a spectrum. J Pediatr Surg 1988; 23:752–754.

65. Fan Y-K, Huang J-K, Sheu C-Y, et al. MR imaging characteristics of cervical neurenteric cysts: two case reports. Chin J Radiol 2001; 26:39–44.

Cloacal anomalies

66. McLaughlin JF, Marks WM, Jones G. Prospective management of exstrophy of the cloaca and myelocystocele following prenatal ultrasound recognition of neural tube defects in identical twins. Am J Med Genet 1984; 19:721–727.

67. Casale P, Grady RW, Waldhausen JH, et al. Cloacal exstrophy variants. Can blighted conjoined twinning play a role? J Urol 2004; 172:1103–1106, discussion 1106–1107.

68. Qureshi F, Jacques SM, Yaron Y, et al. Prenatal diagnosis of cloacal dysgenesis sequence: Differential diagnosis from other forms of fetal obstructive uropathy, Fetal Diagn Ther 1998; 13:69–74.

69. Robinson HB, Tross K. Agenesis of the cloacal membrane: A probable teratogenic anomaly. Perspect Pediatr Pathol 1984; 1:79–96.

70. Sahinoglu Z, Mulayim B, Ozden S, et al. The prenatal diagnosis of cloacal dysgenesis sequence in six cases: can the termination of pregnancy always be the first choice? Prenat Diagn 2004; 24:10–16.

71. Wheeler PG, Weaver DD. Partial urorectal septum malformation sequence: A report of 25 cases. Am J Med Genet 2001; 103:99–105.

72. Liang X, Ioffe OB, Sun CCJ. Cloacal dysgenesis sequence: observations in four patients including three fetuses of second trimester gestation. Pediatr Dev Pathol 1998; 1:281–288.

73. Hendren WH. Cloacal malformations: experience with 105 cases. J Pediatr Surg 1992; 27:890–901.

74. Adams MC, Ludlow J, Brock JWI, et al. Prenatal urinary ascites and persistent cloaca: risk factors for poor drainage of urine or meconium. J Urol 1998; 160:2179–2181.

75. Jaramillo D, Lebowitz RL, Hendren WH. The cloacal malformation: radiologic findings and imaging recommendations. Radiology 1990; 177:441–488.

76. Twinning P. Genitourinary malformations. In: Nyberg DA, McGahan JP, Pretorius DH, et al, eds. Diagnostic imaging of fetal anomalies. Philadelphia: Lippincott Williams & Wilkins; 2003.

77. Bear JW, Gilsanz V. Calcified meconium and persistent cloaca. AJR Am J Roentgenol 1981; 137:867–868.

78. Zaccara A, Gatti C, Silveri M, et al. Persistent cloaca: are we ready for a correct prenatal diagnosis? Urology 1999; 54:367.

78. Taipale P, Heinonen K, Kainulainen S, et al. Cloacal anomaly simulating megalocystis in the first trimester. J Clin Ultrasound 2004; 32:419–422.

80. Cook WA, Stephens FD. Pathoembryology of the urinary tract. In: King L, ed. Urological surgery in neonates and young infants. Philadelphia: WB Saunders; 1988:1–22.

81. Grady RW, Mitchell M. Exstrophy and epispadias anomalies. In: Gillenwater JY, Grayhack JT, Howards SS, et al, eds. Adult and pediatric urology. 4th edn. Philadelphia: Lippincott Williams & Wilkins; 2002:2270–2310.

82. Culp DA. The histology of the exstrophied bladder. J Urol 1964; 91:538–548.

83. Martinez-Frias ML, Bermejo E, Rodriguez-Pinilla E, et al. Exstrophy of the cloaca and exstrophy of the bladder: two different expressions of a primary developmental field defect. Am J Med Genet 2001; 99:261–269.

84. Lattimer J, Smith M. Exstrophy closure: a follow-up on 70 cases. J Urol 1966; 95:356–359.

85. Lancaster P. Epidemiology of bladder exstrophy and epispadias: a communication from the International Clearinghouse for Birth Defects Monitoring Systems. Teratology 1987; 36:221–227.

86. Shapiro E, Lepor H, Jeffs RD. The inheritance of the exstrophy-epispadias complex. J Urol 1984; 132:308–310.

87. Ives E, Coffey R, Carter CO. A family study of bladder exstrophy. J Med Genet 1980; 17:139–141.

88. Froster UG, Heinritz W, Bennek J, et al. Another case of autosomal dominant exstrophy of the bladder. Prenat Diagn 2004; 24:375–377.

89. Reutter H, Shapiro E, Gruen JR. Seven new cases of familial isolated bladder exstrophy and epispadias complex (BEEC) and review of the literature. Am J Med Genet 2003; 120A:215–221.

90. Lee DH, Cottrell JR, Sanders RC, et al. OEIS complex (omphalocele-exstrophy-imperforate anus-spinal defects) in monozygotic twins. Am J Med Genet 1999; 84:29–33.

91. Ambrose SS, O'Brien DPI. Surgical embryology of the exstrophy-epispadias complex. Surg Clin North Am 1974; 54:1379–1390.

92. Muecke E. The role of the cloacal membrane in exstrophy. The first successful experimental study. J Urol 1964; 92:659–667.

93. Mildenberger H, Kluth D, Dziuba M. Embryology of bladder exstrophy. J Pediatr Surg 1988; 23:166–170.

94. Paulhac P, Maisonnette F, Bourg S, et al. Adenocarcinoma in the exstrophic bladder. Urology 1999; 54:744.

95. Smeulders N, Woodhouse CR. Neoplasia in adult exstrophy patients. BJU Int 2001; 87:623–628.

96. Cordonnier JJ, Spjut HJ. Vesical exstrophy and transitional cell carcinoma: unusual longevity following ureterosigmoidostomy. J Urol 1957; 78:242–244.

97. Kliment J, Luptak J, Lofaj M, et al. Carcinoma of the colon after ureterosigmoidostomy and trigonosigmoidostomy for exstrophy of the bladder. Int Urol Nephrol 1993; 25:339–343.

98. Strachan JR, Woodhouse CR. Malignancy following ureterosigmoidostomy in patients with exstrophy. Br J Surg 1991; 78:1216–1218.

99. Curry CJR, Honore L, Boyd E. The ventral wall of the trunk. In: Stevenson RE, Hall JG, Goodman RM, eds. Human malformations and related anomalies. New York: Oxford University Press; 1993:869–891.

100. Carey JC. Exstrophy of the cloaca and the OEIS complex: one and the same. Am J Med Genet 2001; 99:270.

101. Manzoni GA, Ransley PG, Hurwitz RS. Cloacal exstrophy and cloacal exstrophy variants: a proposed system of classification. J Urol 1987; 138:1065–1068.

102. Muecke EC. Exstrophy, epispadias and other anomalies of the bladder. In: Walsh P, Gittes R, Perlmutter A, et al, eds. Campbell's urology. 5th edn. Philadelphia: WB Saunders; 1986:1856–1880.

103. Carey JC, Greenbaum B, Hall BD. The OEIS complex (omphalocele, exstrophy, imperforate anus, spinal defects). Birth Defects Orig Artic Ser 1978; 14:253–263.

104. Koffler H, Aase JM, Papile L-A, et al. Persistent cloaca with absent penis and anal atresia in one of identical twins. J Pediatr 1978; 93:821–823.

105. Wyburn GM. The development of the infra-umbilical portion of the abdominal wall, with remarks on the aetiology of ectopia vesicae. J Anat 1937; 71:201–231.

106. Vermeij-Keers C, Hartwig NG, van der Werff JF. Embryonic development of the ventral body wall and its congenital malformations. Semin Pediatr Surg 1996; 5:82–89.

107. Marshall VF, Muecke EC. Variations in exstrophy of the bladder. J Urol 1962; 88:766–796.

108. Kluth D, Lambrecht W. Current concepts in the embryology of anorectal malformations. Semin Pediatr Surg 1997; 6:180–186.

109. Nievelstein RA, van der Werff JF, Verbeek FJ, et al. Normal and abnormal embryonic development of the anorectum in human embryos. Teratology 1998; 57:70–78.

110. Paidas CN, Morreale RF, Holoski KM, et al. Septation and differentiation of the embryonic human cloaca. J Pediatr Surg 1999; 34:877–844.

111. Bruch SW, Adzick NS, Goldstein RB, et al. Challenging the embryogenesis of cloacal exstrophy. J Pediatr Surg 1996; 31:768–770.

112. Lakshmanan Y, Bellin PB, Gilroy AM, et al. Antenatally diagnosed cloacal exstrophy variant with intravesical phallus in a twin pregnancy. Urology 2001; 57:1178xii–1178xv.

113. Langer JC, Brennan B, Lappalainen RE, et al. Cloacal exstrophy: prenatal diagnosis before rupture of the cloacal membrane. J Pediatr Surg 1992; 27:1352–1355.

Urachal anomalies

114. Hammond G, Yglesias L, Davis JE. The urachus, its anatomy and associated fasciae. Anat Rec 1941; 80:271–287.

115. Noe HN. Urachal anomalies and related umbilical disorders. In: Glenn's Urologic Surgery; 5th ed. Edited by SD Graham. Philadelphia: Lippincott-Raven; 1998:769–776.

116. Cilento BGJ, Bauer SB, Retik AB, et al. Urachal anomalies: defining the best diagnostic modality. Urology 1998; 52:120–122.

117. Maruschke M, Kreutzer HJ, Seiter H. Bladder rupture caused by spontaneous perforation of an infected urachal cyst. Urologe A 2003; 42:834–839.

118. Suita S, Nagasaki A. Urachal remnants. Semin Pediatr Surg 1996; 5:107–115.
119. Amundsen G. Urachal cyst as a cause of ileus. Nord Med 1959; 62:1484–1485.
120. Yamazaki T, Sakai Y, Hatakeyama K, et al. Urachal hernia: an unusual intra-abdominal hernia caused by incarceration into a urachal cyst. Dig Dis Sci 2000; 45:2365–2366.
121. Rubin A. Handbook of congenital malformations, Philadelphia: WB Saunders; 1967.
122. Kubota K, Nomura S, Kawahara M, et al. Familial urachal sinus associated with a possible congenital malformation: report of a case. Surg Today 2003; 33:237–239.
123. Rich RH, Hardy BE, Filler RM. Surgery for anomalies of the urachus. J Pediatr Surg 1983; 18:370–372.
124. Gearhart JP, Jeffs RD. Urachal abnormalities. In: Walsh PC, Retik AB, Vaughan ED, eds. Campbell's urology. Philadelphia: WB Saunders; 1998:1984–1987.
125. Montemarano H, Bulas DI, Rushton HG, et al. Bladder distention and pyelectasis in the male fetus: causes, comparisons, and contrasts. J Ultrasound Med 1998; 17:743–749.
126. Stevens FD. Congenital malformations of the urinary tract. New York: Praegez Publishers; 1983.
127. Moore K, Russell S, Wilson L, et al. Allantoic cysts of the umbilical cord in trisomy 21. Prenat Diagn 1997; 17:883–890.
128. Smith GN, Walker M, Johnston S, et al. The sonographic finding of persistent umbilical cord cystic masses is associated with lethal aneuploidy and/or congenital anomalies. Prenat Diagn 1996; 16:1141–1147.
129. Beck AD, Gaudin HJ, Bonham DG. Carcinoma of the urachus. Br J Urol 1970; 42:555–562.
130. Hertzberg GS, Nyberg DA, Neilsen IR. Ventral wall defects. In: Nyberg D, McGahan J, Pretorius DH, et al, eds. Diagnostic imaging of fetal anomalies. Philadelphia: Lippincott Williams & Wilkins; 2003:507–546.

Anorectal malformations

131. Haddad ME, Corkery JJ. The anus in the newborn. Pediatrics 1985; 76:927–928.
132. McCann J, Reay D, Siebert JR, et al. Postmortem perianal findings in children. Am J Forensic Med Pathol 1996; 17:289–298.
133. Shaul DB, Harrison EA. Classification of anorectal malformations – initial approach, diagnostic tests, and colostomy. Semin Pediatr Surg 1997; 6:187–195.
134. Landau D, Mordechai J, Karplus M, et al. Inheritance of familial congenital isolated anorectal malformations: case report and review. Am J Med Genet 1997; 71:280–282.
135. Winkler JM, Weinstein ED. Imperforate anus and heredity. J Pediatr Surg 1970; 5:555–558.
136. Mo R, Kim JH, Zhang J, et al. Anorectal malformations caused by defects in sonic hedgehog signaling. Am J Pathol 2001; 159:765–774.
137. Pinsky L. The syndromology of anorectal malformation (atresia, stenosis, ectopia). Am J Med Genet 1978; 1:461–474.
138. Stephens FD. Congenital malformations of the rectum, anus and genito-urinary tracts. Edinburgh: E & S Livingstone Ltd; 1963.

Prune-belly syndrome

139. Volmar KE, Fritsch MK, Perlman EJ, et al. Patterns of congenital lower urinary tract obstructive uropathy: relation to abnormal prostate and bladder development and the prune belly syndrome. Pediatr Dev Pathol 2001; 4:467–472.
140. Froelich F. Der Mangel der Muskeln, insbesondere der Seitenbauchmuskeln. Wurzburg: CA Zurn; 1839.
141. Osler W. Congenital absence of the abdominal muscles with distended and hypertrophied urinary bladder. Bull Johns Hopkins Hosp 1901; 12: 331–333.
142. Binder A. Muskelsystem. Jena: G Fischer; 1927.
143. Gruber GB. Harnorgane. Jena: G Fischer; 1927.
144. Stumme EG. Ueber die symmetrischen kongenitalen Bauchmuskeldefekte und ueber die Kombination derselben mit anderen Bildungsanomalien des Rumpfes. Mitt Grenzgebieten Med Chir 1903; 11:548.
145. Bellah RD, States LJ, Duckett JW. Pseudoprune-belly syndrome. Am J Radiol 1996; 167:1389–1393.
146. Jennings RW. Prune belly syndrome. Semin Pediatr Surg 2000; 9:115–120.
147. Manivel JC, Pettinato G, Reinberg Y, et al. Prune belly syndrome: clinicopathologic study of 29 cases. Pediatr Pathol 1989; 9:691–711.
148. Reinberg Y, Shapiro E, Manifel JC, et al. Prune belly syndrome in females: a triad of abdominal musculature deficiency and anomalies of the urinary and genital systems. J Pediatr 1991; 118:395–398.
149. Chan YC, Bird LM. Vertically transmitted hypoplasia of the abdominal wall musculature. Clin Dysmorphol 2004; 13:7–10.
150. Woodward JR. Prune-belly syndrome. Philadelphia: WB Saunders; 1985.
151. Druschel CM. A descriptive study of prune belly in New York State, 1983 to 1989. Arch Pediatr Adolesc Med 1995; 149:70–76.
152. Loder RT, Guiboux JP, Bloom DA, et al. Musculoskeletal aspects of prune-belly syndrome. Description and pathogenesis. Am J Dis Child 1992; 146:1224–1229.
153. Carey JC, Eggert L, Curry C. Lower limb deficiency and the urethral obstruction sequence. Birth Def Orig Art Ser 1982; 18:19–28.
154. Perez-Aytes A, Graham JM, Hersh JH, et al. Urethral obstruction sequence and lower limb deficiency: evidence for the vascular disruption hypothesis. J Pediatr 1993; 123:398–405.
155. Lockhart JL, Reeve HR, Bredael JJ, et al. Siblings with prune belly syndrome and associated pulmonic stenosis, mental retardation and deafness. Urology 1979; 14:140–142.
156. Berdon WE, Baker DH, Blanc WA, et al. Megacystis-microcolon-intestinal hypoperistalsis syndrome: a new case of intestinal obstruction in the newborn: report of radiologic findings in five newborn girls. Roentgenology 1976; 126:957–964.
157. Levin T, Soghier L, Blitman N, et al. Megacystis-microcolon-intestinal hypo-peristalsis and prune belly: overlapping syndromes. Pediatr Radiol 2004; 34:995–998.
158. Anneren G, Meurling S, Olsen L. Megacystis-microcolon-intestinal hypo-peristalsis syndrome (MMIHS), an autosomal recessive disorder: clinical reports and review of the literature. Am J Med Genet 1991; 41:251–254.
159. Garber A, Shohat M, Sarti D. Megacystis-microcolon-intestinal hypo-peristalsis syndrome in two male siblings. Prenat Diagn 1990; 10:377–387.
160. Piotrowska AP, Rolle U, Chertin B, et al. Alterations in smooth muscle contractile and cytoskeleton proteins and interstitial cells of Cajal in megacystis-microcolon-intestinal hypoperistalsis syndrome. J Pediatr Surg 2003; 38:749–755.
161. Rolle U, O'Briain S, Pearl R, et al. Microcystis-microcolon-intestinal hypoperistalsis syndrome: evidence of intestinal myopathy. Pediatr Surg Int 2002; 18:2–5.
162. Wigger HJ, Blanc WA. The prune belly syndrome. Pathol Annu 1977; 12:17–39.
163. Pinto T, Baithun SI, Giwan YA, et al. The prune belly syndrome – a possible pathogenesis. Diagn Histopathol 1982; 5:197–203.
164. Hoagland MH, Frank KA, Hutchins GM. Prune-belly syndrome with prostatic hypoplasia, bladder wall rupture, and massive ascites in a fetus with trisomy 18. Arch Pathol Lab Med 1988; 112:1126–1128.
165. Nunn IN, Stephens FD. The triad syndrome: a composite anomaly of the abdominal wall, urinary system and testes. J Urol 1961; 86:782–794.
166. Palmer JM, Tesluk H. Ureteral pathology in the prune belly syndrome. J Urol 1974; 111:701–707.
167. Siebert JR, Kapur RP. Congenital anomalies in the fetus: approaches to examination and diagnosis. Pathol Case Rev 2000; 5:3–13.
168. Hoagland M, Hutchins G. Obstructive lesions of the lower urinary tract in the prune belly syndrome. Arch Pathol Lab Med 1987; 111:154–156.
169. Moerman P, Fryns J-P, Goddeeris P, et al. Pathogenesis of the prune-belly syndrome: a functional urethral obstruction caused by prostatic hypoplasia. Pediatrics 1984; 73:470–475.
170. Orvis BR, Bottles K, Kogan BA. Testicular histology in fetuses with the prune belly syndrome and posterior urethral valves. J Urol 1988; 139:335–366.

171. Uehling DT, Zadina SP, Gilbert E. Testicular histology in triad syndrome. Urology 1984; 23:364–336.

172. Woodhouse C, Snyder Hr. Testicular and sexual function in adults with prune belly syndrome. J Urol 1985; 133:607–609.

173. Massad CA, Cohen MB, Kogan BA, et al. Morphology and histochemistry of infant testes in the prune belly syndrome. J Urol 1991; 146:1598–1600.

174. Parra RO, Cummings JM, Palmer DC. Testicular seminoma in a long-term survivor of the prune belly syndrome. Eur Urol 1991; 19:79–80.

175. Sayre R, Stephens R, Chonko AM. Prune belly syndrome and retroperitoneal germ cell tumor, Am J Med 1986; 81:895–897.

176. Woodhouse C, Ransley P. Teratoma of the testis in the prune belly syndrome. Br J Urol 1983; 55:580–581.

177. Fryns J, Vandenberghe K, Van den Berghe H. Prune-belly anomaly and large interstitial deletion of the long arm of chromosome 6. Ann Genet 1991; 34:127.

178. Harley LM, Chen Y, Rattner WH. Prune belly syndrome. J Urol 1972; 108:174–176.

179. Petersen DS, Fish L, Cass AS. Twins with congenital deficiency of abdominal musculature. J Urol 1972; 107:670–672.

180. Riccardi VM, Grum CM. The prune belly anomaly. J Med Genet 1977; 14:266–270.

181. Greene C, Wilson A, Shapira E. Prune belly syndrome and heart defect in one of monozygotic twins, following exposure to Tigan and Bendectin. Acta Genet Med Gemellol (Roma) 1985; 34:101–104.

182. Pramanik AK, Altshuler G, Light IJ, et al. Prune-belly syndrome associated with Potter (renal nonfunction) syndrome. Am J Dis Child 1977; 131:672–674.

183. Ikeda K, Stoesser AV. Congenital defect in the musculature of the abdominal wall: case. Am J Dis Child 1927; 33:286.

184. Barr M, Jr, Hanson JW, Currey K, et al. Holoprosencephaly in infants of diabetic mothers. J. Pediatr 1983; 102:565–568.

185. Pagon RA, Smith DW, Shepard TH. Urethral obstruction malformation complex: a cause of abdominal muscle deficiency and the 'prune belly'. J Pediatr 1979; 96:900–906.

186. Podesta E, di Rovasenda E, Sangiorgio L, et al. Obstructive urethral disease in neonates. Cir Pediatr 1991; 4:8–11.

187. King CR, Prescott G. Pathogenesis of the prune-belly anomalad. J Pediatr 1978; 93:273–274.

188. Silverman FN, Huang N. Congenital absence of the abdominal muscles associated with malformation of the genitourinary and alimentary tracts; Report of cases and review of literature, Am J Dis Child 1950; 80:91–124.

189. Ives EJ. The abdominal muscle deficiency triad syndrome-experience with ten cases. Birth Defect Orig Artic Ser 1974; 101:127–135.

190. Woolf AS, Thiruchelvam N. Congenital obstructive uropathy: its origin and contribution to end-stage renal disease in children. Adv Ren Replace Ther 2001; 8:157–163.

191. Freid S, Appelman Z, Caspi B. The origin of ascites in prune belly syndrome – early sonographic evidence (2). Pren Diagn 1995; 15:876–877.

192. Buntinx IM, Bourgeois N, Buytaert PM, et al. Acardiac amorphous twin with prune belly sequence in the co-twin. Am J Med Genet 1991; 39:453–457.

Caudal duplication

193. Nielsen OH, Nielsen R, Parvinen T. Duplicate exstrophy of the bladder. Ann Chir Gynaecol 1980; 69:32–36.

194. Hunter TB, Tonkin IL. Complete duplication of the colon in association with urethral duplication. Gastrointest Radiol 1979; 4:93–95.

195. Payne CE, Deshon GE, Jr, Kroll JD, et al. Colonic duplication: an unusual cause of enterovesical fistula. Urology 1995; 46:726–728.

196. Evans JA, Chudley AE. Tibial agenesis, femoral duplication, and caudal midline anomalies. Am J Med Genet 1999; 85:13–19.

197. La Torre R, Fusaro P, Anceschi MM, et al. Unusual case of caudal duplication (dipygus). J Clin Ultrasound 1998; 26:163–165.

198. Ulman I, Avanoglu A, Erdener A, et al. Evaluation of the lower urinary tract function in caudal duplication (dipygus) anomaly. J Pediatr Surg 1996; 31:1680–1681.

199. Azmy AF. Complete duplication of the hindgut and lower urinary tract with diphallus. J Pediatr Surg 1990; 25:647–649.

200. Dominguez R, Rott J, Castillo M, et al. Caudal duplication syndrome. Am J Dis Child 1993 ; 147:1048–1052.

201. Ravitch MM, Scott WW. Duplication of the entire colon, bladder, and urethra. Surgery 1953; 34:843–858.

202. Bannykh SI, Bannykh GI, Mannino FL, et al. Partial caudal duplication in a newborn associated with meningomyelocele and complex heart anomaly. Teratology 2001; 63:94–99.

203. Gastol P, Baka-Jakubiak M, Skobejko-Wlodarska L, et al. Complete duplication of the bladder, urethra, vagina, and uterus in girls. Urology 2000; 55:578–581.

204. Gyftopoulos K, Wolffenbuttel KP, Nijman RJM. Clinical and embryologic aspects of penile duplication and associated anomalies. Urology 2002; 60:675–679.

205. Jimenez SG, Oliver MR, Stokes KB, et al. Case report: colonic duplication: a rare cause of obstruction. J Gastroenterol Hepatol 1999; 14:889–892.

206. Salman AB. Cloacal duplication. J Pediatr Surg 1996; 31:1587–1588.

207. Currie AB, Hemalatha VH, Doraiswamy NV. Duplications of the alimentary tract. J R Coll Surg Edinb 1978; 23:347–354.

208. Potter EL. Pathology of the fetus and infant. 2nd edn. Chicago: Yearbook Medical Publishers; 1969.

209. Soper RT. Tubular duplication of the colon and distal ileum: case report and discussion. Surgery 1968; 63:998–1000.

210. Collins DC. A study of 50,000 specimens of the human vermiform appendix. Surg Gynecol Obstet 1955; 101:437–445.

211. Griffith CM, Wiley MJ, Sanders EJ. The vertebrate tail bud: three germ layers from one tissue. Anat Embryol 1992; 185:101–113.

212. Keppler-Noreuil KM. OEIS complex (omphalocele-exstrophy-imperforate anus-spinal defects): a review of 14 cases. Am J Med Genet 2001; 99:271–279.

213. Bajpai M, Das K, Gupta AK. Caudal duplication syndrome: more evidence for theory of caudal twinning. J Pediatr Surg 2004; 39:223–225.

214. Siebert JR, Rutledge JC, Kapur RP. The association of cloacal anomalies, caudal duplication, and twinning. Pediatr Dev Pathol 2005; 8:339–354.

215. Alles AJ, Sulik KK. A review of caudal dysgenesis and its pathogenesis as illustrated in an animal model. Birth Defects Orig Art Ser 1993; 29:83–102.

216. Rutledge JC, Shourbaji AG, Hughes LA, et al. Limb and lower-body duplications induced by retinoic acid in mice. Proc Natl Acad Sci USA 1994; 91:5436–5440.

217. Kroes HY, Takahashi M, Zijlstra RJ, et al. Two cases of the caudal duplication anomaly including a discordant monozygotic twin. Am J Med Genet 2002; 112:390–393.

218. Telmesani A. A rare association of myelomeningocele with cloacal duplication malformation. Ann Trop Paediatr 1994; 14:253–256.

219. Yucesan S, Zorludemir U, Olcay I. Complete duplication of the colon. J Pediatr Surg 1986; 21:962–963.

Sacral dysgenesis

220. Martucciello G, Torre M, Belloni E, et al. Currarino syndrome: proposal of a diagnostic and therapeutic protocol. J Pediatr Surg 2004; 39:1305–1311.

221. Wilmshurst JM, Kelly R, Borzyskowski M. Presentation and outcome of sacral agenesis: 20 years' experience. Dev Med Child Neurol 1999; 41:806–812.

222. Duncan PA, Shapiro LR, Klein RM. Sacrococcygeal dysgenesis association. Am J Med Genet 1991; 41:153–162.

223. Lynch SA, Wang Y, Strachan T, et al. Autosomal dominant sacral agenesis: Currarino syndrome. J Med Genet 2000; 37:561–566.

224. Hagan DM, Ross AJ, Strachan T, et al. Mutation analysis and embryonic expression of the HLXB9 Currarino syndrome gene. J Hum Genet 2000; 66:1504–1515.

Sacral dysgenesis with lower extremity anomalies/symmelia

225. Padmanabhan R, Naruse I, Shiota K. Caudal dysgenesis in staged human embryos. Am J Med Genet 1999; 87:115–127.

226. Stocker JT, Heifetz SA. Sirenomelia: a morphological study of 33 cases and review of the literature. Perspect Pediatr Pathol 1987; 10:7–50.

227. Padmanabhan R. Retinoic-acid induced caudal regression syndrome in the mouse fetus. Reprod Toxicol 1998; 12:139–151.

228. Boklage CE. The organization of the oocyte and embryogenesis in twinning and fusion malformations. Acta Genet Med Gemellol (Roma) 1987; 36:421–431.

229. Kapur RP, Mahony BS, Nyberg DA, et al. Sirenomelia associated with a 'vanishing twin'. Teratology 1991; 43:103–108.

230. Davies J, Chazen E, Nance WE. Symmelia in one of monozygotic twins. Teratology 1971; 4:367–368.

231. Jones KL, Benirschke K. The developmental pathogenesis of structural defects: the contribution of monozygotic twins. Sem Perinatol 1983; 7:239–243.

232. Kalter H. Case reports of malformations associated with maternal diabetes. Clin Genet 1993; 43:174–179.

233. Chan BWH, Chan K, Koide T, et al. Maternal diabetes increases the risk of caudal regression caused by retinoic acid. Diabetes 2002; 51:2811–2816.

234. Chandebois R, Brunet C. Origin of abnormality in a human simelian fetus as elucidated by our knowledge of vertebrate development. Teratology 19897; 36:11–22.

235. Hoornbeek EK. A gene producing sirenomelia in the mouse. Teratology 1970; 3:1–10.

Index